MW01106884

Cherry and Merkatz's

Complications of Pregnancy

Fifth Edition

Cherry and Merkatz's *Complications of Pregnancy*

Fifth Edition

Editor

Wayne R. Cohen, M.D.

Visiting Professor
Department of Obstetrics & Gynecology and Women's Health
Albert Einstein College of Medicine
Bronx, New York
Obstetrician and Gynecologist-in-Chief
Sinai Hospital of Baltimore
Baltimore, Maryland

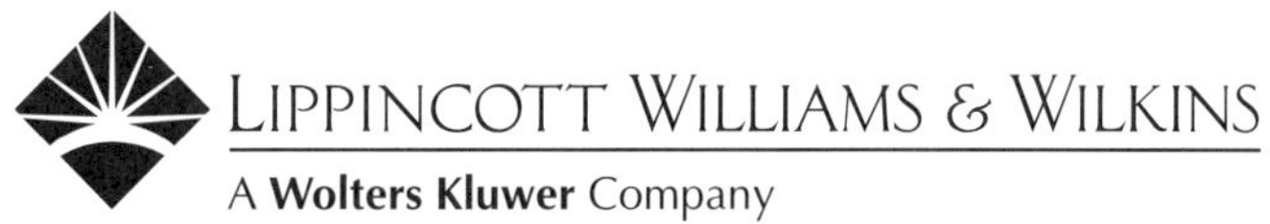

Philadelphia • Baltimore • New York • London
Buenos Aires • Hong Kong • Sydney • Tokyo

Acquisitions Editor: Lisa McAllister
Developmental Editor: Leah Ann Kiehne Hayes
Production Editor: Mary Ann McLaughlin
Manufacturing Manager: Tim Reynolds
Cover Designer: Mark Lerner
Compositor: Lippincott Williams & Wilkins Desktop Division
Printer: Maple Vail

227 East Washington Square
Philadelphia, PA 19106-3780 USA
LWW.com

Chapter 2 is excerpted in part from Worthington-Roberts B, Williams SR. Nutrition in pregnancy and lactation. 4th ed. Dubuque, Iowa: Brown and Benchmark, 1997.

Library of Congress Cataloging-in-Publication Data

Cherry and Merkatz's complications of pregnancy. —5th ed. / editor,
Wayne R. Cohen ;
p. cm.
Rev. ed. of: Complications of pregnancy. 4th ed. ©1991.
Includes bibliographical references and index.
ISBN 0-683-01673-3 (alk. paper)
1. Pregnancy—Complications. I. Cohen, Wayne R. II. Cherry, Sheldon H.
III. Merkatz, Irwin R. (Irwin Richard), 1934– .
IV. Title: Complications of pregnancy.
[DNLM: 1. Pregnancy Complications. WQ 240 C522 1999]
RG571.M45 1999
618.3—dc21
DNLM/DLC
For Library of Congress 98-32438
CIP

Care has been taken to confirm the accuracy of the information presented and to describe generally accepted practices. However, the authors, editors, and publisher are not responsible for errors or omissions or for any consequences from application of the information in this book and make no warranty, expressed or implied, with respect to the currency, completeness, or accuracy of the contents of the publication. Application of this information in a particular situation remains the professional responsibility of the practitioner.

The authors, editors, and publisher have exerted every effort to ensure that drug selection and dosage set forth in this text are in accordance with current recommendations and practice at the time of publication. However, in view of ongoing research, changes in government regulations, and the constant flow of information relating to drug therapy and drug reactions, the reader is urged to check the package insert for each drug for any change in indications and dosage and for added warnings and precautions. This is particularly important when the recommended agent is a new or infrequently employed drug.

Some drugs and medical devices presented in this publication have Food and Drug Administration (FDA) clearance for limited use in restricted research settings. It is the responsibility of health care providers to ascertain the FDA status of each drug or device planned for use in their clinical practice.

10 9 8 7 6 5 4 3 2 1

To Mannie,

for substrate

To Sharon, Daniel, and Giselle

for sustenance

Contents

Section IV Cardiopulmonary Disorders

Section V Genitourinary Disorders

Section VI Gastrointestinal Disorders

Section VII Hematopoietic Disorders

Section VIII Endocrine Disorders

Section IX Neurologic Disorders

Contributing Authors

Fouad M. Abbas, M.D.
Director, Division of Gynecologic Oncology
Sinai Hospital of Baltimore
Baltimore, Maryland

Lindsay Staubus Alger, M.D.
Professor of Obstetrics, Gynecology, and Reproductive Sciences
University of Maryland School of Medicine
Medical Director, Labor and Delivery
University of Maryland Medical Systems
Baltimore, Maryland

Jean R. Anderson, M.D.
Associate Professor of Gynecology and Obstetrics
The Johns Hopkins University School of Medicine
Baltimore, Maryland

Raul Artal, M.D.
Professor and Chairman
Department of Obstetrics and Gynecology
St. Louis University School of Medicine
St. Louis, Missouri

David A. Baker, M.D.
Professor of Obstetrics, Gynecology, and Reproductive Medicine
Director, Division of Infectious Diseases
State University of New York at Stony Brook
Health Science Center School of Medicine
Stony Brook, New York

Gregory T. Bales, M.D.
Assistant Professor of Surgery
Section of Urology
University of Chicago Pritzker School of Medicine
Chicago, Illinois

Brian Berman, M.D., Ph.D.
Professor of Dermatology and Cutaneous Surgery and Internal Medicine
University of Miami School of Medicine
Director, In-patient Consultations
Department of Dermatology and Cutaneous Surgery
University of Miami/Jackson Memorial Center
Miami, Florida

David H. Berman, M.D.
Mount Sinai Medical Center
New York, New York

Peter S. Bernstein, M.D.
Assistant Professor of Obstetrics & Gynecology, and Women's Health
Albert Einstein College of Medicine
Director
Department of Obstetrics and Gynecology
Montefiore Medical Group-Morris Park
Bronx, New York

Hugh F. Biller, M.D.
Professor Emeritus of Otolaryngology
The Mount Sinai School of Medicine
Attending Physician
Department of Otolaryngology
The Mount Sinai Hospital
New York, New York

Allan T. Bombard, M.D.
Professor of Obstetrics and Gynecology and Women's Health
Albert Einstein College of Medicine
Director, Division of Reproductive Genetics
Montefiore Medical Center
Bronx, New York

Deborah Bowers, M.D.
Attending Obstetrician-Gynecologist
Sinai Hospital of Baltimore
Baltimore, Maryland

Frank A. Chervenak, M.D.
Professor of Obstetrics and Gynecology
Cornell University Medical College
Director of Obstetrics and Maternal-Fetal Medicine
The New York Hospital
New York, New York

Ronald A. Chez, M.D.
Professor of Obstetrics and Gynecology
Professor of Community and Family Medicine
University of South Florida
Chief of Obstetrics and Gynecology
Tampa General Hospital
Davis Islands
Tampa, Florida

Christopher F. Ciliberto, M.D.
Assistant Professor of Anesthesiology
Columbia University College of Physicians and Surgeons
Columbia Presbyterian Medical Center
New York, New York

Rhoda H. Cobin, M.D.
Associate Clinical Professor of Medicine
Division of Endocrinology and Medicine
The Mount Sinai School of Medicine
New York, New York

Brian L. Cohen, M.D., F.R.C.O.G., F.A.C.O.G.
Associate Professor of Obstetrics and Gynecology and Women's Health
Albert Einstein College of Medicine
Montefiore Medical Center
Bronx, New York

Charmaine D. Cohen, M.D., F.A.C.P., F.A.A.C.E.
Assistant Attending Physician in Medicine
Montefiore Medical Center-Weiler Division
Albert Einstein College of Medicine
Bronx, New York

Wayne R. Cohen, M.D.
Visiting Professor
Department of Obstetrics & Gynecology and Women's Health
Albert Einstein College of Medicine
Bronx, New York
Obstetrician and Gynecologist-in-Chief
Sinai Hospital of Baltimore
Baltimore, Maryland

Bonnie Joan Dattel, M.D.
Professor of Maternal-Fetal Medicine
Department of Obstetrics and Gynecology
Eastern Virginia Medical School
Norfolk, Virginia

Efraim P. David, M.D.
Fellow
Department of Neurology
University of Maryland
Baltimore, Maryland

James David, M.D.
Associate Professor of Psychiatry
Associate Dean of Students
Albert Einstein College of Medicine
Bronx, New York

Terry F. Davies, M.D., F.R.C.P.
Florence and Theodore Baumritter Professor of Medicine
Director, Division of Endocrinology and Metabolism
The Mount Sinai School of Medicine
Attending Physician
The Mount Sinai Hospital
New York, New York

Warren Dotz, M.D.
Former Assistant Clinical Professor of Dermatology
University of California School of Medicine
Davis, California
Director, Berkeley Dermatology Center
Berkeley, California

Richard Eastell, M.D.
Professor of Clinical Sciences
Bone Metabolism Group
University of Sheffield
Northern General Hospital Trust
Sheffield, England

Rene Elkin, M.D.
Assistant Professor of Neurology
Albert Einstein College of Medicine
New York Medical College
Bronx, New York
Co-Director, Multiple Sclerosis Comprehensive Care Center
St. Agnes Hospital
White Plains, New York

Hervé Fernandez, M.D.
Professor of Gynecology and Obstetrics
Université Pierre et Marie Curie
Paris, France
Hôpital Antoine Béclère
Clamart, France

Jose C.P.B. Ferreira, M.D.
Clinical Fellow in Reproductive Genetics
Department of Obstetrics & Gynecology and Women's Health
Albert Einstein College of Medicine
Montefiore Medical Center
Bronx, New York

Harold E. Fox, M.D., M.Sc.
Dr. Dorothy Edwards Professor and Director
Department of Gynecology and Obstetrics
The Johns Hopkins University School of Medicine
Director and Gynecologist and Obstetrician-in-Chief
The Johns Hopkins Hospital
Baltimore, Maryland

Margaret Comerford Freda, Ed.D., R.N., C.H.E.S., F.A.A.N.
Associate Professor of Obstetrics & Gynecology and Women's Health
Albert Einstein College of Medicine
Director of Patient Education Programs
Montefiore Medical Center
Bronx, New York

Alan H. Friedman, M.D.
Clinical Professor of Ophthalmology and Pathology
The Mount Sinai School of Medicine
New York, New York

Sonia Friedman, M.D.
Fellow in Gastroenterology
The Mount Sinai Medical Center
New York, New York

Glenn S. Gerber, M.D.
Associate Professor of Surgery/Urology
The University of Chicago
Chicago, Illinois

James M. Gilchrist, M.D.
Professor
Department of Clinical Neurosciences
Brown University School of Medicine
Senior Vice-Chairman
Department of Neurology
Rhode Island Hospital
Providence, Rhode Island

Gary L. Goldberg, M.D.
Professor of Obstetrics and Gynecology and Women's Health
The Albert Einstein College of Medicine
Director of Gynecology
Associate Director of Gynecologic Oncology
Department of Obstetrics & Gynecology and Women's Health
Albert Einstein College of Medicine and Montefiore Medical Center
Bronx, New York

Martin E. Goldman, M.D.
Dr. Arthur and Hilda A. Master Professor of Medicine
Department of Medicine (Cardiology)
The Mount Sinai School of Medicine
Director of Echocardiography
Department of Cardiology
The Mount Sinai Medical Center
New York, New York

Martin S. Goldstein, M.D.
Associate Clinical Professor of Obstetrics, Gynecology, and Reproductive Sciences
The Mount Sinai School of Medicine
New York, New York

Glenn S. Hammer, M.D.
Clinical Assistant Professor of Medicine
The Mount Sinai School of Medicine
The Mount Sinai Medical Center
New York, New York

Ellen S. Harrison, M.D.
Associate Professor of Medicine
Assistant Professor of Obstetrics & Gynecology and Women's Health
Albert Einstein College of Medicine
Associate Director of Medicine
Director of Obstetrical Medicine
Jack D. Weiler Hospital
Montefiore Medical Center
Bronx, New York

Cassandra E. Henderson, M.D.
Associate Professor of Obstetrics and Gynecology and Women's Health
Albert Einstein College of Medicine
Bronx, New York
Attending Physician
Department of Maternal-Fetal Medicine
Montefiore Medical Center
Bronx, New York

Steven M. Hollenberg, M.D.
Assistant Professor of Medicine
Departments of Cardiology and Critical Care Medicine
Rush Medical College
Chicago, Illinois
Associate Director
Medical Intensive Care Unit
Rush-Presbyterian-St. Luke's Medical Center
Chicago, Illinois

Iffath Abbasi Hoskins, M.D.
Associate Professor of Obstetrics and Gynecology
New York University School of Medicine
Chief of Obstetrics and Gynecology
New York University Downtown Hospital
New York, New York

Nancy A. Hueppchen, M.D.
Instructor in Obstetrics and Gynecology
Johns Hopkins University School of Medicine
Johns Hopkins Hospital
Baltimore, Maryland

Henry D. Janowitz, M.D.
Clinical Professor Emeritus of Medicine
The Mount Sinai School of Medicine
New York, New York

Sara Kaffe, M.D.
Associate Clinical Professor of Human Genetics and Pediatrics
The Mount Sinai Services of The Mount Sinai School of Medicine
Elmhurst Hospital Center
Elmhurst, New York

Andrew S. Kaplan, D.M.D.
Associate Clinical Professor of Dentistry
The Mount Sinai School of Medicine
The Mount Sinai Hospital
New York, New York

Robert F. Keating, M.D.
Assistant Professor of Neurosurgery and Pediatrics
George Washington University School of Medicine
Vice Chairman
Department of Neurosurgery
Children's National Medical Center
Washington, D.C.

Virginia S. Kelly, M.D.
Instructor in Clinical Obstetrics and Gynecology
Northwestern University School of Medicine
Chicago, Illinois

Susan H. Kim-Lo, M.D.
Clinical Assistant Professor of Anesthesiology
Columbia University College of Physicians and Surgeons
Columbia Presbyterian Medical Center
New York, New York

Jack Klatell, D.D.S.
Professor and Chairman of Dentistry
The Mount Sinai School of Medicine
Director of Dentistry
The Mount Sinai Hospital
New York, New York

Wayne B. Kramer, M.D.
Assistant Professor of Maternal-Fetal Medicine
Department of Obstetrics, Gynecology and Reproductive Sciences
University of Maryland School of Medicine
Baltimore, Maryland

Oded Langer, M.D.
Jane and Roland Blumberg Professor of Obstetrics and Gynecology
Chief, Division of Obstetrics and Maternal-Fetal Medicine
University of Texas Health Sciences Center at San Antonio
San Antonio, Texas

Jan M. Lanouette, M.D.
Sinai Hospital of Baltimore
Institute of Maternal Fetal Health
Baltimore, Maryland

William Lawson, M.D.
Professor of Otolaryngology
The Mount Sinai School of Medicine
New York, New York
Chief, Division of Otolaryngology
Bronx Veterans Administration Hospital
Bronx, New York

Marvin Lesser, M.D.
Associate Professor of Medicine
The Mount Sinai School of Medicine
Director, Division of Pulmonary Medicine
Bronx Veterans Administration Hospital
New York, New York

Roger N. Levy, M.D.
Professor of Orthopaedic Surgery
The Mount Sinai School of Medicine
Chief of Arthritic Surgery
Department of Orthopaedic Surgery
The Mount Sinai Medical Center
New York, New York

Pamela S. Lewis, M.D.
Department of Obstetrics and Gynecology
Sinai Hospital of Baltimore
Baltimore, Maryland

Charles J. Lockwood, M.D.
Stanley H. Kaplan Professor and Chair of Obstetrics and Gynecology
New York University School of Medicine
New York, New York

Laurence B. McCullough, Ph.D.
Professor of Medicine and Medical Ethics
Center for Medical Ethics and Health Policy
Baylor College of Medicine
Houston, Texas

Jose Meller, M.D., F.A.C.C.
Associate Professor of Clinical Medicine
The Mount Sinai School of Medicine
Attending Physician, Cardiology
Department of Medicine
The Mount Sinai Medical Center
New York, New York

Irwin R. Merkatz, M.D.
Professor and Chairman
Department of Obstetrics & Gynecology & Women's Health
Albert Einstein College of Medicine
Montefiore Medical Center
Bronx, New York

John Meyerhoff, M.D., F.A.C.R.
Assistant Professor of Medicine
The Johns Hopkins University School of Medicine
Clinical Scholar in Rheumatology
Sinai Hospital of Baltimore
Baltimore, Maryland

Laurey G. Mogil, M.D.
Assistant Clinical Professor of Ophthalmology
The Mount Sinai School of Medicine
New York, New York

Kim Naylor, Ph.D.
Research Associate in Bone Metabolism Group
University of Sheffield
Sheffield, England

François Olivennes, M.D., Ph.D.
Director, Assisted Reproductive Technologies Unit
Department of Obstetrics and Gynecology
Antoine Béclère Hospital
Clamart, France

Christopher O'Reilly-Green, M.D.
Assistant Professor of Obstetrics & Gynecology and Women's Health
Albert Einstein College of Medicine
Bronx, New York
Attending Perinatologist
Department of Obstetrics and Gynecology and Women's Health
Lenox Hill Hospital
New York, New York

Michael J. Paidas, M.D.
Assistant Professor of Obstetrics and Gynecology
Director, New York University School of Medicine Program in Maternal and Fetal Medicine
New York, New York

Emile Papiernik, M.D.
Professor of Obstetrics and Gynecology
Universite René Descartes
Hôpital Cochin
Paris, France
Stony Brook, New York

Page B. Pennell, M.D.
Assistant Professor
Department of Neurology
Emory University School of Medicine
Director of Epilepsy Monitoring Unit
Department of Neurology
Emory University Hospital
Atlanta, Georgia

Mark E. Pruzansky, M.D.
Assistant Professor of Clinical Orthopaedics
The Mount Sinai School of Medicine
Assistant Attending Physician
Department of Orthopaedic Surgery
Mount Sinai-New York University Medical Center
New York, New York

Bruce A. Rabin, M.D., Ph.D.
Assistant Professor of Neurology
The Johns Hopkins School of Medicine
Co-Director, Division of Neurology
Sinai Hospital of Baltimore
Baltimore, Maryland

Anthony J. Reino
Department of Otolaryngology
Mount Sinai School of Medicine
New York, New York

Todd Rosen, M.D.
Assistant Professor and Attending Physician
Department of Obstetrics and Gynecology
New York University Medical Center
New York, New York

Peter H. Rubin, M.D.
Associate Clinical Professor of Medicine
The Mount Sinai School of Medicine
Attending Physician
The Mount Sinai Hospital
New York, New York

Gay S. Sachs, M.A.
Genetic Counselor
Associate in Reproductive Genetics
Department of Obstetrics and Gynecology and Women's Health
Albert Einstein College of Medicine
Montefiore Medical Center
Bronx, New York

Gregory J. Schilero, M.D.
Assistant Professor of Medicine
The Mount Sinai School of Medicine
New York, New York
Associate Director of the Medical Intensive Care Unit
Pulmonary and Critical Care Division
The Bronx Veterans Affairs Medical Center
Bronx, New York

Ronald E. Schneider, M.D.
Department of Oral Surgery
The Mount Sinai Hospital
New York, New York

Martin Sedlacek, M.D.
Fellow in Nephrology
The Mount Sinai Hospital
New York, New York

Meira Shaham, Ph.D.
Laboratory Director
Cytogenetics Laboratory
Genzyme Genetics
Yonkers, New York

Stephen D. Silberstein, M.D., F.A.C.P.
Professor of Neurology
Thomas Jefferson University
Director,
Jefferson Headache Center
Thomas Jefferson University Hospital
Philadelphia, Pennsylvania

Richard M. Smiley, M.D., Ph.D.
Associate Professor of Anesthesiology
Columbia University College of Physicians and Surgeons
Director, Obstetric Anesthesia
Columbia Presbyterian Medical Center
New York, New York

Babill Stray-Pedersen, M.D., Ph.D.
Head Professor and Senior Consultant
Department of Obstetrics and Gynecology
University of Oslo
Senior Consultant
National Hospital
Oslo, Norway

Alvin S. Teirstein, M.D.
Florette and Ernst Rosenfeld and Joseph Solomon Professor of Medicine
Director, Division of Pulmonary and Critical Care Medicine
The Mount Sinai Medical Center
New York, New York

Marc R. Toglia, M.D.
Assistant Clinical Professor of Obstetrics and Gynecology
Thomas Jefferson University
Philadelphia, Pennsylvania

Gina M. Villani, M.D.
Department of Medical Oncology
Albert Einstein College of Medicine
Montefiore Medical Center
Bronx, New York

Carl P. Weiner, M.D.
Professor and Chairman
Department of Obstetrics, Gynecology and Reproductive Sciences
University of Maryland School of Medicine
Baltimore, Maryland

Sandra Welner, M.D.
Clinical Assistant Professor of Obstetrics and Gynecology
Georgetown University School of Medicine
Department of Obstetrics and Gynecology
Sibley Memorial Hospital
Washington, D.C.

Robert E. Wenk, M.D.
Professor of Pathology
Pennsylvania State University College of Medicine
Hershey, Pennsylvania
Assistant Chief of Pathology
Sinai Hospital of Baltimore
Baltimore, Maryland

Clifford Roberts Wheeless, Jr., M.D.
Associate Professor of Gynecology and Obstetrics
The Johns Hopkins University School of Medicine
Director, Institute for Special Pelvic Surgery
Sinai Hospital of Baltimore
Baltimore, Maryland

Jonathan A. Winston, M.D.
Clinical Associate Professor of Medicine
The Mount Sinai School of Medicine
New York, New York

Robert J. Wityk, M.D.
Assistant Professor of Neurology
The Johns Hopkins University School of Medicine
Director, Clinical Stroke Service
Johns Hopkins Hospital
Baltimore, Maryland

Bonnie S. Worthington-Roberts, Ph.D.
Retired Professor
Nutritional Sciences Program
University of Washington
Seattle, Washington

Joan R. Youchah, M.D.
Department of Psychiatry
Albert Einstein College of Medicine
Bronx, New York

James B. Young, M.D.
Professor of Medicine
Northwestern University Medical School
Chicago, Illinois

Foreword

The interplay between obstetrics and the other fields of medicine is more extensive and intimate than found in any other specialty.

Guttmacher and Rovinsky
1960

When the first edition of *Medical, Surgical and Gynecologic Complications of Pregnancy,* edited by Alan Guttmacher and Joseph Rovinsky, was published in 1960, it represented a landmark text for obstetric literature. It was the first effort to examine the application of broad medical principles to the physiologic and pathophysiologic alterations of pregnancy and, as such, presaged the development of maternal-fetal medicine as a major subspecialty of obstetrics and gynecology. The intervening four decades have witnessed revolutionary changes in attitudes concerning the management of serious pregnancy complications affecting either or both mother and fetus. These changes have been associated with marked improvements in perinatal outcome and with a continued decline in the incidence of maternal mortality.

The immediate success of the first edition prompted the editors to provide an accelerated, updated second edition within five years. However, by the time the subsequent edition was ready for publication in the mid-1980's, the concept of specialized obstetrical care for high-risk women had evolved so extensively that many other texts in maternal-fetal medicine had also become available. The challenge then was to maintain a unique perspective as a work focused primarily on complications of pregnancy. Drs. Cherry, Berkowitz, and Kase, as third edition editors, picked up this challenge and produced a greatly expanded volume. Their efforts served subsequently as a complete reference source for the myriad of intercurrent problems impacting on the well-being of the pregnant woman and/or her unborn child. The unique composition of that editorship reflected a growing realization that a combination of clinical obstetrics, academic orientation, and educational expertise was required for optimal transmission of rapidly expanding new knowledge to the contemporary physician. Both editors and contributors brought to that third edition a clear message that the obstetrician-gynecologist was leading a team responsible not only for the welfare of the mother but also for that of a second patient, the fetus. A broad range of medical consultants needed to be potential members of that team.

Over the recent past, the obstetrical profession and its public have evolved a new set of parameters with which to evaluate pregnancy outcomes and disparate rates of perinatal mortality. Short- and long-term morbidities for mother and child, together with high hospitalization costs for the acute care of the sick newborn, are complications that have now assumed central importance. Public policy decisions with respect to future funding of the maternity care delivery system await creative solutions for these newer problems. Prevention has become the watchword. The contemporary obstetrician now must be even more concerned with a body of information previously not adequately appreciated for its impact on overall maternal and fetal health. The psychosocial complications of pregnancy are now recognized as no less significant than the more traditional medical-surgical complications. To address this new reality upon assuming our editorship of the fourth edition in 1991 we added contributors with a greater public health expertise to the volume's previously excellent clinical and perinatal orientations. Futhermore, the earlier single institutional base was modified to bring a broadened perspective and the resources of a wider contributorship. Nevertheless, the basic concept of an amalgam between clinical and academic communities was preserved and enhanced.

As the direction of obstetrical practice evolves into the 21st century, proudly we now pass this book on to the next generation of editorship so that the collection of authoritative, up-to-date contributions can continue to provide readers with a singular reference source for the care of pregnant women. It is our intent that the current and future volumes of the text continue a 40-year-old unique tradition of excellence and expertise. Concomittantly, we hope that there will continue to be fewer complications of pregnancy and, for those that do occur, the broad skills of our profession will continue to evolve to create successful outcomes for the maternal-newborn dyad.

Sheldon H. Cherry, M.D.
Clinical Professor of Obstetrics and Gynecology
The Mount Sinai School of Medicine, New York

Irwin R. Merkatz, M.D.
Professor and Chairman
Department of Obstetrics & Gynecology and Women's Health
Albert Einstein College of Medicine
Montefiore Medical Center, New York

Preface

I met the opportunity to edit a text of such distinguished editorial patrimony with enthusiasm and great respect for the daunting task at hand. The emergence of this book in 1960 was a cardinal event and a bellwether in obstetric literature: it was the first modern text to address the impact of medical and surgical disease on pregnancy, an interest area that has since spawned dozens of books in the same and related fields.

All books, even scholarly texts, have a character that defines them through generations of editors and authors. I have endeavored to preserve (and, in some instances, to restore) those qualities that Drs. Guttmacher and Rovinsky imparted to the first edition 39 years ago: readability, clinical pertinence, and accessible scholarship. In so doing, I have made several changes in the text that I hope make the volume manageable and focused. These changes reflect the expanding interface (which, more correctly, is an overlap) between obstetrics and allied medical and surgical specialities, and the fact that multiple edition texts must evolve in form and substance in parallel with the advancement of their subject matter. The book is shorter than the previous edition (56 vs. 78 chapters), mostly by virtue of my having eliminated several contributions that, however well written and erudite, had limited practical relevance to today's practitioner. The authorship of chapters has been broadened to include expert physicians from many specialities in academic and clinical practice settings. They work in medical centers across this country and in Europe, a reflection of the widening and increasingly international foundation of expertise in this area.

The book departs from the approach of other texts that address similar ground primarily in the breadth of coverage of some topics. It can serve as a source of extensive and current knowledge about common medical complications of pregnancy, such as hypertension, diabetes, or anemia, but it is also a repository of information not readily available elsewhere about many uncommon but important complications. For example, pertinent and detailed information about neurologic and muscular disorders, sense organ abnormalities, and pheochromocytoma is provided. Chapters are included on issues of general importance to the care of seriously ill pregnant women. Thus, management of septic or hemorrhagic shock, approaches to anesthesia and surgery, and risks of medications are addressed in detail. In addition, I asked all authors to emphasize the importance of grasping basic physiologic concepts in understanding disease processes, and in crafting plans of care. It was, of course, necessary to be selective in the choice of topics covered. I hope the reader finds the array of included subjects to be useful.

An emphasis has been placed on preconceptional counseling, an emerging concept that focuses on prevention of pregnancy complications. The virtues of this approach are spotlighted by devoting the book's first chapter to general principles of preventive obstetric care. In addition, preconceptional care for women with specific medical risks or problems is addressed where relevant throughout the text.

The publisher has named this text to honor the editors of the fourth edition, Sheldon H. Cherry and Irwin R. Merkatz, both influential and respected leaders in obstetrics. This is an especially appropriate encomium because, in addition to the emblem of clinical and academic excellence they lend to the volume, each is a talented teacher, writer, and communicator.

I wish to express my profound appreciation to the chapter authors, each of whom labored to produce work of singular excellence in an era when professional time for such pursuits is shrinking everywhere. I am boundlessly grateful to my secretary, Faye Snyder. Without her stalwart and uncomplaining perseverance through innumerable chapter revisions, incompatible word processing programs, our publisher's merger, several changes in copy editors, and her tolerance of a (perhaps overly) compulsive boss, this edition would still exist only as a good idea.

The book should serve as a source of accessible clinical information for established or aspiring obstetricians, perinatologists, internists, family physicians, and many subspecialists—in short, for anyone who would have the occasion to render medical care to a pregnant woman. I hope that the aggregate of my efforts and those of the chapter authors and the fine staff at Lippincott Williams & Wilkins has resulted in an edition that will contribute to an understanding of what is required to provide competent and compassionate care to pregnant women with medical or surgical complications. They deserve no less.

Wayne R. Cohen, M.D

SECTION I

Prevention of Complications

Cherry and Merkatz's Complications of Pregnancy,
Fifth Edition, edited by W. R. Cohen.
Lippincott Williams & Wilkins, Philadelphia © 2000.

CHAPTER 1

Preconceptional and Prenatal Care

Peter S. Bernstein, Ellen S. Harrison, and Irwin R. Merkatz

From an initial narrow focus on preventing eclampsia, the discipline of prenatal care has evolved to become a pillar of preventive care. It has been expanded from a temporal focus on occurrences during late pregnancy to encompass preconceptional preparation for pregnancy and to include goals for the mother and infant that stretch well beyond the peripartum period. The scope has broadened from an original emphasis on preventing maternal and neonatal mortality to an in-depth concern with short-term and longer-term morbidities that embrace the mother, child, and family. Similarly, the goals of prenatal care have grown beyond the purely biological to include the psychosocial influences on pregnancy outcome.

Whereas later chapters in this text will address care for women with specific problems, this chapter provides an overview of the history, goals, scope, and content of prenatal care. By understanding the goals, it will be easier to judge the value of each component of services delivered to women who may be considering conceiving or, alternatively, to those who are already pregnant.

P.S. Bernstein, E.S. Harrison, I.R. Merkatz: Department of Obstetrics and Gynecology, and Women's Health, Albert Einstein College of Medicine, Montefiore Medical Center, Bronx, NY 10467.

BACKGROUND AND HISTORY

Historically, the concept of prenatal care dates back only to the beginning of the 20th century in Europe and the United States. Prior to this period, care rendered to the pregnant woman related primarily to addressing her physical and emotional hygiene. The first major event in the evolution of the biomedical aspects of prenatal care came with the observation of J.C. Lever in 1843 in England that albumin in the urine of pregnant women was associated with the subsequent development of eclampsia. Gradually, others uncovered the hallmark signs of preeclampsia and eclampsia, including edema, headaches, and elevated blood pressure (1).

In 1858 Sinclair and Johnston founded the world's first prenatal clinic at the Dublin Maternity Hospital (2). Taussig (3) later explained that this resulted from an accident of circumstances. In Dublin, a pregnant woman had to register to see a physician before giving birth in the hospital; overcrowded conditions necessitated that she apply several months before her expected delivery date. Physicians took the opportunity to take a brief history on each woman, perform a physical examination, and check her urine. Those women with edema, headaches, or proteinuria were empirically treated with bed rest, light nourishment, and purges. The incidence of eclampsia was reduced among those women who attended the dispensary, an unanticipated finding (2).

Organized prenatal care in the United States was largely the result of efforts of nurses and social reformers. In 1901, Mrs. William Lowell Putnam of the Boston Infant Social Service Department began a program of home nurse visits to some of the pregnant women who were enrolled in the home delivery service of the Boston Lying-In Hospital. The work of this program expanded, and by 1911 an outpatient clinic was established. Women were urged to enroll as early as possible (1).

Mrs. Putnam subsequently convinced J. Whitridge Williams to support systematic prenatal care. In a 1914 study of 705 fetal deaths that occurred among 10,000 consecutive admissions to the Johns Hopkins Hospital, he estimated that prenatal care could have reduced this mortality rate by 40% (4). His emphasis was on the detection and treatment of syphilis.

In New York City, a program of organized prenatal care was begun in 1907 by Dr. Josephine Baker (5). Interestingly, services were only offered after the seventh month of pregnancy. The first maternity center opened in 1917. In 1918, the Maternity Center Association was founded under the direction of Frances Perkins to oversee the establishment of multiple centers for all of Manhattan (6). A review of 8,743 records of women who received prenatal and postnatal care through these centers demonstrated a 30% decrease in neonatal deaths and a 21.5% reduction in maternal mortality (7). Prenatal care at this time consisted of a physical examination by a physician, home and district clinic visits with public health nurses, and education about preparation for delivery and care of the infant. If seen in the office, the woman's blood pressure was recorded as part of the physical examination, whereas at home visits a nurse analyzed the urine and auscultated the fetal heart. Women were seen twice each month until the seventh month of pregnancy and then weekly (8).

Ann Stevens, the Director of the Maternity Center Association in 1920 noted that the goal of prenatal care was "to bring the woman through the pregnancy with the minimum of mental and physical discomfort, so that she may arrive at the termination of that pregnancy in the maximum of mental and physical fitness with the reward of a truly well baby who has a 100% chance to live and develop and enjoy the life of a useful citizen" (9).

The focus of federal efforts at the time was toward reducing infant mortality. In 1909, Theodore Roosevelt convened what came to be known as the White House Conference on Children. The conference recommended the establishment of the United States Children's Bureau, which was eventually created in 1912. In 1924, the bureau published a report entitled *Prenatal Care* (10) and created a committee whose charge was to establish standards of prenatal care. Its report (11), published in 1925, set standards of prenatal care and outlined a series of medical and educational components for each visit that have changed surprisingly little to the present day.

Thus, although the modern practice of prenatal care developed in response to efforts to control mortality and morbidity associated with preeclampsia, its focus has been expanded to foster the well-being of a mother and her fetus in order to ensure healthy outcomes for both.

In 1989, the U.S. Public Health Service Expert Panel on the Content of Prenatal Care issued its report *Caring for Our Future: The Content of Prenatal Care.* In it, contemporary goals of prenatal care were outlined (Table 1-1). In addition to setting goals for the pregnant woman and her infant, the panel broadened the objective of prenatal care to encompass goals for the family as well. These included the explicit mention of parenting skills, family violence, and child abuse or neglect. In recommending that a woman planning a pregnancy should have a preconceptional visit and that primary care providers of various backgrounds should be prepared to make appropriate recommendations to optimize the conditions in which pregnancy begins, the panel also broadened the time frame encompassed by prenatal care. While expanding its view to include the period prior to pregnancy, the panel also extended its vantage point well beyond pregnancy, asserting that services delivered during prenatal care can affect the well-being of a woman beyond the current pregnancy, into her future pregnancies, and indeed even beyond her childbearing years. The recommendations expand past a medical model and incorporate a full

TABLE 1-1. *Objectives of prenatal care*

For the pregnant woman:
1. To increase her well-being before, during, and after pregnancy and to improve her self-image and self-care.
2. To reduce maternal mortality and morbidity, fetal loss, and unnecessary pregnancy interventions.
3. To reduce the risks to her health prior to subsequent pregnancies and beyond childbearing years.
4. To promote the development of parenting skills.

For the fetus and infant:
1. To increase well-being.
2. To reduce preterm birth, intrauterine growth restriction, congenital anomalies, and failure to thrive.
3. To promote healthy growth and development, immunization, and health supervision.
4. To reduce neurologic, developmental, and other morbidities.
5. To reduce child abuse and neglect, injuries, preventable acute and chronic illness, and the need for extended hospitalization after birth.

For the family:
1. To promote family development and positive parent-infant interaction.
2. To reduce unintended pregnancies.
3. To identify for treatment behavior disorders leading to child neglect and family violence.

From the United States Public Health Service Expert Panel on the Content of Prenatal Care. Caring for Our Future: The Content of Prenatal Care. Washington, DC: US Department of Health and Human Services,1989.

range of psychosocial issues. Without losing its central focus on the traditional elements of care provided during pregnancy, prenatal care as currently envisioned constitutes a much broader preventive health concept.

PLANNING FOR PREGNANCY AND THE INITIATION OF CARE

Preconceptional Care

A woman's health prior to pregnancy is a major determinant of her health during pregnancy and of the outcome of the pregnancy both for her and her child. Disparate factors—including diet, occupational exposure, parity, medical history, immunization, medications, marital status, socioeconomic class, genetic endowment, habits, and access to health care—all contribute to her condition before pregnancy.

Preconceptional care is predicated on the understanding that some useful options to optimize health, safety, and well-being of a woman and her offspring may already be foreclosed or limited by the time of entry into routine prenatal care. Preconceptional care aims to find reducible or potentially reversible risks to a woman's health or her pregnancy outcome, with emphasis on factors that can or must be acted upon before conception in order to have greatest impact.

One major aim of preconceptional care is the protection of the embryo during organogenesis. Because organogenesis begins at about 17 days after conception (just about the time that a woman may suspect that she has conceived) interventions that improve the environment for the developing gestation need to occur prior to conception if they are to be maximally effective. With the mean time of entry into prenatal care in the third month of gestation, most women enter prenatal care after the completion of organogenesis. Therefore, the first visit after the start of the pregnancy is often too late to avert irreversible environmental risks. Preconceptional identification of a medical condition or an unhealthy personal behavior provides the opportunity for more timely intervention, and thus may have a substantial impact on both the outcome of pregnancy and the long-term health of the mother and her offspring.

Failure to identify medical conditions that can affect pregnancy may result in a higher rate of adverse outcomes. For example, one multisite observational study suggested that racial disparities in the incidence of very-low-birth-weight babies could in part be explained by disparities in maternal conditions that require comprehensive interventions initiated long before the onset of pregnancy (12). In fact, programs that have expanded health care services for underserved women limited only to care provided during pregnancy have reported only minimal impact on preventing adverse pregnancy outcomes such as low birth weight and preterm delivery (13).

For these reasons, the U.S. Public Health Service Expert Panel on the Content of Prenatal Care emphasized preconceptional care as potentially the most significant element of prenatal care (14). Unfortunately, the Public Health Service also estimated in its *Healthy People 2000* report that only 20% to 50% of primary care providers were routinely providing appropriate preconceptional care.

As identified by the Expert Panel, the major components of preconceptional care are risk assessment, health promotion, and targeted medical and psychosocial interventions. Risk assessment includes history, physical examination, and laboratory measures. The goal for physician and patient is to identify alterable risks for poor maternal health and adverse pregnancy outcome and to jointly plan interventions designed to decrease those risks. Table 1-2 lists the risk assessment and health promotion activities recommended by the Expert Panel on the Content of Prenatal Care (14). These elements of preconception care are directed at improving the health and well-being of both the woman and her future pregnancies.

A focus of preconceptional care is to address in all women those common areas where collective benefit can be anticipated. Focus on the following areas is thus important: tobacco, alcohol and illicit drug use, domestic violence, infection screening, immunization, nutrition, optimal weight, genetic screening, over-the-counter and prescription medication use, and family planning. The detection of any medical, obstetric, or psychosocial abnormality by careful history and physical examination with appropriate laboratory testing is a central thrust of a preconceptional visit. What sets this kind of evaluation apart from other periodic examinations is the emphasis on potential pregnancy and on reframing the meaning of gathered information in this light. It is also necessary to attend not only to the woman's static condition in the nongravid state but to anticipate how pregnancy may change that condition over 9 months' time. The focus on pregnancy issues changes the perspective on many elements of data collection. A history of genetic disease in either prospective parent's family becomes newly relevant. A physical abnormality that causes no problem for the nonpregnant woman may deserve increased attention as pregnancy is contemplated.

Many of the elements of preconceptional care, such as encouraging the cessation of tobacco or other drug use, improving diet, and screening for treatable medical conditions, can prove beneficial to a woman's health whether or not pregnancy is planned. Other components of preconceptional care, such as genetic counseling and reducing barriers to early initiation of prenatal care, become of significant value only after a pregnancy is anticipated. Consideration should be given as to whether an intervention should be completed prior to conception or whether it can be equally effective if it is performed subsequently. Examples of those that should be completed prior to conception include counseling about the

TABLE 1-2. *Preconceptional risk assessment: history and physical examination*

Content	Evidence of association	Recommended population	Need for research
Medical			
Sociodemographic data	G	All	N
Menstrual history	G	All	N
Past obstetric history	G	All	N
Contraceptive history	NA	All	M
Sexual history	NA	All	M
Medical/surgical history	G	All	N
Infection history	G	All	N
Family and genetic history	G	All	N
Nutrition	G	All	N
Psychosocial			
Smoking	G	All	N
Alcohol	G	All	H
Drugs	G	All	N
Social support	F	All	H
Stress levels	F	All	H
Physical abuse	G	All	H
Mental illness/status	NA	All	H
Pregnancy readiness	F	All	H
Exposure to teratogens	G	All	N
Housing, finances, etc.	G	All	N
Extremes of physical work, exercise, and other activity	F	All	H
Physical examination			
General physical examination	NA	All	N
Blood pressure/pulse	G	All	N
Height	G	All	N
Weight	G	All	H
Height/weight profile	F	All	H
Pelvic examination and clinical pelvimetry	P	All	M
Breast examination	NA	All	N
Laboratory tests			
Hemoglobin or hematocrit	G	All	N
Rh factor	G	All	N
Rubella titer	G	All	N
Urine dipstick			
Protein	G	All	M
Sugar	G	All	M
Pap smear	NA	All	M
Tuberculosis screen	F	Some	N
Gonococcal culture	G	All	N
Chlamydia culture or rapid screen	G	Some	N
Syphilis test	G	All	N
Hepatitis B	G	All	N
Toxoplasmosis	G	Some*	H
CMV	G	Some*	H
Herpes simplex	F	Some*	H
Varicella	F	Some*	H
HIV	G	All (offer)	H
Hemoglobinopathies	G	Some	N
Tay-Sachs	G	Some	N
Parental karyotype	G	Some	N
Illicit drug screen	G	All (offer)	H

*Panel was unable to reach agreement on whether screening for these infections should be recommended for some or all women.

G, good; F, fair; P, poor; NA, not applicable; H, high; M, medium; N, not recommended for research.

impact of pregnancy and parenthood for the woman and her family, reducing exposure to teratogens, and altering medication regimens.

A key component of preconceptional care is family planning, because couples who plan their pregnancies are presumed to be more likely to obtain appropriate prenatal care. There also may be improved outcomes for the entire family with appropriate intervals between births. For example, Lieberman and colleagues reported that a short pregnancy interval may be associated with the birth of a small-for-gestational-age infant in a subsequent pregnancy (15). Hobcraft and colleagues noted that a child born within 2 years of an older sibling had an increased risk of dying in the neonatal period (16). Basso and colleagues in their Danish birth registry study found that there was an increased risk of preterm birth in a subsequent pregnancy if the interpregnancy interval was less than 8 months (17). Huttly and colleagues studied 3,500 urban Brazilian children; after attempting to control for several maternal and socioeconomic factors, they found that children born within 24 months of the birth of a previous child had lower birth weights, greater postneonatal mortality, and worse anthropometric measures at an average age of 19 months (18). The lower birth weights that Huttly and colleagues observed in children born after a short interconceptional interval may be the result of the pregnant woman's inability to build up her nutritional reserves when conceiving a pregnancy within 2 years of her previous one; this may also have an impact on subsequent maternal health. Furthermore, a short interconceptional interval may limit the length of time that an older child has the opportunity to breastfeed and may therefore impact on that child's overall health.

Unfortunately, it has been reported that up to 49% of pregnancies in the United States are unintended—either mistimed or unwanted—and the rates are even greater for adolescents and women over the age of 40 (19). As a result, it becomes practical to recommend that preconceptional care be incorporated as a part of routine primary care for all reproductive age individuals, and that implies participation by a broad range of physicians and other health care specialists.

Furthermore, special mention should be made of the importance of focusing on two areas of preconceptional care where, unfortunately, health care providers have not traditionally been effective. Although these subjects are addressed elsewhere in this text, it is important to highlight them here. They concern modifying high-risk social situations and improving health habits. Relevant examples are discussed in the ensuing sections.

Domestic Violence

Domestic violence is often overlooked, yet its consequences are severe (see Chapter 10). It is widely recognized to lead to depression and substance abuse, among other things. Unfortunately, women are not likely to volunteer the information that they are being emotionally, physically, or sexually abused and are often afraid to have their situation discovered. Dietz and colleagues noted that women who were physically abused were nearly twice as likely to delay entry into prenatal care as those who were not subjected to abuse (20). In addition, Parker and colleagues in their study of more than 1,200 African-American, Hispanic, and white women found that those who were abused were at significantly higher risk of delivering a low-birth-weight baby, low maternal weight gain, infections, anemia, smoking, and use of alcohol or drugs (21). In addition, McKay noted that women who are the victims of abuse are also at greater risk of having children who are themselves abused in childhood (22).

It is estimated that 3 to 4 million women each year are abused by their partner (23), and 29% of these women report an escalation of their abuse during pregnancy (24). All providers of care for women should therefore routinely screen for domestic violence and be prepared to offer assistance to an abused woman.

Tobacco

Smoking contributes to many problems surrounding pregnancy, including low birth weight, placenta previa, and spontaneous abortion (25). A 1980 report issued by the Surgeon General stated that 21% to 39% of the incidence of low-birth-weight infants could be attributed to smoking during pregnancy (26). Although no study has demonstrated that stopping smoking prior to conception is superior to stopping early in pregnancy, common sense dictates that women planning a pregnancy should avoid tobacco smoke. Women who smoke should be encouraged to quit prior to pregnancy at a time when they may be more successful with the assistance of nicotine gum or patches, neither of which is commonly used in pregnancy, even though they may be acceptable treatments given the significant risks associated with cigarette smoking. Nicotine gum was graded by the Food and Drug Administration as pregnancy category C (risk cannot be ruled out) in 1992, and transdermal systems are graded as pregnancy category D (positive evidence of risk).

Physicians often feel powerless to effect change in the smoking behavior of their patients. However, the results of randomized controlled trials showed that even with brief physician training, intervention protocols produced smoking cessation rates of up to 15% at 1 year of follow-up (27).

Alcohol

Alcohol consumption during pregnancy is an often unrecognized problem that warrants more attention (see Chapter 8). Alcohol can cause a variety of problems both for the fetus and the woman, including fetal alcohol syndrome, which may be the leading preventable cause of mental retardation (28). Serdula and colleagues suggested that approximately 25% of pregnant women report continuing to consume alcohol during pregnancy (29). Several screening methods have been studied to aid providers in identifying women who consume alcohol, such as the CAGE or T-ACE questionnaires (30). Proper identification of women who drink prior to conception may allow effective intervention before a child is conceived.

Rosett and colleagues reported that with proper counseling, alcohol consumption can be decreased and birth outcomes improved. They studied 49 women who were heavy drinkers and compared the birth outcomes of the 25 who were able to reduce their drinking significantly or abstain from alcohol completely with those of the women who continued to drink. Continued drinking during pregnancy was significantly associated with impaired fetal growth and other abnormalities (31). This study, however, was small, and further research is needed in this area.

Illicit Drugs

Other drugs, such as cocaine, are associated with poor maternal health and poor pregnancy outcome (see Chapter 8). Often women who frequently use illicit drugs do not seek prenatal care. Examples of some of the most commonly used drugs include opiates, such as heroin, which can cause neonatal drug withdrawal, and cocaine, which may be associated with congenital anomalies, placental abruption, and low birth weight (32).

The harmful effects of drug use during pregnancy have led some to advocate punishing women specifically for using drugs during their pregnancies. Unfortunately, no studies have demonstrated programs that effectively prevent drug abuse among women prior to or during pregnancy. Clearly, the preferred solution would be one that prevented the use of these harmful drugs prior to conception. Given that few interventions have been shown to be effective at treating illicit drug addictions, punishing pregnant women for drug abuse would seem to be counterproductive and serve to alienate women from the health care system.

Nutrition

A woman's nutritional status prior to pregnancy may have a significant impact on the outcome of her pregnancy (see Chapter 2). Women with low prepregnancy weight and inadequate weight gain during pregnancy are at greater risk of having preterm deliveries and delivering a low-birth-weight infant (33).

Additional data are being accrued that suggest women whose diets are deficient in vitamins such as folate are at greater risk of delivering a child with a neural tube defect (NTD). For example, Werler and colleagues in their case-control study compared the vitamin intake history of 436 women with pregnancies affected by NTDs with 2,615 women whose pregnancies were affected by other major malformations. Their study found a 60% reduction in the risk of carrying a fetus with an NTD when 0.4 mg of folate was taken daily (34). Thus, it has been recommended by the Public Health Service, the Centers for Disease Control and Prevention, and the American College of Obstetricians and Gynecologists that all women of childbearing age consume 0.4 mg of folate each day; toward this end, the Food and Drug Administration issued rules in 1996 that required the fortification of certain grain products with folate (35).

For women with a prior pregnancy that was affected by an NTD, the recommendation is that they consume 4 mg of folate in the periconceptional period. This is based on studies such as the one performed by the Medical Research Council of the United Kingdom that found a 70% decrease in the risk of the recurrence of an NTD among the women who received folic acid (36).

Folate is not the only vitamin that has recently drawn attention for its role during pregnancy. Semba and colleagues, in their study of 338 women with human immunodeficiency virus, found that those who were vitamin A deficient were at higher risk of transmitting the virus to their children (37).

Preconceptional Care of Women with Medical Illness

Although preconceptional care can be beneficial for all women contemplating a future pregnancy, it holds special benefits for those women with preexisting medical illness. In addition to the benefits that well women may receive from addressing nutrition, alcohol, smoking, licit and illicit drug use, immunization, genetic screening, occupational hazards, home environment, and psychological state, care of women with medical illness can focus on those diagnostic or therapeutic interventions specific to their history.

Moutquin and colleagues found that 13.9% of women presenting for prenatal care had a medical problem identified at their first visit (38). This prevalence of recognized conditions is not surprising when the incidence of common conditions is considered: asthma (4–5%) (39), hypertension (5%) (40), diabetes (1–2%) (41), mitral valve prolapse (3–8%) (42), epilepsy (0.45–2.65%) (43–45), migraine (10–15%) (46). Furthermore, the advances that make pregnancy a possibility for women with chronic illnesses, who in an earlier era would not have had this option, and the scientific and societal changes that now permit women to conceive later in life also contribute to the population of women with medical problems who attempt pregnancy.

A preconceptional visit affords an opportunity to detect previously unidentified disease. Conditions that cause few or no symptoms and those whose symptoms are so insidious in onset that patients are inured to them and do not recognize them as abnormal are particularly likely to go undetected. These may include hypertension, diabetes, many anemias, renal insufficiency, proteinuria, rheumatic heart disease, goiter, abnormalities of thyroid function, and infections, including chronic hepatitis, human immunodeficiency virus, and tuberculosis.

It is not solely by promoting contact with the health care system that a preconceptional visit contributes to the identification of problems that might have an impact on pregnancy. A designated preconceptional visit is not just an extra opportunity to conduct the same history and physical and laboratory screening tests that would have been performed to the same effect in the course of regular primary care. Beyond some tailoring of the recommended examinations to address pregnancy-related issues, the nature of the inquiry is transformed by the prospect of pregnancy. A unique feature of the preconceptional visit is the reframing of data in this light. Although the knowledge that a woman has several alcohol-containing drinks most weekends or that she has a sister with cystic fibrosis or that she and her partner are both Ashkenazi Jews would have little impact on usual adult medical care, each of these takes on wholly new implications as pregnancy is anticipated. So too, details of the patient's past medical history need to be reframed to extract the new meanings imparted by the prospect of pregnancy. Conditions relegated to the past medical history may move to the fore when reconsidered in light of a proposed pregnancy. A woman born with a ventricular septal defect that closed spontaneously in early life, leaving her asymptomatic with no evident sequelae, nonetheless has an increased risk of bearing a child with congenital heart disease, for which screening can be performed during the gestation (47). A woman whose successful treatment for childhood malignancy included abdominal radiation might consider her disease a closed chapter, but its ongoing implications for fertility and for ability to sustain a pregnancy give it a new meaning in a preconceptional evaluation (48). Quiescent conditions that require little attention in usual primary care may have profound implications for future pregnancies. A woman who received ablative therapy (i.e., thyroidectomy or radioactive iodine) for florid Graves hyperthyroidism may be rendered incapable of responding to a persistently elevated thyroid-stimulating antibody and thus may be little affected; her fetus with its pristine thyroid gland could be a new target of its mother's antibodies which cross the placenta and in rare cases, when the titer is sufficiently high, cause fetal Graves disease, a condition that is often fatal if unrecognized, but easily treatable.

Many medical conditions such as asthma or hypothyroidism will warrant the same care regardless of the prospect of pregnancy. Nonetheless, the anticipation of pregnancy can serve to focus consideration on medical issues that deserve attention in their own right, but are lent a new sense of urgency when the outlook for a child is added. The treatment of epilepsy provides the best example of this. Irrespective of pregnancy, it is appropriate to consider discontinuation of anticonvulsants in selected patients who have been seizure free for 2 or more years on therapy. In nine pooled studies representing 1,580 adults discontinued from anticonvulsants with differing duration of follow-up (1,380 patients were followed for 5 or more years), the recurrence rate was 39.4% (49). The American Academy of Neurology published guidelines in 1996 to help select appropriate patients (49). It can only be surmised to what extent the application of these selection criteria will further improve the 61% success rate in the pooled studies. Although withdrawing anticonvulsants from appropriate patients would be good care in any case, preconceptional discontinuation is even more compelling because of the teratogenicity of all anticonvulsants (50). When discontinuation is not an option, simplification to monotherapy from multidrug regimens is an alternative to consider. Because sudden cessation of anticonvulsants is a frequent precipitant of status epilepticus and because the success of withdrawal is enhanced by phased withdrawal over months, this should be done slowly and gradually. In this case it would be impossible to both prevent the embryo's exposure to the teratogenic drugs and to avoid precipitating seizures by too rapid withdrawal if the intervention began only after pregnancy was known. This illustrates another principle of preconceptional care: not all options that are available in advance of pregnancy can be used once pregnancy is underway; those interventions that take time to accomplish may be foreclosed once conception has occurred.

Preconceptional care provides an opportunity to evaluate medical conditions free of the strictures that pregnancy might later impose and to assess what pregnancy will mean for the individual. Having the opportunity to perform radiologic procedures and nuclear scans with impunity may be valuable. Interpreting tests unencumbered by the sometimes confounding changes that pregnancy adds allows a fuller evaluation. Testing that would not otherwise be warranted may be indicated expressly to determine how pregnancy will be tolerated. For example, in evaluating mitral stenosis, the focus must extend beyond the patient's current state and extrapolate how the increased cardiac output, heart rate, and blood volume typical of normal pregnancy will change her status; sometimes exercise testing may be performed expressly to anticipate whether pregnancy changes will be tolerated.

The evaluation will not always lead to a change in therapy prior to conception. Often its value may be in preparing a patient and her family for what can be expected during pregnancy, what surveillance or testing or treatment regimens she will be asked to follow, and what outcomes are likely.

But for many conditions, medical care before conception offers unique opportunities to affect outcome. It allows medical input into the decision to attempt conception and permits selection of a propitious time for conception. It creates an opportunity to optimize the woman's condition as she enters pregnancy. It allows protection of the fetus during the initial critical weeks of intrauterine life.

It is only before pregnancy that decisions about conception itself can be made. Some medical illnesses raise diverse issues that may influence some women's decisions about attempting pregnancy. These may include concerns about the woman's prospect for survival independent of pregnancy (e.g., AIDS); concerns about pregnancy posing a threat to maternal survival (e.g., Marfan syndrome with aortic dilation, pulmonary hypertension, inoperable cerebral aneurysm) (51); concerns about the mother's disability; conflicts between needed maternal treatment and fetal well-being (e.g., oncologic treatment); transmission of a grave genetic or infectious disease to the offspring; exacerbation of the mother's disease by pregnancy (e.g., congestive heart failure or mitral stenosis); and poor chances of having a successful pregnancy or bearing a healthy baby.

The timing of conception may be an important determinant of outcome. For progressive inexorable diseases, opting to have children earlier in reproductive life may be an important way to optimize safety and success of pregnancy. Long-standing diabetes mellitus and Marfan syndrome would fall into this category. In some cases delay is advisable, such as shortly after renal transplantation or following a lupus flare (52,53). Delay also may be warranted awaiting interventions to be completed to make pregnancy safer. Helping patients to find an appropriate and effective means of contraception until conception is desired can be an important component of care.

Optimization of the woman's care as she enters pregnancy can be valuable in several ways. It can safeguard maternal health; correcting a cerebral arteriovenous malformation prior to pregnancy helps avoid the increased risk of intracranial hemorrhage in pregnancy and beyond. It may increase the chances that pregnancy will be achieved and sustained. Treating hypothyroidism will both improve the mother's health and eliminate a known cause of infertility. Similarly, untreated hyperthyroidism is associated with increased pregnancy loss; its treatment is beneficial to the woman and to the maintenance of the gestation. Preconceptional care can optimize the milieu of the embryo's development. Reinstituting a restricted diet for women with phenylketonuria who abandoned it after their own neurologic development was complete will help prevent the devastating neurologic damage that befalls the offspring of these women.

Medication management presents a major opportunity for preventing teratogenicity. Drugs may be discontinued if not essential (e.g., isotretinoin for acne). Dosage may be changed: maintaining levels of glycemia similar to nondiabetic women is important in preventing the congenital anomalies seen in the infants of pregestational diabetic mothers. In order to achieve tighter control, it is usually necessary to alter the dose of administered insulin. Drugs may be substituted for alternatives that are safer in pregnancy; heparin, which is not the best option for long-term treatment, may be substituted for the teratogenic coumadin. Preconceptional care can be used to educate patients about early diagnosis of pregnancy and to facilitate early entry into prenatal care when appropriate.

Relying on a designated visit to gain the potential benefits that preconceptional care can provide is insufficient, especially for women with chronic medical illnesses. The concerns that preconceptional care highlight need to be built into primary care of all women with childbearing potential. As detailed earlier in this chapter, the fact that only half of pregnancies are intended makes it evident that awaiting an announcement on the part of a patient about her plans to conceive would be decidedly misguided. To the extent that the benefits of preconceptional care are understood and embraced, the need to introduce these ideas into women's health care in other ways becomes evident. Whoever delivers it, primary care needs to include inquiry about pregnancy plans, selection of acute and chronic medications with unintended pregnancy clearly in mind, education about optimal timing of pregnancy, education about need for preconceptional reevaluation or change in treatment when appropriate, offering of contraception whenever pregnancy would be inadvisable, and anticipatory stance toward pregnancy and its effect on the patient's medical condition.

PRENATAL CARE TO REDUCE MEDICAL RISK

The focus of the services offered during prenatal care is to identify medical risks and attempt to reduce their impact on the pregnancy both for the mother and her fetus. This can be enhanced and expedited if a thorough preconceptional consultation has occurred, but needs to be detailed at the first visit after pregnancy has commenced. The major goal of subsequent prenatal care visits is to determine the health status of the fetus and the pregnant woman and to initiate a plan of care for the remainder of the pregnancy and peripartum period that will maximize the chances of a healthy outcome for both.

At the first visit after pregnancy has commenced, a similar history is taken as outlined in Table 1-2 if it was not done as part of the preconceptional consultation. For the woman who had a preconceptional consultation, the history is updated to reflect any changes that have occurred in the interim. Particular attention should be placed on confirming the duration of the pregnancy. This is first accomplished by a careful documentation of the menstrual history. For the woman who menstruates every 28 to 30 days and is certain when the start of her last menstrual period occurred, the gestational (menstrual) age of the pregnancy can be assumed to be the number of weeks since the onset of the last menses. For the woman whose cycle is significantly longer than 28 to 30 days or is irregular, it can not be assumed that ovulation occurred 14 days after her last menstrual period, and the gestational age may not correspond to the number of weeks since the onset of the last menses. In this case it may be necessary to undertake an ultrasonographic examination to help determine the gestational age of the pregnancy because reliance on physical examination is difficult. Accurately determining gestational age allows for more discriminating detection later in the pregnancy of problems related to fetal growth as well as more precise diagnosis of which pregnancies have progressed beyond 42 completed weeks of gestation and may therefore be at increased risk of the complications associated with postterm pregnancy.

A less extensive physical examination can be performed at the first pregnancy visit if a preconceptional visit has been well documented. Otherwise, a complete examination should be performed as outlined in Table 1-2. In either case, particular attention should be directed to the patient's blood pressure, weight, breast examination, and pelvic examination because each of these areas may have undergone significant changes since conception. The pelvic examination should screen for uterine size,

TABLE 1-3. *Pregnancy revisits: risk assessment activities*

Content	Evidence of association	Recommended population	Timing	Need for research
History				
Continuing assessment of pregnancy to date	NA	All	Each visit	N
Physical examination				
Blood pressure	F	All	24 wk and after[a]	N
Weight	P	All	Each visit	N
Fundal height/growth	G	All	16 wk and after	N
Fetal lie/presentation/engagement/FHR	NA	All	24 wk and after	N
Cervical examination	P	All	Begin 41 wk	N
Laboratory tests				
Repeat hemoglobin or hematocrit	G	All	After 24 wk	N
Repeat Rh antibody screen	G	Some	26–28 wk	N
Diabetic screen	G	All	26–28 wk	M
Repeat syphilis test	G	Some	3rd trimester	N
Repeat gonococcal culture	G	Some	36 wk	N
Repeat HIV screen	G	Some	36 wk	H
Maternal serum alpha-fetoprotein or "triple screen"	G	All	14–16 wk	M
Obstetric ultrasonography	NA	Some	When indicated	M

[a]Panel was unable to reach agreement on the frequency of blood pressure measurement.
G, good; F, fair; P, poor; NA, not applicable; H, high; M, medium; N, not recommended for research.

possible gestational age discrepancy, ovarian cysts, myomata, and other pertinent pathology.

Similarly, the laboratory tests obtained at the first pregnancy visit can be limited to urine culture and a hemoglobin or hematocrit if the tests recommended in Table 1-2 were obtained during a preconceptional visit. A screen for antibodies to red blood cell antigens also may be indicated. In a patient at high risk for type II diabetes mellitus, a blood glucose screen is particularly important even if appropriate testing was performed preconceptionally.

Subsequent visits during the course of prenatal care are used to pursue all issues that were revealed at previous visits. If a medical or behavioral risk factor that could lead to a complication is identified during the course of the preconceptional or prenatal care appropriate intervention and surveillance should be undertaken as necessary to mitigate its effects. The content of the subsequent visits during the course of prenatal care as recommended by the Expert Panel on the Content of Prenatal Care is given in Tables 1-3 and 1-4.

TABLE 1-4. *Pregnancy revisits: health promotion activities*

Content	Evidence of association	Recommended population	Timing	Need for research
Counseling to promote and support healthful behavior				
Avoidance of teratogens	P	All	Each visit	H
Safer sex	NA	All	Each trimester	H
Maternal seatbelt use	G	All	Each trimester	N
Support for smoking cessation	G	Some	Each visit	
Work counseling	G	Some	Each visit	H
Nutrition counseling	G	Some	Each visit	M
Signs and symptoms of preterm labor	F	All	2nd and 3rd trimester	H
General knowledge of pregnancy and parenting				
Physiologic and emotional changes	NA	All	1st and 3rd trimesters	H
Sexuality counseling	NA	All	Last half of pregnancy	H
Fetal growth and development	P	All	Each visit	H
Self-help strategies for discomforts	P		Each visit	M
General health habits (hygiene, exercise, rest, and sleep patterns)	F	All	Each visit	H
Promotion of breast feeding	F	All	26 weeks and after	H
Infant car seat safety	G	All	Each visit	H
Classes—preparation for childbirth, parenting	G	All	32 weeks	H
Family roles and adjustment	G	All	38 weeks	H
Information on Proposed Care				
Laboratory tests	NA	All	Before testing	N
Discussion of birth plan	NA	All	3rd trimester	N
When to call, where to go when in labor	NA	All	3rd trimester	M

G, good; F, fair; P, poor; NA, not applicable; H, high; M, medium; N, not recommended for research.

The utility of subsequent visits during the course of prenatal care include detecting and managing medical problems such as anemia, urinary tract infections, diabetes, hypertension, asthma, or exacerbation of other preexisting illnesses, all of which may have significant impact on pregnancy outcome for both the mother and her fetus. Concomitantly, the caregiver should be alert to developing obstetric conditions such as abnormal placentation, isoimmunization, fetal growth abnormalities, multiple gestation, and postterm pregnancy.

PRENATAL CARE TO REDUCE PSYCHOSOCIAL AND ENVIRONMENTAL RISK

In the rush to see more and more patients, an area of prenatal care that is often neglected is efforts to screen for and reduce psychosocial and environmental risks, although these areas may have a significant impact on pregnancy outcome. This is in contrast to the attention that providers focus on elements discussed in the previous section concerning medical risks. Peoples-Sheps and colleagues found in their review of 147 prenatal charts that providers were relatively vigilant about adhering to the recommendations of the Expert Panel on the Content of Prenatal Care concerning physical examination, history taking, and laboratory testing, but were relatively poor in the areas of behavioral risk assessment and health promotion activities (54).

For example, providers of prenatal care should be inquiring about their patients' exercise habits because women with an appropriate exercise regimen may have shorter lengths of labor and less meconium-stained fluid, and may need fewer cesarean sections (55–57).

The relationship of employment to women's health status during pregnancy has been of considerable interest in recent years as the participation of women in the workforce has increased. Unfortunately, good studies on the safety of working during pregnancy are difficult to construct; as a result, we do not have a good understanding of the effects of different jobs on pregnancy outcome. Some researchers, after attempting to control for confounding factors, have found that heavy work may increase a woman's risk of poor pregnancy outcome (58–60).

In addition, a woman's place of employment or even her home environment may expose her pregnancy to teratogens, with effects ranging from increased risk of spontaneous abortions to congenital and chromosomal anomalies. A large body of data exists regarding the teratogenicity of various substances; however, it remains unclear to what degree these data can be extrapolated to workplace exposures. Exposures that have been implicated as potential teratogens include radiation, organic solvents, pesticides, anesthetic gases, antineoplastic drugs and lead (61,62).

Despite substantial interest in the area of nutrition during pregnancy, much of the research has been based on large epidemiologic studies that leave numerous questions unanswered. These studies have included, for example, wartime famine observations. The conclusions drawn from these studies is, not surprisingly, that good nutrition has a positive impact on pregnancy outcome, especially birth weight and neonatal mortality (63).

Although meaningful clinical studies of nutrition during pregnancy have been difficult to design, it has been demonstrated that maternal prepregnancy weight and weight gain during pregnancy are associated with neonatal weight. Underweight women or women with poor weight gain during pregnancy have a greater risk of delivering an infant weighing less than 2,500 g (64). Conversely, obesity places a woman at higher risk of complications such as gestational diabetes. Women also may benefit from iron and vitamin supplementation, especially those with iron deficiency anemia or poor nutritional status.

It is now recognized that screening for domestic violence in pregnancy needs to be incorporated as an integral part of the prenatal consultation because it is reported to occur more frequently during pregnancy. In fact, in 1992 Richard Jones III, as president of the American College of Obstetricians and Gynecologists, made the reduction of domestic violence against women his presidential initiative in order to focus more attention on the subject. Domestic violence may occur more frequently during pregnancy as a result of the following factors: stress related to family transition, including economic changes; sexual frustration of the male perpetrator; history of child abuse in the perpetrator's family of origin as well as the current family; and the defenselessness of the pregnant woman (65). The stress of pregnancy can be an additional precipitating factor in families in which there is already a high degree of stress. The magnitude of the problem is astounding when one considers that some have estimated that 25% to 30% of all married women are beaten at least once during their marriage by their spouses (66). Physical and sexual abuse during pregnancy can have significant implications for the health and well-being of both the woman and her fetus.

Domestic violence, in addition to jeopardizing maternal and fetal physical well-being, generates stress and anxiety in pregnant women. Evaluations of the effectiveness of prenatal care have generally focused on the biological and physiologic aspects of pregnancy, but the psychosocial environment also may have a significant impact on pregnancy outcome as well as maternal and familial welfare. Thus, prenatal care offers an opportunity to attempt to decrease psychosocial stressors. By assessing the need for and then offering social supports, from classes that help women prepare for childbirth and those that provide health education to referrals to social service agencies and programs such as Women, Infants and Children, providers may have a substantial impact on not only the biological outcome of pregnancy but also the health and happiness of an entire family. For example, childbirth education classes have been shown to diminish maternal anxiety and the need for medication and other interventions in labor as well as improve parenting skills and overall parental self-esteem (67).

More recently, it has been found that psychosocial stress is associated with preterm birth. In a multicenter observational study of nearly 2,600 pregnant women, Copper and colleagues found that stress was an independent risk factor for preterm birth (68). Similarly, Hedegaard and colleagues in their study of more than 5,800 Danish women found that stressful life events experienced during pregnancy were associated with an increased risk of preterm delivery (69).

Focus of attention on psychosocial and environmental risks should take place during the course of preconceptional care as well as during prenatal care. Once a pregnancy has been conceived, however, the focus of the counseling changes slightly. It still includes items discussed above, such as nutrition and avoidance of teratogens, as well as safe sex practice. In addition, counseling should now be provided to foster the patient's knowledge about pregnancy and parenthood; this includes discussion of topics such as the physiologic and emotional changes of pregnancy, sexuality during pregnancy, fetal growth and development, and dealing with the discomforts of pregnancy. Finally, providers should talk with patients during the course of prenatal care about the screening and diagnostic tests that are offered, the content and timing of prenatal visits, and warning signs of possible problems that may develop in the pregnancy that should be reported.

PRENATAL CARE TO REDUCE LOW BIRTH WEIGHT

Preterm birth and low birth weight is one of the most significant factors leading to perinatal and neonatal morbidity and mortality in the United States. Because it is easily measured, birth weight is often used as a proxy for gestational age; therefore, low birth weight becomes an indicator of premature birth. However, this blurs the distinction between two distinct problems: fetal growth restriction and preterm birth. Taffel reported that 55% of all low-birth-weight infants were born prematurely and 45% were full-term deliveries (70). Numerous studies have demonstrated associations between various factors and low birth weight, some of which may be amenable to management with appropriate prenatal care. Table 1-5 lists the factors identified by the Institute of Medicine in its 1985 publication *Preventing Low Birthweight.*

Because the largest single contributor to the problem of low birth weight is preterm delivery, a great deal of effort has been made to identify women at greatest risk for this complication. Investigators such as Papiernik-Berkhauer (71) and, later, Creasy (72), developed scoring systems based on risk factors such as those listed in Table 1-5 to predict preterm births. More recent studies have looked at other risk factors including bacterial vaginosis (73), cervical length (74), and biochemical markers.

TABLE 1-5. *Risk factors for low birth weight*

I. Demographic risks
   A. Age (<17, >34)
   B. Race (black)
   C. Low socioeconomic status
   D. Unmarried
   E. Low level of education
II. Medical risk predating pregnancy
   A. Parity (zero or more than four)
   B. Low weight for height
   C. Genitourinary anomalies/surgery
   D. Selected diseases, such as diabetes or chronic hypertension
   E. Nonimmune status for selected infections, such as rubella
   F. Poor obstetric history, including previous low birth weight infant and multiple spontaneous abortions
   G. Maternal genetic factors, such as low maternal weight at own birth
III. Medical risks in current pregnancy
   A. Multiple pregnancy
   B. Poor weight gain
   C. Short interpregnancy interval
   D. Hypotension
   E. Hypertension/preeclampsia/toxemia
   F. Selected infections, such as symptomatic bacteriuria, rubella, and cytomegalovirus
   G. First- or second-trimester bleeding
   H. Placental problems, such as placenta previa and placental abruption
   I. Hyperemesis
   J. Oligohydramnios/polyhydramnios
   K. Anemia/abnormal hemoglobin
   L. Isoimmunization
   M. Fetal anomalies
   N. Incompetent cervix
   O. Spontaneous premature rupture of membranes
IV. Behavioral and environmental risks
   A. Smoking
   B. Poor nutritional status
   C. Alcohol and other substance abuse
   D. Diethylstilbesterol exposure and other toxic exposures, including occupational hazards
   E. High altitude
V. Health care risks
   A. Absent or inadequate prenatal care
   B. Iatrogenic prematurity
VI. Evolving concepts of risk
   A. Stress, physical and psychosocial
   B. Uterine irritability
   C. Events triggering uterine contractions
   D. Cervical changes detected before the onset of labor
   E. Selected infections, such as mycoplasma and Chlamydia
   F. Inadequate plasma volume expansion
   G. Progesterone deficiency

From the Institute of Medicine. *Preventing Low Birthweight.* Washington, DC: National Academy Press, 1985.

Some of the most promising biochemical markers investigated thus far include maternal serum C-reactive protein (75), salivary estriol (76), and cervicovaginal human chorionic gonadotropin (77). The most attention has been focused on cervicovaginal fetal fibronectin (78).

Although the clinical relevance of identifying which woman is at greatest risk of preterm delivery has not been adequately elucidated, the investigation of markers such as the biochemical ones is particularly exciting because they may help us to understand the etiology of preterm delivery. With a better understanding of the etiology, as well as an increased ability to identify women at the highest risk, investigation of potential interventions to decrease the incidence of preterm delivery becomes possible. Already this area of research is bearing fruit. For example, in a randomized, controlled trial involving 624 women at high risk for preterm delivery, it was found that women treated with oral metronidazole and erythromycin for bacterial vaginosis in the second trimester had significantly lower rates of premature delivery (79).

Studies to evaluate the effectiveness of prenatal care to reduce problems such as low birth weight have been limited by the widespread belief that prenatal care is effective in reducing infant morbidity and mortality; as a result, randomized controlled trials of prenatal care versus no care would be considered unethical. Thus, studies of the value of prenatal care for reducing the incidence of low birth weight have necessarily been observational studies and, therefore, limited by confounding factors and selection bias.

Although reports such as *Preventing Low Birthweight* (80) have had the effect of improving funding for prenatal care, the result has been to isolate prenatal care from the remainder of women's health care. Unfortunately, the results of the expansion of prenatal care availability have been disappointing. For example, Haas and colleagues found that changes in rates of women obtaining satisfactory prenatal care in Massachusetts did not correlate with birth outcomes (13). Increased use of prenatal care, particularly among black women in the United States, has not been associated with a decrease in the low birth weight rates. During the 1970's, the use of prenatal care by black women increased by 40% without any reduction in the rate of very-low-birth-weight infants in this population and only a slight reduction (6%) in the rate of low-birth-weight deliveries (81–83).

If prenatal care is to have an impact on the incidence of low birth weight, it must do so by reducing the rate of preterm delivery or fetal growth restriction. Although it may be plausible that prenatal care may be able to reduce the rate of preterm delivery, it would depend on the existence of effective interventions to modify risk factors for premature birth. One estimate is that less than 10% of all preterm births are preventable (84). The possibility of reducing the incidence of fetal growth restriction is even more bleak. At present, there are no proven interventions to prevent fetal growth restriction. Reduction in rates of smoking during pregnancy may be the only broad intervention that might have an impact because effective smoking cessation programs have demonstrated an effect on birth weight (85). Unfortunately, standard prenatal care has never been shown to have a significant impact on the rate of smoking during pregnancy.

The conclusions of several researchers who have reviewed the subject of whether prenatal care can reduce the incidence of low-birth-weight deliveries have differed. Some have argued that prenatal care does improve birth outcomes (80,86), whereas others have found that there are insufficient data to support this judgment (87). This does not lessen the need for appropriate and broadly accessible prenatal care because preventing low birth weight is only one of the goals of prenatal care. Moreover, hypotheses regarding the effectiveness of prenatal care in reducing the incidence of low-birth-weight deliveries have not been adequately tested. The studies that have been done do not have a standardized protocol governing the content of the prenatal care provided. For example, if preconceptional care is considered an integral component of appropriate prenatal care, then few if any of the studies of the effectiveness of prenatal care have delivered complete prenatal care to their study population. Thus, more work remains to be done to demonstrate the effectiveness of prenatal care in reducing the incidence of low birth weight.

APPROACHES TO PRENATAL CARE

Timing of Visits

Traditionally, the timing of repeat visits for women obtaining prenatal care has been one visit every 4 weeks for the first 28 weeks of pregnancy, then every 2 weeks until 36 weeks, and weekly thereafter as long as the pregnancy is progressing normally. More frequent visits can be scheduled as necessary if any significant issues arise. The Expert Panel on the Content of Prenatal Care recommended a schedule of fewer visits for healthy, low-risk women, and this schedule encompassed all of the risk assessment and health promotion activities discussed earlier (14). For these patients, they recommended a total of nine visits during an uncomplicated pregnancy, as opposed to the usual 14 visits that a woman starting care at 6–8 weeks of pregnancy would have. The visits the panel endorsed are outlined in Table 1-6.

More recently, McDuffie and colleagues performed a randomized controlled trial to determine if the reduced visit schedule recommended by the Expert Panel had any effect on perinatal outcome among a group of more than 2,700 pregnant women judged to be at low risk. They found no difference in perinatal outcomes or in patient satisfaction despite the schedule of fewer visits (88). In a follow-up study they also found there was no increase in the use of other medical services by these women seeking additional care that they were not getting as part of the reduced visit schedule (89).

TABLE 1-6. *Timing of the risk assessment component of prenatal care*

	Preconceptional or first visit	Weeks								
		6–8[a]	14–16	24–28	32	36	38	39	40	41
History										
Medical	X									
Psychosocial	X									
Update medical and psychosocial		X	X	X	X	X	X	X	X	X
Physical examination										
General	X									
Blood pressure/pulse	X	X		X	X	X	X	X	X	X
Height	X									
Weight	X	X	X	X	X	X	X	X	X	X
Height/weight profile	X									
Pelvic examination/pelvimetry	X	X								
Breast examination	X	X								
Fundal height			X	X	X	X	X	X	X	X
Fetal position/heart rate				X	X	X	X	X	X	X
Cervical examination										X
Laboratory tests										
Hemoglobin or hematocrit	X	X		X						
Rh factor	X									
Pap smear	X									
Diabetic screen				X						
MSAFP or triple screen			X							
Urine dipstick	X									
Protein	X									
Sugar	X									
Urine culture		X								
Infection										
Rubella titer	X									
Syphilis test	X									
Gonococcal culture	X	X								
Hepatitis B	X									
HIV (offered)	X	X								
Illicit drug screen (offered)	X									

[a]If preconceptional care has preceded.

CONCLUSION

Efforts to improve perinatal outcomes have adhered to a model of maternal-fetal separation that implicitly elevates the fetus over the mother. However, historically the two were seen as interdependent, with the experiences of the fetus mediated through the mother. Efforts to isolate the period of pregnancy as the best time to intervene in order to improve perinatal outcomes fail to consider the preconceptional period. As indicated by the Expert Panel on the Content of Prenatal Care, a better conceptualization of the objectives of prenatal care involves not only efforts to ensure the delivery of a healthy infant but also to see it as an opportunity to improve the health and well-being of the woman and the rest of her family. Prenatal care offers a window of opportunity to provide for the long-term health of a woman and to assist her with caring for her entire family.

REFERENCES

1. Speert H. Obstetrics and gynecology in America: a history. Chicago, IL: American College of Obstetricians and Gynecologists, 1980.
2. Sinclair E, Johnston G. The practice of midwivery. Dublin: 1858.
3. Taussig F. The story of prenatal care. Obstet Gynecol 1937;34: 731–739.
4. Williams J. The limitations and possibilities of prenatal care. JAMA 1915;44:95–101.
5. Heaton C. Fifty years of progress in obstetrics and gynecology. NY State J Med 1951;51:83–85.
6. Maternity Center Association, Log 1915–1975. New York: Maternity Center Association, 1980.
7. Thompson J, Walsh L, Merkatz I. The history of prenatal care: cultural, social, and medical contexts. In: Merkatz I, Thompson J, eds. New perspectives on prenatal care. New York: Elsevier, 1990.
8. Stevens A. Maternity center work. Am J Nurs 1920;20:455–462.
9. Stevens A. The public health nurse and the extension of maternity nursing. Public Health Nurs 1920;12:497.
10. Children's Bureau. Prenatal care. Washington, DC: Department of Labor, US Government Printing Office, 1924.
11. Children's Bureau. Standards of prenatal care: an outline for the use of physicians. Washington, DC: Department of Labor, US Government Printing Office, 1925 (Bureau Publication No. 153).
12. Kempe A, Wise P, Barkan S, et al. Clinical determinants of the racial disparity in very low birthweight. N Engl J Med 1992;327:969–973.
13. Haas J, Udvarhelyi S, Morris C, Epstein A. The effect of providing health coverage to poor uninsured pregnant women in Massachusetts. JAMA 1993;269:87–91.
14. United States Public Health Service Expert Panel on the Content of Prenatal Care. Caring for our future: the content of prenatal care. Washington, DC: United States Department of Health and Human Services, 1989.

15. Lieberman E, Lang J, Ryan K, Monson R, Schoenbaum S. The association of inter-pregnancy interval with small for gestational age births. Obstet Gynecol 1989;74:1–5.
16. Hobcraft J, McDonald W, Rutstein S. Childspacing effects on infant and child mortality. Population Index 1984;50:60–64.
17. Basso O, Olsen J, Knudsen L, Christensen K. Low birth weight and preterm birth after short interpregnancy intervals. Am J Obstet Gynecol 1998;178:259–263.
18. Huttly SR, Victora CG, Barros FC, Vaughan JP. Birth spacing and child health in urban Brazilian children. Pediatrics 1992;89:1049–1054.
19. Henshaw S. Unintended pregnancy in the United States. Family Planning Perspect 1998;30:24–29.
20. Dietz P, Gazmararian J, Goodwin M, Bruce F, Johnson C, Rochat R. Delayed entry into prenatal care: effect of physical violence. Obstet Gynecol 1997;90:221–224.
21. Parker B, McFarlane J, Soeken K. Abuse during pregnancy: effects on maternal complications and birth weight in adult and teenage women. Obstet Gynecol 1994;84:323–328.
22. McKay MM. The link between domestic violence and child abuse: assessment and treatment considerations. Child Welfare 1994;73: 29–39.
23. National Clearinghouse on Domestic Violence. Wife Abuse in the Medical Setting and Introduction for Health Personnel. Rockville, MD: The Clearinghouse, 1981 (monograph series no. 7).
24. McFarlane J. Battering during pregnancy: tip of an iceberg revealed. Women Health 1989;15:69–84.
25. Stillman R, Rosenberg M, Sachs B. Smoking and reproduction. Fertil Steril 1986;46:545–566.
26. United States Department of Health and Human Services. The health consequences of smoking: a report of the Surgeon General. Washington, DC: Department of Health and Human Services, Public Health Service, Center for Disease Control, Center for Chronic Disease Prevention and Health Promotion, Office of Smoking and Health, 1980.
27. Manley M, Epps R, Husten C, Glynn T, Sholand, D. Clinical interventions in tobacco control: a National Cancer Institute training program for physicians. JAMA 1991;266:3172–3173.
28. Abel E, Sokol R. Fetal alcohol syndrome is now the leading cause of mental retardation. Lancet 1986;2:1222.
29. Serdula M, Williamson D, Kendrick J, Anda RF, Byers T. Trends in alcohol consumption by pregnant women. 1985 through 1988. JAMA 1991;265:876–879.
30. Sokol R, Martier S, Ager J. The T-ACE questions: practical prenatal detection of risk-drinking. Am J Obstet Gynecol 1989;160:863–868.
31. Rosett H, Weiner L, Edelin K. Treatment experience with pregnant problem drinkers. JAMA 1983;249:2029–2033.
32. Chasnoff I, Burns W, Schnoll S, Burns KA. Cocaine use in pregnancy. N Engl J Med 1985;313:666–669.
33. Institute of Medicine, Committee on Nutritional Status during Pregnancy and Lactation, National Academy of Sciences. Nutrition during pregnancy. Washington, DC: National Academy Press, 1990.
34. Werler MM, Shapiro S, Mitchell AA. Periconceptional folic acid exposure and risk of recurrent neural tube defects. JAMA 1993;269: 1257–1261.
35. United States Food and Drug Administration. Folic acid to fortify U.S. food products to prevent birth defects, Press release Feb. 29, 1996.
36. MRC Vitamin Study Research Group. Prevention of neural tube defects: results of the Medical Research Council Vitamin Study. Lancet 1991;338:131–137.
37. Semba RD, Miotti PG, Chiphangwi JD, et al. Maternal vitamin A deficiency and mother-to-child transmission of HIV-1. Lancet 1994;343: 1593–1597.
38. Moutquin JM, Gagnon R, Rainville C, et al. Maternal and neonatal outcomes in pregnancies with no risk factors. Can Med Assoc J 1987;137: 728–732.
39. McFadden EJ. Asthma. In: Fauci A, Braunwald E, Isselbacher K, et al., eds. Harrison's principles of internal medicine. New York: McGraw-Hill, 1998.
40. Burt VL, Whelton P, Roccella EJ, et al. Prevalence of hypertension in the US adult population. Results from the third national health and nutrition examination survey, 1988–1991. Hypertension 1995;25: 305–313.
41. Foster D. Diabetes mellitus. In: Fauci A, Braunwald E, Isselbacher K, et al., eds. Harrison's principles of internal medicine. New York: McGraw-Hill, 1998.
42. Gaasch W, O'Rourke R, Cohn L, Rackley C. Mitral valve disease. In: Schlant R, Alexander R, eds. Hurst's the heart: arteries and veins. New York: McGraw-Hill, 1994.
43. Shackleton D, Westendorp R, Kasteleijn-Nolst Treinte D, de Boer A, Herings R. Dispensing epilepsy medication: a method of determining the frequency of symptomatic individuals with seizures. J Clin Epidemiol 1997;50:1061–1068.
44. Kurtz Z, Tookey P, Ross E. Epilepsy in young people: 23 year follow up of the British national child development study. Br Med J 1998;316: 339–342.
45. Cockerell O, Eckle I, Goodridge D, Sander J, Shorvon S. Epilepsy in a population of 6000 re-examined: secular trends in first attendance rates, prevalence, and prognosis. J Neurol Neurosurg Psychiatry 1995; 58:570–576.
46. Ferrari M. Migraine. Lancet 1998;351:1043–1051.
47. Whittemore R, Hobbins J, Engle M. Pregnancy and its outcome in women with and without surgical treatment of congenital heart disease. Am J Cardiol 1982;50:641–651.
48. Li FP, Gimbrere K, Gelber R, et al. Outcome of pregnancy in survivor's of Wilms' tumor. JAMA 1987;257:216–219.
49. Practice parameter: a guideline for discontinuing antiepileptic drugs in seizure-free patients—summary statement. Report of the Quality Standards Subcommittee of the American Academy of Neurology. Neurology 1996;47:600–602.
50. Delgado-Escueta A, Janz D. Consensus guidelines: preconception counseling, management, and care of the pregnant woman with epilepsy. Neurology 1992;42(suppl 5):149–160.
51. McAnulty J, Morton M, Ueland K. The heart and pregnancy. Curr Probl Cardiol 1988;13:589–665.
52. Lindheimer M, Grunfeld J-P, Davison J. Renal disorders. In: Barron W, Lindheimer M, eds. Medical disorders during pregnancy. St. Louis: CV Mosby, 1995.
53. Hayslett J, Lynn R. Effect of pregnancy in patients with lupus nephropathy. Kidney Int 1980;18:207–222.
54. Peoples-Sheps M, Hogan V, Ng'andu N. Content of prenatal care during the initial workup. Am J Obstet Gynecol 1996;174:220–226.
55. Clapp JF 3d. The effects of maternal exercise on early pregnancy outcome. Am J Obstet Gynecol 1989;161:1453–1457.
56. Clapp JF 3d. The course of labor after endurance exercise during pregnancy. Am J Obstet Gynecol 1990;163:1799–1805.
57. Clapp JF 3d. Neonatal morphometrics after endurance exercise during pregnancy. Am Obstet Gynecol 1990;163:1805–1811.
58. Mamelle N, Laumon B, Lazar P. Prematurity and occupational activity during pregnancy. Am J Epidemiol 1984;119:309–322.
59. Mamelle N, Munoz F. Occupational working conditions and preterm birth—a reliable scoring system. Am J Epidemiol 1987;126:150–152.
60. McDonald AD, McDonald JC, Armstrong B, Cherry NM, Nolin AD, Robert D. Prematurity and work in pregnancy. Br J Indust Med 1988; 45:56–62.
61. Taskinen HK. Effects of parental occupational exposures on spontaneous abortion and congenital malformation. Scand J Work Environ Health 1990;16:297–314.
62. Roeleveld N, Zielhuis GA, Gabreels F. Occupational exposure and defects of the central nervous system in offspring: review. Br J Indust Med 1990;47:580–588.
63. Worthington-Roberts B, Klerman L. Maternal nutrition. In: Merkatz I, Thompson J, eds. New perspectives on prenatal care. New York: Elsevier, 1990.
64. Abrams BF, Laros RK. Prepregnancy weight, weight gain, and birth weight. Am J Obstet Gynecol 1986;154:503–509.
65. Gelles R. Violence and pregnancy: a note on the extent of the problem and needed services. Family Coordin 1975;24:81–86.
66. Pagelow M. Family violence. New York: Praeger, 1984.
67. Thompson J. Health education during pregnancy. In: Merkatz I, Thompson J, eds. New perspectives on prenatal care. New York: Elsevier, 1990.
68. Copper RL, Goldenberg RL, Das A, et al. The preterm prediction study: maternal stress is associated with spontaneous preterm birth at less than thirty-five weeks' gestation. National Institute of Child Health and Human Development Maternal-Fetal Medicine Units Network. Am J Obstet Gynecol 1996;175:1286–1292.
69. Hedegaard M, Henriksen TB, Secher NJ, Hatch MC, Sabroe S. Do stressful life events affect duration of gestation and risk of preterm delivery? Epidemiology 1996;7:339–345.

70. Taffel S. Factors associated with low birth weight. Vital Health Stat 21 1976;37:1–37.
71. Papiernik-Berkhauer E. Coefficient de risque d'accouchement prématuré. Presse Med 1969;77:793–794.
72. Creasy R, Gummer B, Liggins G. System for predicting preterm birth. Obstet Gynecol 1980;55:692–695.
73. Hillier SL, Nugent RP, Eschenbach DA, et al. Association between bacterial vaginosis and preterm delivery of low-birth-weight infant. The Vaginal Infections and Prematurity Study Group. N Engl J Med 1995; 333:1737–1742.
74. Iams J, Goldenberg R, Meis P, et al. The length of the cervix and the risk of spontaneous premature delivery. N Engl J Med 1996;334: 567–572.
75. Kotukl K, Moawad A, Ponto K. The association of subclinical infection with preterm labor: the role of C-reactive protein. Obstet Gynecol 1985;153:642–645.
76. McGregor JA, Jackson GM, Lachelin GC, et al. Salivary estriol as risk assessment for preterm labor: a prospective trial. Am J Obstet Gynecol 1995;173:1337–1342.
77. Bernstein P, Stern R, Lin N, et al. Beta-hCG in cervical/vaginal secretions as a predictor of preterm delivery. Am J Obstet Gynecol 1998; 179:870–873.
78. Lockwood C, Senyei A, Dische MR, et al. Fetal fibronectin in cervical and vaginal secretions as a predictor of preterm delivery. N Engl J Med 1991;325:669–674.
79. Hauth J, Goldenberg R, Andrews W, DuBard M, Copper R. Reduced incidence of preterm delivery with metronidazole and erythromycin in women with bacterial vaginosis. N Engl J Med 1995;333: 1732–1742.
80. Institute of Medicine. Preventing Low Birthweight. Washington, DC: National Academy Press, 1985.
81. National Center for Health Statistics. Vital Statistics of the United States, 1970. Natality. Vol. 1. Hyattsville, MD: Public Health Service, 1975.
82. National Center for Health Statistics. Vital Statistics of the United States, 1980. Natality. Vol. 1. Hyattsville, MD: Public Health Service, 1984.
83. National Center for Health Statistics. Health, United States, 1993. Hyattsville, MD: Public Health Service, 1994.
84. Mittendorf R, Herschel M, Williams MA, Hibbard JU, Lee K-S. Reducing the frequency of low birth weight in the United States. Obstet Gynecol 1994;83:1056–1059.
85. Sexton M, Hebel JR. A clinical trial of change in maternal smoking and its effect on birth weight. JAMA 1984;251:911–915.
86. Klein L, Goldenberg RL. Prenatal care and its effect on preterm birth and low birth weight. In: Merkatz IR, Thompson JE, eds. New perspectives on prenatal care. New York: Elsevier, 1993.
87. Fiscella K. Does prenatal care improve birth outcomes? A critical review. Obstet Gynecol 1995;85:468–479.
88. McDuffie RS Jr, Beck A, Bischoff K, Cross J, Orleans M. Effect of frequency of prenatal care visits on perinatal outcome among low-risk women. A randomized controlled trial. JAMA 1996;275:847–851.
89. McDuffie RS, Jr., Bischoff KJ, Beck A, Orleans M. Does reducing the number of prenatal office visits for low-risk women result in increased use of other medical services? Obstet Gynecol 1997;90:68–70.

Cherry and Merkatz's Complications of Pregnancy,
Fifth Edition, edited by W. R. Cohen.
Lippincott Williams & Wilkins, Philadelphia © 2000.

CHAPTER 2

Nutrition

Bonnie S. Worthington-Roberts

Food is essential to life and growth. Without an adequate supply of food and the nutrients it contains, an organism cannot grow and develop normally. Eventually it dies.

Despite these simple and well-established facts, the role that nutrition plays in the course and outcome of pregnancy has not always been appreciated. In the controlled conditions of the laboratory, researchers have been able to demonstrate harmful effects of deficient diets on pregnant animals and their offspring in a number of species. However, studies of human populations have not always demonstrated direct relationships between what a mother eats during gestation and the course and outcome of her pregnancy. Consequently, the emphasis that nutrition has received in prenatal care has varied. At times, when researchers have been able to show positive effects, nutrition has received a great deal of attention; when studies produced equivocal results, nutrition has slipped to a position of indifference and neglect.

By reviewing how the emphasis of research has changed as more has become known about nutrition, reproduction, and human growth, health professionals can gain a sense of perspective that helps in understanding why different dietary recommendations for pregnant women have been made.

EARLY BELIEFS AND PRACTICES

During the 19th century, much of what was recommended about diet during pregnancy was based on casual observation rather than controlled studies. Because little information was available on the nutrient composition of foods or their biological value, dietary advice was influenced by beliefs that obvious physical properties of different foods could produce specific effects on the mother or the child. These beliefs were often colored by the emotional and mystical aura surrounding the pregnant state. For example, pregnant women were sometimes forbidden to eat salty, acidic, or sour foods for fear the infant would be born with a "sour" disposition. Eggs were sometimes restricted because of their association with reproductive function. Certain foods were encouraged for their presumed beneficial effects. Pregnant women were often advised to eat broths, warm milk, and ripe fruits to soothe the fetus and ease the birth process.

At this time dietary recommendations for pregnancy also were influenced by problems current in obstetric practice. In the days of the industrial revolution, children in Europe had poor diets and worked long hours in dark factories. Rickets was a common nutritional disorder that impaired normal bone formation during the growing years. His experience in the 1880's led the German physician Prochownick to advocate a fluid-restricted, low-carbohydrate, high-protein diet for women with contracted pelvis to be followed for 6 weeks prior to birth. Women using such a diet produced smaller infants who were easier to deliver. The diet may have had some justification in the 1880's, but it later gained in popularity and became a standard recommendation for women throughout a pregnancy even when the original rationale for it no longer applied.

The importance of a pregnant woman's diet for the health of her infant has long been emphasized in customs and practices. However, there was little specific information available about diet and pregnancy before the 1930's, other than the reports on effects of food shortages during and after World War I. After the war there was a great deal of evidence that related food shortages to the size of the baby, although much of it was inconclusive and even contradictory.

Over the past 100 years, efforts have been made to determine the specific roles that nutrition plays in embryonic and fetal development. Much information has been

B. S. Worthington-Roberts: Nutritional Services Program, University of Washington, Seattle, WA 98195.

Excerpted in part from Worthington-Roberts B, Williams SR. *Nutrition in pregnancy and lactation,* 6th ed. Dubuque, IA: Brown & Benchmark, 1997.

gleaned from animal models, where clear-cut adverse impacts on pregnancy course and outcome can be reproduced when nutrient deficiencies or excesses are studied. Data from human populations derive from observational efforts because frank experimentation is rarely possible. Epidemiologic data support the concept of detrimental pregnancy course and outcome when nutritional conditions are suboptimal. However, it is clear that a biological force is in place that tends to protect the fetus (to some extent) when maternal diet is inadequate. Nutritional interventions prove to be effective when employed in circumstances of obvious need. We have much to learn about the more subtle effects of poor prenatal nutrition on development of the human fetus.

THE WOMEN, INFANTS, AND CHILDREN PROGRAM

In the United States the major food program for pregnant women is the Special Supplemental Food Program for Women, Infants, and Children, better known as WIC (1). This program is sponsored by the Food and Nutrition Service of the Federal Department of Agriculture. WIC was originally authorized in 1972. Current legislation lists the target population as pregnant and postpartum women (up to 6 months after delivery if not breastfeeding and up to 12 months if breastfeeding), and infants and children up to 5 years old. To be eligible, women, infants, and children must be nutritionally at risk and members of low-income families (i.e., gross family income cannot exceed 185% of the nonfarm poverty income defined by the Office of Management and Budget).

Legislation mandates that applicants are automatically income eligible for WIC if they receive benefits under Medicaid, Aid to Families with Dependent Children (AFDC), or the Food Stamp Program. Applicants are also income eligible if they are members of a family that includes an AFDC recipient or a pregnant woman or infant receiving Medicaid assistance. The program is administered by state health departments, and regulations require that eligible women, infants, and children receive nutrition education and health services as well as food.

Congress appropriates a fixed amount of program funds each year. Federal regulations provide a participant priority system to ensure that program benefits are directed to persons at greatest nutritional risk when the demand for program benefits exceeds available resources. This system recognizes that pregnant and breastfeeding women and infants with documented nutrition-related medical conditions are the highest risk groups of the WIC population.

In 1984 the General Accounting Office (GAO) published an analysis of 54 evaluations of WIC. The GAO conclusions of interest are listed as follows:

1. The six birth-weight studies of high or medium quality gave some support but not conclusive evidence that WIC increased infant birth weight. About 7.9% of the WIC mothers bore infants who were less than 2,500 g, as compared with about 9.5% of the control mothers. Average birth weights were between 30 and 50 g greater for WIC than for mothers in the control group.
2. The studies of fetal and neonatal mortality were insufficient to support claims about WIC's effectiveness.
3. WIC appeared to have a great positive effect on the birth weights of babies of mothers who were teenagers, blacks, or who had several health- and nutrition-related risks.
4. Participation in WIC for more than six months was associated with increases in birth weights and decreases in the proportion of low-birth-weight infants.

In 1986, the Department of Agriculture issued a report on the latest and largest evaluation of WIC, based on three contemporary studies (a longitudinal study of pregnant women, a study of infants and children, and a food expenditure study) and a historical study of pregnancy outcomes.

For the longitudinal study of pregnant women, more than 5,000 pregnant women at 174 WIC sites who were first-time registrants became the experimental subjects. Only 1,358 control women were entered into the study. The controls were low-income women receiving antenatal care for the first time in hospital or health department clinics in countries where WIC programs served less than 30% to 40% of eligible women. In addition to the smaller-than-desired size of the control group and the incomplete record survey, the evaluation suffered from major differences between the socioeconomic characteristics of the WIC and the control group. The latter were more often white, had higher incomes, were more likely to be married, and had higher status occupations.

The historical study was undertaken to determine the effectiveness of the program over its entire history and to permit a sample size large enough to study fetal and infant death rates. It related WIC participation during pregnancy to both extent and quality of prenatal care and perinatal outcome for the WIC program from 1974 to 1980. The proportion of eligible pregnant women served by WIC each year in each county (penetration) was linked to the level of maternal antenatal care and to perinatal outcome rates for the same county and year, as determined by linked birth and infant death certificates.

The longitudinal study showed no significant effect of WIC on mean birth weight or percentage of low-birth-weight or very-low-birth-weight infants, perhaps a result of the lower health risks and greater social privilege of control group women, differences that could only partially be accounted for by statistical adjustment. The historical study, however, showed a significant increase in mean birth weight of 23 g. In the total population, WIC penetration was not significantly related to the proportion of low-birth-weight or very-low-birth-weight infants. A substantial, but not statistically significant, reduction in low birth weight, however, was found among less-educated whites and more-educated blacks. In addition, a special study of the quality of local WIC programs, as perceived by state WIC directors, showed a relationship between quality and increased mean birth weight and reduced frequency of low birth weight.

The longitudinal study showed no significant effect of WIC on either mean duration of pregnancy or frequency of prematurity. In the historical study, however, mean pregnancy duration was significantly longer for those served by the WIC program (1.4 days). WIC participation also reduced preterm delivery in the total population by 9 per 1,000 births. There were also statistically significant reductions in very preterm (under 33 weeks) delivery in the white, less-educated group, in preterm delivery among less-educated white and black women, and longer mean pregnancy duration among less-educated whites.

In the longitudinal study the fetal death rate was 9.7/1000 versus 14.8/1,000 in the control group. Although the magnitude of difference was substantial, the numbers were not large enough to reach statistical significance. The historical study, however, showed a statistically significant reduction of 2.3 fetal deaths per 1,000 births.

It was concluded from these studies that WIC had a significant effect on duration of pregnancy, birth weight, head growth, fetal mortality, and perhaps neonatal mortality.

It is believed that among the most positive effects of WIC are related directly to nutrition education that all participants get as a part of WIC benefits. Each participant receives assessment and counseling geared to individual needs and problems. Monthly contacts allow for reinforcement of education and recommendations.

The Special Supplemental Food Program for Women, Infants, and Children provides selected foods, nutrition education, counseling and support, and referral to or coordination with health care. In so doing, it has become an extremely important program for fostering food security and increasing access to health services for the youngest and most vulnerable members of society (2).

Costs and Costs-Benefits of Nutrition Services

With the increasing focus on demonstrating that federally funded services are cost effective, researchers have approached prenatal nutrition care services with this goal in mind. There is little argument that the greatest costs are associated with the consequences of low birth weight. The Office of Technology Assessment estimated the admission rate to neonatal intensive care units to be 6% of all live births. In 1978 dollars, the average estimated expenditure per patient was $8,000.

Disbrow (3,4) and Splett and colleagues (5) have made an effort to estimate the direct costs of nutrition services in prenatal settings. Disbrow calculated the costs of personnel, space, materials, transportation, and child care. He showed that the direct costs of nutrition services throughout pregnancy for a low-income prenatal population are about $41 per client. Splett and colleagues reported the 1987 costs of prenatal nutrition care delivered at the city health department to be $72 for 3.9 visits and $121 for six visits at the county hospital. Indirect costs of care have rarely been evaluated. Disbrow (4) estimated indirect costs for prenatal nutrition services to be $21.37 per client.

The studies that have addressed cost issues and cost-benefit ratios have generally found an increase in birth weight along with an increase in weight gain of the mother. Reduction in low-birth-weight percentage is associated with the greatest cost savings. A study of the impact of WIC participation on Medicaid costs (6) further verified net benefits attributable to nutrition intervention in pregnancy.

Not all intervention/supplementation programs provided to high-risk pregnant women have demonstrated a strong positive impact. This varied response should certainly be expected given the different populations served, the different supplements employed, the various methods of supplement administration, and a variety of other differing variables. Overall, the findings appear to suggest that the worse the nutritional condition of the mother entering pregnancy, the more valuable the prenatal diet and/or nutritional supplement will be in improving her pregnancy course and outcome.

A general conclusion that can be drawn after review of all published reports on prenatal supplementation studies is that although poor women in developing countries often suffer some degree of malnutrition before and during pregnancy, only a minority of women from low socioeconomic groups in developed countries are truly undernourished. Dietary counseling and nutritional supplementation of the latter will clearly yield less dramatic measurable improvements in outcome. In developed countries, nutrition intervention should focus on women whose prepregnancy status is judged to be inferior. Refined processes of clinical evaluation and monitoring may allow for the establishment of a nutritional milieu supportive of optimal pregnancy course and outcome in the majority of these women.

This finding was confirmed when researchers linked Medicaid and WIC files to birth certificates for live births in North Carolina in 1988 (7). Women who had Medicaid benefits and prenatal WIC services had substantially lower rates of low and very low birth weight than did women who received Medicaid but not prenatal WIC. From these data, it was estimated that for each dollar spent on WIC services, Medicaid savings in costs of newborn medical care were $2.91. A high level of WIC participation was associated with better birth outcomes.

PRECONCEPTIONAL CARE

Preconceptional assessment of nutritional status should identify individuals who are underweight or overweight; those with conditions such as bulimia, anorexia, pica, or hypervitaminosis; and those with special dietary habits such as vegetarianism. Nutrition counseling may prove useful; this may include information about dietary control of chronic diseases such as diabetes mellitus or phenylketonuria.

Underweight

Underweight women are at increased risk for reproductive problems. Not only is fertility compromised, but the likelihood of premature delivery and intrauterine growth retardation is increased; Apgar scores of offspring are more frequently low. The condition of underweight is potentially modifiable because it is often related to abusive dieting practices or exercise programs.

Obesity

Women who exceed their desirable body weight by more than 35% are at greater risk than normal-weight women for an unsatisfactory pregnancy course and outcome. Obese women are at higher risk for antenatal complications, especially pregnancy-induced hypertension, gestational diabetes, urinary tract infections and pyelonephritis; they also are more likely to demonstrate prolonged labor followed by difficult vaginal delivery and thus more frequently deliver by cesarean section. Perinatal mortality is likewise higher. Theoretically, reducing the degree of maternal obesity before conception should improve pregnancy progress and outcome.

Folic Acid Deficiency

Maternal folic acid deficiency in experimental animals is associated with increased incidence of congenital malformations in the offspring. Malformations also have been described in the offspring of women who use drugs that are folate antagonists, and evidence in humans also suggests that deficiency of this vitamin may be associated with spontaneous abortion and neural tube defects (NTDs).

The Centers for Disease Control and Prevention and the U.S. Public Health Service (PHS) have recommended that all women of childbearing age who are capable of becoming pregnant should consume 0.4 mg of folic acid per day for the purpose of reducing their risk of having a pregnancy affected with spina bifida or other NTDs. This recommendation was followed by similar recommendations by several other countries.

Fortification of grain products with folic acid was approved in 1996. This practice took effect in 1998 and should improve folic acid status of women who use these foods. The subject of folic acid deficiency and pregnancy course and outcome will be discussed in detail later in this chapter.

Vitamin A Teratogenesis

Excessive consumption of vitamin A appears to be teratogenic. A number of case reports of adverse pregnancy outcome have been associated with a daily ingestion of 25,000 IU or more. These data derive from Adverse Drug Reaction Reports filed with the Food and Drug Administration (FDA) concerning the use of vitamin A during pregnancy. In addition, epidemiologic evidence indicates that the drug isotretinoin, a vitamin A analogue, causes major malformations. The Terotology Society urges that women in their reproductive years be informed that the excessive use of vitamin A shortly before and during pregnancy could be harmful to their babies. They further support the practice of labeling products containing vitamin A to indicate that consumption of excessive amounts of vitamin A may be hazardous to the embryo or fetus when taken during pregnancy and that women of childbearing age should consult with their physician before consuming these products.

Proof of the potential hazards of excessive doses of vitamin A came recently from researchers who interviewed more than 20,000 pregnant women. Questions were asked about diet and supplemented use, specifically focusing on retinol. Results indicated that retinol intake in excess of 15,000 IU daily was associated with a significantly increased risk of birth defects, specifically those that related to development of neural crest derivatives (Table 2-1).

TABLE 2-1. *Teratogenicity of vitamin A: defects related to cranial neural crest development*

	No. of defects	% Defects
Daily retinol intake (IU)		
0–5,000	33	0.51
5,001–10,000	59	0.47
10,001–15,000	20	0.63
>15,001	9	1.8
Retinol intake from food (IU)		
0–5,000	114	0.52
5,001–10,000	5	0.62
10,001–15,000	2	1.06
Retinol intake from supplements		
0.5000	51	0.46
5,001–8,000	54	0.51
8,001–10,000	9	1.18
>10,001	7	2.21

From Rothman KJ et al. Teratogenicity of high vitamin A intake. N Engl J Med 1995;333:1369.

Control of Chronic Disease

Abundant data support the value for the fetus of preconceptional or very early prenatal control of certain chronic diseases. Good examples of the effectiveness of these early interventions are maternal phenylketonuria (PKU) and insulin-dependent diabetes mellitus (IDDM). Metabolic control of both diseases involves conscientious dietary manipulation well before the critical period of embryonic development. In the case of PKU, restriction of dietary phenylalanine is mandatory, while satisfying the protein and other nutrient requirements of mother and fetus; data indicate that the IQ of the offspring is inversely related to maternal serum phenylalanine concentration during pregnancy.

Women with IDDM must control blood glucose levels through careful food selection and scheduled meal timing in concert with the administration of insulin. In a nonrandomized study of diabetic women in Europe, preconceptional control was associated with a reduction in birth defects in comparison with a nondiabetic control population (9). In a large multicenter study in the United States during the early 1980's, very early prenatal intervention for management of IDDM was associated with a marked reduction in the congenital malformation rate in comparison with pregnant women counseled late in pregnancy (6% versus 13%) but not to the low level of the nondiabetic women (35%) (10). The incidence of spontaneous abortion also was reduced significantly in this early-counseled population, presumably a result of the improved metabolic control (11).

It makes sense, therefore, that efforts should be made preconceptionally to motivate women with controllable diseases to prepare themselves for conception by initiating dietary and other necessary life-style changes to optimize the maternal metabolic state. This can certainly be said for women with IDDM and PKU, but it also applies to women with other chronic diseases. Not only will such efforts reduce morbidity and mortality of offspring, but they also may improve the health and well-being of the mother during the prenatal period.

ENERGY NEEDS

Supplying sufficient energy to maintain life is the principal task of the body's metabolism. All other metabolic processes are subservient to this aim. During pregnancy two factors that determine energy requirements are changes in the mother's usual physical activity and the increase in her basal metabolism to support the work required for growth of the fetus and accessory tissues. The cumulative cost of this extra work has been estimated at about 85,000 kcal. This is derived from the caloric equivalents of protein and fat stored in the products of conception (about 41,000 kcal) and from increased oxygen consumption of the mother (36,000 kcal). An additional 8,000 kcal are needed to convert food to metabolizable energy.

The energy demand is thought to be distributed fairly equally throughout the first three quarters of pregnancy. Deposition of about 3.5 kg of fat in the maternal compartment accounts for two thirds of the total energy need during the second and third quarters of pregnancy. Fetal growth needs are greatest in the fourth quarter.

The total of 85,000 kcal for support of a pregnancy translates into an extra 300 kcal per day throughout pregnancy. A portion of the energy increment may be offset by the tendency of women to reduce their physical activity, especially in the last trimester. Several investigators have clearly shown a reduction in work pace as weight gain proceeds. Women who must continue a previous work pace or have chosen to do so will gradually build up their energy needs associated with movement of their larger body mass.

The energy demand is not distributed equally through the course of pregnancy. Energy expenditure gradually increases over the course of pregnancy, virtually all directly related to the increasing resting metabolic rate.

The energy expenditure for basal or resting metabolism has been measured in several groups of pregnant women. If the original estimates of resting energy needs are correct, a total of 36,000 kcal should be recorded during the course of a pregnancy. In reality, much variability has been observed. The biggest net change was seen in Swedish women (46,500 kcal), whereas the unsupplemented women in the Gambia had the lowest change (1000 kcal). The longitudinal studies of Durnin (12) showed that resting metabolic rate decreased in early gestation and remained below pregravid levels until the 30th week. If this phenomenon is true, researchers assessing resting metabolic rate only in the later weeks of pregnancy may have grossly overestimated the total resting energy needs for pregnancy.

Observations made in the Gambia suggest that maternal nutritional status influences the change in resting metabolism during gestation. The unsupplemented women who were consuming only 1,500 kcal per day had lower resting metabolic rates in the second and third trimesters than did the women receiving supplements and consuming about 1,950 kcal per day. Calculations revealed that the supplemented women required an additional 13,000 kcal for resting metabolism; only 1,000 kcal was required by the unsupplemented women. It is logical that a smaller increase in resting metabolism may enable underfed pregnant women to sustain adequate fetal growth and development even with their limited energy stores.

In light of the substantial controversy about the energy requirements of pregnancy and the degree to which these needs are met by extra food, a series of studies has been carried out in five countries. This integrated undertaking took place in two developed countries (Scotland and the

Netherlands) and three developing countries (the Gambia, Thailand, and the Philippines). Throughout each study, pregnancy, body weight and body fat, energy intake, basal metabolic rate, and daily energy expenditure were determined.

The characteristics of the study populations were diverse, but the results among them were not when variables were expressed as a proportion of the initial body mass. The most startling observation is related to the Gambian women, who seem to be the beneficiaries of a remarkable physiologic adjustment; by becoming pregnant, they save so much energy in basal metabolism that they end with a positive energy balance over the whole of pregnancy of about 11,000 calories. Pregnancy, far from requiring extra energy, is a positive benefit to their state of energy balance.

Several important conclusions of this project should be emphasized (12).

1. Although weight gain and body fat percentage differed substantially among the populations, when expressed as a proportion of initial weight of the mother, more similarity was seen.
2. Dutch women, who were bigger and slightly fatter than the Scottish women, deposited only about two-thirds the amount of fat despite their higher energy intake and similar energy expenditure.
3. In none of the groups did fat gains come close to the values proposed by Hytten and Chamberlain (13) of 3.5 kg.
4. The total increase in basal metabolic rate over the whole pregnancy differed by at least a factor of 10 between the Gambian women and those from the other centers. This enormous difference demonstrates a quite remarkable physiologic adaptation, presumably to pregnancy in the face of severe nutritional stress.
5. The net energy cost of performing a given physical activity (calculated as energy per unit body weight) decreased slightly in most groups, but the change was small and never resulted in a reduced energy expenditure in absolute terms; even though a pregnant woman in the third trimester expends less energy doing a task per kilogram of her body weight than she did in the first trimester, she still expends more total energy.
6. There were apparent differences in the data on the energy cost of pregnancy from the different centers, but if they are standardized for body weight, total energy costs were about 59,750 kcal for all groups except the Gambian women, and the small differences between the other groups were mostly the result of the variable amounts of maternal fat stored during pregnancy.
7. With the exception of the Thai groups, energy intakes did not conform, even remotely, to the theoretically expected quantities. There is no doubt that this result raises difficulties in relation to general recommendations of the energy requirements of pregnancy.

The overall conclusion from these studies is that energy costs of pregnancy are about 59,750 kcal. These studies also showed that this cost is not usually reflected in 59,750 extra kcal being consumed in the diet. The usefulness of virtually all current guidelines for exogenous kcal requirements for pregnant women therefore must be questioned.

FURTHER OBSERVATIONS ON ENERGY COSTS

Gambian women have provided an outstanding example of energy sparing during pregnancy. This was illustrated using whole body calorimetry. Components of daily energy expenditure were measured before and serially during pregnancy. Weight gain was 15 lb (6.8 kg), fat deposition was 4.4 lb (2 kg), and lean tissue deposition was 11 lb (5 kg). Basal metabolic rate was depressed during the first 18 weeks of gestation. Individual responses to pregnancy correlated with changes in body mass. There was no significant increase in the cost of treadmill exercise, 24-hour energy expenditure, activity, or diet-induced thermogenesis during pregnancy despite body weight gain. Total energy costs over 36 weeks were markedly lower than reported for well-nourished Western populations.

A Cross-Country Analysis

To test whether energy-sensitive adjustments in gestational metabolism occur in women other than those studied in the Gambia and England, researchers from the United Kingdom conducted a retrospective analysis of data on basal metabolic rate and fat deposition in 360 pregnancies from 10 studies in a wide range of nutritional settings (14). The energy costs of pregnancy varied widely between different communities. Total costs were correlated with prepregnancy fatness and pregnancy weight gain. Marginally nourished women conserved energy by suppressing metabolic rate and by gaining little fat. They also delivered smaller babies.

Assessing the Adequacy of Energy Intake

Comparing the estimated intake to a recommended intake is not desirable during pregnancy because energy needs differ from one woman to another. Requirements vary with prepregnancy weight and body composition, amount and composition of weight gain, stage of pregnancy, and activity level. It is therefore inappropriate to make a single energy recommendation for all pregnant women. Energy status may be estimated instead by evaluating the rate of weight gain. If the rate of weight gain is appropriate for the stage of pregnancy, it is assumed that the energy supply is adequate.

Theoretically the body can derive all of its energy from dietary or stored protein and fat. Carbohydrates are used preferentially by some cells and are required for intermediaries of the citric acid cycle, but they can be synthesized from protein. The exclusion of carbohydrate from the diet, however, has harmful effects. Because energy production is of primary importance, the body will use protein to manufacture citric acid cycle intermediaries and glucose if no preformed sources are available. This can impair growth. If the body must depend solely on dietary or stored fat for energy, metabolic products of fat oxidation accumulate in excess. These products, known as ketone bodies, cannot be metabolized when their concentrations reach high levels. Because they are acidic in nature, ketones disrupt the body's acid-base balance and can eventually lead to coma and death.

DIETING, FASTING, AND FOOD RESTRICTION

The degree to which the mother is parasitized by the fetus has been the subject of debate for many decades. Although the fetus can draw on maternal stores when maternal dietary input is limited, the extent and duration of this process is unknown. The known effects of food restriction on body composition of pregnant and nonpregnant rats have provided new insights into the nature of maternal-fetal interactions. At term, pregnant rats fed 50% of the food consumed by control animals had a body composition similar to that of pair-fed nonpregnant rats, whereas the mean body weight of the fetus was significantly reduced. These results support the idea that the pregnant, food-restricted rat is not extensively parasitized by the fetus. In addition, data suggest that important metabolic adjustments must occur to allow the mother to prevent fetal parasitism.

Human data are obviously limited, but the Dutch famine experience supports the idea that the malnourished mother is able to protect her body stores of nutrients from fetal parasitism. Mean infant birth weight was reduced by 10%, but most mothers were estimated to lose less than 3% of their initial body weight during the stress of famine during pregnancy. Thus, optimal fetal growth occurs only when the mother is able to accumulate a critical amount of extra body stores during pregnancy. Evidence clearly contradicts the concept that the fetus is protected by the mother when nutritional status is less than optimal or that the fetus can protect itself by parasitizing the mother.

The fact that nature protects the mother more than the fetus seems reasonable from the point of view of survival of the species. During a famine caused by a serious crop failure, for example, a normal-sized newborn delivered by a nutritionally depleted mother would have little chance to survive if the mother could not initiate lactation, protect herself and her young, and cover enough ground during the day to secure food. A stronger or healthier mother who produces a small baby or few offspring probably has a better chance to survive and conceive again.

PROTEIN REQUIREMENTS

The promotion of optimal growth during pregnancy requires adequate supplies of energy and raw materials. Protein is essential because it forms the structural basis for all new cells and tissues in the mother and fetus. Vitamins and minerals participate in the biochemical reactions that build amino acids into new protein molecules and maintain the structural and functional properties of the cells.

Nitrogen is the key element in protein that makes it different from carbohydrate and fat. Protein requirements therefore are usually determined by measuring the amount of nitrogen retained in the body for metabolic use. One gram of nitrogen is equivalent to 6.25 g of protein.

In the factorial method, protein needs are estimated by totaling all the ways that nitrogen can be lost from the body. This gives an indication of how much protein nitrogen must be replaced each day. When these losses are calculated for the average woman used as a reference, requirements are 2.84 g of nitrogen or 18 g of protein per day.

Protein requirements during pregnancy are based on the needs of the nonpregnant woman used as a reference plus the extra amounts needed for growth. The easiest way to determine how much extra protein is needed daily to support the synthesis of new tissue is to divide the amounts contained in the products of conception by the average length of gestation. About 925 g of protein are deposited in a normal-weight fetus and in the maternal accessory tissues. When this is divided by the 280 days of pregnancy, the average is 3.3 g of protein that must be added to normal daily requirements. The rate at which new tissue is synthesized, however, is not constant throughout gestation.

Maternal and fetal growth do not accelerate until the second month, and the rate progressively increases until just before term. The need for protein follows this growth rate. Only about an extra 0.6 g of protein is used each day for synthesis in the first month of pregnancy, but by 30 weeks' gestation, protein is being used at the rate of 6.1 g/day. If this is added to the normal maintenance needs of the reference women, one finds that 18.6 to 24.1 g per day of protein are required during pregnancy.

These calculations would equal dietary allowances if 100% of the protein eaten could be used in the body. In actuality the efficiency of protein utilization depends on its digestibility and amino acid composition. Proteins that do not contain all eight essential amino acids in amounts proportional to human requirements are utilized less efficiently, but the utilization of even a high-quality protein, such as that from eggs, is only about 70%. Utilization from a mixed diet or from one in which protein is supplied totally from vegetable sources is less efficient.

Protein utilization also depends on caloric intake. It has been shown that an extra 100 kcal during pregnancy will have the same effect on nitrogen retention as an additional 0.28 g of nitrogen itself. This means that calories from nonprotein sources (i.e., carbohydrate and fat) have a sparing effect. If these calories are inadequate, protein requirement would increase.

Overall the efficiency of protein utilization has not been quantitated in pregnant women. Assuming that only 70% of the dietary protein is retained in pregnancy, the National Research Council proposed that pregnant women consume an additional 10 to 12 g of protein per day in order to retain 6 to 8 g per day in the last half of pregnancy.

PROTEIN DEFICIENCY

Adverse consequences of protein deficiency during pregnancy are difficult to separate from the effects of calorie deficiency in other situations. Almost all cases of limited protein intake are accompanied by limitation in availability of calories; under such circumstances, decreased birth weight and a greater incidence of preeclampsia have been reported. Provision of supplemental calories alone to patients with deficient levels of protein intake is just as effective as provision of both protein and calories in influencing birth weight of babies.

The notion that protein deficiency causes pregnancy-induced hypertension (PIH) is a highly controversial issue, and the role of protein deficiency in the cause of preeclampsia has not been satisfactorily proved or disproved. Attempts to produce an animal model of PIH using a protein-deficient diet have proven unsuccessful. Given the body of evidence available to evaluate, encouraging sound dietary patterns among pregnant women is a justifiable practice, but use of a protein supplement for prevention of PIH is not justifiable.

ESSENTIAL FATTY ACIDS

Deficiency of essential fatty acids is unlikely in a dietary environment rich in lipids. However, their importance in neural development suggests that a deficiency during the critical period of brain development can occur under adverse dietary circumstances. The brain is 60% structural lipid; it universally uses arachidonic acid and docosahexanoic acid (DHA) for growth, function, and integrity. Evidence from experimental animals has demonstrated that the effects of essential fatty acid deficiency during early brain development are deleterious and permanent. Babies born of low birth weight are more likely to have been born to mothers who are inadequately nourished, and the babies tend to be born with arachidonic acid and DHA deficits.

To test the hypothesis that maternal diet during pregnancy may impact fetal brain development, researchers in London studied 513 pregnancies in a population with a high incidence of low birth weight (15). They tracked 44 nutrients using a computerized nutrition database. Results indicated that the diets of mothers who produced low-birth-weight babies were inferior to those of other mothers in many respects; among the dietary deficits was essential fatty acids. Also, reduced concentrations of arachidonic acid in maternal and cord blood were associated with low birth weight, head circumference, and placental weight. Much remains to be learned about the importance of maternal dietary intake of essential fatty acids and the quality of the neonatal brain. This applies equally to the importance of human milk fatty acid composition and postnatal brain development.

Interest has developed recently in the role of essential fatty acids in the maintenance of normal vascular integrity and the prevention of preeclampsia. The pathogenesis of preeclampsia remains obscure, but dysfunction of the maternal vascular endothelial cells is thought to play a major role. It has been proposed that alterations in circulating lipids may contribute to the induction of endothelial dysfunction in patients with preeclampsia. However, recent data from Scandinavia do not support this idea (16). This randomized controlled trial evaluated the impact of fish oil supplementation in late pregnancy on blood pressure. In the 30th week of pregnancy, over 500 women were assigned to receive fish oil supplementation. No difference was observed among the groups in blood pressure changes during the third trimester.

VITAMIN REQUIREMENTS

Thiamin, Riboflavin, and Niacin

The process of energy production involves several other nutrients in addition to those that yield calories. The oxidation of carbohydrates proceeds in a series of reactions that convert glucose to pyruvic acid and then to acetylcoenzyme A. This last step depends on a coenzyme, thiamin pyrophosphate (TPP). As its name implies, TPP contains the B vitamin thiamin, and its availability can limit the rate at which energy from glucose is produced.

Riboflavin and niacin are also concerned with energy production. These two B vitamins are parts of the coenzymes flavin adenine dinucleotide and niacin adenine dinucleotide, which assist in transferring hydrogen atoms through the respiratory chain in the cells. If protein must be used for energy, riboflavin is also needed as part of the coenzyme that helps to remove nitrogen from the amino acids.

Because thiamin, riboflavin, and niacin are all part of the reactions that produce energy in the body, requirements are related to caloric intake. The adult recommended daily allowances (RDAs) are 0.5, 0.6, and 6.6 mg per 1,000 kcal for thiamin, riboflavin, and niacin, respectively. Because caloric requirements increase during pregnancy, the allowance for thiamin, riboflavin, and niacin automatically increase too.

Thiamin, riboflavin, and niacin are found in almost all foods, but only a few are exceptionally good sources. Whole grains, legumes, organ meats, and pork are high in thiamin, whereas riboflavin is more plentiful in milk, cheese, lean meats, and leafy green vegetables. Foods that are high in thiamin and riboflavin are also good sources of niacin. Niacin is not only found preformed in food but it can also be made in the body from the amino acid tryptophan. For every 60 mg of tryptophan in the diet, 1 mg of niacin will be formed. Foods that are sources of good-quality protein are therefore good sources of niacin as well. Foods that contain only fat or sugar have no thiamin, riboflavin, or niacin.

In animals, severe deficiencies of thiamin, riboflavin, or niacin during pregnancy result in fetal death, reduced growth, and congenital malformations. The skeleton and organs that arise from the ectoderm appear to be especially susceptible to riboflavin deficiency.

Researchers also have evaluated the thiamin status of pregnant women at various stages of gestation and have found that 25% to 30% have values that would be considered deficient by nonpregnant standards. Although there have been some reported cases of congenital beriberi from maternal thiamin deficiency, there is no evidence of functional impairment at the levels described.

The niacin status of pregnant women has been investigated; however, there are no cases that indicate that niacin deficiency in humans produces the malformations noted in animal experimentations.

Folic Acid

The central place that protein occupies in the synthesis of new tissue sometimes obscures the emphasis that should be given to other nutrients. Growth, however, is a complex process that requires more than an adequate supply of protein and energy. To make new cells, DNA must replicate and transmit its genetic information to RNA intermediaries. RNA acts as a template for every new protein synthesized in the body.

Both DNA and RNA are composed of purines and pyrimidines. These ringlike substances are synthesized in the body from one-carbon (methyl) fragments and nitrogen. Derivatives of the B vitamin folic acid accept the carbon fragments from their biochemical donors and transfer them to their sites in the purine and pyrimidine rings. Folic acid also acts as a coenzyme in the synthesis of a nonessential amino acid, glycine. Gycine, in its turn, is a carbon and nitrogen donor in the synthesis of purines. Thus, folic acid is involved in almost all aspects of DNA and RNA synthesis. If it is lacking, cell division cannot proceed normally. The effects are most detrimental in cells that have high turnover rates in the body.

One of the first signs of folic acid deficiency is megaloblastic anemia, which is caused by the production of abnormal red blood cells. These cells are arrested in their development so that bone marrow contains a large number of immature megaloblasts, and hemoglobin levels are reduced.

The dietary availability of folic acid is somewhat limited, and its content in specific foods is inherently variable. A large fraction of folate consumed each day comes from foods that are often ingested but are not particularly concentrated sources of the vitamin (Table 2-2) (17). Orange juice is the largest contributor of folate in the American diet. Those foods with the highest content of folate per serving are listed in Table 2-3.

TABLE 2-2. *Major contributions of folate in the U.S. diet (NHANES II data, 1976–1980)*

Ranking	Description	Total % folate in daily diet
1	Orange juice	9.70
2	White bread, rolls, crackers	8.61
3	Pinto, navy and other dried beans (cooked)	7.08
4	Green salad	6.85
5	Cold cereal, not bran or super-fortified	4.96
6	Eggs	4.63
7	Alcoholic beverages	3.85
8	Coffee, tea	3.40
9	Liver	3.07
10	Superfortified cereals	3.06
11	Whole milk, whole milk beverages	2.90
12	Bran and granola cereals	2.48
13	Whole-wheat, rye, and other dark breads	2.43
14	Corn	1.89
15	Spaghetti with tomato sauce	1.51

From Picciano MF, Green T, O'Connor DL. The folate status of women and health. Nutr Today 1994;29:20.

TABLE 2-3. *Folate content of food sources high in folate*

Ranking	Description	Folate per serving (μg)
1	Liver	383
2	Superfortified cereals	242
3	Cold cereals, not bran or superfortified	112
4	Pinto, navy and other dried beans (cooked)	84
5	Asparagus	82
6	Spinach	70
7	Instant breakfast, diet bars, supplements	65
8	Bran and granola cereals	58
9	Broccoli	53
10	Avocados	49
11	Okra	49
12	Brussels spouts	47
13	Orange juice	43
14	Artichokes	43
15	Chili	36

From Picciano MF, Green T, O'Connor DL. The folate status of women and health. Nutr Today 1994;29:20.

Several factors are known to affect negatively the availability of dietary folate. These include overcooking, long-term thermal processing procedures, and high-fiber diets. The forms of folate found in foods (polyglutamylated folates) are used less effectively than synthetic folic acid.

Low serum folate levels have been reported in as many as 60% of patients in some clinical studies, but only a few of those women exhibit signs of megaloblastic anemia. The low serum values of folic acid are believed to result from a number of factors. Problems with food selection, storage, and cooking losses, which place nonpregnant women in marginal status, are compounded in pregnancy by increased needs for folate. In addition, defects in the utilization of folic acid may be inherent in pregnancy because of the effects of steroid hormones. Folic acid absorbed from food is converted by a series of reduction reactions to its active coenzyme form in the liver. High sex steroid levels may interfere with this process because the liver is also the site where progesterone and estrogen are deactivated before excretion. The reactions for both the activation of folic acid and the deactivation of steroids involve similar biochemical mechanisms. A relationship is suspected because folic acid deficiency sometimes develops in women taking oral steroid contraceptives.

Excitement in recent years has been centered on the recognition that folic acid deficiency may have a role to play in the cause of NTDs (Fig. 2-1). NTDs appear to have some genetic base. That is, although they occur in about 0.1% of all pregnancies, the risk of occurrence is 0.3% to 1% if there is a close relative with an NTD, and the recurrence risk is 2% to 3%. Chromosomal aberrations, gene mutations, and teratogenic drugs (e.g., valproic acid) account for a small fraction of the cases. Most cases may have multifactorial origins such as polygenic liability triggered by environmental factors (18).

Among triggering environmental contributors, undernutrition has been found to be a factor in the well-known association between NTDs and poverty, seasonality, and in the rapid changes in the prevalence of NTDs.

Based on promising hints from available studies, in the early 1980s, the United Kingdom Medical Research Council (MRC) decided to organize a multicenter dou-

A 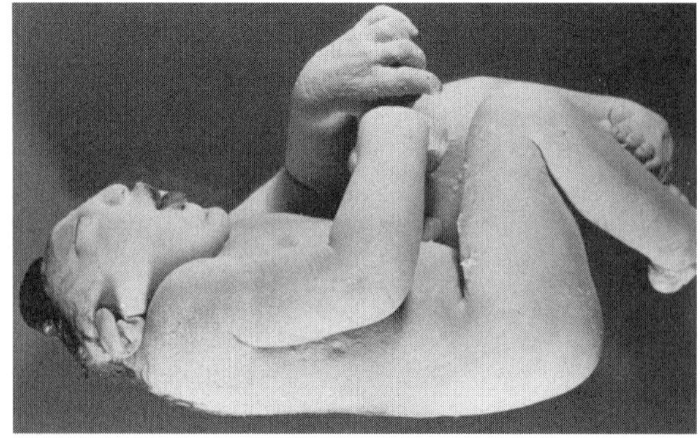

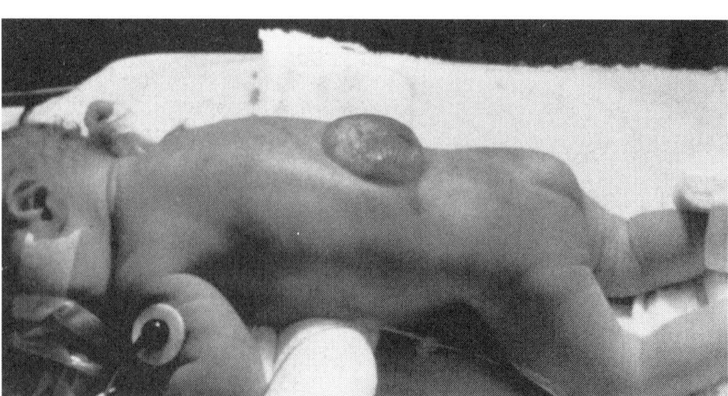 B

FIG. 2-1. Neural tube defects. **A:** Anencephaly. **B:** Spina bifida. (From Worthington-Roberts B, Williams SR. Nutrition in pregnancy and lactation, 6th ed. Dubuque, IA: Brown & Benchmark, 1997.)

ble-blind randomized trial (18,19); 43% of the participants came from Hungary. Women who had already had an infant with an NTD were randomly divided into four supplementation groups:

- Folic acid (4 mg) only
- Folic acid and other vitamins
- Other vitamins
- Neither folic acid nor other vitamins

A total of 1,195 pregnancies was sufficient to conclude that folic acid supplementation alone reduced NTD recurrences by 71%. Other vitamins did not have a significant protective effect.

Research in Cuba provided similar results (20). Folic acid supplementation at the level of 5 mg daily was provided to 81 women with a history of giving birth to babies with NTD. This product was taken before and throughout pregnancy; the control group of women did not follow this practice. The results indicated that there was no recurrence of NTDs among the group of offspring whose mothers chose to use periconceptional folic acid supplementation. In the 114 women who became pregnant without folic acid supplementation, there were four recurrences of NTDs.

The goal of clinical trial of Czeizel and Dudas (21) was to determine the efficacy of folic acid supplementation in the reduction in first occurrences of NTDs. Women planning a pregnancy were randomly assigned to receive a single tablet of a multivitamin, including a physiologic dose (0.8 mg) of folic acid, or a placebo-like trace element supplement daily for at least a month before conception and until at least the date of the second missed menstrual period. Overall, there were six children with NTDs out of 2,391 offspring in the trace element groups compared with none out of 271 offspring in the multivitamin group. The difference was statistically significant.

These intervention trials provided valuable data, and observational studies added confirmatory evidence. In these studies, women were interviewed about their use of nutritional supplements before and during early pregnancy. Mothers of NTD offspring were compared with mothers of control infants. All but one of the studies showed fairly strong protective effects of using vitamin supplements around the time of conception. That is, mothers reporting that they had chosen to do so before and during early pregnancy had a significantly reduced risk of delivering a baby with NTDs. The negative study by Mills and colleagues (22) was well-executed and had a large sample size. However, it was conducted using a population from an area where NTD prevalence is low. Folate intervention may not be beneficial in such circumstances; alternatively, benefits may simply be more difficult to demonstrate statistically in low-incidence populations.

Of considerable interest is the observation that in seven studies of serum or red blood cell concentration of folic acid, less than impressive differences were found between mothers of NTD offspring and mothers of normal infants. If folic acid status makes a difference in pregnancy outcome, why might it be that serum and red blood cell folate levels are not routinely low in mothers of NTD babies?

The underlying mechanisms of periconceptional multivitamin or folic acid supplementation in the prevention of NTD are still not understood. In general, women who have NTD-affected pregnancies have not been found to have lower serum or red blood cell folate values during pregnancy. Available data can be summarized by stating that the risk of NTD is not dramatically altered by raising the red blood cell folate status from very low to a more normal value, whereas the risk is significantly reduced by attaining a red blood cell folate status of >300 or 400 μg/L. Thus, a small change in folate status may profoundly reduce risk.

Recent epidemiologic and biochemical evidence has suggested that the problem is not primarily a lack of sufficient dietary folate; rather the problem appears to be rooted in changes in metabolism of folate in maternal and fetal cells. (Absorption of folate is normal in women with NTD pregnancies, and all pregnant women experience accelerated breakdown to folate during pregnancy.) It is proposed that there is an interaction between a vitamin dependency (i.e., an inborn error of folate metabolism) and nutrition (e.g., a dietary vitamin deficiency) that may have a causal role in the origin of folic acid–related NTDs. The effect on the embryo may be a localized folate deficiency. The supply of folate may be limited even in women with normal folate nutrition, resulting in impaired embryonic cell division at the crucial time of neural tube closure. Folate supplementation may cause an increase in folate concentrations in tissue fluids, and it may overcome this failure of local folate supply.

Although the pathogenesis of NTD is still unproven, three studies shed some light on the subject (23–25). One (23) found a possible role of methionine deficiency in the origin of NTDs, based on cultures of whole rat embryos. Methionine is an essential amino acid, which is converted to *S*-adenosylmenthionine; it is the ultimate methyl donor in human metabolism.

Methionine deficiency may cause NTDs during the phase when the folds of the neural tube first become elevated and have started to oppose opposite ridges. Other researchers reported that 31% of infants with NTDs had methionine intolerance (with abnormally high serum homocysteine concentrations after an oral methionine load), whereas only 1% of the general population had such intolerance. This finding may indicate a metabolic block of demethylation of homocysteine to methionine. Bunduki and colleagues (24) reported a study of 14 NTD mothers and 14 controls. Mothers of NTD offspring had a significantly lower folate methylation rate than did mothers of normal infants. Plasma vitamin B_{12} level is an independent risk factor for NTD offspring. Only one function in humans is independently influenced by both plasma folate and plasma vitamin B_{12}, and that is the action of the enzyme methionine synthase (25).

Mills and colleagues (25) obtained blood during the pregnancies of 81 women who produced infants with NTDs and 323 women who produced normal infants. Mothers of children with NTDs had significantly higher homocysteine values than matched controls. The difference was significant in the 50% of women with the lowest plasma B_{12} concentrations. These researchers propose that an abnormality in homocysteine metabolism, apparently related to methionine synthase, is present in many women who give birth to children with NTDs (Fig. 2-2). They also suggest that the most effective preconceptional prophylactics to prevent NTDs may require B_{12} as well as folic acid.

The mechanism of NTD prevention is the subject of much research. An example of this is a report by Irish and American investigators who studied 550 pregnant and nonpregnant women (26). They found that a substantial number of women carried a gene mutation for an enzyme defect that leads to folate deficiency. They suggested that people who carry two copies of the abnormal gene may need additional folate to reduce their risk of abnormal fetal development. Other American researchers also have reported that providing extra folate to women during the later stages of pregnancy may reduce risk of preterm delivery and low birth weight (27).

What do women know about folic acid and birth defects? A Gallup poll was taken in early 1995 with the sponsorship of the March of Dimes Birth Defects Foundation (28). This telephone survey of women 18 to 45 asked questions about vitamins and birth defects. Overall, 52% of women reported ever hearing of or reading about folic acid. Of these, 9% answered that folic acid helps to prevent birth defects and 6% that folic acid helps reduce the risk of spina bifida; 45% were unable to recall what they had heard or read. Fifteen percent of respondents reported having knowledge of the PHS recommendation regarding the use of folic acid; 4% reported that the recommendation was for prevention of birth defects and 1% for the prevention of spina bifida.

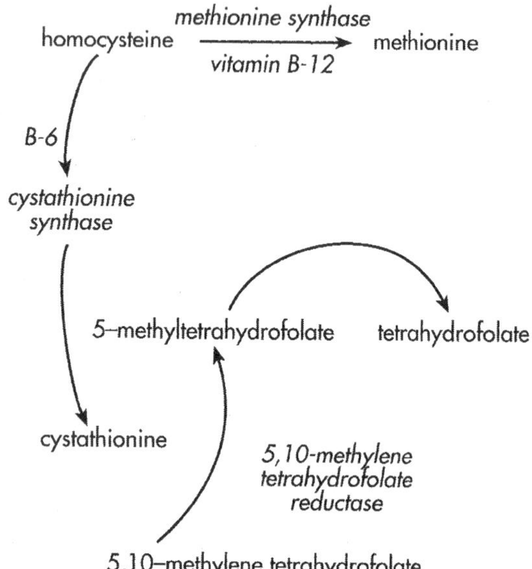

FIG. 2-2. Pathways of homocysteine metabolism. (From Worthington-Roberts B, Williams SR. Nutrition in pregnancy and lactation, 6th ed. Dubuque, IA: Brown & Benchmark, 1997.)

Another important and unexpected finding of the Hungarian NTD occurrence trial was a lower prevalence of birth of major congenital abnormalities other than NTD diagnosed during pregnancy and at birth after periconceptional multivitamin supplementation (9.0 per 1,000 versus 16.6 in the trace element of placebo group). Some congenital abnormality groups such as congenital cardiovascular malformations, defects of the urinary tract, and congenital limb deficiencies, occurred less often in the multivitamin group than in the trace element group. Shaw and colleagues reported in 1995 (29) a reduced risk of orofacial clefts if a mother used multivitamins containing folic acid periconceptionally (overall risk reduction 25% to 50%). Hayes and colleagues reported on such benefit from folate supplementation (30). Also in 1995, Li and colleagues (31) reported a case-control study using the Washington State Birth Defect Registry. Their results indicated that early prenatal multivitamin use was associated with a reduced risk of congenital urinary tract defects. It appears that folic acid (or some other vitamin) may play a role in the prevention of birth defects other than those related to neural tube closure. Czeizel (32) pointed out that the hour may have come for a more effective and primary prevention of birth defects.

In the United States, the current National Research Council RDA for females over 14 years of age is 180 μg of folic acid, and the RDA during pregnancy is 400 μg (0.4 mg). Folic acid is available over the counter in doses of up to 0.8 mg and is also available by prescription in 1-mg tablets. Prenatal vitamins contain 0.8 or 1.0 mg of folic acid. Folic acid is water soluble, with no known toxicity; however, at high doses (more than 1.0 mg/day) the anemia of vitamin B_{12} deficiency (pernicious anemia) can be obscured, with progression of neurologic sequelae. Because pernicious anemia is rare before the age of 50, this is likely to be a rare occurrence among women receiving folic acid during the reproductive years. Studies that definitively address the question of maternal and fetal safety of folic acid are not available. However, folic acid has been used extensively during later pregnancy without adverse effects.

Based on the evidence available, the PHS has recommended that all women of childbearing age who are capable of becoming pregnant take 0.4 mg of folic acid daily.

Implementation of this recommendation is believed to have the potential to reduce the rate of NTD pregnancies by 50%. Regular and continuous ingestion of folic acid is necessary so that offspring of unplanned pregnancies benefit from this intervention. The PHS also points out that this recommendation should be followed by women who have previously had an affected pregnancy, even though they are not planning a pregnancy; by couples with a close relative with an NTD; women with insulin-dependent diabetes mellitus; and women with seizure disorders being treated with valproic acid or carbamazepine.

Is it practical to expect that women will be able to select foods to allow them to ingest 400 μg of folate daily? If the diet is meticulously designed according to the U.S. Food Guide Pyramid or Canada's Food Guide to Healthy Eating, it is possible to provide the level of folate currently recommended to reduce the risk of an NTD-affected pregnancy. However, women in the United States and Canada consistently select diets with less than 400 μg/day of folate. Nutrition education may help. The FDA recently authorized a health claim on food labels relating diets adequate in folate to reduction in risk of NTD pregnancies. They also require fortification of cereal grain products with folate at a level of 140 μg/100 g and to allow fortification of breakfast cereals at 100 μg/serving. Grain product fortification was approved in 1996 (Table 2-4).

Vitamin B_{12}

Vitamin B_{12} deficiency causes megaloblastic anemia. It also can cause irreparable damage to the nervous system. Nevertheless, a dietary deficiency of vitamin B_{12} is rare because it is present in all foods of animal origin. It is also manufactured in small amounts by microorganisms in the gastrointestinal tract. The most common cause of deficiency in humans comes from the inherited or acquired absence of intrinsic factor needed for the absorption of vitamin B_{12}. This occurs most often in older individuals, usually beyond reproductive age. In younger persons, a strict vegetarian diet may eventually be associated with vitamin B_{12} deficiency.

Vitamin B_{12} has been used in the prenatal treatment of a fetus with methylmalonic acidemia. A fetus can be treated nutritionally by supplementing the mother with the appropriate nutrient for the special needs of the offspring. Methylmalonic acidemia is diagnosed prenatally by measuring the levels of methylmalonic acid in amniotic fluid and maternal urine and by measuring the incorporation of propionate labeled with carbon-14 into protein or by assaying methylmalonyl-coenzyme A mutase activity in chorionic villi or amniocytes. Some of these babies are responsive *in utero* to large doses of vitamin B_{12}. That is, the early postnatal problems (lethargy, recurrent vomiting, dehydration, respiratory distress, and muscular hypotonia) may be prevented, and with institution of the appropriate low-protein diet and supplementation program, normal growth and development can be anticipated. Prenatal treatment with appropriate nutrient supplements may allow for much improvement in the prognosis of these infants with inborn defects.

Vitamin B_6

Vitamin B_6, or pyridoxine, is another important nutrient concerned with amino acid metabolism and protein synthesis. In its active form as pyridoxal phosphate, the vitamin is a cofactor in reactions involving a group of enzymes known as *transaminases*. These enzymes transfer the nitrogen-containing portion of certain amino acids to ketoacid intermediaries from the Krebs cycle to synthesize some of the nonessential amino acids. Vitamin B_6 also functions in the reactions that convert tryptophan to niacin. Niacin, in turn, works as nicotinamide adenine dinucleotide along with pyridoxal phosphate in some of the transamination reactions. This is another example of how interdependent the nutrients are in normal metabolism. Vitamin B_6 requirements increase in pregnancy not only because of the greater need for nonessential amino acids in growth but also because the body is making more niacin from tryptophan.

Urinary excretion of vitamin B_6 metabolites during pregnancy is 10 to 15 times higher than in nonpregnant women, whereas blood values are typically reduced. Investigators are not sure what the clinical significance of this is. There have been efforts to link vitamin B_6 to preeclampsia because urinary excretion is even higher in patients with preeclampsia than it is in normal pregnant women. It is far more likely that the observed values are the result of preeclampsia rather than a cause of it.

TABLE 2-4. *Criteria to be considered before instituting a vitamin/mineral prevention/intervention program preconceptionally or prenatally*

1. The condition to be prevented is an important public health problem.
2. There is a safer and acceptable preventive method for women at high risk.
3. High-risk groups can be identified in a way that is acceptable to the population.
4. There is a known time period during which the treatment should be administered.
5. The natural history of the condition is understood.
6. The cost of identifying those at risk is economically feasible.
7. The cost of supplementation is insignificant as compared with the alternative, which is the possible cost of medical care.

From Murphy SP, Abrams BE. Changes in energy intakes during pregnancy and lactation in a national sample of U.S. women. Am J Pub Health 1993;83:1082–1084; and Committee on Drugs. Retinoid therapy for severe dermatological disorders. Pediatrics 1992;90:119.

The placenta concentrates vitamin B_6, and levels in cord blood are much higher than in the maternal circulation. This could mean that the reduced maternal blood levels are simply the result of physiologic adjustments. On the other hand, there is also evidence that the fetus takes up more vitamin B_6 and that maternal levels increase when oral supplements are given.

In neonatal animals and human infants, vitamin B_6 deficiency produces neurologic impairment manifested by marked irritability, ataxia, tremor, abnormal gait, and seizures. Even though much has been learned about the metabolic and neurochemical alterations associated with neonatal vitamin B_6 deficiency, the mechanism(s) underlying the neurologic abnormalities are not clearly known. New and sensitive analytical and behavioral methods are now being applied to determine, at the molecular level, how the lack or the excess intake of a dietary component such as vitamin B_6 can influence brain chemistry and ultimately brain function and behavior.

The dietary allowance of 2.2 mg per day recommended in pregnancy is less than the amounts used by clinical investigators to bring blood levels up to nonpregnant standards, but few clinically significant conditions can be attributed to the levels of vitamin B_6 that are commonly observed. Although some data suggest adverse pregnancy outcome in the presence of vitamin B_6 deficiency, the meaning of these observations remains to be determined because lack of a relationship between vitamin B_6 status and maternal or fetal status also has been reported.

Although the precise cause of the nausea and vomiting common during early pregnancy remains unknown, vitamin B_6 may be important. Vitamin B_6 is known to catalyze a number of reactions involving neurotransmitter production, but a clear connection between vitamin B_6 status and pregnancy nausea remains to be observed.

The first use of pyridoxine for severe nausea and vomiting of pregnancy was reported in 1942; satisfactory relief was obtained in most cases. Other clinicians subsequently reported successful treatment of nausea with injected or oral doses of this vitamin. Fifty-nine women completed a randomized, double-blind placebo-controlled study of vitamin B_6 supplementation for treatment of nausea and vomiting of pregnancy (33). Thirty-one patients received 25-mg vitamin B_6 tablets orally every 8 hours for 72 hours, and 28 patients received placebo in the same regimen. Women with mild to moderate nausea did not benefit from B_6 supplementation. However, women with severe nausea and vomiting showed a substantial reduction in their symptoms.

Most recently, Thai investigators conducted a trial in which women in early pregnancy received either 30 mg of vitamin B_6 daily or a placebo for 5 consecutive days. Patients graded the severity of their nausea. Pyridoxine proved quite effective in decreasing both the severity of nausea and the number of vomiting episodes (34).

Vitamin A

Vitamin A is an essential nutrient for all animal species because of its critical role in reproduction, the immune system, and vision, as well as in the maintenance of cellular differentiation. Although the need for vitamin A in pregnancy is increased above the nonpregnant state, this additional amount is relatively small and confined mostly to the last trimester. Maternal reserves are generally adequate (at least in developed countries) to meet the need. Therefore, the RDA during pregnancy is not different from that of the nonpregnant state. A chronically inadequate intake below the basal requirement must take place to critically deplete maternal body stores before detrimental effects occur in the mother.

In Indonesia, the influence of vitamin A and iron supplementation was studied in anemic pregnant women (35). Subjects were randomly assigned to a supplement routine that provided vitamin A, iron, or both. Maximum improvement in the anemic state was seen when both vitamin A and iron were provided. It was concluded that improvement in vitamin A status may contribute to the control of anemia in pregnant women.

A recent study in Malawi showed that vitamin A status is an important risk factor for the mother-to-child transmission of human immunodeficiency virus (HIV) (36). Among mothers with HIV infection, an association was observed between serum vitamin A and subsequent mother-to-child transmission rates. The relative risk of HIV transmission was four times greater in mothers with a serum vitamin A level of less than 0.7μmol/L compared with a serum vitamin A level of greater than 1.40 μmol/L. This study suggests that vitamin A supplementation may be an economic and relatively simple intervention to reduce mother-to-child transmission of the virus.

Excessive consumption of vitamin A is teratogenic in both experimental animals and humans (37). At least seven case reports of adverse pregnancy outcome have been associated with a daily ingestion of 25,000 IU or more.

Since 1990, two epidemiologic studies addressed the issue. Werler and colleagues (38) examined 2,658 cases of birth defects derived at least in part from neural crest cells. These cases were compared with 2,609 infants with other malformations. Risk of neural crest–related birth defects was increased with reported vitamin A supplement use. Martinez-Frias and Salvador (39) reported the results of an epidemiologic study of prenatal exposure to high doses of vitamin A in Spain. Results suggested that a teratogenic effect might exist for exposures of 40,000 IU or more.

Evans and Hickey-Kwyer (40) reported a case of hourglass cornea and iris with reduplicated lens in the left eye of an infant girl. Her mother's estimated average daily dose of vitamin A was 25,000 IU in the first trimester.

The most impressive report to date on the teratogenicity of retinol derived from data collected by researchers at Boston University (8). Of the 22,748 women interviewed, 339 had babies with birth defects; 121 of these babies had defects occurring in sites that originated in the cranial neural crest. Results indicated that the higher the intake of vitamin A during the first trimester, the greater the risk of a birth defect associated with neural crest cells (e.g., craniofacial, cardiac, thymic, and central nervous system structures) (Table 2-1). The increased frequency of defects was concentrated among the babies whose mothers consumed high levels of vitamin A before the seventh week of gestation. Among the babies born to mothers who took more than 10,000 IU of performed vitamin A per day in the form of supplements, it was estimated that about 1 infant in 57 would have a malformation attributable to the supplement. Topical application of retinoids does not appear to pose a problem (41).

Vitamin C

Vitamin C functions in reactions that oxidize proline, a nonessential amino acid, to hydroxyproline. Hydroxyproline is used to form the collagen matrix in connective tissue, skin, tendons, and bones.

Vitamin C deficiency has not been shown to affect the course or outcome of pregnancy in humans. Questions have arisen, however, about its possible association with several specific conditions made known through isolated clinical observations; low plasma levels of vitamin C have been reported to be associated with premature rupture of the membranes and preeclampsia. An extra 15 mg of vitamin C is recommended daily for the pregnant woman; this total recommendation of 60 mg daily is easily met by the average U.S. diet. Massive intake of vitamin C supplements may adversely influence fetal metabolism. Metabolic dependency on high doses may develop in the offspring such that scurvy may arise in the neonatal period.

Vitamin E

The most active form of vitamin E is alphatocopherol. Its principal function is to prevent the oxidation of unsaturated fatty acids, which make up the structure of cell membranes. Vitamin E also prevents the oxidation of vitamin A in the gastrointestinal tract so that more vitamin A in the diet can be absorbed.

Vitamin E needs are believed to increase somewhat during pregnancy, but deficiency in humans rarely occurs and has not been linked with either reproductive causality or reduced fertility. Because vitamin E deficiency in experimental animals has long been associated with spontaneous abortion, interest in the use of vitamin E for prevention of abortion has been a popular idea. In general, however, studies in humans have not supported the value of this preventive measure.

Although the vitamin E level in the infant at birth is significantly less that than in the mother, the infant's level has been shown to correlate directly with the maternal concentration. Nevertheless, parenteral vitamin E administration to the mother before delivery is not enough to prevent an infant from having the hemolytic anemia of vitamin E deficiency. Because this problem develops within 6 weeks after birth, it can best be prevented by oral supplementation of the infant during the postnatal interval.

Vitamin D

Vitamin D has long been appreciated for its positive effects on calcium balance during pregnancy. Evidence suggests that vitamin D may be involved in neonatal calcium homeostasis. Indeed, the peak season for neonatal hypocalcemia coincides with the time of least sunlight. In addition, serum vitamin D levels are often low in such infants, suggesting that some cases of neonatal hypocalcemia and/or enamel hypoplasia may relate to maternal vitamin D deficiency and subsequent limitation in placental transport of vitamin D to the fetus. Vitamin D supplementation during the third trimester may be associated with improved perinatal handling of calcium.

Clinical osteomalacia is found in 10% to 30% of the Asian immigrant population in northern Europe; 25% to 53% have biochemical disease. Pregnancy is a serious risk factor because of its increased requirements for calcium and vitamin D. Unfortunately, failure to recognize the clinical features of maternal osteomalacia still occurs. Problematic features include a small, deformed pelvis, which often precludes vaginal delivery; other musculoskeletal complications are also common, with bone pain and proximal myopathy both producing impairment in mobility. Routine biochemical screening for osteomalacia in this high-risk population is justified; other routine procedures might be vitamin D supplementation, placental function testing, predelivery pelvimetry and neonatal monitoring for hypocalcemia.

Maternal ingestion of excessive amounts of vitamin D may be harmful to the developing fetus, resulting in infantile hypercalcemia and possibly vascular lesions.

MINERAL REQUIREMENTS

Iron

The importance of folic acid and vitamin B_{12} in the production of red blood cells has been discussed. These two nutrients must be accompanied by adequate amounts of protein and other vitamins and minerals for normal erythropoiesis. Adequacy of these supplies is indicated by the concentration of hemoglobin in the blood.

During pregnancy, iron is needed for the manufacture of hemoglobin in both maternal and fetal red blood cells. The fetus accumulates most of its iron during the last trimester. At term a normal-weight infant has about 246 mg of iron in blood and body stores. An additional 134 mg is stored in the placenta, and about 290 mg is used to expand the volume of the mother's blood (Table 2-5).

Maintenance of erythropoiesis is one of the few instances during pregnancy when the fetus acts as a true parasite. It ensures its own production of hemoglobin by drawing iron from the mother. Maternal iron deficiency therefore does not usually result in an infant who is anemic at birth. The most common cause of iron deficiency anemia in the infant is prematurity. The infant who has a short gestation does not have time to accumulate sufficient iron during the last trimester.

Iron deficiency in the mother may have adverse effects on her obstetrical performance. A reduction in hemoglobin concentration means that the mother must increase her cardiac output to maintain adequate oxygen delivery to placental and fetal cells. This extra work fatigues the mother and makes her more susceptible to other sources of physiologic stress. A very low hemoglobin level places the mother's survival at risk should she hemorrhage on delivery.

Setting requirements for iron during pregnancy is complicated by changes in the erythropoietic system. Even when women have adequate iron status at conception, the plasma volume increases faster than the number of red blood cells so that hemodilution occurs. However, erythropoiesis is stimulated in the last half of pregnancy, and the rate of hemoglobin production increases. If sufficient iron is available, hemoglobin levels should rise to at least 11.5 mg/100 mL by term (Fig. 2-3).

It is generally conceded that the initial decreases in hemoglobin is a normal physiologic phenomenon, but there is concern that the usual iron intakes of pregnant women may not support increased erythropoiesis and fetal demands in the last half of pregnancy. Iron absorption from the gastrointestinal tract increases during pregnancy, possibly to as much as 50% compared with the usual 10% to 20% absorption from the diet, and this may help satisfy the iron needs of the pregnant women.

TABLE 2-5. *Iron "cost" of a normal pregnancy*

Iron contributed to the fetus	200–370 mg
Iron in placenta and cord	30–170 mg
Iron in blood lost at delivery	90–310 mg
Total	310–850 mg[a]

[a]These figures are in addition to the normal excretory loss of 0.5 to 1.0 mg/day and ignore the demand during the second half of pregnancy for iron to support the expansion of red-cell mass. This latter (200–600 mg) is not included as an iron "cost" because it is largely conserved (and not lost from the body) when the red-cell mass returns to normal after delivery.

From Bothwell TH et al. Iron metabolism in man. Oxford, England: Blackwell, 1979.

The pregnant woman probably needs 18 to 21 mg of iron in her diet each day. This can be achieved if large servings of iron-rich foods are eaten; unfortunately, such foods are limited in the average U.S. diet. From an average mixed diet, approximately 6 mg of iron are obtained from each 1,000 kcal of food. At this rate a pregnant woman would have to eat 3,000 to 5,000 kcal per day to meet her iron needs. Furthermore, studies have shown that most women enter pregnancy with low iron stores so they have little to draw on to maintain normal hemoglobin concentrations in the later months. For these reasons the National Research Council recommends that pregnant women receive an oral iron supplement of 30 mg/day. This amount should maintain hemoglobin levels in normal pregnant women, but those who are anemic when they enter pregnancy will need a larger dose. Simple ferrous salts should be used. There are no advantages gained by using compounds purported to have unique properties that increase absorption or enhance erythropoiesis.

In a population of women who opt not to take iron supplements, evidence of iron deficiency without anemia has been reported. The most significant known consequence of maternal iron deficiency is reduced fetal iron storage followed by increased risk of anemia during infancy. This may be prevented by maternal iron supplementation by about 20 to 24 weeks' gestation. In the absence of iron supplements, it may to take up to 2 years after pregnancy before prepregnancy serum ferritin values are regained.

However, the routine need for iron supplementation during pregnancy remains controversial (43,44). One trial of routine iron prophylaxis during pregnancy showed that among well-nourished Finnish women, such prophylaxis is not crucial for the health of mothers or infants during pregnancy and through the first 8 weeks after delivery (42). In a subsequent seven year follow-up, a randomized trial was conducted comparing women who were given iron only if needed and those given iron prophylactically. The outcomes of the two groups were similar—there were not statistically significant differences in deaths after birth, the number or timing of infants' or mothers' hospitalization, reasons for mothers' first hospitalization, number or timing of subsequent miscarriages or births, or problems or outcomes in the next birth. This study did not support routine iron prophylaxis for well-nourished pregnant women (43).

If iron supplements were completely innocuous, a rationale might be that so long as they are relatively inexpensive and the studies about effectiveness are equivocal, supplements might do some good. However, there are important questions about the safety of medicinal iron. A substantial number of prenatal patients develop diarrhea or more commonly constipation, which improves when they discontinue their iron supplements. Iron has been shown to depress the absorption of dietary zinc, and the greatest danger of iron supplements for prenatal patients

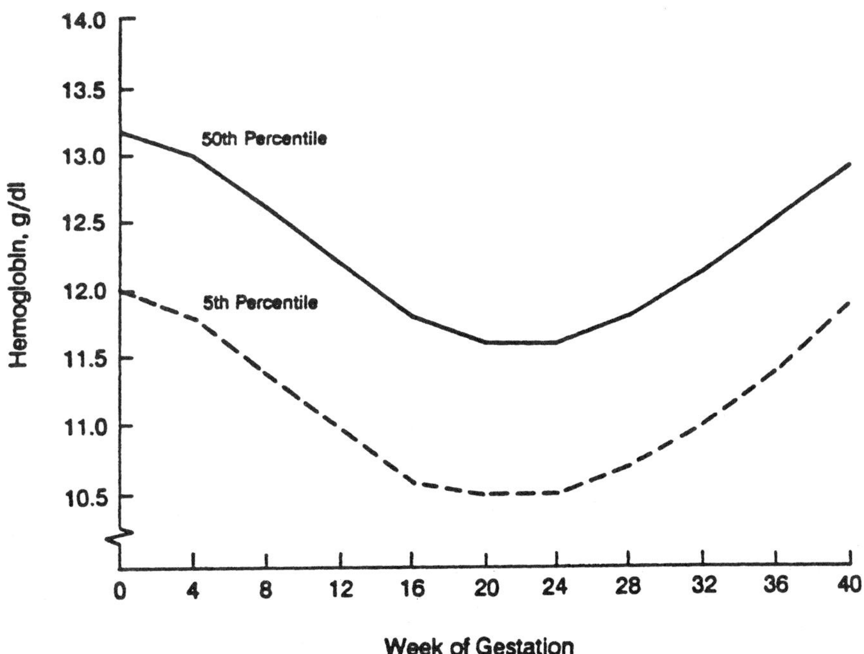

FIG. 2-3. Normal changes in hemoglobin concentration during course of pregnancy. (From the Institute of Medicine. Nutrition during pregnancy. Part II: Nutrient supplements. Washington, DC: National Academy Press, 1990.)

is that iron pills often resemble candy and are the leading cause of poisoning deaths in children under the age of six. The FDA has proposed that packages of capsules and tablets containing iron be labeled with warnings not to leave the packages open or within the reach of children to prevent poisoning.

It seems practical, however, to monitor hemoglobin levels at the onset of pregnancy and at about 26 to 28 weeks' gestation. If hemoglobin levels are less than 10 g/100 mL, a ferritin level should be drawn to determine whether there is iron deficiency. If the ferritin level is below normal, iron-rich foods or iron supplements should be added on a case-by-case basis. Response to therapy should be assessed with subsequent blood tests. All prenatal patients should be instructed about iron-rich foods, foods rich in vitamin C, and foods that inhibit bioavailability of iron.

Iron Deficiency Anemia

Maternal anemia is the major clinical consequence of iron deficiency, but its effects on pregnancy outcome are poorly understood. Because both high altitudes and smoking normally elevate hemoglobin and hematocrit levels, adjustments are necessary in these situations for diagnosis of anemia.

An anemic woman is less able to tolerate hemorrhage with delivery, and she is more prone to development of puerperal infection. Data suggest that the fetal effects of maternal iron deficiency are relatively mild, but several reports suggest that pregnancy outcome may be compromised. Observations in India in the early 1970s showed that moderate to severe anemia in pregnant women was associated with increased incidence of spontaneous abortion, premature and low-birth-weight delivery, stillbirth, and perinatal death.

The pregnant woman with iron deficiency anemia should be treated with iron supplements of appropriate dosage (100 mg or more per tablet). In most anemic women treated in this fashion, an upward shift in the hematocrit level can be achieved easily. However, 15% or 20% of such women will not respond to typical iron therapy; this group is suspected to have markedly expanded plasma volume, such as occurs in multiple pregnancy. Supplementation with iron in excess of need has not been evaluated through critical research; unnecessary use of iron supplements has led to macrocytosis in a small number of pregnant women. Efforts to reduce the prevalence of iron deficiency anemia may not work because of low compliance with an iron-supplementation program (45).

Calcium

Although ionic calcium and phosphorus both have important regulatory functions in the cells and blood, about 99% of the body's calcium and over 80% of its phosphorus are bound as hydroxyapatite, the primary structural component of bones and teeth. The importance of calcium and phosphorus during pregnancy is to promote adequate mineralization of the fetal skeleton and deciduous teeth.

The fetus acquires most of its calcium in the last trimester, when skeletal growth is maximum and teeth are being formed. The fetus draws 13 mg/h of calcium from the maternal blood supply, or 250 to 300 mg/day. At birth the infant has accumulated approximately 25 g. Additional calcium is believed to be stored in the maternal skeleton as a reserve for lactation.

Recommendations for Calcium Intake

In the United States, the current RDA for calcium during pregnancy is 1,200 mg daily, a level 400 mg higher than recommended for the nonpregnant woman over 24 years of age. Some argue that this allowance is set too high because apparently successful pregnancies occur in many other cultures with calcium intakes substantially below those recommended (Fig. 2-4). The explanation likely relates to the large calcium reservoir in the maternal skeleton, of which the total requirement of pregnancy (30 g) amounts to about 2.5%. It should also be noted that in many other cultures, diets are consumed that contain less phosphorus and protein; this factor might reduce the degree of calcium loss in the urine. If maternal intake of calcium is less than 2 g/day, stores of calcium will be depleted to meet the needs of the fetus. If this is the case, frequent pregnancies and consistently low calcium intakes throughout the childbearing years could contribute to osteoporosis in later life. Clinical manifestations of osteomalacia in multiparous women do occur. Neonatal bone density also may relate to adequacy of maternal calcium consumption during pregnancy.

Milk and milk products constitute the most important sources of calcium in the diet, but additional amounts are supplied by legumes, nuts, and dried fruits. Dark leafy green vegetables such as kale, cabbage, collards, and turnip greens contain calcium in high amounts that can be well absorbed, but some of the calcium in spinach, chard, and beet greens is bound with oxalic acid, which makes it unavailable to the body.

Calcium Intake and Hypertensive Disorders

In 1980, an inverse relationship was reported between calcium intake and hypertensive disorders of pregnancy. It was proposed that satisfactory calcium intake may be protective against elevation in blood pressure during pregnancy. The hypothesis was based on the observation that Mayan Indians in Guatemala, who traditionally soak their corn in lime before cooking, had a high calcium intake and a low incidence of preeclampsia and eclampsia. If calcium intake through food or supplements can significantly lower the risk of preeclampsia, strategies to achieve this goal are attractive interventions (46). Most, but by no means all, available data support this benefit (47–49) (Figs. 2-5 and 2-6).

Phosphorus

The RDA for phosphorus is the same as that for calcium—800 mg with an extra 400 mg during pregnancy. It is so widely available in foods that a dietary deficiency is rare. In fact, there is a possibility that the problem may be too much phosphorus rather than too little.

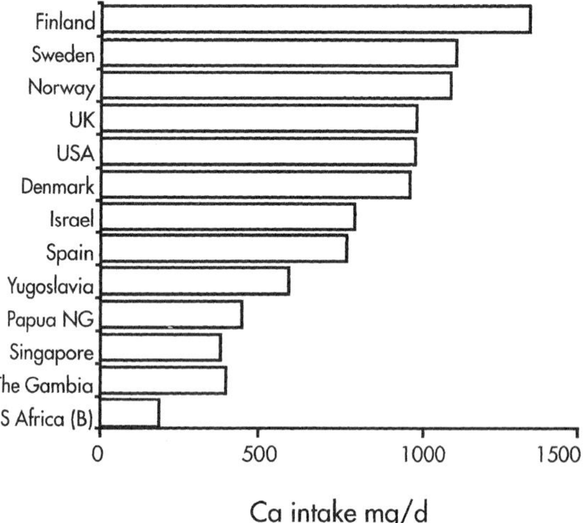

FIG. 2-4. Comparison of average calcium intakes in different countries. (Used with permission from Worthington-Roberts B, Williams SR. Nutrition in pregnancy and lactation, 6th ed. Dubuque, IA: Brown & Benchmark, 1997.)

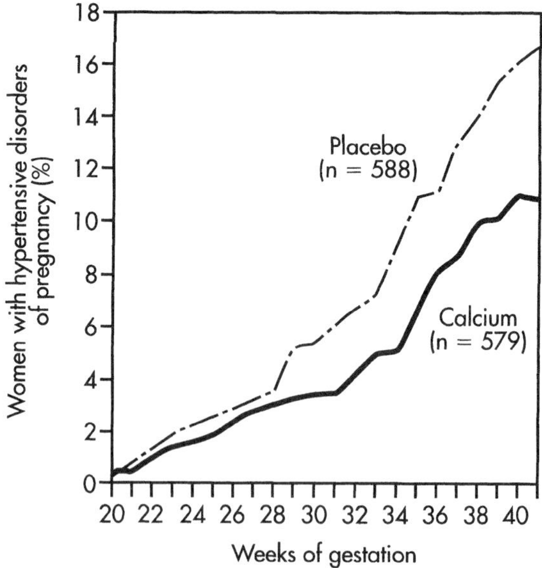

FIG. 2-5. Percentage of women in the calcium-treated and placebo groups in whom hypertensive disorders of pregnancy (gestational hypertension and preeclampsia) developed, according to the week of gestation. (Data from Belizan JM et al. Calcium supplementation to prevent hypertensive disorders of pregnancy. N Engl J Med 1991;325:1399. From Worthington-Roberts B, Williams SR. Nutrition in pregnancy and lactation, 6th ed. Dubuque, IA: Brown & Benchmark, 1997.)

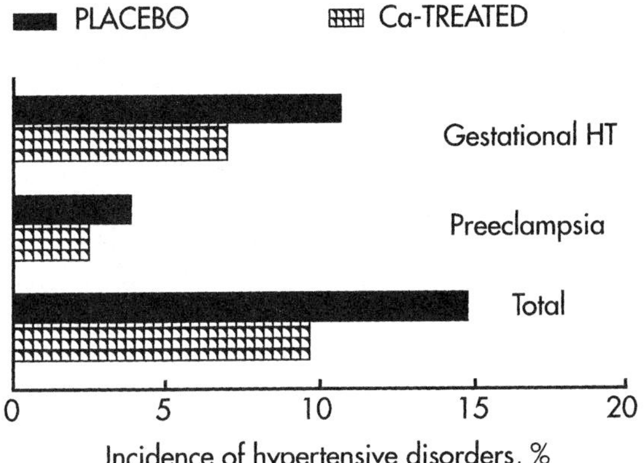

FIG. 2-6. Effect of calcium supplemention on the incidence of hypertensive disorders of pregnancy. Gestational hypertension was defined as a blood pressure greater than or equal to 140/90 mm Hg. Preeclampsia was defined as the presence of both gestational hypertension and proteinuria. Calcium supplementation significantly reduced the risk of developing hypertensive disorders of pregnancy. (Data from Belizan JM et al. Calcium supplementation to prevent hypertensive disorders of pregnancy. N Engl J Med 1991;325: 1399. From Worthington-Roberts B, Williams SR. Nutrition in pregnancy and lactation, 6th ed. Dubuque, IA: Brown & Benchmark, 1997.)

Calcium and phosphorus exist in a constant ratio in the blood. This ratio can be disturbed by the amounts of calcium and phosphorus in foods. If, for example, phosphorus is in excess, it will bind calcium in the gastrointestinal tract and limit the amount of calcium absorbed. A higher phosphorus:calcium ratio in the blood causes more calcium to be excreted in the urine.

The average U.S. diet is high in phosphorus. In addition to the naturally high levels in most animal protein foods, even greater amounts are found in processed meats, snack foods, and carbonated beverages. With the exception of dairy products, foods that are high in phosphorus contain only small amounts of calcium.

Most adults can tolerate relatively wide variations in dietary calcium:phosphorus ratios when vitamin D is adequate. However, pregnancy is a time when calcium reserves are severely stressed. Lowered serum calcium concentrations and the mild alkalosis from the mother's reduced P_{CO_2} tend to increase muscular irritability. When this is compounded by exceptionally high phosphorus intakes, a disturbance of the calcium:phosphorus ratio in the body could result.

Calcium-phosphorus balance is often discussed in relation to maintenance of neuromuscular normality. Many years ago, it was suggested that sudden clonic or tonic contractions (often at night) of the gastrocnemius muscle are caused by a decline in serum phosphate. Prevention or relief was reportedly achieved through reduction in intake of milk (a high-phosphorus, high-calcium beverage). Supplementation with nonphosphate calcium salts was also recommended, along with regular ingestion of aluminum hydroxide to promote formation of insoluble aluminum phosphate salts in the gut. Several studies confirmed the benefit of these measures in the total serum calcium level in affected women. It is clear, however, that the clinical correlation of these observations is far from perfect because some controlled and double-blind studies have failed to indicate a correlation between leg cramps and either intake or dairy products or the type of calcium supplement employed.

Magnesium

Magnesium is much like calcium and phosphorus in that most of it is stored in bones. The amounts that are biochemically active are concentrated in nerve and muscle cells. Deficiencies of magnesium produce neuromuscular dysfunctions characterized by tremors and convulsions. However, there are no convincing data that magnesium supplementation of pregnant women improves pregnancy course or outcome.

Studies of leg cramps have included both magnesium and calcium treatment. Leg cramps have been reported in 5% to 30% of all pregnant women, most often during the latter months of pregnancy and with no relationship to other complications or to unfavorable fetal outcome.

Dahle and colleagues (50) determined that oral magnesium substitution decreased leg cramp distress significantly in pregnant women but did not increase serum magnesium levels; excess magnesium was excreted as measured by an increase in urinary magnesium levels. These researchers concluded that magnesium supplementation seems to be a valuable tool in the treatment of pregnancy-related leg cramps, even if pretreatment serum magnesium levels are low.

Not much is known about the need for magnesium during pregnancy. The RDA is based on estimates of the amounts accumulated by the mother and fetus. Green vegetables are good sources of magnesium because the element is part of the green pigment chlorophyll; but the best sources are nuts, wheat bran, soybeans, and wheat germ. Animal products and fruits are relatively poor sources of magnesium.

Iodine

Iodine deficiency is by far the most common preventable cause of mental deficits in the world. The most severe form of endemic cretinism is characterized by a combination of mental deficiency, deaf-mutism, motor rigidity, and sometimes hypothyroidism. It occurs in parts of the world where iodine deficiency is sufficiently severe to cause goiter in 30% of the population. It is found in southern and eastern Europe and is common in Asia, Africa, and Latin America. Iodine injections in the form of iodized oil before but not during pregnancy will prevent cretinism. Studies in China showed that 2% of the infants of mothers who had injections in the second trimester of pregnancy compared with 9% of those whose mothers had injections in the second trimester had moderate or severe neurodevelopmental abnormalities.

In 1990, the World Health Organization (WHO) estimated that 20 million people in the world had preventable brain damage resulting from the effects of iodine deficiency on fetal brain development. They also set at 1 billion people the number at risk for iodine deficiency caused by low levels of iodine in the soil. Of these, 20% have goiter. Prevalence of neonatal hypothyroidism varies from 1% to 10% in these areas.

Zinc

Zinc has an active role in metabolism because it is a component of insulin. It also is part of the carbonic anhydrase enzyme system that helps to maintain tissue acid-base balance. The action of zinc in the synthesis of DNA and RNA makes it a highly important element in reproduction.

Zinc Deficiency

Zinc is a known constituent of a number of important metalloenzymes and a necessary cofactor for other enzymes. Zinc deficiency is highly teratogenic in rats and leads to the development of a variety of congenital malformations. Other adverse outcomes also have been reported (Table 2-6). Nonhuman primates are affected, and abnormal brain development and behavior have been described in offspring of zinc-deficient monkeys. Unfortunately, it seems that a zinc-deficient diet does not effectively move zinc from maternal bones. This storage pool appears somewhat unavailable so that dietary deficiency can quickly have an impact on the mineral balance of the maternal organism.

TABLE 2-6. *Relationship between plasma zinc and antenatal and intrapartum complications*

	Plasma Zinc		
	Low (n=144) (%)	High (n=35) (%)	P
Mild toxemia	5.6	0.7	0.02
Vaginitis	12.6	4.4	0.01
Postterm >42 wk	4.2	0	0.01
Prolonged latent phase	2.8	0	0.05
Protracted active phase	28.7	18.2	0.04
Labor >20 hr	6.3	1.5	0.03
Second stage >2.5 hr	6.3	0.7	0.01
Lacerations >3rd degree	7.0	1.5	0.02

From Lazebnik N, Kuhner BR, Thompson KL. Zinc status, pregnancy complications and labor abnormalities. Am J Obstet Gynecol 1988;158:161.

Potential adverse pregnancy outcomes have been explored in human pregnancies with regard to their association with zinc deficiency. There is evidence that maternal leukocyte zinc deficiency at the start of the third trimester is a predictor of fetal growth retardation.

One approach to determining whether zinc status is related to the outcome of pregnancy is to supplement women suspected of having zinc inadequacy and look for improved pregnancy outcome. Low-income Mexican-American women supplemented with 20 mg of zinc daily had a lower incidence of PIH than did unsupplemented women; no difference in complications was associated with zinc supplementation. Supplementation of low-income women in India with a much larger amount of zinc, 300 mg $ZnSO_4$ daily, was stopped after three premature births and one stillbirth occurred consecutively. Supplementation of a small number of presumably well-nourished women with a large amount of zinc (90 mg) had no deleterious effects.

Zinc supplementation during pregnancy was recently evaluated in a randomized, double-blind, placebo-controlled trial at the University of Alabama (51). In the trial, 580 medically indigent, but otherwise healthy, pregnant African-American women with plasma zinc levels below the median at enrollment in prenatal care were randomized at 19 weeks' gestation to receive either a daily dose of 25 mg of zinc or a placebo until delivery. (All women were taking a non–zinc-containing multivitamin-mineral tablet daily.) Daily zinc supplementation was associated with greater infant birth weights and head circumferences; the effect occurred predominantly in women who were not overweight. However, Mahomed and colleagues (52), in a study in northern Europe involving zinc supplementation during much of the second and third trimesters, did not observe any impact on outcome.

Until more information is available about the potential value or lack of zinc supplementation during pregnancy, routine supplementation is not advocated. The Institute of Medicine indicated in their summary of recommendations about nutrient supplements during pregnancy that at this time, there is little justification for their use. It is certainly reasonable, however, for prenatal nutrition counseling to include workable recommendations about food choices that maintain proper zinc status. The RDA for zinc during pregnancy is 15 mg, about 30% to 40% higher than the estimated intake of most pregnant women. It is also of interest that high levels of iron supplementation may suppress plasma zinc levels. Ideal levels of both iron and zinc have not yet been defined for prenatal vitamin and mineral supplements. However, attempting to counterbalance a large supplement of one trace element with a correspondingly large supplement of another may lead to unforeseen complications and should not be undertaken.

General Comments about Nutrient Supplementation

Common sense supplementation of pregnant women with vitamins and minerals is justifiable. Time taken to pursue information about dietary patterns is indicated for high-risk women; use of a registered dietitian may be cost effective. Whether or not nutrient supplementation can be clearly justified or is simply suspected to be advantageous, care should be taken to provide recommendations for safe levels of daily intake (Table 2-7).

Recommended Dietary Allowances

The Food and Nutrition Board of the National Research Council is aware of the problems of determining nutrient requirements during pregnancy and takes them in consideration when setting dietary allowances and making recommendations about the need for supplementation. RDAs are based on the best available evidence from metabolic balance studies and from indirect estimates. Requirements for most nutrients are set at levels that prevent signs of deficiency and maintain intake in balance with urinary excretion. When making dietary recommendations, the requirements are adjusted upward to ensure that the amounts derived from experimental subjects will cover individual variations in digestion, absorption, and utilization in the general population. As new evidence concerning requirements becomes available, the allowances are revised.

The 1989 edition of the RDA for pregnant and nonpregnant adult women is presented in Table 2-8. Women may need more or less of the amounts listed for calories and protein depending on body size, activity, and health status. The allowances for vitamins and minerals provide sufficient room for individual variations so that they can be applied to all healthy women. They may not be adequate for women who enter pregnancy in poor nutritional status or who have chronic diseases or other complicating conditions, or for the primigravida who conceives for the first time after 35 years of age.

RDAs have been set for only 18 of the 40 or so nutrients known to be needed to promote growth and maintain health. Strict attention to only those nutrients listed in Table 2-8 without regard for the general quality and variety of foods in the diet can lead to a false sense of security. Intakes can be inadequate when highly fortified foods or vitamin pills are relied on as the primary source of nutrition, even though they contain 100% of the RDA. Daily consumption of foods from all of the food groups is recommended to make sure that nutrient needs, including those for which there is presently no RDA, are met.

TABLE 2-7. *Recommended nutrients for supplementation when diet is inadequate during pregnancy*

Vitamins and minerals	Supplemental dose (per day)
Vitamin B_6	2 mg
Folate	0.4 mg
Vitamin C	50–70 mg (RDA 70 mg)
Vitamin D	400 IU
Iron	30–60 mg (RDA 30 mg)
Zinc	15 mg
Calcium	250–1,200 mg (RDA 1,200 mg)

From Kolasa KM, Weismiller DG. Nutrition during pregnancy. Am Family Physician 1997;56:205–212.

Recommendations for Weight Management

The goal of weight management during pregnancy should be to promote optimal nutrition for the mother and the child. Weight gain is considered a satisfactory measure of adequacy of prenatal nutrition. Although the Committee on Maternal Nutrition in 1970 recommended an optimal weight gain during pregnancy of 24 pounds, that recommendation was based on data from a longitudinal study of only 60 pregnant women in the mid-1950's. Data from the Perinatal Collaborative Study, which described over 50,000 women and their pregnancies between 1959 and 1965, suggest that the best obstetrical outcomes occur among normal-weight women who gain 27 lb (±20%); using perinatal mortality rate as an index of pregnancy outcome, optimum weight gain for underweight women was about 30 lb and for overweight women it was about 15 lb. Newer data from the 1980 National Fetal Mortality Survey indicate that the lowest fetal mortality rate and the lowest rate of low birth weight occur with a weight gain of 26 to 35 lb.

A committee appointed by the National Academy of Sciences (NAS) (54) undertook a thorough review of available data related to weight gain and pregnancy outcome. The conclusions of this expert panel derive from data obtained from women in the United States and may not apply to women living in less-developed countries or recent immigrants from developing countries to the United States. The subcommittee concluded that gestational weight gain has an important relationship to fetal growth and that this relationship appears to vary according to prepregnancy weight for height. Recommended relative weight-for-height categories for pregnant women are defined in Table 2-9. Recommended total weight gain ranges for pregnant women are summarized in Table 2-10.

The NAS Committee on Nutritional Status in Pregnancy and Lactation recommended that health care providers adopt and implement standardized procedures for obtaining and recording anthropometric measurements to serve as a basis for classifying women according to weight for height, setting weight-gain goals, and monitoring weight gain over the course of pregnancy. Clinicians are advised to direct attention to the following:

1. During health care prior to conception, accurately measure and record in the medical record the

TABLE 2-8. *Recommended dietary allowances for women of reproductive age (1989)*

Nutrient	Age 11–14	15–18	19–24	25–50	Pregnancy
Energy (kcal)	2200	2200	2200	2200	+300 (2nd and 3rd trimesters)
Protein (g)	46	48	46	50	60
Vitamin A (RE)	800	800	800	800	800
Vitamin D (μg)	10	10	10	5	10
Vitamin E (mg)	8	8	8	8	10
Vitamin K (μg)	45	55	60	60	65
Vitamin C (mg)	50	60	60	60	70
Folic Acid (μg)	150	180	180	180	400
Niacin (mg)	15	15	15	15	17
Riboflavin (mg)	1.3	1.3	1.3	1.3	1.6
Thiamin (mg)	1.1	1.1	1.1	1.1	1.5
Vitamin B_6 (mg)	1.4	1.5	1.6	1.6	2.2
Vitamin B_{12} (μg)	2.0	2.0	2.0	2.0	2.2
Calcium (mg)	1,200	1,200	1,200	800	1,200
Phosphorus (mg)	1,200	1,200	1,200	800	1,200
Iodine (μg)	150	150	150	150	175
Iron (mg)	15	15	15	15	30
Magnesium (mg)	280	300	280	280	320
Zinc (mg)	12	12	12	12	15
Selenium (μg)	45	50	55	55	65

RE, retinol equivalent.
From National Research Council, Food and Nutrition Board. Recommended Dietary Allowances. Washington, DC: National Academy Press, 1989.

woman's weight and height without shoes, using standardized procedures.

2. Measure weight and height at the first prenatal visit using rigorously standardized procedures.
3. Use standardized procedures to measure weight at each visit.
4. Record weight on a table and plot it in the obstetric record.

The NAS Committee recommended that a weight-gain goal be set, preferably beginning at the comprehensive initial prenatal examination, by the gravida and the professional mutually. A range of desirable total gestational weight gain and rate of weight gain should be identified and accompanied by appropriate counseling. The recommended range for total weight gain and pattern of gain should be based mainly on relative prepregnancy weight for height and height. Adjustments are recommended for women within 2 years of menarche and for short women. Women carrying twins should probably have a goal in the range of 35 to 45 lb. The literature provides no basis for special recommendations for women of different ethnic backgrounds or for older mothers. It is likely that differences in prepregnancy weight-for-height and height account for most differences among ethnic groups. In the case of black women, shorter gestational duration may account for part of the lower mean weight gain.

TABLE 2-9. *Recommended relative weight-for-height categories for pregnant women*

Prepregnancy weight-for-height category(%)[a]	Ideal BMI[b] range	Weight-for-height range
Light or low	<19.8	<90
Normal	19.8–26	90–120
Heavy or high	>26–29	120–135
Extreme obesity	>29	>235

[a]Percentage of the 1959 Metropolitan Life Tables ideal weight for height.
[b]Body mass index [weight (in kilograms) divided by height (in meters) squared].
From National Academy of Science. Nutrition during pregnant: weight gain and nutrient supplement. Washington, DC: National Academy Press, 1990.

TABLE 2-10. *Optimal weight gain in pregnancy*

Maternal classification (prepregnant BMI)	Weight Gain (lb) Total (lb)	Rate (lb/wk)[a]
Underweight (<19.8)	28–40	1.25
Normal weight (19.8–26.0)	25–35	1.00
Overweight (26.1–290)	15.25	0.70
Obese (>29.0)	15	0.50
Twin gestation	35–45	1.50

BMI, body mass index.
[a]Rate during second and third trimester.
Adapted from ACOG Technical Bulletin, 179. April 1993.

By monitoring weight gain throughout the pregnancy, abnormal patterns of gain can be identified and appropriate interventions chosen. Reasons for marked or persistent deviations from the expected pattern of gain should be investigated (Table 2-11).

Special Subgroups of Women

Although underweight and overweight women represent two major subgroups deserving special consideration during pregnancy, other subgroups such as morbidly obese women (>135% of ideal body weight), adolescents, and women carrying more than one fetus (multiple gestation) are also of interest. With morbidly obese women, adverse pregnancy course and outcome are very common, and preconceptional weight loss is highly desirable. However, because this is often not accomplished, prenatal care must include especially careful monitoring. Some data suggest that no ideal weight gain can be recommended for this population; these women tend to produce big babies at all levels of gain. The goal in nutrition counseling should be to emphasize food choices of high nutritional quality with avoidance of unnecessary calorie-rich foods. Ideally, the present pregnancy will not be associated with further augmentation in the already abundant fat stores.

Healthy pregnant teens should gain about 35 lb during pregnancy. Recommendations obviously should be individualized to include attention to prepregnancy weight and gynecologic age (years since menarche).

Women pregnant with twins, triplets, or greater numbers of offspring should gain more weight than women with singleton pregnancies. Observations of large numbers of such women, however, have not been reported such that standards of weight gain can be recommended. One study addressed weight gain patterns in women pregnant with twins; women with optimal outcome (defined as both babies weighing at least 2,500 g at birth, gestational age exceeding 37 weeks, and Apgar scores at 5 minutes of 7 or greater) gained means of 44 lb.

Weight-gain Charts

A variety of usable weight-gain charts are now available that reflect the current guidelines (Fig. 2-7) In most cases, prepregnancy weight status is determined by use of body mass index (weight in kg multiplied by the square of the height in meters. The Institute of Medicine provided its official chart in 1992.

Efforts have been made to evaluate the most recent weight gain recommendations for pregnant women, which were developed in the early 1990s by the Institute of Medicine of the NAS. Evaluations of these recommendations have sought to determine if the recommended weight gains are associated with the least perinatal mortality and morbidity. To date, the follow-up studies indicate that the relatively new standards are appropriate for the general population of U.S. women. In addition, limited weight gain during specific periods of pregnancy may be predictive of later outcome. For example, weight gain during the second trimester is strongly related to fetal birth weight.

Much of the past confusion about weight gain during pregnancy and the misguided attempts to restrict it are the results of the failure to appreciate that the components and rate of weight gain are more important than the actual number of pounds a woman puts on. Pregnancy should be a positive period of growth in which most of the gain is in lean body (protein) tissue.

Postpartum Weight Retention

In evaluating the adequacy of current weight gain recommendations for pregnant women, attention has been drawn to the consequences of level of prenatal weight gain on postpartum weight retention. Since weight gain recommendations today exceed those proposed in the past, concern has been expressed about the potential of the new guidelines to contribute to the growing level of obesity in the United States.

TABLE 2-11. *What to look for if weight gain is very rapid*

Is there a measurement or recording error?
Is the overall pattern acceptable? Was the gain preceded by weight loss or a lower than expected gain?
Is there evidence of edema?
Has the woman stopped smoking recently? The advantages of smoking cessation offset any disadvantages associated by gaining some extra weight.
Are twins or triplets a possibility? (A large increase of fundal height may be the earliest sign.)
Are there signs of gestational diabetes?
Has there been a dramatic decrease in physical activity without an accompanying decrease in food intake?
Has the woman greatly increased her food intake? (Get a diet recall, making special note of high-fat foods. However, rapid weight gain often is accompanied by normal eating patterns, which should be continued. If intake of high-fat or high-sugar foods is excessive, encourage substitutions.)
If serious overeating is occurring, explore why (stress, depression, eating disorder, boredom). Is there a need for special support or a referral?

From Institute of Medicine. Nutrition during pregnancy: weight gain and nutrient supplements. Washington, DC: National Academy of Sciences, 1990.

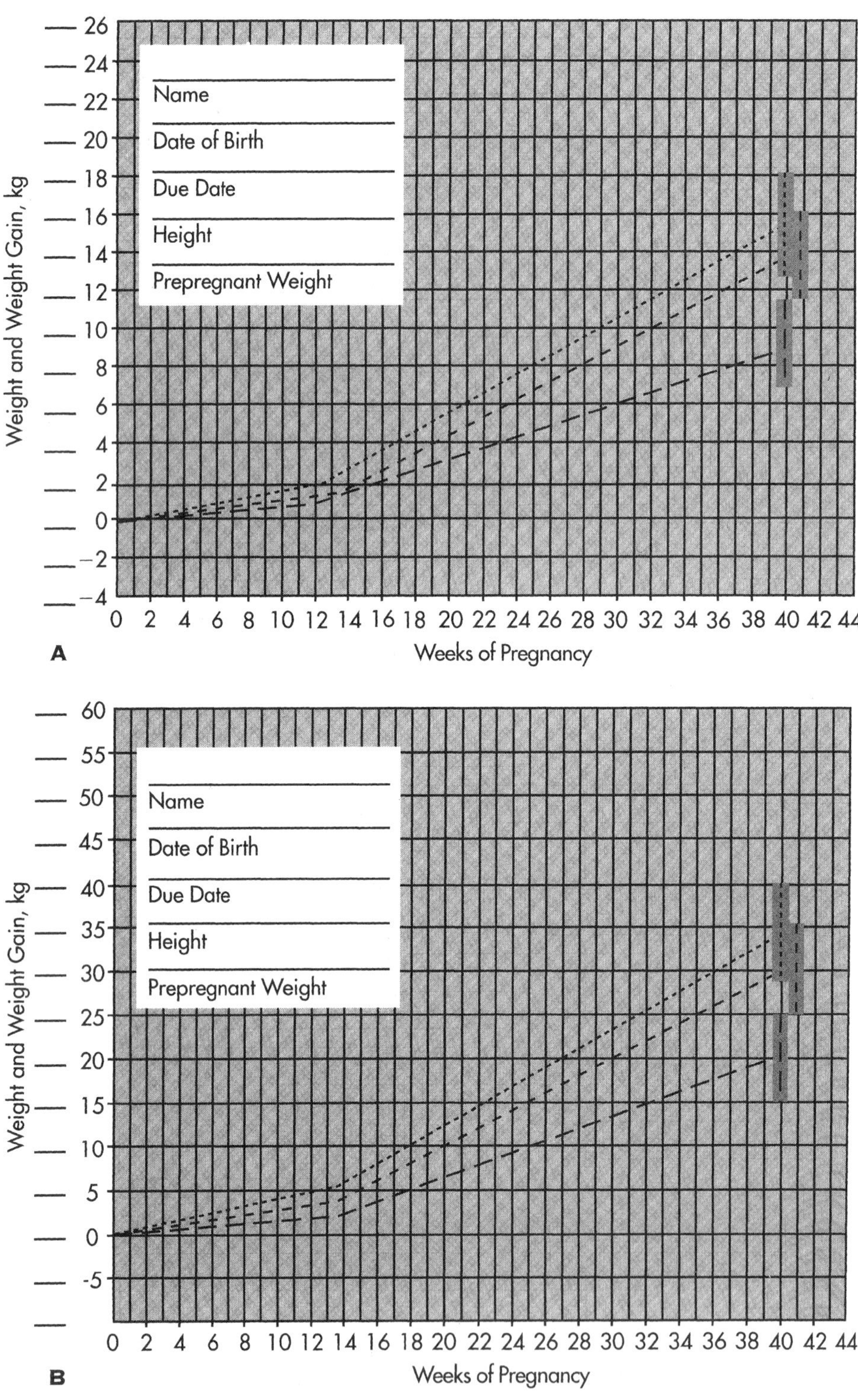

FIG. 2-7. Prenatal weight gain charts in kilograms **(A)** and pounds **(B)**. Underweight (-----), normal weight (- - - - -), overweight (— — — —). (From the Food and Nutrition Board, Institute of Medicine. Nutrition during pregnancy: weight gain and nutritient supplements. Washington, DC: National Academy of Sciences, 1990.)

Gradual weight loss generally occurs during the year following delivery. Rates of weight loss vary considerably among women, but in general the majority of the postpregnancy fat pad is lost during the first 6 months postpartum. In a study of nearly 800 women (55), the average total weight loss was 27 lb, corresponding to an average weight retained from the first obstetric visit to the last weight retained at 6 months postpartum of 3.1 lb. Of these women, 22% had returned to their prepregnancy weight or less by 6 weeks and 37% by 6 months postpatum. Figure 2-8 illustrates the cumulative weight loss pattern of this population.

Recent research focused on evaluating body composition change during this time by use of magnetic resonance imaging (MRI) (56). This technique allows for the approximation of changes in adipose tissue volume (ATV). Fifteen Swedish women were assessed before pregnancy and at intervals after delivery (from two months to 1 year). The women had more ATV postdelivery than before pregnancy. Of the ATV gained during pregnancy, 76% was placed subcutaneously, and the postpartum decrease was due to a loss of subcutaneous ATV. During pregnancy, 68% of the increased ATV was located in the torso and 16% in the thighs. Postpartum adipose tissue was mobilized more completely from the thigh than from the trunk. The results also indicated that women with a high weight gain during pregnancy retained lean tissue in their bodies (Fig. 2-9).

Pregnancy-related weight gain and postpartum retention also were evaluated by researchers in the United States. In the 1988 National Maternal and Infant Survey (57), one group observed weight retention 10 to 18 months following delivery in selected women who had live births. The actual weight gains of these women during pregnancy were retrospectively classified according to the Institutes of Medicine guidelines. The results indicated that weight retention following delivery increased as weight gain increased; black women retained more weight than white women with comparable weight gain. The mean retained weight was 1.6 lb for white women, who gained the amount of weight currently recommended, whereas it was 7.2 lb for black women. Thus, if pregnant women gain weight according to the Institute's guidelines, they need not be concerned about retaining a substantial amount of weight postpartum. However, black women are in need of advice about how to lose weight following delivery.

A further analysis of data from the 1988 National Maternal and Infant Survey focused on retention of 20 lb or more among 990 black and 1,129 white women who began pregnancy at normal weight for height (58). In this case, black mothers were twice as likely to retain 20 lb than white mothers. This difference between races did not differ substantially by socioeconomic status. Interestingly, many factors affecting postpartum weight retention

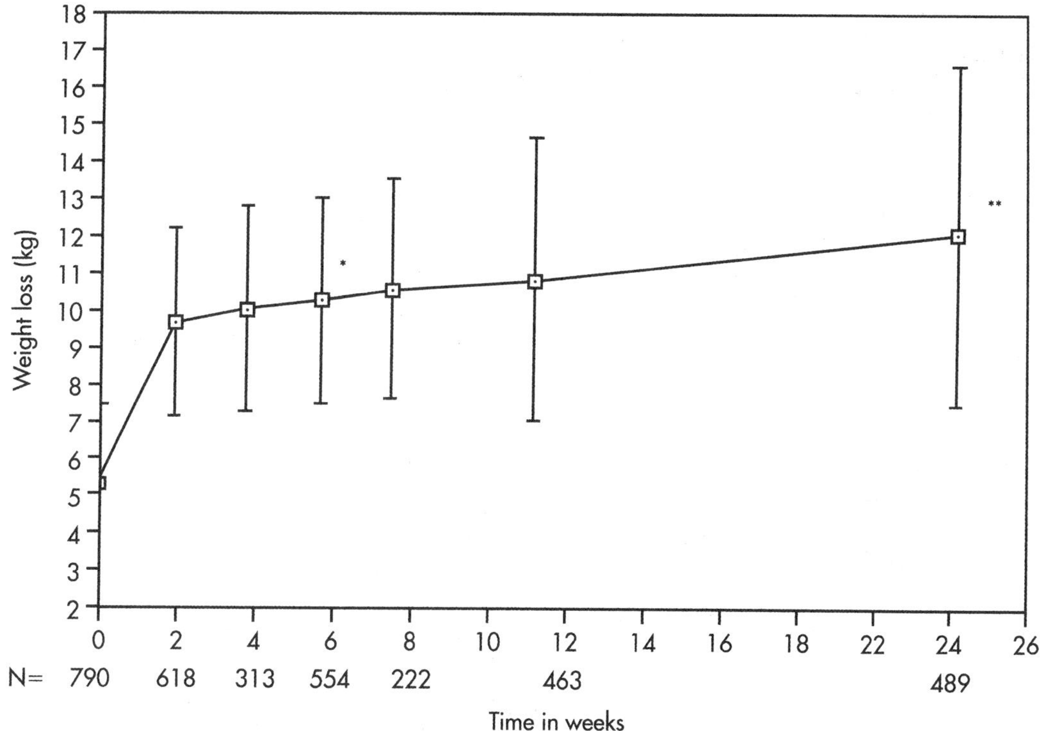

FIG. 2-8. Cumulative weight loss from last antepartum visit to 6 months postpartum. (From Schauberger CW, Rooney BL, Brimer LM. Factors that influence weight loss in the puerperium. Obstet Gynecol 1992;79:424.)

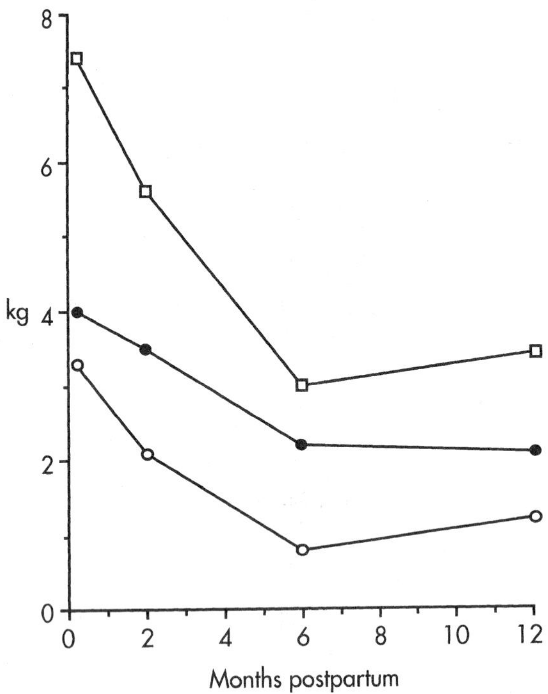

FIG. 2-9. Body weight (□), total body fat (●), and fat-free body weight (○) of Swedish women through the first year postpartum. The figures given are averages and represent differences from the corresponding prepregnant figures. (From Sohlstrom A, Forsum E. Changes in adipose tissue volume and distribution during reproduction in Swedish women as assessed by magnetic resonance imaging. Am J Clin Nutr 1995;61:287–295.)

differed by maternal race. For example, unmarried status was associated with weight retention among white mothers, whereas high parity was associated with weight retention among black mothers. Low socioeconomic status and high prenatal weight gain were associated with an increased risk of weight retention for both black and white mothers. Population-specific strategies may be needed to help mothers return to their prepregnancy weight.

A related observation was made in a study of the rate of gestational weight in a sample of 274 young, low-income, and primarily minority women (ages 12 to 29) with pregravid body mass indices in the normal range (19.8–26.0) (59). Excessive weight gain was defined as one greater than 1.5 lb/wk. Weight gained at an excessive rate by women with normal weight-for-height did not greatly enhance fetal growth and gestation duration, but contributed instead to postpartum overweight.

An effort was made to define factors that influence weight loss in the puerperium. A group of 795 women was followed with frequent weight measurements and questionnaires about their activities for 6 months postpartum. The mean net weight gain from the first prenatal visit to 6 months postpartum was 3.1 lb. Weight gain during the prenatal period was the variable most highly correlated with weight loss. Breastfeeding, exercise, season of the year, age, and marital status were not correlated. An early return to the workplace was associated with greater weight loss at 6 months, possibly because of increased caloric expenditure or less access to food during the week.

Does experiencing one or more pregnancies have any direct bearing on percentage body fat later in life? This question was evaluated in a group of 2,788 women who participated in a prepaid health care plan (60). Women who remained nulligravid were compared with those who had been pregnant at least once over 5 years. Overall, those women who had experienced pregnancy during the 5-year interval weighed 4.5 to 7 lb more than did those who had never been pregnant. Multiparas did not differ from nulliparas in adipose tissue change in either racial group. At each level of parity, black women demonstrated greater adverse changes in percentage of adipose tissue than did white women. These data suggest that women tend to experience modest increases in body weight after a first pregnancy and that these changes are persistent.

Another study reported that the more children a woman has, the higher her weight is likely to be at age 50 (61). A steady increase in body mass index was seen as parity increased from three to eight live births. Parity was associated with an increase of 1.21 lb per live birth.

It was also found that women gained 0.77 lb per year between the ages of 18 and 50 for a total of 24 lb. A difference of 2.3 lb less was recorded, as education increased from less than high school to high school and another 2.2 lb for greater than high school. Never-married women gained nearly 4.4 lb less than did married women, and smokers gained 7.3 lb less than nonsmokers.

These findings derive from a population of women living in an affluent society; the weight gain scenario may be different in other societies. The tendency for increased percentage adipose tissue with reproductive experience may be preventable in the United States. Until more data are available, this question cannot be answered satisfactorily.

Food Beliefs, Cravings, Avoidances, and Aversions

Most women change their diets during pregnancy. Some changes are based on medical advice, others on folk medical beliefs, and others on changes in preference and appetite that may be idiosyncratic or culturally patterned. Because food intake choices and patterns are in part culturally sanctioned, the health care provider should be sensitive to their existence because they will affect a woman's willingness to follow prescribed dietary regimens.

Many folk beliefs about prenatal diet still exist, such as the idea that the mother can mark her child before birth by eating specific foods. Overuse of a craved food during pregnancy is said to explain physical and behavioral peculiarities of the infant. Unsatiated cravings are thought to explain birthmarks that mimic the shape of the desired food (such as strawberry or drumstick-shaped marks). Eating behaviors also have been thought to derive from the prenatal diet; that is, the mother's consumption of certain foods has been said to cause the child to like such foods after birth.

Another group of false beliefs concerns dietary means by which the mother can ensure an easier delivery. Most laypeople know that a smaller weight gain during pregnancy produces a smaller infant; because a smaller baby may be easier to deliver, low weight gain has been proposed as desirable, especially because it is commonly believed that the baby can catch up after birth.

Food avoidances are those foods that the mother consciously chooses not to consume during her pregnancy, usually for a reason she can articulate and that seems reasonable to her. The four most commonly avoided foods are sources of animal protein: milk, lean meats, pork, and liver. Cravings and aversions are powerful urges toward or away from foods. The most commonly reported craved foods are sweets and dairy products. The most common aversions are to alcohol, caffeinated drinks, and meats. However, cravings and aversions are not limited to any particular foods or food groups.

It is difficult to quantify the nutritional effect of restrictive beliefs, avoidances, cravings, or aversions. The nutritional importance of such practices cannot be assessed without reference to the rest of the woman's diet. Overall, most cravings result in increased intakes of calcium and energy, whereas aversions often result in decreased intake of alcohol and caffeine but also decreased intake of animal protein. Cravings and aversions are not necessarily deleterious.

Pica

Pica (62) is the compulsion for persistent ingestion of unsuitable substances having little or no nutritional value. Pica of pregnancy most often involves consumption of dirt and/or clay (geophagia) or starch (amylophagia). However, compulsive ingestion of a variety of nonfood substances has been noted, such as ice, burnt matches, hair, gravel, charcoal, soot, cigarette ashes, mothballs, antacid tablets, milk of magnesia, baking soda, coffee grounds, and tire inner tubes. The practice of pica is not limited to any one geographical area, race, creed, culture, gender, or status within a culture.

The medical implications of pica are not well understood, although several speculations have been put forward. The displacement effect of pica substances could result in reduced intake of nutritious foods, leading to inadequate dietary intakes of essential nutrients. Alternatively, substances that provide calories (e.g., starch) could lead to obesity if ingested in amounts above the usual dietary intakes. Some pica substances may contain toxic compounds or quantities of nutrients not tolerated in disease states, or could interfere with the absorption of certain mineral elements (such as iron). Other less commonly reported complications of pica are congenital lead poisoning, fecal impaction, fetal hemolytic anemia (caused by maternal ingestion of mothballs and toilet air fresheners), parotid enlargement and gastric and small bowel obstruction (from ingestion of excessive laundry starch), and parasitic infection (from ingestion of contaminated soil or clay).

The etiologic factors of pica are poorly understood, although several proposals have been put forth. One theory suggests that the ingestion of nontraditional substances relieves nausea and vomiting. Pica is a normal behavioral response to gastrointestinal tract upset in rats. It has also been hypothesized that a deficiency of an essential nutrient such as calcium or iron results in the eating of nonfood substances that contain these nutrients.

Health care professionals who counsel pregnant women need to be alert to the potential practice of pica in each patient. Anemia and poor pregnancy outcomes may occur as a result of excessive intake of these nonfood items. Consequently, all pregnant patients need to be asked about pica behavior; if present, they should be counseled about the possible effects and monitored for anemia and poor fetal development. Because our knowledge about adverse effects is limited, continued observation of patients with these interesting behaviors is warranted.

POTENTIALLY HARMFUL DIETARY COMPONENTS

Alcohol

In 1973 a University of Washington group described a unique set of characteristics of infants born to women who were chronic alcoholics (see Chapter 8). These infants exhibited specific anomalies of the eyes, nose, heart, and central nervous system that were accompanied by growth retardation, small head circumference, and mental retardation. The investigators named the condition *fetal alcohol syndrome (FAS)* (Table 2-12).

There is a high rate of mortality among fetuses with FAS. Those who survive generally show irritability and hyperactivity after birth, symptoms attributable to alcohol withdrawal. Physical and mental development is impaired. The mental and growth deficits seen at birth persist into later life.

The impact of more moderate levels of alcohol consumption on fetal development has been the focus of much research. It is now recognized that moderate drinkers may produce offspring with fetal alcohol effects (FAE); this term refers to the more subtle features of FAS. Diagnosis of FAE is not easy. For this reason the term *possible fetal alcohol effects* (PFAE) has been suggested to describe individuals who have been exposed to alcohol prenatally and

TABLE 2-12. *Facial characteristics in fetal alcohol syndrome*

	Features necessary to characteristic face	Associated features
Eyes	Short palpebral fissures	
Nose	Short and upturned in early childhood; hypoplastic philtrum	Flat nasal bridge; epicanthal folds
Maxilla	Flattened	
Mouth	Thinned upper vermilion	Prominent lateral palatine ridges; cleft lip with or without cleft palate; small teeth
Mandible		Retrognathia in infancy; micrognathia or relative prognathia in adolescents
Ears		Posterior rotation; abnormal concha

From Clarren SK. Recognition of fetal alcohol syndrome. JAMA 1981;245:2436.

present with cognitive and behavioral problems, but do not have the facial characteristics of FAS. In the absence of the characteristic facial features, the cognitive/behavioral dysfunction in an individual cannot be directly and exclusively linked to the prenatal alcohol exposure. Therefore, FAE is not a medical diagnosis at this time, and it is more accurate to use the term PFAE. PFAE is also not a mild form of FAS. In fact, individuals with PFAE can be just as severely affected cognitively and behaviorally as those with FAS. However, it is often difficult for affected individuals to access social and medical services because they do not have a medical diagnosis.

The mechanisms by which alcohol produces such widespread effects on the fetus are not completely understood. Because alcohol can cross the placenta, the current hypothesis is that high levels build up in the fetus and produce direct toxic effects that are most adverse in the early phases of pregnancy during blastogenesis and cell differentiation. Another theory is that some of the effects of alcohol may be caused by maternal malnutrition. Women who derive a substantial portion of their daily caloric needs from alcohol may not have an appetite for more nutritious foods. Micronutrient deficiencies are often seen in alcoholics.

In the developed world, FAS is the major cause of significant lifetime disabilities. Unlike many other birth defects, however, it is preventable. Prevention of FAS is a national health priority included in the Healthy People 2000 objectives for health promotion and disease prevention. The specific health objective is to reduce the rate of FAS to no more than 1.2 cases per 10,000 live births by the year 2000.

The impact of binge drinking on the outcome of pregnancy has never been satisfactorily evaluated in human populations. Recently, however, use of a monkey model has allowed researchers to study the effects of one binge a week on pregnancy course and outcome. At doses of 2.5 g/kg, pregnancy failure was seen in the early weeks of pregnancy; lower doses were associated with increased risk of spontaneous abortion. Viable offspring of the binge-drinking mothers are currently under study. Preliminary data suggest permanent damage to the central nervous system manifested by abnormal behavior.

It is imperative to identify alcohol and other drug use in pregnant women as early as possible during the course of prenatal care so that interventions may be applied (63,64). Recent estimates suggest that alcohol and drug use continues to escalate, and as many as 10% to 15% of women of childbearing age (15–44 years) are actively using alcohol or other drugs. Prospective studies in large metropolitan areas have reported drug use in approximately 15% of the pregnant women evaluated, often with no substantial differences between clinic and private patients or between black and white patients.

The Maternal Addiction Project at St. Francis Medical Center in Pittsburgh has been treating pregnant women who use alcohol and other drugs since 1979. A major objective of this group is to improve identification of pregnant women using drugs in their geographic areas. The following principles of identification have been put forward (65):

1. All pregnant women should be asked about their use of alcohol and other drugs.
2. An identification method should not disrupt the flow of the prenatal clinic or office or be overly time consuming.
3. An interview style that incorporates respect and encourages trust will yield more truthful responses.
4. Specific questions about alcohol and other drug use can be readily incorporated into the usual history-taking process.
5. Drug and alcohol use during pregnancy has been associated with a number of risk factors in various studies. Determination of the presence of three risk factors can assist in identifying pregnant women who need further assessment.
6. Some women will need to be asked about alcohol and other drug use repeatedly for an honest answer to be obtained.
7. Some women who abuse alcohol and other drugs need to be confronted about their use to help them recognize that such use is a problem for them.
8. Identification can best be accomplished by combining a comprehensive interview and drug screening. Urine screening for drugs should be used in combi-

nation with an interview, with the knowledge that some women who admit to use will have negative results on urine screening and some women who deny use will have positive results on urine screening. The presence of risk factors for alcohol and other drug use can be used to assist in determining which women should have their urine screened.

9. Risk factors associated with use of alcohol and other drugs may differ between pregnant teenagers and pregnant adult women. A separate identification method is necessary for use with teenagers.
10. Many women who abuse alcohol and other drugs do not use prenatal care. Some of these women seek medical care only for a pregnancy-related problem (e.g., pain or bleeding) or at the time of delivery.

Caffeine

In 1980 the FDA warned pregnant women to restrict or even eliminate consumption of coffee based on studies showing teratogenic effects in rodents. Although this advisory remains in effect, the implications of caffeine consumption during pregnancy remain controversial.

The results of studies in rodents indicate that caffeine administered in large single doses has teratogenic effects. In addition to fetal resorptions, the most commonly seen malformations are those of the limbs and digits, as well as cleft lips and palates. Such malformations are observed, however, only in relatively high doses. Teratogenic effects usually appear only at doses high enough to cause toxicity in the mother and far higher than those consumed by humans, even those who drink large amounts of coffee. For example, a woman weighing 60 kg would have to drink about 10 to 14 cups of coffee in one sitting to achieve plasma caffeine concentrations comparable with those associated with teratogenic effects in the rat. Animal studies in which more moderate doses were administered over the course of a day (to mimic the typical pattern of human caffeine intake) have not shown teratogenic effects.

Of significance is the reality that caffeine may have detrimental interactions with other substances that are harmful to the developing fetus, such as alcohol and tobacco.

The European Multicenter Study conducted between 1991 and 1993 found strong evidence for delayed conception among fertile women who consumed more than 500 mg caffeine/day; this effect was augmented by cigarette smoking (66). In addition, Yugoslavian investigators reported impressive evidence of reduced birth weight in offspring of nonsmoking caffeine users (>71 mg/day) (67).

Just how caffeine may interfere with the reproductive process is uncertain. Of interest is a recent report by Norwegian researchers interested in the relationship between plasma homocysteine and risk of cardiovascular disease (68). In a population of over 15,000 men and women there was a strongly positive dose-response relationship between coffee consumption and plasma homocysteine. The combination of cigarette smoking and high caffeine intake was associated with particularly high homocysteine concentrations. Because elevated levels of plasma homocysteine have been mentioned as a distinct risk factor for adverse pregnancy outcome, this observation is particularly provocative.

A recent review of this issue by Nehlig and Debry (69) concluded that in the absence of more precise data and to avoid any fetotoxic risk, women should moderate their consumption of coffee during pregnancy and avoid tobacco and alcohol.

Herbal Teas

Herbal teas and herbal remedies have been part of folk medicine for centuries. There are currently more than 400 distinct herbs and spices commercially available to use either alone or in blended mixtures as tea. Many commercially prepared drugs originated from plants. Consumers interested in natural food often turn to these products; other consumers looking for alternatives to caffeine-containing beverages find herbal teas attractive.

Pregnant women should be discouraged from unlimited consumption of herb teas. The reason is that the composition and safety of most of them is unknown. Rather than seek FDA approval, most manufacturers of herbal tea preparations stopped marketing the mixtures as medicine and simply list the ingredients on the label.

In 1983 the FDA officially designated 28 plants as unsafe to consume: "We cannot conclude that all herbal teas are safe nor that it's safe to consume large amounts of any herbal tea over extended periods" (70). It is likely that many herbal teas are safe, but some (lobelia, sassafras, coltsfoot, comfre, and pennyroyal) have been shown to have potentially harmful side effects. Depressed breathing, convulsions and, in mice, malignancies have been reported.

Because of the lack of safety testing, pregnant women should be advised to choose only products in filtered tea bags, and in order to avoid displacing more nutritious beverages, to limit herbal tea consumption to two 8-oz servings per day.

Aspartame

Since the approval of aspartame for use in carbonated beverages, there has been much debate about the safety of the additive in the diets of pregnant women. Major concern has been voiced about the added phenylalanine load because high circulating levels of phenylalanine (as are seen in women with poorly controlled phenylketonuria) are known to damage the fetal brain. However, individuals who do not have phenylketonuria have markedly lower serum phenylalanine levels, even those who are heterozygous carriers of the phenylketonuria gene. Phenylalanine-induced embryopathy is likely only if the phenylalanine values are continuously 1,200 μmol/L.

In normal persons fed 200 mg/kg aspartame, or the equivalent of 60 12-oz cans of diet soda at one time (or in heterozygotes fed 100 mg/kg), blood phenylalanine concentrations peak well below the sustained concentration level deemed harmful. In view of the practical considerations and the fact that no data exist to suggest that use of aspartame-containing products is associated with adverse pregnancy outcome, it seems unreasonable to direct pregnant women to avoid this artificial sweetener.

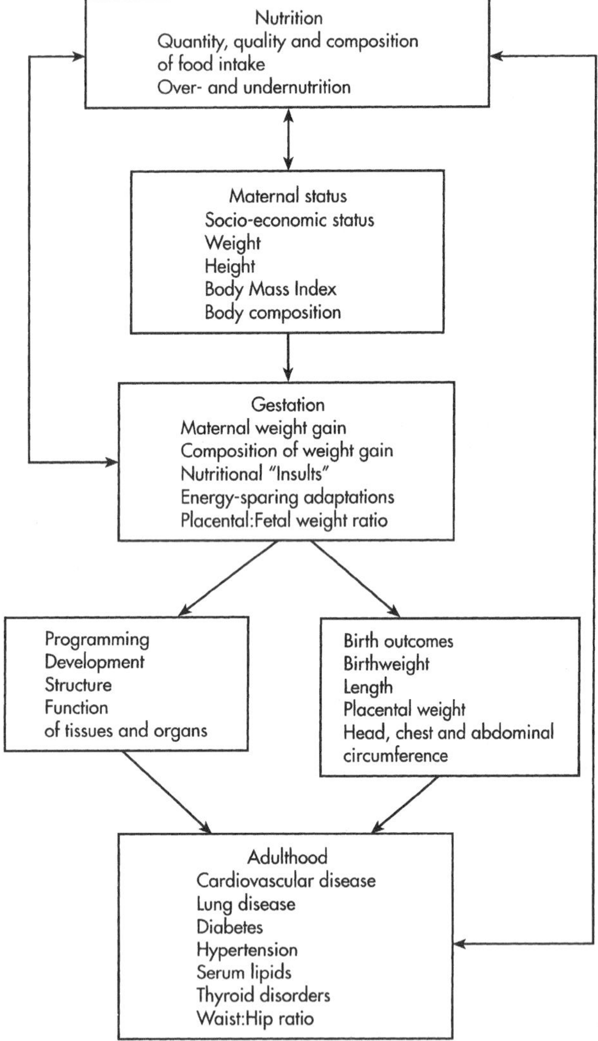

FIG. 2-10. The maternal and *in utero* nutritional influences on the fetus, and the subsequent effects of programming relevant to nutrition. (From Goldberg GR, Prentice AM. Maternal and fetal determinants of adult diseases. Nutr Rev 1994;52: 191–200.)

MATERNAL AND FETAL DETERMINANTS OF ADULT DISEASE

The notion that events occurring during the time of gestation might predispose an individual to chronic diseases later in life has recently been supported by epidemiologic data (71–74). Observations made in the United Kingdom have led to the hypothesis that adverse nutritional experiences *in utero* have a powerful influence on the development of degenerative diseases in adulthood. Poor fetal growth appears to be a strong predictor of hypertension, diabetes, hyperlipidemia, alteration in clotting factors, syndrome X (the combination of noninsulin-dependent diabetes, hypertension, and hyperlipidemia), and mortality from cardiovascular disease and chronic obstructive airway disease. The theory of fetal origins of adult disease proposes that early defects in the development, structure, and function of organs lead to programmed susceptibility, which interacts with later diet and environmental stresses to cause overt disease many decades after the original insult.

Barker and colleagues have proposed that there are five testable hypotheses that deserve attention (71). These are that (a) undernutrition in early life has permanent effects; (b) undernutrition has different effects at different times in early life; (c) rapidly growing fetuses and neonates are more vulnerable to undernutrition than those growing more slowly; (d) undernutrition results from inadequate maternal intake, transport, or transfer of nutrients; and (d) the permanent effects of undernutrition include reduced cell numbers, altered cell structure, and resetting of hormonal axes. Prospective studies in humans and animal models are underway in many laboratories with a view to more clearly define the detailed mechanisms (Fig. 2-10).

SUMMARY

Nutrition is one aspect of pregnancy management over which a woman has considerable control. It is a fact that optimizing nutritional status during this time (and often earlier) will reduce the risk of an adverse reproductive experience. The role of the health care provider is to expose each pregnant or prepregnant client to resources that will aid her in achieving the best possible nutritional status. This includes (as appropriate) individualized nutritional assessment and counseling; referral to available prenatal and/or parenting classes; prescription of specific nutritional supplements; and referral to WIC or other community resources for food assistance. The ideal pregnancy outcome is one in which a healthy term infant is delivered to a mother whose nutritional status is not compromised. The clinician who embraces this goal should take the necessary steps to assist the woman and her family to achieve this end.

APPENDIX: *Overview of initial nutrition assessment*

History, medical record

Sociodemographic

- Age
- Ethnic background
- Living arrangements
- Financial situations
- Support system (spouse or partner, family, friends)

Lifestyle

- Use of cigarettes, alcoholic beverages, illegal drugs
- Use of vitamin/mineral supplements and other over-the-counter medications
- Physical activity

Health history

- Medical, physical, and psychologic conditions that could affect nutrition adversely
- Prescription drug use
- Obstetric history

Dietary

- Usual intake of food and beverages
- Food avoidances
- Dieting and weight history, attitude toward weight gain
- Pica (the ingestion of nonfood substances)

Physical examination

Anthropometric

- Height
- Weight
- Body mass index

Laboratory tests

- Hemoglobin or hematocrit

Clinical

- Physical signs of health; hair, face, eyes, lips, tongue, teeth, gums, neck, skin, nails, musculoskeletal system, etc.

From Suitor CW. Nutritional assessment of the pregnant women. Clin Obstet Gynecol, 1994;37:501–514.

REFERENCES

1. Owen AL, Owen GM. Twenty years of WIC: a review of some effects of the program. J Am Diet Assoc 1997;97:777–782.
2. Brown HL, Watkins K, Hiett AK. The impact of women, infants, and children food supplement program on birth outcome. Am J Obstet Gynecol 1996;174:1279–1283.
3. Disbrow DD. The economic cost of nutrition service for a low income prenatal population. I. Direct costs. J Pediatr Perinat Nutr 1987;1: 35–40.
4. Disbrow DD. The economic costs of nutrition service for a low income prenatal population: indirect and intangible costs. J Pediatr Perinat Nutr 1988;2:17–21.
5. Splett PL, Caldwell HM, Holey ES, Arton IR. Prenatal nutrition services: a cost analysis. J Am Diet Assoc 1987;87:204–208.
6. Mathematics Policy Research Inc. The savings in Medicaid costs for newborn and their mothers from prenatal participation in the WIC Program. Washington, DC: USDA, Food and Nutrition Services, 1990.
7. Buescher PA, Larson LC, Nelson MD Jr, Lenihan AJ. Prenatal WIC participation can reduce low birth weight and newborn medical costs: a cost:benefit analysis of WIC participation in North Carolina. J Am Diet Assoc 1993;93:163–166.
8. Rothman KJ, Moore LL, Singer MR, Nguyen US, Mannino S, Milunsky A. Teratogenicity of high vitamin A intake. N Engl J Med 1995; 333:1369–1373.
9. Fuhrmann K, Reiher H, Semmler K, Fischer F, Fischer M, Glockner E. Prevention of congenital malformations in infants of insulin-dependent diabetic mothers. Diabetes Care 1983;6:219–223.
10. Mills JL, Knopp RH, Simpson JL, et al. Lack of relation of increased malformation rates in infants of diabetic mothers to glycemic control during organogenesis. N Engl J Med 1988;318:671–676.
11. Mills JL, Simpson JL, Driscoll SG. Incidence of spontaneous abortion among normal women and insulin-dependent diabetic women whose pregnancies were identified within 21 days of conception. N Engl J Med 1988;319:1617–1623.
12. Durnin JV. Energy requirements of pregnancy: an integration of the longitudinal data from the five-country study. Lancet 1987;2: 1131–1133.
13. Hytten FF, Chamberlain G. Clinical physiology in obstetrics. Oxford, England: Blackwell Scientific Publications, 1980.
14. Poppitt SD, Prentice AM, Goldberg GR, Whitehead RG. Energy sparing strategies to protect human fetal growth. Am J Obstet Gynecol 1994; 171:118–125.
15. Doyle W, Crawford MA, Wynn AHA, Wynn SW. Maternal nutrient intake and birthweight. J Human Nutr Diet 1989;2:415–422.
16. Salvig JD, Olsen SF, Secher NJ. Effects of fish oil supplementation in late pregnancy on blood pressure: a randomized controlled trial. Br J Obstet Gynaecol 1996;103:529–533.
17. Picciano MF, Green T, O'Connor DL. The folate status of women and health. Nutr Today 1994;29:20–29.
18. Czeizel AE. Folic acid in the prevention of neural tube defects. J Pediatr Gastroent Nutr 1995;10:4–16.
19. MRC Vitamin Study Research Group. Prevention of neural tube defects: results of the Medical Research Council Vitamin Study. Lancet 1991; 338:131–137.
20. Vergel RG, Sanchez LR, Heredero BL, Rodriguez, PL, Martinez AJ. Primary prevention of neural tube defects with folic acid supplementation: Cuban experience. Prenat Diagn 1990;10:149–152.
21. Czeizel AE, Dudas I. Prevention of the first occurrence of neural tube defects in periconceptional vitamin supplementation. N Engl J Med 1992;327:1832–1835.
22. Mills JL, Rhoads GG, Simpson JL, et al. and the NICHD Neural Tube Defects Study Group. The absence of a relation between the periconceptional use of vitamins and neural tube defects. N Engl J Med 1989; 321:430–435.
23. Steegers-Theunissen RP, Boers GH, Blom HJ, et al. Neural tube defects

and elevated homocysteine levels in amniotic fluid. Am J Obstet Gynecol 1995;172:1436–1441.
24. Bunduki V, Dommergues M, Zittoun J, Marguet J, Miller F, Dumez Y. Maternal-fetal folate status and neural tube defects: a case-control study. Biol Neonate 1995;67:154–159.
25. Mills JL, McPartlin JM, Kirke PN, Lee YJ, Conley MR, Weir DG, Scott JM. Homocysteine metabolism in pregnancies complicated by neural tube defects. Lancet 1995;345:149–151.
26. Molloy AM, Daly S, Mills JL, et al. Thermolabile variant of 5,10-methylene tetrahydrofolate reductase associated with low red cell folates: indications for folate intake recommendations. Lancet 1997; 349:1591–1593.
27. Scholl TO, Heidiger ML, Schall JL, Khos CS, Fischer RL. Dietary and serum folate: their influence on the outcome of pregnancy. Am J Clin Nutr 1996;63:520–525.
28. Morbidity and Mortality Weekly Report. Knowledge and use of folic acid by women of childbearing age—United States, 1995. JAMA 1995; 174:1190.
29. Shaw GM, Lammer EJ, Wasserman CR, O'Malley CD, Tolarova MM. Risks of orofacial clefts in children born to women using multivitamins containing folic acid periconceptionally. Lancet 1995;346:393–396.
30. Hayes C, Werler MM, Willett WC, Mitchell AA. Case-control study of periconceptional folic acid supplementation and oral clefts. Am J Epidemiol 1996;143:1229–1234.
31. Li D, Daling JR, Mueller BA, Hickok DE, Fantel AG, Weiss NS. Periconceptional multivitamin use in relation to the risk of congenital urinary tract anomalies. Epidemiology 1995;6:212–218.
32. Czeizel AE. Congenital abnormalities are preventable. Epidemiology 1995;6:205–206.
33. Sahakian V, Rouse D, Sipes S, Rose N. Niebyl J. Vitamin B-6 is effective therapy for nausea and vomiting of pregnancy: a randomized double-blind placebo-controlled study. Obstet Gyneocl 1991;78:33–36.
34. Vutyavanich T, Wongtrangan S, Ruangsri R. Pyridoxine for nausea and vomiting of pregnancy: a randomized, double-blind, placebo-controlled trial. Am J Obstet Gynecol 1995;173:881–884.
35. Suharno D, West CE, Muhilal, Karyadi D, Hautuast JG. Supplementation with vitamin A and iron for nutritional anemia in pregnant women in West Java, Indonesia. Lancet 1993;342:1325–1328.
36. Semba RD, Miotti PG, Chiphangwi JD, et al. Maternal vitamin A deficiency and mother-to-child transmission of HIV-1. Lancet 1994;343: 1593–1597.
37. Hathcock JN, Hattan DG, Jenkins MY, McDonald JT, Sundaresan PR, Wilkening VL. Evaluation of vitamin A toxicity. Am J Clin Nutr 1990;52:183–202.
38. Werler MM, Lammer EJ, Rosenberg L, Mitchell AA. Maternal vitamin A supplementation in relation to selected birth defects. Teratology 1990;42:497–503.
39. Martinez-Frias ML, Salvador J. Epidemiological aspects of prenatal exposure to high doses of vitamin A in Spain. Eur J Epidemiol 1990;6: 118–123.
40. Evans K, Hickey-Kwyer MU. Cleft anterior segment with maternal hypervitaminosis. Br J Ophthalmol 1991;75:691–692.
41. Jick SS, Terris BZ, Jick H. First trimester topical tretinoin and congenital disorders. Lancet 1993;341:1181–1182.
42. Hemminki E, Merileinen J. Longterm follow-up of mothers and their infants in a randomized trial of iron prophylaxis during pregnancy. Am J Obstet Gynecol 1995;173:205–209.
43. Goldenberg RL, Tamura T, DuBard M, Johnston KE, Copper RL, Neggers Y. Plasma ferritin and pregnancy outcome. Am J Obstet Gynecol 1996;175:1356–1359.
44. Tamura T, Goldenberg RL, Johnston KE, Cliver SP, Hickey CA. Serum ferritin: a predictor of early spontaneous preterm delivery. Obstet Gynecol 1996;87:360–365.
45. Yip R. Iron supplementation during pregnancy: is it effective? Am J Clin Nutr 1996;63:853–855.
46. Belizan JM, Villar J, Gonzalez L, Campodonico L, Bergel E. Calcium supplementation to prevent hypertensive disorders of pregnancy. N Engl J Med 1991;325:1399–1405.
47. Carroll G, Duley L, Belizan JM, Villar J. Calcium supplementation during pregnancy: a systematic review of randomized trials. Br J Obstet Gynecol 1994;101:753–758.
48. Bucher HC, Guyatt GH, Cook RJ, Hatala R, Cook DJ, Lang JD, Hunt D. Effect of calcium supplementation on pregnancy-induced hypertension and preeclampsia. A meta-analysis of randomized controlled trials. JAMA 1996;275:1113–1117.
49. DeCherney AH, Koos B. Obstetrics and gynecology. JAMA 1997;277: 1878–1879.
50. Dahle LO, Berg G, Hammer M, Hurtig M, Larsson L. The effect of oral magnesium substitution on pregnancy-induced leg cramps. Am J Obstet Gynecol 1995;173:175–180.
51. Goldenberg RL, Tamura T, Neggers Y, Copper RL, Johnston KE, DuBard MB, Hauth JC. The effect of zinc supplementation on pregnancy outcome. JAMA 1995;274:463–468.
52. Mahomed K, James DK, Golding J, McCabe R. Zinc supplementation during pregnancy: a double-blind randomized controlled trial. Br Med J 1989;299:826–830.
53. National Research Council, Food and Nutrition Board. Recommended dietary allowances. Washington, DC: National Academy Press, 1989.
54. Institute of Medicine. Nutrition during pregnancy: weight gain and nutrient supplements. Washington, DC: National Academy Press, 1990.
55. Schauberger CW, Rooney BL, Brimer LM. Factors that influence weight loss in the puerperium. Obstet Gynecol 1992;9:424–429.
56. Sohlstrom A, Forsum E. Changes in adipose tissue volume and distribution during reproduction in Swedish women as assessed by magnetic resonance imaging. Am J Clin Nutr 1995;61:287–295.
57. Parker JD, Abrams B. Differences in postpatum weight retention between black and white mothers. Obstet Gynecol 1993;81:768–774.
58. Parker JD, Abrams B. Prenatal weight gain advice: an examination of recent weight gain recommendations of the Institute of Medicine. Obstet Gynecol 1992;79:664–669.
59. Siega-Riz AM, Adair LS, Hobel CJ. Institute of Medicine maternal weight gain recommendations and pregnancy outcome in a predominantly Hispanic population. Obstet Gynecol 1994;84:565–573.
60. Smith DE, Lewis CE, Cuveny JL, Perkins LL, Buke GL, Bild DE. Longitudinal changes in adiposity associated with pregnancy. The Cardia Study. JAMA 1994;271:1747–1751.
61. Brown JE, Kaye SA, Folsom AR. Parity-related weight changes in women. Intern J Obes 1992;16:627–631.
62. Horner RD, Lackey CJ, Kolasa K, Warren K. Pica practices of pregnant women. J Am Diebetic Assoc 1991;91:34–38.
63. Russell M, Martier SS, Sokol RJ, Mudor P, Jacobson S, Jacobson J. Detecting risk drinking during pregnancy: a comparison of four screening questionnaires. Am J Public Health 1996;86:1435–1439.
64. Kaufman E. Diagnosis and treatment of drug and alcohol abuse in women. Am J Obstet Gynecol 1996;174:21–27.
65. Hinderliter SA, Zelenak JP. A simple method to identify alcohol and other drug use in pregnant adults in a prenatal care setting. J Perinatol 1993;13:93–102.
66. Bolumar F, Olsen J, Rebagliato M, Bisanti L. Caffeine intake and delayed conception: a European multicenter study on infertility and subfecundity. Am J Epidemiol 1997;145:324–330.
67. Vlajinac HD, Petrovic RR, Marinkovic JM, Sipetic SB, Adanja BJ. Effect of caffeine intake during pregnancy on birthweight. Am J Epidemiol 1997;145:335–338.
68. Nygard O, Refsum H, Ueland PM, et al. Coffee consumption and plasma homocysteine: The Hordaland Homocysteine Study. Am J Clin Nutr 1997;65:136–143.
69. Nehlig J, Debry G. Potential teratogenic and neurodevelopmental consequences of coffee and caffeine exposure: a review of human and animal data. Neurotoxicol Teratol 1994;16:531–543.
70. American Pharmacy. Herbs hazardous to your health. Am Pharm 1984; NS24:20–21.
71. Barker D, Martyn CN, Hales CHD. Growth *in utero* and serum cholesterol concentrations in adult life. Br Med J 1993;307:1524–1527.
72. Bunin GR, Kuijten RR, Buckley JD, Rorke LB, Meadows AT. Relation between maternal diet and subsequent primitive neuroectodermal brain tumors in young children. N Engl J Med 1993;329:536–544.
73. Godfrey KM, Forrester T, Barker DJ, et al. Maternal nutritional status in pregnancy and blood pressure in childhood. Br J Obstet Gynaecol 1994;101:398–403.
74. Goldberg GR, Prentice AM. Maternal and fetal determinants of adult diseases. Nutr Rev 1994;52:191–200.

Cherry and Merkatz's Complications of Pregnancy,
Fifth Edition, edited by W. R. Cohen.
Lippincott Williams & Wilkins, Philadelphia © 2000.

CHAPTER 3

Exercise

Raul Artal

In recent years, the general population has increased its awareness of the importance of maintaining a healthy lifestyle by improving physical fitness and nutrition. The goal of these tasks is to attain metabolic and cardiopulmonary benefits. Physical activity has gained recognition as an important health behavior for maintaining caloric balance and preventing coronary heart disease (1). Pregnancy should not preclude women from maintaining an active lifestyle. It would be expected that pregnant women who maintain a moderate level of physical fitness in pregnancy will derive the same health benefits as those potentially attained by a nonpregnant adult population. Recent epidemiologic studies also suggest that for obese women, exercise may play a role in reducing the risk that they will develop gestational diabetes during pregnancy (2).

Current medical knowledge supports the concept that physically fit women may attain better pregnancy outcomes and that sedentary women may have a higher incidence of complicated pregnancies and deliveries related to, for example, obesity and diabetes. The desirable intensity of physical training varies with different segments of the population. In a technical bulletin published in 1994, The American College of Obstetricians and Gynecologists (ACOG) provided the background and guidelines for exercise in pregnancy (3). Safe exercise guidelines and prescriptions must consider all the potential associated risks and the individual's work capacity to estimate and recommend the training intensity required to induce conditioning. As stated in a position paper by the American College of Sports Medicine, the level of training necessary to induce health benefits does not have to be strenuous; it can be minimal to moderate (4). No matter how beneficial exercise may be, it must be borne in mind that the risks of exercise are amplified in pregnancy by the normal anatomic and physiologic changes that gestation induces.

R. Artal: Department of Obstetrics and Gynecology, St. Louis University School of Medicine, St. Louis, MO 63117.

This chapter reviews the medical aspects of normal maternal and fetal responses to maternal exercise, the potential maternal and fetal risks, principles of exercise prescription in pregnancy, and potential clinical applications for exercise in pregnancy.

MATERNAL PHYSIOLOGICAL RESPONSES TO EXERCISE IN PREGNANCY

Pregnancy is associated with progressive anatomic changes; the most significant change that can impact the ability to exercise is the progressive shift in the body's center of gravity, which shifts anteriorly and cephalad. These changes result in compensatory lordosis, which frequently contributes to acute or chronic low back pain. This anatomic adaptation also causes the pelvic bones to rotate progressively on the femur to prevent falling forward. There is consequently increased strain on the sacroiliac and hip joints, which in turn causes additional strain on the back and creates balance problems, increasing the risk of falls and injury. Certain types of exercises could help to prevent or ameliorate the lordosis or kyphosis associated with pregnancy by strengthening both the abdominal and back muscles (3).

Pregnancy is associated with a progressive increase in progesterone and elastin synthesis that affects the biomechanical properties of connective tissue, resulting in various degrees of laxity of joints and ligaments (5,6), a potential risk for soft-tissue injuries. In addition to these factors, the progressive increase in weight and the accumulation of interstitial fluid play important roles in the various anatomic and biomechanical adaptations to pregnancy and contribute to complications such as peripheral nerve compressions and, more rarely, pathologic separation of the symphysis pubis.

All the aforementioned changes place pregnant women, particularly those who are less fit, at increased risk for musculoskeletal injuries. Exercise guidelines and prescription in pregnancy should be considered against this background and should exclude routines that involve sudden shifts in direction or ballistic movements. Physiologic cardiovascular adaptations to pregnancy can affect exercise significantly. Some of these adaptations could lead to orthostatic hypotension, particularly after prolonged standing or after positioning or exercising in the supine position. Positioning pregnant women in the supine position frequently results in the aortocaval syndrome as a result of mechanical compression of the aorta and vena cava by the pregnant uterus. This compression results in diminished blood return to the heart, potential hypotension, and reduced blood perfusion of visceral organs. These hemodynamic changes could be magnified during exercise by the preferential diversion of blood to the exerting muscles and away from the visceral organs, including the uterus. Symptomatic reduction in cardiac output affects about 5% or more of pregnant women in the supine position (7); asymptomatic women still may have a relative decrease in uterine blood flow.

Cardiac output increases significantly in pregnancy by at least 40% and resting heart rate by approximately 16 beats per minute (8,9). The cardiac output exceeds the peripheral venous capacity. Both cardiac output and heart rate responses are dependent on venous return, which is in turn modulated by catecholamines, the peripheral muscles, thermogenesis, body position, or blood vessel patency. The lower hematocrit level during pregnancy also contributes markedly to the reduction of the cardiorespiratory reserve during increased physical activity.

The relative increase in cardiac output in response to mild and moderate exercise is similar in pregnant and nonpregnant subjects regardless of the type of exercise for either weight-bearing or non-weight-bearing activities (10–13). Using the CO_2 rebreathing technique, it was determined that cardiac output during cycle ergometry exercise in pregnancy has different kinetic adjustments that are, in part, related to the progressive increase in maternal weight (12). At lower exercise intensities, the increase in cardiac output is made possible through a combination of higher heart rates and stroke volumes, whereas during high-intensity exercise the hemodynamics involve predominantly higher stroke volumes. These responses reflect limited functional capacity and a decrease in cardiovascular reserve available for exercise. The main concern related to maternal exercise is that cardiac output distribution to different organs is altered to favor the exercising muscles (14), thus limiting blood flow to the visceral organs including the uterus and possibly affecting transplacental transport of oxygen.

Human and animal research (15–18) data are available to demonstrate that indeed there is a significant impact on uterine blood flow during exercise in pregnancy. Uterine blood flow in the human reaches at least 500 to 600 mL/min, of which 90% perfuses the placenta and the remaining 10% perfuses the myometrium. Such abundant blood flow may be more than sufficient to supply the physiologic needs of the fetus during mild to moderate exercise. Studies conducted in pregnant ewes suggest an approximately 25% reduction in blood flow during light exercise (16). A further progressive reduction occurs as the intensity of exercise increases. These hemodynamic changes can find confirmation in studies conducted in the nonpregnant adult human (14). It has nevertheless been demonstrated (18) that uterine blood flow in the laboratory animal depends on the intensity and duration of the exercise and inversely correlates with the heart rate. Uterine blood flow decreases by 13% during a 10-minute exercise period at 70% $V0_2$ maximum, by 17% during a 10-minute period at 100% $V0_2$ maximum, and by 24% near the end of a 40-minute period at 70% VO_2 maximum.

Studies conducted in pregnant laboratory animals should be interpreted cautiously when applied to humans, especially because most animals are customarily restrained and catheterized during the experiments and, consequently, significantly stressed. Responses to the additional stress of exercise may be limited or inconsequential.

Pulmonary adaptations in pregnancy undergo significant changes that result in the expansion of the chest circumference. These adaptations lead to an increase in inspiratory capacity of 300 mL (inspiratory volume + tidal volume) and a reduction in functional residual capacity. The resting oxygen consumption increases in pregnancy by 10% to 20%. The physiologic purpose of this state of hyperventilation in pregnancy is to reduce arterial pCO_2 while the arterial pH is maintained at 7.44. This mild maternal alkalosis facilitates placental gas exchange. The combined alterations could be reduced or compromised, primarily during strenuous exercise, and result in a lower oxygen reserve.

During exercise, pregnant or nonpregnant subjects experience an increase in respiratory frequency, minute ventilation, and tidal volume. During light to moderate exertion, no significant differences in oxygen uptake are seen between pregnant and nonpregnant subjects.

The single most essential laboratory paramenter used in evaluating the physiological response to exercise is the test of maximal aerobic capacity or the $V0_2$ max test. $V0_2$ max is the maximal rate at which oxygen can be used by the body. It relates to the capacity of the heart, lungs, and blood vessels to provide oxygen to the working muscles and to the ability of the peripheral muscles to extract and use the oxygen provided. Several reports are available in the literature on $V0_2$ max measurements during pregnancy (Table 3-1). These indicate that during $V0_2$ maximum testing, or strenuous exercise, the $V0_2$ is significantly decreased in pregnant subjects compared with nonpregnant subjects when indexed for weight (Fig. 3-1).

TABLE 3-1. *Measurement of maximal oxygen consumption during pregnancy*

Modality (direct measure)	Gestation (wk)	VO_2max	Reference
Bicycle; treadmill	16, 25, 35	2.20; 2.19 L/min	Lotgering et al. (91)
Bicycle	26	1.89 L/min 27 ml/kg/min	Sady et al. (92)
Bicycle ergometer	25	1.97 L/min 30.1 mL/kg/min	Sady et al. (13)
Bicycle ergometer	26	1.91 L/min	Sady et al. (13)
Bicycle	33	1.39; 1.21 L/min 19.2; 16.8 mL/kg/min	Artal et al. (75)
Bicycle	29	1.930 L/min	Khodiguian et al. (93)
Bicycle/swim	25,35	1.94 L/min	McMurray et al. (94)
Bicycle ergometer	29	37.9 mL/kg/min	Artal et al. (unpublished)

It has been demonstrated that there is a tendency for higher respiratory exchange ratios (*R*) during exercise in pregnancy, which suggests a preferential utilization of carbohydrates (19). *R* is a respiratory variable that reflects the ratio between carbon dioxide output (CO_2) and oxygen uptake (VO_2). *R* provides information about the proportion of substrate derived from various foodstuffs. For carbohydrates to be completely oxidized to $C0_2$ and H_20, one volume of $C0_2$ is produced for each volume of 0_2 consumed. An *R* value of 1.0 would indicate that only carbohydrates are being used. Comparative measurements by indirect calorimetry indicate preferential use of carbohydrates in pregnancy during exercise (Fig. 3-2) (20). Assessing fuel use during exercise in pregnancy is essential because of the possible effects of exercise-induced maternal hypoglycemia. Normoglycemia is a guarded function during light and moderate exercise in pregnancy, whereas during prolonged or stren-

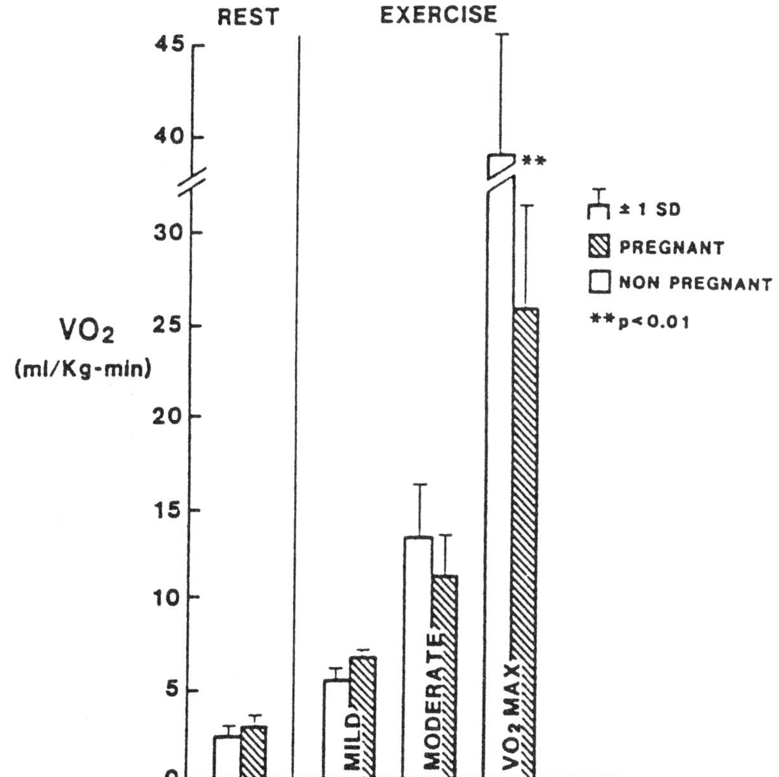

FIG. 3-1. Oxygen consumption (VO_2) determined at rest and at the peak of mild, moderate, and maximal oxygen consumption exercise.

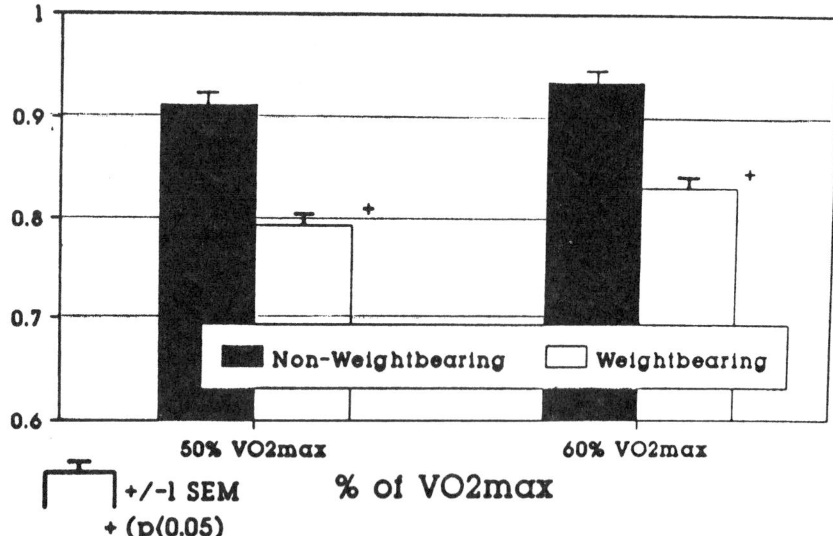

FIG. 3-2. Respiratory exchange ratio during non-weight-bearing (bicycle ergometry) and weight-bearing (treadmill) exercise at incremental workloads.

uous exercise, plasma glucose concentrations may decline significantly (Fig. 3-3) (21).

The energy cost of pregnancy is estimated at about 80,000 kcal, or 300 kcal per day; women exercising need proportionately more calories. Activity of the sympathoadrenal system is important in governing energy metabolism. The heavier the workload, the more sustained the sympathoadrenal activity. Catecholamines promote both glycogenolysis and lipolysis. Epinephrine modulates the release of glucagon and free fatty acids (FFA). The increments of epinephrine during exercise in pregnancy appear to be smaller than in nonpregnant controls, whereas the norepinephrine responses appear to be more pronounced in pregnancy. The increases in norepinephrine blood concentrations have clinical relevance in that norepinephrine has restrictive effects on visceral, renal, and uterine blood flow and can precipitate uterine activity (22).

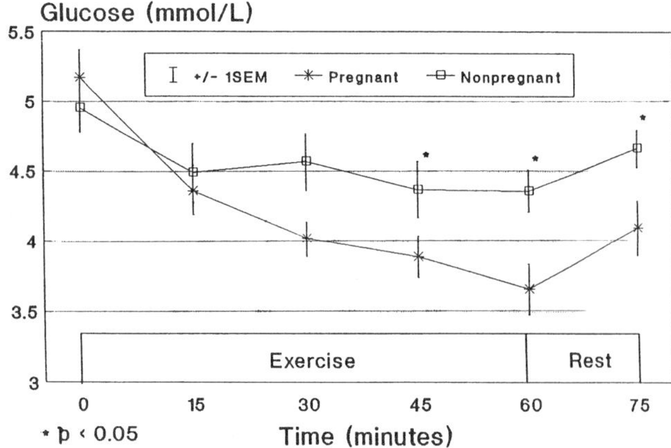

FIG. 3-3. Blood glucose concentrations during prolonged exercise in pregnant and nonpregnant women.

FETAL RESPONSES TO MATERNAL EXERCISE

In the past, the main concerns related to exercise in pregnancy focused on the fetus and any potential maternal benefits that might be offset by fetal injuries. In the uncomplicated pregnancy, such events are highly unlikely. Most potential risks are hypothetical; however, health care providers that prescribe exercise should be cognizant of all the potential complications.

The principal physiologic question that remains to be answered is, to what extent does the selective redistribution of blood flow during exercise in pregnancy reduce the transplacental transport of oxygen, $C0_2$, and nutrients, and what are the lasting effects, if any? The indirect evidence is that there are no lasting effects.

It is recognized that during certain obstetric events transient hypoxia can result initially in fetal tachycardia and an increase in fetal blood pressure. These fetal responses are protective mechanisms for the fetus to facilitate transfer of oxygen and carbon dioxide across the placenta. Acute alterations in fetal oxygenation can result in fetal heart rate (FHR) changes, whereas chronic effects may result in intrauterine growth restriction. Though fetal demise may be associated with either of the above events, there is no report in the literature to link fetal death or growth restriction definitively with maternal exercise. Nevertheless, given this theoretical concern, water exercise during pregnancy has been advocated by some as the preferred form of exercise because, during immersion, a centripetal shift in blood volume occurs.

The FHR responses to exercise have been the focus of numerous studies (23–41). Most studies demonstrate a minimum or moderate increase in FHR by 10 to 30 beats per minute over baseline during or following maternal exercise. FHR decelerations and bradycardia have been reported to occur with a frequency of 8.9% (23). The mechanism leading to fetal bradycardia during maternal exercise is not understood; most likely, a vagal reflex, cord compression, or fetal head malposition is the provocation. It is not known whether these transient events have any lasting effects on the fetus, because no long-term studies have been conducted to address this specific question.

Several studies (42–44) have attempted to assess umbilical blood flow during maternal exercise with Doppler velocimetry; they demonstrated inconsistent or no changes. Doppler velocimetry studies are technically difficult to conduct during exercise; so most measurements are taken before and after exercise, by which time any changes could have returned to normal.

The presence of fetal activity often has been interpreted as a reflection of well-being. The same is true for fetal breathing, which is related to the stage of gestation, diurnal variations, maternal plasma glucose, and plasma catecholamine concentrations. A direct relationship has been demonstrated between the sympathetic activity of the mother and the frequency of occurrence of both fetal breathing movements and fetal body movements (Fig. 3-4) (22).

Many epidemiologic studies have suggested that a link exists between strenuous physical activities, deficient diets, and the development of intrauterine growth restriction (45–47). This association appears to be particularly true for mothers engaged in physical work. Working mothers have a tendency to deliver earlier and have smaller-for-gestational-age infants (47). Corroborating data have been obtained in laboratory animals that engaged in strenuous physical activities throughout gestation and who then delivered smaller offspring (48,49). At least one study conducted in pregnant women arrived at similar conclusions (50). Uncontrolled studies done in elite athletes indicate conflicting evidence (51,52). Prolonged exercise in pregnancy has been demonstrated to result in significant hormonal changes and alterations in available circulating substrates (53). One hour of prolonged exercise has resulted in blood glucose levels of 3.66 mmol/L. Most investigations conducted in pregnant athletes report a low incidence of complications, but one study (52) found that Olympic athletes had a greater number of newborn infants weighing 2,600 to 3,000 g (potentially growth restricted or born prematurely) than newborn infants weighing in excess of 3,500 g. The information available in the literature is too limited to allow quantitative risk assignment for either premature labor or fetal growth restriction for exercising mothers, and the link to deficient diets has not been sufficiently addressed. Clinical observations indicate that patients at risk for premature labor may have labor triggered by exercise. Women who are diet conscious often do not receive the minimum required nutrients. The combined energy requirements of pregnancy and exercise coupled with poor weight gain may lead to fetal growth restriction.

One theoretical fetal risk that has received considerable attention is the possible teratogenic effect of heat

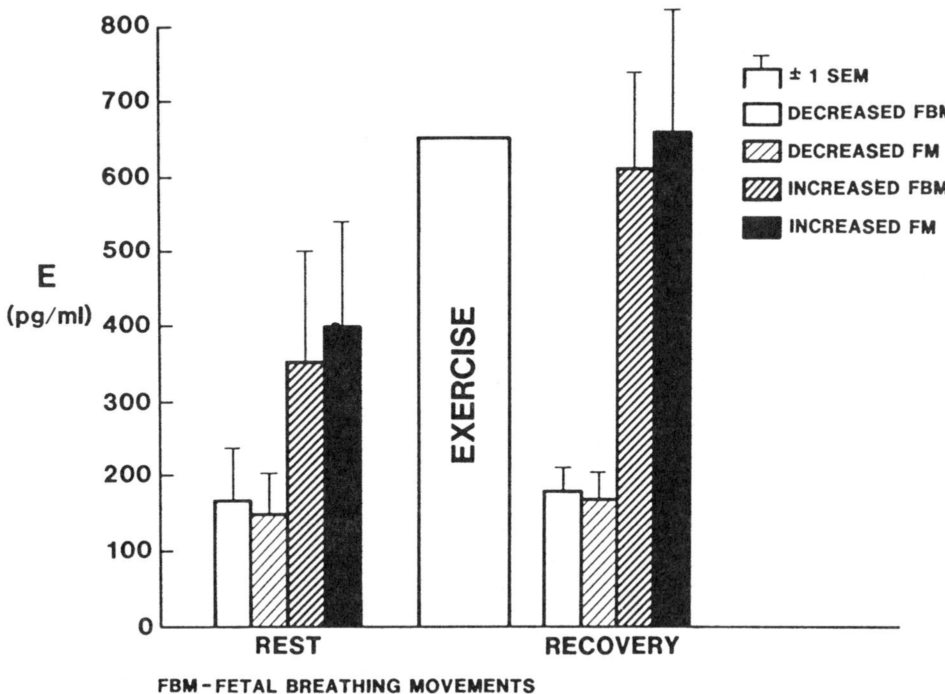

FIG. 3-4. Fetal breathing movements and fetal body movements in relation to maternal plasma epinephrine (*E*) levels before and after exercise.

stress generated by exercise. Data obtained in laboratory animals demonstrate that hyperthermia is teratogenic and can result in neural tube defects (54–56). A few case reports have suggested that this adverse effect is likely to occur in the human as well (57–61); however, the only prospective study examining women exposed to hyperthermia in their first trimester failed to confirm this association (62). The teratogenic threshold in the human is believed to be 39° C during the first 45 to 60 days gestation. Core temperatures for recreational runners have been shown to exceed 39° C at high training intensities, indicating a potential for human teratogenesis (63).

EXERCISE PRESCRIPTION IN PREGNANCY

Safety considerations always should be a primary concern when prescribing exercise, particularly during pregnancy. The potential maternal and fetal risks have been described and are summarized in Table 3-2. Based on these theoretical risks, the goal of exercise during pregnancy is to maintain the highest level of fitness consistent with maximum safety. The quantity and quality of exercise necessary to derive general health benefits is not different in pregnancy compared with the nonpregnant state.

The ideal exercise program should offer a variety of options: walking, swimming, stationary cycling, modified forms of dancing, or calisthenics. No single exercise or exercise program will be able to meet the needs of all women. It is thus incumbent on the physician to assess each woman's ability to engage in physical activities and then to advise on a program that maintains the highest level of fitness consistent with maximum safety.

The essentials of exercise prescription in pregnancy promulated by the American College of Obstetricians and Gynecologists (3) are summarized as follows:

1. Any exercise program offered to pregnant women must be safe and fun to do. In the absence of clear benefits for the mother or pregnancy outcome, safety is a main concern. It certainly can be assumed that the same exercise-related health benefits derived by nonpregnant women could be derived by pregnant women as well.

2. Before prescribing exercise, patients should be screened for any concurrent obstetric or medical complications. The contraindications to exercise in pregnancy are listed in Table 3-3. Health care providers should be especially concerned about women whose oxygen-carrying capacity is compromised by anemia and women who are morbidly obese. It is important to recognize that because of individual physiologic adaptations to pregnancy, some patients may not be able to continue to train for part or all of the components of fitness (i.e., cardiovascular endurance, flexibility, and ideal body composition.) The potential long-term impact of any detraining period in pregnancy is unknown. Guidelines available from the ACOG and the American College of Sports Medicine help to distinguish between the active pregnant woman interested in maintaining a *healthy lifestyle* and the very active pregnant athlete interested in *performance*. The guidelines are based on a physiologic rationale intended to minimize both maternal and fetal injury.

3. Exercise programs for pregnant women can effect benefits of promoting strength and coordination, both of which decrease in pregnancy. By strengthening the abdominal and back muscles, women can prevent the low back pain that is common in pregnancy.

4. Regular exercise at least three times weekly is preferable to intermittent activity. Nevertheless, sedentary women are not discouraged from engaging in physical activities, although moderation is advised. Pregnancy is a particularly suitable time to introduce behavior modification.

5. Women should avoid exercise in the supine position after the first trimester. Throughout pregnancy, 5% or more of all pregnant women may experience symptomatic supine hypotension. The supine position after midpregnancy is associated with decreased cardiac output in pregnant women. Because the remaining cardiac output will be preferentially distributed away from splanchnic beds (including the uterus) during vigorous exercise, such regimens are best avoided during pregnancy. Prolonged periods of motionless activity also are associated with a significantly decreased cardiac output and hypotension and thus should be avoided.

6. Women should be aware of the relatively decreased oxygen availability for aerobic exercise during pregnancy. Thus, pregnant women should be encouraged to modify the intensity of their exercise according to symptoms. Pregnant women should stop exercising when fatigued and should not exercise to exhaustion. The effects of strenuous and prolonged exercise on the fetus have not been sufficiently studied. Weight-bearing or non-weight-bearing exercise routines should be individualized and adjusted to the patient's work capacity and abilities. Non-weight-bearing exercises such as cycling or swimming will minimize the risk of injury and facilitate the continuation of exercise during the entire pregnancy. Currently, there is no physiologic or health-related rationale for strenuous activities; however, if pregnant women engage in such activities, additional medical supervision would be indicated.

TABLE 3-2. *Theoretical maternal and fetal risk of exercise in pregnancy*

Maternal	Fetal
Premature labor	Prematurity
Musculoskeletal injuries	Fetal distress
Heat stress	Congenital malformations
Cardiovascular complications	Fetal injury
Hypoglycemia	Intrauterine growth restriction

TABLE 3-3. *Contraindications to exercise in pregnancy*

Relative contraindications	Absolute contraindications
Anemia or other blood disorders	Cardiac disease
Breech presentation in last trimester	Restrictive lung disease
Cardiac arrhythmia or palpitations	History of three or more spontaneous abortions
Chronic bronchitis	Incompetent cervix/cerclage
Diabetes	Multiple gestation
Excessive obesity	Persistent second- or third-trimester bleeding
Extreme underweight	Placenta previa
History of bleeding during present pregnancy	Premature labor during a prior or current pregnancy
History of extremely sedentary lifestyle	Ruptured membranes
History of intrauterine growth restriction	Additional contraindications should be left for the physician to determine on individual basis.
History of precipitate labor	
Hypertension	
Orthopedic limitations	
Seizure disorder	
Thyroid disease	

7. Morphologic changes in pregnancy should serve as a relative contraindication to types of exercise in which loss of balance could be detrimental to maternal or fetal well-being, especially in the third trimester. Furthermore, any type of exercise involving the potential for even mild abdominal trauma should be avoided.

8. Pregnancy requires an additional 300 kcal daily to maintain metabolic homeostasis. Thus, women who exercise during pregnancy should be particularly careful to ensure an adequate diet. Breastfeeding adds an additional 300 kcal per day or more. Published studies indicate that after strenuous exercise there is a twofold to fourfold increase in breast milk lactic acid and a decrease in the nutritional quality; however, moderate exercise does not affect the quality of milk (64–66).

9. Pregnant women who exercise should augment heat dissipation by ensuring adequate hydration, appropriate clothing, and optimal environmental surroundings during exercise. Such precautions are particularly important during the first trimester.

10. Many of the physiologic and morphologic changes of pregnancy persist for 4 to 6 weeks postpartum.

11. Because monitoring maternal heart rates is impractical, it has been suggested that exercise be guided by rates of perceived exertion. The need for intensive and strenuous training is limited to only a few women, and for them recommendations should be individualized.

12. To prevent musculoskeletal injuries, warm-ups and cool-downs are recommended. The progressive laxity of joints and ligaments predisposes pregnant women to injuries.

RECREATIONAL AND SPORTS ACTIVITIES

Consistency is the most important part of any exercise program; if the woman is not willing to exercise regularly, it probably would be better to reduce markedly the intensity of the exercise routine. By doing so, she can prevent injuries associated with sporadic exertion. Pregnancy is an ideal time for behavior modification, and the introduction of sedentary women to principles of an active lifestyle is warranted for its long-term benefits.

Activities such as softball, volleyball, and racquet sports can be performed by pregnant women who want to remain active throughout pregnancy. Such activities have an unknown incidence of injuries. The number of potentially untreated, or self-treatable, injuries is most likely considerably greater than the treated injuries. Whether the risk of strains and sprains in pregnant women is appreciably greater than in the general population is not known. Nevertheless, it should be obvious that where there is an orthopedic risk associated with some of these activities, continuous activity may increase that risk. Exercise programs should be modified during the pregnancy to allow for the physical and mental changes taking place and then resumed after delivery to facilitate recovery to prepregnancy conditions. I recommend that pregnant women engaged in fitness programs be examined periodically to assess the effect of their exercise program on the developing fetus and have their programs readjusted to their level of tolerance or discontinued if necessary.

Jogging

Many women find jogging an excellent form of exercise and want to continue jogging as long as possible into pregnancy. This activity is not one that should be initiated after the pregnancy has begun. For those who continue their jogging programs, special precautions should be taken during the first trimester if certain common complications occur, for example, nausea, vomiting, or poor weight gain.

Ketosis and hypoglycemia are more likely to occur during prolonged strenuous exercise in pregnancy. Because of nausea, vomiting, or the feeling of fatigue that is prevalent in pregnancy, women may be unable to run long distances. In pregnancy, we advise the recreational athlete to reduce mileage to no more than 2 miles per day. This is a precautionary step intended to prevent complications such as hyperthermia or dehydration. Studies of women who averaged between 1.5 and 2.5 miles per day throughout pregnancy have shown no deleterious effects (67).

Because pregnant women are running to maintain fitness rather than training for competition, shorter distances should suffice. During the first trimester, if patients would like to exceed 2 miles per day, such activity should be coordinated with physician supervision.

If pregnant women are unable to jog, they can engage in a brisk walking program. Such a program could include a 4- to 6- mile walk, depending on terrain and climatic conditions. This could be a reasonable alternative to a jogging program; the same precautions should be taken to avoid hyperthermia and dehydration. A summary of recommendations for the patients include the following admonitions:

- Do not begin a jogging program while pregnant; the risk for musculoskeletal injuries is increased.
- Reduce jogging mileage to less than 2 miles per day.
- If temperature or humidity is high, do not exercise. Adverse conditions may cause fetal loss.
- Give special attention to terrain and running surface because of connective tissue changes associated with pregnancy.
- Wear running shoes that have proper support.

Aerobics Programs

In the past 5 to 10 years, women who have wanted to derive the benefit of the aerobic workout associated with jogging but who did not like running alone searched for another way to exercise. This spawned, in part, the "aerobics" enthusiasm, which combined dance with an aerobic workout. Women could work out in groups using a form of exercise they enjoyed, thus keeping them exercising long enough to improve their aerobic capacity. The number of women who wanted to continue an aerobic activity during their pregnancy has led to a proliferation of aerobics classes specifically for pregnant women. Unfortunately, many of these programs are conducted by unqualified exercise leaders who are unaware of the basic physiology of pregnancy and have no formal training in physical education.

Because aerobics is a weight-bearing exercise, the same concerns associated with jogging should be considered by the pregnant mother (i.e., heat stress, potential joint and ligament injuries, and unrecognized fetal distress). If necessary, these programs should be modified. I recommend close obstetric follow-up for these women to determine how they and their fetuses are responding to the program. Such programs should be supervised by a certified exercise leader who is qualified to conduct programs for pregnant women. Exercise leaders should be required to maintain a record of injuries and to modify programs to lower the incidence of injuries. There are four additional considerations:

- Programs should have a scientific basis.
- Specific exercises that should be avoided include overextension and exercises performed in the supine position.
- Women should avoid hard surfaces during exercise and limit repetitious movements to 10.
- Warm-up and cool-down should be done gradually.

Bicycling

Several aerobic exercises do not involve weight-bearing, of which bicycling is one; but bicycling is not without risk. With a stationary bicycle, heat dissipation may become a problem, and exercising outdoors in traffic and smog might have negative effects on both mother and fetus. Bicycling may strain the lower back if the rider is in the aerodynamic position while using a multispeed unit, because the weight of the abdomen accentuates the lordosis. This problem can be reduced by using a more upright position and exercising to strengthen the abdominal wall. Also, the extra weight of pregnancy, especially its altered distribution, could make the woman less stable and more susceptible to falls.

Cycling on a stationary bicycle (with a fan) could provide a reasonable alternative to all those who wish to continue this type of exercise. This exercise has several advantages:

- The program can be started during pregnancy.
- A stationary cycle is preferable to standard bicycling because of weight and balance changes during pregnancy.
- Bicycling should be avoided outdoors during high temperatures and high pollution levels.

Swimming

Swimming, another non-weight-bearing aerobic exercise, may be the most adequate and reasonable aerobic exercise for pregnant women (68). The changing body composition makes the mother more buoyant and swimming easier; however, with a change in weight distribution during the second and third trimesters, breathing may be more difficult. Lap swimming is one means of maintaining aerobic capacity. Also, as long as the temperature of the water is not too high (above 85°F to 90°F), thermoregulation is not a problem in a swimming pool (69). Water calisthenics and wading-in-water programs can augment swimming as an aquatic activity.

Throughout the pregnancy, the mother may be able to maintain a given distance but take longer to complete it. General guidelines for swimmers are as follows:

- Respiratory changes may make swimming difficult in late pregnancy.
- Calisthenic exercise in water is encouraged for maintenance of strength and flexibility.
- Swimming in water that is too cold or too hot should be avoided.
- Jacuzzi temperatures above 38.5°C should be avoided.

Scuba Diving

Based on available information, it is recommended that women who are or may become pregnant not dive (70,71). The risks of diving during pregnancy are not justified. Both experimental and case reports indicate that the fetus may be at greater risk than the diving mother. The potential effects include decompression sickness, hyperoxia, hypoxia, hypercapnia, and asphyxia. There are insufficient data to establish safe diving tables for the pregnant woman and her fetus. The Undersea Medical Society recommends that pregnant women who, against medical advice, choose to dive should be informed that the potential risk to the fetus apparently increases as the no-decompression limits are approached, as the oxygen tension of the inspired gas increases, and perhaps also as a function of other factors that remain to be identified (70).

Muscular Strength and Endurance Activities

For many years, weight lifting was not recommended for women in general; for pregnant women, it was an unheard-of activity. As more and more health clubs opened, weight lifting became a complementary exercise for whatever form of aerobic activity was being undertaken. Because women who become pregnant may not want to give up any part of their usual fitness routine, they need to know how to lift weights safely.

Weight machines are used more frequently than free weights; therefore, the fear of damage to the fetus by dropping a weight is alleviated. This is not to say that free weights cannot be used, but rather that "spotting" is even more necessary to avoid injury at this time. The fetus is well protected by the maternal anatomic structures, but there is evidence that blunt trauma to the abdomen could damage the uterus or cause placental abruption. Weight-lifting programs may place pregnant women at high risk for spinal and disc injuries facilitated by the relaxation of ligaments and joints in pregnancy. Any program that works the entire body, promoting toning and flexibility, can be recommended but only within certain limits.

One possible problem that could arise for the inexperienced weight lifter is transient hypertension caused by the Valsalva maneuver, which causes a marked decrease in venous return to the heart, an increase in arterial pressure, and increased work for the heart. The decreased cardiac output and blood flow to the brain may cause orthostatic hypotension. It also may cause decreased perfusion of the uterus. Breathing properly (that is, exhaling during a lift) will keep this from happening.

Low weights and moderate repetitions should constitute the program to maintain flexibility while toning the muscles. Using light weights (2–5 kg) as the pregnancy progresses is recommended to prevent injuries to ligaments and joints. Exercise should not be performed in the supine position. Heavy weight lifting or high-resistance activities should be limited or avoided in pregnancy and done only under strict prescription and supervision. The following is a summary of the recommendations pertaining to weight lifting:

- Training with light weights can be cautiously continued throughout pregnancy.
- Heavy resistance on weight machines should be avoided.
- The use of heavy free weights should be avoided.
- Proper breathing is necessary to avoid the Valsalva maneuver, that is, exhaling while lifting and inhaling when returning the weight load to its original position.
- All sporting events include some inherent danger to participants. When a pregnant woman desires to engage in such activities, she must be advised, consider the dangers, and decide whether she can modify her activities accordingly or elect to avoid the activity altogether. Contact sports such as basketball are better avoided not just for fear of potential trauma to the abdomen from falling but also because of the unpredictability of the opponent's movements. Volleyball, gymnastics, and horseback riding follow closely on the list of potentially dangerous sports for gravid women.
- Sports such as tennis, racquetball, and squash are considered fairly safe sports, within limits. The intensity should be reduced as the pregnancy progresses to prevent injuries resulting from impaired coordination secondary to the new weight distribution and change in center of gravity. Especially in racquetball and squash, heat stress should be considered because these activities are played in a confined area with little air circulation.
- Certain winter sport activities also can be enjoyed by the pregnant woman, provided appropriate clothing is worn to protect against cold exposure. Cross-country skiing at a moderate pace will promote a high fitness level. Downhill skiing or ice skating are two particular winter activities that should be discouraged during pregnancy, particularly for unskilled women. The muscle and joint injuries associated with sports activities are less likely if a woman is skilled and in good physical condition.

Physical Activity at Altitude in Pregnancy

Pregnant women frequently engage in physical activity at high altitudes. The following are the most commonly encountered activities by pregnant women at high altitude (72).

- Recreational: Hiking and skiing at standard resort altitudes or, more rarely, high-altitude trekking in early pregnancy at more than 4,000 m (13,000 ft), both largely involving acute exposure
- Occupational: Flight attendants in pressurized cabins at a maximum of about 2,500 m (8,250 ft) (73,74) involving semiacute exposure
- Residential: Dwellers at high altitude, conventionally defined as higher than 3,000 m (9,750 ft), combining long-term exposure with occupational and generally life-sustaining activity

The response to exercise during short exposure to altitude was studied by several investigators as summarized in Table 3-4.

To simulate exposure to brief exercise at altitude and exposure to commercial flights, we compared the maternal and fetal responses to exercise at sea level [50 m (180 ft)] and at 1,800 m (6,000 ft) without prior acclimatization. Seven sedentary pregnant women, mean gestational age 34 weeks, performed a symptom-limited maximal exercise test and a submaximal cardiac output exercise test at sea level and altitude at intervals of 2 to 4 days (75). After a 30-minute acclimatization, exercise was performed on a bicycle ergometer in 5-minute periods at 25, 50, and 75 W followed by 2-minute periods at workloads increasing by 25-W increments until volitional fatigue was reached. Measures comprised maternal and fetal heart rates, oxygen consumption, ventilation (tidal volume and respiratory rate) and cardiac output, together with blood sampling before and after each exercise level for determination of glucose, lactate and catecholamines, and monitoring of uterine contractions.

The results (Table 3-5) showed a higher capacity to perform work at sea level. Aerobic capacity at altitude, as shown by the significantly lower work at peak VO_2, was 13% lower than at sea level, which exceeds the difference seen in nonpregnant women similarly exposed to altitude. In submaximal exercise, no alternations in exercise efficiency or response were seen in most of the variables when altitude and sea level were compared. Both cardiac output and stroke volume were elevated at altitude at rest but not during exercise, suggesting a lower reserve for both variables at altitude. Plasma glucose, lactate, and catecholamine concentrations did not differ significantly at sea level and altitude. With the exception of one episode of a 2-minute bradycardia after exercise at altitude, all FHR patterns were reactive. We concluded that mothers and fetuses were not adversely affected by this level of moderate altitude stress combined with relatively intensive exercise but, given the decrease observed in peak aerobic capacity at altitude, using sea level maximal exercise testing results to advise on exercise at altitude may not accurately reflect an individual's exercise potential.

Based on the published literature on exertion at altitude, the following could be used as guidelines for short-term altitude exposure and exercise at altitude during pregnancy:

- In the first 4 to 5 days limit exposure to altitudes of less than 2,500 m (8,250 ft).
- The higher the altitude, the briefer the exercise bouts should be.
- In the presence of obstetric or medical complications of pregnancy, exercise should be limited or avoided.

TABLE 3-4. *Studies of short-term altitude exposure with or without exercise in human pregnancy*

Study no.	Author/year (no.)	Altitude: Feet	Altitude: Meters	Mode of altitude exposure	Variables: Maternal	Variables: Fetal	Exercise
1	Baumann et al., 1985 (74)	3,500/7,300	1,080/2,228	Cable car	Yes	Yes	25 W bicycle ergometer
2	Baumann and Huch, 1986 (86) Bung et al., 1987 (87)	3,600/7,200	1,100/2,200	Low-pressure chamber	Yes	Yes	50 W bicycle ergometer
3	Huch et al., 1986 (73)	7,850	2,400	Aircraft	Yes	Yes	None
4	Bung, 1992 (88)	11,500	3,500	Low-pressure chamber	No	Yes	None
5	Elliott and Trujillo, 1992 (89)	1,100–7,000	335 to 2,150	Aircraft	No	Yes	None
6	Artal et al., 1996 (75)	6,000	1,800	Car	Yes	Yes	Symptom-limited max exercise (82 ± 10.5 W) bicycle ergometer

TABLE 3–5. *Cardiopulmonary parameters of symptom-limited maximal exercise in seven pregnant women at sea level versus 6,000 feet*

Variable	No	Sea level	Altitude	Significance (p value)
Maximal work (W)	7	98.86 ± 5.57	82.14 ± 10.51[a]	0.03
Peak VO_2				
L/min	7	1.39 ± 0.07	1.21 ± 0.12[b]	0.03
mL/kg/min	7	19.21 ± 1.46	16.82 ± 2.05[b]	0.04
Maximal heart rate (beats/min)	7	167.86 ± 5.89	161.64 ± 7.03	NS
Ve_{max} (L/min)	7	52.84 ± 1.66	47.36 ± 5.05	NS
Tidal volume (L)	7	1.30 ± 0.07	1.23 ± 0.12	NS
Ventilatory frequency (breaths/min)	7	41.14 ± 2.20	38.50 ± 1.98	NS
Vco_2max (L/min)	7	1.54 ± 0.08	1.28 ± 0.14[b]	0.03
Maximal RER	7	1.11 ± 0.02	1.05 ± 0.03	NS

RER, respiratory exchange ratio (Vco_2/Vo_2); NS, not significant.
[a]Data are presented as mean ± 1 SE.
[b]Significant difference ($p < 0.05$).
From Lotgering FK, van Doorn MB, Struijk PC, Pool J, Wallenburg HC. Maximal aerobic exercise in pregnant women: heart rate, O_2 consumption, CO_2 production and ventilation. J Appl Physiol 1991;70:1016–1023.

CLINICAL APPLICATIONS TO EXERCISE IN PREGNANCY

Exercise is being routinely prescribed for various clinical conditions in the nonpregnant woman, but it has not been offered to pregnant women in the past because of the fear that the potential maternal benefits could be offset by fetal risks. Exercise prescription requires a thorough knowledge of exercise physiology and recognition of potential risks associated with exercise during pregnancy. Risks are amplified in pregnancy by normal gestational anatomic and physiologic changes.

Pelvic floor exercises (Kegel or levator exercises) and their benefits in subsequent labor are overrated in the lay literature; they were originally prescribed for pregnant women to increase the elasticity and tonicity of the perineum and to prevent perineal tears at delivery. There is no scientific evidence to support this view. The only possible benefit of pelvic floor exercises is for the postpartum period, when they may help the pelvic muscles return to the prepregnancy condition. Viewed from this perspective, the exercises may offer some advantage.

Many proposed but unproved benefits of exercise for the pregnant woman have been suggested: shorter labor; fewer complications during pregnancy; faster recovery from labor and delivery; prevention of varicose veins, thrombosis, and leg cramps; and improved mental outlook for these patients (76–83). Certain toning exercises may have some benefit in pregnancy in maintaining proper posture and preventing lower back pain and may facilitate recovery after birth. Some of the stretching routines, however, may need to be modified to prevent injuries.

Exercises are generally divided into areas of the body, first emphasizing the upper body, next the legs, and, finally, the abdomen. Some exercises may be combined with yoga, dance, and calisthenic routines to the patient's benefit.

Exercises for Pregnant Diabetics

The Second International Conference on Gestational Diabetes Mellitus endorsed the concept of exercise as an adjunct therapy for the pregnant diabetic: "Available evidence indicates that women with active lifestyles may continue a program of moderate exercise conducted under medical supervision" (84). Along with the exercise program, these patients should follow a balanced diet of 30 kcal/kg ideal body weight.

A previously published clinical protocol (85) appears to be particularly suited for patients with gestational diabetes. Patients entering such a program initially are screened to rule out intercurrent medical or obstetric complications. Then they undergo a symptom-limited $V0_{2max}$ bicycle ergometer test to determine the individual's work capacity. (In the clinical office situation, this step is not necessary.) The patient then is instructed to follow this program: before each meal (breakfast, lunch, and dinner) she rests for 30 minutes, during which time she monitors fetal activity and records the number of perceived fetal movements. After each meal she exercises for 30 minutes at a mild to moderate pace. The patients are instructed to count fetal movements for 30 minutes after each exercise session and instructed not to proceed with the next exercise session if the fetus did not move during the 30 minutes postexercise period. Furthermore, the physician is to be notified if the fetus moved fewer than 10 times in 24 hours. The patient checks her blood glucose level with a home blood glucose monitoring device. If the blood glucose is above 250 mg/dL or below 60 mg/dL or if ketonuria is present, she must not proceed with the exercise session and must notify the physician.

In the absence of these conditions, the patient will have her prescribed meal and then exercise on a stationary cycle ergometer at 50% of her predetermined maximum aerobic capacity. Immediately after the exercise, she will again check her blood glucose, rest for 30 minutes, and count fetal movements. The patient should be aware of uterine activity, and if uterine contractions become regular or occur at intervals of 15 minutes or less, she should inform her obstetrician. I inform patients of potential complications and have them sign an informed consent. Patients also are required to keep accurate records of their blood glucose determinations, food intake, fetal movements, and physical activities. Beginning after about 32 weeks, FHR reactivity (nonstress testing) is conducted weekly. Further fetal testing is done as indicated.

Other exercise programs may be suitable for pregnant diabetics. There are indications that 45 minutes of moderate exercise every 48 hours may suffice to induce upregulation of insulin receptors in these patients.

Benefits of Walking

Several studies on the possible benefits that walking may have on labor are inconclusive. Few past studies have shown such benefit, (78,79). A recent study by Bloom et al. (77) failed to show that the effect of walking in active labor either enhances or impairs the course of labor. Although this was a large study, the results may have been affected by poor compliance (22% of the patients assigned to the walking group did not comply). In our own work, we found that exertion in labor definitely enhances the quality of uterine contractions; however, the effect on the progress of labor is inconclusive. Definitive studies should be designed to address these issues.

SUMMARY

Much information has accumulated from which we can conclude that the risk of exercise for both mother and fetus in the uncomplicated pregnancy is reasonably low. The available medical literature does not allow us to assign a quantitative risk for exercising in pregnancy. It indicates, however, a certain trend that can be summarized as follows:

- Women who exercise before pregnancy and continue to do so in pregnancy without proper caloric replacement weigh less, gain less weight, and deliver smaller babies than controls.
- No definitive information is available to assess whether active women have better pregnancy outcomes than sedentary women, although indirect evidence suggests that this is the case.
- The exact incidence of fetal injury related to exercise is not known but is probably low.
- Fit women appear to cope better with labor, although they do not have shorter or easier labors.
- The medical need for intensive and strenuous training is limited in pregnancy, especially because it has been demonstrated in nonpregnant women that health benefits can be derived from moderate exercise.
- The goal of exercise in pregnancy is to balance the highest level of fitness against maximum safety.
- Elite athletes may engage in strenuous activities in pregnancy, but they should be doing so under strict medical supervision (83).
- Exercise prescription in pregnancy should be individually tailored.

REFERENCES

1. Blair SN, Chandler JY, Ellisor DB, Langley J. Improving physical fitness by exercise training programs. South Med J 1980;73:1594–1596.
2. Dye TD, Knox KL, Artal R, Aubry RH, Wojtowycz MA. Physical activity, obesity and diabetes in pregnancy. Am J Epidemiol 1997;146: 961–965.
3. ACOG Technical Bulletin no. 189. Washington DC: American College of Obstetricians and Gynecologists, Feb 1994.
4. American College of Sports Medicine. Position stand: The recommended quantity and quality of exercise for developing and maintaining cardiorespiratory and muscular fitness in healthy adults. Med Sci Sports Exer 1990;22:265–274.
5. Calganeri M, Bird HA, Wright Y. Changes in joints occurring during pregnancy. Ann Rheum Dis 1982;41:126–128.
6. Dumas GA, Reid JG. Laxity of knee cruciate ligaments during pregnancy. Journal of Physical Therapy 1997;26:2–6.
7. Kerr MG. The mechanical effects of the gravid uterus in late pregnancy. J Obstet Gynaecol Br Commonw 1965;72:513–529.
8. Morton MJ, Metcalfe J. Changes in maternal hemodynamics during pregnancy. In: Artal R, Wiswell RA, eds. Exercise in pregnancy. Baltimore: Williams & Wilkins, 1986:113.
9. Clapp JF. Maternal heart rate in pregnancy. Am J Obstet Gynecol 1985;152:659–660.
10. Pivarnik JM, Lee W, Clark SL, Cotton DB, Spillman HT, Nliller JF. Cardiac output responses of primigravid women during exercise determined by the direct Fick technique. Obstet Gynecol 1990;75:954–959.
11. Artal R, Khodiguian N, Kammula R, Rutherford S, Wiswell RA. Cardiopulmonary adaptations to graded exercise in pregnancy. Proc Soc Gynecol Invest 1986:66.
12. Artal R, Khodiguian N, Rutherford S, Wiswell RA. Cardiopulmonary and metabolic responses to bicycle ergometry in pregnancy. Proc Soc Gynecol Invest 1987:48.
13. Sady SP, Carpenter MW, Thompson PD, Sady MA, Heydon B, Coustan DR. Cardiovascular response to cycle exercise during and after pregnancy. J Appl Physiol 1989;66:336–341.
14. Rowell LB. Human circulation: regulation during physical stress. New York: Oxford University Press, 1986:232.
15. Morris N, Osborne SB, Wright HP, Hart A. Effective uterine blood flow during exercise in normal and pre-eclamptic pregnancies. Lancet 1956;2:481–484.
16. Clapp JF. Acute exercise stress in the pregnant ewe. Am J Obstet Gynecol 1980;136:489–494.
17. Hohimer AR, Bissonnette JM, Metcalf J, McKean TA. Effect of exercise in uterine blood flow in the pregnant pygmy goat. Am J Physiol 1984;246:H2O7–H212.
18. Lotgering FK, Gilbert RD, Longo LD. Exercise responses in pregnant sheep: oxygen consumption, uterine blood flow and blood volume. J Appl Physiol 1983;55:834–841.
19. Artal R, Wiswell R, Romem Y, Dorey F. Pulmonary responses to exercise in pregnancy. Am J Obstet Gynecol 1986;154:378–383.
20. Clapp JF, Wesley M, Sleamaker RH. Thermoregulatory and metabolic responses prior to and during pregnancy. Med Sci Sports Exerc 1987; 29:124–130.
21. Soultanakis HN. Glucose homeostasis during pregnancy in response to prolonged exercise. Postdoctoral thesis, University of Southern California, 1989.
22. Artal Mittelmark R. Hormonal responses to exercise in pregnancy. In:

Artal R, Wiswell RA, Drinkwater B, eds. Exercise in pregnancy. 2nd ed. Baltimore: Williams & Wilkins, 1990.
23. Artal R, Posner M. Fetal responses to maternal exercise. In: Artal R, Wiswell RA, Drinkwater B, eds. Exercise in pregnancy. 2nd ed. Baltimore: Williams & Wilkins, 1990.
24. Soiva K, Salmi A, Gronroos M, Peltonen T. Physical working capacity during pregnancy and effect of physical tests on fetal heart rate. Ann Chir Gynaecol 1963;53:187.
25. Pokorny J, Rotis J. The effect of mother's work on foetal heart sounds. In: Horsky J, Stembera ZK, eds. Intra-uterine dangers to the foetus. Amsterdam: Excerpta, Medica Foundation, 1967:359.
26. Pomerance JJ, Gluck L, Lynch VA. Maternal exercise as a screening test for uteroplacental insufficiency. Obstet Gynecol 1974;44:383–387.
27. Eisenberg de Smoler P, Karchmer S, Castelazo-Ayala L, Dominguez J. El electrocardiograma fetal durinte el ejercicio materno. Ginecol Obstet Mex 1974;35:521–534.
28. Pernoll ML, Metcalf J, Paul M. Fetal cardiac response to maternal exercise. In: Longo LD, Reneau DD, eds. Fetal and newborn cardiovascular physiology, vol 2. New York: Garland Press, 1978:389.
29. Dale E, Mullinax KM, Bryan DH. Exercise during pregnancy: effects on the fetus. Can J Appl Sport Sci 1982;7:98–103.
30. Hauth JC, Gilstrap LC, Widmer K. Fetal heart rate reactivity before and after maternal jogging during the third trimester. Am J Obstet Gynecol 1982;142:545–547.
31. Collings CA, Curet LB, Mullin JP. Maternal and fetal responses to a maternal aerobic exercise program. Am J Obstet Gynecol 1983;145: 702–707.
32. Artal R, Romem Y, Wiswell R. Fetal heart responses to maternal exercise. Am J Obstet Gynecol 1986;155:729–733.
33. Pijpers L, Wladimiroff W, McGhie Y. Effect of short-term maternal exercise on maternal and fetal cardiovascular dynamics. Br J Obstet Gynaecol 1984;91:1081–1086.
34. Clapp JF. Fetal heart rate response to running in midpregnancy and late pregnancy. Am J Obstet Gynecol 1985;153:251–252.
35. Jovanovic L, Kessler A, Peterson CM. Human maternal and fetal responses to graded exercise. J Appl Physiol 1985;58:1719–1722.
36. Rauramo L. Effect of short-term physical exercise on fetal heart rate and uterine activity in normal and abnormal pregnancies. Ann Chir Gynaecol 1987;76:1–6.
37. Paolone AM, Shangold M, Paul D, Minnitti J, Weiner S. Fetal heart rate measurements during maternal exercise-avoidance of artifact. Med Sci Sports Exerc 1987;19:605–609.
38. Carpenter MW, Sady SS, Hoegsberg B, et al. Fetal heart rate response to maternal exertion. JAMA 1988;259:3006–3009.
39. Wolfe LA, Lowe-Wylde SJ, Tranmer JE, McGrath MJ. Fetal heart rate during maternal static exercise. Can J Sport Sci 1988;13:95—96P.
40. Artal R, Khodughian N, Paul RH. Intrapartum fetal heart rate responses to maternal exercise. Case reports. J Perinat Med 1993;21:499–502.
41. Artal R, Romem Y, Paul RH, Wiswell R. Fetal bradycardia induced by maternal exercise. Lancet 1984;2:258–260.
42. Moore DH, Jarrett JC, Bendick PJ. Exercise induced changes in uterine artery blood flow, as measured by Doppler ultrasound, in pregnant subjects. Am J Perinatol 1988;5:94–97.
43. Morrow RJ, Ritchie WK, Bull SB. Fetal and maternal hemodynamic responses to exercise in pregnancy assessed by Doppler ultrasonography. Am J Obstet Gynecol 1989;160:138–140.
44. Veille JC, Bacevice AE, Wilson B, Janos J, Hellerstein HK. Umbilical artery waveform during bicycle exercise in normal pregnancy. Obstet Gynecol 1989;73:957–960.
45. Fox ME, Harris RE, Brekken AL. The active-duty military pregnancy: a new high-risk category. Am J Obstet Gynecol 1984;129:705–707.
46. Tafari N, Naeye RL, Gobezie A. Effects of maternal undernutrition and heavy physical work during pregnancy on birth weight. Br J Obstet Gynaecol 1980;87:222–226.
47. Naeye RL, Peters E. Working during pregnancy; effects on the fetus. Pediatrics 1982;69:724–727.
48. Terada M. Effect of physical activity before pregnancy on fetuses of mice exercised forcibly during pregnancy. Teratology 1974;10: 141–144.
49. Nelson PS, Gilbert RD, Longo L. Fetal growth and placental diffusing capacity in guinea pigs following long-term maternal exercise. J Dev Physiol 1983;5:1–10.
50. Clapp JF, Dickstein S. Endurance exercise and pregnancy outcome. Med Sci Sports Exerc 1984;16:556–562.
51. Erdelyi GJ. Gynecological survey of female athletes. J Sports Med Phys Fit 1962;2:174–175.
52. Zaharieva E. Olympic participation by women; effects on pregnancy and childbirth. JAMA 1972;221:992–995.
53. Soultanakis HN, Artal R, Wiswell RA. Prolonged exercise in pregnancy: glucose homeostasis, ventilatory and cardiovascular responses. Semin Preinatol 1996;20:315–327.
54. Edwards MJ. Congenital defects in guinea pigs: fetal resorptions, abortions and malformations following induced hyperthermia during early gestation. Teratology 1969;2:313–328.
55. Skreb N, Frank Z. Developmental abnormalities in the rat induced by heat shock. J Embryo Exp Morphol 1983;11:445.
56. Kilham L, Ferm VH. Exencephaly in fetal hamsters exposed to hyperthermia. Teratology 1976;14:323–326.
57. Miller P, Smith DW, Shepard TH. Maternal hyperthermia as a possible cause of anencephaly. Lancet 1978;1:519–521.
58. Shiota K. Neural tube defects and maternal hyperthermia in early pregnancy. Epidemiology in a human embryonic population. Am J Med Genet 1982;12:281–288.
59. Edwards MJ. Hyperthermia as a teratogen. Teratol Carcinog Mutagen 1986;6:563–582.
60. Halperin LR, Wilroy RS Jr. Maternal hyperthermia and neural tube defects. Lancet 1978;2:212–213.
61. Harvey MAS, McRorie, Smith DW. Suggested limits to the use of hot tubs and saunas by pregnant women. Can Med Assoc J 1981;125: 50–54.
62. Clarren SK, Smith DW, Harvey MAS, Ward RH, Myrianthopoulos NC. Hyperthermia—a prospective evaluation of a possible teratogenic agent in man. J Pediatr 1979;95:81–83.
63. Katz VL. Water exercise in pregnancy. Semin Perinatol 1996;20: 285–291.
64. Wallace JP., Inbar G, Ernsthausen K. Infant acceptance of post exercise breast milk. Pediatrics 1992;89:1245–1247.
65. Wallace JP, Inbar G, Ernsthausen K. Lactate concentrations in breast milk following maximal exercise and a typical workout. Journal of Women's Health 1994;3:91–96.
66. Carey GB, Quinn TJ, Goodwin E. S. Breast milk composition after exercise of different intensities. J of Human Lactation 1997;13: 115–120.
67. Jarrett JC II, Spellacy WN. Jogging during pregnancy: an improved outcome? Obstet Gynecol 1983:61:705–709.
68. Katz J. Swimming through your pregnancy, the perfect exercise for pregnant women. New York: Dolphin Books, Doubleday, 1983:1:59.
69. McMurray RG, Katz VL, Berry MJ, Cefalo RC. The effect of pregnancy on metabolic responses during rest immersion and aerobic exercise in the water. Am J Obstet Gynecol 1988;158:481–486.
70. Camporesi EM. Diving and pregnancy. Semin Perinatol 1996;20: 292–302.
71. Newhall JF. Scuba diving during pregnancy: a brief review. Am J Obstet Gynecol 1981;140:893–894.
72. Huch R. Physical activity at altitude in pregnancy. Semin Perinatol 1996;20:303–314.
73. Huch, R, Baumann H, Fallenstein F, Schneider KT, Holdener F, Huch A. Physiologic changes in pregnant women and their fetuses during jet air travel. Am J Obstet Gynecol 1986;154:996–1000.
74. Bauman H, Bung P, Fallenstein F, Huch A, Huch R. Reaktion von mutter und Fet auf die Korperliche Belastung in der Hohe. Geburtshilfe Frauenheilkd 1985;45:869–876.
75. Artal R, Fortunato V, Welton A, et al. A comparison of cardiopulmonary adaptations to exercise in pregnancy at sea level and altitude. Am J Obstet Gynecol 1996;175:505–506.
76. Stevenson L. Exercise in pregnancy. Part I: Update on pathophysiology. Can Fam Physician 1997;43:97–104.
77. Bloom SL, McIntire DD, Kelly MA, et al. Lack of effect of walking on labor and delivery. N Engl J Med 1998;339:76–79.
78. Flynn AM, Kelly J, Hollins G, Lynch PF. Ambulation in labor. BMJ 1978;2:591–593.
79. Read JA, Miller FC, Paul RH. Randomized trial of ambulation versus oxytocin for labor enhancement; a preliminary report. Am J Obstet Gynecol 1981;139:669–672.
80. Hemminki E, Saarikoski S. Ambulation and delayed amniotomy in the first stage of labor. Eur J Obstet Gynecol Reprod Biol 1983;15:129–139.
81. Danforth DN. Pregnancy and labor from the vantage point of the physical therapist. Am J Phys Med 1967;46:653–658.

82. Blankfield A. Is exercise necessary for the obstetric patient? Med J Aust 1967;1:163–165.
83. Hale RW, Artal MR. Pregnancy in the elite and professional athlete—a stepwise clinical approach. In: Artal MR, Wiswell RA, Drinkwater BL, eds. Exercise and pregnancy. Baltimore: Williams & Wilkins, 1991.
84. Second International Workshop—Conference on Gestational Diabetes Mellitus. Summary and recommendations: therapeutic strategies. Diabetes 1985;34:1–130.
85. Bung P, Artal R, Khodiguian N, Kjos S. Exercise in gestational diabetes. An optional therapeutic approach? Diabetes 1991;40(Suppl 2):182–185.
86. Baumann H, Huch R. Hohenexposition und Hohenaufenthalt in der Schwangerschaft: Auswirkungen auf Mutter und Fet. Zentralbl Gynakol 1986;108:889–899.
87. Bung P, Baumann H, Huch R, Huch A. Fetale Herz-frequenz bei mutterlicher Hohenexposition und Korperlicher Belastung. Gynakol Prax 1987;11:217–226.
88. Bung P. Korperliche Belastung und Sport in der Schwangerschaft-Moglichkeiten und Gefahren unter besonderer Bercksichtigung der klinischen Wertigkeit. Habilitationsschrift Med. Fakultat Universitat Bonn, 1992.
89. Elliott JP, Trujillo RN. Fetal monitoring during emergency obstetric transport. Am J Obstet Gynecol 1987;157:245–247.
90. Clapp JF, Capeless E. The VO_2 max of recreational athletes before and after pregnancy. Med Sci Sports Exer 1991;23:1128–1133.
91. Lotgering FK, van Doorn MB, Struijk PC, Pool J, Wallenburg HC. Maximal aerobic exercise in pregnant women: heart rate, 0_2 consumption, CO_2 production and ventilation. J Appl Physiol 1991;70:1016–1023.
92. Sady SP, Carpenter MW, Sady MA, et al. Prediction of VO_2 max during cycle exercise in pregnant women. J Appl Physiol 1988;65:657–661.
93. Khodiguian N, Jaque-Fortunato SV, Wiswell RA, Artal R. A comparison of cross-sectional and longitudinal methods of assessing the influence of pregnancy on cardiac function during exercise. Semin Perinatol 1996;20:232–241.
94. McMurray RG, Hackney AC, Katz VL, Gall M, Watson WJ. Pregnancy-induced changes in the maximal physiological responses during swimming. J Appl Physiol 1991;71:1454–1459.
95. Artal R, et al. VO_2 max in pregnant professional athletes (unpublished observations).

Cherry and Merkatz's Complications of Pregnancy,
Fifth Edition, edited by W. R. Cohen.
Lippincott Williams & Wilkins, Philadelphia © 2000.

CHAPTER 4

Maternal-Fetal Ethics

Frank A. Chervenak and Laurence B. McCullough

TWO BASIC ETHICAL PRINCIPLES

Ethics is the disciplined study of morality, which concerns both right and wrong behavior (i.e., what one ought and ought not to do) and good and bad character (i.e., virtues and vices). Ethics asks, "What ought morality to be?" This question can be broken down into two further questions: "What ought our behavior to be?" and "What virtues ought to be cultivated in our moral lives?" Ethics in maternal-fetal medicine deals with these same questions, focusing on what morality ought to be for obstetric practitioners.

For centuries the basis for what morality ought to be in clinical practice has been the obligation to protect and promote the interests of the patient. This general clinical ethical obligation needs to be considered in more specific terms if it is to be useful. This can be accomplished by interpreting two perspectives by which the patient's interests can be understood: that of the physician and that of the patient (1).

The Principle of Beneficence

The older of these two perspectives on the interests of patients in the history of medical ethics is the perspective of the medical caregiver. On the basis of scientific knowledge, shared clinical experience, and a careful, unbiased evaluation of the patient, the physician identifies those clinical strategies that will likely serve the health-related interests of the patient and those that will not. The health-related interests of the patient include preventing premature death and preventing, curing, or at least managing disease, injury, handicap, or unnecessary pain and suffering (2). That these matters are constitutive of any patient's health-related interests is a function of the competencies of medicine as a social institution (3). The identification of a patient's interests should not be a function of the personal or subjective outlook of a particular physician, but rather of rigorous clinical judgment.

The ethical principle of beneficence structures this rigorous clinical perspective in the interests of the patient. This principle obliges the physician to seek the greater balance of advantages over harms for the patient as the consequence of the physician's and the patient's behaviors. On the basis of rigorous clinical judgment, physicians should identify those strategies expected to result in the greater balance of goods (i.e., the protection and promotion of health-related interests) over harms with the potential to impair those interests. The principle of beneficence has an ancient pedigree in Western medical ethics, at least back to the time of Hippocrates (2).

The principle of beneficence in obstetric ethics must be sharply distinguished from the principle of nonmaleficence, commonly known as *primum non nocere* or "first, do no harm." It is important to note that *primum non nocere* does not appear in the Hippocratic Oath or in the texts that accompany the Oath. Instead, the principle of beneficence was the primary consideration of the Hippocratic writers. For example, in "Epidemics," the text reads, "As to diseases, make a habit of two things—to help or to at least do no harm" (4). In fact, the historical origins of *primum non nocere* remain obscure.

There are more than historical reasons to reject *primum non nocere* as a principle of obstetric ethics because virtually all medical interventions involve unavoidable risks of harm. If *primum non nocere* were the primary principle of obstetric ethics, virtually all of obstetric practice would be unethical.

Primum non nocere is therefore superseded in obstetric ethics by the principle of beneficence. The latter is sufficient to alert the physician to those circumstances in which a clinical intervention has the potential to harm the

F. A. Chervenak: Department of Obstetrics and Gynecology, Cornell University Medical College, The New York Hospital, New York, NY 10021; L. B. McCullough: Center for Medical Ethics and Health Policy, Baylor College of Medicine, Houston, TX 77030.

patient. When a clinical intervention is on balance likely to be harmful to a patient, it should not be performed.

The Principle of Respect for Autonomy

A well-formed clinical perspective on the interests of the patient is not the only legitimate one. The perspective of the patient on her own interests is equally worthy of consideration by the physician (1). This is because the patient has developed a set of values and beliefs according to which she should be presumed capable of making judgments about what will and will not protect and promote her interests. It is commonplace that in other aspects of her life the patient regularly makes such judgments concerning matters of considerable complexity (e.g., choosing a professional calling, rearing children, entering into contracts, and writing a will of property). Despite the complexity of these decisions, she is rightly assumed to be competent to make them, with the burden of proof on anyone who would challenge her competence.

The same is true about health care decisions made by the patient. She must be assumed by her physician to be competent to determine which clinical strategies support her interests and which do not. In making such judgments it is important to note that the patient uses values and beliefs that can range far beyond the scope of health-related interests (e.g., religious beliefs or beliefs about how many children she wants to have). Beneficence-based clinical judgment, because it is limited by the competencies of medicine, gives the physician no authority to assess the worth or meaning to the patient of her non–health-related interests. Therefore, these are matters solely for the patient to determine.

The ethical significance of this perspective is captured by the ethical principle of respect for autonomy. This principle obligates the physician to respect the integrity of the patient's values and beliefs, to respect her perspective on her interests, and to implement only those clinical strategies authorized by her as the result of the informed consent process.

Respect for autonomy is put into clinical practice by the informed consent process. This process has three elements: (a) disclosure by the physician to the patient of adequate information about the patient's condition and its management; (b) understanding of that information by the patient; and (c) a voluntary decision by the patient to authorize or refuse clinical management (5).

Beneficence and Respect for Autonomy Applied to the Pregnant Woman and Fetus

There are obviously beneficence-based and autonomy-based obligations to the pregnant patient (6). The physician's perspective on the pregnant woman's interests provides the basis for beneficence-based obligations owed to her. Her own perspective on those interests provides the basis for autonomy-based obligations owed to her.

Because of an insufficiently developed central nervous system, the fetus cannot meaningfully be said to possess values and beliefs. There is thus no basis for saying that a fetus has a perspective on its interests. There can therefore be no autonomy-based obligations to any fetus (1,6,7). Hence, the language of fetal rights has no meaning and therefore no application to the fetus in obstetric ethics, despite its popularity in public and political discourse in the United States and other countries. Obviously, the physician has a perspective on the fetus's health-related interests and the physician can have beneficence-based obligations to the fetus, but only when the fetus is a patient. Because of its importance for obstetric ethics, the topic of the fetus as patient requires detailed consideration.

TWO SENSES OF THE CONCEPT OF THE FETUS AS PATIENT

The concept of the fetus as patient has recently come to prominence, largely because of developments in fetal diagnosis and management strategies to optimize fetal outcome (3,8–11) and has become widely accepted (12–19). This concept has clinical significance because when the fetus is a patient, directive counseling (i.e., recommending a form of management) for fetal benefit is appropriate. When the fetus is not a patient, nondirective counseling (i.e., offering but not recommending a form of management) is appropriate. These apparently straightforward roles for directive and nondirective counseling are, however, often difficult to apply in actual obstetric practice because of uncertainty about when the fetus is a patient. One approach to resolving this uncertainty has been to argue that the fetus is or is not a patient by virtue of personhood (20–25) or some other form of independent moral being (26–29). This approach fails to resolve the uncertainty, and we will therefore defend an alternative approach that does resolve it.

The Independent Moral Status of the Fetus

A prominent approach for establishing whether or not the fetus is a patient has involved attempts to show whether or not the fetus has independent moral status. This is the first sense of the concept of the fetus as patient. Such status for the fetus means that one or more characteristics that the fetus possesses in and of itself (independently of the pregnant woman), generate obligations to the fetus on the part of the pregnant woman and her physician.

A striking variety of characteristics has been nominated for this role: moment of conception, implantation, central nervous system development, quickening, and the moment of birth (30–32). It should come as no surprise that, given the diversity of proposed characteristics, there is marked variation among ethicists about when the fetus acquires independent moral status. Some take the view that the fetus has independent moral status from the moment of conception or implantation (33–35). Others believe that independent moral status is acquired in degrees, thus resulting in "graded" moral status (26,28). Still others hold, at least by implication, that the fetus never has independent moral status so long as it is *in utero* (27).

Despite an ever-expanding theological and philosophical body of literature on this subject, there has been no closure on a single authoritative account of the independent moral status of the fetus (36,37). This is not a surprising outcome because, given the absence of a single methodology that would be authoritative for all of the markedly diverse theological and philosophical schools of thought involved in this endless debate, closure is impossible. For closure ever to be possible, debates about such a final authority within and between theological and philosophical traditions would have to be resolved in a way satisfactory to all, an inconceivable intellectual and cultural requirement. It is prudent therefore to abandon futile attempts to understand the fetus as patient in terms of the independent moral status of the fetus and turn to an alternative approach that makes it possible to identify ethically distinct senses of the fetus as patient and their clinical implications for directive and nondirective counseling. In its first sense, the independent moral status of the fetus—the fetus as patient—has no stable or clinically applicable meaning. We therefore consider a second sense of the concept of the fetus as patient.

The Dependent Moral Status of the Fetus

Our analysis of this second sense of the concept of the fetus as patient begins with the recognition that being a patient does not require that one possess independent moral status (29). Rather, being a patient means that one can benefit from the applications of the clinical skills of the physician. Put more precisely, a human being without independent moral status is properly regarded as a patient when two conditions are met: that person (a) is presented to the physician (b) and there exist clinical interventions that are reasonably expected to be efficacious (i.e., they will result in a greater balance of benefits over harms for the human being in question) (38). This is the second sense of the concept of the fetus as patient, what we call the dependent moral status of the fetus.

We have argued elsewhere that beneficence-based obligations to the fetus exist when the fetus is reliably expected later to achieve independent moral status (sometime during the second year postpartum) (1). That is, the fetus is a patient when the fetus is presented for medical interventions, whether diagnostic or therapeutic, that reasonably can be expected to result in a greater balance of goods over harms for the person the fetus can later become during early childhood. The ethical significance of the concept of the fetus as patient therefore depends on links that can be established between the fetus and the child later achieving independent moral status.

The Viable Fetal Patient

One such link is viability. Viability is not, however, an intrinsic property of the fetus because viability must be understood in terms of both biological and technological factors (37,39,40). It is only by virtue of both factors that a viable fetus can exist *ex utero* and thus later achieve independent moral status. Moreover, these two factors do not exist as a function of the autonomy of the pregnant woman. When a fetus is viable (i.e., when it is of sufficient maturity so that it can survive into the neonatal period and later achieve independent moral status given the availability of the requisite technological support), and when it is presented to the physician, the fetus is a patient.

Viability exists as a function of biomedical and technological capacities, which vary in different parts of the world. As a consequence, there is presently no worldwide, uniform gestational age at which to define viability. In the United States, the authors believe, viability presently occurs at approximately 24 weeks of gestational age (41,42).

When the fetus is a patient, directive counseling for fetal benefit is ethically justified. In clinical practice, directive counseling for fetal benefit involves one or more of the following: recommending against termination of pregnancy; recommending against nonaggressive management; or recommending aggressive management. Aggressive obstetric management includes interventions such as fetal surveillance, tocolysis, cesarean delivery, or delivery in a tertiary-care center when indicated. Nonaggressive obstetric management excludes such interventions. Directive counseling for fetal benefit must, however, take into account the presence and severity of fetal anomalies, extreme prematurity, and obligations to the pregnant woman.

It is very important to appreciate in clinical practice that the strength of directive counseling for fetal benefit varies according to the presence and severity of anomalies. As a rule, the more severe the fetal anomaly, the less directive counseling should be for fetal benefit (7,43). In particular, when there is "(1) a very high probability of a correct diagnosis and (2) either a very high probability of death as an outcome of the anomaly diagnosed or a very high probability of severe irreversible deficit of cognitive or developmental capacity as a result of the anomaly diagnosed" (44), counseling should be nondirective in recommending between aggressive and nonaggressive management. By contrast, when lethal anomalies can be diagnosed with certainty, there are no beneficence-based obligations to provide aggressive management (43,45). Such fetuses are not patients; they are appropriately regarded as dying fetuses, and the counseling should be nondirective in recommending between nonaggressive management and termination of pregnancy, but directive in recommending against aggressive management for the sake of maternal benefit (43).

The strength of directive counseling for fetal benefit in cases of extreme prematurity of viable fetuses does not vary. This is the case for what we term just-viable fetuses (3), those with a gestational age of 24 to 26 weeks, for whom there are significant rates of survival but high rates of mortality and morbidity (41,42). These risks can be increased by nonaggressive obstetric management, whereas aggressive obstetric management may favorably influence outcome. Thus it would appear that there are substantial beneficence-based obligations to just-viable fetuses to provide aggressive obstetric management. This is more evident in pregnancies beyond 26 weeks gestational age (41,42). Therefore, directive counseling for fetal benefit is justified in all cases of extreme prematurity of potentially viable fetuses. Of course, such directive counseling is appropriate only when it is based on documented efficacy of aggressive obstetric management for each fetal indication. For example, such efficacy has not been demonstrated for routine cesarean delivery to manage extreme prematurity (41).

Any directive counseling for fetal benefit should occur in the context of balancing beneficence-based obligations to the fetus against beneficence-based and autonomy-based obligations to the pregnant woman (1,6). Any such balancing must recognize that a pregnant woman is obligated only to take reasonable risks of medical interventions that are reliably expected to benefit the viable fetus or child later. The unique feature of obstetric ethics is that whether, in a particular case, the viable fetus ought to be regarded as presented to the physician is, in part, a function of the pregnant woman's autonomy.

Obviously, any strategy for directive counseling for fetal benefit that takes account of obligations to the pregnant woman must be open to the possibility of conflict between the physician's recommendation and a pregnant woman's autonomous decision to the contrary. Such conflict is best managed preventively through informed consent as an ongoing dialogue throughout the pregnancy, augmented as necessary by negotiation and respectful persuasion (1,46).

The Previable Fetal Patient

The only possible link between the previable fetus and the child it can become is the pregnant woman's autonomy. This is because technologic factors cannot result in the previable fetus becoming a child. This is simply what previable means. The link, therefore, between a fetus and the child it can become, when the fetus is previable, can be established only by the pregnant woman's decision to confer the status of being a patient on her previable fetus. The previable fetus, therefore, has no claim to the status of being a patient independent of the pregnant woman's autonomy. The pregnant woman is free to withhold, confer, or, having once conferred, withdraw the status of being a patient on or from her previable fetus according to her own values and beliefs. The previable fetus is presented to the physician solely as a function of the pregnant woman's autonomy.

Counseling a woman regarding the management of her pregnancy when the fetus is previable should be nondirective in terms of continuing the pregnancy or having an abortion, if she refuses to confer the status of being a patient on her fetus. If she does confer such status in a settled way, at that point beneficence-based obligations to her fetus come into play and directive counseling for fetal benefit becomes appropriate for these situations. Just as for viable fetuses, such counseling must take into account the presence and severity of fetal anomalies, extreme prematurity, and obligations owed to the pregnant woman.

For pregnancies in which the woman is uncertain about whether to confer such status, the authors propose that the fetus be regarded provisionally as a patient (1). This justifies directive counseling against behavior that can harm a fetus in significant and irreversible ways (e.g., substance abuse) until the woman settles on whether to confer the status of patient on the fetus.

Nondirective counseling is particularly appropriate in cases of what we term near-viable fetuses (1) (i.e., those at 22-23 weeks gestational age and for which there are only anecdotal reports of survival) (41). In the authors' view, aggressive obstetric and neonatal management at this age should be regarded as clinical investigation (i.e., a form of medical experimentation and not standard of care). There is no obligation on the part of a pregnant woman to confer the status of being a patient on a near-viable fetus because the efficacy of aggressive obstetric and neonatal management has yet to be proven.

The *In Vitro* Embryo Patient

A subset of previable fetuses as patient concerns *in vitro* embryos. It might at first seem that the *in vitro* embryo is a patient because such an embryo is presented to the physician. However, for there to be beneficence-based obligations to a human being, it also must be the case that there exist medical interventions that are reliably expected to be efficacious.

Recall that, in terms of beneficence, whether the fetus is a patient depends on links that can be established between the fetus and its later achieving independent moral status. Therefore, the reasonableness of medical interventions on the *in vitro* embryo depends on whether that embryo later becomes viable. Otherwise, no benefit of such intervention can meaningfully be said to result.

An *in vitro* embryo, therefore, becomes viable only when it survives *in vitro* cell division, transfer, implantation, and subsequent gestation to such a time that it becomes viable. This process of achieving viability occurs only *in vivo* and, should assisted conception successfully result in the gestation of the previable fetus, is therefore entirely dependent on the woman's decision regarding the status of the fetus as a patient. Whether an *in vitro* embryo will become a viable fetus and whether medical intervention on such an embryo will benefit the fetus are both functions of the pregnant woman's autonomous decision to withhold, confer, or, having once conferred, withdraw the moral status of being a patient on the previable fetus that might result from assisted conception.

It therefore is appropriate to regard the *in vitro* embryo as a previable fetus rather than as a viable fetus. As a consequence, any *in vitro* embryo should be regarded as a patient only when the woman into whose reproductive tract the embryo will be transferred confers that status. Thus, counseling about how many *in vitro* embryos should be transferred and about preimplantation diagnosis should be nondirective (47). Information should be presented about prognosis for a successful pregnancy and the possibility of confronting a decision about selective reduction, depending on the number of embryos transferred. However, no definitive recommendation should be made about these matters because directive counseling for fetal benefit is not appropriate until the woman confers the status of patient on the *in vitro* embryo. In short, the woman should have the final say about how many embryos are to be transferred. Preimplantation diagnostic counseling should be nondirective because the woman may elect not to implant abnormal embryos. These embryos are not patients, so there is no basis for directive counseling.

HOW TO READ THE OBSTETRIC ETHICS LITERATURE CRITICALLY

Inquiry into various issues pertinent to obstetric ethics is sure to continue and expand. We therefore provide the reader with tools appropriate to the task of evaluating the literature on obstetric ethics critically.

A Basic Distinction: Descriptive Versus Normative Obstetric Ethics

The first tool involves recognizing the basic distinction between descriptive and normative obstetric ethics. Descriptive obstetric ethics employs the long-established methods of the quantitative and qualitative social sciences to obtain data about actual ethical beliefs and practices regarding the ethical dimensions of obstetrics. Normative obstetric ethics, by contrast, is concerned with what ethical beliefs and practices in obstetrics ought to be. Normative obstetric ethics employs the qualitative methods of rigorous ethical analysis and argument. Descriptive obstetric ethics provides an important reference point for normative ethics, but descriptive ethics can never tell us what beliefs and practices of obstetricians ought to be, only—and importantly—what they actually are. Articles on descriptive obstetric ethics are becoming increasingly common in the literature (48).

Criteria for Rigorous Ethical Analysis and Argument in Normative Obstetric Ethics

The main qualitative methods of normative obstetric ethics are ethical analysis and argument. Ethical analysis identifies component elements of ethical principles such as beneficence and respect for autonomy, as well as virtues such as compassion and integrity (1). Ethical argument uses ethical principles and virtues as premises from which conclusions can reliably be drawn. Over the centuries, philosophical ethics has developed a number of criteria for intellectually rigorous ethical analysis and argument in normative ethics. Our reading of that history is that six criteria are relevant for evaluating ethical analysis and argument for their intellectual rigor.

The first of these is clarity, which requires that terms and concepts be provided precise meanings. Consider for example the popular phrase "right to life" (33). This phrase does not refer to a single right but to at least three. These are the right not to be killed unjustly; the right not to have technological or biological supports discontinued unjustly; and the right to have such supports continued for as long as it is reasonable to do so. These rights, however, make different demands upon the pregnant woman. For example, the first version seems limited by very few exceptions, whereas the third version must admit to many exceptions because no person has an overriding right to the property or body of another. Yet another clarification can be made about the "right to life." In the first two senses just identified, the right is a negative right, that is, a right to noninterference. In the third sense indicated above, the right to life is a positive right, that is, a claim to the resources of others. There is a temptation to trivialize the criterion of clarity as a definition of terms. As the preceding example illustrates, clarity involves much more than mere definition (e.g., careful explanation and the introduction of relevant distinctions).

A second criterion is consistency. Consistency makes two requirements of ethical analysis and argument. First, once key terms and phrases have been clarified, they should always be used with the same meaning. Consistency also requires that arguments be free of contradiction. That is, the conclusion of an argument should logically follow from its premises. For example, an inconsistent argument about abortion might be one in which different senses of the "right to life" are introduced into the premises and the conclusion of an argument. An example would be asserting the first version of the right to life as the sole premise of an argument and concluding that abortion in the case of rape or incest is permissible because the fetus does not have an overriding right to continue to exist under those circumstances. The problem is that this conclusion does not follow from a premise that asserts the right of the fetus not to be killed unjustly. This is because such a right stands independently of how the fetus is conceived. Hence, the exceptions claimed in the conclusion, rape and incest, are inconsistent with the first sense of a fetal right to life. The argument thus fails because of a lack of consistency.

A third criterion is coherence. Coherence requires the premises of an argument join into a meaningful whole. For example, simply listing ethical principles without demonstrating their connection to each other fails to satisfy the criterion of coherence. If, for example, one were to say that criminal penalties for drug use during pregnancy were ethically unjustified on the grounds of the principles of autonomy and beneficence, but not show how in clinically meaningful terms, then the two principles complement each other regarding this topic, and such a stringing together of principles would fail the criterion of coherence.

A fourth criterion is clinical applicability. Clinical applicability requires that normative obstetric ethics can actually be used to guide and direct clinical judgment and behavior in obstetrics. That is, normative obstetric ethics worthy of the name is never an "ivory tower" enterprise because normative obstetric ethics should be solidly grounded in clinical reality.

A fifth and related criterion is clinical adequacy. Clinical applicability means that normative obstetric ethics applies to present clinical realities. Clinical adequacy means that normative obstetric ethics will be applicable in future, as yet unforeseen, clinical situations.

Finally, all of the preceding criteria presuppose a well-known criterion of scholarship, namely, completeness. Just as in clinical research so, too, in normative ethics, no ethical analysis and argument in obstetric ethics is complete unless it takes account of and responds to the existing literature on the subject being addressed.

Readers may conveniently recall these criteria for intellectual rigor in normative obstetric ethics as the six C's: clarity, consistency, coherence, clinical applicability, clinical adequacy, and completeness (49).

Pitfalls To Be Avoided

Critical evaluation of the literature in obstetric ethics involves the identification of pitfalls to be avoided. These occur when the inherent limitations in the several disciplines that contribute to normative obstetric ethics are ignored. Because of their prominence, we will consider law, religion, professional consensus, uses of authority, and philosophy.

The main limitations of the law—common, statutory, regulatory, and administrative—are its incomprehensibleness and possible inconsistency. Although the law is surely clinically applicable and clinically adequate to many areas of obstetric practice, it is silent or virtually silent in many other areas. For example, some state courts have issued court orders for cesarean delivery for fetal distress or placenta previa.

However, no court has addressed, or is likely to address, a pregnant woman's disinclination to appear for prenatal care until she is in labor, although there would be justified ethical doubts about such behavior on beneficence-based grounds concerning both the woman's and the fetal patient's interests. Moreover, the law is largely silent on the virtues that physicians in obstetric practice ought to cultivate. Yet, attention to virtues such as compassion and integrity is critical for any adequate response to society's concerns about the dehumanization of obstetric practice (1).

The law is also at risk for internal conflict and thus possible inconsistency. On the one hand, statutory and regulatory law governing publicly funded health care seems to obligate physicians to do less for their patients. On the other hand, the common law of malpractice seems to obligate physicians to do more. Ignoring the incomprehensibleness or possible inconsistency of the law involves a pitfall.

The main limitations of religion are its potential lack of clinical applicability and clinical adequacy. This is because obstetric ethics based on religious belief requires all to accept the existence of a deity or some transcendent reality and a particular interpretation within a faith community of what the deity or transcendent reality deems to be the ultimate good of human beings—two conditions that can never be satisfied in a pluralistic society that includes people of different religions as well as atheists or agnostics (21). In addition, because the intellectual warrant of medicine, the biomedical sciences, and because the legal warrant of medicine, licensure by the state, are secular in character, obstetric ethics based on religion cannot be presumed to be clinically applicable or clinically adequate. To suggest otherwise involves a serious pitfall.

The main limitation of consensus (50) concerns the distinction drawn earlier between descriptive and normative ethics. The limitation of consensus is that it is a version of descriptive ethics. Taking consensus to be normative obstetric ethics involves a serious pitfall.

Uses of authorities are also subject to limitations (51). The problem here is that the intellectual authority of any expert view in obstetric ethics depends on the quality and rigor of the analysis and argument that supports the view (i.e., satisfying the six C's) and not on the prestige of an individual, an academic institution, professional association, or government commission or agency. These individuals or institutions may well have produced well-reasoned analysis and argument. The pitfall of inappropriate uses of authorities occurs when one overlooks the need to evaluate critically the statements of authorities according to the six C's. Such statements therefore should not be taken at face value.

The main limitation of philosophic ethics is a function of its subject matter. Aristotle noted that a science or area of knowledge can only be as exact as its subject matter (52). The subject matter of philosophic ethics comprises human beliefs and behaviors, which are notoriously inexact. From this fact Aristotle concluded correctly that philosophic argument in ethics cannot ever be exact in the sense that geometric proofs are exact. The lesson of Aristotle for our time is that the aims of any endeavor in normative obstetric ethics should be intellectually rigorous ethical analysis and argument that acknowledge intellectually rigorous competing ethical analysis and argument. This should not be a disabling shortcoming provided that the ethical analysis and argument in question satisfy the six C's. The pitfall of philosophic ethics is to treat one's ethical analysis and argument as final and irrefutable and thus above the necessity to acknowledge competing ethical analysis and argument.

Accepting this limitation of philosophic ethics has great clinical value because doing so obliges one to be willing to receive, and respond in a thoughtful way to, the critical evaluation of others. Every experienced clinician knows that failure to be open to critical evaluation of one's clinical judgment and practice in scientific matters more often than not leads to preventable problems in the care of patients. The same is true for clinical judgment and practice in ethical matters. In other words, the lack of finality that at first appears to be a serious limitation turns out on closer consideration to be an intellectual and clinical virtue and thus a powerful antidote to narrow-mindedness and inflexibility.

REFERENCES

1. McCullough LB, Chervenak FA. Ethics in obstetrics and gynecology. New York: Oxford University Press, 1994.
2. Beauchamp TL, Childress JF. Principles of biomedical ethics, 3rd ed. New York: Oxford University Press, 1989.
3. American Academy of Pediatrics Committee on Bioethics. Fetal therapy: ethical considerations. Pediatrics 1988;81:898–899.
4. Hippocrates. Epidemics i:xi [WHS Jones, translator]. Loeb Classical Library, vol. 147. Cambridge. MA: Harvard University Press, 1923.
5. Faden RR, Beauchamp TL. A history and theory of informed consent. New York: Oxford University Press, 1986.
6. Chervenak FA, McCullough LB. What is obstetric ethics? J Perinat Med 1996;23:331–341.
7. Chervenak FA, McCullough LB. Does obstetric ethics have any role in the obstetrician's response to the abortion controversy? Am J Obstet Gynecol 1990;163:1425–1429.
8. American College of Obstetricians and Gynecologists. Committee on Ethics. Patient choice: maternal-fetal conflict. Washington, DC: American College of Obstetricians and Gynecologists, 1987.
9. American College of Obstetricians and Gynecologists. Technical Bulletin. Ethical decision-making in obstetrics and gynecology. Washington, DC: American College of Obstetricians and Gynecologists, 1989.
10. Harrison MR, Golbus MS, Filly RA. The unborn patient. New York: Grune & Stratton, 1984.
11. Liley AW. The foetus as a personality. Aust N Z J Psych 1972;6:99–105.
12. Fletcher JC. The fetus as patient: ethical issues. JAMA 1981;246: 772–773.
13. Mahoney MJ. Fetal-maternal relationship. In: Reich WT, ed. Encyclopedia of bioethics. New York: Macmillan, 1978:485–489
14. Mahoney MJ. The fetus as patient. West J Med 1989;150:517–540.
15. Murray TH. Moral obligations to the not-yet born: the fetus as patient. Clin Perinatol 1987;14:313–328.
16. Newton ER. The fetus as patient. Med Clin North Am 1989;73:517–540.
17. Pritchard JA, MacDonald PC, Gant NF. Williams obstetrics, 17th ed. Norwalk, CT: Appleton-Century-Crofts, 1985:xi.
18. Shinn RL. The fetus as patient: a philosophical and ethical perspective. In: Milunsky A, Annas GJ, ed. Genetics and the law III. New York: Plenum Press, 1985:317–324.
19. Walters L. Ethical issues in intrauterine diagnosis and therapy. Fetal Ther 1986;1:32–37.
20. Anderson G, Strong C. The premature breech: Cesarean section or trial of labor? J Med Ethics 1988;14:18–24.
21. Engelhardt HT Jr. The foundations of bioethics. New York: Oxford University Press, 1986.
22. Fleming L. The moral status of the fetus: a reappraisal. Bioethics 1987; 1:15–34.
23. Ford NM. When did I begin? Conception of the human individual in history, philosophy and science. Cambridge, England: Cambridge University Press, 1988.
24. Strong C. Ethical conflicts between mother and fetus in obstetrics. Clin Perinatol 1987;14:313–328.
25. Strong C, Anderson G. The moral status of the near-term fetus. J Med Ethics 1989;15:25–27.
26. Dunstan GR. The moral status of the human embryo. A tradition recalled. J Med Ethics 1984;10:38–44.
27. Elias S, Annas GJ. Reproductive genetics and the law. Chicago: Year Book Medical Publishers, 1987.
28. Evans MI, Fletcher JC, Zador IE, Newton BW, Quigg MH, Struyk CD. Selective first-trimester termination in octuplet and quadruplet pregnancies: clinical and ethical issues. Obstet Gynecol 1988;71:289–296.
29. Ruddick W, Wilcox W. Operating on the fetus. Hastings Cent Rep 1982; 12:10–14.
30. Curran CE. Abortion: contemporary debate in philosophical and religious ethics. In: Reich WT, ed. Encyclopedia of bioethics. New York: Macmillan, 1978:17–26.
31. Hellegers AE. Fetal development. Theol Studies 1970;31:3–9.
32. Noonan JT, ed. The morality of abortion. Cambridge, MA: Harvard University Press, 1970.
33. Bopp J, ed. Restoring the right to life: the Human Life Amendment. Provo, UT: Brigham Young University, 1984.
34. Bopp J, ed. Human life and health care ethics. Frederick, MD: University Publications of America, 1985.
35. Noonan JT. A private choice. Abortion in America in the seventies. New York: Free Press, 1979.
36. Callahan S, Callahan D, eds. Abortion: understanding differences. New York: Plenum Press, 1984.
37. Roe v. Wade, 410 US 113 (1973).
38. Chervenak FA, McCullough LB. The fetus as patient: implications for directive versus nondirective counseling for fetal benefit. Fetal Diagn Ther 1991;6:93–100.
39. Fost N, Chudwin D, Wikker D. The limited moral significance of fetal viability. Hastings Cent Rep 1980;10:10–13.
40. Mahowald M. Beyond abortion: refusal of cesarean section. Bioethics 1989;3:106–121.
41. Hack M, Fanaroff AA: Outcomes of extremely-low-birth-weight infants between 1982 and 1988. N Engl J Med 1989;321:1642–1647.
42. Whyte HE, Fitzhardinge PM, Shennan AT, Lennox K, Smith L, Lacy J. External immaturity: outline of 568 pregnancies of 23–26 weeks' gestation. Obstet Gynecol 1993;82:1–7.
43. Chervenak FA, McCullough LB. An ethically justified, clinically comprehensive management strategy for third-trimester pregnancies complicated by fetal anomalies. Obstet Gynecol 1990;75:311–316.
44. Chervenak FA, McCullough LB. Nonaggressive obstetric management: an option for some fetal anomalies during the third trimester. JAMA 1989;261:3430–3439.

45. Chervenak FA, Farley MA, Walters L, Hobbins JC, Mahoney MJ. When is termination of pregnancy during the third trimester morally justifiable? N Engl J Med 1984;310:501–504.
46. Chervenak FA, McCullough LB. Clinical guides to preventing ethical conflicts between pregnant women and their physicians. Am J Obstet Gynecol 1990;162:303–307.
47. Grifo JA, Boyle A, Tang YX, Ward DC. Preimplantation genetic diagnosis. Arch Pathol Lab Med 1992;116:393–397.
48. Wertz DC, Fletcher JC. Ethics and human genetics: a cross-cultural perspective. Heidelberg: Springer-Verlag, 1989.
49. Chervenak FA, McCullough LB. How to critically evaluate positions on obstetric ethics. Reprod Med 1993;38:281–284.
50. Moreno J. Ethics by committee: the moral authority of consensus. J Med Phil 1988;14:411.
51. Rachels J. When philosophers shoot from the hip. Bioethics 1991;5:67.
52. Aristotle: Nichomachean ethics. Indianapolis: Bobbs-Merrill, 1962.

SECTION II

Identification of Risk

Cherry and Merkatz's Complications of Pregnancy,
Fifth Edition, edited by W. R. Cohen.
Lippincott Williams & Wilkins, Philadelphia © 2000.

CHAPTER 5

Prenatal Diagnosis

Sara Kaffe and Meira Shaham

The ability to diagnose genetic diseases in the fetus has improved greatly during the past two decades. Extensive experience has been acquired with ultrasonography and amniocentesis, both of which have become important tools for the diagnosis of congenital abnormalities. The advent of chorionic villus sampling (CVS) made prenatal diagnosis possible in the first trimester, with the opportunity for earlier diagnosis and decision making. The progress in understanding the molecular basis of disease made it possible to develop tests for direct analysis of specific mutations in many disorders. Recently developed techniques allow simultaneous analysis of multiple samples and make possible accurate, rapid testing for disease-causing mutations. Much of the growth in demand for genetic counseling and prenatal diagnosis has resulted from the availability of population-based genetic screening, which provides the patient options for family planning and reproductive alternatives. Carrier testing based on ethnic background or family history (optimally implemented prior to conception) is routinely offered for Tay-Sachs disease, Gaucher's disease, Canavan's disease, and cystic fibrosis (CF) to the Jewish population of northeastern European ancestry, and sickle-cell disease in patients of African origin. Heterozygote screening programs for β- and α-thalassemia are well received in various parts of the Mediterranean and are also appropriate for couples from eastern Asia. When prenatal diagnosis is requested because of a previously affected child or family history of a hereditary disorder, a precise diagnosis is of utmost importance. Only when the specific protein, enzyme, or gene mutation is known can adequate counseling and prenatal testing be provided.

The increasing number of genetic diseases amenable to prenatal diagnosis makes it practically impossible to include all the information in a brief review. The discussion in this chapter will pertain to some common aspects of prenatal diagnosis, focusing primarily on practical issues in prenatal cytogenetic diagnosis and will outline briefly selected topics as they relate to the diagnosis of genetic disease at the DNA level.

TECHNIQUES USED IN PRENATAL DIAGNOSIS

The procedures used for prenatal diagnosis may be classified as invasive and noninvasive. The invasive procedures include amniocentesis, CVS, fetoscopy, and fetal biopsy. These procedures are performed to obtain cells or cell-free amniotic fluid. The common noninvasive procedure, ultrasonography, is especially valuable for the intrauterine diagnosis of a variety of congenital anomalies not associated with known chromosomal or metabolic defects.

S. Kaffe: Private Practice, New York, NY 10021; M. Shaham: Genzyme Genetics, Yonkers, NY 10701.

Amniocentesis

Amniocentesis is the most common means of obtaining amniotic fluid and fetal cells for analysis of a variety of genetic disorders: chromosomal, metabolic, neural tube defects (NTDs), and those detectable by DNA studies. Transabdominal needle aspiration under ultrasonographic guidance can provide 20 to 40 mL of amniotic fluid for cell culture and cell-free fluid. Traditionally, the procedure is performed at 15 to 20 weeks' gestation. At this stage, sufficient amniotic fluid is present and the ratio of viable to nonviable cells is greatest. Because only a small percentage of amniotic fluid cells are viable, and the different cell types grow at different rates, the viable amniotic fluid cells must be cultured to provide sufficient quantities of actively dividing cells for analysis.

The safety, accuracy, and efficacy of amniocentesis has been studied in the United States and Europe (1–6). These studies concluded that the procedure is relatively safe and complications such as fetal injury and bacterial infection are extremely infrequent. The U.S. study documented that rates of fetal loss in amniocentesis and nonrandom controls were not significantly different (3.5% versus 3.2%) (3). Amniocentesis at an earlier stage of pregnancy was reported by several groups (7–9). According to those studies, amniocentesis can be performed at 9 to 14 weeks, when 1 mL of amniotic fluid per gestational week can be withdrawn. Early amniocentesis may provide an alternative for CVS when passage through the cervical canal is not advisable because of cervical-vaginal infections or myomas. It also has an advantage over CVS in that it allows the determination of α-fetoprotein (AFP), which is important for the diagnosis of NTDs, ventral wall defects, and other malformations associated with elevated amniotic fluid α-fetoprotein (AFAFP). However, the safety of early amniocentesis has been debated. Shulman and colleagues (10) and Brumfield and colleagues (11) reported a greater number of complications and pregnancy loss with early amniocentesis when compared with transabdominal CVS and second-trimester amniocentesis. Others also questioned the accuracy of cytogenetic analysis with an increased number of cases of pseudomosaicism (9.9%) and structural anomalies reported (2.8%) (12).

Chorionic Villus Sampling

First-trimester genetic diagnosis by CVS has been developed to overcome the need to wait until the 16th week of pregnancy for prenatal testing. The introduction of CVS permitted the diagnosis of numerous genetic disorders by the use of DNA from fetal tissue samples in the first trimester and reduced the maternal risk when pregnancy termination was chosen. It also made prenatal diagnosis feasible for those ethnic groups in which religious and social objections to mid-trimester amniocentesis made prenatal diagnosis unacceptable, even for families at high risk.

Chorionic villus sampling can be performed by a transcervical or transabdominal approach. Both techniques involve aspiration of chorionic villi under ultrasonographic guidance (13–15). A single good aspiration could yield 10 to 25 mg of wet tissue, which provides abundant material for cytogenetic, enzymatic, and DNA analysis (16–19). Transcervical CVS was first attempted by Hahnemann and Mohr in 1968 (20). Their studies suggested that the 9th to 11th weeks of gestation are the most suitable for obtaining placental biopsy samples.

Chorionic villus sampling is currently performed in an increasing number of specialized centers in the United States and Europe. An international registry, a CVS newsletter, World Health Organization (WHO) sponsorship, and other clinical studies have made it possible to evaluate CVS as a standard fetal-diagnostic approach (21–28). As with amniocentesis, the main considerations were whether the procedure is safe for the patient, the fetus, and continuation of the pregnancy, as well as how accurately the chorionic villi represent the fetal condition. Most published reports have demonstrated that first-trimester diagnosis by CVS is safe and reliable enough to be offered in specialized centers. Comparisons of the transcervical and transabdominal approaches showed no difference in rates of pregnancy loss between the two techniques (2.5% versus 2.3%) (29). Furthermore, a prospective randomized study by Smidt-Jensen and colleagues showed no difference in pregnancy loss between transabdominal CVS and second-trimester amniocentesis (30). In 1991, a report by Firth and colleagues (31) identified five cases of severe limb abnormalities in children whose mothers had CVS at 56 to 66 days of gestation. This report was followed by several others, which raised the concern that previous studies might have missed this specific malformation (32). To address this concern, in 1992 the WHO initiated an international registry of post-CVS limb defects. The analysis of data from 138,996 pregnancies has indicated no increased risk of limb defects after CVS compared with the incidence in the general population (33).

Fetal Blood Sampling, Fetoscopy, and Fetal Biopsy

Prior to the availability of direct DNA analysis, fetal blood sampling was the only method by which sickle cell anemia, thalassemia, and hemophilia A could be diagnosed prenatally (34). At present, fetal blood sampling does not require fetoscopy. It is performed by ultrasound-directed percutaneous umbilical cord blood sampling (PUBS) at 18 to 20 weeks. Fetal blood sampling can help distinguish most cases of true mosaicism from pseudomosaicism in amniotic fluid cultures. It also can be used when workup is initiated late in the second trimester and there is a need for rapid karyotyping, or in twin pregnancies (with a single amniotic sac), where it may be especially important when one twin is found to be abnormal by ultrasonographic evaluation (35,36).

Fetoscopic visualization has facilitated sampling of fetal skin and liver for diagnoses that could not be made by cytogenetic or biochemical analysis of cultured amniotic cells or amniotic fluid (37–39). It is known to cause complications to both fetus and mother and carries a high rate of sampling failure. Even experienced fetoscopists have reported a 5% risk of spontaneous abortion within 48 hours of the procedure and a 2% to 4% risk for prematurity. Amniotic fluid leakage occurs in about 4% of cases.

The introduction of DNA technology and direct gene analysis for prenatal diagnosis has significantly decreased the need for fetoscopic sampling. Fetal liver biopsies were used in the past for the diagnosis of disorders resulting from the deficiency of liver-specific enzymes such as ornithine transcarbamylase deficiency (OTC), phenylketonuria (PKU), and glycogen storage disease type I (Von Gierke's disease) (40,41). Most of these disorders can now be diagnosed by DNA techniques if the specific mutation is known. Approximately 90 different mutations associated with OTC deficiency have been identified (42,43), and an even larger number of mutations are known for PKU (44–46). Some of the mutations seem to be recurrent, but the majority are private mutations; therefore, family studies of the affected and carrier status of the parents are essential before prenatal diagnosis is attempted. Once a mutation is identified, prenatal diagnosis can be offered.

At present, fetoscopy is limited to prenatal diagnosis of severe congenital autosomal-recessive forms of epidermolysis bullosa and ichthyosis, which require morphologic examination of fetal skin (47–50). Bakharev and colleagues (51) have reported that fetal skin biopsies can be successfully obtained by an endoscopic needle introduced transabdominally under ultrasonographic guidance. This procedure might reduce the unfavorable outcome in pregnancies at risk for the various genodermatoses as well.

Ultrasonography

State-of-the-art real-time ultrasound scanners provide detailed dynamic images of the fetus. In a routine level I examination, when no fetal abnormality is suspected, gestational age is assessed by measurement of the biparietal diameter and femur length. Confirmation of multiple gestations, assessment of the quantity of amniotic fluid, and localization of the placenta are also performed. A discrepancy in any one of these parameters or the detection of a gross fetal abnormality are indications for additional diagnostic evaluation.

Level II scans are performed to evaluate pregnancies in which an abnormality is suspected or prenatal diagnosis is indicated. High-resolution ultrasonography has led to the rapid expansion of the number of diagnoses that can be made by indirect visual evaluation of the fetal anatomy. Abnormalities such as small facial clefts, polydactyly, and defects in the fetal spine can be visualized (52). Disproportionate growth can be readily assessed for the prenatal diagnosis of skeletal dysplasias (53). Filling and emptying of the fetal bladder in response to maternal diuretic ingestion can be used to assess the functional integrity of the fetal urinary tract. The need for amniocentesis has been the subject of ongoing debate when choroid plexus cysts are seen on ultrasonographic examination because of the association with trisomy (54). Generally, the finding of more than one anomaly increases the risk of a chromosome abnormality, in which case amniocentesis should be offered for cytogenetic studies.

Fetal gender can be determined by about 20 menstrual weeks. In cases in which sex determination is performed for diagnostic reasons (e.g., prenatal diagnosis of X-linked disorders), ultrasonographic determination of sex is suggestive but not conclusive. Karyotype confirmation of fetal gender must be performed in these cases.

The simultaneous use of ultrasonography with other prenatal diagnostic techniques has reduced the associated risk and facilitated the performance of these procedures. Ultrasonographic localization of the placenta, fetus, and amniotic fluid pool prior to amniocentesis has reduced the number of bloody taps. It has also made the assessment of twin pregnancies by amniocentesis feasible. When fetoscopy is performed, ultrasonographic localization of the placenta, cord, and head significantly shortens the time of the procedure and improves fetal tissue sampling. Ultrasonography is also used for visual guidance during chorionic villus biopsy.

Fetal echocardiography has been successful in diagnosing congenital heart disease and dysrhythmias (55). Both M-mode and real-time echocardiograms may be necessary for adequate interpretation of cardiac anatomy (56). Serial echocardiography is performed at mid-gestation on fetuses with a family history of congenital heart disease as well as for the evaluation of fetal ascites and dysrhythmias appreciated by auscultation of fetal heart tones. The association of maternal nongestational diabetes and congenital heart disease makes this group of high-risk patients candidates for fetal echocardiography. Echocardiography also should be performed as part of a complete diagnostic evaluation of fetuses found to have a major structural anomaly, such as an omphalocele. The finding of additional malformations may alert physicians to the possibility of a chromosomal anomaly and optimize intrapartum decision making. The rapid development of high-resolution ultrasonography has made other forms of radiologic imaging virtually obsolete. Amniography, using water-soluble dye to outline the fetus, and fetography, which uses a fat-soluble dye that is miscible with the vernix caseosa, have been replaced by safer, noninvasive ultrasonography.

INDICATIONS FOR PRENATAL CYTOGENETIC DIAGNOSIS

Advanced Maternal Age

Of requests for prenatal diagnosis, more than 90% are for the diagnosis of chromosome abnormalities in the fetus by cytogenetic techniques. The risk of having a child with trisomy 21, trisomy 18, trisomy 13, and sex chromosome aneuploidies such as 47,XXX or 47,XXY increases with maternal age as a result of the increased tendency toward meiotic nondisjunction in oogenesis (57–59). It was suggested by Hook and Cross that an association exists between maternal age and supernumerary marker chromosomes (60). Advanced maternal age is therefore the most common indication for cytogenetic prenatal diagnosis.

The criteria for determining at what age to offer amniocentesis were derived largely from several surveys (61,62). Most centers in the United States now offer amniocentesis to women who will be over 35 at the time of delivery. However, this cutoff reflects the age at which the risks for the procedure are balanced by the risks of finding an abnormality. Increasing numbers of younger patients request amniocentesis because of maternal anxiety. Table 5-1 lists estimated maternal age-specific risks for trisomy 21 and other chromosome anomalies. It has been estimated by Hook and colleagues that 30% of trisomy 21, 68% of trisomy 18, and 43% of trisomy 13 fetuses are lost during the first half of pregnancy. This accounts for the greater detection rate of chromosome abnormalities at prenatal diagnosis (CVS and amniocentesis) than at term (63).

Balanced Structural Rearrangements in One Parent

Structural aberrations are derived from chromosome breakage and rearrangement or unequal crossing over at meiosis. A balanced structural rearrangement implies that the entire genome is present but certain chromosomes are structurally rearranged. An individual with a balanced translocation is at risk for recurrent abortions, infertility, or phenotypically abnormal offspring. The risk of having a chromosomally unbalanced fetus depends on three contributing factors: (a) the type of structural rearrangement, (b) the specific chromosome involved with specific breakpoints on the chromosomes in question, and (c) whether the balanced rearrangement is maternal or paternal in origin.

Reciprocal Translocation

A reciprocal translocation results from the exchange of segments between two nonhomologous chromosomes, or two homologous chromosomes at different breakpoints. If no genetic material is lost or duplicated, the translocation is balanced, and the individual is phenotypically normal. However, such an individual is at increased risk for early miscarriages, stillbirths, or offspring with malformation syndromes because of the formation of gametes with unbalanced chromosome complements. At meiosis I, the four chromosomes with segments in common form a quadrivalent (Fig. 5-1). When the first meiotic cell divi-

TABLE 5-1. *Maternal age-specific risks for chromosome anomalies: incidence in live born, amniocentesis, and CVS*

	% in live born[a]		% at amniocentesis[b]				% at CVS[c]
Maternal age (yr)	47, + 21	All chromosome abnormalities	47, + 21	47, + 18	47, + 13	All chromosome anomalies	All chromosome anomalies
33	0.16	0.29	0.24	0.06	0.04	0.50	—
34	0.20	0.36	0.31	0.08	0.04	0.65	—
35	0.26	0.49	0.40	0.10	0.05	0.76	0.78
36	0.33	0.60	0.52	0.13	0.06	0.97	0.80
37	0.44	0.77	0.67	0.16	0.06	1.21	2.58
38	0.57	0.97	0.87	0.21	0.07	1.54	3.82
39	0.73	1.23	1.12	0.26	0.09	1.95	2.67
40	0.94	1.59	1.45	0.33	0.10	2.50	3.40
41	1.23	2.00	1.89	0.42	0.11	3.10	6.11
42	1.56	2.56	2.41	0.53	0.13	4.00	8.05
43	2.00	3.33	3.11	0.66	0.15	5.25	5.15
44	2.63	4.17	4.00	0.84	0.18	6.60	10.00
45	3.33	5.26	5.18	1.06	0.20	8.30	7.14

[a]Estimated live-born statistics (59).
[b]Adapted from Hook EB. Chromosome abnormalities and spontaneous fetal death following amniocentesis. Further data and associations with maternal age. Am J Hum Genet 1983;35:110–116.
[c]Data derived from Mikkelsen M, Ayme S. Cytogenetic findings in chorionic villi. A collaborative study. Presented at the 7th International Congress of Human Genetics, Berlin, 1986.

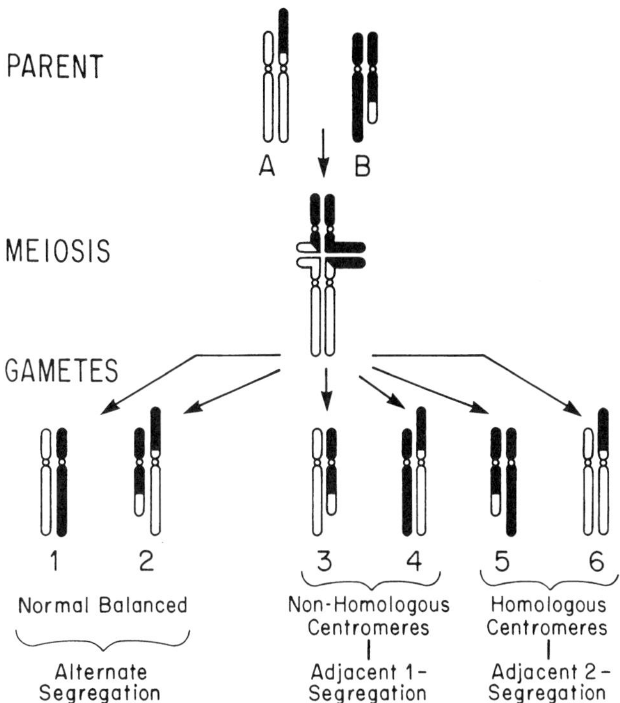

FIG. 5-1. Inheritance of reciprocal translocations. The meiotic segregation in the germ cells of a balanced translocation carrier indicates how the six major types of gametes may be produced. The translocation chromosomes and their homologues form a quadrivalent configuration in meiotic prophase I. Subsequently, these chromosomes segregate in different combinations outlined. (From Wilson JG, Fraser FC, eds. Handbook of teratology. Vol 2. Mechanisms and pathogenesis. New York: Plenum Press, 1977:56.)

sion occurs, the four chromosomes may be distributed to the two daughter cells in a number of ways. When two chromosomes go to one cell and two to the other, it is referred to as 2:2 segregation. Of the possible combinations, four will have a duplication or deficiency of chromosome material in their daughter cells, one will have a normal constitution, and one will contain the balanced translocation like the parent. When the balanced translocation detected in the fetus is identical to that in the parent, most geneticists would believe it to confer no increased risk of phenotypic abnormalities in the fetus. Although a submicroscopic rearrangement at the breakpoints cannot be excluded, it would be extremely exceptional. In 3:1 segregation (or 3:1 nondisjunction), three chromosomes go to one daughter cell and only one to the other. This rare mode of segregation results in the formation of gametes with 24 and 22 chromosomes, and the fetal cells will have 47 or 45 chromosomes. The 4:0 segregants are never viable.

The overall risk of a reciprocal translocation carrier to have a child with an unbalanced chromosome complement depends on the mode of ascertainment of the family, the predicted type of segregation leading to the viable gamete, the size of the chromosome segment involved, and the sex of the transmitting parent. Boué and Gallano (64) and Daniel and colleagues (65) suggested risk estimates of 10% to 13%, whether maternal or paternal in origin. In a subsequent analysis (66), Daniel and colleagues derived figures of approximately 20% for female and 24% for male carriers to have an offspring with an unbalanced karyotype when ascertainment of the parental translocation was through a previous child with an unbalanced karyotype, and 3.5% and 1.5%, respectively, when ascertainment was through recurrent miscarriage. When parental translocation was detected incidentally, the risk for an unbalanced karyotype was about 5%. Slightly higher overall risk figures were presented by Mikkelsen and Ayme, who detected 17 unbalanced progeny in a CVS study group that included 75 carrier parents (25).

Robertsonian Translocation

A Robertsonian or centric fusion translocation results from breakage and rearrangement of two acrocentric chromosomes in their centromere region. Individuals with a balanced Robertsonian translocation therefore have 45 chromosomes in each cell, with the translocation chromosome containing two complete long arms and no short arms. The loss of short arms appears not to be clinically significant, and individuals with such translocations are usually phenotypically normal. The most frequent balanced Robertsonian translocation is der(13;14), which occurs in approximately 1:1,500 live births and is followed by der(14;21) at a frequency of 1:5,000 live births. Carriers of such balanced translocations are at risk for producing abnormal offspring. Depending on the chromosomes involved, the risk may vary from 2% to 100% (Table 5-2). Robertsonian translocations involving chromosomes 21 and 13 have been implicated in about 5% of newborns with Down syndrome and approximately 20% of those with trisomy 13.

TABLE 5-2. *Risk for abnormal offspring in carriers of balanced Robertsonian translocations.*

Translocation	Carrier	% Risk
der(21;21)	Either parent	100
der(22;22)	Either parent	100
der(21;22)	Either parent	5
der(14;22)	Mother	10
	Father	4
der(13;14)	Mother	2
	Father	0
der(14;21)	Mother	14
	Father	0

Adapted from Milunsky A. Genetic disorders and the fetus. New York: Plenum Press, 1979: Boué A, Gallan P. A collaborative study of the segregation of inherited chromosome structural rearrangements in 1356 prenatal diagnoses. Prenat Diagn 1984;4 (special issue):45–47; Mikkelsen M, Ayme S. Cytogenetic findings in chorionic villi. A collaborative study. Presented at the 7th International Congress of Human Genetics, Berlin, 1986.

Inversion

An inversion involves two breaks within a chromosome and subsequent rejoining of the segments in reverse. The normal banding pattern is altered, as is the order (i.e., linkage) of the genes in the chromosome. If the centromere is included in the segment between the breaks, the inversion is termed pericentric. If the segment is on one side of the centromere, the inversion is termed paracentric. Individuals carrying an inversion are phenotypically normal. They are at risk for abnormal offspring as a consequence of crossing over during meiosis, which may result in duplication or deficiency of chromosomal material. The risk for an inversion carrier to have an offspring with an abnormal karyotype was reported to be 5% to 9% in one survey (64) and 10% to 15% according to a survey by Daniel and colleagues (66). Prenatal diagnosis should be recommended to couples when one is a carrier, with the exception of inversion of chromosome 9, which involves only the secondary constriction region, and is considered a chromosome heteromorphism with no clinical significance.

Previous Child with Chromosome Abnormality

The history of a previous pregnancy with a *de novo* chromosome aneuploidy increases the risk for the same or different chromosome abnormality in future pregnancies to 1% to 2% if the mother is under 35 years of age (67). Statistical data indicate that women over 35 maintain the age-related risk figures, regardless of past history. Prenatal diagnosis also should be considered following a pregnancy with a *de novo* structural rearrangement because of the possibility of parental gonadal mosaicism.

Maternal Serum Multiple Marker Screening for Chromosome Anomalies

The association between low maternal serum α-fetoprotein (MSAFP) level and autosomal trisomies, particularly Down syndrome, was first noted by Merkatz and colleagues in 1984 (68) and documented repeatedly since then (69–73). In 1987, Bogart and coworkers reported that the maternal serum human chorionic gonadotropin (MS-hCG) level is elevated in pregnancies with Down syndrome (74–76). Others have reported an elevated MS-hCG level with sex-chromosome aneuploidy and decreased MS-hCG level in cases of trisomy 18 (77). Some suggestion was made that the beta subunit of hCG is a more accurate indicator than total hCG (78). Another analyte, maternal serum unconjugated estriol (MS-uE3), was reported to be low in both Down syndrome and trisomy 18 (79). In an attempt to improve the detection rate of chromosome anomalies, Haddow and colleagues (80) recommended the use of multiple-marker screening, which could lead to the detection of 60% of Down syndrome as compared with a 15% to 20% detection rate by MSAFP alone. Although there is still no uniformly accepted protocol for second-trimester maternal serum screening, the most widely used are the combination of MSAFP and hCG, or a triple screen including MSAFP, hCG, and uE3. Variables that affect MSAFP are age, weight (dilution factor), ethnic background (black women have an MSAFP level about 10% higher than that of white or Asian women), and other factors such as insulin-dependent diabetes (15% lower values). For most gestational ages, median AFP, hCG, and uE3 levels for white, black, Asian, and Hispanic women have now been established (81). Because all three analytes are gestational-age dependent, it is essential to confirm or revise the gestational age by ultrasonography in order to calculate accurately the adjusted risk. Repeat sampling is not recommended in Down syndrome screening. An initial positive result when gestational age has been confirmed should be followed by counseling and consideration of amniocentesis. Cytogenetic prenatal diagnosis is now recommended to younger women whose risk for Down syndrome is equal to or greater than the age-related risk of a 35-year-old (i.e., 1:270) (82).

Most laboratories now process serum samples at 14 to 20 weeks' gestation, and both the American College of Obstetricians and Gynecologists and the American College of Medical Genetics have issued guidelines recommending that women who are not at increased risk because of their age should be counseled as to the purpose of the test and its limitations and should be offered testing with the understanding that the test does not guarantee the birth of a normal baby, but serves as a screen to make amniocentesis accessible for further diagnostic testing in younger women at risk (83).

A number of additional biochemical markers in serum and urine are being evaluated for their potential for prenatal screening. Dimeric inhibin-A in serum as well as degradation products in maternal urine have been reported (84). The combination of free βhCG with pregnancy associated plasma protein A (PAPP-A) holds promise to become a suitable screen for Down syndrome during the first trimester (85).

Previous Stillborn or Spontaneous Abortion

About 40% of first-trimester spontaneous abortuses and 5% of stillborn infants have a chromosome abnormality (86). Couples who experience recurrent abortions or have a history of a stillborn or malformed child should undergo cytogenetic studies to rule out the possibility that one of the partners is a carrier of a balanced translocation or inversion that predisposes them to frequent pregnancy loss or phenotypically abnormal offspring. If abortuses or stillborn infants in prior pregnancies were known to have a chromosome abnormality, prenatal diagnosis should be offered. However, because chromosome analysis is rarely performed on abortion tissue or stillborn infants, it might be of benefit to offer prenatal cytogenetic diagnosis even when no aneuploidy was documented.

Parental Aneuploidy

Individuals with numerical chromosome abnormalities can be functionally fertile but are at an increased risk of having abnormal offspring. Bovicelli and colleagues (87) have listed 27 reports of women with Down syndrome having given birth. In that group the ratio of Down syndrome to normal offspring was 10 to 17. No male with Down syndrome has ever been reported to be a father. Parental trisomy 21 mosaicism was found in both mothers and fathers of trisomy 21 patients, and it was also reported for trisomy 18 (86–88). These individuals usually are first documented because they have had more than one child with autosomal trisomy, and less frequently because they have subtle phenotypic features suggestive of Down syndrome. Prenatal diagnosis is advisable for these individuals, even though no accurate risk figures can be provided. Infertility is practically inevitable in Klinefelter syndrome (47, XXY) and very common in Turner syndrome (45,X). However, a parent may have a sex chromosome aneuploidy that does not affect fertility, such as 47,XXX or 47,XYY. These abnormalities are usually not associated with any increased risk for chromosomally abnormal offspring. Mosaic forms of sex chromosome anomalies may result in chromosome abnormalities in the fetus, and amniocentesis is therefore recommended.

Disorders of DNA Repair and Chromosome Breakage

Several disorders inherited in an autosomal-recessive manner have an underlying defect of DNA repair and are characterized by chromosome breakage *in vivo* and *in vitro.* Included in this group are Fanconi's anemia, ataxia telangiectasia, Bloom syndrome, xeroderma pigmentosum, and others. The prenatal diagnosis of Fanconi's anemia is based on an increased number of chromosome breaks induced by diepoxybutane in an affected fetus as compared with normal controls (89). The chromosome preparations from ataxia telangiectasia exhibit a wide range of chromosome abnormalities. They are diagnosable by a combined scoring of spontaneous breakage and the clastogenic effect of culture media in which the at-risk amniotic fluid cells were grown on normal lymphocytes (90).

Bloom syndrome can be diagnosed by the increased frequency of sister chromatid exchanges in cultured amniotic fluid cells (91). In xeroderma pigmentosum, DNA repair mechanisms are faulty, but no abnormality is detected at the cytogenetic level.

DNA studies have identified the genes responsible for some Fanconi's anemia subgroups, ataxia telangiestasia, and Bloom syndrome. A number of mutations were identified in patients with these disorders. Further characterization of the mutations involved should allow for carrier identification as well as prenatal diagnosis (92–94). At present, cytogenetic analysis in combination with DNA tests are being attempted.

PRACTICAL PROBLEMS IN PRENATAL CYTOGENETIC DIAGNOSIS

Greater than 99% accuracy is achieved in prenatal cytogenetic diagnosis. Patients should nonetheless be aware that the procedure is not infallible. Amniotic fluid cells may not grow, requiring a repeat amniocentesis. Routine microscopy cannot always detect small amounts of missing or additional chromosomal material. Studies such as fluorescence *in situ* hybridization (FISH) may be helpful for more conclusive evaluation when subtle deletions are suspected. FISH is a technique in which cloned DNA sequences are labeled with fluorescent tags and then hybridized to chromosome preparations and visualized under a microscope. FISH probes consisting of cocktails of chromosome-specific DNA probes also allow for whole chromosomes to be painted. Thus, it has become a powerful diagnostic tool when routine cytogenetic methods are insufficient. When ultrasonographic findings suggest a specific microdeletion syndrome, such as the group of velo-cardio-facial syndromes, specific probes may be used to detect the suspected deletion.

Maternal Cell Contamination

Both amniotic fluid and chorionic villus samples may occasionally include maternal cells because of the way these samples are obtained. Maternal cell contamination (MCC) is usually identified when an admixture of male and female cells is observed in one culture. A European collaborative study gave an admixture detection incidence of 0.315% (95), and data from several North American laboratories suggest a detection rate of 0.23% (2,5,96). Because contamination of female cultures will usually go unnoticed, the actual frequency should be estimated as twice that observed with male fetuses alone. Amniotic fluid cultures affected by MCC may yield a variable proportion of maternal to fetal cells and are therefore a potential source of error in prenatal diagnosis. At least four cases of trisomy 21 were misdiagnosed and considered normal because of an overgrowth of maternal cells in culture, whereas in others the wrong fetal sex was determined (86).

The following recommendations were made to reduce the occurrence rate of MCC with amniocentesis:

1. Amniocentesis should be performed under ultrasonographic monitoring.
2. A small-gauge (21-gauge) needle with stylet in place should be used.

3. The first few milliliters of amniotic fluid should be discarded, and the syringe changed to obtain fluid for culture.

When suspecting MCC, it may be useful to obtain the mother's karyotype in order to compare chromosome polymorphisms of maternal blood cells with those of the female fetal cells. This will allow identification of maternal cells in most instances. It is also important to exclude the possibility of a twin pregnancy or the extremely rare possibility of chimerism (97).

The risk for MCC has been a major concern in CVS prenatal diagnosis as well. During the first years of experience with CVS, there were numerous reports of discrepancies between the chromosome complement of the villi and those of the fetus. Tissue culture trials by Simoni showed occasional overgrowth of maternal cells resulting in a female karyotype in a male fetus (98,99). This has been reduced considerably by careful dissection of visible decidual tissue and microscopic identification of chorionic fetal tissue (16,100) and the use of direct preparations for chromosome analysis if sufficient material is available (101,102). The direct method produces metaphases from actively mitotic cells that are found in villi and not in maternal decidua, thus carrying a lesser risk for MCC compared with the long-term cultures. Although some investigators did not find cultivation time a significant determining factor for MCC (103), the vast majority of reported cases were in long-term CVS cultures in which as many as 10% of cases were involved (104). The current recommendations therefore include both direct CVS preparation and long-term culture for cytogenetic analysis, as well as comparison of chromosome polymorphism of the XX cells in CVS to maternal chromosomes if MCC is suspected.

Chromosome Mosaicism

Chromosomal mosaicism is defined as the presence of two or more distinct cell lines of different karyotypes in an individual. When different cells from amniotic fluid culture show different chromosome complements (usually one normal and one abnormal), interpretation is important because true chromosome mosaicism can be the cause of abnormal development in the fetus, whereas pseudomosaicism does not have clinical significance.

Criteria for diagnosis of true (i.e., constitutional) mosaicism were first defined by Boué and colleagues in 1979 (105). They suggested that true mosaicism should be diagnosed only when two cell populations with different karyotypes are detected in at least two independent cell cultures. When cells with an abnormal chromosome complement are found in only one culture and two additional cultures show only normal chromosome complements, pseudomosaicism is assumed. Most likely the cells with abnormal karyotype arose in culture and are of no clinical significance, whether a single cell or multiple cells are found in the one culture vessel. The risk that a case diagnosed as pseudomosaicism actually represents a true mosaic is not known. Benn and colleagues have estimated that a minimum of 7% of true mosaics could be misdiagnosed as pseudomosaicism, and about 4.5% of true mosaics may go completely undetected, even when the currently required protocols for cytogenetic prenatal diagnosis are followed (106). Repeat amniocentesis is not helpful in resolving this issue. A normal second result does not make the first result invalid, and when the first mosaic result is duplicated, it could represent resampling of the same extraembryonal tissue. Fetal blood sampling may be more useful in resolving such a situation. It must be emphasized, however, that true mosaicism can never be ruled out completely. Hsu and colleagues proposed laboratory guidelines for diagnosis of chromosome mosaicism in amniocytes based on a series of 22,000 cases and review of the literature (107). They recommended that emphasis be placed on autosomes known to be associated with phenotypic abnormalities. They concluded that genetic counseling be provided for cases with established chromosome mosaicism and information regarding single-cell/single-colony pseudomosaicism be retained in the laboratory.

The importance of timing the event that leads to mosaicism has been extensively reviewed by Kalousek, who suggested a distinction of three different types of constitutional chromosome mosaicism: (a) generalized mosaicism involving all tissues of the conceptus (i.e., embryo, fetus, and placenta) and tissue-specific chromosome mosaicism, which can be (b) confined to the placenta, or (c) confined to the embryo (108,109). Generalized chromosome mosaicism arises when an error in cell division occurs in the first or second postzygotic division, affecting all fetal tissues and detectable in amniotic fluid and fetal blood cells. This type of mosaicism often results in an abnormal phenotype and has been described in most autosomal trisomies, as well as sex chromosome trisomies and monosomy X.

The existence of confined placental mosaicism (CPM) in the placentas of full-term infants with unexplained intrauterine growth retardation was recognized before the introduction of CVS as a prenatal diagnostic test (108, 110,111). CPM is most commonly considered when a diagnosis of chromosome mosaicism is made on a CVS sample, but not found in confirmatory studies of amniotic fluid or umbilical blood sampling. CPM may account for some cases of pseudomosaicism and discrepancy in pregnancy outcome. The most common aneuploidy observed with CPM is trisomy 16. Other frequently reported cases involve trisomies 2, 7, 9, 15, and 22.

Confined placental mosaicism can be the result of a mitotic error after fertilization occurring in the trophoblast or extraembryonic mesoderm progenitor cells. Alternatively, it may derive from an originally trisomic conceptus that has undergone selective loss of the extra chromosome in some, but not all, cells (zygote rescue). Theoretically, one third of such "trisomic rescue" cases may have a chromosome pair in which both chromosomes originate from the same parent. This is defined as *uniparental disomy* (maternal or paternal) and may be the cause of phenotypic abnormality even though the karyotype appears normal. Today, it is recognized that the phenotypic outcome of a prenatally diagnosed trisomy mosaic may be influenced by the potential effects of uniparental disomy because some genes are preferentially expressed depending on whether they are maternally or paternally inherited. This phenomenon is known as *genomic imprinting* (112).

Three large surveys of chromosome mosaicism in amniotic fluid cultures, with data compiled from close to 119,000 amniocenteses, were published in 1984 (113–115). The frequency of true mosaicism was established to be 0.1% to 0.3% and did not differ whether a closed flask system with trypsinized cells or open petri dishes and *in situ* harvesting were used. The frequency of multiple-cell pseudomosaicism ranged from 0.64% in a U.S. survey to 1.1% in a Canadian study. [All three groups reported even higher frequency rates for pseudomosaicism when only a single cell with a chromosome abnormality was detected (2.4–7.0%).]

The most frequent autosomal trisomy considered to occur as an *in vitro* event (pseudomosaicism) is trisomy 2, followed by trisomy 20, trisomy 17, and trisomy 7 (86). Follow-up of these cases at birth has revealed no phenotypic abnormalities. True mosaicism involving an autosome accounts for close to 50% of all mosaic cases diagnosed in amniocytes. Fetuses with true mosaicism involving trisomy of chromosomes 21, 8, 9, 13, and 18 appear to be phenotypically abnormal and compatible with the respective clinical syndromes. Trisomy 20, which is the most frequently diagnosed true autosomal mosaicism, is unique because it is usually associated with an apparently normal phenotype (85%). The cases that did present with phenotypic abnormalities showed no consistent pattern of malformations. Thus, it is likely that they represent a fortuitous association, rather than a well-defined syndrome. Fetal blood sampling is not helpful for further evaluation of trisomy 20 mosaic pregnancies because the trisomic cells do not appear in blood. They have been recovered from specific fetal tissues such as kidney, lung, and esophagus (116). Similar situations can be seen with trisomies 9 and 17, as well as tetrasomy 12p, which is known as Palister-Killian syndrome.

Karyotype/phenotype correlations of rare trisomy mosaicism cases were recently reported by Hsu and colleagues (117). Mosaic autosomal monosomy was diagnosed prenatally in 13 cases (Hsu, personal communication). Autosomal monosomy is usually considered pseudomosaicism, but rare cases with abnormal phenotypic outcome have been reported.

The most commonly diagnosed sex chromosome mosaics are 45,X/46,XX, 46,XX/47,XXX, 46,XY/47,XXY, and 45,X/46,XY. With the exception of 45,X/46,XY, all other sex chromosome mosaicism detected in amniotic fluid culture reflected true fetal mosaicism. The percentage of notable dysmorphology in sex chromosome mosaicism is generally lower when compared with autosomal mosaicism. Special attention needs to be given to 45,X/46,XY mosaicism. Although postnatally diagnosed cases of 45,X/46,XY present a spectrum of phenotypic abnormalities ranging from mixed gonadal dysgenesis to phenotypic female, most cases diagnosed prenatally (90%) resulted in phenotypically normal male newborns (118,119). Ultrasonographic visualization of male external genitalia might be used as an additional diagnostic test for prenatal sex determination in these fetuses.

Cytogenetic errors and inconclusive results are more common with CVS than with amniocentesis. Discrepancies between CVS findings and the fetal karyotype can be attributed to the fact that chorionic villus samples may contain extraembryonic tissue only, and that chromosome mosaicism can be confined to placental tissue or chorionic tissue, thus not reflecting the actual fetal status (108,109). A possible nonrandom involvement of certain chromosomes in forming mosaic trisomies has been suggested in several studies. The chromosomes most frequently involved in numerical aberrations were chromosomes 18, 16, 3, 13, and 7. Other abnormal cell lines frequently observed were 45,X and tetraploidy. In these situations the patient frequently has to undergo additional testing by amniocentesis or fetal blood sampling to distinguish true mosaicism from pseudomosaicism.

De Novo Structural Rearrangement

Although chromosome analysis of cultured amniotic fluid cells (and to a lesser degree CVS) has been used for many years, there are still occasions when the clinical significance of certain findings is not clear. The most obvious examples of such difficulties are the *de novo* structural rearrangements and the *de novo* marker chromosomes.

The term *de novo* implies that the chromosome aberration is present in fetal cells while both parents have apparently normal karyotypes. The rate of all *de novo* abnormalities diagnosed at amniocentesis was reported to be 2 per 1,000 (120). This included 1 per 1,000 *de novo* balanced rearrangements, 0.5 per 1,000 *de novo* unbalanced structural rearrangements, and about 0.5 per 1,000 *de novo* markers. These frequencies are slightly greater than rates reported in the newborn, probably because some abnormal conceptions are lost during pregnancy (121,122).

De novo structural chromosome rearrangements may be balanced or unbalanced. Unbalanced rearrangements have a visible deletion or show additional chromosomal material. Abnormal outcome can therefore be predicted even when the origin of the extra material cannot be identified. It is nevertheless important to determine (using a special staining technique) that the segment involved is actually euchromatin and not heterochromatin, which does not have an obvious effect on the phenotype.

When an apparently balanced *de novo* structural rearrangement is detected, the outcome is difficult to predict. There is a possibility that a submicroscopic deletion or duplication, undetectable at the level of resolution achieved by currently used cytogenetic techniques, may be overlooked. Several studies in newborns have suggested that balanced *de novo* rearrangements can be associated with an increased risk of mental retardation and physical abnormalities. This is especially true with non-Robertsonian translocations (121,122). When a *de novo* X-autosome translocation is detected, the recombinant chromosome may contain the X-inactivation center, and the inactivation can spread into the autosomal segment, resulting in chromosomal imbalance and phenotypic abnormalities.

Warburton has collected information on breakpoints and outcome of *de novo* balanced rearrangements ascertained through amniocentesis, including only malformations recognizable at birth or fetal autopsy (123,124). A risk estimate of 8% to 10% of an offspring with phenotypic abnormalities was derived. *De novo* balanced Robertsonian translocations are usually associated with normal phenotypic outcome.

Recent studies suggest that an unusually high proportion of the *de novo* structural rearrangements are of paternal origin. Using multiple staining techniques and heterochromatin markers to establish the parental origin of rearranged chromosomes, Olson and Magenis (125) determined that of 32 cases, 27 (84%) were paternal in origin and only 5 (16%) were maternal.

Supernumerary Marker Chromosomes

Marker chromosomes comprise a mixed collection of structurally rearranged chromosomal regions, usually unidentifiable by routine cytogenetic techniques. Chromosome fragments that do not retain a centromere are usually lost during meiosis or mitosis. Those that do retain a centromere may segregate as supernumerary marker chromosomes. Because markers have been detected in normal individuals as well as patients with dysmorphic features and mental retardation, they pose a serious problem in counseling and decision making when detected in cultured amniotic fluid cells or CVS. The incidence of prenatal diagnosis of supernumerary marker chromosomes varies from 0.6 to 1.5 per 1,000 (126–128). Some are inherited and others are *de novo* in nature. The marker may be present in all cells or be limited to only a portion of cells (mosaic).

About half the markers are satellited or bisatellited. This means that they have derived from the short arm regions of the acrocentric autosomes (126) and therefore suggest a better prognosis than markers without satellites.

A review of the literature suggests that in most inherited cases and in some of the nonfamilial cases, the additional material has no apparent phenotypic effect (124, 127). However, some of the nonfamilial cases have been associated with malformation syndromes or neurologic and behavioral problems. Therefore, when a supernumerary marker is diagnosed in amniotic fluid, it is important to perform a chromosome analysis of parental blood, regardless of the characteristics of the marker, so that proper counseling can be provided. If one parent carries the marker chromosome, it can be assumed that there is no increased risk of fetal abnormalities. When neither parent is a carrier, the marker is considered *de novo,* and the outcome of such a pregnancy is more difficult to predict. Various attempts have been made to correlate phenotypic outcome to staining characteristics of the marker. Several markers have been identified as inversion duplication of chromosome 15. These markers have been associated with mental retardation and seizures. Other metacentric markers were considered to be isochromosomes derived from the short arms of chromosome 12 or 18 (129). In most cases it is now possible to determine the origin of the supernumerary marker by using the FISH technique. However, the clinical implications cannot always be predicted. Several ongoing surveys have suggested risk figures for abnormal outcome of about 10% to 14%, regardless of whether mosaicism for the abnormal cell line was found. It is our impression that a fragmentlike marker, with mostly centromeric heterochromatin, generally carries a better prognosis and that the extent of euchromatic material rather than the presence or absence of satellites per se is the crucial factor in determining the deleterious effect of a *de novo* marker.

Tetraploidy

Tetraploidy is observed frequently in cultured amniotic fluid cells, with frequencies of 10% to 80% reported. Several published cases of liveborns with tetraploidy mosaicism have aroused some concern (130), but most cytogeneticists consider tetraploidy to be an *in vitro* event that has no clinical significance.

CONGENITAL DISORDERS ASSOCIATED WITH ELEVATED AFP

Elevated Amniotic Fluid AFP

Brock and Sutcliffe first observed elevated amniotic fluid α-fetoprotein (AFAFP) concentrations in a pregnancy in which the fetus had an open NTD (131). Confirmation of this observation soon followed from many other laboratories, and the AFP assay was introduced as a routine test for prenatal diagnosis of open NTDs (132).

Alpha-fetoprotein, a major protein in fetal serum by the third month of gestation, is measured immunologically in cell-free amniotic fluid. Its structure is similar to that of albumin in molecular weight and charge, but it has a different primary configuration and is antigenically distinct. Its gene is located on chromosome 4, and the primary structure was extensively studied by the use of cDNA clones. It is synthesized in the yolk sac, gastrointestinal tract, and fetal liver and can be detected as early as 30 days after conception. Fetal serum AFP is normally filtered by the fetal kidney and excreted into the amniotic fluid with peak concentrations of AFAFP reached at 13 weeks' gestation, then decreasing by about 10% a week until 20 weeks' gestation and declining steadily thereafter to become almost undetectable by 30 weeks' gestation. Normal ranges for AFAFP have been established for each week of gestation. Because greater than 95% of NTDs occur sporadically, AFP levels are now determined routinely in every amniotic fluid sample regardless of the indication for the tap.

The recurrence rate for an NTD following the birth of an affected child has been determined to be about 2%, and following the birth of two previously affected children about 6%. No reliable recurrence risks can be given for an affected parent because some studies included parents with spina bifida occulta, which is associated with a normal AFAFP. A 2% risk is usually quoted in this situation as well.

The demonstration of elevated AFAFP levels [greater than 3.0 standard deviations from the mean, or over 2.0 multiples of the median (MoM) for gestational age] will detect 98% to 100% of fetuses with NTD. Errors in estimation of gestational age account for the majority of false-positive results and can be resolved by ultrasonographic reassessment of fetal measurements. Increased AFAFP levels are usually the result of exudation of fetal serum proteins through skin defects or across fetal membranes. This mechanism accounts for the elevated AFAFP in anencephaly, open spinal cord lesions, and ventral wall defects such as omphalocele and gastroschisis. Abnormal renal filtration of protein, as is found in the Finnish type of congenital nephrosis, also results in high AFAFP. Gastrointestinal obstruction or swallowing defects make it impossible for the fetus to reabsorb the AFP in the small intestine, thus resulting in polyhydramnios and elevated AFAFP. Twin gestations, missed abortion, impending fetal demise, and fetal blood contamination also can result in false-positive AFAFP determinations. Table 5-3 lists the various disorders that may be the cause of elevated AFAFP.

TABLE 5-3. *Conditions associated with elevated amniotic fluid α-fetoprotein*

Open neural tube defects	Anencephaly, meningomyelocele, meningocele, encephalocele, spina bifida (open)
Ventral wall defects	Omphalocele, gastroschisis, exstrophy of the bladder, viscerocutaneous fistula
Renal anomalies	Finnish type nephrosis
Swallowing defects	CNS malformation, cleft palate
Gastrointestinal obstruction	Duodenal atresia, tracheoesophageal fistula, volvulus, large or small bowel obstruction
Miscellaneous	Chromosome anomalies, cystic hygroma, sacrococcygeal teratoma, intrauterine fetal demise, fetal distress (infants of diabetic mothers, Rh isoimmunization)
Dermatological disorders	Epidermolysis bullosa, fetus papyraceus
Nonpathologic	Incorrect gestational age, multiple gestations, fetal blood contamination

Amniotic Fluid Acetylcholinesterase

The diagnostic nonspecificity of AFAFP, with its possible elevation by fetal blood contamination, led to a search for a more specific indicator of neural tissue exposure *in utero.* Smith and colleagues (133) demonstrated that acetylcholinesterase (AchE), which is produced by neuronal axons, could be distinguished from nonspecific cholinesterases in neural tissues. They also showed it could be suppressed by a specific inhibitor. This assay approach has been recommended to distinguish elevations of AFP associated with NTDs from those that are not. However, it was later shown that the AchE assay is also nonspecific, with about 67% of fetuses with omphalocele/gastroschisis and 57% of cases of fetal cystic hygroma being AchE positive. Other fetal abnormalities, fetal demise, and fetal blood contamination have been reported to show a positive AchE band (134,135). High-resolution ultrasonography is at present the procedure of choice for confirmation of lesions in the spinal column and ventral wall or other defects and should be performed even when the possibility of fetal blood contamination is seriously considered as the cause of elevated AFP and positive AchEs.

MSAFP Screening

Seppala and Ruoslahti first noted significantly higher than normal levels of MSAFP in cases of fetal death or spontaneous abortion (136). Similar observations were made in pregnancies with anencephalic fetuses by Brock and colleagues in 1972 (131). Because 90% to 95% of NTDs are sporadic and would not be detected if family history were used as an indicator for evaluation, it was important to develop a strategy to identify the pregnancies at risk. The discovery that MSAFP levels are elevated with fetal NTDs led to a multicenter study that established its feasibility for screening purposes.

MSAFP screening at 16 to 18 weeks' gestation has now become standard practice in screening pregnancies for open NTDs. The detection rate of NTD pregnancies does vary according to cutoff levels used. Most screening programs established a cutoff of 2.0 to 2.5 times the median value (MoM). When the cutoff used is 2.5 MoM (about 97th percentile), close to 90% of anencephalies will be detected, and 69% of open NTDs, with 3% to 4% false-positive value (132). With a lower cutoff, a higher percentage of false-positive results will occur. The most common reason for a false-positive MSAFP is an underestimation of gestational age or twin pregnancy. However, it also can be the result of blood-group sensitization (Rh, Kell), placental factors such as placental lakes, hemangiomas, or retroperitoneal bleeds. On rare occasions MSAFP is elevated with maternal acute viral hepatitis or a tumor of the liver. For high-risk patients, such as diabetics for whom the incidence of NTDs is increased tenfold, and individuals whose risk of NTD is increased because of periconceptional ingestion of agents such as valproic acid or retinoic acid, MSAFP screening is especially important. Defects other than NTDs that can be detected as a result of elevated MSAFP are listed in Table 5-3. A protocol for MSAFP testing is shown in Fig. 5-2.

Patients with one or more elevated MSAFP results are advised to undergo an ultrasonographic examination, which provides a 95% sensitivity for detecting NTDs. However, because the identification of NTDs may be limited by the location and extent of the lesion, and because some of the structural defects are due to a chromosome abnormality, amniocentesis for chromosome analysis should be recommended as well (137).

Several studies have shown that the use of folic acid supplements during pregnancy decreases the rate of NTDs. In 1991, the Medical Research Council (MRC) reported that folic acid supplementation had decreased the recurrence rate of NTDs by 71% in women who had a previously affected child (138). Other studies indicated that use of folic acid has decreased the rate of first occurrence of NTDs by about 50% in families not considered at increased risk.

The U.S. Public Health Service recommends that women at reproductive age consume 0.4 mg of folic acid daily to reduce their risk of having an affected pregnancy. In those with a previously affected child, a periconcep-

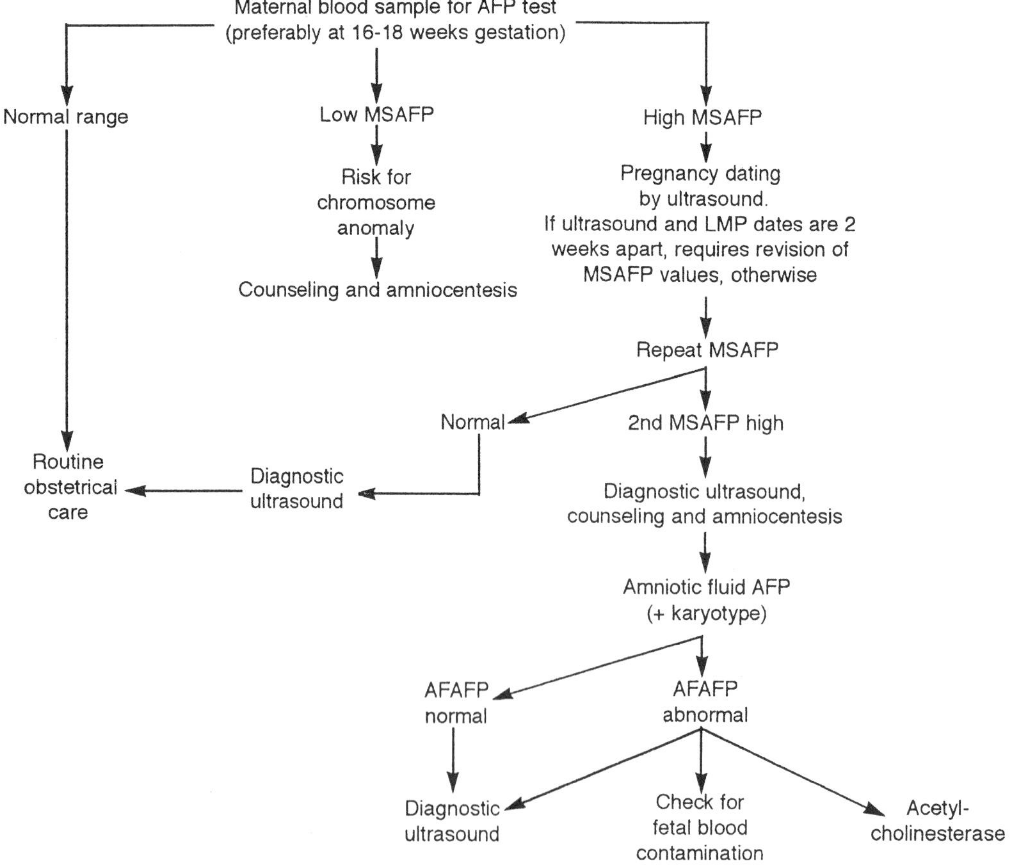

FIG. 5-2. Proposed clinical management protocol for MSAFP testing.

tional dosage of 4.0 mg/day beginning 3 months prior to conception and extending through the first trimester is recommended. This does not preclude the need for MSAFP screening because a residual risk of 30% for NTDs still exists for patients taking folic acid supplementation.

PRENATAL DIAGNOSIS OF METABOLIC DISORDERS

Specific enzymatic defects have been identified in over 200 inborn errors of metabolism. The laboratory diagnosis in these disorders is based on the demonstration of specific enzyme deficiencies or protein characterization. Essentially, all enzyme assays developed for cultured fibroblasts can be performed on amniotic fluid cells or tissue obtained by CVS, which is rich in enzymes and can be used for rapid prenatal diagnosis. However, fibroblast culture techniques may not apply to the study of all inborn errors of metabolism.

Disorders of mucopolysaccharide metabolism can all be diagnosed prenatally. Tay-Sachs disease, Krabbe's disease, metachromatic leukodystrophy, and Niemann-Pick disease are some examples of diagnosable disorders that involve sphingolipid metabolism. Copper accumulation in Menke's disease and cystine accumulation in cystinosis have been successfully used for prenatal diagnosis of these diseases. Similarly, ultrastructural examination for abnormal intracellular accumulation of material in mucolipidosis IV and Pompe's disease has been used in addition to specific enzyme analysis. A compendium listing the inherited metabolic disorders in which prenatal diagnosis has been reliably made and those for which prenatal diagnosis is feasible was published by Desnick and associates in 1985 (139). The number of single-gene disorders for which prenatal diagnosis is available continues to grow, and the techniques involved in making the diagnosis depend on the condition, particular enzyme deficiency, or specific mutation involved.

Because different mutations or enzyme deficiencies can lead to similar clinical manifestations, each case should be individually evaluated so that proper monitoring of the pregnancy can be offered, and misdiagnosis due to heterogeneity can be avoided.

PRENATAL DIAGNOSIS BY DNA ANALYSIS

A variety of genetic disorders are caused by mutations at the DNA level (140). The use of DNA analysis for prenatal diagnosis has become an integral part of routine prenatal care. Because molecular diagnosis does not require that the gene product (protein or enzyme) be expressed in fetal cells, it is possible to accomplish prenatal diagnosis by analysis of DNA from amniotic fluid cells, chorionic villi, or fetal blood.

Diagnosis by DNA analysis can be achieved through direct detection of the disease-producing mutation or by indirect detection (linkage analysis), studying the patterns of inheritance of DNA polymorphisms closely linked to the disease locus.

Direct detection requires knowledge of the specific mutations in the family. The commonly used techniques for molecular diagnosis include restriction endonuclease analysis and allele-specific oligonucleotide probe analysis.

Restriction endonucleases are bacterial enzymes that cut DNA at specific nucleotide base sequences (4 to 6 base pairs long), generating fragments of reproducible size, which are then separated electrophoretically in agarose gel. The base sequence recognized by a restriction endonuclease is known as the restriction site. Any alteration in the site renders it unrecognizable to the restriction endonuclease and prevents DNA cleavage. This change creates fragment size alterations that can be visualized using Southern blot analysis (141).

Allele-specific oligonucleotide probes (ASOs) are synthesized nucleotide sequences, usually 14 to 30 base pairs long. They are used to detect directly the presence of a specific DNA mutation. Two different oligonucleotides are used: one that is complementary to the normal allele, and the other complementary to the mutant allele. Because the single-stranded DNA probes are very short, they will not hybridize to genomic sequences that differ by even one single nucleotide, but only to completely homologous sequences. Thus, it is possible to diagnose an affected fetus with a specific disorder and distinguish between carriers (heterozygotes) and unaffected normal (homozygotes for the normal allele) individuals. Allele-specific oligonucleotide analysis has been used for the direct detection of a number of disorders for which carrier detection is possible by population screening.

Direct detection gives the least ambiguous results and does not always require the study of other family members. However, it cannot be applied to diagnose disorders in which the mutant gene or the specific mutation has not been identified. For the diagnosis of these disorders it is necessary to use indirect methods of detection involving restriction fragment length polymorphisms (RFLPs) and linkage analysis.

Restriction fragment length polymorphisms are inherited variations in noncoding DNA sequences that result in variable restriction endonuclease sites, thus producing various length DNA fragments with different electrophoretic mobility in different individuals. The occurrence of at least two different alleles at a locus, each having a frequency of at least one percent, is considered polymorphism. Each RFLP is inherited in a simple codominant Mendelian manner. This provides a potentially large number of linkage markers that can be used to trace a mutant gene in a family. Linkage is said to exist when two or more DNA sequences are located closely together. Prenatal diagnosis is accomplished indirectly by the use of RFLPs that cosegregate with the gene in question. If a marker and the mutant gene are closely linked, the two will not be separated during meiosis, and it should be possible to exclude or confirm the presence of the mutant gene in the fetus. Results and conclusions in such a study therefore depend on the degree of linkage and on whether recombination (interchromosome exchange of homologous DNA sequences during meiosis) between the marker and the disease gene has occurred. If recombination has occurred, association between the disease gene and a linked polymorphism will be disrupted and lead to an error in diagnosis. The use of several RFLPs near the gene in question reduces the risk of erroneous result interpretation.

For both direct and indirect analysis techniques, sufficient amounts of DNA can be obtained by using a technique called polymerase chain reaction (PCR). This involves the use of a heat-stable DNA polymerase (the enzyme that synthesizes new copies of individual DNA strands) to amplify a short segment of genomic DNA and produce large quantities of the DNA from the region of interest. Utilization of PCR greatly reduces the need for time-consuming tissue culture and shortens turn-around time for reporting results (142–144).

DNA analysis was initially offered for the diagnosis of the various hemoglobinopathies (thalassemias and sickle cell anemia). The first RFLP described in association with a specific gene defect was reported in sickle cell disease, where a single nucleotide substitution results in the loss of a restriction site. Kan and colleagues reported that the normal β^A-globin gene was found in a 7.6-kb fragment, whereas the abnormal β^S-globin gene was found in a 13-kb fragment produced by the loss of the restriction site at the normal position (145–147). Sickle-cell anemia can be diagnosed today by PCR amplification along with restriction enzyme digest or by ASOs (148). Most laboratories prefer to use the PCR technique because a relatively small amount of DNA is necessary for the analysis.

Unlike sickle cell or hemoglobin E disease, which are caused by the formation of a variant hemoglobin, the thalassemias are a group of autosomal-recessive hemoglobin disorders involving gene mutations that lead to insufficient production of globin chains. (There are two α-globin genes on each chromosome 16 and one β-globin gene on each chromosome 11.) The α-thalassemias are caused by deletions involving any number of the four normal genes. With the exception of hydrops fetalis, which is a lethal fetal disorder, the α-thalassemias are a more benign clinical entity than the β-thalassemias. They are extremely common in the Southeast Asian population and parts of Africa, the Mediterranean, and the Middle East.

Beta-thalassemia causes severe anemia in an affected individual; therefore, prenatal diagnosis has been targeted at identification of homozygous β-thalassemia. It is most common in the Mediterranean, but also in Southeast Asia and Africa. Because of the severity of these disorders, the American College of Obstetricians and Gynecologists issued a recommendation to screen pregnant women by complete blood count and hemoglobin electrophoresis followed by DNA analysis when indicated. Once it has been established that both parents are carriers, and the fetus is therefore at risk, prenatal diagnosis can be offered (149,150).

Prenatal diagnosis of CF has been attempted in informative families for several years. Genetic markers on chromosome 7 (RFLPs), linked tightly with the CF locus, were described simultaneously by several groups in 1985 and 1986 (151–154). Prenatal diagnosis was achieved with the use of multiple polymorphic sites in combination with assays for fetal intestinal enzyme activity in amniotic fluid (alkaline phosphatase and gammaglutamyl-transpeptidase) (155). A major breakthrough was accomplished by the cloning of the CF gene and the demonstration that a three-base deletion, designated ΔF508, is the predominant mutation that causes CF in 70% of the white population and 30% of Ashkenazi Jewish families (156–158). More than 500 different mutations have been identified to date, and screening for 70 of them is currently offered by selected laboratories (159). Direct detection of the CF mutation represents a major improvement in prenatal diagnosis for families with a history of CF, and for couples identified through population screening.

To date, the list of disorders that can be diagnosed prenatally by DNA analysis is growing rapidly. For most mendelian disorders, it is essential to test the parents first. When both parents are identified as carriers (heterozygotes) for an autosomal-recessive disorder, prenatal diagnosis can be performed. Examples of such disorders are listed in Table 5-4.

An important practical addition to the molecular diagnosis of autosomal-recessive inheritance is determination of the Rh genotype of the fetus of Rh-negative women. Administration of Rh-immune globulin to Rh-negative women has reduced the frequency of elevated Rh-antibody titer and fetal anemia. However, some pregnancies remain at risk. Prenatal DNA testing for Rh is recommended for pregnancies of Rh-negative women with Rh-heterozygote partners (160).

Linkage analysis using intragenic and flanking RFLPs made it possible to diagnose prenatally Duchenne's and Becker's muscular dystrophy in over 70% of at risk pregnancies (161,162). Duchenne's and the milder Becker's muscular dystrophies are both X-linked disorders that result from mutations in the same gene, located on the short arm of the X chromosome. In a significant proportion of cases, the mutations are caused by deletions in the gene. In both disorders, the deletions are distributed throughout the gene. Large and small deletions were described in both disorders. The molecular difference between the two disorders can be explained in most cases by the "reading-frame hypothesis." Depending on the breakpoints of the deletions, it can be determined

TABLE 5–4. *Examples of genetic disorders prenatally diagnosed by DNA analysis*

Disorder	Mode of inheritance	Carrier frequency	Ethnicity
Sickle cell anemia	AR	1:10	African-American, Mediterranean
Gaucher disease	AR	1:15	Ashkenazi Jewish
Tay-Sachs disease	AR	1:27	Ashkenazi Jewish, French Canadian
		1:150–1:300	Other than above
Cystic fibrosis	AR	1:25	Caucasian
		1:65	African-American
		1:150	Asian
α-Thalassemia	AR		Asian
α-Thalassemia	AR		Mediterranean
Canavan disease	AR	1:40	Ashkenazi Jewish
Spinal muscular atrophy	AR	1:40–1:80	
Congenital adrenal hyperplasia (21 hydroxylase deficiency)	AR		
Adult polycystic kidney disease	AD	1:1000	
Duchenne/Becker muscular dystrophy	XLR	1:3000	
Hemophilia A	XLR	1:5,000–1:10,000	
Hemophilia B	XLR	1:30,000	

AD, autosomal dominant; AR, autosomal recessive; XLR, X-linked recessive.

whether transcription of DNA into messenger RNA will maintain the reading frame, producing the milder Becker's dystrophy, or will change the reading frame, producing a truncated protein and the more severe Duchenne's muscular dystrophy (163).

Other X-linked disorders amenable to prenatal diagnosis by DNA techniques are hemophilia A and B. Hemophilia A, or factor VIII deficiency, occurs in approximately 1 in 5,000 males. In the past, prenatal diagnosis was achieved by determining the factor VIII activity in fetal blood. Since the isolation of the factor VIII gene, almost all prenatal diagnosis is made at the molecular level. DNA probes for the factor VIII gene itself, for closely linked markers, and for intragenic polymorphisms are used for diagnosis (164). The database for known mutations is regularly updated. The mutation most commonly screened for is a large gene inversion that leads to severe hemophilia, with no detectable factor VIII activity (165). Hemophilia B is also an X-linked recessive disorder with a defect causing deficiency of factor IX. Unlike hemophilia A, no common recurrent mutation has been identified; therefore, it is difficult to offer prenatal diagnosis. It is essential to test the parent or affected relative for their specific mutation, and prenatal diagnosis can be recommended only when the mutation is identified or the polymorphisms are informative (166,167).

In instances in which an autosomal-dominant disorder is suspected because of an affected parent or ultrasonographic examination results of the fetus, diagnosis by DNA is feasible for conditions in which the mutation is known, such as adult-onset polycystic kidney disease (168,169), Marfan syndrome (170), osteogenesis imperfecta type I (171), or neurofibromatosis type I (172).

TRINUCLEOTIDE REPEAT EXPANSIONS

A growing number of hereditary disorders are now considered to be caused by nontraditional modes of inheritance. One novel mechanism of human gene mutation involves instability in the area around certain trinucleotide repeats and results in trinucleotide repeat expansion in or near an expressed sequence (gene) (173).

The first disorder in which expansion of trinucleotide repeats was reported is the fragile X syndrome, a common cause of mental retardation. The expansion of a segment of DNA containing a specific three base pair sequence has now also been determined to be the molecular basis for a number of neurologic conditions including Huntington's disease, myotonic dystrophy, spinocerebellar ataxia 1, and others (Table 5-5). A common phenomenon in these disorders is *anticipation* (i.e., earlier onset and more severe symptoms in subsequent generations).

The number of copies of a repeat sequence can be detected by Southern blot and PCR analyses. A direct

TABLE 5–5. *Examples of trinucleotide repeat expansion disorders*

Disorder	Chromosome	Triplet repeat
Fragile X	Xq27.3	CGG (5′ untranslated region of gene)
Huntington disease	4p16.3	CAG (coding region)
Myotonic dystrophy	19q13.2	CTG (3′ untranslated region of gene)
Spinocerebellar ataxia I	6p22-23	CAG (coding region)
Friedrich ataxia	9q13	GAA (first intron)

correlation can be established between the number of triple repeat sequences and the clinical manifestations (i.e., affected, asymptomatic carrier, and normal). Only when a clear family history and diagnosis are available can prenatal diagnosis be attempted.

Fragile X

The fragile X syndrome is a common cause of inherited mental retardation seen in about 1 in 1,200 males and 1 in 2,500 females. Males often exhibit characteristic facial features, postpubertal macroorchidism, and, in some cases, autistic behavior. Although most hemizygous males are mentally retarded, 20% of males carrying the mutation may be phenotypically normal. Such individuals are considered to be transmitting males (174). There is also evidence that some heterozygous females may be affected, but exhibit a less severe phenotype. The diagnosis of fragile X was originally based on the expression of a folate-sensitive fragile site on the long arm of the X chromosome at Xq27.3. This chromosome abnormality was induced in culture when cells were grown in media deprived of folic acid. Prenatal diagnosis of fragile X in amniotic fluid cells by the above technique was difficult because the cytogenetic abnormality could not always be readily detected, and the interpretation was complicated by the presence of other fragile sites in the same region. In 1991, it was shown that the fragile X syndrome is caused by an unstable expansion of a tandemly repeated trinucleotide sequence (CGG) in the 5′-untranslated region of the FMR1 gene (175). The number of CGG repeats in the FMR1 gene in the normal population ranges from 6 to 50. Patients with premutations show 50 to 200 repeats, and the full mutations have more than 200 repeats. DNA analysis has therefore become the method of choice for prenatal diagnosis of fragile X syndrome. When the mother is proven to be a carrier, trinucleotide repeat analysis can help determine whether the fetus inherited the normal or mutant FMR1 gene (176).

FUTURE PROSPECTS IN PRENATAL DIAGNOSIS

Prenatal diagnosis using the previously described approaches is now an accepted component of routine obstetric care. With the exception of ultrasonography, the diagnostic techniques used are invasive in nature and are performed at a time when organogenesis is virtually complete. Attempts are currently directed at developing procedures that would make diagnosis of genetic disease possible during early stages of development and by noninvasive techniques. Steps toward achieving these goals were recently made in the areas of preimplantation genetic diagnosis and analysis of fetal cells derived from maternal blood.

The field of preimplantation genetic diagnosis has undergone significant advances in the past decade and has been successfully applied in more than 100 pregnancies at risk for single-gene and chromosome disorders. This approach to prenatal diagnosis is currently offered mostly to couples who are infertile and have to use *in vitro* fertilization or intracytoplasmic sperm injection in order to become pregnant. It is also a more attractive option for couples who would not consider a termination of pregnancy under any circumstances (177–179).

The source of cells for DNA or cytogenetic diagnosis can be the polar body, the blastomere (i.e., the removal of one to two cells at the eight-cell-stage embryo), or the blastocyst (i.e., removing 10–30 cells from the trophoectoderm, which is a component of the 200-cell blastocyst).

Each of these techniques has advantages and disadvantages. The advantage of preconception diagnosis by removal of the polar body is that it has no known function in embryonic development. Its disadvantages are that no paternal alleles are examined, the fetal sex cannot be determined, and there is a small amount of DNA. The use of PCR will therefore increase the risk of error through contamination or technical failure. Biopsy of the blastocyst provides a greater amount of tissue, but there are reports of diagnostic error, and there is still insufficient experience as to long-term effects on the developing embryo.

With refinement of available techniques and the development of more accurate and less expensive assays, preimplantation genetic diagnosis has the potential to become an important tool for prenatal diagnosis.

Another attractive potential approach to noninvasive prenatal diagnosis is the analysis of fetal cells retrieved from maternal blood. The presence of fetal cells in maternal circulation during pregnancy has been well documented, but enrichment and purification procedures are necessary for their detection.

The most promising cell type for the purpose of prenatal diagnosis is the nucleated red blood cell (180). The ratio of fetal to maternal nucleated red blood cells is estimated as $1{:}1 \times 10^7$ or 10^8. They may be present in maternal circulation as early as 10 weeks' gestation. Their short life span reduces the likelihood that they originated in prior pregnancies. Simpson and Elias (181) reported a high frequency of fetal erythroblasts in the maternal circulation of pregnancies complicated by chromosome anomalies (74%), suggesting an unusually high transplacental transfer in these cases. Valerio and colleagues (182) showed that fetal erythroid cells can be successfully cultured reliably and reproducibly *in vitro*. This makes noninvasive prenatal genetic diagnosis in the first trimester a realistic prospect for the near future.

ACKNOWLEDGMENT

We thank Yuval Rosenberg for his assistance in the preparation of this manuscript.

REFERENCES

1. Crandall BF, Lebherz TB, Rubinstein L. Chromosome findings in 2500 second trimester amniocenteses. Am J Med Genet 1980;5: 345–356.
2. Golbus MS, Loughman WD, Epstein CJ, Halbasch G, Stephens JD, Hall BD. Prenatal genetic diagnosis in 3000 amniocenteses. N Engl J Med 1979;300:157–163.
3. Lowe CU, Alexander D, Bryla D, Seigel D. The NICHD amniocentesis registry. The safety and accuracy of mid-trimester amniocentesis. Bethesda, MD: National Institutes of Health, DHEW publication (NIH), 1978:78–90.
4. NICHD National Registry for Amniocentesis Study Group. Midtrimester amniocentesis for prenatal diagnosis. Safety and accuracy. JAMA 1976;236:1471–1476.
5. Simpson NE, Dallaire L, Miller JR, et al. Prenatal diagnosis of genetic disease in Canada: report of a collaborative study. Can Med Assoc J 1976;115:739–748.
6. Tabor A, Philip J, Madsen M, Bang J, Obel EB, Norgaard-Pederson B. Randomized controlled trial of genetic amniocentesis in 4000 low risk women. Lancet 1986;1:1287–1293.
7. Elejalde BR, de Elejalde MM, Acuna JM, Thelen D, Trujillo C, Karrmann M. Prospective study of amniocentesis performed between weeks 9 and 16 of gestation: its feasibility, risks, complications and the use in early genetic prenatal diagnosis. Am J Med Genet 1990;35: 188–196.
8. Evans MI, Koppitch FC, Nemitz B, Quigg MH, Zador IE. Early genetic amniocentesis and chorionic villus sampling: expanding the opportunities for prenatal diagnosis. J Reprod Med 1988;33:450–452.
9. Hanson FW, Zorn M, Tennat FR, Marianos S, Samuas S. Amniocentesis before 15 weeks gestation: outcome, risks and technical problems. Am J Obstet Gynecol 1987;156:1524–1531.
10. Shulman LP, Meyers CM, Simpson JL, Andersen RN, Tolley EA, Elias S. Fetomaternal transfusion depends on amount of chorionic villi aspirated but not on method of chorionic villus sampling. Am J Obstet Gynecol 1990;162:1185–1188.
11. Brumfield CG, Lin S, Conner N, Cosper P, Davis RO, Owen J. Pregnancy outcome following genetic amniocentesis at 11–14 weeks gestation. Obstet Gynecol 1996;88:114–118.
12. Eiben B, Goebel R, Hansen S, Aammans W. Early amniocentesis—a cytogenetic evaluation of over 1500 cases. Prenat Diagn 1994;146: 487–501.
13. Bovicelli L, Rizzo N, Montacuti V, Morandi R. Transabdominal versus transcervical routes for chorionic villus sampling. Lancet 1986; 2:290.
14. Brambati B, Lanzani A, Tului L. Transabdominal and transcervical chorionic villus sampling: efficiency and risk evaluation of 2411 cases. Am J Med Genet 1990;35:160–164.
15. Hahnemann JM, Vejerslev LO. European collaborative research on mosaicism in CVS (EUCROMIC)—fetal and extrafetal cell lineage in 192 gestations with CVS mosaicism involving single autosomal trisomy. Am J Med Genet 1997;70:179–187.
16. Grebner EE, Wapner RJ, Barr NA, Jackson LG. Prenatal Tay-Sachs diagnosis by chorionic villi sampling. Lancet 1983;2:286–287.
17. Simoni G, Brambati B, Danesino C, et al. Efficient direct chromosome analyses and enzyme determinations from chorionic villi samples in the first trimester of pregnancy. Hum Genet 1983;63:349–357.
18. Smidt-Jensen S, Hahnemann N. Transabdominal chorionic villus sampling for fetal genetic diagnosis. Technical and obstetrical evaluation of 100 cases. Prenat Diagn 1988;8:7–17.
19. Williamson R, Eskdale J, Coleman DV, Niazi M, Loeffler FE, Modell BM. Direct gene analysis of chorionic villi: a possible technique for first trimester antenatal diagnosis of haemoglobinopathies. Lancet 1981;2:1125–1127.
20. Hahnemann N, Mohr J. Genetic diagnosis in the embryo by means of biopsy from extra embryonic membranes. Bull Eur Soc Human Genet 1968;2:23–29.
21. Canadian Collaborative CVS-Amniocentesis Clinical Group. Multiple center randomized clinical trial of chorion villus sampling and amniocentesis. First report. Lancet 1989;1:1–6.
22. Evans MI, Drugan A, Koppitch FC, Zador IE, Sacks AJ, Sokol RJ. Genetic diagnosis in the first trimester: the norm for the 1990s. Am J Obstet Gynecol 1989;160:1332–1339.
23. Jahoda MGJ, Pijpers L, Reuss A, Los FJ, Wladimiroff JW, Sachs ES. Evaluation of transcervical chorionic villus sampling with a completed follow-up of 1550 consecutive pregnancies. Prenat Diagn 1989; 9:621–628.
24. Kazy Z, Rozovsky IS, Bakharev VA. Chorion biopsy in early pregnancy. A method of early prenatal diagnosis for inherited disorders. Prenat Diagn 1982;2:39–45.
25. Mikkelsen M, Ayme S. Cytogenetic findings in chorionic villi. A collaborative study. Presented at the 7th International Congress of Human Genetics, Berlin, 1986.
26. Rhoads GG, Jackson LG, Schlesselman SE, et al. The safety and efficacy of chorionic villus sampling for early prenatal diagnosis of cytogenetic abnormalities. N Engl J Med 1989;320:609–617.
27. Vejerslev LO, Mikkelsen M. The European collaborative study on mosaicism in chorionic villus sampling: data from 1986 and 1987. Prenat Diagn 1989;9:575–588.
28. MRC Working Party on the evaluation of chorionic villus sampling: Medical Research Council European Trial of chorionic villus sampling. Lancet 1991;337:1491–1499.
29. Chueh JT, Goldberg JD, Wohlferd MM, Golbus MS. Comparison of transcervical and transabdominal CVS loss rate in 9000 cases from a single center. Am J Obstet Gynecol 1995;173:1277–1282.
30. Smidt-Jensen S, Permin M, Philip J, et al. Randomized comparison of amniocentesis and transabdominal and transcervical chorionic villus sampling. Lancet 1992;340:1237–1244.
31. Firth HV, Boyd PA, Chamberlain P, MacKenzie IZ, Lindenbaum RH, Huson SM. Severe limb abnormalities after chorion villus sampling at 56–66 days gestation. Lancet 1991;337:762–763.
32. Burton BK, Schultz CJ, Burd LJ. Spectrum of limb disruption defects associated with chorionic villus sampling. Pediatrics 1993;91: 989–993.
33. Foster UG, Jackson L. Limb defects and chorionic villus sampling: results from an international registry, 1992–1994. Lancet 1996;347: 489–494.
34. Rodeck CH. Fetoscopy guided by real-time ultrasound for pure fetal blood samples, fetal skin samples and examination of the fetus in utero. Br J Obstet Gynaecol 1980;87:449–456.
35. Cordesius E, Gustavii B, Mitelman F. Prenatal chromosomal analysis of fetal blood obtained at fetoscopy. Br Med J 1980;280:1107.
36. Hobbins JC, Grannum PA, Romero R, Reece EA, Mahoney MJ. Percutaneous umbilical blood sampling. Am J Obstet Gynecol 1985; 152:1–6.
37. Golbus MS. Special report: the status of fetoscopy and fetal tissue sampling. Prenat Diagn 1984;4:79–81.
38. Rodeck CH. Fetoscopy and the prenatal diagnosis of inherited conditions. J Genet Hum 1980;28:41–47.
39. Rodeck CH, Nicolaides KH. Fetoscopy and fetal tissue sampling. Br Med Bull 1983;39:332–337.
40. Hogge WA, Koresawa M, Simpson T, Golbus MS. Prenatal diagnosis of glycogen storage disease (von Gierke) by fetal liver biopsy. Am J Hum Genet 1983;35:97A.
41. Hozygrove W, Golbus MS. Prenatal diagnosis of ornithine transcarbamylase deficiency. Am J Hum Genet 1984;36:320–328.
42. Tuchman M, Morizon OH, Reish O, Allewell NM. The molecular basis of ornithine transcarbamylase deficiency: modelling the human enzyme and the effects of mutations. J Med Genet 1995;32:680–688.
43. Tuchman M, Plante RJ, Garcia-Perez MA, Rubio V. Relative frequency of mutations causing ornithine transcarbamylase deficiency in 78 families. Hum Genet 1996;97:274–276.
44. Lidsky AS, Guttler F, Woo SLC. Prenatal diagnosis of classical phenylketonuria by DNA analysis. Lancet 1985;1:549–551.
45. Lidsky AS, Ledley FD, DiLella AG, Kwok SC, Daiger SP, Robson KJ, Woo SL. Extensive restriction site polymorphism at the human phenylalanine hydroxylase locus and application in prenatal diagnosis of phenylketonuria. Am J Hum Genet 1985;37:619–634.
46. Huang I, Byck S, Prevost I, Scriver CR. PAH mutation analysis consortium database: a database for disease-producing and other allelic variation at the human PAH locus. Nucleic Acids Res 1996;24: 127–131.
47. Dale BA, Perry TB, Holbrook KA, Hamilton EF, Senikas V. Biochemical examination of fetal skin biopsy specimens obtained by fetoscopy: use of the method for analysis of keratins and filaggrin. Prenat Diagn 1986;6:37–44.
48. Elias S. Use of fetoscopy for the prenatal diagnosis of hereditary skin disorders. Curr Probl Dermatol 1987;16:1–13.

49. Elias S, Mazur M, Sabbagha R, Esterlyn B, Simpson JL. Prenatal diagnosis of harlequin ichthyosis. Clin Genet 1980;17:275–280.
50. Rodeck CH, Eady RA, Gosden CM. Prenatal diagnosis of epidermolysis bullosa letalis. Lancet 1980;1:949–952.
51. Bakharev VA, Aivazyan AA, Karetnikova NA, Mordovtsev YN, Yantovsky YR. Fetal skin biopsy in prenatal diagnosis of some genodermatoses. Prenat Diagn 1990;10:1–12.
52. Nicolaides KH, Campbell S. Ultrasound diagnosis of congenital abnormalities. In: Milunsky A, ed. Genetic disorders and the fetus: diagnosis, prevention, and treatment, 3rd ed. Baltimore: Johns Hopkins University Press, 1992:593–648.
53. Hobbins JC, Bracken MB, Mahoney MJ. Diagnosis of fetal skeletal dysplasias with ultrasound. Am J Obstet Gynecol 1982;142:306–312.
54. Reinsch RC. Choroid plexus cysts—association with trisomy: prospective review of 16,059 patients. Am J Obstet Gynecol 1997; 176:1381–1383.
55. Allan LD, Tynan MJ, Campbell S, Anderson RH. Identification of congenital cardiac malformations by echocardiography in midtrimester fetus. Br Heart J 1981;46:358–362.
56. Allan LD, Joseph MC, Boyd EG, Campbell S, Tynan M. M-mode echocardiography in the developing human fetus. Br Heart J 1982;47: 573–583.
57. Hook EB, Cross PK. Interpretation of recent data pertinent to genetic counseling for Down syndrome: maternal age-specific rates, temporal trends, adjustments for paternal age, recurrence risks, risks after other cytogenetic abnormalities, recurrence risk after remarriage. In: Willey AM, Carter TP, Kelly S, Porter IH, eds. Clinical genetics: problems in diagnosis and counseling. New York: Academic Press, 1982:119–139.
58. Hook EB. Chromosome abnormalities and spontaneous fetal death following amniocentesis. Further data and associations with maternal age. Am J Hum Genet 1983;35:110–116.
59. Schreinemachers DM, Cross PK, Hook EB. Rates of trisomies 21, 18, 13 and other chromosome abnormalities in about 20,000 prenatal studies compared with estimated rates in live births. Hum Genet 1982; 61:318–324.
60. Hook EB, Cross PK. Extra structurally abnormal chromosomes (ESAC) detected at amniocentesis: frequency in approximately 75,000 prenatal cytogenetic diagnoses and association with maternal and paternal age. Am J Hum Genet 1987;40:83–101.
61. Ferguson-Smith MA, Yates JRW. Maternal age specific rates for chromosome aberrations and factors influencing them: report of a collaborative European study on 52,965 amniocenteses. Prenat Diagn 1984; 4(special issue):5–44.
62. Hook EB, Cross PK, Schreinemachers DM. Chromosomal abnormality rate at amniocentesis and in liveborn infants. JAMA 1983;249: 2034–2038.
63. Hook EB, Cross PK, Jackson L, Pergament E, Brambati B. Maternal age-specific rates of 47, +21 and other cytogenetic abnormalities diagnosis in the first trimester of pregnancy in chorionic villus biopsy specimens: comparison with rates expected from observations at amniocentesis. Am J Hum Genet 1988;42:797–807.
64. Boué A, Gallano P. A collaborative study of the segregation of inherited chromosome structural rearrangements in 1356 prenatal diagnoses. Prenat Diagn 1984;4(special issue):45–67.
65. Daniel A, Boué A, Gallano P. Prospective risk in reciprocal translocation heterozygotes at amniocentesis as determined by potential chromosome imbalance sizes. Data of the European collaborative prenatal diagnosis centers. Prenat Diagn 1986;6:315–350.
66. Daniel A, Hook EB, Wolf G. Risks of unbalanced progeny at amniocentesis to carriers of chromosome rearrangements: data from United States and Canadian laboratories. Am J Med Genet 1989;31:14–53.
67. Stene J, Stene E, Mikkelsen M. Risk for chromosome abnormality at amniocentesis following a child with a non-inherited chromosome aberration. Prenat Diag 1984;4:81–95.
68. Merkatz IR, Nitowsky HM, Macri JN, Johnson WE. An association between low maternal serum α-fetoprotein and fetal chromosome abnormalities. Am J Obstet Gynecol 1984;148:886–891.
69. DiMaio MS, Baumgarten A, Greenstein RM, Saal HM, Mahoney MJ. Screening for fetal Down's syndrome in pregnancy by measuring maternal serum alpha-fetoprotein levels. N Engl J Med 1987;317: 342–346.
70. New England Regional Genetics Group Prenatal Collaborative Study of Down Syndrome Screening. Combining maternal serum alpha-fetoprotein measurements and age to screen for Down syndrome in pregnant women under age 35. Am J Obstet Gynecol 1989;160: 575–581.
71. Palomaki GE, Knight GJ, Kloza EM, Haddow JE. Maternal weight adjustment and low serum alpha-fetoprotein values. Lancet 1985,1: 468.
72. Palomaki GE, Haddow JE. Maternal serum alpha-fetoprotein, age, and Down syndrome risk. Am J Obstet Gynecol 1987;156:460–463.
73. Cuckle HS, Wald NJ, Lindenbaum RH. Maternal serum alpha-fetoprotein measurement: a screening test for Down syndrome. Lancet 1984;1:926-929.
74. Bogart MH, Golbus MS, Sorg ND, Jones OW. Human chorionic gonadotropin levels in pregnancies with aneuploid fetuses. Prenat Diagn 1989;9:379–384.
75. Bogart MH, Jones OW, Felder RA, et al. Prospective evaluation of maternal serum human chorionic gonadotropin levels in 3428 pregnancies. Am J Obstet Gynecol 1991;165:663–667.
76. Bogart MH, Pandian MR, Jones OW. Abnormal maternal serum gonadotropin levels in pregnancies with fetal chromosome abnormalities. Prenat Diagn 1987;7:623–630.
77. Canick JA, Palomaki GE, Osathanondh R. Prenatal screening for trisomy 18 in the second trimester. Prenat Diagn 1990;10:546–548.
78. Spencer K, Mallard AS, Coombes EJ, Macri JN. Prenatal screening for trisomy 18 with free beta human chorionic gonadotrophin as a marker. Br Med J 1993;307:1455–1458.
79. Canick JA, Knight GJ, Palomaki GE, Haddow JE, Cuckle HS, Ward NJ. Low second trimester maternal serum unconjugated oestriol in pregnancies with Down syndrome. Br J Obstet Gynaecol 1988;95: 330–333.
80. Haddow JE, Palomaki GE, Knight GJ, et al. Prenatal screening for Down's syndrome with use of maternal serum markers. N Engl J Med 1992;327:588–593.
81. Benn PA, Clive JM, Collins R. Medians for second-trimester maternal serum α-fetoprotein, human chorionic gonadotropin, and unconjugated estriol: differences between races or ethnic groups. Clin Chem 1997;43:333–337.
82. Knight GJ, Palomaki GE, Haddow JE. Use of maternal serum alpha-fetoprotein measurements to screen for Down's syndrome. Clin Obstet Gynecol 1988;31:306–327.
83. American College of Obstetricians and Gynecologists Educational Bulletin. Maternal serum screening. 1996;228:1–9.
84. Aitken DA, Wallace E, Crossley JA. Dimeric inhibin A as a marker for Down's syndrome in early pregnancy. N Engl J Med 1996;334: 1231–1236.
85. Aitken DA, McCaw G, Crossley JA, Berry E, Connor JM, Spencer K, Macri JN. First-trimester biochemical screening for fetal chromosome abnormalities and neural tube defects. Prenat Diagn 1993;13: 681–689.
86. Hsu LYF. Prenatal diagnosis of chromosome abnormalities through amniocentesis. In: Milunsky A, ed. Genetic disorders and the fetus: diagnosis, prevention, and treatment, 3rd ed. Baltimore: Johns Hopkins University Press, 1992:155–190.
87. Bovicelli L, Ornisi LF, Rizzo N, Montacuti V, Bacchetta M. Reproduction in Down syndrome. Obstet Gynecol 1982;59(suppl):13–17.
88. Kohn G, Shohat M. Trisomy 18 mosaicism in an adult with normal intelligence. Am J Med Genet 1987;26:929–931.
89. Auerbach AD, Sagi M, Adler B. Fanconi anemia: prenatal diagnosis in 30 fetuses at risk. Pediatrics 1985;76:794–800.
90. Schwartz S, Flannery DB, Cohen MM. Tests appropriate for the prenatal diagnosis of ataxia telangiectasia. Prenat Diagn 1985;5:9–14.
91. Ray JH, German J. The chromosome changes in Bloom's syndrome, ataxia telangiectasia and Fanconi's anemia. In: Arrighi FE, Rao PN, Stubblefield E, eds. Genes, chromosomes and neoplasia. New York: Raven Press, 1981:351–378.
92. Auerbach AD. Fanconi anemia: genetic testing in Ashkenazi Jews. Genet Test 1997;1:27–33.
93. Savitsky K, Bar-Shira A, Gilad S, et al. A single ataxia telangiectasia gene with a product similar to PI-3 kinase. Science 1995;268: 1749–1753.
94. Ellis NA, Groden J, Ye TZ, et al. The Bloom's syndrome gene product is homologous to Rec Q helicases. Cell 1995;83:655–666.
95. Therkelsen AJ. Cell culture and cytogenetic technique. In: Murkin JD, Stengel-Rutkowski S, Swinger E, eds. Prenatal diagnosis: proceedings of 3rd European conference on prenatal diagnosis of genetic disorders. Stuttgart: Ferdinand Euke, 1979:258–270.

96. Benn PA, Schonhaut AG, Hsu LYF. A high incidence of maternal cell contamination of amniotic fluid cell cultures. Am J Med Genet 1983; 14:361–365.
97. Freiberg AS, Blumberg B, Lawce H, Mann J. XX/XY chimerism encountered during prenatal diagnosis. Prenat Diagn 1988;8:423–426.
98. Simoni G, Gimelli G, Cuoco C. Discordance between prenatal cytogenetic diagnosis after chorionic villi sampling and chromosomal constitution of the fetus. In: Fraccaro M, Simoni G, Brambati B, eds. First trimester fetal diagnosis. Berlin: Springer-Verlag, 1985:137–143.
99. Simoni G, Rossella F, Lalatta F, Fraccaro M. Maternal metaphases on direct preparation from chorionic villi and in cultures of villi cells [Letter]. Hum Genet 1986;72:104.
100. Elles RG, Williamson R, Niazi M, Coleman DV, Horwell D. Absence of maternal contamination of chorionic villi used for fetal gene analysis. N Engl J Med 1983;308:1433–1435.
101. Simoni G, Gimelli G, Cuoco C, et al. First trimester fetal karyotyping: one thousand diagnoses. Hum Genet 1986;72:203–209.
102. Simoni G, Terzoli G, Rossella F. Direct chromosome preparation and culture using chorionic villi: an evaluation of the two techniques. Am J Med Genet 1990;35:181–183.
103. Roberts E, Duckett DP, Lang GD. Maternal cell contamination in chorionic villus samples assessed by direct preparations and three different culture methods. Prenat Diagn 1988;8:635–640.
104. Williams J III, Medearis AL, Chu WH, Kovacs GD, Kaback MM. Maternal cell contamination in cultured chorionic villi: comparison of chromosome Q-polymorphisms derived from villi, fetal skin and maternal lymphocytes. Prenat Diagn 1987;7:315–322.
105. Boué J, Nicholas H, Barichard F, Boué A. Le clonage des celluies du liquide amniotique, aide dans l'interpretation des mosaiques chromosomiques en diagnostic prenatal. Ann Genetique 1979;22:3–9.
106. Benn PA, Hsu LYF, Perlis T, Schonhaut AG. Prenatal diagnosis of chromosome mosaicism. Prenat Diagn 1984;4:1–9.
107. Hsu LYF, Kaffe S, Jenkins EC, et al. Proposed guidelines for diagnosis of chromosome mosaicism in amniocytes based on data derived from chromosome mosaicism and pseudomosaicism studies. Prenat Diagn 1992;12:555–573.
108. Kalousek DK, Dill FJ. Chromosomal mosaicism confined to the placenta in human conceptions. Science 1983;221:665–667.
109. Kalousek DK. The role of confined chromosome mosaicism in placental function and human development. Growth Genet Horm 1988; 4:1–3.
110. Kalousek DK, Dill FJ, Pantzar T, McGillivray BC, Yong SL, Wilson RD. Confined chorionic mosaicism in prenatal diagnosis. Hum Genet 1987;77:163–167.
111. Kalousek DK, Barrett IJ, McGillivray BC. Placental mosaicism and intrauterine survival of trisomies 13 and 18. Am J Hum Genet 1989; 44:338–343.
112. Ledbetter DH, Engel E. Uniparental disomy in humans: development of an imprinting map and its implications for prenatal diagnosis. Hum Mol Genet 1995;4:1757–1764.
113. Bui TH, Iselius L, Lindsten J. European collaborative study on prenatal diagnosis: mosaicism, pseudomosaicism and single abnormal cell in amniotic fluid cell cultures. Prenat Diagn 1984;4(special issue): 145–162.
114. Hsu LYF, Perlis TE. United States survey on chromosome mosaicism and pseudomosaicism in prenatal diagnosis. Prenat Diagn 1984;4(special issue):97–130.
115. Worton RG, Stern R. A Canadian collaborative study of mosaicism in amniotic fluid cell cultures. Prenat Diagn 1984;4(special issue): 131–144.
116. Hsu LYF, Kaffe S, Perlis TE. Trisomy 20 mosaicism in prenatal diagnosis—a review and update. Prenat Diagn 1987;7:581–596.
117. Hsu LYF, Yu MT, Neu RL, et al. Rare trisomy mosaicism diagnosed in amniocytes, involving an autosome other than chromosomes 13, 18, 20, and 21: karyotype/phenotype correlations. Prenat Diagn 1997;17: 201–242.
118. Chang HJ, Clark RD, Bachman H. The phenotype of 45,X/46,XY mosaicism: an analysis of 92 prenatally diagnosed cases. Am J Hum Genet 1990;46:156–167.
119. Hsu LYF. Prenatal diagnosis of 45,X/46,XY mosaicism a review and update. Prenat Diagn 1989;9:31–48.
120. Hook EB, Cross PK. Rates of mutant and inherited structural cytogenetic abnormalities detected at amniocentesis: results on about 63,000 fetuses. Ann Hum Genet 1987;51:27–55.
121. Evans JA, Canning N, Hunter AGW, et al. A cytogenetic survey of 14,069 newborn infants. III. An analysis of the significance and cytologic behavior of the Robertsonian and reciprocal translocations. Cytogenet Cell Genet 1978;20:96–112.
122. Tierney I, Axworthy D, Smith L, Ratcliffe SG. Balanced rearrangements of the autosomes: results of a longitudinal study of a newborn survey population. J Med Genet 1984;21:45–51.
123. Warburton D. Outcome of cases of *de novo* structural rearrangements diagnosed at amniocentesis. Prenat Diagn 1984;4(special issue):69–80.
124. Warburton D. *De novo* balanced chromosome rearrangements and extra marker chromosmes identified at prenatal diagnosis: clinical significance and distribution of breakpoints. Am J Hum Genet 1991; 49:995–1013.
125. Olson SB, Magenis RE. Preferential paternal origin of de novo structural chromosome rearrangements. In: Daniel A, ed. The cytogenetics of mammalian autosomal rearrangements. New York: Alan R. Liss, 1988:583–599.
126. Benn PA, Hsu LYF. Incidence and significance of supernumerary marker chromosomes in prenatal diagnosis. Am J Hum Genet 1984; 36:1092–1102.
127. Kaffe S, Hsu LYF. Supernumerary marker chromosomes in a series of 19,000 prenatal diagnoses: pregnancy outcome of satellited vs. nonsatellited *de novo* markers [Abstract]. Am J Hum Genet 1988;43: A237.
128. Sachs ES, Van Hemel JO, Den Hollander JC, Jahoda GJ. Marker chromosomes in a series of 10,000 prenatal diagnoses. Cytogenetic and follow-up studies. Prenat Diagn 1987;7:81–89.
129. Shivashankar L, Whitney E, Colmorgen G, et al. Prenatal diagnosis of tetrasomy 47,XY,+i(12p) confirmed by *in situ* hybridization. Prenat Diagn 1988;8:85–91.
130. Scarbrough PR, Hersh J, Kukolich MK, et al. Tetraploidy: a report of three live-born infants. Am J Med Genet 1984;19:29–37.
131. Brock DJH, Sutcliffe RG. Alpha-fetoprotein in the antenatal diagnosis of anencephaly and spina bifida. Lancet 1972;2:197–199.
132. Milunsky A. Maternal serum screening for neural tube and other defects. In: Milunsky A, ed. Genetic disorders and the fetus: diagnosis, prevention, and treatment, 3rd ed. Baltimore: Johns Hopkins University Press, 1992:507–564.
133. Smith AD, Wald NJ, Cuckle HS, Stirrat GM, Bebrow M, Lagercrantz H. Amniotic-fluid acetylcholinesterase a possible diagnostic test for neural-tube defects in early pregnancy. Lancet 1979;1:685–688.
134. Barlow RD, Cuckle HS, Wald NJ, Rodeck CH. False positive gel-acetylcholinesterase results in blood-stained amniotic fluids. Br J Obstet Gynaecol 1982;89:821–826.
135. Crandall BF, Kasha W, Matsumoto M. Prenatal diagnosis of neural tube defects: experiences with acetylcholinesterase gel electrophoresis. Am J Med Genet 1982;12:361–366.
136. Seppala M, Ruoslahti E. Alphafetoprotein in maternal serum: a new marker for detection of fetal distress and intrauterine death. Am J Obstet Gynecol 1973;115:48–53.
137. Platt LD, Feuchtbaum L, Filly R, Lustig L, Simon M, Cunningham GC. The California maternal serum α-fetoprotein screening program: the role of ultrasonography in the detection of spina bifida. Am J Obstet Gynecol 1992;166:1328–1329.
138. MRC Vitamin Study Research Group. Prevention of neural tube defects: results of the Medical Research Council vitamin study. Lancet 1991;338:131–137.
139. Desnick RJ, Grabowski GA, Hirschhorn K. Prenatal metabolic diagnosis: a compendium. In: Filkins K, Russo JF, eds. Clinical and biochemical analysis. Vol. 18. Human prenatal diagnosis. New York: Marcel Dekker, 1985:59–108.
140. Antonarakis SE. Diagnosis of genetic disorders at the DNA level. N Engl J Med 1989;320:153–163.
141. Southern EM. Gel electrophoresis of restriction fragments. Methods Enzymol 1979;68:152–176.
142. Eisenstein BI. The polymerase chain reaction: a new method of using molecular genetics for medical diagnosis. N Engl J Med 1990;322: 178–183.
143. Saiki RK, Gelfand DH, Stoffel S, et al. Primer-directed enzymatic amplification of DNA with a thermostable DNA polymerase. Science 1988;239:487–491.
144. Saiki RK, Scharf S, Faloona F, et al. Enzymatic amplification of B-globin genomic sequences and restriction site analysis for diagnosis of sickle cell anemia. Science 1985;230:1350–1354.

145. Chang JC, Kan YW. A sensitive new prenatal test for sickle cell anemia. N Engl J Med 1982;307:30–32.
146. Kan YW, Dozy AM. Polymorphism of DNA sequences adjacent to human beta-globin structural gene: relationship to sickle mutation. Proc Natl Acad Sci U S A 1978;75:5631–5635.
147. Kan YW, Dozy AM. Antenatal diagnosis of sickle cell anemia by DNA analysis of amniotic fluid cells. Lancet 1978;2:910–912.
148. Wang X, Seaman C, Paik M, Chen T, Bank A, Piomelli S. Experience with 500 prenatal diagnoses of sickle cell disease: the effect of gestational age on affected pregnancy outcome. Prenat Diagn 1994;14: 851–857.
149. ACOG Technical Bulletin: an educational aid to obstetrician-gynecologists. Hemoglobinopathies in pregnancy. 1996;220:1–9
150. Gay JC, Phillips JA, Kazazian HH. Hemoglobinopathies and thalassemias. In: Rimoin DL, Connor MJ, Pyeritz RE, eds. Emery and Rimoin's principles and practice of medical genetics. 1996: 1599–1626.
151. Beaudet AL, Rosenbloom C, Spencer JE. Linkage of cystic fibrosis (CF) and the met oncogene [Abstract]. Pediatr Res 1986;20:470.
152. Knowlton RG, Cohen-Haguenauer O, Cong NV, et al. A polymorphic DNA marker linked to cystic fibrosis is located on chromosome 7. Nature 1985;318:380–382.
153. Tsui LC, Buchwald M, Barker D, et al. Cystic fibrosis locus defined by a genetically linked polymorphic DNA marker. Science 1985;230: 1054–1057.
154. White R, Woodward S, Leppert M, et al. A closely linked marker for cystic fibrosis. Nature 1985;318:382–384.
155. Brock DJH, Clarke HA, Barron L. Prenatal diagnosis of cystic fibrosis by microvillar enzyme assay on a sequence of 258 pregnancies. Hum Genet 1988;78:271–275.
156. Kerem B, Rommens JM, Buchanan JA. Identification of cystic fibrosis gene: genetic analysis. Science, 1989;245:1073–1080.
157. Riordan JR, Rommens JM, Kerem B, et al. Identification of the cystic fibrosis gene: cloning and characterization of complementary DNA. Science 1989;245:1066–1073.
158. Feldman GL, Lewiston N, Fernbach SD, et al. Prenatal diagnosis of cystic fibrosis by using linked DNA markers in 138 pregnancies at 1 in 4 risk. Am J Med Genet 1989;33:238–241.
159. The Cystic Fibrosis Genetic Analysis Consortium (CFGAC). Population variation of common cystic fibrosis mutations. Hum Mutat 1994; 4:167–177.
160. Spence WC, Maddalena A, Demers DB, Bick DP. Molecular analysis of the RhD genotype in fetuses at risk for RhD hemolytic disease. Obstet Gynecol 1995;85:296–298.
161. Monaco AP, Bertelson CJ, Middleworth W, et al. Detection of deletions spanning the Duchenne muscular dystrophy locus using a tightly linked DNA segment. Nature 1985;316:842–845.
162. Ward PA, Hejtmancik JF, Witkowski JA, et al. Prenatal diagnosis of Duchenne muscular dystrophy: prospective linkage analysis and retrospective dystrophin cDNA analysis. Am J Hum Genet 1989;44: 270–281.
163. Monaco AP, Bertelson CJ, Liechti-Gallati S, Moser H, Kunkel LM. An explanation for the phenotypic differences between patients bearing partial deletions of the DMD locus. Genomics 1988;2:90–95.
164. Naylor J, Brinke A, Hassock S, Green PM, Gianelli F. Characteristic mRNA abnormality found in half the patients with severe hemophilia A is due to large DNA inversions. Hum Mol Genet 1993;2: 1773–1778.
165. Antonarakis SE, Rossiter JP, Young M. Factor VIII gene inversions in severe hemophilia A. Results of an international consortium study. Blood 1995;86:2206–2212.
166. Giannelli F, Choo KH, Rees DJG, Boyd Y, Rizza CR, Brownlee GG. Gene deletions in patients with haemophilia B and anti-factor IX antibodies. Nature 1983;303:181–182.
167. Giannelli F, Green PM, High KA, et al. Hemophilia B: database of point mutations and short additions and deletions—5th edition. Nucleic Acids Res 1994;22:3534–3546.
168. Harris PC, Ward CJ, Peral B, Hughes J. Autosomal dominant polycystic kidney disease: Molecular analysis. Hum Mol Genet 1995;4: 1745–1749.
169. Reeders ST, Breuning MH, Davies KE, et al. A highly polymorphic DNA marker linked to adult polycystic kidney disease on chromosome 16. Nature 1985;317:542–544.
170. Wang M, Mata J, Price CE, Iverson PL, Godfrey M. Prenatal and presymptomatic diagnosis of the Marfan syndrome using fluorescence PCR and an automated sequencer. Prenat Diagn 1995;15: 499–507.
171. Byers PH. Osteogenesis imperfecta. In: Royce PM, Steinmann B, eds. Connective tissue and its heritable disorders: molecular genetic and medical aspects, 10th Ed. New York: John Wiley & Sons, 1993: 317–350.
172. Barker D, Wright E, Nguyen K, et al. Gene for von Recklinghausen neurofibromatosis is in the pericentromeric region of chromosome 17. Science 1987;236:1100–1102.
173. Timchenko LT, Caskey CT. Trinucleotide repeat disorders in humans: discussions of mechanisms and medical issues. FASEB J 1996;10: 1589–1597.
174. Sherman SL, Jacobs PA, Morton NE, et al. Further segregation analysis of the fragile X syndrome with special reference to transmitting males. Hum Genet 1985;69:289–299.
175. Fu Y-H, Kuhl DPA, Pizzuti A, et al. Variation of the CGG repeat at the fragile X site results in genetic instability: resolution of the Sherman paradox. Cell 1991;67:1047–1058.
176. Nolin SL, Lewis FA, Ye LL, et al. Familial transmission of the FMR1 CGG repeat. Am J Hum Genet 1996;59:1252–1261.
177. Adinolfi M, Polani P. Prenatal diagnosis of genetic disorders in preimplantation embryos: invasive and non-invasive approaches. Hum Genet 1989;83:16–19.
178. Grifo JA, Tang YX, Munne S, Krey L. Update in preimplantation genetic diagnosis: successes, advances and problems. Curr Opin Obstet Gynecol 1996;8:135–138.
179. Handyside AH, Delhanty JDA. Preimplantation genetic diagnosis: strategies and surprises. Trends Genet 1997;13:270–275.
180. Bianchi DW, Shuber AP, DeMaria A, Fougner AC, Klinger KW. Fetal cells in maternal blood: determination of purity and yield by quantitative polymerase chain reaction. Am J Obstet Gynecol 1994;171: 922–926.
181. Simpson JL, Elias S. Isolating fetal cells in maternal circulation for prenatal diagnosis. Prenat Diagn 1994;14:1229–1242.
182. Valerio D, Aiello R, Altieri V Malato AP, Fortunato A, Cauazio A. Culture of fetal erythroid progenitor cells from maternal blood for noninvasive prenatal genetic diagnosis. Prenat Diagn 1996;16:1073–1082.

Cherry and Merkatz's Complications of Pregnancy,
Fifth Edition, edited by W. R. Cohen.
Lippincott Williams & Wilkins, Philadelphia © 2000.

CHAPTER 6

Environmental and Occupational Hazards

Todd Rosen and Iffath Abbasi Hoskins

In this century, women have attained freedoms in the social, economic, scientific, military, and political spheres that in previous generations were accessible only to men. During this revolution, technology and industry also have grown tremendously, as have the number of potential hazards to women and their pregnancies. Whereas advances in medicine, surgery, and pharmacology have led to significantly improved overall maternal and neonatal health in the twentieth century, individuals must cope with a new set of reproductive hazards. These hazards include numerous synthetic chemicals, many of which became widespread in the marketplace and environment before sufficient testing was performed to assess their impact on human health and reproduction. The widespread use of nuclear technology has increased the number of women at risk from exposure to ionizing radiation. Pregnant women in certain occupations are subject to physical exertion, psychologic stressors, or both. Even in the home, women are becoming engaged in an increasingly diverse range of activities, each of which may present a danger to pregnancy.

It is important for the clinician caring for pregnant women or for women considering pregnancy to recognize that there are potential occupational and environmental risks that may affect these patients adversely. It is not reasonable to expect every primary care physician to become an expert in occupational medicine, but every physician should include a screening occupational history as part of the initial evaluation of all women. This history should include an assessment of the home and of hobbies that might present a danger to pregnancy. For example, many female artists and wives of male artists may be exposed to hazardous art materials in home studios (1). Ceramics artists may be exposed to a variety of toxic heavy metals, including lead, and to toxic gasses such as carbon monoxide from a kiln; painters may be exposed to lead and a variety of solvents. Health care providers also should become familiar with the potential environmental hazards in their community, such as proximity to hazardous waste sites or other sources of pollution. If a potential occupational or environmental hazard is identified, an occupational medicine specialist may be consulted. Depending on the nature of the hazard, a clinical intervention or increased surveillance of an at-risk pregnancy may be indicated.

Almost any biologically active substance can behave as a potential toxin and, in turn, affect pregnancy adversely. The first list of such agents was prepared after passage of the United States Occupational Safety and Health Act (OSHA) in 1970 to establish standards to provide a workplace free of hazards that are known to, or are likely to, cause serious physical harm or death to workers. Listings containing these standards have been used as guidelines to make recommendations for workers. The National Institute for Occupational Safety and Health (NIOSH) (2) also monitors the problems of occupational exposures and performs scientific investigations to identify hazards, determine methods to control them, and recommend federal standards to limit these dangers. In this chapter, a strong effort has been made to address the most significant reproductive toxicities facing women, but because of the vast scope of this topic, the reader may require additional information. In this instance, the reader is referred to the excellent, comprehensive text edited by Paul (3).

GENERAL CONSIDERATIONS

In the United States, most women are employed, and more than 80% continue their employment into the third trimester of pregnancy (4). More than one half of women continue their employment until less than one month before their expected date of confinement. In 1991, the U.S. Department of Labor reported that 44.4% of women worked in technical, sales, and administrative positions;

T. Rosen and I. A. Hoskins: Department of Obstetrics and Gynecology, New York University School of Medicine, New York, NY 10016.

26.2% in managerial jobs; 17.7% in service; and the remainder in blue-collar jobs such as machine operators, laborers, and farming (5). Studies have had conflicting conclusions, but, overall, work during pregnancy does not appear to increase the risk for adverse pregnancy outcomes (6). Women who must stand for long periods or whose job requires heavy lifting may be at risk for preterm labor and delivery as well as low-birth-weight infants.

Studies on occupational risk may be confounded by what has been termed the *healthy worker effect* (7), which describes the favorable sociodemographic profile of women who work compared with those who do not. Women who work tend to be white, married, have higher income and education levels, are less likely to smoke, and more often have a planned, desired pregnancy. All these factors are associated with improved perinatal outcome and can confound the analysis of studies comparing pregnancy outcomes between workers exposed to a given hazard and nonworkers.

With the high rate of female employment, correlations between occupational hazards and increasing rates of adverse pregnancy outcomes are being drawn. Limited data are available on the potential hazardous effects of most occupational chemicals to which pregnant women are exposed. To date, fewer than 1% of the thousands of industrial agents have been identified as perinatal toxins or teratogens (8). The American College of Obstetricians and Gynecologists, in conjunction with the American Academy of Pediatrics, developed guidelines in an attempt to help protect pregnant women and their fetuses (9,10).

Generally, most environmental and occupational agents will affect pregnant women much as they would affect any other adults; however, the physiologic alterations of pregnancy may modify susceptibility to these agents (11). For example, increased ventilation may enhance the absorption of volatile toxins and gases. Progesterone-induced hypomotility of the gut may result in enhanced absorption of toxins. Increased blood volume and body fat may result in increased distribution and sequestration of some agents. Hypoalbuminuria may result in decreased protein binding and increased bioavailability of toxins. Placental metabolism and biotransformation of substances may detoxify or enhance their fetal teratogenic effects (12). Additionally, the increased glomerular filtration rate seen in pregnancy may help to eliminate potentially hazardous metabolites of toxins (13).

Despite the possible increased sensitivity of the fetus to environmental and occupational hazards, well-defined, separate safety standards and exposure limits for pregnant women have not been developed for most substances. Most previously established standards were intended to prevent acute toxicity in exposed or at-risk workers (14). Thus, although complying with available standards may protect pregnant women from possible adverse sequelae, their fetuses still may be vulnerable.

Susceptibility

The final outcomes of teratogenesis include death, malformations, growth retardation, and functional disorders, all of which depend on the developmental stage at which the insult occurs. Often a teratogen may have one effect if exposure occurs during embryogenesis and another if it occurs later in pregnancy. Exposures occurring during the critical period of embryogenesis, that is, at 2 to 8 weeks' gestation, may lead to severe structural abnormalities and result in fetal death. If exposures occur later, functional deficits and growth retardation are the likely results.

In the early first trimester, the embryo contains few undifferentiated cells, each with the potential for extensive proliferation, but with immature repair, detoxification, and defense mechanisms (15). Furthermore, because the placental barrier is not yet fully formed, the susceptibility of the embryo to potential harm is further enhanced. Most insults at this critical period result in an all-or-nothing damage phenomenon; either there is such severe damage as to cause death, or the insult is overcome by the unexposed, normal cells and normal development ensues (16).

Other factors that influence the ability of toxins to affect the fetus are the nature, dose, and duration of exposure of the agent. The manifestations of noxious agents increase proportionately with the dose and duration, varying from no effect to total lethality.

Evaluation of Data

Much of the data regarding the potential dangers of occupational and environmental hazards are based on animal experiments. Caution should be exercised in interpretation and extrapolation to humans, because obvious biologic differences and the effects of dose and route of exposure of the agent.

Although most substances have been tested inadequately in humans, increasing the knowledge of interspecies physiologic variations improves the ability of animal tests to predict human effects. Human susceptibility in some cases may be identical to, if not greater than, that of certain animals (16). Chronic exposure of pregnant workers may result in body-tissue levels far in excess of the acute short-term exposure of most animal experiments. Finally, currently available information is often inaccurate and incomplete on the subject of potential hazards to the fetus.

ALTITUDE

The physiologic effects of high altitude begin when the oxygen saturation of arterial blood falls below that of sea level. The altitude at which this change occurs depends primarily on a person's preexisting medical conditions and the duration of high-altitude exposure. Permanent residents of high-altitude areas become acclimatized after a variable amount of time, which raises arterial oxygen saturation. Oxygen saturations fall below 90% for permanent residents at about 8,400 feet and 5,800 feet for visitors to high-altitude locations before acclimatization occurs (17).

Altitude-specific disorders that affect both pregnant and nonpregnant persons are acute mountain sickness (AMS), high-altitude pulmonary edema (HAPE), and chronic mountain sickness (CMS). AMS is characterized by symptoms including headache, insomnia, dyspnea, anorexia, and fatigue, which develop during the first 24 hours at altitude (18). Persons with HAPE, a potentially fatal disorder, present with tachypnea, tachycardia, frothy pink sputum, and may be obtunded or unconscious (19). CMS is characterized by severe headaches and confusion after a prolonged exposure to high altitude.

The normal physiologic changes that occur with pregnancy result in an increased demand for oxygen that predisposes the pregnant woman to altitude-aggravated disorders. Minute ventilation increases by 30% to 40% by late pregnancy, primarily as a result of an increase in tidal volume (20), with oxygen consumption increasing 15% to 20% percent. Cardiac output increases by about 30% by the end of the second trimester (21,22). The primary mechanisms by which the woman compensates for the relative hypoxia encountered at high altitude already have been employed in response to pregnancy, making her more susceptible to disease. Data from pregnancies that occur at high altitude demonstrate that inadequate oxygen delivery may influence pregnancy outcome.

Pregnancy at high altitude is associated with intrauterine growth restriction (IUGR) (23). Data collected from more than 300,000 pregnancies at altitudes ranging from sea level to 5,030 m document a decrease of approximately 100 g for neonatal birth weight per 1000 m of elevation for term pregnancies (24,25). In a study by Moore and colleagues, infants born to mothers averaged 3,186 g at 3,110 m and 2920 g at 4,329 m (23). The average birth weight at sea level was 3409 g. Smoking appears to exacerbate the effects of high altitude on fetal growth. In the same study, the authors found a 2.5-fold greater depressant effect from smoking on infant birth weight at 3,110 m than in women who smoked but resided at sea level. In a 1977 study, McCullough and colleagues (25) reported a twofold increased risk for infant mortality for women living at high altitude in Colorado, but not all investigators have confirmed this relationship.

It has been reported that the incidence of pregnancy-induced hypertension was increased among women living at high altitude, but this has not been confirmed in other studies (23). Recent reports document that total blood volume and uterine blood flow in humans are decreased during pregnancies at high altitude and that alterations in uteroplacental blood flow precede hypertension in preeclampsia at high altitude (26–28). A recent epidemiologic study linked an increased risk of craniosynostosis in the fetus with maternal high-altitude exposure (29). The authors hypothesized that because the cranial sutures are *acral*, that is, they are supplied by vessels at the terminus of an arterial tree, they have increased susceptibility to altitude-induced hypoxemia.

A paucity of data exists about pregnant women visiting high altitude for short periods. Information on 12 pregnancies from U.S. embassy personnel stationed at La Paz, Bolivia, at 3,597 m suggested that women who arrived there during pregnancy experienced more complications than women who conceived after arrival. Five of the six women who arrived during pregnancy experienced complications such as eclampsia, preterm delivery, and threatened abortion (30).

Most modern aircraft cruise at altitudes of 20,000 to 40,000 feet above sea level. Even though they maintain a self-contained pressurized cabin environment, this pressure is corrected only to an atmospheric pressure equivalent to 5,000 to 8,000 feet above sea level. For most passengers, this exposure to a moderate high-altitude environment is short lived and unlikely to have an adverse effect on pregnancy. Air travel industry employees such as pilots and flight attendants have a more prolonged exposure to this environment and may be subject to the same pregnancy risks as women living at these altitudes. A 1973 study found that flight attendants were at increased risk for spontaneous fetal loss and birth defects (31), but more recent data (32) suggest that these risks may have been overestimated.

In addition to the effects of chronic hypoxia, high-altitude air travel workers are subject to increased ozone concentrations in their environment. Chronic exposure to levels greater than 1 part per million (ppm) is considered hazardous in humans, producing ophthalmologic and respiratory irritation. OSHA recommends that the peak cutoff level for ozone exposure is 0.3 ppm for up to 2 hours. Airline personnel have developed symptoms traceable to ozone when levels reach four times the standards recommended by OSHA. Other potential hazards to personnel of the air travel industry include cosmic radiation exposure and disruption of circadian patterns to travelers across time zones.

One additional risk to passengers on long flights may be the *economy class syndrome*, which describes deep vein thrombosis, presumably caused by prolonged venous stasis in the lower limbs (33). The likelihood of venous thromboembolism is increased fivefold in healthy pregnant women compared with nonpregnant women of similar age (34); so they are likely to be more susceptible during flight. Women should be advised to perform frequent leg and body exercises with regular walks down the aisles during airplane flights.

ARSENIC

Occupational exposure to arsenic occurs in mining and smelting and also in the pesticide, pharmaceutical, electronics, and chemical industries. Populations without occupational exposure may ingest arsenic via contaminated seafood and drinking water (35). Acute poisoning usually occurs after the consumption of tainted food or drink but has occurred after an industrial exposure (36). Symptoms are related to severe gastrointestinal inflammation and cardiogenic shock (37). Chronic exposure can result in a myriad of symptoms affecting multiple organ systems. It is known to be a lethal toxicant as well as a neurotoxicant and human carcinogen. Studies on the effects of arsenic on pregnant women and their developing offspring are limited, however.

Two case reports (38,39) involved poisoning of pregnant women, one resulting in a fetal demise and the other one a study by Nordstrom and colleagues that linked occupational exposure to arsenic around a smelter in Sweden to spontaneous abortions and infants of low birth weight (40). Two epidemiologic studies have been published on environmental exposure to drinking water contaminated by arsenic. The first found that when arsenic was detected at any level, it was associated with an elevated risk of developing coarctation of the aorta in affected fetuses (41); however, the risk of neural tube defects or renal agenesis, anomalies seen most frequently in laboratory animals exposed to arsenic (42), was not found, which calls these results into question. The second study associated arsenic in drinking water with an increased frequency of spontaneous abortion. Subsequent studies have not been performed to confirm this report.

Most data about the developmental toxicity of arsenic come from animal studies, primarily with rodents as subjects. There are multiple natural forms of arsenic. Arsenite has been found in most studies to have the greatest toxicity for both mother and fetus. Arsenate has approximately one fourth the toxicity of arsenite, and organic arsenic forms are substantially less toxic than the inorganic forms. Data from rodent species demonstrated that arsenic causes a reproducible set of congenital anomalies: neural tube defects and renal agenesis. These effects could be produced without maternal toxicity, and malformation incidence was greatest when arsenic was given at days 9 or 10 of development, suggesting specific teratogenic events related to arsenic. In a 1994 analysis of the reproductive toxicity of arsenic, Golub concluded that arsenic is a developmental toxicant because it produces characteristic anomalies in a dose- and stage-specific manner (42). The applicability of these studies to human pregnancies is not certain. It seems prudent, nevertheless, to advise patients with a history of arsenic exposure of the potential adverse effects. Immediate removal of the patient from this environment should ensue, and a targeted ultrasound examination should be offered to assess for anomalies.

ASBESTOS

Asbestos is a term used to describe six different fibrous mineral silicates with various biological effects (43). Demand for asbestos has decreased significantly in the United States, but worldwide production has not decreased because of less stringent regulation of its use and production in other parts of the world. Persons most at risk for developing asbestos-related disease are involved in industries in which the processed fiber is handled and maintained. Chronic exposure to asbestos leads to *asbestosis*, which manifests initially as dyspnea and a nonproductive cough. The disease may progress with an increase in the severity of symptoms and the development of a productive cough (44). *Cor pulmonae* may develop in severe cases and is a frequent cause of death from asbestosis. Asbestos is also a carcinogen responsible for adenocarcinoma and mesothelioma of the lung; the former is the most common. Evidence also has been found that asbestos is associated with gastrointestinal cancers. In most patients, prolonged exposure to asbestos of 20 to 30 years is required before the onset of either symptomatic benign disease or malignancy.

Sparse data are available on the reproductive toxicity of asbestosis. In two recent studies, transplacental passage of asbestos fibers to lung, liver, and skeletal muscle was documented in stillborn infants born to exposed women (45,46). The most recent of these reports compared the asbestos fiber counts in the placentas of 40 stillborn infants with 45 full-term, liveborn controls; a highly significant difference was found in the asbestos fiber counts between the two groups (46). Mesotheliomas have been documented in children (47), perhaps the consequence of transplacental passage of asbestos, but they may have been caused by nonoccupational exposure to asbestos from fibers brought into the home by an exposed household member.

When chrysotile asbestos was added to the drinking water of pregnant mice, neither an increase in congenital anomalies nor an increased rate of fetal loss was seen (48). In the same study, *in vitro* administration of asbestos to mouse blastocysts resulted in a decreased postimplantation survival, but no teratogenic effects were noted.

AGRICULTURAL WORKERS

Although these workers do not appear to be at increased risk for adverse pregnancy outcomes, low sperm counts have been reported by Henderson and co-workers (49), Strohmer and colleagues (50), and Figa-Talamanca and colleagues (51). No increase in spontaneous abortion rates has been described (52), nor have there been any associated increases in congenital abnormality rates (53–55). Sanjose and colleagues (56) found no increase in the incidence of low birth weight.

BERYLLIUM AND SELENIUM

Before 1950, beryllium was used in fluorescent lamp manufacturing, and most cases of beryllium-related disease were noted in workers occupationally exposed in this industry. Today, beryllium is used in nuclear technologies, defense industries, and manufacture of heat shields. It is also used as an alloying agent for copper (57). Estimates of the total number of workers at risk in the United States vary widely, from 30,000 to 800,000 (58,59).

Chronic beryllium disease is a granulomatous disease characterized by exertional dyspnea with cough, chest pain, fatigue, weight loss, and arthralgias. Differentiation from sarcoidosis may be difficult. The primary treatment is complete avoidance of beryllium and medication with corticosteroids if necessary.

Beryllium crosses the placenta and has been found in neonatal urine. There have been no reports of adverse pregnancy outcome resulting from beryllium disease; however, children have been indirectly exposed to beryllium when this substance has been brought home inadvertently by an exposed household member (60).

Selenium is an essential trace element required for the production of glutathione peroxidase. When present in excessive amounts, it can be toxic to humans. Exposure to airborne selenium may irritate mucous membranes, causing eye irritation, coughs, sneezes, and respiratory distress. There is a report of a fatal exposure to selenium (61).

Although strong evidence exists that selenium is embryotoxic and teratogenic in nonmammalian species, data are less conclusive in mammals (62). Some data suggest that selenium may be teratogenic in mammals, but this may be a result of the maximum tolerated dose protocol rather than a direct teratogenic effect of this agent. Epidemiologic evidence has failed to demonstrate a relationship between selenium and teratogenesis or reproductive toxicity (63,64).

CADMIUM

Like many heavy metals, cadmium has toxic effects in humans. Primary adverse effects are due to pulmonary and renal toxicity. There is evidence that cadmium may be a carcinogen, although this evidence is considerably weaker than that for other metals. Cadmium is present in the environment and may present a danger by occupational exposure. It is used in nickel-cadmium batteries, electroplating, smelting, and mining. Shellfish are a dietary source of cadmium and may contain from 100 to 1,000 mg per kilogram of this metal (65). Estimated daily intake in the United States from all sources is 10 to 40 mg per day. Cigarette smoke is another source of exposure, and it is estimated that smoking one or two packs per day doubles daily intake of cadmium (65).

Animal and human studies show that cadmium has a special affinity for the placenta (66) and suppresses mitochondrial succinic dehydrogenase and cytochrome oxidase activities. Its concentrations in the placenta far exceed those in cord blood, suggesting that the placenta serves as a barrier against fetal exposure (67).

Animal data reveal that when injected into rodents in early gestation, cadmium may be highly teratogenic. In a series of studies, facial malformations, undescended testes, hydrocephalus, and resorptions were noted in exposed fetuses (65). Other researchers have found evidence of severe growth retardation, fetal death, and neonatal anemia under similar experimental conditions. In a recent study (68), female rats exposed to 5 and 10 mg per kilogram of cadmium before fertilization demonstrated a dose-dependent increase in infertility. No effects on pregnancy were seen in the rats that had litters after such an exposure, however. It has been reported that multiple skeletal defects and abnormal bone formation may occur secondary to effects on calcium metabolism following cadmium exposure (67).

Single doses of cadmium administered to male rodents resulted in marked testicular atrophy (69). Similar exposures in humans do not appear to have the same result, possibly because of the protective effect of the testicular protein metallothionein, which preferentially binds cadmium.

Human data are limited, and much of it is anecdotal; but some studies suggest a decrease in the birth weight of exposed neonates (70). The most recent study on occupational exposure to cadmium was a retrospective epidemiologic study conducted by Berlin and co-workers (71) on female workers in a nickel-cadmium battery plant. When 157 children born to exposed mothers were compared with 109 children born to unexposed controls, no differences in mean birth weight were detected. Only smoking had a negative effect on birth weight in this study. Interestingly, it has been suggested that cadmium in cigarette smoke contributes significantly to the increased incidence of low birth weight in infants born to women who smoke. One of the main effects of cadmium toxicity is decreased absorption and metabolism of nutrients like iron in the gastrointestinal tract. Even though they may not significantly decrease nutrient absorption in the mother, low levels of cadmium may cause a significant decrease in the availability of nutrients to the fetus, resulting in IUGR.

Counseling patients with cadmium exposure during pregnancy may be difficult. Both OSHA and the American Conference of Governmental Industrial Hygienists (ACGIH) have set occupational limits for cadmium exposure. Whereas the data from animal experiments indicate that cadmium in high doses injected parenterally is highly teratogenic, insufficient data are available to suggest that cadmium presents a major hazard to pregnant women. Cadmium's poor absorption from the gastrointestinal tract or protection of the fetus by the placental barrier may account for this scarcity of data. Certainly, a targeted ultrasound examination should be offered to pregnant women who have had known exposure, and cadmium toxicity may be explored in infertile couples. Currently, insufficient evidence exists to offer termination of pregnancy based solely on a history of cadmium exposure.

CARBON DISULFIDE

More than half of the carbon disulfide used in the United States is involved in the manufacture of viscose rayon and cellophane (72). Carbon disulfide also is used in the production of carbon tetrachloride, neoprene cement, and rubber accelerators; in paint and varnish products; and in rocket fuel. It produces symptoms in affected persons similar to those produced by other solvents, but it also produces a characteristic group of toxic effects. It is a neurotoxicant that is capable of causing peripheral neuropathy and global central nervous system (CNS) dysfunction. Outcomes of acute poisonings may be fatal or may cause irreversible CNS injury. Prolonged exposure also has been linked to an increase in atherosclerotic heart disease and retinal microangiopathy (73).

Only a limited number of studies have implicated carbon disulfide as a reproductive toxicant. A 1972 study by Lancranjan found that male workers exposed to carbon disulfide had significantly lower sperm counts and a greater incidence of abnormal morphology than controls (74). In a more recent study, investigators found no difference in the semen analysis of exposed workers compared with controls, but the workers had decreased libido and potency.

Carbon disulfide is known to be transmitted transplacentally and through breast milk (75). Two epidemiologic studies (76,77) have linked carbon disulfide to spontaneous abortions in exposed women, but this relationship is far from certain, and more work is needed to verify this effect. There is a paucity of animal data on carbon disulfide and its effect in pregnancy. Fetal toxicity was demonstrated in pregnant rats by an increase in congenital malformations but only at concentrations about 100 times the current federal standard for a permissible level of carbon disulfide exposure (78). In a study that may be more applicable to typical human exposures, pregnant rats exposed to inhaled concentrations of 3 ppm of carbon disulfide did not show an increased rate of spontaneous abortions or offspring with congenital anomalies, but their offspring did demonstrate behavioral abnormalities (79). This finding could be consistent with the known neurotoxicant effects of this agent.

CARBON MONOXIDE

Carbon monoxide (CO) is the most common pollutant present in the lower atmosphere (80). It is a colorless, odorless gas that is produced by the incomplete combustion of hydrocarbons. Most of the CO in the atmosphere results from natural pollution, produced primarily by forest fires, atmospheric oxidation of methane, and ocean life. About 10% of environmental CO is derived from man-made sources (81). Exposure in industry and to sources in the home are often the cause of poisoning in humans. Occupational exposure to CO may occur in the steel and mining industries; firefighters, cooks, garage mechanics, chauffeurs, and furnace repairers are nonindustrial workers at risk of CO toxicity. Most cases of CO poisoning are not workplace exposures. Although asphyxiation by CO may be used as an instrument for suicide, most poisonings during pregnancy are accidental (82). Poisoning can occur during winter from faulty heaters or in any season from a variety of causes, such as sleeping in a motor home with the motor running. The greatest nonnatural source of CO is the automobile. Concentrations of CO in heavy traffic can reach 115 ppm, 75 ppm in vehicles on the highway, and 23 ppm in residential areas. In contrast, the average atmospheric CO concentration is 0.1 ppm (81).

CO is an asphyxiant; it causes its toxic effects mainly by reducing oxygen delivery to tissue. Poisoning from CO is not uncommon in the United States. The U.S. Centers for Disease Control and Prevention (CDC) reported in 1982 (83) that 3,500 to 4,000 deaths annually were attributable to CO intoxication. In 1986, Marzella and Myers (84) reported that CO was responsible for half of the fatal poisonings in the United States. By 1990, 60 case reports of pregnant women who suffered from CO poisoning had appeared, only one resulting from an occupational exposure. Severe exposures in the chemical industry in nonpregnant workers have been reported, however (85).

A patient with acute CO poisoning may present with symptoms of weakness, dizziness, nausea, and vomiting and, in severe cases, cardiovascular collapse. Blood carboxyhemoglobin (COHb) levels generally correlate with the severity of disease, and acute intoxications are generally seen with COHb levels of 30% to 40%. When COHb levels reach 50%, syncope, seizures, and death may result (86). In cases of severe intoxication, the cherry-red color of COHb may be visible in the skin, mucous membranes, and fingernails, but this color is often absent and diagnosis may be difficult. In cases of chronic exposure to low CO concentrations, patients are likely to exhibit cyanosis and pallor, and the clinician often must have a high degree of suspicion to make the diagnosis of chronic poisoning (81).

CO causes its toxicity primarily by two mechanisms. It binds reversibly to hemoglobin (Hb) with an affinity that is 250 times greater than oxygen (O_2) (87). CO competes with O_2 for binding to Hb and, in addition, causes a left shift of the Hb dissociation curve, reducing O_2 delivery to tissues. The second mechanism by which CO may cause toxicity is by poisoning the machinery of intracellular respiration. CO has been demonstrated to bind to mitochondrial enzymes that contain non-Hb ferroproteins (80).

In addition to exposure from exogenous sources, CO is produced endogenously from the breakdown of heme pigments. Endogenous production is doubled in the pregnant versus the nonpregnant state, with 15% of CO production coming from the fetus. Normal maternal COHb levels, in the absence of environmental pollution, vary between 0.5% and 1%.

CO is a component of cigarette smoke and is likely the most common exogenous source of fetal exposure to this agent. COHb levels in the blood of women who smoke and their infants at the time of delivery have been measured to be as high as 14%. Actual levels during most of pregnancy may be even higher because it is likely that women reduce their cigarette smoking during parturition (87). Fetal COHb levels tend to be 10% to 15% higher than maternal levels, which in part accounts for the fetus's increased susceptibility to CO intoxication. A well-established relation exists between maternal smoking and low birth weight, and it has been proposed that CO intoxication contributes to IUGR by decreasing O_2 delivery to the fetus.

Studies in rodents indicate that fetal damage can occur with relatively low levels of CO inhalation. Pregnant rats exposed to an environment containing 125 to 150 ppm of CO demonstrated IUGR and neurobehavioral deficits. Pregnant monkeys exposed to higher doses of CO gave birth to fetuses with severe brain damage (81).

Norman and Halton, in a review of 60 case reports of maternal CO poisonings (88), found that the degree of fetal toxicity correlated well with the amount of CO exposure. Of 27 women who suffered toxicity that was severe enough to cause unconsciousness, 15 fetal deaths occurred and 10 survived but with impairments. Of 12 first-trimester exposures, six fetuses suffered from congenital malformations, although this was a heterogenous group of disorders. Acute, severe CO poisoning is associated with a maternal mortality of approximately 20% and fetal mortality up to 67% (80).

One study assessed the contribution of environmental CO to infant birth weight in Denver, Colorado, which had the highest levels of CO exposure in the United States (89). The researchers investigated whether the relative hypoxia due to chronic CO poisoning in this setting would result in adverse fetal outcome. They did not demonstrate a strong relationship between ambient levels of CO and fetal birth weight, but the study had several limitations, including its retrospective design and an inability to control for maternal smoking.

The definitive therapy for CO intoxication is administration of high-dose O_2, which displaces CO from Hb and causes its diffusion out of tissues. Hyperbaric oxygen therapy (HBO) is the treatment of choice when available. The half-life of CO in the blood of the adult is approximately 280 minutes; it is longer in the fetus. When 100% O_2 is administered via nonrebreathing face mask, this half-life is reduced to 90 minutes. The half-life of CO may be reduced to 23 minutes using HBO at an equivalent depth of 60 feet of sea water (80). There is a theoretic risk of causing ophthalmologic abnormalities in the fetus with HBO, specifically retrolental fibroplasia; but because of the high risk of fetal and maternal mortality, the possible disastrous consequences of CO poisoning in the pregnant woman clearly outweigh the theoretic morbidity associated with HBO treatment (80). Exchange transfusions have been used in moribund patients (81), and measures to minimize O_2 consumption, such as relative hypothermia and intubation followed by paralysis, could be considered in a severely affected patient.

DIOXIN

Chlorinated dioxin derivatives are polyhalogenated compounds like polychlorinated and polybrominated biphenyls (PCBs and PBBs). They are among the most potent human toxins. They are fat soluble, stable, and cause adverse effects when concentrations measure in parts per billion (ppb) and even parts per trillion (ppt). Dioxins are toxic by-products created during the manufacture of chlorinated phenols such as herbicides. There are a large number of dioxin isomers, with 2,3,7,8-tetrachlordibenzo-para-dioxin (2,3,7,8-TCDD) being the most toxic; its use was banned in 1989 by the U.S. Environmental Protection Agency (EPA) (90). Dioxin became a source of national attention and controversy when Vietnam war veterans alleged birth defects in their offspring after exposure to Agent Orange. Not all studies have supported this association (91).

Well-conducted studies of human toxicities from dioxins have been conducted following accidental exposures involving large populations. The most notable industrial accident occurred when an explosion in Seveso, Italy, in 1976 contaminated more than 700 acres and affected more than 25,000 inhabitants. In the exposed population, an increased incidence of chloracne, polyneuropathy, and hepatomegaly occurred, and on long-term follow-up, cancer rates in the exposed population were increased (92). TCDD is a potent carcinogen in animal models (93), thought to exert its effect by tumor promotion rather than by mutagenesis.

Dioxin derivatives are potent teratogens in animals (94), but studies of human exposures have not clearly demonstrated an adverse effect on pregnancy outcome. No major congenital malformations were found in infants born to 26 women in Seveso who were in their first trimester at the time of the explosion (95). In a heavily contaminated region of Missouri from 1971 through 1973, a trend toward increased neonatal death rates, low birth weight, and birth defects was seen, but none of these outcomes reached statistical significance (90). Exposure to Agent Orange in Oregon in the early 1970s was associated with an increased risk of spontaneous abortion in a study by the EPA (94), and a recent study from the Netherlands (96) showed that infants who were exposed to low levels of dioxins through breastfeeding had elevated liver enzymes and decreased platelet levels. Investigators were able to measure maternal and fetal dioxin levels and were able to establish a dose-response relationship between dioxin and its toxic effects.

Dioxin has been postulated to exert at least some of its biological effect by acting as an antiestrogen (97). It does not block binding of estrogen to its receptor, but it may alter the metabolism of estrogen, thereby modifying its effects. Dioxin belongs to a class of pollutants that includes pesticides and labeled endocrine disrupters, whose effects on the ecology and on human disease are just beginning to be explored. Endocrine disrupters have been postulated to affect human fertility adversely and to increase the incidence of endometriosis, hypospadias, and various teratogenic events. Work on the effects of endocrine disrupters is in its infancy, and it is hoped that studies will help to define the risk that these agents pose to human health.

ELECTROMAGNETIC FIELDS

Over the past few years, the possibility that electromagnetic fields (EMF) emitted from various appliances may have deleterious effects has aroused public concern. Despite several reviews that have provided reassurances regarding their safety, EMF emissions continue to incite public anxiety. All people are subjected to EMF exposure from numerous sources. EMF exposures can result from the use of water beds, electric blankets, home heating devices, and video display terminals (VDTs) and occupation in the electric and electronics industry. The types of exposure can be *very low frequency* or *extremely low frequency*. The amount of EMF emissions from VDTs is usually lower than from other office equipment such as printers and copiers.

Lindbohm and Hietanen (98) found that the magnetic fields emitted by VDTs were not associated with adverse pregnancy outcomes. Parazzini and colleagues (99) performed a metaanalysis of nine published case–control studies on the relation between VDT exposure during pregnancy and adverse outcomes. The odds ratio (OR) for spontaneous abortions was 1.0 (95% CI, 0.9–1.0). No consistent evidence of increasing risk with duration of exposure to VDT was found. The OR for low birth weight was 1.0 and for congenital malformations, also 1.0. No specific malformation pattern was seen. Thus, this metanalysis provided reassuring evidence on the absence of any major risk of adverse pregnancy outcome following VDT exposure, including spontaneous abortions, low birth weight, and congenital malformations.

In a related study, Bracken and co-workers (100) reviewed the effects of high (60 Hz) residential exposure to EMF from electric blankets or water beds on fetal growth and found no adverse effects. There was no relationship even with longer exposures and higher settings. Dlugosz and colleagues (101) and Milansky and colleagues (102) found no increase in the congenital anomaly rates following maternal use of electric blankets, nor was there any evidence of an increase in mutagenicity rate following EMF exposure. All these studies showed a uniform lack of adverse outcomes across all three trimesters.

Paternal EMF exposure has not been associated with any adverse pregnancy outcomes (103); however, Nordstrom and colleagues (104) described altered sex ratios (fewer male children) in the offspring of fathers exposed to EMF.

HEALTH CARE WORKERS

The term *health care worker* encompasses a large number of different professions, many engaged in quite different activities involved in the care of patients. Positions range from physicians and nurses to radiology technicians to home health aides and even veterinarians; thus, it is difficult to assess risks to this group as a whole. Many common exposures are shared, however, and we have attempted to detail the risks of the best studied reproductive hazards. The risks of anesthetic agents, antineoplastic drugs, residency training for physicians, infectious diseases, and sterilization media are discussed herein.

In addition to these risks, health care workers face a significant risk of job-related violence. In a 1996 report, OSHA (105) stated that more assaults occurred against workers in the health care and social services fields than in any other industry. Most nonfatal assaults occurred in nursing homes, hospitals, and institutions providing residential care. Pregnancy would not appear to be any protection against violence. OSHA has made recommendations for prevention and control of this unfortunate hazard (105).

Anesthetic Agents

Between 50,000 and 250,000 health care workers are exposed to inhalational anesthetics on a regular basis each year (106,107). These agents are found not only in the operating room but also in dentists' offices, delivery rooms, emergency rooms, and recovery rooms from the expired breath of postoperative patients. Because exposure to these agents is widespread, occupational exposure is of serious concern.

Currently, the most widely used inhalation anesthetic agents in the United States are nitrous oxide (N_2O), enflurane, halothane, and isoflurane. Data published in 1969 and 1970 documented peak levels of 27 ppm of halothane and 428 ppm of N_2O in an operating room, with significantly higher concentrations in the work space of an anesthesiologist when a nonrebreathing system was used (108). For reference, the current NIOSH recommended exposure limits are 2 ppm halothane over 1 hour and 25 ppm N_2O over 8 h (109). In facilities with newer equipment, lower ambient levels of these agents have been measured (110).

Data from work with laboratory animals indicate that the commonly used inhalational anesthetic agents may be teratogenic. It has been established that anesthetic agents inhibit cell division (111). In a 1988 review of the topic, Friedman reported that N_2O was shown to cause increases in the frequency of fetal resorption, growth restriction, and malformations in the offspring of animals exposed to pharmacologic doses of this drug (112). Anomalies of the CNS, ocular, and skeletal anomalies were the most commonly observed malformations. A similar effect was not seen in mice or hamsters given N_2O alone. Halothane was noted to cause malformations, growth retardation, and fetal death in mice, but these treatments often resulted in death of the mother. Other researchers did not find evidence of teratogenic effects in rabbits or rats. Isoflurane was associated with increased frequencies of fetal anomalies and growth retardation in pregnant mice in one study but not in others. Enflurane was associated with an increase in limb and abdominal wall defects in the offspring of rabbits by one group, but a similar effect was not seen in mice or rabbits by other researchers. The applicability of these studies to human pregnancies is uncertain. No epidemiologic data to date have linked a specific anesthetic agent to adverse pregnancy outcome in humans.

A large number of retrospective cohort studies of reproductive outcome in health care workers with regular exposure to anesthetics have been published. The primary outcome variables in these studies were spontaneous abortion and congenital malformations of exposed fetuses. The results of these studies are summarized in Table 6-1. To date, a large prospective trial studying the relationship between occupational exposure to anesthetic agents and adverse pregnancy outcome has not been conducted.

When interpreting the results of these studies, the methodologic limitations of this work must be appreciated. All these studies are retrospective studies, and most were based solely on questionnaire data, which is highly susceptible to recall bias. For example, in the studies that reported the greatest increase in spontaneous abortions among exposed women, the spontaneous abortion rates in the control populations were remarkably low. In the large study by the American Society of Anesthesiologists (7), the spontaneous abortion rates in the control group was approximately 7%, which is significantly lower than the reported population rate of at least 15%. Additional criticisms of these works are that in most studies outcome data were accepted as reported by the respondent without further validation, and potential confounding variables may not have been studied adequately (113).

Keeping these limitations in mind, most of these studies demonstrated an increased risk for spontaneous abortion among women with occupational exposure to anesthetic gases. Many investigators reported a 1.5- to 2-fold increased risk for spontaneous abortion for exposed groups versus controls. The absolute frequency of spontaneous abortion in exposed groups does not appear to vary widely from the expected rate in the general population.

Several authors also reported an increased risk of congenital anomalies in affected fetuses, although in only two of the reviewed studies did these risks achieve statistical significance. No consistent difference in the type or pattern of congenital anomalies has been found in children born to women with occupational anesthetic exposure.

Several investigators studied the possibility that paternal exposure to anesthesia may be a reproductive hazard. Most studies were unable to link this exposure to adverse pregnancy outcome.

This body of literature, taken as a whole, suggests a slightly increased risk of spontaneous abortion in women with occupational exposure to anesthetic gases during pregnancy, but this risk is not substantially greater than that of the general population. A link between exposure and congenital malformations or between paternal exposure and adverse pregnancy outcome is not supported by the current literature.

Workers exposed to excessive amounts of anesthetic gases may demonstrate symptoms of drowsiness, irritability, depression, headache, and impaired judgment or coordination. Hepatic and renal toxicity has been reported with certain agents, and the use of laboratory assessment of liver and kidney function should be considered. Sufficient evidence has not been found to support a risk to the fetus of an affected pregnant woman.

Another hazard for pregnant patients may be that of exposure to high anesthetic concentrations over short periods, as for surgery. This finding is in contrast to the chronic, low-dose exposure encountered in the work setting. Most information on this subject is based on either animal data or retrospective epidemiologic work.

The largest controlled epidemiologic study of reproductive outcome in women who received general anesthesia during pregnancy was the Collaborative Perinatal Project (114). In this study, no specific link could be made between a specific agent and a teratogenic effect. In one series of 287 women who underwent surgery during the first and second trimesters of pregnancy, the rates of pregnancy loss were increased (115). A later study by Duncan and coworkers (116) examined 2,565 pregnancies of women undergoing surgical procedures during pregnancy and found an increased risk of spontaneous abortion compared with controls; however, the risk of abortion was linked to the type of surgery performed, which underscores the point that the risk of spontaneous abortion is related not only to the anesthetic given but also to the underlying disease process. Neither of these studies found an increased risk of congenital malformations in infants born of exposed pregnancies.

TABLE 6-1. *Pregnancy outcomes following exposure to anesthetic gases*

Study	Design	Exposed group	Controls	Rates of miscarriage			Rates of congenital anomalies		
				Exposed	Controls	RR (95% CI)	Exposed	Controls	RR (95% CI)
Knill-Jones et al, 1972 (357)	Cohort, retrospective	Anesthesiologists (n=563)	Other MDs (n=828)	180/1073 (16.8%)	315/2150 (14.7%)	1.2 (0.9 –1.4)	46/893 (5.2%)	89/1835 (4.9%)	1.1 (0.7 –1.5)
		Working anesthesiologists	Unexposed anesthesiologists	134/737 (18.2%)	46/336 (13.7%)	1.4 (0.9 –1.9)	39/599 (5.6%)	7/284 (2.5%)	2.6 (0.5 –4.7)
Corbett et al., 1972 (358)	Cohort, retrospective postal survey	Nurse anesthetists who practiced during pregnancy	Nurse anesthetists who did not practice during pregnancy				71/434 (16.4%)	15/261 (5.7%)	3.1 (1.3 –4.9)
American Society of Anesthesiologists, 1974 (359)	Cohort, retrospective postal survey	Anesthesiologists (n=1,059)	Pediatricians (639)	80.0/468 (17.1%)	27.4/308 (8.9%)	2.1 (1.1 –3.0)	22.7/384 (5.9%)	8.3/276 (3.0%)	2.0 (0.4 –3.5)
		Working anesthesiologists	Unexposed anesthesiologists	80.0/468 (17.1%)	21.7/138 (15.7%)	1.1 (0.5 –1.6)	22.7/384 (5.9%)	3.9/116 (3.4%)	1.6 (0–3.3)
		Anesthesia and OR nurses (n=19,408)	Other nurses (n=6,560)	852.7/4607 (18.5%)	294.1/1948 (15.1%)	1.3 (1.1 –1.5)	312.2/3690 (8.5%)	123.8/1629 (7.6%)	1.1 (0.9 –1.4)
		Working anesthesia and OR nurses	Unexposed anesthesiologists and OR nurses	852.7/4607 (18.5%)	328.8/2209 (14.9%)	1.3 (1.1 –1.5)	312.2/3690 (8.5%)	122.6/1841 (6.7%)	1.3 (1.0 –1.6)
Knill-Jones et al. 1975 (360)	Cohort, retrospective postal survey	Physicians' wives who worked in OR during 1st trimester of pregnancy	Matched wives, neither spouse worked in OR	65/435 (14.9%)	24/435 (5.5%)	3.0 (1.5 –4.4)	20/366 (5.5%)	6/408 (1.5%)	3.7 (0.4 –6.9)
Pharoah et al., 1977 (361)	Cohort, retrospective postal survey	Physicians with appointments in anesthesiology	Physicians with other medical appts. or no appt.	93/670 (13.8%)	1120/8375 (13.4%)	1.0 (0.8 –1.3)	16/541 (3.0%)	130/6829 (1.9%)	1.6 (0.8 –2.4)
Ericson and Kallen, 1979 (362)	Cohort, retrospective record linkage	OR personnel (n=541)	All health care workers				7/541 (1.3%)	267/19.127 (1.4%)	1.0 (0.3 –1.7)
Cohen et al., 1980 (363)	Cohort, retrospective postal survey	Dental assistants exposed to anesthetics	Dental assistants not exposed to anesthetics	134.2/807 (16.6%)	257.9/3184 (8.1%)	2.3 (1.8 –2.8)	35.8/657 (5.4%)	103.8/2882 (3.6%)	1.6 (0.9 –2.2)
Axelsson and Rylander, 1982 (364)	Cohort, retrospective postal survey with abnormalities confirmed by medical records	Exposed medical personnel (n=152)	Unexposed medical personnel (n=172)	21/133 (15.8%)	43/470 (9.1%)	1.9 (0.8 –2.9)			
Hemminki et al., 1985 (355)	Cohort retrospective postal survey	Nurses with adverse pregnancy outcome	Nurses with normal pregnancy outcome	N/A	N/A	1.2	N/A	N/A	0.9
Guirguis et al., 1990 (356)	Cohort retrospective postal survey	Exposed OR personnel	Other hospital employees	15.6% (726/4659)	12.6% (266/2213)	1.98 (1.53 –2.56)	N/A	N/A	2.24 (1.69 –2.97)

CI, confidence interval.
OR, operating room; RR, relative risk.

Antineoplastic Drugs

Many antineoplastic drugs have been reported to be mutagenic, carcinogenic, and teratogenic in both animal and human studies. Antineoplastic drugs include multiple classes of drugs, including alkylating agents, antibiotics, hormones, antimetabolites, and antimitotic agents, each with different mechanisms of action, but most with documented reproductive toxic effects.

Antineoplastic agents may have adverse effects on both male and female fertility (117). In men, oligospermia and azoospermia have been noted in cancer patients treated with a variety of agents. These changes are often reversible with cessation of therapy. Freckman and colleagues (118) discovered a loss of ovarian primordial follicles along with amenorrhea in women treated with chlorambucil for breast cancer. The alkylating agents and vinca alkaloids were the types of agents associated with the greatest effect on fertility (117).

The teratogenicity of many antineoplastic agents has been documented in experimental animals. Alkylating agents and antimetabolites appear to be associated with the greatest incidence of congenital malformations in human studies (119). There also may be an association between exposure of men to antineoplastics and congenital malformations in their offspring (117).

Pharmacy personnel and nurses working with antineoplastics may be at risk from the adverse reproductive toxic effects of these agents. Historically, these agents have been prepared without hoods, and detectable levels of the drugs have been noted in workers under these conditions (120). Several studies demonstrated an increase in the mutagenic activity of urine of exposed workers (117), and cyclophosphamide can be detected in the urine of nurses handling this drug. Several studies documented that when vertical laminar-flow hoods were used in the handling and mixing of antineoplastic drugs, worker exposure was significantly decreased and that mutagenic agents were not detectable in the urine of hospital personnel (121). Horizontal laminar-flow hoods, which are used to prevent contamination of medications, are not effective in reducing worker exposure (122).

Selevan and colleagues (121) reported their findings on the association between fetal loss and exposure to antineoplastic agents in nurses in 17 Finnish hospitals. Each of the 124 nurses with fetal loss was compared with three controls who had live births. They found a statistically significant association between exposure to the agents and spontaneous abortions. The implicated agents were cyclophosphamide, doxorubicin, and vincristine. The women who experienced fetal loss were more than twice as likely to have had first-trimester exposures to antineoplastic drugs as those who had liveborn infants. No association was found between fetal loss and cumulative exposure to the drugs.

Hemminki and colleagues (123) found that nurses who gave birth to congenitally abnormal infants were five times as likely to have handled cytotoxic drugs more than once a week during early pregnancy as women who had healthy newborns. They found no association, however, between cytotoxic drug exposure and increased pregnancy wastage. Based on these findings, they suggested that pregnant workers exercise caution when handling antineoplastic drugs.

In 1986, OSHA published guidelines for the handling of antineoplastic agents in the workplace (124). The use of special handling procedures, including a glove-box or vertical laminar-flow hood, was recommended. In addition, OSHA recommends that all workers be given a physical examination that includes a complete blood count before beginning preparation of antineoplastic agents. OSHA also recommends that a record be kept of all drugs along with their doses prepared by individual workers. Male or female workers who are planning pregnancies and breastfeeding women should be offered alternative assignments after being informed of the potential risks of occupational exposure.

Residency

Concern that the rigorous demands made on women during residency training would adversely affect their pregnancies led to a number of studies that investigated pregnancy outcomes of resident physicians. In 1985 Schwartz (125) found that pregnant residents suffered an increased incidence of preterm labor as well as placental abruption. A second study found that children born to women during their residencies had a statistically significant decrease in birth weight compared with controls. In 1990 Klebanoff and colleagues (126) published the outcomes of the pregnancies of resident physicians and compared them to the wives of male residents. They found no increase in preterm births, IUGR, or stillbirths for the study group. An increase in preeclampsia was observed but was not associated with an increase in adverse neonatal outcome or additional maternal morbidity. Also, working more than 100 hours per week was associated with an increase in preterm delivery. Another study published by the same group did not find that the risk for spontaneous abortion was increased among resident physicians (127).

Based on these data, it appears that women are not at significantly increased risk for adverse pregnancy outcome during their residencies. Special accommodations may be needed for those women who develop symptoms of preterm labor or preeclampsia.

Infectious Disease

Congenitally acquired infection is discussed in detail elsewhere in this text and is examined only briefly in this chapter. The biological agents posing a threat to health care workers that have received the most attention are the hepatitis B virus (HBV) and the human immunodeficiency virus (HIV). The most common occupational routes of exposure are through needlestick injury and splash injuries onto mucous membranes. Universal precautions should be followed when working with any patient. Other agents to which health care workers may be exposed include tuberculosis, hepatitis C, cytomegalovirus, parvovirus B19, and varicella.

Both the CDC (128) and OSHA (129) recommend hepatitis B vaccine for susceptible workers with no contraindication cited for pregnant women. In an HBV-susceptible woman exposed to HBV, the CDC recommends administration of hepatitis B immune globulin (0.06 mL/kg i.m.) within 24 hours and initiation of a vaccine series.

Recent evidence demonstrated that following exposure to HIV by needlestick or splash injury, prophylaxis with zidovudine may be effective in reducing the risk of transmission. Pregnant workers exposed to HIV should be counseled and offered this therapy. Little is known about the teratogenic effects of zidovudine given in the first trimester, but in the large AIDS Clinical Trial Group 076 Study, women with HIV were given zidovudine after 14 weeks' gestation, and no teratogenic effects were noted (130).

Veterinarians are at additional risk from toxoplasmosis infection. Almost all species of warm-blooded animals are susceptible to infection by toxoplasma, but the principal risk in small-animal practice is through contact with cat feces. Whereas it is unlikely for infection to occur through ingestion, infection has occurred via inhalation in dusty environments. Women veterinarians who are considering pregnancy should be screened for toxoplasmosis, and if susceptibility is found, protective masks may be effective in preventing transmission of this agent (131).

Sterilization Media

Chemical sterilants are widely used in operating rooms, pharmacies, and laboratories. They include a number of suspected mutagens and carcinogens, including formaldehyde, propylene oxide, and glutaraldehyde, but little is known of their reproductive toxic effects.

In the late 1970's hexachlorophene, a polychlorinated biphenyl compound used for topical sterilization, was implicated as a teratogen in humans and received a significant amount of media attention. Halling (132) suggested that hand washing with hexachlorophene soap was teratogenic in exposed pregnant workers. Of 460 neonates he studied who were born to female health care workers using hexachlorophene for hand washing 10 to 60 times per day, 25 were born with major malformations and 46 with minor malformations, corresponding to a malformation rate of 15.4%, which was significantly greater than expected. No specific type or group of major or minor malformations was described. Criticisms of this study have been published (133,134) that focused primarily on how the study and control groups were selected. A subsequent study by Baltzar and colleagues (135) found no correlation between maternal hexachlorophene use and congenitally malformed offspring. The Halling study is the only report to date to document the teratogenic effects of hexachlorophene in a human population (136).

In animal studies, low doses of hexachlorophene were not associated with congenital malformations, but the offspring of rats and rabbits exposed to higher doses suffered from cleft palate, microphthalmia, anophthalmia, and rib anomalies (136). Oral and vaginal administration resulted in maternal blood concentrations that were six to ten times higher than when applied dermally. Hexachlorophene crossed the placenta and accumulated in neural tissue of fetal mice exposed early in gestation. Later in gestation, in both mice and monkeys, there was less accumulation in the brain of affected fetuses, presumably secondary to development of the blood–brain barrier (136).

Hexachlorophene has been found to produce short-term reversible neurotoxic effects in exposed human neonates (137). To prevent systemic toxicity, current FDA restrictions prohibit the bathing of neonates with hexachlorophene soap.

Ethylene oxide, which is used to clean plastic medical equipment, is a known mutagen and carcinogen. Occupational exposure has been linked to an increased risk of spontaneous abortions and malformed offspring (138). It is one of the few chemicals, along with dibromochloropropane and lead, that have specific OSHA standards based on reproductive effects (139).

LEAD

Lead is one of the most abundant metals on earth and has been used by man for a variety of applications since early civilization. By the time of ancient Greek civilization, its toxic effects were suspected. Hippocrates described a severe attack of abdominal pain, probably lead colic, in a man employed as a metal extractor. Lead was used in ancient Rome and through the Middle Ages for improving the taste of poor vintages of wine, and in 1965 Gilfillan wrote that lead poisoning may have been a factor in the decline of the Roman empire (140).

Lead has been suspected to pose a reproductive hazard since at least the 1800's. Sterility, abortion, stillbirth, premature delivery, low birth weight, failure to thrive, and mental retardation of infants born to men and women working in the lead industry were reported many years ago. Animal studies have since confirmed that when animals are exposed to high levels of lead, they suffer reproductive toxicity and their offspring have an increase in congenital malformations (141).

Lead is used extensively in modern industry. It is the most widely used nonferrous metal (142). Occupational exposures occur in the smelting and refining of lead.

Sixty percent of the lead used in this country is used to produce storage batteries, making this industry a frequent source of occupational exposure. Red lead (Pb_3O_4) is used as a weather-resistant coating on metals, and workers in shipbuilding and demolition or similar occupations are susceptible to lead toxicities. Other hazardous industries and occupations are small workshops, cable and wire manufacturing, firearms instruction, pottery and crystal glass manufacture, and production of tin cans with lead-based solder (142).

Until recently, leaded gasoline was the primary source of environmental lead pollution. Between 1930 and 1960, 90% of atmospheric lead resulted from the use of leaded gasoline in automobiles (143), but the introduction of lead-free gasoline has reduced environmental pollution in many areas (142). Soil contamination is primarily a result of the weathering of lead-based exterior paints (144) and is often the source of childhood lead poisoning. Blood lead levels in industrialized nations are significantly higher than those in more remote or agricultural regions, implicating man-made environmental pollution as the primary source of lead exposure.

In adults, lead can cause disease in multiple organ systems, with prominent effects in the CNS, gastrointestinal tract, kidneys, joints and reproductive system. Toxic effects of lead in adults are generally seen with blood levels above 25 mg/dL. Anemia becomes apparent at blood level 80 mg/dL, encephalopathy has been reported with blood levels greater than 50 mg/dL, and chronic levels greater than 40 mg/dL are associated with chronic nephropathy (145). Death can occur with blood lead levels of 300 mg/dL. The CDC defined 25 mg/dL as an elevated blood lead level (146). Of great concern is that between 1976 and 1980 it was estimated that at least 1.5 million North American children had blood levels higher than this cutoff (147). There is evidence that children are more susceptible to the effects of lead than adults with toxicity at lower levels, meaning that significantly more children may be at risk for lead-related disease.

Four recent prospective studies (148–151) addressed the effects of low-level lead exposure *in utero,* that is, levels below 25 mg/dL. These studies consistently identified a link between neurobehavioral performance in the infant and maternal or umbilical cord blood lead levels. In three of the four studies, the Bayley Scales of Infant Development were primarily the tests used to assess infants under study, and these scores have been shown to correlate with later childhood intelligence quotient (IQ) scores (152). The studies suggested that lead levels of maternal blood of 10 to 15 mg/dL are grounds for concern. Follow-up assessments of most of these cohorts indicated that the effects of low-level *in utero* lead exposure were transient and undetectable when children were of school age (153). One study that was conducted in children living near a smelter who had mean cord blood levels of 22.4 mg/dL reported residual developmental delay in exposed children (154). In Bellinger's study of affected children in Boston (153), the greatest improvement in the neurodevelopmental performance of children aged between 2 and 5 years with antenatal cord blood lead levels was associated with low postnatal blood levels. Upper family socioeconomic status and female sex also were correlated with improvements in performance.

These findings are alarming but demonstrate that, with proper attention, therapeutic interventions are effective. In 1984, in the United States, more than 400,000 pregnant women had blood levels of lead greater than 10 mg/dL (146); so *in utero* exposure to low levels of lead represents a large public health hazard. The World Health Organization (WHO) concluded from a metanalysis of available data that the decline in IQ for each 10 mg/dL in lifetime mean blood level is likely to be in the range of 1 to 3 points (153). In neonates exposed to low levels of lead *in utero*, lowering lead exposure in childhood may be associated with normal neurologic function by school age.

Although the association between *in utero* exposure and developmental delay is consistent across many studies, results from studies vary in terms of the ability of lead to cause structural malformations in affected infants. In 1984, Needleman and colleagues (155) reported an increased risk of a variety of minor and seemingly unrelated congenital malformations in infants with high cord blood lead levels. More recently, Aschengrau and colleagues (156) conducted a case–control study of more than 14,000 women and assessed their exposure to chemicals and metals in drinking water. They found that detectable lead levels in drinking water were associated with anomalies of the head and neck and cardiovascular system and that the risk of stillbirth was greatest in women who had the highest levels of lead in their drinking water. The other prospective studies cited here did not find an association between lead and structural congenital anomalies, but in his 1994 review (153), Bellinger pointed out that these studies may not have had the power to detect such a difference because of small sample sizes. Studies also demonstrated a possible association between low-level lead exposure and preterm labor, decreased birth weights, and spontaneous abortions.

In the United States, there is no blood lead standard for pregnant women. The blood lead level must exceed 50 mg/dL before medical removal of an exposed person from the suspected source can be ordered (153). This current OSHA standard predates the most recent literature on the hazards of low-level lead exposure during pregnancy. The CDC considers a blood level of 10 mg/dL in children to constitute lead poisoning, and because fetal blood levels tend to be equivalent to maternal blood levels in the case of chronic exposures, it would be reasonable to remove a pregnant woman from the source of exposure at these considerably lower blood lead levels.

Primary prevention of lead exposure is the best approach for lead-related toxicities. At-risk couples should be screened during the preconceptional period and advised to delay pregnancy if maternal blood lead levels are high. In a person at risk from personal behavior, such as hobbies or projects like home remodeling, behavior modification may result in decreased exposure. Occupational exposure may be reduced by improved engineering methods or transfer to a lower-exposure position.

If elevated lead levels are detected as part of prenatal screening, treatment options are limited. During pregnancy, the main treatment consists of removing the patient from the source of exposure. Chelation therapy has been found to be teratogenic in animal studies (157) and should be avoided except in the case of overt maternal toxicity. Chelating agents are unlikely to reduce lead levels in an affected fetus (146). In addition, even though chelation is effective at removing lead from the blood compartment of an individual, 95% of lead is stored in bone, and it is unclear whether lowering blood lead levels can impact neonatal outcome favorably.

Counseling a patient with elevated lead levels is a difficult task. Persons who have sufficiently high lead levels could be offered termination of pregnancy as an option. Women with lower-level exposures (10–40 mg/dL) might be counseled that whereas early infant testing may indicate a developmental delay, school-age performance for the child is unlikely to be affected significantly. Again, prompt removal of the woman from the source of lead exposure is appropriate.

MERCURY

Although evidence about the potential reproductive toxicities of many environmental hazards is often tenuous, there is clear evidence from animal studies and human exposures that document the toxic and teratogenic effects of mercury. During this century, numerous reports of antenatal mercury ingestion have appeared (158–160). Exposed infants demonstrate severe psychomotor retardation, cerebral palsy, and microcephaly.

It is important to distinguish between inorganic and organic forms of mercury exposure. Organic mercury, primarily methylmercury, is responsible for outbreaks of disease in humans and has been documented to cause large-scale ecologic damage. In the late 1960's, an outbreak of disease occurred around an acetaldehyde manufacturing plant in Minamata, Japan, which had released methylmercury into Minamata Bay. Methylmercury accumulated in fish, which were consumed by the population and caused serious toxicity. A second well-documented exposure occurred in Iraq in 1971 through 1972, when grains treated with methylmercury- and ethylmercury-containing fungicides intended for planting were instead used to bake bread. All signs and symptoms in adults in these outbreaks were related to neurologic toxicity.

Today the principal and probably only route of human exposure is thought to occur through the consumption of fish and fish products. Methylmercury enters the aquatic food chain when environmental inorganic mercury, half of which is produced industrially and half naturally, is deposited in bodies of water and then is methylated by certain microorganisms. The highest concentrations are found in the longest-lived, top predatory fish, such as shark, swordfish, pike, and bass. No overt cases of poisoning from this type of exposure have been reported, but populations that consume large quantities of fish have had blood mercury levels that overlap the lowest levels associated with symptoms in the outbreaks in Japan and Iraq (161). In 1976, Koos and Longo (162) recommended that consumption of fish by pregnant women be limited to 350 g per week, and the WHO advises monitoring hair levels for methylmercury in persons who consume more than 100 g of fish daily (163).

A dose-response relationship for the effects of methylmercury on adults has been established, with paresthesias occurring at the lowest levels. Ataxia, dysarthria, deafness, and eventually death manifest at progressively higher levels. Overt signs and symptoms of organic mercury poisoning generally take weeks or months to occur, even in cases of lethal doses.

Evidence that prenatal exposure was the most hazardous form of exposure came from Minamata, when women who experienced only mild paresthesias or were asymptomatic gave birth to severely affected infants (164). Approximately 6% of the children born over a 10-year period in this area had cerebral palsy (162). Increased sensitivity of the fetus to methylmercury poisoning was later demonstrated in animal experiments (165). Large exposures to methylmercury in Japan and Iraq resulted in infants who were severely brain damaged with microcephaly, cerebral palsy, mental retardation, and blindness. A milder form of prenatal damage also was identified with lesser exposures, which resulted in psychomotor retardation (161). Whereas mercury poisoning resulted in selective cortical damage in adults, damage to the developing brain was widespread (166).

It has been determined, primarily from animal studies, that there is a species-dependent constant brain-to-blood ratio for mercury that is 5:1 in primates. Scalp hair is an excellent indicator of blood levels and can be used to assess individual exposures to mercury. From studies done by Clarkson and colleagues during the Iraqi outbreak, a threshold in the adult response was determined to be 50 to 100 mg Hg per gram of hair; the prenatal threshold was 10 to 20 mg Hg per gram of hair, indicating that the fetus may be five to ten times more sensitive to the effects of methylmercury than the adult.

Inorganic mercury is also toxic to humans, but its reproductive toxicities are not certain. Exposure to inorganic mercury is largely an occupational hazard. Workers involved in the production of electrolytic chlorine, electric apparatus catalysts, paint, and amalgamations may be exposed. Ceramic workers, neon-light makers, dentists and their assistants, and thermometer makers are all at risk from mercury exposure (167). Acute mercury poisoning, which is rare today, manifests with respiratory symptoms of chest tightness, dyspnea, cough, gingivitis, headaches, and fever (168). Chronic mercurialism is associated with oral cavity disorders, renal damage resulting in nephrotic syndrome, and neurologic symptoms such as a fine tremor and psychologic disturbances.

There are two case reports of maternal exposure to elemental mercury (169,170). In both cases, apparently normal children without any neurologic sequelae were born. Both cases were due to inhalation of mercury vapor, the primary route of poisoning from inorganic mercury. Mercury vapor is poorly absorbed from the digestive system and across the skin. It is known from animal studies that inorganic mercury crosses the placenta less readily than organic forms (171). In both cases, appreciable levels of mercury were detectable in the neonate of exposed women, but the levels of mercury detectable in the hair of the neonate in the case reported by Thorp and colleagues (170) after a significant maternal exposure were below those thought to cause motor retardation or other CNS signs in the exposed infant (172). Epidemiologic studies on dental personnel from Denmark with occupational exposure to inorganic mercury did not find an increase in spontaneous abortion or congenital malformations among exposed personnel (170). These data cannot be interpreted to mean that exposure to inorganic mercury does not have reproductive toxicity, but the patient exposed to inorganic mercury should be counseled that the risk from this type of exposure is significantly lower than exposure to organic mercury compounds.

NIOSH and ACGIH both recommend that exposure to organic mercury be limited to 50 mg/m^3 as an 8-hour time-weighted average (TWA). The OSHA standard for inorganic mercury is a ceiling level of 100 mg/m^3. Melkonian and Baker wrote that these guidelines may not be sufficient to ensure fetal protection and recommended that women of childbearing age not be exposed to mercury vapor concentrations greater than 10 mg/m^3 (169).

The results of methylmercury poisoning can be irreversible after destruction of neuronal cells. Treatment is directed toward early removal of methylmercury from the body before this damage may occur. Both D-penicillamine and *N*-acetyl-D-penicillamine are chelating agents effective in reducing blood levels of mercury (161). Oral administration of these drugs affects the enterohepatic circulation of mercury. Dialysis with a diffusible thiol compound can be highly effective in reducing blood levels of mercury (161). Dimercaptosuccinic acid and dimercaptopropane sulfonate are dithiocomplexing agents, which may be superior to currently used chelating agents.

MICROWAVES

Microwaves are a form of electromagnetic radiation, but they differ from x-rays and gamma rays in that they do not produce ionization in tissue. Although microwave energy is nonionizing, it can cause teratogenic effects when given in large enough doses as a result of thermal effects; however, persons working or living with microwaves in their environment are not exposed to levels anywhere near the maximal allowable levels of electromagnetic energy for occupational or medical exposures (173).

Through animal studies, a hazardous effect level of 4 W per kilogram was determined, and the National Council on Radiation Protection (NCRP) set an occupational exposure limit of 0.4 W per kilogram, that is, one tenth of the level known to cause adverse effects (174). The limit for casual, nonoccupational exposure is 0.08 W per kilogram.

Several safety mechanisms were designed to prevent accidental exposure to microwaves. A metal screen or foil is 100% effective in shielding all emissions (173). Theoretically, it is possible to be exposed to such energy by direct contact with a door leak; however, electromagnetic energy dissipates at a rate related to the square root of the distance traveled. Therefore, even if leakage occurred from a device such as a household microwave oven, no significant danger occurs several feet from the device.

The eye and developing fetus are the structures most vulnerable to the thermal effects of microwave radiation because they have the least capacity to dissipate heat (173). There are no known mutagenic or carcinogenic effects of this form of electromagnetic energy. Properly manufactured and functioning microwave equipment does not appear to present a hazard to pregnant women.

MAGNETIC RESONANCE IMAGING

Magnetic resonance imaging (MRI) requires the simultaneous application of intense static magnetic fields to align the nuclei of tissue, matched radiofrequency fields that excite the nuclei into a resonance state, and pulsed magnetic fields that create different resonant frequencies in different tissues so they may be recognized by the imaging technology. When considering the possible deleterious reproductive effects of MRI, each of these types of magnetic fields must be considered separately. Whether any of these types of magnetic fields is a reproductive hazard is unclear. There were early reports that static, pulsed, and radiofrequency magnetic fields had biological effects *in vitro* and in animal studies, but recent well-controlled experiments have not confirmed these data (175).

The National Radiological Protection Board (NRPB) (176) recommends that patients should not be exposed to more than 2500 mT for static magnetic fields and not more than 20,000 mT s^{-1} for longer than 10 msec for time-varying magnetic fields. Exposure to radiofrequency fields should not raise body temperature by more than 1°C. Additional recommendations were that patients with metal aneurysm clips should not undergo MRI and that care should be taken when examining patients with cardiac pacemakers or metallic prostheses. They also recommended that women in their first 3 months of pregnancy be excluded from MRI examinations; however, insufficient evidence exists about the teratogenic effects of an MRI examination to recommend termination of pregnancy after inadvertent exposure.

It is well known that current passing through a magnetic field creates electric potential; therefore, consideration must be given to the effects of MRI on neural and muscle tissues, specifically the myocardium. Because of the concern for the induction of cardiac arrhythmias, the NRPB adopted limits on the intensity and duration of pulsed magnetic fields to one tenth of the threshold current known to produce fibrillation for pulses longer than 10 msec. Monkeys exposed to static magnetic fields greater than 5000 mT were observed to undergo behavioral changes with emesis in some of the animals. These experiments led the NRPB to recommend using MRI on epileptic patients with caution (177). Smith (175) wrote that the use of MRI need not be inhibited in patients with a history of cardiac or CNS abnormalities, but the clinician should act with caution until more experience is gained with these patients.

To date, one epidemiologic study has assessed the potential reproductive toxicity of occupational exposure to female MRI technologists and nurses. Workers in this field are shielded from radiofrequency and pulsed magnetic fields, and the primary concern is the potential adverse effects caused by the powerful static magnetic field. In 1993 Evans and colleagues (178) received responses to questionnaires from 1,915 women, of whom 287 were pregnant while working as an MRI operator. When MRI workers were compared with other workers, no statistically significant differences between the two groups in time to pregnancy, spontaneous abortion, preterm delivery, or low birth weight was observed. When MRI workers were compared with homemakers for the same outcomes, MRI workers were three times as likely to miscarry, but this may have been due to an unusually low rate of spontaneous abortions of 6% among homemakers. The authors concluded that there did not appear to be a major reproductive hazard associated with MRI work.

MILITARY SERVICE

The number of women in the military has increased with the creation of an all-volunteer force. New regulations prohibit the automatic discharge of pregnant women from military service. In fact, these women are required to complete their assigned tasks.

They face unique problems, however, because not only are they subject to many of the usual pregnancy-related concerns but also to the stresses and demands created by a need for "military readiness." Sometimes this results in the inability to ensure the safety and well-being of the fetus and the mother (179). Military women may be subjected to long periods of standing, heavy lifting, and exposure to high noise levels. In addition, long hours spent sitting at computers (which are essential on many ships, planes, and tanks) can lead to exposure to low-level EMF and also to repetitive stress syndromes (e.g., carpal tunnel syndrome, tendinitis). To aggravate the situation, most of these women must do shift work, which disrupts their normal diurnal patterns (180). Often, the women's duties require exposure for long periods to extremes of temperature. Exposure to intense heat during the first trimester (such as the 130–140°F temperatures in a ship's boiler room or after donning heat-trapping protective gear) results in increased rates of neural tube defects and exposure to excessive noise if transmitted through the abdominal wall to the developing fetus *in utero*. Lalande and colleagues (181) studied the effects of increased noise levels (>95 dB) in pregnant municipal bus workers and found evidence of hearing loss in the children up to age 5 years following *in utero* exposure. The permissible noise levels are shown in Table 6-2. Meyer and colleagues (182) reported increased rates of neural tube defects in the offspring of mothers exposed to high noise levels. Often, however, in addition to noise, there is also exposure to whole-body vibration, which has been associated with increased rates of sperm abnormalities and spinal cord injuries (51,183,184).

The requirements for peak physical fitness require aerobic training and thus can pose increased risks for adverse pregnancy outcomes, such as IUGR and perinatal mortality (185,186). McGann and colleagues (187) studied pregnancy outcomes in women Marines and compared them to pregnancy outcomes in dependent wives of male Marines at the same base. The pregnant Marines had a 23% cesarean section rate compared with a rate of 15% in the dependent wives. The incidence of preeclampsia was 7% in the Marine women compared with 3.2% in the dependent wives. Preterm labor (or birth) occurred in

TABLE 6-2. *Permissible noise levels*

Decibels	Permissible duration of exposure (hr)
90	8
92	6
95	4
97	3
100	2
102	1½
105	1
110	½
115	¼

3% of the Marine women compared with 0.24% in the dependent wives.

Many investigators (188–190) have described increased rates of preterm labor, preterm delivery, and low birth weight as a result of prolonged standing, heavy lifting, and working long hours, all common conditions in the military. Klebanoff and colleagues (126) showed that enlisted nonwhite women had higher rates of preterm delivery and postulated that these may be due to the psychological stresses associated with the high-demand, low-control situations common in the enlisted military.

The risks of preterm delivery have been studied extensively in this population. Special characteristics of these women include their homogeneity with regard to access to care and extremely low incidence of drug abuse (126). Also, they are uniformly healthier than civilian women. Adams and colleagues (191) found that black enlisted women had a 31% higher preterm delivery rate than white enlisted women. If the women's partners were also black, the rate increased to 47%. Fox and associates (185) and McGann and Nolan (187) found similar rates.

Lavitz and colleagues (193) reviewed the etiologic heterogeneity of preterm delivery and found that black women had a higher rate of preterm premature rupture of membranes, whereas white women with higher socioeconomic status appeared to have idiopathic preterm labor. Shiono and Klebanoff (194) also found three times higher rates of delivery between 33 and 36 weeks.

Possible explanations after correcting for access to care, drug use, and overall health are the socioeconomic disparity between blacks and whites, which may affect the mother's own early environment. Klebanoff and Yip (195) described patients in Tennessee whose own low maternal weights were associated with higher rates of growth restriction and prematurity regardless of maternal race. Similarly, Baird (196) found that a woman's risk of delivering a low-birth-weight infant was associated most closely with the social class of the mother's father than that of her husband. Thus, it appeared that a woman's childhood environment affected her reproductive outcomes.

Pregnancy-induced hypertension also was studied in active-duty Navy women (197). Interestingly, nulliparous women engaged in high levels of physical activity had a significantly lower risk compared with those whose activity was considered low level.

Paternal military service often has been considered a risk factor for adverse pregnancy outcomes. Most of these concerns resulted from exposure to Agent Orange, a chemical defoliant that was sprayed extensively during the Vietnam War. It contains esters of 2,4-dichlorophenoxyacetic acid and 2,4,5-trichlorophenoxyacetic acid in addition to small amounts of dioxin (198). Controversy still exists about the possible effects of Agent Orange on pregnancy outcomes. An increased risk of adverse pregnancy outcomes was found in the offspring of fathers with prior military service in Vietnam (199). The risk for major malformations was 1.7 (95% CI, 0.8–3.5) compared with veterans who did not serve in Vietnam. No specific pattern to the types of abnormalities was noted, however. No such association was found with the perinatal mortality rate (stillbirths and neonatal deaths).

In a prior study (200), investigators found no increase in the spontaneous abortion rate for wives of Vietnam veterans compared with that of veterans who did not serve in Vietnam. In another study (201), Vietnam veterans interviewed by telephone reported increased rates of spontaneous abortion (OR, 1.7; 95% CI, 1.3–1.4) and neural tube defects; review of the birth and hospital records revealed no such increase. Other investigators also found no increase (202).

NICKEL

Nickel and nickel compounds are used in electroplating, ceramics, permanent magnets, batteries, and fuel cells. They also are used as chemical catalysts, in the construction industry, in making machine parts, and in the production of certain metals and alloys (203). The primary route of occupational nickel exposure is through inhalation, which has been associated with a number of cancers of the respiratory tract (204). Nickel can produce disease in many organ systems, the most common insult being nephrotoxicity. Repeated cutaneous exposure causes a contact dermatitis in about 5% of the population.

Until recently, information on the reproductive toxicity of nickel was derived exclusively from animal experiments. Weischer and colleagues exposed rats to 1.6 mg/m^3 of nickel oxide gas throughout gestation and noted an association with fetal growth restriction but no other anomalies (205). Mice exposed to 160 mg of nickel per kilogram daily from day 2 to day 17 of gestation had an increase in the rate of spontaneous abortion, but this effect was not seen in another study with about half that dose (205). Recently, Smith and colleagues (206) found a dose-dependent perinatal toxicity in rats exposed to nickel chloride drinking water solutions, with the lowest observed adverse effect occurring at concentrations of 10 ppm of nickel. No studies have been conducted on developmental effects after dermal exposures. For comparison, OSHA recommends inhalational exposure limits of 0.1 mg/m^3 for soluble nickel compounds and 1 mg/m^3 for insoluble ones (205). The EPA has stated that long-term exposure to 0.02 mg of nickel per kilogram daily in drinking water is safe.

Only one study of nickel toxicity during pregnancy in humans could be located. In 1994, a Russian group (207) reporting on workers in a nickel-refining plant found an increased risk of spontaneous and threatened abortion (17% versus 9%) and congenital malformations (17% versus 6%) compared with construction workers used as controls. These results have not been replicated, and evidence of an increase in the incidence of congenital malformations has not been seen in most animal studies.

NOISE

Chronic exposure to noise between 60 and 80 dB may invoke a stress response, and noise louder than 80 dB may be harmful to hearing. The most thoroughly documented pathologic effect of chronic exposure to excessive noise is hearing loss (208).

With society becoming more industrialized and women gaining access to the workplace in a variety of fields, increasing numbers of women are subjected to increased high noise levels. A suggested mechanism for noise effects on pregnancy is a stress-induced increase of catecholamine levels and vasoconstriction in placental vasculature (209). The potential for noise as a reproductive hazard has been studied over the past 20 years without conclusive evidence that noise is indeed harmful during pregnancy. Numerous retrospective studies have linked excessive noise exposure with adverse pregnancy outcomes including low birth weight (210–212), teratogenic risk (213,214), spontaneous abortion (215), stillbirth (214), and infertility or delayed conception (216). These studies have been criticized because they did not control for confounding variables (217). Other studies found no adverse pregnancy outcomes related to excessive noise exposure (218,219). It is interesting to note that although studies found an association between adverse pregnancy outcome and noise exposure, no consistently documentable pathologic response to noise has been found. If a more homogeneous group of outcomes was seen across studies, it would give stronger support to the hypothesis that noise affects pregnancy outcome adversely.

One recent prospective study assessed the effect of noise exposure during pregnancy on birth weight (217). The noise exposure of 200 women was sampled during each trimester of pregnancy with a personal data log and compared against birth outcome. The study was limited by a small sample size and by the fact that the level of noise experienced by the participants ranged from only 52.4 dB to 86.8 dB, which may have been too narrow a range to detect an effect. Keeping these limitations in mind, no adverse pregnancy outcomes were noted in the women with the greatest exposures.

It is unclear whether acoustic stimulation used in antepartum testing can interfere with normal fetal development or whether the inner ear of the fetus is vulnerable to acoustic trauma. During acoustic stimulation, sound levels of 100 dB can reach the inner ear of the fetus (220). The fetus responds to this stimulation, as evidenced by an increase in the heart rate and fetal movements, but adverse effects have not been described in the literature.

ORGANIC SOLVENTS

Organic solvents are one of the most prevalent sources of chemical exposure in working populations (221). Tossavaineu and colleagues (222) found organic solvents to be one of the top 12 most hazardous agents. Exposure to organic solvents occurs in many types of manufacture, painting, graphics, glue, plastics, lamination, dry cleaning, electronics manufacture, textiles, laboratories, printing, building, handicrafts, and others. Exposure occurs mainly through inhalation of fumes or absorption through skin contact. Sometimes patients are exposed because they sniff glue or paint intentionally. A concentration exceeding 110% of the present occupational exposure limit in the workroom air is considered too high (223). The proposed federal industrial standard is 0.55 ppm (224).

Ethylene glycol ethers are activated by alcohol dehydrogenase to alkoxyacetic acid metabolites (225). They are rapidly absorbed through the skin. The metabolites have a long half-life, lasting 1 to 2 days. Therefore, daily exposure to low levels can result in accumulation in the tissues. Continued toxicity can occur even after the exposure has ceased.

The mechanism of action for toxicity is unknown. One possibility is that the alkoxyacetic acids interfere with nucleic acid formation (226,227). These effects may be more apparent in areas of rapid cell proliferation such as spermatogenesis and embryogenesis.

Information about their reproductive toxicity is controversial, but a "fetal solvent syndrome" has been reported. Like fetal alcohol syndrome, the stigmata include microcephaly, short palpebral fissures, midline facial abnormalities, micrognathia, limb and CNS defects, and IUGR (228–230).

Many investigators suggest an association between exposure to multiple organic solvents and increased risks of adverse pregnancy outcomes (230–235). These risks include increased rates of spontaneous abortions, birth defects, and low birth weight. Most investigators agree, however, that it is difficult to estimate the specific effect of a single compound because most workers are exposed to multiple agents.

Ethylene glycol ethers are used in electronics and photochemical processing. They have been classified by NIOSH as reproductive hazards (236). The solvents used in the dry-cleaning and garment industry are methylene chloride, perchlorethylene, and formaldehyde; all are known teratogens. Methylene chloride is metabolized to carbon monoxide, which is an asphyxiant. Perchlorethylene accumulates in fatty tissue and can cause liver damage and is excreted in breast milk.

Correra and colleagues (237) studied workers in the semiconductor industry and found that exposed women had increased rates of spontaneous abortion (relative risk, 2.8). In addition, a statistically significant dose-response relationship with increasing ethylene glycol ether exposure was noted. The wives of male exposed workers, however, did not exhibit any such increase. Of note, the investigators found that the rates of spontaneous abortion were similar among formerly and currently exposed women.

Many investigators (238–240) describe the occurrence of facial clefts (241) and other congenital anomalies that include anencephaly (242–244), urethral atresia, and clubfoot. Toluene, xylene, and formalin exposures occur in hospital laboratories and in the pharmaceutical industry. Toluene crosses the placenta, and data from animal studies reveal that fetal blood has 75% of the concentration in maternal blood. Even though no teratogenic effects have been found, decreased birth weights have been reported from studies in animal models. Formalin and xylene also cross the placenta. Workroom air concentration of these solvents is approximately 0.45 ppm. Formaldehyde is a known mutagen that acts with amino groups to form ethynol adducts with nucleic acids, proteins, and amino acids (245).

Tikkanen and Heinonen (231) studied the effects of solvent exposure on reproductive outcomes and found that exposed women had a slight but nonsignificant increase in spontaneous abortions (OR, 1.4; 95% CI, 0.9–2.2) compared with controls (OR, 0.9; 95% CI, 0.5–1.7). When they studied individual solvents, they found that exposure to toluene three times a week gave a spontaneous abortion OR of 4.7 (95% CI, 1.4–15.9). With xylene, the OR was 3.1 (95% CI, 1.3–7.5), and with formalin, 3.5 (95% CI, 1.1–11.2). One study reported more CNS defects in children born to mothers exposed to industrial organic solvents (246).

The vast majority of investigators report increased spontaneous abortion rates after exposure to organic solvents (222,247–249). A few also report increased rates of low birth weight and preterm delivery. Heidam (250), however, found no increase in spontaneous abortion rates among histopathology laboratory workers who had frequent exposure to solvents. Other investigators have reported similar results (251). Because of these data and also because most patients are exposed to more than one solvent at any time, the results should be interpreted with care. A good policy would require the transfer of pregnant workers who are in areas with levels exceeding 10% of the threshold limit value to other areas.

Paternal exposure to organic solvents has been considered to be associated with increased pregnancy risks. Kristensen and colleagues (252) reviewed the pregnancy outcomes of partners of men in printing industries and found increased rates of adverse pregnancy outcomes. The small for gestational age (SGA) rate was 67 in 1,000 births in the study population compared with 54 per 1,000 in controls. No increase was found in the rate of low birth weight in these patients. The OR for preterm delivery was 5.4 (95% CI, 1.7–17.4). The exposed patients had a fivefold increased stillbirth rate over that of controls. The OR for perinatal mortality was 1.4 (95% CI, 0.49–4.1). In a similar study, Matanoski (253) found no increase in the stillbirth rates of partners after exposure to solvents in printers. Chandley (254) suggests that the possible mechanism for adverse outcomes may be the occurrence of mutations in sperm DNA. Jager (255) suggests that it may be due to changes in the chromatin stability of maturing spermatozoa.

PBBs and PCBs

Polychlorinated diphenyls and their bromine analogues have the property of heat transfer and thermal stability. They are used as fire retardants, heat-exchange fluids, and plasticizers; they are used extensively for commercial purposes in electric appliances, hydraulic oils, and additives for printing inks and are found ubiquitously because improper disposal has resulted in environmental contamination. These compounds are highly lipid soluble and accumulate in fat depots. Fish are the primary source of dietary PCBs. The highest concentrations are found in fish caught from rivers and lakes contaminated from industrial areas (256). They can become bioconcentrated in the food chain whereby animals higher in the food chain may have levels severalfold higher than those in lower marine life. These agents can enter the environment from leakage of PCB-containing liquids from transformers, heat-exchanger systems, and hydraulic systems (257).

PCBs have been found in breast milk and body fat (258,259). Rogan (260) described "cola-colored babies" who were born with discolored skin following maternal exposure to PCBs in cooking oil. These children exhibited lung abnormalities, short stature, failure to thrive, developmental delay, mental retardation, and abnormal behavior patterns. Kuratsune and colleagues (261) described an epidemic called "Yusho disease" in Japanese infants whose mothers consumed PCB-contaminated cooking oil. They had transient (up to 6 months) dark-brown pigmentation of the skin and mucosa; IUGR in 17%; skull, dental, and bone abnormalities in most infants; but no residual neurological sequelae.

Fein and colleagues (262) described infants with microcephaly and low birth weight whose mothers consumed PCB-contaminated fish. Once a mother accumulates PCBs in her tissues, she may continue to be a source of contamination to her fetus and neonate, either through placental transfer or in the breast milk. This risk persists each time she mobilizes body fat and has fluctuations in weight.

PESTICIDES

Pesticides contaminate the environment with chemical agents, many of which may have long-term effects on health and reproduction. The EPA has classified fewer than 0.1% of the active ingredients in pesticides as toxic; about 25% are considered mutagenic and carcinogenic (263). Exposure to these agents is inherent not only in agricultural jobs but also for those who work in forestry and as florists, fruit handlers, or fisherman. Once pesticides that contain organic chlorine enter the food chain, they are almost impossible to eliminate and persist in soils, lake sediments, and even fish. Toxicity may result from acute high-concentration or chronic occupational exposures.

The most commonly used pesticides, in both homes and industries, are organophosphates and carbamates. Both are acetylcholinesterase (ACE) inhibitors that act by binding to ACE, allowing it to accumulate at the motor end plates, myoneural junction, and autonomic ganglia. These pesticides include malathion, parathion, and mipafox. They do not persist for long periods in the environment but do persist in contaminated clothing and containers. They are readily absorbed through the skin and often cannot be washed away by a brief scrub with soap and water. Because many workers and their families live near the fields where they work, exposure can result not only from occupational skin contact but also from aerial and ground exposures.

Malthion was used in California in the early 1980's for low-level spraying of agricultural areas. Thomas and colleagues (264) studied its effect on pregnancy outcomes and found no increase in the spontaneous abortion or IUGR rates in exposed mothers. They did, however, find an increased incidence of stillbirths and limb reduction defects. Orofacial and gastrointestinal tract abnormalities also were increased.

Willis and colleagues (265) studied the effects of pesticide exposure on birth outcomes in Hispanic agriculture workers and found an increased rate of stillbirths in both exposed female workers (OR, 1.5–1.6) and partners of exposed males (OR, 1.2–1.4). In addition, partners of exposed males gave birth to more SGA babies (OR, 1.4–2.0). Similarly, Goulet (266) found increased stillbirth rates (OR, 3.1) in Canadian workers exposed to herbicides and pesticides. Munger and colleagues (267) in an earlier study on the same subject, however, found no association between malathion exposure and birth defects or low birth weight.

Matos and colleagues (268) reported that Argentinean pregnant gardeners who were exposed to organophosphates and carbamates had a RR of 1.96 for spontaneous abortions and 1.86 for preterm delivery. Similarly, Restrepo and coworkers (269) studied female floriculture workers and partners of male workers and also found moderately increased rates of spontaneous abortions, preterm delivery, and congenital anomalies.

Other investigators (264,270) found that low level, occasional exposure to malathion in workers of urban communities resulted in no increase in either birth defects or stillbirths. Nurminen (271) studied the effects of pesticide exposure during the periconceptional period and found increased rates of neural tube defects (spina bifida and hydrocephaly; RR, 2.3; 95% CI, 1.2–4.5). The stillbirth risk also was increased following second-trimester exposure (OR, 1.9; 95% CI, 1.2–3.1).

The Bhopal, India gas disaster occurred as a result of leakage of a toxic gas called methylisocyanate (MIC), which is used in the pesticide manufacturing process. MIC is a small molecule that reacts rapidly with sulphydryl, carboxyl, and hydroxyl groups to cause tissue damage (198). The patients who were exposed to MIC had a fourfold increased spontaneous abortion rate (24.2% versus 5.6% in controls; $p < 0.001$). The perinatal mortality rate was 69.5% in the exposed pregnancies compared with 50.5% in the unexposed ones ($p < 0.001$). The congenital abnormality rates were similar: 14.2 per 1,000 births in the exposed group versus 12.6 per 1,000 births in the unexposed group. The fetal demise rate was similar in the two groups (27.2% versus 23.6% in controls).

Zhang and colleagues (214) found an increased rate of SGA babies when they reviewed maternal occupational exposure to pesticides; however, many investigators have stated that no such increased risks occur for any adverse pregnancy outcomes (267,272). It appears that there is some increased reproductive risk of adverse reproductive outcomes, but at present the epidemiologic evidence does not allow any clear inferences.

The association between male pesticide exposure and reproductive outcomes was studied by deCock and coworkers (273) and Potashnik and Porath (274); both studies found an increased rate of infertility as assessed by time to pregnancy; this increase in infertility resulted from suppressed spermatogenesis. No increases in the spontaneous abortion or the congenital abnormality rates were found. Interestingly, Potashnik and Porath (274) also found that exposed men fathered fewer male babies, 17% during the exposure period compared with 53% for the period before the exposure. Once the exposure had ended and sperm production improved, the number of male babies conceived increased to 41%.

Recently, Rupa and colleagues (275) reviewed 1,006 exposed men compared with 1,020 unexposed men and reported increased complications in pregnancies fathered by exposed males. They also found an increased spontaneous abortion rate (26%) compared with controls (15%). Neonatal deaths occurred in 9% of the study group and in 2% in controls. Stillbirths occurred in 9% versus 3%, respectively, and congenital abnormalities were found in 3% of exposed versus 0.07% of the unexposed workers' offspring.

PHYSICAL AND PSYCHOLOGIC STRESS

Many professions involve either long hours of work or severe psychologic stress or both. These professions include workers in hospitals, assembly plants, factories, retail, physical fitness, and others. Pronounced physical stress and exertion are known to have a deleterious effect on body functions such as intraabdominal pressure, uterine blood flow, and nutritional status, all of which affect optimal fetal development (276). Strenous long hours of standing and walking during pregnancy are associated with increased rates of premature and low-birth-weight newborns. A possible explanation may be muscle work resulting in decreased uteroplacental blood flow. There is no increase in the spontaneous abortion rate, however. Heavy lifting and frequent bending have not been associated with adverse pregnancy outcomes by some investigators (188,189), whereas others (277,278) have suggested increased preterm delivery rates with heavy lifting that is performed frequently (more than 20 to 50 times weekly). Therefore, pregnant women should avoid strenuous physical stresses and have adequate rest periods, especially during the third trimester.

Psychologic stress has been defined as high mental demands coupled with low control over the demand (279). Animal and human studies show increased production of catecholamines and steroids in response to severe psychologic stress.

Many authors (280,281) found no increase in the spontaneous abortion rates of women with increased levels of self-perceived stress; however, Cohen and co-workers (282) suggested that stressful work was associated with increased spontaneous abortion rates if the woman was aged over 35 years, a smoker, or worked more than 40 hours a week. Similarly, increased spontaneous abortion rates were reported in women who described increased levels of stress in relation to their work in the semiconductor industry (283) and bank clerical workers (284). Williamson and colleagues (285) found that increased stress levels in the latter half of pregnancy were associated with increased rates of low birth weight babies and low Apgar scores. The neonatal mortality in these women was 9.2% compared with 3.9% in the controls. Klebanoff and co-workers (286) suggested that strong social supports at work can, to some extent, ameliorate the adverse effects of the perceived stresses.

RADIATION

Ionizing radiation has been studied more extensively than any other environmental hazard (173). X-rays and gamma-rays are forms of ionizing radiation composed of short-wavelength electromagnetic waves that are highly penetrating, capable of producing ionization within living tissue that breaks chemical bonds, and can cause subsequent damage (287). Exposures to ionizing radiation can produce cell death, mutation, cancer, and developmental defects in a dose-related manner (173). Microwaves, shortwave, powerline transmissions, radiowaves, and diathermy are composed of a longer wave, low-energy form of radiation that does not possess the ability to produce ionization and should not be considered in the following discussion. The potential reproductive effects of these agents are considered elsewhere in this chapter.

Natural background radiation accounts for more than 80% of the exposure to the U.S. population, the major source being radon gas. Approximately 20% of ionizing radiation exposure is from man-made sources, most of which comes from medical radiography and nuclear medicine studies (288). The dose of natural background radiation in the United States is approximately 3 milliSeiverts (mSv) or 300 mrem per year. It is not believed that this level of natural background radiation presents a reproductive hazard. Seiverts or rem are terms used to quantify the degree of biologic effect of a given dose of radiation, taking into account a quality factor based on the linear energy transfer of that type of radiation (289). Because the quality factor for x-rays and gamma rays is 1, the dose equivalent of these types of radiation is equal to the amount of absorbed radiation, measured in Grays or rads. To put this dose of radiation in perspective, in 1989 Brent (173) reviewed the literature concerning low-level radiation exposures in both animals and humans throughout pregnancy and concluded that continuous exposures below 2,000 millirad per day had no effect on fertility, growth, mortality, or the incidence of congenital malformations in the offspring of affected pregnancies. Two thousand millirads per day is more than 10,000 times the amount of background radiation in the United States.

There is ample evidence from studies in experimental animals and humans that ionizing radiation is capable of causing serious deleterious effects in living organisms. In developing mammals, the classic effects of radiation are embryonic death, IUGR, and gross congenital malformations. In humans, growth retardation and CNS system effects are seen with significant intrauterine radiation exposures (173). Each of these effects demonstrates a dose-response relationship and a threshold below which teratogenic effects are not observed.

The evidence for potential teratogenic effects of radiation in humans comes principally from two sources. The first is from women treated with pelvic radiation for indications ranging from malignancy to therapeutic abortion. In 1929, Goldstein and Murphy reported on 28 infants born to women who underwent radium therapy for uterine cancer during pregnancy. Each of these women received a minimum radiation dose of 100 rads (173). Sixteen of these children developed microcephaly, sometimes accompanied by mental retardation. Dekaban reported on 22 infants who had microcephaly or mental retardation or both born to women who had radiation exposure of approximately 250 rads in their first half of pregnancy (290). Brent wrote that there has not been a *bona fide* radiation-induced morphologic malfunction in a human being that has not exhibited either a CNS abnormality or growth retardation (173).

The second series of human data related to the effects of ionizing radiation on pregnancy comes from studies of atomic bomb survivors from Nagasaki and Hiroshima. Yamakazi and Schull recently summarized the results of the many studies carried out under the auspices of a joint effort between the governments of the United States and Japan (291). Initial studies demonstrated an excess of fetal loss and brain injury resulting in microcephaly and mental retardation in children born to mothers within 2,000 m of the hypocenter of the bombings. The gestational age at which the fetus appeared to be most susceptible to the effects of radiation was between 7 and 15 weeks. In studies after 1972, because of improvements in technology, it became possible to estimate maternal radiation doses and relate them to fetal effects. The minimum dose at which a clearly observable increase of microcephaly occurred was in the group exposed to 100 to 190 cGy of radiation. A dose-related increase in microcephaly was noted at 1500 cGy, at which point microcephaly was often accompanied by mental retardation. Data from these studies revealed that maximum vulnerability to the effects of radiation occurred from the 8th through the 15th week after fertilization. From the 16th through 25th week after fertilization, a period of diminished vulnerability existed. Before 8 weeks' gestation, no radiation-related cases of mental retardation were seen. From the atomic bomb survivor data, it was not clear whether a threshold exists below which teratogenic effects do not occur; however, the data did suggest that a threshold between 120 and 230 cGy between 8 and 15 weeks and again between 21 cGy and 70 cGy between 2 and 8 weeks may be present, below which mental retardation does not occur.

Whereas there is general agreement that the doses of background radiation and those used in diagnostic imaging techniques are considerably less than those associated with teratogenesis, this does not rule out the possibility of an association with oncogenesis either in childhood or later in adult life. There is a large body of evidence linking diagnostic radiation with an increased risk of childhood leukemia. In 1966, Lilienfeld (292) reviewed nine studies, of which six demonstrated an association and by metanalysis demonstrated an increase in leukemia risk of 1.3 to 1.8 from *in utero* diagnostic radiation exposure. Brent (173) questioned the validity of this association and stated that it is not clear whether radiation exposure in either preconception or postconception cases is a causative or associative factor in the increased incidence of leukemia. The risk of childhood leukemia in the general population is 1 in 3,000; so if a relative risk of 1.5 is assumed for children exposed to *in utero* diagnostic radiation, their risk would be 1 in 2,000 for developing this malignancy after exposure, representing one additional case of leukemia per 6,000 children.

The amount of radiation delivered to the fetus by different diagnostic radiographic procedures varies widely by the type of study and the anatomy being studied. The American College of Radiology has stated that no single procedure would irradiate a patient enough to threaten the well-being of the developing embryo or fetus (293). Brent has called the risk of less than 5 rads of radiation to the fetus minuscule. Multiple procedures, however, may result in doses of radiation that could potentially be responsible for an adverse outcome. In addition, if the embryo is shielded, even when giving high doses of radiation to the mother, no increase in the incidence of congenital malformations has been seen.

The most common plain film used in pregnant women is the chest radiograph, which results in 0.07 mrad of exposure to the fetus. The average exposure from an abdominal film is 100 mrads, and this exposure increases with the number of films taken. Multiple exposures are generally required for an intravenous pyelogram (IVP) and radiation dose to the fetus can reach a dose as high as 1.4 rads. A one-shot retrograde pyelogram delivers substantially less radiation to the fetus than an IVP (294).

Fluoroscopic procedures potentially can deliver more radiation to the fetus than plain films, but doses vary widely with the time and type of the study. Total uterine dosing can reach 4 rads during a barium enema, and endoscopy can be considered an alternative modality. An upper gastrointestinal series delivers substantially less radiation (<100 mrad) to the fetus than studies of the lower abdomen (294).

Computed tomography (CT) delivers doses of radiation that can range from approximately 5 rad to the skin to 2 rad in the center of the slice. Maximal fetal doses of radiation from CT studies of the head and chest are minimal, but studies of the abdomen and lumbar spine can range from 2.6 to 3.5 rad, depending on gestational age (295). CT pelvimetry can result in a dose of 1.5 rad to the fetus; using the techniques described by Moore and Shearer (296), however, this dose can be reduced to 250 mrad.

Radionuclide imaging may be used in pregnancy. The amount of radiation delivered to the fetus depends on the type of radioisotope used and the agent to which it is tagged. Of the commonly used studies, the highest dose of radiation to the fetus is caused by a gallium scan, which is used to localize inflammatory or neoplastic disease, and the dose delivered to the fetus is estimated to be less than 1 rad. Ventilation-perfusion lung scans are among the most common radionuclide studies ordered in pregnancy, and they deliver little radiation to the fetus. Technetium, which is bound to macroaggregated albumin during the perfusion scan, is sequestered in the lung, and exposure is limited to approximately 40 mrad to the fetus. Xenon is used for pulmonary ventilation scans, has a short half-life, and delivers approximately 10 mrad to the fetus (297).

Radioiodine (^{131}I) can cause fetal hypothyroidism (298), is considered a category X drug, and is contraindicated in pregnancy. Uptake is minimal before 12 weeks of gestation (299), however. Sodium iodide delivers less than 10 mrad to the fetal thyroid, and its uptake into the fetal thyroid may be blocked by administering stable iodide to the mother, making administration during pregnancy feasible.

Protection standards for occupational and environmental exposures to radiation are based on data from atomic bomb survivors and patients who underwent radiation therapy; however, extrapolation of data from a single high-intensity exposure to a low-level chronic exposure is necessarily accurate. Occupational exposure to ionizing radiation is limited to 100 mSV over 5 years, not to exceed 50 mSV in 1 year, by recommendation of the International Commission on Radiological Protection (300).

Probably the best estimate of cancer mortality resulting from low doses of radiation comes from the IARC Study Group on cancer risk among nuclear industry workers (301). In this study, researchers combined mortality data from seven cohort studies on nearly 100,000 workers and developed a dose-response relationship between radiation exposure and excess cancer risks. The authors demonstrated an excess of leukemias (excluding chronic lymphocytic leukemia) in exposed workers and estimated an excess relative risk for developing cancer of 2.6 per Sv. There was no demonstrable increase in risk for other malignancies. The potential reproductive toxicities of radiation exposure were not examined in this study, as more than 80% of study subjects were men, and they received more than 90% of the exposure. Ambach (302) wrote that these estimates of carcinogenic risk should be applicable to other workers, such as hospital staff exposed to ionizing radiation. He wrote that the occupational exposure of hospital staff is about 1 mSv per year, which amounts to about 30 mSv over a worker's life. He calculated a 1.17 relative risk for death from leukemia based on this exposure.

Roman and associates (303) studied the health of children born from 9,208 pregnancies of 6,730 medical radiographers. Rates of major congenital malformations, chromosomal anomalies, and cancer in offspring were not found to differ significantly from baseline population rates. When the exposed workers were analyzed separately by sex, they demonstrated an increase in chromosomal anomalies among children of exposed females and an increase in cancers among children of exposed males; however, the authors of the study cautioned that these results were based on small numbers (five cases in each group) and must be interpreted cautiously.

SPACE

Many medical effects of travel into space have been studied, but possible effects of space travel on pregnancy have not been addressed. If long-term stays in space are planned, the effects on the developing fetus and any interactions with the normal physiologic changes of pregnancy need to be studied. The environmental factors of most concern are motion sickness, microgravity, radiation exposure, and long-term use of closed life support systems (304–307) (Table 6-3).

Motion sickness in space is due to alterations in the normal relationships between the vestibular, ocular, and cortical areas (308–310) and occurs in 50% of astronauts. Motion sickness could exacerbate the effects of the nausea and vomiting of early pregnancy, thus resulting in dehydration, ketonuria, and electrolyte abnormalities (311).

TABLE 6-3. *Reproductive effects of outer space environments*

Environmental conditions	Effects
Motion sickness	Nausea, vomiting, hyperemesis Electrolyte imbalances Pregnancy loss
Radiation	Microcephaly, mental retardation Pregnancy loss Mutations, malignancy Amenorrhea, azoospermia
Microgravity	Infertility Uteroplacental insufficiency: IUGR, SGA, fetal demise Osteoporosis
Closed-life support system	Decompression sickness Death Hypoxia SGA, IUGR

IUGR, intrauterine growth restriction; SGA, birth weight small for gestational age.

Cosmic radiation exposure is a known hazard of travel to outer space and may well become a limiting factor to reproduction in space. The average person is exposed to 125 mrem of radiation per year. Of this, approximately one third is from cosmic radiation and two thirds from a combination of medical exposures and radiation from the earth's surface (312). Acute radiation effects usually occur after an exposure of 400 to 500 mrem over one month (313). Acute exposure usually does not produce any systemic effects, but the cumulative effects of continued exposure over time may result in an increased chance of teratogencity, mutations, cancers, cataract formation, infertility, and decreased life span (314–316). Acute high-dose radiation exposure during the first half of pregnancy can result in microcephaly and mental retardation (317–319) or decreased IQ. Spermatogenesis can be affected with doses as low as 10 mrem. Therefore, the higher doses of radiation exposure that would result from travel to outer space could result in long-term (6 months to 3 years) sterility in men (320). The current lifetime exposure of astronauts is 400 mrem, which may result in a decrease of 1 to 3 years in life span and a doubled rate of cancers (321).

The weightlessness that occurs in microgravity can have adverse effects if allowed to continue over a long period, including muscle wasting, bone demineralization, anemia, and oculovestibular changes (322–324). Approximately 0.4% of the total body calcium is lost per month of exposure to microgravity, an effect that might potentiate the risk of osteoporosis when combined with the fetal demands on body calcium stores (323,325). The physiologic demands of pregnancy, when compounded with the effects of microgravity, may result in uteroplacental insufficiency. Paradoxically, the usual complications of pregnancy that are caused by the effects of gravity on the vasculature may improve, and include hemorrhoids, varicosities, and pedal edema. Paternal exposure to microgravity, however, does not appear to have any deleterious effects on fertility.

Use of closed life support systems is essential in outer space to avoid the adverse effects of exposure to decreased barometric pressures. Such exposures can quickly (within 1–2 minutes) result in respiratory distress, abdominal distension, tissue hemorrhage and swelling, lacrimation, incontinence, and hypotension. If left uncorrected, death ensues. It is obvious that such changes would be detrimental to a developing pregnancy. The cardiorespiratory system is exquisitely sensitive to the effects of microgravity. Cardiac output increases by approximately 20%, stroke volume by approximately 50%. Alveolar diffusing capacity increases by approximately 30%. Airway closing volume does not change (326).

Decompression sickness (DS) results when the body is exposed to differences in saturation pressures. Inert gases such as N_2 and CO escape into tissue spaces including fatty tissue. Women are four times more likely to develop these complications because of their higher adipose tissue content (327,328). N_2 bubbles accumulate in the pulmonary vasculature, especially the veins. The patent foramen ovale and ductus arteriosus allow rapid and fatal systemic embolization of the bubbles. The treatment for DS involves the administration of hyperbaric oxygen, which might be teratogenic in the first trimester. The risk of DS is a major hazard restricting safe reproduction in outer space.

ULTRASOUND

The increased use of diagnostic ultrasound has resulted in concerns about its effects on fetal health. It is estimated that more than half of all pregnant woman in the United States are examined with ultrasound (329). In laboratory animals, exposure to sufficiently high levels of ultrasound energy induced a variety of abnormalities in developing fetuses, including CNS, hematologic, genetic, and structural anomalies as well as IUGR (330,331). Energy levels used in diagnostic ultrasonography are substantially lower, however, and there are no confirmed reports of adverse effects in humans at these levels (332).

There are two potential mechanisms by which ultrasound can produce harmful effects in tissue. The first is by raising tissue temperature secondary to dissipation of ultrasound energy. Serious tissue damage is known to occur with prolonged elevation of the body temperature by 2.5°C or more (333); however, it has been demonstrated that during diagnostic ultrasonography, body temperatures increase by less than 1°C (329). Temperature elevations of this magnitude have not been associated with either fetal structural anomalies or spontaneous abortions.

The second method by which ultrasound may cause tissue damage is by a process called *cavitation*. When ultrasound energy interacts with microscopic gas bubbles, the bubbles collapse, causing a release of energy, a sudden rise in temperature, and the release of free radicals. The free radicals diffuse into tissue and can have biological action. This phenomenon is thought not to be significant at the energy levels used in diagnostic ultrasound but cannot be excluded completely as a possible mechanism for fetal injury.

Conflicting results have been reported in the literature regarding the effect of diagnostic ultrasound on *sister chromatid exchanges*, a term that refers to the exchange of portions of genetic material between two chromatids in the same chromosome. These changes occur spontaneously, but mutagenic agents can increase the frequency of this phenomenon (333). In 1979 Liebeskind and coworkers (334) described an increase in sister chromatid exchanges in human lymphocytes after exposure to diagnostic ultrasound. A subsequent study by Barnett and coworkers (335), however, could not reproduce these results. Studies in animal models on the effects of ultrasound on bone marrow, nervous system function, and embryonic growth have not yielded consistent results; but in a 1991 review of the literature, Brent and colleagues (336) concluded that in animal studies, temperature elevation in the region of the embryo was not significant enough to be deleterious.

Epidemiologic studies in humans have not demonstrated adverse fetal effects of diagnostic ultrasonography. Stark and colleagues (337) found similar perinatal outcomes in exposed and unexposed infants. They also had similar neurologic, cognitive, and behavioral outcomes. Segall and colleagues (338) found higher rates of adverse pregnancy outcomes following long-term occupational paternal exposure to ultrasound, but this finding has not been corroborated. When 1,114 newborns were studied after *in utero* exposure to ultrasound, 2.7% had congenital malformations, a rate that was similar to the general population; thus, no increases in abnormalities were observed to result from diagnostic ultrasound. The gestational age at the time of the study had no effect on neonatal outcome.

Serr and colleagues reported an increased rate of chromosome breaks diagnosed on amniocentesis following diagnostic ultrasound exposure (339). Others found no increase in chromosomal aberrations in lymphocytes, amniotic fluid cells, cultured fibroblasts, and neonatal karyotypes (340–342).

Studies to date have indicated that diagnostic ultrasound does not have any measurable or significant biologic effects, with low exposure presenting either minimal or no risk to pregnancy. The American Institute of Ultrasound in Medicine reviewed reports on the biological effects of ultrasound and concluded that there were no confirmed adverse biological effects on patients or instrument operators caused by currently used ultrasound intensities (i.e., less than 100 mW/cm) (329); however, Reece and colleagues stated that despite the large number of studies on the bioeffects of ultrasound, unequivocal conclusions cannot be drawn regarding its safety (333).

OCCUPATIONAL HAZARDS FOR MALES

Approximately 15% of couples have no children, and another 10% have fewer children than they desire. In about half of these cases, the underlying cause is due to the man. Of these, the role of occupational and environmental factors remains controversial. Possible mechanisms include direct effects on sperm quantity and production, mutations in sperm cells, transmission of toxins through seminal fluid, and direct exposure of the mother or fetus to agents brought home by the partner. Evidence suggesting potential maternal or fetal harm resulting from paternal occupational exposures exists for a number of agents outlined here. Many problems pertaining to interpretation of the data exist, however, and these should be evaluated when assessing relevant information. Small sample size, recall bias, confounding variables (e.g., the number of agents being evaluated), overlapping between various occupations, and differences between exposure levels are some examples of potential problems.

In addition, the accuracy of the sources of obtaining the information is often questionable. Sources can vary between reviews of birth and death records to parental interviews and even sometimes malformation registries. The information entered varies with the expertise and accuracy of the person(s) providing the information.

Response bias also can occur as a result of varying participation rates in surveys, questionnaires, and studies. Small sample sizes limit the ability to generate risk estimates. In many studies, data are lacking on the many extraneous confounding factors.

Many physical and chemical occupational agents have been shown to affect male reproduction in animals and humans; however, human data are often conflicting, and it is difficult to identify a single agent because most exposures result from combinations of agents and confounding effects related to lifestyle (343). In addition, many factors affect the extent of the exposures (Table 6-4). Thus, counseling exposed pregnant women about the possible effects of occupational exposures is difficult.

It is well known that exposure to different toxins such as metals, solvents, welding, heat exposure, and others may result not only in abnormalities of sperm production and morphology but also in ejaculation abnormalities in males and increased rates of adverse pregnancy outcomes in partners of exposed men (344). Welding of stainless steel is associated with the release of mutagenic agents such as hexavalent chromium and therefore has been thought to result in adverse in pregnancy outcomes. Hjollund and colleagues (345) found no increase in the spontaneous abortion rate in 2,520 pregnancies in women whose partners were welders, whereas Bonde and associates (346) reported that steel welders have increased rates of abnormal sperm and lower sperm quantity. This effect appears to be irreversible (347). Olshan and associates (348) found an increased risk for cleft lip/cleft palate in the offspring of welders.

TABLE 6-4. *Factors affecting potential occupational exposures to hazardous agents*

Nature of the chemical
Pharmacokinetics and half-life
Concentrations in tissues with both high and low affinities for the agent
Possible human exposure dose
Route of entry of agent
Absorption of agent
Transportation within the body
Metabolic degradation of the agent
Route and rate of excretion of the agent

A slightly increased risk for childhood cancers has been found in these offspring (349). Involved organs include brain and Wilm's tumor. This association is more significant if the exposure occurred during early pregnancy than if exposure was prior to the onset of pregnancy. In contrast, neither Olsen and colleagues (350) nor Bonde and colleagues (351) found an increase in the childhood cancer rate.

An additional hazard for welders is exposure to excessive heat (especially of the male genital area), which can result in altered spermatogenesis (352). Scrotal temperature remains 3°C lower than core body temperature. An increase of every degree Centigrade in the scrotal temperature results in a 14% drop in sperm count (353). Sperm quality also decreases, but this change is reversible.

Other occupations that are associated with heat exposure include cooks, firefighters, and ceramics and foundry workers. Sanjose and colleagues (354) found an increased risk of low birth weight (RR, 1.8) and preterm birth (RR, 1.9) in pregnancies in which the fathers worked in the ceramics industry.

REFERENCES

1. Paul M. Common household exposures. In: Paul M, ed. Occupational and environmental reproductive hazards. Baltimore: Williams & Wilkins, 1993;361–378.
2. National Institute for Occupational Safety and Health. Rockville, MD. United States Department of Health Education and Welfare, 1978.
3. Paul M, ed. Occupational and environmental reproductive hazards. Baltimore: Williams & Wilkins, 1993.
4. Gabbe SG, Turner LP. Reproductive hazards of the American lifestyle: work during pregnancy. Am J Obstet Gynecol 1997;176:826–832.
5. US Department of Labor. Household data: annual averages. Washington, DC: Dureau of Labor Statistics, 1991.

6. Gabbe SG, Turner LP. Reproductive hazards of the American lifestyle: Work during pregnancy. Am J Obstet Gynecol 1997;176:826–832.
7. Wen CP, Tsai SP, Gibson RL. Anatomy of the healthy worker effect: A critical review. J Occup Med 1983;24:283–289.
8. World Health Organization. Health hazards of the human environment. Geneva: World Health Organization, 1972.
9. American Academy of Pediatrics. The susceptibility of fetus and child to chemical pollutants. Pediatrics (Suppl) 1974;53:77.
10. American College of Obstetricians and Gynecologists. Guidelines on pregnancy and work. Washington, DC: ACOG, 1977.
11. Pritchard J, MacDonald PC, Gant NF., eds. Williams obstetrics, Norwalk, CT: Appleton-Century-Crofts, 1985;181.
12. Juchau MR. Drug biotransformation with placenta. Pharmacol Ther 1980;8:501.
13. Miller RK. Perinatal toxicology: its recognition and fundamentals. Am J Ind Med 1983;4:205.
14. Hemminki K. Occupational chemicals tested for teratogenicity. Int Arch Occup Environ Health 1980;47:191–207.
15. Pries C. Reproductive effects of occupational exposures. Am Family Physician 1981;24:161:165.
16. Nordstrom S, Beckman L, Nordcusen I. Occupational and environmental risks in and around a smelter in northern Sweden. III. Frequencies of spontaneous abortion. Hereditas 1978;88:41.
17. Moore LG. Altitude-aggravated illness: examples from pregnancy and prenatal life. Ann Emerg Med 1987;16:965–973.
18. Johnson TS, Rock PB. Acute mountain sickness. N Engl J Med 1988; 319:841–845.
19. Rom WN. High-Altitude environments. In Rom WN, ed. Environmental and occupational medicine, 2nd ed. Boston: Little Brown and Company, 1992:1143–1151.
20. Cugell DW, Frank NR, Gaensler ER, Badger TL. Pulmonary function in pregnancy. Am Rev Tuberc 1953;67:568.
21. Hytten FE, Lind T. Indices of cardiovascular function. In: Hytten FE, Lind T, eds. The physiology of human pregnancy. Oxford: Blackwell, 1971:234.
22. Elkayam U, Gleicher N. Cardiovascular physiology of pregnancy. In: Elkayam U, Gleicher N, eds. Cardiac problems in pregnancy: diagnosis and management of maternal and fetal disease. New York: Alan R. Liss, 1982;5.
23. Moore LG, Rounds SS, Jahnigen D, et al. Infant birth weight is related to maternal arterial oxygenation at high altitude. J Appl Physiol 1982; 52:695–699.
24. Lichty JA, Ting RY, Bruns PD, et al. Studies of babies born at high altitude: relation of altitude to birth weight. Am J Dis Child 1957;93: 666–669.
25. McCullough RE, Reeves JT, Liljegren RL. Fetal growth retardation and infant mortality at high altitude. Arch Environ Health 1977; 32:36–39.
26. Zamudio S, Palmer SK, Dahms TE, et al. Blood volume expansion, preeclampsia, and infant birth weight at high altitude. J Appl Physiol 1993;74:1566–1573.
27. Zamudio S, Palmer SK, Droma T, Stamm E, Coffin C, Moore LG. Effect of altitude on uterine artery blood flow during normal pregnancy. J Appl Physiol 1995;79:7–14.
28. Zamudio S, Palmer SK, Dahms TE, Berman JC, Young DA, Moore LG. Alterations in uteroplacental blood flow precede hypertension in preeclampsia at high altitude. J Appl Physiol 1995;79:15–22.
29. Alderman BW, Zamudio S, Barron AE. Increased risk of craniosynostosis with higher antenatal maternal altitude. Int J Epidemiol 1995; 24:420–426.
30. Flak LJ. Intermediate sojourners in high altitude: Selection and clinical observations. In: Adjustment to high altitude. Bethesda, MD: NIH pub 83-2496, 1983.
31. Cameron RG. Should air hostesses continue flight duty during the first trimester of pregnancy? Aerospace Medicine 1973;44:552–556.
32. Daniell WE, Vaughan TL, Millies BA. Pregnancy outcomes among female flight attendants. Aviat Space Environ Med 1990;61:840–844.
33. Cruickshank JM, Gorlin R, Jennett B. Air travel and thrombotic episodes: the economy class syndrome. Lancet 1988;2:497–498.
34. National Institutes of Health Consensus Development Conference. Prevention of venous thrombosis and pulmonary embolism. JAMA 1986;256:744–749.
35. McKone TE, Daniels JI. Estimating human exposure through multiple pathways from air, water, and soil. Regul Toxicol Pharmacol 1991; 12:36–61.
36. Gerhardsson L, Dahlgren E, Eriksson E, Lagerkvist BE, Lundstrom J, Nordberg GF. Fatal arsenic poisoning—a case report. Scand J Work Environ Health 1990;14:130–133.
37. National Academy of Sciences Committee on Medical and Biological Effects of Environmental Pollutants. Arsenic. Washington, DC: National Academy of Sciences, 1977.
38. Lugo G, Cassady G, Palmisano P. Acute maternal arsenic intoxication with neonatal death. Am J Dis Child 1969;117:328–320.
39. Bollinger CT, Van Zijl P, Louw JA. Multiple organ failure with the adult respiratory distress syndrome in homicidal arsenic poisoning. Respiration 1992;59:57–61.
40. Nordstrom S, Beckman L, Nordenson L. Occupational and environmental risks in and around a smelter in northern Sweden. III. Frequencies of spontaneous abortion. Hereditas 1978;88:41.
41. Zierler S, Theodore M, Cohen A, Rothman KJ. Chemical quality of maternal drinking water and congenital heart disease. Int J Epidemiol 1988;17:589–594.
42. Golub MS. Maternal toxicity and the identification of inorganic arsenic as a developmetnal toxicant. Reprod Toxicol 1994;8:283–295.
43. Levy SA. Asbestosis. In: Zenz C, Dickerson OB, Horvath EP Jr, eds. Ocupational medicine, 3rd ed. St. Louis: Mosby, 1994;179–184.
44. Kleinfeld M, Messie J, Shapiro J. Clinical, radiological, and physiological findings in asbestosis. Arch Intern Med 1966;117:813.
45. Haque AK, Mancuso MG, Williams MG, Dodson RF. Asbestos in organs and placenta of five stillborn infants suggests transplacental transfer. Environ Res 1992;58:163–175.
46. Haque AK, Vrazel DM, Burau KD, Cooper SP, Downs T. Is there transplacental transfer of asbestos? A study of 40 stillborn infants. Pediatr Pathol Lab Med 1996;16:877–892.
47. Wassermann M, Wassermann D, Steinitz R, Katz L, Lemesch C. Mesothelioma in children. IARC Sci Publ 1980;30:253–257.
48. Scheider U, Maurer RR. Asbestos and embryonic development. Teratology 1977;15:273–280.
49. Henderson J, Rennie GC, Baker HWG. Association between occupational group and sperm concentration in infertile men. Clin Reprod Fertil 1986;4:275.
50. Strohmer H, Boldizsar A, Plöcinger B, Feldner-Bustzin M, Feichtinger W. Agricultural work and male infertility. Am J Ind Med 1993;24:587.
51. Figa-Talamanca I, Dondero F, Gandini L, Lenzi A, Lombardo F, Osborn J, Simeone M. Expositions professionalles et environmentales et spermatogenèse: une enquête cas-témoins. Arch Mal Prof 1992;52: 614.
52. McDonald AD, McDonald JC, Armstrong B, Cherry NM, Nolin AD, Robert D. Fathers' occupation and pregnancy outcome. Br J Ind Med 1989;46:329.
53. Lin S, Marshall EG, Davidson GK. Potential parental exposure to pesticides and limb reduction defects. Scand J Work Environ Health 1994;20:166.
54. Olshan AF, Teschke K, Baird PA. Paternal occupation and congenital anomalies in offspring. Am J Ind Med 1991;20:447.
55. Brender JD, Suarez L. Paternal occupation and anencephaly. Am J Epidemiol 1990;131:517.
56. Sanjose S, Roman E, Beral V. Low birth weight and preterm delivery, Scotland 1981–84: effect of parents' occupation. Lancet 1991;338: 428.
57. Sprince NL, Kazemi Homayoun. Beryllium disease. In: Rom WN, ed. Environmental and occupational medicine, 2nd ed. Boston: Little Brown and Company, 1992;781–790.
58. Criteria for a Recommended Standard. Occupational Exposure to Beryllium. Washington, DC: U.S. Government Printing Office, 1972 DHEW publication (NIOSH)72-10268.
59. National Occupational Hazard Survey. Washington, DC. U.S. Government Printing Office, 1977. DHEW publication (NIOSH)78–114.
60. Knishkowy B, Baker E. Transmission of occupational disease to family contacts. Am J Ind Med 1986;9:543–550.
61. Schellmann B, Raithel H, Schaller KH. Acute fatal selenium poisoning: toxicologic and occupational medicine aspects. Arch Toxicol 1986;59:61–63.
62. Willhite CC. Selenium teratogenesis. Species-dependent response and influence on reproduction. Ann NY Acad Sci 1993;678:169–177.
63. Shamberger RJ. Is selenium a teratogen? Lancet 1971;2:1316.
64. Elwood JM, Coldman AJ. Water composition in the etiology of anencephalus. Am J Epidemiol 1981:113:681–690.
65. Miller RK, Bellinger D. Metals. In: Paul M, ed. Occupational and

environmental reproductive hazards. Baltimore: Williams & Wilkins, 1992:233–252.

66. Parizek J. Vascular changes at sites of oestrogen biosynthesis produced by parenteral injection of cadmium salts: the destruction of placenta by cadmium salts. J Reprod Fertil 1964;7:263.
67. Barlow SM, Sulivan FM. Reproductive hazards of industrial chemicals. New York: Academic Press, 1982.
68. Palsy K, Varga B, Lazar P. Effect of cadmium on female fertility, pregnancy and postnatal development in the rat. Acta Physiol Hung 1996; 84:119–130.
69. Goyer RA. Toxic effects of metals. In: Amdur MO, Doull J, Klaasen CD, eds. Casarett and Doull's toxicology, 4th ed. New York: Pergamon Press, 1991:623–680.
70. Sullivan FM, Barlow SM. Congenital malformations and other reproductive hazards from encironmental chemicals. Proc R Soc Lond Biol Sci 1979;205:91–110.
71. Berlin M, Blanks R, Catton M. Birth weight of children and cadmium accumulation in placentas of female nickel-cadmium (long-life) battery workers. IARC Sci Publ 1992;118:257–262.
72. National Institute for Occupational Safety and Health. Criteria for a recommended standard: occupational exposure to carbon disulfide. Washington, DC U.S. Government Printing Office. DHEW publication (NIOSH), 1977.
73. Lilis R. Carbon disulfide. In: Rom WN, ed. Environmental and occupational medicine, 2nd ed. Boston: Little Brown and Company, 1992: 993–998.
74. Lancranjan I. Alterations of spermatic liquid in patients chronically poisoned by carbon disulfide. Med Lav 1972;63:29.
75. Cai Sx, Bao YS. Placental transfer, secretion into mother's milk of carbon disulfide and the effects on maternal function of female viscose rayon workers. Indust Health 1981;19:15–29.
76. Petrov MV. Some data on the course and termination of pregnancy in female workers of the viscose industry. Pediatr Akushersvo Ginekol 1969;3:50.
77. Hemminki K; Niemi ML. Community study of spontaneous abortions: relation to occupation and air pollution by sulfur dioxide, hydrogen sulfide, and carbon disulfide. Int Arch Occup Environ Health 1982;51:55–63.
78. Saillenfait AM, Bonnet P, de Ceaurriz J. Effects of inhalation exposure to carbon disulfide and its combination with hydrogen sulfide on embryonal and fetal development in rats. Toxicol Lett 1989;48: 57–66.
79. Tabacova S, Balabaeva L. Subtle consequences of prenatal exposure to low carbon disulfide levels. Arch Toxicol Suppl 1980;4:252–254.
80. Gabrielli A, Layon AJ, Gallagher TJ. Carbon monoxide intoxication during pregnancy: a case presentation and pathophysiologic discussion, with emphasis on molecular mechanisms. J Clin Anesth 1995;7: 82–87.
81. Sorokin Y. Asphyxiants. In: Paul M, ed. Occupational and environmental reproductive hazards. Baltimore: Williams & Wilkins, 1992: 253–266.
82. Norman CA, Halton DM. Is carbon monoxide a workplace teratogen? A review and evaluation of the literature. Ann Occup Hyg 1990;34: 335–347.
83. Centers for Disease Control. Carbon monoxide intoxication—a preventable environmental health hazard. MMWR 1982;31:529–531.
84. Marzella L, Myers R. Carbon monoxide poisoning. Pract Therap 1986;34:186–94.
85. Norman CA, Halton DM. Is carbon monoxide a workplace teratogen? A review and evaluation of the literature. Ann Occup Hyg 1990;34: 335–347.
86. Farrow JR, Davis GJ, Roy TM, McCloud LC, Nichols GR II. Fetal death due to nonlethal maternal carbon monoxide poisoning. J Forensic Sci 1990;35:1448–1452.
87. Longo LD. The biological effects of carbon monoxide on the pregnant woman, fetus, and newborn infant. Am J Obstet Gynecol 1977;129: 69–103.
88. Norman CA, Halton DM. Is carbon monoxide a workplace teratogen? A review and evaluation of the literature. Ann Occup Hyg 1990;34; 335–347.
89. Alderman BW, Baron AE, Savitz DA. Maternal exposure to neighborhood carbon monoxide and risk of low infant birth weight. Pub Health Rep 1987;102;410–414.
90. Moses M. Pesticides. In: Paul M, ed. Occupation and environmental reproductive hazards. Baltimore: Williams & Wilkins, 1993:296–305.
91. Erickson JD, Mulinaire J, McClain PW, et al. Vietnam veterans risks for fathering babies with birth defects. JAMA 1984;252:903–912.
92. Rosenman KD. Dioxin, polychlorinated biphenyls, and dibenofurans. In: Rom WN, ed. Environmental and occupational medicine 2nd ed. Boston: Little, Brown and Company 1992:927–933.
93. Esposito MP. Dioxins. Cincinnati, OH: United States Environmental Protection Agency. EPA publication 600/2-80-197, 1980.
94. Longo LD. Environmental pollution and pregnancy: Risks and uncertainties for the fetus and infant. Am J Obstet Gynecol 1980;137: 162–173.
95. Mastroiacovo P, Spangnolo A, Marni E, et al. Birth defects in the Seveso area after TCDD contamination. JAMA 1988;259:1668–1672.
96. Pluim HJ, Koppe JG, Olie K, et al. Clinical laboratory manifestations of exposure to background levels of dioxins in the perinatal period. Acta Paediatr 1994;83:583–587.
97. Birnbaum LS. Developmental effects of dioxins. Environ Health Perspect 1995;103:89–94.
98. Lindbohm ML, Hietanen M. Magnetic fields of video display terminals and pregnancy outcome. J Occup Environ Med 1995;37: 952–956.
99. Parazzini F, Luchini L, LaVecchia C, Crosignani PG. Video display terminal use during pregnancy and reproductive outcome-a meta-analysis. J Epidemiol Community Health 1993;47:265–268.
100. Bracken MB, Belanger K, Hellenbrand K, et al. Exposure to electromagnetic fields during pregnancy with emphasis on electrically heated beds: association with birthweight and intra uterine growth retardation. Epidemiology 1995; 6:263–270.
101. Dlugosz L, Vena J, Byers T, Sever L, Bracken MB, Marshall E. Congenital defects and electric bed heating in New York State: a register based case control study. Am J Epidemiol 1992;135:1000–1011.
102. Milansky A, Ulcickas M, Rothman RJ, Willett W, Jick SS, Jick H. Maternal heat exposure and neural tube defects. JAMA 1992;268: 882–885.
103. Pearn JH. Teratogens and the male: an analysis with special reference to herbicide exposure. Med J Aust 1983;2:16–20.
104. Nordstrom S, Birke E, Gustavson L. Reproductive hazards during workers at high voltage substations. Bioelectromagnetics 1983;4: 91–101.
105. Occupational Safety and Health Administration. Guidelines for preventing workplace violence for health care and social service workers. OSHA publication no. 3148-1996.
106. National Institute for Occupational Safety and Health. Criteria for a recommended standard: occupational exposure to waste anesthetic gases and vapors. DHEW (NIOSH) publication no. 77-140. Cincinnati, OH: U.S. Department of Health, Education and Welfare, 1977.
107. Spence AA. Chronic exposure to trace concentrations of anaesthetics. In: Gray TC, Nuff JF, Utting JE, eds. General anaesthesia, 4th ed. London: Butterworths, 1980;189–201.
108. McDiarmid M. Occupational exposure to pharmaceuticals: antineoplastics, anesthetic agents, sex steroid hormones. In: Paul M, ed. Occupational and environmental reproductive hazards. Baltimore: Williams & Wilkins, 1993;280–295.
109. National Institute for Occupational Safety and Health. Rockville, MD: United States Department of Health Education and Welfare, 1978.
110. Vainio H. Inhalation anesthetics, anticancer drugs and sterilants as chemical hazards in hospitals. Scand J Work Environ Health 1982;8: 94–107.
111. Anderson NB. The effect of CNS depressants on mitosis. Acta Anaesth Scand 1966;10:2–36.
112. Friedman JM. Teratogen update: anesthetic agents. Teratology 1988; 37:69–77.
113. Tannenbaum TN, Goldberg RJ. Exposure to anesthetic gases and reproductive outcome. J Occup Med 1985;27:659–668.
114. Heinonen OP, Slone D, Shapiro S. Birth defects and drugs in pregnancy. Littleton, MA: Publishing Sciences Group, 1977.
115. Brodsky JB, Cohen EN, Brown BW Jr, Wu ML, Whitcher C. Surgery during pregnancy and fetal outcome. Am J Obstet Gynecol 1980;138: 1165.
116. Duncan PG, Pope WD, Cohen MM, Greer N. Fetal risk of anesthesia and surgery during pregnancy. Anesthesiology 1986;64:790–794.
117. McDiarmid M. Occupational exposure to pharmaceuticals: antineoplastics, anesthetic agents, sex steroid hormones. In: Paul M, ed. Occupational and environmental reproductive hazards. Baltimore: Williams & Wilkins, 1993:280–295.
118. Freckman HA, Fry HL, Mende FL, Maures ER. Chlorambucil-pred-

nisolone therapy for disseminated breast carcinoma. JAMA 1964;189: 23–26.
119. Gililland J, Weinstein L. The effects of cancer chemotherapeutic agents on the developing fetus. Obstet Gynecol Surv 1983;38:6–13.
120. deWerk Neal A, Wadden RA, Chiou WL. Exposure of hospital workers to airborne antineoplastic agents. Am J Hosp Pharm 1983;40: 587–601.
121. Selevan SG, Lindbohm ML, Hornung RW, Hemminki K. A study of occupational exposure to antineoplastic drugs and fetal loss in nurses. N Engl J Med 1985;313:1173–1178.
122. Health hazard evaluation report: Emanuel Hospital, Portland, Oregon. Cincinnati: National Institute of Occupational Safety and Health.
123. Hemminki K, Kyronen P, Lindbohm M-L. Spontaneous abortions and malformations in the offspring of nurses exposed to anesthetic gases, cytostat drugs, and other potential hazards in hospitals based on registered information of outcome. J Epidemiol Community Health 1985;39:141.
124. Yodaiken RE. OSHA work practice guidelines for personnel dealing with cytotoxic drugs. Am J Hosp Pharm 1986;43:1193–1204.
125. Schwartz R. Pregnancy in physicians: characteristics and complications. Obstet Gynecol 1985;66:673–676.
126. Klebanoff MA, Shiono PH, Rhoads GG. Outcomes of pregnancy in a national sample of resident physicians. N Engl J Med 1990;323: 1040–1045.
127. Klebanoff MA, Shiono PH, Rhoads GG. Spontaneous and induced abortion among resident physicians. JAMA 1991;265:2821–2825.
128. Centers for Disease Control. Hepatitis B virus: a comprehensive strategy for eliminating transmission in the United States through universal childhood vaccination: recommendations of the Immunization Practices Advisory Committee. MMWR 1991;40:1–24.
129. U.S. Department of Labor, Occupational Safety and Health Administration. Occupational exposure to bloodborne pathogens; final rule. 29 CFR Part 1910.1030, 1991.
130. Connor EM, Sperling RS, Gelber R, et al. Reduction of maternal-infant transmission of human immunodeficiency virus type 1 with zidovudine treatment. Pediatric AIDS Clinical Trials Group Protocol 076 Study Group. New Engl J Med 1994;331:1173–1180.
131. Moore RM Jr, Davis YUM, Kaczmarek RG. An overview of occupational hazards among veterinarians, with particular reference to pregnant women. Am Ind Hyg Assoc J 1993;54:113–120.
132. Halling H. Suspected link between exposure to hexachlorophene and malformed infants. Ann NY Acad Sci 1979;320:426–435.
133. Kallen B. Hexachlorophene teratogenicity in humans disputed. JAMA 1978;240:1585–1586.
134. Janerich DT. Environmental causes of birth defects: the hexachlorophene issue. JAMA 1979;241:830–831.
135. Baltzar B, Ericson A, Kallen B. Pregnancy outcome among women working in Swedish hospitals. N Engl J Med 1979;300:627–628.
136. Briggs GG, Freeman RK, Yaffe SJ. Drugs in pregnancy and lactation, 4th ed. Baltimore, MD: Williams & Wilkins, 1994;415–418.
137. Hansson E, Jansa S, Wande H, Kallen B, Ostlund E. Pregnancy outcome for women working in laboratories in some of the pharmaceutical industries in Sweden. Scand J Work Environ Health 1980;6:131.
138. Hemminki K, Mutanen P, Saloniemi I, Naimi ML, Vainjo H. Spontaneous abortion in hospital staff engaged in sterilizing instruments with chemical agents. Br Med J Clin Res Ed 1982;285:1461–1463.
139. Bertin JE, Werby EA. Legal and policy issues. In: Paul M, ed. Occupational and environmental reproductive hazards. Baltimore: Williams & Wilkins, 1993;280–295.
140. Gilfillan SC. Lead poisoning and the fall of Rome. J Occup Med 1965;7:53–60.
141. Wong GP, Ng TL, Martin TR, Farquharson DF. Effects of low-level lead exposure in utero. Obstet Gynecol Surg 1992;47:285–289.
142. Fischbein A. Occupational and environmental lead exposure. In: Rom WN, ed. Environmental and occupational medicine, 2nd ed. Boston: Little Brown and Company, 1992;735–758.
143. Murozumi, Chow TJ, Patterson CC. Chemical concentrations of pollutant lead aerosols, terrestrial dusts and sea salt in Greenland and Antarctic snow strata. Geochim Cosmochim Acta 1969;33: 1247–1294.
144. Yaffe Y, Flessel CP, Weselowski JJ, et al. Identification of lead sources in California children using the stable isotope ratio technique. Arch Environ Health 1983;38:227–245.
145. Toxicological Profile for Lead. Atlanta: US Department of Health and Human Services, Agency for Toxic Substances and Disease Registry. ATSDR publication TP-88/17, 1990.
146. Wong GP, Ng TL, Martin TR, Farquharson DF. Effects of low-level lead exposure in utero. Obstet Gynecol Surg 1992;47:285–289.
147. Mahaffey KR, Annest JL, Roberts J, Murphy RS. National estimates of blood lead levels: United States, 1976–1980. N Engl J Med. 1982; 307:573–579.
148. Bellinger D, Leviton A, Wateraux C, Needleman HL, Rabinowitz M. Longitudinal analyses of prenatal and postnatal lead exposure and early cognitive development. N Engl J Med 1987;316:1037–1043.
149. Dietrich KN, Kraft KM, Bornschein RL, et al. Low-level fetal lead exposure effect on neurobehavioral development in early infancy. Pediatrics 1987;80:721.
150. Ernhart CB, Wolf AW, Kennard MJ, Erhard P, Filipowich HF, Sokol RJ. Intrauterine exposure to low level of lead: the status of the neonate. Arch Environ Health 1986;41:287.
151. McMichael AJ, Baghurst PA, Wigg NR, Vimpani GV, Robertson EF, Roberts EJ. Port Pirie cohort study: environmental exposure to lead and children's abilities at the age of four years. N Engl J Med 1988; 31:468–475.
152. Bayley N. Bayley scales of infant development. New York: Psychological Corporation, 1969.
153. Bellinger D. Teratogen update: lead. Teratology 1994;50:367–373.
154. Wasserman G, Graziano J, Factor-Litvak, P, et al. Consequences of lead exposure and iron supplementation on childhood development at age 4 years. Neurotoxicol Teratol 1994;16:23–40.
155. Needleman H, Rabinowitz A, Leviton S, Linn S, Schoenbaum S. The relationship between prenatal exposure to lead and congenital anomalies. JAMA 1984;251:2956–2959.
156. Aschengrau A, Zierler S, Cohen A. Quality of community drinking water and the occurrence of late adverse pregnancy outcomes. Arch Environ Health 1993;48:105–113.
157. Miller RK, Bellinger D. Metals. In: Paul M, ed. Occupational and environmental reproductive hazards. Baltimore: Williams & Wilkins, 1992:233–252.
158. Alfonso J, DeAlvarez R. Effects of mercury on human gestation. Am J Obstet Gynecol 1960;80:145–54.
159. Bakir F, Damluji SF, Amin-Zaki L, et al. Methylmercury poisoning in Iraq: an interuniversity report. Science 1973;181:230–241.
160. Snyder RD. Congenital mercury poisoning. N Engl J Med 1971;18: 1014–1016.
161. Clarkson TW. Mercury: major issues in environmental health. Environ Health Perspect 1992;100:31–38.
162. Koos BJ, Longo LD. Mercury toxicity in the pregnant woman, fetus, and newborn infant. Am J Obstet Gynecol 1976;126:390.
163. Miller RK, Bellinger D. Metals. In: Paul M, ed. Occupational and environmental reproductive hazards. Baltimore: Williams & Wilkins, 1992:233–252.
164. Harada Y. Study group on Minamata disease. In: Katsuma M, ed. Minamata disease. Kumamato, Japan: Kumatoto University, 1966: 93–117.
165. Spyker JM, Sparber SB, Goldberg AM. Subtle consequences of methylmercury exposure: Behavioral deviations in offspring of treated mothers. Teratology 1972;5:267.
166. Choi B. Effects of methylmercury on the developing brain. In: Suzuki T, Imura N, Clarkson TE, eds. Advances in mercury toxicology. New York: Plenum Press, 1991:315–558.
167. Melkonian R, Baker D. Risks of industrial mercury exposure in pregnancy. Obstet Gynecol Surv 1988;637–641.
168. National Institute for Occupational Safety and Health: NIOSH/OSHA Occupational Health Guidelines for Chemical Hazards. National Institute for Occupational Safety and Health, Cincinnati, OH. (DBBS (NIOSH) publication no. 81-123), 1981.
169. Melkonian R, Baker D. Risks of industrial mercury exposure in pregnancy. Obstet Gynecol Surv 1988;637–641.
170. Thorp JM, Boyette DD, Watson WJ, Cefalo RC. Elemental mercury exposure in early pregnancy. Obstet Gynecol 1992;79:874–875.
171. Kuhnert PM, Kuhnert BR, Erhaud P. Comparison of mercury levels in maternal blood, fetal cord blood, and placental tissues. Am J Obstet Gynecol 1981;139:209–213.
172. Cox C, Clarkson TW, Marsh DO, Amin-Zaki L, Tikriti S, Myers GC. Dose-response analysis of infants prenatally exposed to methylmercury: an application of a single compartment model to single strand hair analysis. Environ Res 1989;49:318–332.

173. Brent RL. The effects of embryonic and fetal exposure to x-ray, microwaves and ultrasound. Clin Perinatol 1986;13:615.
174. National Council on Radiation Protection and Measurements (NCRP). Biological effects and exposure criteria for radiofrequency electromagnetic fields. NCRP report no. 86. Bethesda, MD:NCRP, 1986.
175. Smith H. On the safety of nuclear magnetic resonance imaging and spectroscopy systems. In: Partain Cl, Price RR, Patton JA, et al., eds. Magnetic resonance imaging, 2nd ed. Philadelphia: WB Saunders, 1988:1467–1482.
176. National Radiological Protection Board. Exposure to nuclear magnetic resonance clinical imaging. Radiography 1981;47:258–260.
177. National Radiological Protection Board ad hoc Advisory Group on Nuclear Magnetic Resonance Clinical Imaging. Revised guidance on acceptable limits of exposure during nuclear magnetic resonance clinical imaging. Br J Radiol 1982;56:974–977.
178. Evans JA, Savitz, DA, Kanal E, Gillen J. Infertility and pregnancy outcome among magnetic resonance imaging workers. J Occup Med 1993;35:1191–1195.
179. Fox ME, Harris RE, Brekken AL. The active duty military pregnancy: a new high risk category. Am J Obstet Gynecol 1977;129:707–709.
180. McGann EF, Nolan TE. Pregnancy outcome in an active duty population. Obstet Gynecol 1991;78:391–393.
181. Lalande NM, Hetu R, Lambert J. Is occupational noise exposure during pregnancy a risk factor of damage to the auditory system of the fetus? Am J Ind Med 1986;10:427–435.
182. Meyer RE, Aldrich TE, Easterly CE. Effects of noise and electromagnetic fields on reproductive outcomes. Environ Health Perspect 1989; 81:193.
183. Johanning E, Wilder DG, Landrigan PJ, Pope MH. Whole body vibration exposure in subway cars and review of adverse health effects. J Occup Med 1991;33:605.
184. Sas M, Szllösi J. Impaired spermatogenesis as a common finding among professional drivers. Arch Androl 1979;3:57.
185. Fox ME, Harris RE, Brekken AL. The active duty military pregnancy: a new high risk category. Am J Obstet Gynecol 1977;129:707–709.
186. Hauth JC, Gilstrap LC, Brekken AL, Hauth JM. The effect of 17 hydroxy-progesterone caproate on pregnancy outcome in an active duty military population. Am J Obstet Gynecol 1983;146:187–190.
187. McGann EF, Nolan TE. Pregnancy outcome in an active duty population. Obstet Gynecol 1991;78:391–393.
188. Mamelle N, Laumon B, Lazar P. Prematurity and occupational activity during pregnancy. Am J Epidemiol 119:309–322.
189. Saurel-Cubizolles MJ, Kaminski M, Llado-Arkhipoff J, et al. Pregnancy and its outcome among hospital personnel according to occupation and working conditions. J Epidemiol Community Health 1985; 39:129–134.
190. Tafari N, Naeye RL, Gobezie A. Effects of maternal undernutrition and heavy physical work during pregnancy on birth weight. Br J Obstet Gyneacol 1980;87:222–226.
191. Adams MM, Read JA, Rawlings JS, Harlass FB, Sarno AP, Rhodes PH. Preterm delivery among black and white enlisted women in the United States Army. Obstet Gynecol 1993;81:65–71.
192. Buttemiller R. Prematurity among United States Air Force active duty gravidas. Milit Med 1984;149:665–668.
193. Lavitz DA, Blackmore CA, Thorp JM. Epidemiologic characteristics of preterm delivery: etiologic heterogeneity. Am J Obstet Gynecol 1991;164:467–471.
194. Shiono PH, Klebanoff MA. Ethnic differences in preterm and very preterm delivery. Am J Public Health 1986;76:1317–1321.
195. Klebanoff MA, Yip R. Influence of maternal birth weight on rate of fetal growth and duration of gestation. J Pediatr 1987;111:287–292.
196. Baird D. The epidemiology of prematurity. J Pediatr 1964;64: 909–924.
197. Irwin DE, Savitz DA, St Andre KA, Hertz-Piciotto I. Study of occupational risk factors for pregnancy-induced hypertension among active duty enlisted navy personnel. Am J Ind Med 1994;25:349–359.
198. Bajaj JS, Misra A, Rajalakshmi M, Madan R. Environmental release of chemicals and reproductive ecology. Environ Health Perspect 1993; Suppl2:125–130.
199. Aschengrau A, Monson RR. Paternal miliary service in Vietnam and risk of late adverse pregnancy outcomes. Am J Public Health 1990;80: 1218–1224.
200. Aschengrau A, Mon RR. Paternal military service in Vietnam and the risk of spontaneous abortion. J Occup Med 1989;31:618–623.
201. Centers for Disease Control and Prevention (CDC). Vietnam Experience Study, health status of Vietnam veterans III. Reproductive outcomes and child health. JAMA 1988;259:2715.
202. Sterling TD, Arundel A. Review of recent Vietnamese studies on the carcinogenic and teratogenic effects of phenoxy herbicide exposure. Int J Health Serv 1986;16:265.
203. Snow ET, Costa M. Nickel toxicity and carcinogenesis. In: Rom WN, ed. Environmental and occupational medicine, 2nd ed. Boston: Little, Brown and Company, 1992;807–813.
204. Health Assessment Document for Nickel and Nickel Compounds. EPA publication 600/8-83/012FF, NTIS PB86-232212, 1986.
205. U.S. Department of Health and Human Services. Toxicological profile for nickel. ATSDR/TP-92/14. Syracuse Research Corporation, 1993.
206. Smith MK, George EL, Stober JA, Feng HA, Kimmel GL. Perinatal toxicity associated with nickel chloride exposure. Environ Res 1993; 61:200–211.
207. Chashschin VP. Artunina GP. Norseth T. Congenital defects, abortion and other health effects in nickel refinery workers. Sci Total Environ 1994;148:287–291.
208. Dickman DM. Noise and its effect on human health and welfare. Ear Nose Throat 1977;56:61–72.
209. Nurminen T. Female noise exposure, shift work, and reproduction. J Occup Environ Med 1995;37:945–950.
210. Ando Y, Hattori H. Statistical studies on the effects of intense noise during human fetal life. J Sound Vib 1973;27:101–110.
211. Knipschild P, Meijer H, Salle H. Aircraft noise and birth weight. Int Arch Occup Environ Health 1981;48:131–136.
212. Xu X, Ding M, Li B, Christiani DC. Association of rotating shiftwork with preterm births and low birth weight among never smoking women textile workers in China. Occup Environ Med 1994;51: 470–474.
213. Jones FN, Tausher J. Residence under an airport landing pattern as a factor in teratism. Arch Environ Health 1978;33:10–12.
214. Zhang J, Cai W, Lee DJ. Occupational hazards and pregnancy outcomes. Am J Ind Med 1992;21:397–408.
215. McDonald AD, McDonald JC, Armstrong B, et al. Fetal death and work in pregnancy. Br J Ind Med 1988;45:148–157.
216. Rachootin P, Olsen J. The risk of infertility and delayed conception associated with exposures in the Danish workplace. J Occup Environ Med 1983;24:394–402.
217. Wu TN, Chen LJ, Lai JS, Ko GN, Shen CY, Chang PY. Prospective study of noise exposure during pregnancy on birth weight. Am J Epidemiol 1996;143:792–796.
218. Kurppa K, Ranala K, Nurminen T, Holmberg PC, Stark J. Noise exposure during pregnancy and selected structural malformations in infants. Scand J Work Environ Health. 1989;15:111–116.
219. Peoples-Sheps MD, Siegel E, Suchindran CM, Origasa H, Ware A, Barakat A. Characteristics of maternal employment during pregnancy: effects on low birthweight. Am J Public Health 1991;81:1007–1012.
220. Dwornicka B, Jasineske A, Smolarz W, et al. Attempt of determining the fetal reaction to acoustic stimulation. Acta Otolaryngol 1964;57: 571–574.
221. Lindbohm ML. Effects of parental exposure to solvents on pregnancy outcome. JOEM 1995; 37:908–914.
222. Tossavaineu A, Jaakkola J. Occupational exposure to chemical agents in Finland. Appl Occup Environ Hyg 1994;9:28–31.
223. Taskinen HK, Olsen J, Bach B. Experiences developing legislation protecting reproductive health. J Occup Environ Med 1995;37: 974–979.
224. Browning RG, Curry SC. Clinical toxicology of ethylene glycolmonoalkyl ethers. Hum Exp Toxicol 1994;13:325–335.
225. Jonsson AK, Pederson J, Steen G. Ethoxyacetic acid and *N*-ethoxyacetyl glycine: metabolites of ethoxy ethanol (ethylcellosolve) in rats. Acta Pharmacol Toxicol 1982;50:358–362.
226. Stedman DB, Welsch F. Inhibition of DNA Synthesis in mouse whole embryo culture by 2 methoxyacetic acid and alternation of the effects by simple physiological compounds. Toxicol Lett 1989;45:111–117.
227. Mebus CA, Welsch F. The possible role of one carbon moieties in 2 methoxy ethanol and 2 methoxyacetic acid induced developmental toxicity. Toxicol Appl Pharmacol 1989;99:98–109.
228. Taskinen H, Kyyrönen P, Hemminki K, Hoikkala M, Lajunen K, Lindbohm ML. Laboratory work and pregnancy outcome. J Occup Environ Med 1994;36:311–319.
229. Loutant C, Lipman S. Fetal solvent syndrome. Lancet 1979;2:1356.

230. Jelnes JE. Effects on reproduction of styrene, toluene and xylene. Part II. Toluene. Summary and evaluation of effects on reproduction. In: Nordic council of Ministers. KEMI reports N 02/90 Solna, Sweden: The Swedish National Chemicals Inspectorate, 1990:37–53.
231. Tikkanen J, Heinonen OP. CV malformations and organic solvents exposure during pregnancy in Finland. Am J Ind Med 1988;14:1–8.
232. Lindbohm ML, Taskinen H, Sallmen M, Hemminkikl. Spontaneous abortions among women exposed to organic solvents. Am J Ind Med 1990;17:449–463.
233. Windham GC, Schusterman D, Swan SH, Fenster L, Eskenatai B. Exposure to organic solvents and adverse pregnancy outcome. Am J Ind Med 1991;20:241–259.
234. Pastides H, Calabrese EJ, Hosmer DW Jr, Harris DR. Spontaneous abortion and general illness symptoms among semiconductor manufacturers. J Occup Med 1988;30:543–551.
235. Lipscomb JA, Fenster L, Wrensch M, Schusterman D, Swan S. Pregnancy outcomes in women potentially exposed to occupational solvents and women working in the electronics industry. J Occup Med 1991;33:597–604.
236. NIOSH. Current Intelligence Bulletin 39. Glycol ethers: 2 Methoxyethanol and 2-Ethoxyethanol. DHSS (NIOSH). Publication 83-112 Cincinatti: National Institute for Occupational Safety and Health, 1983.
237. Correra A, Gray RH, Cohen R, et al. Ethylene glycol ethers and risk of spontaneous abortion and sub-fertility. Am J Epidemiol 1996;143: 707–714.
238. Bloniquist U, Ericson A, Kallen B, Westerholm P. Delivery outcome for women working in the pulp and paper industry. Scand J Work Environ Health 1981;7:114–118.
239. Holmberg PC, Hermberg S, Kurppak K, Rautala K, Riala R. Oral clefts and organic solvent exposure during pregnancy. Int Arch Occup Environ Health 1982;50:371–376.
240. Cordier S, Ha MC, Aynre S, Gonjard J. Maternal exposure and congenital malformations. Scand J Work Environ Health 1992;18:11–17.
241. Erickson JD, Cochran WM, Anderson CE. Parental occupation and birth defects: a preliminary report. Contrib Epidemiol Biostat 1979;1: 107–117.
242. Olshan AF, Teschke K, Baird PA. Paternal occupation and congenital anomalies in offspring. Am J Ind Med 1991;20:447–475.
243. Fredrick J. Anencephalus in the Oxford Record Linkage Study area. Dev Med Child Neurol 1976;18:643–656.
244. Brender JD, Suarez L. Paternal occupation and anencephaly. Am J Epidemiol 1990;131:517–521.
245. Gibson JE, ed. Formaldehyde toxicity. Washington DC: Hemisphere Publishing Company, 1983.
246. Holmberg PC. Central nervous system defects in children born to mothers exposed to organic solvents during pregnancy. Lancet 1979; 2:177–179.
247. Kyyronen P, Taskineor H, Lindbohm M-L, Hemminki K, Heinomen OP. Spontaneous abortions and congenital malformations among women exposed to tetrachloroethylene in dry cleaning. J Epidemiol Community Health 1989;43:346–351.
248. Olsen J, Hemminki K, Ahlborg G, et al. Low birth weight, congenital malformations, and spontaneous abortions among dry cleaning workers in Scandinavia. Scand J Work Environ Health 1990;16:163–168.
249. Lindbohm M-L, Taskinen H, Sallmen M, Hemminki K. Spontaneous abortions among women exposed to organic solvents. Am J Ind Med 1990;17:449–463.
250. Heidam LZ. Spontaneous abortions among laboratory workers: a follow-up study. J Epidemiol Commun Health 1984;300:627–628.
251. Ahlborg G. Pregnancy outcome among women working in laundries and dry cleaning shops using tetrachloroethylene. Am J Ind Med 1990;17:567–575.
252. Kristensen P, Irgens LM, Daltveit AK, Andersen A. Perinatal outcome among children of men exposed to lead and organic solvents in the printing industry. Am J Epidemiol 1993;137:134–144.
253. Matanoski GM. Final report: Occupational exposures and selected congenital defects. December 1, 1978–January 31, 1980. (Unpublished Report). Baltimore, MD: Dept of Epidemiology, School of Hygiene and Public Health, The Johns Hopkins University, 1980.
254. Chandley AC. On the parental origin of de novo mutations in man. J Med Genet 1991;28:217–223.
255. Jager S. Sperm nuclear stability and male infertility. Arch Androl 1990;25:253–259.
256. Stelling DL, Mayer FL. Toxicities of PcBs on fish and environmental residues. Environ Health Perspect 1972;1:159–164.
257. Rogan WJ, Gladen BC, Wilcox AJ. Potential reproductive and postnatal morbidity from exposure to polychlorinated biphenyls: epidemiologic considerations. Environ Health Perspect 1985;60:233.
258. Acker L, Schulte E. Uber das Vorkommern chlorierter Kohlen wasserstoffe im meschlichen Fett-gewebe Und in Humanmilch. Dtsch Lebensm-Rdsch 1970;66:385–390.
259. Acker L, Schulte E. Chlorkohlen wasserstoffe im menschlichen. Fett Naturwissenschaften 1974;61:32.
260. Rogan WJ. PCBs and cola colored babies: Japan 1968 and Taiwan 1979. Teratogen Update 1982;26:259–261.
261. Kuratsune M, Yoshimura T, Masuzaka J, Yamaguchi A. Yusho, a poisoning caused by rice oil contaminated with polychlorinated biphenyls. HSMHA Health Report 2 1971;86:1083–1091.
262. Fein GG, Jacobson JL, Jacobson SW, Schwartz PM, Dowler JK. Prenatal exposure to polychlorinated biphenyls: effects on birth size and gestational age. J Pediatr 1984;105:315.
263. Smith AH, Matheson DP, Fisher DO, Chapman CJ. Preliminary report of reproductive outcomes among pesticide applicators using 2, 4, 5-T. N Z Med J 1981;93:277–279.
264. Thomas DC, Petitti DB, Goldhaber M, Swan SH, Rappaport EB, Hertz-Picciotto I. Reproductive outcomes in relation to malathion spraying in the San Francisco Bay area. 1981–1982 Epidemiology 1992;3:32–39.
265. Willis WO, de Peyster A, Molgaard CA, Walker C, MacKendrick T. Pregnancy outcome among women exposed to pesticides through work or residence in an agricultural area. J Occup Environ Med 1993; 35:943–949.
266. Goulet L, Theriault G. Stillbirth and chemical exposure of pregnant workers. Scand J Work Environ Health 1991;17:25–31.
267. Munger R, Isacson P, Kramer M, et al. Birth defects and pesticide contaminated water supplies in Iowa. Am J Epidemiol 1992;136:959.
268. Matos EL, Loria DI, Albiano N, Sobel N, deBujan EL. Pesticides in intensive cultivation: effects on working conditions and workers health. Pan Am Health Org Bull 1987;21:405–416.
269. Restrepo M, Munoz N, Day NE, Parra JE, deRomero L, Ngugen-Dink X. Prevalence of adverse reproductive outcomes in a population occupationally exposed to pesticides in Columbia. Scand Work Environ Health 1990;16:232–238.
270. Grether JK, Harris JA, Neutra R, Kizer KW. Exposure to aerial malathion application and the occurrence of congenital anomalies and low birth weight. Am J Public Health 1987;77:1009–1010.
271. Nurminen T. Maternal Pesticide exposure and pregnancy outcome. J Occup Environ Med 1995;37:935–940.
272. Lin S, Marshall EG, Davidson GK. Potential parental exposure to pesticides and limb reduction defects. Scand J Work Environ Health 1994;20:166–179.
273. deCock J, Westveer K, Heederick D, Le Velde E, Van Kooij R. Time to pregnancy and occupational exposure to pesticides in fruit flowers in The Netherlands. Occup Environ Med 1994;51:693–699.
274. Potashnik G, Porath A. Dibromochloro-propane (DBCP): a 17 year reassessment of testicular function and reproductive performance. J Occup Environ Med 1995;37:1287–1292.
275. Rupa DS, Reddy PP, Reddi OS. Reproductive performance in populations exposed to pesticides in cotton fields in India. Environ Res 1991; 55:123.
276. Ahlborg G. Physical Work Load and Pregnancy Outcome. J Occup Environ Med 1995;37:941–944.
277. Ahlborg G, Bodin L, Hogstedt C. Heavy lifting during pregnancy–a hazard to the fetus? A prospective Study. Int J Epidemiol 1990;19: 90–97.
278. McDonald AD, McDonald JC, Armstrong B, Cherry NM, Nolin AD, Robert D. Prematurity and work in pregnancy. Br J Ind Med 1988;45: 56–62.
279. Marbury MC, Linn S, Monson RR, et al. Work and pregnancy. J Occup Med 1984;26:415–421.
280. Ahlborg G, Hogstedt C, Bodin L, Bárány S. Pregnancy outcome among working women. A prospective study. Scand J Work Environ Health 1989;15:227–233.
281. Kleinbaum DG, Kupper LL, Morgenstern H. Epidemiologic research: principles and quantitative methods. New York: Van Nostrand Reinhold, 1982:146.
282. Cohen E, Brown B, Bruce DL, et al. Occupational disease among

operating room personnel: a national study. Anesthesiology 1974;41: 321–340.
283. Magnus P. Causes of variation in birthweight. A study of offspring of twins. Clin Genet 1984;25:15–24.
284. Goulet L, Thériault G. Association between spontaneous abortion and ergonomic factors: a literature review of the epidemiologic evidence. Scand J Work Environ Health 1987;13:399–403.
285. Williamson H, Le Fevre M, Hector M. Association between life stress and serious perinatal complications. J Fam Pract 1989;29:489–496
286. Klebanoff MA, Shiono PH, Carey JC. The effect of physical activity during pregnancy on preterm delivery and birth weight. Am J Obstet Gynecol 1990;163:1450–1456.
287. Hall EJ. Scientific view of low-level radiation risks. Radiographics 1991;11:509.
288. National Council on Radiation Protection and Measurements (NCRP). Ionizing radiation exposure of the population of the United States. MNCRP report no. 93. Bethesda: NCRP, 1987.
289. Brent R, Meistrich M, Paul M. Ionizing and nonionizing radiations. In: Paul M, ed. Occupational and environmental reproductive hazards. Baltimore: Williams & Wilkins, 1993;165–189.
290. Dekaban AS. Abnormalities in children exposed to x-irradiation during various stages of gestation: Tentative timetable of radiation injury to the human fetus. J Nucl Med 1968;9:471.
291. Yamakazi JN, Schull WJ. Perinatal loss and neurological abnormalities among children of the atomic bomb. Nagasaki and Hiroshima revisited, 1949 to 1989. JAMA 1990;264:605–609.
292. Lilienfeld AM. Epidemiological studies of the leukemogenic effects of radiation. Yale J Biol Med 1966;39:143–164.
293. Hall EJ. Scientific view of low-level radiation risks. Radiographics 1991;11:509.
294. Imaging modalities during pregnancy. In: Cunningham FG, MacDonald PC, Gant NF, et al., eds. Williams obstetrics, 19th ed. Norwalk, CT. Appleton & Lange 1993;981–989.
295. Ragozzino MW, Breckle R, Hill LM, Gray JE. Average fetal depth in utero: Data for estimation of fetal absorbed radiation dose. Radiology 1986;158:513–515.
296. Moore MM, Shearer DR. Fetal dose estimates for CT pelvimetry. Radiology 1989;171:265–267.
297. Ginsberg JS, Hirsh J, Rainbow AJ, Coates G. Risks to the fetus of radiologic procedures used in the diagnoses of maternal venous thromboembolic disease. Thromb Haemost 1989;61:189.
298. Fisher WD, LoVorhees M, Gardener LT. Congenital hypothyroidism in infants following maternal ^{131}I therapy. J Pediatr 1963;62:132.
299. Mettler FA, Guiberteau MJ. Essentials of nuclear medicine imaging, 3rd ed. Philadelphia: WB Saunders, 1991.
300. IRCP 60: International Commission on Radiological Protection. Recommendations of the International Commission on Radiological Protection. Oxford: Pergamon, 1991.
301. IARC Study Group on Cancer Risk among Nuclear Industry Workers. Direct estimates of cancer mortality due to low doses of ionizing radiation: an international study. Lancet 1994;344:1039–1043.
302. Ambach W. Occupational low-dose exposure to ionizing radiation. Lancet 1994;344:1037.
303. Roman E, Doyle P, Ansell P, Bull D, Beral V. Health of children born to medical radiographers. Occup Environ Med 1996;53:73–79.
304. Santy PA, Jennings RT, Cralgie D. Reproduction in the space environment: Part I. Animal reproductive studies. Obstet Gynecol Surv 1989; 45:1–6.
305. Jennings RT, Santy PA. Reproduction in the space environment. Part II. Concerns for human reproduction. Obstet Gynecol Surv 1989;45: 7–17.
306. Serova L, Denisova L. The effect of weightlessness on the reproductive function of mammals. The Physiologist 1982;25:9–13.
307. Rock JA, Fortney SM. Medical and surgical considerations for women in space flight. Obstet Gynecol Surv 1984;39:525–528.
308. Lackner JR, Graybiel A. Etiological factors in space motion sickness. Aviat Space Environ Med 1983;54:675–681.
309. Lackner JR,Graybie A. Head movements in non-terrestrial force environments elicit motion sickness. Aviat Space Environ Med 1986;57: 443–448.
310. Triesman M. Motion sickness: an evolutionary hypothesis. Science 1977;1971:493–495.
311. Cunningham FG, MacDonald PC, Gant NFG. Williams obstetrics, 18th ed. Prentice Hall International, 1989:829–830.
312. Sullivan R. The hazards of reproduction in space. Acta Obstet Gynecol Scand 1996;75:372–377.
313. Letow JR, Silberberg R, Tsao CH. Radiation hazards on space missions. Nature 1987;330:709–710.
314. Wood DH. Long term mortality and cancer risk in irradiated rhesus monkeys. Radiat Res 1991;126:132–140.
315. Searle AG, Edwards JH. The estimation of risks from the induction of recessive mutation after exposure to ionizing radiation. J Med Gene 1986;23:220–224.
316. Fanton JW, Golden JG. Radiation induced endometriosis in *Macaca mulatta.* Radiat Res 1991;126:141–146.
317. Mole RH. consequences of prenatal radiation exposure for postnatal development Int J Radiat Biol 1982;42:1–5.
318. Beeke GW. The atomic bomb survivors and the problems of low dose radiation effects. Am J Epidemiol 1981;114:761–764.
319. Otake M, Schnu WJ. *In utero* exposure to A bomb radiation and mental retardation: a reassessment. Br J Radiol 1984;57:409–414.
320. MacLeod J, Hotchkiss RS, Sitterson BW. Recovery of male fertility after sterilization by nuclear radiation. JAMA 1964;187:637–641.
321. Peterson LE, Naeltwey DS. Radiological health risks to astronauts from space activities and medical procedures. NASA tech memorandum 102164. Springfield: Nat Tech Info Service, 1990.
322. Leach CS. An overview of the endocrine and metabolic changes in manned space flight. Acta Astronautica 1981;8:977–1001.
323. Leach CS, Altchaler SI, Cintron-Trevino NM. The endocrine and metabolic responses to space flight. Med Sci Sports Exerc 1983;15: 432–437.
324. Sandler H, Winters DL. Physiological responses of women to simulated weightlessness: a review of the significant findings of the first female bed rest study. NASA Sp 430. Washington, DC: Scientific Office, 1978.
325. Drinkwater BL, Nilson K, Chesnut CH. Bone mineral content of amenorrheic adults. N Engl J Med 1984;311:277–281.
326. Rambaut PC, Goode AW. Skeletal changes during space flight. Lancet 1985;2:1052–1052.
327. Behnke AR. Physique and exercise. In: exercise physiology 3rd ed, New York: Academic Press, 1968.
328. Bassett B. Twelve year survey of the susceptibility of women to attitude decompression sickness. Aerospace Med Assoc Ann Meeting 1978:31–40.
329. American Institute of Ultrasound in Medicine. Bioeffects Committee. Bioeffects consideration for the safety of diagnostic ultrasound. J Ultrasound Med 1988;7(Suppl):53–56.
330. Shoji R, Murakami U, Shimizu T. Influence of low intensity ultrasound irradiation on prenatal development of two inbred mouse strains. Teratology 1975;12:227
331. Stratmeyer ME. Effects on animals: an overview of ultrasound: theory, measurement, medical applications and biological effects. FDA Publ 82-8190. Rockville, MD: Department of Health and Human Services, 1982;77.
332. Thompson HE. Introduction. First symposium on safety and standardization of ultrasound in obstetrics. Ultrasound Med Biol 1986;12: 679–684.
333. Reece EA, Assimakopoulos E, Zheng X, Hagay Z, Hobbins JC. The safety of obstetric ultrasonography: concern for the fetus. Obstet Gynecol 1990;76:139–146.
334. Liebeskind D, Bases R, Mendez F, Elequin F, Koehigsberg M. Sister chromatid exchanges in human lymphocytes after exposure to diagnostic ultrasound. Science 1979;205:1273–1275.
335. Barnett SB, Barnstable SM, Kossoff G. Sister chromatid exchange, frequency in human lymphocytes after long duration exposure to pulsed ultrasound. J Ultrasound Med 1987;6:637–642.
336. Brent RL, Jensh RP, Beckman DA. Medical sonography: Reproductive effects and risks. Teratology 1991;44:123–146.
337. Stark CR, Orleans M, Haverkamp AD, Murphy J. Short and long term risks after exposure to diagnostic ultrasound in utero. Obstet Gynecol 1984;63:194.
338. Segall A, MacMahon B, Hannigan M. Congenital malformations and background radiation in northern New England. J Chron Dis 1964; 17:915.
339. Serr DM, Padet B, Zakett H. Studies on the effects of ultrasonic waves on the fetus. In: Huntingford PJ, Beard RW, Hytten F, et al. eds. Proceedings of the Second European Congress in Perinatal Medicine, London, 1971. New York: Karger, 1971.

340. Abdulla U, Dewhurst C, Campbell S, Talbert D, Lucas M, Mullarkey M. Effects of diagnostic ultrasound on maternal and fetal chromosomes. Lancet 1971;2:829
341. Falus M, Korany G, Sobel M, Resti E, Trinh vanBao. Follow-up studies on infants examined by ultrasound during fetal age. Orv Hetil 1972;113:2119.
342. Wegner RO, Myenberg M. The effects of diagnostic ultrasonography on frequencies of sister chromatid exchanges in Chinese hamster cells and human lymphocytes. J Ultrasound Med 1982;1:355.
343. Tas S, Lauwerys R, Lison D. Occupational hazards for the male reproductive system. Crit Rev Toxicol 1996;26:261–307.
344. Baranski B. Effects of the workplace on fertility and related reproductive outcomes. Environ Health Persp Suppl 1993;101:81–90.
345. Hjollund NH, Bonde JP, Hansen KS. Male mediated risk of spontaneous abortion with reference to stainless steel welding. Scand J Work Environ Health 1995;21:272–276.
346. Bonde JP. Semen quality and sex hormones among mild steel and stainless steel welders: a cross-sectional study. Br J Ind Med 1990;47: 508–514.
347. Bonde JP. Semen quality among welders before and after three weeks on non exposure. Br J Ind Med 1990;47:515–518.
348. Olshan AF, Teschke K, Baird PA. Paternal occupation and congenital anomalies in offspring. Am J Ind Med 1991;20:447–475.
349. Wilkins JR III, Sinks TH Jr. Occupation exposures among fathers of children with Wilms tumor. J Occup Med 1984;26:427–435.
350. Olsen JH, Brown PN, Schlugen G, Jensen OM. Parental employment at time of conception and risk of cancer in offspring. Eur J Cancer 1991;27:958–965.
351. Bonde JP, Olsen JH, Hansen KS. Adverse pregnancy outcome and childhood malignancy with reference to paternal welding exposure. Scand J Work Environ Health 1992;18:169.
352. Rachootin P, Olsen J. The risk of infertility and delayed conception associated with exposures in the Danish Workplace. J Occup Med 1983;25:394–402.
353. Robinson D, Rock J. Intrascrotal hyperthermia induced by scrotal insultation: effect on spermatogenesis. Obstet Gynecol 1967;29: 217–223.
354. Sanjose S, Roman E, Beral V. Low birthweight and preterm delivery, Scotland, 1981–84; effect of parents occupation. Lancet 1991;338: 428–431.
355. Hemminki K, Pentti K, Lindbohm M. Spontaneous abortions and malformations in the offspring of nurses exposed to anaesthetic gases, cytostatic drugs, and other potential hazards in hospitals, based on registered information of outcome. J Epidemiol Community Health 1985;39:141–147.
356. Guirguis SS, Pelmear PL, Roy ML, Wong L. Health effects associated with exposure to anaesthetic gases in Ontario hospital personnel. Br J Ind Med 1990:47:490–497.
357. Knill-Jones RP, Rodrigues LV, Moir DD, Spence AA. Anaesthetic practice and pregnancy: controlled survey of women anaesthetists in the United Kingdom. Lancet 1972;1:1326–1326.
358. Corbett TH. Exposure to anesthetic gases in the operting room. J Am Assn N Anest 1972;40:347–350.
359. American Society of Anesthesiologists. Occupational disease among operating room personnel: a national study. Anesthesiology 1974;41: 321–340.
360. Knill-Jones RP, Newman BJ, Spence AA. Anaesthetic practice and pregnancy: controlled survey of male anaesthetists in the United Kingdom. Lancet 1975;2:807–809.
361. Pharoah PO, Alberman E, Doyle P, Chamberlain G. Outcome of pregnancy among women in anaesthetic practice. Lancet 1977;1:34–36.
362. Ericson A, Kallen B. Survey of infants born in 1973 or 1975 to Swedish women working in operating rooms during their pregnancies. Anesth Analg 1979;58:302–305.
363. Cohen EN, Gift HC, Brown BW, et al. Ocupational disease in dentistry and chronic exposure to trace anaesthetic gases. J Am Dent Assoc 1980;101:21–31.
364. Axelsson G, Rylander R. Exposure to anaesthetic gases and spontaneous abortion: response bias in a postal questionnaire study. Int J Epidemiol 1982;11:250–256.

Cherry and Merkatz's Complications of Pregnancy,
Fifth Edition, edited by W. R. Cohen.
Lippincott Williams & Wilkins, Philadelphia © 2000.

CHAPTER 7

Teratogenic Drugs

Jose C. P. B. Ferreira, Gay S. Sachs, and Allan T. Bombard

In recent years, for legal as well as medical reasons, teratogens have been of growing interest and concern to patients and physicians. Since the thalidomide disaster of the 1960's, when an antinauseant prescribed during pregnancy resulted in devastating birth defects, there has been an awareness of the possible deleterious effects of medications on the fetus. At times that awareness has escalated to near paranoia such that pregnant women are reluctant, even fearful, of taking any drug. Moreover, many physicians are similarly reluctant and fearful of prescribing.

As physicians and genetic counselors in a reproductive/medical genetics unit, we provide teratogen counseling for many patients, all of whom are quite anxious. Some may be considering interruption of pregnancy, with wholly inadequate information, for the putative teratogen exposure. Most of these patients find that such a decision is unwarranted. Indeed, in many instances, the exposure was trivial.

In this chapter, we provide a brief overview of the history and biology of teratology and describe what drugs are currently proved to be teratogens, how to assess others, and how best to deliver this information to patients.

DEFINITIONS

Teratology (Greek, *teras, terat*—monster) is the study of abnormal embryonic and fetal development. *Teratogens* classically are defined as any chemical or environmental agent that at usual pharmacologic doses* has the potential to disrupt normal development, damage embryonic primordia, and ultimately result in one or more congenital malformations (the latter defined as abnormalities in form or function that are detectable in the newborn period).

A broader definition of teratogen encompasses agents acting in the prenatal period that also can cause pathologic, functional, and behavioral alterations, some of which may be recognized only later in life. A classic example is the prenatal exposure of the female fetus to diethylstilbestrol and the subsequent risk for developing, among other things, benign and malignant epithelial alterations in the vagina and cervix. With cause and effect often difficult to identify, unforeseen outcomes are always a source of concern when dealing with drugs in pregnancy.

Some amusing definitions have also been proffered; for example, *litogen*, an agent that has no proven harmful effect on the embryo or fetus but results in a lawsuit (1). Although meant to be humorous, litogens (such as Bendectin) have become an unfortunate reality and a source of growing concern among physicians.

Two other terms, *carcinogen* and *mutagen*, deserve mention because they are sometimes employed erroneously in the context of teratology. A carcinogen is an agent capable of inducing or promoting the malignant transformation of a cell. An environmental agent sometimes can act either as a teratogen or a carcinogen because the same mechanisms of action can have either or both effects (Table 7-1). Whereas teratogens and carcinogens are defined by their effect (i.e., malformation or malignancy), a mutagen is defined by its mechanism of action, the induction of alterations in the DNA. A mutagen has the potential for causing either teratogenic or carcinogenic effects if it acts on a somatic cell. If a mutagen acts on a germline cell, however, it can result in a monogenic disorder in the offspring of the exposed individual.

J. C. P. B. Ferreira, G. S. Sachs, and A. T. Bombard: Department of Obstetrics and Gynecology, Albert Einstein College of Medicine, Montefiore Medical Center, Bronx, NY 10461.

*According to some authors, this is a requirement; supposedly, all drugs will have a threshold above which they can behave as teratogens. Only the ones whose threshold is at or below pharmacologic doses should be considered teratogens.

TABLE 7-1. *Teratogens vs carcinogens*

Teratogen	Carcinogen
Multicellular injury required for effects to be expressed	One damaged cell can result in disease
Acts at many levels, affects many processes	Acts at DNA level causing gene mutation(s)
Results in malformation, impaired growth, or chemical toxicity	Results in overgrowth neoplasia
Absence of effects below threshold dose	Can induce mutation at all doses
Greater doses result in more severe and frequent disease	Greater doses result in more frequent disease, but same severity

From Brent RL, Beckman DA. Principles of teratology. In: Evans MI, ed. Reproductive risks and prenatal diagnosis, Stamford, CT: Appleton & Lange, 1991, with permission.

Not all teratogens or carcinogens are mutagenic, but mutagens can be teratogens or carcinogens. Although many different types of teratogens exist, including physical and infectious agents and maternal illnesses, this chapter deals with exposures to chemicals, with an emphasis on drugs.

HISTORICAL BACKGROUND

Hippocrates and Soranus of Ephesus (4th century AC, 2nd century AD) were already aware of the influence of substances ingested by the pregnant woman and the possible consequences for her offspring. In *Aphorisms*, Hippocrates wrote:

> Drugs may be administered to pregnant women from the fourth to the seventh month of gestation. After that period, the dose should be less (2).

In *Gynecology*, Soranus wrote:

> Even if a woman transgresses some or all of the rules mentioned (re: administration of drugs, sternutatives, pungent substances, and drunkenness, especially during the first trimester) and yet miscarriage does not take place, let no one assume that the fetus has not been injured at all. For it has been harmed: it is weakened, becomes retarded in growth, less well nourished, and in general, more easily injured and susceptible to harmful agents; it becomes misshapen and of ignoble soul (3).

These ancient wisdoms seem to have disappeared by the Middle Ages and were replaced by the superstition that punishment by a divinity or a particular behavior during pregnancy was the cause of congenital anomalies. Unfortunately, even as we approach the 21st century, many patients still cling to these medieval notions.

In modern literature, the first environmental agent shown to be teratogenic in humans was ionizing radiation (4–7). Subsequently, Gregg described fetal rubella syndrome in 1941 (4,8–13) demonstrating the teratogenicity of an infectious agent. Yet it was only after the thalidomide tragedy that occurred almost 50 years ago (4,9–14) that the potential teratogenicity of drugs was fully appreciated.

Thalidomide was evaluated in several animal species with no apparent harmful effect and then was prescribed in Europe for hyperemesis in pregnancy. Despite severe and characteristic limb malformations and the 20% to 30% incidence of this or other abnormalities in an exposed fetus, it was several years and the births of thousands of malformed children before the link between drug and defect was finally recognized.

The fear of overlooking a teratogenic agent notwithstanding, jumping to conclusions about teratogenicity also can have disastrous consequences. In the 1970's, a report of an association of chromosome breakage and birth defects with spray adhesive exposure resulted in nationwide warnings and a ban on the sale of these popular arts and crafts products. Six months later, when the findings failed to be confirmed, the ban was lifted. Meanwhile, nine women had terminated a pregnancy because of the exposure (15).

Although the awareness and understanding of the effects of drugs and various environmental agents in pregnancy have increased among health professionals, data based on systematic studies that would permit accurate assessments of teratogenicity are still woefully lacking.

EPIDEMIOLOGY OF CONGENITAL DEFECTS

Human reproduction and embryonic development are complex processes that are highly susceptible to error. It is estimated that up to 75% of all conceptions are lost before term, 50% within the first 3 weeks (9,16). Of pregnancies that result in a live birth, about 2% to 3% of newborns possess congenital abnormalities of structure or function, which constitute the leading cause of perinatal mortality in the United States today (17,18). This 2% to 3% malformation rate is considered the background risk for all pregnancies against which the effects of a potential teratogenic agent must be weighed. The vast majority of these malformations (60%–65%) have no definable etiology; approximately 20% to 25% are considered to be genetically determined (monogenic or chromosomal); about 10% are attributable to environmental agents, and most of these are thought to be related to maternal disease, including infections (17–21). Thus, only about 1% can be attributed directly to the effect of drugs, chemicals, or radiation (17–18,20) (Table 7-2).

Although only a small percentage of congenital anomalies are drug related, these are the birth defects most amenable to primary prevention. In that regard, the study of the mechanisms involved in teratogenesis may help to elucidate the pathophysiology of malformations in general as well as the factors (most likely genetic) that increase susceptibility to the harmful effects of environmental agents. Such insights may make it possible to identify the woman and her fetus at greatest risk and,

TABLE 7-2. *Etiology of birth defects*

No definitive etiology (multifactorial, polygenic, synergistic interactions of teratogens, spontaneous errors of development)	60%–65%
Pure genetic causes (monogenic or chromosomal)	20%–25%
Environmental agents (maternal disease and infections)	10%
Drugs, chemicals, or radiation	1%

therefore, the patients most likely to benefit from intervention and prevention strategies during and before pregnancy.

PHARMACOLOGY, BIOLOGY, AND MECHANISM OF ACTION OF DRUGS IN PREGNANCY

The damaging effects of noxious external agents on an embryo or fetus may include death, congenital malformation, growth restriction, functional deficit, cognitive or behavioral dysfunction, or malignancy. It appears, however, that only a small proportion of these outcomes can be directly attributable to *in utero* exposure to environmental toxicants during pregnancy (22).

Although proven teratogens usually elicit a specific phenotype, there is great variability in the expression of these effects. Indeed, even with exposure to known teratogens, most outcomes are normal. Teratogenic effects depend not only on the action of the agent per se but also the timing and stage of development, the dosage and length of exposure, the susceptibility to the agent of mother and fetus, and interaction with other agents that can moderate or exacerbate the end result (e.g., cigarette smoking with alcohol) (Table 7-3).

Mechanism of Action

The processes of embryonic development, although not completely understood, seem to be determined at the cellular level by programmed cell replication, migration, differentiation, and death (*apoptosis*). These actions are dependent on and coordinated by both intracellular and intercellular control mechanisms. The intracellular mechanisms rely on perfect DNA replication, correct and sequential expression of genes, integrity of enzymatic pathways, and cellular structure maintenance. Intercellular communication relies on gap junctions for the exchange of morphogenetic signaling substances (direct cell–cell communication), the ability to send information through secretory products, and receiving and processing external information through receptor systems (indirect communication). Finally, distant intercellular communication and the delivery of energy sources and substrates depend on an efficient transport system represented by the vascular network and the intercellular milieu. The biochemical and pharmacologic effects of a drug effectively can interfere with all these functions through the following mechanisms (23):

At the cellular level:

- Gene mutation, altered nucleic acid synthesis and function, mitotic interference, chromosome breakage, or nondisjunction (24)
- Enzyme inhibition
- Changes in intracellular milieu secondary to osmolar imbalance, alterations in fluid pressures, viscosities, and osmotic pressures
- Altered membrane characteristics (23)

At the intercellular level:

- Inhibition of intercellular communication (25–26)
- Modulation of hormone receptors (23)
- Depletion of precursors, substrates, or coenzymes for biosynthesis
- Depletion of energy sources

The disruption of such basic cellular functions can lead to a myriad of deleterious effects: reduced or increased cell division; abnormal cell migration; slowing or cessation in the process of differentiation; excessive cell death beyond the recuperative capacity of the embryo or fetus with necrosis, calcification, or scarring; interfering with histogenesis; failure of cell death; physical constraint; vascular insufficiency with secondary disruption of developing structures (9,12); and alteration of control mechanisms (25–26).

The effect of these insults at the tissue and organ levels can be hyperplasia, hypoplasia, and aplasia. (If the critical mass necessary for induction or continuation of differentiation is lacking, the organ system can fail to develop) (27). Other adverse effects include asynchronous growth with an absence of fusion, abnormal fusion between structures, aberrant morphology, and, especially later in the development process, neoplasia. The noxious agent would not be considered a teratogen, however, unless the final result is a physical or functional defect (13). It must be appreciated that birth defects also can occur as a result of constraint, disruption, or destruction in the absence of any teratogenic insult.

A drug also can cause embryo lethality without direct embryotoxic effects by influencing maternal homeostasis

TABLE 7-3. *Factors that influence teratogenic effects*

Mechanism of action of the agent
Stage of development of the embryo or fetus
Amount of the exposure to the agent
Susceptibility to the agent of mother and fetus
Interaction with other agents

adversely and disrupting physiologic support of the embryo (28). Each of the above mechanisms of action will not predict, by itself, what effect a particular agent will have. Moreover, as emphasized earlier, exposure to a putative teratogenic agent does *not* ensure that maldevelopment will occur (9); other factors can modify or mitigate potential adverse effects.

Stages of Development

Because the teratogenic effects of external agents are expressed through a disruption of the normal processes of tissue and organ growth, these effects will depend on what processes are occurring at the time of exposure. It is possible to predict the likelihood of an adverse outcome caused by a teratogenic exposure based on when during the three main stages of the embryonic and fetal development the exposure occurs (Table 7-4).

The first lunar month (i.e., the 2 weeks before and after conception) is often termed the *predifferentiation stage* (12). At this stage, the embryo appears relatively resistant to teratogenic effects although particularly susceptible to lethal ones. This is often referred to as an *all-or-none phenomenon*; in other words, the propensity is for embryo death rather than survival of malformed liveborn infants. The rationale behind this phenomenon is different for the preimplantation and postimplantation periods. In the former, the possibility of a drug affecting a dividing zygote not yet implanted is unlikely. In the latter, a major insult may destroy most of the cells of the embryo, compromising its survival. However, a lesser postimplantation insult may allow the totipotential cells to replace the damaged cells without causing any disturbance in the normal developmental process. Thus, compared with unexposed liveborn infants, malformation rates of surviving embryos will not be increased.

The organogenesis stage (weeks 3 to 8 after fertilization, menstrual weeks 5 to 10), in which the differentiation of most of the organ systems takes place, is the period of highest susceptibility to teratogenesis and the developmental stage when most major malformations can be induced (9).

After week 8, in the histogenesis and maturation stages, development is characterized principally by increasing organ size (9). Thus, a noxious agent likely will affect the overall growth of the embryo (intrauterine growth restriction), or it will modify the proper development of a particular organ. The occurrence of structural malformations attributable to teratogens is unlikely at these stages because most organs already are formed, but functional defects may be induced. Exceptions include the genitourinary system, the palate, the brain, the auditive apparatus, and the eye, all of which require longer periods to complete their full development. Central nervous system (CNS) maturation continues even after birth. Given the length of this developmental process, it is easy to appreciate that this is the organ system most frequently exhibiting congenital abnormalities, including mental retardation. Throughout its development, the CNS is vulnerable to the effects of environmental agents that may disrupt cell proliferation, migration, and differentiation over a longer period (29). Effects such as cell depletion or functional abnormalities in the CNS may be evident only later in life and could be manifest as changes or abnormalities in behavior (9).

TABLE 7-4. *Teratogenicity and gestational age*[a]

First 2 wk	Predifferentiation stage	Low susceptibility: "all or none" effect
3–8 wk	Organogenesis	Susceptible
8–32 wk	Histogenesis	Less susceptible
32–48 wk	Functional maturation	Least susceptible

[a]Weeks from conception.

Thus, the developmental period at which an exposure occurs will determine which structures are most susceptible to a given deleterious effect (9). An agent may affect one organ system at one stage of development but another system at a different stage. In addition, an agent may act as a teratogen when the exposure occurs early in pregnancy and be carcinogenic when the exposure is later in gestation, suggesting that there may be a continuum of teratogenesis and carcinogenesis (30). Thus, defects caused by drugs in the developing embryo or fetus are not random events but result from specific biochemical and pharmacologic interactions that reflect the mechanism of teratogenesis. An interesting and illustrative example is the warfarin (Coumadin) embryopathy.

As a vitamin K antagonist, warfarin inhibits the formation of carboxyglutamyl residues, decreasing the ability of proteins to bind calcium. This action prevents the calcium binding not only of coagulation factors but also of particular bone-molding proteins (31). These cellular actions explain both the unusual skeletal findings in the exposed fetus as well as the other malformations related to the drug's anticoagulant properties.

The warfarin embryopathy also illustrates potential differences in outcome depending on when in development an adverse exposure occurs. Exposures between 6 and 9 weeks after conception, a critical period of embryonic ossification, inhibit the formation of vitamin-K-dependent calcium-binding proteins (*osteocalcins*) and result in nasal hypoplasia and stippled epiphyses, which are clinical hallmarks of this syndrome (31). Warfarin exposure later and throughout the pregnancy most often results in CNS anomalies, probably the consequences of hemorrhagic events.

Dose or Magnitude of Exposure

Teratogenic agents typically manifest a *threshold effect*, operationally defined as the amount of exposure below which the incidence of adverse effects in exposed pregnancies does not differ from unexposed controls. The threshold is usually one third the dose that kills or malforms 50% of the embryos. Exposures at greater levels exhibit a dose-response relationship, in contrast to mutagens or carcinogens, which have a stochastic dose-response curve (see Table 7-1) (9,24). Theoretically, there is a dose for all drugs above which the embryo or fetus will be affected in some fashion. Most experts consider a drug to be a teratogen only if adverse effects occur at or below usual pharmacologic doses.

Several factors influence the dose of agent that reaches the developing fetus, all of which may modulate potential teratogenic effects. These factors include drug pharmacokinetics, placental transfer rate, and the stage of fetal development (9).

Drug Pharmacokinetics

Drug pharmacokinetics in pregnancy are influenced by the route of administration, absorption rate, body distribution and half-life (both of which are dependent on protein-binding properties and lipid solubility of the drug), metabolic excretion rate, and the activity of metabolites. These physical characteristics may be further modified by the pregnant state, which enhances absorption, dilutes the concentration of the drug, decreases binding to albumin or other transport proteins, and increases excretion.

Placental Transfer

Most drugs and chemicals cross the placenta. The rate of transfer depends on both placental and drug related factors. Placental factors include uterine and umbilical blood flow, pH gradient between maternal and fetal circulation, and the dependence of the embryo or fetus on histiotrophic (local macromolecules are chiefly responsible for the maintenance of the embryo) and hemotrophic nutrition (the transfer of material between the maternal and fetal circulations) (32). Drug characteristics that increase placental transfer include increased lipid solubility, decreased polarization, low molecular weight (most drugs weigh between 250 and 400 daltons; compounds less than 600 daltons cross the placenta, and those greater than 1,000 D do not), decreased protein binding, the presence of transport receptors, and decreased placental bioconversion (9).

Fetal Physiology

In fetal physiologic development, changes occur in the amount and distribution of fat, the plasma protein level, drug receptors, and excretion capacity through placenta. The complexity and variations resulting from these many interacting factors that serve to maximize or limit the exposure of the embryo or fetus to an external agent explain some of the difference in susceptibility and outcome in pregnancies exposed to teratogens.

Susceptibility

Outcomes following teratogenic exposures are explained not only by the intrinsic characteristics and mechanisms of action of the drug in question but also by the differences in susceptibility of the individual or species. Most factors affecting susceptibility are under genetic control.

Genetic polymorphisms in drug-metabolizing enzymes and in drug targets that affect drug efficacy and toxicity are well recognized. Indeed, genetic variation in metabolizing enzymes and increased susceptibility to carcinogens and teratogens have been reported (33). An individual's susceptibility to chemical carcinogenesis or teratogenesis is also influenced by diet, lifestyle, and other environmental exposures (34). An understanding of these interacting factors could be helpful in predicting and possibly controlling the action of some teratogens. For instance, Torchinsky and colleagues (1994), using intrauterine immunopotentiation with allogenic paternal splenocytes, were able to enhance the tolerance of mice embryos to cyclophosphamide and 2,3-quinoxalinedimetanol,1,4-dioxide. The authors showed that the embryo's response to environmental teratogens is influenced by fetomaternal immune interactions (35) and that it was therefore possible to manipulate some teratogenic effects.

Sex differences also appear to modulate susceptibility to the action of teratogens. Watanabe and colleagues found that in mice at day 14.4 of gestation, digital and palatal formation was more advanced in female embryos than in males. They concluded that the period for digit development is longer in male embryos than in female embryos, and male embryos would be more likely to manifest defects in this organ system when exposed to specific teratogens. That is, if the mouse dams were exposed to the appropriate teratogen, a sex difference in incidence of digital defects could be produced (36).

IDENTIFYING TERATOGENS

The need for efficient methods to screen new chemicals, drugs, and environmental pollutants for teratogenic activity is obvious (37). It is not, however, an easy task to evaluate the teratogenic potential of a specific chemical or environmental agent. If the adverse effects of a teratogen were always or almost always manifest in a severe outcome or a specific spectrum of abnormalities, its teratogenic potential would be readily appreciated. More common, however, are findings in exposed persons that are partial, mild, and nonspecific. Still, it is important to recognize that even some nonspecific effects following prenatal exposure to a chemical or drug may raise the suspicion of teratogenicity.

Under ideal circumstances, each new chemical or drug to which a pregnant woman could be exposed should be evaluated by prospective randomized controlled trials to test for teratogenicity, including testing in pharmacologic doses at different stages of pregnancy. Because such studies are ethically inconceivable in humans, and well-designed animal studies may not correlate directly with human outcomes (e.g., thalidomide), other assessments such as case reports are often relied on, but they are obviously more susceptible to bias than are randomized trials. Thus, they provide less reliable conclusions.

Relative risk could be quantified with some confidence by retrospective analyses if (a) the incidence of a particular birth defect was significantly higher in the exposed group compared with nonexposed controls, (b) different studies gave consistent results, and (c) there was a probable biological rationale for the effect. With other than prospective controlled studies, definitive conclusions are usually not possible, although if several such studies result in similar findings, it may be deduced that the drug is likely or unlikely to be teratogenic. In reality, many results will be contradictory, providing little or no guidance in assessing true risk.

Methods of assessing teratogenic potential in humans include *case reports* of a malformation following a prenatal exposure, which may raise the suspicion of (but not prove) teratogenicity; *animal toxicologic studies*, which are required for any drug to be approved for clinical use; *surveillance registry systems*, which are valuable during the clinical evaluation process and provide summary statistics concerning the effects (*congenital defects*) and exposures after the introduction of a new drug; *case–control studies*, which usually are motivated by suggestive case reports and compare the incidence of exposure between groups cases and controls; and *cohort studies*, which compare the incidence of cases between exposed and nonexposed fetuses and may permit definitive, quantifiable conclusions (Table 7-5).

TABLE 7-5. *Studies used to determine the teratogenic character of a drug*

Toxicologic studies	*In vivo* models	Animal studies
	In vitro models	Embryo culture Organ culture Tissue culture
Case reports		
Epidemiologic studies	Descriptive	Surveillance systems of exposures Surveillance systems of effects
	Analytical	Case–control studies (retrospective) Retrospective cohort studies Prospective cohort studies

Case Reports

Case reports provide the initial suspicion that a specific agent may be a human teratogen and serve as the basis for further study (38). Although a case report does not prove a causal relationship between exposure to a specific agent and a pregnancy outcome (39), most human teratogens have been identified initially as a result of case reports rather than through epidemiologic studies (40). For example, Robert (1996) described the identification of valproic acid as a teratogen, specifically the induction of spina bifida, as an example of the combined use of both clinical experience and epidemiologic analysis (40).

Case reports are particularly useful if they reveal a recurrent, unique, or rare idiopathic pattern of birth defects in persons exposed at similar times during pregnancy (39). A compelling and relatively recent example is the finding of hypoplasia of the calvarium, an extremely unusual defect, with maternal use of angiotensin converting enzyme (ACE) inhibitors (9,41–44).

Toxicologic Studies (*In Vivo* and *In Vitro* Models)

Animal and *in vitro* studies can be particularly helpful in determining the etiologic mechanisms and pharmacokinetics related to teratogenesis (9). Although animal studies cannot be directly extrapolated to human reproduction, adverse results may alert the investigator to the need for confirmation (possibly in other species) and follow-up with human data. Indeed, most agents that are well accepted as human teratogens also have been shown to be teratogenic in one or more laboratory species (45). By contrast, many agents shown to be teratogenic in animals (often at extraordinarily large dosages) have not been proven to be damaging in humans.

Schardein and colleagues (1985) reviewed the different species used in the detection of human teratogens to determine the optimal animal model. They concluded that no single species is more advantageous than any other (45).

Many of the inadequacies of animal models can be reduced or eliminated by using *in vitro* culture techniques (37). Embryo culture, organ culture, and tissue culture allow maternal and placental effects to be bypassed and permit manipulation of both the concentrations of the suspected teratogen and the duration of the exposure. Because maternal physiology is eliminated in these experiments, it is necessary to introduce drug-metabolizing additives to the culture medium.

According to Kochhar (1980), organ culture, whole embryo culture, and a combination of the two offer the best potential for screening suspected teratogens. These techniques provide a better simulation of *in vivo* situations than isolated cells grown as monolayers (37). Limb buds (37) and embryonic palates (46) are examples of organs that already have been used as culture systems.

Epidemiologic Studies

Descriptive Studies

A summary of epidemiologic methods employed to assess drug influences in pregnancy is relevant to understanding the documentation and proof of teratogenicity of specific agents (see Table 7-5). Surveillance systems of congenital anomalies have been developed in several countries as sources for epidemiologic studies of possible teratogens. Hungary (Hungarian Congenital Malformation Register) (47), Europe (EUROCAT program) (48), U.S. [Metropolitan Atlanta Congenital Defects Program (MACDP), Birth Defects Monitoring Program (BDMP)] (49), Sweden (50), and Australia (51) are some of the countries with such programs. These programs establish a baseline rate (48) for the incidence of congenital anomalies, which facilitates the rapid identification of new birth defect clusters (47) or variations in the background rate (48) that could be attributed to a new teratogen. Surveillance systems also can be a source of data for case–control studies and other investigations of the epidemiology of birth defects (49). Having such systems in place should decrease the time before potent teratogens such as thalidomide or the rubella virus are recognized. These surveillance systems have some disadvantages, however, as noted by Holtzman and Khoury and associates (52–57). Teratogenic agents whose widespread use antedates monitoring will not cause rate changes or clusters detectable by monitoring, as will incomplete reporting. In addition, the statistical power of data drawn from surveillance systems is frequently insufficient to allow meaningful conclusions to be drawn. The weakness of many suspected teratogens, the low population frequency of exposure to a new teratogen, the relatively small population size (fewer than 50,000 to 100,000 births per year) of many monitoring programs, the low background rate, and the etiologic heterogeneity in the measured defects all could be factors responsible for increases in birth defects to go unnoticed through those programs. For example, in a system that monitors 25,000 births per year, a potent new teratogen such as thalidomide [Relative risk (RR) = 175] can lead to a significant increase in the number of observed cases in 1 to 2 weeks of monitoring. Even proven teratogens such as valproic acid and isotretinoin (RR = 20–25) have required more than 20 years of monitoring to demonstrate a statistically significant increase in the number of cases because of low exposure frequency. Moreover, teratogens manifesting minimal risk and effect (RR = 2–5) can be totally missed (55).

To improve the capability of birth defects monitoring programs to detect new teratogens, it would require that surveillance systems examine subsegments of the population with maximal exposure potential, classify birth defects into more etiologically homogeneous groups, and expand the sample size of the monitored population.

Congenital malformations in newborns are only one indicator of teratogenicity. At least 20% of all conceptions end in spontaneous abortion. Monitoring the spontaneous abortion rate or chromosomal and other abnormalities in abortuses would be an important adjunct to monitoring newborns; however, inadequate ascertainment of affected newborns is far less a problem than monitoring affected abortuses.

Analytical Studies

Most frequently, case–control studies are invoked to raise or strengthen the suspicion of a teratogenic effect related to a particular exposure. A number of inherent biases exist that can result in erroneous assessment regarding risk. For example, case–control studies rely heavily on maternal recall. Feldman and co-workers assessed the magnitude of recall of early pregnancy exposure as well as determinants likely to affect it in 145 consecutive cases. The mean recall of exposure identity was 62%; accurate recall of timing of exposure was 37%; and of dosage 24% (58). Factors and methods that can strengthen the conclusions drawn from case–control studies include the rarity of the defect pattern, the rarity of the exposure in the population, the small source population, short time for the study, and biological plausibility for the association (59).

Cohort studies, conducted either retrospectively or prospectively, should include both exposed and nonexposed populations. Elimination of biases is essential. Two types are particularly relevant to teratogenic epidemiologic analytic studies: observation and confounding bias.

Observation bias occurs in cohort studies when the occurrence of birth defects is measured differently in children of exposed and unexposed women. In case–control studies, this bias occurs if drug exposure is ascertained differently when the risk of malformation is different.

Confounding bias occurs when a third underlying risk factor either is responsible for an indirect association between an exposure and a defect or conceals a direct one. An example is the reason for the administration of the drug. For example, epilepsy itself is thought to have a teratogenic effect that is independent of the effects of the drugs used to control the disease. Other confounding variables besides maternal disease states include maternal age, cigarette smoking, illicit drug consumption, other adverse health habits, and socioeconomic factors.

The main disadvantage of cohort studies is the difficulty and cost involved. One of the largest prospective cohort studies actually completed involved 50,000 pregnancies surveyed between 1959 and 1965 [The Collaborative Perinatal Project registry; Heinonen and colleagues (4)] and required the long-term support of the federal government. This is a landmark study not only because of the information it contains regarding the most frequently prescribed drugs at that time but also because it constitutes a model for all cohort studies.

TABLE 7-6. *Criteria for human teratogenicity*

1. Consistent findings by two or more epidemiologic studies of high quality showing an association between an exposure and an effect
2. The exposure occurred during the organogenesis of the affected organs
3. There is a specific defect or syndrome related to the agent
4. Rare environmental exposures are associated with a rare defect
5. There is an animal model that duplicates the effects in humans
6. There is a plausible biological explanation for the mechanism of action of the teratogen
7. There is evidence that the agent acts directly, in its unaltered state, on the embryo or fetus
8. A dose-response relationship has been observed
9. The reason for the medical use of the agent is not associated with the effect
10. There is a genetically more susceptible group of potentially exposed individuals
11. The anomaly was less common before the time the potential teratogen was available

1, 2, and 3 or 1, 2, and 4 are necessary conditions. The rest of the conditions strengthen our assumptions about the teratogenic character of the drug.

From Shepard TH. Catalog of teratogenic agents; 8th ed. Baltimore: The Johns Hopkins University Press, 1995, with permission.

Criteria to Demonstrate Teratogenicity

Consistent findings in two or more epidemiologic studies of high quality (control of confounding factors, sufficient numbers of exposed pregnancies, exclusion of positive and negative bias factors) that demonstrate an association between an exposure and an adverse effect are necessary to support the assessment that an environmental agent is a teratogen. Other criteria also should be met and are outlined in Table 7-6 (13,60). The greater the extent to which a particular agent meets these criteria, the greater the likelihood of true teratogenicity. Schardein nicely sums up the contemporary view of testing and surveillance for teratogens:

> The facts demonstrate conclusively that ingestion of certain drugs during pregnancy can induce adverse effects in the unborn child. However, few new teratogens or epidemics of birth defects have been identified since the thalidomide disaster, which attests both to effective laboratory testing of drugs in animals prior to clinical use and the extensive surveillance of use of new therapeutic agents in women during pregnancy. It is clear that these practices should continue in order to protect the pregnant woman and her conceptus, and benefits and risks should be carefully weighed before administration of a drug during pregnancy (61).

SOURCES OF INFORMATION ON DRUGS IN PREGNANCY

Two common scenarios generally prompt the clinician to obtain information about the potential teratogenic effects of a specific medication. In one scenario, the clinician is providing care for the pregnant woman who has a condition that requires medical therapy. The second scenario involves counseling the pregnant woman who takes a drug inadvertently, usually unaware of the pregnancy, and is concerned with possible deleterious effects in her offspring. The latter situation is common and is the cause of substantial anxiety to the patient and often to the physician as well. Reaching for *The Physician's Desk Reference* (PDR) becomes almost reflexive, and although it may be appropriate for prescribing a drug for a pregnant patient, the PDR should *not* be the sole source of information for inadvertent exposures.

The U.S. Food and Drug Administration (FDA) developed a set of guidelines for assessing risk of teratogenicity of specific agents: *The Food and Drug Administration Categorization of Drugs and Medications with Regards to Possible Fetal Effects* (62). These ratings are summarized in Table 7-7. Assessments are based on the degree to which available information has ruled out risk to the fetus and

TABLE 7-7. *Definitions for FDA risk classification*

Category	Definition
A	Controlled studies in women fail to demonstrate a risk to the fetus in the first trimester (and there is no evidence of a risk in later trimesters), and the possibility of fetal harm appears remote.
B	Either animal-reproduction studies have not demonstrated a fetal risk but there are no controlled studies in pregnant women or animal-reproduction studies have shown an adverse effect (other than a decrease in fertility) that was not confirmed in controlled studies in women in the first trimester (and there is no evidence of risk in later trimesters).
C	Either studies in animals have revealed adverse effects on the fetus (teratogenic, embryocidal, or other) and there are no controlled studies in women, or studies in women and animals are not available. Drugs should be given only if the potential benefit justifies the potential risk to the fetus.
D	There is positive evidence of human fetal risk, but the benefits from the use in pregnant women may be acceptable despite the risk (e.g., if the drug is needed in a life-threatening situation or for a serious disease for which safer drugs cannot be used or are ineffective).
X	Studies in animals or human beings have demonstrated fetal abnormalities or there is evidence of fetal risk based on human experience or both, and the risk of the use of the drug in pregnant women clearly outweighs any possible benefit. The drug is contraindicated in women who are or may become pregnant.

FDA, U.S. Food and Drug Administration.

From U.S. Food and Drug Administration. Pregnancy labeling. FDA Drug Bull. 1979;9:23–24 (Level III), with permission.

newborn (including perinatal risks), balanced against the drug's potential benefits in pregnant women. These ratings are designed to provide therapeutic guidance, but they are *not* intended to be the basis for counseling about the potential teratogenic effect of a drug taken inadvertently before a pregnancy was recognized. Much better resources are teratogen databases, such as Reprotox or TERIS (The Teratogen Information System). They address the germane question of what the chance is that exposure to this agent during pregnancy harmed the developing baby (63) rather than the benefit-risk approach of the FDA ratings. This database consists of summaries of the agent based on a review of the literature and other sources.

An illustrative and not uncommon example is inadvertent conception occurring in a woman taking oral contraceptives. In the PDR, ethinyl estradiol (a common component of birth control pills) is listed as (FDA) Category X—contraindicated in pregnancy, thus assigning risk that would exceed benefit; however, according to TERIS, the drug has no proven teratogenic risk. Geneticists regularly counsel patients referred for oral contraceptive ingestion during pregnancy. Regrettably, many women, uninformed about true risks, have undergone elective terminations of their pregnancies before receiving complete and up-to-date genetic counseling, making decisions based solely on information gleaned from the PDR.

TABLE 7-8. *Teratogen reference resources*

Books	*Drugs in Pregnancy and Lactation: A Reference Guide to Fetal and Neonatal Risk,* 1994, GG Briggs, RK Freeman, SJ Yaffe *Catalog of Teratogenic Agents,* 9th ed., 1998, T Shepard *Chemically Induced Birth Defects,* 1993, JL Schardein *Reproductive Hazards of Industrial Chemicals,* 1982, SM Barlow, F Sullivan *Occupational and Environmental Reproductive Hazards: A Guide for Clinicians,* 1992, M Paul
Electronic	National Library of Medicine, MEDLARS Service Desk (Grateful med TOXLINE, TOXNET, DART and Medline—sources of bibliographic search), Bethesda, MD, 800-638-8480—for information and access: http://www.nlm.nih.gov/pubs/factsheets/toxlinfs.html http://www.nlm.nih.gov/pubs/factsheets/dartfs.html http://www.nlm.nih.gov/pubs/factsheets/toxnetfs.html Teratogen Information System (TERIS and Shepard's Catalog of Teratogenic Agents—catalogs of teratogenic agents), University of Washington, Seattle, WA, 206-543-2465—for information and access: http://weber.u.washington.edu/~terisweb/teris/index.html http://weber.u.washington.edu/~terisweb/computer_info.html Micromedex, Inc. (Reprorisk—CD-ROM system including the following teratogenic agents catalogs: Reprotext, Reprotox, Shepard's Catalog of Teratogenic Agents and TERIS) Englewood, Colorado, 800-525-9083 Reproductive Toxicology Center (Reprotox), Columbia Women's Hospital, Washington, DC, 202-293-5137
Information centers	Organization of Teratology Information Services—OTIS, Information Pregnancy Riskline, Box 144270, Salt Lake City, Utah 84114-4270, Tel.-801-328-BABY; Fax-801-538-6510—Organization that informs which are the Teratogen information services available in each area of the U.S. and Canada. Available on line at: http://orpheus.ucsd.edu/ctis/index.html
Drug registries	Mefloquine (Lariam)—617-787-4957 Acyclovir (Zovirax)—800-722-9292 or 919-248-8465 Fluoxetine (Prozac)—317-276-7047 or Prozac registry in Utah, 801-548-8488 Lithium—US and Canadian Collaborative Project, 416-598-6780 Zidovudine (AZT)—Burroughs Welcome Co, 800-722-9292, x4865 Alprazolam (Xanax)—Upjohn Co., 616-329-3686 ACE inhibitors: Teratogen information Services Collaborative Project, Pregnancy Riskline, 801-583-2229 Methotrexate: Investigating maternal and paternal use, preconceptional and prenatal—Pregnancy Healthline—215-829-3601 Antiepileptic drugs—AED Pregnancy Registry—Genetics and Teratology Unit, Massachusetts General Hospital—1-888-233-2334; aedregistry@helix.mgh.harvard.edu; http://neuro-www2.mgh.harvard.edu/aed/registry/nclk
Others	
Books	*Birth Defects and Drugs in Pregnancy,* 1977, OP Heinonen, D Slone, S Shapiro. *Peace of Mind During Pregnancy,* 1988, C. Kelly-Buchanan
Centers	Occupational and Environmental Reproductive Hazards Center—general information about occupational exposures, 508-856-6162 Regional Occupational Safety and Health Administration (OSHA) and Occupational Medicine Specialists

Friedman and colleagues evaluated 157 frequently prescribed drugs and compared TERIS ratings of 83 of these with FDA pregnancy categories assigned to the same agents. The correlation between the two rating systems was no greater than that expected by chance, suggesting that each has a different objective in its evaluation of a drug (63). The FDA ratings serve an important purpose but are not a substitute for databases and studies from the literature that provide information directly related to teratogenic risks.

Another concern with the FDA ratings in the PDR as the basis for teratogen counseling is the ubiquitous designation of category C, which indicates risk cannot be ruled out. There are more than 1,000 drugs listed in the PDR and some 20 known teratogens, and yet 66% of the drugs have a C rating, which raises the specter of possible birth defects and termination. Certainly, there is a dearth of data on many of these drugs, but an investigation of other sources almost always will supply more information and help to clarify the ambiguity of this rating.

Resources for Information on Teratogens

With the growing interest of both the public and health professionals in teratogens, a concomitant increase has occurred in the availability of resources and data on drug effects in pregnancy. Summarized in Table 7-8, these resources include computer databases, teratogen information services, the teratology literature, and various other sources.

Teratology Databases

Information provided usually includes a summary of available data, interpretation, and references. These services, which are regularly updated, are available on-line through bulletin board systems or the Internet and usually by subscription.

Teratogen Information Services

These programs, mostly operating like telephone hot lines, generally are affiliated with a medical school or hospital and offer services statewide but may serve nonresidents as well. They are staffed by knowledgeable personnel, are available to patients and doctors, and will refer a patient for evaluation or counseling if indicated. Most of these services are members of the Organization of Teratogen Information Services (OTIS).

Miscellaneous Resources

- The Birth Defects, Infectious Disease, and Immunization sections of the Centers for Disease Control in Atlanta may be helpful for prenatal exposures in these categories.
- The regional offices of the Occupational Safety and Health Agency (OSHA) as well as Occupational Medicine specialists are increasingly utilized as the numbers of women in the workplace increase.
- NIOSH (National Institute of Occupational Safety and Health) can be helpful with evaluations of maternal and fetal health hazards.
- Poison Control Centers are an invaluable resource to identify chemicals contained in most medications and products and for toxicity information on obscure substances such as homeopathic remedies.
- Drug Registries compiled by manufacturers contain data based on voluntary reporting and thus have all the biases and limitations inherent in a registry (i.e., defects get reported and normal outcomes may not). Still, registries often include significant numbers of patient exposures; on occasion, they include prospectively obtained data.
- Pharmaceutical companies may be the only source of information for recently introduced drugs (e.g., premarketing data).
- Finally, reference texts about teratogens should be on the desk of every obstetrician as a supplement to the PDR.

COUNSELING FOR DRUGS IN PREGNANCY

Patients seeking advice on teratogenic risks often have feelings of anxiety and guilt and may have been frightened by misinformation from friends, the media, and even health care personnel. Counseling in this situation should be sympathetic, supportive, and fully informative (64). Obtaining information that is as complete as possible about the exposure and the patient's health and family history is the initial phase in counseling for teratogenic risks. The following information is key to a complete assessment of pregnancy risk:

- *Health history.* The patient's medical condition may constitute a significant risk factor and may be an indication for the drug in question. All drugs taken by the patient should be identified.
- *Family history.* The paternal as well as the maternal side of the family should be questioned about birth defects, mental retardation, significant pregnancy wastage, and consanguinity, all of which could increase the risk for a poor outcome unrelated to a teratogen.
- *Work history.* Occupations that involve exposure to potential teratogens such as radiation, toxic chemicals and gases, chemotherapeutic agents, pesticides, and so forth may be risk factors that have not been considered by a patient concerned with a drug exposure; paternal exposures may be relevant as well as those of the pregnant woman.

- *Drug name and ingredients* (if a compound). The half-life and pharmacokinetics must be considered because the drug or its metabolites may be present in the maternal milieu even if ingested before conception.
- *Timing of exposure.* The date from ovulation/conception rather than menstrual age is considered. Dates of the last two menstrual periods, regularity of cycles, and contraception may be relevant. Ultrasound dating should be used for accuracy.
- *Dose and route of exposure.* Most teratogenic effects are dose related; the route of entrance may help to estimate the amount of embryo or fetal exposure.
- *Maternal symptoms related to exposure.* Symptoms are particularly important in workplace or accidental exposures.

After evaluating these pertinent details in terms of any impact on risks, the information available on the drug in question should be shared with the patient at a level commensurate with her educational background. Most patients cannot be expected to sort through the results of differing studies. Therefore, the clinician must summarize these findings and provide the assessment of risk to the patient, which of necessity may be based on a paucity of data or on data that are inconclusive *(indeterminate risk)*. What this kind of information means and how it is interpreted can and should be explained. For example, as often is the case with any widely used drug, some birth defects will have been reported following maternal exposure. The defects reported often include a range of malformations that affect different organ systems and may include Down syndrome or a genetic disorder that is clearly of a nonteratogenic etiology. The physician or counselor can explain that these kinds of data suggest these defects occurred at random and probably represent the 2% to 3% background risk faced by all couples rather than a systematic teratogenic effect. The patient can be told that a true teratogen usually produces a particular defect or a constellation of anomalies, such as the warfarin embryopathy.

We believe it is inappropriate to base counseling solely on case reports or animal studies, especially if these show teratogenesis, and particularly at suprapharmacologic doses. Corticosteriods and aspirin, for example, are teratogenic in mice but not in humans. Conversely, thalidomide appeared benign in several species that had a higher threshold for its potent teratogenic effects than humans or primates. Some data on human exposures to a drug such as premarketing evaluation are usually available. Even soft information, such as how long the drug has been on the market or how many prescriptions have been written without reports of adverse outcomes, can lend a measure of reassurance to a patient.

It is always important to provide teratogen counseling in the framework of the 2% to 3% background risk and the concept that no pregnancy can be guaranteed a normal outcome. The risk or absence of risk from an exposure always should be related to this background risk, which patients understand and accept as part of childbearing.

Ideally, if the data exist, teratogen counseling should include these points:

- *The absolute risk for the patient,* that is, the chances of having a baby with a birth defect
- *The absolute risk for the general population,* the chance that a woman who was not exposed will have a child with the same condition. As noted earlier, this often is referred to as the *background risk* against which all probabilities are measured.
- *The relative risk.* How much greater the risk is of having an affected infant than someone who was not exposed.
- *Description of the birth defects* for which a teratogenic risk has been demonstrated, including prognosis and treatment possibilities
- *Availability of prenatal testing* for some teratogenic effects. Because most defects induced by teratogens are morphologic, our practice has been to offer a comprehensive (targeted) ultrasound examination, although no statistically significant, long-term, prospective studies yet support the efficacy of this approach.

Whereas normal findings on these tests can decrease the likelihood of the malformation in question, it is important that the patient understand that no test can rule out with absolute certainty all the potential teratogenic effects. With valproic acid (VPA), for example, the risk for spina bifida is significantly increased, which can be effectively diagnosed with amniotic fluid alphafetoprotein (AFP) determination (and less reliably with ultrasound and a serum AFP). However, VPA exposure also carries a risk for subtle craniofacial dysmorphology as well as developmental defects that are not amenable to prenatal detection. In regard to prenatal testing, fetal chromosome studies are almost never appropriate for detecting birth defects caused by environmental teratogens (64) with the possible exception of periconceptional radiation exposure.

Physicians often are confronted with anxious questions about drugs such as diet pills, psychotropics, nonsteroidal antiinflammatory agents, and over-the-counter (OTC) medications taken before the pregnancy was recognized. As the data on the specific drug will indicate, the vast majority of these agents have *not* been proven to be human teratogens. The problem with these presumed nonteratogens is that in most cases systematic studies have not been performed. Nonteratogenicity is inferred, more from the absence of proven teratogenicity than from a significant body of data that indicate that a particular exposure has not increased the risk for fetal malformation beyond the risk faced by all pregnant couples. For such exposures, comprehensive counseling and normal ultrasound results usually serve to allay concerns.

Rarely would it be appropriate to advise a patient to terminate a pregnancy based on limited data. The decision to interrupt a pregnancy belongs to the patient and her partner and is influenced not only by the risk (actual or perceived) but also by a myriad of factors such as the level of anxiety, the perception of a handicap, the family constellation, and sometimes a hidden agenda not intended to be shared with the physician or counselor.

Although most drugs are not proven human teratogens, this does not imply such drugs should be prescribed freely in pregnancy. It is always necessary to balance the unknown potential risks (either maternal, embryonic, fetal, or perinatal) with the risk of no treatment. In some instances, even a drug that has some potential for teratogenesis may be necessary for maternal well being, and the patient should be involved in such decisions.

SPECIFIC DRUG EXPOSURES IN PREGNANCY

For ease of reference, we have listed the drugs currently considered teratogens with a brief summary of relevant information in Table 7-9. For some drugs, because of their importance or frequency of use, we have included additional information in the text. Besides prescription drugs, we will refer briefly to illicit drugs as well as environmental and work exposures. *Possible teratogens*, drugs that are currently suspected of being teratogens and are still under scrutiny, as well as unlikely *teratogens*, drugs that have not been demonstrated to be teratogenic, are listed in Table 7-10. Most drugs fall into the latter category, but we have listed the ones most frequently requested for counseling and for which evidence of non-teratogenicity is available.

The management of pregnancies with exposure to possible teratogens should follow the same general guidelines as those for which insufficient data exist, but the counseling should reflect the higher likelihood of risk. It is important to note, that at our present state of knowledge, paternal exposures have not been shown to be teratogenic. Although radiation and chemotherapy can theoretically affect the male germ cells, several reports suggest that there is little teratogenic risk from such exposures (65–66).

Topical applications also do not appear to present a risk. Concern about Retin-A cream recently surfaced because defects suggestive of the isotretinin embryopathy have been reported. Absorption of the topical agent is minimal, and there is some question as to the cause-effect relationship in these cases of topical use (Table 7-9).

Anticonvulsants

The teratogenic effects of anticonvulsants are well known. It is generally appreciated that women with seizures have a twofold to threefold greater risk for congenital malformations compared with the general population (67–69). Phenytoin (PHT), phenobarbital (Pb), and carbamazepine (CBZ) are relatively mild teratogens compared with VPA (70). All data available about this issue are based on chronic therapy; thus, risks cannot be assessed for the sporadic use of these drugs.

The fetal hydantoin or phenytoin syndrome (growth restriction, microcephaly, facial dysmorphism, fingernail hypoplasia, and mild developmental delay) is well recognized (71,72). Full expression of the syndrome is encountered rarely; it is more common to find isolated findings in affected children (73,74). With the exception of the nail hypoplasia, most effects noted with PHT exposure also are shared with the other anticonvulsants (e.g., CBZ) (69). In addition, spina bifida has been described in fetuses exposed *in utero* to both CBZ and VPA (75,76). The effects of VPA seem to manifest a broader spectrum, including not only growth restriction, craniofacial abnormalities, and spina bifida, but also heart and limb defects as well as other CNS lesions not associated with spina bifida (77).

The incidence of specific malformations is difficult to ascertain. According to Holmes (70), the risk for fetal malformations in pregnancies exposed to single-agent regimens for any of the anomalies (isolated or associated) can be cited as double the incidence of the general population. Quoted risks should be less for Pb and greater for VPA. In patients undergoing multidrug treatments for epilepsy that include VPA, risks for one or several drug-specific defects may be threefold that of the general population (69). The risk for spina bifida is more firmly established. The risk for fetal neural tube defects in women being treated with CBZ is approximately 0.5 to 1% and with VPA is 1% to 2% (76,77).

Data regarding neurobehavioral development in children exposed to PHT and CBZ in pregnancy are less clear. Exposed children manifest a slight decrease in mean IQ compared with unexposed children (78). One study, however, found 7 of 35 (20%) infants exposed *in utero* to CBZ manifested developmental delay (79). Thus, although the magnitude of the alterations in cognitive function is not firmly established, it seems there may be a risk for at least mild deleterious action in this regard (80).

The mechanism of teratogenic action of PHT seems related to its oxidative metabolites and not directly to the drug itself. Buehler and colleagues (1990) measured epoxide hydrolase activity in PHT-exposed infants with and without features of the fetal hydantoin syndrome and found that *in utero* exposed infants with the syndrome had lower levels than infants without the syndrome. In further evaluating the parents of the affected infants, the authors concluded that the activity of this enzyme was regulated by one recessive gene. They hypothesized that measurement of enzyme activity could be employed in the prenatal diagnosis of the fetus at risk or in the preconceptional assessment of parental enzymatic activity.

TABLE 7-9. *Drugs that present problematic counseling issues*

Drug and fetal effects	Comments	Counseling: Retrospective counseling	Counseling: Prospective counseling
Antibiotics			
Tetracycline			
Yellow-brown discoloration of deciduous teeth (if exposure occurs during second half of pregnancy) (135–136) Staining of the crowns of the permanent teeth (if exposure occurs close to term) (137–138). Enamel hypoplasia (with very high dosages) (138)	Tetracycline complexes with calcium and the organic matrix of newly forming bone without altering the crystalline structure of hydroxyapatite (138)	Low severity of the anomalies; no modification of care in patients in whom exposure to this drug occurred They must be warned about the possible anomaly and the transient character of it	Given the availability of other equivalent drugs, tetracycline is relatively contraindicated in pregnancy
Streptomycin and kanamycin (?)			
Sensorineural hearing loss related to eighth-nerve damage	This effect is seen postnatally; Reports about this effect related to prenatal exposure are conflicting; estimated risks of fetal toxicity range from 3% to 11%; some reports concluded no risk Gentamicin and vancomicin are safer alternatives (139–140)	Women exposed should be informed of the conflicting results of different studies and the hypothetical, even if small, risk for deafness; after birth, the child should be screened to rule out this effect	Given the availability of alternative drugs with, apparently, no proven risks, streptomycin or kanamycin should be used only if resistance to the other agents exists; for tuberculosis, use the other agents (avoid also ethionamide)
Angiotensin converting enzyme inhibitors (ACEI): *captopril, enalapril, lisinopril*			
Lack of cranial ossification, patent ductus arteriosus (141) Fetal hypotension Renal tubular dysplasia Anuria/oligohydramnios Growth restriction Neonatal renal failure and death (142,143)	Risk can be as great as 30% during the second and third trimester of pregnancy; some of the effects result from the profound hypotension (144); no reports of teratogenic effects in first trimester exposure and in a report recently published of 66 women with first trimester exposure, none of whom had affected offspring (145); there are, however, contrary reports (143)	Evaluate pregnancies by targeted ultrasound scans (US); suggest enrollment in the ACEI Registry (see Table 7-8)	ACE inhibitors should not be used in pregnancy; however, if a child is born with ACE inhibitor fetopathy, aggressive therapy with dialysis to remove the inhibitor may mitigate the profound hypotensive effects; there are reports of residual renal impairment in affected newborns (146–147)
Anticonvulsants (AC) (see text)			
Carbamazepine (CBZ), phenytoin (PHT), phenobarbital (Pb)			
Intrauterine growth restriction Decreased cranial circumference (which may develop only after birth) Facial features: midface hypoplasia with inner epicanthal folds, short nose, broad depressed nasal bridge, anteverted nostrils and long upper lip Fingernail hypoplasia (with PHT exposure)–hypoplasia of distal phalanges and nails with stiff distal interphalangeal joints (148) Congenital malformations: spina bifida (with CBZ exposure),	Monotherapy doubles the frequency of microcephaly, growth retardation and major malformations; greatest risk seems to be for the facial features and minor abnormalities; polytherapy [including Valproic acid (VPA)] triples risk Additional risk of CBZ: 0.5 to 1% for spina bifida; both the incidence and the severity of the effects on development and intelligence (either in the presence or absence of microcephaly) have not been determined with certainty (68); overall, the risk for any anomaly is usually accepted as slightly lower than 10% (149)	Consult a neurologist for the possibility of (a) suspending the medication, (b) reducing to monotherapy and/or (c) reducing the dose to the minimum effective; add 4 mg folate/day for patients taking CBZ or VPA, starting 1 mo prior to conception, if possible (68,86–87) If a decision is made to pursue pregnancy, for CBZ and VPA exposure, offer spina bifida prenatal diagnosis in addition	Work up etiology of seizures; use minimal medical therapy to keep patient seizure-free; after the first trimester the risks for most defects are reduced except growth restriction, microcephaly, and subtle effect on cognitive function

continued

TABLE 7-9. *Continued.*

Drug and fetal effects	Comments	Counseling: Retrospective counseling	Counseling: Prospective counseling
cleft lip, heart defects, hypospadias and undescended testis, polydactyly Possible mild developmental delay		to the general targeted ultrasound; suggest the patient enroll in the Antiepileptic Drug Pregnancy Registry (see Table 7-8)	
Valproic acid (VPA)			
Facial features, as above Congenital malformations: spina bifida and other central nervous system (CNS) structural abnormalities not secondary to spina bifida	Valproic acid has the highest risk for spina bifida (1%–2%); overall, the risk for any anomaly is usually accepted as ~10%	See above	See above
Antineoplastics (see text)			
Folic acid antagonists: aminopterin and methotrexate (MTX)			
Miscarriage, intrauterine growth restriction, stillbirth, neonatal death Neural tube defects (NTD) Facial features: ocular hypertelorism, shallow orbits, midfacial hypoplasia, micrognathia, and facial assymetry. Skeletal anomalies: vertebral segmentation abnormalities with anomalous ribs, abnormalities of ossification of sacral structures, ectrodactyly, syndactyly, longitudinal limb reduction malformations Other malformations: cleft palate Mental retardation (150–151)	These are the only antimetabolites with proven teratogenicity, when used in large doses in first trimester; data are insufficient to substantiate an exact risk for each individual anomaly, but the risk for having any anomaly is most likely high; no specific pattern of malformations characteristically and uniquely repeated among exposed fetuses; for small dose exposures, such as treatment for psoriasis, data are less compelling (152)	In cases of accidental exposure in the first trimester, the risk of malformations is high; if pregnancy continues, offer ultrasound examination and prenatal diagnosis of NTD Suggest to the patient to enroll in the MTX registry (see Table 7-8)	These drugs are contraindicated during pregnancy; the use of MTX as an abortifacient represents a presumed risk for the cases with failure of therapy, although both the risk of failure and the risk of exposure, at those doses, are unknown
Alkylating agents: cyclophosphamide (CP), busulfan, chlorambucil, and nitrogen mustard			
Miscarriage, intrauterine growth restriction, stillbirth Microphthalmia, cleft palate, genitourinary anomalies, renal anomalies, limb malformations (ectrodactyly, oligodactyly, terminal longitudinal limb reduction)	All reported effects based on anecdotal reports (153); risks are 10% to 35% (11) Mechanism of action is related to the inactivation of DNA through the formation of crosslinks (12); effects need activation mediated by microsomal cytochrome P-450 mono-oxygenases, and resultant metabolites thought to be responsible for the antineoplastic and mutagenic effects (154)	For first trimester accidental exposure, monitor the pregnancy with ultrasound examination	These agents are contraindicated during pregnancy
Antithyroid drugs: *Inorganic iodides, thioureas, propylthiouracil, methimazole, iodine (131)*			
Hypothyroidism and congenital goiter	Antithyroid drugs can cause neonatal goiter and hypothyroidism; there is not enough data for quantitation of risk but it seems low; propylthiouracil and methimazole seems to be the safest (155–157). Thiourea causes minimal goiter and signs of neonatal hypothyroidism disappear in 2 to 6 wk; iodides, also used in mucolytics, if used for long periods can	In patients anticipating pregnancy, switch to safer alternative therapies; do not stop therapy; on exposure to antithyroid drugs, reassurance and supplementation to the newborn with transitory hypothyroidism can be given; if long exposure	For hyperthyroidism use preferentially propylthiouracil (157); Diagnostic tests using I^{131} should be postponed to the end of pregnancy

TABLE 7-9. *Continued.*

Drug and fetal effects	Comments	Counseling: Retrospective counseling	Counseling: Prospective counseling
	cause massive thyroid enlargement, hydramnios and respiratory obstruction after birth (12); a high percentage of survivors develop cretinism (158); iodine (131), if used after 10 wk, can destroy fetal thyroid tissue (12)	to iodides occurs, anticipate hydramnios and be prepared to perform tracheostomy at the time of birth (12); amniotic fluid thyroid-stimulating hormone (TSH) may prove useful in the diagnosis and treatment of a hypothyroid fetus. Intraamniotic injections of L-thyroxine have proven successful for fetal therapy (159); accidental exposure to I^{131} after 10 wk may necessitate treatment of hypothyroidism for life (12)	
Lithium			
Congenital heart disease, especially Ebstein anomaly	Risks are much less then previous reported: (relative risk) (RR) 1.2–7.7 (160–162); absolute risk 1% to 8% and relate to exposures in first trimester; some kidney, thyroid and neuromuscular toxic effects in exposure near delivery have been reported, most self-limiting	When possible, taper medication or use alternative therapy before pregnancy occurs; reinitiate, if necessary, after 10 wk; in first trimester exposure, consider a fetal echocardiogram to rule out anomalies. Suggest the patient to enroll in the lithium registry (see Table 7-8)	If lithium therapy is needed during pregnancy, consider decrease in dose before delivery
Oral anticoagulants: *warfarin and other coumarin derivatives*			
Nasal hypoplasia with upper airway obstruction related to choanal atresia, lag in skeletal maturation with stippled calcification of epiphyses of long bones (most common) Broad short hands and phalanges Anomalies of the eye (optic atrophy), neck and CNS (microcephaly and others) Developmental delay, hypotonia and seizures Intrauterine growth restriction Spontaneous abortion, stillbirth, abruptio placentae, fetal or neonatal hemorrhage (163–166)	Period of greatest risk is 8–14 wk; exposures at 8–10 wk for bone and nasal anomalies and developmental delay (risk: 10%–25%) (9); exposures at 10–14 wk for CNS, ophthalmologic anomalies, and also for developmental delay; exact risk figures are unknown. If exposure occurs later in pregnancy, effects are related to hemorrhage; The appearance of vitamin K-dependent clotting factors occurs later in pregnancy (9,11)	If exposure occurs between 8 and 14 wk of gestation, the risk of anomalies is very high; few anomalies of surviving pregnancies are amenable to ultrasound diagnosis, with the exception of hemorrhagic sequelae in the CNS	Contraindicated in pregnancy; if anticoagulation necessary, use heparin
Penicillamine (?)			
Cutis laxa	Penicillamine is a copper-chelating agent, used for the treatment of Wilson's disease, cystinuria, and rheumatoid arthritis; although the data that raised the suspicion are anecdotal and based on case reports, the mechanism of action of penicillamine can explain this	For accidental exposure to this drug during first trimester, there should be no change in management of pregnancy	For Wilson's disease the continuation of therapy throughout pregnancy is indicated

continued

TABLE 7-9. *Continued.*

Drug and fetal effects	Comments	Counseling: Retrospective counseling	Counseling: Prospective counseling
	effect (167–168); however, there is no consistent proof of teratogenicity and prospective studies did not find this effect (169–170)		
Sex hormones			
Androgenic drugs: androgenic progestins (19-nortestosterone derivatives) and testosterone derivatives (e.g., danazol)			
Virilization of female fetus: labioscrotal fusion and clitoromegaly No effect on male fetus	The severity of the effects depend of the drug, dose, and time of exposure (labioscrotal fusion with exposure before 9 wk gestation; clitoromegaly at any gestational age); risks are low, especially for androgenic progestins and only with high doses (~1%–2%) (11–12,171)	Accidental first trimester exposure is unlikely to be associated with those effects if the drug is stopped early in pregnancy	Contraindicated in pregnancy; no valid indication for use; progestogens are not effective for threatened abortion
Diethylstilbestrol			
Female fetus: vaginal adenosis, clear-cell carcinoma of vagina and cervix, cervix and uterine anomalies. Male: epididymal cysts, capsular induration of testes and hypotrophy, abnormal spermatozoa with possible infertility.	Risk for vaginal adenosis has been reported between 30% and 90% if exposure occurs before 9 wk gestation; the fact that the altered epithelium has increased carcinogenic susceptibility has been considered the reason for an increased risk for carcinoma (172); absolute risk is very low (173); the reproductive organ anomalies can cause infertility; risks for male genitalia can be as great as 25% (174,175)	Accidental exposure should be rare because its former indications for use are no longer valid; use now limited to some research protocols in the treatment of cancer	Contraindicated in pregnancy; no valid indication for use
Thalidomide			
Limb reduction malformations, anotia and microtia, facial hemangiomas, esophageal or duodenal atresia, cardiac anomalies, renal agenesis	One of the most powerful known teratogens; the risk for any of the reported anomalies, if exposure occurred between 22 and 36 days after conception, is 20% (9,11,176–177)	It is unlikely to be faced with first trimester exposure because its use is restricted to experimental protocols in very specific conditions (178–180). Now it is used for the treatment of leprosy (181); in exposed fetuses, ultrasound examination is appropriate (182)	Exposures may occur in women of reproductive age undergoing therapy for leprosy; contraception is essential in these women; thalidomide is contraindicated in pregnancy
Vitamin derivatives			
Vitamin A (retinol) and derivatives: all-trans-retinoic acid (tretinoin-Retin-A, topical), 13-cis-retinoic acid (isotretinoin-Accutane), etretinate			
Characteristic pattern similar to 22q11 deletion syndromes-DiGeorge and velocardiofacial syndrome CNS anomalies: microcephaly, developmental anomalies consequent to hydrocephaly, holoprosencephaly, cerebellar hypoplasia, posterior fossa cysts, cortical blindness and facial nerve palsies Craniofacial defects: maldevelopment of the facial and cal-	This group of drugs is one of the strongest teratogens; differences in teratogenic potency of various retinoids linked to their metabolism and placental transfer Risk period for teratogenic effects is between 4 and 7 wk gestational age; risks may exceed 50% in exposed pregnancies; only systemic agents are implicated in fetal effects; topical agents, (retinol, tretinoin) are *not* teratogenic (183–184)	Although indications for these medications are specific (psoriasis etretinate; severe acne, isotretinoin) and the patients are informed of the strong teratogenic risks, first trimester accidental exposure may occur, usually by failure of contraception (190); in exposed pregnancies, ultrasound examination	Absolute contraindication in pregnancy and in sexually active reproductive age women without effective contraception which should be maintained up to 1 mo after the suspension of therapy; for etretinate this period should be longer (up to 2 yr?) (192–193);

TABLE 7-9. *Continued.*

Drug and fetal effects	Comments	Counseling: Retrospective counseling	Counseling: Prospective counseling
varial bones with facial asymmetry, midfacial hypoplasia, micrognathia, cleft palate, microphthalmia, oculomotor palsies, microtia and anomalies of the ear canal Cardiovascular anomalies: conotruncal and aortic arch defects Thymic hypoplasia Many other isolated defects have been reported Spontaneous abortion	Daily doses for which risk exists: Isotretinoin (half-life of less than one day); 0.4–1.5 mg/kg per day Etretinate (half-life of 100–120 days); 0.4–1.5 mg/kg per day Vitamin A (retinol) (half-life of weeks to mos)—megadoses of 0.2–1.5 mg/kg, 15,000 U, although this is still subject of discussion; regular doses of vitamin A supplementation are safe (185–188) Acitretin, the carboxylic acid derivative of etretinate, has a much shorter half-life (50 hr), the same efficacy, and is therefore considered a good substitute for etretinate (189)	is warranted Cases of use of etretinate and isotretinoin before conception should be managed as "insufficient data" The same should be applied to high-dose (>15,000 U) exposure to vitamin A (188,191)	The Teratology Society recommends maximum daily doses of 8,000 IU of vitamin A during pregnancy (191,194)
Vitamin D (?)			
Syndrome consisting of supravalvular aortic stenosis, elfin facies and mental retardation (195)	This syndrome appeared in some fetuses exposed to very high doses of vitamin D administered for rickets prophylaxis; those doses are no longer used (9)	Such high doses exposure not likely to occur nowadays	Supplementation of vitamin D in pregnancy, if needed, is safe
Substance abuse (see text)			
Ethanol			
Fetal alcohol syndrome (196)—Intrauterine growth restriciton, microcephaly, short palpebral fissures, maxillary hypoplasia with short philtrum, thin upper lip, and developmental delay Varying degrees of mental compromise, from learning disabilities to moderate mental retardation (fetal alcohol effects) (197,198).	The fetal alcohol effects are well documented. The risk for fetal alcohol syndrome is related to continued ingestion and is highly dose-dependent (199); if one includes all the possible effects, including the learning disabilities, no dose is completely safe (200,201), although the risks are probably greater for greater exposures (197,198)	Any regular ingestion should be strongly discouraged during the pregnancy (202); exposure to a small dose of ethanol in an occasional social event is not, most likely, reason for excessive anxiety (197,198)	No alcohol during pregnancy
Cocaine (see text)			
Fetal vascular related conditions (101–203): bowel atresia, limb defects, cerebral infarctions, microcephaly (110–112), genitourinary anomalies (100,204) Nonfetal vascular related conditions (110–112): amniotic membrane syndrome, intrauterine growth restriction, abruptio placentae,	Quantitation of risks not appropriately determined; likelihood of direct fetotoxic effects probably small	Avoid illicit medications in pregnancy (see text)	No illicit drug exposures during pregnancy
Toluene abuse (see text)			
Occupational exposures: Lead, organic mercury (see text and Table 7–10)			

Fetal effects are effects currently accepted as proven
Comments: when data exist, we present the calculated relative and/or absolute risks for the effects described
Retrospective counseling refers to the management and counseling in pregnancies complicated by exposure to the drug
Prospective counseling refers to the possible indications for the use of the drug in pregnancy

TABLE 7-10. *Commonly used medications*

Possible teratogens	Unlikely teratogens
Amphetamines	Acetylsalicylic acid (?)
Disulfiram	Acetaminophen
Ergotamine	Anesthetics
Ethionamide	Antiemetics (phenothiazines, trimethobenzamide, bendectin)
Oral hypoglycemic agents	Antihistamines (doxylamine)
Primidone	Aspartame
Quinine	Corticosteroids
Vitamin A (high doses)	Metronidazole
Abused substances (cigarette smoking)	Minor tranquilizers (meprobamamate, fluoxetine, chlordiazepoxide)
	Oral contraceptives
	Penicillin, cephalosporins
	Thyroid hormones
	Tricyclic antidepressants
	Trimethropin-sulfamethoxazole
	Spermicides
	Zidovudine, acyclovir
	Abused substances (cannabis, LSD, opiates)
	Others (caffeine, hairspray)

LSD, D-lysergic acid diethylamide.

From Brent RL, Beckman DA. Principles of teratology. In Evans MI, ed. Reproductive risks and prenatal diagnosis. Stamford, CT: Appleton & Lange, 1991; Briggs GG, Freeman RK; Yaffe St. Drugs in pregnancy and lacation—a reference guide to fetal and neonatal risk, 4th ed. Baltimore: Williams & Wilkins, 1994; Hanson JW. Human teratology. In: Rimoin DL, Connor JM, Pyeritz RE; eds. Principles and practice of medical genetics, 3rd ed. New York: Churchill-Livingstone, 1997; Simpson JL, Golbus MS. Genetics in obstetrics and gynecology, 2nd ed. Philadelphia: WB Saunders Company, 1992; Shepard TH. Catalog of teratogenic agents, 8th ed. Baltimore: The Johns Hopkins University Press, 1995, with permission.

Medical therapy could be modified in at-risk couples who manifest decreased levels of epoxide hydrolase activity (81,82). CBZ and Pb are metabolized by the same mechanism as PHT; thus, these agents may have similar mechanisms of action (83). The teratogenic action of VPA, based in animal models, seems mediated by the inhibition of tetrahydrofolate reductase (84).

When maternal seizure activity must be controlled, Pb seems to be the safest drug for use in pregnancy. An assessment of seizure activity while the patient is not pregnant and off medication is ideal but frequently is not possible. Patients who have been free of seizures for 2 years may be considered for discontinuation of therapy (85).

Little can be offered the pregnant woman on anticonvulsant medication in the way of assessment for fetal defects, with the exception of comprehensive ultrasound examination and genetic amniocentesis to assess amniotic fluid for open fetal defects (measurement of amniotic fluid AFP and acetylcholinesterase). Maternal serum alphafetoprotein (MSAFP) is used as a screening test for these anomalies, and is employed in low-risk patients (86). It is recommended currently that all women of reproductive age receive dietary folate supplementation; this public health policy may ameliorate the increased risk for fetal neural tube defects in patients on anticonvulsant medications (69,87,88). It is hoped that some of the new anticonvulsants becoming available may show better outcomes in the offspring of women needing this therapy (89).

Antineoplastic Agents

Given that antineoplastic agents are designed to kill rapidly dividing cells, it is not surprising that these agents may be teratogens (12). Not all antineoplastic agents are proven teratogens (maybe just because of lack of data), however, and not all fetuses exposed to antineoplastic agents that are proven teratogens have birth defects. Variations in metabolizing and detoxification mechanisms likely play a role in determining which fetus will be affected.

Agents currently accepted as having teratogenic effects include alkylating agents (busulfan, chlorambucil, cyclophosphamide, nitrogen mustard, triethylene melamine, and triethylene thirophosphoramide) and folic acid antagonists (aminopterin and methotrexate) (90). Other antimetabolites (e.g., 5-fluorouracil, 6-mercaptopurine, azathioprine) are not yet proven teratogens (12).

Data regarding exposures to any neoplastic agent are minimal for several reasons. First, even though cancer is the second leading cause of death of women during the reproductive years, cancer is rare in pregnancy (0.07–0.1%) (91). Second, treatment usually involves more than one drug; thus, it is difficult to assign specific risks to specific drugs. Third, the disease itself can have noxious effects to the fetus, although the principal outcome is usually spontaneous abortion, stillbirth, intrauterine growth restriction, and prematurity rather than infants with defects (92,93). Thus, putative effects ascribed to these drugs are based on series with small numbers of patients or case reports.

The prudent course of action for the clinician treating a woman of reproductive age for cancer is to ensure that she does not become pregnant while on therapy. If a first-trimester exposure occurs, she should be informed of the potential for teratogenicity, and genetic counseling should be offered expeditiously.

Substance Abuse

Ethanol, tobacco, and street drugs such as opiates, amphetamines, benzodiazepines, barbiturates, lysergic acid (LSD), other hallucinogens, cocaine (and crack), and cannabis (marijuana) are exogenous agents that, if consumed by the pregnant woman, may affect the developing fetus. With the exception of ethanol, which is probably the best studied substance of abuse and the one with the most clearly defined risks, appropriate and correct information about the vast majority of social drugs is simply not available (94). There are several reasons for this (95–98): consumers often use more than one of these agents concurrently (99); abusers of social drugs may have many other socioeconomic influences that may increase the risk for adverse perinatal outcome (i.e., the effect of confounding variables) (100); consumed substances are often mixed (laced or diluted) with other ingredients, with their own inherent effects preventing both the possibility of establishing an accurate dose-effect relationship for the primary agent as well as preventing the attribution of responsibilities for any putative teratogenic effects to either the primary or secondary agent(s); denial of use as well as ignorance of specific agents precludes accurate assessment and counseling; and testing performed on neonates may not accurately reflect fetal exposure.

A few additional comments regarding specific abused chemical agents are relevant, however. Cocaine abuse has been shown to result in teratogenic effects, the poor outcomes being related to its maternal vasoactive properties (101). Despite an understanding of the likely underlying mechanism (disruption anomalies), exact risk estimates for defects following fetal exposure are not available (97, 102,103). Practically speaking, risks are probably minimal given the prevalence of use among women of reproductive age (104) and the relative paucity of reported malformations (94,105–107).

Toluene, an industrial solvent, has been used as a drug of abuse and is linked to a characteristic pattern of growth and development (toluene embryopathy) (108). Fetal toluene exposures from abuse far exceed the infrequent, minimal exposures occasionally noted in pregnant women who work in industrial environments, where the risk for toluene embryopathy is small.

Even though teratogenic effects have not been proven for most socially abused substances, the incidence of miscarriage, intrauterine growth restriction, stillbirth, preterm delivery, and neonatal death is higher among pregnant substance abusers. Thus, women should be strongly advised to avoid exposure to any medically unnecessary agent if they are pregnant or anticipating pregnancy (109–112).

Environmental Exposure to Chemicals

Industrial agents for which teratogenicity has been claimed are presented in Table 7-11. Except for organic mercury compounds and lead, there is no definitive proof of teratogenicity for any of these agents because of the lack of adequate, statistically significant data. For the most part, only animal studies, anecdotal reports, and ret-

TABLE 7-11. *Environmental agents and teratogenesis*

Agent	Source of exposure	Quality of evidence
Organic mercury compounds: CNS deficits and cerebral palsy with maternal poisoning.	Ingestion of grain or fish contaminated through concentration along the food chain	Effects occur at or near maternal toxic levels; considered teratogen
Polychlorinated biphenyls (PCBs) and polybrominated biphenyls (PBBs)	Ingestion of contaminated food	Anecdotal information; considered "possible" teratogens (124)
Organic industrial solvents (aromatic hydrocarbons; benzene, xylene, toluene; aliphatic hydrocarbons: propane, some aerosol propellants; glycols: ethylene glycol, antifreeze; isopropyl alcohol; rubbing alcohol)	Professional or hobby activity contact with gasoline, motor oil, spray paint, aerosol sprays, nail polish remover, many cleaning products	Retrospective case–control studies; conflicting results; considered "possible" teratogen or reproductive toxic (113,115,117,125)
Dioxins	Component of agent orange, used as herbicide in Vietnam	Not proved to be a teratogen (126–128)
Heavy metals (lead, cadmium): neurobehavioral effects, growth deficits	Ingestion of contaminated food	Even small exposures to lead may affect the central nervous system adversely; Considered teratogenic (129–131)
Polyvinyl chloride	Industry and construction professional inhalation	Although chronic toxicity and carcinogenesis has been proven, teratogenic effects were not. Considered "not teratogen"
Pesticides	Farm professionals inhalation	Although acute toxicity is very well known, there is no proof of teratogenicity; considered "not teratogen" (126)
Anesthetic gases	Health professionals inhalation	Anecdotal evidence, not proven, of risk for miscarriage. Considered "possible" teratogen or 'reproductive toxic' (113)
Laboratory exposures	Health professional exposures.	Anecdotal evidence, not proven; considered 'not teratogen' (132)
Electromagnetic fields from video display terminals	Professional exposure	Anecdotal evidence, not proven; considered "not teratogen" (133,134)

CNS, central nervous system

From Paul M. Occupational reproductive hazards. Lancet 1997;349:1385–1388.

rospective case–control studies are available. Such data, like exposures to drugs of abuse, are sensitive to many ascertainment biases (e.g., identification of specific offending agents, accurate assessment of dosage) and study deficiencies (e.g., quality of the control population) (113–116). It is likely that the most common adverse reproductive outcome following substantial exposure to a harmful industrial agent is infertility (both male and female) or spontaneous abortion rather than teratogenic effects (117).

It should be intuitive that significant single, multiple, or complex exposures to pollutants might have an adverse effect on fetal development. This, after all, is consistent with theories on the multifactorial etiology of many birth defects (118). Some facts do provide general reassurance regarding day-to-day exposures to the environment. Thousands of new chemical entities are synthesized each year worldwide, and of the seven million chemicals recorded, 100,000 substances are currently estimated in commercial use (119). Despite the continuous development of new chemicals, the incidence of congenital anomalies has not increased for many decades.

It is worth remembering that most chemicals to which humans are exposed (including pesticides) are natural, produced by plants for their protection and are present in many common foods. Furthermore, the dose exposure is insignificant compared with the toxic level of the substance (120–122).

Information about potential chemical exposures during pregnancy, whether by inhalation, dermal contact, or ingestion, should be part of any prepregnancy counseling and should be included in the overall evaluation of the patient during the first prenatal visit. For example, If potential exposure to lead is found, blood lead levels should be monitored. If maternal lead levels exceed 10 µg per milliliter, removal from exposure and chelation therapy should be considered (123). Management of workplace or domestic exposures may require removal from current job or home environments.

CONCLUSION

The increasing interest and concern of both patients and clinicians about the effects of drugs in pregnancy has led to the greater availability of teratology information from a variety of sources. Epidemiologic approaches have succeeded in identifying the significant human teratogens. For some of these proven teratogens, the underlying biologic mechanisms have been elucidated, which indicate why a particular anomaly or syndrome results. More problematic are the possible teratogens, and the largest group, those drugs that are not suspected teratogens but for which there are only sparse data. Even so, risks must be assessed and appropriate counseling and clinical management provided so that such exposures do not result in severe anxiety or unwarranted terminations of pregnancy.

REFERENCES

1. Mills JL, Alexander D. Teratogens and "litogens." N Engl J Med 1986; 19:1234–1236.
2. Chadwick J, Mann WN. The medical works of Hippocrates. Springfield, IL: Charles C Thomas, 1935:158.
3. Ephesus S, Owsei T (Translators). Soranus's Gynecology. Baltimore, MD: The Johns Hopkins University Press, (reprint) 1991:48.
4. Heinonen OP, Slone D, Shapiro S. Birth defects and drugs in pregnancy, 1st ed. Littleton Massachusetts: Publishing Sciences Group, 1977:1–7.
5. Warkany J. Congenital malformations: notes and comments. Chicago: Year Book Medical Publishers, 1971:82
6. Murphy DP. Outcome of 625 pregnancies in women subjected to pelvic radium or roentgen irradiation. Am J Obstet Gynecol 1929;18: 179–187.
7. Goldstein L, Murphy DP. Microcephalic idiocy following radium therapy for uterine cancer during pregnancy. Am J Obstet Gynecol 1929; 18:189–195.
8. Gregg NM. Congenital cataract following German measles in the mother. Trans Ophtalmol Soc Aust 1941;3:35.
9. Brent RL, Beckman DA. Principles of teratology. In: Evans MI, ed. Reproductive risks and prenatal diagnosis. Stamford, CT: Appleton & Lange, 1991.
10. Briggs GG, Freeman RK, Yaffe SJ. Drugs in pregnancy and lactation—a reference guide to fetal and neonatal risk, 4th ed. Baltimore: Williams & Wilkins, 1994.
11. Hanson JW. Human teratology. In: Rimoin DL, Connor JM, Pyeritz RE, eds. Principles and practice of medical genetics, 3rd ed. New York: Churchill-Livingstone, 1997.
12. Simpson JL, Golbus MS. Genetics in obstetrics and gynecology, 2nd ed. Philadelphia: WB Saunders Company, 1992.
13. Shepard TH. Catalog of teratogenic agents, 8th ed. Baltimore: The John Hopkins University Press, 1995.
14. McBride WG. Thalidomide and congenital malformations. Lancet 1961;2:1358.
15. Hook EB, Healy KM. Consequences of a nationwide ban on spray adhesives alleged to be human teratogens and mutagens. Science 1976;191:566–567.
16. Hertig AT. The overall problem in man. In: Benirschke K, ed. Comparative aspects of reproductive failure. Berlin: Springer-Verlag, 1967.
17. Dicke JM. Teratology: principles and practice. Med Clin North Am 1989;73:567–582.
18. Zacharias J. A rational approach to drug use in pregnancy. J Obstet Gynecol Neonatal Nurs 1983;12:183–187.
19. Brent RL. Beckman DA. Landel CP. Clinical teratology. Curr Opin Pediatr 1993;5:201–211.
20. Brent RL. Beckman DA. Environmental teratogens. Bull NY Acad Med 1990;66:123–163.
21. Seaver LH, Hoyme HE. Teratology in pediatric practice. Pediatr Clin North Am 1992;39:111–134.
22. Brent RL, Beckman DA. The contribution of environmental teratogens to embryonic and fetal loss. Clin Obstet Gynecol 1994;37: 646–70.
23. Wilson JG. Environment and birth defects. New York: Academic Press, 1973.
24. Vainio H. Carcinogenesis and teratogenesis may have common mechanisms. Scand J Work Environ Health 1989;15:13–17.
25. Trosko JE, Chang CC, Netzloff M. The role of inhibited cell-cell communication in teratogenesis. Teratog Carcinog Mutagen 1982;2:1–45.
26. Welsch F, Stedman DB, Carson JL. Effects of a teratogen on [3H]uridine nucleotide transfer between human cells and on gap junctions. Exp Cell Res 1985;159:1–102.
27. Sáxen L. Defective regulatory mechanisms in teratogenesis. Int J Gynecol Obstet 1970;8:798.
28. Black DL, Marks TA. Role of maternal toxicity in assessing developmental toxicity in animals: a discussion. Regulat Toxicol Pharmacol 1992;16:89–201.

29. Rodier PM. Vulnerable periods and processes during central nervous system development. Environ Health Persp 1994;102(Suppl 2): 121–124.
30. Gordis L. Geographic and environmental factors in pediatric cancer. Cancer 1986;58(2 Suppl):546–549.
31. Pauli RM, Lian JB, Mosher DF, Suttie JW. Association of congenital deficiency of multiple vitamin K-dependent coagulation factors and the phenotype of the warfarin embriopathy: Clues to the mechanism of teratogenecity of coumarin derivatives. Am J Hum Genet 1987;41: 566–583.
32. Beck F. Comparative placental morphology and function. Environ Health Persp 1976;18:5–12.
33. May DG. Genetic differences in drug disposition. J Clin Pharmacol 1994;34:881–897.
34. O'Brien PJ, Hales BF, Josephy PD, Castonguay A, Yamazoe Y, Guengerich FP. Chemical carcinogenesis, mutagenesis, and teratogenesis. Can J Physiol Pharmacol 1996;74:565–571.
35. Torchinsky A, Fein A, Carp HJ, Toder V. MHC-associated immunopotentiation affects the embryo response to teratogens. Clin Exp Immunol 1994;98:513–519.
36. Watanabe T. Endo A. Sex difference in digit and palate formation of mouse embryos at midgestation. Teratology 1989;40:359–364.
37. Kochhar DM. *In vitro* testing of teratogenic agents using mammalian embryos. Teratog Carcinog Mutag 1980;1:63–74.
38. Goldberg JD, Golbus MS. The value of case reports in human teratology. Am J Obstet Gynecol 1986;154:479–482.
39. Rosenwasser SK. Critical issues in teratology for prenatal counselors. In: Zellers N, ed. Strategies in genetic counseling, 1st ed. New York: Human Sciences Press, 1989.
40. Robert E. Un exemple de détection de tératogene dans le cadre d'un registre de malformations: depakine et spina bifida. Rev Epidemiol Sante Publique 1996;44(Suppl 1):S78–S81.
41. Rothberg AD, Lorenz R. Can captopril cause fetal and neonatal renal failure? Pediatr Pharm 1984;4:189–192.
42. Barr M. Teratogen update: angiotensin converting enzyme inhibition. Teratology 1995;50:399–409.
43. Duminy PC. Fetal abnormality associated with the use of captopril during pregnancy. S Afr Med J 1981;60:805.
44. Schardein JL. Chemically induced birth defects. New York: Marcel Dekker, 1985.
45. Schardein JL. Schwetz BA. Kenel MF. Species sensitivities and prediction of teratogenic potential. Environ Health Perspect 1985;61: 55–67.
46. Abbott BD, Buckalew AR. Embryonic palatal responses to teratogens in serum-free organ culture. Teratology 1992;45:369–382.
47. Czeizel A. Surveillance of congenital anomalies in Hungary. Acta Paediatr Acad Sci Hung 1976;17:123–134.
48. De Wals P, Dolk H, Bertrand F, Gillerot Y, Weatherall JA, Lechat MF. La surveillance epidemiologique des anomalies congenitales par le registre EUROCAT. Rev Epidemiol Sante Publique 1988;36:273–282.
49. Edmonds LD, Layde PM, James LM, Flynt JW, Erickson JD, Oakley GP Jr. Congenital malformations surveillance: two American systems. Int J Epidemiol 1981;10:247–252.
50. Kallen B. Search for teratogenic risks with the aid of malformation registries. Teratology 1987;35:47–52.
51. Lancaster PA. Health registers for congenital malformations and *in vitro* fertilization. Clin Reprod Fertil 1986;4:27–37.
52. Holtzman NA, Khoury MJ. Monitoring for congenital malformations. Ann Rev Public Health 986;7:237–266.
53. Khoury MJ, Adams MM, Rhodes P, Erickson JD. Monitoring for multiple malformations in the detection of epidemics of birth defects. Teratology 1987:36:345–353.
54. Khoury MJ, Stewart W, Weinstein A, Panny S, Lindsay P, Eisenberg M. Residential mobility during pregnancy: implications for environmental teratogenesis. J Clin Epidemiol 1988;41:15–20.
55. Khoury MJ, Holtzman NA. On the ability of birth defects monitoring to detect new teratogens. Am J Epidemiol 1987;126:136–143.
56. Khoury MJ, Waters GD, Erickson JD. Patterns and trends of multiple congenital anomalies in birth defects surveillance systems. Teratology 1991;44:57–64.
57. Khoury MJ, Botto L, Waters GD, Mastroiacovo P, Castilla E, Erickson JD. Monitoring for new multiple congenital anomalies in the search for human teratogens. Am J Med Genet 1993;46:460–466.
58. Feldman Y, Koren G, Mattice K, Shear H, Pellegrini E, MacLeod SM. Determinants of recall and recall bias in studying drug and chemical exposure in pregnancy. Teratology 1989;40:37–45.
59. Khoury MJ, James LM, Lynberg MC. Quantitative analysis of associations between birth defects and suspected human teratogens. Am J Med Genet 1991;40:500–505.
60. Brent RL. Editor's note. Teratology 1978;17:183–184.
61. Schardein JL. Current status of drugs as teratogens in man. Prog Clin Biol Res 1985;163C:181–190.
62. U.S. Food and Drug Administration. Pregnancy labeling. FDA Drug Bull 1979;9:23–24 (Level III).
63. Friedman JM, Little BB, Brent RL, Cordero JF, Hanson JW, Shepard TH. Potential human teratogenicity of frequently prescribed drugs. Obstet Gynecol 1990;75:594–599.
64. American College of Obstetricians and Gynecologists. Teratology. ACOG Educational Bulletin. Washington, DC: ACOG (Level III), 1997:236.
65. Senturia YD, Peckham CS, Peckham MJ. Children fathered by men treated for testicular cancer. Lancet 1985;2:766–769.
66. Hinkes E, Plotkin D. Reversible drug-induced sterility in a patient with acute leukemia. JAMA 1973;223:1490–1491.
67. Steegers-Theunissen RP, Renier WO, Borm GF, et al. Factors influencing the risk of abnormal pregnancy outcome in epileptic women: a multi-centre prospective study. Epilepsy Res 1994;18:261–269.
68. Kaneko S, Otani K, Kondo T, et al. Malformation in infants of mothers with epilepsy receiving antiepileptic drugs. Neurology 1992;42(4 Suppl 5):68–74.
69. Holmes LB, Harvey EA, Brown KS, Hayes AM, Khoshbin S. Anticonvulsant teratogenesis: I. A study design for newborn infants. Teratology 1994;49:202–207.
70. Fedrick J. Epilepsy and pregnancy: a report from the Oxford Record Linkage Study. Br Med J. 1973;2:442–448.
71. Hanson JW, Myrianthopoulos NC, Harvey MA, Smith DW. Risks to the offspring of women treated with hydantoin anticonvulsants, with emphasis on the fetal hydantoin syndrome. J Pediatr 1976;89: 662–668.
72. Hanson JW, Buehler BA. Fetal hydantoin syndrome: current status. J Pediatr 1982;101:816–818.
73. Leavitt AM, Yerby MS, Robinson N, Sells CJ, Erickson DM. Epilepsy in pregnancy: developmental outcome of offspring at 12 months. Neurology 1992;42(4 Suppl 5):141–143.
74. Gaily E, Granstrom ML. Minor anomalies in children of mothers with epilepsy. Neurology 1992;42(4 Suppl 5):128–131.
75. Rosa FW. Spina bifida in infants of women treated with carbamazepine during pregnancy. N Engl J Med 1991;324:674–677.
76. Omtzigt JG, Los FJ, Grobbee DE, et al. The risk of spina bifida aperta after first trimester exposure to valproate in a prenatal cohort. Neurology 1992;42(Suppl 5):119–125.
77. Martinez-Frias ML. Clinical Manifestations of prenatal exposure to valproic acid using case reports and epidemiologic information. Am J Med Genet 1990;32:277–282.
78. Scolnik D, Nulman I, Rovet J, et al. Neurodevelopment of children exposed *in utero* to phenytoin and carbamazepine monotherapy. JAMA 1994;271:767–770.
79. Jones KL, Lacro RV, Johnson KA, Adams J. Pattern of Malformations in the children of women treated with carbamazepine during pregnancy. N Engl J Med 1989;320:1661–1666.
80. Vanoverloop D, Schnell RR, Harvey EA, Holmes LB. The effects of prenatal exposure to phenytoin and other anticonvulsants on intellectual function at 4 to 8 years of age. Neurotoxicol Teratol 192;14: 329–35.
81. Buehler BA, Delimont D, Van Waes M, Finnell RH. Prenatal prediction of risk of the fetal hydantoin syndrome. N Engl J Med 1990;322: 1567–1572.
82. Srickler SM, Dansky LV, Miller MA, Seni MH, Andermann E, Spielberg SP. Genetic predisposition to phenytoin-induced birth defects. Lancet 1985;2:746–749.
83. Wells PG, Nagri MK, Grego GS. Inhibition of trimethadione and dimethadione teratogenicity by the cyclooxygenase inhibitor acetylsalicilic acid: a unifying hypothesis for the teratogenic effects of hydantoin anticonvulsants and structurally related compounds. Toxicol Appl Pharmacol 1989;97:406–414.
84. Wegner C, Nau H. Valproic acid-induced neural tube defects: disturbance of the folate metabolism in day 9 mouse embryo. Teratology 1989;39:488.

85. Callaghan N, Garrett A, Goggin T. Withdrawal of anticonvulsant drugs in patients free of seizures for two years: a prospective study. N Engl J Med 1988;318:942–946.
86. Omtzigt JG, Los FJ, Hagenaars AM, Stewart PA, Sachs ES, Lindhout D. Prenatal diagnosis of spina bifida aperta after first-trimester valproate exposure. Prenat Diagn 1992;12:893–897.
87. Biale Y, Lewenthal H. Effect of folic acid supplementation on congenital malformations due to anticonvulsive drugs. Eur J Obstet Gynecol Reprod Biol 1984;18:211–216.
88. Lindhout D, Omtzigt JG. Teratogenic effects of antiepileptic drugs: implications for the management of epilepsy in women of childbearing age. Epilepsia 1994;35(Suppl 4):S19–S28.
89. Morrell MJ. The new antiepileptic drugs and women: efficacy, reproductive health, pregnancy, and fetal outcome. Epilepsia 1996;37 (Suppl)6:S34–S44.
90. Sorosky JI, Sood AK, Buekers TE. The use of chemotherapeutic agents during pregnancy. Obstet Gynecol Clin North Am 1997;24: 591–599.
91. Zemlickis D, Lishner M, Degendorfer P, Panzarella T, Sutcliffe SB, Koren G. Fetal outcome after in utero exposure to cancer chemotherapy. Arch Intern Med 1992;152:573–576.
92. Zemlickis D, Lishner M, Degendorfer P, et al. Maternal and fetal outcome after breast cancer in pregnancy. Am J Obstet Gynecol 1992; 166:781–787.
93. Zemlickis D, Lishner M, Degendorfer P, Panzarella T, Sutcliffe SB, Koren G. Maternal and fetal outcome after invasive cervical cancer in pregnancy. J Clin Oncol 1991;9:1956–1961.
94. Zimmerman EF. Substance abuse in pregnancy: teratogenesis. Pediatr Ann 1991;20:541–544.
95. Rizk B, Atterbury JL, Groome LJ. Reproductive risks of cocaine. Hum Reprod Update 1996;2:43–55.
96. Slutsker L. Risks associated with cocaine use during pregnancy. Obstet Gynecol 1992;79:778–789.
97. Gingras JL, Weese-Mayer DE, Hume RF Jr, O'Donnell KJ. Cocaine and development: mechanisms of fetal toxicity and neonatal consequences of prenatal cocaine exposure. Early Hum Dev 1992;31:1–24.
98. Singer LT, Garber R, Kliegman R. Neurobehavioral sequelae of fetal cocaine exposure. J Pediatr 1991;119:667–672.
99. Little BB, Snell LM, Gilstrap LD III, Johnston WL. Patterns of multiple substance abuse during pregnancy: implications for mother and fetus. South Med J 1990;83:507–509.
100. Lutiger B, Graham K, Einarson TR, Koren G. Relationship between gestational cocaine use and pregnancy outcome: a meta-analysis. Teratology 1991;44:405–414.
101. Hoyme HE, Jones KL, Dixon SD, et al. Prenatal cocaine exposure and fetal vascular disruption. Pediatrics 1990;85:743–747.
102. Singer L, Arendt R, Minnes S. Neurodevelopmental effects of cocaine. Clin Perinatol 1993;20:245–262.
103. Kain ZN, Kain TS, Scarpelli EM. Cocaine exposure in utero: perinatal development and neonatal manifestations. J Toxicol Clin Toxicol 1992;30:607–636.
104. Neerhof MG, MacGregor SN, Retzky SS, Sullivan TP. Cocaine abuse during pregnancy: peripartum prevalence and perinatal outcome. Am J Obstet Gynecol 1989;161:633–638.
105. Koren G, Graham K, Feigenbaum A, Einarson T. Evaluation and counseling of teratogenic risk: the motherisk approach. J Clin Pharmacol 1993;33:405–411.
106. Kain ZN, Kain TS, Scarpelli EM. Cocaine exposure *in utero*: perinatal development and neonatal manifestations—review. J Toxicol Clin Toxicol 1992;30:607–636.
107. Koren G, Graham K, Shear H, Einarson T. Bias against the null hypothesis: the reproductive hazards of cocaine. Lancet 1989;16: 1440–1442.
108. Pearson MA, Hoyme HE, Seaver LH, Rimsza ME. Toluene embryopathy: delineation of the phenotype and comparison with fetal alcohol syndrome. Pediatrics 1994;93:211–215.
109. Hoegerman G, Wilson CA, Thurmond E, Schnoll SH. Drug-exposed neonates. West J Med 1990;152:559–564.
110. Ryan L, Ehrlich S, Finnegan L. Cocaine abuse in pregnancy: effects on the fetus and newborn. Neurotoxicol Teratol 1987;9:295–299.
111. Chasnoff IJ, Lewis DE, Griffith DR, Willey S. Cocaine and pregnancy: clinical and toxicological implications for the neonate. Clin Chem 1989;35:1276–1278.
112. Bateman DA, Ng SK, Hansen CA, Heagarty MC. The effects of intrauterine cocaine exposure in newborns. Am J Public Health 1993; 83:190–193.
113. Baranski B. Effects of the workplace on fertility and related reproductive outcomes. Environ Health Perspect 1993;101(Suppl) 2:81–90.
114. Lemasters GK. Epidemiologic methods for evaluating the effects of occupational exposure on pregnancy outcome. Med Pr 1994;45: 419–433.
115. Lipscomb JA, Fenster L, Wrensch M, Shusterman D, Swan S. Pregnancy outcomes in women potentially exposed to occupational solvents and women working in the electronics industry. J Occup Med 1991;33:597–604.
116. Zhang J, Cai WW, Lee DJ. Occupational hazards and pregnancy outcomes. Am J Int Med 1992;21:397–408.
117. Gold EB, Tomich E. Occupational hazards to fertility and pregnancy outcome. Occup Med 1994;9:435–469.
118. Cordier S, Goujard J. Occupational exposure to chemical substances and congenital anomalies: state of the art. Rev Epidemiol Sante Publique 1994;42:144–159.
119. Rhodes C, Purchase IF, Pemberton MA, Oliver GJ. A balanced approach to the detection, characterisation and mechanism of toxicity of industrial chemicals. J Toxicol Sci 1987;12:243–251.
120. Ames BN, Gold LS. Animal cancer tests and cancer prevention. J Natl Cancer Inst Monographs 1992;12:125–132.
121. Ames BN, Gold LS. Natural chemicals, synthetic chemicals, risk assessment, and cancer. Princess Takamatsu Symposia 1990;21: 303–314.
122. Ames BN, Profet M, Gold LS. Nature's chemicals and synthetic chemicals: comparative toxicology. Proc Nat Acad Sci 1990;87: 7782–7786.
123. Paul M. Occupational reproductive hazards. Lancet 1997;349: 1385–1388.
124. Exon JH. A review of chlorinated phenols. Vet Hum Toxicol 1984;26: 508–520.
125. Lindbohm ML. Effects of parental exposure to solvents on pregnancy outcome. Occup Environ Med 1995;37:908–914.
126. Ames BN. Natural carcinogens and dioxin. Sci Total Environm 1991;104:159–166.
127. Kaye CI, Rao S, Simpson SJ, Rosenthal FS, Cohen MM. Evaluation of chromosomal damage in males exposed to agent orange and their families. J Craniofacial Genet Devel Biol 1985;1(Suppl):259–265.
128. Pearn JH. Herbicides and congenital malformations: a review for the paediatrician. Aust Paediatr J 1985;21:237–242.
129. Miller RK, Belinger D. Metals. In: Paul M, ed. Occupational and environmental reproductive hazards: a guide for clinicians. Baltimore: Williams & Wilkins, 1993:233–252.
130. Bellinger D, Sloman J, Leviton A, Needleman H, Rabinowitz M, Waternaux C. Low-level lead exposure and children's cognitive function in the preschool years. Pediatrics 1991;87:219–227.
131. Deitrich KN, Sucoop PA, Bornschein RL, et al. Lead exposure and neurobehavioral development in later infancy. Environ Health Prospect 1990;89:13–19.
132. Axelsson G, Rylander R. Outcome of pregnancy in women engaged in laboratory work at a petrochemical plant. Am J Ind Med 1989;16: 539–545.
133. Bramwell RS, Davidson MJ. Visual display units and pregnancy outcome: a prospective study. J Psychosom Obstet Gynaecol 1993;14: 197–210.
134. Parazzini F, Luchini L, La Vecchia C, Crosignani PG. Video display terminal use during pregnancy and reproductive outcome, a meta-analysis. J Epidemiol Commun Health 1993;47:265–268.
135. Davies PA, Little K, Aherne W. Tetracycline and yellow teeth. Lancet 1962;1:743.
136. Genot MT, Golan HP, Porter PJ, Kass EH. Effect of administration of tetracycline in pregnancy on the primary dentition of the offspring. J Oral Med 1970;25:75–79.
137. Anthony JR. Effect on deciduous and permanent teeth of tetracycline deposition *in utero*. Postgrad Med 1970;48:165–168.
138. Baden E. Environmental pathology of the teeth. In: Gorlin RJ, Goldman HM, eds. Thomas oral pathology, 6th ed. St Louis: Mosby, 1970:189–191.
139. Rasmussen F. The ototoxic effects of streptomycin and dihydrostreptomycin on the fetus. Scand J Respir Dis 1969;50:61–67.

140. Warkany J. Teratogen update: antituberculous drugs. Teratology 1979; 20:133–138.
141. Barr M Jr, Cohen MM Jr. ACE inhibitor fetopathy and hypocalvaria: the kidney–skull connection. Teratology 1991;44:485–495.
142. Pryde PG, Sedman AB, Nugent CE, Barr M Jr. Angiotensin-converting enzyme inhibitor fetopathy. J Am Soc Nephrol 1993;3: 1575–1582.
143. Shotan A, Widerhorn J, Hurst A, Elkayam U. Risks of angiotensin-converting enzyme inhibition during pregnancy: experimental and clinical evidence, potential mechanisms, and recommendations for use. Am J Med 1994;96:451–456.
144. Barr M Jr. Teratogen update: angiotensin-converting enzyme inhibitors. Teratology 1994;50:399–409.
145. Anonymous. Postmarketing surveillance for angiotensin-converting enzyme inhibitor use during the first trimester of pregnancy—United States, Canada, and Israel, 1987–1995. MMWR 1997;46:240–242.
146. Sedman AB, Kershaw DB, Bunchman TE. Recognition and management of angiotensin converting enzyme inhibitor fetopathy. Pediatr Nephrol 1995;9:382–385.
147. Bhatt-Mehta V, Deluga KS. Fetal exposure to lisinopril: neonatal manifestations and management. Pharmacotherapy 1993;13:515–518.
148. Barr M, Pozanski AK, Schmickel RD. Digital hypoplasia and anticonvulsants during gestation, a teratogenic syndrome. J Pediatr 1975; 86:459.
149. Buehler BA, Rao V, Finnell RH. Biochemical and molecular teratology of fetal hydantoin syndrome. Neurol Clin 1994;12:741–748.
150. Milunsky A, Graef JW, Gaynor MF Jr. Methotrexate induced malformations with a review of the literature. J Pediatr 1968;72:790–795.
151. Warkany J. Aminopterin and methotrexate: folic acid deficiency. Teratology 1978;17:353.
152. Kozlowski RD, Steinbrunner JV, MacKenzie AH, Clough JD, Wilke WS, Segal AM. Outcome of first-trimester exposure to low-dose methotrexate in eight patients with rheumatic disease. Am J Med 1990;88:589–592.
153. Schardein JL. Cancer chemotherapeutic agents. In: Chemically induced birth defects. New York: Marcel Dekker, 1985:467–520.
154. Mirkes PE. Cyclophosphamide teratogenesis: a review. Teratog Carcin Mutagen 1985;5:75–88.
155. Momotani N, Ito K, Hamada N, Ban Y, Nishikawa Y, Mimura T. Maternal hyperthyroidism and congenital malformation in the offspring. Clin Endocrinol (Oxf) 1984;20:695–700.
156. Wing DA, Millar LK, Koonings PP, Montoro MN, Mestman JH. A comparison of propylthiouracil versus methimazole in the treatment of hyperthyroidism in pregnancy. Am J Obstet Gynecol 1994;170:90–95.
157. Anonymous. Thyroid disease in pregnancy. ACOG Technical Bulletin Number 1993;181. Int J Gynaecol Obstet 1993;43:82–88.
158. Carswell F, Kerr MM, Hutchinson JH. Congenital goiter and hypothyroidism produced by maternal ingestion of iodides. Lancet 1970; 1:1241.
159. Perelman AH, Clemons RD. The fetus in maternal hyperthyroidism. Thyroid 1992;2:225–228.
160. Leonard A, Hantson P, Gerber GB. Mutagenicity, carcinogenicity and teratogenicity of lithium compounds. Mutat Res 1995;339: 131–137.
161. Cohen LS, Friedman JM, Jefferson JW, Johnson EM, Weiner ML. A reevaluation of risk of in utero exposure to lithium. JAMA 1994;271: 146–150.
162. Jacobson SJ, Jones K, Johnson K, et al. Prospective multicentre study of pregnancy outcome after lithium exposure during first trimester. Lancet 1992;339:530–533.
163. Pettiflor JM, Benson R. Congenital malformations associated with the administration of oral anticoagulants during pregnancy. J Pediatr 1975;86:459.
164. Holzgreve W, Carey JC, Hall BD. Warfarin-induced fetal abnormalities. Lancet 1976;2:914.
165. Pauli RM, Hall JG, Shaul WL. Spectrum of intrauterine effects of warfarin. In: Motulsky AG, Lenz W, eds. Birth defects. Amsterdam: Excerpta Medica, 1977.
166. Hall JG, Pauli RM, Wilson RM. Maternal and fetal sequelae of anticoagulation during pregnancy. Am J Med 1980;68:122.
167. Mjolnerod OK, Rasmussen K, Dommerud SA, Gjeruldsen ST. Congenital connective-tissue defect probably due to D-penicilllamine treatment in pregnancy. Lancet 1971;1:673.
168. Solomon L, Abrahams G, Dinner M, Berman L. Neonatal abnormalities associated with D-penicillamine treatment during pregnancy. N Engl J Med 1977;296:54.
169. Lyle WH. Penicillamine in pregnancy. Lancet 1978;1:606.
170. Scheinberg IH, Sternlieb I. Pregnancy in penicillamine treated patients with Wilson's disease. N Engl J Med 1975;293:1300–1302.
171. Raman-Wilms L, Tseng AL, Wighardt S, Einarson TR, Koren G. Fetal genital effects of first-trimester sex hormone exposure: a meta-analysis. Obstet Gynecol 1995;85:141–149.
172. Vessey MP. Epidemiological studies of the effects of diethylstilboestrol. IARC Sci Publ 1989;96:335–348.
173. Edelman DA. Diethylstilbestrol exposure and the risk of clear cell cervical and vaginal adenocarcinoma. Int J Fertil 1989;34:251–255.
174. Giusti RM, Iwamoto K, Hatch EE. Diethylstilbestrol revisited: a review of the long-term health effects. Ann Intern Med 1995;122:778–788.
175. Gill WB, Schumacher GFB, Bibbo M. Pathological semen and anatomical abnormalities of the genital tract in human male subjects exposed to diethylstilbestrol in utero. J Urol 1977;117:477.
176. Lenz W, Knapp K. Thalidomide embryopathy. Arch Environ Health 1962;5:100.
177. Lenz W. A short story of thalidomide embryopathy. Teratology 1988; 38:203.
178. Anonymous. New uses of thalidomide. Med Lett Drugs Ther 1996; 38:15–16.
179. Tseng S, Pak G, Washenik K, Pomeranz MK, Shupack JL. Rediscovering thalidomide: a review of its mechanism of action, side effects, and potential uses. J Am Acad Dermatol 1996;35:969–979.
180. Stirling D, Sherman M, Strauss S. Thalidomide: a surprising recovery. J Am Pharm Assoc (Wash) 1997;NS37:306–313.
181. Castilla EE, Ashton-Prolla P, Barreda-Mejia E, et al. Thalidomide, a current teratogen in South America. Teratology 1996;54:273–277.
182. Gollop TR, Eigier A, Guidugli Neto J. Prenatal diagnosis of thalidomide syndrome. Prenat Diagn 1987;7:295–298.
183. Buchan P. Evaluation of the teratogenic risk of cutaneously administered retinoids. Skin Pharmacol 1993;6:45–52.
184. Johnson EM. A risk assessement of topical tretinoin as a potential human developmental toxin based on animal and comparative human data. J Am Acad Dermatol 1997;36:s86–90.
185. Rothman KJ, Moore LL, Singer MR, Nguyen UDT, Mannino S, Milunsky A. Teratogenicity of high vitamin A intake. N Engl J Med 1995;333:1369–1373.
186. Brent RL, Hendrickx AG, Holmes LB, Miller RK. Teratogenicity of high vitamin A intake. [Letter]. N Engl J Med 1996;334:1196.
187. Challem JJ. Teratogenicity of high vitamin A intake [Letter]. N Engl J Med 1996;334:1196–1197.
188. Mills JL, Simpson JL, Cunningham GC, Conley MR, Rhoads GC. Vitamin A and birth defects. Am J Obstet Gynecol 1997;177:31–36.
189. Bouvy ML, Sturkenboom MC, Cornel MC, De Jong-Van den Berg LT, Stricker BH, Wesseling H. Acitretin (Neotigason): a review of pharmacokinetics and teratogenicity and hypothesis on metabolic pathways. Pharmaceutisch Weekblad Scientific Edition 1992;14:33–37.
190. Trussell J. Contraceptive efficacy. Arch Dermatol 1995;131: 1064–1068.
191. Underwood BA. Teratogenicity of vitamin A. Int J Vitam Nutr Res Suppl 1989;30:42–55.
192. Geiger JM, Baudin M, Saurat JH. Teratogenic risk with etretinate and acitretin treatment. Dermatology 1994;189:109–116.
193. Sturkenboom MC, de Jong-Van Den Berg LT, van Voorst-Vader PC, Cornel MC, Stricker BH, Wesseling H. Inability to detect plasma etretinate and acitretin is a poor predictor of the absence of these teratogens in tissue after stopping acitretin treatment. Br J Clin Pharmacol 1994;38:229–235.
194. Anonymous. Teratology Society position paper: recommendations for vitamin A use during pregnancy. Teratology 1987;35:269–275.
195. Friedman WF. Vitamin D and the supravalvular aortic stenosis syndrome. In: Woollan DHM, ed. Advances in teratology, vol 3. New York: Academic Press, 1968:83–86.
196. Jones KL. Recognition of the fetal alcohol syndrome in early infancy. Lancet 1973;2:999–1001.
197. Brown RT, Coles CD, Smith IE, et al. Effects of prenatal alcohol exposure at school age. II: attention and behavior. Neurotoxicol Teratol 1991;13:369–376.
198. Coles CD, Brown RT, Smith IE, Platzman KA, Erickson S, Falek A.

Effects of prenatal alcohol exposure at school age. I. Physical and cognitive development. Neurotoxicol Teratol 1991;13:357–367.
199. Spagnolo A. Teratogenesis of alcohol. Ann Ist Super Sanita 1993;29: 89–96.
200. Pietrantoni M, Knuppel RA. Alcohol use in pregnancy. Clin Perinatol 1991;18:93–111.
201. Pieters JJ. Nutritional teratogens: a survey of epidemiological literature. Prog Clin Biol Res 1985;163B:419–429.
202. Elhassani SB, Purohit DM, Ferlauto JJ. Maternal use of alcohol during pregnancy is a risky lifestyle. J S C Med Assoc 1996;92:128–132.
203. Plessinger MA, Woods JR Jr. Maternal, placental, and fetal pathophysiology of cocaine exposure during pregnancy. Clin Obstet Gynecol 1993;36:267–278.
204. Chavez GF, Mulinare J, Cordero JF. Maternal cocaine use during early pregnancy as a risk factor for congenital urogenital anomalies. JAMA 1989;262:795–798.

Cherry and Merkatz's Complications of Pregnancy,
Fifth Edition, edited by W. R. Cohen.
Lippincott Williams & Wilkins, Philadelphia © 2000.

CHAPTER 8

Alcohol and Substance Abuse

Cassandra E. Henderson

Abundant data exist documenting the correlation between maternal prenatal substance use and adverse perinatal outcome (1–3). In contrast, the predictive value of various patterns of drug use, such as binge, frequent or occasional, has not been established. Similarly, although it is clear that the fetus is more vulnerable to most insults early in gestation, perinatal risks of substance abuse for specific gestational ages also have not been established. Several other important clinical variables that confound the study of the effects of perinatal substance abuse include the use of multiple substances and the prevalence of psychiatric comorbidity in 56% to 92% of female substance users (4–6).

ALCOHOL ABUSE AND FETAL HEALTH

The association between maternal alcohol use and fetal malformation had been suspected by clinicians for decades; however, the syndrome was not delineated until Lemoine and colleagues published a series of 127 affected infants (7). Subsequently, Jones and Smith labeled these congenital abnormalities as fetal alcohol syndrome (FAS) in their description of a cluster of congenital birth defects observed in children born to women who were known to be addicted to alcohol (8). The constellation of FAS features consisted of growth retardation at birth and delayed growth in the postnatal period, a small head circumference, flattened midface, sunken nasal bridge, and flattened and elongated philtrum.

Despite the plethora of reports identifying the classic features of FAS, diagnosis in the neonatal period remains difficult. The characteristic facial features are often difficult to recognize and the central nervous system (CNS) dysfunction may not be evident until the infant is several years old (9,10). These delayed and subtle CNS dysfunctions caused by *in utero* alcohol exposure are perhaps the most debilitating component of FAS. Detection of developmental delays and behavioral and intellectual impairment often are detected at a time remote from the occurrence of the insult (11). These developmental and behavioral impairments can occur following consumption even of limited quantities of alcohol. Women should be aware that there is no certain level of alcohol consumption below which no risk to the fetus exists. It now appears that infants with the findings supporting a diagnosis of FAS represent only the tip of the iceberg. Most infants affected by alcohol do not demonstrate the classic findings of FAS but rather have mild dysmorphic findings accompanied by subtle developmental problems (12). These mildly affected children are described as having alcohol-related disorders (ARD). The incidence of mildly affected children who weigh less than 2,500 g at birth has been reported to be twice that in women who consume between one and two drinks per day compared with rates in infants of nondrinkers (13). Even though FAS apparently is limited to women who consume large quantities of alcohol during pregnancy, neurobehavioral deficits and intrauterine growth retardation have been reported in infants born to mothers who drink moderate quantities of alcohol during pregnancy (14). Therefore, to affect public health positively in this area, concerted efforts must be made to identify all reproductive-age, at-risk drinkers.

Extrapolation from several reports supports the supposition that the 6.7 cases per 10,000 live births incidence of FAS is an underestimate (15). In 1984, Mills and coworkers documented that one drink per day could result in neonatal alcohol-related disorders (16), a finding that is especially disturbing because 20% of all women consume some alcoholic beverage during pregnancy (17). Despite the issuance of a recommendation by the Surgeon General and the Secretary of Health and Human Services to abstain from alcohol consumption in the preconceptional and prenatal period, the Centers for Disease Control and Prevention (CDC) reported that between

C. E. Henderson: Jack D. Weiler Hospital, Bronx, NY 10461.

1991 and 1995 the percentage of women who consumed more that seven drinks per week or more than five drinks per occasion increased from 0.8% to 3.5% (18).

This increase in prenatal alcohol use may be attributable to improved self-reporting or improved detection by health care professionals. The combination of an increase in illicit drug use and the known use of alcohol as a secondary drug of abuse probably makes the reported increase in prenatal alcohol use a reliable statistic.

ALCOHOL ABUSE AND MATERNAL HEALTH

Excessive alcohol use in adults has been associated with an increased risk of premature mortality (19). Well-documented health consequences of alcohol abuse include malnutrition, trauma, hepatitis, and aspiration pneumonia. For the 20% of women who continue to use alcohol during pregnancy, drinking not only jeopardizes their health but also threatens the health of their fetus (19). Stratton and colleagues reported the results of a recent survey conducted by the Institute of Medicine suggesting that alcohol use during pregnancy may be most prevalent among girls aged 12 to 17 (17). This survey found that alcohol was preferred to cocaine or marijuana as the recreational drug of choice for both males and females in this age group.

SCREENING

Screening tests for a disease are designed to be administered to large populations not identified as being at risk for the disease. *At-risk drinking* during pregnancy (defined as having more than one ounce of alcohol per day) is not always obvious to a woman's family or health care provider. Identifying pregnancy risk drinking is difficult and requires that women in all segments of the population be screened, because such drinking is not confined to women who reside in lower socioeconomic urban areas (20). Concern about social stigmatization or disapproval from health care professionals may cause pregnant women to deny drinking or not to report accurately their total daily consumption of alcohol (21). Although obtaining a medical history through patient interviews is a time-honored tradition, several investigators have shown convincingly that this method is an insensitive method by which to determine perinatal substance use.

To enhance the ability to assess risk drinking, a four-item screening questionnaire known as T-ACE has been developed (20). This screen has been tested in minority indigent populations (22) and in an ethnically and socioeconomically diverse population (23). In contrast, three other screens used during the prenatal period—TWEAK (24), MAST (25), and CAGE—have not been evaluated in diverse populations (26).

T-ACE adds an assessment of alcohol tolerance to the three questions posed by the CAGE Screen. CAGE is more widely used on medical and surgical services. T-ACE is a mnemonic for the following questions. A total score of two or more is considered evidence of problem drinking.

Tolerance: How many drinks do you need to get high?
2 points are given if more than two drinks are needed.
Annoyance: Have you ever felt annoyed by criticism of your drinking?
1 point is given for a positive response.
Cut-down: Have you ever felt a need to cut-down on your drinking?
1 point is given for a positive response.
Eye-Opener: Have you ever taken a morning eye-opener?
1 point is given for a positive response.

T-ACE, like most clinical screening tools, sacrifices specificity and sensitivity for improved clinical simplicity. None of the screening tools currently in use is designed to identify the occasional drinker. Adding this screening tool and a nonjudgmental question that has a yes or no answer to the routine intake interview can be an effective way to identify pregnant women who drink alcoholic beverages.

TREATMENT OF ALCOHOL ADDICTION

As a special population, the gender- and situation-specific needs of women generally are not addressed by traditional alcohol treatment programs (27). Since 1970, however, the National Institute on Alcohol Abuse and Alcoholism (NIAAA) has attempted to address the dearth of research and health care services available for this population. These initiatives by NIAAA and other set-aside grants have increased gender-specific investigations of alcohol abuse and its treatment. This increased gender-specific focus, however, has not adequately addressed the unique needs of pregnant alcohol users (28).

Many pregnant women find it difficult to find a facility that will provide treatment for their addiction. Once accepted in a facility, it is unlikely that the program will be able to meet effectively the specific treatment needs and limitations presented by the pregnancy. Furthermore, concern about criminal charges and prosecution for child abuse or neglect is an obvious disincentive to seek treatment during the prenatal period. All these barriers are frequently superimposed on the woman's psychologic denial of having a drinking problem.

To date there are no well-documented successful alcohol treatment programs for pregnant women. The primary mechanism to prevent fetal and maternal alcohol-related disease is education and counseling. Women need to be aware that drinking anytime during pregnancy is dangerous. Unplanned pregnancies create even more dangers for the fetus, because drinking may occur during the most vulnerable stages of the gestation, when many women do not know they are pregnant. Although the risk of congenital malformations is greater following alcohol exposure earlier in pregnancy, there is no time during the gestation when it is safe to consume alcoholic beverages. Women unable to abstain should be encouraged to decrease their intake as much as possible. If withdrawal is likely, hospitalization is indicated. The appearance of single-sex public and private treatment programs for women may soon provide a mechanism to address the unique problems of this prenatal population (29).

TOBACCO

In 1957 Simpson and Loma reported that maternal smoking was directly correlated to the risk of low birth weight and intrauterine growth retardation (30). Subsequent data suggest that maternal smoking increases the relative risk of intrauterine fetal demise and neonatal death to 1.4 and 1.2, respectively. Obstetric complications associated with maternal tobacco use include higher rates of spontaneous abortion and preterm delivery. Women who smoke during pregnancy also have children who are more likely to have respiratory tract infections and sudden infant death syndrome. Physiologic mechanisms responsible for the perinatal risks associated with maternal tobacco use include fetal hypoxia from decreased uteroplacental perfusion and lower maternal blood pressure, which leads to decreased placental oxygenation (31).

Although the national use of tobacco has declined, the prevalence of cigarette smoking among women increased from 1990 to 1992 (32). To prevent prenatal exposure to nicotine, women contemplating pregnancy should be encouraged to stop smoking or at least to decrease the amount of tobacco used. Attempts to quit smoking are more likely to be successful if accompanied by an endorsement from a health care provider. For many persons, nicotine replacement therapy has been more effective than placebo or counseling alone (33). The safety and efficacy of nicotine replacement has not been established for pregnant women, however. Parturients who continue to smoke while using nicotine replacement may inadvertently expose their fetus to excessively high levels of nicotine. Nevertheless, for women motivated to stop smoking, the risk of continued tobacco use in pregnancy probably will outweigh the risk associated with nicotine replacement therapies that are currently marketed.

American women are exposed to ubiquitous messages alerting them to the hazards of smoking in pregnancy. Despite these warnings, many women who are seriously concerned about the well-being of their fetus continue to smoke during gestation. Published studies of smokers treated with counseling and self-help interventions have indicated that fewer than 20% of pregnant women are able to quit smoking (34,35). Hypnosis does not appear to be an effective intervention for pregnant smokers. A report from Norway compared the smoking cessation rate in a control group of pregnant women (no intervention) and a study group who received hypnosis sessions during the study period. These investigators found the smoking cessation rates were the same for the hypnosis and the control groups (36).

Although it is preferable to eliminate tobacco use before conception, many women are still smoking when they present for prenatal care. These women have continued to smoke for a variety of reasons, including an unplanned pregnancy, concern about weight gain, and the need to use tobacco during periods of stress. In a small observational study, pregnant women were found no more likely to quit smoking than nonpregnant women (37). In this same study, however, it was observed that women who did quit during pregnancy were more likely to do so in the first trimester. The greatest risk factor for continued smoking during pregnancy appears to be the number of cigarettes smoked (38). This finding is important because many smokers often increase the number of cigarettes smoked after switching to a low-tar and low-nicotine product. Despite the reported low success rate, smoking cessation should be promoted at any gestational age. There is no stage in the pregnancy when stopping or decreasing tobacco use ceases to benefit the fetus. Quitting later in gestation still has value to the growing fetus (33,39).

ILLEGAL SUBSTANCE USE

Illegal substance use during pregnancy is associated with scores of deleterious maternal and fetal effects. These adverse perinatal conditions are direct results of both drug toxicity and the lifestyle required to procure street drugs. Informing women of the risks associated with drug use is complicated by their frequent use of multiple legal and illegal drugs. For many chemically dependent women, comprehending the concept of perinatal risk is difficult because they are aware that the prenatal use of one or several substances does not always lead to undesirable perinatal outcome. To effect a change in the use of illegal substances during pregnancy, details and admonishments about perinatal risks must be accompanied by information about community treatment programs.

Statistical information presented in this chapter on the use of illegal drugs is referenced in the National Household Survey on Drug Abuse conducted by the federal government and sponsored by the Substance Abuse and Mental Health Services Administration. The survey covers residents of households; noninstitutional group quarters, such as shelters or rooming houses; and civilians living on military bases. Excluded from the survey are homeless persons who never use shelters, active military personnel, and residents of institutional group quarters such as jails and hospitals.

The frequent concurrent use of tobacco and alcohol by users of illegal substances was documented by Vega and colleagues (40). Data based on self-reports and urine toxicology from a longitudinal study of a human immunodeficiency virus (HIV) cohort indicated that, among the 42% who used hard-core drugs, 44% admitted to using multiple drugs (41). Therefore, suspected or documented use of any illegal substance should be considered a marker for the use of other licit or illicit substances.

ASSOCIATED INFECTIOUS DISEASES

Current or previous use of any illicit substance is associated with a higher risk for an infectious disease. Tuberculosis, hepatitis, HIV, and other sexually transmitted diseases cause significant maternal and neonatal morbidity. The lifestyle of this population has been characterized as "drug-seeking behavior." Activities to secure drugs include employment in the sex industry, sharing needles, or engaging in sexual activities with multiple partners. A recent report indicated that maternal cocaine, opiates, or methadone use increases the mother's risk of HIV seropositivity at delivery [odds ratio (OR), 3.08] (41). Several studies have shown that a history of crack cocaine use is an independent risk factor for HIV infection (42–44).

All women with a history of current or previous illegal substance use certainly should be screened for these associated infectious diseases. Because it is clear that the prevalence of substance abuse in all populations is underreported, however, all women should be offered and encouraged to accept screening for tuberculosis, hepatitis, HIV, gonorrhea, and syphilis during their first prenatal encounter.

MARIJUANA

The use of marijuana by adolescents continues to increase despite major efforts to decrease its use and availability. Like alcohol and tobacco, marijuana is a substance often abused by users of cocaine and opiates (45). No evidence exists that marijuana is teratogenic. In the 1980's, conflicting reports that addressed the association between marijuana use and preterm delivery were published. Fried and colleagues (46) found that an increased risk of prematurity accompanied perinatal use of marijuana. In the same year, Tennes and co-workers (47) found no increase in preterm deliveries for women using marijuana during pregnancy. These conflicting findings may be due to the confounding presence of known risk factors for prematurity. The most commonly encountered of these risks for preterm delivery are poverty and the use of other legal and illegal substances. No association has been found between perinatal marijuana use and early fetal loss (48).

Unlike the screening tests for most illicit substances, the high lipid solubility of cannabis makes urine screening tests sensitive for several days after its use. The best use of marijuana screening tests in perinatal risk assessment models is as a marker for likely use of other substances, such as tobacco, alcohol, and cocaine. Although controversy exists concerning the specific hazards of marijuana use in pregnancy, it is clear that perinatal outcome is adversely affected by the use of the other licit and illicit substances.

In a study of 143 postpartum women, Singer and colleagues observed that women who used cocaine during pregnancy were likely to have started marijuana use by their midteen years (49). This finding, accompanied by lay press reports of increased marijuana use among adolescents, has obvious implications for the efforts of public health and law enforcement officials to control the supply and use of illicit substances.

COCAINE

In 1990 it was estimated that 10% to 15% of pregnant women used cocaine (50). Cocaine consumption peaked in 1985, when the national estimate by the annual National Household Survey on Drug Abuse (NHSD) was 5.7 million users. The most recently released NHSD report from 1996 indicates that the rate of use remained mostly the same between 1995 and 1996 at 1.45 million and 1.75 million, respectively. A dramatic increase in cocaine-affected pregnancies accompanied the widespread use of alkaloidal (crack) cocaine. In contrast to the heat-labile form of the drug, which is administered across mucous membranes or parenterally, this potent heat stable form of the drug can be smoked and is easily manufactured using ammonia or sodium bicarbonate and water. Smoking crack cocaine leads rapidly to a high serum-drug level. This almost instantaneous euphoria often lasts for only 5 to 10 minutes and is quickly addictive.

Despite widespread educational campaigns, cocaine use remains a significant contributor to adverse perinatal outcome. Physiologic effects of its use include euphoria, vasoconstriction, and tachycardia. In numerous uncontrolled descriptive studies, maternal use of cocaine was associated with adverse perinatal outcome. Affected pregnancies were reported to have higher rates of low-birth-weight infants, premature delivery, and premature rupture of membranes (51,52). Perinatal cocaine use also is associated with higher rates of maternal morbidity and mortality. Case reports have associated prenatal cocaine use with *abruptio placentae* and maternal cerebral vascular accidents (53,54). In a controlled study comparing prenatal marijuana, tobacco, and alcohol use with cocaine use, Martin and colleagues observed that the infants exposed to cocaine *in utero* had a lower mean birth weight, smaller mean head circumference, and shorter mean gestational age. This study also found that cocaine exposure resulted in significant alteration in the infants' sucking, reflexes, and behavioral state (55). In another study that controlled for confounding substances, infant neurobehavioral changes considered to be associated with perinatal cocaine exposure were observed to persist for 6 years in a targeted pediatric population (56). Newborns exposed *in utero* to cocaine may exhibit symptoms consistent with cocaine withdrawal. These affected infants have tremulousness, irritability, and an inability to suck properly (57).

Drug-seeking activities and cocaine-induced vasculopathy may increase the risk of vertical HIV transmission. It is hypothesized that vasculitis associated with cocaine administration may reduce natural barriers to vertical transmission by altering the maternal-fetal interface (placentitis or chorioamnionitis) or affecting the fetal blood–brain barrier (58).

Urine screening for cocaine is a valuable clinical and research tool for assessing recent use. In contrast, more remote use of cocaine can be determined by analyzing cocaine bound to hair. Recent reports indicate, however, that the hair test results may be affected by hair type. Joseph and co-workers found binding to be affected by gender and racial differences in density of melanin binding sites (59). The clinical significance of this report remains to be evaluated.

OPIATES

Opium is a mixture of alkaloids derived from the seeds of the poppy plant. Morphine and codeine are derived from opium. Heroin and hydromorphone (Dilaudid) are semisynthetic opiates. Heroin was developed in 1874 as a presumed nonaddicting treatment for morphine addiction. As crack and other forms of cocaine are decreasing in popularity, abuse of other opiates is increasing. The 1995 NHSD estimated that 1.4 million people have used heroin in their lifetime, double the estimate from 1994. Pure heroin is rarely sold on the street. Rather, the 100-mg bags of powder that are sold as heroin have a purity that previously ranged from 1% to 10% but recently has been reported to range between 1% and 98%. The various diluents include sugar, starch, powdered milk, or quinine. The higher purity of currently available heroin has allowed users to snort or smoke the drug rather than use the more dangerous parenteral administration. Smoking purer forms of heroin has created a more socially acceptable means by which heroin cravings can be satisfied. In addition, users can avoid HIV exposure from sharing needles by smoking the drug. This combination of characteristics probably led to the dramatic resurgence of heroin use in recent years.

The primary psychologic effects of opiate use include analgesia, sedation, feelings of well-being, and euphoria. Tolerance develops to these effects, and higher doses are required to prevent withdrawal. Signs and symptoms of narcotic withdrawal include lacrimation, rhinorrhea, yawning, sweating, restlessness, abdominal cramps, tremor, insomnia, hypertension, and muscle spasms. In pregnancy, signs and symptoms of abrupt cessation of narcotics may be accompanied by intrauterine fetal death (60).

The use of heroin during pregnancy is associated with higher rates of stillbirths, intrauterine growth retardation, prematurity, and neonatal mortality (61). Enrollment in a methadone maintenance program is associated with improved perinatal outcome for pregnant heroin users. This improvement is manifested by longer gestational age and increased birth weight; however, infants exposed to methadone *in utero* have a lower birth weight and smaller head circumference than neonates not exposed to any opiates *in utero* (62). Findings consistent with narcotic withdrawal are observed in 30% to 90% of infants born to narcotic-addicted women. These affected infants may present with high-pitched cry, poor feeding, hypertonicity, tremors, irritability, sneezing, sweating, vomiting, diarrhea, and seizures (63). Signs of withdrawal appear in infants of heroin-addicted women within 24 to 72 hours. Appearance of withdrawal signs in infants of methadone-addicted women may not occur for up to 10 days after birth. It is important that infants of methadone-addicted mothers be under medical supervision for at least this period. No long-term effect on development has been found in the offspring of narcotic-addicted women (64).

Synthetic derivatives of narcotics such as fentanyl or meperidine are used to manufacture designer drugs as a substitute for controlled opiates. The street names of these substances change frequently and vary by geographic location. The current street names of some fentanyl analogs include China White, synthetic heroin, Tango and Cass, and Goodfella. MPPP (1-methyl-4-phenyl-4-propionoxypiperidine) and PEPAP (1-[2-phenylethyl]-4-acetyloxypiperdine) are meperidine analogs known on the street as *new heroin*. The toxic effects of smoking, intravenous or intranasal administration of designer drugs mirror the complications of opiate use.

HALLUCINOGENIC AND INHALED SUBSTANCES

Several times per year, the National Institute of Drug Abuse at the National Institutes of Health provides data on national trends in drug abuse. Epidemiologic data provided in the following section were abstracted from the February 1998 Directors Report from Epidemiology, Etiology and Prevention Research Branch of the National Institute of Drug Abuse.

AMPHETAMINES

Amphetamines have vasoconstrictive properties similar to those of cocaine. They can be smoked, taken orally, intranasally, or intravenously. The smoking of crystalline methamphetamine ("ice" or "blue ice") in pregnancy is associated with perinatal complications similar to those observed with perinatal cocaine use. *In utero* exposure to amphetamines has been associated with reduced fetal head circumference, *abruptio placentae*, intrauterine growth restriction, and intrauterine fetal demise (65). Methylenedioxymethamphetaine (MDMA) know as "ecstasy," "Adam," or "X-TC," is an amphetamine-like compound. Another related ephedrine-based product, known as herbal ecstasy, is widely available in convenience stores and truck stops. Although no information is available concerning the use of MDMA in pregnancy, it is believed the effects are similar to those observed with perinatal amphetamine use.

TOLUENE

Toluene (methylbenzene) is an aromatic hydrocarbon used as an organic solvent in common products such as gasoline, glue, and paint (66). "Glue sniffing," or "huffing," is an intentional form of exposure to toluene vapors that results in mind-altering experiences. Users exhibit confusion, auditory and visual hallucinations, and incoordination (67). The low cost and wide availability of substances containing toluene have resulted in the continued abuse of this substance. Reports from the early 1980's indicated that 10% of adolescents surveyed occasionally inhaled toluene as a recreational drug (68). More recent data from a national survey documented that 20% of recent high school students admitted to abusing toluene at least once (69).

Animal studies have shown a positive association between toluene exposure and intrauterine growth restriction (70). In humans, intrauterine toluene exposure has been associated with a craniofacial dysmorphogenesis similar to those reported after prenatal alcohol exposure (71). Toluene-exposed fetuses are described as having small palpebral fissures, thin upper lip, and midface hypoplasia (72).

Although human and animal studies suggest that toluene is a teratogen, conclusive evidence does not exist. Establishing that toluene is a human teratogen is complicated by maternal abuse of multiple agents, particularly alcohol. Furthermore, the effect of toluene on perinatal outcome may be mediated in part by maternal acidosis caused by toluene-induced renal damage. Maternal acidosis may result in decreased uterine perfusion and lead to fetal hypoperfusion and ischemia (73).

SUBSTANCE ABUSE TREATMENT

Pregnancy offers a unique opportunity to engage substance-abusing women in cessation programs. Studies have shown that 17% to 40% of smokers were able to quit during pregnancy, although many resumed smoking after delivery (74). Similarly, most alcohol users have been found to reduce or cease consumption during pregnancy (46). Effective treatment of cocaine dependence during pregnancy using a mutifaceted approach has been reported recently (75). This comprehensive regimen of contingency management interventions (CMI) has been reviewed in multiple reports. CMI as described by Elk and colleagues includes weekly prenatal care visits and semiweekly individual and weekly group behavioral-based drug counseling sessions (75). Prenatal care visits encompass serial nutritional and HIV counseling sessions. In addition, the CMI provides monetary gifts for cocaine-free urine samples. This intensive treatment program appears to be effective in promoting cocaine abstinence and prenatal care compliance. Using case management, Laken and Ager reported a similar effect on abstinence and retention in outpatient drug treatment (76). In a subsequent study, Laken and colleagues found that the use of case management and the threat of involving child protective services increased retention in substance abuse treatment during pregnancy (77). This higher retention rate was associated with a decrease in illicit drug use and a higher infant birth weight. The reports by the Elk and colleagues and the Laken and Ager group suggest that improved access to comprehensive compassionate substance abuse treatment programs is required to interrupt long-term use of substances by women. Hser and colleagues found that prior treatment experience and legal coercion motivated pregnant women to seek treatment for substance abuse (78). Although these effective treatment programs are labor intensive, involving social workers, the case manager, and the primary health care provider, the reported outcome is desirable. Pregnancy appears to present an excellent opportunity to engage substance users in such community-based programs.

Interventions for treatment and prevention have engendered lively political and community discussions. A 1995 report of national policies and practices of state directors of substance abuse services documented a lack of coordination among public health substance initiatives directed at reproductive and infant health (79). Subsequent to this report, budget cuts have led to a reduction in federally funded treatment programs. Concurrently, we have witnessed the implementation of state required mandatory reporting of positive maternal or neonatal toxicology results (80). Punitive measures are unlikely to reduce the incidence of substance use or abuse by pregnant women.

In an effort to control quality and cost, many managed care organizations (MCOs) regulate the provision of substance abuse services. Larson and colleagues presented data describing the potential opportunities MCOs have to impact positively the services provided to a substance-abusing population. MCOs could use case managers effectively to facilitate the provision of comprehensive services by teams of psychiatric and primary care providers. Prevention and treatment protocols established by MCO may lead to the development of model programs for the health care of addicted persons (81). Using their own infrastructure, local organizations modeled on successful MCOs could coordinate many of the necessary health care systems needed for community-wide perinatal substance abuse programs (82,83).

Prevention and treatment plans must be grounded in the fact that addiction is not a voluntary condition but a chronic illness. Intervention programs must become more widely available and accepting of women whether they are pregnant or not pregnant. Intervention plans for addicted women should be developed to address gender differences in the etiology and manifestations of addiction. Women who abuse substances are more likely than men to give specific reasons for starting drug use. Women, unlike men, do not often start drug use as a part of an overall pattern of antisocial behavior, but rather women begin abusing substances following an event such as a divorce, job loss, health problems, or sexual abuse. Several investigators reported that a substantial proportion of chemically dependent women have been raped (84), have been victims of childhood sexual abuse (85), or have been been victims of domestic violence (86).

To be effective, interventions for substance abuse and other undesirable social activity must ensure that basic housing, food, and clothing needs are fulfilled (87). This approach is consistent with the psychotherapy proposition described by Maslow, who showed that higher-order psychological growth cannot be accomplished until survival needs have been met (88). Demographic variables considered by Haller and colleagues in an evaluation of perinatal substance abuse treatment were housing status and trimester of pregnancy at the time of enrollment in the treatment program. Psychologic outcome variables in this study included treatment resistance and the presence or absence of an antisocial personality disorder. Haller and colleagues found that women who were provided housing were less likely to discontinue treatment prematurely (87).

Methadone is the only medical addiction treatment for which there are meaningful perinatal outcome data; however, a new treatment for opiate addiction, levomethadyl acetate hydrochloride (LAAM), was approved in 1993. The long half-life of LAAM prevents withdrawal using a weekly administration of only three times. Methadone, in contrast, must be ingested daily. As a group, pregnant women may be excellent candidates for this long-acting drug treatment of opiate addiction. Although women respond to LAAM as well as do men, currently no data are available concerning the use of LAAM in pregnancy (89).

Despite the paucity of trials that demonstrate effective methods to treat substance abuse in pregnancy, there is evidence that early and regular prenatal care is effective in improving perinatal outcome for this group of women. Information about the benefit of prenatal care for this population is provided in the 1988 National Maternal and Infant Health Survey conducted by the National Center for Health Statistics. Data from this survey suggest that prenatal care may alleviate some of the adverse perinatal outcomes associated with abuse of multiple substances, such as alcohol, tobacco, and cocaine. This modulating effect of prenatal care was observed even if women continued to use substances throughout their pregnancy (90). Clearly, improving access to prenatal care services by developing community prenatal care sites and increasing perinatal outreach services for high-risk obstetric and pediatric care is likely to benefit groups of chemically dependent women.

To treat substance users effectively before and during pregnancy, clinicians must be diligent in making the diagnosis by maintaining a high index of suspicion. In addition, health care providers must be nonjudgmental and become acquainted with appropriate treatment facilities in each community they serve.

REFERENCES

1. Roland EG, Volpe JJ. Effect of maternal cocaine use on the fetus and newborn: review of the literature. Pediatr Neurosci 1995;15:88–94.
2. Wolman I, Niv D, Yovel I, Pauser D, Geller E, David MP. Opioid-addicted parturient, labor and outcome: a reappraisal. Obstet Gynecol Surv 989;44:592–597.
3. Zuckerman B, Frank DA, Hingson R, et al. Effects of maternal marijuana and cocaine use on fetal growth. N Engl J Med 1989;320:762–768.
4. Haver B, Dahlgren L. Early treatment of women with alcohol addiction (EWA): a comprehensive evaluation and outcome study. I. Patterns of psychiatric comorbidity at intake. Addiction 1995;90:101–109.
5. Rowe MG, Gleming MF, Barry KL, Manwell LB, Kroop S. Correlates of depression in primary care. Fam Pract 1995;41:551–558.
6. Regier DA, Farmer ME, Rae DS, et al. Comorbidity of mental disorders with alcohol and other drug abuse: results from the Epidiological Catchment Area (ECA) study. JAMA 1990;254:2511–2518.
7. Lemoine P, Harouseau H, Borteyra JP, Menuet JC. Les enfants de parents alcoliques anomalites observées: apropos de 127 cas. Oues Med 1968;2:476–482.
8. Jones KL, Smith DW. Recognition of the fetal alcohol syndrome in early infant. Lancet 1973;2:999–1001.
9. Sokol, RJ, Clarren SK. Guidelines for use of terminology describing the impact of prenatal alcohol on the offspring. Alcohol Clin Exp Res 1989;13:597–598.
10. Little BB, Snell LM, Rosenfeld, CR, Gilstrap LC, Gant NF. Failure to recognize fetal alcohol syndrome in newborn infants. Am J Dis Child 1990;144:1142–1146.
11. Sokol RJ, Clarren SK. Guidelines for use of terminology describing the impact of prenatal alcohol on the offspring. Alcohol Clin Exp Res 1989;13:597–598.
12. Jacobson JL, Jacobson SE. Prenatal alcohol exposure and neurobehavioral development. Alcohol Health Res World 1994;18:30–36.
13. Cook, et al. Alcohol, tobacco and other drugs may harm the unborn. USDJJS Pub. No 90-1711, 1990:16.
14. Little RE, Asker RL, Sampson PD, Renwick JH. Fetal growth and moderate drinking in early pregnancy. Am J Epidemiol 1989;123:270–278.
15. Centers for Disease Control and Prevention. Update: frequent alcohol consumption among women of childbearing age—behavior risk factor surveillance system, 1991. MMWR 1994;43:328–329,335.
16. Mills JL, Graubard BI, Harley EE, Rhoads GG, Berendes HW. Maternal alcohol consumption and birthweight. JAMA 1984;252:1875–1879.
17. Stratton K, Howe C, Battaglia F, eds. Institute of Medicine summary: fetal alcohol syndrome. Washington, DC: National Academy Press, 1996.
18. Centers for Disease Control and Prevention. Alcohol consumption among pregnant and childbearing-aged women—United States, 1991 and 1995. MMWR 1997;46:346–349.
19. U.S. Department of Health and Human Services. Eight Special Report to the US Congress on Alcohol and Health from the Secretary of Health and Human Services, September 1993. Washington, DC: U.S. Department of Health and Human Services, Public Health Service, National Institutes of Health, National Institute on Alcohol Abuse and Alcoholism, Publication ADM-281-91-003, 1993.
20. Sokol RJ, Martier SS, Ager JW. T-ACE questions: practical prenatal detection of risk-drinking. Am J Obstet Gynecol 1989;160:863–871.

21. Verkerk PH. The impact of alcohol misclassification on the relationship between alcohol and pregnancy outcome. Int J Epidemiol 1992;21: S33–S37.
22. Russell M, Martier SS, Sokol RJ, Mudar P, Jacobson S, Jacobson J. Detecting risk drinking during pregnancy: a comparison of four screening questionnaires. Am J Public Health 1996;86:1435–1439.
23. Chang G, Wilkins-Haug L, Berman S, Goetz MA, Heidi Behr, Hiley A. Alcohol use and pregnancy: improving identification. Obstet Gynecol 1998;91:892–898.
24. Russell M, Bigler L. Screening for alcohol-related problems in an outpatient obstetric-gynecologic clinic. Am J Obstet Gynecol 1979;134:4–12.
25. Selzer MI. The Michigan alcoholism screening test: the quest for a new diagnostic instrument. Am J Psychiatry 1971;127:1653–1558.
26. Ewing JA. Detecting alcoholism: the CAGE questionnaire. JAMA 1984;252:1905–1907.
27. National Council on Alcoholism. A federal response to a hidden epidemic. alcohol and other drug problems among women. Washington, DC: National Council on Alcoholism, 1987.
28. United States General Accounting Office. ADMS Block Grant: Women's set-aside does not assure drug treatment for pregnant women. Washington, DC: US General Accounting Office, 1991.
29. Sandmaier M. Women helping women: opening the door to treatment. Alcohol Health Res World 1977;2:17–23.
30. Simpson WJ, Loma LA. Preliminary report on cigarette smoking and its effect on birth weight. Am J Obstet Gynecol 1957;73:808–815.
31. Morrow RJ, Ritchie JK, Bull SB. Maternal cigarette smoking: the effects on umbilical and uterine blood flow velocity. Am J Obstet Gynecol 1988;159:1069–1071.
32. Fiore MC, Novotny TE, Pierce JP, Hatziandreu EJ, Patel KM, Davis RM. Trends in cigarette smoking in the United States: the changing influence of gender and race. JAMA 1989;261:49–55.
33. The Smoking Cessation Clinical Practice Guideline Panel. The Agency for Health Care Policy and Research smoking cessation clinical practice guideline. JAMA 1996;275:1270–1280.
34. Hjalmarson A, Hahn L, Svanberg B. Stopping smoking in pregnancy: effect of a self-help manual in controlled trial. Br J Obstet Gynaecol 1991;98:260–264.
35. Windsor RA, Cutter G, Morris J, et al. The effectiveness of smoking cessation methods for smokers in public health maternity clinics: a randomized trial. Am J Public Health 1985;75:1389–1392.
36. Valbo A, Eide T. Smoking cessation in pregnancy: the effect of hypnosis in a randomized study. Addict Behav 1996;21:29–35.
37. Hutchison KE, Stevens VM, Collins FL. Cigarette smoking and the intention to quit among pregnant smokers. J Behav Med 1996;19; 307–316.
38. Cnattingius S. Smoking habits in early pregnancy. Addict Behav 1989; 14:453–457.
39. Gloyd RL, Rimer BK, Giovino GA, Mullen PD, Sullivan SE. A review of smoking in pregnancy: effects on pregnancy outcomes and cessation efforts. Annu Rev Publ Health 1993;14:379–411.
40. Vega WA, Kolody B, Hwang J, Noble A. Prevalence and magnitude of perinatal substance exposures in California. N Engl J Med 1993;329: 850–854.
41. Rodiquez EM, Mofenson LM, Chang BH, et al. Association of maternal drug use during pregnancy with maternal HIV transmission. AIDS 1996,10:273–282.
42. Fullilove RE, Fullilove MT, Bower BP, Gross SA. Risk of sexually transmitted disease among black adolescent crack users in Oakland and San Francisco, California. JAMA 1990;263:851–855.
43. Ellerbrock TV, Lieb S, Harrington PE, et al. Heterosexually transmitted human immunodeficiency virus infection among pregnant women in a rural Florida community. N Engl J Med 1992;327:1704–1709
44. Lindsay MK, Peterson HB, Boring J, Gramling J, Willis S, Klein L. Crack cocaine: a risk factor for human immunodeficiency virus infection type 1 among inner-city parturients. Obstet Gynecol 1992;80:981–984.
45. National Institute of Drug and Alcohol Abuse. National pregnancy and health survey-drug use among women delivering livebirths. Rockville, MD: NCADI Publication no. BKD192, 1992.
46. Fried PA, Barnes MV, Drake ER Soft drug use after pregnancy compared to use before and during pregnancy. Am Obstet Gynecol 1985; 151:787–792.
47. Tennes K, Avitable N, Blockard C, Bogles C, Hassoun B, Holmes L, Kreye M. NIDA Res Monogr 1985;59:48–60.
48. Wilcox AJ, Weinberg CR, Baird DD. Risk factors for early pregnancy loss. Epidemiology 1990;1:382–385.
49. Singer L, Arendt R, Minnes S, Farkas K, Yamashita T, Kliegman R. J Subst Abuse 1995;7:265–274.
50. Centers for Disease Control and Prevention. Statewide prevalence of illicit drug use by pregnant women—Rhode Island. MMWR 1990;14: 225–227.
51. Chasnoff IJ, Burns WJ, Schnoll SH, Burns KA. Cocaine use in pregnancy. N Engl J Med 1985;313:666–669.
52. Chasnoff IJ, Griffith DR, MacGregor S, Dirkes D, Burns KA. Temporal patterns of cocaine use in pregnancy: perinatal outcome. JAMA 1989;261:1741–1744.
53. Acker E, Sachs BP, Tracey KJ, Wise WE. Abruptio placentae associated with cocaine use. Am J Obstet Gynecol 1983;146:220–221.
54. Henderson CE, Torbey M. Rupture of intracranial aneurysm associated with cocaine use during pregnancy. Am J Perinatol 1988;5:142–143.
55. Martin JC, Barr HM, Martin DC, Streissguth AP. Neonatal neurobehavioral outcome following prenatal exposure to cocaine. Neurotoxicol Teratol 1996;18:617–625.
56. Richardson GA, Conroy ML, Day NL. Prenatal cocaine exposure: effects on the development of school-age children. Neurotoxicol Teratol 1996;18:627–634.
57. Chasnoff IJ. Newborn infants with drug withdrawal symptoms. Pediatr Rev 1988;9:273–277.
58. Lyman WD. Perinatal AIDS: drugs of abuse and transplacental infection. Adv Exp Med Biol 1993;325:211–217.
59. Joseph RE, Tsai WJ, Tsao LI, Su TP, Cone EJ. In vivo characterization of cocaine binding sites in human hair. J Pharmacol Exp Ther 1997;282;1228–1241.
60. Zuspan FP, Gumpel JA, Mejia-Zelaya A, Madden J, Davis R. Fetal stress from methadone withdrawal. Am J Obstet Gynecol 1975;122: 43–46.
61. Fricker HS, Segal S. Narcotic addiction, pregnancy, and the newborn. Am J Dis Child 1978;132:360–366.
62. Newman RG, Bashkow S, Calko D. Results of 313 consecutive live births of infants delivered to patients in the New York City Methadone Maintenance Treatment Program. Am J Obstet Gynecol 1975;121: 233–237.
63. Ostrea EM, Chavez CJ, Strauss ME. A study of factors that influence the severity of neonatal narcotic withdrawal. J Pediatr 1976;88: 642–645.
64. Chasnoff IJ. Effects of maternal narcotic vs nonnarcotic addiction on neonatal neurobehavior and infant development. In: Pinkert TM, ed. Consequences of maternal drug abuse. Rockville, MD: Department of Health and Human Services. DJJS publication no. (ADM) 85-1400, 1985:84–95.
65. Oro AS, Dixon SD. Perinatal cocaine and methamphetamine exposure: maternal and neonatal correlates. J Pediatr 1987;111:571–578.
66. U.S. Public Health Service, Agency for Toxic Substances and Disease Registry. Toxicological profile for toluene. (In collaboration with U.S. Environmental Protection Agency), Atlanta, GA: USPHS, 1989.
67. Winkler M. Glue sniffing in children and adolescents. NY State Med J 1965;65:1984–1989.
68. Lowenstein LF. Recent research into glue-sniffing: extent of the problem, its repercussions and treatment approaches. Int J Soc Psychol 1985;31:93–97.
69. National survey results on drug use from the Monitoring the Future Study, 1975–1991, vol 1. Secondary school and college students study, NIDA 93-3480 Rockville, MD: NIDA.
70. Ungvary G, Tatrai E. On the embryotoxic effects of benzene and its alkyl derivatives in mice, rats and rabbits. Arch Toxicol 1985;8: 425–430.
71. Goodwin TM. Toulene abuse and renal tubular acidosis. Obstet Gynecol 1988;71:715–718.
72. Pearson MS, Hoyme LE, Seaver LH, Rimsza ME. Toluene embryopathy: delineation of the phenotype and comparison with fetal alcohol syndrome. Pediatrics 1994;93:211–215.
73. Blechner JN, Stenger VG, Prystowsky H. Blood flow to the human uterus during maternal metabolic acidosis. Am J Obstet Gynecol 1975; 121:789–794.
74. Quinn VP, Mullen PD, Ershoff DH. Women who stop smoking spontaneously prior to prenatal care and predictors of relapse before delivery. Addict Behav 1991;16:29–40.
75. Elk R, Mangus L, Rhoades H, Andres R, Grabowski J. Cessation of cocaine use during pregnancy: effects of contingency management interventions on maintaining abstinence and complying with prenatal care. Addict Behav 1998;23:57–64.

76. Laken MP, Ager J. Effects of case management on retention in prenatal substance abuse treatment. Am J Drug Alcohol Abuse 1996;22:439–448.
77. Laken MP, McComish JF, Ager J. Predictors of prenatal substance use and birth weight during outpatient treatment. J Subst Abuse Treat 1997; 14:359–366 .
78. Hser YI, Maglione MA, Polinsky ML, Anglin MD. Predicting treatment entry among treatment-seeking drug abusers. J Subst Abuse Treat 1997;14:1–8.
79. Chavkin W, Breitbart V, Wise PH. Efforts to reduce perinatal mortality, HIV, and drug addiction: surveys of the states. J Am Med Wom Assoc 1995;50:164–166.
80. Chavkin W, Breitbart V, Elman D, Wise PH. National Survey of States: policies and practices regarding drug-using pregnant women. Am J Public Health 1998;88:117–119 .
81. Larson MJ, Samet JH, McCarty D. Med Clin North Am 1997;81: 1053–1069.
82. DeLeon G, Jainchill N. Residential therapeutic communities for female substance abusers. Bull NY Acad Med 1991;67:277–290.
83. Giles W, Patterson T, Sanders RN, Batey R, Thomas D, Collins J. Aust N Z J Obstet Gynaecol 1989;29:225–229.
84. Teets JM. The incidence and experience of rape among chemically dependent women. J Psychoacitve Drugs 1997;29:331–336.
85. Teets JM. Childood sexual trauma of chemically dependent women. J Psychoactive Drugs 1995;27:231–238.
86. Stark E, Filcraft A, Zuckerman D, Grey A, Robison J, Frazier W. Wife abuse in the medical setting: an introduction for health personnel. Rockville, MD: National Clearinghouse on Domestic Violence.
87. Haller DL, Kinisely JS, Elswick RK, Dawson KS, Schnoll SH. Perinatal substance abusers: factors influencing treatment retention. J Subst Abuse Treat 1997;12:513–519.
88. Maslow AH. Some basic propositions of growth and self actualizing psychology. In: Perceiving, behaving, becoming: a new focus for education. Washington, DC: Yearbook of the Association for Supervision and Curriculum Development, 1962.
89. Eissenberg T, Bigelow GE, Strain EC, et al. Dose-related efficacy of levomethadyl acetate for treatment of opioid dependence. JAMA 1997; 277:1945–1951.
90. Faden VB, Hanna E, Graubard BI. The effect of positive and negative health behavior during gestation on pregnancy outcome. J Subst Abuse 1997;9:63–76.

SECTION III

Psychiatric Disorders

Cherry and Merkatz's Complications of Pregnancy,
Fifth Edition, edited by W. R. Cohen.
Lippincott Williams & Wilkins, Philadelphia © 2000.

CHAPTER 9

Psychosocial and Psychiatric Issues

Joan R. Youchah and James David

The practice of obstetrics and gynecology frequently includes diagnosing and treating or referring patients with psychological and psychiatric difficulties. As the scope of practice for women's health care providers is broadened to include functions formerly expected of traditional primary care physicians, even greater emphasis is warranted on screening for mental disorders (1–3). This chapter endeavors to assist clinicians in obstetrics and gynecology in reviewing and referencing the material that will support the improved identification of psychiatric symptoms and disorders, as well as to encourage a heightened awareness of the complex psychosocial concomitants and stressors associated with the health and development of women (4,5).

The expectation of a thorough physician, regardless of one's area of specialization, is to elicit and directly address issues of emotional distress. The initial evaluation of the severity of this distress is immediate, and the decision as to reassurance versus treatment versus referral, or a combination of these, is warranted at the time of visit. At a minimum, all clinicians must screen for the presence of suicidality or psychosis in all patients who appear to be experiencing moderate or severe emotional pain or turmoil or other visible indications of mental decompensation. A majority of completed suicides occur in patients who have visited physicians in the previous 6-month period (1,6,7).

J. R. Youchah and J. David: Department of Psychiatry, Albert Einstein College of Medicine, Bronx, NY 10461.

PSYCHIATRIC DISORDERS

The lexicon of psychiatry and psychology is often imprecise, and the jargon that has evolved further obscures clear communication between patient and clinician, and even between clinicians. Those of us who are not primarily mental health experts are often confronted by the resultant schism, which operates at the level of language and vocabulary, and interferes with optimal patient evaluation and care. *The Diagnostic and Statistical Manual of Mental Disorders,* now in its fourth major revision—the so-called DSM-IV—reflects a tremendous effort to standardize, on an international basis, the terms applied and the disorders and syndromes recognized in the modern practice of psychiatry. For example, the syndrome of schizophrenia, paranoid type, is defined in specific detail. The diagnostic criteria for this disease are delineated in sufficient detail so that a clinician in New York City and one in Tierra del Fuego, if presented with the same patient, would assign the same diagnosis. Similarly, terms such as "obsession," "delusion," and "flight of ideas" are defined in the DSM-IV's Appendix C: Glossary of techical terms. The critical role of the DSM series in research, education, and the practice of psychiatry cannot be overemphasized, and arguably, all health providers would benefit from an available copy (8).

DSM-IV consists largely of the descriptions of the DSM-IV–recognized disorders. As such, one can read the diagnostic criteria required to assign the diagnosis of obsessive-compulsive disorder; the associated descriptive features and comorbid mental disorders; associated laboratory findings, physical examination findings, and general medical conditions (if any); culture, age, and gender features; prevalence; course; and familial patterns. Treatment information, around which consensus is far more variable, is not addressed in the DSM series. Information concerning some of the more prevalent disorders likely to be encountered in pregnant women is briefly reviewed:

MOOD DISORDERS

The DSM-IV precisely defines the criteria signs and symptoms that constitute a major depressive episode, a manic episode, and a mixed episode. These episodes do not constitute disorders, but are elements of establishing a diagnosis of major depressive disorder, bipolar disorder, and other disorders.

A major depressive episode is defined as at least a 2-week period of patient-reported depressed mood or the patient's loss of interest or pleasure in virtually all activities. Four or more additional symptoms also must be endorsed from a list of seven possible symptom areas, which include appetite disturbance or significant weight change; insomnia or hypersomnia; restlessness or conspicuous physical appearance of motionlessness; loss of energy; feeling worthless or guilty; diminished concentration or marked indecisiveness; or persistent thoughts of death or suicidality. The full DSM-IV criteria are provided in Table 9-1 and are included because of the importance of this particular constellation of symptoms and to illustrate criterion-based diagnostic methodology. The criteria for making a diagnosis of major depressive disorder, either recurrent or single episode, are then simply counting the major depressive episodes to date. Of note, when the symptoms are attributable to a general medical condition etiology (e.g., hypothyroidism), the diagnosis is clearly distinguished from the above and is established as a mood disorder due to hypothyroidism, with depressive features (8).

The DSM-IV does not recognize postpartum depressions as a separate diagnostic category among the mood disorders, but expects the diagnosing clinician to modify a diagnosis of major depressive disorder, bipolar disorders, or brief psychotic disorder to include the specifier "with postpartum onset" if the episode begins within 4 weeks of giving birth. Note that the diagnostic criteria for the clinical syndrome itself are otherwise the same; a major depressive episode in an elderly man versus one in a young postpartum woman are not symptomatically distinguishable syndromes, other than by the temporal proximity to childbirth in the latter. The recommendations for treatment are essentially the same in both cases (1,9).

TABLE 9-1. *Major depressive episode*

To diagnose a major depressive episode, five (or more) of the following symptoms must have been present during the same 2-week period, representing a change from previous functioning. At least one of the symptoms must be (1) depressed mood or (2) loss of interest or pleasure.

1. depressed mood most of the day, nearly every day, as indicated by either subjective report or observation made by others
2. markedly diminished interest or pleasure in all, or almost all, activities most of the day, nearly every day
3. significant weight loss when not dieting, or weight gain (e.g., a change of more than 5% of body weight in a month), or decrease or increase in appetite nearly every day
4. insomnia or hypersomnia nearly every day
5. psychomotor agitation or retardation nearly every day (observable by others, not merely subjective feelings of restlessness or being slowed down)
6. fatigue or loss of energy nearly every day
7. feelings of worthlessness or excessive or inappropriate guilt (which may be delusional) nearly every day (not merely self-reproach or guilt about being sick)
8. diminished ability to think or concentrate, or indecisiveness, nearly every day
9. recurrent thoughts of death (not just fear of dying), recurrent suicidal ideation without a specific plan, or a suicide attempt, or a specific plan for committing suicide

In addition, the symptoms must cause clinically significant distress or impairment in social or occupational functioning; and cannot be due to the direct physiological effects of a substance (e.g., alcohol or another drug of abuse, a medication) or a general medical condition (e.g., hypothyroidism).

From the American Psychiatric Association. Diagnostic and statistical manual of mental disorders, 4th ed. Washington, DC: American Psychiatric Association, 1994.

The lifetime incidence of a major depressive disorder is approximately 20% in women (10% in men), and in women of reproductive age the prevalence is approximately 8%, with a mean age of onset at 40 years. Fewer than one third of these women receive appropriate medical treatment despite the incontrovertible efficacy of antidepressants (with or without psychotherapy), with two thirds of treated patients showing remission or marked improvement. The population risk for postpartum depressions is reported to be on the order of 1 in 10; however, after an initial episode, this risk climbs fivefold to 1 in 2 after subsequent pregnancies (8,10–15).

Postpartum depressed mood incidence peaks at 10 weeks postpartum; however, major depressive episodes in the postpartum period may have an insidious onset and come to clinical attention 4 to 6 months postpartum, which correlates with the peak incidence of postpartum hypothyroidism. Thyroid dysfunction is implicated in depression in women far more often than in men, and the postpartum period (or treatment with lithium) are provocative of thyroid hypofunction with sufficient frequency to warrant endocrine evaluations in depressed women in general, and more so in the postpartum period. Major depressions refractory to antidepressants, especially in postpartum women, should be considered for thyroxine augmentation of the antidepressant medication. The "maternity blues" is a relatively mild and transient phenomenon, is not considered a disorder per se, and is thought to occur in a majority of women within the first 2 weeks postpartum with a duration of 3 to 10 days. Associated symptoms include labile mood, crying spells, nervousness, and sadness. Studies of fluctuating hormone levels have to date not identified a relationship between this symptom complex and circulating levels of luteinizing hormone, follicle-stimulating hormone, estrogen, or progesterone (16–20).

Bipolar disorder, often referred to in the vernacular as manic depression, has several subtypes and is defined behind specific criteria for major depressive episodes, manic episodes, and mixed episodes. The criteria for a manic episode are provided in Table 9-2, and most bipolar patients experience a combination of these three types of episodes during the course of their illness. The postpartum period is considered a higher risk period for manic episodes in particular, and for relapse in general, for bipolar patients. The use of lithium, even during pregnancy, and the reestablishment of lithium maintenance shortly after parturition may be advisable in some patients (see discussion of lithium below); and the antepartum and postpartum treatment of these patients with neuroleptics is often warranted, even for a breastfeeding mother. Full-blown manic episodes are dangerous to the mother and to the fetus or baby, not only because of the risks of suicide or harm to others, but because of the impulsive and even psychotic affect and thinking that supervene. Others with antecedent bipolar disorders should be monitored closely throughout pregnancy and in the subsequent months. Unlike most depressive syndromes, mania can more often arise abruptly and in full force. This risk is multiplied by the fact that many manic patients are not aware of their condition, whereas most depressed patients know all too well that they are ill (21–23).

TABLE 9-2. *Manic episode*

A manic episode is a distinct period of abnormally and persistently elevated, expansive, or irritable mood, lasting at least 1 week (or any duration if hospitalization is necessary).

During the period of mood disturbance, three (or more) of the following symptoms have persisted (four if the mood is only irritable) and have been present to a significant degree:

1. inflated self-esteem or grandiosity
2. decreased need for sleep
3. more talkative than usual or pressure to keep talking
4. flight of ideas or subjective experience that one's thoughts are racing
5. distractibility, i.e., attention too easily drawn to unimportant or irrelevant external stimuli
6. increase in goal-directed activity (either socially, at work or school, or sexually) or psychomotor agitation (i.e., visible physical restlessness).
7. excessive involvement in pleasurable activities that have a high potential for painful consequences (e.g., engaging in unrestrained buying sprees, sexual indiscretions, or foolish business investments).

In addition, the mood disturbance is sufficiently severe to cause marked impairment in occupational functioning or in usual social activities or relationships, or to necessitate hospitalization to prevent harm to self or others. Lastly, the symptoms must not be due to the direct physiological effects of a substance (e.g., amphetamines or another drug of abuse, a medication) or a general medical condition (e.g., hyperthyroidism).

From the American Psychiatric Association. Diagnostic and statistical manual of mental disorders, 4th ed. Washington, DC: American Psychiatric Association, 1994.

SCHIZOPHRENIA AND OTHER PSYCHOTIC DISORDERS

The term "psychotic" is defined as a gross impairment in reality testing (as conspicuously occurs in delusions or hallucinations), and one must always bear in mind that this particular symptom may be present in a major depressive episode, in a manic episode, in alcohol intoxication or withdrawal deliria, or in dementias and is not generally indicative, in and of itself, of a nominally psychiatric disorder, such as schizophrenia. Indeed, in a general hospital population, the majority of the "psychotic" patients are medically or neurologically acute patients in varying states of delirium consequent to a legion of etiologies. In the specific context of "psychiatric" patients, one thinks of schizophrenia (several variations), delusional (or paranoid) disorder, and brief psychotic disorder as accounting for the majority of cases (24,25).

In schizophrenic women of childbearing age, one must expect that conception often occurs while the patient is receiving neuroleptic medication. Many patients warrant maintenance on these medications despite the low-level risk of teratogenicity (see below). The lifetime prevalence of schizophrenia, worldwide, is estimated to be between 0.5% and 1.0%, a tremendous cohort (6,8,14,26). The more severe subset of these patients will be terribly stressed by pregnancy, childbirth, and the role obligations that follow, and the ongoing involvement of mental health providers is essential. This illness is well known for the patient's poor compliance with medical care and medication treatment that attends it, so all health providers must be cognizant of the need to support these patients' capacity to remain in continuous treatment and to comply with prophylactic and acute medication regimens.

The sudden onset of delusions, hallucinations, or disorganized speech, or grossly disorganized or catatonic behavior—with a duration of from 1 day up to 1 month followed by full recovery—constitutes the diagnostic criteria for a brief psychotic disorder. The key differential here is from a similar-appearing syndrome caused by a general medical condition or from the use of or withdrawal from alcohol or drugs. Most postpartum psychoses have an acute onset within the first 2 weeks postpartum, and fully 80% have their onset within the first month. Women with a history of any psychotic condition are at significantly greater risk for postpartum relapse, and early identification and treatment has been found to correlate with improved outcomes. Low-dose neuroleptics, instituted early, can sometimes abort full-blown decompensations that would have required admission and higher dose medication(s). In the general population, a woman's risk of postpartum psychosis is approximately 1 in 500; however, after the first such episode, subsequent risk climbs dramatically to 1 in 3. Compared with antepartum data, psychiatric admission rates have been reported to increase six-fold in the first month postpartum (11,23,27,28).

PREMENSTRUAL SYNDROME

Commonly referred to as PMS, the DSM-IV includes this so-called disorder in Appendix B, which consists of criteria sets that represent proposed disorders needing further study. The current research criteria for premenstrual dysphoric disorder (PMDD) are presented in Table 9-3, and the provisional status of this syndrome in the DSM at least partly reflects controversy as to the role of cultural (negative) bias in the consensual definition of what is psychopathology and what is arguably within the "accepted-as-normal" bell curve within a more broadly conceived human condition. PMS is not as yet consensually defined, and as such, data describing its diagnosis or treatment are difficult to compare and interpret. Commonly included physical complaints include breast tenderness, headache, and edema. Irritable or depressed mood and mood lability are considered hallmarks, yet a long list of psychological and behavioral symptoms have been included in the controversial literature of PMS. A cyclical pattern, with symptoms predominantly present in the luteal phase and abolished or much-reduced after menses, is classic, and most definitions or descriptions of PMS require an identifiable symptom-free interval with most cycles.

Impairment of social or occupational functioning is a threshold required in order to diagnose most psychiatric disorders, to aid in demarcation from the many symptoms that constitute day-to-day life for most persons, and the proposed criteria for PMDD apply this requirement. It has been reported, using this threshold, that more than one third of women may report PMDD symptoms, but that less than 10% evidence severe symptoms accompanied with functional impairments. Although a variety of treatments have been proposed and studied, no definitive improvement over placebo has been consistently shown for any compound. It has been reported that exercise, reduced caffeine intake, and reduced salt in the diet has a positive result in many women. Targeting specific symptoms, rather than the full pattern, may be beneficial. Edema often responds to diuretics, and breast tenderness to bromocriptine. Headaches respond to nonsteroidal antiinflammatory drugs and severe insomnia or anxiety to low-dose, long-acting benzodiazepines, such as clonazepam (Klonopin), prescribed on a short-term basis (8,10,11,18,20,28,29). Selective serotonin reuptake inhibitors may be effective for PMDD as well.

TABLE 9-3. *Premenstrual dysphoric disorder (research criteria)—"PMS"*

In most menstrual cycles during the past year, five (or more) of the following symptoms were present for most of the time during the last week of the luteal phase, begin to remit within a few days after the onset of the follicular phase, and were absent in the week postmenses. At least one of the symptoms were (1), (2), (3), or (4):

1. markedly depressed mood, feelings of hopelessness, or self-deprecating thoughts
2. markedly anxiety, tension, feelings of being "keyed up," or "on edge"
3. marked affective lability (e.g., feeling suddenly sad or tearful or increased sensitivity to rejection)
4. persistent and marked anger or irritability or increased interpersonal conflicts
5. decreased interest in usual activities (e.g., work, school, friends, hobbies)
6. subjective sense of difficulty in concentrating
7. lethargy, easily fatigued, or marked lack of energy
8. marked change in appetite, overeating, or specific food cravings
9. hypersomnia or insomnia
10. a subjective sense of being overwhelmed or out of control
11. other physical symptoms, such as breast tenderness or swelling, headaches, joint or muscle pain, a sensation of "bloating," weight gain

In addition, the disturbance markedly interferes with work or school or with usual social activities and relationships; and the syndrome should be confirmed by prospective monitoring of at least two consecutive symptomatic cycles.

From the American Psychiatric Association. Diagnostic and statistical manual of mental disorders, 4th ed. Washington, DC: American Psychiatric Association, 1994.

ANXIETY DISORDERS

A complex group of disorders, the DSM-IV anxiety disorders, include panic disorder (with or without agoraphobia); different types of phobias, including social phobia; obsessive-compulsive disorder; and posttraumatic stress disorder, and the related acute stress disorder, among others. The current discussion will be limited to the varieties of panic disorder, the most significantly prevalent of the above. The others are beyond the scope of this chapter (26).

Panic attacks (not synonymous with panic disorder) are the hallmark of several different anxiety disorders, much as a major depressive episode is a component of both major depressive disorders and bipolar disorders. Door-to-door community surveys turned up a surprisingly high rate of panic attacks in the general population, with the 1-year prevalence rates of panic disorder in the range of 1% to 2%, a significant minority of the population. The criteria for a panic attack are included in Table 9-4, and the diagnosis of panic disorder consists primarily of the presence of recurrent unexpected panic attacks and one of several associated psychological concomitants, such as fear of impending panic attacks, altered behavior as a result of the attacks, and so forth. Panic attacks are quite different from a complaint of generalized anxiety or nervousness, being dramatically episodic in nature, reaching peak intensity within minutes, and abating substantially in 20 to 30 minutes (6,8,14,30).

Agoraphobia is strongly associated with panic disorder and is defined as avoidance of places or situations from which escape might be difficult or embarrassing. This commonly translates into fearing or avoiding riding in elevators, airplanes, buses, trains, crowded supermarkets, congested highways, bridges, tunnels, movie theatres, and similar. Many individuals who avoid plane trips are not at all afraid of a plane crash but have panic attack–associated agoraphobia because an airplane is a crowded, enclosed area from which escape is literally impossible once airborne (6,8).

The treatments for panic disorder, with or without agoraphobia, include cognitive-behavioral psychotherapies and medications. Importantly, the benzodiazepines are commonly prescribed for these patients (although antidepressants have been shown to have greater primary efficacy) yet should be avoided, if possible, during pregnancy, especially during the first trimester. Most patients with this disorder can tolerate several months unmedicated with antidepressants, or can remain on selective serotonin reuptake inhibitor (SSRI) antidepressants, which, when clinically indicated, are generally continued during pregnancy. However, reducing or discontinuing benzodiazepines often exacerbates anxiety symptoms, including panic attacks and agoraphobia, and pose a challenge in patients maintained on these habit-forming medicines. The SSRI antidepressants (however misnamed given their efficacy for a number of anxiety disorders) are greatly preferred agents during pregnancy and are generally the medications of choice for anxiety-spectrum disorders, partly because addiction is a well-known risk with benzodiazepines that has not been found to occur with antidepressants (6,30–32).

TABLE 9-4. *Criteria for a panic attack*

A discrete period of intense fear or discomfort, in which four (or more) of the following symptoms developed abruptly and reached a peak within 10 minutes:

1. palpitations, pounding heart, or accelerated heart rate
2. sweating
3. trembling or shaking
4. sensations of shortness of breath or smothering
5. feeling of choking
6. chest pain or discomfort
7. nausea or abdominal distress
8. feeling dizzy, unsteady, lightheaded, or faint
9. derealization (feelings of unreality) or depersonalization (being detached from oneself)
10. fear of losing control or going crazy
11. fear of dying
12. paresthesias (numbness or tingling sensations)
13. chills or hot flushes

From the American Psychiatric Association. Diagnostic and statistical manual of mental disorders, 4th ed. Washington, DC: American Psychiatric Association, 1994.

SUBSTANCE-RELATED DISORDERS

Perhaps the most common mental disorders (as currently defined), some would suggest that these syndromes be taken as somewhat separate phenomena. The DSM-IV designates in excess of 100 separately defined substance-related disorders: from alcohol-induced persisting dementia to opioid-induced sexual dysfunction. The substances covered, which include drugs of abuse, medications, and toxins, are divided into 11 classes: alcohol, amphetamines, caffeine, cannabis, cocaine, hallucinogens, inhalants (e.g., glue), nicotine, opioids, phencyclidine (PCP), and the sedative/hypnotic/anxiolytics (primarily the benzodiazepines and barbiturates). The notion of drug abuse or addiction as a useful wholesale category of diagnosis is long past, with many different syndromes (differing with different drugs and even within the same drug class but with a different route of administration, e.g., cocaine versus crack) now distinguished. A full review of these disorders is beyond the scope of this discussion (see Chapter 8), but several issues relevant to pregnancy and reproduction will be discussed.

The fetal alcohol syndrome (33) is considered a common cause of mental retardation, notable as a theoretically preventable etiology of this tragic outcome (see Chapter 8). Approximately one third of infants born to heavy drinkers have demonstrable congenital findings, twice the rate found in moderate drinkers, and roughly four times the rate of abstinent women. There is evidence that suggests that pregnant alcoholics are at their most receptive to recommended treatment interventions, and clinicians in regular contact with these women are strongly encouraged to make a priority of screening and referring these patients. Many physicians have grown pessimistic as to their influence on drinking behavior (and smoking behavior) in their patients; however, one must note that even several months of sobriety or reduced alcohol intake during pregnancy would greatly reduce the likelihood of morbidity for the infant at hand (34). Some alcohol-dependent women who are not ready to give up drinking altogether are able to abstain temporarily or cut down on the frequency or severity of drinking while they are pregnant. Given the terrifically high prevalence of alcohol use and abuse in all socioeconomic groups the world over, sensible prenatal care includes a high index of suspicion for an alcohol-related disorder. The lifetime prevalence for alcohol dependence in the United States has been reported to be 14% in community samples, and one can safely assume statistical error to be in the direction of underreporting (14,35). Alcohol is correlated with suicides, homicides, child abuse and neglect, vehicle accidents, and a host of medical complications, including dementia. Because the well-being of a fetus or newborn is meaningful leverage with an alcoholic mother, clinicians who provide prenatal care are in a unique position to take the best advantage of these conditions.

Elevated serum γ-glutamyltransferase (>30 U), in two thirds of cases, is indicative of heavy drinking and, given the dearth of laboratory indicators of alcohol dependence, should be sent as a screening test as a matter of routine. An unexplained delirium or seizures should be considered alcohol withdrawal related until proven otherwise, especially if the time course fits (i.e., a patient who by dint of hospital admission has not had a drink in 24–72 hours). Delirium tremens (DTs) carries a mortality rate in excess of 1 in 10 cases and occurs in relation to alcohol and in relation to abrupt discontinuation of benzodiazepines or barbiturates (6,36–38).

Opioid dependence, primarily heroin, has risen in recent years, partly due to the increased availability of lower-priced, higher purity heroin on the street. Pregnant heroin addicts should be maintained on methadone, at least through the pregnancy, as the risks associated with withdrawal or detoxification are not justified by the benefits; especially given the high initial relapse rate for detoxified patients. Heroin use (as opposed to methadone) is attended by the risks of injected adulterants, contaminated needles (hepatitis, HIV, etc.), thrombophlebitis, cellulitis, abscesses, septic pulmonary emboli, premature labor, decreased birth weights, and an increased frequency of toxemia and hemorrhage (33,38).

Pregnancies in addicts (including to alcohol) are by definition high risk, and infants are frequently born in the throes of withdrawal. In addition, there is an increased rate of sexually transmitted diseases (including AIDS and the hepatitides), abruptio placentae, premature membrane rupture, toxemia, prolapsed cords and limbs, and breech presentations. Newborns may be extremely irritable and may have seizures, tremors, tachypnea, diarrhea, vomiting, and disturbed sleep patterns. The babies of cocaine-addicted mothers may manifest intrauterine growth retardation, microcephaly, intracranial hemorrhage, and gastrointestinal and renal tract anomalies and are at higher risk for sudden infant death syndrome (33).

The immediate availability of addiction treatment systems to prenatal caregivers is of paramount public health importance; and concentrated intervention efforts with pregnant addicts are especially warranted. Even short-lived periods of abstinence impact directly on the well-being of newborns, especially when alcohol use is curtailed or methadone can be substituted for heroin use.

SUICIDE

One of the harshest outcomes for a physician is the suicide of a patient, yet completed suicides occur in all practices and in all varieties of clinical settings, even when vigilant surveillance for warning signs is in place.

Annually, roughly 30,000 people die in the United States by their own hand, reflecting a relatively stable rate of approximately 12 per 100,000, with suicide consistently ranking at the lower end of the ten most common causes of death. Provocatively, suicide rates vary considerably from country to country, with approximately double the U.S. rate recorded in Eastern European and Scandinavian countries and in Japan. Demographic statuses that may reflect social relatedness profoundly affect suicide rates. Never-married persons are twice as likely to commit suicide than married persons. Divorced persons are at higher relative risk, and divorced men are four times more likely to commit suicide than their female counterparts. In general, white males are four times more likely to commit suicide than are white females; however, female physicians are several-fold more likely to commit suicide than are age-matched and sex-matched controls (6,20,22,28).

Demographic risk factors for suicide are often quoted, yet clinical efficacy has not been demonstrated in applying this information to clinical decision making. These data are retrospective and largely drawn from death certificates and therefore have questionable utility for the forward-looking practice of screening for potentially suicidal patients. Nonetheless, these risk factors should serve to raise the clinician's index of suspicion when they are present, yet should not lower the level of concern when they are absent.

Increasing age strongly correlates with increased suicide risk, with a concomitant increase in the likelihood that a given attempt will be lethal. Men are three times more likely to succeed in a given suicide attempt than are women, overall, partly related to their greater use of more lethal methods—gunfire, hanging, and so forth. Women are, however, several-fold more likely to make suicide attempts. The colloquial interpretation of an unsuccessful suicide attempt as a dramatic "cry for help" may be correct in some cases, but too often fails to appreciate the actual risk of suicide that remains for these individuals.

White race strongly correlates with increased suicide risk and is roughly twice the mean rate. Native Americans are at significantly higher risk, with the confound of a higher rate of alcoholism possibly contributing to this statistic. Religious orthodoxy is considered protective, overall. Medical illness correlates with increased suicide risk. The majority of female cancer patients who commit suicide carry diagnoses of gender-associated cancers (i.e., breast, uterine, etc.). Loss of physical mobility and disfiguring procedures are considered to contribute to suicide risk.

Substance abuse and alcoholism are strongly correlated to increased suicide risk. Perhaps one in ten alcoholics commit suicide, a tenfold rate increase compared with matched controls, keeping in mind that mood disorders are quite frequent in this population and that this group is mostly male. Roughly one in three suicides involves alcohol. Heroin addicts, as a group, commit suicide at an even higher rate than do alcoholics, keeping in mind that a lethal method is immediately at hand for these individuals (2,35,39).

Pregnant women rarely commit suicide, but disordered mood, alcohol or drug abuse, and other intervening factors make this generalization unreliable. AIDS increases suicide risk, as does social isolation, and younger persons in urban areas typically contradict the overall population trends that increased age and white race are good predictors of suicidal behavior.

It is terribly important to remember that the majority of patients who complete suicide do so on their first attempt. Again, prior attempts should raise the index of suspicion, but the absence or prior attempts cannot be considered necessarily reassuring in a patient who provokes concern for other reasons.

PSYCHOTROPIC MEDICATIONS

There is emphatically not a one-to-one correspondence between categories of psychiatric disorders and the classes of psychotropic medications. The antidepressants are not used simply in the treatment of depression; the antipsychotics [haloperidol (Haldol) and others] are not used only in the treatment of the schizophrenic disorders; and the antianxiety agents [diazepam (Valium) and others] are not confined to the treatment of the so-called anxiety disorders. The discrepancies here are not minor but reflect the fact that patients commonly suffer from symptoms and even full syndromes that are described in different chapters of the psychiatric textbooks; and that the medication groupings do not adequately indicate the actual clinical use of these potent (and often puzzling) psychotropic agents. For example, a patient experiencing a major depressive episode may be simultaneously prescribed an antidepressant, an antianxiety agent, and possibly an antipsychotic medication, if mood-congruent psychotic features are present. In other words, three classes of medications are treating: disturbed mood, severe insomnia and anxiety, and delusional thinking, respectively. In time, given a good treatment response, the benzodiazepine (antianxiety) and antipsychotic (for the delusions) would be tapered and discontinued, with ongoing antidepressants prescribed on a prophylactic basis.

LITHIUM

Lithium has been the mainstay of the treatment of bipolar disorder since the 1950's, and two generations of psychiatrists have been trained to eschew the use of this effective medication in pregnant women, particularly during the first trimester, to avoid the cardiovascular anomalies reported to result from its use (specifically, Ebstein's anomaly). This congenital defect is characterized by a downward-located tricuspid valve (into the right ventricle) with redundancy of the valve, and possible adherence of the septal and posterior cusps to the ventricular wall (6,36).

More recent data have called this historical caution into question, and prospectively collected data suggest that the earlier reports of greatly increased risk ratios are flawed. These new data revise the risk-to-benefit calculation for many women of childbearing age who are maintained on lithium, particularly those more prone to frequent or severe manic relapses (40,41).

Ebstein's anomaly is often lethal; in one series, approximately half of the newborns died within the first week of life. This anomaly occurs in approximately 1 in 20,000 live births in the general population, and it had been estimated that this risk was increased several hundred-fold in women receiving lithium during the early, critical stages of cardiac development. The International Register of Lithium Babies was the primary data source upon which lithium's reputation as a potent and specific teratogen was based. The registry consisted of voluntary reports from physicians, and these data have guided practice for decades, until recent and more epidemiologically sound methodologies corrected for the case-finding ascertainment error of the register (42,43).

Current thinking is that lithium carries only a moderately increased risk of congenital malformations. This has relaxed the stringent conditions under which women were once discouraged from childbearing rather than discontinue lithium maintenance. Even women with moderately severe bipolar disorder can be managed with a minimum risk to both fetus and mother. This approach illustrates the cost-to-benefit clinical reasoning attendant to the use of marginally teratogenic medications that nonetheless offer substantial benefits with regard to psychotropic utility (32):

> . . . [Temporary] discontinuation of lithium after tapering the dosage over ten days may provide a limited window of time during which the pregnancy could be undertaken without any risk of exposure. Ideally, this window should cover the entire embryonic period, which extends from about four weeks to twelve weeks after the patient's last menstrual period. Tapering of the lithium dosage can coincide with dis-

continuation of contraception and a conscious attempt to become pregnant. Lithium use can also be continued until the first missed menstrual period. Immediately following confirmation of the pregnancy, lithium treatment would be discontinued over the next ten days. Although the latter approach involves some exposure to lithium after cardiac embryogenesis has begun, the risk of inducing malformations prior to the first missed menses is small. Thus, treatment during most of embryogenesis may be avoided while providing the patient with a long period of antimanic prophylaxis. Discontinuation of lithium may pose an unacceptable risk of increased morbidity in women with bipolar disorder who have had multiple episodes of affective instability. If such women become pregnant, they should continue their lithium therapy, but appropriate reproductive risk counseling and prenatal diagnosis should be offered (44).

In the not so distant past, many women with bipolar disorder were counseled to defer childbearing, sometimes indefinitely, and even encouraged to terminate pregnancies. The present evidence suggests that the teratogenic risks of lithium had been overestimated by roughly two orders of magnitude, and that with prudent clinical supervision, lithium maintenance (or its brief interruption) is clinically advisable, if it is the patient's wish to bear a child.

Breast milk will contain a significant lithium concentration (approximately one half the mother's serum concentration), and it is recommended that mothers maintained on lithium not breastfeed their infants (45,46).

ANTIDEPRESSANTS

A heterogenous group of medications (chemically speaking), the so-called antidepressants have many other uses, including the treatment of pain, headache, bed-wetting, insomnia, obsessive-compulsive disorder, narcolepsy, and so forth. As a group, these pharmaceuticals are widely prescribed. Most patients receiving antidepressant medicines are prescribed them by nonpsychiatrists, and many of these patients do not have clinical pictures that meet the DSM-IV criteria for major depressive episodes. There is an important dichotomy present with the use of these medicines, in that the research diagnostic criteria that fueled the robust evidence of efficacy for antidepressants are not applied to most of the patients who are given antidepressants. The newest class of antidepressants, SSRIs [the most well known of which is Prozac (fluoxetine)], are routinely dispensed at a low threshold of patient complaint, far below the DSM-IV criteria of symptoms that technically constitute a major depression. This is important to keep in mind when deciding to continue or discontinue antidepressants (SSRI or otherwise) in a woman who is pregnant or is intending to become pregnant (8,36).

In order of historical appearance, the first major class of antidepressants were the monoamine oxidase inhibitors (MAOIs), defined by their ability to block oxidative deamination of naturally occurring monoamines (e.g., norepinephrine, serotonin, etc.) by irreversible suicide inhibition of the MAO enzyme. Examples of MAOIs include phenelzine (Nardil) and tranylcypromine (Parnate). Not commonly used, but still present in clinical practice, these potentially highly toxic medications are contraindicated during pregnancy and would not be responsibly prescribed other than by a psychiatrist in exceptional cases, where the severity of the psychiatric illness tips the cost-to-benefit analysis in favor of MAOIs. The notorious toxicities are (a) hypertensive crisis, provoked classically by foods containing tyramine, or by other pressor amines (e.g., over-the-counter decongestants); and (b) life threatening CNS and circulatory symptoms, if combined with meperidine (Demerol) or a number of other medications, including the tricyclic antidepressants (36,47).

The tricyclic antidepressants—amitriptyline (Elavil), desipramine (Norpramin), doxepin (Sinequan), nortriptyline (Pamelor), imipramine (Tofranil), and others—had been the mainstay of the pharmacologic treatment of major depressive disorders over the past four decades, until the advent of the SSRIs, as described below. The clinical evidence for the efficacy of the tricyclics is indisputable, and imipramine, the best-studied member of this class, is the gold standard against which newly developed compounds are compared in clinical trials. A great improvement over the MAOIs (notably, no tyramine-free diet is required), the tricyclics retain sufficient toxicity and a low enough therapeutic index such that many depressed patients have committed suicide by taking an overdose of this class of antidepressants. Cardiac toxicity is the usual cause of death in these unfortunate cases. Many patients warrant short-term prescriptions (as little as 1 week's supply) at the outset or during symptomatic periods of a longer course of treatment to reduce the morbidity and mortality should a patient ingest his or her entire medication supply. Emergency rooms still routinely test serum for this class of antidepressants in lethargic or comatose patients in whom an overdose is suspected.

Past studies have shown an increase in the frequency of congenital malformations in the babies of women who received tricyclics during pregnancy, but more recent data do not support this association and suggest otherwise. The Finnish Registry of Congenital Malformations, with thousands of cases reported, has not shown the use of tricyclic antidepressants to correlate with malformation risk. Current practice should preferentially avoid the unnecessary use of tricyclics during pregnancy, especially during the first trimester; but discontinuation of these medicines in patients at significant risk of relapse is not warranted by the relatively low risk of teratogenic effect (48–50).

The SSRIs, although no more efficacious on a case-by-case basis than the preceding classes of antidepressants, are far less toxic in overdose and have fewer unpleasant side effects, and on this basis alone represent a major advance in the treatment of depression. These medications, partly because of this highly favorable safety profile, are prescribed frequently at a low threshold of patient complaint. Many physicians who had not previously felt comfortable prescribing antidepressants now find themselves writing prescriptions for fluoxetine (Prozac) or sertraline (Zoloft) to patients who fall far short of the level of symptoms meeting DSM-IV criteria for major depression. Patients routinely request these medications, which are often prescribed on a "why not" basis. Studies of women on SSRIs during pregnancy have generally not shown untoward effects on the fetus. One must note, however, that the rate of miscarriage has been reported to be increased in women receiving SSRIs or tricyclic antidepressants, as compared with unexposed pregnancies. The popularity of SSRIs has provided a large database in a short period of time, and the absence of data correlating malformations with fetal exposure is consistent and has been demonstrated in large, prospective samples (36,51,52).

Women who are receiving antidepressant medications and become pregnant should be reassured that there is no cause for alarm. However, given the low threshold at which these medicines are prescribed, one should encourage women who are planning to become pregnant, if there is little if any evidence of benefit from their antidepressant use, to taper and discontinue these medicines. If a clinical benefit is apparent, especially if depressive or other symptoms have been moderate to severe, the SSRIs need not be discontinued in the setting of conception, pregnancy, or breast-feeding. In the majority of cases in which clinical benefit is apparent in the history, this benefit far outweighs the low risk of teratogenicity or miscarriage (53,54).

ANTIPSYCHOTICS

The antipsychotic agents, commonly referred to as neuroleptics, are used in the treatment of schizophrenias, delusional disorders, tic disorders, bipolar disorders (usually in the acute management of mania), severe personality disorders, depressive episodes (if psychotic features are present), dementias, deliria, and in the acute management of agitated states from almost any cause. Repressive government regimes have given these medications, known in pharmacologic circles for their taming effect on laboratory animals, to political dissident prisoners. Residents of nursing homes and facilities for the mentally retarded are frequently maintained on neuroleptics for a variety of reasons, some of which are debatable. High-potency neuroleptics include haloperidol (Haldol), fluphenazine (Prolixin), trifluoperazine (Stelazine), and thiothixene (Navane); low-potency neuroleptics include chlorpromazine (Thorazine), thioridazine (Mellaril), and others. These medicines are potent antiemetics; prochlorperazine (Compazine) is commonly prescribed postoperatively for this purpose and is not otherwise in use for the treatment of psychiatric symptoms (6,36).

Given the high population prevalence of schizophrenia (0.5–1.0%), many women of childbearing age are receiving antipsychotic medications. In schizophrenia, the median age at onset for women is in the late 20's (slightly later than men), although prodromal behavioral changes and a deterioration in social and occupational functioning can often be elicited that precede this first onset of prominent psychotic symptoms. Hospitalized schizophrenics may become pregnant while on neuroleptics, partly due to the impaired judgment and social skills that often characterize this disorder, especially during more symptomatic periods. Similarly, institutionalized mentally retarded women may become pregnant while on neuroleptics, again with mental incapacity contributing to this intended or unintended turn of events (6,8).

Phenothiazine neuroleptics have been used in the treatment of hyperemesis gravidarum, and an increased rate of congenital anomalies was reported. In general, one does not prescribe neuroleptic agents during the first trimester, and, if manageable, patients are given drug holidays from neuroleptics when they plan to conceive a child, through the first trimester if practical, and ideally until after childbirth. Although not absolutely contraindicated, without a countervailing risk of clinical decompensation (which might include psychosis, agitated and impulsive behavior, substance abuse, suicidal behavior) one avoids prescribing these agents to pregnant women. When using these agents during pregnancy, chlorpromazine (Thorazine) is not the agent of choice because the teratogenicity data implicate this phenothiazine at a greater frequency than the high-potency neuroleptics. Patients with significant clinical histories are better remedicated shortly after childbirth (or after an abbreviated course of breastfeeding, possibly) rather than awaiting the signs of an impending psychotic decompensation (55–57).

Breast milk contains neuroleptics. Concentrations are low, but a sedating effect (lethargy) on the infants has been reported. It is not recommended, although it is not absolutely contraindicated, for mothers receiving neuroleptics to breastfeed their children (33,45,46).

ANTIANXIETY MEDICATIONS

Also known as sedative-hypnotics, or as anxiolytics, this class of medications includes the benzodiazepines, the barbiturates, and many miscellaneous medications with similar properties, such as chloral hydrate. The anxiolytic effect versus the hypnotic effect (encouraging sleep) is largely a function of dosage, not of the unique properties of one of these compounds over another. Nonetheless, common practice has one thinking of temazepam (Restoril) as a sleep medication and alprazolam (Xanax) as an anxiolytic. Chlordiazepoxide (Librium) is associated with detoxification from alcohol and treatment of alcohol withdrawal symptoms, and diazepam (Valium) is associated with sleep induction, anxiety reduction, and addiction. Yet pharmacologically, most of the benzodiazepines can be cross-utilized if dosages are properly adjusted and if one is cognizant of a given compound's rate of absorption, metabolism, and elimination; and the presence or absence of active metabolites (6,36).

The data regarding congenital malformations and benzodiazepine use are conflicting. Some reports are sufficiently positive so as to have these medicines contraindicated during pregnancy (especially during the first trimester), unless the clinical indication for their use is compelling. However, there is not a compelling reason to assume these drugs are teratogenic. Unlike the antidepressants or the antipsychotics, the physiologic dependence on sedative-hypnotics may make tapering or discontinuation of these medicines problematic in some patients, keeping in mind that this class of medications is frequently prescribed, especially to women and often for extended periods of time. The long-term efficacy of benzodiazepines (or barbiturates) is controversial in the treatment of many anxiety disorders (or insomnia, stress, or nerves), yet they are prescribed on a grand scale, and pregnant women (or women intending to become pregnant) should not be overly alarmed if they conceive while on these medications, or if they cannot successfully discontinue their use during pregnancy. Alprazolam (Xanax) may be particularly difficult to wean patients from. It is sometimes possible to switch an alprazolam-dependent patient to a longer acting sedative-hypnotic [e.g., clonazepam (Klonopin)] and then gradually taper the new medication. Slower tapers are generally better tolerated, especially after extended use (32,48,53,58,59).

ADAPTATION TO PREGNANCY

Browse any large bookstore and you will find a variety of books written for pregnant women. Especially during the first pregnancy, there is mystery, anxiety, excitement, even a hint of experiencing the magical for many women. For the majority of women, this is a positive context, and even moderate discomfort in the first and second trimesters is met with positive adaptation. The second and third trimesters are generally accompanied by a positively modified social status, replete with total strangers smiling, opening doors, and so on. These first months of first pregnancies are very special and positive times for most women. One must acknowledge, however, that the final weeks of the first pregnancy, and subsequent pregnancies, are not necessarily suffused with the same glow.

Having endorsed the above stereotype, a critical principle must be introduced. There is a fundamental tension between cultural ideals and individual personalities throughout life. One's role expectations (e.g., to be beaming proudly at one's college graduation) cannot always be met. Increasing stress predictably reduces a given person's ability to meet role obligations, which include feeling and appearing to feel the way one is expected to feel by one's family and social context. In relation to the archetypal first pregnancy, the physical exhaustion and chronic sleep deprivation that can characterize the final trimester is frequently when the cheerful stereotype loses its shine. This deglorification of childbearing varies tremendously from woman to woman. Some women glow throughout five closely spaced pregnancies, juggling child rearing and all the rest of it smiling all the way. Some women start vomiting within weeks of conception and suffer miserably with much of their first and subsequent pregnancies. The interposition of child rearing work in the background of later pregnancies cannot be overlooked; nor can the myriad stressors of life that do not magically evaporate while one is busy being pregnant. Money, marriage, work in and out of the home, medical illness, family care-taking duties, and other stressors remain (22,60).

In general, clinicians should expect a given patient to cope with pregnancies as adaptively or maladaptively as she has coped so far with life in general. Women who are anxious in the course of day-to-day life are often more so during pregnancy. Women who have labile mood as a base trait will likely bring this temperament, possibly amplified, to their pregnancy and childbearing experiences. Women who have frequent physical complaints will more than likely have this pattern exacerbated by the tremendous physical changes of pregnancy and childbirth, and so on. It is more the exception than the rule for things to be so very different for a woman when she is pregnant or when she is raising children.

In general terms, stressors tax psychological defenses, and it is these defenses that allow us to cope with our day-to-day lives, generally without our being aware of them. Taxed defenses fail more frequently, so our typically better managed affects (e.g., anger, sadness, and worrying) become less well-managed and come to the fore and become more public more often. For example, on some days one is more likely to lose one's temper than on another given day. The latter is a day when our defenses are said to be functioning more optimally. Chronic sleep deprivation is a simple example of a stressor (quite apropos of pregnancy and the round-the-clock feeding and rearing of young children) that provokes affective instability, interpersonal conflict, and diminished social and occupational functioning in many persons. Chronic nausea, back pain, or difficulty breastfeeding are all discrete stressors, to name only a few, that tax the functional and characterological reserves of women during these times in their lives, which are both magical and very stressful. Clinicians are better positioned to provide meaningful support when they appreciate the ambivalent and dialectical nature of positive and negative life events and stages. We must not expect our patients to be happy when they are not; conversely, we must not demand the stereotyped signs of grief when they are not forthcoming.

The overarching principle is to regularly ask patients about their psychosocial lives, i.e., their emotional and interpersonal functioning; and having asked, to then refer those in moderate to severe distress (at least for an initial consultation, not necessarily for ongoing treatment) and to reassure effectively those with milder, more normal distress. The word "normal" is quite important in this context, and it is a thorough clinician's duty to normalize the subjective experiences of patients. If a patient speaks of her fear of bearing a malformed baby, the appropriate clinical response is to say that "many women have fearful thoughts about this . . ." and so on. If a woman expresses the feeling that she resents the major changes in her life that her pregnancy and imminent motherhood entail, a similar reassurance may be offered. One goes on to assess whether the fear and anger are such that referral is warranted, but the reframing of the woman's experience as one that is shared by many women is a fundamental and all-purpose intervention. In addition, one makes a note of the patient's concern for follow-up at subsequent visits. When a clinician asks, a month or two later, about a psychosocial concern raised at a previous visit, rapport is nourished and it greatly increases the likelihood that the patient would confide (rather than conceal) possibly critical information such as thoughts of committing suicide, or of hurting the baby, or of abuse taking place in the home (33,61,62).

Pregnant women either will or will not have experiences that match the expectations of the maternity books, their families' expectations, or their own expectations, but they must not be made to feel that they are failing to meet the expectations of their health providers. We are to take our patients wherever they are—"boom or bust," emotionally speaking—and are to listen patiently and support their adaptation, however characterized, to these life changes. A clinician's acknowledgment and acceptance that one is sad, frightened, or frustrated, or feeling hopeless, is a powerful medicine that we must not be too busy to dispense.

LOSS

The flip side of the coin of pregnancy are the losses, broadly defined, associated with reproduction. Infertility issues confront 10% to 20% of couples, and many are not able to be helped despite the explosive growth of assisted reproductive technologies. The protracted attempts of infertility patients to conceive and carry to term are fraught with loss, the anticipation of loss, and the loss of the expected life that did not include these difficulties on such a large scale. Abortions, intentional or spontaneous, are losses (4,17,27,60).

Even successful and uneventful pregnancies entail (difficult for some women) losses, for example, of one's prior life-style, of one's previous physical appearance, of one's full-time (or more) dedication to one's career, of the undivided attention of one's spouse, of financial flexibility, of time for socializing, of less-pressured time spent with older siblings, and so forth. A baby born with a malformation or other medical disorder, especially those that affect mental development, reflect immense losses, not only of time, financial resources, and the like, but the loss of one's imagined future as well. Loss, in this context, is personally and subjectively defined and is not limited to the losses that attend more straightforward medical mortality or morbidity. Women with healthy children may be terribly distressed by their losses, although the childless woman in the next room who has experienced yet another in a series of miscarriages is much more obviously faced with loss.

Responses to loss obviously vary greatly from woman to woman, and vary in the same person at different times of life and depending on the type of loss encountered. Coping with a mastectomy, coping with the miscarriage of a long-awaited pregnancy, coping with a postpartum separation and divorce, coping with a Down syndrome baby, coping with the stigmata of a baby born with fetal alcohol syndrome—all will be variably managed by different women. A sexual assault can lead to the loss of a subjective sense of control over one's life, and the loss of the general feeling that something violent and nightmarish would not happen at a moment's notice. Having acknowledged the great variability in responses to loss, some generalizations and historical background are in order.

Elizabeth Kubler-Ross, based substantially on work with cancer patients, disseminated the view that the response to loss moves through identifiable stages, in sequence: denial, anger, bargaining, depression, and acceptance. One envisioned a patient told of his or her terminal cancer diagnosis, and the initial shock or numbness, possibly without even registering what they had been told. This is followed by anger, perhaps in the form of a "why me" reaction or that it is not fair that this is happening. Some patients then try to bargain for more time, perhaps pledging greater religious adherence in exchange for a modified prognosis. This classic pattern then leads to a deep sadness, as the true gravity of the terminal diagnosis sinks in. The final stage, acceptance, is characterized by Kubler-Ross as a very positive adaptation, in which patients make peace with loved ones, put their affairs in order, and make the most of the time remaining (63).

When this work was first published, it flew in the face of common practice, in that Dr. Kubler-Ross advocated openly discussing death with cancer patients, in contrast to the prevailing wisdom of the time, which was inclined to minimize (even conceal) terminal conditions from patients, and often avoided forthright communication with dying patients. It had been more the rule than the exception that a doctor's visit to a hospitalized cancer patient would not involve any mention of the patient's actual prognosis; and survival likelihoods that were nearly negligible were discussed quite optimistically. The patient, the family, and the doctor, in concert, would make believe that everything was going to be just fine. Kubler-Ross and others asserted that this avoidance was not really in the patient's best interests, but reflected the others' fear of death and dying and of the emotions evoked by these losses. Many clinicians prefer to avoid provoking painful emotions in their patients and have historically distorted or withheld information (bad news) in this spirit.

The medical care culture and the culture as a whole shifted with regard to the above, and it became more accepted doctrine that patients would benefit from more honest discussions of their conditions, their treatment options, and so forth. Some would say that the pendulum has swung too far in the other direction, with clinicians being overly confrontational with some types of bad news. Specifically, women who miscarry, especially in the third trimester, are sometimes pressured to hold the lost fetus, save photographs, locks of hair, and so forth in the new view that avoidance of painful emotions necessarily interferes with the successful progression of grief to a stage of acceptance or completion. Some women may be traumatized by these experiences, whereas others find them useful in moving on with their lives. It is critical that we, as clinicians, appreciate that different women relate to loss in different ways, and that some benefit from frankness and some from indirectness, some from extensive discussion and some from much more abbreviated reassurance. Some are greatly relieved at the suggestion of a referral for counseling, and some may consider going for counseling an embarrassment, something not done in their family or social circle. Some request medications and others consider them an insult to their self-esteem.

In summary, loss is best broadly defined, not confined to strictly medical losses such as fetal demise. The responses to loss are very individual, although some patterns are discernible, and no cookbook approach is applicable to all patients, other than to ask, listen, normalize, possibly refer for consultation, and follow up the patient's concern at a later visit.

CONCLUSION

In actual practice the statistics are quite beside the point. Taking a thorough history is the key to good clinical work, and, arguably, the most efficacious intervention is to identify successfully and refer those patients in need of psychiatric evaluation and treatment. This is a two-step process: (a) eliciting the appropriate history of psychosocial or psychiatric difficulties, and (b) a well-chosen referral. The ready availability of a mental health professional is absolutely critical to this process. If a practitioner (nonpsychiatric) knows exactly whom to call for consultation and referral of patients, he or she can be quite intrepid in asking patients about their emotional distress, their personal problems, whether they are contemplating suicide, if they are drinking heavily, and so forth. If one has not developed a ready consultation and referral path, the nonpsychiatric practitioner will come to avoid the probing questions that might open the Pandora's box of a patient's psychosocial and psychiatric material. Busy clinicians, being human, are less likely to say, "You look terribly sad and exhausted . . . is there anything bothering you?" when the patient's response might immediately provoke a time-consuming dialogue in which the physician experiences greater and greater duty to help and no familiar clinical method at hand. Without a psychiatrist or similar clinician at arm's length to pick up the ball, most of us come to neglect the historical information that we are not truly prepared to deal with. This may seem like "putting the cart before the horse," but the destination (for the patient) clarified will lead to it's frequent use and increasing utility over time. Without this, only the most florid clinical presentations will trigger interventions for patients' psychosocial and psychiatric suffering, and this high threshold is inherently an invitation for a tragic outcome.

REFERENCES

1. Agency for Health Care Policy and Research Depression Guideline Panel. Depression in primary care: detection, diagnosis, and treatment. Quick reference guide for clinicians, no. 5. AHCPR publication no. 93-0552. Rockville, MD: US Department of Health and Human Services, Public Health Service, 1993.
2. Chang G, Wilkins-Haug L, Berman S, Goetz MA, Behr H, Hiley A. Alcohol use and pregnancy: improving identification. *Obstet Gynecol* 1998;91:892–898.
3. Ewing JA. Detecting alcoholism: the CAGE questionnaire. *JAMA* 1984;252:1905–1907.
4. Downey J, Yingling S, McKinney M, Husami N, Jewelicz R, Maidman J. Mood disorders, psychiatric symptoms, and distress in women presenting for infertility evaluation. *Fertil Steril* 1989;52:425–432.
5. Kumar R, Brockington IF, eds. *Motherhood and mental illness*, 2nd ed. Boston: Butterworth & Co, 1988.
6. Kaplan HI, Sadock BJ. Synopsis of psychiatry, 8th ed. Baltimore, MD: Williams & Wilkins, 1988.
7. Feldman MD, ed. Behavioral medicine in primary care: a practical guide, 1st ed. Stamford, CT: Appleton & Lange, 1997.
8. American Psychiatric Association. *Diagnostic and statistical manual of mental disorders*, 4th ed. Washington, DC: American Psychiatric Association, 1994.
9. American College of Obstetricians and Gynecologists. Depression in women. *ACOG Tech Bull* no. 182, July 1993.
10. Gard PR, Handley SL, Parsons AD, Waldron G. A multivariate investigation of postpartum mood disturbances. *Br J Psychiatry* 1986;148: 567–575.
11. Nott PN. Extent, timing and persistence of emotional disorders following childbirth. *Br J Psychiatry* 1987;151:523–527.
12. O'Hara MW, Neunober DJ, Zekoski GH. Prospective study of postpartum depression: prevalence and predictive factors. *J Abnorm Psychol* 1984;93:158–171.
13. Parry BL. Mood disorders linked to the reproductive cycle in women. In: Bloom FE, Kupfer DJ, eds. *Psychopharmacology: the fourth generation of progress*. New York: Raven Press, 1995.
14. Robins LN, Regier DA, eds. Epidemiologic catchment area study. New York: Free Press, 1991.
15. Weissman MM, Klerman GL. Sex differences and the epidemiology of depression. *Arch Gen Psychiatry* 1977;34:98–111.
16. Hamilton M. A rating scale for depression. *J Neurol Neurosurg Psychiatry* 1960;23:56–62.
17. Lloyd C. Life events and depressive disorder reviewed. I: Events as predisposing factors. *Arch Gen Psychiatry* 1980;37:529–535.

18. Nott PN, Franklin M, Armitage C, Gelder MG. Hormonal changes and mood in the puerperium. *Br J Psychiatry* 1976;128:379–383.
19. Pop VJM, Essed GGM, de Geus CA, van Son MM, Komproe IH. Prevalence of postpartum depression—or is it post-puerperium depression?; *Acta Obstet Gynecol Scand* 1993;72:354–358.
20. Stotland N. Obstetrics and gynecology. In: Rundell JR, Wise MG, eds. *Textbook of consultation-liaison psychiatry*. Washington, DC: American Psychiatric Press, 1996.
21. Reich T, Winokur G. Postpartum psychosis in patients with manic depressive disease. *J Nerv Ment Dis* 1970;151:60–68.
22. Kumar R, Brockington IF, eds. Motherhood and mental illness, 2nd ed. Boston: Butterworth & Co., 1988.
23. Kendell RE, Wainwright S, Hailey A, Shannon B. The influence of childbirth on psychiatric morbidity. Psychol Med 1976;6:297–301.
24. Brockington IF, Cernik KF, Schofield EM, Downing AR, Francis AF, Keelan C. Puerpueral psychosis. *Arch Gen Psychiatry* 1981;38:829–833.
25. Kendell RE, Chalmers JC, Platz C. Epidemiology of puerperal psychoses. *Br J Psychiatry* 1987;150:662–673.
26. Myers JK, Weissman MM, Tischler GL, et al. Six-month prevalence of psychiatric disorders in three communities, 1980–1982. *Arch Gen Psychiatry* 1984;41:959–967.
27. Gitlin MJ, Pasnau RO. Psychiatric syndromes linked to reproductive function in women: a review of current knowledge. *Am J Psychiatry* 1989;146:1413–1422.
28. Peterson J. Obstetrics and gynecology. In: Stoudemire A, Fogel BS, eds. *Psychiatric care of the medical patient*. New York: Oxford University Press, 1993:637–656.
29. Logue CM, Moos RH. Perimenstrual symptoms: prevalence and risk factors. *Psychosom Med* 1986;48:388–414.
30. Northcott CJ, Stein MB. Panic disorder in pregnancy. *J Clin Psychiatry* 1994;55:539–542.
31. Kulin N, Pastuszak A, Sage SR, et al. Pregnancy outcome following maternal use of the new selective serotonin reuptake inhibitors: a prospective controlled multi-center study. *JAMA*1998;279:609–610.
32. Miller LJ. Psychiatric medication during pregnancy: understanding and minimizing risks. *Psychiatric Ann* 1994;24:2.
33. Nelson EW, Behrman RE, Kleigman RM, Arvin AM. *Textbook of pediatrics*, 15th ed. Philadelphia: WB Saunders, 1996.
34. Mills JL, Graubard BI, Harley EE, Rhoads GG, Berendes HW. Maternal alcohol consumption and birthweight. *JAMA*1984:252:1875–1879.
35. Williams GD, Grant BF, Hartford TC, Noble J. Population projections using DSM-III criteria for alcohol abuse and dependence, 1990–2000. Epidemiologic bulletin no. 23. *Alcohol Health Res World* 1989;366–369.
36. Gilman AG, Rall TW, Nies AS, Taylor P, eds. *The Pharmacological basis of therapeutics*, 8th ed. New York: Pergamon Press, 1990.
37. Moore RA, Bone LR, Geller G, Mamon JA, Stokes EJ, Levine DM. Prevalence, detection and treatment of alcoholism in hospitalized patients. *JAMA*1989;261:403–407.
38. Isselbacher KJ, et al. *Harrison's principles of internal medicine*. New York: McGraw-Hill, 1994.
39. Sokol RJ, Martier SS, Ager JW. The T-ACE questions: practical prenatal detection of risk-drinking. Am J *Obstet Gynecol* 1989;160:863–871.
40. Altshuler LL, Szuba MP. Course of psychiatric disorders in pregnancy: dilemmas in pharmacologic management. *Neurol Clin* 1994;12:613–635.
41. Altshuler LL, Cohen L, Szuba MP, Burt VK, Gitlin M, Mintz J. Pharmacologic management of psychiatric illness during pregnancy: dilemmas and guidelines. *Am J Psychiatry* 1996;153:592–606.
42. Kirklin JW, Barratt-Boyes BG, eds. *Cardiac surgery*. New York: John Wiley & Sons, 1986:889–907.
43. Zalstein E, Koren G, Einarson T, Freedom RM. A case-control study on the association between first trimester exposure to lithium and Ebstein's anomaly. *Am J Cardiol* 1990;65:817–818.
44. Cohen LS, Friedman JM, Jefferson JW, Johnson EM, Weiner ML. A reevaluation of risk of in utero exposure to lithium. *JAMA* 1994;271: 146–150.
45. Committee on Drugs, American Academy of Pediatrics. The transfer of drugs and other chemicals into human milk. *Pediatrics* 1994;93: 137–150.
46. Committee on Drugs, American Academy of Pediatrics. The transfer of drugs and other chemicals into human breast milk. *Pediatrics* 1983;72: 375–383.
47. Poulson E, Robson JM. Effect of phenelzine and some related compounds on pregnancy. *J Endocrinol* 1964;30:205–215.
48. Goldberg HL, Nissim R. Psychotropic drugs in pregnancy and lactation. *Int J Psychiatry Med* 1994;24:129–149.
49. Greden JF. Antidepressant maintenance medications: when to discontinue and how to stop. *J Clin Psychiatry* 1993;54:39–45.
50. Idanpaan-Keikkila J, Saxen L. Possible teratogenicity of imipramine/chloropyramine. *Lancet* 1973;282–284.
51. Kuller JA, Katz VL, McMahon MJ, Wells SR, Bashford RA. Pharmacologic treatment of psychiatric disease in pregnancy and lactation: fetal and neonatal effects. *Obstet Gynecol* 1996;87:789–794.
52. Pastuszak A, Schick-Boschetto B, Zuber C, et al. Pregnancy outcome following first-trimester exposure to fluoxetine (Prozac). *JAMA* 1993; 269:2246–2248.
53. Miller LJ. Clinical strategies for the use of psychotropic drugs during pregnancy. *Psychiatry Med* 1991;9:275–298.
54. Nulman I, Rovet J, Stewart DE, et al. Neurodevelopment of children exposed *in utero* to antidepressant drugs. *N Engl J Med* 1997;336: 258–262.
55. Edlund MJ, Craig TJ. Antipsychotic drug use and birth defects: an epidemiologic reassessment. *Compr Psychiatry* 1994;25:32–38.
56. Rumeau-Rouquette C, Goujard J, Huel G. Possible teratogenic effects of phenothiazines in human beings. *Teratology* 1977;15:57–64.
57. Slone D, Siskind V, Heinonen OP, Monson RR, Kaufman DW, Shapiro S. Antenatal exposure to phenothiazines in relation to congenital malformations, perinatal mortality rate, birth weight, and intelligence quotient score. *Am J Obstet Gynecol* 1977;128:486–488.
58. Herman JB, Rosenbaum JF, Brotman AW. The alprazolam to clonazepam switch for treatment of panic disorder. *J Clin Psychopharmacol* 1987;7:175–178.
59. Saxen I, Saxen L. Association between maternal intake of diazepam and oral clefts. *Lancet* 1975;2:498.
60. Holahan CJ, Moos RH. Social support and psychological distress: a longitudinal analysis. *J Abnorm Psychol* 1981;90:365–370.
61. Amaro H, Fried LE, Cabral H, Zuckerman B. Violence during pregnancy and substance abuse. *Am J Public Health* 1990;80:575–579.
62. O Hara MW. Social support, life events, and depression during pregnancy and the puerperium. *Arch Gen Psychiatry* 1986;43:569–573.
63. Kubler-Ross E. On death and dying. New York: Macmillan, 1969.

Cherry and Merkatz's Complications of Pregnancy,
Fifth Edition, edited by W. R. Cohen.
Lippincott Williams & Wilkins, Philadelphia © 2000.

CHAPTER 10

Battering

Bonnie Joan Dattel and Ronald A. Chez

Domestic violence can be defined as physical, sexual, or psychological abuse between family members and intimate partners. Subcategories of domestic violence include child abuse, elder abuse, sexual assault, incest, and child-parent abuse. Woman battering is another subcategory. It can be defined as a relationship in which a woman is coerced, intimidated, and dominated by her partner via psychological, sexual, or physical abuse. The abuse results in behaviors that physically harm the woman and arouse fear. It prevents her from doing what she wishes to do, or forces her to behave in a way she does not want.

Battering is not just the threat of or even the attack per se. Rather, it is a series of traumatic interactions outside of the boundaries of human experience that is expected in relationships. The result is persistent severe stress with energy directed at survival and avoiding or minimizing further abuse.

It is estimated that as many as 6 million women experience at least one act of battering per year (1,2). Abuse of women occurs throughout society. It cannot be predicted by any demographic feature related to age, race, ethnicity, education, religious denomination, socioeconomic status, or class (3,4). Battered women are cared for by all types of clinicians; most do not recognize that the abuse exists (5,6).

PREGNANCY

It is estimated that 4% to 8% of women are hit at least once during their pregnancy (7–9). Battering that precedes pregnancy continues during pregnancy in 25% to 45% of cases (7–9). Indeed, battering may be one of the most common complications of pregnancy.

Despite these statistics, our knowledge about abuse during pregnancy is limited. This is due to a lack of data on frequency, timing, and severity of injuries during pregnancy as well as a lack of stratified data on ethnic and other demographic variables (9,10). Abuse during pregnancy can pose significant risk for both mother and fetus. The adverse effects of abuse during pregnancy can be direct or indirect. Direct causes of adverse perinatal effect include abruptio placentae, fetal fractures, rupture of maternal organs, and antepartum hemorrhage (9).

It is clinically intuitive to believe that living in an environment of unremitting emotional stress can indirectly result in adverse perinatal outcome. The generic basis for this idea can be derived from Selye's three phases of adaptation elicited by stress (10). The stress syndrome is associated with changes in hormonal levels as well as alterations in cardiac output and its distribution. Furthermore, there is evidence that once a woman has been battered, the threat of repetition is always present, and that leads to a heightened state of stress that can indirectly compromise maternal and fetal health (11). These indirect effects of domestic violence on pregnancy can include elevated maternal stress, isolation of the mother, inadequate health care, behavioral risks such as substance abuse, and inadequate nutrition. The presence of domestic violence also determines the trimester during which women will initially seek prenatal care during pregnancy (9,11,12). Abused women are three times more likely to seek care during the third trimester (13). In fact, the abuser may force the woman not to seek earlier prenatal care by denying transportation, nutrition, and access to medications (vitamins, antibiotics). Similarly, because injuries around the head and neck are so visible, the victim's embarrassment or shame may contribute to missed prenatal appointments.

Postpartum, abused women are less likely to breastfeed (14). In addition, women experiencing abuse may be

B. J. Dattel: Department of Obstetrics and Gynecology, Eastern Virginia Medical School, Norfolk, VA 23507-1912; R.A. Chez: Departments of Obstetrics and Gynecology and Community and Family Medicine, University of South Florida, Department of Obstetrics and Gynecology, Tampa General Hospital, Tampa, FL 33606.

unable to negotiate reasonable family planning strategies with their partners. This in turn may contribute to unwanted or unplanned pregnancies. Women with unintended pregnancies are at greater risk of physical violence from their partners (15), completing a cycle of domestic abuse. It is crucial that clinicians are aware of the implications of abuse for their pregnant patients. Opportunities for identification, assessment, and intervention may be limited. Pregnancy nevertheless provides an important window of opportunity for the health care provider because the woman may be motivated to seek help to escape from the abusive relationship. It also may be the only time that a woman seeks medical attention. The fetal consequences of the abuse may motivate her to take steps to remove herself from the abusive situation.

DIAGNOSIS: ASSESSMENT BY HISTORY AND PHYSICAL EXAMINATION

Most battered women feel isolated and alone. Many do not recognize that there can be alternatives to their way of life, or that help is available. A major key to the recognition and seeking of alternatives is the clinician, who can recognize that the problem exists, inform the patient of tangible options, and support her decision making. An organized clinical construct leading to diagnosis and medical intervention will ensure that this therapeutic opportunity is made available to the pregnant woman. Providers of health care to women are particularly well situated to identify those who suffer from domestic violence because most women seek annual examinations, family planning, gynecologic, and obstetric care during their lives.

Battering results in a range of responses. They can include physical injury, a medical illness as a result of the injury, or the recurrent stress, social isolation, and overt emotional illness. The composite medical picture can change over time as a function of the relative frequency and severity of the abuse, as well as the amount of fear and isolation engendered by it.

There are some women who state directly as their chief complaint that they have been abused. However, most women conceal the history of an abusive relationship. In the latter situation, the chief complaint is not straightforward. Because there are no pathognomonic symptoms, attention is directed to subtle and indirect clues present in the history.

When an injury is present, some of the indicators of abuse in the medical history include vagueness about or an inconsistent explanation of the cause of the injury, and a time delay from the event to the presentation. When there is no overt physical injury, the complaint may relate to stress-induced symptoms including headache, insomnia, choking sensations, hyperventilation, dysphasia, back, chest, and chronic pelvic pain, and dyspareunia. When an emotional illness is manifested, the physician may detect signs of overt depression, suicidal ideation, anxiety, agitation, exhaustion, and substance abuse.

A diagnostic clue obtained from an overview of the medical chart is the tendency for abused patients to be labeled. These labels include accident prone, hysterical, help-rejecting, immature personality, and hypochondriac. These labels are not necessarily initiated by the clinician; many times the abused woman will self-label as an explanation for her injuries (accident prone, careless, clumsy).

A separate diagnostic clue can be the overly solicitous partner. This is the individual who stays close to the woman and answers questions directed to her. He will need to be separated from the patient if she is to provide a valid and candid history. This is particularly difficult if the partner serves as the translator for a non–English-speaking or hearing-impaired woman.

A pregnant woman who misses prenatal appointments and childbirth education classes, or one who increases the frequency of appointments because of minor complaints, requires follow-up for the possibility of battering. Marital discord, particularly separation and divorce during a pregnancy, are also associated with an increased likelihood of battering. All suicide attempts must be evaluated as a possible response to abuse. Approximately 25% of female suicides have a history of battering. In addition, unwanted or unplanned pregnancy also may be associated with the abusive relationship because the woman is unable to negotiate family planning options successfully or she seeks pregnancy as a haven from the abuse.

Any injury during pregnancy requires investigation. Frequently, there are multiple injuries out of phase with each other. The dominant distribution of physical abuse injuries tends to be head and neck, breasts, abdomen, and genitalia. The latter three have been referred to as the one-piece bathing suit pattern. These areas can be the main targets of assault in pregnant women (9). True home injuries, such as burns, cuts, and bruises, usually involve the extremities. A central location of injuries, covered by clothing, is less likely to be accidental. Importantly, the severity of the injury may not reflect the extent of the danger. For instance, the lack of injury or a minor injury may be associated with a failed attempted murder. Indeed, because some injuries are visible so readily during the obstetric examination, their presence may contribute to missed appointments because the woman is fearful of having them discovered.

In the absence of injuries, there is no specific clue to abuse on physical examination. A patient who has a flat affect or is hesitant, fearful, embarrassed, shy, or evasive may have a concern that her abuse will be identified. Certainly, this type of behavior plus an injury or the history described above begs exploration of the possible diagnosis of abuse.

There are no laboratory tests to validate a diagnosis of battering. Colored photographs of injuries are valuable not only for documentation in the medical record, but also for the patient's potential future needs in court actions. The use of medical photography requires a signed patient consent form, preferably identification of the patient with her face or hand included in the photograph, sealing the pictures in a labeled envelope, and filing it appropriately. These recommendations are standard and described elsewhere in detail (16).

ESTABLISHING THE DIAGNOSIS

The diagnosis of battering can be confirmed by direct questioning. Examples of such direct questioning include, "Did someone cause these injuries?" and "Are you in a relationship with a person who threatens or physically hurts you?" Each clinician needs to develop a comfortable method for initiating these questions as part of routine history taking for women.

The question is the first step on the path to enhanced patient well-being. Furthermore, if the patient is presenting with the express hope of being diagnosed, ignoring of the obvious by the clinician and the failure to ask the question will further dehumanize and isolate the patient.

Many women will respond truthfully when they are asked by a health care professional if they are being battered. When affirmation is given, it is important not to evidence disbelief, surprise, or irritation. It is also true that some women in whom battering is evident may deny its existence (5). When this happens, it is a challenge to remain nonjudgmental, supportive, and available (17). There are patients who are not emotionally ready to admit the need for help. Whether this is because of the belief that admission equates to the failure of the relationship or family, to the fantasy that the abuse will not happen again, or to feelings of shame, guilt, and embarrassment, it is necessary to respect the patient's pace in this process.

Sometimes denial of battering or nonacceptance of counseling is a function of the patient's present home life situation. Although not found invariably in victims' lives, most domestic violence evolves in three main phases: a time of tension building; the act of battering; and a phase of remorse, calm, and kindness (7). When present, the last phase can support the hope that violence will not recur. Unfortunately, the cycle is repetitive and may in fact escalate (11,17). It is necessary for the clinician to understand where the woman is in this behavioral cycle of violence. For example, during the period immediately after battering when the batterer is showing remorse (honeymoon phase), the woman has hope that the battering will not recur and may be reluctant to leave the relationship. Similarly, if the patient believes that there are no viable alternatives and is unaware of the resources in the community, she may not expose herself to an offer of help.

When a patient learns there are no reporting requirements to the police and that the clinician will maintain confidentiality in this interaction, she is more likely to talk. Specifically, unless the state's laws require it, the abuse should not be reported to the police without the patient's permission. To do so may jeopardize her safety if resultant government intervention is taken before she has a plan of action. In fact, the only consistent reporting law requirement for family violence in the United States is when minor children are suspected of being abused.

TREATMENT OF THE ABUSED WOMAN: IMMEDIATE

The physician's initial responsibility is to make a determination of the patient's safety (18). Attention is first directed to the patient's immediate needs related to protection from physical injury. Some injuries may require that the patient be hospitalized. The physician's response may be less defined when an emotional injury exists. When in doubt, the physician needs to ask the woman about the value of sheltering or hospitalization. One of the questions that also must be included relates to the safety of any children in the home. In one study, half of the children of battered wives were also abused (7). All children are adversely affected emotionally and behaviorally. There is evidence that witnessing parental violence may effectively prevent a child's understanding of the role of violence in family interactions. It is one of the factors consistently related to subsequent husband-to-wife violence in offspring of families with domestic abuse (19). Therefore, decisions about not returning to an unsafe home must include provisions for other family members in that home who are real or potential victims.

The patient is the best judge of the risks and safety in her present environment. She will choose a course that she believes most likely will ensure her survival. This may mean she will return to an unsafe home. If this occurs, it is necessary for the clinician to remain nonjudgmental. A positive approach is to encourage the patient to make necessary preparations for a fast and safe escape when the violence occurs (9). A contingency plan of action is provided in the following checklist:

1. Access to important documents that identify the woman and validate her presence in society (driver's license, birth certificate, titles, leases, income tax forms, pay slips, and social security card)
2. Access to transportation
3. Keys to house, car, bank vault
4. Emergency money, check and savings books
5. Important phone numbers, including the police, rescue squad, and domestic violence hotline
6. Safe haven for the night

7. Clothing, toilet articles, and medications for herself and the children packed in a suitcase and stored safely
8. Practice dry runs

TREATMENT OF THE ABUSED WOMAN: LONG-TERM

Pertinent for most battered women is the opportunity to obtain long-term help toward emotional healing. This type of help can result in lifelong change. Its goals for the patient are to identify safer viable alternatives to her current life-style and then to build a support system to help her achieve the alternatives chosen.

The clinician can start this process by encouraging the patient to talk and then listening in a supportive manner. The initial focus is to give permission for the woman to want her life to change, to need help, and to seek support. Once the patient's needs and wishes are identified, most of the specific treatment will be defined through community-based programs designed to protect and assist her. The second focus is to inform the patient how to access this array of available resources.

The most effective way to do so is use the domestic violence hotline. The number in the United States is 1-800-333-7233 (SAFE). It is a toll-free call and available 24 hours a day. This resource will provide the caller with local numbers in each state and most communities. Local hotline numbers also are listed in the information section of the phone book. The hotline number is answered by people with experience in providing information about sheltering, legal advocacy, financial advocacy, and child services. They also provide emotional support. Most local hotlines answer 24 hours a day. For many, both English and Spanish is spoken, and communication devices for the deaf are available.

An additional resource for the patient is office brochures and pamphlets on battering published by various organizations, including hospitals and state coalitions against domestic violence. These brochures encourage the patient to seek alternatives and support that decision making. Placing these materials in holders in the privacy of patient dressing areas and bathrooms will increase patient confidentiality.

Counseling is the critical focus of care. Although this type of counseling is not usually in the province or the experience of the obstetric-gynecologic clinician, he or she can be a strong advocate of its value. The source of the counseling (individual, group, self-help) is less important than the content. There appears to be no optimal forum and no optimal duration. Some patients require long-term counseling because of severe and long-standing emotional trauma, and others may require none once the violence itself ends. The thrust of counseling is to help the woman learn and then understand that she need not isolate herself because of shame, that her problem is not unique and many women share it, that she is not to blame for the violence, that no person deserves to be beaten, and that violence is the responsibility of the batterer. The overall goal of counseling is to empower the victim to take control of her life, develop a support system, plan independently, and restore her self-esteem.

This is not marital or family counseling. Battering is not the couple's problem. Rather, it is a problem precipitated by the batterer on a victim. These are issues of coercive control and abuse of power. This is not a fight between equals, but rather an imposition of one person's will on another in which violence is the tactic. Individual counseling is required to increase the woman's candor and to decrease the possibility of reprisal by the batterer.

In some communities, counseling also is available for the motivated abuser. Just as there is no typical social profile of a battered woman, there is no typical abuser. They have no identifiable traits in society. They do not usually have criminal records. They are sensitive to the realities of status and power, and are usually law-abiding outside of the home. In other words, they have different public and private images (19).

The thrust of abuser counseling is to stop the man from refusing to take responsibility for his actions. That is, because violence is learned, it can be unlearned and changed as a basic behavior response pattern. This includes the ability to tolerate the woman's autonomy and to stop blaming the victim as a rationalization for his actions. The abuser learns that he provokes himself and is solely responsible for his violent actions.

Temporary sheltering with safe living space is another important resource of the community. A shelter is a non-profit emergency housing facility; there are about 13,000 shelters in the United States. Therefore, many counties do not have one. On average, shelters turn away approximately 25% of petitioners because of lack of space. The shelter is established to provide food, clothing, transportation, counseling, child care services, and advocacy to other services in the community. Many have access to alternative permanent housing as well. In some communities, there also may be private safe homes offered by volunteers. Also, the regulations of some states allow the domestic violence victim to be designated for emergency eligibility in welfare-designated motel and hotel housing.

Legal action can be necessary to accelerate change and minimize continued harm. However, the legal system can be difficult to manage. Both the hotlines and shelters provide advocates who understand the system and can work through its processes. The battered woman has access to civil actions that set restraints protective of her and her family's safety at home and at work. One such action is a temporary restraining order. This order can be extended, vacated, or made into a permanent restraining order. It is a legal document that does not result in a criminal record. It does not preclude the potential filing of a criminal action, nor does it preclude the potential filing of other civil actions such as legal separation, divorce, and petitions for child custody and financial support. Battering per se can result in criminal charges. A conviction will result in a criminal record and sentencing that may include some combination of jail, fine, probation, and parole.

There is the expectation that a battered woman can just leave her chaotic and violent home life. Although many women do leave after the first incident or eventually, many women feel trapped, isolated, and alone and do not leave.

There are strong incentives to stay. There can be formidable personal, social, and economic impediments to starting a new life. There is the potential loss of income, shelter, and custody of the children coupled with a relative lack of money, job training, employment opportunities, affordable quality child care, and decent housing. Going to a shelter may mean giving up one's possessions, life-style, and personal home. These potential losses can reinforce a reluctance to leave. Furthermore, leaving may not stop the stress or the violence because the threat of harm and actual reprisal can continue. For some women, not leaving an unsafe home can be interpreted as normative and responsible behavior given the alternatives and benefit-risk ratios.

Women do leave their partners and their environment. They do so for a number of reasons, including the fact that the children are being directly affected by the abuser or by an escalation of the violence. A different and pertinent reason for a victim to leave is the gaining of knowledge of local community resources and getting an effective and understanding response from these resources. This fact emphasizes the therapeutic value of the clinician actively encouraging the woman to use the domestic violence hotline in the community to access these resources.

CONCLUSIONS

Woman battering is prevalent in our society. It has adverse impact on the patient and her children's well-being. It is necessary to be alert to and aware of battering in any woman seeking health care. Because the presenting signs and symptoms of battering during pregnancy can be difficult to identify, the recommendation is that all pregnant women be assessed for battering routinely in prenatal care. Furthermore, when battering is identified, the clinician should be prepared to offer intervention through supporting the patient's access and use of counseling and advocacy groups (7,17).

Consistent, replicable scientific data about most facets of woman battering is just now becoming available. As a relatively new area of social science research, a number of hypotheses continue to require objective proof. An increased focus on the husband/partner/batterer is a critical area of research need.

The clinician's role and responsibility is to act as an agent of change for the patient. The active steps include identifying the presence of abuse by awareness of the problem; informing the victim of her rights by acknowledging the unacceptability of the violence; supporting her decision making; and encouraging the woman to initiate change by providing appropriate community referrals, including the domestic violence hotline.

REFERENCES

1. Plichta S. The effects of woman abuse on health care utilization and health status. A literature review. *Women's Health Issues* 1992;2: 154–163.
2. Bachman R, Saltzman L. Violence against women. US Department of Justice Statistics. Washington, DC: US Department of Justice, 1992.
3. Hotaling GT, Sugarman DB. An analysis of risk markers in husband to wife violence: the current state of knowledge. *Violence Victims* 1986;1: 101–122.
4. Sugg NK, Innui T. Primary care physician's response to domestic violence: opening Pandora's box. *JAMA* 1992;267:3157–3160.
5. Abbott J, Johnson R, Kozial-McLain J, Lowenstein SR. Domestic violence against women. Incidence and prevalence in an emergency department population. *JAMA* 1995;269:1763–1767.
6. Jecker NS. Privacy beliefs and the violent family. Extending the ethical argument for physician intervention. *JAMA* 1993:269:776–780.
7. Gelles RJ. Violence in pregnancy: are pregnant women at greater risk of abuse? *J Marriage Family* 1988;50:841–847.
8. Gazmararian JA, Lazorick S, Spitz AM, Ballar TJ, Saltzman LE, Marks JS. Prevalence of violence against pregnant women. *JAMA* 1996;275: 1915–1920.
9. Dattel BJ. Women, domestic violence and the obstetrician-gynecologist. In: Sciarra JJ, ed. Gynecology and obstetrics. New York: Lippincott-Raven, 1997:1–7.
10. Selye H. Physiology and pathology of exposure to stress. Montreal: ACTA Medical Publishers, 1950.
11. Brookoff D, O'Brien KK, Cook CS, Thompson TD, Williams C. Characteristics of participants in domestic violence. Assessment at the scene of domestic assault. *JAMA* 1997;277:1369–1373.
12. Martin SL, English KT, Clark KA, Cilenti D, Kupper LL. Violence and substance use among North Carolina pregnant women. *Am J Public Health* 1996;86:991–998.
13. Taggart L, Mattson S. Delay in prenatal care as a result of battering in pregnancy: cross-cultural implications. *Health Care Women Int* 1996; 17:25–34.
14. Acheson L. Family violence and breastfeeding. *Arch Fam Med* 1995;4: 650–652.
15. Gazmararian JA, Adams MM, Saltzman LE, et al. The relationship between pregnancy intendedness and physical violence in mothers of newborns. The PRAMS Working Group. *Obstet Gynecol* 1995;85: 1031–1038.
16. Bullock LFC. Battering and pregnancy: effect on infant birth weight [Dissertation]. Denton, TX: Texas Woman's University, 1987.
17. ACOG Technical Bulletin. The battered woman. Number 124. Washington, DC: American Congress of Obstetricians and Gynecologists, 1989.
18. Helton AS, Snodgrass G. Battering during pregnancy: intervention strategies. *Birth* 1987;14:142–147.
19. Surgeon General's Workshop on Violence and Public Health Report. US Public Health Service Publication HRS-D-MC 86-1.

Cherry and Merkatz's Complications of Pregnancy,
Fifth Edition, edited by W. R. Cohen.
Lippincott Williams & Wilkins, Philadelphia © 2000.

CHAPTER 11

Educational Interventions in High-Risk Pregnancy

Margaret Comerford Freda

Although patient education is an integral component of the care of women with high-risk pregnancies, health care providers have little formal training in its provision. Women who find themselves in the midst of a pregnancy that has been labeled high risk are understandably concerned and apprehensive about the myriad changes occurring within their bodies. This apprehension is compounded by worry about the possible impact of their condition on the fetus (1). Health care providers barrage women with information about their high-risk condition and expect that they will follow our well-meaning directions for the sake of their health and that of their fetus. They sometimes do not. It is important, therefore, that we consider how we deliver information and education to our patients, because teaching and communication methods can influence how well women understand their condition and affect their ability to make informed choices about how to proceed (2–4).

Every encounter with a woman experiencing a high-risk pregnancy should be an educational encounter (5). Despite the fact that formal instruction in patient education is not usually included in the education of physicians, it is he or she who is generally charged with informing the pregnant woman that she has developed a high-risk condition and with teaching her all she needs to know. Physicians might need to tell the patient that she has developed gestational diabetes or pregnancy-induced hypertension, and they must ask for and obtain informed consent for complicated screening tests such as triple marker screening, or for HIV testing. By witnessing the signing of the informed consent, you are affirming that your patient understands enough about the ramifications of her diagnosis, procedure, or test in question to make an informed decision. Does she possess that understanding? Confronted with disturbing news about her condition, the woman may be frightened or shocked at her diagnosis. She is surely anxious. In many cases the woman and her family must absorb an overwhelming amount of new information in a short period of time and must learn unfamiliar skills and behaviors to assist in the treatment of the high-risk condition. When we teach our patients, we assume that the patients have learned. But have they? Do we know how much they actually hear of our explanations?

There are many cogent issues regarding patient education that the provider of high-risk pregnancy care should ponder. The first concerns how much you know about the basic principles of patient education, and whether you use teaching methods known to be most effective in promoting knowledge gain and behavior change. What is your usual method of teaching your patients? Do you provide all the information yourself, one-to-one? Do you use a multidisciplinary team to provide teaching? If you use a team approach, who is the most appropriate member of your team to do the teaching? Do you use written handouts, films, videotape, or computer-assisted program information? Are your ancillary written or audiovisual materials appropriate for the patients in your population? Do you include the family in the teaching? Do you teach the woman in a group, along with other patients with the same diagnosis?

The next issue concerns how you can assure that the material you teach is actually learned by the woman. When she leaves your office or clinic, how much does she remember about what you taught? After your teaching, does she know enough to make choices in life-style changes needed to improve her chance of an optimal outcome? What are her misconceptions, and will those misconceptions prevent her from carrying out the plan of care? Will her family assist, or hinder? Will her cultural

M. Comerford Freda: Albert Einstein College of Medicine, Bronx, NY 10461.

This chapter contains selected original text from Freda MC. Cultural competence in patient education. *Am J Maternal Child Nurs* 1997;22;219–220.

beliefs interfere with or enhance the plan of care? Is she physically, emotionally, and cognitively capable of performing the tasks you ask of her? All of these questions are essential to understanding the appropriate provision of health education to your patients.

GOAL OF PATIENT EDUCATION

It is important for health care providers to understand why engagement in the education of their patients is important. It is tempting to think that we educate our patients in order to help them follow our instructions more fully, but that is not the case. The goal of patient education for women with high-risk pregnancies is to assist our patients in the improvement of their own health. This is accomplished by educating them about their condition and their options, thus helping them to make informed decisions concerning treatment.

Although there are numerous studies concerning this general concept, the application of it specifically to high-risk pregnancies has received little attention in the literature. Available studies on a similar concept—informed consent—are applicable.

Patient Education and Informed Consent

One of the reasons health care providers teach patients is to obtain informed consent for tests or procedures. Although what patients understand before informed consent is requested has not been studied extensively, there is evidence that our patients rarely comprehend or recall what we have taught them (6–11). Despite this dismal outcome exposed by patient learning research, the medical community has done little to improve the teaching of patients from whom we request informed consent. Braddock, for instance, found recently that discussions in the primary care setting rarely assessed the patient's understanding of information presented by a physician (6). Hekkenberg studied what patients understood after a teaching session about surgical complications and found that half of the surgical patients taught had a flawed understanding of the complications from surgery (11). Other authors have suggested that the emotional distress associated with a medical decision makes comprehension difficult when informed consent is requested (10–16). In a recent study on whether pregnant women who were taught about maternal serum alpha fetoprotein testing understood enough to fulfill the criteria for informed consent, it was found that although 80% of the women who were educated agreed to have the screening test, 38% of those women could not describe the purpose of the test, and 72% of the women thought that a negative test meant that their baby would be healthy in all respects (17). Similar misconceptions also were found in other studies of this subject (8,9,18).

There is no agreement in the literature or in the legal system on what actually constitutes understanding of topics that require informed consent (17,19). Until further study of this issue is undertaken, therefore, providers have no standards to guide them as to how much comprehension is acceptable. Thus, it is incumbent upon us who teach our patients and then request informed consent to evaluate what our patients really understand. It has been suggested that providers should alter the way they think about informed consent, and that it should actually be considered an interactive process through which two people come to an understanding (20), and that informed consent be the vehicle through which an ongoing dialogue between pregnant women and their care providers can be fostered (21). Searight (22) recommended that informed consent be considered strictly a method for educating patients, and that providers use this set of five questions to evaluate patients learning every time a new treatment, test, or procedure is suggested:

What do you call your condition?
Which treatment is being recommended?
What is the treatment supposed to do for you?
Are there risks associated with the treatment?
What alternatives are there to the treatment?

Because the goal of patient education is to assist the patient to understand enough about her condition to be able to make informed choices about treatment, and because research shows that patients generally do not understand the complicated issues we teach them, it seems that changes should be made in the way we request informed consent. Searight's suggestion to use an interactive dialogue between provider and patient during which the patient is asked to restate the education given, describing the test or treatment and its ramifications, seems appropriate and long overdue. Unfortunately, the time required of such interactive processes involving dialogues between patients and providers through which evaluation of patient learning can be assessed may not be congruent with the goal of cost cutting in today's health care environment. Health care providers need to work toward devising more effective and efficient ways to permit patients to have an educated voice in their own health care. One way of doing this is to become more knowledgeable themselves about how best to educate their patients.

TEACHING AND LEARNING

Motivation to Learn

One of the difficulties in the provision of patient education is determining whether our patients are motivated to learn, because although we can teach any time we perceive a need, learning requires motivation on the part of the learner. In preventive health, we might choose, for example, to suggest that our patients stop smoking, or lose weight, or start exercising. Whether the patient is ready to learn that lesson, and act on it, is the key to whether the behavior we target will change. We in perinatal health are fortunate, however, for pregnancy has been called the teachable moment, that special time when most pregnant patients are interested in learning and are willing to modify behaviors that could impact on pregnancy outcome (23–25).

Motivation to learn cannot be assumed, however, even during pregnancy. Although most women are motivated by the hope of an optimum pregnancy outcome, there are women with high-risk pregnancies who may be unwilling or unable to change their behaviors. Women who use illicit drugs in pregnancy, for example, may avoid prenatal care and the educational interventions inherent therein. Yet these women, too, can be motivated. Kearney (26,27) found that women who are actively using illicit drugs will be more likely to attend prenatal care when they think that the prenatal care is an asset to improve fetal outcome, and when they do not feel threatened with loss of child custody. By understanding the motivation for learning in high-risk pregnancy situations such as this, providers are better able to structure educational experiences that emphasize motivating factors.

Adult Learning Principles

Most high-risk pregnant patients we target for teaching are adults. Before we can understand how best to teach them the information they need to know, it is important that we appreciate the general principles of adult learning. Adults learn differently from children, and principles developed for classroom teaching of children are not necessarily useful in teaching adults. The classic reference in adult learning is Knowles (28), who taught us that adults learn best under certain circumstances. These adult learning principles (Table 11-1) are important for all patient educators to understand if we hope to assist our patients to learn as much as is needed during a high-risk pregnancy.

The principles set forth in Table 11-1 need to be understood before patient teaching for women with high-risk pregnancies can be planned. For example, these principles can be used as follows when developing a teaching plan about preterm labor symptoms.

TABLE 11-1. *Adult learning principles*

Adults learn best in response to a perceived need.
Teaching of adults should progress from what they already know to the unknown.
Teaching of adults should progress from simple concepts to the more complex.
Active participation, rather than passive listening, promotes learning.
Adults require opportunities to practice new skills with the teacher.
Reinforcement of the desired behavior enhances learning.
Immediate feedback and correction of misconceptions increases learning.

Because adults learn best in response to a perceived need, the patient first needs to be engaged in a discussion of the problem of preterm birth and her risk. The severe health implications of preterm birth need to be emphasized so the woman understands that although she might not perceive herself to be at risk, that risk does exist in her pregnancy as it does in all pregnancies.

She should then be assessed for what she already knows about the topic. Has she ever had a preterm birth? Does she know anyone who has? Is there a prevailing myth in her family or culture that needs to be addressed? Myths are powerful pieces of information that are often internalized at an early age and understood to be the absolute truth (29–31). Because the patient considers them truths, it is not likely that the myths will be discussed in the context of a patient education session unless the provider of care specifically asks what the patient knows about this topic. Myths need to be addressed in a direct and forthright manner. When teaching about preterm birth, for example, the provider should ask what the patient's family or friends have told her about babies being born too early. In this author's 15 years of teaching about this topic, for instance, she has found that there is a predominating myth among some cultural groups that a baby born at 7 months' gestation is healthier than a baby born at 8 months. This myth, which we providers recognize as false as well as dangerous, is passed from grandmother to mother to daughter, making it difficult to convince women who have preterm symptoms at 28 weeks' gestation that they should seek care in order to avoid delivery at that time. When teaching the woman about preterm birth, the lesson should proceed from the simple concept of why babies need at least 37 weeks of gestation to have the best chance of health, to teaching the subtle symptoms of preterm labor, to the instructions for what to do if symptoms develop, and then to the more complex concepts of how to access care if symptoms develop, and what treatments might be offered.

Because active participation, rather than passive listening, promotes learning in adults, each concept in the teaching should be addressed in a discussion form with the patient, not in a lecture format. The patient should be asked meaningful questions throughout the lesson to encourage active participation. The health care provider should not ask, "Do you understand?" but rather ask open-ended questions that require the patient to restate the portion of the lesson that just occurred ("Now, please tell me the symptoms of preterm labor").

Because preterm labor teaching requires that the patient be taught to palpate for contractions, that skill should be practiced during the lesson so the patient feels confident that she truly understands where to place her fingers and what she is feeling for.

Reinforcement of the behavior can be encouraged by asking the patient to tell you just how she would go about dealing with preterm symptoms in specific conditions (e.g., while at work, or while in the park with her other children). Invent a scenario in which the patient experiences symptoms, and elicit her response.

Providing immediate feedback to the patient on how she handled the hypothetical situation will help to correct any misconceptions she might have and reassure the provider that the teaching session has provided the patient with needed decision-making skills should the symptoms appear.

Use of a Multidisciplinary Team to Provide Patient Education

Providing comprehensive teaching such as that illustrated here is difficult to achieve when physicians are the only professionals working with the patients in an office, because time constraints are the reality of patient care. We also know that when patient education is the purview of only one provider, there is a lack of congruence between what physicians think their patients want to learn about pregnancy and what the patient themselves want to learn (32). Use of a multidisciplinary team to provide comprehensive care and education that meets the individual needs of high-risk pregnant patients is therefore ideal. Because physicians are responsible for actually delivering the complex high-risk care, the use of registered professional nurses to provide high-quality patient education in offices or clinics is appropriate. Registered nurses consider patient education one of their major professional responsibilities and are trained in its provision. When working as a team to provide quality education to high-risk pregnant women, the physician institutes the teaching by providing the diagnosis and the initial discussion with the patient, and the registered nurse uses her or his expertise to deliver the comprehensive education the patient needs to cope with her illness both in individual and in group class settings.

Models of Behavior Change

There are numerous models to assist us in understanding how and why people change their behavior (33–38). One cited most commonly is the Health Belief Model (33), which has been used since the 1950's and helps us to understand why patients take or do not take action to improve their health. In this model, behavior change is theorized to be a balance among the patient's perceived susceptibility to the disease, her perceived benefits from performing the behavior asked of her, and her perceived barriers to performing the behavior. For example, a woman diagnosed with gestational diabetes first has to believe that the disease is a reality (if she is not experiencing symptoms, stressing objective findings such as the laboratory reports and the ultrasonographic findings of fetal macrosomia helps to make the condition more tangible), then has to understand what benefits she will gain from learning to test her blood sugar and inject insulin several times a day, and balance that with the barriers in her life that would interfere with compliance with the treatment plan. These barriers might include difficulty in obtaining the appropriate equipment, learning the tasks, or working with syringes, a motion that is frightening to most adults and might be equated with the illicit drug culture for others. Only when the perceived benefits outweigh the perceived barriers in her own mind will she learn the tasks and perform the behavior. When examined for effect size, perceived barriers have been shown to be the most powerful of the dimensions of the Health Belief Model (34). Knowing this, the health care provider attempting to help a high-risk pregnant woman alter her behavior can spend time discussing the barriers to treatment that the woman perceives. This could help in proactively averting problems with the medication regimen. This model has been studied with hypertension, asthma, obesity, medication taking, adhering to regimens, and keeping appointments, among other health issues (35). The Health Belief Model helps us to understand that our patients will respond if they perceive they are susceptible, that the risk is serious, that they will benefit, and that the barriers to adherence are not too great.

A newer theoretical framework that attempts to explain why and how people change their behavior is the Transtheoretical Stages of Change Model, which assists the provider to anticipate the patient's readiness for change (37,38). In this model, change is seen as a series of stages. Before one can move to the next level, one must have accomplished the stage before it. The stages of change are precontemplation, contemplation, preparation, action, and maintenance. In this model, the provider first assesses the apparent stage of the patient in question. If, for example, a patient is in the precontemplative stage, it is virtually impossible to ask them to move directly to an action mode. An example of this is the patient who does not perceive her smoking to be a problem for her or for her fetus. The patient's mother might have told her, for instance, that she smoked while she was pregnant and she had no problems. For a patient in this precontemplation stage, time must be spent educating the patient about the dangers of cigarette smoke to her and to the fetus. If, however, a patient has moved past precontemplation when you meet her and is in the preparation stage, there is little need for the provider to spend time and effort teaching about the dangers of cigarettes. Furnishing that patient with the telephone numbers of smoking cessation clinics or programs might be the most appropriate use of the provider's time and efforts.

Self-efficacy theory (36) is a third theory of behavior change useful to the provider of high-risk pregnancy care. This theory states that a patient must first feel that change is possible before change can occur. A person with high self-efficacy will be more likely to change a behavior. For example, when discussing domestic violence with an affected patient, it might be clear to the provider that the patient does not think it is possible for her to live a life free of violence, and she cannot get away from her abuser. In this instance, helping the patient to increase her self-efficacy is the appropriate course of action to help activate behavior change. It is the health care provider's task to make the behavior change seem possible by partitioning the task into smaller, easier subtasks. Asking (or worse, telling) the patient with low self-efficacy to leave the abuser will not promote behavior change. One strategy that uses self-efficacy theory to promote behavior change for such a patient would be for the provider to assist the patient in developing an escape plan as a first step. The patient would not be told that she must leave the abuser; she would be asked just to start thinking about it. The next time she is seen in the office or clinic, the provider can ask about her plan and discuss it. In this way, the patient can be recognized and rewarded for taking a first step toward eventual success. Each succeeding visit would elicit one more small step, until the small behavioral changes become additive, self-efficacy grows, the escape plan is completed, and the patient is able to contemplate acting on it.

Readability and Literacy

Written information that accompanies oral teaching enhances understanding of complicated topics. Therefore, every patient education session should end with the provision of appropriate written information for the patient to take home (4,39,40). Conversely, a patient education booklet or information sheet written at an inappropriate reading level will not educate patients (41). It is incumbent upon us as providers to be sure that the materials we provide for our patients are at the appropriate reading level. Literacy does not equate with grade level; in fact, most patients' reading levels are 3 to 5 years below their completed grade level (40). The average reading level of citizens of the United States is 8th grade, and about one in five people in the United States read at the 5th grade level or below (40). It is illustrative to learn that most newspapers in the United States are written at the 9th to 12th grade reading levels; about 20% of Americans, therefore, cannot read them. It has been shown that most health education materials are written at readability levels that are far above the average reader's 6th grade reading level and are therefore incomprehensible to a significant number of patients (39–45). Davis (46) found that 80% of materials produced by the American Academy of Pediatrics, the Centers for Disease Control and Prevention, and pharmaceutical companies were written at the 10th grade reading level; analysis of consent forms from the National Cancer Institute found all to be at readability levels of grades 12 to 17 (47). Similarly, patient information booklets from the American College of Obstetrics and Gynecology have been analyzed, and readability evaluated at grades 11 and higher (48). We know that receiving written information helps patients to increase their recall of health education material (39), and we also know that materials written at a lower readability level are more effective (23,49). Therefore, all of us who provide patient education should be aware of the issue of readability and should not be using patient education materials written above the 6th grade level, so that the majority of women can comprehend them (41).

There are many different formulas used for testing the readability of written materials. Computer programs are available to calculate the readability of patient educational materials according to several standardized formulas such as FOG, FLESCH, Dale-Chall, and FRY (50), but probably the easiest formula to use is the SMOG formula (51), which requires no computer software and is used frequently by health care providers. Tables 11-2, 11-3, and 11-4 describe the SMOG formula and how it can be used to evaluate the readability of patient education materials.

Because one in five Americans is functionally illiterate, it is important as well to consider the patient education needs of high-risk pregnant women with low literacy skills (52). When planning educational materials for women with low literacy, the following techniques have proven effective (24):

TABLE 11-2. *SMOG testing*

The SMOG formula predicts the grade level difficulty of a passage within 1.5 grades. Its advantages include its simplicity and how fast it is to use. It is useful for evaluating readability for materials from grade 5 through college.

Instructions:

You need 30 sentences (see below if you have less than 30 sentences). Count out 10 sentences near the beginning, 10 from the middle and 10 from the end.

Count the words containing three or more syllables in the 30 sentences.
Count hyphenated words as one word.
Proper names are counted.
Abbreviations should be sounded out and counted (Oct. = October = 3 syllables).
Numbers should be sounded out and counted (573 = 7 syllables).
Use the SMOG Conversion Table to see the grade level.

If you have less than 30 sentences:

If you do not have 30 sentences, you can still use SMOG. Count the number of sentences you have and the number of words with three or more syllables. Use the table showing SMOG Conversion for Samples with Less than 30 Sentences to convert to grade level. For instance, if you have 15 sentences and 12 words with three or more syllables, look for 15 in the first column of the table showing SMOG Conversion for Samples with Less than 30 Sentences, then find the conversion number opposite it (2.0). Multiply your word count (12) by the conversion number (2.0). That equals 24. Now look at the SMOG Conversion Table. For a word count of 24, the grade level is 8.

TABLE 11-3. *SMOG conversion table*

Word count of words with three or more syllables	Grade level
0–2	4
3–6	5
7–12	6
13–20	7
21–30	8
31–42	9
43–56	10
57–72	11
73–90	12
91–110	13
111–132	14
133–156	15
157–182	16
183–210	17
211–240	18

Use larger print.
Do not use all capital letters (more difficult to read).
Use boldface type to emphasize important facts.
Use short sentences and words with few syllables.
Use illustrations wherever possible.
Use the active voice.
Use cues such as underlining, circles, and color to help guide the eye.
Leave much blank space on each page.
Use a question-and-answer format for written information.
Use no more than seven items in lists.
Avoid double negatives.

TABLE 11-4. *SMOG conversion for samples with less than 30 sentences*

No. of sentences	Conversion number
29	1.03
28	1.07
27	1.1
26	1.15
25	1.2
24	1.25
23	1.3
22	1.36
21	1.43
20	1.5
19	1.58
18	1.67
17	1.76
16	1.87
15	2.0
14	2.14
13	2.3
12	2.5
11	2.7

Adapted from Redman B. *The process of patient education,* 8th ed. St. Louis: Mosby Year Book, 1996:55–56.

Cultural Competence in Patient Education

There is no doubt that culture influences the behavior of our patients. When teaching women with high-risk pregnancies, providers must be cognizant of the cultural values and mores of their patients, or they risk losing an opportunity to enhance the patients' knowledge base. In previous decades this was called cultural sensitivity; this terminology has been replaced by the term "cultural competence." This change has come about because it is perceived that when one is sensitive to another culture, the implication is that the health care provider's culture is dominant (or even superior), and he or she must be sensitive to others. The newer concept of cultural competence suggests that no one culture is superior to another, and that we must all be competent to work with people of many cultures (53,54).

As the American public becomes ever more diverse ethnically, we are all faced with providing care and patient education to patients from cultures with which we may be completely unfamiliar. How can patient education be accomplished in a culturally competent manner? The first step is to develop an understanding of the target audience's subjective culture, including some of the major beliefs, attitudes, roles, social norms, and values of the group. This can be accomplished by talking to members of the cultural group you want to reach. Health care providers should make an effort to learn more about the cultural groups likely to come to their offices because the methods used to teach one cultural group may not be effective with a different ethnic or cultural group. Sabogal and colleagues, for instance, found that the use of scare tactics (generally felt to be of little value in health education) were very effective in working with a Vietnamese population, for their belief system includes a strong requirement to visualize the results of disease (53). Sabogal's group has offered suggestions for how to gain an understanding of a target audience's culture:

- Work with a multicultural team to develop educational programs. If you have no colleagues from the culture you are targeting, find patients or community members with whom you can consult before you develop your program. Use community members who have approximately the same years of education and acculturation as your patient population. Involvement of the target audience from the beginning of the development of the program significantly improves your success.
- Be aware of your own assumptions, biases, and prejudices. Unless you know something directly from members of the cultural group, do not assume it to be true. Most generalizations we make about cultural groups are unfounded.
- Understand the core cultural values of the group. For instance, Latinos in Sabogal's study described a strong sense of family (*familismo*). This was used to be sure that family was included in the education they pro-

vided, and the material taught included the implications of treatment options on the family. Another Latino cultural value identified was *fatalismo*, a belief that little can be done to alter one's fate. This could have significantly reduced the impact of the health teaching, but instead was addressed forthrightly as a part of the teaching. The Latino patients studied needed to be reminded repeatedly that treatment and cure were possible; stories from other affected Latino community members who had been treated successfully significantly improved the effectiveness of the teaching.
- Develop the written materials in the native language of the target audience. Do not develop them in English and have them translated. Translations from English to another language are often impossible and culturally irrelevant.
- Use testimonials of persons within the target audience as role models. If you or your colleagues are not of the target ethnic group, talk to one of your patients or community members who could come to your session and vouch for your credibility. Testimonials build confidence, and an interested community member can be your best ally.

SOME GENERAL GUIDELINES FOR THE PROVISION OF EFFECTIVE PATIENT EDUCATION

Once providers understand the principles of how adults learn, learn how adults can change behavior, acknowledge the importance of cultural competence, and develop an awareness of literacy and readability issues, some general guidelines for how best to provide effective patient education can be better understood. Three guidelines that are most helpful in conducting patient education are simplicity, reinforcement, and sensitivity.

Simplicity

- Assess what the patient knows about the topic before teaching.
- Do not overteach. When planning a teaching session, choose the three or four most important things for the patient to know, and teach only those topics.
- Teach the simple concepts about the diagnosis and treatment before the complex ones.
- Communicate at the patient's level of understanding. Do not use medical terminology.
- Be aware of literacy issues and the educational level of your patients. Check the readability of the materials you hand out. Are they written at too high a level?
- Be aware of the words you use. To the general public, for instance, the word positive is a good thing, whereas in health care it often is not (e.g., HIV positive). The term "intrauterine growth retardation" is another frequently used term that can be easily misunderstood by patients. We should make every effort to use the word "restriction," not "retardation," because patients hear "retarded" and assume that their child will be mentally retarded (55).
- Be concrete. Tell the patient exactly what you mean and exactly what she needs to do.

Reinforcement

- Present the most important information first and then again last.
- Always reinforce what you have taught with written materials. Patients typically forget half of everything you tell them, so written materials they can take home enhance learning.
- Look for myths and misinformation, and correct them.

Sensitivity

- Be aware of your patients' culture. Culture can be a profound factor in learning.
- Involve the family in the education if possible.
- Be alert for emotional cues. Patients who are crying or distracted cannot listen or learn.

Methods of Providing Patient Education

There is no one method of patient education that is superior to any other. Individual teaching, group teaching, and computer-aided teaching are all useful but are most effective when chosen for the appropriate patient, with the appropriate diagnosis, using the appropriate materials (56–67). No matter which method is chosen, the principles presented earlier in this chapter need to be kept in mind. All patient education should be planned to meet the individual learner's abilities, using the optimal personnel and materials.

One-to-one Teaching

The most commonly used method of teaching pregnant patients is one-to-one education, in which the provider teaches the patient about one particular topic in the midst of an office visit. This method is effective in increasing knowledge and promoting behavior change and is ideally performed by a knowledgeable provider who uses the principles of patient education to inform the teaching (4). One-to-one teaching is especially appropriate when sensitive or private topics need to be discussed, or when the topic is not complex and requires little time. Providers who wish to teach patients about how to disclose positive HIV status to a loved one, for instance, might appropriately choose individual, one-to-one teaching with role playing rather than assembling a group of similar patients for instruction. In addition, for a simple concept such as teaching fetal movement counting, it has been shown that teaching women this skill within the context of an obstetrical visit is effective not only in promoting the counting of fetal movements, but also in the added benefit of increasing maternal-fetal attachment, which fosters positive postpartum attachment behaviors (68–70).

The major disadvantage of one-to-one teaching is that it is not cost effective because it is the most time-consuming method for the provider (4). When pregnancy-related topics must be taught to many patients, more efficient methods should be considered. Because one-to-one teaching is the method most often used in physicians' offices, it is instructive to consider whether that approach results in comprehensive education during pregnancy. In one study that examined the difference between what private care and public care patients were taught in pregnancy, it was found that the public care patients were taught a greater variety of pregnancy-related topics. Because public care settings generally offer more group teaching opportunities than private office settings, these results suggest we should rethink the customary one-to-one method of teaching women and consider using methods that more effectively educate pregnant women about topics of importance in pregnancy (71).

Group Teaching

For most topics of interest to high-risk pregnant women, group teaching of patients is a method that has been shown to be very effective (61,72). The results of studies of women being taught about preterm labor symptoms, diabetes management, contraception, smoking cessation, parenting, breastfeeding, and childbirth preparation showed that knowledge and behavior change was increased when they were taught in groups (73–80). Group teaching is generally planned, executed, and evaluated by registered professional nurses, working as a part of a multidisciplinary team in the care of pregnant women. This use of registered nurses for patient education is generally seen more often in public care settings and in some health maintenance organizations, but is increasingly common in multiphysician private practices (4). Some additional advantages of group teaching include the availability of support from the other group members, questions asked by group members that might not have been considered by each individual patient, and the modeling of behaviors and skills by the teacher and by the group members. Group teaching is best used for general topics of interest to most patients. Early prenatal care education, for instance, which includes nutrition education, genetic screening tests, and common discomforts of pregnancy, are topics often covered in group instruction (17,56,74).

Videotape Teaching

Recent years have witnessed the proliferation of videotape patient education programs. There are several companies that produce such videos, and although the video genre in general has been found to be an effective method of delivering standardized information to patients during individual or group teaching sessions, certain caveats must be heeded when using this method (62,74,81–83). Audiovisual materials such as videotapes should be no longer than 11 minutes because information presented after that time period is not retained well (4). Providers considering the use of videotapes should always arrange to preview the video before using it for patients because it is important that the video portray situations and conditions that are culturally relevant to the group for which it is intended (83). During the preview process, the provider also should be cognizant of the language used in the video and should determine if the literacy level is appropriate for the designated population. Videotaped patient education has been shown to be more effective when followed by facilitation by a professional who can clarify information and answer questions than when used as a stand-alone method of teaching. In O'Donnell's study (67), videotaped information with an imbedded suggestion for obtaining coupons and redeeming them was used for teaching about the prevention of sexually transmitted diseases. When a video alone was used for teaching, 27.6% of the patients used the information to redeem coupons. When facilitation with a provider answering questions was furnished after the video, 36.9% of the patients used the information. When just oral teaching without a video was used, 21.2% of the patients redeemed coupons. These differences were statistically significant.

In recent years there has been an expansion of videotaped educational programs being provided in medical waiting rooms, with the express intention of teaching patients through this method. When this phenomenon was studied by Freda and colleagues, the use of passive waiting room teaching with videotapes was found to be ineffective in teaching the patients most in need of quality patient education: nulliparas, African-American women, and teenaged pregnant women (25). Videotapes should always be considered an adjunct to enhance patient education, not a primary method.

Computers for Patient Education

Computers are being used for patient education in a variety of ways. Pregnant patients use computers in their homes to access information not previously available to them, and health care providers use computers to design health education materials for their patients and as an adjunct to structured health education classes.

Computer-aided instruction (CAI) is a recent entry into the teaching tool armament of patient educators (84,85). To date, most computer programs developed for patient education have been didactic in nature, with little or no tailoring of the material to the specific needs of the individual patient. As the use of computers for education increases in the next decade, we can expect that software companies will be increasingly tapping the market of adults wanting to learn more about pregnancy, especially issues in high-risk pregnancy. Computer-aided instruction is a rapidly expanding method for patient education; but it should be remembered that, as with videotaped information, CAI should not be considered a replacement of the teacher/learner interaction, but rather an enhancer of that interaction.

Computers also can be used for patient education through the use of CD-ROMs, which are available from many educational companies and are designed to teach pregnant women about what to expect in pregnancy, just as popular books have for decades. One such CD-ROM popular with patients is *Your Pregnancy and Newborn from Parenting Magazine.* There are literally hundreds of products available in this category. It is always a good idea for providers of high-risk pregnancy care to preview what advice is being proffered in the most popular CD-ROMs, in anticipation of the questions that will be asked by their patients.

Another important use of computers in patient education is for the development of patient educational materials, which can be tailored to the specific needs of a patient population. The widespread use of desktop publishing has made this practice practical for even the small office setting.

For the sophisticated patient who is familiar with computers and the Internet, there are now myriad health education outlets available through the World Wide Web and its many search engines. For the patient interested in the latest research findings about any aspect of her high-risk pregnancy, the National Library of Medicine now provides public access to MEDLINE for those patients who have Internet capability (http://www.ncbi.nlm.nih.gov/PubMed). Interesting and informative sites are being added to the World Wide Web daily and can be found easily by using YAHOO, LYCOS, InfoSeek, or any other search engine provided by the Internet service provider company used by the patient. A LYCOS search by this author in preparation for writing this chapter, using the words "high-risk pregnancy," yielded 4,967 separate sites where information could be gathered on every conceivable aspect of high-risk pregnancy. Providers who want to suggest useful World Wide Web sites for their patients might first preview the following three commonly used sites. The URL (Universal Resource Locator, or web site address) for The March of Dimes Birth Defects Foundation is http://www.modimes.org; for Geo Health Web, an international site offering a full range of health care information and networking for consumers, professionals and educators, it is http://geohealthweb.com; and for Healthfinder, a consumer oriented information source run by the US government, it is http://www.healthfinder.gov.

SUMMARY

The appropriate provision of patient education is a task every health care provider must assume, whether or not he or she is formally prepared to do so. It is our responsibility, therefore, to educate ourselves about the most effective ways to provide that patient education. This chapter has presented basic information about health education for providers of care to high-risk women that will assist them in performing this task. By reviewing this chapter, providers can better understand the general principles of teaching and learning, the concepts of motivation to learn and change behavior, and how adults learn best. In addition, the concepts of cultural competence in patient education and how to assure that the patients literacy level is acknowledged have been presented. The various methods currently in use for patient education were discussed so the provider could best decide which method is most useful in each circumstance. Individualizing the teaching plan for each patient based on her diagnosis, culture, educational level, and family situation, using the principles set forth in this chapter, will provide the best chance for effective education of high-risk pregnant women about their conditions, their options, and their treatment choices.

REFERENCES

1. Mercer RT, Ferketich SL. Stress and social support as predictors of anxiety and depression during pregnancy. *Adv Nurs Sci* 1988;10:26–39.
2. Blankson ML, Goldenberg RL, Keith B. Noncompliance of high risk pregnant women in keeping appointments at an obstetric complications clinic. *South Med J* 1994;87:634–638.
3. Healton C, Taylor S, Burr C, Dumois A, Lowenstein N, Kaye J. The impact of patient education about the effect of zidovudine on HIV perinatal transmission: knowledge gain, attitudes, and behavioral intent among women with and at risk of HIV. *Am J Prev Med* 1996;12:47–52.
4. Redman BK. The process of patient education, 8th ed. St. Louis: Mosby Year Book, 1996.
5. US Public Health Service. Caring for our future: the content of prenatal care. Washington, DC: US Public Health Service, 1989.
6. Braddock CH, Fihn SD, Levinson W, Jonsen AR, Perlman RA. How doctors and patients discuss routine clinical decisions: informed decision making in the outpatient setting. *J Gen Int Med* 1997;12:339–345.
7. Marteau TM, Johnston M, Plenicar M, Shaw R, Slack J. Development of a self-administered questionnaire to measure women's knowledge of prenatal screening and diagnostic tests. *J Psychosom Res* 1988;23: 403–408.
8. Marteau TM, Kidd J, Michie S, Cook R, Johnston M, Shaw RW. Anxiety, knowledge and satisfaction in women receiving false positive results on routine prenatal screening: a randomized controlled trial. *Obstet Gynecol* 1993;14:185–196.
9. Faden RR, Chwalow J, Orel-Crosby E, Holtzman NA, Chase GA, Leonard CO. What participants understand about a maternal serum alpha-fetoprotein screening program. *Am J Public Health* 1985;75: 1381–1384.
10. Earley KJ, Blanco JD, Prien S, Willis D. Patient attitudes toward testing for maternal serum alpha-fetoprotein values when results are false-positive or true-negative. *South Med J* 1991;84:439–441.
11. Hekkenberg RJ, Irish JC, Rotstein LE, Brown DH, Gullane PJ. Informed consent in head and neck surgery: how much do patients actually remember? *J Otolaryngol* 1997;26:155–159.
12. Klepatsky A, Mahlmeister L. Consent and informed consent in perinatal and neonatal settings. *J Perinat Neonat Nurs* 1997;11:34–51.
13. Kuba LM. The prenatal testing roller coaster: one mother's story. *J Perinat Educ* 1995;4:19–22.

14. Pape T. Legal and ethical considerations of informed consent. *Assoc Operating Room Nurses J* 1997;65:1122–1127.
15. Charles C, Gafni A, Whelan T. Shared decision making in the medical encounter: what does it mean? *Social Sci Med* 119;44:681– 692.
16. Sandelowski M & Jones LC. Couples evaluations of foreknowledge of fetal impairment. *Clin Nurs Res* 1996;5:81–96.
17. Freda MC, DeVore N, Valentine-Adams N, Bombard A, Merkatz IR. Informed Consent for MSAFP screening in an inner city population: how informed is it? *J Obstet Gynecol Neonat Nurs* 1998;27:99–105.
18. Sikkink J. Patient acceptance of prenatal alpha-fetoprotein screening: a preliminary study. *Fam Practice Res J* 1990;10:123–131.
19. Lurvey LD, Nager CW, Johnson DD. Informed consent: a review. *Primary Care Update Obstet Gynecol* 1996;3:192–196.
20. Andre J. Commentary: ethical dimensions of informed consent. *Women's Health Issues* 1993;3:24.
21. Chervenak FA, McCullough LB. Clinical guidelines to preventing ethical conflicts between pregnant women and their physicians. *Am J Obstet Gynecol* 1990;162:303–306.
22. Searight HR, Barbarash RA. Informed consent: clinical and legal issues in family practice. *Fam Med* 1994;26:244–249.
23. Calabro K, Taylor WC, Kapadia A. Pregnancy, alcohol use and the effectiveness of written health education materials. *Patient Educ Counsel* 1996;2:301–309.
24. Corrarino J, Freda MC, Barbara M. Development of a health education booklet for pregnant women with low literacy skills. *J Perinat Educ* 1995;4:23–28.
25. Freda MC, Abruzzo M, Davini D, DeVore N, Damus K, Merkatz IR. Are they watching? are they learning? prenatal video education in the waiting room. *J Perinat Educ* 1994;3:20–28.
26. Kearney M, Murphy S, Irwin K, Rosenbaum M. Salvaging self: a grounded theory of pregnancy on crack cocaine. *Nursing Research* 1995;44:208–213.
27. Kearney M. Drug treatment for women: traditional models and new directions. *J Obstet Gynecol Neonat Nurs* 1997;26:459–468.
28. Knowles M. The modern practice of adult education. New York: Cambridge University Press, 1980.
29. Myhre P. Myths and facts . . . about how your patient views her diabetes. *Nursing* 1996;26:17–20.
30. Koff E, Rierdan J. Early adolescent girls understanding of menstruation. *Women's Health* 1995;22:1–21.
31. Levinson RA. Reproductive and contraceptive knowledge, contraceptive self-efficacy, and contraceptive behavior among teenage women. *Adolescence* 1995;30:65–85.
32. Freda MC, Andersen HF, Damus KH, Merkatz IR. What do pregnant women really want to know? A comparison of client and provider perceptions. *J Obstet Gynecol Neonat Nurs* 1993;22:237–244.
33. Becker MH. The health belief model as predictor of preventive health behavior. *Am J Public Health* 1974;64:205–216.
34. Janz NK, Becker MH. The health belief model, a decade later. *Health Educ Q* 1984;11:1–47.
35. Becker MH, Janz NK. The health belief model applied to understanding diabetes regimen compliance. *Diabetes Educ* 1985;11:41–47.
36. Bandura A, Adams NE. Analysis of self efficacy theory in behavior change. *Cognitive Ther Res* 1982;1:287–310.
37. Grimley DM, Prochaska JO, Velicer WF, Prochaska GE. Contraceptive and condom use adoption and maintenance: a stage paradigm approach. *Health Educ Q* 1996;22:20–35.
38. Prochaska JO. The transtheoretical model of change and HIV prevention: a review. *Health Educ Q* 1994;21:471–486.
39. Arthur VA. Written patient information: a review of the literature. *Adv Nurs* 1995;21:1081–1086.
40. Doak C, Doak L, Root J. Teaching patients with low literacy skills, 2nd ed. New York: JB Lippincott, 1996.
41. Estey A, Musseau A, Keehan L. Patient's understanding of health information: a multihospital comparison. *Patient Educ Counsel* 1994;24: 73–78.
42. Albright J, deGuzman C, Acebo P, Paiva D, Faulkner M, Swanson J. Readability of patient education materials: implications for clinical practice. *Appl Nurs Res* 1996;9:139–143.
43. Dowe MC, Lawrence PA, Carlson J, Kerserling TC. Patients use of health teaching materials at three readability levels. *Appl Nurs Res* 1997;10:86–93.
44. Ayello EA. A critique of the AHCPR's preventing pressure ulcers—a patient's guide as a written instructional tool. *Decubitus* 1993;6:44–46.
45. Beaver K, Luker K. Readability of patient information booklets for women with breast cancer. *Patient Educ Counsel* 1997;31:95–102.
46. Davis TC. Reading ability of parents compared with reading level of pediatric patient education materials. *Pediatrics* 1994;93:460–468.
47. Meade CD, Howser DM. Consent forms: how to determine and improve readability. *Oncol Nurs Forum* 1992;19:1523–1528.
48. Zion AB, Aiman J. Level of reading difficulty in the American College of Obstetricians and Gynecologists patient education pamphlets. *Obstet Gynecol* 1989;74:955–960.
49. Meade C, Byrd J, Lee M. Improving patient comprehension of literature on smoking. *Am J Public Health* 1989;79:1411–1412.
50. Micro Power and Light. Readability Calculator. Dallas, TX, 1996.
51. Jiminez SL. Evaluating the readability of written patient education materials. *Perinat Educ* 1994;3:188–193.
52. Weiss BD, Coyne C. Communicating with patients who cannot read. *N Engl J Med* 1997;337:272–274.
53. Sabogal F. Printed health education materials for diverse communities: suggestions learned from the field. *Health Educ Q* 1996;23:123–141.
54. Freda MC. Cultural competence in patient education. *Am J Mat Child Nurs* 1997;22:219–220.
55. Freda MC. Arrest, trial and failure. *J Obstet Gynecol Neonat Nurs* 1995;24:393–394.
56. Lindeman CA. Patient education. *Nurs Res* 1988;6:29–60.
57. Padgett D. Meta analysis of the effects of educational and psychoeducational interventions on management of diabetes mellitus. *J Clin Epidemiol* 1988;41:1007–1030.
58. Mullen PD, Ramirez G, Groff JY. A meta analysis of randomized trials of prenatal smoking cessation interventions. *Am J Obstet Gynecol* 1994;171:1328–1334.
59. Mullen PD, Green LW, Persinger GS. Clinical trials of patient education for chronic conditions: a comparative meta analysis of intervention types. *Prev Med* 1985;14:753–781.
60. Theis SL, Johnson JH. Strategies for teaching patients: a meta analysis. *Clin Nurse Specialist* 1995;9:100–120.
61. Leff E. Comparison of the effectiveness of videotape versus live group infant classes. *J Obstet Gynecol Neonat Nurs* 1988;17:338–344.
62. Long C. Teaching parents about infant CPR—lecture or audiovisual tape? *Am J Maternal Child Nurs* 1992;17:30–32.
63. Tomaino-Brunner C, Freda MC, Damus K, Runowicz CD. Can precolposcopy education increase knowledge and decrease anxiety? *J Obstet Gynecol Neonat Nurs* (in press).
64. Freda MC, Damus K, Merkatz IR. What do pregnant women know about the prevention of preterm birth? *J Obstet Gynecol Neonat Nurs* 1991;20:140–145.
65. Freda MC, Andersen HF, Damus K, Poust D, Brustman L, Merkatz IR. Lifestyle modification as an intervention for inner city women at high risk for preterm birth. *J Adv Nurs* 1990;15:364– 372.
66. Freeman HP, Orlandi MA. A self help smoking cessation program for inner city African Americans: results from the Harlem Health Connection project. *Health Educ Behav* 1997;24:201–217.
67. O'Donnell LN, San Doval AS, Duran R, O'Donnell C. Video-based sexually transmitted disease patient education: its impact on condom acquisition. *Am J Public Health* 1995;85:817–822.
68. Bloom KC. The development of attachment behaviors in pregnant adolescents. *Nurs Res* 1995;44:284–289.
69. Freda MC, Mikhail M, Polizzotto R, Mazloom E, Merkatz IR. Fetal movement counting: which method? *Am J Maternal Child Nurs* 1993; 18:314–321.
70. Mikhail M, Freda MC, Merkatz RB, Polizzotto R, Mazloom E, Merkatz IR. The effect of fetal movement counting on maternal attachment to the fetus. *Am J Obstet Gynecol* 1991;165:988–991.
71. Freda MC, Andersen HF, Damus KH, Merkatz IR. Is there a difference in the information being given to private vs. public prenatal patients? *Am J Obstet Gynecol* 1993;169:155–160.
72. Likar LL, Panciera TM, Erickson AD, Rounds S. Group education sessions and compliance with nasal CPAP therapy. *Chest* 1997;111: 1273–1277.
73. Freda MC, Damus K, Merkatz IR. What do pregnant women know about the prevention of preterm birth? *J Obstet Gynecol Neonat Nurs* 1991;20:140–145.
74. Freda MC, Damus K, Andersen HF, Merkatz IR. A PROPP for the Bronx: preterm birth prevention education in the inner city. *Obstet Gynecol* 1990;76:93–96.
75. Waller CS, Zollinger TW, Saywell RW, Kubisty KD. The Indiana Pre-

natal Substance Use Prevention Program: its impact on smoking cessation among high risk pregnant women. *Indiana Med* 1996;89: 184–187.

76. Mullen P, Ramirez G, Groff JY. A meta analysis of randomized trials of prenatal smoking cessation interventions. *Am J Obstet Gynecol* 1994; 171:1328–1334.
77. Lowe NK. Maternal confidence in coping with labor: a self-efficacy concept. *J Obstet Gynecol Neonat Nurs* 1991;20:457–463.
78. Koniak-Griffin D, Verzemnieks I, Cahill D. Using videotaped instruction and feedback to improve adolescents mothering behaviors. *J Adolesc Health* 1992;13:570–575.
79. Jones LC. A meta analysis study of the effects of childbirth education on the parent infant relationship. *Health Care Women Int* 1986;7:357–370.
80. Hobel CJ. The West Los Angeles Preterm Birth Prevention Project. *Am J Obstet Gynecol* 1994;170:54–62.
81. Brown SA. Studies of educational interventions and outcomes in diabetic adults: a meta analysis revisited. *Patient Educ Counsel* 1990;16:189–215.
82. Healton CG, Messeri P. The effect of video interventions on improving knowledge and treatment compliance in the sexually transmitted disease clinic setting. *Sexually Transmitted Diseases* 1993;20:70–76.
83. O'Donnell L, San Doval A, Vornfett R, DeJong W. Reducing AIDS and other STDs among inner city Hispanics: the use of qualitative research in the development of video-based patient education. *AIDS Educ Prev* 1994;6:140–153.
84. Skinner CS, Siegfried JC, Kegler MC, Strecher VJ. The potential of computers in patient education. *Patient Educ Counsel* 1993;22:27–34.
85. Consoli SM, Ben Said M, Jean J, Menard J, Plouin PF, Chatellier G. Benefits of a computer assisted education program for hypertensive patients compared with standard education tools. *Patient Educ Counsel* 1995;26:343–347.

SECTION IV

Cardiopulmonary Disorders

Cherry and Merkatz's Complications of Pregnancy,
Fifth Edition, edited by W. R. Cohen.
Lippincott Williams & Wilkins, Philadelphia © 2000.

CHAPTER 12

Cardiovascular Disease

Jose Meller and Martin E. Goldman

The pregnant woman who has heart disease presents complex medical problems to her physicians. Because normal pregnancies produce cardiorespiratory symptoms that mimic the symptoms of patients who have organic heart disease, it is important to differentiate normal physiologic changes of pregnancy from the pathophysiologic problems of pregnancy. In addition, the circulatory changes of pregnancy may unmask heart disease in a previously asymptomatic woman. Moreover, preexisting cardiac pathology can affect the pregnant mother and the fetus, especially in women who have cyanotic congenital heart diseases.

In this chapter, we discuss the normal circulatory changes that occur in pregnancy as well as different cardiovascular disorders, their diagnoses, and their management during pregnancy.

CARDIOCIRCULATORY CHANGES DURING PREGNANCY

During pregnancy there is a marked increase in cardiac output that begins to rise in the tenth week and peaks by the twentieth week (1). At that point, the cardiac output may increase 30% to 50% above the nonpregnant levels, and is maintained until term. If cardiac output is measured in the supine position during the last trimester, however, it may be found to be decreased because of mechanical compression of the inferior vena cava by the uterus with subsequent decreased venous return to the heart.

Cardiac output is the product of stroke volume and heart rate, and both variables contribute to increased cardiac output during pregnancy. Stroke volume is increased in early pregnancy, whereas later in pregnancy, increased heart rate is the more important factor producing the increase in cardiac output. In labor, uterine contractions cause a 20% increase in stroke volume because of the blood squeezed into the circulation from the uterine venous network. This augmentation in stroke volume is augmented by the increased sympathetic tone that results from pain and anxiety (2).

Blood Volume

Blood volume, which can increase up to 40% during pregnancy, begins to increase in the first trimester of pregnancy and continues to increase progressively until term (3). The increase in plasma volume is greater than the increase in red cell volume, which explains the physiologic anemia of pregnancy (4). There have been studies that correlate the changes in blood volume with fetal weight or placental weight. Blood volume is greater in

J. Meller and M. E. Goldman: Department of Medicine, Mount Sinai Medical Center, New York, NY 10029.

twin pregnancies than in singleton pregnancies (5). The blood volume postdelivery depends on the amount of blood lost at the time of delivery and the volume of fluids reabsorbed from the third space (accumulated during pregnancy), as well as from blood squeezed from the uterine vessels once uterine contraction has occurred.

These circulatory changes occur before the fetal metabolic demands become evident and before the placenta is developed well enough to function as an arteriovenous fistula. The increased cardiac output and blood volume are thought to be caused by sodium retention secondary to an increase in aldosterone and to increased sex steroids released by the ovaries or the placenta, with subsequent increased total body water (6,7). This explains why hypervolemia can be seen in cases of hydatidiform mole without the presence of a fetus. The changes in late pregnancy are also caused by the presence of a larger uterus, the increased blood flow to the placenta and breasts, and the increased metabolic demands of the fetus.

The maternal heart rate begins to increase (around 10–15 beats/min) early in pregnancy and remains high through term. Twin pregnancies may cause a greater tachycardia than single pregnancies (8). Systemic vascular resistance tends to decrease during the first two trimesters, with a subsequent decrease in systolic and diastolic blood pressures. During the last trimester, inferior vena caval obstruction caused by the mechanical effect of the larger gravid uterus tends to reduce venous return with a subsequent increase in peripheral vascular resistance to maintain blood pressure. The pulmonary vascular resistance also tends to decrease throughout the pregnancy, but there is a mild increase in right-sided cardiac chamber pressures and pulmonary artery pressures because of the increase in pulmonary blood flow. The peripheral and pulmonary vasodilation is possibly caused by the increased endothelial release of vasodilating prostaglandins (i.e., E_2, prostacyclin), estrogen, and progesterone. In the later stages of pregnancy, placental arteriovenous shunting becomes a more important factor. The blood pressure is maintained by an activated renin-angiotensin system.

Echocardiographic studies performed during pregnancy reflect the blood volume increase and show a progressive mild dilatation of all cardiac chambers' diastolic dimensions without change at end systole (9). There is also an increased velocity in circumferential fiber shortening seen throughout pregnancy, implying that the volume overload of a normal pregnancy may be responsible for the increased myocardial contractility and the increased left ventricular ejection fraction.

Cardiovascular Findings During Normal Pregnancy

The cardiovascular changes previously mentioned are responsible for a series of physical findings that can mimic cardiac pathology. Because of the increased blood volume, the peripheral pulse is bounding, and because of the decreased peripheral resistance, the pulse occasionally can collapse, as seen in aortic regurgitation. Also, because of the hypervolemia, the neck veins may be distended and a cervical venous hum can be heard.

The large uterus produces a change in the heart position, which is responsible for a more horizontal heart than in the nonpregnant state. This will mimic cardiac enlargement because the apex beat will be palpated more to the left and cephalad of its normal nonpregnant position. The hypervolemia is also responsible for an increase in intensity of the first sound (S1), an apical S3 sound, an occasional S4 sound (10), and the functional systolic ejection murmur commonly heard at the apex or left sternal border (11). Rarely, a mammary soufflé can be heard as a continuous murmur superficially over the breast. With the increase in pulmonary flow, the second pulmonic sound can be increased in intensity. Diastolic murmurs have been reported as physiologic findings during pregnancy and are thought to be caused by dilatation of the pulmonary artery and resultant pulmonic insufficiency.

Radiographic studies of the chest performed during pregnancy show a more horizontal heart with a cardiothoracic ratio greater than 50%. Also, straightening of the left upper cardiac border can mimic left atrial enlargement. Moreover, increased vascular markings can be seen in the lungs, simulating the findings of mitral stenosis (12). The electrocardiogram may show a shift of axis to the left with a deeper Q wave in lead three. All other changes reported in the electrocardiogram during pregnancy may have been caused by incidental cases of labile repolarization changes or by mitral valve prolapse. Transient S-T segment and T-wave changes, arrhythmias, and heart block, therefore, are as common during pregnancy as in nonpregnant women. An echocardiogram will demonstrate mildly dilated chambers with normal or hypercontractile ventricular function.

Finally, a healthy woman who has a normal pregnancy often has symptoms identical to those of persons with cardiac disorders and mild heart failure. The hyperventilation of a normal pregnancy that begins very early because of increased progesterone (13) is responsible for a compensated maternal respiratory alkalosis that favors renal excretion of bicarbonate to enhance the transfer of fetal CO_2 (14) to maternal blood. Also, as the gravid uterus elevates the diaphragm, the functional respiratory reserve capacity decreases. A pregnant woman, therefore, normally would complain of dyspnea, easy fatigability, and a reduction in exercise tolerance.

SPECIFIC CARDIAC DISORDERS

Although heart disease is the leading nonobstetric cause of maternal death during and immediately after pregnancy (15,16), there has been a marked reduction in the total number of maternal deaths in the United States in the past few decades. This lower maternal mortality rate is related to the decrease in rheumatic heart disease in this country, despite the fact that more potential high-risk women with surgically corrected congenital heart disease or older women with potential coronary artery disease are becoming pregnant. Half of the cardiac deaths during pregnancy are caused by rheumatic heart disease; one fifth are attributable to bacterial endocarditis, and another fifth to coronary artery disease. An average of three maternal deaths per year in the United States are caused by congenital heart disease in cases equally divided among patients who have Eisenmenger's syndrome, interatrial and interventricular septal defects, patent ductus arteriosus, and other disorders. The marked reduction in maternal mortality has been attributed to better general medical management of cardiac conditions as well as to prevention and termination of high-risk pregnancies.

Mitral Stenosis

Mitral stenosis is the leading cause of maternal cardiac mortality during pregnancy (17). The characteristic increased blood volume and heart rate of pregnancy are particularly dangerous in patients who have significant obstruction to left ventricular filling because of mitral stenosis. The increase in heart rate shortens the left ventricular filling time, one of the factors leading to higher left atrial pressure and consequent pulmonary congestion. The increase in pulmonary blood flow in patients who have mitral stenosis and pregnancy also may cause severe symptoms because of pulmonary congestion. During labor, with increased blood volume secondary to uterine contractions that force blood into the venous circulation, combined with tachycardia, transient pulmonary edema may develop if the stenosis is severe.

If the patient who has mitral stenosis is in cardiac functional class 1 before pregnancy, it is unlikely that pregnancy will add any risk to the mother. Patients in classes 3 and 4, however, may have mortality rates as high as 5%. If atrial fibrillation is present, the mortality rate can reach 15% (17). If the functional class is unclear because the patient has been asymptomatic but is relatively sedentary, symptoms could develop under stress. For these patients, we recommend an exercise treadmill test for objective functional evaluation before pregnancy or during the first trimester to determine whether the pregnancy should be allowed to continue.

A two-dimensional (2-D) echocardiogram can evaluate the mitral valve area accurately, as well as determine left ventricular size and function. When excessive calcification of the valve and subvalvular apparatus distort visualization of the valve, pulsed- or continuous-wave Doppler can calculate mitral valve area based on transmitral flow velocity (pressure half-time). Color-flow Doppler can estimate the severity of valvular regurgitation.

The medical management of pregnant women with symptomatic mitral stenosis should be directed to the reduction of blood volume and to the increase of left ventricular diastolic filling time by slowing the heart rate. The reduction in blood volume can be achieved by a reduced sodium intake and by the use of diuretics (18). Increase in diastolic filling time of the left ventricle can be achieved with bed rest and beta blockers. If atrial fibrillation is present, anticoagulation is mandatory in patients with mitral stenosis because of the high risk of systemic embolization.

If the mother's life is at risk at any point in the pregnancy, emergent intervention, balloon valvuloplasty, or cardiac surgery should be performed. Closed commissurotomy does not carry an increased risk for the mother or for the fetus (19). Cardiopulmonary bypass may have deleterious effects on the fetus, however, especially in the first trimester. Miscarriage and mental retardation have been reported. Short perfusion times at high flow rates for optimal placental perfusion should be attempted. Cardiopulmonary bypass has no higher risk for the mother who is pregnant than similar surgery for the nonpregnant patient. Currently, mitral balloon valvuloplasty performed during cardiac catheterization by inserting a deflated balloon into the mitral orifice and expanding it can successfully dilate a stenotic mitral valve as successfully as open surgical commissurotomy. A preprocedure 2-D echocardiogram can score the mitral valve by four criteria (valve mobility, leaflet thickness, leaflet calcification, and subvalvular apparatus) to determine if catheter mitral balloon valvuloplasty is a viable alternative. Transesophageal echocardiography is usually necessary to evaluate the valve for a potential valvuloplasty. Significant valvular regurgitation, marked valvular calcification and presence of left atrial thrombi are contraindications to valvuloplasty. Mitral valvuloplasty by balloon during cardiac catheterization should carry no extra risk during pregnancy, except for the fetal radiation. To minimize radiation exposure, transesophageal 2-D echography can guide the valvuloplasty catheter. Left lateral uterine displacement is important if the procedure is performed in the third trimester. Dommisse et al. reported on 11 pregnant patients who underwent balloon valvuloplasty, increasing their mitral valve area from a mean of 0.9 cm^2 to 2.1 cm^2 with all subsequently having normal pregnancies (20).

Patients who have mitral stenosis should generally be allowed to enter into labor spontaneously at term. Induction may be appropriate to allow for establishment of invasive monitoring techniques. Lumbar epidural analgesia is recommended for the first stage of labor. During the second stage, the use of forceps may be indicated to limit maternal straining efforts. Following delivery, excessive fluid replacement should be avoided to prevent pulmonary congestion.

Mitral Regurgitation

Mitral regurgitation is usually well tolerated by pregnant women. The reduced systemic vascular resistance characteristic of pregnancy may even reduce the intensity of the murmur of mitral regurgitation because of increased forward flow and less backward flow. In asymptomatic patients, even with marked cardiomegaly on chest x-ray but with normal left ventricular size, pregnancy presents no increased risk for the mother. An echocardiogram can precisely determine the pathophysiologic mechanism of the valve lesion and assess right and left atrial and ventricular sizes. If the left ventricle is markedly dilated with an end-systolic diameter of ≥5 cm, or left ventricular systolic dysfunction is present, a higher risk should be expected for the mother and termination of the pregnancy should be considered if recognized early. If atrial fibrillation is present, anticoagulation should be considered to reduce the risk of systemic embolization. In symptomatic patients, the approach should be similar to that for nonpregnant persons, with the expectation that the symptoms will only progress with the continuation of the pregnancy. If by echocardiography or cardiac catheterization the pulmonary artery pressure is increased significantly, or if the left ventricle is markedly dilated, surgical repair should be considered, even if the patient is pregnant.

Aortic Stenosis

Although usually a problem of the elderly, aortic stenosis can present in younger patients secondary to congenital bicuspid leaflets or rheumatic heart disease. Aortic stenosis of mild or moderate severity is usually well tolerated by pregnant women. An echocardiogram can determine the precise valve area, the degree of ventricular hypertrophy, and ventricular diastolic compliance. Severe aortic stenosis (aortic valve area ≤0.75 cm^2) carries a reported 17% maternal mortality rate (14). In these circumstances, patients should be thoroughly counseled about the options of avoiding or terminating a pregnancy. Balloon aortic valvuloplasty is a potential option, but there is little documentation on the effects of the procedure on the fetus. Of note, therapeutic abortion can be responsible for maternal mortality in patients who have severe aortic stenosis. In severe aortic stenosis, excessive fluid administration can result in pulmonary edema; however, excessive diuretic administration can result in hypotension and death. When a pregnant woman with severe aortic stenosis is going to have an induced abortion or is first diagnosed close to the delivery date, a pulmonary artery catheter should be used for hemodynamic monitoring of these extremely difficult cases. The left ventricular filling pressure should be maintained at relatively high levels (around 18 mm Hg) to prevent a decline in cardiac output. Immediately following delivery or abortion, compulsive fluid replacement should be achieved to maintain left ventricular filling pressures. In general, if severe aortic stenosis is diagnosed, an aggressive approach to the valvular problem should be taken. If an abortion is planned, it is better to correct the stenosis first by surgery and then perform the abortion. If surgery is refused or is not advisable, a balloon valvuloplasty should be considered as a temporary measure to improve the hemodynamics to make an abortion or the continuation of pregnancy safer for the mother.

Aortic Regurgitation

Aortic regurgitation may be attributable to valvular (bicuspid leaflets, rheumatic, prolapse, healed endocarditis) or aortic (root dilatation) causes and produces left ventricular volume overload. Aortic regurgitation is a usually well-tolerated disorder during pregnancy. The reduced systemic vascular resistance during pregnancy favors forward flow into the aorta and a decrease in the regurgitant flow back into the left ventricle. If moderate or marked left ventricular dysfunction is present before pregnancy, or if left ventricular echocardiographic end systolic dimension is above 5.5 cm, pregnancy should be counseled against, or if already present, therapeutic abortion should be considered by the patient. In all other cases, pregnancy should be well tolerated, although diuretics may be indicated for mild symptoms. During the last trimester in patients who have severe aortic regurgitation, afterload-reducing agents should be used if pulmonary congestion develops. If acute aortic regurgitation (usually because of bacterial endocarditis) precipitates severe congestive failure, emergency cardiac surgery is indicated at any time during the pregnancy.

Anticoagulation in Pregnancy

The most common cardiac indications for anticoagulation during pregnancy are mitral stenosis with atrial fibrillation and mechanical prosthetic valvular heart disease. These conditions also have an increased risk of thromboembolism in nonpregnant individuals.

The presence of atrial (and especially left atrial appendage) thrombi can be detected best by transesophageal echo. Occasionally, patients who have supraventricular arrhythmias and a history of systemic embolization also are anticoagulated at the time of pregnancy. Some noncardiac conditions also require anticoagulation (e.g., pulmonary emboli and deep venous thrombosis).

During pregnancy there normally is an increase in factors II, VII, VIII, IX, and X. There also is decreased thrombolytic activity (21). These changes may predispose pregnant women to thrombosis. Most likely, these alterations in the clotting factor levels are not of great significance during the pregnancy itself; however, there is a definite increased risk of thromboembolic disease during the first weeks following delivery.

The warfarin-like drugs that lower the plasma levels of proteins involved in the coagulation cascade are not often used during pregnancy. They decrease factors II, VII, IX, and X—all vitamin K–dependent factors. In one study of 418 reported cases of warfarin use during pregnancy collected in the literature, two thirds of the fetuses were born as normal infants (22), 9% resulted in abortions, and another 9% resulted in stillbirths. The other 17% were abnormal, liveborn infants who had different types of anomalies. When warfarin was used in the first trimester of pregnancy, there was a 4% incidence of warfarin embryopathy, primarily nasal hypoplasia and stippled epiphyses. When warfarin was used in the last trimester, 3% of patients had a hemorrhagic event associated with the trauma of delivery; therefore, when a woman taking warfarin begins labor, fresh frozen plasma should be given if more than 24 hours will elapse until delivery time. If delivery is imminent, cesarean section is safer than vaginal delivery to avoid cerebral hemorrhage in the anticoagulated fetus. Because the fetus is sensitive to warfarin (due to the immaturity of its clotting system), the fetus may remain anticoagulated from 7 to 10 days after cessation of warfarin therapy. In the 135 cases of heparin therapy without other anticoagulants during pregnancy, there were three cases of maternal death (one from hemorrhage and two from treatment failure) and a 10% incidence of maternal hemorrhage. Surprisingly, fetal morbidity and mortality were 36%, despite the fact that heparin does not cross the placenta (22). The reason for these fetal problems is unclear, but may be attributable to the heparin-related chelation of calcium.

There is no completely safe method of anticoagulation during pregnancy for either the mother or the fetus. Both warfarin and heparin carry hazards during pregnancy; warfarin brings risk to the fetus, whereas heparin compromises the mother. A recent article suggested that warfarin treatment should not be interrupted during pregnancy in women with mechanical valves (23). Another approach is to use warfarin throughout pregnancy until 2 weeks before the expected delivery date and then switch to heparin until the delivery time. A mother who follows this approach should be aware that there is an approximately 30% chance of fetal morbidity or mortality because of warfarin. An alternative is to use heparin throughout pregnancy, with careful monitoring of the partial thromboplastin time, to avoid complications from thrombus formation or hemorrhage. However, in a recent study, adjusted-dose subcutaneous heparin failed to prevent thromboembolic phenomena in pregnant patients with mechanical cardiac valve prostheses. Activated partial thromboplastin times were adjusted between 1.5 and 2.5 times control. The incidence of spontaneous abortion was 37.5%. There was one neonatal death, one maternal death from gastrointestinal bleeding, and two fatal massive thromboses of mitral tilting disk prostheses (24). It is hoped that problems will become less frequent in better controlled patients with the use of heparin during pregnancy. In the future, low molecular weight heparin may prove to be more efficacious, or new oral agents may be available.

Coronary Artery Disease in Pregnancy

Coronary artery disease is rare in women of childbearing age. Acute myocardial infarction occurs in fewer than 1 in 10,000 deliveries (25); however, when it occurs in a pregnant woman, the maternal mortality rate is 25% to 50% (26), related to the marked increase in the myocardial oxygen demands in a woman during pregnancy or immediately following delivery. Since the first well documented case by Katz in 1922, 136 peripartum patients with acute myocardial infarction have been reported. In 42.6% of patients, no coronary risk factors were observed, but when present, hypertension and cigarette smoking were the most common. The maternal mortality rate was 19.1% and was higher during the third trimester, labor, and puerperium. The fetal mortality rate was 16.9%; however, in only 52% was death coincidental with that of the mother. The researchers felt that coronary artery spasm and a hypercoagulable state of pregnancy were likely precipitants (27).

Coronary atherosclerosis is still the most common cause of coronary artery disease, and myocardial infarction can occur in pregnant women as often as in other persons. A recent review of 125 collected cases of acute myocardial infarction associated with pregnancy by Roth and Elkayam reported that the highest incidence was in the third trimester in multigravidas over 33 years of age. Most commonly, the anterior wall was involved. Coronary atherosclerosis was the most frequent etiology (43%), followed by coronary thrombus without atherosclerosis (21%), and coronary dissection (16%); normal coronary arteries were found in 29% (28). Other less common causes of ischemic heart disease that are proportionately more prevalent in these young women include coronary artery dissection, cocaine use, and coronary spasm. Coronary artery dissection tends to occur near term or within 3 weeks postpartum. Most cases involve the left anterior descending artery, but more than one artery may be involved (29,30). Although there are only 103 cases of spontaneous dissection of a coronary artery in the English-language literature, a recent review reported 28 cases of peripartum spontaneous coronary artery dissection (31). In only 11 of these was the diagnosis made antemortem. Therapeutic approaches ranged from heart transplant in two subjects and coronary bypass surgery, percutaneous angioplasty, and conservative care in four. Hormonal changes, hemodynamic stress, and genetic predisposition to cystic medial necrosis have been proposed as etiologies. Early diagnosis and surgical treatment may improve the outcome.

Among 11 other cases of postpartum myocardial infarction without previous history of heart disease, five patients had the preeclampsia-eclampsia syndrome, two had received ergotamine, three demonstrated coronary heart disease at autopsy, and two had normal coronary arteries shown on angiography (32).

Oral contraceptives used by women over age 30 increase the risk for myocardial infarction by three- to sixfold, compared with women not taking contraceptives. This risk is synergistic with other risk factors for coronary heart disease (33). Also, having six or more pregnancies is associated with an increase in the risk of coronary artery disease.

Obviously, women who have other known risk factors for coronary artery disease should be carefully observed for the symptoms of coronary artery disease. These include women who have hypercholesterolemia or are heavy smokers, diabetics, or hypertensives. An exercise stress test (and occasionally a stress echocardiogram to reduce the moderate incidence of false-positive tests due to high circulating estrogen) should be part of their routine medical evaluations.

If a woman with known coronary heart disease becomes pregnant, an early decision regarding continuation of pregnancy should be made. Even if her angina is stable or she is asymptomatic, the development of unstable angina pectoris in the later stages of pregnancy is a possibility. If her coronary anatomy is known and she is considered to have a low risk of mortality and her exercise treadmill test is negative for myocardial ischemia and arrhythmias, probably pregnancy will be safe for both mother and fetus (34). If unstable angina develops early in pregnancy, termination of pregnancy should be considered; but it may be safer to perform a coronary angiogram and potential angioplasty or surgery without termination the pregnancy. If unstable angina develops in the later stages of pregnancy, the mother should be treated in the same manner as a nonpregnant person. In patients not easily stabilized with nitrates, beta blockers, and calcium blockers, intravenous nitroglycerin should be used. Even an intraaortic balloon pump should be considered as a way of stabilizing the patient who is extremely unstable. We would consider coronary bypass or coronary angioplasty or alternative catheter techniques in the severely unstable pregnant woman as a safer approach than the major stress of delivery with the high mortality of acute myocardial infarction at delivery or immediately after. Recent reports of successful management of acute myocardial infarction during pregnancy treated with angioplasty, intracoronary stent, or even bypass surgery using a cardiopulmonary bypass pump with good outcome for mother and fetus emphasize that an aggressive approach may be appropriate in individual cases (35–37).

A small acute myocardial infarction during pregnancy should be well tolerated and is not an indication for pregnancy termination. With a larger infarction in a pregnant woman, management should be individualized to separate those patients who could be managed with medication from those who require surgery even while pregnant or those who have to be stabilized while the uterus is being emptied.

We believe that the general management of stable angina and myocardial infarction in pregnant patients is similar to that in nonpregnant patients. The treatment of unstable angina should take precedence over emptying the uterus. There are few case reports of thrombolytic agents and percutaneous transluminal coronary angioplasty used in pregnant patients.

Peripartum Cardiomyopathy

Peripartum cardiomyopathy is a congestive cardiomyopathy with an incidence ranging from 1 in 1,000 to 1 in 4,000 pregnancies (38). Usually the patient presents during the last month of pregnancy or within the first few months after delivery with symptoms of heart failure because of significant left ventricular dysfunction. No other cause for left ventricular dysfunction should be present.

Several risk factors have been proposed for the development of peripartum cardiomyopathy, including malnutrition, race (more prevalent among blacks), twin pregnancy, age over 30, primigravidity, multigravidity, toxemia, and family history (39).

At the time of presentation, the symptoms and signs of peripartum cardiomyopathy are the same as those for any congestive cardiomyopathy, with complaints of dyspnea, weakness, orthopnea, chest pain, palpitations, paroxysmal nocturnal dyspnea, and edema. The physical findings include jugular vein distention, peripheral edema, and hepatic and pulmonary congestion. On cardiac auscultation, gallop rhythms may be present and a murmur of mitral regurgitation (due to a dilated left ventricle) may be heard.

The electrocardiogram may show abnormal Q waves, ST segments, and T-wave changes, as well as a left ventricular hypertrophy pattern or conduction disturbance patterns. Arrhythmias are common, especially atrial fibrillation. Chest x-ray will show cardiomegaly and signs of pulmonary venous congestion. The echocardiogram is diagnostic, demonstrating severe left ventricular dysfunction in the absence of primary valvular heart disease. The left ventricle will appear dilated and have poor wall excursion. Commonly, the other cardiac chambers also will be enlarged. Additional diagnostic tests are not usually necessary, but if the diagnosis is equivocal, radionuclear tests and cardiac catheterization may be useful to exclude coronary or congenital heart disease.

The cause of peripartum cardiomyopathy is still unknown. The pathologic findings in these cases are indistinguishable from those in other congestive cardiomyopathies. Immune studies have given negative results in these cases. Reports of cases of myocarditis diagnosed by endomyocardial biopsy in patients who had peripartum cardiomyopathy supports a viral cause for this disorder (40). Of importance, these patients may improve with therapy consisting of steroids and azathioprine (40). Rare cases of peripartum heart failure associated with prolonged tocolytic therapy have been reported. In these patients, the left ventricular function will normalize after stopping the terbutaline therapy (41).

The treatment of patients who have peripartum cardiomyopathy is similar to that for any patient with congestive cardiomyopathy. Restriction of sodium intake and diuretics are important, with careful monitoring of potassium replacement. Treatment includes digitalis, vasodilators, and anticoagulation if ventricular function is poor (42). All arrhythmias should be treated. Anticoagulation should be continued postpartum as long as severe left ventricular dysfunction persists. Prolonged bed rest is a controversial therapy to which we do not subscribe (43).

Because of the possibility of underlying myocarditis, patients with rapid deterioration and ectopy should have viral titers measured and an endomyocardial biopsy. Therapy with steroids and azathioprine if acute inflammation is found, however, is controversial. Even if this aggressive therapy is not followed, half of the patients will have regression of their left ventricular dysfunction in 3 to 6 months, with disappearance of all the symptoms even without medications (44). If cardiomegaly persists after 6 months postdelivery, the prognosis of these patients is as poor as that of patients who have congestive cardiomyopathy. Future pregnancies are potentially life threatening in these patients, and therapy with ACE inhibitors and beta blockers should be tried for improvement of cardiac output and pulmonary congestion.

An occasional patient may present with symptoms of heart failure around the time of delivery, and review of past clinical evaluations will reveal that left ventricular dysfunction was present before the pregnancy. The stress of pregnancy may have precipitated symptoms, but these patients should not be classified as having peripartum cardiomyopathy.

A rare patient with severe cardiomyopathy will present in heart failure earlier in pregnancy, owing to the pregnancy burden. The approach to these cases is difficult. A therapeutic abortion would reduce the extra hemodynamic stress to the heart, but the stress of the abortion itself could result in the death of the patient. An intraaortic balloon and a Swan-Ganz catheter to monitor the administration of vasodilators (i.e., nitroprusside) and inotropic drugs (i.e., dopamine) may be indicated. In sicker patients, cardiac transplantation may be necessary.

The long-term prognosis of these patients cannot be predicted at the time of diagnosis, but once endomyocardial biopsies are performed in more patients, we will learn the value in altering the therapy and will be able to predict the outcome of the patients. As histologic abnormalities are found, even when the heart size has returned to normal, it seems advisable to counsel against future pregnancies in recovered patients. A dobutamine echocardiogram challenge has been used to assess the left ventricular contractile reserve in patients with normalized ventricular function. In most patients the contractile reserve is significantly impaired. If persistent severe cardiomyopathy is present and the patient is significantly symptomatic, cardiac transplantation should be considered. Survival rates in these transplanted patients are similar to those of patients with idiopathic cardiomyopathy despite a propensity for increased rate of rejection in the first 3 weeks. Patients with peripartum cardiomyopathy are more immune reactive, and their rejections following transplant are more aggressive in nature. There is a trend for the patients who survive without a transplant to be initially less symptomatic and to have smaller left ventricular end-diastolic diameters and higher ejection fractions. Biopsy results were more often normal or showed only mild abnormalities in the survivors without transplantation.

Pericarditis and Pregnancy

There is no special association between pericarditis and pregnancy, and there are relatively few cases reported of their coincidence. The cause, symptoms, physical and laboratory findings, and management are exactly the same for all patients who have acute pericarditis, whether or not they are pregnant. In cases of chronic constrictive pericarditis, if there is only a mild increase in venous pressure, surgical stripping should not be performed and pregnancy will follow a benign pattern. In cases of more significant systemic congestion, surgery should be delayed until after delivery, if considered safe. If tamponade is present, however, pericardiocentesis could be performed with 2-D echographic guidance of the needle insertion and fluid removal. If necessary, pericardiectomy for constrictive pericarditis can be performed successfully during pregnancy (45).

Hypertrophic Cardiomyopathy

Hypertrophic cardiomyopathy, or idiopathic hypertrophic subaortic stenosis (IHSS), manifested by global or focal primary hypertrophy of the left ventricle and hypercontractility, is one of the leading causes of sudden death in young male athletes. However, pregnant women with IHSS tend to tolerate the condition well. Patients who have hypertrophic cardiomyopathy often are asymptomatic and come to medical attention because of the presence of a systolic murmur, arrhythmias, or an abnormal electrocardiogram. Some patients have angina pectoris or dyspnea because of the noncompliant left ventricle with elevated diastolic pressures. Others have palpitations, dizziness, or syncope caused by arrhythmias. On physical examination, if left ventricular outflow obstruction is present, a systolic murmur will be heard at the apex and left sternal border, with accentuation during the Valsalva maneuver or after extrasystoles. If there is no resting left ventricular outflow obstruction, physical examination may be remarkable only for an S_4 gallop. In more advanced stages of the condition, however, signs of left-sided and right-sided congestion may be present.

On chest radiography, the heart size may be normal or enlarged. In severe cases, the lungs will show varying degrees of pulmonary venous congestion. The right-sided chambers also may be dilated. The electrocardiogram may be normal but frequently will show left ventricular hypertrophy. Abnormal Q waves suggestive of myocardial infarction as well as ventricular conduction disturbances and P-wave abnormalities reflective of atrial dilation or hypertension may be seen. The echocardiogram is used to make the definitive diagnosis of hypertrophic cardiomyopathy by the pathognomonic findings of asymmetric septal hypertrophy (less commonly the pattern of hypertrophy may involve the entire septum, the entire left ventricle, or the apex), systolic anterior motion of the anterior mitral valve leaflet, and mid-systolic notching of the aortic valve if left ventricular outflow obstruction is present. The left ventricular contractility tends to be increased with mid-cavity obliteration. One or more of these echocardiographic findings may be present in hypertrophic cardiomyopathy. Obviously, secondary left atrial dilation or right-sided chamber dilation may be seen. Rarely, right ventricular outflow obstruction attributable to hypertrophic cardiomyopathy can be detected. Importantly, pulsed or continuous-wave Doppler can localize and quantify the severity of left ventricular outflow obstruction and its response to therapy. If 24-hour electrocardiographic monitoring is performed, frequent atrial and ventricular arrhythmias will be seen—usually premature atrial contractions or ventricular extrasystoles.

The management of the asymptomatic patient who has hypertrophic cardiomyopathy is controversial. Because sudden death can occur even in the asymptomatic person, antiarrhythmic therapy is suggested for those patients in whom significant arrhythmias are detected by electrocardiographic monitoring. Even in the absence of such arrhythmias, treatment with beta blockers or calcium channel blockers has been advocated for the asymptomatic patient who has hypertrophic cardiomyopathy. In an asymptomatic pregnant woman with this condition who has been on no medication, however, we prefer to continue without medication until the time of delivery. If at any point tachyarrhythmias are detected or symptoms appear, therapy can be initiated. For symptomatic persons who have hypertrophic cardiomyopathy, therapy with calcium channel or beta blockers is indicated for improvement in left ventricular compliance, decrease in left ventricular outflow tract obstruction, and for prevention of rapid ventricular rates if supraventricular tachycardias develop. For patients who have serious ventricular arrhythmias, the addition of antiarrhythmic therapy is necessary. If signs of pulmonary congestion are present and left atrial dilatation is seen, diuretics are indicated, with care to avoid hypovolemia and hypokalemia. If symptoms develop during delivery, intravenous beta blockers may be used. Esmolol, a short-acting beta-adrenergic antagonist, with extradural anesthesia and invasive cardiovascular monitoring can be used to achieve an assisted vaginal delivery with minimal hemodynamic disturbance in patients with significant hypertrophic cardiomyopathy (46).

In general, because of volume expansion, pregnancy should be tolerated well by patients who have hypertrophic cardiomyopathy. Death because of this condition during pregnancy is extremely rare (47).

Primary Pulmonary Hypertension

Fortunately, primary pulmonary hypertension is an uncommon disorder. It has a grave prognosis for those patients who become pregnant. Because of a reported 50% mortality rate for patients who have pulmonary hypertension during pregnancy, abortion should be considered as soon as pregnancy is confirmed (48).

Patients who have primary pulmonary hypertension have medial constriction of the arteriolar vessels in the lungs. Although pulmonary function may be normal, because of the intimal fibrosis and arteriolar obstruction, elevated pulmonary artery pressure develops. This results in right ventricular hypertension, right ventricular hypertrophy and dilatation, and, eventually, right ventricular failure with tricuspid regurgitation and systemic congestion.

Primary pulmonary hypertension is a progressive idiopathic disease that tends to occur primarily in young women (48)—with an increased incidence of Raynaud's phenomenon—and may be a collagen vascular disease. One theory suggests recurrent pulmonary embolism, another cause of pulmonary hypertension, as either as a potential etiology or exacerbating underlying disease.

The symptoms of this condition are dyspnea, occasional chest pain, fatigue, and, eventually, ascites and edema. On physical examination a loud second pulmonic valve closure (P_2) sound will be heard together with the presence of a right ventricular heave caused by right ventricular hypertrophy. If systemic congestion is present, jugular venous distension will be seen; hepatomegaly, ascites, and edema may be present. Usually murmurs are absent; however, a systolic ejection murmur may be present at the level of the pulmonary area, and when tricuspid regurgitation occurs, a loud systolic murmur will be present at the lower left sternal border.

A chest x-ray may show right ventricular and right atrial dilatation and dilatation of the proximal pulmonary vessels, but the peripheral pulmonary vasculature is decreased. The electrocardiogram shows right ventricular hypertrophy and, occasionally, P pulmonale related to right atrial enlargement. An echocardiogram should be performed to exclude causes of secondary pulmonary hypertension (i.e., congenital heart disease, valvular lesions). The echocardiogram will show normal left-sided structures but right ventricular hypertrophy and enlargement with varying degrees of right ventricular dysfunction. In later stages, paradoxical motion of the interventricular septum can be seen. Right atrial enlargement also may be significant. The pulmonic valve motion has changes on m-mode echo that are consistent with pulmonary hypertension, such as horizontalization of the E-to-F interval, decrease or disappearance of the A wave, and mid-systolic notching of the pulmonic valve. Doppler studies may allow the measurement of pulmonary artery pressure when tricuspid regurgitation is present; color Doppler may detect any cardiac shunt. A Swan-Ganz catheter may corroborate the diagnosis of pulmonary hypertension with normal pulmonary capillary wedge pressure and, at the same time, exclude the presence of a cardiac shunt.

In a review of 38 pregnancies in 21 patients who had primary pulmonary hypertension, 50% of them died during pregnancy or in the early postdelivery period (48,49). Even if the patient is asymptomatic with this condition, a 42% mortality rate has been observed during pregnancy. Half of the deaths occur during the early postpartum period; the sudden loss of blood volume may be responsible for this.

The medical management of pregnant women who have primary pulmonary hypertension and who do not choose abortion should include close monitoring, elastic hose when ambulating, avoidance of the supine position late in pregnancy, compulsive replacement of blood loss, and early ambulation immediately following delivery to prevent pooling of blood. Because of the risk of intravascular pulmonary thrombosis, anticoagulation is indicated. Oxygen should be administered to the mother to prevent hypoxemia. Epidural anesthesia has been suggested to offer hemodynamic stability at the time of labor. Prolonged infusion of prostacyclin in individuals with primary pulmonary hypertension (nonpregnant) is done nowadays in specialized centers. In some patients significant reduction in pulmonary vascular resistance is found; in others, the progression of the illness is slowed. In many, this therapy is considered palliation until a lung transplant becomes available.

Despite the occasional reports of successful pregnancies in patients who have primary pulmonary hypertension, we feel that early abortion should be recommended and, more importantly, prevention of pregnancy is indicated. Patients who have primary pulmonary hypertension should be candidates for potential heart-lung transplant. This surgery has a high mortality rate, however, and its long-term prognosis is still unknown.

Mitral Valve Prolapse

Mitral valve prolapse is probably one of the most common cardiac conditions among the general population (50), with an incidence of 5% to 10% of normal women. The incidence in men is probably only half of that in women. Persons who have this condition may have no symptoms, variable symptoms, or, rarely, total disability. The most common complaint is palpitations; other symptoms include different types of chest pains, dyspnea, easy fatigability, anxiety, and even panic attacks.

The diagnosis is provided during the physical examination by the auscultation of a nonejection systolic click at the apex and frequently a mid-to-late systolic murmur that may or may not increase with the Valsalva maneuver or with standing up. The electrocardiogram usually is normal, but some of these patients tend to have nonspecific ST-segment and T-wave changes. The chest x-ray usually is normal. The echocardiogram will corroborate the diagnosis by demonstrating systolic hammocking of the mitral valve and variable degrees or absence of mitral regurgitation. Occasionally tricuspid valve prolapse also occurs, and, rarely, aortic valve prolapse can be seen. Electrocardiographic monitoring will reveal frequent atrial and ventricular arrhythmias among these patients.

The prognosis of patients who have mitral valve prolapse is excellent. Most of them require only reassurance and encouragement to continue normal lives. Some may require beta blockers to decrease palpitations and chest pain. If a murmur and mitral regurgitation are present, bacterial prophylaxis for dental and other procedures is indicated as noted above.

The blood volume increase of pregnancy is well tolerated by women who have mitral valve prolapse (51). Some of them may be extremely sensitive to occasional palpitations, whereas others may be less aware of them. There is no special medical management for these women during pregnancy, and antibiotic prophylaxis for normal deliveries is not indicated, as noted above.

Women who have mitral valve prolapse and documented ventricular tachycardia or syncope represent a small minority that requires more careful attention. Electrophysiologic studies may be necessary in these women before allowing pregnancy. Sudden death is extremely rare in patients who have mitral valve prolapse, and some of the reported cases might be attributed to associated conditions such as the prolonged QT interval syndrome. More commonly, patients have significant mitral regurgitation because of mitral valve prolapse; they should be treated and followed like any other patient who has mitral regurgitation.

Aortic Dissection

Aortic dissection is a rare disorder, but it tends to occur slightly more frequently during pregnancy. Type A involves the proximal aorta, whereas type B is limited to the distal aorta, below the left subclavian artery. When type A aortic dissection occurs, it will be the cause of death in the majority of cases if not immediately treated aggressively.

The patient who has aortic dissection usually presents with excruciating chest pain, usually in the back, with sudden onset of dyspnea and even cyanosis. If cerebral vessels are involved, a cerebrovascular accident will occur. If a coronary vessel is involved, acute myocardial infarction and death will occur. If a renal vessel is involved, increasing renal failure will occur. If a mesenteric vessel is involved, the patient will present with signs of an acute abdomen caused by ischemia of the bowel. The differential diagnosis of patients who have aortic dissection includes myocardial infarction, pneumothorax, acute aortic valve rupture, and pulmonary embolism. In pregnant women, the differential diagnosis should also include rupture of the uterus and abruptio placentae. If a new murmur of aortic regurgitation is present, the diagnosis of aortic dissection is almost certain. A chest x-ray may show widening of the mediastinum because of dilatation of the aorta. An echocardiogram may show a dilated aorta with a double lumen or intimal flap and signs of aortic regurgitation. In these patients a definitive diagnosis is essential as soon as possible. At the same time that their blood pressure is stabilized and (if necessary) lowered, transesophageal echocardiography can be performed rapidly at the bedside and should be diagnostic without radiation exposure. If a diagnosis of type A dissection (involving the ascending aorta) is made, the patient should be taken immediately for surgical repair of the aorta. If the dissection is distal to the origin of the left subclavian artery, medical management should be considered unless symptoms continue. Medical therapy usually includes good control of the blood pressure with nitroprusside and the addition of propranolol or other beta blockers to prevent increased force of ejection of the blood from the left ventricle.

The reason for a slight increase in aortic dissections during pregnancy is unclear. Hormonal changes may be a risk factor; however, women who use birth control pills do not have an increased incidence of aortic dissections (52). In nonpregnant persons, hypertension is a major factor in aortic dissection, but it is seen in only 25% of cases during pregnancy. Malformations of the aorta, and especially Marfan syndrome, seem to account for a large number of the aortic dissections that occur during pregnancy.

Pregnancy in Marfan syndrome is associated with two primary problems: potential catastrophic aortic dissection and the risk for having a child with the syndrome (53). Marfan syndrome during pregnancy has an associated 50% rate of mortality (54). Any woman with this diagnosis, with marked dilatation of the aorta, should be counseled about this risk as soon as the diagnosis of pregnancy is made. Ideally, thorough preconceptional counseling should be given to these women. Of note, a person may have no "marfanoid" appearance but may have all the cardiovascular findings of Marfan syndrome, putting this person at the same high risk as those who have full expression of the syndrome. Pregnant women who have relatives with Marfan syndrome should therefore have echocardiographic studies for evaluation of their aortas. If dilatation of the aorta is present, especially if it measures more than 4 cm, pregnancy should be avoided or terminated. Of interest, in 106 pregnancies in 26 women followed at the John Hopkins University, only one maternal death was seen and it was attributable to endocarditis (55). This low rate of mortality was attributed to counseling against pregnancy if the aorta was over 4 cm in diameter with or without the presence of aortic regurgitation. The aortic diameter did not change during pregnancy with serial echocardiography (56). However, an occasional increase in aortic root size has been observed during pregnancy. If a woman who has Marfan syndrome continues her pregnancy, beta blockers will reduce the incidence of cardiovascular complications and should be continued throughout pregnancy. If she develops an aortic dissection during the pregnancy, surgery should be performed. The approach to aortic dissection during pregnancy, therefore, should be exactly the same as that in the nonpregnant person. If the cardiovascular involvement is mild, the pregnant woman with Marfan syndrome will likely have a safe pregnancy, but there is a 50% chance of bearing an affected offspring.

Congenital Heart Disease

Because of better surgical techniques and better medical management, large numbers of women who have diverse congenital heart diseases are reaching childbearing age. No large experience exists in many types of complicated congenital heart disease. More experience exists regarding patients who have atrial septal defect, ventricular septal defect, and patent ductus arteriosus. Most patients with uncomplicated left-to-right shunts tolerate their pregnancies well. Occasionally, heart failure and arrhythmias will occur and require management. Most patients who have acyanotic congenital heart disease will tolerate pregnancy safely. Some conditions, such as Eisenmenger syndrome, carry an extremely high rate of maternal mortality. Women at particular risk are those with left-sided obstruction, pulmonary hypertension, poor ventricular function, potentially fragile aortas, valve prostheses, and cyanosis (57).

Atrial Septal Defect

Most women who have an atrial septal defect tolerate pregnancy without complications. Not uncommonly, this condition will be first diagnosed during pregnancy in an asymptomatic woman. The hypervolemia of pregnancy will further increase pulmonary blood flow in patients who have atrial septal defect, but the pulmonary artery pressure will remain normal or will be only minimally elevated. In rare cases of systemic congestion caused by large atrial septal defects, surgical closure must be considered even during pregnancy (58). Nowadays, small defects, the same as patent foramen ovales, can be closed with percutaneous techniques, but it is not necessary to do this during the pregnancy unless there is significant risk of paradoxical embolism. In the future larger defects also may be closed using similar techniques (59).

Patients who have an atrial septal defect are exposed to paradoxical embolization, even if only the left-to-right shunt exists. This is caused by transient, hemodynamically nonsignificant right-to-left shunts induced by Valsalva, deep cough, or straining. If thrombophlebitis of the lower extremities occurs, the risks of pulmonary embolism with subsequent elevation of the pulmonary artery pressure and systemic embolization are high. Also, atrial arrhythmias, especially atrial fibrillation, may occur in patients who have atrial septal defect, and they should be treated the same as any other patient who has atrial arrhythmias.

Most patients who have an atrial septal defect do not have significant hemodynamic problems until after age 40, remaining at low risk during the childbearing age. Cardiac chamber size, ventricular function, and, occasionally, the septal defect itself can be visualized by 2-D echography. Transesophageal echography is the technique of choice to define the septal defect accurately. Doppler can estimate the relative shunt flow noninvasively.

Patients who have repaired atrial septal defects should be considered normal. Pregnancy will be as safe for them as for any healthy woman: however, it should be delayed for at least 6 to 12 months after surgery for complete healing and recovery.

Ventricular Septal Defect

The risk of pregnancy in a patient who has a ventricular septal defect depends mostly on the size of the defect. With a small defect, pregnancy is well tolerated; with large ventricular septal defects, most pregnancies also will be uncomplicated (60); however, in cases of borderline bidirectional flow caused by elevated pulmonary artery and right ventricular pressures, pregnancy will favor right-to-left shunting of blood because the decrease in systemic vascular resistance will be greater than the decrease in pulmonary vascular resistance. This group of ventricular septal defect patients carries a high rate of mortality during pregnancy. Most of the symptoms will be caused by congestive heart failure. Occasional patients may have paradoxical embolism and infective endocarditis. When ventricular septal defect is complicated by Eisenmenger syndrome (pulmonary pressures equal left-sided pressures, and the shunt is right to left), pregnancy carries a 50% chance of mortality for the mother (61).

The diagnosis of ventricular septal defect is relatively simple by physical examination, with a thrill and holosystolic murmur over the left parasternal area radiating to the rest of the precordium. Patients commonly have a third heart sound, and the pulmonic component of the second heart sound will be louder during pregnancy. Depending on the size of the defect, patients will have electrocardiograms and echocardiograms consistent with left and right ventricular enlargement. Two-dimensional echocardiography may show the interventricular septum defect itself; however, this sign is unreliable. Contrast echocardiography with microbubbles (usually obtained by injection of dextrose and water or normal saline solution through a peripheral vein) may demonstrate noninvasively the passage of bubbles from the left ventricle to the right ventricle. Color flow Doppler can usually identify the precise location, estimate the defect size and determine if there are multiple defects. Doppler echocardiography can estimate right ventricular systolic pressures. The chest x-ray will show varying increases in pulmonary vascularity, depending on the size of the defect.

In a woman who has a complicated ventricular septal defect during pregnancy with symptoms of heart failure unresponsive to medical management, surgical closure of the ventricular septal defect during pregnancy could be performed safely for the mother. (Women with Eisenmenger syndrome will be discussed separately.)

Patent Ductus Arteriosus

Today, few women who have a patent ductus arteriosus reach the childbearing age without repair. Most of them undergo surgery in earlier years, especially because the operation is so simple. Moreover, currently available percutaneous closure of a ductus is also simple (59).

Patients who have a small patent ductus arteriosus are asymptomatic, have an excellent prognosis, and tolerate pregnancy extremely well. Occasional patients with a large patent ductus will develop heart failure during pregnancy. If Eisenmenger syndrome already is present at the time of pregnancy, the maternal mortality rate reaches 50% (61).

Pulmonic Stenosis

Valvular pulmonic stenosis is usually well tolerated with pregnancy (58). Mild pulmonic stenosis gives no symptoms, a normal or minimally abnormal electrocardiogram, a normal echocardiogram, and relatively normal hemodynamics. The circulatory changes of pregnancy do not change any of these findings. Patients who have severe pulmonic stenosis still will tolerate pregnancy relatively well; however, right heart failure can develop and there is an increased incidence of abortion and premature deliveries.

The physical examination will reveal a systolic ejection murmur in the upper left sternal border, varying in intensity, depending on the severity of the stenosis. With milder forms of stenosis, a systolic ejection click will be heard, especially during expiration. With more severe pulmonic stenosis, the pulmonic component of the second sound becomes delayed and soft and eventually disappears. With significant pulmonic stenosis, a right ventricular parasternal heave will be palpable, a right-sided fourth heart sound can be heard, and prominent A waves in the jugular venous pulse can be seen. The electrocardiogram will be normal in mild pulmonic stenosis and will have varying evidence of right ventricular hypertrophy in more severe cases according to the severity of the stenosis. The x-ray will show poststenotic pulmonary artery dilatation with normal pulmonary vascularity, or reduced vascularity in very severe cases. The echocardiogram will be normal in mild pulmonic stenosis but will show systolic doming of the pulmonic valve plus right ventricular hypertrophy in severe cases. Importantly, echography may be used to differentiate valvular from muscular infundibular pulmonic stenosis.

In cases of severe pulmonic stenosis, most of the medical therapy is intended to maintain normal or increased volume in the circulation of the mother. This will avoid hypotension that could be fatal. Paradoxical emboli is a rare complication of "pure" pulmonic stenosis facilitated by concomitant patent foramen ovale. This is another condition that can be easily corrected with percutaneous transluminal techniques (valvuloplasty) and should be advised to any patient with severe stenosis before pregnancy is contemplated (59).

Tetralogy of Fallot

Because there is increased survival following the surgery for tetralogy of Fallot (pulmonic stenosis, ventricular septal defect, overriding aorta, and right ventricular hypertrophy), large numbers of women are reaching childbearing age who have had previous palliative or total correction of their tetralogy of Fallot. Thus far, few women with tetralogy of Fallot have been reported to have had pregnancies, although these few have been mostly successful (62). Poor prognostic signs are reported to be marked arterial oxygen desaturation, residual right ventricular outflow obstruction with severe right ventricular pressure elevation, and maternal hematocrits over 62%. Women who have had successful total correction should tolerate pregnancy very well.

Physical examination of the woman who has tetralogy of Fallot will reveal cyanosis, clubbing of the fingers and toes, signs of right ventricular hypertrophy, and a systolic murmur consistent with right ventricular outflow obstruction. The electrocardiogram usually will show right ventricular hypertrophy. The 2-D echocardiogram is diagnostic, showing a dilated aorta overriding the ventricular septum in which there is a defect, and right ventricular enlargement and hypertrophy. Doppler can be used to localize and measure the right ventricular outflow obstruction.

Patients who have tetralogy of Fallot commonly complain of dyspnea, syncope, and fatigue. Significant ventricular arrhythmias may be seen, especially in the postsurgical cases. Rare cases present with cerebrovascular accidents or brain abscesses because of paradoxical emboli.

Coarctation of the Aorta

Coarctation of the aorta is one of the treatable causes of arterial hypertension. In cases of severe coarctation of the aorta, pregnancy presents a high risk of death for the mother.

The usual presentation is hypertension with a systolic blood pressure that is higher in the arms than in the legs. A systolic murmur usually will be present at the left sternal border, and an S_4 sound may be present because of left ventricular hypertrophy and decreased left ventricular compliance. The electrocardiogram will show varying degrees of left ventricular hypertrophy if the coarctation is significant. The chest x-ray may show a "3" sign along the left mediastinal area. Rib notching on the inferior edges of the ribs secondary to dilated intercostal vessels is considered pathognomonic of this condition. The echocardiogram will show varying degrees of left ventricular hypertrophy, possibly a bicuspid aortic valve frequently associated with this condition and the gradient across the coarctation. For women who have mild coarctation of the aorta and no hypertension or minimal hypertension, pregnancy is safe; however, in more significant coarctation, there is an increased incidence of aortic dissection or rupture during pregnancy. Congestive heart failure may occur. There is a potential risk of infective endocarditis of a bicuspid aortic valve or cerebral hemorrhage caused by rupture of a saccular aneurysm, two conditions associated with coarctation of the aorta. In women who have coarctation of the aorta and a systolic blood pressure over 200 mm Hg or significant heart failure, surgical correction of the coarctation should be performed even during pregnancy (63). In milder cases, surgery should be delayed until after delivery. Aggressive therapy against hypertension is imperative, and these patients require marked limitation of their physical activities. In patients with restenosis of the aorta following previous surgical repair of a coarctation, a percutaneous correction of the stenosis is currently feasible with significant reduction in gradient (59).

Pregnancy After Congenital Heart Disease Surgery

Each year more cases are reported of women with different types of operated congenital heart disease having uncomplicated pregnancies. For many years patients with simple congenital lesions (i.e., atrial and ventricular septal defects) have been known to tolerate pregnancy well following surgery. Nowadays, women with complex abnormalities corrected surgically also tolerate pregnancy well. These include Ebstein's anomaly, tricuspid atresia, tetralogy of Fallot, and transposition of the great vessels. Pregnancy after the Fontan operation for univentricular heart disease is well tolerated, but carries a moderately increased risk of miscarriage (64).

Eisenmenger Syndrome

Eisenmenger syndrome is characterized by markedly elevated pulmonary pressure caused by intracardiac shunting and is associated with a high rate of maternal mortality during pregnancy (8). Occasional cases are reported with successful outcome during pregnancy, but they should not encourage physicians to advise women with this condition to continue their pregnancies. Termination of pregnancy or ideally its avoidance if medical consultation is obtained prior to pregnancy may be necessary to preserve the mother's life.

The most common cause of Eisenmenger syndrome is ventricular septal defect; other patients may have atrial septal defect and patent ductus arteriosus. They all carry the same poor maternal and fetal prognosis during pregnancy.

Because the majority of the deaths are caused by hypovolemia or thromboembolic episodes, the treatment of women who continue to be pregnant with this syndrome is directed to prevent hypovolemia, with assistance of invasive hemodynamic monitoring if necessary. Anticoagulation is also recommended during and, especially, immediately following delivery. Elastic stockings and compulsive replacement of fluids are the mainstays of therapy. High concentrations of oxygen during labor are recommended. Anticoagulation with heparin, especially after delivery, is important. Regardless of the therapy, this diagnosis still carries a high rate of mortality for the mother and the fetus. Although termination of pregnancy is often recommended for pregnant women with Eisenmenger syndrome, 13 pregnancies in 12 women with this syndrome were recently reported. Their mean systolic and diastolic pulmonary artery pressures were 112.7 and 61.7 mm Hg, respectively. There were three spontaneous abortions, and two maternal deaths during the 23rd and 27th weeks of gestation. Caesarean section was performed in all patients due to worsening maternal or fetal condition. Prolonged bed rest, the use of heparin, and oxygen therapy presumably positively influenced maternal and infant outcomes (65).

ARRHYTHMIAS AND CONDUCTION DISTURBANCES DURING PREGNANCY

In a patient who has an arrhythmia, the most important factor in the approach to the arrhythmia is determining the presence or absence of underlying organic heart disease. Most arrhythmias will be well tolerated and will not require any therapy in the absence of disease. In the presence of organic heart disease, however, different arrhythmias may require therapy because they will bring symptoms. The treatment of arrhythmias during pregnancy is similar to the treatment of arrhythmias in the nonpregnant person. A recent study comparing 110 consecutive patients without organic heart disease who had complaints of palpitations, dizziness, and syncope with 52 control patients confirms a mild increase in arrhythmias during pregnancy, mostly atrial and ventricular premature beats. However, there was no correlation between the incidence of arrhythmias and symptoms, and only 10% of symptomatic episodes were accompanied by documented arrhythmias (66).

Supraventricular Arrhythmias

In women who have sinus tachycardia, therapy is not indicated and correction of the cause of the tachycardia will restore normal heart rate. The most common cause of tachycardia is anxiety, and in other patients it may be anemia, fever, hypotension, or hyperthyroidism. Intravenous tocolytics also may cause atrial arrhythmias. Terbutaline prescribed for preterm labor resulted in cardiac complications in 47 of 8,709 of patients (0.54%), including pulmonary edema, hypertension, irregular heart beats, and electrocardiogram changes (67).

Rarely a pregnant woman will present with sick sinus syndrome, with marked sinus brachycardia and signs of cerebral hypoperfusion. These patients commonly also have paroxysmal tachycardias. A portable electrocardiographic recording will detect paroxysmal tachyarrhythmias alternating with bradyarrhythmias. If the symptoms are mild, no therapy is necessary; however, if syncope has occurred or dizziness can be found secondary to marked bradycardias, a permanent pacemaker will be necessary. If the pacemaker is implanted, medications still may be needed for concurrent paroxysmal tachycardias.

Atrial premature beats are frequent in normal nonpregnant women as well as in pregnancy. They are thought of as benign arrhythmias that do not require medication. In women who complain of palpitations caused by atrial premature beats, reassurance should be the most effective therapy.

Paroxysmal atrial tachycardias are more likely to occur during pregnancy in susceptible women. If a patient has no underlying organic heart disease, this tachycardia will be well tolerated. If it occurs in a patient who has organic heart disease, symptoms of heart failure or cerebral or coronary insufficiency may develop. Vagal maneuvers are helpful in the identification of the arrhythmia and also in its therapy. If conversion to normal rhythm is not achieved with vagal maneuvers, a decision should be made regarding the importance of the arrhythmia. If the ventricular rate is rapid and there is danger of serious consequences, electric shock cardioversion could be indicated. Some patients will convert rapidly after parasympathomimetic drugs such as edrophonium chloride (Tensilon) are given intravenously. This drug should not be given if hypotension is present. In the latter case, pressor drugs in intravenous drips should be given until the systolic blood pressure increases to around 180 mm Hg. These patients will convert by reflex stimulation of the vagal nerve. Most patients respond to adenosine or verapamil intravenously, but verapamil should not be administered to patients who have hypotension. In patients who have paroxysmal atrial tachycardia, slowing of the ventricular rate can be achieved with digitalis, beta blockers, or calcium blockers in different combinations, or with any of those drugs individually. Occasionally these patients require medications to prevent further attacks. The same medications can be used, or combinations with quinidine, procainamide hydrochloride, or disopyramide can be used. Complicated cases involving paroxysmal atrial tachycardia may require electrophysiologic testing and possible ablation of conduction pathways under sonographic guidance to interrupt the arrhythmias. Those procedures are usually elective and are preferably performed in the nonpregnant state.

Atrial flutter is not a common arrhythmia during pregnancy. This is a difficult arrhythmia to convert into normal sinus rhythm. When the ventricular rate is relatively rapid, therapy with electrocardioversion with direct countershock or rapid atrial pacing should be performed. Digitalis or beta blockers in combination with quinidine are commonly used to prevent recurrence of atrial flutter.

Atrial fibrillation is a common arrhythmia seen in patients who have mitral valve disease, coronary artery disease, and cardiomyopathy. Occasionally, patients will have no organic heart disease. This arrhythmia is associated with risk of systemic embolization, especially in patients who have organic heart disease. The rapid ventricular rate that usually accompanies this arrhythmia is controlled easily with digitalis, beta blockers, or calcium channel blockers. Rarely will patients require cardioversion to normal sinus rhythm, especially if they have had this arrhythmia for a short time and the left atrium is not enlarged. Ibutilide administered intravenously may convert new-onset atrial fibrillation into sinus rhythm in up to 50% of cases. In patients who have mitral valve disease, anticoagulation is indicated. In patients who have no evidence of organic heart disease, and normal echocardiographic findings, anticoagulation is not necessary.

Ventricular Arrhythmias

Occasional ventricular premature beats are common in normal persons and are equally common in pregnancy. They do not require any therapy in pregnant women who have no underlying organic heart disease. If a woman is aware of palpitations, reassurance usually is adequate. The most common underlying organic heart disease in young women is mitral valve prolapse; much less frequently women may have hypertrophic cardiomyopathy. Rarely will they have congestive cardiomyopathy or coronary artery disease. Only when ventricular premature beats are very frequent, or when bigeminy with resultant symptomatic bradycardia occurs, or when the premature beats are multifocal, or occur in couplets or longer salvos will therapy be required. Procainamide hydrochloride, quinidine, disopyramide, and sotalol are the most frequently used medicines to suppress or reduce the number of ventricular premature beats. In women who have mitral valve prolapse, beta blockers seem to reduce the frequency or awareness of the arrhythmia.

Ventricular tachycardia is an arrhythmia that may cause death; therefore, it requires therapy in most of the patients who have it. Most patients are symptomatic, especially when the ventricular rate is over 150 beats/min. The most frequent hemodynamic problem is hypotension, and, occasionally, it also will produce heart failure. Ventricular tachycardia is a rare arrhythmia during pregnancy and usually is associated with underlying organic heart disease (e.g., hypertrophic cardiomyopathy, mitral valve prolapse, coronary artery disease, right ventricular dysplasia and congestive cardiomyopathy). Rarely it will be seen in the prolonged Q-T interval syndrome. Digitalis intoxication also may be responsible for ventricular tachycardia.

In women who have ventricular tachycardia and hemodynamic compromise, emergency therapy is mandatory. Intravenous lidocaine can be attempted first while preparing for electric countershock. Usually low-energy countershock is necessary. If hemodynamic derangement is not present, the patient should be hospitalized in an intensive care unit, and a rapid evaluation of the underlying heart condition should be made. An attempt to terminate the arrhythmia as rapidly as possible is still indicated because many of these patients can deteriorate into ventricular fibrillation. If the prolonged Q-T syndrome is present, a beta blocker or permanent ventricular pacemaker is indicated.

Newer antiarrhythmics are effective in suppressing ventricular arrhythmias; however their effects on the fetus are unknown. Lidocaine-type medications (mexiletine and tocainide), type IC antiarrhythmics (flecainide, encainide, and propafenone), and sotalol and amiodarone all are useful (in different degrees); but in pregnant women they should be used only in life-threatening arrhythmias or in those with hemodynamic derangement not responsive to other antiarrhythmics. Gestational exposure to amiodarone may be complicated by perinatal hypothyroidism, hyperthyroidism, and possibly neurologic abnormalities, intrauterine growth restriction, or fetal bradycardia (68). Electrophysiologic testing with echocardiographic guidance has been performed in pregnant patients. Pregnancy after implantation of an automatic cardiac defibrillator also has been reported (69).

Heart Block

First-degree atrioventricular block usually is benign and requires no special management. Second-degree atrioventricular block (Mobitz type I) usually requires no therapy in women, with or without underlying heart disease and who takes no medications. If digitalis has been used, this may be a sign of digitalis intoxication and the drug should be withheld. In Mobitz type II second-degree atrioventricular block, a permanent pacemaker usually is indicated. This is a rare condition generally associated with underlying heart disease. Patients who have third-degree atrioventricular block and narrow QRS complexes usually have only mild to moderate ventricular bradycardias, and such patients tolerate these arrhythmias well. If the patient is symptomatic because of a slow ventricular rate, a permanent pacemaker is indicated; however, most patients, including pregnant women, will tolerate complete heart block with narrow QRS complexes extremely well. When the third-degree atrioventricular block is below the His bundle, the escape ventricular rate usually is slow (below 40 beats/min), the QRS complexes are wide, and patients are always symptomatic. A ventricular pacemaker is indicated as soon as the diagnosis is made.

Bundle-Branch Block

The approach to bundle-branch blocks is the same in the pregnant patient as in the nonpregnant one. If the patient has complaints of dizziness or syncope, she requires ambulatory electrocardiographic recording or electrophysiologic studies. If complete heart block is found at the time of the symptoms, a permanent pacemaker is indicated. Some of these patients will have ventricular tachycardia as an explanation for the symptoms, and the therapy is antiarrhythmic medications. Bundle-branch block can be seen without underlying organic heart disease or complicating any form of organic heart disease.

Wolff-Parkinson-White Syndrome

Patients who have Wolff-Parkinson-White syndrome are more susceptible to arrhythmias during pregnancy (70). If the supraventricular arrhythmia has a relatively slow ventricular rate, no special therapy is indicated; however, if the ventricular rate is over 150 beats/min (it may reach as high as 200 to 300 beats/min), serious hemodynamic consequences can develop. If the patient presents with tachycardia and severe hypotension, emergency cardioversion is indicated. Otherwise, drugs such as procainamide and beta blockers (usually in combination) could be successful in preventing further attacks. Cardioversion is safe during pregnancy, as has been reported in several cases (71). The approach to cardioversion during pregnancy is exactly the same as that for any person. It should be avoided in persons suspected of having digitalis intoxication, unless the procedure is an emergency one. The patient should be fasting, sedated, relaxed, and, in specific cases, anticoagulated. After cardioversion, the patient should be monitored for several hours to watch for any new arrhythmias that may develop after cardioversion. Most patients with preexcitation syndromes with a history of arrhythmias should undergo electrophysiologic testing and curative ablation, ideally before planning pregnancy.

In patients who have no underlying organic heart disease, most arrhythmias should require no therapy. Reassurance should be used for benign arrhythmias that produce only palpitations. Of note, most palpitations during pregnancy are caused by sinus rhythm. With serious arrhythmias, the therapy should be similar to that for nonpregnant patients. If cardioversion is necessary, it is a safe procedure that should not be avoided. Pregnancy itself rarely makes an arrhythmia more refractory to therapy.

Antiarrhythmics

Lidocaine is safe during pregnancy for the mother and the fetus when given in usual therapeutic doses (72). Quinidine crosses the placenta, but it does not seem to have any teratogenetic effect (73). Rarely, it may cause premature labor or thrombocytopenia in the fetus (74). Procainamide is relatively safe in pregnancy, but because more experience has been accumulated with quinidine, procainamide is reserved as a second-line drug, used if quinidine has been unsuccessful or not tolerated (75). Disopyramide crosses the placenta but does not produce any teratogenic effect. Digitalis crosses the placenta and it has been found safe during pregnancy (76). The fact that it crosses the placenta readily has been used in a therapeutic way for treatment of fetal arrhythmias. Propranolol has been thought to be responsible for intrauterine growth retardation of the fetus, neonatal hypoglycemia (77), and hyperbilirubinemia (78). Maternal and fetal brachycardia have been reported, but they do not carry any hemodynamic problems. The largest experience with propranolol is in pregnant women who have hypertension, in whom it has proved beneficial, with few serious side effects. Verapamil seems to be safe for use during pregnancy, but this is a relatively new drug and we do not have a large experience with it.

SUMMARY

The medical care of a pregnant cardiac patient is a considerable challenge. Good communication between obstetrician and cardiologist is essential for the successful management of these patients. Whereas some patients require only reassurance, others require in-depth counseling concerning the risks of pregnancy and the available options, especially patients in cardiac class 3 or 4, patients who have severe pulmonary hypertension of any kind, and patients who have cardiomyopathy and Marfan syndrome with dilatation of the aortic root.

Occasionally, patients may require cardiac surgery during their pregnancy. These include women who have acute aortic dissection, coarctation of the aorta and severe hypertension, or refractory pulmonary edema caused by valvular insufficiency. Patients who have severe mitral stenosis and those rare patients who have aortic or pulmonic stenosis may require balloon valvuloplasty. Patients who have severe, symptomatic coronary artery disease may require angioplasty or surgery.

Pregnant women have a slightly higher incidence of some diseases, some serious (such as aortic or coronary dissection), others more benign (paroxysmal atrial tachycardia). In general, however, their management is similar to that of nonpregnant patients.

Just as important as the treatment of pregnant cardiac patients is the counseling against pregnancy in extremely high-risk cases. It is also important to reassure women who have minor cardiac pathology about their benign condition, thus eliminating unnecessary anxiety.

REFERENCES

1. Lees MM, Taylor SH, Scott DB, Kerr MG. A study of cardiac output at rest throughout pregnancy. *J Obstet Gynaecol Br Commonw* 1967;74: 319–328.
2. Henricks CH, Quilligan RJ. Cardiac output during labor. *Am J Obstet Gynecol* 1965;71:953–972.
3. Rovinsky JJ, Jaffin N. Cardiovascular hemodynamics in pregnancy. I: Blood and plasma volume in multiple pregnancy. *Am J Obstet Gynecol* 1965;93:1–15.
4. Hytten FE, Leitch I. The physiology of human pregnancy, 2nd ed. Oxford, England: Blackwell, 1971:1–111.
5. Adams JQ. Cardiophysiology in normal pregnancy: studied with dye dilution technique. *Am J Obstet Gynecol* 1954;67:741–759.
6. MacGillivray I. Hypertension in pregnancy and its consequences. *J Obstet Gynaecol Br Commonw* 1961;68:557–569.
7. Seitchik JJ. Total body water and total body density of pregnant women. *J Obstet Gynecol* 1967;29:155–166.
8. Roy BS, Malkani PK, Vivik R, Bhatia ML. Circulatory effects of pregnancy. *Am J Obstet Gynecol* 1966;96:221–225.
9. Katz R, Karliner JS, Resnick R. Effects of a natural volume overload state (pregnancy) on left ventricular performance in normal human subjects. *Circulation* 1978;58:343–441.
10. Perlof JK. Pregnancy and cardiovascular disease. In: Braunwald E, ed. Heart disease. Philadelphia: WB Saunders, 1980:1871–1891.
11. Cutforth R, Macdonald MB. Heart sounds and murmurs in pregnancy. *Am Heart J* 1966;71:741–747.
12. Turner AF. The chest radiograph in pregnancy. *Clin Obstet Gynecol* 1975;18:65–74.
13. Lyons HA, Antonio R. The sensitivity of the respiratory center in pregnancy and after the administration of progesterone. *Trans Assoc Am Phys* 1959;72:173–180.
14. Arias F, Pineda J. Aortic stenosis and pregnancy. *J Reprod Med* 1970; 20:229–232.
15. Hibbard LT. Maternal mortality due to cardiac disease. *Clin Obstet Gynecol* 1975;18:27–36.
16. Rush RW, Verjans M, Sprecklen FH. Incidence of heart disease in pregnancy. *S Afr Med J* 1979;55:808–810.
17. Szekely P, Snaith L. Atrial fibrillation and pregnancy. *Br Med J* 1961: 1407.
18. Ueland K, McAnulty JH, Ueland FR, Metcalfe J. Special considerations in the use of cardiovascular drugs. *Clin Obstet Gynecol* 1981;24: 809–823.
19. Szekely P, Turner R, Snaith L. Pregnancy and the changing pattern of rheumatic heart disease. *Br Heart J* 1973;35:1293–1303.
20. Dommisse J, Commerford PJ, Levetan B. Ballon valvuloplasty for severe mitral valve stenosis in pregnancy. *S Afr Med J* 1996;86(suppl): 1194–1196.
21. Graeff H, Kuhn W, eds. Coagulation disorders in obstetrics. Philadelphia: WB Saunders 1980:7–9.
22. Hall JG, Paull RM, Wilson KM. Maternal and fetal sequelae of anticoagulation during pregnancy. *Am J Med* 1980;68:122–140.
23. Oakley C. Pregnancy and congenital heart disease. *Heart* 1997;78:12–14.
24. Salazar E, Izaquirre R, Verde J, Mutchinick O. Failure of adjusted dose of subcutaneous heparin to prevent thromboembolic phenomena in pregnant patients with mechanical cardiac prostheses. *J Am Coll Cardiol* 1996;27:1698–1703.
25. Guiz B. Myocardial infarction in pregnancy. *J Obstet Gynaecol Br Commonw* 1972;63:381–390.
26. Husani MH. Myocardial infarction during pregnancy. *Postgrad Med J* 1971;47:660–665.
27. Badui E, Encisco R. Acute myocardial infarction during pregnancy and puerperium: a review. *Angiology* 1996;47:739–756.
28. Roth A, Elkayam U. Acute myocardial infarction associated with pregnancy. *Ann Intern Med* 1996;125:751–762.
29. Engleman DT, Thayer J, Derossi J, Scheinerman J, Brown L. Pregnancy related coronary artery dissection. A case report and collective review. *Conn Med* 1993;7(suppl):135–139.
30. Euror T, Goto Y, Maeda T, Chiba Y, Haze K. Multiple coronary artery dissections diagnosed in vivo in a pregnant woman. *Chest* 1993;104: 289–290.
31. Bac DJ, Lotyering FK, Verkaaik APK, Deckers JW. Spontaneous coronary artery dissection during pregnancy and postpartum. *Eur Heart J* 1995;16:136–138.
32. Shaver P, Corrig T, Baker W. Postpartum coronary artery dissection. *Br Heart J* 1978;40:83–86.
33. Mann JI, Vessey MP, Thorogood M, Doll R. Myocardial infarction in young women with special reference to oral contraceptive practice. *Br Med J* 1975;2:241–245.
34. Shalev Y, Ben-Hur H, Hagay Z, et al. Successful delivery following myocardial ischemia during the second trimester of pregnancy. *Clin Cardiol* 1993;16:754–756.
35. Ascarelli MH, Grider AR, Hsu HW. Acute myocardial infarction during pregnancy managed with immediate percutaneous transluminal coronary angioplasty. *Obstet Gynecol* 1996;88:655–657.
36. Klutstein MW, Tzivoni D, Britran D, Mendzelevski B, Ilan M. Almagory. *Cathet Cardiovasc Diagn* 1997;40:372–376.
37. Garry D, Leikin E, Fleisher AG, Tejani N. Acute myocardial infarction in pregnancy with subsequent medical and surgical management. *Obstet Gynecol* 1996;87:802–804.
38. Demakis JG, Rahimtoola SH. Peripartum cardiomyopathy. *Circulation* 1971;44:964–968.
39. Burch GE, Giles TD, Tsui C-Y. Post partum cardiomyopathy. *Cardiovasc Clin* 1972;4:270–282.
40. Stuart KL. Cardiomyopathy of pregnancy and the puerperium. *Q J Med* 1968;37:463–477.
41. Lampert MB, Hibbard J, Weinert L, Briller J, Lindheimer M, Lang RM. Peripartum heart failure associated with prolonged tocolytic therapy. *Am J Obstet Gynecol* 1993;168:493–495.
42. Lampert M, Lang R. Peripartum cardiomyopathy. *Am Heart J* 1995; 130:860–870.
43. Burch GE, McDonald CD, Walsh JJ. The effect of prolonged bed rest on post partum cardiomyopathy. *Am Heart J* 1971;81:186–201.
44. Melvin KR, Richardson PJ, Olsen EGJ, Daly K, Jackson G. Peripartum cardiomyopathy due to myocarditis. *N Engl J Med* 1982;307:731–734.
45. Richardson PM, LeRoux BT, Rogers MA, Cootsman MS. Pericardiectomy in pregnancy. *Thorax* 1970;25:627–630.
46. Fairley C, Clarke J. Use of esmolol in a parturient with hypertrophic obstructive cardiomyopathy. *Br J Anesth* 1995;75:801–804.
47. Oakley GDG, McGarry K, Limb DG, Oakley CM. Management of pregnancy in patients with hypertrophic cardiomyopathy. *Br Med J* 1975;37:305–312.
48. Elkayam U, Gleicher N. Primary pulmonary hypertension and pregnancy. In: Elkayam U, Gleicher N, eds. Cardiac problems in pregnancy. New York: Alan R. Liss, 1982.
49. Walcott G, Burcell HB, Brown AL. Primary pulmonary hypertension. *Henry Ford Hosp Bull* 1961;9:271–311.
50. Schlandt RC, Felner JM, Miklozek CL, Lutz JF, Hurst JW. Mitral valve prolapse. *Dis Mon* 1980;26:1–51.
51. Rayburn WF, Fontana ME. Mitral valve prolapse and pregnancy. *Am J Obstet Gynecol* 1981;141:9–11.
52. Manolo-Estrella P, Barko AE. Histopathogic findings in human aortic media associated with pregnancy. *Arch Pathol* 1967;83:336–341.

53. Elkayam U, Ostrzega E, Shotan A, Mehra A. Cardiovascular problems in pregnant women with the Marfan syndrome. *Ann Intern Med* 1995; 127:117–122.
54. Elias S, Berkowitz RL. Marfan syndrome and pregnancy. *Obstet Gynecol* 1976;47:358–361.
55. Pyeritz RE. Maternal and fetal complications of pregnancy in the Marfan syndrome. *Am J Med* 1981;71:784–790.
56. Rossiter J, Repke J, Morales a, Murphy E, Pyeritz R. A prospective longitudinal evaluation of pregnancy in the Marfan syndrome. *Am J Obstet Gynecol* 1995;71:784–790.
57. Oakley C. Pregnancy and congenital heart disease. *Heart* 1997; 78:12–14.
58. Mendelson CL. Cardiac disease in pregnancy. Philadelphia: FA Davis, 1960:150–151.
59. Allen HD, Beekman RH, Garson A, et al. Pediatric therapeutic cardiac catheterization. *Circulation* 1998;97:609–625.
60. Schaefer G, Arditi LI, Solomon HA, Ringland JE. Congenital heart disease in pregnancy. *Clin Obstet Gynecol* 1968;11:1048–1063.
61. Gleicher N, Midwall J, Hochberger D, Jaffin H. Eisenmenger's syndrome in pregnancy. *Am J Obstet Gynecol* 1979;34:721–741.
62. Loh TF, Tan NC. Fallot's tetralogy and pregnancy: a report of a successful pregnancy after complete correction. *Med J Aust* 1971;2: 141–145.
63. Cobb T, Gleicher N, El Kayam U. Congenital heart disease in pregnancy. In: El Kaydam U, Gleicher N, eds. Cardiac problems in pregnancy. New York: Alan R. Liss, 1982.
64. Canobbio M, Mair D, Van-Der-Velde M, Koos B. Pregnancy outcomes after the Fontan procedure. *J Am Coll Cardiol* 1996; 28:763–767.
65. Avila W, Grinberg M, Snitcowsky R, et al. Maternal and fetal outcome in pregnant women with Eisenmenger's syndrome. *Eur Heart J* 1995;16:460–464.
66. Shotan A, Ostrzega E, Mehra A, Johnson J, Elkayam U. Incidence of arrhythmias in normal pregnancy and relation to palpitations, dizziness and syncope. *Am J Cardiol* 1997;79:1061–1064.
67. Perry KG, Morrison JC, Rust OA, Sullivan CA, Martin RW, Naef RW. Incidence of adverse cardiopulmonary effects with low dose continuous terbutaline infusion. *Am J Obstet Gynecol* 1995;173:1273–1277.
68. Magee LA, Downar E, Semer M., Coulton BC, Allen LC, Koren G. Pregnancy outcome after gestational exposure to amiodarone in Canada. *Am J Obstet Gynecol* 1995:172:1307–1311.
69. Isaacs JD, Mulholland DH, Hess LW, Albert JR, Martiu RW. Pregnancy in a woman with an automatic implantable cardioverter defibrillator. A case report. *J Reprod Med* 1993;57:487–488.
70. Gleicher N, Meller J, Sendler RZ, Sullem S. Wolff-Parkinson-White syndrome in pregnancy. *Am J Obstet Gynecol* 1981;58:748–752.
71. Finley AY, Edmurds V. DC Cardioversion in pregnancy. *Br J Clin Pract* 1979;33:88–94.
72. Biehl D, Shnider SM, Levinson G. The direct effects of circulatory lidocaine on uterine blood flow and foetal well-being in the pregnant ewe. *Can Anaesth Soc J* 1977;24:445–451.
73. Metcalfe J, Ueland K. The heart and pregnancy. In: Hurst JW, ed. The heart, 4th ed. New York: McGraw-Hill, 1978:1721.
74. Bellet S. Essentials of cardiac arrhythmias. Philadelphia: WB Saunders, 1972.
75. Merx W, Effert S, Heinrich KW. Heart disease in pregnancy, intra- and postpartum. *Z Geburtshilfe Perinat* 1974;178:317–336.
76. Aronson JK. Clinical pharmacokinetics of digoxin. *Clin Pharmocokinet* 1980;5:137–149.
77. Cottrill CM, McAllister RG, Gettes L, Noonan JA. Propranolol therapy during pregnancy. *J Pediatr* 1977;91:812–814.
78. Pruyn SC, Phelan JP, Buchanen GC. Long-term propranolol therapy in pregnancy. Maternal and fetal outcome. *Am J Obstet Gynecol* 1979; 135:485–489.

Cherry and Merkatz's Complications of Pregnancy,
Fifth Edition, edited by W. R. Cohen.
Lippincott Williams & Wilkins, Philadelphia © 2000.

CHAPTER 13

Preeclampsia and Hypertensive Disorders

Charles J. Lockwood and Michael J. Paidas

The origin and pathogenesis of preeclampsia (PE) have been pondered since antiquity. However, from a phylogenetic perspective the disease has only recently emerged, since the human is the only animal clearly affected. Some form of the disorder complicates 3% to 7% of all pregnancies. PE complicates 30% of multifetal gestations, 30% of pregnancies in diabetic patients, and 20% of gestations in patients with chronic hypertension, although two-thirds of all cases occur in otherwise healthy nulliparous patients. It is a leading cause of maternal and perinatal morbidity and is associated with a 20-fold increase in perinatal mortality (1–3).

DEFINITION

Preeclampsia is classically defined as the occurrence of hypertension, proteinuria, and edema in the second half of gestation. Unfortunately, much controversy surrounds the precise classification of hypertensive and proteinuric disorders in pregnancy (4,5). A comprehensive scheme has been proposed based on the onset and severity of hypertension and proteinuria (Table 13-1) (5). However, such taxonomic paradigms belie the complex multisystemic nature of PE. Indeed, patients may show initial signs of thrombocytopenia and liver dysfunction and only subsequently experience hypertension and proteinuria (6). A simplified, more useful classification scheme has been suggested by the National Institutes of Health Working Group on Hypertension in Pregnancy (Table 13-2) (2,7).

Normal and retarded fetal growth can occur in conjunction with either severe or minimal maternal disease. PE is, however, consistently characterized by (a) a failure of physiologic placental bed vascular change, followed by progressive uterine spiral artery damage; (b) maternal platelet hyperaggregation; (c) a reduction in maternal and fetal vascular prostacyclin production and/or effect in the microcirculation; (d) a loss of systemic arterial vasoregulation, with pathologic vasodilation followed by vasoconstriction; and (e) evidence of endothelial cell perturbation or damage.

TABLE 13-1. *Classification of hypertensive and proteinuric syndromes in pregnancy including preeclampsia*

Gestational hypertension (HTN) and/or proteinuria (PTN)
Hypertension and/or proteinuria developing during pregnancy, labor, or the puerperium in a previously normotensive, nonproteinuric woman, including
Gestational HTN without PTN
developing antenatally after 20 weeks
developing intrapartum
developing postpartum
Gestational PTN without HTN
developing antenatally after 20 weeks
developing intrapartum
developing postpartum
Gestational HTN with PTN (preeclampsia)
developing antenatally after 20 weeks
developing intrapartum
developing postpartum
Chronic HTN and chronic renal disease
HTN and/or PTN in pregnancy in a woman with chronic hypertension or chronic renal disease (Diagnosed prior to 20 weeks), including
Chronic HTN without PTN
Chronic renal disease PTN with or without HTN
Chronic HTN with superimposed preeclampsia (PTN >20 weeks in patient with Chronic HTN)
Unclassified HTN and/or PTN
Unclassified HTN without PTN
Unclassified PTN without HTN
Unclassified HTN with PTN (preeclampsia cannot be diagnosed because of late registration for prenatal care)

C. J. Lockwood and M. J. Paidas: Department of Obstetrics and Gynecology, New York University School of Medicine, New York, NY.

TABLE 13-2. *Hypertensive disorders of pregnancy*

Chronic hypertension	Known hypertension before pregnancy or rise in blood pressure to >140/90 mm Hg before 20 weeks
Preeclampsia/ eclampsia	Rise in blood pressure of >15 mm Hg diastolic or >30 mm Hg systolic from measurement in early pregnancy or to >140/90 mm Hg in late pregnancy if no early reading available, with proteinuria (>0.3 g per 24 h) and /or edema
Transient hypertension	Rise in blood pressure as for preeclampsia, no proteinuria (>3 g per 24 h)

From Roberts JM, Redman CW. *Pre-eclampsia: more than pregnancy-induced hypertension.* Lancet 1993;341: 1447–1451.

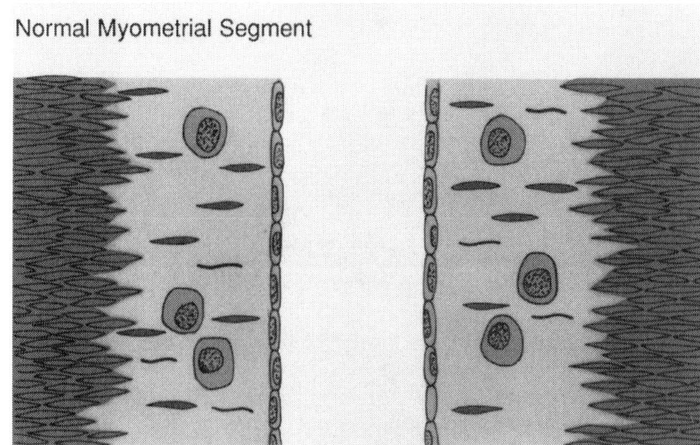

FIG. 13-2. Schematic representation of the myometrial segment of a placental bed spiral artery in an uncomplicated pregnancy. Note that trophoblast invasion is limited to the inner media.

ETIOLOGY

The Placenta in Preeclampsia

Physiologic Placentation

Pregnancy is associated with a tenfold increase in uterine blood flow, 90% of which is directed to the intervillous space (8). At term, intervillous blood flow may be as high as 750 mL/min (9–11). Despite this increase in intervillous blood flow, the number of spiral arteries supplying the placental bed is fixed relatively early in pregnancy at approximately 120 (12). To accommodate the increasing blood flow, these placental bed spiral arteries undergo extensive morphologic changes (13–18) mediated by trophoblast invasion into the media of the vessels (14,16,19). The process occurs in two phases (20,21). In the first trimester the decidual segments of the spiral arteries are apparently "invaded" by trophoblasts. There is subsequent degeneration of the internal elastic lamina and denuding of smooth muscle and elastin in the inner and outer media. This is accompanied by replacement of normal vessel wall architecture with hyalin and fibrin (13–18,20–22) (Fig. 13-1). During the second trimester there is a second phase of endovascular trophoblastic invasion into the myometrial segments of the spiral arteries, but it is limited to the inner media (13–18,20–22) (Fig. 13-2).

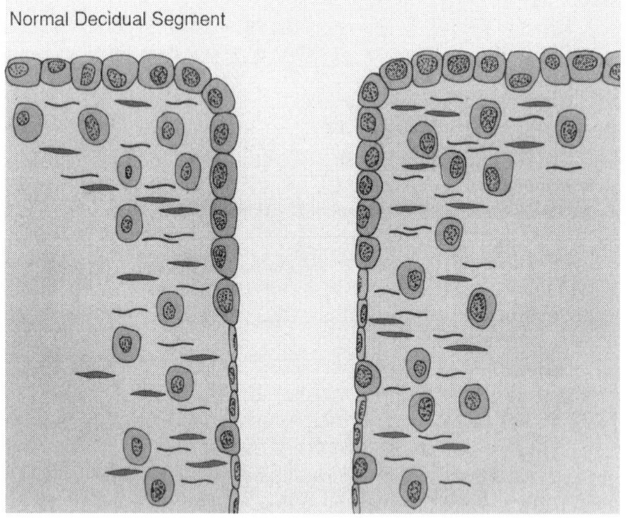

FIG. 13-1. Schematic representation of the decidual segment of a placental bed spiral artery in an uncomplicated pregnancy. Note the extensive invasion of the entire media by trophoblasts (*large cuboidal cells*). The maternal endothelium (*flat cells*) is replaced by trophoblasts only in the distal portion of the vessel at term. The vascular smooth muscle (*spindle-shaped cells*) and reticulum (*curved black lines*) have been extensively denuded and replaced by fibrin and hyalin (*background*).

Physiologic placentation is thus accompanied by profound morphologic changes in placental bed arteries that allow for maximal blood flow at low resistance through widely patent vessels. The principal consequence of this architectural rearrangement is that placental vascular resistance is fixed and not variable, as is the case in the remainder of the maternal and fetal vasculature. Therefore, increases in maternal perfusion pressure will directly augment intervillous blood flow, whereas decreases in maternal perfusion pressure will reduce intervillous blood flow.

Preeclamptic Placentation

In PE, trophoblast-induced physiologic changes are incomplete and restricted to the decidual segments of the placental bed spiral arteries. Endovascular trophoblasts do not extend into the myometrial segments (23–27). Moreover, the myometrial segments and, to a lesser extent, the decidual segments of the spiral arteries demonstrate a distinctive lesion termed "acute atherosis" (28,29). The latter is characterized by endothelial cell discontinuity, focal interruption of the basement membrane, platelet deposition, mural thrombi, and fibrinoid necrosis

(23–27). There are haphazard proliferative changes of intimal cells (myointimal cell hyperplasia) and hyperplasia of smooth-muscle cells in the media, both of which could reflect the mitogenic effects of platelet-derived growth factor (30). There is also extensive lipid necrosis of myointimal and smooth-muscle cells (foam cells) (23–27) (Figs. 13-3 and 13-4). Subendothelial fibronectin is depleted from fetal villous vessels in PE, which is perhaps indicative of concomitant fetal endothelial injury (31). Vascular smooth muscle undergoes hyperplasia with concomitant vasospasm. Acute atherosis is the pathognomonic lesion of idiopathic PE in primigravid patients, but it is also present in the placentas of PE patients with preexisting chronic hypertension, diabetes, renal disease, and lupus (32–33).

Examination of placental bed biopsies from preeclamptic pregnancies suggests that adhesion molecule switching by invasive trophoblasts is abnormal in PE, favoring a less invasive phenotype of integrins, which are cell-extracellular matrix receptors. In normal pregnancies, downregulation of integrins α_6 and β_4 and upregulation of integrins α_1 and β_1 occur, whereas in PE there is persistent expression of the integrins α_6 and β_4, without upregulation of the receptors α_1 and β_1 (34,35). In addition, placental bed biopsy examinations of third trimester placentas reveal that there is focal disruption of endothelial cells lining the uteroplacental arteries by intraluminal endovascular trophoblast cells in placentas of preeclamptic pregnancies. In normal pregnancies, complete reendothelialization of the uteroplacental arteries occurs (36). These persistent endovascular trophoblast cells might be responsible for the elevated levels of fetal fibronectin seen in asymptomatic women destined to experience PE (37).

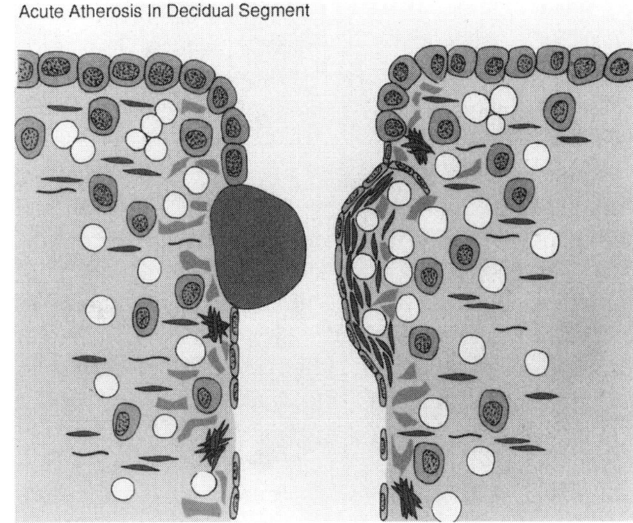

FIG. 13-4. Schematic representation of preeclampsia-induced changes in the decidual segments of a placental bed spiral artery. Note the extensive endothelial cell disruption, myointimal cell hyperplasia, and lipoid necrosis of muscle cells–foam cells. There are focal areas of fibrinoid necrosis (*dark brown background*) and both recent thrombi (*large dark brown mass in vessel lumen*) and acute atherotic plaques (*mixture of foam cells and smooth muscle cells protruding into the lumen*). Nonetheless, the physiologic changes induced by endovascular trophoblast invasion remain evident. (From Romero R, Lockwood CJ, Oyarzun E, Hobbins JC. Toxemia: new concepts in an old disease. Semin Perinatol 1988;4:302–323.)

Acute Atherosis In Myometrial Segment

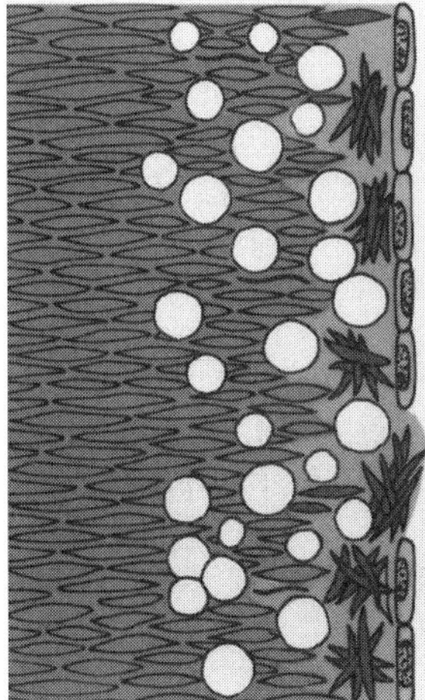
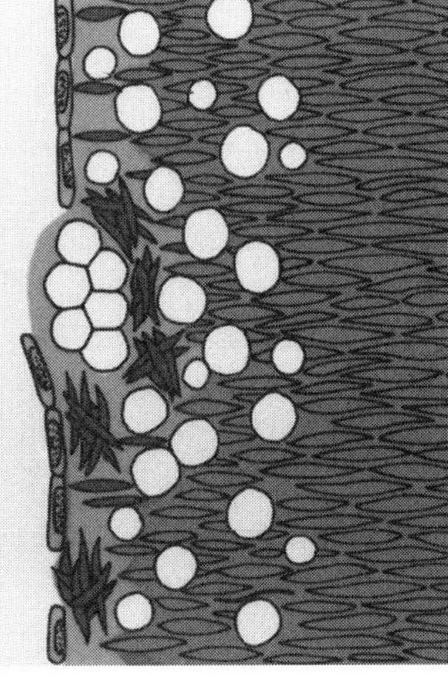

FIG. 13-3. Schematic representation of preeclampsia-induced acute atherosis in the myometrial segment of a spiral artery. Note the extensive endothelial cell disruption, fibrinoid necrosis (*dark brown background*), myointimal cell hyperplasia (*clusters of overlapping dark brown spindle cells*), lipoid necrosis of muscle cells–foam cells (*clear white vacuoles*), and reduction in vessel-lumen diameter stemming from smooth-muscle hypertrophy and vasospasm. (From Romero R, Lockwood CJ, Oyarzun E, Hobbins JC. Toxemia: new concepts in an old disease. Semin Perinatol 1988;4: 302–323.)

Evidence of Enhanced Platelet Turnover in Preeclampsia

Absence of Disseminated Intravascular Coagulation in Toxemia

There is little evidence to support the previously held view that disseminated intravascular coagulation is a primary hemostatic abnormality in PE. Many studies suggest that fibrinogen concentrations are unchanged in PE (38–44). In addition, fibrin degradation products are not a prominent feature of the disorder (43,45,46). Plasma fibrinopeptide A levels, an excellent index of fibrinogen turnover (45), are modestly increased in the third trimester of uncomplicated pregnancies (46), and PE is associated with only a further modest elevation (47,48). Levels of thrombin–antithrombin III complexes, a marker for thrombin generation, are increased in PE, and these levels inversely correlate with platelet counts (r = -0.53) (50). Thus, the excess fibrin and thrombin generation present in PE appears to be predominantly associated with platelet aggregation.

Romero and associates (51) reviewed coagulation parameters in 355 patients with PE, 12% of whom had thrombocytopenia. Fibrinogen concentrations were normal in both thrombocytopenic (495 mg/dL) and nonthrombocytopenic patients (496 mg/dL). Only thrombocytopenic patients with PE showed signs of fibrin degradation products. Thrombocytopenia was found by regression analysis to be an independent risk factor for maternal multiorgan system dysfunction, fetal growth restriction, preterm delivery, and fetal distress. It is worth noting that in five patients, the development of thrombocytopenia preceded the onset of hypertension and proteinuria. These observations suggest that enhanced platelet aggregation is the primary coagulation abnormality in PE and contributes to the pathogenesis of the disorder (51).

Enhanced Platelet Aggregation

There is abundant evidence linking increased platelet turnover with PE.

Increased mean platelet volume (52,53) as well as increased responses to platelet agonists have been found from one to several weeks before the onset of disease (52). Recently, flow cytometric analysis of platelet activation has been studied in normal pregnant women and in women with PE. In a cross-sectional study, Nicolini and colleagues found no difference across gestational ages in women without PE, but platelets from pregnant women were less responsive to selective agonist stimulation (U44619:9, a stable analogue of thromboxane A_2) (54). Janes and Goodall investigated dense and lysosomal granule release (cluster domain 63 antigen), as well as fibrinogen receptor exposure compared with controls (55). Proteinuric patients with PE expressed the highest levels of CD63 antigen.

In a prospective study evaluating platelet activation in the first and second trimester, Konijnenberg and colleagues found that women who experienced PE (n = 17) had elevated median levels of anti-GP53 (lysosomal secretion), a marker of platelet activation, expression in the first trimester compared with controls (n = 227) (56). In another study, this same group of investigators found that women with PE (n = 10) expressed higher levels of P-selectin, anti-GP53 (lysosomal secretion), and platelet endothelial cell adhesion molecule type 1 compared with women without PE (n = 10) (57).

Paidas and colleagues found that preeclamptic women exhibited significantly higher levels of P-selectin and CD63 antigen expression and that P-selectin expression increased with disease severity (58). In a follow-up study, soluble circulating P-selectin in plasma was found to be significantly elevated at 15 weeks' gestation in women destined to experience PE (59). Infusion of a platelet-specific nitric oxide donor, *S*-nitrosoglutathione, in women with severe preterm PE, was associated with reduced mean arterial pressure, platelet activation, and uterine artery resistance (60). In addition, the platelets taken from women with PE appeared to be more sensitive to the inhibitory effects of nitric oxide donors when the platelet release reaction and peak cyclic GMP responses to sodium nitroprusside were studied (61) The expression of activation-specific antigens likely represents the end result of distinct intracellular events mediated by guanine nucleotide binding proteins, G-proteins. When G-protein-mediated platelet inhibition was studied, the greatest inhibition of platelet activation occurred with administration of inhibitors of the initial phase of platelet activation (sodium/hydrogen transport) (62). This finding suggests that early inhibition in the cascade of platelet activation will be more effective in platelet inhibition, later than inhibitors such as aspirin, which inhibit platelets through dense granule release subsequent to surface membrane activation.

Platelet counts are consistently reduced in patients with PE (39–41,43,45). Platelet size and production time are increased in PE, whereas platelet half-life is decreased. There is also a greater proportion of young platelets detected in the circulation. Each of these observations suggests increased platelet turnover (63–65). The platelets of women with PE are less responsive to aggregating agents, suggesting that they have undergone repeated aggregation and disaggregation within the circulation (66). Beta-thromboglobulin (BTG) is a platelet-specific protein stored in α-granules and secreted during the platelet-release reaction. BTG is an excellent index of intravascular platelet aggregation (67). Elevated plasma levels and increased urinary excretion of BTG are noted in PE (47,68,69). PE is also associated with a reduction in serum inhibition of platelet-activating factor (PAF) activity (70). Since PAF promotes platelet aggregation, alters vascular smooth-muscle tone, and increases capillary permeability, this reduction in PAF inhibitory activity might contribute to the observed platelet hyperaggregability in PE.

Reduced Vascular Prostacyclin and Enhanced Thromboxane Effect in Preeclampsia

Prostacyclin Production in Normal Pregnancy

Uncomplicated pregnancy is associated with increases in plasma renin, angiotensin, and aldosterone, and yet a reduction in systemic vascular resistance occurs (71).

Pregnant patients are resistant to the pressor effect of infused angiotensin II (72,73), and this resistance is dependent on prostaglandin production (74,75). Pretreatment with both indomethacin and high-dose aspirin enhances sensitivity to infused angiotensin in uncomplicated pregnancies (74,75). Conversely, infusion of prostaglandin E_2 and prostacyclin (PGI_2) decreases the pressor effect of infused angiotensin II (76). Therefore, a likely candidate for this vasodilating prostanoid is PGI_2, since it is the primary product of arachidonic acid metabolism in vascular tissue (77). PGI_2 is the most potent inhibitor of platelet aggregation and avidly induces vasodilation (78). The half-life of PGI_2 is 1.5 to 3 minutes in an aqueous medium, although albumin prolongs half-life modestly (77,79). It is nonenzymatically degraded to the stable, but inactive metabolite 6-oxo-$PGF_1\alpha$ (78). Plasma levels of PGI_2 are extremely low (<3 pg/mL), suggesting that it exerts its effect at a microcirculatory level and not as a "hormone" (80).

There is evidence of an enhanced systemic PGI_2 effect in pregnancy. Studies assessing plasma concentrations have identified increases using a gas/liquid chromatography–mass spectrometry method (GCMS) (81). Given the evanescent nature of PGI_2 and evidence that it is not a circulating hormone in humans (80), an appropriate estimate of total vascular production can be derived by measuring the dinor and 15-kd dinor urinary metabolites of PGI_2 (81). Using GCMS, uncomplicated pregnancies were associated with a fivefold increase in dinor metabolite excretion. The normal placenta appears to be capable of producing large quantities of PGI_2 (82). Maximal placental production rates are reported to range from 0.12 to 0.64 ng/min/g (82,83); thus, a 500-g placenta in a 60-kg woman would yield 1 to 5 ng/min/kg of PGI_2. Biological effects are seen with intravenous PGI_2 infusions of less than 2 to 4 ng/min/kg (84). Therefore, it appears that placental production contributes significantly, though perhaps not predominantly, to the increased PGI_2 level noted in uncomplicated pregnancies.

Prostacyclin and Thromboxane in Preeclampsia

There is a loss of refractoriness to infused angiotensin II as early as 18 weeks' gestation in patients destined to experience PE (72,73). It is worth noting that PGI_2 production appears to decrease in the disorder. Urinary dinor metabolites of PGI_2 are reduced in patients with PE compared with those patients with uncomplicated pregnancies (81). Placental production of PGI_2 is diminished significantly in PE, and this reduction does not result from impaired arachidonic acid substrate availability (82). Placental PGI_2 production is also limited by hypoxia (81), suggesting that the reduction in intervillous blood flow accompanying acute atherosis results in diminished placental PGI_2 production. Umbilical PGI_2 production, as measured by assay for 6-oxo-$PGF_1\alpha$, is also depressed in PE (85–91). Impaired production appears to be a consequence of decreased enzyme quantity (decreased V_{max}) rather than decreased enzyme activity (normal K_m) (90).

A reduction in endothelial vascular PGI_2 production will create an enhancement of platelet thromboxane effect. Thromboxane A_2 (TxA_2) is a product of platelet arachidonic acid metabolism (92). It is a potent stimulant of platelet aggregation and vasospasm. Thromboxane has a half-life of 30 seconds and is nonenzymatically degraded to thromboxane B_2 (92). A microcirculatory TxA_2 predominance would promote vasoconstriction and platelet aggregation, contributing to the focal ischemia and platelet deposition present in PE. Placental tissue also produces TxA_2 in abundance (6.3 ng/g/h), and production is significantly increased in PE (22.9 ng/g/h) (93). The progressive proteinuria of PE might be exacerbated by excess TxA_2 (94). Moreover, the resultant hypoalbuminemia, in turn, reduces systemic PGI_2 half-life (77,79), establishing a pathologic cycle.

Loss of Arterial Vasoregulation: Pathologic Vasodilation Followed by Vasoconstriction

Dramatic elevations in systemic vascular resistance (SVR), frequently exceeding 2,000 dyne/s/cm, accompany clinical evidence of PE. This finding has led to the theory that PE is a vasospastic state; however, often preclinical disease is associated with a reduction in SVR (95). Easterling and associates carried out serial evaluations of blood pressure, cardiac output, and SVR in 120 nulliparous patients, 5% of whom experienced overt PE and 36% of whom had isolated hypertension (94). Significant elevations in cardiac output were noted throughout gestation in the group with combined PE and hypertension compared with unaffected controls. Before 26 weeks, the group with combined PE and hypertension had a significantly lower SVR compared with controls. Presumably, elevations in SVR are late consequences of the disease. While patients with PE are more sensitive to pressor agents, the autoregulation of resistance vessels may be impaired, facilitating hypertensive end-organ damage.

Whereas the initial stages of endothelial cell damage are accompanied by increased vascular PGI_2 (78) and endothelium-derived relaxing factor (EDRF), i.e. nitric oxide production, later stages are associated with reduced PGI_2 and EDRF synthesis and release of the microcirculatory vasoconstrictive peptide endothelin (96). The observation of an initial decrease in SVR in preclinical PE followed by SVR increases during the course of overt disease might parallel variations in arteriolar PGI_2, EDRF, or endothelin synthesis and therefore mirror the natural history of vascular damage in this disorder. Concomitant platelet hyperaggregability could result from primary placental or systemic endothelial-vascular damage or from an imbalance in the circulatory ratio of TxA_2/PGI_2, promoting platelet deposition with secondary endothelial damage. Regardless of the precise sequence of events, it is clear that platelet hyperaggregability, aberrant vasoregulation, and derangements in vascular prostanoid homeostasis are integral components of the pathogenesis of PE.

Evidence for Endothelial Perturbation in Preeclampsia

The characteristic placental lesion of PE, acute atherosis, provides direct histologic evidence for local endothelial-vascular disruption in the disorder. There is also growing indirect evidence for PE-associated endothelial-vascular injury. While concentrations of both factor VIII and von Willebrand factor (vWF) are increased in uncomplicated pregnancies, there is a greater relative increase in the vWF concentration in PE, leading to an increase in the vWF/factor VIII ratio (40,65,97–99). Endothelial cells synthesize and store vWF and release it as a consequence of endothelial cell perturbations (100). The activity of plasminogen activator inhibitor type 2 (PAI-2) (placental derived) is decreased in PE and intrauterine growth restriction (101–107), whereas plasminogen activator inhibitor type 1 (PAI-1), which is derived from endothelium and platelets, is increased (101–105,107–116).

Paidas and colleagues prospectively evaluated PAI-1 and PAI-2 levels in pregnancy (117). PAI-1 levels were increased (164.2 ± 84.6 ng/mL vs. 123.9 ± 63.5 ng/mL, $p = 0.01$), and PAI-2 levels were decreased (102.6 ± 63.5 vs. 144.9 ± 80.0 ng/mL, $p = 0.02$) in asymptomatic women destined to experience PE compared with those patients without PE. Delta PAI (PAI-1 minus PAI-2) was significantly different between the two groups (61.6 ± 92.9 vs. 21.0 ± 95.0, $p = 0.0003$). Collectively, these studies support the presence of endothelial damage and decreased placental function in PE. Serum samples from women with PE have been found to be cytotoxic to endothelial monolayer cultures by some, but not all, investigators (118,119). Taylor and colleagues found selective effects of preeclamptic sera in human endothelial cell procoagulant protein expression, with increased expression of cellular fibronectin and no increases in tissue factor or vWF expression (120,121). Platelet-poor sera from patients with PE induce potent vasoconstriction in an *in vivo* mouse mesenteric arteriolar preparation, whereas sera from patients with uncomplicated pregnancies do not have such an effect (122). Similarly, the clinical response of patients with severe preeclampsia to delivery and to plasmapheresis with plasma infusions (123,124) suggests that a trophoblast-associated effect (induced or produced) is responsible for the multisystemic side effects.

Lockwood and Peters noted that clinical signs of PE were preceded by accumulation in the circulation of a cellular-derived fibronectin bearing an extra type III domain (ED1) (125). Given immunohistochemical evidence that ED1+ fibronectin is normally localized within the endothelium of larger blood vessels (126), the intravascular accumulation of ED1+ fibronectin associated with PE could be the result of accelerated release from sites of placental bed or systemic endothelial injury. Consistent with this mechanism of action, intravascular release of this protein has been shown to specifically reflect vascular injury in experimental *in vivo* and platelet-free *in vitro* models (127,128). Plasma levels of ED1+ fibronectin are also significantly elevated in individuals with clinical evidence of vasculitis (129). Embryonic capillary basement membranes contain ED1+ fibronectin (126), and, as noted, PE is associated with denudement of fetal intervillous fibronectin (28). Plasma levels of ED1+ fibronectin, or fetal fibronectin, are not elevated in the first half of pregnancy in women destined to experience PE (130), but they are elevated in the third trimester in asymptomatic women in whom PE develops (37).

THE COMPLEX CLINICAL PRESENTATION OF PREECLAMPSIA

Definitions

As has been noted, hypertension is but one of the many side effects of PE. Nonetheless, hypertension remains the primary diagnostic sign and the principal clinical concern of the obstetrician caring for the patient with PE. By definition, hypertension in pregnancy is diagnosed by a rise of >30 mm Hg in systolic blood pressure or >15 mm Hg in diastolic blood pressure. Alternatively, the diagnosis is present when blood pressures exceed 139/89 mm Hg on at least two occasions 6 hours apart (131). Mean arterial pressures (MAPs) in the second trimester (MAP-2), calculated as the average of all second trimester blood pressures, are considered elevated at >90 mm Hg (132). Third trimester MAP (MAP-3) values of >105 mm Hg on two occasions separated by at least 6 hours are considered abnormal (132). Page and Christianson noted increased perinatal mortality at MAP-2 and MAP-3 values above these limits (132,133). The precise diagnosis of PE also requires coexisting proteinuria, defined as more than 0.3 g of protein in a 24-hour urine collection. Alternatively, proteinuria can be diagnosed by the presence >1 g/L (quantitative more than +2) in a random urine specimen. The exact mechanism of action of hypertension in PE is not known. Increased cardiac output with normal systemic vascular resistance has been documented in some cases, whereas decreased cardiac output and greatly increased systemic vascular resistance have been found in other patients. The condition is considered severe when any of the signs outlined in Table 13-3 are present (134).

Chronic hypertension in a pregnant patient is defined as persistent pressures of >140/90 mm Hg appearing before pregnancy or 20 weeks' gestation and persisting after the puerperium. Hypertension before 20 weeks' gestation is not always chronic hypertension. True PE in the early second trimester can result from the lupus anticoagulant/antiphospholipid antibody syndrome, gestational trophoblastic neoplasia, and fetal hydrops. PE superimposed on chronic hypertension is diagnosed by a sharp increase in blood pressure (30 mm Hg systolic or 15 mm Hg diastolic or more) and the presence of proteinuria. Superimposed PE carries the highest risk for perinatal morbidity and mortality (135). As noted, a precise classification of hypertensive and proteinuric syndromes in pregnancy is outlined in Table 13-1.

End-Organ Damage

The view that PE is exclusively a hypertensive disorder is, of course, incorrect. As has been shown, PE is a consequence of progressive maternal and placental endothelial cell perturbations, platelet hyperaggregability, altered prostacyclin–thromboxane balance, and aberrant vasoregulation. However, an individual mother's susceptibility to specific vascular derangements will vary greatly, adding to the confusing and enigmatic clinical signs and symptoms of the disease.

TABLE 13-3. *Clinical manifestations of severe disease in patients with pregnancy-induced hypertension*

Blood pressure >160–180 mm Hg systolic or >110 mm Hg diastolic
Proteinuria >5 g/24 h (normal, <300 mg/24 h)
Elevated serum creatinine
Grand mal seizures (eclampsia)
Pulmonary edema
Oliguria <500 mL/24 h
Microangiopathic hemolysis
Thrombocytopenia
Hepatocellular dysfunction (elevated alanine aminotransferase, aspartase aminotransferase)
Intrauterine growth restriction or oligohydramnios
Symptoms suggesting significant end-organ involvement: headache, visual disturbances, or epigastric or right-upper-quadrant pain

From *Hypertension in Pregnancy.* The American College of Obstetricians and Gynecologists Technical Bulletin January 1996, no. 219.

Renal Disease

The characteristic renal lesion of PE occurs in the glomerular endothelial cell. Its cytoplasm swells with an as yet uncharacterized substance (136). This lesion, glomeruloendotheliosis, correlates best with the presence of proteinuria. While proteinuria and elevated serum urate are the best predictors of perinatal morbidity and mortality (45,137,138), 20% to 40% of patients with PE have no antecedent proteinuria (139,140).

Liver Disease

Severe abnormalities in liver function indexes are well-known components of the syndrome of hemolytic anemia, elevated liver function test results, and low platelet counts (HELLP), which complicates <10% of severe PE (141). However, Minakami and associates identified increased microvascular fat deposition in 41 of 41 patients with severe PE, including 13 patients with normal liver function indexes (142). Moreover, the density of hepatocellular fat deposition directly correlates with plasma uric acid levels and inversely correlates with platelet count (142). These data suggest that subclinical hepatic damage is a common occurrence in PE. Expansion of the liver parenchyma as the result of microvesicular fat deposition or edema, with consequent swelling of Glisson's capsule, is one explanation for the epigastric pain characteristic of severe disease. Microvesicular fat deposition is also the characteristic lesion of acute fatty liver, suggesting a relationship between these two disorders (142). Liver biopsies have also found hemorrhage and architectural deformation as well as infarcts, suggestive of both vasodilation and vasoconstriction (143). Immunofluorescence studies have discovered hepatic sinusoid fibrin deposition.

Pancreatic Disease

DeVore and associates (144) have described elevations in the ratio of amylase to creatinine clearance in preeclamptic patients with abdominal pain:

$$\text{Cam/Ccr\%} = \frac{\text{Amylase clearance}}{\text{Creatinine clearance}} \times 100$$

They postulated that pancreatitis stemming from pancreatic ischemia could also cause epigastric pain in severe PE.

CNS Disease

Seizure activity (eclampsia) is the most dreaded clinical manifestation of the preeclamptic process. The precise mechanism of seizure activity, however, remains a mystery. Malignant hypertension might account for some cases, but seizures frequently occur in patients with antecedent mild elevations in blood pressure. Sibai and colleagues noted that 78% of eclamptic patients had MAP-2 of <85 mm Hg (145). Electroencephalograms (EEGs) are abnormal in 75% of eclamptic patients, but this group did not have statistically significant elevations in blood pressure when compared with patients with eclampsia with normal EEG findings (146). Moreover, in patients with persistent abnormal EEG recordings 6 weeks postpartum, blood pressure readings were normal (146). It is unlikely, therefore, that hypertension is the sole cause of seizure activity.

Further confusing the clinical picture of eclampsia is the observation, noted earlier, that about 20% of eclamptic patients have no preceding proteinuria, headache, or hyperreflexia (147). Computerized axial tomography (CT) fails to show specific focal or diffuse abnormalities (e.g., edema) in the vast majority of eclamptic patients (146). Localized or generalized retinal arteriolar vasospasm is found in half of all patients with PE, and such findings correlate with renal biopsy data (148). Perhaps similar cerebral microvascular changes induce widespread, though discrete cerebral ischemia with resultant seizure activity and EEG abnormalities but with normal CT images.

Pulmonary Disease

Pulmonary edema is another dreaded complication of PE. Compared with patients with uncomplicated pregnancies, patients with PE have dramatic reductions in colloid oncotic pressure (COP) as the result of renal losses (18 vs. 22 mm Hg) (149,150). Elevations in pulmonary capillary wedge pressure (PCWP) (an indicator of pulmonary vascular hydrostatic pressure) in excess of COP predict pulmonary edema in PE (151). However, not all preeclamptic patients with pulmonary edema will manifest this symptom (152). Consequently, the origin of pulmonary edema in PE is multifactorial. Large elevations in pulmonary vascular hydrostatic pressure (the PCWP) compared with plasma oncotic pressures can produce pulmonary edema in some patients, particularly in the postpartum period. In other patients pulmonary vascular damage might compromise capillary integrity, resulting in fluid shifts with or without adult respiratory distress syndrome.

COUNSELING BEFORE CONCEPTION

The relevant issues regarding implications for PE are related to incidence, recurrence risk, and remote prognosis.

Incidence

The incidence of PE is estimated to be 5% to 7%. There are a variety of predispositions that significantly affect this risk. Table 13-4 summarizes the relevant risk factors for the development of PE (134). Multiple fetuses are associated with an increased risk of PE (153), and the risk is greater with higher-order multiple fetuses (triplets or more), where the incidence is about 70% (154). Patients with thrombophilia have a propensity for PE. For example, when three thrombophilic mutations (resistance to activated protein C caused by an adenine-to-guanine mutation at nucleotide 506 in the factor V gene, or factor V Leiden mutation; the mutation of cytosine to thymine at nucleotide 677 in the gene encoding for methylenetetrahydrofolate reductase; and the mutation of guanine to adenine at nucleotide 20210 in the prothrombin gene) were examined in a group of women with poor pregnancy outcome, one of these mutations was present in more than 50% of cases of severe PE (155). Routine screening in cases of severe early-onset PE has been advocated by some investigators, with testing for protein S deficiency, activated protein C resistance, hyperhomocysteinemia, and anticardiolipin antibodies (156). Prospective studies are required to assess the risk of development of PE in women with genetic predispositions to thrombophilia. Our current evaluation for unexplained early-onset severe PE includes screening for deficiencies of protein S, protein C, antithrombin III, activated protein C resistance, factor V Leiden mutation, the prothrombin gene mutation, hyperhomocysteinemia, anticardiolipin antibody, and lupus anticoagulant.

Recurrence Risk

The recurrence risk of some form of PE depends on the nature of the initial episode of PE and the presence of underlying medical conditions. Prospective series have yielded different results, which probably reflect varying genetic predispositions in different populations and the

TABLE 13-4. *Risk factors for the development of pregnancy-induced hypertension*

Factor	Risk ratio
Nulliparity	3:1
Age >40 y	3:1
African-American race	1.5:1
Family history of pregnancy-induced hypertension	5:1
Chronic hypertension	10:1
Chronic renal disease	20:1
Antiphospholipid syndrome	10:1
Diabetes mellitus	2:1
Twin gestation	4:1
Angiotensinogen gene T235	
Homozygous	20:1
Heterozygous	4:1

presence of disparate underlying medical conditions. For example, Chesley reported a rate of 5% for recurrence of eclampsia in a group of 187 women who had eclampsia in their first pregnancy (157). Sibai and colleagues reported a recurrence risk of 45% in primiparas who had experienced severe PE in a previous pregnancy (158). In their respective series, both researchers have recorded an increase in some form of hypertensive event in subsequent pregnancies. The recurrence risk for the HELLP syndrome varies from 3% to 27% (159,160).

Remote Prognosis

The principal concern for long-term prognosis is the future risk of cardiovascular disease and hypertension. Chesley and co-workers' long-term follow-up (40 years) data of patients with eclampsia in their first pregnancy suggest that there is no excess of hypertension, cardiovascular mortality, or death (161). Chesley also reviewed 53 publications with follow-up on 2,637 women with eclampsia and found the average prevalence of hypertension to be 23.8% (range 0%–78%) (162). Sibai and associates found that 67% of patients who had severe PE before 28 weeks experienced chronic hypertension (163). Underlying chronic hypertension or renal disease might account for this increased risk of chronic hypertension. One other interesting finding from Chesley's data is that women who are normotensive throughout their pregnancies have a lower rate of chronic hypertension (157).

CLINICAL MANAGEMENT

Rational management of the patient with PE must be based on an understanding of the known pathogenetic features of the disorder—placental and systemic microvascular damage, abnormal vascular prostanoid homeostasis, excessive platelet aggregation, and aberrant vasoregulation. However, truly effective therapy awaits an understanding of the origin of the disease. The "cure" of PE through delivery and the transient response of patients with severe PE to bed rest and to plasmapheresis with plasma infusions provide vital clues to the source of the disorder. These observations suggest that a trophoblast-associated, -induced, or -produced substance directly provokes endothelial perturbations, platelet aggregation, and aberrant vasoregulation.

Paradoxically, this trophoblast-derived "product" might serve to enhance intervillous blood flow by augmenting maternal perfusion pressure. However, in susceptible hosts, or at higher concentrations, it could damage both the placental bed and the systemic endothelium (Fig. 13-5). The

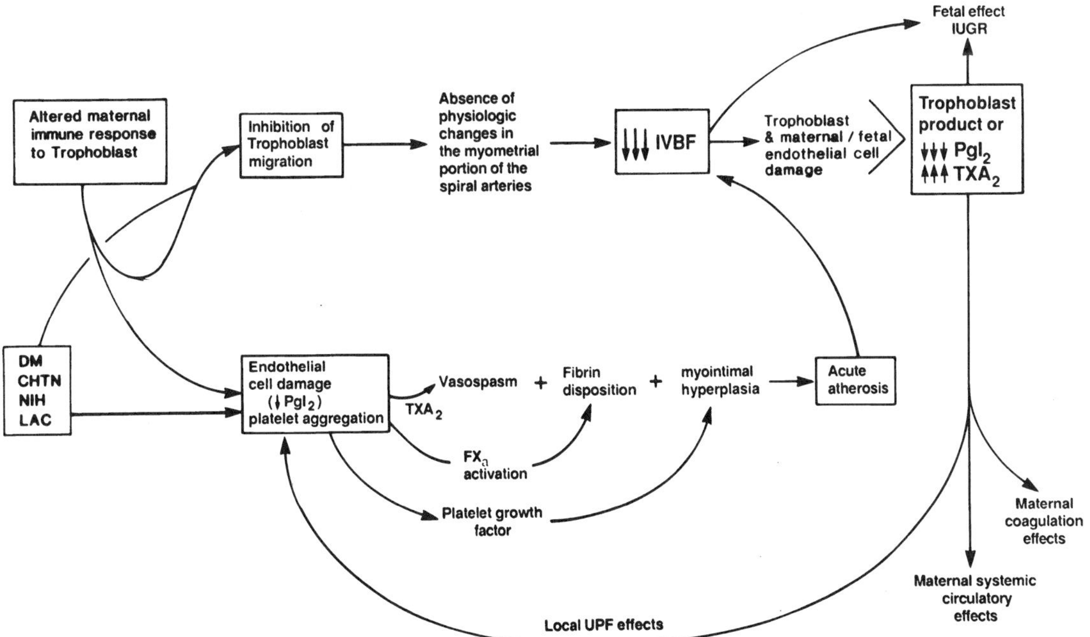

FIG. 13-5. The pathogenesis of preeclampsia. Aberrant trophoblast invasion and/or placental bed endothelial damage give rise to acute atherosis and decreased intervillous blood flow (IVBF). Impaired IVBF causes fetal intrauterine growth retardation (IUGR) and may elicit a "signal" that impairs placental, maternal, and fetal vascular prostacyclin production and enhances thromboxane effect, perhaps by damaging endothelial cells. This leads to the observed multisystemic maternal side effects of toxemia as well as further compromise of uteroplacental blood flow (UPF). (DM, diabetes mellitus; CHTN, chronic hypertension; NIH, nonimmune hydrops; LAC, lupus anticoagulant/antiphospholipid antibodies; FXa, activated factor X; TXA_2, thromboxane A_2; PgI_2, prostacyclin.

product could be toxic to the endothelium or bind to a critical circulating endothelial cytoprotective protein. Alternatively, the product could simply represent reduced placental PGI_2 and enhanced TxA production stemming from impaired intervillous blood flow–induced hypoxia. In any case, this theory accounts for the clinical improvement induced by measures that increase intervillous blood flow (e.g., bed rest in the left lateral decubitus position). Plasmapheresis with albumin infusion could eliminate the product or simply increase the half-life of PGI_2 sufficiently to exert beneficial effects.

Taken together, these observations on the pathogenesis and origin of PE provide support for our current rather limited management schemes. These schemes are predicated on expeditious delivery at term. In less severe preterm cases, the goal is to maximize uteroplacental blood flow and avoid maternal morbidity, with expeditious delivery carried out when either of these goals is in jeopardy.

Management of Preeclampsia at Term

When patients have signs and symptoms of mild or severe PE after 36 weeks' gestation, both mother and fetus should be stabilized and delivery expedited. Initial steps include confirmation of the diagnosis through (a) a blood pressure reading of >140/90, or systolic pressure >30 mm Hg and/or diastolic pressure >15 mm Hg, and/or MAP-3 >105 mm Hg on at least two occasions separated by 6 hours and (b) >2+ proteinuria on urine dipstick or >300 mg/day of protein in a 24-hour urine collection. After admission, blood pressure readings should be obtained every 15 minutes to 4 hours, depending on the severity of the elevations, and urine protein should be assessed at least every 8 hours.

To rule out multisystemic involvement, one should obtain the following maternal blood laboratory test results: aspartate aminotransferase, alanine aminotransferase, amylase, total protein and albumin, and complete blood count with platelet count, creatinine, blood urea nitrogen, and urate levels. Evidence of HELLP syndrome mandates immediate action. Severe thrombocytopenia might require platelet transfusions if counts drop precipitously below 50,000 or should excessive maternal bleeding be encountered between 50,000 and 100,000.

Antiseizure prophylaxis must be promptly instituted. Although some investigators have suggested that anticonvulsant therapy might not be indicated routinely in patients with PE (164), the administration of anticonvulsant therapy is a cornerstone of peripartum treatment in the United States. A selective approach for placing patients on anticonvulsant therapy is unreasonable, since accurate prediction of those patients who will experience seizures is not possible at this time. Magnesium sulfate ($MgSO_4 \cdot 7H_2O$) therapy as prophylaxis for seizures (145), remains the standard treatment for this purpose. Most data suggest that magnesium sulfate is the anticonvulsant of choice for the prevention of eclampsia or recurrent eclamptic seizures. In 1995, Lucas and colleagues reported that magnesium sulfate was superior to phenytoin in preventing eclamptic seizures. Ten of 1,089 women who received phenytoin had an eclamptic seizure compared with none of 1,049 in the group who received magnesium sulfate (165). Magnesium sulfate was also found to be superior to diazepam in preventing the recurrence of seizures and maternal death in patients with eclampsia.

In the Eclampsia Trial Collaborative Group, 1,687 women with eclampsia were randomly given one of three anticonvulsant medications: magnesium sulfate, phenytoin, or diazepam (166). In one arm of the study, 453 women were randomized to receive magnesium sulfate, and 452 were given diazepam. There was a 50% reduction in seizures (60 vs. 126 seizures) and a lower maternal mortality rate (3.8% vs. 5.1%) in those patients receiving magnesium therapy. In the other arm of the trial, 309 patients received magnesium sulfate, and 319 received phenytoin. There were fewer recurrences of convulsions (22 vs. 66) and a lower mortality rate (2.6 vs. 5.2%) with magnesium sulfate compared with phenytoin. Women randomized to receive magnesium sulfate experienced a 50% reduction in the incidence of seizures. If a patient has a seizure while on magnesium sulfate, a second anticonvulsant should be added to terminate the seizure, such as 5 mg diazepam administered intravenously.

A 4-g intravenous loading dose of $MgSO_4$ is given over 15 minutes, followed by an infusion of 1 to 2 g/h titrated to maintain serum concentrations between 4 and 7 mEq/L. If serum magnesium levels are not rapidly available from the hospital laboratory, the infusion dose should be titrated to preserve deep tendon reflexes. A Foley catheter should be inserted to follow urinary output. Since magnesium excretion by the kidney results from magnesium delivery to the proximal tubules in excess of its transport maximum (T_m), a reduction of renal blood flow and glomerular filtration rate, as evidenced by a fall in urinary output, could necessitate a reduction in the $MgSO_4$ infusion rate. Following magnesium levels will assist the clinician in titrating the infusion dose when urinary output falls below 50 mL/h. Respiratory depression and arrest can occur with magnesium levels >10 to 15 mEq/L, and calcium gluconate (10 mL of a 10% solution) should be given intravenously over 3 minutes to reverse magnesium toxicity. The $MgSO_4$ infusion should be maintained for 24 to 48 hours after delivery. However, Sibai and colleagues have noted that the initial seizure occurs in the postpartum period in 27% of patients, with half occurring >48 hours after delivery (145).

The development of progressive oliguria in PE despite prudent fluid challenge (up to 2,000 mL of crystalloid over 2 hours) is an indication for central hemodynamic assessment via a Swan-Ganz catheter (167) (see Chapter 48). Evidence of hypovolemia in the form of depressed PCWP should be treated with colloid and/or crystalloid infusion to maintain urinary output of >30 mL/h and PCWP below 12 to 16 mm Hg, depending on the COP and clinical situation. Following improvement in urinary output, further fluid management should be directed toward correcting electrolyte and serum osmolarity imbalances. Oliguria in the context of elevated PCWP must be treated only after full assessment of cardiac output and SVR and an evaluation of cardiac function. The latter can be derived by graphing the left ventricular stroke work index versus PCWP. This modified Starling curve can be used to evaluate and subsequently maximize left ventricular function. In the patient with PE and oliguria with a normal or increased PCWP, increased SVR, and decreased cardiac output, vasodilators might improve renal perfusion (167,168). However, if the SVR is normal and the cardiac output is increased, a preload reducer, such as nitroglycerin, may be beneficial. Meticulous fetal surveillance is required in the context of antepartum PE-induced oliguria, since uteroplacental blood flow might be compromised.

Care must be taken not to overhydrate patients in the postpartum period, since delivery results in a significant redistribution of extracellular fluid into the intravascular space. The greatest risk of pulmonary edema occurs 15 hours after delivery (152). These patients should be followed for clinical evidence of pulmonary edema (tachypnea, tachycardia, cyanosis, and rales on pulmonary auscultation). Should urine output fall below 30 mL/h in a patient with a normal or elevated PCWP, 20 mg of furosemide should be administered intravenously. If there is no response, 40 mg should be given. Continued oliguria can be treated with vasodilators, although oliguria can be evidence of acute tubular necrosis. In the absence of central hemodynamic monitoring during the postpartum period, intravenous infusion rates should be minimized to maintain urine output >30 mL/h. If no central hemodynamic monitoring is available in the postpartum period for a patient with PE and oliguria who is unresponsive to modest fluid challenge (<500 mL/h), a single dose of furosemide, 20 to 40 mg, can be given intravenously. Continued oliguria is an indication for central hemodynamic monitoring.

In patients with eclampsia, a padded tongue blade should be inserted and their airways maintained during seizures. Oxygen should be administered and the airway kept clear of secretions. If they are not being treated with intravenous $MgSO_4$, such treatment should be instituted as described earlier. Seizure activity that develops during the course of $MgSO_4$ administration or recurrent seizure activity unresponsive to $MgSO_4$ necessitates assessment of the magnesium level, with adjustment of the infusion accordingly. In the interim, administration of intravenous diazepam, 5 mg, or pentobarbital, 125 mg, should be considered. Other causes of seizures should be ruled out by history and physical examination. CT scans and EEG appear to have limited efficacy in these patients (146).

Severe persistent hypertension (blood pressure of >160/110 mm Hg) should be treated with an antihypertensive agent. A number of antihypertensive agents are available, but the direct vasodilator hydralazine has been the most widely administered agent. Its principal advantage is that while it effectively lowers blood pressure, it also results in increased cardiac output through a reflex mechanism, thus augmenting uteroplacental perfusion. Intravenous hydralazine therapy is instituted with a 1-mg test dose. If there is no adverse effect after 1 minute, 4 mg is administered over 4 minutes. Additional 5- to 10-mg boluses can be given every 20 minutes, as needed.

Since intervillous blood flow is critically dependent on maternal perfusion pressure, diastolic pressures should be maintained above 90 mm Hg in the antepartum period, to avoid uteroplacental insufficiency with resultant fetal distress. Hydralazine has an onset of action of 10–20 minutes, and its dosage and frequency of administration should not exceed 20 mg every 20 minutes. Hydralazine should never be used in an infusion, since its hypotensive effect may persist for hours (169). Should higher and more frequent dosages be required, consideration should be given to administration of a sodium nitroprusside infusion. Nitroprusside's mechanism of action includes dilation of both resistance and capacitance blood vessels. Nitroprusside must be given by meticulously monitored intravenous infusion and has an immediate (<2 minutes) onset. The infusion dose is generally 30 to 500 µg/min and should not exceed 800 µg/min (170).

Since cyanide is produced by the interaction of nitroprusside with protein sulfhydryl groups, prolonged administration can lead to cyanide toxicity in the mother. This agent crosses the placenta and selectively accumulates in sheep fetuses (171). Low rates of nitroprusside infusion appear to prevent cyanide accumulation in the sheep model (171,172). There is conflicting evidence of an adverse effect of nitroprusside on uterine blood flow (172–174). Careful surveillance of uteroplacental function by fetal heart rate monitoring and fetal umbilical artery Doppler flow studies, when available, is mandated by a nitroprusside infusion in the antepartum period.

Other potentially useful agents include the calcium channel blocker nifedipine, which has quick onset of action (5–10 minutes). The starting dose is 10 mg, and it can be given every 4 to 8 hours. It is well tolerated, but the principal concern is the potential synergistic action with magnesium, leading rapidly to hypotension (175,176) and skeletal muscle blockade (177). Labetalol, another frequently administered antihypertensive agent in the context of PE, has been our drug of choice for prolonged therapy. Labetalol is a mixed α- and β-adrenergic antagonist and is administered intravenously for rapid lowering of blood pressure. It is useful to begin with a bolus infusion of 20 mg; repeated doses of 10 to 50 mg can be given every 10 minutes (177). Labetalol does not reduce afterload, which is a theoretical disadvantage, particularly in severe PE. It also can be administered orally, beginning at a dose of 100 mg p.o. b.i.d. Usually, no more than 1,600 mg per day is required for blood pressure control.

Vaginal delivery is the preferred route in PE. Abdominal delivery is, of course, indicated for obstetric indications, fetal distress, and rapidly deteriorating maternal status. The latter category includes rapidly progressive thrombocytopenia, rising liver function indices, status epilepticus, and refractory malignant hypertension. In the absence of these potentially ominous findings, pitocin induction with or without preceding prostaglandin gel administration should be carried out. Epidural anesthesia is preferred for abdominal delivery and is an effective analgesic for labor (179). It should be employed after blood pressure stabilization, with a platelet count above 100,000/mm^3 and no evidence of fetal distress.

Management of Preterm Preeclampsia

The leading cause of perinatal morbidity and mortality in PE is prematurity. Therefore, conservative management might be appropriate for patients with PE who are preterm and who have stable, mild disease. By contrast, the perinatal salvage rate is low (12%), prolongation of gestation is short, and maternal morbidity is high for patients with persistent evidence of severe disease remote from term

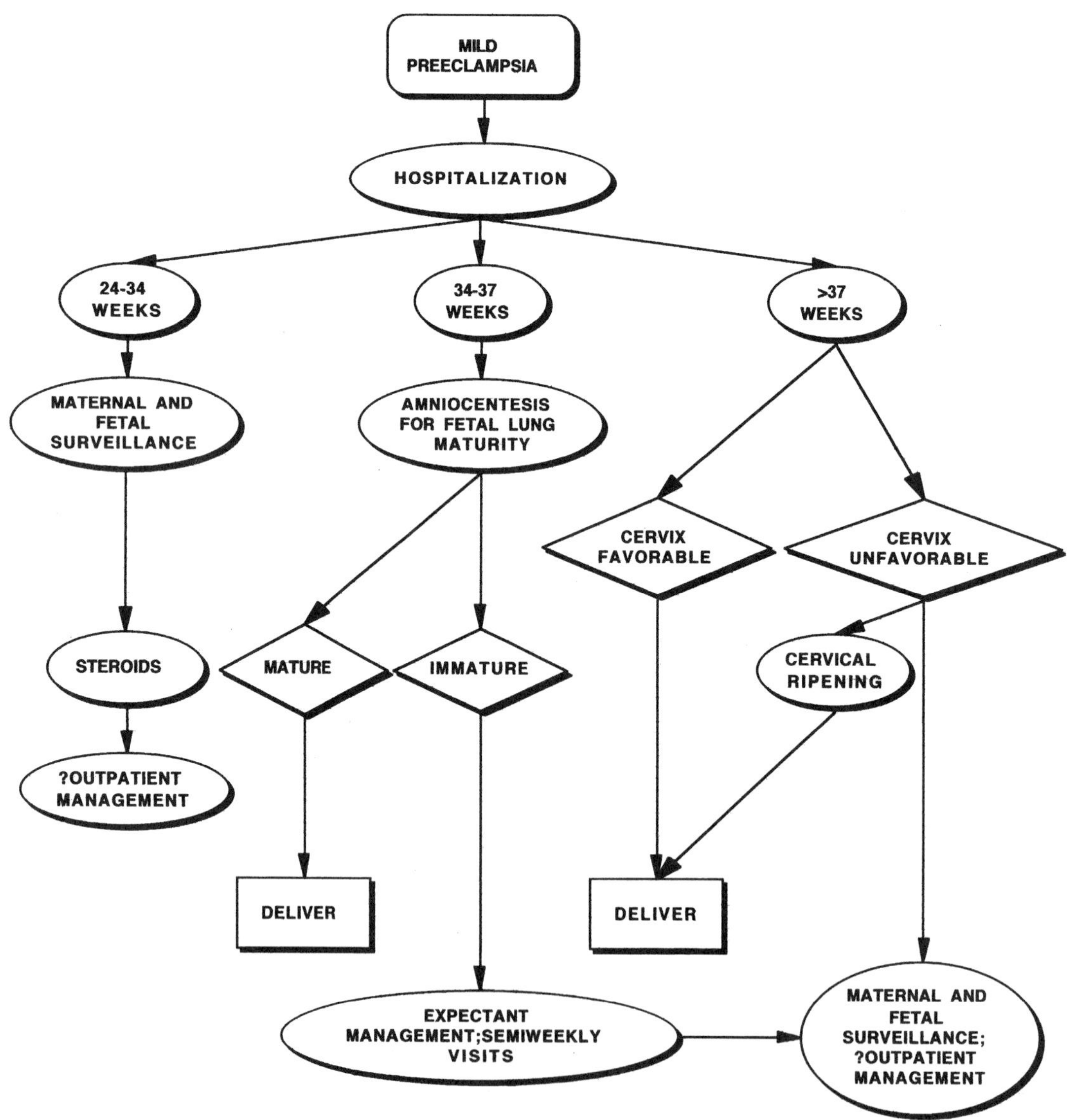

FIG. 13-6. Management approach for mild preeclampsia.

(18–27 weeks) (180). These patients should be stabilized and delivered to optimize maternal outcome (180). Patients with persistent signs and symptoms of severe disease between 28 and 36 weeks should also be expeditiously delivered, but the perinatal survival rate is significantly higher in this group, and vigilance in fetal surveillance during labor is indicated. A strategy for treating the patient with PE is outlined in Figs. 13-6 and 13-7.

Conservative management includes hospitalization with bed rest in the left lateral recumbent position. The

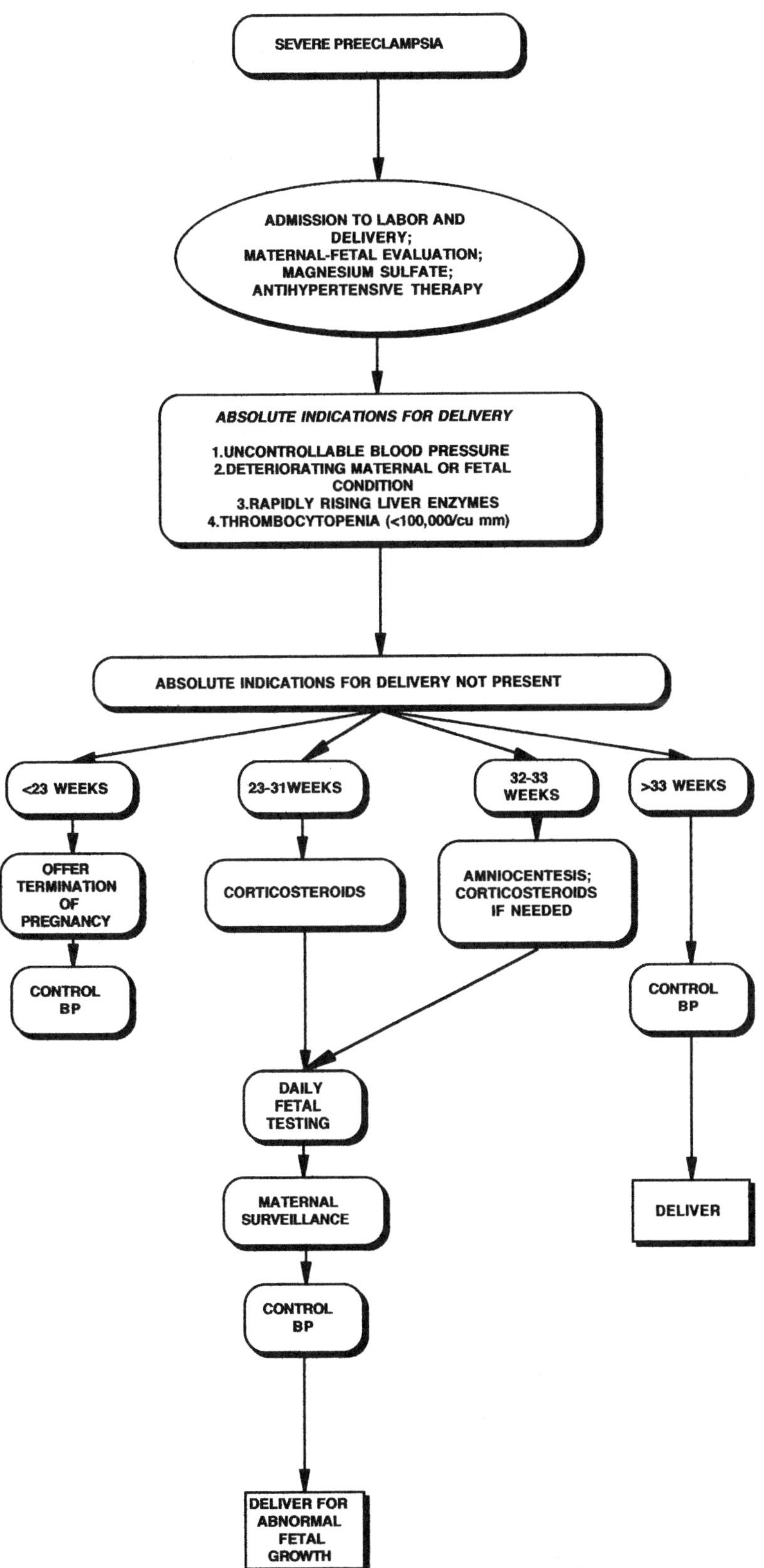

FIG. 13-7. Management approach for severe preeclampsia.

TABLE 13-5. *Conservative treatment of the patient with preeclampsia*

Maternal surveillance
- Maternal weight (daily)
- Blood pressure (q 4–8 h)
- Urine protein (q 8 h)
- Laboratory studies including
  - AST/ALT/amylase (q 2–7 d)
  - Creatinine, BUN, urate (q 2–7 d)
  - Platelet count (q 2–7 d)
  - 1-h glucose screen
- 24-h urine collection for total protein and creatinine clearance (q 7 d)

Fetal surveillance
- Detailed (level II) ultrasound to rule out multiple gestations, fetal hydrops, and partial hydatidiform mole
- Fetal testing at diagnosis or after 26 wk gestation
  - Nonstress tests (twice weekly)
  - Contraction stress tests (weekly)
  - Biophysical profile or amniotic fluid volume assessment (q 7 d)
  - Ultrasound for fetal growth assessment (q 10–14 d)
  - Doppler flow studies of the fetal umbilical artery if fetal growth restriction is present (q 7 d)
  - Amniocentesis for pulmonary maturity indexes at 34–37 wk and, if immature, weekly thereafter until mature or until 37 wk is reached in a nondiabetic patient

AST, aspartate aminotransferase; ALT, alanine aminotransferase; BUN, blood urea nitrogen.

protocol for conservative treatment of patients with PE is outlined in Table 13-5. When PE develops early in the second trimester, the patient should be evaluated for the underlying cause, as previously outlined. The presence of lupus anticoagulant can be tested via the kaolin clotting time or activated partial thromboplastin time on platelet-poor plasma. Abnormal results should be further evaluated by mixing studies (adding normal control plasma in a 1:1 dilution to eliminate the possibility of factor deficiencies) and by the platelet neutralization procedure, which confirms the phospholipid dependency of the inhibitor. Anticardiolipin antibodies should also be searched for. Finally, PE in the second trimester should prompt a detailed sonographic evaluation of the placenta to rule out a partial mole or normal gestation coexisting with a complete mole. Multiple gestations and fetal hydrops can be excluded by a careful targeted ultrasound study. Blood pressure elevations >150/100 or MAP values >110 should be managed with antihypertensive therapy (Table 13-6).

Delivery is indicated at 37 weeks' gestation or more or between 34 and 37 weeks when there is confirmation of fetal maturity. Delivery is, of course, indicated with evidence of either maternal deterioration or fetal compromise. Fetal compromise includes fetal heart rate evidence of fetal distress or a persistent biophysical profile of <6. A more subtle sign of fetal compromise is the cessation of fetal growth between two ultrasound evaluations 10 to 14 days apart. In this context, delivery should be considered when there is documentation of fetal maturity or a gestational age >34 weeks. If fetal growth is not confirmed at <34 weeks' gestation and immature pulmonary indexes are evident, one can administer two doses of betamethasone, 12 mg i.m. every 24 hours, or dexamethasone, 6 mg i.m. every 12 hours, for four doses (181,182). Daily or twice daily fetal testing should also be initiated. If fetal testing remains reassuring, another ultrasound can be performed in 10 days; continued absence of fetal growth is an indication for delivery in all but the most preterm gestations. Alternatively, if adequate fetal growth is confirmed, routine management can be resumed. Finally, less than optimal fetal growth should prompt daily testing and repeated ultrasound evaluation every 10 days.

Occasionally, a preterm patient with mild PE can be treated as an outpatient. These patients should have diastolic pressures <95 mm Hg, normal liver function indices, platelet counts of >100,000/mm^3, creatinine clearance >100 mL/min, adequate fetal growth with normal amniotic fluid volume, reassuring fetal heart rate testing, and acceptable fetal umbilical artery waveform patterns (i.e., systolic to diastolic peak velocity waveform ratios not elevated for gestational age), if this testing method is available. The patient must be able to maintain bed rest in the left lateral position and have a family member in constant attendance. The recording of blood pressures and urine protein dipstick results twice daily by a family member is quite useful. Home nursing services are increasingly available to assess vital signs, obtain laboratory tests, and even conduct nonstress tests. Patients should be seen weekly in the physician's office, undergo twice-weekly nonstress tests and/or assessment of biophysical profiles, and have fetal growth ultrasound evaluations every two weeks.

TABLE 13-6. *Antihypertensive therapy*

Agent	Usual oral dose	Maximal daily oral dose	Time to peak concentration	Half-life (h)
Methyldopa	250 mg b.i.d.	2,000 mg	2–3 h	—
Clonidine	0.3 mg q.d.	0.8 mg q.i.d.	1–3 h	10 h
Atenolol	50 mg q.d.	100 mg q.i.d.	—	8 h
Hydralazine	25 mg q.i.d.	200 mg q.i.d.	0.5 h	6 h
Nifedipine	10 mg t.i.d.	180 mg	1 h	2–3 h
Labetalol	100 mg b.i.d.	2,400 mg	2–4 h	6–8 h

When aggressive management and delivery are indicated in a previously conservatively treated preterm patient with PE or in a preterm patient with severe, refractory PE, the protocol described earlier for the management of PE at term should be implemented. Special considerations in the latter case include the higher probability of fetal growth retardation, the greater susceptibility to fetal distress in labor, and the increased risk of breech presentation. In light of these factors, a higher incidence of abdominal delivery can be anticipated.

Management of Chronic Hypertension

In the case of a pregnant patient with chronic hypertension, the primary concern of the obstetrician is the early identification of superimposed PE. A careful medical and genetic history should be taken. The use of tricyclic and monoamine oxidase inhibitor antidepressants can be associated with exacerbation of hypertension, as can excessive use of decongestants and glucocorticoids. A physical examination should be performed to rule out symptoms of Cushing's and Graves syndromes. Blood pressure should be assessed in both arms (sitting, supine, and in the left lateral decubitus position), with the diastolic pressure assessed at disappearance of sound (phase V). Fundoscopic examination should be undertaken to exclude retinal hemorrhages, arteriolar spasm, exudates, and papilledema. The thyroid, abdomen (<16 weeks), and carotids should be auscultated for bruits. Early in pregnancy, the kidneys should be palpated to dismiss the possibility of masses suggestive of adult-onset polycystic kidney disease. Femoral pulses should be evaluated; a delay or absence suggests aortic coarctation.

Initial laboratory tests include assessment of serum electrolytes, calcium, uric acid, creatinine, and blood urea nitrogen. A baseline 24-hour urine sample should be obtained to evaluate creatinine clearance and total protein. These renal function tests should be repeated every 4 to 8 weeks. Urinalysis might raise the suspicion of end-organ damage (red blood cells), glomerulonephritis (red cell casts), or chronic interstitial nephritis (crystals, white blood cells, white blood cell casts). Sonographic evidence of renal calculi might also suggest the presence of chronic interstitial nephritis stemming from recurrent infections. Long-standing hypertension necessitates a maternal electrocardiogram, even in younger patients. Serologic testing for antinuclear antibodies and ribonucleoprotein antibodies could aid in excluding lupus, autoimmune vasculitis, and scleroderma. Finally, serum anticardiolipin antibodies and the presence of a lupus anticoagulant, which is accompanied by chronic hypertension in 20% of cases, should be ruled out.

If the source of the chronic hypertension has not been previously established and there is a strong reason to suspect pheochromocytoma, obtain a 24-hour urine sample (acidified collection) for catecholamines, metanephrine, and vanillylmandelic acid (see Chapter 25). Although it is rare, maternal pheochromocytoma carries a high mortality rate. If the family history or physical examination is suggestive, obtain an ultrasound of the mother's kidneys to rule out autosomal dominant adult-onset polycystic disease.

An ultrasound examination should be performed early in gestation to confirm the estimated date of confinement. This is particularly critical in pregnancies complicated by chronic hypertension, since there is a high risk of intrauterine growth retardation (IUGR). The precise diagnosis of IUGR by ultrasound requires an accurate delivery date. A targeted ultrasound should be performed at 15 to 20 weeks to exclude anomalies. Serial ultrasound testing for growth should be done every 4 weeks beginning at 24 weeks. Any evidence of fetal growth lag mandates the initiation of more frequent growth scans (every 10 to 14 days), fetal testing at >24 weeks' gestation, and, if available, fetal umbilical artery Doppler flow studies.

Contemporary treatment of chronic hypertension continues to evolve. The goal of all therapeutic regimens is the maintenance of blood pressures <140/90 mm Hg. In nonpregnant patients, initial efforts can include or be limited to such nonpharmacologic approaches as weight reduction, exercise, avoidance of tobacco and alcohol, and biofeedback techniques. The options for initiating pharmacologic therapy in nonpregnant patients newly diagnosed with hypertension are now quite varied. Diuretics, beta blockers, calcium channel antagonists, and angiotensin-converting enzyme inhibitors can all be used as initial therapeutic agents, depending on the presumed cause of hypertension and the specific characteristics of the patients (183). If the initial therapy is inadequate, three options are available. First, the dosage can be increased. Second, the drug can be discontinued and a new agent begun. Third, a second agent can be added, if the maximum dose of the initial agent does not achieve the desired effect. For a complete discussion of current management recommendations, the reader is referred to "The Sixth Report of the Joint National Committee on Detection, Evaluation, and Treatment of High Blood Pressure" (183).

Unfortunately, this therapeutic repertoire is more limited in pregnancy. Angiotensin-converting enzyme inhibitors have been associated with irreversible fetal–neonatal renal failure (184,185). There is a theoretical concern regarding the effects of calcium channel blockers on uteroplacental blood flow, but evidence suggests that judicious use of nifedipine is not associated with a reduction in uteroplacental blood flow (186). Nonetheless, the effects of long-term therapy in pregnancy are not yet known. There is no clear evidence that long-term diuretic therapy will result in untoward side effects on the fetus. While there is a well-described association between reduction in plasma volume and fetal growth inhibition (187), the intravascular volume reduction caused by diuretic therapy is transient. It lasts only weeks. Furthermore, the reduction in renal blood flow and glomerular filtration caused by diuretics is minimized by the addition of methyldopa (188). In general, methyldopa, atenolol, clonidine, and hydralazine appear to be safe and effective when used for the treatment of chronic hypertension in pregnancy.

Methyldopa is the most commonly prescribed drug for the treatment of hypertension in pregnancy. Its antihypertensive effects are mediated centrally by stimulation of central nervous system α-adrenergic receptor sites and peripherally by inhibition of dopa-decarboxylase. Peripheral conversion of α-methyldopa to α-methylnorepinephrine also diminishes the effects of norepinephrine. Administration of methyldopa without a diuretic expands plasma volume and limits its antihypertensive effectiveness (189). Side effects include lethargy, depression, sodium retention, and constipation. Results of Coombs' test are positive in 20% of nonpregnant patients receiving methyldopa after at least 6 months of treatment (190). Methyldopa does not appear to result in adverse effects on the fetus (191,192).

Propranolol, timolol, and nadolol are nonselective β-adrenergic blockers. Atenolol, labetalol and metoprolol are β_1-selective adrenergic blockers. An additional advantage of atenolol is its longer half-life and single daily dose (193,194). Atenolol's antihypertensive action results from reductions in cardiac output and in renal renin production. Atenolol therapy appears to be safe in pregnancy (195). Caution must be exercised with the use of all beta blockers, because they can precipitate cardiac failure by virtue of their negative inotropic effect and can induce bronchospasm through their β_2-antagonist activity. Beta blockers blunt counter-regulatory catecholamine responses to hypoglycemia, particularly in recent-onset diabetes, and can mask hypoglycemic symptoms. These agents are also contraindicated in Raynaud's syndrome because unopposed alpha stimulation will worsen vasoconstriction. Side effects of beta blockers include sleeplessness, depression, nightmares, hallucinations, and neurologic dysfunction. Paradoxical hypertensive reactions are also possible in rare patients, owing to the potential vasoactivity of the methyldopa metabolite α-methylnorepinephrine (196). Reports of fetal growth restriction in mothers receiving beta blockers are, of course, subject to ascertainment biases; however, these agents can certainly produce transient neonatal hypoglycemia, bradycardia, and respiratory depression (197–199). In general, their judicious use in pregnant hypertensive patients appears to be warranted (200).

Clonidine also exerts its antihypertensive actions by stimulation of α-adrenergic receptor sites in the central nervous system, but, unlike methyldopa, it does not act on peripheral α-adrenergic receptors (190). Important side effects include postural hypotension, sodium retention, and a potential hypertensive crisis upon abrupt discontinuation of the drug (190,201). There is no clear evidence that this agent is teratogenic (202).

Hydralazine directly relaxes arteriolar smooth muscle, decreasing vascular resistance without generating significant orthostasis. Its vasodilation does result in a reflex increase in heart rate and cardiac output. The latter effect can be further potentiated by sodium retention mediated by the renin-angiotensin-aldosterone system and by a direct renal mechanism (203). Hydralazine is metabolized by hepatic *N*-acetyltransferase, and genetic polymorphisms in this enzyme can result in variable serum concentrations at a given dose. Significant side effects include nasal congestion, headaches, dizziness, palpitations, and myocardial ischemia. A lupuslike syndrome occurs with prolonged high-dose (>200 mg/day) therapy in patients with low hepatic *N*-acetyltransferase activity. Additional rare adverse effects include rash, fever, neuropathy, and bleeding dyscrasias (203). A study by Gant et al. (204) noted decreases in the clearance of dehydroisoandrosterone sulfate in patients with chronic hypertension following administration of hydralazine. Since dehydroisoandrosterone sulfate clearance is dependent on placental delivery, those data are taken as evidence of impaired uteroplacental perfusion. Animal studies of the effects of hydralazine on uterine blood flow are equivocal (173,205,206). It should be noted that while antihypertensive therapy reduces blood pressure and might delay the diagnosis of superimposed PE, there is no evidence that it prevents the multisystemic effects of the disorder, and it might lower birth weights (191,192,207,208).

OTHER CAUSES OF HYPERTENSION

Primary hypertension, that is, essential or idiopathic hypertension, accounts for 92% to 94% of hypertension in the general population. The causes of secondary hypertension include renal hypertension (3%–5%) and endocrinologic hypertension (about 1%) (209). Renal hypertension is the result of renovascular and parenchymal diseases. Among the endocrinologic causes of hypertension are primary aldosteronism, Cushing's syndrome, pheochromocytoma, and oral contraceptive–induced hypertension. Miscellaneous problems, such as coarctation of the aorta, account for the remaining 0.2% of causes of hypertension. It is important to consider these rarer sources of hypertension, since they can have a significant impact on maternal and fetal well-being, and most are curable.

Renal Hypertension

Renovascular Hypertension

Renovascular hypertension results from decreased perfusion of renal tissue due to stenosis of a main or branch renal artery, with activation of the renin–angiotensin system. Circulating angiotensin II increases arterial blood pressure by directly causing vasoconstriction, stimulating aldosterone secretion, or stimulating the adrenergic nervous system. Renal artery stenosis is the most common cause of nonessential hypertension (210). Fibromuscular dysplasia is primarily responsible for renal artery stenosis in the younger population (under 40 years of age). The most significant concern regarding renal artery stenosis is the high risk of progression to malignant hypertension. Distinguishing renal artery stenosis from essential hypertension might be difficult. Abdominal bruits are present in more than 50% of patients, but bruits can be difficult to detect in pregnancy.

Definitive diagnosis is made by renal angiography. Arterial narrowing of more than than 50% is considered significant. In pregnancy, the best option for diagnosis is magnetic resonance imaging (211). Digital subtraction angiography is also an option, but it carries the risk of radiation exposure to the fetus. Medical treatment consists of beta blockers. Percutaneous transluminal angioplasty is the treatment of choice, but it, too, risks radiation exposure to the fetus. Angioplasty has been performed in pregnancy (212,213). There are limited data regarding the impact of renal artery stenosis on pregnancy. Sellars et al. reported on a group of three women before and after treatment for renal artery stenosis (214). Before treatment, a total of five pregnancies resulted in two spontaneous abortions, two intrauterine fetal deaths, and one live infant delivered at 37 weeks because of growth restriction. After definitive treatment, four pregnancies resulted in four live births.

Parenchymal Renal Disease

Acute and chronic renal parenchymal disease make up a vast array of disorders, with varying maternal and fetal implications. While maternal and obstetric complication rates are high in patients with significant renal impairment, the chance of neonatal survival is also quite high at present. In 1991, Imbasciati and Ponticelli reported on a large series of patients with renal disease (215). In patients with chronic renal failure and a serum creatinine level >1.4 mg/dL, these investigators found the following incidences: worsening hypertension, 57%; fetal loss, 17%; perinatal loss, 9%; growth restriction, 34%; and preterm delivery, 50%. In patients with primary glomerulonephritis, blood pressure increased in 36% of cases. The spontaneous loss rate was 8%, perinatal loss was 13%, and preterm delivery occurred in 19% of cases. A decline in renal function occurred in 11% of cases.

Arterial hypertension is a significant contributor to adverse perinatal outcome in women with chronic renal failure. Jones and Hayslett reported on the maternal and obstetrical outcomes of 67 women (82 pregnancies) with primary renal disease (216). The underlying renal disease was chronic glomerulonephritis in 51% of women and chronic tubulointerstitial disease in 49%. Hypertension increased in frequency from a baseline of 28% to 48% in the third trimester. There was pregnancy-related loss of maternal renal function in 43% of patients. Preterm delivery was necessary in 59% cases, and growth retardation was present in 37%. The infant survival rate was 93%. Excellent outcomes have been documented in patients with mild renal disease (serum creatinine <1.4 mg/dL). Katz and colleagues reported on 121 pregnancies in 89 women (217). They found that hypertension was present in 23% of pregnancies. A small decline in renal function (usually reversible) was noted in 16% of pregnancies. Preterm delivery occurred in 20%, and growth restriction was seen in 24% of cases. The overall infant survival rate was 89%. Similar findings have been reported by other investigators (218–221).

Endocrinologic Causes of Hypertension

Primary Hyperaldosteronism

Primary hyperaldosteronism is a condition in which there is autonomous production of aldosterone, resulting in elevated aldosterone levels, hypokalemia, hypertension, and depressed renin. Benign adrenal adenomas are most often responsible for cases of primary hyperaldosteronism. Patients can have clinical symptoms of hypokalemia: muscle cramps, weakness, headache, or hypertension. Hypokalemia, either spontaneous or provoked, can provide a clue to the diagnosis. Diagnosing primary hyperaldosteronism in pregnancy can be difficult, since aldosterone levels rise considerably in normal pregnancies. Plasma renin activity rises in pregnancy, but in patients with chronic hypertension, renin activity decreases, making it difficult to differentiate between essential hypertension and primary hyperaldosteronism. Magnetic resonance imaging might be helpful in locating an adrenal lesion. Treatment options include medical and surgical approaches. In pregnancy, pharmacologic treatment options are limited—calcium channel blockers are probably the best option. Spironolactone and angiotensin-converting enzyme inhibitors are contraindicated in pregnancy. A limited number of cases of primary hyperaldosteronism in pregnancy have been documented (222–225). A variety of pregnancy complications have been reported, including superimposed PE, placental abruption and preterm delivery. Medical and surgical treatment approaches have both been reported.

Cushing Syndrome

Cushing syndrome, or hypercortisolemia, can result from a variety of causes in pregnancy (see Chapter 24). Adrenal adenomas account for the majority of cases, while the remaining cases are due to pituitary adenomas, and ectopic corticotropin (ACTH) production from malignancy. Hypercortisolemia manifests in clinical symptoms of central obesity, round facies, excessively rapid weight gain, proximal myopathy, wide striae, hirsutism, acne, spontaneous bruising, and neuropsychiatric disturbances. Diagnosing hypercortisolemia is difficult in pregnancy. Evaluation can include measurement of 24-hour urinary free cortisol in more than one sample, serum cortisol measurement at 0800 and 2300 hours, and a 1-mg dexamethasone suppression test conducted overnight. All three tests are affected by pregnancy.

Definitive biochemical diagnosis is accomplished with a two-day low-dose (0.5 mg every six hours) dexamethasone suppression test. Plasma ACTH levels should be drawn to help differentiate ACTH-dependent (pituitary and ectopic) from ACTH-independent (adrenal) causes. Administration of corticotropin-releasing hormone (CRH) can help differentiate pituitary from adrenal or ectopic sources of ACTH, since ACTH will increase with administration of corticotropin-releasing hormone when the pituitary is the source but will not increase in response to adrenal or ectopic causes. Inferior petrosal sampling has been reported to identify the source of ACTH production (226) in pregnancy.

In the context of pregnancy, treatment options depend upon the location of the tumor, gestational age at diagnosis, and the severity of disease. Transphenoidal resections have been performed in pregnancy (227–229). Adrenal lesions should be removed during pregnancy, unless the diagnosis is made near term (230). Metyrapone might be helpful in terms of blocking cortisol secretion (231). Maternal mortality and adverse effects consisting of aggravated hypertension, gestational diabetes, and congestive heart failure have been documented with Cushing syndrome (232,233). Significant fetal and neonatal side effects have been seen, and increased preterm delivery rates (33%) and spontaneous abortion and stillbirth (17%) have been reported (234).

THE EFFECT OF HYPERTENSION ON THE FETUS AND NEONATE

The fetal and neonatal consequences of hypertensive disease have been recognized for decades. It has long been appreciated that disease severity significantly affects fetal and neonatal outcomes (235). Gestational hypertension alone does not have a significant impact on pregnancy (236), but PE is associated with adverse fetal outcomes (237). Furthermore, increasing proteinuria in the context of PE is correlated with worsening fetal outcomes when the diagnosis is established by renal biopsy (238). PE superimposed on preexisting chronic hypertension continues to carry the worst perinatal prognosis (239). In 1982, Lin and colleagues reported a perinatal mortality rate of 134/1,000 among 157 hypertensive women in whom the underlying source of disease was established by renal biopsy (238). In 1984, Sibai and colleagues reported on the outcome of severe PE in 303 patients (240). Thirty percent of cases (91/303) were complicated by PE superimposed on chronic hypertension. The perinatal mortality rate was 32% for patients with superimposed PE and 7.7% for those with PE alone. The perinatal survival rate was zero when severe PE developed at or before 28 weeks, whereas all fetuses survived when the disease developed after 28 weeks.

Sibai and colleagues randomized patients with severe PE at 28 to 32 weeks to aggressive treatment or expectant treatment (241). Aggressively treated patients were delivered 48 hours after steroid administration. Expectant treatment consisted of bed rest, administration of oral antihypertensive agents, and intensive antenatal testing. The average latency period before delivery was 15.4 days (range, 4–36 days). There were no cases of eclampsia or perinatal death in either group, and there were similar incidences of abruptio placentae. In the expectantly treated group, there was a significantly higher gestational age at delivery, higher birth weights, a lower incidence of admissions to the neonatal intensive care unit, lower mean days of hospitalization in the intensive care unit, and a lower incidence of neonatal complications. Odendaal et al. reported on 58 women with severe PE between 28 and 34 weeks who were randomized to aggressive versus expectant treatment (242). The incidence of abruption was 17% (10 cases)—six in the aggressively treated group (three unexpectedly found) and four in the expectantly treated group.

There is significant perinatal morbidity and mortality associated with pregnancies complicated by the HELLP syndrome. During an 8-year period, 112 patients with HELLP syndrome were evaluated (243). The perinatal mortality rate was 367/1,000. Abruption complicated 20% of cases, and 82% of patients delivered at or before 36 weeks. Fetuses that were small for gestational age complicated 31.6% of pregnancies.

Contemporary data suggest that neonatal outcome in patients delivered preterm for PE is no different than that among patients without PE. In a matched cohort study, Friedman and colleagues found no differences in neonatal death, grades three and four respiratory distress syndrome, grades two and three necrotizing enterocolitis, and culture-proven sepsis (244). The matched patients in the control group consisted of patients who delivered as the result of refractory preterm labor. Paidas et al. also found no significant differences in perinatal mortality rate (32.8/1,000 vs. 42/1,000), incidence of respiratory distress syndrome, bronchopulmonary dysplasia, or intraventricular hemorrhage in newborns delivered at or before 34 weeks whose mothers had PE compared with newborns from pregnancies not complicated by PE (245). Antenatal steroids were routinely administered during this period—nearly all patients (approximately 90%) in both groups received steroids (245).

In 1983, Sibai et al. reported on the pregnancy outcome of 211 patients with mild chronic hypertension (246). Antihypertensive medications were discontinued at the initial visit. The perinatal mortality rate was 28.1/1,000. The incidence of babies who were small for gestational age was 7.9%, but the rate increased to 32% when superimposed PE developed. Indeed, the majority of perinatal deaths occurred in the superimposed PE group. Antihypertensive medications were restarted in 13% of patients. In the remaining 190 patients, there was one perinatal death (5/1,000), five infants who were small for gestational age infants (5.3%), and one abruption (0.5%), suggesting a favorable outcome in the majority of patients with mild chronic hypertension without PE. The findings of one other study in a similar population were in agreement, but this study showed a higher incidence of superimposed PE, which might have been the result of a discrepancy in the definition of superimposed PE (247).

For patients with severe chronic hypertension, perinatal morbidity and mortality are much more significant. In a cohort of 44 consecutive patients with severe hypertension (≥170/110), there was a perinatal mortality rate of 25% (248). Seventy percent of patients were delivered before 37 weeks, and 43% were small for gestational age. Controversy exists regarding the impact of antihypertensive therapy on perinatal outcome. Two early studies suggested a benefit (249,250), while a more recent randomized trial comparing results among no medication, methyldopa, or labetalol did not demonstrate any differences in perinatal outcome (251).

CURRENT STATUS OF THE PREVENTION OF PREECLAMPSIA

Low-dose Aspirin

The concept that PE is the consequence of progressive maternal and placental endothelial cell disruption and platelet hyperaggregability, at least in part, has led to consideration of antiplatelet therapy. Low-dose aspirin (ASA) has been shown to reduce platelet TxA production without impeding endothelial PGI_2 production (252). Low-dose ASA (81 mg/day) increases the effective pressor dose of infused angiotensin and increases the ratio of vascular PGI_2 to TxA (253). Studies in pregnant patients confirm the efficacy of low-dose ASA in selectively blocking TxA synthesis (254).

The first report suggesting that ASA therapy is associated with a lower incidence of PE was published in 1979 (255). Crandon and Isherwood reviewed antenatal salicylate usage in 964 primigravid patients, 98 of whom had no history of ASA or other drug use and 48 of whom had ingested ASA or salicylate-containing medication at least once every two weeks throughout gestation (255). The prevalence of sustained elevations in diastolic blood pressure (>20 mm Hg) was 16% in controls compared with 4% in the salicylate group. Since that initial report, there have been several small prospective trials that have suggested that ASA is beneficial. In 1993, Decker and Sibai reviewed the published trials (256) and found that ASA was effective in reducing the incidence of pregnancy-induced hypertension, PE, and fetal growth retardation (257–262). Several large prospective studies have subsequently been performed. Over 27,000 patients have now been studied, and the results of all these studies, except one, do not prove that ASA lowers the incidence of PE (Table 13-7) (263). Routine prophylactic administration of low-dose ASA for either low-risk or high-risk patients cannot be supported at this time. The one study that found that low-dose ASA was effective in lowering the incidence of PE was performed at a single center, and compliance was recorded and assessed by serum TxB_2 levels (264).

Calcium Supplementation

Interest in calcium supplementation has arisen principally as the result of a few noteworthy observations. Populations with a low calcium intake have a high incidence

TABLE 13-7. *Randomized trials of low-dose aspirin to prevent preeclampsia*

Study (ref.)	Risk factors	Enrollment gestational age (wk)	No. of patients		Preeclampsia (%)	
			Aspirin	Placebo	Aspirin	Placebo
Hauth et al. (264)	Nulliparas	24	302	302	1.7	5.6[a]
Sibai et al. (270)	Nulliparas	13$_2$6	1,485	1,500	4.6	6.3
Italian study (271)	Obstetrical history	16–32	565	477[b]	2.9	2.7
CLASP (272)	Obstetrical history	12–32	4,659	4,650	6.7	7.6
ECPPA (273)	Obstetrical history	12–32	476	494	6.7	6.1
Golding (274)	Nulliparas	12–32	3,022	3,024	7.1	6.3
Caritis et al. (275)	High risk	13–26	1,254	1,249	18.4	20.3
BLASP (276)	None	12–32	1,819	1,822	2.2	2.5

[a]No treatment.
[b]$p = 0.009$.
From Mattar F, Sibai BM. Prevention of preeclampsia. *Semin Perinatol* 1999;23(1):58–64.

of PE, while populations with a high calcium intake have a low incidence of PE (265). In addition, patients with PE were noted to be hypocaliuruc before and when the diagnosis of PE was made (266,267). The rationale for linking calcium metabolism to PE is that a low dietary intake of calcium might result in parathyroid hormone release or renin release, causing increased renal calcium resorption. Calcium is then driven into vascular smooth-muscle cells, increasing vascular tone (268). Several prospective randomized, double-blind, placebo-controlled trials have been performed, with different conclusions. Four studies have shown favorable effects with calcium supplementation, but these studies are limited by either an abnormally high incidence of PE or a small sample size. Levine and associates reported the largest study to date (nearly 2,300 patients in each of two arms, calcium supplementation or placebo) and did not find any significant reductions in the incidence of PE (269). Thus far, routine calcium supplementation cannot be recommended solely for the purpose of reducing the risk of PE.

REFERENCES

1. Friedman EA, Neff RK. Pregnancy hypertension: a systematic evaluation of clinical diagnostic criteria. Littleton, Mass.: PSG, 1977.
2. Robert JM, Redman CW. Pre-eclampsia: more than pregnancy-induced hypertension. Lancet 1993;341:1447–1451.
3. Rochat RW, Koonin LM, Atrash HK, Jewet JF. The Maternal Mortality Collaborative. Maternal mortality in the United States: report from the Maternal Mortality Collaborative. Obstet Gynecol 1988;72: 91–97.
4. Sibai BM. Pitfalls in diagnosis and management of pre-eclampsia. Am J Obstet Gynecol 1988;159:1–5.
5. Davey DA, MacGillivray I. The classification and definition of the hypertensive disorders of pregnancy. Am J Obstet Gynecol 1988;158: 892–898.
6. Goodlin RC. Severe pre-eclampsia: another great imitator. Am J Obstet Gynecol 1976;125:747–753.
7. Consensus Report. National High Blood Pressure Education Program Working Group report on high blood pressure in pregnancy. Am J Obstet Gynecol 1990;163:1689–1712.
8. Pritchard JA, MacDonald PC, Gant NF. Williams obstetrics, 17th ed. Norwalk, Conn.: Appleton-Century-Crofts, 1985.
9. Assali NS, Rauramo L, Peltonen T. Measurement of uterine blood flow and uterine metabolism. VIII. Uterine and fetal blood flow and oxygen consumption in early pregnancy. Am J Obstet Gynecol 1960; 79:86–98.
10. Browne JCM, Veall N. The maternal placental blood flow in normotensive and hypertensive women. J Obstet Gynaecol Br Emp 1953; 60:141–147.
11. Metcalfe J, Romney SL, Ramsey LH, et al. Estimation of uterine blood flow in normal human pregnancy at term. J Clin Invest 1955;34: 1632–1638.
12. Brosens I, Dixon HG. The anatomy of the maternal side of the placenta. Br J Obstet Gynaecol 1963;73:357–372.
13. DeWolf F, DeWolf-Peeters C, Brosens I. Ultrastructure of the spiral arteries in the human placental bed at the end of normal pregnancy. Am J Obstet Gynecol 1973;117:833.
14. Robertson WB, Khong TY, Brosens I, DeWolf F, Sheppard BL, Bonnar J. The placental bed biopsy: review from three European centers. Am J Obstet Gynecol 1986;155:401–412.
15. Brosens I, Robertson WB, Dixon HG. The physiological response of the vessels of the placental bed to normal pregnancy. J Pathol Bacteriol 1967;93:569–579.
16. Pijnenborg R, Dixon G, Robertson WB, Brosens I. Trophoblastic invasion of the human decidua from 8 to 18 weeks of pregnancy. Placenta 1980;1:3–19.
17. Pijnenborg R, Bland JM, Robertson WB, Dixon G, Brosens I. The pattern of interstitial trophoblastic invasion of the myometrium in early human pregnancy. Placenta 1981;2:303–316.
18. Pijnenborg R, Bland JM, Robertson WB, Brosens I. Uteroplacental arterial changes related to interstitial trophoblast migration in early pregnancy. Placenta 1983;4:397–413.
19. Orsini MW. Trophoblastic giant cell and endovascular cells associated with pregnancy in the hamster (*Cricetus auratus*). Am J Anat 1954;94: 273.
20. Robertson WB, Brosens I, Dixon G. Uteroplacental vascular pathology. Eur J Obstet Gynecol Reprod Biol 1975;5:47–65.
21. Pijnenborg R, Robertson WB, Brosens I, Dixon G. Review article: trophoblast invasion and the establishment of haemochorial placentation in man and laboratory animals. Placenta 1981;2:71–91.
22. Sheppard BL, Bonnar J. The ultrastructure of the arterial supply of the human placenta in early and late pregnancy. J Obstet Gynaecol Br Commonw 1974;81:497–511.
23. DeWolf F, Robertson WB, Brosens I. The ultrastructure of acute atherosis in hypertensive pregnancy. Am J Obstet Gynecol 1975;123: 164–174.
24. Robertson WB, Brosens I, Dixon HG. The pathological response of the vessels of the placental bed to hypertensive pregnancy. J Pathol Bacteriol 1967;93:581–592.
25. Sheppard BL, Bonnar J. The ultrastructure of the arterial supply of the human placenta in pregnancy complicated by fetal growth retardation. Br J Obstet Gynaecol 1976;83:948–959.
26. Brosens I, Dixon HG, Robertson WB. Fetal growth retardation and the arteries of the placental bed. Br J Obstet Gynaecol 1977;84:656–663.
27. DeWolf F, Brosens I, Renaer M. Fetal growth retardation and the maternal arterial supply of the human placenta in the absence of sustained hypertension. Br J Obstet Gynaecol 1980;87:678–685.
28. Hertig AT. Vascular pathology in the hypertensive albuminuric toxaemias of pregnancy. Clinics 1945;4:602.
29. Zeek PM, Assali NS. Vascular changes in the decidua associated with eclamptogenic toxemia of pregnancy. Am J Clin Pathol 1950;20:1099.
30. Levin M, Stroobant P, Walters M, Cheng DJ, Waterfield MD, Barratt M. Platelet-derived growth factors as possible mediators of vascular proliferation in the sporadic haemolytic uraemic syndrome. Lancet 1986;2:830–833.
31. Anunciado AN, Stubbs TM, Pepkowitz SH, Lazarchick J, Miller CM 3d, Pilia P. Altered villus vessel fibronectin in preeclampsia. Am J Obstet Gynecol 1987;156:898–900.
32. Abramowsky CR, Vegas ME, Swinehart G, Gyves MT. Decidual vasculopathy of the placenta in lupus erythematosus. N Engl J Med 1980; 303:668–672.
33. Kitzmiller JL, Watt N, Driscoll SG. Decidual arteriopathy in hypertension and diabetes in pregnancy: immunofluorescent studies. Am J Obstet Gynecol 1981;141:773–779.
34. Damsky CH, Fitzgerald ML, Fisher SJ. Distribution patterns of extracellular matrix components and adhesion receptors are intricately modulated during first trimester cytotrophoblast differentiation along the invasive pathway, *in vivo*. J Clin Invest 1992;89:210–222.
35. Zhou Y, Damsky CH, Chiu K, Roberts JM, Fisher SJ. Preeclampsia is associated with abnormal expression of adhesion molecules by invasive cytotrophoblasts. J Clin Invest 1993;91:950–960.
36. Khong TY, Sawyer H, Heryet AR. An immunohistologic study of the endothelialization of uteroplacental vessels in human pregnancy: evidence that endothelium is focally disrupted by trophoblast in preeclampsia. Am J Obstet Gynecol 1992;167:751–756.
37. Paidas MJ, Schwartzman H, Taylor RN, Alvarez MA, Lockwood CJ. Third trimester fetal fibronectin (FNN) levels are associated with the development of pre-eclampsia (PE). Presented at the forty-first annual meeting of the Society for Gynecologic Investigation, Chicago, Illinois, March 22–25, 1994.
38. Pritchard JA, Cunningham FG, Mason RA. Coagulation changes in eclampsia: their frequency and pathogenesis. Am J Obstet Gynecol 1976;124:855–864.
39. Bonnar J, McNichol GP, Douglas AS. Coagulation and fibrinolytic systems in pre-eclampsia and eclampsia. Br Med 1971;2(752):12–16.
40. Howie PW, Prentice CRM, McNichol GP. Coagulation, fibrinolysis and platelet function in pre-eclampsia, essential hypertension and placental insufficiency. J Obstet Gynaecol Br Commonw 1971;78: 992–1003.
41. Davidson EC Jr, Phillips LL. Coagulation studies in the hypertensive toxemias of pregnancy. Am J Obstet Gynecol 1972;113:905–910.

42. Condie RG, Ogston D. Sequential studies on components of the haemostatic mechanism in pregnancy with particular reference to the development of preeclampsia. Br J Obstet Gynaecol 1976;83: 938–942.
43. Kitzmiller JL, Lang JE, Yelenosky PF, Lucas WE. Hematologic assays in preeclampsia. Am J Obstet Gynecol 1974;118:362–367.
44. The Birmingham Eclampsia Study Group. Intravascular coagulation and abnormal lung-scans in pre-eclampsia and eclampsia. Lancet 1971;2:889–891.
45. Dunlop W, Hill LM, Landon MJ, Oxley A, Jones P. Clinical relevance of coagulation and renal changes in preeclampsia. Lancet 1978;2: 346–349.
46. Romero R, Rickles FR, Matthews E, Scott D, Dinan C, Duffy T. Fibrinopeptide A during normal pregnancy. Am J Perinatol 1988;5: 70–73.
47. Douglas J, Shah M, Lowe GDO, Prentice CRM. Fibrinopeptide A and beta-thromboglobulin levels in preeclampsia and hypertensive pregnancy. Thromb Haemost 1981;46:8(abst).
48. Nossel HL, Yudelman I, Canfield RE, et al. Measurement of fibrinopeptide A in human blood. J Clin Invest 1974;54:43–53.
49. Reference 49 deleted in text.
50. de Boer K, ten Cate JW, Sturk A, Borm JJJ, Treffers PE. Enhanced thrombin generation in normal and hypertensive pregnancy. Am J Obstet Gynecol 1989;160:95–100.
51. Romero R, Mazor M, Lockwood C, et al. Observations on the frequency, natural history and clinical significance of thrombocytopenia in pregnancy induced hypertension. Am J Perinatol 1989;6:32–38.
52. Hutt R, Ogunniyi SO, Sullivan MHF, Elder MG. Increased platelet volume and aggregation precede the onset of preeclampsia. Obstet Gynecol 1994;83:146–149.
53. Walker JJ, Cameron AD, Bjornsson S, Singer CR, Fraser C. Can platelet volume predict progressive hypertensive disease in pregnancy? Am J Obstet Gynecol 1989;161:676–679.
54. Nicolini U, Guarneri D, Gianotti GA, Campagnoli C, Crosignami PG, Gatti L. Maternal and fetal platelet activation in normal pregnancy. Obstet Gynecol 1994;83:65–69.
55. Janes SL, Goodall AH. Flow cytometric detection of circulating activating platelets and platelet hyper-responsiveness in pre-eclampsia and pregnancy. Clin Sci 1994;86:731–739.
56. Konijnenberg A, van der Post JA, Mol BW, et al. Can flow cytometric detection of platelet activation early in pregnancy predict the occurrence of preeclampsia? A prospective study. Am J Obstet Gynecol 1997;177:434–442.
57. Konijnenberg A, Stokkers EW, van der Post JA, et al. Extensive platelet activation in preeclampsia compared with normal pregnancy: enhanced expression of cell adhesion molecules. Am J Obstet Gynecol 1997;176:461–469.
58. Paidas MJ, Byrne AMC, Lockwood CJ, et al. Increased surface expression of activation dependent platelet glycoproteins occurs in preeclampsia. Presented at the Tenth World Congress of the International Society for the Study of Hypertension in Pregnancy Seattle, Washington, August 4–8, 1996 (abst 092).
59. Paidas MJ, Dijstra K, Salafia CM, et al. Elevated levels of plasma P-selectin are found in women destined to develop preeclampsia (PE) J Soc Gynecol Invest 1998;5[Supp](abst 381).
60. Lees C, Langford E, Brown AS, et al. The effects of *S*-nitrosoglutathine on platelet activation, hypertension, and uterine and fetal Doppler in severe preeclampsia. Obstet Gynecol 1996;88:14–19.
61. Hardy E, Rubin PC, Horn EH. Effects of nitric oxide donors in vitro on the arachidonic acid–induced platelet release reaction and platelet cyclic GMP concentration in pre-eclampsia. Clin Sci 1994;85: 195–202.
62. Paidas MJ, Byrne AMC, Lockwood CJ, et al. Guanine nucleotide binding protein (G-protein) mediated platelet inhibition in preeclampsia. Am J Obstet Gynecol 1997;176:S103(abst 337).
63. Giles C, Inglis TC. Thrombocytopenia and macrothrombocytosis in gestational hypertension. Br J Obstet Gynaecol 1981;88:1115–1119.
64. Stubbs TM, Lazarchick J, Van Dorsten JP. Evidence of accelerated platelet production and consumption in nonthrombocytopenic preeclampsia. Am J Obstet Gynecol 1986;155:263–265.
65. Rakoczi I, Tallian F, Bagdany S, Gati I. Platelet life-span in normal pregnancy and pre-eclampsia as determined by a non-radioisotope technique. Thromb Res 1979;15.
66. Kelton JG, Hunter DJS, Neame PB. A platelet function defect in preeclampsia. Obstet Gynecol 1985;65:107.
67. Kaplan KL, Owen J. Plasma levels of beta-thromboglobulin and platelet factor 4 as indices of platelet activation in vivo. Blood 1981; 57:199.
68. Redman CWG, Allington MJ, Bolton FG, Stirrat GM. Plasma beta-thromboglobulin in pre-eclampsia. Lancet 1977;2:248.
69. Leiberman JR, Aharon M, Schuster M, Plotnick-Schtadler T, Nathan I, Dvilansky A. Beta-thrombo-globulin in preeclampsia. Acta Obstet Gynecol Scand 1985;64:407–409.
70. Benedetto C, Massobrio M, Bertini E, Abbondanza M, Enrieu N, Tetta C. Reduced serum inhibition of platelet-activating factor activity in preeclampsia. Am J Obstet Gynecol 1989;160:100–104.
71. Symonds EM. The renin–angiotensin system in pregnancy. Obstet Gynecol Ann 1981;10:45.
72. Talledo OE. Renin and angiotensin system in normal and toxemic pregnancy. I. Angiotensin infusion test. Am J Obstet Gynecol 1966; 96:141–143.
73. Gant NF, Daley GL, Chand S, Whalley PJ, MacDonald PC. A study of angiotensin II pressor response throughout primigravid pregnancy. J Clin Invest 1973;52:2682–2689.
74. Everett RB, Worley RJ, MacDonald PC, Gant NF. Effect of prostaglandin synthetase inhibitors on pressor response to angiotensin II in human pregnancy. J Clin Endocrinol Metab 1978;46:1007–1010.
75. Worley RJ, Gant NF, Everett RB, MacDonald PC. Vascular responsiveness to pressor agents during human pregnancy. J Reprod Med 1979;23:115–128.
76. Broughton PF, Hunter JC, Turner SR, et al. Prostaglandin E2 attenuates the pressor response to angiotensin II in pregnant subjects but not in nonpregnant subjects. Am J Obstet Gynecol 1982;142:168–176.
77. Dusting GJ, Moncada S, Vane JR. Prostacyclin: its biosynthesis, actions, and clinical potential. Adv Prostaglandin Thromboxane Leukot Res 1982;10:59–106.
78. Moncada S, Gryglewki R, Bunting S, Vane JR. An enzyme isolated from arteries transforms prostaglandin endoperoxides to an unstable substance that inhibits platelet aggregation. Nature 1976;263: 663–665.
79. Wynalda M, Fitzpatrick F. Albumin stabilizes prostaglandin I-2. Prostaglandins 1980;20:853.
80. Blair IA, Barrow SE, Wadell KA, Branch RA. Prostacyclin is not a circulating hormone in man. Prostaglandins 1982;23:579–580.
81. Goodman RP, Killam AP, Brash AR, Branch RA. Prostacyclin production during pregnancy: comparison of production during normal pregnancy and pregnancy complicated by hypertension. Am J Obstet Gynecol 1982;142:817–822.
82. Walsh SW, Behr MJ, Allen NH. Placental prostacyclin production in normal and toxemic pregnancies. Am J Obstet Gynecol 1985;151: 110–115.
83. Makila UM, Jouppila P, Kirkinen P, Viinikka L, Ylikorkala O. Placental thromboxane and prostacyclin in the regulation of placental blood flow. Obstet Gynecol 1986;68:537–540.
84. FitzGerald GA, Brash AR, Falardeau P, Oates JA. Estimated rate of prostacyclin secretion into the circulation in normal man. J Clin Invest 1981;68:1272–1275.
85. Remuzzi G, Marchesi D, Mecca G, et al. Reduction of fetal vascular prostacyclin activity in preeclampsia. Lancet 1980;2:310.
86. Makila UM, Viinikka L, Ylikorkala O. Evidence that prostacyclin deficiency is a specific feature in preeclampsia. Am J Obstet Gynecol 1984;148:772–774.
87. Bussolino F, Benedetto C, Massobrio M, Camussi G. Maternal vascular prostacyclin activity in preeclampsia. Lancet 1980;2:702.
88. Dadak C, Kefalides A, Sinzinger H, Weber G. Reduced umbilical artery prostacyclin formation in complicated pregnancies. Am J Obstet Gynecol 1982;144:792–795.
89. Carreras LO, Defreyn G, van Houtte E, et al. Prostacyclin and pre-eclampsia. Lancet 1981;1:442.
90. Downing I, Shepherd GL, Lewis PJ. Reduced prostacyclin production in pre-eclampsia. Lancet 1980;2(8208–8209):1374.
91. Stuart MJ, Clark DA, Sunderji SG, et al. Decreased prostacyclin production: a characteristic of chronic placental insufficiency syndromes. Lancet 1981;1:1126–1128.
92. Granstrom E, Diczfalusy U, Hamberg M, et al. In: Oates J, ed. Prostaglandins and the cardiovascular system. New York: Raven Press, 1982:15.
93. Walsh SW. Preeclampsia: an imbalance in placental prostacyclin and thromboxane production. Am J Obstet Gynecol 1985;152:335–340.
94. Pierucci A, Simonetti BM, Pecci G, et al. Improvement of renal func-

tion with selective thromboxane antagonism in lupus nephritis. New Engl J Med 1989;320:421–425.
95. Easterling TR, Benedetti TJ, Schmucker BC. Maternal cardiac output in preeclamptic pregnancies: a longitudinal study. Presented at the Ninth Annual Meeting of the Society of Perinatal Obstetricians, New Orleans, February 1–4, 1989 (abst 2).
96. Vanhoutte PM. The endothelium: modulator of vascular smooth-muscle tone [Editorial]. New Engl J Med 1988;319:512–513.
97. Thornton CA, Bonnar J. Factor VIII-related antigen and factor VI coagulant activity in normal and pre-eclamptic pregnancy. Br J Obstet Gynaecol 1977;84:919–923.
98. Fournie A, Monrozies M, Pontonnier G, Boneu B, Bierme R. Factor VIII complex in normal pregnancy pre-eclampsia and fetal growth retardation. Br J Obstet Gynaecol 1981;88:250–254.
99. Redman CW, Denson KW, Beilin LJ, Bolton FG, Stirrat GM. Factor-VIII consumption in pre-eclampsia. Lancet 1977;2:1249–1252.
100. Stemerman MB, Colton C, Morell E. Perturbations of the endothelium. Prog Hemost Thromb 1984;7:289–324.
101. de Boer K, Lecander I, ten Cate JW, Born JJJ, Treffers PE. Placental-type plasminogen activator inhibitor in preeclampsia. Am J Obstet Gynecol 1988;158:518–522.
102. Estelles A, Gilabert J, Aznar J, Loskutoff DJ, Schleef RR. Changes in the plasma levels of type 1 and type 2 plasminogen activator inhibitors in normal pregnancy and in patients with severe preeclampsia. Blood 1989;74(4):1332–1338.
103. Gilabert J, Estelles A, Ridocci F, Espana F, Aznar J, Galbis M. Clinical and haemostatic parameters in the HELLP syndrome: relevance of plasminogen activator inhibitors. Gynecol Obstet Invest 1990;30:81–86.
104. Reith A, Booth NA, Moore NR, Cruickshank DJ, Aberdeen UK. Plasminogen activator inhibitors (PAI-1 and PAI_2) in normal pregnancies, preeclampsia and hydatidiform mole. Br J Obstet Gynaecol 1993;100: 370–374.
105. Koh SCL, Anadakumar C, Montan S, Ratnam SS. Plasminogen activators, plasminogen activator inhibitors and markers of intravascular coagulation in preeclampsia. Gynecol Obstet Invest 1993;35: 214–221.
106. Lindoff C, Astedt B. Plasminogen activator of urokinase type and its inhibitor of placental type in hypertensive pregnancies and in intrauterine growth retardation: possible markers of placental function. Am J Obstet Gynecol 1994;171:60–64.
107. Halligan A, Bonnar J, Sheppard B, Darling M, Walshe J. Haemostatic, fibrinolytic, and endothelial variables in normal pregnancies and preeclampsia. Br J Obstet Gynecol 1994;101:488–492.
108. Chmielewska J, Ranby M, Wiman B. Evidence for a rapid inhibitor to tissue plasminogen activator in plasma. Thromb Res 1983;31: 427–436.
109. Wiman B, Csemiczky G, Marsk L, Robbe H. The fast inhibitor of tissue plasminogen activator in plasma during pregnancy. Thromb Haemost 1984;52:124–126.
110. Declerk PJ, Alessi MC, Verstrekn M, Kruithof EKO, Juhan-Vague I, Collen D. Measurements of plasminogen activator inhibitor 1 in biologic fluids with aneurine monoclonal antibody–based enzyme linked immunosorbent assay. Blood 1988;71(1):220–225.
111. Aznar J, Gilabert J, Estelles A, Espana F. Fibrinolytic activity and protein C in preeclampsia. Thromb Haemost 1986;55(3):314–317.
112. Estelles A, Gilabert J, Grancha S, et al. Abnormal expression of type 1 plasminogen activator inhibitor and tissue factor in severe preeclampsia. Thromb Haemost 1998;79:500–508.
113. Gilabert J, Estelles A, Aznar J, et al. Contribution of platelets to increased plasminogen activator inhibitor type 1 in severe preeclampsia. Thromb Haemost 1990;63(3):361–366.
114. Cadroy Y, Grandjean H, Pichon J, et al. Evaluation of six markers of haemostatic system in normal pregnancy and pregnancy complicated by hypertension or preeclampsia. Br J Obstet Gynecol 1993;100:416–420.
115. Friedman SA, Schiff E, Emeis JJ, Dekker GA, Sibai BM. Biochemical corroboration of endothelial involvement in severe preeclampsia. Am J Obstet Gynecol 1995;172:202–203.
116. Caron C, Goudemand J, Marey A, Beague D, Ducroux G, Drouvin A. Are haemostatic and fibrinolytic parameters predictors of preeclampsia in pregnancy associated hypertension? Thromb Haemost 1991;66(4):410–414.
117. Paidas MJ, Taylor RN, Schwartzman H, Saleh AA, Alvarez M, Lockwood CJ. Third trimester type 1 and type 2 plasminogen activator inhibitor (PAI 1, PAI 2) levels are associated with preeclampsia. Presented at the forty-first annual meeting of the Society of Gynecologic Investigation, Chicago, Illinois, March 22–25, 1994 (abst 0148).
118. Rodgers GM, Taylor RN, Roberts JM. Preeclampsia is associated with a serum factor cytotoxic to human endothelial cells. Am J Obstet Gynecol 1988;159:908–914.
119. Stoffel M, Morgan MA, Silavin S. The preeclampsia-associated endothelial cytotoxic factor. Presented at the Tenth Annual Meeting of the Society of Perinatal Obstetricians, Houston, Texas, January 1990 (abst 263.119).
120. Taylor RN, Casal DC, Jones LA, Varma M, Martin JN Jr, Roberts JM. Selective effects of preeclamptic sera on human endothelial cell procoagulant protein expression. Am J Obstet Gynecol 1991;165: 1705–1710.
121. Roberts JM, Taylor RN, Musci TJ, Rodgers GM, Hubel CA, McLaughlin MK. Preeclampsia: an endothelial cell disorder. Am J Obstet Gynecol 1989;161:1200–1204.
122. Puffer HW, Cheek SE, Oakes GK, et al. Vasoactive effect of sera from preeclamptic patients. Am J Obstet Gynecol 1982;142:468–470.
123. Schwartz ML. Possible role for exchange plasmapheresis with fresh frozen plasma for maternal indications in selected cases of preeclampsia and eclampsia. Obstet Gynecol 1986;68(1):136–139.
124. Schwartz ML, Brenner W. Severe preeclampsia with persistent postpartum hemolysis and thrombocytopenia treated by plasmapheresis. Obstet Gynecol 1985;65:53s–55s.
125. Lockwood CJ, Peters JH. Increased plasma levels of ED1 + cellular fibronectin precede the clinical signs of preeclampsia. Am J Obstet Gynecol 1990;162:358–362.
126. Vartio T, Laitinen L, Narvanen O, et al. Differential expression of the ED sequence–containing form of cellular fibronectin in embryonic and adult human tissues. J Cell Sci 1987;88:419–430.
127. Peters JH, Ginsberg MH, Case CM, Cochrane CH. Release of soluble fibronectin containing an extra type III domain (ED1) during acute pulmonary injury mediated by oxidants or leukocytes in vivo. Am Rev Respir Dis 1988;138(1):167–174.
128. Peters JH, Ginsberg MH, Bohl BP, Sklar LA, Cochrane CG. Intravascular release of intact cellular fibronectin during oxidant-induced injury of the in vitro perfused rabbit lung. J Clin Invest 1986;78: 1596–1603.
129. Peters JH, Maunder R, Woolf A, Cochrane CG, Ginsberg MH. Increased plasma levels of ED1+ ("cellular") fibronectin in patients with vascular injury. J Lab Clin Med 1989;113:586–597.
130. Friedman SA, de Groot CJM, Taylor RN, Roberts JM. Circulating concentrations of fetal fibronectin do not reflect reduced trophoblastic invasion in preeclamptic pregnancies. Am J Obstet Gynecol 1992; 167:496–497.
131. Gant NF, Worley RJ. Hypertension in pregnancy: concepts and management. New York: Appleton-Century-Crofts, 1980:1.
132. Page EW, Christianson R. Influence of blood pressure changes with and without proteinuria upon outcome of pregnancy. Am J Obstet Gynecol 1976;126:821–833.
133. Page EW, Christianson R. The impact of mean arterial pressure in the middle trimester upon the outcome of pregnancy. Am J Obstet Gynecol 1976;125:740–746.
134. Hypertension in pregnancy. The American College of Obstetricians and Gynecologists Technical Bulletin January 1996, no. 219.
135. Lopez-Llera M, Hernandez-Horta JLH. Perinatal mortality in eclampsia. J Reprod Med 1972;8:281–287.
136. Spargo BH, McCartney CP, Winemiller R. Glomerular capillary endotheliosis in toxemia of pregnancy. AMA Arch Pathol 1959;68: 593.
137. MacGillivray I. Some observations in the incidence of pre-eclampsia. J Obstet Gynaecol Br Commonw 1958;65:536.
138. Redman CWG, Beilin LJ, Bonnar J, Wilkinson RH. Plasma urate measurements in predicting fetal death in hypertensive pregnancy. Lancet 1976;1:1370–1373.
139. Naidoo DV, Moodley J. A survey of hypertension in pregnancy at the King Edward VIII Hospital, Durban. S Afr Med J 1980;58:556–559.
140. Chesley LC. Hypertensive disorders in pregnancy. New York: Appleton-Century-Crofts, 1978.
141. Sibai BM, Taslimi MM, El-Nazer A, Amon E, Mabie BC, Ryan GM. Maternal-perinatal outcome associated with the syndrome of hemolysis, elevated liver enzymes, and low platelets in severe preeclampsia–eclampsia. Am J Obstet Gynecol 1986;155:501–509.
142. Minakami H, Oka N, Sato T, Tamada T, Yasuda Y, Hirota N.

Preeclampsia: a microvesicular fat disease of the liver? Am J Obstet Gynecol 1988;159:1043–1047.
143. Sheehan HL, Lynch JB. Pathology of toxemia in pregnancy. London: Churchill Livingstone, 1973.
144. DeVore GR, Bracken M, Berkowitz RL. The amylase/creatinine clearance ratio in normal pregnancy and pregnancies complicated by pancreatitis, hyperemesis gravidarum and toxemia. Am J Obstet Gynecol 1980;136:747–754.
145. Sibai BM, Abdella TN, Spinnato JA, Anderson GD. Eclampsia. V. The incidence of non-preventable eclampsia. Am J Obstet Gynecol 1986; 154:581–590.
146. Sibai BM, Spinnato JA, Watson DL, Lewis JA, Anderson GD, Eclampsia. IV. Neurological findings and future outcome. Am J Obstet Gynecol 1985;152:184–192.
147. Sibai BM, Lipshitz J, Anderson GD, Dilts PV Jr. Reassessment of intravenous MgSO4 therapy in preeclampsia–eclampsia. Obstet Gynecol 1981;57:199–202.
148. Pollak VE, Nettles JB. The kidney in toxemia of pregnancy: a clinical and pathologic study based on renal biopsies. Medicine 1960;39:469.
149. Nguyen HN, Clark SL, Greenspoon J, Diesfield R, Wu PY. Peripartum colloid osmotic pressure: correlation with serum proteins. Obstet Gynecol 1986;68:807–810.
150. Benedetti TJ, Carlson RW. Studies of colloid osmotic pressure in pregnancy-induced hypertension. Am J Obstet Gynecol 1979;135: 308–311.
151. Cotton DB, Gonik B, Dorman K, Harrist R. Cardiovascular alteration in severe pregnancy-induced hypertension: relationship of central venous pressure to pulmonary capillary wedge pressure. Am J Obstet Gynecol 1985;151:762–764.
152. Benedetti TJ, Kates R, Williams V. Hemodynamic observations in severe preeclampsia complicated by pulmonary edema. Am J Obstet Gynecol 1985;152:330–334.
153. Coonrad DV, Hickok DE, Zhu K, Easterling TR, Daling J. Risk factors for preeclampsia in twin pregnancies: a population based cohort study. Obstet Gynecol 1995;85;645–650.
154. Hardardottir H, Kelly K, Bork MD, Cusick W, Campbell WA, Rodis JF. Atypical presentation of preeclampsia in high-order multifetal gestations. Obstet Gynecol 1996;87:370–374.
155. Kupferminc MJ, Eldor A, Steinman N, et al. Increased frequency of genetic thrombophilia in women with complications of pregnancy. N Engl J Med 1999;340:9–13.
156. Dekker GA, de Vries JIP, Doelitzsch PM, et al. Underlying disorders associated with severe early-onset preeclampsia. Am J Obstet Gynecol 1995;173:1042–1048.
157. Chesley LC. Hypertension in pregnancy: definitions, familial factor, and remote prognosis. Kidney Int 1980;18:234.
158. Sibai BM, el-Nazer A, Gonzalez-Ruiz A. Severe preeclampsia–eclampsia in young primigravid women: subsequent pregnancy outcome and remote prognosis. Am J Obstet Gynecol 1986;155: 1011–1016.
159. Sullivan CA, Magann EF, Perry KG Jr, Roberts WE, Blake PG, Martin JN Jr. The recurrence risk of the syndrome of hemolysis, elevated liver enzymes and low platelets (HELLP) in subsequent gestations. Am J Obstet Gynecol 1994;171:940–943.
160. Sibai BM, Ramadan MK, Chari RS, Friedman SA. Pregnancies complicated by HELLP syndrome (hemolysis, elevated liver enzymes, low platelets) and long term prognosis. Am J Obstet Gynecol 1995;172: 125–129.
161. Chesley C, Annitto JE, Cosgrove RA. The remote prognosis of eclamptic women: sixth periodic report. Am J Obstet Gynecol 1976; 124:446–459.
162. Chesley LC. Hypertensive disorders in pregnancy. New York: Appleton-Century-Crofts, 1978:1–574.
163. Sibai BM, Mercer B, Sarinoglu C. Severe preeclampsia in the second trimester: recurrence risk and long-term prognosis. Am J Obstet Gynecol 1991;165:1408–1412.
164. Burrows RF, Burrows EA. The feasibility of a control population for a randomized control trial of seizure prophylaxis in the hypertensive disorders of pregnancy. Am J Obstet Gynecol 1995;173: 929–935.
165. Lucas MJ, Leveno KJ, Cunningham FG. A comparison of magnesium sulfate with phenytoin for the prevention of eclampsia. N Engl J Med 1995;333:201–205.
166. Eclampsia Trial Collaborative Group. Which anticonvulsant for women with eclampsia? Evidence from the collaborative eclampsia trial. Lancet 1995;346(8969):258.
167. Clark SL, Greenspoon JS, Aldahl D, Phelan JP. Severe preeclampsia with persistent oliguria: management of hemodynamic subsets. Am J Obstet Gynecol 1986;154:490–494.
168. Rafferty TD, Berkowitz RL. Hemodynamics in patients with severe toxemia during labor and delivery. Am J Obstet Gynecol 1980;138: 263–270.
169. Cotton DB, Gonik B, Dorman KF. Cardiovascular alterations in severe pregnancy-induced hypertension with intravenously given hydralazine bolus. Surg Gynecol Obstet 1985;161:240–244.
170. Palmer RF, Lasseter KC. Drug therapy: sodium nitroprusside. N Engl J Med 1975;292:294–297.
171. Naulty J, Cefalo RC, Lewis PE. Fetal toxicity of nitroprusside in the pregnant ewe. Am J Obstet Gynecol 1981;139:708–711.
172. Ellis SC, Wheeler AS, James FM 3d, et al. Fetal and maternal effects of sodium nitroprusside used to counteract hypertension in gravid ewes. Am J Obstet Gynecol 1982;143:766–770.
173. Ring G, Krames E, Shnider SM, et al. Comparison of nitroprusside and hydralazine in hypertensive pregnant ewes. Obstet Gynecol 1977;50:598–602.
174. Lieb SM, Zugaib M, Nuwauhid B, et al. Nitroprusside-induced hemodynamic alteration in normotensive and hypertensive pregnant sheep. Am J Obstet Gynecol 1981;139:925–931.
175. Childress CH, Katz VL. Nifedipine and its indications in obstetrics and gynecology. Obstet Gynecol 1994;83:616–624.
176. Waisman GD, Mayorga LM, Camera MI, Vigndo CA, Martinotti A. Magnesium plus nifedipine: potentiation of hypotensive effect in preeclampsia? Am J Obstet Gynecol 1988;159:308–309.
177. Ben-Ami M, Giladi Y, Shalev E. The combination of magnesium sulfate and nifedipine: a case of neuromuscular blockade. Br J Obstet Gynecol 1994;101:262–263.
178. Mabie WC, Gonzalez AR, Sibai BM, Amon E. A comparative trial of labetalol and hydralazine in the acute management of severe hypertension complicating pregnancy. Obstet Gynecol 1987;70:328–333.
179. Hodgkinson R, Husain FJ, Hayashi RH. Systemic and pulmonary blood pressure during caesarian section in parturients with gestational hypertension. Can Anaesth Soc J 1980;27:389–394.
180. Sibai BM, Taslimi M, Abdella TN, Brooks TF, Spinnato JA, Anderson GD. Maternal and perinatal outcome of conservative management of severe preeclampsia in midtrimester. Am J Obstet Gynecol 1985;152: 32–37.
181. National Institutes of Health Consensus Statement 1994. February 28–March 2, 1994, 1292:1–24.
182. The American College of Obstetricians and Gynecologists Committee Opinion, October 1998, no. 210.
183. National Institutes of Health. The sixth report of the Joint National Committee on Detection, Evaluation, and Treatment of High Blood Pressure. November 1997:23–39.
184. Scott AA, Purohit DM. Neonatal renal failure: a complication of maternal antihypertensive therapy. Am J Obstet Gynecol 1989;160: 1223–1224.
185. Schubiger G, Flury G, Nussberger J. Enalapril for pregnancy-induced hypertension: acute renal failure in a neonate. Ann Intern Med 1988; 108:215–216.
186. Lindow SW, Davies N, Davey DA, Smith JA. The effect of sublingual nifedipine on uteroplacental blood flow in hypertensive pregnancy. Br J Obstet Gynaecol 1988;95:1275–1281.
187. Croall J, Sherrif S, Matthews J. Non-pregnant maternal plasma volume and fetal growth retardation. Br J Obstet Gynaecol 1978;85: 90–95.
188. Kaplan NM. Antihypertensive drugs in combination: effects of methyldopa on thiazide-induced changes in renal hemodynamics and plasma renin activity. Arch Intern Med 1975;135:660–663.
189. Koch-Weser J. Correlation of pathophysiology and pharmacotherapy in primary hypertension. Am J Cardiol 1973;32:499–510.
190. Frohlich ED. The sympathetic depressant antihypertensives. Drug Ther 1975;5:85.
191. Redman CWG, Beilin LJ, Bonnar J, Ounsted MK. Fetal outcome in trial of antihypertensive treatment in pregnancy. Lancet 1976;2:753.
192. Cockburn J, Ounsted M, Moar VA, Redman CWG. Final report of study on hypertension drug pregnancy: the effects of specific treatment on the growth and development of the children. Lancet 1982;1: 647.

193. Frishman WH. Drug therapy. Atenolol and timolol: two new systemic beta-adrenoceptor antagonists. N Engl J Med 1982;306:1456–1462.
194. Frishman WH. Beta-adrenoceptor antagonists: new drugs and new indications. N Engl J Med 1981;305:500–506.
195. Rubin PC, Butters L, Clark DM, et al. Placebo-controlled trial of atenolol in treatment of pregnancy-associated hypertension. Lancet 1983;1:431–434.
196. Nies AS, Shand DG. Hypertensive response to propranolol in a patient treated with methyldopa: a proposed mechanism. Clin Pharmacol Ther 1973;14:823–826.
197. Gladstone GR, Hordof A, Gersony WM. Propranolol administration during pregnancy: effects on the fetus. J Pediatr 1973;56:962–964.
198. Reed RL, Cheney CB, Fearon RE, Hook R, Hehre FW. Propranolol therapy throughout pregnancy: a case report. Anesth Analg (Cleve) 1974;53:214.
199. Tunstall ME. The effect of propranolol on the onset of breathing at birth. Br J Anaesth 1969;41:792.
200. Rubin PC. Current concepts: beta-blockers in pregnancy. N Engl J Med 1981;305:1323–1326.
201. Yudkin JS. Withdrawal of clonidine. Lancet 1977;1:546.
202. Johnston Cl, Aickin DR. The control of high blood pressure during labor with clonidine ("Catapres") Med J Aust 1971;2:132–135.
203. Koch-Weser J. Hydralazine. N Engl J Med 1976;295:320.
204. Gant NF, Madden MD, Siiteri PK, MacDonald PC. The metabolic clearance rate of dehydroisoandrosterone sulfate. IV. Acute effects of induced hypertension, hypotension, and naturesis in normal and hypertensive pregnancies. Am J Obstet Gynecol 1976;124:143–148.
205. Vink GJ, Moodley J, Philpott RH. Effects of hydralazine on the fetus in the treatment of maternal hypertension. Obstet Gynecol 1970;50:519–522.
206. Woods JR Jr, Brinkman CR 3d. The treatment of gestational hypertension. J Reprod Med 1975;15:195–199.
207. Mabie WC, Pernoll ML, Biswas MK. Chronic hypertension in pregnancy. Obstet Gynecol 1986;67:197–205.
208. Fidler J, Smith V, Fayers P, DeSwiet M. Randomized controlled comparative study of methyldopa and oxyprenolol in treatment of hypertension in pregnancy. Br Med J Clin Res Edu 1983;286:1927–1930.
209. Williams GH. Hypertensive vascular disease. In: Harrison's principles of internal medicine, 14th ed. 1998:1380–1394.
210. Heyborne KD, Schultz MF, Goodlin RC, Durham JD. Renal artery stenosis during pregnancy: a review. Obstet Gynecol Surv 1991;46: 509–514.
211. Hertz SM, Holland GA, Baum Rahaska ZJ, Carpenter JP. Evaluation of renal artery stenosis by magnetic resonance angiography. Am J Surg 1994;168:140–143.
212. Le TT, Haskal ZJ, Holland GA, Towsend R. Endovascular stent placement and magnetic resonance angiography for management of hypertension and renal artery occlusion during pregnancy. Obstet Gynecol 1995;85:822–825.
213. McCarron DA, Keller FS, Lundquist G, Kirk PE. Transluminal angioplasty for renovascular hypertension complicated by pregnancy. Arch Intern Med 1982;142.
214. Sellars L, Siamopoulas K, Wilkinson R. Prognosis for pregnancy after correcting renovascular hypertension. Nephron 1985;39:280–281.
215. Imbasciati E, Ponticelli C. Pregnancy and renal disease: predictors for fetal and maternal outcome. Am J Nephrol 1991;11:353–362.
216. Jones DC, Hayslett JP. Outcome of pregnancy in women with moderate or severe renal insufficiency. N Engl J Med 1996;335:226–332.
217. Katz AI, Davison JM, Hayslett JP, Singson E, Lindheimer MD. Pregnancy in women with kidney disease. Kidney Int 1980;18:192–206.
218. Jungers P, Forget D, Henry-Amar M, et al. Chronic kidney disease and pregnancy. Adv Nephrol Necker Hosp 1986;15:103–141.
219. Barcelo P, Lopez-Lillo J, Cabero L, Del Rio G. Successful pregnancy in primary glomerular disease. Kidney Int 1986;30:914–919.
220. Surian M, Imbasciati E, Cosci P, et al. Glomerular disease and pregnancy: a study of 123 pregnancies in patients with primary and secondary glomerular diseases. Nephron 1984;36:101–105.
221. Abe S, Amagasaki Y, Konishi K, Kato E, Sakaguchi H, Iyori S. The influence of antecedent renal disease on pregnancy. Am J Obstet Gynecol 1985;153:508–514.
222. Solomon CG, Thiet MP, Moore FJR, Seely EW. Primary hyperaldosteronism in pregnancy: a case report. J Reprod Med 1996;41: 255–258.
223. Webb JC, Bayliss P. Pregnancy complicated by primary hyperaldosteronism. South Med J 1997;90:243–245.
224. Baron F, Sprauve ME, Huddleston JF, Fisher AJ. Diagnosis and surgical treatment of primary aldosteronism in pregnancy: a case report. Obstet Gynecol 1995;86:644–645.
225. Elterman JJ, Hagen GA. Aldosteronism in pregnancy: associated virilization of female offspring. South Med J 1983;76.
226. Sasaki A, Shinkawa O, Yoshinaga K. Placental corticotropin releasing hormone may be a stimulator of maternal pituitary adrenocorticotropic hormone secretion in humans. J Clin Invest 1989;84: 1997–2001.
227. Ross RJM, Chew SL, Perry L, Erskine K, Medbak S, Afshar F. Diagnosis and selective cure of Cushing's disease during pregnancy by transphenoidal surgery. Eur J Endocrinol 1995;132:722–726.
228. Casson RF, Davis JC, Jeffreys RV, Silas JH, Williams J, Belchetz PE. Successful management of Cushing's disease during pregnancy by transphenoidal adenectomy. Clin Endocrinol 1987;27:423–428.
229. Mampalam TJ, Tyrrell JB, Wilson CB. Transphenoidal microsurgery for Cushing's disease. Ann Intern Med 1988;487–493.
230. Pricolo VE, Monchik JM, Prinz RA, DeJong S, Chadwick DA, Lamberton RP. Management of Cushing's syndrome secondary to adrenal adenoma during pregnancy. Surgery 1990;108:1072–1077.
231. Close CF, Mann MC, Watts JF, Taylor KG. ACTH independent Cushing's syndrome in pregnancy with spontaneous resolution after surgery: control of the hypercortisolism with metyrapone. Clin Endocrinol (Oxf) 1993;39:375–379.
232. Hadden DR. Adrenal disorders of pregnancy. Endocrinol Metab Clin North Am 1995;24:139–151.
233. Aron DC, Schanall AM, Sheeler LR. Cushing's syndrome and pregnancy. Am J Obstet Gynecol 1990;162:244–252.
234. Pickard J, Jochen AL, Sadur CN, Hofeldt FD. Cushing's syndrome in pregnancy. Obstet Gynecol Surg 1990;45:87–93.
235. Taylor HC, Tillman AJB, Blanchard. Fetal losses in hypertension and preeclampsia. Obstet Gynecol 1954;3(3):225–239.
236. Page EW, Christianson E. Influence of blood pressure changes with and without proteinuria upon outcome of pregnancy. Am J Obstet Gynecol 1976;126:821–833.
237. Ferrzzani S, Caruso A, Decarolis S, Martino IV, Mancuso S. Proteinuria and outcome of 444 pregnancies complicated by hypertension. Am J Obstet Gynecol 1990;162:366–371.
238. Lin CC, Lindheimer MD, River P, Moawad AH. Fetal outcome in hypertensive disorders of pregnancy. Am J Obstet Gynecol 1982;142:255–260.
239. McCowan LME, Buist RG, North RA, Gamble G. Perinatal morbidity in chronic hypertension. Br J Obstet Gynecol 1996;103:123–129.
240. Sibai BM, Spinnato JA, Watson DL, Hill GA, Anderson GD. Pregnancy outcome in 303 cases with severe preeclampsia. Obstet Gynecol 1984;64:319–325.
241. Sibai BM, Mercer BM, Schiff E, Friedman SA. Aggressive versus expectant management of severe preeclampsia at 28 to 32 weeks' gestation: a randomized controlled trial. Am J Obstet Gynecol 1994;171: 818–822.
242. Odendaal HJ, Pattinson RC, Bam R, Grove D, Kotze TJVW. Aggressive or expectant management for patients with severe preeclampsia between 28–34 weeks' gestation: a randomized controlled trial. Obstet Gynecol 1990;76:1070–1074.
243. Sibai BM, Taslimi MM, El-Nazer A, Amon E, Mabie BC, Ryan GM. Maternal-perinatal outcome associated with the syndrome of hemolysis, elevated liver enzymes and low platelets in severe preeclampsia–eclampsia. Am J Obstet Gynecol 1986;155:501–509.
244. Friedman SA, Schiff E, Kao L, Sibai BM. Neonatal outcome after preterm delivery for preeclampsia. Am J Obstet Gynecol 1995;172: 1785–1792.
245. Paidas MJ, Turtulici P, Winslow J, et al. Neonatal outcome of preeclamptic (PE) women delivered <34 weeks gestation. Am J Obstet Gynecol 1995;172:375(abst 416).
246. Sibai BM, Abdella TN, Anderson GD. Pregnancy outcome in 211 patients with mild chronic hypertension. Obstet Gynecol 1983;61: 571– 576.
247. Mabie WC, Pernoll ML, Biswas M. Chronic hypertension in pregnancy. Obstet Gynecol 1986;67:197–205.
248. Sibai BM, Anderson GD. Pregnancy outcome of intensive therapy in severe hypertension in first trimester. Obstet Gynecol 1986;67: 517–520.
249. Arias F, Zamora J. Antihypertensive treatment and pregnancy outcome in patients with mild chronic hypertension. Obstet Gynecol 1979; 53(4):489–494.

250. Redman CW. Fetal outcome in trial of antihypertensive treatment in pregnancy. Lancet 1976:753–756.
251. Sibai BM, Mabie WC, Shamsa F, Villar MA, Anderson GA. A comparison of no medication versus methyldopa or labetalol in chronic hypertension during pregnancy. Am J Obstet Gynecol 1990;162: 960–967.
252. Masotti G, Galanti G, Poggesi L, Abbate R, Neri Semeri GG. Differential inhibition of prostacyclin production and platelet aggregation by aspirin. Lancet 1979;2:1213–1217.
253. Spitz B, Magness RR, Cox SM, Brown CEL, Rosenfeld CR, Gant NF. Low-dose aspirin. I. Effect on angiotensin II pressor responses and blood prostaglandin concentrations in pregnant women sensitive to angiotensin II. Am J Obstet Gynecol 1988;159:1035..
254. Ylikorkala O, Makila UM, Kaapa P, Viinikka L. Maternal ingestion of acetylsalicylic acid inhibits fetal and neonatal prostacyclin and thromboxane in humans. Am J Obstet Gynecol 1986;155:345–349.
255. Crandon AJ, Isherwood DM. Effect of aspirin on incidence of preeclampsia. Lancet 1979;1:1356.
256. Dekker GA, Sibai BM. Low dose aspirin in the prevention of preeclampsia and fetal growth retardation: rationale, mechanisms, and clinical trials. Am J Obstet Gynecol 1993;168:214–227.
257. Beaufils M, Uzan S, Donsimoni R, Colau JC. Prevention of pre-eclampsia by early antiplatelet therapy. Lancet 1985;1:840–842.
258. Wallenburg HC, Dekker GA, Makovitz JW, Rotmans P. Low-dose aspirin prevents pregnancy-induced hypertension and pre-eclampsia in angiotensin-sensitive primigravidae. Lancet 1986;1:1–3.
259. Schiff E, Peleg E, Goldenberg M, et al. The use of aspirin to prevent pregnancy-induced hypertension and lower the ratio of thromboxane A-2 to prostacyclin in relatively high risk pregnancies. N Engl J Med 1989;321:351–356.
260. Benigni A, Gregorini G, Frusca T, et al. Effect of low-dose aspirin on fetal and maternal generation of thromboxane by platelets in women at risk for pregnancy-induced hypertension. N Engl J Med 1989;321: 357–362.
261. Wallenburg HCS, Rotmans N. Prevention of recurrent idiopathic fetal growth retardation by low-dose aspirin and dipyridamole. Am J Obstet Gynecol 1987;157:1230–1235.
262. Trudinger BJ, Cook CM, Thompson RS, Giles WB, Connelly A. Low-dose aspirin therapy improves fetal weight in umbilical placental insufficiency. Am J Obstet Gynecol 1988;159:681–685.
263. Mattar F, Sibai BM. Prevention of preeclampsia. Semin Perinatol 1999;23(1):58–64.
264. Hauth JC, Goldenberg RL, Parker CR Jr, et al. Low dose aspirin therapy to prevent preeclampsia. Am J Obstet Gynecol 1993;168: 1083–1093.
265. Ito M, Koyama H, Ohshige A, Maedu T, Yoshimura T, Okamura H. Prevention of preeclampsia with calcium supplementation and vitamin D3 in an antenatal protocol. Int J Gynecol Obstet 1994;47: 115–120.
266. Taufield PA, Ales KL, Resnick LM, Druzin ML, Geertner JM, Laragh JH. Hypocalciuria in preeclampsia. N Engl J Med 1987;316: 715–718.
267. Sanchez-Ramos L, Jones DC, Cullen MT. Urinary calcium as an early marker for preeclampsia. Obstet Gynecol 1991;77:685–689.
268. Belizan JM, Villar J, Repke J. The relationship between calcium intake and pregnancy induced hypertension: up to date evidence. Am J Obstet Gynecol 1988;158:898–902.
269. Levine RJ, Hauth JC, Curet LB, et al. Maternal Fetal Medicine Units Network: trial of calcium to prevent preeclampsia. N Engl J Med 1997;337:69–76.
270. Sibai BM, Caritas SN, Thom E, et al.: Prevention of preeclampsia with low-dose aspirin in healthy, nulliparous pregnant women. The National Institute of Child Health and Human Development Network of Maternal–Fetal Medicine Units. N Engl J Med 1993;329: 1213–1218.
271. Anonymous: Low-dose aspirin in prevention and treatment of intrauterine growth retardation and pregnancy-induced hypertension. Italian study of aspirin in pregnancy. Lancet 1993;341:396–400.
272. Anonymous: CLASP: a randomised trial of low-dose aspirin for the prevention and treatment of pre-eclampsia among 9364 pregnant women. CLASP (Collaborative Low-dose Aspirin Study in Pregnancy) Collaborative Group. Lancet 1994 343:619–629.
273. Anonymous: ECPPA: randomised trial of low dose aspirin for the prevention of maternal and fetal complicatons in high risk pregnant women. ECPPA (Estudo Colaborativo para Prevencao da Pre-eclampsia com Aspirina) Collaborative Group. Br J Obstet Gynaecol 1996;103:39–47.
274. Golding J.: A randomised trial of low dose aspirin for primiparae in pregnancy. The Jamaica Low Dose Aspirin Study Group. Br J Obstet Gynaecol 1998;105:293–299.
275. Caritis S, Sibai B, Hauth J, et al.: Low-dose aspirin to prevent preeclampsia in women at high risk. National Institute of Child Health and Human Development Network of Maternal–Fetal Medicine Units. N Engl J Med 1998;338:701–705.

Cherry and Merkatz's Complications of Pregnancy,
Fifth Edition, edited by W. R. Cohen.
Lippincott Williams & Wilkins, Philadelphia © 2000.

CHAPTER 14

Respiratory Disease

Alvin S. Teirstein, Gregory J. Schilero, and Marvin Lesser

ASTHMA

Definition, Clinical Manifestations, and Diagnosis

Approximately 4% of pregnancies are complicated by bronchial asthma (1). Asthma may be the most common respiratory disorder encountered among obstetric patients requiring prolonged pharmacologic management. Ideal therapy assumes importance in the pregnant woman not only because of the need to maintain optimal maternal health but also because of concern about the effects of maternal asthma on the fetus and the potential fetotoxic effects of drugs used to treat asthma. Uncontrolled asthma is associated with increased risk of perinatal mortality, premature or low-birth-weight infants, and preeclampsia (1).

Asthma is a chronic pulmonary disease characterized by airway obstruction that reverses spontaneously or with treatment, airway inflammation, and increased airway responsiveness to a variety of stimuli (1). Commonly encountered symptoms, which generally occur more often during acute or subacute exacerbations, include cough, wheeze, chest tightness, and dyspnea. Stimuli that provoke worsening of asthma include viral respiratory infections, allergens (pollens, house-dust mites, animal danders), cold air, exercise, food additives (sulfites), drugs (aspirin, nonsteroidal antiinflammatory agents, beta-blockers), irritants (tobacco smoke, ozone, sulphur dioxide), and occupational exposures (toluene diisocyanate, laboratory animals). Among younger adults there is often a family history of asthma or associated atopic conditions, including urticaria, allergic rhinitis, and atopic eczema.

The entire pathogenesis of asthma remains undefined; however, many of the pathologic and clinical features of the disease are attributed to ongoing airway inflammation, which is characterized by increased numbers of mast cells, eosinophils, neutrophils, platelets, and lymphocytes. The cells, in turn, release a variety of mediators, including histamine, leukotrienes, and platelet activating factor, which contribute to bronchial hyperresponsiveness, epithelial damage, and microvascular leakage (2). Associated contributing neural mechanisms may include enhanced cholinergic activity and amplified release of neuropeptides (substance P, neurokinin A), from C-fiber sensory nerve endings. Accumulation of excess mucus and fluid further contributes to airway narrowing and hyperresponsiveness.

A diagnosis of asthma must be considered in any patient who reports episodic wheezing or cough or shortness of breath. The diagnosis may be more difficult to establish in patients who have vague respiratory complaints such as chest tightness, nocturnal breathlessness or cough, or exertional dyspnea. Helpful diagnostic clues include a history of asthma at an earlier age, a history of allergies, a family history of asthma or allergies, and identification of precipitating factors. During exacerbations, physical examination usually reveals diffuse wheezing, hyperventilation, and prolonged duration of expiration. During more severe attacks physical findings may include hyperinflation and use of accessory respiratory muscles. Specific evidence for reversible airway disease can be obtained by pulmonary function testing with and without a bronchodilator. Methacholine or histamine challenge testing establishes the presence of airway hyperreactivity. Associated findings may include sputum and blood eosinophilia and elevated serum immunoglobulin E (IgE) levels. Generally, it is not difficult to differentiate asthma from other causes of obstructive lung diseases (i.e., chronic bronchitis, emphysema, or bronchiectasis), because these entities are encountered much less frequently among women of childbearing age, do not involve a history of allergy, and frequently are associated with cigarette smoking.

A. S. Teirstein and M. Lesser: Mt. Sinai School of Medicine, New York, NY 10029-6574.

G. J. Schilero: Department of Medicine, The Mount Sinai–NYU Medical Center, New York, NY 10029 and Division of Pulmonary and Critical Care, The Bronx Veterans Affairs Medical Center, Bronx, NY 10468.

Effect of Pregnancy

In an early study, Schaefer and Silverman reported that 93% of patients with asthma experienced no change in asthma symptoms during pregnancy (3). In a combined series of 1,087 patients detailed in the literature, Gluck and Gluck reported that during pregnancy asthma improved in 36%, worsened in 23%, and remained unchanged in 41% (4). Although for a specific patient it may be difficult to anticipate how asthma symptoms will respond during pregnancy, the status of asthma activity before pregnancy is of some predictive value. Gluck and Gluck noted that among patients who had mild asthma before pregnancy, 12% improved during pregnancy, 72% remained unchanged, and 16% worsened. Among those with severe asthma before pregnancy, none improved, 17% remained unchanged, and 83% worsened. Similarly, Williams observed that among patients with severe asthma before pregnancy, 44% experienced worsening of symptoms during gestation (5).

For patients whose asthma symptoms worsen during pregnancy, divergent data have been obtained regarding when worsening occurs. Jensen noted that nearly 50% of his patients worsened during the first four months of gestation (6). Gluck and Gluck observed, however, that worsening occurred more often during the sixth month of gestation (4). Improvement of asthma symptoms usually occurs during the first trimester and during weeks 37 to 40 (6,7). Disease activity remains generally stable during labor and delivery (7). In a study that objectively assessed the status of asthma during gestation, Sims and colleagues found that pulmonary-function test parameters did not change significantly during pregnancy (8). Juniper and colleagues performed methacholine challenge studies among 16 women preconception, during pregnancy, and postpartum and found that airway responsiveness exhibited twofold improvement during pregnancy (9). There was an associated improvement in the severity of clinical asthma as indicated by a reduction in minimum medication requirements, although both symptoms and spirometry remained unchanged. Following parturition, the status of asthma activity generally returns to the prepregnancy level or worsens (5,6). In most asthma patients, the change in disease activity associated with pregnancy is repeated during subsequent pregnancies (7). For those whose asthma worsens during pregnancy, symptoms tend to be even more severe during subsequent pregnancies (5,6).

Effect on Mother and Fetus

Data published in 1970 from the Collaborative Perinatal Project revealed a significant increase in perinatal mortality among asthmatic patients (10). There was no increase in prematurity or low-birth-weight infants. During the first year, 5.7% of the survey infants developed asthma, and 18.4% had severe respiratory diseases (seven and two times the expected frequency, respectively). Subsequently, Bahna and Bjerkedal found that patients with asthma had no increase in perinatal mortality but had increased incidences of hyperemesis gravidarum, preeclampsia, and vaginal hemorrhage (11). There was also an increase in prematurity, low birth weight, and neonatal mortality. Malformations were not increased, nor were stillbirths.

In two retrospective studies consisting of a total of 106 women with severe asthma requiring corticosteroids during pregnancy, no maternal, fetal, or neonatal deaths were observed (12,13). There was an overall increase in the incidence of premature and low-birth-weight infants, particularly among women who experienced *status asthmaticus* (12). There was no increase in toxemia, uterine hemorrhage, or congenital malformations (13). In a retrospective, case-controlled study, Perlow and associates observed that steroid-dependent asthmatic subjects had an increased incidence of gestational diabetes mellitus (14). Among all asthmatic subjects, preterm delivery, preterm premature rupture of membranes, cesarean section rate, and cesarean delivery for fetal distress increased. Neonates born to asthmatic subjects had lower birth weights and were admitted more often to the neonatal intensive care unit.

Stenius-Aarniala and colleagues performed a prospective, case-matched study that was designed to investigate whether asthma, when carefully managed, is associated with an increased risk of complications (15). Antiasthma treatment consisted of inhaled beta-2 agonists, beclomethasone, sodium cromoglycate, oral theophylline, and systemic corticosteroids as needed. They observed a higher incidence of preeclampsia and cesarean section among asthmatic subjects, particularly among those with severe asthma. Hypoglycemia occurred more often in infants of mothers with severe asthma. Compared with controls, no difference was found in length of gestation, birth weight, incidence of perinatal deaths, low Apgar scores, neonatal respiratory difficulties, hyperbilirubinaemia, or malformations. Schatz and colleagues also performed a prospective, case-matched study of women actively managed for asthma (16) and found that chronic hypertension was significantly more common in asthmatic subjects. Compared with controls matched for age, smoking status, parity, and year of delivery, no significant differences were found in the incidences of preeclampsia, perinatal mortality, preterm births, low-birth-weight infants, intrauterine growth retardation, or congenital malformations. There was a trend toward increased incidence of preeclampsia and low-birth-weight infants among women requiring emergency therapy or corticosteroids. The authors concluded that the overall perinatal prognosis for women with actively managed asthma during pregnancy is comparable to that for the nonasthmatic population.

Management

As detailed by the Working Group on Asthma and Pregnancy (1), the management of asthma during pregnancy consists of using objective measures to assess and monitor maternal lung function and fetal status, avoidance of environmental allergens and irritants, stepwise administration of pharmacological agents, and patient education.

Maternal and Fetal Monitoring

Maternal respiratory status can be measured at home by use of a portable peak flow meter (17). With daily monitoring, it is possible to detect clinical deterioration and to initiate therapy before obstruction progresses to more serious stages. Following initial training and confirmation of reliable and reproducible measurements, peak flow determinations can be performed at a frequency dictated by the severity of asthma. Following establishment of "personal best" values at times of optimum disease stability, measurements can be performed several times daily, preferably morning and evening. Findings of peak flow values 80% to 100% of personal best indicate disease stability. Findings of values 50% to 80% of personal best suggest cautious concern and possible need for more aggressive pharmacologic intervention. Values below 50% of personal best indicate a medical alert and the need for immediate therapy, with possible consultation with a physician (17).

Fetal evaluation during early gestation can be performed by sonography, which serves as a benchmark against which subsequent fetal growth can be measured. In the third trimester, electronic fetal heart rate monitoring and ultrasonic determinations of fetal behavior should be used, if needed, to ensure fetal well-being. For many third-trimester patients, weekly fetal assessment is sufficient. Intensive fetal heart rate monitoring should be performed at times of maternal asthma exacerbations, if response to therapy is incomplete or poor, or with significant maternal hypoxemia (1).

Environmental Control Measures

Avoidance of environmental irritants and allergens may decrease the need for pharmacologic therapy. Irritants to be avoided include tobacco smoke, offensive fumes and odors, dusts, and air pollutants. Allergens that may worsen asthma include those associated with warm-blooded pets, house-dust mites, indoor mold spores, and cockroaches. Animal allergens are derived from dander, feathers, urine, and saliva. High levels of house-dust mite antigens are found in mattresses, pillows, carpets, bed covers and upholstered furniture. Indoor molds are found in highest numbers in areas of increased humidity.

Pharmacologic Therapy

Pharmacologic treatment of asthma during pregnancy involves a step-care approach based on subjective and objective assessment of disease status. By use of a step-care approach, the number of medications and frequency of administration are increased until disease control and stability are achieved. Then, following sustained control, medication number and concentration are progressively lowered to maintenance levels. Specific goals of asthma therapy are to maintain normal activity levels, maintain near-normal pulmonary function, prevent chronic and troublesome symptoms, prevent recurrent exacerbations, and avoid adverse effects from asthma medications (17). Therapeutic regimens depend largely on the severity and stage of asthma, which are classified as (a) chronic mild asthma, (b) chronic moderate asthma, (c) chronic severe asthma, and, (d) acute exacerbation (1). A step-care approach to asthma management is shown in Table 14-1.

TABLE 14-1. *Recommended steps for treatment of asthma during pregnancy*

Chronic mild asthma (intermittent, brief episodes; asymptomatic between exacerbations; fewer than 2 nocturnal episodes per month)
- Inhaled beta-2 agonist (2 puffs p.r.n. t.i.d./q.i.d.)
- Pretreatment with cromolyn (2 puffs) or inhaled beta-2 agonist for exposure to exercise, allergen, or other stimuli

Chronic moderate asthma (symptoms greater than 1–2 times weekly; exacerbations affect sleep and activity level and may last several days; occasional emergency care)
- Inhaled beta-2 agonist (p.r.n. to t.i.d./q.i.d.) and
- Inhaled corticosteroid (2–4 puffs b.i.d.) or
- Cromolyn (2 puffs q.i.d.) and, if symptoms persist
- Increase inhaled corticosteroid and/or
- Sustained release theophylline

Chronic severe asthma (Continuous symptoms; limited activity levels; frequent exacerbations and nocturnal symptoms; occasional hospitalization and emergency treatment)
- Inhaled beta-2 agonist (p.r.n., q.i.d.) and
- Inhaled corticosteroid (4–6 puffs b.i.d. or 2–5 puffs q.i.d.) with or without
- Cromolyn (2 puffs q.i.d) with or without
- Sustained release theophylline with
- Episodic extra beta-2 agonist (2–4 puffs or nebulized) and
- Oral corticosteroid burst for active symptoms (40 mg a day, single or divided dose for 1 wk, then tapered)

Emergency department management
- Inhaled beta-2 agonist (up to 3 doses over 60–90 min); follow peak expiratory flow rate with therapeutic goal of >70% of baseline
- Supplemental oxygen to maintain saturation >95% and
- Systemic steroids for those not responding immediately to bronchodilator and for those already taking regular oral corticosteroids with incomplete response
- Inhaled beta-2 agonist (every 1–4 hr) and

Consider hospitalization

p.r.n., as required; t.i.d., three times a day; q.i.d., four times a day; b.i.d., twice a day.

Modified from National Asthma Education Program, National Heart, Lung, and Blood Institute, National Institutes of Health Report of the working group on asthma and pregnancy: management of asthma during pregnancy. Bethesda, MD: National Institutes of Health. NIH Publication no: 93-3279, 1993, and National Asthma Education Program Expert Panel on the Management of Asthma. Guidelines for the diagnosis and management of asthma. J Allergy Clin Immunology 1991;88(part 2):431–534.

Specific Pharmacologic Agents

Beta-2 agonists

Inhaled beta-2 agonists are the drugs of first choice for treatment of mild, moderate, or severe chronic asthma. The agents are also first choice for initial treatment of acute exacerbations of asthma. Albuterol, bitolterol, metaproterenol, pirbuterol, and salmeterol are classified as U.S. Food and Drug Administration (FDA) category C agents (risk cannot be ruled out: human studies are lacking, and animal studies are either positive for fetal risk or lacking as well; potential benefits may outweigh the potential risks) (18). Salmeterol has not been evaluated extensively in pregnant women. Terbutaline is considered a category B drug (no evidence of risk in humans: either animal findings show risk but human findings do not, or, if no adequate human studies have been done, animal findings are negative). To assess the safety of inhaled beta-2 agonists during pregnancy, Schatz et al. compared perinatal outcomes in 259 prospectively managed women with asthma using beta-2 agonists during pregnancy with 101 concurrently followed pregnant subjects with asthma not using inhaled bronchodilators and with 295 concurrently followed pregnant control subjects without asthma (19). No significant differences were found in perinatal mortality, congenital malformations, preterm births, low-birth-weight infants, mean birth weight, small for gestational age or low ponderal index infants, Apgar scores, labor and delivery complications, or postpartum bleeding. Epinephrine, which has both alpha- and beta-adrenoreceptor agonist activity, is a frequently used sympathomimetic agent for emergency treatment of acute asthma exacerbations. Concern over its safety during pregnancy arose when Heinonen et al. found in the Perinatal Collaborative Study that among 189 women exposed to the drug, a slight but significant increase in birth defects occurred (20). The Report of the Working Group on Asthma and Pregnancy concluded that the positive findings of the Perinatal Collaborative Study need to be confirmed before they can be considered sufficient evidence of epinephrine toxicity (1).

The most frequently encountered side effects of beta-2 agonists are skeletal muscle tremor and tachycardia. Although beta-2 agonists can be given by subcutaneous, intramuscular, intravenous, oral, and inhalational routes, side effects are reduced by inhalational administration. For acute exacerbations, beta-2 agonists can be given by nebulization. Terbutaline is also used as a tocolytic in women with preterm labor. Delayed labor does not occur with bronchodilators administered by metered-dose inhaler or wet nebulization (21). Major cardiopulmonary side effects include tachycardia, hypotension, arrhythmias, myocardial ischemia, and pulmonary edema (22).

Corticosteroids

Corticosteroids are the most effective antiinflammatory drugs available for the treatment of asthma. Parenteral, oral, or inhaled corticosteroid preparations often are required for maintenance of asthma stability or for treatment of significant symptoms associated with chronic moderate or severe asthma or acute exacerbations. To evaluate the safety of corticosteroids during pregnancy, Fitzsimons and colleagues (12) and Schatz and colleagues (13) assessed the outcome of 126 pregnancies in 106 women with severe asthma requiring systemic or inhaled corticosteroids. One spontaneous abortion occurred (13); there were no fetal deaths and no increase in congenital malformations. The incidence of premature deliveries and low-birth-weight infants was slightly increased (12). Similarly, data from the Perinatal Collaborative Project revealed no congenital malformations in infants from 54 women who took prednisone or hydrocortisone during pregnancy (20). Collectively, these studies indicate that corticosteroids can be used safely during pregnancy.

Fewer studies are available that report on the safety of inhaled corticosteroids during gestation. Beclomethasone, budesonide, and flunisolide are listed by the FDA as category C agents (18). Triamcinolone is listed as a category D agent (positive evidence of risk: investigational or postmarketing data show risk to the fetus; nevertheless, potential benefits may outweigh the potential risk). In a study that evaluated the usefulness of inhaled beclomethasone for treatment of asthma, Brown and colleagues found among 20 women who took the agent during pregnancy that no abortions occurred and all the infants were born normal (23). Because there has been more experience with beclomethasone, it is the preferred agent for use during pregnancy (1).

Hospital management of severe asthma exacerbations requires the use of corticosteroids administered parenterally (see Table 14-1). When disease stability is achieved, oral preparations are provided and maintained after discharge until peak expiratory flow rates are stable near personal best or predicted values (17). Patients with acute exacerbations requiring emergency department management but not hospitalization may be treated with an oral corticosteroid agent, although benefit may not be appreciated before 3 to 12 hours. For chronic maintenance, oral corticosteroid agents must be tapered to the minimum amounts necessary to control symptoms. Occasionally, patients can be tapered to alternate-day therapy, which is associated with fewer systemic side effects. If possible, all patients requiring corticosteroids should be switched to an inhaled preparation. The major problem with inhaled preparations is asymptomatic or symptomatic oropharyngeal candidiasis, which can be reduced or prevented by the use of a chamber or spacer and by rinsing the mouth with water after each use.

Cromolyn Sodium and Nedocromil Sodium

Cromolyn sodium and nedocromil sodium are nonsteroidal antiinflammatory agents that act primarily by preventing mast cell degranulation. Both agents are listed as FDA category B agents (18), although little information is available regarding the safety of nedocromil sodium during human pregnancy. These agents are only effective when used prophylactically and should not be used for treatment of acute exacerbations. They are also effective when inhaled before exercise or anticipated exposure to allergens. Side effects are minimal. Although therapeutic benefits vary, in general, cromolyn sodium and nedocromil sodium are less effective than inhaled corticosteroids. A clinical trial of 4 to 6 weeks may be needed to determine the efficacy of cromolyn sodium in individual patients. For management of chronic severe asthma, patients can be given both inhaled corticosteroid and cromolyn sodium.

Methylxanthines

Theophylline and aminophylline are the principal methylxanthines used in the treatment of asthma. Both are listed as FDA category C drugs (18). No birth defects were associated with the use of theophylline or aminophylline in the Perinatal Collaborative Project (20). Rubin and associates found no increase in congenital heart disease among infants of women who used theophylline during pregnancy (24). Theophylline as a sustained-release preparation is used as additional therapy in patients with chronic moderate and severe asthma whose disease activity is not controlled with an inhaled corticosteroid and an inhaled beta-2 agonist. Sustained-release preparations are occasionally useful for management of nocturnal asthma. Intravenous aminophylline is used as a supplemental agent for hospital management of acute exacerbations.

The therapeutic plasma concentration range for theophylline is 10 to 20 μg/mL. Toxic effects, which generally are associated with elevated serum levels, include nausea, vomiting, cardiac arrhythmias, anxiety, tremor, headache, and grand mal seizure. Because degradation and elimination kinetics vary significantly from patient to patient, theophylline blood levels must be monitored to prevent adverse reactions. Also, several drugs, including cimetidine and erythromycin, decrease elimination. Gastrointestinal absorption of theophylline in some sustained-release preparations is affected by food intake. Because theophylline crosses the placenta and can cause toxicity in the newborn, it is recommended that therapeutic levels during pregnancy should not exceed 12 μg/mL (1). Aminophylline should be used cautiously during labor, because it can inhibit uterine contractions (25).

Anticholinergics

Atropine was used historically to induce bronchodilation through inhibition of intrinsic vagal tone. Local and systemic side effects limited its usefulness in the treatment of asthma. In contrast, ipratropium, a quaternary derivative of atropine, causes few adverse effects because it is poorly absorbed. The role of inhaled ipratropium (a category B agent) in the day-to-day management of asthma remains unclear. Because of minimal side effects, however, it should be considered supplemental to a treatment regimen that includes a beta-2 agonist, corticosteroid, and theophylline. Ipratropium administered by nebulization may provide therapeutic benefit in patients with severe asthma exacerbations.

Additional Pharmacologic Considerations

Medications to be avoided during pregnancy include alpha-adrenergic compounds (other than pseudoephedrine), epinephrine, iodides, sulfonamides (in late pregnancy), tetracyclines, and quinolones (1). Antihistamines and expectorants provide little benefit in the management of asthma. Because bacterial infections rarely, if ever, cause exacerbations of asthma, and atopic persons may react adversely to an antibiotic, an asthma treatment regimen should not include antibiotics. Yellow or green sputum associated with an asthma exacerbation reflects recruitment of polymorphonuclear leukocytes as part of disease activity, not a bacterial infection.

Management during Delivery or Surgery

In general, most medications used to treat asthma can be continued throughout labor and delivery. The status of asthma can be followed by measuring peak expiratory flow. Caution should be exercised, however, with terbutaline and theophylline because these agents can inhibit labor. For patients who have been receiving systemic corticosteroids, supplemental corticosteroids (hydrocortisone) are required during the stress of labor and delivery. If anesthesia is required during labor, it is preferable to use epidural block, local anesthesia, pudendal, or spinal block. For general anesthesia, halogenated agents are preferred because they induce less bronchospasm (26). Fentanyl is preferred to narcotic analgesics, which can cause histamine release. Oxytocin is the drug of choice for labor induction and postpartum hemorrhage. If methylergonovine or ergonovine must be used, pretreatment with methylprednisolone is recommended (27).

COMMON PNEUMONIAS

Pneumonia is encountered during pregnancy and is the most common etiology of nonobstetric infection culminating in maternal death (28). Pregnancy is characterized by increased metabolic demands and diminished ventilatory reserve, both of which conceivably can render the gravid woman less able to combat pulmonary infection. The fetus is vulnerable to the effects of hypoxemia, acidosis, electrolyte imbalance, and dehydration that may accompany pneumonia. Immunologic alterations that occur during pregnancy have been postulated to account for the aggressive nature and increased mortality that may characterize certain types of pneumonia, especially those of viral origin. The epidemiology, bacteriology, clinical course, and management of pneumonia during pregnancy are reviewed, followed by a discussion of the common bacterial, viral, and fungal pathogens that cause pneumonia in this population.

Epidemiology

In the preantibiotic era, Finland and Dublin (29) reported pneumococcal pneumonia as a complication in 0.63% of pregnancies. The infection rate of 0.85% for all cases of pneumonia reported by Hopwood (30) in 1965 was not remarkably different. More recent studies suggest that the overall incidence of pneumonia during pregnancy has decreased. Specifically, Benedetti and colleagues (31) cited one case of pneumonia per 2,288 deliveries (0.04%) between 1972 and 1975. More than a decade later, Madinger and colleagues (32) noted a 0.08% infection rate among 32,179 deliveries. When Berkowitz and La Sala (33) reviewed their experience from a large city university hospital from 1988 to 1989, the frequency of pneumonia had climbed to 1 in 367 deliveries (0.27%). A comparatively lower incidence of antepartum pneumonia (0.12% among 59,656 parturients) was derived from a university-affiliated county hospital setting between 1989 and 1993 (34).

Pneumonia complicating pregnancy thus remains a rare occurrence despite reports suggesting a rising prevalence of underlying disease in the present-day obstetric population. In an era of advanced obstetric care, a willingness to proceed with pregnancy despite advancing age and serious preexisting illness might render pregnant patients more susceptible to pneumonia and explain why pneumonia has been reported in a significant number of gravidas with a history of preexisting respiratory disease (30–34), immunosuppression (32–34) anemia, (31,33–34) illicit drug use, (33–34) tobacco smoking, (30,32,34) and cardiac disease (31).

Pathogenesis of Pneumonia in Pregnant Women

Maternal Aspects

There is little evidence to support the idea that mechanical factors and alterations in pulmonary function predispose to pneumonia in pregnant subjects. Although elevation of the diaphragm as a result of the enlarging uterus results in a decrement in the functional residual capacity of 18% during pregnancy, vital capacity and diaphragmatic function are well retained (35). Nevertheless, normal pregnancy is associated with augmented physiologic demands manifested by an increase in oxygen consumption imposed by the fetoplacental unit and a disproportionate rise in minute ventilation mediated by the respiratory stimulant effect of progesterone (35,36). Circulating blood volume and cardiac output also are increased, especially during the latter stages of pregnancy (36). The prognosis of pneumonia in pregnancy depends on the ability of the gravida to withstand infection despite the excess metabolic stress, tachycardia, dehydration, and hypoxemia that may ensue. The coexistence of underlying disease adds to this burden.

Studies of immune function during pregnancy demonstrated a diminution in cell-mediated immunity (37–39). Impaired cell-mediated immunity probably plays an adaptive role in preventing rejection of the fetal allograft but may be associated with decreased resistance to various pathogens. Indeed, influenza and primary varicella infection complicated by pneumonia often pursue an aggressive course in pregnant patients (40–51). Although defects in cell-mediated immunity also predispose to infection by fungal, protozoan, and intracellular bacterial organisms (37), all of which have been reported to cause pneumonia in pregnant patients (52–55), there is insufficient evidence to suggest that pregnant patients are at increased risk for infection by these pathogens.

The immunologic basis underlying suppression of the maternal immune response has been reviewed (37–39). A decrease in the maternal lymphocyte proliferative response to soluble antigens is demonstrated during the second and third trimesters of pregnancy (37) and seems to coincide with the period when antepartum pneumonia is most frequently diagnosed (30,32–34). Numerous substances in maternal serum known to curtail lymphocyte function include pregnancy-associated glycoproteins, progesterone, estradiol, cortisol, human chorionic gonadotropin, and α-fetoprotein (37–39). Fetal lymphocytes obtained from cord blood appear to suppress maternal lymphocyte function (37,39). Other factors implicated in the altered immune response include circulating IgG antibodies directed against histocompatibility antigens, a decrease in the number of circulating CD4 lymphocytes, and depressed natural killer cell activity (37–38).

Fetal Aspects

The viability of the fetus is threatened by the fever, tachycardia, hypoxemia, acidosis, electrolyte imbalance, and dehydration that may complicate antepartum pneumonia. Premature labor and delivery also occur with increased frequency (32,56), although the underlying mechanisms are unclear. It is possible that by eliciting remote effects on the uterus, the systemic release of phospholipases, proteases, and prostaglandins in response to bacterial infection provokes labor (57).

Outcomes of Pregnancy Complicated by Pneumonia

During the early 1900's, the maternal mortality rate from antepartum pneumonia was approximately 30% (29,58). Following the availability of antibiotics, Oxhorn (56) in

1953 noted a drop in maternal mortality from 20% to 3.5%. A decade later, Hopwood (30) reviewed 23 cases of pneumonia in 2,720 pregnant women referred to a Naval hospital and reported two maternal deaths (8.6%) subsequent to preterm delivery during the acute pneumonia episode, an association recognized by prior investigators (29,56). Maternal outcomes derived from four more recent hospital-based surveys of antepartum pneumonia reveal a mortality rate of less than 2% (31–34). Of the three deaths that occurred in the 161 reported cases of pneumonia, one was in a woman with cystic fibrosis and poor pulmonary function who had been advised against pregnancy (32). With the possible exceptions of viral pneumonia and pulmonary infection in human immunodeficiency virus (HIV)-positive patients, lower maternal mortality rates are being reported at a time when ostensibly older and sicker women are opting for pregnancy. Prompt recognition and treatment of pneumonia coupled with modern day advances in obstetric care are credited with the improved survival; however, maternal morbidity resulting from antepartum pneumonia is not rare. In Madinger's study (32), 12 of 25 pregnant subjects with pneumonia developed complications, which included respiratory failure requiring mechanical ventilation (20%), bacteremia (16%), and preterm delivery during the active phase of pneumonia (36%). Complications were significantly more prevalent in the 24% of patients with pneumonia who had underlying medical conditions (32). Similarly, Berkowitz and La Sala reported pneumonia and respiratory failure requiring mechanical ventilation in two pregnant women with preexisting asthma (33). In another study (34), despite a history of underlying disease in 31 of 71 cases of antepartum pneumonia, no correlation was found between preexisting illness and negative outcomes. Complications were significantly more common in active smokers; in those with a lower mean arterial blood pO_2 on admission; and radiographic evidence of multilobar, bilateral, or diffuse pulmonary involvement (34).

Obstetric outcomes are concerned primarily with preterm delivery and perinatal death, both of which are increased when pneumonia complicates pregnancy. Oxorn (56) reported preterm delivery in the setting of pneumonia in 71% of patients between the 25th and 36th week of gestation. Perinatal mortality occurred in approximately half of these cases. The introduction of antibiotics was not associated with a decrement in preterm delivery but significantly reduced fetal mortality by one third (56). Neonatal death in modern surveys also has been linked to delivery during the acute episode of pneumonia (30,32,34). Madinger and colleagues (32) reported premature labor as a complication of pneumonia in 11 of 25 patients (44%) and premature delivery in 36%. Tocolytic therapy failed to arrest labor in more than half of these cases. Underlying maternal disease was associated with all three neonatal deaths and was a significant risk factor for delivery during the acute pneumonia episode (32). In contrast, better outcomes were reported by Benedetti et al. (31); 2 of 19 women delivered during the acute phase of pneumonia, associated with one fetal death. The favorable outcomes were ascribed to the early institution of antibiotics, absence of significant maternal hypoxemia, and the availability of neonatal intensive care (31). Berkowitz and La Sala (33) similarly attributed modern obstetric and respiratory care to the low incidence of complications they observed, which consisted of one premature delivery unrelated to pneumonia and no perinatal deaths.

Bacteriology

The spectrum of infectious agents reported to cause pneumonia during pregnancy is as diverse as that witnessed in the general population. The true incidence of antepartum pneumonia resulting from a specific pathogen is, however, difficult to ascertain. In many studies, sputum and blood cultures were the primary means of determining the etiology of pneumonia, thus mitigating against the detection of atypical pathogens such as *Mycoplasma*, *Legionella*, *Listeria*, and viruses (31–33). Consequently, pneumonia caused by these agents may be underrepresented in surveys done during pregnancy. In most studies, the use of limited diagnostic techniques explains why the largest subset of patients have pneumonia for which the causative agent is unknown (31–34).

When the cause for pneumonia can be established, a bacterial etiology accounts for most cases, with pneumococcus the most common isolate (31–34). In descending order, *Hemophilus influenzae*, atypical pathogens (*Mycoplasma*, *Legionella*, *Chlamydia*), viruses (influenza A, varicella), fungal/protozoan agents, and enteric bacteria account for the remainder. The relative frequencies of the pathogens that cause pneumonia in the pregnant population therefore mirror that encountered in nonpregnant women (59).

The likelihood that a given pathogen is the cause for pneumonia is also biased by background conditions. Immunocompromised hosts are susceptible to otherwise unusual opportunistic infections. For hospital-acquired pneumonia, staphylococcal and enteric gram-negative bacteria assume a greater etiologic significance. Postpartum pneumonia resulting from anaerobes or gram-negative bacteria may develop following aspiration of oropharyngeal and gastric contents during labor and delivery. Community or epidemic outbreaks of influenza or other viruses should heighten one's suspicion for antepartum pneumonia caused by these pathogens.

Bacterial Pneumonia

General Features

The clinical features of bacterial pneumonia are similar in both pregnant and nonpregnant hosts. Community-acquired pneumonia traditionally has been divided into either a typical or atypical presentation, but this distinction has limitations for narrowing the etiologic spectrum and directing antimicrobial therapy. The typical pneumonia syndrome is characterized by the abrupt onset of fever, shaking chills, productive cough, leukocytosis, focal findings on lung examination, lobar consolidation on chest radiographs, and bacterial etiology. Conversely, atypical pneumonia generally afflicts younger persons and is distinguished by a subacute-onset, lower fever, nonproductive cough, extrapulmonary symptoms, a relative lack of physical findings, and a bronchopneumonic or diffuse radiographic pattern. As previously discussed, *Streptococcus pneumoniae* and *H. influenzae* are the two most common typical bacterial pneumonias encountered in the pregnant population, and atypical pathogens include *Legionella* species, *Mycoplasma pneumoniae*, and *Chlamydia pneumoniae*. Unfortunately, classifying pneumonia in this fashion is confounded by the recognition that typical bacterial pneumonias can present with atypical features and vice versa. For example, *Legionella* pneumonia can evolve rapidly over a few days from an atypical to a typical appearing syndrome with potentially serious sequelae.

There are certain distinguishing features regarding community-acquired pneumonia in the pregnant host. Hopwood (30) reported a preceding upper respiratory infection in all 23 subjects with pneumonia in his series, cough in 20 patients, fever above 101°F in 18, chills in 5, and dyspnea in 3. The low incidence of dyspnea as a presenting symptom could be related to the subjectively high sensation of breathlessness that is already experienced in up to 75% of pregnant women (35). Whereas dyspnea may not be a reliable symptom in this setting, tachypnea is never normal and should prompt further investigation (60). To avoid misdiagnosis, Hopwood suggested that all pregnant women with a persistent upper respiratory infection undergo chest radiography (30). Indeed, the diagnosis of pneumonia was overlooked in 5 of the 25 patients in Madinger's series (32), and may have contributed to the high incidence of complications reported in that study.

Specific Bacterial Pathogens (Table 14-2)

S. pneumoniae accounts for 25% to 60% of community-acquired pneumonia in the general population (59). Gram stain of sputum may be helpful in the diagnosis. It will reveal gram-positive lancet-shaped diplococci in a background of polymorphonuclear cells. More commonly contracted during the winter and early spring, the onset of illness is usually abrupt and is heralded by high fever, rigors, purulent and often blood-streaked sputum, pleuritic chest pain, focal physical findings, and lobar consolidation on chest radiograph. Leukocytosis is the norm, although leukopenia may be seen in severe infections. Bacteremia or parapneumonic effusion is present in 25% of cases. Empyema is a rare complication. Defects in humoral immunity, as in asplenic persons or those with lymphoproliferative disorders, is associated with more fulminant infection and greater morbidity and mortality (59).

H. influenzae, a pleomorphic gram-negative coccobacillus, is the next most common isolate in pregnant patients and accounts for 4% to 15% of community-acquired pneumonia in the general population (59). Findings on Gram stain are inconsistent, and the organisms are frequently misidentified. The onset of illness may be more insidious than that for pneumococcal pneumonia, but in general the presenting features and natural history are similar. Pleural effusion is seen in up to 50% of cases, whereas bacteremia complicates 10% (59). As with pneumococcus, underlying illness and immunocompromised status predispose to infection.

Rarer causes of community-acquired pneumonia include *Klebsiella pneumoniae* and *Staphylococcus aureus*. The former is a large gram-negative rod with a predilection for infection in the setting of decreased host resistance, as in alcoholics. Cavitation, abscess formation, and tissue destruction are not uncommon. Bacteremia is seen in up to 70% of cases (59). *S. aureus* is a gram-positive coccus that may appear in pairs, tetrads, clusters, or short chains on Gram stain. This organism has historical importance as a cause for secondary bacterial pneumonia during influenza epidemics, second in incidence to pneumococcus in this regard (45). Multilobar infiltrates and parapneumonic effusions occur in 50% of patients. Bacteremia is seen in 33%, empyema in 25%, and abscess formation in 20% of cases (59).

Of the atypical pneumonias, *Mycoplasma* and *Chlamydia pneumoniae* often pursue a mild course with prodromal flulike symptoms. The diagnosis of these pathogens relies on appropriate serologic testing, although treatment is often empiric and infection self-limited. Conversely, *L. pneumonia* may be life-threatening in the pregnant patient with rapidly progressive multilobar consolidation and respiratory failure, especially in the setting of previous cardiopulmonary disease (54). Systemic manifestations are commonly present and include headache or altered sensorium, the syndrome of inappropriate antidiuretic hormone secretion, liver function test abnormalities, diarrhea, hematologic abnormalities, and renal insufficiency. Extrapulmonary involvement, however, is not exclusive to *Legionella* infection but also may be encountered in other types of bacterial pneumonia. A Gram stain revealing polymorphonuclear cells but lacking an identifiable pathogen is a clue to the diagnosis. Recently, *Legionella* and pneumococcal pneumonia were found to be the most common etiologies of severe community-acquired pneumonia in nonpregnant patients requiring intensive care unit admission and also were complicated by the highest incidence of the adult respiratory distress syndrome (61).

Management in Pregnant Patients

Supportive measures in the management of antepartum pneumonia are no different from those in nonpregnant patients and include hydration, supplemental oxy-

TABLE 14-2. *Summary of pneumonia during pregnancy*

Organism	Incidence	Gram stain	Clinical features	Other	Treatment[a]
Streptococcus pneumoniae	25%–60% of CAP; also most common cause during pregnancy	Gram+ lancet-shaped diplococci, PMNs	Abrupt onset of fevers, shaking chills, purulent sputum, pleuritic chest pain; leukocytosis or leukopenia Chest x-ray; lobar consolidation or bronchopneumonia	Bacteremia 25%, pleural effusion 25%, empyema rarely	Ampicillin ± β-lactamase inhib.; 1st or 2nd-generation cephalosporin
Hemophilus influenzae	4%–15% of CAP, second most common cause during pregnancy	Pleomorphic gram-coccobacilli, PMNs	Slightly more insidious onset than pneumococcus with many similar features	Bacteremia 10%, pleural effusion 50%	Ampicillin ± β-lactamase inhib.; 2nd-generation cephalosporin
Mycoplasma pneumoniae	30%–60% of CAP in 5 to 20 yr age group; common in pregnancy	Mononuclear cells outnumber PMNs, no predominant organism	Community outbreaks "Atypical" presentation after 1 to 3 wk incubation period Diagnosis: Cold agglutinins in 50% (titer ≥ 1:64) 4-fold rise in complement fixation antibody titers between acute and convalescent serum or single titer > *1:64*	Empyema and cavitation do not occur; rare severe infection with systemic manifestations	Erythromycin
Legionella pneumophila	1%–15% of CAP; occasionally reported in pregnancy	PMNs, few organisms	Contaminated water may serve as reservoir; high fever 20%; scant sputum that may be blood tinged; rapid radiographic progression with multilobar; involvement possible; Diagnosis: Direct fluorescent antibody of sputum (sensitivity 50%); legionella urinary antigen; indirect fluorescent antibody titer ≥ 1:128	Pleural effusion 50% Extrapulmonary involvement.[b] SIADH, CNS symptoms, ↑ liver enzymes, diarrhea, hematologic	Erythromycin
Chlamydia pneumoniae	≈10% of CAP; ? incidence in pregnancy	Nondiagnostic	Often mild or asymptomatic disease; Diagnosis: nasopharyngeal swab (species-specific monoclonal antibodies); direct fluorescent antibodies of respiratory secretions		Erythromycin
Influenzae	Most common viral etiology of pneumonia in pregnancy	Nondiagnostic	Winter outbreaks; epidemics; type A most common; asymptomatic to severe infections; Diagnosis: throat washings, viral titers	Increased maternal mortality during influenza epidemics	Supportive care, amantadine; aerosolized ribavirin
Varicella-Zoster	Uncommon	Nondiagnostic	Household contacts; highly contagious; pneumonia is associated with primary varicella infection; tobacco smoking is a risk factor for pneumonia; characteristic vesicular skin eruption; Diagnosis: characteristic viral inclusions in skin lesions	Fetal complications: congenital varicella syndrome, neonatal varicella infection	Acyclovir
Klebsiella pneumoniae	Rare cause of CAP in pregnancy	Gram-bacilli, PMNs	Decreased host resistance, i.e., alcoholics; "currant-jelly" sputum; nosocomial pneumonia	Necrotizing pneumonia, abscess formation; bacteremia 70%	2nd or 3rd-generation cephalosporin + aminoglycoside[d]
Staphylococcus aureus	Rare cause of CAP in pregnancy	Gram+ cocci, PMNs	Superinfection after influenza pneumonia; nosocomial pneumonia; associated with intravenous drug abuse and endocarditis	Lung abscess 20%, multilobar 50%, pleural effusion 50%, empyema 25%, bacteremia 33%, mortality 50%	Nafcillin; 1st-generation cephalosporin
Fungi	Rare	Variable	Endemic or opportunistic infection	Species specific	Amphotericin B
Anaerobes (Aspiration)	Uncommon	Mixed flora, PMNs	Complication of labor and delivery; foul-smelling sputum	Abscess formation	Penicillin; clindamycin

CAP, community-acquired pneumonia; PMN, polymorphonuclear leukocytes; CNS, central nervous system; SIADH, syndrome of inappropriate antidiuretic hormone.

[a]Treatment refers to the antibiotics of choice for the pregnant patient.

[b]Extrapulmonary involvement can also be seen in other etiologies of pneumonia.

[c]The use of amantadine and ribavirin are reserved only for severe influenza pneumonia.

[d]The use of aminoglycosides must be weighed against the potential for ototoxicity in the newborn.

gen, antipyretics, chest physiotherapy, and bronchodilators, as required. Given the overlapping features that characterize many etiologies of pneumonia, the initial choice of antibiotics is often empiric. The antibiotic regimen subsequently may be tailored depending on the results of a diagnostic evaluation consisting of sputum Gram stain and culture, serologic studies, blood and urine cultures, chemistry profile, complete blood count, and chest roentgenogram. For uncomplicated community-acquired pneumonia, initial antimicrobial therapy should be directed against common offending pathogens including pneumococcus and *H influenzae* as well as atypical agents, depending on the clinical assessment. For severe community-acquired pneumonia, the empiric addition of *Legionella* coverage is recommended (61,62). For cases in which aspiration pneumonia is suspected, coverage of gram-negative and anaerobic pathogens is warranted. Management of bacterial superinfection complicating influenza pneumonia requires broad-spectrum gram-positive and gram-negative coverage. Antibiotics with activity against enteric gram-negative organisms are recommended for the treatment of hospital-acquired pneumonia.

The initial choice of antibiotics for the management of antepartum pneumonia also must take into account the potential for harm to the developing fetus. Penicillins and cephalosporins are considered safe in pregnancy and are first-line agents for the treatment of community-acquired pneumonia resulting from pneumococcus and *H influenzae*. Resistance to penicillins conferred by β-lactamase producing organisms can be circumvented without demonstrable fetal toxicity by the use of penicillin-β-lactamase inhibitor conjugates (63). Erythromycin and clindamycin are macrolides that also are considered safe during pregnancy, the former effective against atypical pathogens including *Legionella*, the latter for management of anaerobic infections. When broader gram-negative coverage is desired, third-generation cephalosporins, some with antipseudomonal activity, can be employed. Because of the risk of fetal ototoxicity, the use of aminoglycosides should be reserved for the treatment of severe infections. Similarly, vancomycin may be necessary to manage resistant gram-positive infections, although its use must be weighed against the potential for fetal renal and ototoxicity. Judicious monitoring of serum drug levels is required if aminoglycosides or vancomycin are used (63). Tetracyclines should be avoided during pregnancy because of their association with abnormal fetal bone growth and teeth discoloration. Folate antagonists have been associated with fetal malformations, whereas sulfonamides administered during late pregnancy may cause hyperbilirubinemia in the newborn. For this reason, combinations of sulfa and trimephoprim have potential adverse effects in pregnancy. Because fluoroquinolones have unknown teratogenic potential, their use is also discouraged during pregnancy (63).

Continuous fetal monitoring is recommended for patients beyond the 24th week of gestation and in cases of severe pneumonia (62,64). Impending respiratory failure marked by refractory hypoxemia, carbon dioxide retention, metabolic acidosis, or other signs of sepsis may dictate the need for mechanical ventilation. In situations in which maternal status continues to decline, it is unclear whether emergent delivery will confer beneficial effects on pulmonary mechanics or gas exchange (64). Indeed, the converse may be true, given reports of increased maternal mortality when delivery occurs during the acute pneumonia episode (29,30,56). Most authorities advocate delivery only for obstetric or fetal indications. A similar debate surrounds the use of tocolytic therapy to arrest premature labor. Rodrigues and Niederman (62) recommended attempts at tocolysis in cases in which no signs of fetal distress are seen and the mother can continue to compensate for the physiologic stresses imposed by pregnancy. In contrast, Goodrum (64) warned against the use of tocolytic agents such as β-2 agonists and magnesium sulfate, which can cause pulmonary edema. The pregnant patient with pneumonia may be at particular risk for this complication given the decreased plasma oncotic pressure that occurs during pregnancy and the increases in pulmonary capillary permeability mediated by infection (64).

Viral Pneumonia (see Table 14-2)

Influenza Virus

The influenza viruses are RNA orthomyxoviruses consisting of three antigenically distinct types, of which type A is responsible for most epidemic outbreaks and severe infections. Influenza type B is associated with rarer outbreaks and generally milder infections, whereas type C is the least clinically significant. These viruses are further characterized by surface antigens that include four hemagglutinin (H0, H1, H2, and H3) and two neuroaminidase (N1 and N2) subtypes (45,65). Epidemics occur every several years and result from major changes, or shifts, in these surface antigens. Antigenic drifts result from minor changes in these surface antigens, occur commonly, and are classified by their year and location. Presumably because partial immunity is still conferred to drifted strains, they are not considered to give rise to epidemics (45).

Influenza is contracted during the winter months, and following a short 1- to 4-day incubation, is heralded by the abrupt onset of cough, coryza, sore throat, high fever, headache, and generalized malaise. Person-to-person transmission is thought to occur via aerosolization of infected respiratory secretions. The diagnosis can be confirmed by viral isolation from throat washings or by a fourfold or greater rise in antibody titers. In uncomplicated cases, physical findings are limited to inflammation of the upper respiratory tract, and symptoms resolve in a self-limited fashion within 3 to 5 days (45,65). More serious infection is characterized by persistence of symptoms beyond 5 days, and in these situations superimposed pneumonia should be suspected. Rapid decompensation due to hemorrhagic bronchopneumonia of solely viral origin is possible, although secondary bacterial pneumonia can supervene. In descending order of frequency, these bacterial pathogens include pneumococcus, *S. aureus, H. influenzae*, and enteric gram-negative organisms (45,62,65).

Influenza in pregnant hosts had been associated with a high incidence of complications and increased mortality in the past (40,41). The maternal mortality rate during the influenza pandemic of 1917 through 1918 was 27%, with deaths reported exclusively in the 50% of cases whose infection was complicated by pneumonia (41). Mortality also correlated with pregnancy duration and reached 61% if infection was contracted during the ninth month of gestation. During the 1957 through 1958 epidemic, nearly half of all women of childbearing years who died of influenza were pregnant, representing 10% of all fatal cases (46).

Since 1958, however, influenza in pregnant patients has not been associated with increased morbidity and mortality, although rare fatalities are still reported (42–43,46). Regarded as the most common viral etiology for pneumonia in the pregnant population, the true incidence of infection is difficult to ascertain as many cases are asymptomatic, not reported, or unrecognized (45). In one study, 60% of asymptomatic pregnant women had serologic evidence of recent influenza infection, whereas 35% of women with typical flulike symptoms were found to be serologically negative (66). Uncertainty therefore has arisen as to the diagnostic accuracy and prevalence of true disease during influenza epidemics and reinforces the rationale by the Centers for Disease Control and Prevention (CDC) not to recommend routine influenza immunization to all pregnant women (46,65,67). Exceptions are those with underlying medical conditions that include cardiac disease, chronic pulmonary disorders (including asthma), diabetes mellitus, immunosuppression, severe anemia, hemoglobinopathy, and renal dysfunction (68). The vaccine is best administered after the first trimester to avoid the theoretic risk of teratogenicity, although vaccination should not be delayed in high-risk patients who are in the first trimester when flu season begins (45,62,68). Because the vaccine is made from virus grown in embryonated hen's eggs, immunization is contraindicated in persons allergic to eggs (68).

When pneumonia complicates influenza broad spectrum antibiotics are indicated to cover for potential secondary bacterial infection. Successful treatment was reported with oral amantadine and aerosolized ribavirin in one pregnant woman with suspected viral pneumonia (44). Amantadine blocks the release of viral nucleic acids, and when given prophylactically in high risk patients is effective in preventing influenza A infection (68). Administration to nonpregnant subjects within the first 48 hours after symptom onset can decrease the duration of fever and systemic symptoms. Amantadine is teratogenic in rats, has a poorly understood safety profile during pregnancy, and is secreted in breast milk; therefore its use in gravid subjects should be restricted to life-threatening infection (45). Ribavirin is virustatic against influenza types A and B, and no teratogenicity has been reported in limited experience (44).

Transplacental passage of influenza virus has been documented, although the virus has never been isolated from fetal blood. Maternal IgG antibodies can also cross the placenta, and probably confer protection (45). While early reports suggested that influenza was a cause for congenital malformations, most investigators now feel this association is unlikely (45).

Varicella Virus

Varicella is a highly contagious DNA-herpes virus that presents with a characteristic pustular exanthem in more than 90% of children before adolescence (47,69). Although primary infection occurs in fewer than 2% of adults, nearly 30% of deaths resulting from varicella occur in this age group (70). Pneumonia is the most common serious complication and varies greatly in its presentation. Clinically apparent varicella pneumonia occurs in 0.3% (71) to 1.8% (72) of adults. It is likely that many more cases of pneumonia go unrecognized. In a study of military recruits with primary varicella infection, only 2 of 18 patients with radiographic evidence of pneumonia manifested symptoms (71); however, varicella pneumonia can be fulminant, leading to respiratory failure and death (49,50,73–75). The mortality rate is less than 1% in uncomplicated cases, but it increases to approximately 11% when pneumonia supervenes (75,76). Cigarette smoking, perhaps by impairing mucociliary clearance and the phagocytic function of alveolar macrophages, is an important risk factor for the development of varicella pneumonia (76).

Primary varicella infection during pregnancy is rare, with an estimated incidence of 0.5 to 0.7/1000 pregnancies (77). Nevertheless, it has been suggested that pregnancy predisposes to and enhances the virulence of varicella pneumonia. Composite mortality rates in pregnant patients derived from individually reported cases have been quoted to be as high as 35% to 44% (73,76). In contrast, other investigators have found mortality to be no greater than that witnessed in the general adult population (49,74,78). Despite there being no apparent difference in mortality rates between pregnant and nonpregnant subjects reported by Esmonde et al. (49), the morbidity of varicella pneumonia seemed greater in pregnant women, 46% of whom required assisted ventilation. Infection contracted during the third trimester is more likely to be complicated by pneumonia, an observation hypothetically linked to suppression of cell-mediated immunity during the latter stages of pregnancy (76).

Following an incubation period of 10 to 21 days (47), primary varicella infection is heralded by the onset of rash, fever, and malaise. Pneumonia, often in conjunction with oral mucosal lesions (62), develops between the 2nd and 6th days after the first appearance of rash. Respiratory symptoms may include chest pain, cough, dyspnea, and hemoptysis (73). Auscultatory findings are often minimal and correlate poorly with the severity of pneumonia. Radiographic changes include diffuse miliary and nodular infiltrates in a peribronchial distribution that usually resolve within 2 weeks (73). The peak in severity of the mucocutaneous eruption often coincides with maximal radiographic abnormalities (48). Discrete diffuse pulmonary calcifications have been reported 3 to 10 years following varicella pneumonia (49).

Hospitalization and commencement of antiviral therapy are advised for all pregnant patients with varicella pneumonia given the potential for rapid disease progression. A recent study found that institution of acyclovir, a DNA polymerase inhibitor, within the first 36 hours of hospitalization was associated with a reduction in fever and tachypnea by the 5th hospital day and improved oxygenation by the sixth day (76). The use of acyclovir in pregnant patients was associated with no increase in birth defects or consistent pattern of abnormalities in 312 acyclovir-exposed pregnancies (79).

The incidence of fetal infection resulting from intrauterine varicella has been estimated at 25% following maternal exposure in which one half of cases are symptomatic (74). The risk of varicella embryopathy has been estimated at 2.2% when primary maternal varicella infection occurs between the 8th and 20th week of gestation (77). The congenital varicella syndrome is characterized by cutaneous scars, limb hypoplasia, microcephaly, cortical atrophy, chorioretinitis, cataracts, autonomic dysfunction, and other abnormalities (47,69,74,77). The risk of disseminated neonatal varicella is highest when the infant is born within 1 day before to 4 days after the onset of maternal varicella, which corresponds to the interval prior to the development of specific maternal antibodies that might otherwise confer passive immunity (47). The mortality rate for infants with disseminated neonatal varicella born within this time window is 21% (47). Congenital zoster of infancy is another complication that has been reported following 2nd trimester infection (62). Varicella-zoster immunoglobulin may have a role in decreasing the incidence of disease in susceptible pregnant women who have been exposed to the virus. For prevention of fetal complications, the benefits of varicella-zoster immunoglobulin are unknown (74).

Rubeola Virus

Rubeola (measles), a paramyxovirus, is a relatively rare infection in pregnancy since the introduction of widespread immunization in 1963 (65). Following an incubation period of 8 to 13 days, patients experience 1 to 2 days of fever, coryza, cough, and conjunctivitis followed on day 3 by the appearance of pathognomonic Koplik spots. Rash is seen at the height of the illness around day 4 (80). Pneumonia complicates 3.5% to 50% of adult measles cases with a high incidence of superimposed bacterial infection (80). Other complications include otitis media, encephalitis, and liver dysfunction. Rubeola virus is not a teratogen, although infections complicated by pneumonia are associated with an increased risk of spontaneous abortion, premature delivery, and perinatal mortality (65,80). Because the measles vaccine is a live attenuated form of the virus, its use in pregnancy is not recommended. Hyperimmune globulin may be efficacious if administered to susceptible pregnant women within 6 days of known exposure.

Fungal Pneumonia

Coccidioidomycosis

Fungal pneumonia is rare during pregnancy but includes cases of cryptococcosis (81), blastomycosis (82,83), and, most notably, coccidioidomycosis (52). The latter has received the most attention because it is the most common deep mycosis reported in the pregnant population and because infection is associated with a high incidence of maternal and fetal complications (52,84). *Coccidioides immitis* is a soil saprophyte endemic to the southwestern United States. Infection occurs via inhalation of airborne arthrospores that elicit a neutrophilic exudative response in lung tissue (85). As with other fungal pneumonias, control of infection requires cell-mediated immunity, which in this case usually develops within 2 weeks of primary infection. Primary infection is exceedingly common in endemic areas and is asymptomatic in 60% of cases. The remaining 40% have a febrile flulike illness lasting 1 to 3 weeks. Pleuritic chest pain is common, as are symptoms of cough, myalgias, arthralgias, headache, and fatigue. The chest roentgenogram may reveal a focal alveolar consolidation or small nodular-appearing densities (85). A positive coccidioidin skin test develops within approximately 2 weeks, but it cannot discern acute infection from prior exposure. Diagnostic tools for detection of recent infection include serum measurement of specific IgM antibodies, complement-fixing antibodies (IgG), and direct examination of respiratory secretions or tissue specimens. In 95% of cases, primary infection resolves without sequelae. Persistent pneumonia defined by pulmonary symptoms lasting beyond 6 weeks is associated with cavitary pulmonary infiltrates, endobronchial spread, and, rarely, dissemination, the most feared complication (85). The onset of dissemination is often insidious, with verrucous skin lesions, bony lesions, and meningitis the most common extrapulmonary manifestations.

Coccidioidomycosis complicates about 1 in 5,000 pregnancies, an incidence fivefold less than that reported in the 1940's (52,84). The mortality rate from disseminated disease was reported to be as high as 90% in the past, but it appears to have dropped markedly in recent years (52,84). Possibly, this decrease is related to improved treatment strategies, alternative study designs, or differences in the exposure risk and demographics of the populations studied (52,84). Past and present investigators agree that the risk of disseminated disease is greatest when coccidioidal infection occurs during the third trimester (84). The numbers are too small to assess whether fetal mortality also has fallen in recent years. In a recent survey, no fetal deaths attributable to infection occurred in the ten cases described and included the delivery of two healthy term infants in women with disseminated disease (84). Catanzaro (52) reviewed mechanisms in addition to suppression of cell-mediated immunity that may be of greater importance in predisposing pregnant women to serious coccidioidal infection. In vitro assays demonstrating proliferation of coccidioidal forms in the presence of 17-β-estradiol suggest that the hormonal milieu in pregnancy may play a role in potentiating coccidioidal infection.

Amphotericin B is the treatment of choice for severe coccidioidal infections and disseminated disease. No teratogenic effects have been reported in limited experience with the use of this agent (83). Care should be taken in monitoring renal function and blood counts, because amphotericin B is nephrotoxic and may exacerbate the anemia of pregnancy (52,83).

Aspiration Pneumonia

Aspiration of oropharyngeal and gastric contents as a complication of labor and delivery has long been recognized as an important cause of maternal morbidity and mortality. In a recent comprehensive review of the subject (86), the term *aspiration-induced lung injury* was coined in place of aspiration pneumonia to emphasize that many of the pathophysiologic correlates of this syndrome are of noninfectious origin. Since Mendelson's original description of 66 women with witnessed or highly suspected aspiration during labor and delivery (87), a number of investigators have corroborated in animal studies that destruction of the bronchial mucosa and chemical pneumonitis follow aspiration of low pH solutions (pH < 2.5) and liquid gastric contents (86). Although the importance of highly acidic aspirated material has been emphasized by many authors, other proinflammatory factors also must be involved because animal models reveal acute lung injury following aspiration of relatively alkaline solutions. Cytokines, neutrophil chemotactic factors, and adhesion molecules have been implicated in the pathogenesis of lung injury at the cellular level.

Aspiration of solid particulates can result in acute airway obstruction, cough, dyspnea, cyanosis, and death from asphyxia (88). When gastric juice is aspirated, symptom onset is usually more insidious, with dyspnea, wheezing, cyanosis, and hypotension developing 6 to 8 hours after the event. The chest radiograph in this circumstance often resembles bronchopneumonia and, in severe cases, diffuse pulmonary edema. Occasionally, a period of stabilization or improvement is followed by renewed symptoms and new or progressive radiographic changes. Superimposed bacterial pneumonia is usually the cause, most often resulting from gram-negative and anaerobic organisms (87).

In pregnancy, several risk factors predispose to aspiration during labor and delivery: elevations in intragastric pressure, progesterone-mediated relaxation of the lower gastroesophageal sphincter, delayed gastric emptying, vigorous abdominal palpation, and reduced consciousness secondary to anesthesia (62). Suspicion of aspiration should arise when respiratory failure occurs in the early postpartum period. Management of aspiration is supportive and includes supplemental oxygen, bronchodilators, and assisted ventilation. When superimposed bacterial infection is suspected, antibiotics should be initiated.

The major emphasis should be focused on primary prevention of aspiration. Forms of analgesia that preserve maternal consciousness and maintain the integrity of upper airway reflexes are optimal. Heavy sedation or analgesia may lead to obtundation and occasionally induce nausea and vomiting. Regional anesthesia is preferred to general anesthesia, but if the latter is required, rapid-sequence induction with application of cricoid pressure is advised at the time of endotracheal intubation. If possible, the patient also should have received nothing by mouth for at least 8 hours before anesthesia induction. Pharmacologic intervention has included attempts at raising intragastric pH with the use of liquid antacids and histamine-2 receptor antagonists (89), often given in combination. To promote gastric emptying, dopamine antagonists such as meclopropamide and domeperidone may be added to the acid prophylaxis regimen (89). Decreased maternal mortality from these pharmacologic interventions has yet to be demonstrated.

Summary

Pneumonia is not a common complication of pregnancy, but it may pose serious problems for the expectant mother and child. Pathogens implicated in antepartum pneumonia are commonly of bacterial or viral origin, and their relative frequencies mirror those seen in the general population. Suppression of cell-mediated immunity may predispose to and increase the severity of pneumonia caused by certain viruses and fungi. The physiologic stresses imposed by pregnancy may compromise the mother's ability to withstand the rigors of infection, and fetal loss may result. Despite these concerns, and the suggestion that sicker and older women are now opting for pregnancy, maternal mortality from antepartum pneumonia has not increased in recent years. Improvements in modern obstetric and respiratory care may account for this observation. Besides supportive measures, treatment of antepartum pneumonia requires a thorough understanding of the potential toxicity of the antibiotic regimen utilized.

TUBERCULOSIS

It seems that humans are destined to battle with the tubercle bacillus forever. Since the days of the Pharaohs, the white plague has been a presence for civilized mankind. The discovery of the tubercle bacillus by Robert Koch was followed by almost a century of study, until effective antituberculous therapy emerged. With the institution of specific treatment, the frequency of tuberculosis in the United States receded each year, spurring hope for eventual liberation from this scourge. In 1985, however, the frequency of tuberculosis began to increase and the number of cases of active disease grew until 1994 (90–92). Ominously, the increase in the numbers of cases was compounded by the appearance of a significant number of patients with multidrug-resistant organisms (MDR) (93). The unexpected rise in new patients with active tuberculosis could be attributed to the influx of immigrants from countries with a high rate of tuberculosis and the large numbers of immunosuppressed patients, especially those with acquired immunodeficiency syndrome (AIDS), who are uniquely susceptible to tuberculosis as an opportunistic infection (90,94,95). MDR was attributable to haphazard adherence to treatment regimens, resulting in inadequate therapy and thus promoting the emergence of tubercle bacilli resistant to isoniazid and rifampin (96). The result of this increase in tuberculosis is the increased exposure of the entire population to tuberculosis and MDR organisms. Even immunocompetent persons may succumb to tuberculosis if the organism is MDR. The introduction of directly observed therapy has been important, and since 1994 the frequency of tuberculosis has begun to diminish. It would be foolhardy, however, to believe that tuberculosis will be eradicated in our lifetime.

National surveillance for tuberculosis in the United States began in 1953. Through 1984, incidence rates decreased about 6% each year. That steep decline ended in 1985 and increased until 1992, reaching a peak incidence of 10.5 cases per 100,000 population in 1986 (97). In 1993 and 1994, the incidence began to decrease but was still higher than the rate in 1985. Importantly, with therapy the mortality rate for tuberculosis has declined, reaching 0.6 deaths per 100,000 in 1993 compared with 12.4 deaths per 100,000 population 40 years earlier (98). Unfortunately, with recent improvement in prevalence rates, innovative programs, such as direct observed therapy, which have been effective in regaining control of the tuberculosis epidemic, are currently being phased out. Some fear we are condemning our communities to further increases in tuberculosis patients by curtailing these efforts. More than half of all cases of tuberculosis in the United States occur in five states: California, Florida, Illinois, New York, and Texas. During 1985 through 1990, the number of persons aged 25 to 44 years developing tuberculosis increased by 44%, suggesting that tuberculosis was increasing in women of childbearing age (99). The increase was verified in a study of pregnant women in two public hospitals in New York City. Most, but not all, of this increase occurred in patients who were drug abusers or were HIV positive (100).

In 1985 in the United States, 22,201 cases of tuberculosis were reported (95). The overall case rate was 9.3 per 100,000, 5.7 per 100,000 for whites, 26.7 per 100,000 for blacks, and 49.6 per 100,000 for Asian/Pacific Islanders (95). In the United States, it is estimated that approximately 10% of all women of childbearing age have a positive tuberculin skin test. A positive skin test indicates infection, not disease; however, approximately 10% of all persons with a positive tuberculin test will develop tuberculosis during their life. The vast majority of pregnant women who develop active tuberculosis disease come from this large reservoir of positive skin test reactors.

Effect of Pregnancy

Prechemotherapy Era

From the beginning of the twentieth century until 1950, tuberculosis was thought to be aggravated by pregnancy. Freeth (101) observed worsening in all pregnant patients who had active tuberculosis. Twenty-two of Cromie's patients worsened with pregnancy (102), and all patients reported by Selikoff and Drofman (103) who had active untreated pulmonary tuberculosis manifested progression of their lung disease. Whether these studies represented a real difference from the course of untreated active tuberculosis in the general population is questionable. In early studies of nonpregnant women and men who had untreated active pulmonary tuberculosis, Ames and Schuck (104) reported that 30% of patients who had minimal pulmonary tuberculosis deteriorated in the prechemotherapy era. Two reports in the German literature emphasized that tuberculosis worsened during the first postpartum year (105,106). Studies from England and the United States (107,108), however, reported no increased risk in the postpartum period compared with a control group.

Postchemotherapy Era

Much better data are available concerning the effects of pregnancy on tuberculosis since the advent of effective antituberculosis chemotherapy. In 1975, DeMarch (109) compared the course of 120 pregnant patients who had pulmonary tuberculosis with 108 nonpregnant tuberculosis patients. All were treated with standard antituberculosis medications. No greater number of relapses occurred in the pregnant group than in the nonpregnant group. Although noting a comparable frequency of tuberculosis in pregnancy before and after the era of chemotherapy, Schaefer et al. (110) reported fewer than 1% having deterioration of tuberculosis in the post-chemotherapy age compared with a 3% to 4% worsening before chemotherapy. Reactivation of preexisting inactive tuberculosis by pregnancy has not been specifically studied. The question is of particular interest when addressing pregnancy in women whose only manifestation of prior tuberculosis infection is a positive purified protein (PPD) skin test, with or without previous isoniazid prophylaxis. Snider stated that pregnancy does not cause activation of inactive tuberculosis (111). Therefore, abortion is not indicated in the treatment of a pregnant woman with tuberculosis. With proper antituberculosis chemotherapy, pregnancy poses no additional hazard to the woman who has tuberculosis.

Effects on Pregnancy

Little reliable data are available on the effects of tuberculosis on pregnancy. Bjerkedal and associates (112) noted an increase in toxemia and vaginal hemorrhage in pregnant women who had tuberculosis. They also reported 20.1 per 100 miscarriages in tuberculosis patients compared with only 2.3 per 100 in pregnant women without tuberculosis. Ratner and colleagues reported increased prematurity in women with tuberculosis (113). Increased congenital malformations were noted by Varpela in tubercular women receiving antituberculosis medications compared with pregnant women not receiving such therapy (114). In 1975, Schaefer and colleagues stated that at present the probability of a tuberculous mother giving birth to a normal healthy infant is excellent (110). They could find no evidence to support the presumption of fetal wastage, prematurity, or medical complications of pregnancy in their patients who had tuberculosis. Jana and colleagues observed a twofold increase in adverse perinatal problems and a sixfold increase in perinatal mortality in pregnant women with active tuberculosis (111). Nevertheless, whereas maternal tuberculosis confers a high-risk status on pregnancy, Schaefer's statement is still the current view in the United States.

Clinical Presentation and Diagnosis

The diagnosis of pulmonary tuberculosis depends on the demonstration of tubercle bacilli in body fluid smears, cultures, or tissues. Several clinical procedures are extremely helpful in leading to the correct diagnosis, beginning with the history and physical examination. Most young patients with tuberculosis are asymptomatic at presentation. In most patients, the diagnosis is suggested by a positive tuberculin skin test or abnormal chest radiograph. When symptomatic, as with other pulmonary infections, fever, diaphoresis, malaise, anorexia, weight loss, cough, and chest pain are common. Occasionally, hemoptysis is the first presenting symptom. Physical examination is often normal. In chronically ill patients, especially those with underlying immunosuppressed states, the patient may be debilitated and febrile. Cervical lymphadenopathy and hepatosplenomegaly may be present in disseminated disease. Posttussic upper-lobe rales or pleural effusions may be detected. When chest radiographs are normal in patients who have a positive tuberculin skin test, the patient is a candidate for prophylactic therapy with isoniazid (INH). Patients with active tuberculosis almost always have an abnormal chest radiograph, usually characterized by upper zone infiltrations and cavities. These patients require multidrug antituberculosis therapy. Rarely, usually in immunosuppressed patients, the diagnosis of tuberculosis is made from specimens obtained from an extrathoracic source, such as peripheral lymph node. Pulmonary tuberculosis in these patients often presents with an atypical chest radiographic presentation.

Because most asymptomatic patients who have tuberculosis can be detected by routine chest radiography or tuberculin skin test, these two procedures being done in pregnancy have been the focus of special attention and discussion. Studies have shown depression of cell-mediated immunity in pregnancy (115,116). It has been proposed that lymphocyte unresponsiveness protects the embryo from rejection by the pregnant woman's immunologic system. Rocklin and colleagues (117) demonstrated a deficiency of factors that inhibit lymphocyte function in patients who experience repeated miscarriages. Although it is true that a lymphocyte depression factor has been shown to increase and lymphocyte response to PPD is depressed in pregnancy, PPD skin sensitivity appears to remain intact, at least during the first trimester (118). Of 1,420 pregnant women, 172 (12.2%) were noted to be tuberculin positive by Covelli and Wilson (115), an incidence about the same as that of the nonpreganant young population in the United States. Present and Comstock noted similar results (119). A positive tuberculin skin test does not indicate the presence of active tuberculosis. It is evidence of infection with the tubercle bacillus and that the immunologic system is recalling that encounter, past or present. Indeed, of the 172 women with a positive PPD in the series reported by Covelli and Wilson, only one had active tuberculosis (115). The enormous value of the PPD rests on its incomparable ability to identify persons who require additional surveillance. Carter and Mates reported that pregnant women with tuberculosis are usually asymptomatic, and their diagnosis is first suspected by a positive Mantoux tuberculin skin test (120). The Tine test is a less sensitive indicator of tuberculin sensitivity. All pregnant women should therefore have a tuberculin skin test, preferably PPD 5 TU, performed during the first trimester of pregnancy, unless they are known to have a previous positive PPD or active tuberculosis. In the occasional patient who presents with a clinical picture suggesting active tuberculosis, skin testing should be performed initially with PPD 1 TU. The tuberculin test is performed by intracutaneous injection of 0.1 mL of the test suspension (usually 5 TU) into the volar surface of the forearm. Although there are no specific guidelines for reading the tuberculin test in pregnant women, the occurrence of the AIDS epidemic and recognition of other diseases that blunt immunologic responses have led to complicated standards for declaring a PPD as positive. All are based on the size of induration, not erythema, arising 48 to 72 hours after injection. The American Thoracic Society and the CDC recommend a positive reading as greater than 5-mm induration in high- risk groups (e.g., HIV-positive patients), greater than 10 mm in moderate-risk groups (e.g., patients who have diabetes mellitus), and greater than 15 mm in low-risk groups (121). Because pregnancy may depress tuberculin sensitivity, it would appear prudent to initiate confirmatory studies for the presence of active tuberculosis when a pregnant woman exhibits greater than 5-mm induration at a PPD site (122).

The second major case-finding tool in tuberculosis is chest radiography. Because of fear of radiation, the use of chest radiography in pregnancy has been controversial. Importantly, a routine 6-foot posterior-anterior chest radiograph gives only 50 mrads to the target, far less than the dose thought to be hazardous to the fetus when given directly to the uterus. It is appropriate to assume that chest radiography in pregnancy is safe, especially when the maternal abdomen is shielded (123). Recognizing the safety of a chest radiograph, many have questioned its utility in pregnancy. Bonebrake et al. (124), in a study of 11,725 consecutive prenatal chest roentgenograms, found only one patient who had tuberculosis, and it was inactive. In a similar investigation of 5,422 pregnant women, Hadlock et al. (125) encountered 19 patients who had tuberculosis, three suspected on the basis of history and physical examination, and only two who had active tuberculosis. It can be concluded that routine prenatal chest radiographs are not indicated, not because of danger to the fetus, but because they are nonproductive and not cost-effective. Far more effective surveillance is achieved through prenatal routine PPD skin testing. In the event of a positive PPD in which recent conversion is suspected, previous status of PPD sensitivity is unknown, or the patient has symptoms or signs suggestive of tuberculosis, a chest radiograph is indicated.

The diagnosis of active tuberculosis is not established by a tuberculin skin test or chest radiograph. Whereas a chest radiograph that exhibits an upper lobe cavity strongly suggests the presence of active tuberculosis, activity should be proved by the demonstration of tubercle bacilli in sputum, organ aspirates, or tissues, either by smear or culture of *Mycobacterium tuberculosis*. If sputum cannot be obtained spontaneously, inhalation of superheated water may induce an adequate specimen. Occasionally, the patient's clinical status does not allow the 8-week delay required for growth of tubercle bacilli on culture media. In that event, fiberoptic bronchoscopy can be performed with safety, and biopsy smears and culture material can be obtained directly from the area of radiographic abnormality (126). In smear-negative patients with a strong suspicion for active tuberculosis, several new techniques are available for rapid diagnosis. These involve new rapid culture media or the identification of *M. tuberculosis* DNA by polymerase chain reaction (126,127). It must be remembered that atypical mycobacteria (usually *M. avium-intracellulare* complex) are causing lung disease in increasing numbers of patients. Most of these patients are in an older age group, often with underlying lung or systemic disease. Therefore, a positive smear for acid-fast bacilli is presumptive evidence of tuberculosis but always should be confirmed by culture of *Mycobacterium tuberculosis*.

Treatment

Treatment of tuberculosis is divided into therapy of the patient who has clinically active tuberculosis and those with a positive tuberculin skin test with no evidence of active tuberculosis.

Patients with Clinically Active Tuberculosis

Previously, strains of *M. tuberculosis* resistant to antituberculosis drugs were relatively uncommon in the United States, and a salutary outcome with appropriate treatment for tuberculosis was expected. With the advent of increasing numbers of patients with MDR tuberculosis, therapy has changed significantly, and the prognosis for cure in some high-risk groups has worsened. The general increase in the prevalence of tuberculosis in patients with HIV infection and immigrants from countries with a high frequency of tuberculosis and limited treatment facilities has been paralleled by an increase in the presence of MDR organisms in these high-risk groups. MDR tuberculosis is defined as resistance to isoniazid (INH) or rifampin (RIF). Therefore, in considering treatment for tuberculosis, one must ensure that sensitivity studies are performed on the culture-isolated tubercle bacillus, that four-drug therapy is administered to patients at high risk for MDR tuberculosis (e.g., health care workers), and that the patient complies with the treatment regimen. The recent downward trend in tuberculosis and MDR tuberculosis is attributable to the strict adherence to these guidelines. Directly observed therapy (DOT) may be necessary to ensure compliance with treatment regimens. There is no unanimity of opinion about the number of drugs, the frequency of administration, and the length of therapy. The CDC recommends that pregnant women should receive at least INH 10 to 30 mg per kilogram daily (usually 300 mg four times daily), RIF 600 mg daily, and ethambutol (EMB) 25 mg per kilogram daily. Most authorities continue treatment for 9 months, although some will stop EMB after 2 months if drug sensitivity studies fail to show resistance to INH or RIF. In high-risk groups and in nonpregnant tuberculous patients in cities with a high frequency of MDR (New York, Miami, Houston, Los Angeles, San Francisco) a four-drug regimen incorporating pyrazinamide (PZA) 250 mg four times daily is the rule. PZA is not routinely prescribed for pregnant women because of lack of data concerning teratogenicity. When indicated, PZA has been used safely around the world and in the United States in pregnant and nonpregnant patients. Streptomycin is the fifth first-line drug for the treatment of tuberculosis; however, it must be given by intramuscular injection and has major toxicity for the eighth cranial nerve, leading to deafness or vestibular dysfunction. Most importantly, there are numerous reports of fetal eighth-nerve damage when the pregnant woman is given streptomycin. Therefore, streptomycin is given in pregnancy only in life-threatening circumstances (128).

Drug toxicity is common in patients receiving antituberculosis medications. Understandably, as the number of medications increases, the frequency of complications rises. INH may cause a chemical hepatitis and must be monitored by measurement of serum alanine aminotransferase (ALT), aspartate aminotransferase (AST), and bilirubin levels. Central nervous system symptoms and peripheral neuropathies may occur and can be prevented by the simultaneous administration of pyridoxine, 50 mg daily. RIF also may cause hepatitis, mandating monitoring blood tests. Liver toxicity for INH and RIF is more common in patients with prior liver disease. Prescription of these medications is another strong reason for interdicting alcoholic beverages during pregnancy. Rarely, both INH and RIF may cause pancytopenia. RIF may turn bodily fluids orange, and patients should be warned about this discoloration of their tears and urine. EMB may cause optic neuritis and requires an ophthalmologic examination every 6 months. PZA may cause hepatotoxicity, but it does not increase liver disease in patients receiving INH or RIF. PZA may raise serum uric acid levels and cause gout.

Several newer and infrequently used older medications are available to treat tuberculosis. These medications include clarithromycin, azithromycin, clofazamine, rifambutin, ofloxacin, and other more toxic medications such as ethionamide, cycloserine, kanamycin, amikacin, and capreomycin. Their selection should be based on intolerance to one of the four first-line therapeutic drugs and sensitivity studies.

Patients Who Have a Positive Tuberculin Skin Test and No Clinically Active Tuberculosis

In the course of practice, the obstetrician is more likely to encounter patients who have positive tuberculin skin tests (PPD 5 TU) and no evidence of active tuberculosis than patients who have clinically active pulmonary or extrapulmonary disease. Every person with a positive PPD 5 TU is at some risk to develop clinically active tuberculosis. The rate of progression depends on the clinical setting. Active tuberculosis occurs at the rate of 5% per year in the following patients, and these nonpregnant patients should receive prophylactic isoniazid (300 mg daily) for 9 months to 1 year.

1. Recent converters from a negative to a positive PPD 5 TU skin test, regardless of age, with a normal chest radiograph
2. Positive PPD 5 TU skin test in a person younger than 35 years of age with a normal chest radiograph
3. Close contacts, household members, and newborns of a patient who has active tuberculosis
4. Persons with a positive PPD 5 TU skin test and chest radiographic evidence of healed pulmonary tuberculosis with negative bacteriology
5. Persons with a positive tuberculin skin test and a disease or clinical state with a high prevalence for tuberculosis (e.g., AIDS, diabetes mellitus, corticosteroid or immunosuppressive therapy, and subtotal gastrectomy)

Whether such prophylaxis should be given during pregnancy is debatable. Some authorities have stated that a pregnant patient falling into any of the aforementioned categories should receive prophylactic INH during pregnancy. Others contend that prophylaxis can await termination of the pregnancy. Even though evidence for tetragenicity of INH is weak and the drug usually is well tolerated in young patients, it may be prudent to delay prophylactic INH at least until completion of the first trimester of pregnancy in patients who belong to one of the high risk groups (129,130)

Suggested Regimen for Treatment of Pregnant Women (131,132)

1. Patients with smear- or culture-positive active tuberculosis in low-risk populations use INH, RIF, EMB, and pyridoxine for 9 months; add PZA in high-risk areas.
2. Patient with positive PPD 5 TU and abnormal chest radiograph, but negative smear and cultures for acid-fast bacilli:
   a. If chest radiograph suggests activity (e.g., cavity) use INH, RIF, EMB, and pyridoxine for 9 months.
   b. If chest radiograph suggests healed disease (calcified lymph nodes or calcified parenchymal lesions), observe, treat appropriately after pregnancy, or treat with prophylactic INH and pyridoxine for 9 months, beginning in the second trimester of pregnancy;
3. Patients with recent conversion to a positive PPD 5 TU skin test and normal chest radiograph and negative bacteriology, observe during pregnancy and treat appropriately after pregnancy or treat prophylactic INH and pyridoxine for 9 months, beginning in the second trimester of pregnancy.

4. Patients with resistant organisms, INH, RIF, EMB, and PZA, alter according to sensitivity studies;
5. In patients unable to tolerate INH or RIF, use of EMB or other available drugs of unproven fetal safety may be necessary (Table 14-3).

Bacillus of Calmette and Guerin (BCG) vaccination for control of tuberculosis

Bacillus of Calmette and Guerin (BCG) vaccination for the prevention of clinical tuberculosis has been the rule in Europe and most of the developed countries of Asia, Africa, and South America for decades; however, the routine use of BCG vaccination has never been recommended in the United States. Because of the unique value of the tuberculin skin test in the diagnosis of tuberculosis in 1988, the Practice Advisory Committee and the Advisory Committee for the Elimination of Tuberculosis recommended BCG vaccine only for uninfected children who are at high risk for infection. Because of the resurgence of tuberculosis, these two groups reviewed the use of BCG vaccine again, especially for children and health care workers. They concluded that BCG vaccination should be considered for infants and children who reside in settings in which the likelihood of *M. tuberculosis* transmission and subsequent infection is high, provided no other measures can be implemented (e.g., removing the child from the source of infection). They also concluded that BCG vaccination may be considered for high-risk health care workers. In the United States, BCG vaccination is rarely indicated (133).

Effect of Antituberculous Medication on the Fetus

Isoniazid crosses the placental barrier, and neonatal seizures have been reported, but these may be prevented by the addition of pyridoxine. Snider et al. (134) reported that only slightly more than 1% of the infants and fetuses of 1,480 pregnant patient receiving INH were abnormal. It is concluded that INH is the most effective and safest of the antituberculous drugs in pregnancy. No birth defects have been linked to its use. No large series has attained statistical significance regarding RIF and fetal toxicity. Fetal limb reduction has been reported in one of 150 pregnancies of mothers who received RIF compared with one of 435 pregnancies in which the mother was taking other antituberculous medications (135). Because of the small number of subjects studied, however, no conclusions can be drawn, and RIF remains a mainstay of treatment for tuberculosis in

TABLE 14-3. *Antituberculosis drugs and adverse and teratogenic effects*

Drug	Usual adult dosage and route of administration	Adverse effect of drug in host	Teratogenic effects	Comments
Isoniazid	300 mg/d orally	Gastrointestinal disturbance, peripheral neuropathy, hepatitis	Not teratogenic but may be embryocidal in rabbits and rats	Crosses placenta and found in breast milk Nursing infants have been reported pyridoxine response seizures
Rifampin	600 mg/d orally	Gastrointestinal disturbance, headache, rarely hepatitis	Rodents; spina bifida and cleft palates	Crosses placenta, alleged to interfere with contraceptive agents
Ethambutol	25 mg/kg for 1 mo, then 10–15 mg/kg/d orally	Decreased visual acuity (optic neuritis)	Rats—decreased fertility; mice—cleft palate and exencephaly; rabbits: monophthalmia	No human teratogenic effects recommended for children <1 difficulty in testing visual acuity
Pyrazinamide	20–35 mg/kg/d orally	Hepatic toxicity, hyperuricemia	Unknown	
Streptomycin	0.75; 1 daily for 14–21 days, then 1 g 3 times per wk, i.m.	Otoxicity (vestibular and cochlear), headache, pain at site of injection, rare nephrotoxicity	Unknown	Crosses placenta and associated with ototoxicity in newborns
Capreomycin	0.75–1 g/d for 60–120 d, then 1 g 3 times per wk, i.m.	Nephrotoxicity and ototoxicity	"Wavy ribs" in litter of female rats	Possibly crosses placenta and is associated with ototoxicity in newborn
Kanamycin	15 mg/kg 3–5 times per wk, i.m.	Otoxicity (auditory), nephrotoxicity	Unknown	Variable cross-resistance with and viomycin
Ethionamide	0.5–1 g/d in divided doses orally	Gastrointestinal disturbances, hepatitis, optic and peripheral neuritis	Teratogenic effects in rabbits and rats	Side effects similar to those of isoniazid
Cycloserine	250 mg twice a day, not to exceed 1 g/d orally	Central nervous system; psychoses, drowsiness, headache, convulsions	Unknown	Toxicity usually related to high blood levels

i.m., intramuscularly.

From Goode JT, Iseman MD, Davidson PT, et al: Tuberculosis in association with pregnancy. Am J Obstet Gynecol 140:492–498, 1981.

pregnant women. EMB is teratogenic in laboratory animals. Snider cited its extensive use in pregnancy without fetal damage, however, and it is proving a valuable drug in the age of MDR tuberculosis. Streptomycin toxicity has been reported regularly in fetuses and in the newborns of women who take this medication. The toxicity is not related to the stage of pregnancy, however, and streptomycin remains hazardous to the fetus throughout gestation (134). Streptomycin should be used only in the rare instance in which no other first-line drug is available. A list of the commonly used antituberculous medications and their potential toxicities is presented in Table 14-3.

Treatment of the Newborn

Fortunately, congenital tuberculosis is rare. When it does occur, however, the outcome often is disastrous (136). Congenital tuberculosis occurs when the fetus becomes infected with *M. tuberculosis in utero*. In the fetus, the disease usually is disseminated with lung, liver, spleen, lymph node, and kidney involvement (137–139). Three avenues for infections have been suggested: fetal ingestion of infected amniotic fluid, fetal aspiration of amniotic fluid, and infection with dissemination through the umbilical vein. The infant usually is premature, but signs of infection may not appear until weeks after delivery. The child may exhibit fever, malaise, irritability, hepatosplenomegaly, and tachypnea. A few cases of fetal tuberculous otitis with mastoiditis have been reported. With rapid, prompt diagnosis, therapy is lifesaving in approximately 50% of afflicted infants. The mother may appear well, and her infection may go undetected until after delivery (140). This rare, devastating form of tuberculosis strongly buttresses the necessity for careful tuberculosis screening of pregnant women with skin tests and chest radiographs when the tuberculin skin test is positive, for INH prophylaxis, and for therapy of clinically active tuberculosis during pregnancy. The diagnosis of congenital tuberculosis requires the presence of a proven tuberculous lesion, usually in the liver, in a newborn infant with tuberculosis infection of the placenta or maternal genitalia and no evidence of postnatal contact with tuberculosis. Mortality is high, and treatment for the infant is four antituberculous drugs (136).

Kendig (141) noted that among 75 infants born to women who had active tuberculosis, 38 infants became infected and three died. In contrast, among 30 infants of mothers who had active tuberculosis and the newborn was given BCG postpartum, no infant contracted tuberculosis. Kendig strongly recommended that infants of mothers who have active tuberculosis be given BCG vaccination immediately postpartum. The infants should be isolated from the mothers until the infants' PPD skin test has become positive or the mother has been treated and is no longer infectious. Good et al. (142) pointed out that none of the infants in Kendig's series was given INH prophylaxis. Treatment of the infant with INH is an alternative to BCG, but when there is reason to suspect that the infant will not receive the required INH therapy, BCG should be administered. Raucher and Gribetz (143) suggested that a mother who has tuberculosis of unknown activity should be separated from her neonate until it is determined that she is no longer contagious or that she has been receiving adequate therapy for tuberculosis. They advise observation of the newborn with repeated tuberculin skin testing before instituting prophylactic or therapeutic antituberculous therapy for the child. Although no large studies on the effects of antituberculous medication on breast-fed infants exist, the milk levels of medication appear to be too low to affect the infant adversely (144).

In our current age of excellent antituberculous chemotherapy, tuberculosis carries no additional risk to the pregnant woman, because appropriate antituberculous therapy can be administered to pregnant women without fear of major fetal toxicity. Infants born to women who have active tuberculosis should be isolated from the mothers until the disease no longer is infectious, and the infants should receive BCG vaccination, or prophylactic isoniazid if their tuberculin skin tests become positive.

SARCOIDOSIS

Sarcoidosis is a multiorgan disease characterized by noncaseating epithelioid granulomas with no histologic, bacteriologic, or historical evidence of a known etiologic granulomagenic agent in a patient with a compatible clinical picture. Sarcoidosis occurs most frequently in the 20- to 40-year age group. Although there is a propensity for sarcoidosis in black Americans, sarcoidosis occurs in all races (145). Because sarcoidosis occurs most frequently in childbearing age, pregnancy is common in patients with it.

For most patients, sarcoidosis pursues a benign course with little functional impairment. The most common presentation is an abnormal chest radiograph performed for reasons unrelated to the disease, for example, routine medical examination, preoperative or preemployment examinations, or major insurance policy application. The most frequently afflicted organs are hilar and mediastinal lymph nodes, lungs, eyes, skin, peripheral lymph nodes, and lacrimal and parotid glands (146). Sarcoidosis may significantly affect any organ, however. Pulmonary, neurologic, and cardiac sarcoidosis may be especially disabling and difficult to treat. Whereas most patients have no symptoms, when present, the most prevalent complaints are dyspnea and cough; blurred vision, photophobia, and eye pain resulting from uveitis; swollen lacrimal and salivary glands; and enlarged peripheral lymph nodes. Skin lesions are common and range from nonspecific erythema nodosum, which is a nongranulomatous marker of the acute onset of sarcoidosis, to granulomatous lesions presenting in any location. Lupus pernio is a particularly disfiguring nasal skin lesion that is unique to sarcoidosis. Sarcoidal granulomas may elaborate a precursor of vitamin D, resulting in increased calcium absorption from the intestines, hypercalciuria, hypercalcemia, and nephrolithiasis. Liver and splenic enlargement are common and may cause disabling symptoms. Cardiac sarcoidosis occurs in two major patterns. The most common is tachyarrhythmias or bradyarrhythmias. Heart block with syncope or sudden death may occur in otherwise apparently healthy young patients. Sarcoidal cardiomyopathy with chronic congestive heart failure is rare in most of the Western world but is common in Japan. Neurologic sarcoidosis may present in an almost infinite variety of manifestations. The most common is a peripheral VIIth nerve palsy; however, all the cranial nerves may be affected. Peripheral neuropathy, myopathy, and myositis may occur. Brain and spinal cord sarcoidosis can exhibit the entire gamut of central nervous system clinical syndromes, including leptomeningeal manifestations, leukoencephalopathy, cerebral masses, seizures, pituitary dysfunction, and paralysis. Bone and joint sarcoidosis are granulomatous manifestations of chronic sarcoidosis and almost always are accompanied by skin lesions.

The diagnosis of sarcoidosis is established in most patients by the demonstration of noncaseating epithelioid granulomas with negative stains, smears, and cultures for acid-fast bacilli and fungi in a patient with a compatible clinical picture. The latter clause is essential because the histologic appearance of sarcoidosis is nonspecific and the presence of granulomas involving a single organ, in the absence of additional clinical evidence of sarcoidosis, does not establish the diagnosis. Validated Kveim-Siltzbach (KS) test suspensions are available in most of the world but rarely in the United States. Using validated antigen, a positive KS test is diagnostic of sarcoidosis (147). Tissue biopsy sites depend on the clinical presentation. Bronchoscopy, lymph node, and skin biopsies are the most common diagnostic procedures. Any involved tissue may yield confirmatory histology, however, for example, conjunctiva, lacrimal gland, liver, spleen, and bone marrow.

The typical chest radiograph of sarcoidosis exhibits well- recognized patterns: bilateral hilar and right paratracheal lymph node enlargement and clear lung fields (stage I); hilar lymph node enlargement with pulmonary infiltrations (stage II); pulmonary infiltrations with no adenopathy (stage III); evidence of pulmonary fibrosis such as retraction of the hilar areas, bullous transformation, linear streaks, and tented diaphragm (stage IV). A normal chest radiograph in a patient with extrathoracic sarcoidosis is stage 0 (146).

Despite the presence of an abnormal chest radiograph, most patients with sarcoidosis have little pulmonary dysfunction. In the dyspneic patient, the most common pattern of dysfunction is restrictive, with decreased lung volumes, vital capacity (FVC), and forced expiratory volume in one second (FEV_1). The single-breath diffusing capacity is often diminished. When pulmonary fibrosis complicates sarcoidosis, the chest radiograph is usually stage IV, and evidence of obstructive dysfunction supervenes. The ratio of FEV_1/FVC decreases and the patient's dyspnea may be accompanied by cough and wheezing (148).

Most patients with pulmonary sarcoidosis require no therapy. Most will experience a spontaneous cure or will remain asymptomatic with a persisting abnormal chest radiograph. Indeed, a minority of patients with sarcoidosis require therapy. Anterior uveitis, central nervous system involvement, cardiac sarcoidosis, hypercalcemia, and progressive pulmonary dysfunction are absolute indications for therapy. Lesser degrees of involvement that do not threaten to produce organ failure are relative indications for treatment (e.g., cutaneous granulomas, enlarged peripheral lymph nodes and lacrimal and parotid glands, liver enlargement with abnormal liver chemistries, and splenomegaly with pancytopenia. The most effective medication for the treatment of sarcoidosis is prednisone, usually 30 to 40 mg daily. Central nervous system disease and cardiac sarcoidosis usually require larger doses, up to 80 mg daily, for longer periods. In most patients, the course of treatment is 6 to 18 months. Relapse after discontinuation of prednisone occurs in approximately 25% of patients. In some patients, treatment is required for several years. Hydroxychloroquine or chloroquine and methotrexate have attained recognition as second-line medications for patients who have relative indications for therapy, for example, disfiguring skin lesions. They may be substituted for prednisone in patients with contraindications for steroid therapy or in patients whose sarcoidosis requires prolonged treatment. Cyclophosphamide, azathioprine, colchicine, cyclosporine, radiotherapy and a variety of other cytotoxic or immunosuppressive agents have been administered to patients with sarcoidosis, with varying degrees of success (149); however, prednisone is the only medication approved for treatment of sarcoidosis during pregnancy.

There are several reports of the effects of sarcoidosis in pregnancy and the effects of pregnancy on sarcoidosis. There appears to be no effect of sarcoidosis on fertility. One of Siltzbach's patients had nine pregnancies in 10 years (150). O'Leary reported 28 pregnancies in 23 patients (151) and found no maternal deaths, two neonatal deaths, and one premature birth. One patient with sickle cell disease had premature separation of the placenta. There were no toxemias. He concluded that no special management of labor was required. Thirteen sarcoidosis patients reported by de Regt experienced no negative effect on pregnancy (152). Two premature deliveries and one stillbirth were reported by Mayock and colleagues in ten sarcoidosis patients (153). Three fetal abnormalities occurred in this group. In a review of 52 pregnancies in 35 patients with sarcoidosis, Given and DiBenedetto reported two spontaneous abortions, one premature delivery, and one antepartum death of a 34-week-gestation infant (154). Three patients had a hysterotomy to interrupt pregnancy. They also reported a single sarcoidosis patient who developed preeclampsia during the seventh month of pregnancy who died from cardiorespiratory failure resulting from severe pulmonary sarcoidosis and eclampsia.

The effect of pregnancy on sarcoidosis has been reported to be variable, and most patients tolerate pregnancy well; however, several patients have suffered life-threatening worsening of sarcoidosis during pregnancy and a few have died. Mayrock and colleagues noted improvement in sarcoidosis during pregnancy in eight of ten patients (153) and concluded that pregnancy has a beneficial effect on sarcoidosis. In four of these patients, sarcoidosis relapsed within 4 months of delivery. Most of O'Leary's 23 patients experienced no change in their sarcoidosis during pregnancy, whereas five improved (151). In another study, six of 18 patients had improved sarcoidosis during pregnancy (155). It has been proposed that improvement in sarcoidosis during pregnancy may be related to increased levels of circulating corticosteroid hormones during gestation; however, there are several reports of worsening of respiratory function during pregnancy in patients with pulmonary sarcoidosis, and most of these patients responded to increased adrenocorticosteroid steroid therapy. Grossman and Littner reported a patient with hemoptysis, dyspnea, and rapidly progressive restrictive pulmonary dysfunction (156) who responded to steroid therapy and promptly improved after delivery. A similar patient was reported by Reisfeld and colleagues (157) who presented at term with dyspnea. She had been taking prednisone, but this medication was discontinued. Her course was complicated by pneumonia, and she suffered rapidly progressive cardiopulmonary failure. There was dramatic improvement after induced delivery. The patient reported by Given and DiBenedetto who had sarcoidosis and preeclampsia was the first pregnancy-related death attributable to respiratory failure (154). De Regt reported two deaths, one complicated by lung abscesses and the other with hemoptysis (152). Seballos et al. reported a patient who developed acute postpartum cardiomyopathy thought at first to be due to peripartum cardiomyopathy (158); however, endomyocardial and bronchoscopic biopsies revealed granulomas, and autopsy 16 months later confirmed the diagnosis of sarcoidosis.

Whereas sarcoidosis is not a contraindication to pregnancy, and even patients with severe pulmonary sarcoidosis have successfully completed pregnancy, many young women with sarcoidosis present with severe pulmonary dysfunction. The physician cannot assume that these patients will have an uncomplicated course, especially during the last trimester, when the normal hypervolemia of pregnancy imposes an additional burden on patients with diminished respiratory function and, occasionally, myocardial dysfunction. All pregnant patients with sarcoidosis should have complete pulmonary function evaluation performed, particularly as they approach term. Adrenocorticosteroid therapy should be administered if there is significant worsening of pulmonary function. The obstetrician and anesthesiologist must be aware that the patient has diminished cardiopulmonary reserve. Judicious management of fluid balance, use of oxygen, and shortening of labor are indicated.

CYSTIC FIBROSIS

Serious concerns beset young women with cystic fibrosis who are contemplating pregnancy. Thirty years ago, pregnancy in these patients was a rare occurrence, as relatively few women with cystic fibrosis reached adulthood. When pregnancy was realized, the incidence of complications was high (159,160). Today, the median survival for persons with cystic fibrosis exceeds 30 years (161) compared with ten years in 1960 (162), and an increasing number of adult women with this disease are having healthy children. The dramatic improvement in survival in cystic fibrosis is attributed to earlier diagnosis and intervention; to better management options, especially antibiotics and nutrition; and to an enhanced appreciation of disease pathophysiology, highlighted by the discovery of the cystic fibrosis gene (163–165). Pregnant patients with cystic fibrosis often have significant underlying pulmonary disease, however, and suffer from malnutrition. The clinician must have a thorough understanding of the disease process and the attendant risks to mother and fetus.

Overview

Cystic fibrosis is the most common genetic disease in the white population with an autosomal recessive pattern of inheritance. Approximately 4% of the white population is heterozygous for the cystic fibrosis gene (166), with an incidence of disease of one in 3,200 live white births. The gene is comparatively rare in black Americans and Asians (166).

Through the use of laborious chromosomal mapping techniques, the gene responsible for cystic fibrosis was discovered in 1989 (163–165) and isolated to a single locus on the long arm of chromosome seven. A deletion of three base pairs (-F508) that would normally encode for a phenylalanine residue results in translation of an abnormal protein, the cystic fibrosis transmembrane conductance regulator (*CFTR*). Roughly 90% and 50% of patients with cystic fibrosis are heterozygous and homozygous for the -F508 mutation, respectively. Other comparatively rare mutations of the *CFTR* gene, of which more than 700 have been identified (167), account for the remainder of cystic fibrosis chromosomal abnormalities.

The discovery of *CFTR* led to an enhanced understanding of the pathogenesis of cystic fibrosis. A membrane glycoprotein that acts as an apical chloride conductance channel with regulatory function, *CFTR* has been linked to the widespread epithelial cell and mucous gland dysfunction that is the hallmark of this disease. The exact mechanism by which *CFTR* exerts deleterious effects in different tissues remains unclear. In respiratory epithelium, mutant *CFTR* is believed to interfere with chloride ion efflux from cells while sodium transport into cells is enhanced. Water is drawn intracellularly, resulting in relative dehydration of the airway lumen, and to the formation of thick, tenacious airway secretions. Ineffective clearance of airway mucus attracts bacteria and inflammatory cells and sets the stage for recurrent respiratory infections and chronic inflammation. Pancreatic insufficiency, especially common in subjects with the -F508 mutation, arises via similar mechanisms, leading to obstruction of exocrine pancreatic ducts. Defects in chloride conductance account for the characteristic elevations in sweat chloride that are diagnostic of the illness.

Cystic fibrosis primarily affects the lungs, sinuses, pancreas, sweat glands, gastrointestinal tract, hepatobiliary system, and reproductive tract. Patients with cystic fibrosis are predisposed to recurrent sinopulmonary infections, pancreatic insufficiency, and male infertility. Less frequently, meconium ileus or meconium ileus equivalent, diabetes mellitus, pancreatitis, cholestatic biliary tract disease, and cirrhosis complicate the clinical picture (166).

Chronic progressive pulmonary disease is the major cause of morbidity and mortality in patients with cystic fibrosis. Recurrent bouts of bronchitis and sinopulmonary infections herald the development of bronchiectasis and pulmonary fibrosis. Thick, inspissated secretions obstruct airways and provide the nidus for bacterial colonization and recurrent infection. Whereas *H. influenzae* and *S. aureus* tend to colonize the airway early, inevitably infection by resistant strains of *Pseudomonas aeruginosa* and occasionally *Burkholderia cepacia* occurs. *Aspergillus* species, mycobacteria, and viruses are also potential airway pathogens. In addition to infection, life-threatening pulmonary complications include massive hemoptysis and pneumothorax. Cor pulmonale is often seen in far advanced cases and portends a poor prognosis.

Chest roentgenographic findings initially may be subtle, with upper lobe involvement and normal-sized or hyperinflated lung fields. With disease progression, the chest radiograph may reveal bronchiectatic changes, peribronchial thickening, bullae, and mucus plugging. Hilar retraction toward the lung apices, hilar adenopathy, fibrosis, and enlargement of the pulmonary arteries are late findings (166).

Pulmonary function abnormalities include airflow obstruction, air trapping, and, in advanced disease, a combined obstructive and restrictive pattern. An FEV_1 of less than 30% of predicted, a pO_2 of less than 55 mm Hg, and a pCO_2 greater than 50 mm Hg are poor prognostic signs and are associated with an estimated 2-year mortality of 50% (168).

Management of bronchopulmonary disease in cystic fibrosis has traditionally included chest physiotherapy, bronchodilators, physical exercise, and intravenous antibiotics for respiratory infections. Aerosolized antibiotics such as tobramycin are used for treatment of airway infection by *P. aeruginosa* (169). Maintenance therapy with nebulized dornase alfa (rh-DNase), an enzyme capable of degrading DNA derived from dead airway leukocytes, is associated with decreased mucus viscoelasticity and improved pulmonary function (170). Ion-channel modifiers including aerosolized amiloride and uridine 5'-triphosphate also favorably alter the rheology of airway secretions and improve mucociliary clearance (171,172). Gene therapy using adenoviral vectors holds promise for the transmission of normal *CFTR* to airway epithelium (173). Recently, patients with mild disease receiving anti-inflammatory therapy with ibuprofen were found to have better preservation of pulmonary function and percent ideal body weight, a delay in the progression of chest roentgenographic findings, and a reduced need for hospitalizations (174). Finally, lung or heart–lung transplantation is a treatment option for patients with end-stage disease (175).

Pancreatic enzyme supplements, fat-soluble vitamins, and a high-calorie, high-protein, non-restricted fat diet are recommended for patients with pancreatic insufficiency. Recognition that malnutrition correlates with poorer survival of children and adolescents and that improved nutrition is associated with a slower decline in pulmonary function (176,177) and enhanced respiratory muscle strength (178) underscores the rationale for meeting the nutritional needs of patients with cystic fibrosis. For a more comprehensive discussion of these management options and cystic fibrosis in general, the reader is directed to recently published reviews (162,166).

Fertility Issues

Men with cystic fibrosis are infertile in more than 95% of cases (179,180). The absence or atresia of embryonic mesonephric derivatives including the vas deferens, seminal vesicles, and body and tail of the epididymis prohibits the passage of spermatozoa from the testes to the urethra (179). It is now recognized that male infertility may be the sole clinical manifestation of cystic fibrosis (181). Some men with long-standing sinopulmonary involvement and pancreatic insufficiency have been found to have normal reproductive anatomy and function, (180) as have persons with comparatively mild disease (182). Consequently, semen analysis is indicated for all men with cystic fibrosis to assess their reproductive potential adequately.

Whether the anatomic derangements seen in the vast majority of men with cystic fibrosis are congenital or secondary to localized inflammation is unclear. A developmental abnormality seems likely given that morphologic changes are restricted to structures of similar embryologic origin. It is also conceivable that lumenal obstruction of mesonephric derivatives by inspissated secretions, analogous to events taking place in other tissues, leads secondarily to focal inflammation and fibrosis (183). In addition, semen analysis in infertile men is characterized by a decrease in the volume of ejaculate, a decrease in fructose concentration, and an increase in acidity, citrate concentration, and acid phosphatase activity (179). The testes are usually normal in appearance, although on cut section the number of spermatozoa is reduced and an increased number of immature forms is seen (179).

Unlike men, the reproductive tract in women with cystic fibrosis is structurally normal. Analysis of cervical mucus, however, reveals certain physicochemical abnormalities. Kopito et al. (184) found that cervical mucus in women with cystic fibrosis is relatively dehydrated and, in dry-weight specimens, has a decreased sodium concentration. These women failed to exhibit the midcycle surge in sodium concentration required to thin cervical mucus and facilitate passage of spermatozoa across the cervical os (184). Whereas these observations may lead one reasonably to conclude that fertility in this population is decreased, the extent to which this is true has not been well studied. In addition, malnutrition and advanced disease are associated with infertility by predisposing to anovulatory cycles and secondary amenorrhea (183). Pregnancy is no longer a rarity in women with cystic fibrosis (183,185–187) and carries significant risks. Sexually active women with cystic fibrosis who do not desire pregnancy warrant counseling regarding contraception. Combination birth control pills are the most reliable and frequently used contraceptive method among women with cystic fibrosis (188). One report of their use in this setting noted deterioration in pulmonary function in two of four women. The authors postulated that the progestogen component might have stimulated a deleterious increase in airway mucus production mediated by goblet cell hyperplasia (189). Other potential adverse effects of birth control medications in patients with cystic fibrosis include exacerbation of preexisting conditions such as diabetes mellitus and malabsorption. Despite these concerns, Fitzpatrick and colleagues (190) followed ten patients who received combination birth control drugs while undergoing serial pulmonary function testing. They failed to observe any major deterioration in lung function over a 6-month period, but they advised periodic monitoring of liver function tests and routine gynecologic examinations given the increased incidence of cholelithiasis, polypoid cervicitis, and *Candida* vaginitis associated with oral contraceptive use (190). Barrier methods of contraception are reasonable alternatives in motivated patients, although compliance may prove troublesome, with reported failure rates twice that of oral contraceptives (190).

Cardiopulmonary and Nutritional Demands Associated with Pregnancy

Normal pregnancy is characterized by multiple physiologic alterations in pulmonary function. Mechanical alteration of the thoracic cage induced by the enlarging uterus results in an elevation of up to 4 cm of the diaphragm and an increase in the transverse diameter of the chest (191). During the latter half of pregnancy, these changes are manifested by a reduction in the expiratory reserve volume, residual volume, and functional residual capacity (FRC) of 18% (191,192). The decrement in FRC may result in airway closure during tidal breathing and could account for the slight increase in the alveolar-arterial gradient noted in the sitting position near term (191). Oxygen consumption also increases by 20% during pregnancy and is associated with a disproportionate 40% increase in minute ventilation. The resultant respiratory alkalosis is presumed secondary to the respiratory stimulant effect of progesterone (192). Although these physiologic adaptations are well tolerated in normal gravidas, pregnant patients with cystic fibrosis are conceivably more susceptible to hypoxemia and pulmonary decompensation as a result of the excessive metabolic burden imposed by the work of breathing in the setting of chronic pulmonary infection and diminished gas-exchange efficiency. Maternal hypoxemia may jeopardize fetal well-being with the associated increased risk of abortion and premature delivery (183).

A number of cardiovascular changes also accompany normal pregnancy. Plasma volume increases by 40% to 50%, beginning at approximately 6 to 8 weeks' gestation. Cardiac output increases by 30% to 50%, especially during the third trimester. During parturition, the cardiac output acutely increases an additional 13% and represents the time of greatest hemodynamic stress (192). Patients who have cystic fibrosis and pulmonary hypertension associated with advanced pulmonary disease are particularly limited in their ability to compensate for the cardiovascular stresses imposed by pregnancy and delivery and are at high risk for developing right ventricular failure and circulatory collapse. The inability of cystic fibrosis patients with cor pulmonale to augment their cardiac output effectively during pregnancy also may compromise uterine blood flow, resulting in fetal hypoxemia (183). Ideally, the normal gravida should gain between 11 and 12 kg during pregnancy to ensure normal fetal growth and development (193). Pregnant patients with cystic fibrosis are often unable to achieve adequate weight gain due to malabsorption, the increased work of breathing, and the catabolic state induced by chronic lung infection.

Outcome of Pregnancy (see Table 14-4)

Early reports of pregnancy in patients who have cystic fibrosis were not encouraging for mother or child. In 1960, Siegel and Siegel reported the first case of pregnancy in a 19-year-old woman with cystic fibrosis who contracted pneumonia during the last few months of pregnancy and died in the early postpartum period (159). The infant was delivered prematurely at 34 weeks with subsequently normal development and normal sweat chloride determinations. Grand and colleagues, in 1966 (160), summarized the outcomes of all known pregnancies in women with cystic fibrosis up to that time, amounting to 13 pregnancies in 10 women. Five women developed progressive pulmonary decompensation during and following pregnancy with two deaths in the early postpartum period. Four of the infants were born prematurely, one stillborn (160). Drawing from this limited experience and that of others (194), Larsen (195) recommended therapeutic abortion for subjects with extensive pulmonary involvement and a vital capacity below 50% predicted. Progressive cor pulmonale, pneumonitis, or hypoxemia were considered indications for termination of pregnancy (195).

In a national survey of 119 cystic fibrosis centers in North America, Cohen and colleagues (185) in 1980 reviewed 129 pregnancies in 100 women with cystic fibrosis. No maternal deaths occurred antepartum, and the postpartum 2-year maternal mortality rate of 18% did not appreciably differ from the 10% to 11% 1-year mortality projected for nonpregnant women with cystic fibrosis of similar age. Maternal morbidity, however, was significant, with congestive heart failure developing in 13% of gravidas and suboptimal weight gain (<10 pounds) in 41% of subjects. Seventy-five percent of pregnancies were completed, with therapeutic abortions performed in 19% of cases. The spontaneous abortion rate of 5% was no greater than that seen in the control population. Preterm delivery (26.8%) correlated with perinatal mortality (11.3%) in 10 of the 11 infant deaths, the incidence of both occurring at rates significantly greater than that observed in unselected pregnancies. Perinatal deaths also were linked to antepartum maternal respiratory compromise and to inadequate maternal weight gain. One infant was born with cystic fibrosis (0.8%), a finding consistent with an autosomal recessive mode of transmission. On the basis of this large series, the authors recommended against pregnancy for women with a Shwachman-Kulczycki (196) or Taussig score (197) less than 80, lower values being associated with serious pulmonary disease based on clinical, radiologic, and pulmonary function criteria (185).

Other investigators also found a significant correlation between maternal pulmonary and nutritional status and pregnancy outcome (186,198,199). In a small series of eight women who completed 11 pregnancies, Palmer and colleagues (199) identified four factors predictive of a favorable outcome for mother and child: a high Shwachman-Kulczycki clinical score, good nutritional status, a nearly normal chest roentgenogram, and well-preserved pulmonary function. In a review from one institution of 38 pregnancies in 25 subjects, Canny and colleagues (186) reported fewer complications than those cited by Cohen et al. (185). The study population had generally mild pulmonary disease with pregravid forced vital capacities of greater than 70% of predicted in 17 of the 26 subjects in whom pulmonary function tests were performed. Consistent with prior reports (185), the mean age at which cystic fibrosis was diagnosed in these pregnant women was significantly higher compared with their nonpregnant counterparts, implying a less severe disease presentation. Preexisting pulmonary hypertension was assumed to be unlikely in this cohort given the absence of significant pregravid hypoxemia, and this finding may have accounted for the observed absence of antepartum cardiac failure. Twelve of the 25 gravidas were pancreatic sufficient, reflecting the overall good nutritional status of the group, and maternal weight gain was appropriate in most cases. A significant decline in pulmonary function was noted when prepartum and postpartum spirometry rates were compared, although this may have reflected disease progression rather than a direct effect of pregnancy (186). The single maternal death in this study occurred 2 years postpartum. In all cases, maternal labor and delivery were well tolerated. With regard to fetal outcome, there was one neonatal death from sepsis. Preterm delivery occurred in only 5.9% of pregnancies, and infant weights were appropriate for gestational age. In two cases, therapeutic abortion was performed on the basis of Larsen's (195) recommendation to terminate pregnancy in cases in which the forced vital capacity falls below 50% of predicted. These women subsequently carried pregnancies successfully to term. The authors suggested that when pulmonary function is significantly compromised but otherwise stable over the long term, pregnancy may successfully proceed to completion (186).

Clearly, milder pulmonary disease and better nutritional status bode well for expectant mothers who have cystic fibrosis. Corroboration comes from the analysis of specific outcome data on pregnancy submitted annually since 1990 by approved centers to the Cystic Fibrosis Foundation. Kotloff and colleagues (183) reviewed the outcomes of 111 pregnancies reported to the Cystic Fibrosis Data Registry in 1990, representing 4% of all women with cystic fibrosis aged 17 to 37 years. Pregnant women were statistically

TABLE 14-4. *Outcome of pregnancy in cystic fibrosis*

Author/ year (ref.)	No. of cases/no. of pregnancies	Maternal pulmonary function	Maternal mortality	Abortion	Preterm delivery (%)	Perinatal mortality	Other
Grand et al. 1966 (160)	10/13	5 of 13 (38%): serious progressive pulmonary decompensation during and following pregnancy	2 of 13 (15%): both died in early postpartum period	None	5/13 (38%)	2 of 13 (15%): one stillborn, one death 20 hours after delivery)	Study consisted of all known pregnancies in women with cystic fibrosis up to that time.
Cohen et al. 1980 (185)	100/129	The 15 women who died within 6 mo of delivery had moderate to severe pulmonary dysfunction and pulmonary infections during pregnancy	15 of 84 (18%) died within 24 mo of delivery; 10 (12%) died within 6 mo	31 (25%): 6 (5%) spontaneous, 25 (19%) therapeutic	26 of 97 (27%)	11 of 97 (11.3%): 6 stillborn, 5 neonatal deaths; 10 of 11 deaths associated with preterm gestation	Maternal dyspnea and cyanosis associated with increased maternal and fetal death; congestive heart failure was seen in 9 (13%) of gravidas. Insufficient maternal weight gain was predictive of prematurity and stillbirth
Corkey et al. 1981 (198)	7/11	Five of 7 patients had a stable gradual decline in pulmonary function followed over several years	None	1 of 11 (9%) therapeutic	None	None	The two patients with a rapid decline in pulmonary function had respiratory problems during pregnancy and were the only two with pancreatic insufficiency
Palmer et al. 1983 (199)	8/11 (only completed pregnancies assessed)	The patients stratified into two groups: Group 1 (5 patients): no maternal deterioration during pregnancy (associated with higher S-K clinical scores, better nutritional status, near normal chest x-ray findings, and preserved pulmonary function) Group 2 (3 patients): maternal deterioration during pregnancy	Two maternal deaths in group 2 within two years postpartum	13 pregnancies not evaluated due to interruption by abortion (2 spontaneous, 11 therapeutic)	Preterm delivery in all 3 group 2 patients.	None	
Canny et al. 1991 (186)	25/38	Mean pregravid pulmonary function in this cohort well preserved	None	4 of 38 (10.5%); 2 therapeutic, 2 spontaneous	2 of 34 (5.9%)	1 of 38 (2.6%); died of sepsis after 31 week gestation.	Cesarean section rate (21%) no higher than in general population
Kotloff et al. 1992 (183)	111 pregnancies	Pregnancy occurred in women with all levels of pulmonary function	None	24 (21.6%) therapeutic	≈25%	N/A	The risk of premature delivery and therapeutic abortion was higher in women with more severe pulmonary dysfunction
Edenborough et al. 1995 (187)	20/22	FEV_1 correlated with maternal survival, maternal weight gain, and birth weight. FVC% correlated with birth weight	4 of 20 (20%); 2 deaths at 1.8 and 3.2 yr postpartum, 2 deaths shortly after delivery	4 of 22 (18%); 3 of 22 (13.6%) therapeutic, 1 of 22 (4.5%) spontaneous	6 of 18 (33%); 5 of 6 delivered by cesarean section	None	Moderately to severely decreased FEV_1 correlated with preterm delivery

S-K, Shwachman-Kulczycki score (see ref. 38); FEV_1, percent predicted forced expiratory volume in 1 sec; FEV_1, forced expiratory volume in one second; FVC%, percent predicted forced vital capacity.

more likely to be of minority extraction, to be diagnosed with cystic fibrosis at a later age, and less likely to have pancreatic insufficiency and diabetes mellitus compared with nonpregnant controls. In contrast, the distribution of pulmonary dysfunction did not differ significantly between the pregnant and nonpregnant groups and was defined as mild (FEV_1 70% of predicted, 37% of pregnant women), moderate (FEV_1 50% to 69% of predicted, 26% of pregnant women), and severe ($FEV_1 < 50\%$ of predicted, 36% of pregnant women) (183). Pregnancy was not biased toward those with mild pulmonary disease but rather was seen in women with all levels of pulmonary impairment. When pregnancy outcomes were stratified, term deliveries were more prevalent in those with mild pulmonary impairment, whereas premature deliveries and therapeutic abortions were skewed toward those with more severe pulmonary dysfunction. The incidence of hospitalizations, home intravenous antibiotic therapy, supplemental oxygen, and supplemental feedings was similar between pregnant and nonpregnant subjects, implying that intensification of therapy for disease-related complications was not altered by pregnancy. No maternal deaths were reported. Overall, 53% of pregnancies were completed, with premature deliveries in one fourth of cases; 30.6% of pregnancies were ongoing. Therapeutic abortions were performed in 21.6% of patients, suggesting to the authors that counseling may have been suboptimal with regard to the advisability of pregnancy and the use of effective contraceptive methods (183). Alternatively, the ability to predict outcomes effectively in these patients may have been inadequate. To this end, prospective studies by the Cystic Fibrosis Data Registry are anticipated that will compare pregnant and nonpregnant cohorts matched for age and disease severity.

In a published series from the United Kingdom, 22 pregnancies in 20 women with cystic fibrosis were reviewed by Edenborough et al. (187). Analysis of pulmonary function revealed a decrease in both the FEV_1 (13%) and FVC (11%) during pregnancy that was almost completely regained in the postpartum period. Live births occurred in 81.8% of pregnancies, one third of which were premature deliveries. The abortion rate was 18.2% (one spontaneous and three therapeutic). In keeping with prior studies, mothers with comparatively mild pulmonary dysfunction tolerated pregnancy well, whereas those with more severe disease fared worse. Specifically, a pregravid FEV_1 of <60% was the best predictor of pregnancy outcome and correlated with preterm delivery, a greater decline in maternal lung function, and maternal mortality. Of the four maternal deaths that occurred within 3.2 years after delivery, all had prepregnancy FEV_1% values of 50% or less. Birth weight correlated with baseline FEV_1% and FVC% but not percent ideal body weight (187).

Respiratory infections during pregnancy in women who have cystic fibrosis are a frequent occurrence and often require multidrug antimicrobial therapy. Between 48% and 65% of pregnant patients have been reported by various investigators to have received systemic antibiotics to manage pulmonary exacerbations (185–186,199). Many antibiotics have uncertain teratogenic potential. Caution regarding their use in the first trimester of pregnancy is warranted (187).

Counseling the Patient with Cystic Fibrosis about Pregnancy

The counseling of women with cystic fibrosis contemplating pregnancy should include a discussion of the potential risks to the mother and child. An understanding of the limitations that presently exist to predict outcomes in any given patient should be emphasized, although certain caveats with respect to risk stratification deserve attention. Significant maternal risk factors can be identified by the presence of comorbidities such as diabetes mellitus and cirrhosis and by pregravid clinical assessment using Shwachman-Kulczycki scoring, pulmonary function testing, arterial blood gas analysis, and estimates of ideal body weight (183). Experience extrapolated from the literature suggests that patients with rapidly progressive pulmonary disease, especially those with coexistent hypoxemia, carry greater risk. The presence of pulmonary hypertension or cor pulmonale should be a strong deterrent to pregnancy. Although it may seem relatively straightforward to endorse pregnancy in women with well-preserved pulmonary function, pancreatic sufficiency, and absence of comorbidities, and equally as prudent to advise against pregnancy in those with disease at the opposite end of the spectrum, for many patients these lines of distinction are obscured, rendering firm recommendations difficult. Indeed, subjects with chronically stable yet severe pulmonary impairment have carried pregnancies successfully to term (186). A rapid decline in pulmonary function over the short term may be more deleterious to pregnancy outcome than the absolute level of pulmonary function as assessed by spirometric parameters. The prospective parents should be made cognizant of the increased risk for preterm delivery, low infant birth weight, and perinatal mortality. Indications regarding the potential need for therapeutic abortion must be discussed (183).

Genetic counseling is warranted for all women who have cystic fibrosis and desire children. At a minimum, all offspring will be carriers of the cystic fibrosis gene. The probability that an infant will be afflicted with cystic fibrosis depends on the carrier state of the father. For a white man with unknown carrier status, the probability of a child being born with cystic fibrosis is approximately 1 in 50. If the father carries the cystic fibrosis gene, the infant's risk of having cystic fibrosis increases to 1 in 2. Genetic testing of the father is therefore advised to assess more accurately the risk of disease transmission. Genetic analysis is sensitive enough to detect 90% of carriers

(188), although rare mutations of the cystic fibrosis gene will go undetected. Should the prospective father test negative by DNA screening, the risk of having a child with cystic fibrosis drops to 1 in 492 (188).

Psychosocial assessment is also an important facet of preconceptional counseling. Pregnancy is undertaken with the realization that the mother has a foreshortened life span and that the rearing of her child may be compromised by failing health. An understanding is essential by the prospective father and other family members that they may need to lend physical and emotional support and assist in the upbringing of the child in the event of declining maternal health. A decision regarding who should raise the child in case of maternal death is also advised.

Management of Pregnancy in Women with Cystic Fibrosis

To minimize the risks imposed by pregnancy, meticulous attention should be given to the expectant mother with cystic fibrosis. Optimally, care should be orchestrated through a multidisciplinary team consisting of an obstetrician specializing in high-risk pregnancy, a pulmonologist, a nutritionist, and a respiratory therapist (183). Maintenance respiratory care, including postural drainage, inhaled bronchodilators, and possibly rotational antibiotics, should be continued throughout pregnancy. Each office visit should include an assessment of respiratory symptoms, objective spirometric measurements of pulmonary function, and pulse oximetry. Pulmonary exacerbations should be suspected when there is an increase in cough or sputum production coupled with a decline in pulmonary function or hypoxemia. With exacerbations, prompt institution of antibiotics directed toward pathogens cultured from the sputum is indicated. Oral antibiotics or home intravenous therapy may suffice in milder cases, although hospitalization is advised for more severe exacerbations that require treatment with multidrug regimens (183). Improvement can be assessed by resolution of symptoms and return of pulmonary function toward pretreatment values (188).

The choice of antibiotics to manage pulmonary infection during pregnancy requires discretion. Beta-lactam antibiotics, including the penicillins and cephalosporins, are relatively safe during pregnancy and are the first-line agents for management of bacterial infections. Aminoglycosides are effective as part of a multidrug regimen to treat resistant pseudomonal infections, but their use must be weighed against the risk of potential fetal ototoxicity. Tetracyclines should be avoided during pregnancy because of their known ability to cause fetal teeth discoloration and abnormal bone growth. The use of trimethoprim/sulfamethoxazole is similarly discouraged, because folic acid antagonists are associated with fetal anomalies and sulfonamides with hyperbilirubinemia in the newborn. Too little information is available to recommend the use of fluoroquinolones during pregnancy (200).

Women should be encouraged to reach 90% of their ideal body weight at the onset of pregnancy, and with each office visit they should have an assessment of their nutritional status by ascertaining caloric intake, monitoring symptoms related to maldigestion or malabsorption, and obtaining objective weight measurements. Given that malabsorption and the use of antibiotics also may predispose to vitamin K deficiency, periodic measurements of the prothrombin time are recommended with parenteral supplementation of vitamin K as required. Adjustment of pancreatic enzymes may be required in some cases. When caloric intake and weight gain are suboptimal, oral nutritional supplements may suffice. In more extreme cases, enteral nasogastric tube feedings may be attempted. This method must be counterbalanced against the increased risk of aspiration that is especially relevant in the latter stages of pregnancy, when intragastric pressure increases as a result of the enlarging uterus (183,188). Continuous enteral feedings rather than bolus feedings are better tolerated. In severe cases of malnutrition, parenteral hyperalimentation may be required (183).

Besides routine maternal-fetal monitoring, pulse oximetry should be used to dictate the need for supplemental oxygen during labor and delivery. In patients with tenuous cardiopulmonary function, invasive hemodynamic monitoring allows for a more precise assessment of right- and left-sided filling pressures. For surgical deliveries, the use of inhaled anesthetic agents that are associated with elevations in pulmonary arterial pressures should be avoided. Similarly, the preoperative administration of anticholinergic agents that may result in drying of respiratory secretions is contraindicated (183).

Summary

As the life span of patients with cystic fibrosis continues to increase, more and more women with this disease are seeking advice regarding pregnancy. Whereas men with cystic fibrosis are infertile in the vast majority of cases, an undefined but significant number of women are fertile and conceiving in increasing numbers. Review of the literature suggests that women with better underlying cardiopulmonary and nutritional status tolerate pregnancy well; however, the absence of large prospective studies precludes the ability to predict pregnancy outcomes for many of these patients with any degree of certainty. Advice regarding the use of contraceptive methods should be offered to all women of childbearing years who have cystic fibrosis. Preconceptional counseling should seek to educate the prospective parents of the maternal and fetal risks, and recommendations should be based on clinical and pulmonary function criteria. Management of the gravida with cystic fibrosis requires close observation with periodic assessments of pulmonary function and nutritional status. Firmer recommendations regarding the advisability of pregnancy and management of expectant mothers with cystic fibrosis will be forthcoming as prospective data are compiled by the Cystic Fibrosis Data Registry.

PNEUMOTHORAX

Spontaneous pneumothorax occurs almost exclusively in patients younger than 40 years (201). Although it occurs more commonly in men, young women are also susceptible. Hsu et al. published the first report of pneumothorax in pregnancy in 1959 (202). Since that time, several reports have addressed the problems of preexisting lung disease, bilateral and tension pneumothoraces, pneumomediastinum, and therapy during pregnancy. Occasionally, pneumothorax occurs secondary to underlying chronic lung disease (i.e., asthma, pulmonary fibrosis, sarcoidosis, tuberculosis, emphysema). The common spontaneous pneumothorax of young patients is due to apical subpleural blebs that rupture, causing a bronchopleural fistula with no other complicating lung disease. As air accumulates in the pleural space, the lung is compressed. Adhesions to the chest wall may prevent complete collapse. Pneumothoraces are reported by radiologists as a percentage of lung that has been compressed by the intrapleural air. These estimations are quite gross, and therapy should not be based on radiographic evaluations other than the presence of a tension pneumothorax. With continued air leakage and no egress for the air entering the pleural space, the intrapleural pressure may exceed the atmospheric pressure and displace the mediastinum to the contralateral side. Such a tension pneumothorax may become life-threatening because of the compromise of normal expansion of the contralateral lung and, most importantly, because of decreased venous return to the heart.

All degrees of pneumothorax may occur in any stage of pregnancy. Most reported cases occurred at term, during labor, or in the immediate postpartum period (203–206); however, considering the marked elevation of intrathoracic pressure generated during the Valsalva-like maneuvers of the second stage of labor, it is surprising how few episodes of pneumothorax occur at parturition. Several pregnant patients have presented with simultaneous bilateral pneumothoraces (207,208). The most common preexisting lung disease in patients with pneumothorax occurring in pregnancy is a history of previous pneumothorax, usually occurring when the patient is not pregnant. Pneumothorax also may occur with any chronic inflammatory lung disease but rarely in neoplasms.

Most patients with pneumothorax complain of the sudden onset of pleuritic chest pain and dyspnea. The differential diagnosis of chest pain and dyspnea in a young woman is broad. Pneumonia, pulmonary emboli, noninfectious pleuritis, pericarditis, and chest wall trauma must be considered. When the pneumothorax causes greater than 25% collapse of the underlying lung, physical diagnosis should allow early diagnosis. The patient has tachypnea. The affected hemithorax exhibits restricted motion with marked resonance to percussion. Breath sounds and fremitus are markedly diminished on the affected side; however, the patient may be relatively comfortable with mild symptoms present for several days, even with a large pneumothorax. Tension pneumothorax always causes severe chest pain and dyspnea with rapid respiratory and heart rates. When under marked tension, the affected hemithorax may bulge with loss of the intercostal spaces and deviation of the trachea and heart to the contralateral side. With tension pneumothorax, cyanosis and circulatory collapse may ensue (209).

Occasionally, the first sign of pneumothorax is the presence of neck and facial subcutaneous emphysema, which has been reported in pregnancy (210–212) and usually occurs when a small intrapulmonary air space ruptures into a bronchovascular bundle and dissects retrograde to the hilum and mediastinum. A rough sound (Hammond's crunch) synchronous with the heart beat may be heard. Chest radiograph reveals mediastinal and subcutaneous air and a pneumothorax. The pneumothorax may not be visible because of obscuration by the shadows of subcutaneous air. Rarely, no pneumothorax is seen despite the presence of mediastinal air, but computed tomography scan of the chest usually shows a pneumothorax accompanying the pneumomediastinum.

The diagnosis of pneumothorax is confirmed by a single upright position anterior chest radiograph performed with the uterus shielded. An expiratory radiograph may be required. The amount of radiation received by the fetus is well within the limits of safety. Hypoxemia is common in larger pneumothoraces and tension pneumothorax with reductions in arterial PO_2 and lesser reductions in arterial oxygen saturation. Because many patients hyperventilate with chest pain, arterial PCO_2 is often diminished.

Treatment of pneumothorax in pregnancy was reviewed by Van Winter and colleagues (213). Some authors recommend that all pneumothoraces be treated by placement of a surgical chest tube attached to underwater drainage or syringe aspiration of air. Others prefer to tailor the treatment to the clinical state of the patient. Most authorities are content to observe patients with small pneumothoraces (less than 30%) without specific treatment. In most of these patients, the lung will expand spontaneously within 1 to 2 weeks. If the lung does not expand, a chest tube should be placed. Because recurrence of pneumothorax on the ipsilateral or contralateral side occurs in 25% to 30% of all patients after their first spontaneous pneumothorax, treatment often is required to prevent recurrence. The therapies available range from intrapleural instillation of an irritative agent such as doxycipline to thoracotomy with resection of the usual apical pleural blebs and attempts at pleurodesis by mechanical or laser abrasion of the pleura (214). The latter procedure can be accomplished using a thorascope and has been performed successfully during pregnancy with the patient under single lung anesthesia and a muscle relaxant (206,215).

Although spontaneous pneumothorax can be fatal, death occurs almost exclusively in patients with severe underlying lung disease with markedly impaired pulmonary function or tension pneumothorax. This is rare in pregnant women. The major threat of pneumothorax during pregnancy is the effect of hypoxemia on the fetus. The immediate administration of oxygen to the dyspneic and tachypneic pregnant patient and prompt diagnosis and treatment of pneumothorax should obviate fetal damage and wastage. Pneumothorax should have no bearing on the choice of vaginal delivery or cesarean section. Pneumothorax, including recurrent pneumothorax, is not an indication to interrupt pregnancy (209).

ACUTE RESPIRATORY FAILURE

Acute respiratory failure is a clinical state in which gas exchange and delivery of oxygen are no longer adequate to support body function (216). Physiologic correlates may include an increase in dead space (VD/VT), a reduction in compliance, an increase in shunt (Qs/Qt), reduced PaO_2, elevated $PaCO_2$, reduced pH, increased respiratory rate, and increased work of breathing (216). Acute respiratory failure is a significant cause of morbidity and mortality during pregnancy and following delivery (217). Causes of acute respiratory failure in pregnancy are shown in Table 14-5. Aspiration of gastric contents occurs with increased frequency during labor and delivery. Venous air embolism has been associated with normal labor or delivery of patients with placenta previa (218). Signs and symptoms of beta-adrenergic-induced pulmonary edema usually develop within 24 to 48 hours after initiation of therapy (218). Two review articles provide detailed discussions of acute respiratory failure associated with pregnancy (218,219).

Adult Respiratory Distress Syndrome

Many of the entities that cause acute respiratory failure associated with pregnancy do so because of progression to the adult respiratory distress syndrome (ARDS), which is characterized by accumulation of interstitial and alveolar fluid resulting from injury to pulmonary endothelial cells. Cell injury has been attributed to the release of toxic oxygen metabolites and proteinases from activated polymorphonuclear leukocytes and to the toxic effects of other proinflammatory mediators. Numerous predisposing conditions have been associated with ARDS. Those more often associated with pregnancy are listed in Table 14-6. The signs and symptoms of ARDS are nonspecific and include dyspnea, tachypnea, anxiety, tachycardia, and cyanosis. More specific findings include diffuse pulmonary edema pattern on chest roentgenograms, hypoxemia with a need to maintain oxygenation with positive end-expiratory pressure, reduced pulmonary compliance, and an absence of findings of left ventricular dysfunction. Occasionally, the predisposing condition cannot be identified.

Treatment of Acute Respiratory Failure

Treatment of acute respiratory failure is best provided in an intensive care unit under the supervision of a critical care specialist. In general, the overall goals of treatment of acute respiratory failure regardless of cause are to provide ventilatory, hemodynamic, and nutritional support; to treat the underlying disease process; and to prevent iatrogenic complications (218). In addition, the fetus must be provided with adequate oxygenation and protected from potential damaging effects of roentgenographic procedures and medications (218). Endotracheal intubation and mechanical ventilation with supplemental oxygen are required when the PaO_2 cannot be maintained above 65 mm Hg with supplemental oxygen or when arterial blood gases demonstrate acute respiratory acidosis. Intubation and possible mechanical ventilation may be indicated in the presence of hemodynamic or neurologic decompensation. It is recommended that maternal PaO_2 be maintained at a level of 65 mm Hg or greater to provide sufficient oxygen for the fetus (218).

Specific treatment for ARDS is directed toward identifying and treating the underlying cause. There is no specific pharmacologic agent that effectively reverses endothelial cell injury. Therefore, supportive measures are required until acute lung injury resolves. Following initiation of mechanical ventilation, it is necessary to

TABLE 14-5. *Causes of acute respiratory failure in pregnancy*

Adult respiratory distress syndrome (ARDS)
Pneumonia
Amniotic fluid embolism
Pulmonary embolism
Aspiration pneumonia
Severe asthma
Venous air embolism
Pneumothorax
Beta-adrenergic tocolytic therapy

TABLE 14-6. *Predisposing diseases causing adult respiratory distress syndrome*

Pneumonia or sepsis or both
Amniotic fluid embolism
Aspiration pneumonia
Venous air embolism
Multiple blood transfusions
Eclampsia
Abruptio placentae
Dead fetus syndrome

avoid large tidal volumes and high peak airway pressures to decrease the risk of barotrauma. Positive end expiratory pressure is indicated when greater than 50% inspired oxygen is required to achieve a PaO_2 of greater than 65 mm Hg. Positive end-expiratory pressure should be provided in increasing small increments to achieve acceptable oxygenation without significantly reducing cardiac output. Diuresis and fluid restriction should be maintained as dictated by hemodynamic status. Specific agents—including corticosteroids, antioxidants, nitric oxide, eicosanoids, and pentoxifylline—have shown no therapeutic value in controlled studies or have not been sufficiently evaluated (220). The routine use of antibiotics without evidence of infection must be avoided because the practice allows the emergence of antibiotic-resistant organisms that cause nosocomial pneumonias associated with high mortality. The overall outcome of ARDS depends on underlying cause, comorbid conditions, and coexistence of multiorgan system failure.

REFERENCES

1. National Asthma Education Program, National Heart, Lung, and Blood Institute, National Institutes of Health. Report of the working group on asthma and pregnancy: management of asthma during pregnancy. Bethesda, MD: National Institutes of Health. NIH Publication no. 93-3279, 1993.
2. Barnes PJ. New concepts in the pathogenesis of bronchial hyperresponsiveness and asthma. J Allergy Clin Immunol 1989;83:1013–1026.
3. Schaefer G, Silverman F. Pregnancy complicated by asthma. Am J Obstet Gynecol 1961;82:182–191.
4. Gluck JC, Gluck PA. The effects of pregnancy on asthma: a prospective study. Ann Allergy 1976;37:164–168.
5. Williams DA. Asthma and pregnancy. Acta Allergologica 1967;22: 311–323.
6. Jensen K. Pregnancy and allergic diseases. Acta Allergol 1953;6:44–53.
7. Schatz M, Harden K, Forsythe A, et al. The course of asthma during pregnancy, post partum, and with successive pregnancies: a prospective analysis. J Allergy Clin Immunol 1988;81:509–517.
8. Sims CD, Chamberlain GVP, de Swiet M. Lung function tests in bronchial asthma during and after pregnancy. Br J Obstet Gynaecol 1976;83:434–437.
9. Juniper EF, Daniel EE, Roberts RS, Kline PA, Hargreave FE, Newhouse MT. Improvement in airway responsiveness and asthma severity during pregnancy. Am Rev Respir Dis 1989;140:924–931.
10. Gordon M, Niswander KR, Berendes H, Kantor AG. Fetal morbidity following potentially anoxigenic obstetric conditions: bronchial asthma. Am J Obstet Gynecol 1970;106:421–429.
11. Bahna SL, Bjerkedal T. The course and outcome of pregnancy in women with bronchial asthma. Acta Allergol 1972;27:397–406.
12. Fitzsimons R, Greenberger PA, Patterson R. Outcome of pregnancy in women requiring corticosteroids for severe asthma. J Allergy Clin Immunol 1986;78:349–353.
13. Schatz M, Patterson R, Zeitz S, O'Rourke J, Melam H. Corticosteroid therapy for the pregnant asthmatic patient. JAMA 1975;233:804–807.
14. Perlow JH, Montgomery D, Morgan MA, Towers CV, Porto M. Severity of asthma and perinatal outcome. Am J Obstet Gynecol 1992;167:963–967.
15. Stenius-Aarniala B, Piirila P, Teramo K. Asthma and pregnancy: a prospective study of 198 pregnancies. Thorax 1988;43:12–18.
16. Schatz M, Zeiger RS, Hoffman CP, et al. Perinatal outcomes in the pregnancies of asthmatic women: a prospective controlled analysis. Am J Respir Crit Care Med 1995;151:1170–1174.
17. National Asthma Education Program Expert Panel on the Management of Asthma. Guidelines for the diagnosis and management of asthma. J Allergy Clin Immunology 1991;88(part 2):431–534.
18. Hornby PJ, Abrahams TP. Pulmonary pharmacology. Clin Obstet Gynecol 1996;39:17–35.
19. Schatz M, Zeiger RS, Harden KM, et al. The safety of inhaled B-agonist bronchodilators during pregnancy. J Allergy Clin Immunol 1988;82:686–695.
20. Heinonen OP, Slone D, Shapiro S. Drugs affecting the autonomic nervous system. In: Kaufman DW, ed. Birth defects and drugs in pregnancy. Littleton, MA: Publishing Sciences Group, 1977:345–398.
21. McDonald CF, Burdon JGW. Asthma in pregnancy and lactation. Med J Aust 1996;165:485–488.
22. Hankins GDV. Complications of tocolytic therapy. Curr Obstet Med 1983;1:301–325.
23. Brown HM, Storey G, Jackson FA. Beclomethasone dipropionate aerosol in long-term treatment of perennial and seasonal asthma in children and adults: a report of five-and-half years experience in 600 asthmatic patients. Br J Clin Pharmacol 1977;4:259S–267S.
24. Rubin JD, Loffredo C, Correa-Villasenor A, Ferencz C. Prenatal drug use and congenital cardiovascular malformations. Teratology 1991; 43:423A.
25. Dombrowski MP, Bottoms SF, Boike GM, Wald J. Incidence of preeclampsia among asthmatic patients lower with theophylline. Am J Obstet Gynecol 1986;155:265–267.
26. Coutinho EM, Lopes ACV. Inhibition of uterine motility by aminophylline. Am J Obstet Gynecol 1971;110:726–729.
27. Marx GF. Obstetric anesthesia in the presence of medical complications. Clin Obstet Gynecol 1974;17:165–181.
28. Kaunitz AM, Hughes JM, Grimes DA, Smith JC, Rochat RW, Kafrissen ME. Causes of maternal mortality in the United States. Obstet Gynecol 1985;65:605–612.
29. Finland M, Dublin TD. Pneumococcal pneumonias complicating pregnancy and the puerperium. JAMA 1939;112:1027–1032.
30. Hopwood HG. Pneumonia in pregnancy. Obstet Gynecol 1965;25: 875–879.
31. Benedetti TJ, Valle R, Ledger WJ. Antepartum pneumonia during pregnancy. Am J Obstet Gynecol 1982;144:413–417.
32. Madinger NE, Greenspoon JS, Ellrodt AG. Pneumonia during pregnancy: has modern technology improved maternal and fetal outcome? Am J Obstet Gynecol 1989;161:657–662.
33. Berkowitz K, La Sala A. Risk factors associated with the increasing prevalence of pneumonia during pregnancy. Am J Obstet Gynecol 1990;163:981–985.
34. Richey SD, Roberts SW, Ramin KD, Ramin SM, Cunningham SG. Pneumonia complicating pregnancy. Obstet Gynecol 1994;84: 525–528.
35. Weinberger SE, Weiss ST, Cohen WR, Weiss JW, Johnson TS. Pregnancy and the lung. Am Rev Respir Dis 1980;121:559–581.
36. Parisi VM, Creasy RK. Maternal biologic adaptations to pregnancy. In: Reece EA, Hobbins JC, Mahoney MJ, et al., eds. Medicine of the fetus and mother. Philadelphia: JB Lippincott, 1995:831–848.
37. Lederman MM. Cell-mediated immunity and pregnancy. Chest 1884;86:6S–9S.
38. Gehrz RC. Immunology and the host response to viral infection. Clin Obstet Gynecol 1982;25:545–554.
39. Sargent IL, Redman CWG. Immunologic adaptations to pregnancy. In: Reece EA, Hobbins JC, Mahoney MJ, et al., eds. Medicine of the fetus and mother. Philadelphia: JB Lippincott, 1995:25–40.
40. Bland PB. Influenza and its relation to pregnancy and labor. Am J Obstet 1919;79:184–197.
41. Harris JW. Influenza occurring in pregnant women. JAMA 1919;72: 978–980.
42. Kort BA, Cefalo RC, Baker VV. Fatal influenza A pneumonia in pregnancy. Am J Perinatol 1986;3:179–182.
43. Ramphal R, Donnelly WH, Small PA. Fatal influenza pneumonia in pregnancy: failure to demonstrate transplacental transmission of influenza virus. Am J Obstet Gynecol 1980;138:347–348.
44. Kirshon B, Faro S, Zurawin RK, Samo TC, Carpenter RJ. Favorable outcome after treatment with amantadine and ribavirin in a pregnancy complicated by influenza pneumonia. J Reprod Med 1988;33:399–401.
45. Larsen JW. Influenza and pregnancy. Clin Obstet Gynecol 1982;25: 599–603.
46. McKinney WP, Volkert P, Kaufman J. Fatal swine influenza pneumonia during late pregnancy. Arch Intern Med 1990;150:213–215.
47. Herrmann KL. Congenital and perinatal varicella. Clin Obstet Gynecol 1982;25:605–609.
48. Duong CM, Munns, RE. Varicella pneumonia during pregnancy. J Fam Pract 1979;8:277–280.

49. Esmonde TF, Herdman G, Anderson G. Chickenpox pneumonia: an association with pregnancy. Thorax 1989;44:812–815.
50. Cox SM, Cunningham FG, Luby J. Management of varicella pneumonia complicating pregnancy. Am J Perinatol 1990;7:300–301.
51. Zambrano MAR, Martinez A, Minguez JA, Vazquez F, Palencia R. Varicella pneumonia complicating pregnancy. Acta Obstet Gynecol Scand 1995;74:318–320.
52. Catanzaro A. Pulmonary mycosis in pregnant women. Chest 1984;86: 14S–18S.
53. Candolfi E, de Blay F, Rey D, et al. A parasitology proven case of *Toxoplasma pneumonia* in an immunocompetent pregnant women. J Infect 1993;26:79–81.
54. Soper DE, Melone PJ, Conover WB. Legionnaire disease complicating pregnancy. Obstet Gynecol 1986;67:10S–11S.
55. Boucher M, Yonekura ML, Wallace RJ, Phelan JP. Adult respiratory distress syndrome: a rare manifestation of *Listeria monocytogenes* infection in pregnancy. Am J Obstet Gynecol 1984;149:686–688.
56. Oxorn H. The changing aspects of pneumonia complicating pregnancy. Am J Obstet Gynecol 1955;70:1057–1063.
57. McGregor JA. Prevention of preterm birth: new initiatives based on microbial-host interactions. Obstet Gynecol Surv 1988;43:1–14.
58. Ramsdell RC. Pneumonia in pregnancy. Am Med 1905;9:237–239.
59. Masters PA, Weitekamp MR. Community-acquired pneumonia. In: Bone RC, Dantzker DR, George RB, et al., eds. Pulmonary and critical care medicine, update 2. St. Louis MO: Mosby Year Book, 1995:1–16.
60. Clinton MJ, Niederman MS, Matthay RA. Maternal pulmonary disorders complicating pregnancy. In: Reece EA, Hobbins JC, Mahoney MJ, et al., eds. Medicine of the fetus and mother. Philadelphia: JB Lippincott, 1995:955–981.
61. Torres A, Serra-Batlles J, Ferrer A, et al. Severe community-acquired pneumonia. Am Rev Respir Dis 1991;144:312–318.
62. Rodrigues JR, Niederman MS. Pneumonia complicating pregnancy. Clin Chest Med 1992;13:679–691.
63. Hedstrom S, Martens MG. Antibiotics in pregnancy. Clin Obstet Gynecol 1993;36:886–892.
64. Goodrum LA. Pneumonia in pregnancy. Semin Perinatol 1997;21: 276–283.
65. Korones SB. Uncommon virus infections of the mother, fetus, and newborn: influenza, mumps, and measles. Clin Perinatol 1988;15: 259–272.
66. Wilson MG, Stein AM. Teratogenic effects of Asian influenza. JAMA 1969;210:336–337.
67. Rigby FB, Pastorek JG. Pneumonia during pregnancy. Clin Obstet Gynecol 1996;39:107–119.
68. Douglas RG. Prophylaxis and treatment of influenza. N Engl J Med 1990;322:443–449.
69. Balducci J, Rodis JF, Rosengren S, Vintzileos AM, Spivey G, Vosseller C. Pregnancy outcome during first-trimester varicella infection. Obstet Gynecol 1992;79:5–6.
70. Preblud SR. Age-specific risk of varicella complications. Pediatrics 1981;68:14–17.
71. Guess HA, Broughton DD, Melton LJ III, Kurland LT. Population-based studies of varicella complications. Pediatrics 1986;78(Suppl): 723–727.
72. Weber DM, Pellecchia JA. Varicella pneumonia: study of prevalence in adult men. JAMA 1965;192:572–573.
73. Pickard RE. Varicella pneumonia in pregnancy. Am J Obstet Gynecol 1968;101:504–508.
74. Paryani SG, Arvin AM. Intrauterine infection with varicella-zoster virus after maternal varicella. N Engl J Med 1986;314:1542–1546.
75. Hockberger RS, Rothstein RJ. Varicella pneumonia in adults: a spectrum of disease. Ann Emerg Med 1986;15:931–934.
76. Haake DA, Zakowski PC, Haake DL, Bryson YJ. Early treatment with acyclovir for varicella pneumonia in otherwise healthy adults: retrospective controlled study and review. Rev Infect Dis 1990;12:788–798.
77. Pastuszak AL, Levy M, Schick B, et al. Outcome after maternal varicella infection in the first 20 weeks of pregnancy. N Engl J Med 1994;330:901–905.
78. Baren JM, Henneman PI, Lewis RJ. Primary varicella in adults: pneumonia, pregnancy, and hospital admission. Ann Emerg Med 1996; 28:165–169.
79. Andrews EB, Yankaskas BC, Cordero JF, Schoeffler K, Hampp S. Acyclovir in pregnancy registry: six years experience. Obstet Gynecol 1992;79:7–13.
80. Stein SJ, Greenspoon JS. Rubeola during pregnancy. Obstet Gynecol 1991;78:925–929.
81. Silverfarb PM, Sarosi GA, Tosh FE. Cryptococcosis and pregnancy. Am J Obstet Gynecol 1972;112:714–720.
82. Neiberg AD, Mavromatis F, Dyke J, Fayyad A. Blastomyces dermatiditis treated during pregnancy: report of a case. Am J Obstet Gynecol 1977;128:911–912.
83. Ismail MA, Lerner SA. Disseminated blastomycosis in a pregnant woman: review of amphotericin usage during pregnancy. Am Rev Respir Dis 1982;126:350–353.
84. Wack EE, Ampel NM, Galgiani JN, Bronnimann DA. Coccidioidomycosis during pregnancy: an analysis of ten cases among 47,120 pregnancies. Chest 1988;94:376–379.
85. Davies SF, Sarosi GA. Pulmonary mycoses. In: Bone RC, Dantzker DR, George RB, et al., eds. Pulmonary and critical care medicine, update 2. St. Louis: Mosby Year Book, 1995:1–26.
86. Nelson JE, Lesser M. Aspiration-induced pulmonary injury. J Intensive Care Med 1997;12:279–297.
87. Mendelson CL. The aspiration of stomach contents into the lungs during obstetric anesthesia. Am J Obstet Gynecol 1946;52:191–205.
88. Baggish MS, Hooper S. Aspiration as a cause of maternal death. Obstet Gynecol 1974;43:327–336.
89. Rowe TF. Acute gastric aspiration: prevention and treatment. Semin Perinatol 1997;21:313–319.
90. Current Trends. Tuberculosis—United States, 1984. MMWR Morb Mortal Wkly Rep 1985;34:299–307.
91. Schramfnagel D. Elimination of tuberculosis in the United States. Chest 1990;97:1283–1284.
92. Murray JF. The white plague: down and out, or up and coming? (J Burns Amberson Lecture.) Am Rev Respir Dis 1989;140: 1788–1795.
93. Frieden TR, Sterling T, Pablos-Mendez A, Kilburn JO, Couthen GM, Dooley SW. The emergence of drug-resistant tuberculosis in New York City. N Engl J Med 1993;328:521–526.
94. Topics in minority health: Tuberculosis in Minorities-United States. MMWR Morb Mortal Wkly Rep 1987;36:77–81.
95. Topics in minority health: tuberculosis in blacks—United States. MMWR Morb Mortal Wkly Rep 1987;36:212–220.
96. Centers for Disease Control and Prevention. Nosocomial transmission of multidrug-resistant tuberculosis to health care workers and HIV-infected patients in an urban hospital. MMWR Morb Mortal Wkly Rep 1991;40:585.
97. Centers for Disease Control and Prevention. Expanded tuberculosis surveillance and tuberculosis morbidity—United States, 1993. MMWR Morb Mortal Wkly Rep 1994;361–366.
98. Centers for Disease Control and Prevention. Reported tuberculosis in the United States. 1994, Atlanta: U.S. Department of Health and Human Services, Public Health Service, CDC, 1995.
99. Epidemiologic notes and reports: tuberculosis among pregnant Women—New York City, 1985–1992. MMWR Morb Mortal Wkly Rep 1993;42:605,611–612.
100. Margono F, Mroueh J, Garley A, White D, Duerr A, Minskoff HL. Resurgence of active tuberculosis among pregnant women. Obstet Gynecol 1994;83:911–914.
101. Freeth A. Routine x-ray examination of the chest at an antenatal clinic. Lancet 1953;1:287–288.
102. Cromie JB. Pregnancy and pulmonary tuberculosis. Br J Tuberc 1954;48:97.
103. Selikoff IJ, Dorfman HL. Pulmonary disease in pregnancy. In Guttmacher AF, Rovinsky JJ (eds): Medical, Surgical and Gynecological Complications of Pregnancy. Baltimore, Williams and Wilkins, 1960, 99–130.
104. Ames WR, Schuck MH. General population roentgenographic surveys: Subsequent course of persons considered to have tuberculosis. Am Rev Tuberc 1953;68:9–23.
105. Schwabe KH, Dobstadt HP. Lungentuberkulose Schwangerschaft. Betr Klin Tuberk 1986;134:75–96.
106. Giercke HW. Tuberkuloseablaufe kurz nach Schwangerschafts-beendigung. Ztschr Tuberk 1983;108:1–8,56.
107. Edge JR. Pulmonary tuberculosis and pregnancy. BMJ 1952;2:845–847.
108. Cohen JD, Patton EA, Badger TL. The tuberculosis mother. Am Rev Tuberc 1952;65:1–23.
109. DeMarch AP. Tuberculosis and pregnancy. Chest 1975;68:800–804.

110. Schaefer G, Zervoudakis JA, Fuchs FF, David S. Pregnancy and pulmonary tuberculosis. Obstet Gynecol 1975;46:706–715.
111. Snider DE. Pregnancy and tuberculosis. Chest 1984;86:510–513.
112. Bjerkedal T, Bahna SL, Lehmann EH. Course and outcome of pregnancy in women with tuberculosis. Scand J Respir Dis 1975;56: 245–250.
113. Ratner B, Rostler AE, Salgado PS. Care, feeding and fate of premature and full-term infants born of tuberculous mothers. Am J Dis Child 1951;81:471–482.
114. Varpela E. On the effect exerted by first-line tuberculosis medicines on the foetus. Acta Tuberc Scand 1964;35:53–69.
115. Covelli HD, Wilson RT. Immunologic and medical considerations in tuberculin-sensitized pregnant patients. Am J Obstet Gynecol 1978; 132:256–259.
116. Smith JK, Caspary EA, Field EJ. Lymphocyte reactivity to antigen in pregnancy. Am J Obstet Gynecol 1972;113:602–606.
117. Rocklin RE, Kitzmiller JL, Carpenter CB, Garovoy MR, David JR. Maternal-fetal relation: absence of an immunologic blocking factor from the serum of women with chronic abortions. N Engl J Med 1976; 295:1209–1213.
118. Smith JK, Caspary EA, Field EJ. Immune responses in pregnancy. Lancet 1972;1:96.
119. Present PA, Constock GW. Tuberculin sensitivity in pregnancy. Am Rev Respir Dis 1975;112:413–416.
120. Carter JE, Mates S. Tuberculosis during pregnancy: the Rhode Island experience, 1987–1991. Chest 1994;106:1466–1470.
121. American Thoracic Society Diagnostic Standards and Classification of Tuberculosis. Am Rev Respir Dis 1990;142:725–735.
122. Purified protein derivative (PPD)—tuberculin anergy and HIV infection: guidelines for anergy testing and management of anergic persons at risk of tuberculosis. MMWR Morb Mortal Wkly Rep 1991;40:27–32.
123. Weinstein L, Murphy T. The management of tuberculosis during pregnancy. Clin Perinatol 1974;1:395–405.
124. Bonebrake CR, Noller KL, Loehnen CP, Muhm JR, Fish CR. Routine chest roentgenography in pregnancy. JAMA 1978;240:2747–2748.
125. Hadlock FP, Park SK, Wallace R. Routine radiographic screening of the chest in pregnant women: is it indicated? Obstet Gynecol 1979; 54:433–436.
126. Jett JR, Cortese DA, Dines DE. The value of bronchoscopy in the diagnosis of mycobacterial disease. Chest 1981;80:575–578.
127. Schluger N, Kinney D, Harkin T, Rom W. Clinical utility of the polymerase chain reaction in the diagnosis and evaluation of infections due to Mycobacterium tuberculosis. Chest 1994;105:1116–1121.
128. Initial therapy for tuberculosis in the era of multidrug resistance. Recommendations of the Advisory Council for the elimination of tuberculosis. MMWR Morb Mortal Wkly Rep 1993;24:1–8.
129. Maccato ML. Obstetric and gynecologic infections: pneumonia and pulmonary tuberculosis in pregnancy. Obstet Gynecol Clin North Am 1989;16:417–430.
130. Medchill MT, Gillum M. Diagnosis and management of tuberculosis during pregnancy. Obstet Gynecol Sur 1989;44:81–84.
131. Miller KS, Miller JM. Tuberculosis in pregnancy: interaction, diagnosis and management. Clin Obstet Gynecol 1996;39:120–142.
132. Vallejo JG, Starke JR. Tuberculosis and pregnancy. Clin Chest Med 1992;13:693–707.
133. The role of BCG vaccine in the prevention and control of tuberculosis in the United States: a joint statement by the Advisory Council for the Elimination of Tuberculosis and the Advisory Committee on Immunization Practice. MMWR Morb Mortal Wkly Rep 1996;45(RR-4): 1–18.
134. Snider DE, Layde PM, Johnson MW, Lyle MA. Treatment of tuberculosis during pregnancy. Am Rev Respir Dis 1980;122:65–79.
135. Myrianthopoulos NC, Chung CS. Congenital malformations in singletons: epidemiologic survey. Birth Defects 1974;10:1–58.
136. Cantwell MF, Shehab ZM, Costello AM, et al. Brief report: congenital tuberculosis. N Engl J Med 1994;330:1051–1054.
137. Snider DE, Bloch A. Congenital tuberculosis. Tubercule 1984;65: 81–82.
138. Nemir RL, O Hare D. Congenital tuberculosis: review and diagnostic guidelines. Am J Dis Child 1985;139:284–287.
139. Bate TW, Sinclair RE, Robinson MJ. Neonatal tuberculosis. Arch Dis Child 1986;11:512–514.
140. Nemir RL, O Hare D. Congenital tuberculosis. Am J Dis Child 1985;139:284–287.
141. Kendig EI. The place of BCG vaccine in the management of infants born of tuberculous mothers. N Engl J Med 1969;281:520–523.
142. Good JT, Iseman MD, Davidson PT, Lakhminarayan S, Sahn SA. Tuberculosis in association with pregnancy. Am J Obstet Gynecol 1981;140:492–498.
143. Raucher HS, Gribetz I. Care of the pregnant woman with tuberculosis and her newborn infant: a pediatrician s perspective. Mt Sinai J Med 1986;53:70–76.
144. Snider DE. Should women taking antituberculous drugs breast-feed? Arch Intern Med 1984;144:589–590.
145. Teirstein AS, Lesser M. Worldwide distribution and epidemiology of sarcoidosis. In: Sarcoidosis and other granulomatous diseases of the lung. In: Fanburg BL, ed. New York: Marcel Dekker, 1983:101–134.
146. Siltzbach LE. Sarcoidosis: clinical features and management. Med Clin North Am 1967;51:483–502.
147. Siltzbach LE. The Kveim test is a reliable means of diagnosing sarcoidosis. In: Ingelfinger FJ, ed. Controversy in internal medicine, vol 2. Philadelphia: WB Saunders, 1974:349–358.
148. Miller A, Chuang MT, Teirstein AS. Pulmonary function in stage I and II pulmonary sarcoidosis. Ann NY Acad Sci 1976;278:292–300.
149. Baughman RP, Lower EE. Alternatives to corticosteroids in the treatment of sarcoidosis. Sarcoidosis 1997;14:121–130.
150. Siltzbach LE. In: Rovinsky JJ, Guttmacher AF, eds. Medical-surgical and gynecological complications of pregnancy. Baltimore: Williams & Wilkins, 1965.
151. O'Leary JA. Ten-year study of sarcoidosis and pregnancy. Am J Obstet Gynecol 1962;84:462–466.
152. De Regt RH. Sarcoidosis and pregnancy. Obstet Gynecol 1987;3: 369–372.
153. Mayrock RL, Sullivan RD, Greening RR, Jones R Jr. Sarcoidosis and pregnancy. JAMA 1957;162:158–163.
154. Given FT, Dibenedetto RL. Sarcoidosis and pregnancy. Obstet Gynecol 1963;22:355–359.
155. Agha FP, Vade A, Amendola MA, Cooper RF. Effects of pregnancy on sarcoidosis. Surg Gynecol Obstet 1982;155:817–822.
156. Grossman JH, Littner MR. Severe sarcoidosis in pregnancy. Obstet Gynecol 1977;50(Suppl 1):81S–84S.
157. Reisfield DR, Yahia C, Laurenzi GA. Pregnancy and cardiorespiratory failure in Boeck s sarcoid. Surg Gynecol Obstet 1959;109:412–416.
158. Seballos RJ, Mendel SG, Mirmiran-Yazdy A, Khoury W, Marshall JB. Sarcoid cardiomyopathy precipitated by pregnancy with cocaine complications. Chest 1994;105:303–305.
159. Siegal B, Siegel S. Pregnancy and delivery in a patient with cystic fibrosis of the pancreas. Obstet Gynecol 1960;16:438–440.
160. Grand RJ, Talamo RC, di Sant'Agnese PA, Scwartz RH. Pregnancy in cystic fibrosis of the pancreas. JAMA 1966;195:993–1000.
161. Patient registry 1995 annual data report. Bethesda, MD: Cystic Fibrosis Foundation, 1996.
162. Fiel SB. Cystic fibrosis. In: Bone RC, Dantzker DR, George RB, et al., eds. Pulmonary and critical care medicine, update 2. St. Louis, MO: Mosby Year Book, 1995:1–12.
163. Rommens JM, Iannuzzi MC, Kerem B, et al. Identification of the cystic fibrosis gene: chromosome walking and jumping. Science 1989;245:1059–1065.
164. Riordan JR, Rommens JM, Kerem B, et al. Identification of the cystic fibrosis gene: cloning and characterization of complementary DNA. Science 1989;245:1066–1073.
165. Kerem B, Rommens JM, Buchanan JA, et al. Identification of the cystic fibrosis gene: genetic analysis. Science 1989;245:1073–1080.
166. Aitken ML, Fiel SB. Cystic fibrosis. Dis Mon 1993;39:1–52.
167. Cystic fibrosis genetic analysis consortium. Website: http://www.genet.sickkids.on.ca/eftr/.
168. Kerem E, Reisman J, Corey M, Canny GJ, Levison H. Prediction of mortality in patients with cystic fibrosis. N Engl J Med 1992;326: 1187–1191.
169. Fiel SB. Aerosol delivery of antibiotics to the lower airways of patients with cystic fibrosis. Chest 1995;107(Suppl):61–64.
170. Fuchs HJ, Borowitz DS, Christiansen DH, et al. Effect of aerosolized recombinant human DNase on exacerbations of respiratory symptoms and on pulmonary function in patients with cystic fibrosis. The Pulmozyme Study Group. N Engl J Med 1994;331:637–642.
171. Knowles RK, Church NL, Waltner WE, et al. A pilot study of aerosolized amiloride for the treatment of lung disease in cystic fibrosis. N Engl J Med 1990;322:1189–1194.

172. Bennett WD, Olivier KN, Zeman KL, Hohneker KW, Boucher RC, Knowles MR. Effect of uridine 5'-triphosphate plus amiloride on mucociliary clearance in adult cystic fibrosis. Am J Respir Crit Care Med 1996;153:1796–1801.
173. Wilson JM. Cystic fibrosis: strategies for gene therapy. Semin Respir Crit Care Med 1994;15:439–445.
174. Konstam MW, Byard PJ, Hoppel CL, Davis PB. Effect of high dose ibuprofen in patients with cystic fibrosis. N Engl J Med 1995;332: 848–854.
175. Kotloff RM, Zuckerman JB. Lung transplantation for cystic fibrosis. Chest 1996;109:787–798.
176. Levy LD, Durie DR, Pencharz PB, Corey ML. Effects of long-term nutritional rehabilitation on body composition and clinical status in malnourished children and adolescents with cystic fibrosis. J Pediatr 1985;107:225–230.
177. Boland MP, Stoski DS, MacDonald NE, Soucy P, Patrick J. Chronic jejunostomy feeding with a non-elemental formula in undernourished patients with cystic fibrosis. Lancet 1986;232–234.
178. Drury DM, Pianosi P, Kopelman H, Charge D, Coates AL. The effect of nutritional status on respiratory muscle strength and work capacity in cystic fibrosis. Pediatr Res 1990;28:104A.
179. Kaplan E, Shwachman H, Perlmutter AD, Rule A, Khaw KT, Holsclaw DS. Reproductive failure in males with cystic fibrosis. N Engl J Med 1968;279:65–69.
180. Taussig LM, Lobeck CC, di Sant Agnese PA, Ackerman DR, Kattwinkel J. Fertility in males with cystic fibrosis. N Engl J Med 1972; 287:586–589.
181. Anguiano A, Oates RD, Amos JA, et al. Congenital bilateral absence of the vas deferens: a primary genital form of cystic fibrosis. JAMA 1992;267:1794–1797.
182. Barreto C, Pinto LM, Duarte A, Lavinha J, Ramsay M. A fertile male with cystic fibrosis: molecular genetic analysis. J Med Genet 1991;28: 420–421.
183. Kotloff RM, FitzSimmons SC, Fiel SB. Fertility and pregnancy in patients with cystic fibrosis. Clin Chest Med 1992;13:623–635.
184. Kopito LE, Kosasky HJ, Shwachman H. Water and electrolytes in cervical mucus from patients with cystic fibrosis. Fertil Steril 1973;24: 512–516.
185. Cohen LF, di Sant Agnese PA, Friedlander J. Cystic fibrosis and pregnancy. A national survey. Lancet 1980;2:842–844.
186. Canny GJ, Corey M, Livingstone RM, Carpenter M, Green L, Levison H. Pregnancy and cystic fibrosis. Obstet Gynecol 1991;77: 850–853.
187. Edenborough FP, Stableforth DE, Webb AK, Mackenzie WE, Smith DL. Outcome of pregnancy in women with cystic fibrosis. Thorax 1995;50:170–174.
188. Hilman BC, Aitken ML, Constantinescu M. Pregnancy in patients with cystic fibrosis. Clin Obstet Gynecol 1996;39:70–86.
189. Dooley RR, Braunstein H, Osher AB. Polypoid cervicitis in cystic fibrosis patients receiving oral contraceptives. Am J Obstet Gynecol 1974;118:971–974.
190. Fitzpatrick SB, Stokes DC, Rosenstein BJ, Terry P, Hubbard VS. Use of oral contraceptives in women with cystic fibrosis. Chest 1984;84:863–867.
191. Weinberger SE, Weiss ST, Cohen WR, Weiss JW, Johnson TS. Pregnancy and the lung. Am Rev Respir Dis 1980;121:559–581.
192. Parisi VM, Creasy RK. Maternal biologic adaptations to pregnancy. In: Reece EA, Hobbins JC, Mahoney MJ, et al., eds. Medicine of the fetus and mother. Philadelphia: JB Lippincott, 1995:831–848.
193. Institute of Medicine. Nutrition During Pregnancy: Part I, weight gain; Part II, nutrient supplements. Washington, DC: National Academy Press, 1990.
194. Novy MJ, Tyler JM, Shwachman H, Easterday CL, Reid DE. Cystic fibrosis and pregnancy: report of a case, with a study of pulmonary function and arterial blood gases. Obstet Gynecol 1967;30: 530–536.
195. Larsen JW. Cystic fibrosis and pregnancy. Obstet Gynecol 1972;39: 880–883.
196. Shwachman H, Kulczycki LL. Long-term study of one hundred five patients with cystic fibrosis. Am J Dis Child 1958;96:6–15.
197. Taussig LM, Kattwinkel J, Friedewald WT, di Sant Agnese PA. A new prognostic score and clinical evaluation system for cystic fibrosis. J Pediatr 1973;82:380–390.
198. Corkey CWB, Newth CJL, Corey M, Levison H. Pregnancy in cystic fibrosis: a better prognosis in patients with pancreatic function? Am J Obstet Gynecol 1981;140:737–742.
199. Palmer J, Dillon-Baker C, Tecklin JS, et al. Pregnancy in patients with cystic fibrosis. Ann Intern Med 1983;99:596–600.
200. Hedstrom S, Martens MG. Antibiotics in pregnancy. Clin Obstet Gynecol 1993;36:886–894.
201. Light RW. Management of spontaneous pneumothorax. Am Rev Respir Dis 1993;148:245–248.
202. Hsu CT, Huang PW, Lin CT. A term delivery complicated by spontaneous pneumothorax. Report of a case. Obstet Gynecol 1959;14: 527–529.
203. Jonas G. Spontaneous pneumothorax at term: report of a case. Obst Gynecol 1964;23:799–801.
204. Bending JJ. Spontaneous pneumothorax in pregnancy and labour. Postgrad Med J 1982;58:711–713.
205. Freedman LJ. Antepartum spontaneous pneumothorax. Diagn Gynecol Obstet 1982;4:151–153.
206. Brodsky JB, Eggen M, Cannon WB. Spontaneous pneumothorax in early pregnancy: successful management by thoracoscopy. J Cardiothorac Vasc Anesth 1993;103:950–951.
207. Brantley WM, Del Valle RA, Schonbucher AK. Pneumothorax, bilateral, spontaneous complicating pregnancy: case report. Am J Obstet Gynecol 1961;81:42–44.
208. Farrel SJ. Spontaneous pneumothorax in pregnancy: a case report and review of the literature. Obstet Gynecol 1983; 62(Suppl):43–45.
209. Vance JP. Tension pneumothorax in labour. Anesthesiology 1968;23: 94–97.
210. Schwartz M, Rusoff L. Pneumomediastinum and bilateral pneumothoraces in a patient with hyperemesis gravidarum. Chest 1994;106: 1904–1906.
211. Dudley DK, Patten DE. Intrapartum pneumomediastinum associated with subcutaneous emphysema. Can Med Assoc J 1988;139:641–642.
212. Karson EM, Saltzman D, Davis MR. Pneumomediastinum in pregnancy: two case reports and a review of the literature, pathophysiology, and management. Obstet Gynecol 1984;64(Suppl):39–43.
213. Van Winter JT, Nichols FC, Pairolero PC, Ney JA, Ogburn PL. Management of spontaneous pneumothorax during pregnancy: case report and review of the literature. Mayo Clin Proc 1996;71:249–252.
214. Dhalla SS, Teskey JM. Surgical management of recurrent spontaneous pneumothorax during pregnancy. Chest 1985;88:301–302.
215. Wakabayashi A, Brenner M, Wilson AF, Tadir Y, Berns M. Thoracoscopic treatment of spontaneous pneumothorax using carbon dioxide laser. Ann Thor Surg 1990;50:786–789.
216. Demling RH, Nerlich M. Acute respiratory failure. Surg Clin North Am 1983;63:337–355.
217. Kaunitz AM, Hughes JM, Grimes DA, Smith JC, Rochat RW, Katrissen ME. Causes of maternal mortality in the United States. Obstet Gynecol 1985;65:605–612.
218. Hollingsworth HM, Irwin RS. Acute respiratory failure in pregnancy. Clin Chest Med 1992;13:723–740.
219. Deblieux PM, Summer WR. Acute respiratory failure in pregnancy. Clin Obstet Gynecol 1996;39:143–152.
220. Kollef MH, Schuster DP. The acute respiratory distress syndrome. N Engl J Med 1995;332:27–37.

Cherry and Merkatz's Complications of Pregnancy,
Fifth Edition, edited by W. R. Cohen.
Lippincott Williams & Wilkins, Philadelphia © 2000.

CHAPTER 15

Venous Disease and Thromboembolism

Marc R. Toglia

Chronic venous disease of the lower extremities and venous thromboembolism (VTE) are common conditions affecting pregnant women that may lead to significant maternal morbidity. Pulmonary embolism, although uncommon, is the leading cause of maternal mortality in the United States (1) and in most developed countries (2,3).

The management of venous disease and thromboembolism during pregnancy remains a significant challenge for the obstetrician. Recent scientific advances in the management of VTE in the nonpregnant patient led to a dramatic reduction in both the mortality and morbidity associated with these conditions. The diagnosis and management of VTE during pregnancy, however, remain controversial and challenging because of the lack of similar studies involving gravid women.

The overall incidence of VTE related to pregnancy is approximately 0.5% (4–6); accurate incidence figures are difficult to obtain because of the lack of studies using objective diagnostic techniques. Deep vein thrombosis (DVT) occurs more commonly than does pulmonary embolism. In one retrospective study using venography as the diagnostic standard, the incidence of DVT was 7 per 1,000 deliveries (24). More recent investigations reported a lower incidence, ranging from 0.5 to 0.7 per 1,000 (5–7). Contrary to traditional teaching and most older reports, recent investigations using rigorous diagnostic criteria indicate that most DVTs occur antenatally rather than postpartum. In the largest study to date, Rutherford and colleagues reported that 75% of DVTs occurred antepartum, with 51% having taken place by the 15th week of gestation (5). Others have reported that DVT occurs with approximately equal frequency in all three trimesters (8–10).

In contrast, pulmonary embolism most commonly occurs postpartum, particularly after cesarean section. Rutherford and colleagues (5) noted that 66% of pulmonary embolism cases occurred postpartum and Aaro and Juergens (11), in a review of 32,000 pregnancies, reported that 77% of documented cases occurred postpartum.

M. R. Toglia: Riddle Memorial Hospital, Media, PA 19063.

PATHOPHYSIOLOGY

It has long been recognized that VTE occurs with an increased frequency during pregnancy; the incidence in gestation is approximately fivefold higher than that of nonpregnant women of a similar age (12). In 1847, Virchow established the triad of venous stasis, hypercoagulability, and vascular wall injury as the major predisposing factors leading to thromboembolic disease. All three are now acknowledged to exist during pregnancy.

Physiologic and anatomic changes associated with pregnancy result in an increase in venous distensibility and capacitance that results in a decrease in venous flow. These changes, apparent from the first trimester, are thought to be hormonally mediated by both estrogen and progesterone. Later in pregnancy, the gravid uterus compresses the pelvic veins and inferior vena cava, resulting in a mechanical obstruction to venous flow (13). This tendency toward venous stasis is likely to be augmented if the patient requires prolonged periods of bed rest.

Pregnancy also is associated with an increased concentration of coagulation factors, decreased levels of coagulation inhibitors, and decreased fibrinolytic capacity, all of which result in a state of hypercoagulability. Increased levels of clotting factors II, VII, VIII, IX, and X are evident by midpregnancy (14–16). Fibrinogen increases markedly, reaching levels that are three times those of the nonpregnant state (15). Antithrombin III, protein C, and protein S are important naturally occurring coagulation inhibitors. Protein S levels significantly decrease throughout pregnancy, whereas protein C and antithrombin III levels remain unchanged (14,15,17). Inhibition of the fibrinolytic system is also thought to occur and is greatest during the third trimester (14,18).

Recent attention has focused on a mutation in the factor V gene (Factor V Leiden) that results in an activated protein C resistance (APCR), which has been associated with a threefold to fivefold increased risk of VTE in nonpregnant subjects (19). It is currently believed that this mutation is the most common hereditary cause of VTE. A few recent studies have implicated APCR as a cause of thromboembolism during pregnancy (20,21). Hellgren and associates found that 60% of pregnant women with thromboembolism had this genetic defect (22).

Injury of the vascular wall endothelium initiates a sequence of fibrin production and platelet aggregation that can result in thrombus formation. Delivery is associated with vascular injury and changes at the uteroplacental interface, which may be further compromised by instrumental and surgical delivery.

Several independent obstetric factors have been associated with an increased risk of VTE, including prolonged bed rest (such as may be required for threatened preterm labor or preeclampsia), hemorrhage, sepsis, instrumental or cesarean delivery, and multiparity (2).

SUPERFICIAL VENOUS THROMBOPHLEBITIS

Superficial thrombophlebitis is seen most frequently in patients who have varicose veins or as a sequela of intravenous catheterization. Superficial thrombophlebitis is diagnosed by the presence of a warm, erythematous, tender, and indurated cord within a superficial and often varicose vein. Ancillary testing is unnecessary unless there is concern about extension to the deep veins. Supportive therapy, including analgesia and elastic support, are all that is necessary, because the inflammatory process should resolve within about a week. An elastic bandage is the most effective way to apply direct external compression. Antibiotics are not indicated. It should be noted that a residual cord may be palpable for several months following resolution of the acute inflammation. Anticoagulant therapy should be reserved for cases that develop deep venous extension.

DEEP VEIN THROMBOSIS

Clinical Diagnosis

Clinical signs and symptoms of DVT are both nonspecific and unreliable, contributing to the difficulty in diagnosis. The intensity of the classic symptoms of pain, tenderness, and swelling of the affected limb depend on the extent of the vascular occlusion, existing collateral circulation, and the associated inflammatory response. Other associated findings are varicosities, increased heat, redness, pitting edema, and a palpable cord over the affected vessel. It is widely recognized that the clinical ability to diagnose DVT is poor and that none of the signs or symptoms is specific. In one study, fewer than half of patients with signs and symptoms strongly suggestive of DVT had the diagnosis confirmed by objective testing (23). The clinical diagnosis of DVT during pregnancy is particularly difficult because physiologic leg swelling and discomfort occur commonly.

During pregnancy, venous thrombosis begins most frequently either in the calf veins or in the iliofemoral segment of the deep venous system (11,24). There is a striking propensity for the left leg, with approximately 80% of DVTs in pregnancy occurring on this side (8,9,24,25). The venous drainage of the left leg follows a more tortuous course through the pelvis, with the left common iliac vein traversed by the right common iliac artery. It has been suggested that this renders the left leg more prone to DVT.

Diagnostic Tests

In the last decade, noninvasive diagnostic studies such as impedance plethysmography (IPG), real-time B mode ultrasonography, and duplex Doppler scanning have replaced venography as the initial screening test in the diagnosis of DVT in nonpregnant patients (26). These diagnostic studies have high sensitivity for the detection of thrombosis in the proximal iliofemoral veins but not in the distal deep veins of the lower extremities. Experience with these techniques during pregnancy is limited, but preliminary studies are promising.

IPG measures changes in electric resistance measured by two electrodes wrapped around the calf in relationship to changes in venous volume. In the nonpregnant patient, IPG has shown high sensitivity and specificity, nearly comparable to venography in diagnosing proximal DVT (27). Serial normal studies performed over 7 to 14 days have shown sufficient sensitivity and specificity to withhold therapy in both nonpregnant (28,29) and pregnant(25) patients. Hull and colleagues (25) reported on 152 pregnant women evaluated for suspected deep vein thrombosis. Thirteen women (9%) had an abnormal IPG, 11 of whom had a DVT confirmed by venography. Of the remaining 139 women, serial testing was performed over the subsequent 2 weeks, and none developed a clinically evident DVT during follow-up.

Real-time B-mode ultrasonography assesses venous compressibility and is currently considered the procedure of choice in the initial evaluation of the nonpregnant patient. When evaluating proximal DVT, a sensitivity and specificity of 91% and 99%, respectively, compared with venography, have been reported (30). Heijboer et al. (31) compared serial IPG with serial compression ultrasonography prospectively in 985 nonpregnant patients with clinically suspected DVT. In each group, approximately 20% had positive findings on the noninvasive testing and underwent venography. Serial ultrasonography had a positive predictive value of 94% compared with 83% for IPG. In addition, 6% of cases were diagnosed on serial scanning. This study also supported the safety of withholding therapy when serial studies remained normal.

Preliminary experience with this modality during pregnancy is promising (32).

Venography remains the diagnostic standard for DVT in both pregnant and nonpregnant patients. Venography has the advantage of accurately evaluating the entire lower extremity from the calf veins to the common iliac vessels. It is also more reliable than noninvasive techniques in differentiating between intraluminal defects and external venous compression. These advantages are offset by potential side effects such as chemical phlebitis, leg swelling and pain, and skin necrosis secondary to dye extravasation. In addition, the procedure is relatively expensive, and the results can be difficult to interpret. Estimated fetal radiation exposure is negligible: approximately 0.314 rad (0.00314 Gy) for a unilateral procedure without abdominal shielding (33). Limited venography using an abdominal shield can reduce the estimated fetal exposure to less than 0.05 rads (0.0005 Gy).

The role of venography in diagnosing DVT during pregnancy remains unresolved. Although venography remains the diagnostic mainstay, a positive noninvasive study such as ultrasound is generally accepted as sufficient evidence to initiate therapy in the nonpregnant patient. Although limited data exist in gravid women, this approach seems reasonable for the pregnant patient as well (34,35). Venography may be helpful when the results of noninvasive imaging studies are equivocal or serial scanning is impractical. Venography is also the preferred technique in patients with a prior history of DVT in the suspected limb.

PULMONARY EMBOLISM

The clinical diagnosis of pulmonary embolism (PE) remains difficult because of the wide spectrum of clinical findings. Commonly reported symptoms include dyspnea, tachypnea, and pleuritic chest pain (Table 15-1). Other signs and symptoms such as apprehension, cough, and pulmonary rales are present in approximately half of patients with a pulmonary embolus (36). Massive PE may be associated with cardiovascular collapse, right-sided heart failure, and jugular venous distention. Clinical findings suggestive of DVT are found rarely in patients with PE. Only 15% of patients in the Prospective Investigation of Pulmonary Embolism Diagnosis (PIOPED) trial had clinical evidence of a DVT (37). Physical findings and symptoms must be interpreted with particular caution during pregnancy because dyspnea, tachypnea, and leg discomfort occur commonly as pregnancy progresses.

TABLE 15-1. *Signs and symptoms in patients with pulmonary embolism*

Finding	(%)
Tachypnea	70
Dyspnea	73
Pleuritic chest pain	66
Cough	37
Tachycardia	30
Hemoptysis	13
Fever	7
Rales	51

From Stein PD, Terrin ML, Hales CA, et al. Clinical, laboratory, roengenographic and electrocardiographic findings in patients with acute pulmonary embolism and no pre-existing cardiac or pulmonary disease. Chest 1991;100:598–603, with permission.

Routine laboratory studies such as chest radiographs, electrocardiograms, and arterial blood gas determination may support the diagnosis or suggest other etiologies for the patient's complaints; however, they lack the specificity and sensitivity to establish the diagnosis of PE. A posterior-anterior chest radiograph with lateral views should be obtained to rule out pneumonia or pulmonary edema. The radiographic study is also necessary for an accurate interpretation of the ventilation-perfusion (V/Q) scan. Nonspecific chest radiograph findings such as atelectasis, unilateral pleural effusions, areas of consolidation, or an elevation of the hemidiaphragm are present in more than 80% of patients with PE. Similarly, nonspecific electrocardiographic changes are found in almost 90% of individuals with PE. Nonspecific abnormalities of the ST-segment or T-wave inversion are the most common findings. The S1Q3T3 pattern often said to be characteristic of PE is rarely present.

Most clinically significant pulmonary emboli are associated with hypoxemia, an arterial PaO_2 less than 85 mm Hg; however, 10 to 15% of patients with a documented PE have a normal PaO_2. During the third trimester of pregnancy, the PaO_2 may be as much as 15 mm Hg lower with the patient in the supine position compared with that obtained with the patient upright (38). Therefore, during the third trimester, arterial blood gases should be measured with the patient sitting upright.

Currently, the V/Q scan is the primary screening technique for the diagnosis of pulmonary embolism. The PIOPED study evaluated the specificity and sensitivity of V/Q scans versus pulmonary angiography in acute PE. This prospective, multicenter study included 933 patients; 33% of the 755 patients studied with angiography had PE (39). The results of this study may be summarized as follows: Most patients with a high probability V/Q scan (88%) had an embolism detected by angiography, but only a minority of patients with PE (13%) had a high probability scan (sensitivity 41%; specificity 97%). Of patients with intermediate probability scans, 33% had a PE detected by angiography. Sixteen percent of patients with a low probability scan had a PE, and only 4% of patients with PE had a scan interpreted as near normal or normal. The study also reported that combining clinical impression with the results of the V/Q scan increased the positive predictive value of the scan. For example, among patients in whom the clinical impression was high and the scan interpretation was low probability, 40% had a PE compared with only 4% of patients with a low probability scan when the clinical suspicion was low. The authors concluded that a V/Q scan permitted a noninvasive diagnosis or exclusion of PE in only a minority (27%) of patients and that the only interpretations that support clinical decision making solely on the basis of the V/Q scan were the high probability and near-normal or normal scans. All other patients require pulmonary angiography to establish or exclude the diagnosis.

Although the PIOPED study excluded pregnant women, many experts believe these results and recommendations can be applied to the pregnant patient (34). The diagnosis of VTE has long-term implications for the pregnant patient: (a) a need for prolonged anticoagulation throughout the pregnancy, (b) a potential need for prophylaxis during subsequent pregnancies, and (c) concern regarding future use of oral contraceptives and estrogen replacement therapy. Given these concerns and the gravity of the diagnosis itself, the author believes that the diagnosis of PE should be pursued aggressively with objective testing when it is suspected. Although there is often great reluctance by clinicians to perform radiologic studies in pregnant patients, Ginsberg and colleagues reported that the estimated radiation exposure from the combination of chest radiograph, V/Q scan, and pulmonary angiography is less than 0.5 rad (0.005 Gy) (33). If pulmonary angiography is not readily available, it is acceptable to initiate heparin therapy following the V/Q scan and to perform the angiography when convenient. Emboli can be detected by angiography up to several weeks after the event.

MANAGEMENT

Once diagnosed, VTE requires rapid and prolonged anticoagulation to prevent extension of the thrombus, to restore venous patency, and to limit the risk of PE or its recurrence. Clinical experience and retrospective cohort studies have established heparin as the safest anticoagulant to use during pregnancy because it does not cross the placenta (40–42). Heparin is a naturally occurring mucopolysaccharide that exerts its antithrombotic and anticoagulant effects by binding to and potentiating antithrombin III, which is a major inhibitor of thrombin (factor II) and other anticoagulation factors such as XIIa, XIa, and Xa. Heparin has minimal effect on platelet function and does not stimulate fibrinolysis or directly lyse formed clots.

Audits of heparin therapy suggest that heparin administration based on clinical intuition is fraught with difficulty and frequently results in prolonged periods of subtherapeutic anticoagulation (43,44). Recent prospective studies have established that failure to reach a therapeutic level of anticoagulation within the first 24 hours is associated with an unacceptably high rate of recurrent VTE (45,46). The pharmacokinetics of heparin are complicated and the dose response curve is nonlinear: The anticoagulation response increases disproportionately as the dose increases (47). A number of nomograms have been developed and prospectively studied in nonpregnant patients to assist in properly managing heparin therapy (44,48,49). In most contemporary studies, the mean daily dose of heparin required to obtain and maintain a therapeutic level is 30,500 to 36,000 IU per 24 hours, which is substantially more than the traditional teaching of starting with 1,000 U of heparin per hour.

Because therapeutic regimens have not been well established in pregnant patients, heparin therapy should be initiated according to the current recommendations for nonpregnant patients (50) (Table 15-2). Heparin can be administered both intravenously and subcutaneously. Continuous intravenous infusion following an initial intravenous loading dose of 5,000 IU (or 80 IU/kg) is currently the most popular method of delivery. For most patients, an initial infusion rate of at least 1300 IU per hour is necessary to reach therapeutic levels. Heparin anticoagulation can be monitored by a variety of laboratory assays. The activated partial thromboplastin time (APTT) is a global coagulation assay and is the method used by most clinical laboratories. An optimal level of anticoagulation is obtained with a prolongation of the APTT that is 1.5 to 2.5 times the patient's baseline value. Alternatively, plasma heparin levels can be determined by protamine titration, with a therapeutic range of 0.2 to 0.4 IU per milliliter.

Prompt achievement of therapeutic levels of heparin is critical. Failure to reach a therapeutic level of anticoagulation within the first 24 hours of treatment is associated with a 15-fold increase in the risk of recurrent thromboembolism (45). Heparin therapy should be monitored frequently (every 4 to 6 hours) in the first few days of therapy to achieve therapeutic levels rapidly. Additionally, heparin requirements are typically greatest immediately after an acute thromboembolic event. Once a steady state is reached, the monitoring test can be obtained daily. The traditional length of intravenous heparin therapy has been 7 to 10 days in nonpregnant patients with DVT or PE. More recent data indicate that 5 days of heparin therapy is equally efficacious (51). In the nonpregnant patient, DVT and PE should be treated with outpatient anticoagulation therapy for at least 3 months. In pregnant patients, the length of anticoagulant therapy should be dictated by when the thromboembolic event occurred in relationship to the pregnancy.

Oral Anticoagulant Therapy During Pregnancy

Oral anticoagulants such as warfarin cross the placenta and may result in significant fetal morbidity. Warfarin use is contraindicated during the first trimester, because its use between the 6th and 9th week of gestation has been associated with a syndrome of congenital malformations.

TABLE 15-2. *Protocol for adjustment of the dose of intravenous heparin*[a]

Activated partial thromboplastin time (sec)[b]	Repeat bolus?	Stop infusion?	New rate of infusion	Repeat measurement of activated partial thromboplastin time
<50	Yes (5000 U)	No	+3 mL/hr (+2880 U/hr)	6 hr
50–59	No	No	+3 mL/hr (+2880 U/hr)	6 hr
60–85[c]	No	No	Unchanged	Next morning
86–95	No	No	–2 mL/hr (–1920 U/24 hr)	Next morning
96–120	No	Yes (for 30 min)	–2 mL/hr (–1920 U/24 hr)	6 hr
>120	No	Yes (for 60 min)	–4 mL/hr (–3840 U/hr)	6 hr

[a]A starting dose of 5000 U is given as an intravenous bolus, followed by 31,000 U per 24 hours, given as a continuous infusion in a concentration of 40 IU/mL. The activated partial-thromboplastin time is first measured 6 hr after the bolus injection, adjustments are made according to the protocol, and the activated partial-thromboplastin time is repeated as indicated.

[b]The normal range, measured with the Dade Actin-FS reagent, is 27 to 35 sec.

[c]The therapeutic range of 60 to 85 sec is equivalent to a heparin level of 0.2 to 0.4 IU/mL by protamine titration or 0.35 to 0.7 U/mL according to the level of inhibition of factor Xa. The therapeutic range varies with the responsiveness of the activated partial-thromboplastin time to heparin.

From Toglia MR, Weg JG. Venous thromboembolism during pregnancy. N Engl J Med 1996;335:100–114.

Fetal warfarin syndrome includes nasal cartilage hypoplasia, stippling of the epiphyses (*chondrodysplasia punctata*), and limb hypoplasia (52–55). The use of warfarin during the second and third trimester of pregnancy remains controversial. Exposure to coumarin derivatives outside the first trimester has been associated with a variety of central nervous system abnormalities, including dorsal midline dysplasia, midline cerebellar atrophy, and mental retardation. Ophthalmic abnormalities including optic disk atrophy, microphthalmia, and blindness also have been reported (53,54,55). Fetal hemorrhage and placental abruption have occurred with the use of warfarin during the second and third trimesters and are thought to be secondary to fetal anticoagulation (55).

Alternative Therapy

Low-molecular-weight heparins (LMWHs) are a new class of antithrombotic agents that are rapidly replacing unfractionated heparin in the treatment and prophylaxis of venous thromboembolism (56,57). They differ from unfractionated heparin in that they more selectively inhibit factor Xa (which results in inhibition of clot formation) than factor IIa (which results in prolongation of bleeding). Other advantages of LMWHs include greater bioavailability and longer half-life, which allow single daily dosing and a more predictable anticoagulant response when administered subcutaneously as a fixed dose. Experimental evidence suggests that LMWHs do not cross the placenta (58,59), and limited clinical experience with LMWH during pregnancy has been encouraging (59–62).

Inferior vena caval filters can be used safely during pregnancy (63,64). Suprarenal placement has been recommended. Indications are the same as in a nonpregnant patient: a contraindication to anticoagulant therapy, prior complication of anticoagulant therapy such as heparin-induced thrombocytopenia, and recurrent pulmonary embolism while adequately anticoagulated. The use of thrombolytic agents has been limited to life-threatening situations because of the risk for significant maternal bleeding, especially at the time of delivery and during the postpartum period (65). The risk of placental abruption and premature labor with these agents is unknown.

Antepartum Thromboembolism

Acute VTE during pregnancy requires prompt anticoagulation with heparin for 5 to 10 days, followed by continued anticoagulation for at least 3 months. Conversion to a subcutaneous adjusted-dose heparin protocol following the initial intravenous course is advisable. Sodium heparin (20,000 IU/mL) should be injected into the lateral abdominal wall using a 25- or 27-gauge needle. Following the injection, the patient should compress the injection site for 5 to 10 minutes to avoid local hematoma formation. Because of the lack of prospective studies, considerable controversy exists regarding the optimal regimen to use for the remainder of the pregnancy, that is, whether to use therapeutic or low-dose heparin.

Well-controlled, randomized trials of long-term treatment of venous thrombosis in nonpregnant patients have reported an unacceptably high rate of recurrence (47%) with low-dose heparin therapy, defined as 5,000 IU administered twice a day, compared to therapeutic anticoagulation for 3 to 6 months (66,67). Recent studies involving pregnant women suggest that the pharmacokinetics and pharmacodynamics of subcutaneous heparin are altered during pregnancy such that peak heparin concentrations are lower and the time to peak concentrations is shorter compared with nonpregnant controls (68,69). Because pregnant women are at high risk for recurrent thrombosis, low- dose heparin is likely to be inadequate to prevent recurrent thromboembolism for the remainder of the pregnancy. It has been the author's recommendation that therapeutic heparin be continued throughout the pregnancy and discontinued after 6 weeks postpartum, assuming that at least 3 months of anticoagulant therapy have been completed (34).

A reasonable approach for adjusted-dose subcutaneous heparin administration is to estimate the initial subcutaneous dose by dividing the total daily intravenous dose in half or in thirds and administering the heparin twice or three times a day, respectively. A midinterval APTT then is measured after four to six injections, and the dose of heparin is adjusted to maintain the APTT at 1.5 to 2.0 times control, or a heparin level of 0.2 to 0.3 U/ml (45). The mean dose of heparin needed to anticoagulate a patient is typically higher when administered subcutaneously rather than intravenously in nonpregnant subjects, presumably because of reduced plasma recovery. Once a stable dosage is reached, a midinterval APTT should be checked weekly at the prenatal visit. It should be anticipated that heparin requirements will increase throughout pregnancy until term. In the postpartum period, this regimen may be continued, or warfarin may be substituted.

Use of the continuous-infusion subcutaneous heparin pump has been described in pregnancy in a limited number of patients (70,71). In one study, significant bleeding complications occurred in 66% of women (70). A randomized multiple crossover study suggested that urticarial reactions occur more commonly with the subcutaneous pump (71).

During Labor

There is no consensus on the appropriate management of anticoagulation for pregnant patients who are receiving therapeutic anticoagulation for a VTE. Rational decisions can be made once one quantifies the risks of a recurrent VTE for a given person. After an acute episode of VTE, the risk of recurrence declines rapidly over the following 3 months in a nonpregnant patient (72). Therefore, if the thromboembolic event occurs 3 or more months before the anticipated delivery, anticoagulation during labor probably is not indicated. Insertion of a vena caval filter should be considered in patients with a recent VTE—within 2 to to 4 weeks of anticipated delivery—as the recurrence rate in nonpregnant patients exceeds 50% (73,74). Alternatively, these patients can be managed with intravenous heparin throughout labor and delivery. The rationale behind these recommendations is based on recent guidelines for the management of anticoagulation before and after elective surgery in nonpregnant subjects (75).

Patients with a history of VTE remote from delivery and patients receiving heparin prophylaxis because of a history of VTE probably do not require anticoagulation during labor and delivery. Heparin therapy should be restarted promptly 4 to 6 hours postpartum. Patients can be instructed to discontinue subcutaneous heparin therapy with the onset of regular contractions. Some authors suggest continuing "low-dose" (defined as 2,500–5,000 U every 8–12 hours) subcutaneous heparin through labor (76,77). The risk of hemorrhage with a spontaneous vaginal delivery is minimal when the heparin level is less than 0.4 U/ml (24,76,77). One report suggests that there is an increased risk of episiotomy hematomas in women on anticoagulant therapy (77). The decision to use regional anesthesia should be made on an individual basis; some authorities believe that regional anesthesia is not contraindicated if the APTT is normal and heparin has not been administered within 4 to 6 hours of the procedure (78). Blood loss at the time of cesarean section has not been increased significantly in the few reports that have addressed this issue (79).

Postpartum Venous Thromboembolism

The postpartum patient who develops VTE can be managed in the same manner as a nonpregnant person (Table 15-3). Intravenous heparin is initiated to maintain the APTT at 1.5 to 2.5 times control or to achieve a blood heparin level of 0.2 to 0.4 IU/mL. Heparin is continued for at least 5 days. Warfarin should be started on the first day of heparin administration (50,51) and adjusted according to the prothrombin time (PT). The dose of warfarin should be adjusted to maintain the International Normalized Ratio (INR) at 2.0 to 3.0 (80). Heparin is continued during the first several days of warfarin therapy until a stable INR of 2.0 to 3.0 is consistently achieved. Warfarin therapy should be continued for at least 3 months to minimize the risk of recurrence. Neither heparin nor warfarin is secreted in significant quantities in breast milk, and they are not contraindicated in breastfeeding mothers (42,81).

Complications of Therapy

The major risk of heparin therapy is hemorrhage, which occurs in 2% to 4% of nonpregnant patients. One retrospective cohort study of 100 pregnancies reported that long-term heparin use during pregnancy had a 2% incidence of clinically significant bleeding (82). Heparin-induced thrombocytopenia can occur in a benign form with platelet counts usually decreasing to a range of 100,000 to 150,000 as the result of platelet aggregation and agglutination. This process is self-limiting and requires no therapy. A more fulminant form can result from an IgG-mediated response and requires the immediate discontinuation of therapy. The onset of either thrombocytopenia usually occurs 3 to 10 days after the initiation of therapy.

Osteoporosis is an uncommon but important complication of long-term heparin therapy. Clinically evident fractures associated with heparin therapy during pregnancy have been reported (83,84). Recent studies suggest that

TABLE 15-3. *Guidelines for anticoagulation*

Obtain baseline complete blood count with platelets, APTT and PT
Give heparin bolus, 5,000 U i.v. or 80 U/kg as a loading dose
Start a maintenance heparin infusion of 1300 U/hr for DVT and 1500 U/hr for PE
Check an APTT at 6 hr and adjust the infusion rate to maintain the APTT between 1.5 and 2.5 times the patient's baseline (or maintain blood heparin level at 0.2 to 0.4 U/mL)
If APTT is not prolonged, rebolus with 5000 U, in addition to increasing the rate
Repeat the APTT every six hr during the first 24 hr of therapy. Thereafter, monitor the APTT daily, unless outside of the therapeutic range
Monitor the platelet count daily or every other day during the first 10 d of heparin therapy to check for heparin induced thrombocytopenia
Begin warfarin therapy on the first day of heparin (in the postpartum patient) at 5 to 10 mg and administer daily at the estimated maintenance dose
Check the PT daily after starting warfarin therapy and adjust therapy to maintain the INR at 2.0 to 3.0
Discontinue heparin after an INR of 2.0 to 3.0 has been achieved for 4 to 7 consecutive days
Continue anticoagulation with warfarin for 3 mo at an INR of 2.0 to 3.0

APTT, activated partial thromboplastin time; DVT, deep venous thrombosis; INR, international normalized ratio; i.v., intravenous; PE, pulmonary embolus; PT, prothrombin time.

From Toglia MR, Nolan TE. Venous thromboembolism during pregnancy: a current review of diagnosis and management. Obstet Gynecol Survey 1997;52:1–13, with permission.

although the incidence of symptomatic fractures is less than two percent, subclinical reduction in bone density occurs in approximately one third of women receiving heparin therapy for longer than one month (85–88). These changes seem to be reversible in most patients, and it is uncertain whether these women are at future risk for developing fractures.

HYPERCOAGULABLE STATES AND THROMBOPROPHYLAXIS

The risk of recurrent VTE in pregnancy for a woman who has a prior episode is not known defitively. Retrospective studies have estimated the risk to be 4% to 15% (10,89). Recent data suggest that these women may have an increased risk of recurrent thrombosis because, compared with controls, they have higher plasma levels of biochemical markers of activation of the coagulation cascade during subsequent pregnancies (90).

Because of the paucity of prospective studies involving pregnant subjects, firm clinical guidelines for antepartum prophylaxis are difficult to establish. A recent consensus conference has recommended that pregnant women with a history of VTE receive 5,000 IU of subcutaneous heparin every 12 hours throughout pregnancy (42). Several authors (34,76,90,91) have expressed concern, however, that higher doses of heparin are likely to be needed for effective prophylaxis during pregnancy to offset the characteristic increases in plasma volume, renal clearance, and blood levels of coagulation factors and to counteract the alterations in metabolism of heparin that occur during pregnancy. A few authorities still advocate giving no prophylaxis (92).

The rationale that low-dose heparin is effective in preventing VTE in nonpregnant patients is based on the concept that a critical concentration of factor Xa is necessary for thrombus formation and that low-dose heparin regimens achieve an effective level of inhibition without a noticeable effect on the APTT. It was recommended recently that pregnant women at risk for VTE be treated with subcutaneous heparin, 7,500 to 10,000 U every 12 hours, during the second and third trimester of pregnancy, because this range of heparin therapy is required during pregnancy to achieve the same level of Xa inhibition that 5,000 U of heparin given subcutaneously every 12 hours achieves in nonpregnant subjects (76). Limited data indicate that following this recommendation is associated with an extremely low incidence of recurrence (86). At present, this recommended approach seems to be a rational one for pregnant women, although data confirming the efficacy of this regimen are lacking.

It has been suggested that antepartum thromboprophylaxis be considered for all pregnant women with a prior history of VTE, regardless of whether it was related to the use of oral contraceptives or a previous pregnancy (34,42, 91). Subcutaneous heparin, 7,500 to 10,000 U, should be administered twice daily beginning in the first trimester and continued until 6 weeks postpartum. More aggressive prophylaxis should be considered for women with a known hypercoagulable state. Patients with congenital antithrombin III, protein C, and protein S deficiencies and those with the factor V Leiden mutation have a 17% to 70% incidence of thrombosis during pregnancy (22,93, 94). Women with a history of antiphospholipid antibody syndrome and thrombosis should also be included in this group (95). These women should receive therapeutic doses of heparin throughout pregnancy, followed by heparin or warfarin for 6 weeks postpartum (34).

OTHER PERIPHERAL VENOUS DISEASE

Septic Pelvic Thrombophlebitis

Septic pelvic thrombophlebitis is a serious but uncommon complication of pyogenic pelvic infections. Because the diagnosis is often one of exclusion, the exact incidence is unknown. One series reported a frequency of 11 in 1,263 consecutive cesarean sections, or 0.9% (96). Other investigators have reported an incidence of 0.05% to 0.18% of all deliveries (97,98). Clinically, septic pelvic thrombophlebitis is seen most commonly in association with post-cesarean endomyometritis.

It is currently believed that septic pelvic thrombophlebitis develops in the background of a pyogenic pelvic infection. The vascular endothelium may be injured as a result of surgical trauma or as a result of inoculation by bacteria. Bacterial infection of the placental site may extend to the venous routes, including the ovarian veins, iliac veins, and even the inferior vena cava. The process is typically unilateral and most commonly involves the right ovarian vein.

Sweet and Gibbs (99) classified pelvic vein thrombophlebitis into two distinct clinical forms. The most commonly described syndrome involves acute thrombosis of the right ovarian vein (100,101). Acute thrombosis of an ovarian vein typically presents with mild to moderate fever the first 48 to 96 hours following delivery, accompanied by worsening abdominal or flank pain localized to the affected side. Nausea and vomiting also may be present. On abdominal and pelvic examination, bowel sounds are typically normal but may be diminished. There is usually direct tenderness on the affected side and a tender, palpable mass may be present in one half of patients (101). The second presentation has been described as enigmatic fever by Dunn and Van Voorhis (102) and is notable for the lack of positive clinical findings. These patients typically do not appear to be clinically ill, but they manifest persistent fever spikes despite broad-spectrum antibiotic therapy.

Although the diagnosis of ovarian vein thrombophlebitis is made largely on the basis of the patient's clinical course and physical examination, recent case reports suggest that diagnostic studies such as ultrasound (103,104) and computerized axial tomography (105–107) are useful adjuncts in confirming the diagnosis. Early investigators advocated the heparin challenge test, in which therapeutic anticoagulation with intravenous heparin was initiated and the diagnosis was confirmed if prompt lysis of fever resulted (97). Subsequent studies have not supported this approach. Brown and colleagues showed that 6 of 11 patients with proven pelvic thrombophlebitis showed clinical resolution with prolonged antimicrobial therapy without the addition of heparin therapy. Conversely, in the remaining five women who were treated with heparin as well as antibiotics, the febrile course was not significantly altered (98).

Standard therapy for pelvic vein thrombophlebitis is based on retrospective data and clinical opinion. Since it is believed that bacterial injury to the vascular endothelium serves as the initiating event in the thrombotic process in most patients, broad spectrum antibiotic therapy should be continued. Anticoagulation with intravenous heparin is the accepted therapy once the diagnosis has been made, although the necessary duration of therapy has yet to be determined (97,108). Some investigators have suggested that heparin anticoagulation be continued only until the patient is afebrile for 48 to 72 hours, whereas most advocate treating these patients in a manner similar to that for deep vein thrombosis-intravenous heparin for 7 to 10 days. Since the real value of anticoagulation therapy in the treatment of thromboembolic disorders is the prevention of the propagation of the thrombosis or its recurrence, the latter approach seems the most reasonable. The benefit of long term anticoagulation is unknown but can be considered in patients with large, clinically evident thrombi or septic pulmonary emboli (109). Surgical ligation or excision of the infected vessel should be reserved for patients who fail to respond to antibiotics and adequate heparinization.

Varicose Veins

Varicose veins are superficial vessels that are abnormally twisted, lengthened, or dilated and usually are caused by inefficient or incompetent valves within the veins. Chronic venous stasis can result in thrombosis and cutaneous disorders such as hyperpigmentation and leg ulcers. The occurrence of varicose veins during pregnancy is commonplace. They are caused by hormonally mediated (estrogen and progesterone) relaxation of the vascular smooth muscle resulting in a decrease in venous tone. The effects of estrogen and progesterone are seen early in the first trimester. Later in pregnancy, compression of the inferior vena cava and iliac vessels by the gravid uterus results in increasing venous obstruction. Consequently, the veins of the lower extremities and the vulva are commonly affected. Venous dilation results in characteristic distended and often tortuous varices, a feeling of heaviness, and often edema. During pregnancy, supportive therapy may be initiated in symptomatic patients. In most cases, elastic stockings or supportive leotards are prescribed to keep the veins compressed and to increase interstitial pressure in the surrounding tissue. This results in a decrease in interstitial edema and venous stasis.

REFERENCES

1. Berg CJ, Atrash HK, Koonin LM, Tucker M. Pregnancy-related morbidity in the United States, 1987–1990. *Obstet Gynecol* 1996;88: 161–167.
2. Report on confidential enquiries into maternal deaths in England and Wales 1986–1988. London: Her Majesty's Stationary Office, 1991.
3. Högberg U, Innala E, Sanström A. Maternal mortality in Sweden. *Obstet Gynecol* 1994;84:240–244.
4. de Swiet M, Fidler J, Howell R, Letsky E. Thromboembolism in pregnancy. In: Jewell D, ed. Advanced medicine. London: Pitman Medical, 1981:309–317.
5. Rutherford S, Montoro M, McGehee W, Strong T. Thromboembolic disease associated with pregnancy: an 11 year review. *Am J Obstet Gynecol* 1991;164(Suppl):286. (Abst)

6. Dixon JE. Pregnancies complicated by previous thromboembolic disease. *Br J Hosp Med* 1987;37:449–452.
7. Kierkegaard A. Incidence and diagnosis of deep vein thrombosis associated with pregnancy. *Acta Obstet Gynecol Scand* 1983;62:230–243.
8. Bergqvist D, Hedner U. Pregnancy and venous thrombo-embolism. *Acta Obstet Scand* 1983;62:449–453.
9. Ginsberg JS, Brill-Edwards P, Burrows RF, et al. Venous thrombosis during pregnancy: leg and trimester of presentation. *Thromb Haemost* 1992;67:519–520.
10. Tengborn L, Bergqvist D, Mätzsch R, Bergqvist A, Hedner U. Recurrent thrombo-embolism in pregnancy and the puerperium. *Am J Obstet Gynecol* 1985;28:107–118.
11. Aaro LA, Juergens JL. Thrombophlebitis associated with pregnancy. *Am J Obstet Gynecol* 1971;109:1128–1133.
12. National Institutes of Health Consensus Development Conference: prevention of venous thrombosis and pulmonary embolism. *JAMA* 1986;256:744–749.
13. Kerr MG, Scott DB, Samuel E. Studies of the inferior vena cava in late pregnancy. *BMJ* 1964;1:532–536.
14. Bremme K, Östund E, Almqvist, I, Heinonen K, Blombäck. Enhanced thrombin generation and fibrinolytic activity in normal pregnancy and the puerperium. *Obstet Gynecol* 1992;80:132–137.
15. Gerbasi FR, Bottoms S, Farag A, Mammen E. Increased intravascular coagulation associated with pregnancy. *Obstet Gynecol* 1990;75: 385–389.
16. Bonnar J. Haemostasis and coagulation disorders in pregnancy. In: Bloom AL, Thomas DP, eds. Haemostasis and thrombosis, 2nd ed. Edinburgh, Scotland: Churchill Livingstone, 1987:570–584.
17. Faught W, Garner P, Jones G, Ivey B. Changes in protein C and protein S levels in normal pregnancy. *Am J Obstet Gynecol* 1995;172: 147–150.
18. Kruithof EKO, Tran-Thang C, Gudinchet A, et al. Fibrinolysis in pregnancy: a study of plasminogen activator inhibitors. *Blood* 1987;69: 460–466.
19. Ridker PM, Hennekens CH, Lindpaintner K, Stamper MJ, Eisenberg PR, Miletich, JP. Mutation in the gene coding for coagulation factor V and the risk of myocardial infarction, stroke, and venous thrombosis in apparently healthy men. *N Engl J Med* 1995;332:912–917.
20. Cook G, Walker ID, McCall F, Conkie J, Greer A. Familial thrombophilia and activated protein C resistance: thrombotic risk in pregnancy? *Br J Haematol* 1994;87:873–875.
21. Vasse M, Leduc O, Borg JY, Chretien MH, Monconduit M. Resistance to activated protein C: evaluation of three functional assays. *Thromb Res* 1994;76:47–59.
22. Hellgren M, Svensson PJ, Dahlbäck B. Resistance to activated protein C as a basis for venous thromboembolism associated with pregnancy and oral contraceptives. *Am J Obstet Gynecol* 1995;173:210–213.
23. Hull R, Hirsh J, Sackett DL, et al. Replacement of venography in suspected venous thrombosis by impedeance plethysmosgraphy and ^{125}I-fibrinogen leg scanning: a less invasive approach. *Ann Intern Med* 1981;94:12–15.
24. Bergqvist A, Bergqvist D, Hallböök T. Deep vein thrombosis during pregnancy. A prospective study. *Acta Obstet Gynecol Scand* 1983;62: 443–448.
25. Hull RD, Raskob GE, Carter CJ. Serial impedance plethysmography in pregnant patients with clinically suspected deep-vein thrombosis: clinical validity of negative findings. *Ann Intern Med* 1990;112: 663–667.
26. Weinmann EE, Salzman EW. Deep-vein thrombosis. *N Engl J Med* 1994;331:1630–1641.
27. Wheeler HB. Diagnosis of deep vein thrombosis: review of clinical evaluation and impedance plethysmography. *Am J Surg* 1985;150:7–13.
28. Hull RD, Hirsh J, Carter CJ, et al. Diagnostic efficacy of impedance plethysmography for clinically suspected deep-vein thrombosis: a randomized trial. *Ann Intern Med* 1985;102:21–28.
29. Huisman MV, Büller HR, ten Cate JW, Heijermans HS, van der Laan J, van Maanen DJ. Management of clinically suspected acute venous thrombosis in outpatients with serial impedance plethysmography in a community hospital setting. *Arch Intern Med* 1989;149:511–513.
30. Lensing AWA, Prandoni P, Brandjes D, et al. Detection of deep-vein thrombosis by real time B-mode ultrasonography. *N Engl J Med* 1989;320:342–345.
31. Heijboer H, Büller HR, Lensing AWA, Turpie AGG, Colly LP, ten Cate JW. A comparison of real-time compression ultrasonography with impedance plethysmography for the diagnosis of deep-vein thrombosis in symptomatic outpatients. *N Engl J Med* 1993;329: 1365–1369.
32. Polak JF, Wilkinson DL. Ultrasonographic diagnosis of symptomatic deep venous thrombosis in pregnancy. *Am J Obstet Gynecol* 1991; 165:625–629.
33. Ginsberg JS, Hirsh J, Rainbow AJ, Coates G. Risks to the fetus of radiologic procedures used in the diagnosis of maternal venous thromboembolic disease. *Thromb Hemost* 1989;61:189–196.
34. Toglia MR, Weg JG. Venous thromboembolism during pregnancy. *N Engl J Med* 1996;335:108–114.
35. Toglia MR, Nolan TE. Venous thromboembolism during pregnancy: a current review of diagnosis and management. *Obstet Gynecol Survey* 1997;52:1–13.
36. Bell WR, Simon TL, DeMets DL. The clinical features of submassive and massive pulmonary emboli. *Am J Med* 1977;62:355–360.
37. Stein PD, Terrin ML, Hales CA, et al. Clinical, laboratory, roengenographic and electrocardiographic findings in patients with acute pulmonary embolism and no pre-existing cardiac or pulmonary disease. *Chest* 1991;100:598–603.
38. Ang CK, Tan TH, Walters WA, Wood C. Postural influence on maternal capillary oxygen and carbon dioxide tension. *BMJ* 1969;4:201–203.
39. The PIOPED Investigators. Value of the ventilation/perfusion scan in acute pulmonary embolism: results of the prospective investigation of pulmonary embolism diagnosis (PIOPED). *JAMA* 1990;263: 2753–2759.
40. Ginsberg JS, Hirsh J, Turner DC, Levine MN, Burrows R. Risks to the fetus of anticoagulant therapy during pregnancy. *Thromb Haemost* 1989;61:197–203.
41. Ginsberg JS, Kowalchuk G, Hirsch J, Brill-Edwards P, Burrows R. Heparin therapy during pregnancy: risks to the fetus and mother. *Arch Intern Med* 1989;149:2233–2236.
42. Ginsberg JS, Hirsh J. Use of antithrombotic agents during pregnancy. *Chest* 1995;108(Suppl):305S–311S.
43. Wheeler AP, Jaquiss RDB, Newman JH. Physician practices in the treatment of pulmonary embolism and deep vein thrombosis. *Arch Intern Med* 1988;148:1321–1325.
44. Cruickshank MK, Levine MN, Hirsh J, Roberts R, Siguenza M. A standard heparin nomogram for the management of heparin therapy. *Arch Intern Med* 1991;151:333–337.
45. Hull R, Raskob G, Hirsh J, et al. Continuous intravenous heparin compared with intermittent subcutaneous heparin in the initial treatment of proximal-vein thrombosis. *N Engl J Med* 1986;315:1109–1114.
46. Basu D, Gallus A, Hirsh J, Cade J. A prospective study of the value of monitoring heparin treatment with the activated partial thromboplastin time. *N Engl J Med* 1972;287:324–327.
47. deSwart CAM, Nijmeyer B, Roelofs JMM, Sixma JJ. Kinetics of intravenously administered heparin in normal humans. *Blood* 1982; 60:1251–1258.
48. Hull RD, Raskob GE, Rosenbloom D, et al. Optimal therapeutic level of heparin therapy in patients with venous thrombosis. *Arch Intern Med* 1992;152:1589–1595.
49. Rasachke RA, Reilly BM, Guidry JR, Fontana JR, Srinivas S. The weight-based heparin dosing nomogram compared with a standard care nomogram: a randomized controlled trial. *Ann Intern Med* 1993;119:874–881.
50. Hyers TM, Hull RD, Weg JG. Antithrombotic therapy for venous thromboembolic disease. *Chest* 1995;108(Suppl):335S–351S.
51. Hull RD, Raskob GE, Rosenbloom D, Panju AA, Brill-Edwards P, Ginsberg JS. Heparin for 5 days as compared with 10 days in the initial treatment of proximal vein thrombosis. *N Engl J Med* 1990;322: 1260–1264.
52. Hall JAG, Paul RM, Wilson KM. Maternal and fetal sequelae of anticoagulation during pregnancy. *Am J Med* 1980;68:122–140.
53. Shaul WL, Hall JG. Multiple congenital anomalies associated with oral anticoagulants. *Am J Obstet Gynecol* 1977;127:191–198.
54. Holzgreve W, Carey JC, Hall BD. Warfarin-induced fetal abnormalities. *Lancet* 1976;2:914–915.
55. Wong V, Cheng CH, Chan KC. Fetal and neonatal outcome of exposure to anticoagulants during pregnancy. *Am J Med Genet* 1993:145;17–21.
56. Simonneau G, Soris H, Charbonnier B, et al. A comparison of low-molecular weight heparin with unfractionated heparin for acute pulmonary embolism. *N Engl J Med* 1997;337:663–669.
57. The Columbus Investigators. Low molecular weight heparin in the

treatment of patients with venous thromboembolism. *N Engl J Med* 1997;337:657–662.
58. Forestier F, Daffos F, Capella-Pavlovsky M. Low molecular weight heparin (PK 10169) does not cross the placenta during the second trimester of pregnancy: study by direct blood sampling under ultrasound. *Thromb Res* 1984;34:557–560.
59. Omri A, Delaloye JF, Anderson H, Bachmann F. Low molecular weight heparin NOVO (LHN-1) does not cross the placenta during the second trimester of pregnancy. *Thromb Haemost* 1989;61:55–56.
60. Gillis A, Shush ANA, Eldor A. Use of low molecular weight heparin for prophylaxis and treatment of thromboembolism in pregnancy. *Int J Gynecol Obstet* 1992;39:296–301.
61. Melissari E, Parker CJ, Wilson NV, et al. Use of low molecular weight heparin in pregnancy. *Thromb Haemost* 1992;68:652–656.
62. Dutlitzki M, Pauzner R, Langevitz P, Pras M, Many A, Schiff E. Low-molecular-weight heparin during pregnancy: preliminary experience with 41 pregnancies. *Obstet Gynecol* 1996;87:380–383.
63. Greenfield LJ, Cho KJ, Proctor MC, Sobel M, Shah S, Wingo J. Late results of suprarenal Greenfield vena cava filter placement. *Arch Surg* 1992;127:969–973.
64. Narayan H, Cullimore J, Krarup K, Thurston H, Macvicar J, Bolia A. Experience with the Cardial inferior vena cava filter as prophylaxis against pulmonary embolism in pregnant women with extensive deep venous thrombosis. *Br J Obstet Gynaecol* 1992;99:637–640.
65. Fagher B, Ahlgren M, Astedt B. Acute massive pulmonary embolism treated with streptokinase during labor and the early pueperium. *Acta Obstet Gynecol Scand* 1990;69:659–661.
66. Hull RD, Delmore TJ, Carter C, Hirsch J, Genton E, Gent M, Turpie G, McLaughlin D. Adjusted subcutaneous heparin versus warfarin sodium in the long term treatment of venous thrombosis. *N Engl J Med* 1982;306:189–194.
67. Hull RD, Raskob GE, Hirsh J, Sackett DL. A cost-effectiveness analysis of alternative approaches for long-term treatment of proximal venous thrombosis. *JAMA* 1984;252;235–239.
68. Barbour LA, Smith JM, Marlar RA. Heparin levels to guide thromboembolism prophylaxis during pregnancy. *Am J Obstet Gynecol* 1995;173:1240–1245.
69. Brancazio LR, Roperti KA, Stierer R, Leifer SA. Pharmacokinetics and pharmacodynamics of subcutaneous heparin during the early third trimester of pregnancy. *Am J Obstet Gynecol* 1995;173:1240–1245.
70. Barss VA, Schwartz PA, Green MF, Philippe M, Saltzman D, Frigoletto FD. Use of the subcutaneous heparin pump during pregnancy. *J Reprod Med* 1985;30:899–901.
71. Anderson DR, Ginsberg JS, Brill-Edwards P, Demers C, Burrows RF, Hirsh J. The use of an indwelling teflon catheter for subcutaneous heparin administration during pregnancy: a randomized cross-over study. *Arch Intern Med* 1993;153:841–844.
72. Coon WW, Willis PW III. Recurrence of venous thromboembolism. *Surgery* 1973;73:823–827.
73. Hull R, Delmore T, Genton E, Hirsh J, Gent M, Sackett D, McLaughlin D, Armstrong P. Warfarin sodium versus low-dose heparin in the long-term treatment of venous thrombosis. *N Engl J Med* 1979;301: 855–858.
74. Bergqvist D. The role of vena caval interruption in patients with venous thromboembolism. *Prog Cardiovasc Dis* 1994;37:25–37.
75. Kearon C, Hirsh J. Management of anticoagulation before and after elective surgery. *N Engl J Med* 1997;336:1506–1511.
76. Dahlman TC, Hellgren MS, Blombäck M. Thrombosis prophylaxis in pregnancy with the use of subcutaneous heparin adjusted by monitoring heparin concentration in plasma. *Obstet Gynecol* 1989;161:420–425.
77. Bonnar J. Venous thromboembolism and pregnancy. *Clin Obstet Gynecol* 1981;8:455–473.
78. Horlocker TT. Central neural blockage for patients receiving anticoagulants. *Clin Anesthesia Updates* 1994;5:1-9.
79. Anderson DR, Ginsberg JS, Burrows R, Brill-Edwards P. Subcutaneous heparin therapy during pregnancy: a need for concern at the time of delivery. *Thromb Haemost* 1991;65:248–250.
80. Hirsh J, Dalen J, Deykin D, Poller L. Oral anticoagulants: mechanism of action, clinical effectiveness, and optimal therapeutic range. *Chest* 1995;108(Suppl):312S–326S.
81. Orme ML, Lewis PJ, de Swiet M, et al. May mothers given warfarin breast-feed their infants? *BMJ* 1977;1:1564–1565.
82. Ginsberg JS, Kowalchuk G, Hirsh J, Brill-Edwards P, Burrows R. Heparin therapy during pregnancy: risks to the fetus and mother. *Arch Intern Med* 1989;149:2233–2236.
83. Wise PH, Hall AJ. Heparin induces osteopenia in pregnancy. *BMJ* 1980;281:110–111.
84. de Swiet M, Ward PD, Fidler J, et al. Prolonged heparin therapy in pregnancy causes bone demineralization. *Br J Obstet Gynecol* 1983; 90:1129–1134.
85. Dahlman T, Lindvall N, Hellgren M. Osteopenia in pregnancy during long term heparin treatment: a radiological study postpartum. *Br J Obstet Gynecol* 1990;97:221–228.
86. Dahlman TC. Osteoporotic fractures and the recurrence of thromboembolism during pregnancy and the puerperium in 184 women undergoing thromboprophylaxis with heparin. *Am J Obstet Gynecol* 1993; 168:1265–1278.
87. Barbour LA, Kick SD, Steiner JF, et al. A prospective study of heparin-induced osteoporosis using bone densitometry. *Am J Obstet Gynecol* 1994;170:862–869.
88. Dahlman TC, Sjöberg HE, Ringhertz H. Bone mineral density during long-term prophylaxis with heparin in pregnancy. *Am J Obstet Gynecol* 1994;170:1315–1320.
89. Badaracco MA, Vessey MP. Recurrence of venous thromboembolic disease and use of oral contraceptive pills. *BMJ* 1974;1:215–217.
90. Bremme K, Lind H, Blombäck M. The effect of prophylactic heparin treatment on enhanced thrombin generation in pregnancy. *Obstet Gynecol* 1993;81:78–83.
91. Barbour LA, Pickard J. Controversies in thromboembolic disease during pregnancy: a critical review. *Obstet Gynecol* 1995;86:621–633.
92. Tengborn L, Bergqvist D, Mätzch T, Bergqvist A, Hedner U. Recurrent thromboembolism in pregnancy and puerperium: is there a need for thromboprophylaxis? *Am J Obstet Gynecol* 1989;160:90–94.
93. Hellgren M, Tengborn L, Abildgaard U. Pregnancy in women with congenital antithrombin III deficiency: experience of treatment with heparin and antithrombin. *Gynecol Obstet Invest* 1982;14:127–141.
94. Trauscht-Van Horn JJ, Capeless EL, Easterling TR, Bovill EG. Pregnancy loss and thrombosis with protein C deficiency. *Am J Obstet Gynecol* 1992;167:968–972.
95. Branch DW, Scott JR, Kochenour NK, Herhgold E. Obstetric complications associated with the lupus anticoagulant. *N Engl J Med* 1985; 313:1322–1326.
96. Malkamy H. Heparin therapy in post cesarean septic pelvic thrombophlebitis. *Int J Gynecol Obstet* 1980;17:564–566.
97. Josey WE, Staggers SR. Heparin therapy in septic pelvic vein thrombophlebitis: a study of 46 cases. *Am J Obstet Gynecol* 1974;120: 228–233.
98. Brown TK, Munsick RA. Puerperal ovarian vein thrombophlebitis: a syndrome. *Am J Obstet Gynecol* 1971;109:263–273.
99. Sweet RL, Gibbs RS. Infectious diseases of the female genital tract. 3rd ed. Baltimore: Williams & Wilkins, 1995:593–597.
100. Derrick FC, Turner WR, House EE, Stresing HA. Incidence of right ovarian vein syndrome in pregnant females. *Obstet Gynecol* 1970;35: 37–38.
101. Munsick RA, Gillanders LA. A review of the syndrome of puerperal ovarian vein thrombophlebitis. *Obstet Gynecol Surv* 1981;36:57–66.
102. Dunn LJ, Van Voorhis LW. Enigmatic fever and pelvic thrombophlebitis. *N Engl J Med* 1967;276:265–268.
103. Baka JJ, Lev-Toaff AS, Friedman AC, Radecki PD, Caroline DF. Ovarian vein thrombosis with atypical presentation: role of sonography and duplex doppler. *Obstet Gynecol* 1989;73:887–889.
104. Grant TH, Schoettle BW, Buchsbaum MS. Postpartum ovarian vein thrombosis: Diagnosis by clot protrusion into the inferior vena cava at sonography. *AJR Am J Roentgenol* 1993;160:551–552.
105. Khurana BK, Rao J, Friedman SA, Cho KC. Computed tomographic features of puerperal ovarian vein thrombosis. *Am J Obstet Gynecol* 1988;159:905–908.
106. Angel JL, Knoppel RA. Computerized tomography in the diagnosis of puerperal ovarian vein thrombosis. *Obstet Gynecol* 1984;63: 61–64.
107. Brown CEL, Lowe TW, Cunningham FG, Weinreb JC. Puerperal pelvic thrombophlebitis: impact on diagnosis and treatment using x-ray computed tomography and magnetic resonance imaging. *Obstet Gynecol* 1986;68:789–794.
108. Shulman H. Use of anticoagulants in suspected pelvic infection. *Clin Obstet Gynecol* 1969;12:240–247.
109. Collins CG, MacCallum EA, Nelson EW, Weinstein BB, Collins JH. Suppurative pelvic thrombophlebitis: study of 70 patients treated by ligation of the inferior vena cava and ovarian vessels. *Surgery* 1951; 30:298–304.

SECTION V

Genitourinary Disorders

Cherry and Merkatz's Complications of Pregnancy,
Fifth Edition, edited by W. R. Cohen.
Lippincott Williams & Wilkins, Philadelphia © 2000.

CHAPTER 16

Renal Function and Renal Disease

Martin Sedlacek and Jonathan A. Winston

Kidney function and body fluid composition are altered in normal pregnancy. Blood pressure changes, as do glomerular and tubular function. An understanding of these physiologic events allows early detection of abnormalities, thereby avoiding serious morbidity and mortality. Women with renal disease face difficult choices in pregnancy. The possibility of a late pregnancy loss, progressing to end-stage renal failure or of a shortened life span must be considered. Fortunately, the prospect for a successful pregnancy has improved in this patient population thanks to a multidisciplinary approach to medical care.

RENAL FUNCTION IN PREGNANCY

Anatomic Changes

Kidney mass increases modestly during gestation as the interstitial space fills and renal water content rises (1,2). Normal kidney length increases approximately 1 cm during pregnancy; so a reduction in kidney size postpartum does not necessarily signify a pathological process. These are important considerations when performing imaging studies.

The most striking anatomic change in the genitourinary system occurs in the renal pelvis and upper collecting system (3,4). By the first trimester, there is sonographic evidence of dilatation of the renal pelvis (5) and by midtrimester well over 60% of gravidas have a characteristic hydronephrosis that extends to the pelvic brim (6). In more than 90% of pregnant women, right-sided hydronephrosis predominates. The finding of isolated left-sided dilatation should make one suspicious of an abnormal process, such as obstruction from a congenital stricture, stone, or sloughed papilla (7). Both hormonally induced smooth-muscle atony and mechanical obstruction from the gravid uterus are responsible for ureteral dilatation. The propensity to right-sided hydronephrosis is ascribed to the physiologic dextroversion of the uterus and the crossing of the right ureter by the ovarian veins and iliac artery at the pelvic brim (8,9). The dilated ureters can contain significant amounts of urine, which may introduce dead-space errors in collection of timed urine volumes. It is recommended to start and end 24-hour urine collections after having the patient lying for an hour in the lateral recumbent position (10). Because the dilatation of the collecting system may last up to 6 weeks postpartum, it is wise to wait at least 2 months postpartum or beyond before evaluating anatomic urinary tract abnormalities.

Renal Hemodynamics

Pregnancy-induced alterations in renal blood flow (RBF) and glomerular filtration rate (GFR) have been studied extensively (11–14). Before the third trimester,

M. Sedlacek: Department of Nephrology, Mount Sinai Hospital, New York, NY 10029; J. A. Winston: Department of Medicine, Mount Sinai School of Medicine, New York, NY 10029.

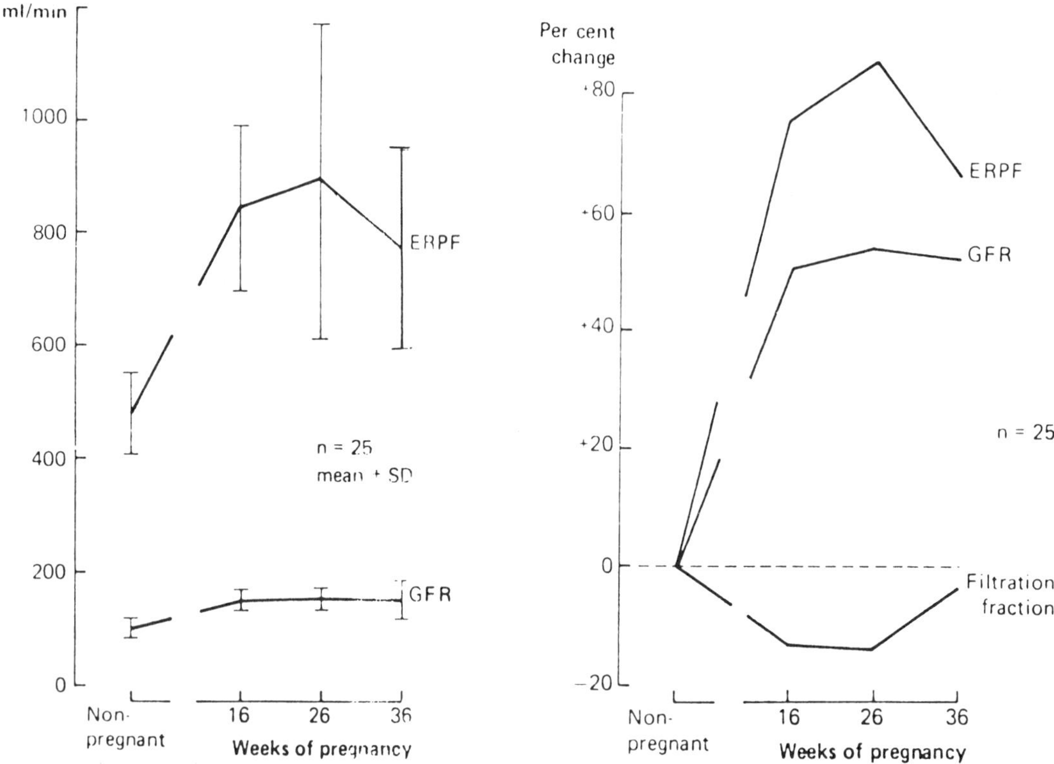

FIG. 16-1. Absolute and percentage changes in glomerular filtration rate (*GFR*), effective renal plasma flow (*ERPF*), and filtration fraction measured serially during pregnancy. (From Dunlop W. Serial changes in renal hemodynamics during normal human pregnancy. Br J Obstet Gynaecol 1981;88:1–9, with permission.)

RBF and GFR increase appreciably (15–17) (Fig. 16-1). When measured by endogenous creatinine clearance, GFR increases progressively from conception to peak levels that are 45% greater than in nonpregnant controls at approximately the ninth week of gestation (18). When measured by inulin clearance during an infusion protocol, the adaptation in GFR is temporally similar but of a greater magnitude. RBF measured by the clearance of infused para-aminohippuric acid (PAH) increases by 80% compared with nonpregnant controls by week 26 of gestation (19,20).

In the third trimester, hemodynamics are more controversial, in part because of the effects of changes in posture on renal function. Early experiments showed a 20% decrease in GFR and RBF in the near-term gravid patient when studied in the supine position compared with levels in lateral recumbency (21). This finding may represent the effects of the gravid uterus compressing the inferior vena cava and diminishing venous return to the heart. Not all investigators have agreed on the effects of posture on renal function. In any event, if they exist, their relevance under normal daily living conditions is not clear (17,22). When measured by endogenous creatinine clearance under normal ambulatory conditions, GFR decreases from its peak in the midtrimester to a value at term not significantly different from that of controls (23). The discrepancy in methodology for measurements of GFR is exemplified in a report that shows that although creatinine clearance may fall toward nonpregnant values during the third trimester, the increased inulin clearance found at midtrimester is sustained through term (19). Similar controversy exists with use of PAH clearance to estimate RBF in late gestation (20). Although some authors have shown a decline related to postural changes, one report suggests that there is a significant decrease in RBF in the third trimester that is unrelated to posture (24).

Animal studies using the pregnant rat as a model have confirmed the increase in GFR during the 3-week period of gestation. The onset of the rise in GFR is variable, however, because of its relation to volume expansion and renal blood flow changes (25–27). As in human studies, these variations have been attributed to differences in salt balance and differing infusion protocols. In elegant micropuncture studies of superficial glomeruli in the pregnant Munich-Wistar rat, whole-kidney hemodynamics as well as those in individual glomeruli have been measured and correlated (28). The increase in GFR results from increasing renal and glomerular blood flow. Studies in chronically catheterized conscious animals confirm these findings and extend them to the near-term animal when GFR and RBF return toward nongravid levels (29).

The site of vasodilatation within the glomerular microcirculation is important. Dilatation of the afferent arteriolae increases GFR and hydrostatic pressure in the glomerular capillaries. This phenomenon is called *hyperfiltration* and is believed to be one of the principal mechanisms of progression of renal disease. Importantly, in pregnancy, the concomitant dilatation of both afferent and efferent arterioles increases GFR but not glomerular cpaillary pressure and, in experimental animals, there is no glomerulosclerosis even after repeated pregnancies (30,31).

The specific mechanism of the vasodilatation of the renal and systemic circulation is an area of active investigation. Because some of these changes may be reversed by nitric oxide inhibition in animal models, this substance has been implicated as a key mediator (32). Whereas studies of urinary excretion of nitric oxide breakdown products in human pregnancy have yielded conflicting results, it has been demonstrated that intraarterial nitric oxide inhibition leads to greater vasoconstriction in a regional vascular bed (the hand) in pregnant women compared with nonpregnant human volunteers (33). A recent study of human omental arteries obtained during cesarean section found no effect of nitric oxide inhibition on acetylcholine and bradykinin-induced relaxation, again raising the prospect that other mechanisms are involved (34).

On the basis of the preceding discussion, some generalizations can be made. During normal human pregnancy, GFR rises by approximately 50% of control values by week 10 to 16 of gestation, and this is sustained through term. Late in gestation, however, when measured under the usual clinical circumstances of endogenous creatinine clearance and normal ambulation, GFR estimates may decline to values similar to those in nonpregnant controls. Renal blood flow peaks at values 60% to 80% greater than that of controls by early midtrimester and declines gradually to values 40% greater than those of controls by term (see Fig. 16-1) (14). At the week 10 of gestation, plasma blood urea nitrogen (BUN) and creatinine will have decreased from 13.0 ± 3 and 0.67 ± 0.14 to 8.7 ± 1.5 and 0.46 ± 0.15 mg per day, respectively (17). The implication of these observations is that values considered normal in nonpregnant women may represent a significant reduction in renal function in pregnancy and require further investigation. Thus, the clinician may be alerted to a preexisting unrecognized renal disease. Of note, the standard Crockcroft-Gault formula cannot be used to estimate GFR accurately in the pregnant woman because of changes in protein intake, extracellular fluid volume, and salt balance (35). There is conjecture that the failure to increase GFR early in gestation implies a maladaptive pregnancy with a high incidence of early abortion.(18)

Sodium Balance and Volume Homeostasis

Sodium salts are found in all body fluids. Sodium is actively pumped from the cell's interior; so virtually all total body sodium is found in the extracellular space. Changes in the amount of total body sodium reflect changes in extracellular fluid volume, and changes in the concentration of sodium in plasma water reflect changes in the tonicity of the body fluids.

The kidney is the primary regulator of salt and water excretion by playing a central role in regulating the volume and composition of the extracellular fluid. The amount of sodium excreted daily is the difference between the filtered load (plasma concentration × GFR) and the amount reabsorbed by the renal tubules. In a person who has a GFR of 100 mL/min and a plasma sodium concentration of 140 mEq/L, more than 20,000 mEq will be filtered daily. Assuming this woman is in sodium balance while ingesting 200 mEq sodium daily, she will excrete 200 mEq, or 1% of her filtered load [(200/20,000) × 100]. About 99% of filtered sodium will have been reabsorbed. A significant change in net excretion of, for instance, 50 mEq per day could occur by changing the percentage of reabsorption by only 0.25% [(150/20,000) × 100]. Thus, clinically significant changes in absolute sodium excretion may be the consequence of subtle and virtually unmeasurable changes in the handling of sodium in various nephron segments.

Pregnancy is characterized by marked sodium retention and expansion of the extracellular fluid space (36–40). There is a mean weight gain of approximately 10–12 kg, with an estimated 70% to 75% of this resulting from increases in total body water. Between 500 to 900 mEq of sodium is retained, 60% of which is used by the products of conception. Extracellular fluid volume begins to increase from at about week 6 of gestation and peaks between weeks 24 and 30. Total extracellular fluid accumulation ranges from 1.5 to 4 liters (Fig. 16-2).

The filtered load of sodium increases by as much as 50% during pregnancy. The absolute tubular reabsorption of sodium must increase simply to maintain balance. Tubular avidity must increase even more if it is to generate a positive salt balance. As in all sodium-retaining states, there is more than one mediator of these events. Proximal tubular sodium reabsorption is enhanced, as shown by micropuncture studies in the pregnant rat (36). Sodium-potassium adenosing triphosphatase (ATPase), an enzyme important in salt transport, has been shown to be increased during pregnancy in homogenates of renal tissue (37).

The role of the renin angiotensin system and adrenocortical hormones in this salt retention has received much attention. Plasma renin activity, angiotensinogen, and aldosterone increase during gestation, and aldosterone levels may exceed those measured in primary hyperaldosteronism (41–47). Although basal levels are high, the hormonal axis responds physiologically to changes in sodium balance in much the same way as it does in the nonpregnant state. Plasma renin activity and aldosterone increase after experimentally induced salt deprivation and are suppressed after salt loading (Fig. 16-3). Adrenalectomized

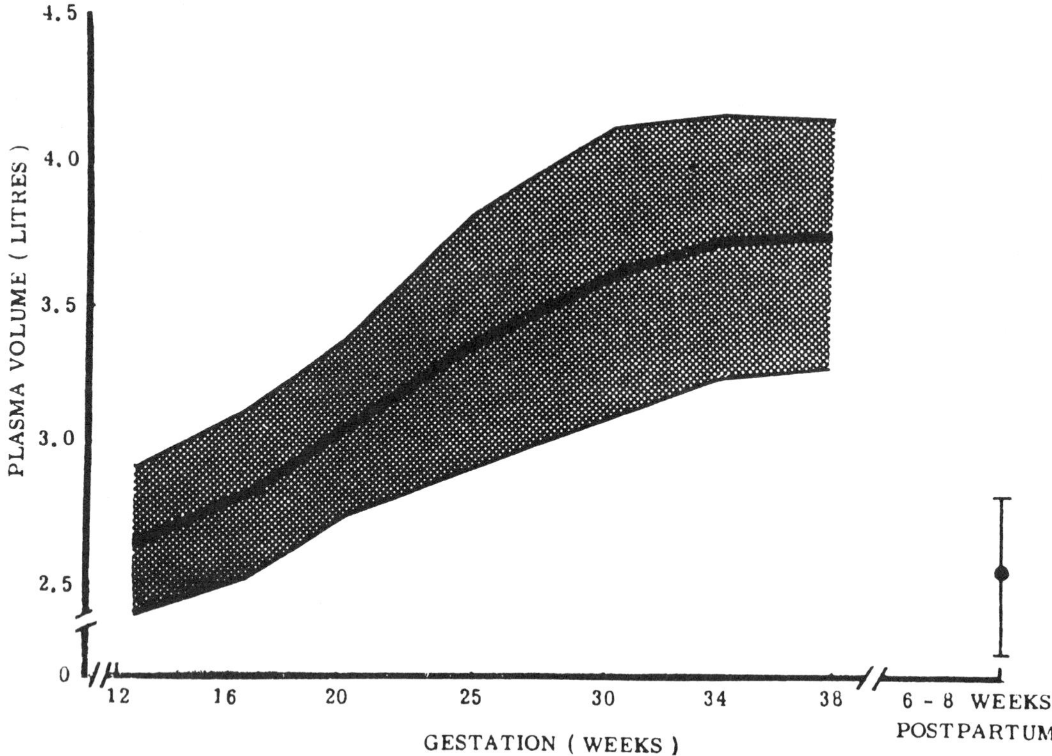

FIG. 16-2. The mean plasma volume ± SD in normal pregnancy and postpartum (**vertical bar**). (From Pirani B, Campbell D, MacGillivroy I. Plasma volume in normal first pregnancy. J Obstet Gynecol Br Communw 1973; 80:884–887, with permission.)

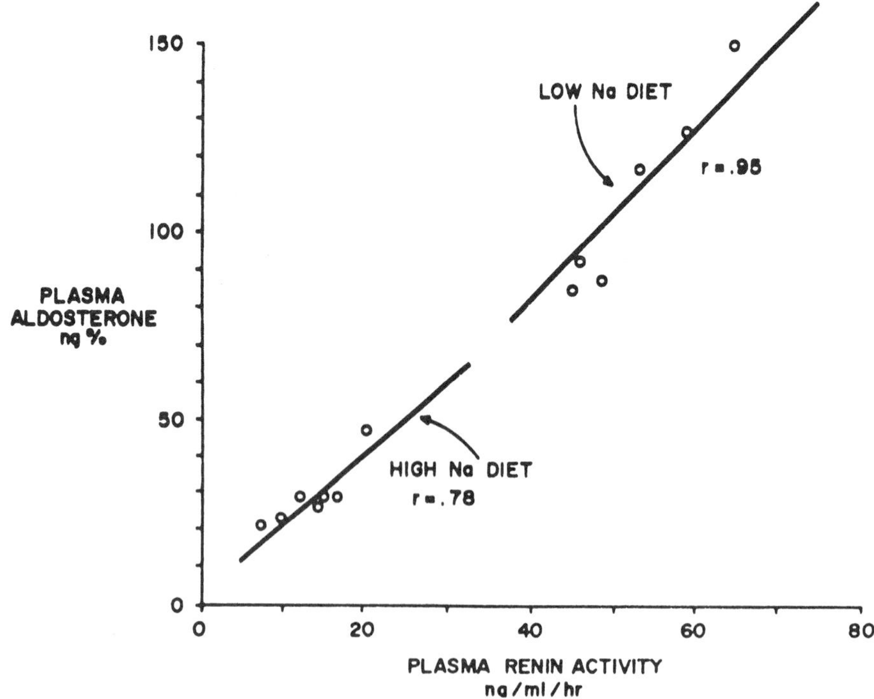

FIG. 16-3. Correlation between plasma renin activity and plasma aldosterone in pregnant women on a low- and high-sodium intake (*r*, coefficient or correlation). (From Bay W, Ferris T. Factors controlling plasma renin and aldosterone during pregnancy. Hypertension 1979;1:410–415, with permission.)

rats or those pretreated with spironolactone retain as much sodium as do gravid controls, suggesting that the high levels of aldosterone seen during gestation are not a requisite for sodium retention in this species (48).

When given exogenous mineralocorticoid or adrenocorticotrophic hormone (ACTH) in the presence of adequate dietary sodium, normal nongravidas retain sodium and gain weight for a relatively short time, until they become refractory to and "escape" from the mineralocorticoid effect. Thereafter, urinary sodium excretion increases and sodium balance is maintained at a new steady state of plasma volume expansion (49). Similarly, third-trimester grivadas are sensitive to exogenous mineralocorticoids or ACTH and retain sodium despite plasma volume expansion and high pretreatment levels of aldosterone (50). The physiologic responses of renin and aldosterone to changes in dietary sodium, the sensitivity of the gravida to exogenous mineralocorticoid, and the tendency to lose sodium when aldosterone is suppressed suggest that hyperaldosteronism in pregnancy is a physiologic adaption to the changes in renal and systemic hemodynamics. This relates to the controversial question of whether the vasodilatation in pregnancy precedes and drives the volume expansion or vice versa. The response of the renin and aldosterone system supports the effective arterial underfilling hypothesis, meaning that vasodilatation is the primary event, and sodium and water reaborption follow.

Signals other than arterial underfilling may stimulate aldosterone hypersecretion. Plasma levels of prostaglandin E increase during gestation, which may stimulate aldosterone secretion directly (51). Nonaldosterone mineralocorticoids, such as desoxycorticosterone acetate (DOCA), also are elevated in plasma during pregnancy. Changes in adrenal or fetoplacental secretion of such hormones or changes in their plasma protein binding during gestation may contribute to salt retention (43,52,53). Recent experiments mating female mice transgenic for human angiotensinogen with male mice transgenic for human renin demonstrated that during pregnancy renin can be secreted from the placental tissue into the maternal circulation and produce a preeclampsia-like syndrome (54). The relevance of these findings for humans is unclear because of the differences of uteroplacental circulation among species. Postural changes affect renal salt handling during gestation (55–57). Assumption of the supine or sitting position from lateral recumbency is associated with salt retention and, in some studies, increases in plasma renin activity and aldosterone. Whereas the uterus, placenta and fetal tissues are potential sources of these hormones, the response is immediate, making the kidney the most likely source.

Water Balance

Water retention in pregnancy accounts for a reduction in plasma osmolarity from a mean of 285 ± 4 to 278 ± 3 mOsm/kg H_2O by week 10 of gestation (Fig. 16-4) (58).

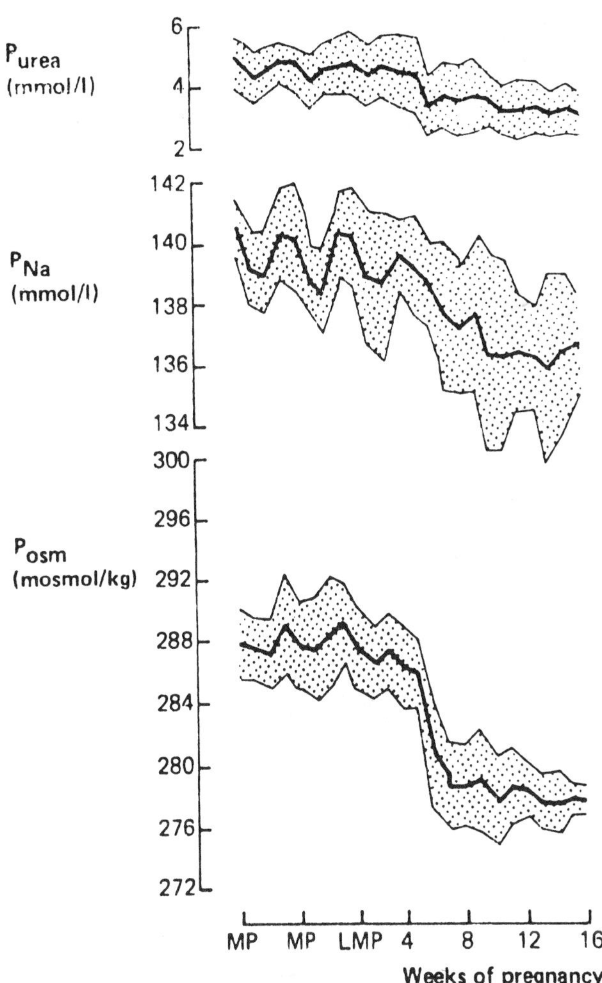

FIG. 16-4. Mean values (–SD) for plasma urea (P_{urea}), sodium (P_{Na}), and osmolality (P_{osm}) measured at weekly intervals from before conception to the first trimester in nine women with successful obstetric outcome. *MP*, menstrual period; *LMP*, last menstrual period. (From Davison J, Vallotton M, Lindheimer M. Plasma osmolality and urinary concentration during and after pregnancy: evidence that lateral recumbency inhibit maximal urinary concentrating ability Br J Obstet Gynaecol 1981;88:472–479, with permission.)

Serum sodium decreases by about 5 mEq/L during gestation; levels of 130 mEq/L being normal; those above 140 mEq/L suggest hypernatremia. Under conditions of water loading, normal gravidas maximally dilute their urine and suppress vasopressin release. They appropriately enhance vasopressin secretion and concentrate their urine when water deprived. Hence arginine vasopressin (AVP) secretion and its effects on renal water excretion are physiologically intact and appropriately sensitive to changes in plasma tonicity. The threshold for vasopressin release is adjusted to accommodate more extracellular water at a lower baseline plasma osmolarity. Equally important, the osmotic threshold for thirst also is reduced, because for any given level of plasma AVP, water retention cannot occur unless a patient is stimulated to drink (59).

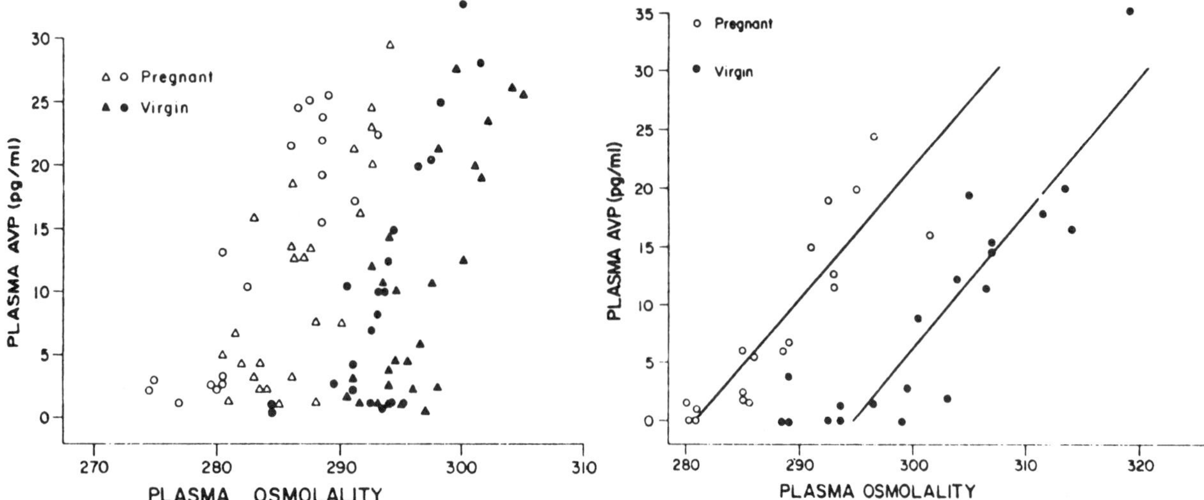

FIG. 16-5. The relationship between plasma osmolality and plasma arginine vasopressin (*AVP*) concentration in pregnant and control rats during water deprivation (**left panel**) and intraperitoneal saline injection (right panel). During dehydration, rats were water restricted for 12, 24, and 48 hours, and the results are from two separate experiemnts (**circles and triangles**). Under both conditions, increases in plasma AVP concentration are correlated to increased plasma osmolality in pregnant and virgin animals; AVP levels are greater in pregnant rats at similar levels of plasma osmolality. (From Durr J, Stamoutsos B, Lindheimer M. Osmoregulation during pregnancy in the rat. J Clin Invest 1981;68:337–346, with permission.)

Pregnant rats have significantly lower plasma osmolarity than virgin litter mates, and they enhance AVP secretion as do their nonpregnant counterparts when volume-deprived or rendered hyperosmolar (Fig. 16.5) (60). AVP secretion is appropriately suppressed under conditions of water loading. At any given plasma tonicity, AVP levels are significantly higher in pregnant rats, again suggesting that the threshold for its release is set for a lower level of baseline plasma tonicity. Administration of gestational hormones to virgin litter mates does not change the threshold for AVP release. Hence, other as yet unknown factors are responsible. Of interest, plasma tonicity is low during gestation in Brattleboro rats, who have a hereditary lack of circulating AVP. Some evidence suggests a role for human chorionic gonadotropin (HCG) in osmoregulation. Infusion of HCG into nonpregnant women lowered the osmotic thresholds for vasopressin release and thirst. In addition, a patient was described with hydatiform mole in whom these thresholds remained decreased postevacuation and normalized in parallel to serum HCG levels (61).

Rare problems with water handling have been recognized in pregnant women. Patients with preexisting central diabetes insipidus may require more replacement therapy during gestation, and inapparent partial central diabetes insipidus may be transiently unmasked by pregnancy. These phenomena are believed to be due to increased metabolism of AVP by placental factors (62).

RENAL TUBULAR FUNCTION

Uric Acid

Renal clearance of uric acid increases and plasma levels decrease during pregnancy from mean nongravid levels from 4 to 6 mg/dL to minimum values of 3 to 4 mg/dL by week 16 of gestation (63,64). Under normal conditions, uric acid is freely filterable at the glomerulus. In the proximal tubule, it is subjected to reabsorption, secretion, and further reabsorption. The relative contribution of each process to the final clearance of uric acid is modified by such factors as filtered load, extracellular fluid volume, amount and distribution of RBF, and the actions of other organic anion transport systems (65). In gravidas who have high GFR and renal blood flow, there is relatively less reabsorption (or enhanced secretion) of uric acid in the proximal tubule, leading to an increased clearance. As gestation proceeds, there is a tendency for uric acid levels to increase toward nongravid controls as the relative rate of reabsorption in the proximal tubule increases. Evidence suggests that this is secondary to the altered hemodynamics and their posturally related changes of late gestation.

The relationship between elevated plasma uric acid and toxemia of pregnancy was described early in this century. Traditionally, this observation has been attributed to enhanced tubular reabsorption because of alterations in renal hemodynamics. It has also been proposed that abnormal implantation resulting in relative hypoxia and increased turnover of trophoblast tissue leads to induction of xanthine oxidase and increased production of uric acid. Because uric acid production by xanthine oxidase is coupled with formation of reactive oxygen species, this mechanism could contribute to increased oxidative stress present in preeclampsia. Alternatively, uric acid itself has antioxidant properties, and some authors link decreased production of uric acid in the first trimester to the subsequent development of preeclampsia (66,67).

Glucose Excretion

Glucose is freely filtered at the glomerulus, and the major portion of the filtered load is actively cotransported with sodium in the proximal tubule. Whole-kidney dynamics of glucose handling have been described in terms of the classic proximal tubule titration curve (68). Below a plasma concentration termed the *threshold*, all filtered glucose is reabsorbed and the net excretion rate is zero. Above the threshold level, as delivery increases, so does net reabsorption, but some glucose is spilled into the urine. When the maximum rate of glucose reabsorption is reached (T_m, transport maximum) all reabsorptive sites are saturated, and there can be no net increase in reabsorption. So, with increasing plasma concentrations and renal delivery, there is a concomitant increase in excretion rate. It is now increasingly clear that whole-kidney glucose reabsorption is intimately associated with extracellular volume and renal salt handling. When given a glucose load under conditions of sodium avidity or minimal volume expansion, a patient can reabsorb glucose beyond the limits described in earlier clearance studies. Conversely, glucose reabsorption may diminish when extracellular fluid volume is expanded (69).

During an infusion of glucose, the net excretion of glucose is greater in gravidas compared with nonpregnant controls (70). When volume expansion and high filtration rate of pregnancy are corrected for, renal tubular threshold is not altered during pregnancy. The T_m for glucose does not increase to the same degree as does GFR; so at high delivery rates, more glucose will be excreted. At similar increments in GFR, women studied postpartum will reabsorb more glucose than they do while pregnancy (71,72).

As many as 50% of women tested during pregnancy have glycosuria (glucose excretion greater than 150 mg/24 hr) (73). There is, however, a large day-to-day variation in glucose excretion, with little correlation between excretion rates and plasma glucose concentrations. Glycosuria during pregnancy is not a reliable estimate of carbohydrate intolerance, and only a small minority of glucosuric subjects display abnormal glucose tolerance curves.(74)

Acid Excretion

Renal bicarbonate reabsorption and hydrogen secretion are intact during normal pregnancy; however, blood pH is increased to 7.42 to 7.44, and arterial PCO_2 is decreased to a mean of 31 torr (75). This respiratory alkalosis is secondary to the stimulatory effects of progesterone on the respiratory center. Consequently, serum bicarbonate levels are normally decreased during pregnancy to 18 to 22 mEq/L. A normal PCO_2 and pH level in a pregnant asthmatic patient thus represents considerable CO_2 retention and acidosis. With decreased bicarbonate and PCO_2 levels, pregnant women also have diminished defenses against acute metabolic acidosis.

RENAL DISEASE IN PREGNANCY

Acute Renal Failure

Acute renal failure (ARF) is defined as an impairment in renal function developing over a period of hours to days. Often, but not always, there is a reduction of urinary volume to below 400 mL/day. Pregnancy-associated renal failure has a bimodal distribution (76–79). The initial peak occurs early in gestation and comprises mostly cases of septic abortion. The later peak occurs toward the end of pregnancy and is mainly a result of bleeding complications and preeclampsia. Thanks to the legalization of abortion and improved social and economic conditions, the intial peak has almost disappeared in the most developed countries, but it remains an important problem in many parts of the world.

Acute Tubular Necrosis

Acute tubular necrosis (ATN) complicates many conditions, most commonly sepsis and hypotension. A variety of nephrotoxins also can cause ATN, but exposure of pregnant women to these agents is limited. In septic abortion, ATN is frequent, especially when shock develops. In early pregnancy, ATN also has been described as a result of hemorrhage complicating spontaneous abortion or as a consequence of severe volume depletion in hyperemesis gravidarum. In late pregnancy, ATN is a common renal complication in preeclampsia, eclampsia, hemorrhage, and acute fatty liver of pregnancy.

Thorough urine analysis is important to diagnose ATN. Typical urinary findings are an increased number of tubular cells and brownish pigmented casts in the sediment and sodium concentrations of greater than 25 mEq/L. Oliguria is present in about one half of patients. The degree of acidosis and hypotension will depend more on the causal event than on the magnitude of the renal failure. Because the patients are generally free of prior heart disease, congestive heart failure does not generally exist unless inordinate fluid loads have been administered. Treatment must be directed toward the control of the underlying infection and bleeding, because these factors may prove lethal.

Depending on the series, the death rate in patients who have ARF complicating septic abortion may approach 50%. Early referrals to a center equipped for comprehensive medical care, including dialysis, can reduce morbidity and mortality substantially (76). Both peritoneal and hemodialysis have been used successfully in ARF in pregnant women.

Occasionally, ARF can develop from some other cause, such as transfusion reaction, acute postinfectious glomerulonephritis, collagen vascular disease, obstruction of a single kidney or both kidneys by a gravid uterus, and even sarcoidosis. A correct diagnosis in these rare situations is important because of the potential reversibility of the underlying disorder, which generally is managed as in a nonpregnant patient (80–85).

Acute Cortical Necrosis (ACN)

Bilateral renal cortical necrosis is likely to occur in association with abruptio placentae. Preeclampsia and prolonged intrauterine fetal death are other associated conditions (76,80). The diagnosis of extensive cortical necrosis is suggested by prolonged anuria and severe renal failure that is slow to reverse. Patchy or incomplete cortical necrosis may present as a wide spectrum of degrees of renal insufficiency, ranging from mild impairment of renal function to an abrupt decline of renal function clinically indistinguishable from acute tubular necrosis. Kidney biopsy, which may miss patchy involvement of the kidney by sampling error, or better, computed tomography or renal angiography generally will confirm the diagnosis. The latter will show delayed filling and poor arborization of interlobar arteries, with complete absence or nonhomogenous filling of the cortical nephrogram (86). Pathologically, the changes can range from focal necrosis of individual glomeruli and tubules with thrombosis of the glomerular tuft, to patchy or total cortical destruction surrounded by areas of congestion, with thrombosis, necrosis, and dilatation of intrarenal arteries and arterioles.

Unlike in ATN, the onset of renal failure is frequently preceded by hypertension (79). In patients who develop ARF late in pregnancy, there is no difference in age, parity, or incidence of premature separation of the placenta in those who develop ACN as opposed to ATN (78,86).

Why some patients develop ACN and others do not is unknown. Normal pregnancy is associated with enhanced capacity to produce fibrin and a diminished facility for removing intravascular fibrin deposition (87). Whereas it has been hypothesized that these changes may constitute an evolutionary adaptation in anticipation of hemorrhage at childbirth, intravascular coagulation phenomena are frequent and have been implicated in preeclampsia, eclampsia, postpartum renal failure, and acute cortical necrosis. It has been suggested that these latter conditions may represent the clinical spectrum of one unifying disease (88–90). Consistent with this proposal is the frequent finding by some investigators of glomerular fibrin deposits in biopsy or autopsy specimens from patients who had these entities (91–93). The increased susceptibility to glomerular thrombosis in pregnancy has been attributed to decreased protein S levels, the presence of activated protein C, resistance, activation of Hageman factor, imbalance between thromboxane and prostacyclin and relative L-arginine deficiency, which compromises NO-dependent antiaggregatory effects. In contrast to virgin rats, normal late pregnant rats develop gomerular thrombosis when given low doses of endotoxin. This effect is prevented by L-arginine treatment but not by D-arginine (94–99).

There are, however, many instances of renal failure in late pregnancy in which evidence of intravascular coagulation is lacking (100). Although intravascular coagulation and glomerular fibrin deposition may be common links between the glomerular lesions that ensue from a variety of stimuli, this phenomenon is inadequate by itself to explain the variety of distinct renal and hypertensive disorders of pregnancy (101,102).

Acute Renal Failure in Preeclampsia

Preeclampsia is a multisystem disorder characterized by hypertension, proteinuria, edema, and central nervous system irritability. It occurs most frequently in young primiparas during the third trimester. In the presence of convulsions, the disorder is referred to as *eclampsia*. Proteinuria almost always accompanies preeclampsia, and historically this association was recognized before the introduction of routine blood pressure measurements. The proteinuria may be minimal or in the nephrotic range, and the magnitude correlates with the severity of the renal lesions (103). Preeclampsia is the most common cause of nephrotic proteinuria in pregnancy, a fact that exemplifies how infrequently women with a nephrotic syndrome of other cause get pregnant. *Proteinuria* is defined as more than 300 mg per day in pregnant women, which is more than the normal upper limit of 150 to 200 mg daily in healthy nonpregnant adults (104). Pregnant women excrete more protein largely because of their increased GFR. About 2% to 5% of healthy young adults have orthostatis proteinuria, which may become apparent only during pregnancy. Thus, proteinuria without hypertension is not always of concern. Even though proteinuria is relatively nonspecific and appears late during the course of preeclampsia, its presence greatly bolsters the diagnosis. These considerations underscore how the availability of baseline measurements may greatly facilitate the diagnosis of pregnancy-related complications.

Histologically, the glomeruli in preeclampsia are large and swollen, with encroachment of the capillary lumen by swollen, vacuolated endothelial cells, a finding referred to as *endotheliosis* (Figs. 16-6 and 16-7) (105). The mesangial cells may be swollen, with an increase in matrix that further impinges on the capillary lumen. Ultrastructurally, the cells are characterized by increases in the amount of cytoplasm, cytoplasmic vacuoles containing lipid droplets, and myelin-like figures within clusters of cytoplasmic lysosomal structures (Figs. 16-8 and 16-9). Immunofluorescent findings are variable. Staining for immunoglobin has been described (105,106) but appears to be caused by nonspecific trapping (100,102). Fibrin and fibrinlike deposits are seen frequently but are not invariably present, nor are they necessary for the development of the pathognomonic endotheliosis (Fig. 16-10). The glomerular lesion of focal segmental glomerulosclerosis (FGS) has been described in persons who have severe preeclampsia. Because this lesion often is accompanied by nephrosclertotic vascular disease, most authorities consider that the combination of endotheliosis and FSGS represents two independent processes in which preeclampsia is superimposed on chronic vascular disease

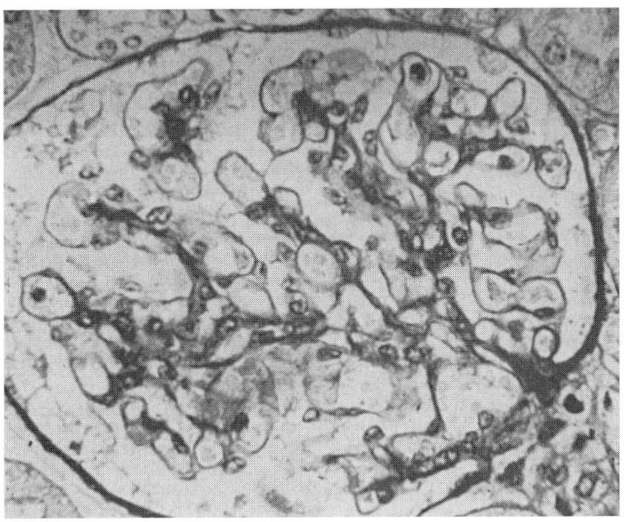

FIG 16-6. Normal glomerulus cut through the hilus. The capillaries are attached to the branching mesangial stalk, forming peripheral capillary loops (periodic acid Schiff's stain × 450). (From Churg J. In: Churg J, Sobin LM, eds. Renal disease classification and atlas of glomerular disease. Tokyo: Igaku-Shoin, 1982.)

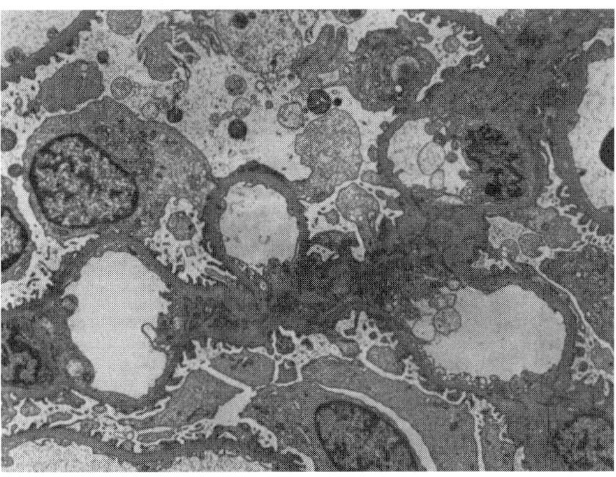

FIG. 16-8. Electron micrograph of a normal glomerulus cut longitudinally. The narrow mesangial area in the center is surrounded by capillaries. (From Churg J. In: Trump BF, Jones RT, eds. Diagnostic electron microscopy of renal diseases. New York, John Wiley & Sons, 1980.)

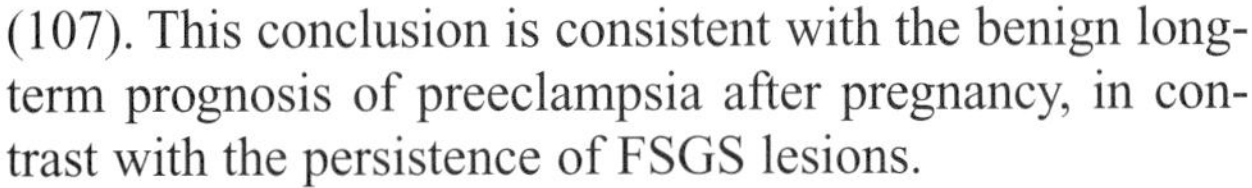

(107). This conclusion is consistent with the benign long-term prognosis of preeclampsia after pregnancy, in contrast with the persistence of FSGS lesions.

The exact incidence of renal insufficiency in patients who have eclampsia or preeclampsia is unknown. GFR may be reduced in all patients, but this is rarely clinically evident (108). In a series of 154 patients with eclampsia, only one is described as having florid renal failure (109), and in another study of 69 patients with eclampsia, 6 had a BUN greater than 20 mg/dL (110). When renal failure develops in preeclampsia, it is often due to superimposed ATN. The association of renal failure with preeclampsia is found more frequently in older multiparas who, late in pregnancy, develop severe hypertension and seizures. The finding of considerable nephrosclerotic arteriolar changes in the kidneys of these patients implies that toxemia is not primarily responsible for the renal disease, but rather that these changes are the result of chronic hypertension or superimposed preeclampsia aggravating chronic vascular disease (107,111). To distinguish between the failing renal function and rising blood pressure of underlying renal disease with hypertension late in pregnancy and superimposed preeclampsia is clinically difficult (112). In a series of 176 hypertensive gravidas in whom kidney biopsies were performed, the clinical diagnosis of preeclampsia without associated nephrosclerosis or glomerulonephritis was correct in only 50% of case (103).

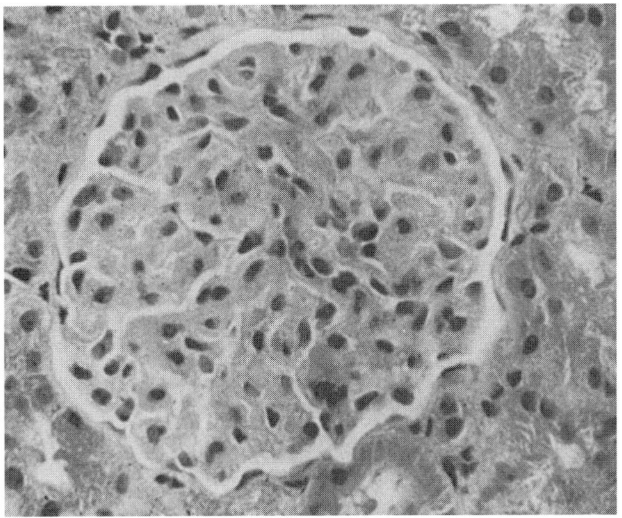

FIG. 16-7. Preeclampsia. The glomerulus is swollen. There is encroachment on the capillary lumen (hematoxylin and eosin stain, × 400). (Courtesy of Dr. Jacob Churg.)

Although the pathophysiology of preeclampsia remains poorly understood, current thinking is that there is abnormal placentation characterized by shallow trophoblastic invasion of the maternal spiral arteries. This leads to placental ischemia and the release of factors into the maternal circulation that cause widespread endothelial damage and the multisystem disorders that characterize the clinical syndrome. Difficulties in studying preeclampsia include the transitory nature of the disease and the absence of good animal models (113). Evidence of platelet activation in the form of increased cytoplasmic calcium concentration after *in vitro* stimulation with AVP or increased CD 63 expression can be detected early in the first trimester, but measuring blood pressure is still of more predictive value (114,115).

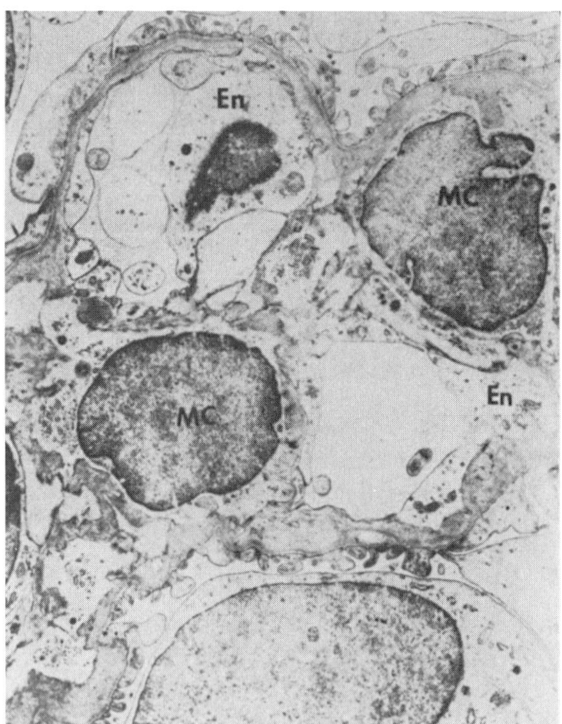

FIG. 16-9. Preeclampsia; electron micrograph; enlargement and edema of endothelial (*En*) and mesangial cells (*MC*). (From Spargo BH. In: Trump BF, Jones RT, eds. Diagnostic electron microscopy of renal diseases. New York: John Wiley & Sons, 1980.)

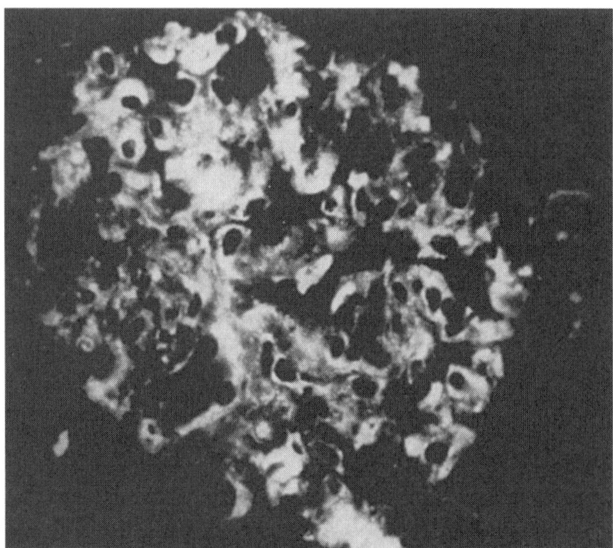

FIG. 16-10. Preeclampsia. Immunoflurescence microscopy. Depositis of fibrinogen along the capillary walls and in the mesangium (×400). (From Churg J. In: Churg J, Sobin LN, eds. Renal disease classification and atlas of glomerular disease. Tokyo: Igaku-Shoin, 1982.)

IDIOPATHIC POSTPARTUM ACUTE RENAL FAILURE

Idiopathic postpartum acute renal failure, also named *postpartum hemolytic–uremic syndrome* (116–119), has been recognized with increasing frequency since the mid-1960's. It develops generally in women who have completed normal pregnancies, and it may appear immediately or even weeks and months after an uneventful pregnancy. Clinically, it mimics the syndrome of the hemolytic–uremic syndrome described first in children, even to the extent that it is preceded by a prodromal, flu-like syndrome. Many authorities feel that the postpartum hemolytic–uremic syndrome is a form of thrombotic thrombocytopenic purpura. The clinical picture characteristically includes varying degrees of oliguric renal failure and microangiopathic hemolytic anemia. The renal failure may vary from brief mild periods of oliguria to sustained anuria lasting for weeks. Generally, the more severe the renal failure, the more evident the associated hematologic disorder, including hemolysis, anemia, numerous schistocytes, thrombocytopenia, and coagulopathy. Hypertension may be absent, mild, or severe and may develop at any time, even months after the development of the hemolytic uremia (120). When this syndrome is severe, as in the hemolytic–uremic syndrome, seizures and coma from brain involvement and cardiac failure may develop. Prognosis is guarded, and this syndrome of renal failure may lead to end-stage renal disease, although some patients have recovered. Becausse retained placental fragments have been implicated as a possible cause, currettage should be considered if this syndrome occurs close to delivery. Most authorities would recommend that patients who have recovered from any form of this syndrome not undergo subsequent pregnancies. Precise data on the outcome of subsequent pregnancies are, however, lacking.

Pathologically, edema, necrosis, and thrombosis of the interlobular and afferent arterioles are present, as well as glomerular thromboses. Mesangial swelling compresses the glomerular capillary lumen, and separation of the endothelium from the glomerular basement membrane has been described (Fig. 16-11). Immunofluorescent staining can show glomerular fibrin deposition. The picture of complete renal cortical necrosis may be seen. When severe hypertension develops, fibrinoid necrosis of many arteries and arterioles can mimic the picture of malignant nephrosclerosis.

Although the cause of this syndrome is not established, it is interesting that women who develop this picture have used oral contraceptives (121,122). This association, although not established as pathogenetically relevant, is intriguing because these agents are known to provoke vasospastic phenomena (123,124). In this syndrome, impaired intrarenal production of vasodilatory prostaglandins may predispose to endothelial damage and intravascular coagulation (125).

It is tempting to speculate that in patients who have acute renal failure late in pregnancy, the kidney may be conditioned for accentuated vasospasm as the renal hyperemia of early pregnancy subsides. This might explain the marked severity of renal failure that occurs at this time when provoked by illnesses associated with hypertension, hypovolemia, and hypoperfusion.

PREGNANCY AND URINARY TRACT INFECTION

Asymptomatic Bacteriuria

In the pregnant woman, asymptomatic bacteriuria has been emphasized as a major cause of ascending pyelonephritis, fetal prematurity, anemia, and hypertension (126,127). Depending on the study, 28% to 40% of pregnant women with asymptomatic bacteriuria will develop acute pyelonephritis. Because there are no symptoms, the diagnosis depends on the presence of more than 100,000 colonies of a single pathogen per milliliter of urine obtained by clean-voided technique. Treatment of bacteriuria diminishes the incidence of ascending pyelonephritis to approximately 3% to 4% (126–131). Early in pregnancy, sulfonamides, nitrofurantoin, cephalosporins, or ampicillin are given orally for 5 to 7 days (132).

SYMPTOMATIC INFECTION

Cystitis

Many women have symptoms of bladder dysfunction throughout pregnancy, with burning, frequency, and urgency. Because leukocytes and microhematuria may be present in the urine of normal pregnant women, cultures are necessary to diagnose cystitis. Many of the bladder symptoms may be caused by pressure and hormonal influences and are not attributable to superimposed infection.

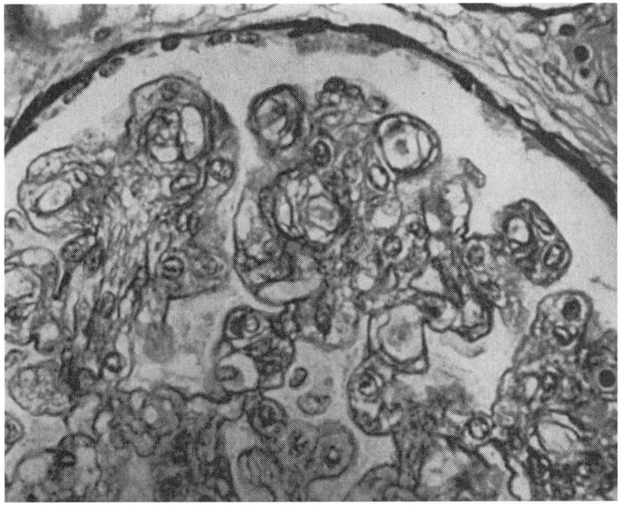

Fig. 16-11. Postpartum renal failure: Part of a glomerulus showing thickening of capillary walls by pale staining material. The capillary lumen are narrowed by patent. The mesangium is expanded (PAS stain x 640). (From Churg J, Koffler D, Paronetto F, Rorat E, Barnett RN. Hemolytic uremic syndrome as a cause of postpartum renal failure. Am J Obstet Gynecol 1970;108:253–261.)

Acute Pyelonephritis

Acute pyelonephritis is a potentially life-threatening complication during pregnancy. In contrast to the nonpregnant patient, pyelonephritis leads more frequently to acute renal failure in the pregnant woman. Complications such as septic shock, renal abscess, and renal vein thrombosis may develop, and patients are generally hospitalized and treated with intravenous antibiotics (126,131). Considering the severe dilatation of the ureters and pelvis that takes place during normal pregnancy and the pressure from the enlarging uterus on the bladder and ureters, the infrequency of ascending symptomatic pyelonephritis attests to the resistance of the pregnant kidney to severe infection. Whereas the single most important risk factor for pyelonephritis is the presence of asymptomatic bacteriuria, only 1% of women will acquire bacteriuria during pregnancy if it is not already present at the time of the original screening culture. In fact, when symptomatic kidney infection does occur, underlying disease may be present. Unrecognized diabetes, analgesic abuse nephropathy, reflux nephropathy, prior stone disease, or congenital obstruction all must be considered. There are instances, however, when women who have congenital urinary tract strictures and other mild or even moderate structural obstruction go through pregnancies without recognizable infections. Often these defects are recognized many years after the childbearing period has passed. Good examples of how an abnormal kidney protects itself against infection are patients with polycystic kidney disease, in whom infection is infrequent.(133)

PREGNANCY AND CHRONIC RENAL DISEASE

The likelihood of a successful pregnancy in women who have chronic stable renal disease and variable degrees of renal insufficiency has been a topic of much debate over the years. Both the effect of pregnancy on the natural history of the kidney disease and the likelihood of a successful pregnancy in the face of underlying kidney disease must be considered. It is now clear that many women with a mild to modest degree of impaired renal function may become pregnant and carry through a successful gestation with a normal infant and no adverse effect on the kidney disease. For example, generally favorable results were reported in a study of 121 pregnancies in 89 women with biopsy-proved renal disease but only minimal impairment of GFR (prepregnancy creatinine ≤1.4 mg/100 mL) (134). Despite a high incidence of gestational hypertension (23%) and transiently increased proteinuria (47%), renal function was not adversely affected by gestation. There was an increased incidence of small-for-date infants (24%), premature delivery (20%), and fetal death (9%). These findings have been confirmed by several subsequent studies (135,136). After a mean follow-up of 15 years, no difference was found in renal survival between 171 women with histologically confirmed primary glomerulonephritis who became pregnant compared with 189 women who did not (135).

It must be emphasized that most patients in these studies had near-normal renal function at conception. If the renal failure is advanced or hypertension is present, rapid deterioration of renal function may be observed. In one series of eight patients with initial creatinine of 1.6 or greater, seven had troublesome gestational hypertension (diastolic ≥90) and, in four, renal function deteriorated during pregnancy (134). Similarly, another series reported that 8 of 11 pregnancies were complicated by deteriorating renal function when the initial BUN was greater than 50 mg/dL (137). Unfortunately, our understanding of the mechanism by which pregnancy can impair residual kidney function is limited because pregnancy does not have adverse effects when superimposed on experimental kidney disease in animal models (138). In women with more advanced renal insufficiency, the recommendation may be made to postpone pregnancy until renal transplantation. To establish a fixed level of renal insufficiency beyond which pregnancy is not recommended is difficult, but it appears that a successful result is unlikely if creatinine clearance is appreciably below 35 to 40 mL/min and serum creatinine is much above 2 or 2.5 mg/dL (139).

In considering the effects of gestation on renal function, the type of renal lesion is also important (140,141). Patients with scleroderma and polyarteritis nodosa, both of which are associated with hypertension, do poorly. Most authorities agree that pregnancy should be discouraged. When albuminuria is sufficient to produce a nephrotic syndrome with edema, hypoalbuminemia, and hyperlipidemia, women only rarely become pregnant, and there is a high rate of spontaneous abortion, intrauterine growth retardation, and prematurity (142–146). Therefore, whenever possible, diagnosis and treatment should be achieved before planning pregnancy.

Two specific causes of chronic kidney disease warrant special consideration because of their propensity to affect women in the childbearing years: systemic lupus erythematosus (SLE) and diabetes mellitus. Convincing evidence now exists to show that when SLE has been in clinical remission for months to a year, pregnancy is feasible and renal function may remain unchanged or become only transiently reduced (147–152). Although in this and in other glomerular diseases there may be increasing proteinuria during gestation, it is not clear whether this represents significant structural renal damage (149,153). If exacerbation does occur during pregnancy or postpartum, it generally can be controlled with steroids or immunosuppressive therapy. In patients in whom renal SLE has been active before pregnancy, exacerbations are more likely, with associated hypertension, renal insufficiency, and a high percentage of fetal death. In some patients, SLE first develops late in pregnancy or postpartum. It may be difficult to distinguish between a new onset of renal lupus and preeclampsia. In most cases, a diagnostic renal biopsy can be postponed until after delivery. If immunosuppressive therapy that may be potentially detrimental to the fetus is considered, a biopsy can be performed under conditions of adequate blood pressure control and normal coagulation parameters before week 32 of gestation to secure the diagnosis and aid in decision making. Beyond week 32 of gestation, decisions for inducing labor are generally made on clinical grounds, and a renal biopsy should be delayed until postpartum (8,154,155).

The management of patients with diabetic nephropathy is similar to that of other patients with chronic glomerular disease. The better the renal function and the less the hypertension, the more likely an uncomplicated pregnancy. Fetal and maternal outcomes are worse with more overt diabetic nephropathy. These observations are similar to the experience with diabetic retinopathy, in which the severity of preexisting disease greatly influences the degree of progression during pregnancy (156). Whereas no rapid onset of renal impairment in patients with near-normal renal function has been observed, several authors have reported accelerated progression of overt nephropathy with pregnancy (157). Angiotensin-converting enzyme inhibitors, which may slow the progression of the disease, are contraindicated in pregnancy because of the risk of fetal loss and malformations associated with their use. With the recognition that the level of glycemia is directly related to the incidence of congenital malformations, the emphasis on the management of diabetic pregnancy has been on the meticulous control of blood sugar (158). Given that the prognosis of diabetic patients on dialysis is worse than of other patients on dialysis, renal transplantation is recommended wherever possible.

The value of dietary protein restriction in patients with renal disease has been debated for years among nephrologists. Most authors agree, however, that dietary protein restriction may be harmful in pregnancy and should therefore be abandoned.

PREGNANCY AND DIALYSIS

The experience of single dialysis centers with pregnant patients is limited. The results of a nationwide survey to which 40% of dialysis centers responded were published recently. In a 4-year period, the infant survival rate was 40.2% in 184 pregnancies conceived after starting dialysis compared with 73.6% of 57 pregnancies conceived prior to dialysis. Thirty-eight percent of all spontaneous abortions occurred in the second trimester. The calculated frequency of conception of the studied population of 6,230 women was 1% to 2% over a 3-year period. Of the infants for whom gestational age was reported, 84% were premature. There was a trend toward better survival and decreased prematurity in patients who received 20 hours of more dialysis per week and a weak correlation (p = 0.05) between number of hours of dialysis and gestational age (159). Similar surveys were conducted in Saudi Arabia and Belgium, reporting 27 and 15 pregnancies in dialysis patients, respectively. Both studies showed a correlation between longer dialysis time and decreased prematurity or increased birth weight (160,161). Most clinicians recommend increasing the dialysis dose in pregnancy.

The diagnosis of pregnancy is difficult in dialysis patients and often made late by ultrasonography. Early symptoms of pregnancy, such as nausea and amenorrhea, are nonspecific and frequently attributed to the renal insufficiency. Single urine and serum HCG measurements cannot be used reliably for diagnosis. Because HCG is produced by extraplacental tissues and normally excreted by the kidneys, nonpregnant dialysis patients may have borderline elevated serum levels (162). The first apparent symptom of pregnancy actually may be worsening of anemia with increased iron and erythropoietin requirements. As a consequence, dialysis patients often come to obstetric care rather late after conception.

One frequent complication of dialysis during pregnancy is hypotension. Because of the weight gain related to the growing fetus and the physiologic volume expansion and edema, the target weight at the end of the dialysis must be increased constantly or hypotension may occur during treatment. An additional cause may be the physiologic decrease in peripheral vascular resistance. For this reason, more frequent treatments with less fluid removal are advised (163,164). It is also recommended to maintain pretreatment blood urea nitrogen low to prevent polyhydramnios, from osmotic diuresis in the fetal kidneys. As the composition of the dialysate has been formulated to meet the needs of thrice-weekly treatments, adjustments are required for daily intensive dialysis to prevent hypokalemia, hypercalcemia, and alkalai overload. Severe maternal anemia can be deleterious to the fetus, and maintenance of a low normal hematocrit usually requires increased erythropoietin doses. Several reports describe erythropoietin use during pregnancy without side effects. Although intravenous iron has been used during pregnancy, it has been reported that in the last trimester most of a given dose is transferred to the fetus. To avoid acute iron toxicity, a recommendation was made to use multiple small doses (163). The requirement for 1,25 dihydroxyvitamin D_3 supplements may decrease during pregnancy because of placental production (165).

Dialysis may trigger preterm labor, and a plan for medical treatment should be in place should this event occur. Because of the severely diminished renal excretion of magnesium, there is a potential for severe life-threatening side effects if magnesium is used to treat preterm labor, and its use has been discouraged by several authorities (163). In peritoneal dialysis patients, however, serum magnesium levels could be titrated by adding magnesium to the dialysate as described in the series of Redrow and colleagues (165).

PREGNANCY AND RENAL TRANSPLANTATION

The first reported successful term delivery following renal transplant occurred in 1958 in a recipient from an identical twin (166). By 1975 a multicenter survey described 406 transplant recipients who accounted for 440 pregnancies (167). To date, the number of pregnancies in women who previously received a renal transplant is several thousand. In a survey of the world literature in 1994, 3,382 gestations were recorded in 2,409 renal allograft recipients (168). Spontaneous and therapeutic abortion occurred in 34%, but more than 90% of pregnancies that passed the first trimester delivered successfully. The incidence of preterm delivery and intrauterine growth retardation was 40% to 50%. The most significant maternal complications are hypertension and preeclampsia, which are reported to occur in about 30% of pregnant transplant recipients. Recent case–control studies did not show adverse long-term effects of pregnancy on renal allograft function or survival after 11 to 15 years (169, 170).

In 1991 the National Transplantation Pregnancy Registry was established at Thomas Jefferson University in Philadelphia to study pregnancy outcome in recipients of all types of transplants. No adverse effects of cyclosporine A on pregnancy have been demonstrated (171,172). Because the bioavailability of cyclosporine changes during pregnancy, close monitoring on doses and graft function is recommended, especially during the third trimester and the immediate postdelivery period.

The experience of individual centers corroborates the data from the large surveys. In one of the larger single series, 56 pregnancies in 37 women were studied (173). Out of 16 pregnancies marked by preexisting hypertension or renal impairment, 10 were complicated by preeclampsia. Five additional cases of preeclampsia were recorded, an overall incidence of 27%. In four instances, deteriorating renal function was attributed to pregnancy, three cases of which had prior hypertension or renal insufficiency. Out of 44 deliveries, 20 infants were born before 37 weeks gestation, although most were of a size appropriate for gestational age.

Thus, the experience of most authors is that hypertension and toxemia are relatively common complications of pregnancy in transplant recipients, occurring in slightly more than 30% of patients (167,173–175). Less common but important complications include bacterial infections, viral infections, aand rejection. The latter is estimated in one series to occur in 9% of cases (174). Mechanical interference between the gravid uterus and the transplanted kidney is a rare event. The indications for cesarean section in renal transplant patients generally do not differ from those of other women (175). For the infant, prematurity and its complications are the most common threats. Less frequent are septicemia, lymphopenia, and adrenocortical insufficiency and congenital anomalies. Renal transplants are performed without regard to rhesus factor compatibility and can lead to rhesus immunization of the mother.

Although the course of pregnancy in the transplant population is, in many instances, uneventful, it carries a high risk to mother and infant. Many agree that the least risk is imposed on both parties when conception occurs after 1 to 2 years of stable renal function posttransplantation and in the absence of significant renal impairment, hypertension, proteinuria, or the need for high doses of immunosuppressive therapy (176,177). As the relative infertility of patients on dialysis recedes rapidly with renal transplantation, the possibility of conception raises the need for appropriate family planning counseling so that pregnancy can be planned in the most favorable conditions.

ACKNOWLEDGMENT

The authors would like to express thanks to Dr. Jacob Churg who reviewed this manuscript and provided us with graphic material.

REFERENCES

1. Bailey R, Rolleston G. Kidney length and ureteric dilatation in the puerperium. *J Obstet Gynaecol Br Commonw* 1971;78:55–61.
2. Lindheimer M, Katz A. The renal response to pregnancy. In: Brenner BM, Rector FC (ed). The kidney, 2nd ed. Philadelphia: WB Saunders, 1981:1762.
3. Fayad M, Youssef A, Zahran M, Kamel M, Badr M. The ureterocalyceal system in normal pregnancy. *Acta Obstet Gynecol Scand* 1973; 52:69–76.
4. Schulman A, Herlinger H. Urinary tract dilatation in pregnancy. *Br J Radiol* 1975;48:638–645.
5. Fried A. Hydronephrosis of pregnancy: ultrasonographic study and classification of asymptomatic women. *Am J Obstet Gynecol* 1979; 135:1066–1070.
6. Erickson LM, Nicholson S, Lewall D, Frischke L. Ultrasound evaluation of hydronephrosis of pregnancy. *J Clin Ultrasound* 1979;7:128–132.
7. Harris R. Correlation of postpartum intravenous pyelograms with clinical localization of antepartum pyelonephritis. *Am J Obstet Gynecol* 1981;141:105–106.
8. Lindheimer MD, Katz AI. Kidney function and disease in pregnancy. Philadelphia: Lea & Febiger, 1977:6–7.
9. Roberts J. Hydronephrosis of Pregnancy. *Urology* 1976;8: 1–4.
10. Lindheimer MD, Katz AI. Renal physiology and disease in pregnancy. In: Seldin DW, Giebisch G, ed. The kidney: physiology an pathophysiology, 2nd ed. New York: Raven Press, 1992:373.
11. Chesley L, Chesley E. The diodrast clearance and renal blood flow in normal pregnant women. *Am J Physiol* 1939;127:731–737.
12. Nice M. Kidney function during normal pregnancy. 1. The increased urea clearance of normal pregnancy. *J Clin Invest* 1935;14:575–578.
13. Chesley L. Renal functional changes in normal pregnancy. *Clin Obstet Gynecol* 1960;3:349–363.
14. Davison J, Dunlop W. Renal hemodynamics and tubuler function in normal human pregnancy. *Kidney Int* 1980;18:152–161.
15. Assali N, Dignam W, Dasgupta K. Renal function in human pregnancy: II. Effects of venous pooling on renal hemodynamics and water, electrolyte, and aldosterone excretion during normal gestation. *J Lab Clin Med* 1959;54:394–408.
16. DeAlvarez R. Renal glomerular tubular mechanisms during normal pregnancy. I. Glomerular filtration rate, renal plasma flow and creatinine clearance. *Am J Obstet Gynecol* 1958;75:931–944.
17. Sims E, Krantz K. Serial studies of renal function during pregnancy and the puerperium in normal women. *J Clin Invest* 1958;37:1764–1774.
18. Davison J, Noble M. Serial changes in 24-hour creatinine clearance during normal menstrual cycles and the first trimester of pregnancy. *Br J Obstet Gynaecol* 1981;88:10–17.
19. Davison J, Hytten F. Glomerular filtration during and after pregnancy. *J Obstet Gynaecol Br Commonw* 1974;81:588–595.
20. Dunlop W. Serial changes in renal hemodynamics during normal human pregnancy. *Br J Obstet Gynaecol* 1981;88:1–9.
21. Chesley L, Sloan D. The effect of posture on renal function in late pregnancy. *Am J Obstet Gynecol* 1964;89:754–759.
22. Dunlop W. Investigations into the influence of posture on renal plasma flow and glomerular filtration rate during late pregnancy. *Br J Obstet Gynaecol* 1976;83:17–23.
23. Davison J, Dunlop W, Ezimokhai M. 24-Hour creatinine clearance during the third trimester of normal pregnancy. *Br J Obstet Gynaecol* 1980;87:106–109.
24. Ezimokhai M, Davison J, Philips P, Dunlop W. Nonpostural serial changes in renal function during the third trimester of normal human pregnancy. *Br J Obstet Gynaecol* 1981;88:465–471.
25. Atherton J, Pirie S. The effect of pregnancy on glomerular filtration rate and salt and water reabsorption in the rat. *J Physiol* 1981;319: 153–164.
26. Davison J, Lindheimer M. Changes in renal hemodynamics and kidney weight during pregnancy in the unanesthetized rat. *J Physiol* 1980;301:129–136.
27. Lindheimer M, Katz A. Kidney function in the pregnant rat. *J Lab Clin Med* 1971;78:633–641.
28. Baylis C. The mechanism of the increase in glomerular filtration rate in the twelve-day pregnant rat. *J Physiol* 1980;305:405–414.
29. Conrad KP. Renal hemodynamics during pregnancy in chronically catheterized, conscious rats. *Kidney Int* 1984;26:24–29.
30. Baylis C, Rennke HG. Renal hemodynamics and glomerular morphology in repetitively pregnant aging rats. *Kidney Int* 1985;28:140–145.
31. Baylis C, Reckelhoff JF. Renal hemodynamics in normal and hypertensive pregnancy: lessons from micropuncture. *Am J Kidney Dis* 1991;17:98–104.
32. Deng A, Engels K, Baylis C. Impact of nitric oxide deficiency on blood pressure and glomerular hemodynamic adaptations to pregnancy in the rat. *Kidney Int* 1996;50:1132–1138.
33. Williams DJ, Vallance PJT, Neild GH, Spencer JAD, Imms FJ. Nitric oxide mediated vasodilatation in human pregnancy. *Am J Physiol* 1997;272:H748–752.
34. Pascoal IF, Lindheimer MD, Nalbantian-Brandt C, Umans JG. Preeclampsia selectively impairs endothelium-dependent relaxation and leads to oscillatory activity in small omental arteries. *J Clin Invest* 1998;101:464–470.
35. Wuadri KH, Bernadini J, Greenberg A, Laifer S, Syed A, Holley JL. Assessment of renal function during pregnancy using a random urine protein to creatinine ratio and Cockcroft-Gault formula. *Am J Kid Dis* 1994;24:416–420.
36. Burg MB. Renal handling of sodium chloride water, amino acids and glucose. In: Brenner BM, Rector FC, eds. The kidney, 2nd ed. Philadelphia: WB Saunders, 1981:328.
37. Stein JH, Reimeck HJ. Regulation of sodium balance. In: Maxwell MH, Kleeman CR, eds. Clinical disorders of fluid and electrolytes metabolism, 3rd ed. New York: McGraw-Hill, 1980:989.
38. Chesley L. Plasma and red cell volumes during pregnancy. *Am J Obstet Gynecol* 1972;112:440–450.
39. Pipe N, Smith T, Halliday D, Edmonds C, Williams C, Cortart T. Changes in fat, fat-free mass and body water in human normal pregnancy. *Br J Obstet Gynaecol* 1979;86:929–940.
40. Pirani B, Campbell D, MacGillivroy I. Plasma volume in normal first pregnancy. *J Obstet Gynecol Br Communw* 1973;80:884–887.
41. Becker R, Hagashi R, Franks R, Speroff L. Effects of positional change and sodium balance on the renin-angiotensin-aldosterone system; big renin and prostaglandins in normal pregnancy. *J Clin Endocrinol Metab* 1978;46:467–472.

42. Ehrlich E. Mineralocorticoids in normal and hypertensive pregnancies. *Semin Perinatol* 1978;2:61–71.
43. Nolten W, Ehrlich E. Sodium and mineralocorticoids in normal pregnancy. *Kidney Int* 1980;18:162–172.
44. Skinner S, Lumbers E, Symonds E. Analysis of charges in the renin-angiotensin system during pregnancy. *Clin Sci* 1972;42:479–488.
45. Weinberger M, Kremer N, Petersen L, Cleary R, Young P. In: Lindheimer M, Katz A, Zuspan F, eds. Hypertension in pregnancy. New York: John Wiley & Sons, 1976:263.
46. Weir R, Brown J, Fraser R, et al. Relationship between plasma renin, renin substrate, angiotensin II, aldosterone and electrolytes in normal pregnancy. *J Clin Endocrinol Metab* 1975;40:108–115.
47. Wilson M, Morganti A, Zervoudakis J, et al. Blood pressure, the renin-aldosterone system and sex-steroid throughout normal pregnancy. *Am J Med* 1980;68:97–104.
48. Churchill S, Bengele H, Melby J, Alexander E. Role of aldosterone in sodium retention of pregnancy in the rat. *Am J Physiol* 1981;240: R175–R181.
49. Relman AS, Schwartz WB. The effect of DOCA on electrolyte balance in normal man and its relation to sodium chloride intake. *Yale J Biol Med* 1952;24:540–558.
50. Ehrlich E, Lindheimer M. Effect of administered mineralocorticoids or ACTH in pregnant women. *J Clin Invest* 1972;51:1301–1309.
51. Bay W, Ferris T. Factors controlling plasma renin and aldosterone during pregnancy. *Hypertension* 1979;1:410–415.
52. Ehrlich E, Biglieri E, Lindheimer M. ACTH-induced sodium retention in pregnancy: role of desoxycorticosterone and corticosterone. *J Clin Endocrinol Metab* 1974;38:701–705.
53. Nolten W, Lindheimer M, Oparil S, Rueckert P, Ehrlich E. Desoxycorticosterone in normal pregnancy. *Am J Obstet Gynecol* 1979;133: 644–648.
54. Takimoto E, Ishida J, Sugiyama F, Horiguchi H, Murakami K, Fukamizu A. Hypertension induced in pregnant mice by placental renin and maternal angiotensinogen. *Science* 1996;274:995–998.
55. Brandes J, Abramovici H, Katz M, Diengott D, Spindel A, Kahana L. The effect of postural changes on plasma renin activity during normal and pathologic pregnancies. *Obstet Gynecol* 1978;52:530–532.
56. Lindheimer M, Ehrich E. Postural effects on renal function and volume homeostasis during pregnancy. *J Reprod Med* 1979;23:135–141.
57. Lindheimer M, Del Greco F, Ehrlich E. Postural effects on Na and steroid excretion, and serum renin activity during pregnancy. *J Appl Physiol* 1973;35:343–348.
58. Davison J, Vallotton M, Lindheimer M. Plasma osmolality and urinary concentration during and after pregnancy: evidence that lateral recumbency inhibits maximal urinary concentrating ability. *Br J Obstet Gynaecol* 1981;88:472–479.
59. Lindheimer MD, Barron WM, Davison JM. Osmoregulation of thirst and vasopressin release in pregnancy. *Am J Physiol* 1989;257: F159–F169.
60. Durr J, Stamoutsos B, Lindheimer M. Osmoregulation during pregnancy in the rat. *J Clin Invest* 1981;68:337–346.
61. Davison JM, Shiells EA, Philips PR, Lindheimer MD. Serial evaluation of vasopressin release and thirst in human pregnancy: role of human chorionic gonadotrophin on the osmoregulatory changes of gestation. *J Clin Invest* 1988;81:798–806.
62. Lindheimer MD, Katz AI. Renal physiology and disease in pregnancy. In: Seldin DW, Giebisch G, eds. The kidney: physiology and pathophysiology, 2nd ed. New York: Raven Press, 1992:3381.
63. Boyle J, Campbell S, Duncan A, Greig W, Buchanan W. Serum uric acid levels in normal pregnancy with observations on the renal excretion of urate in pregnancy. *J Clin Pathol* 1966;19:501–503.
64. Dunlop W, Davison J. The effect of normal pregnancy upon the renal handling of uric acid. *Br J Obstet Gynaecol* 1977;84:13–21.
65. Chonko AM, Granthem J. Disorders of urate metabolism and excretion. In: Brenner BM, Rector FC, eds. The kidney, 2nd ed. Philadelphia: WB Saunders, 1981:1033.
66. Many A, Huel CA, Roberts JM. Hyperuricemia and xanthine oxidase in preeclampsia, revisited. *Am J Obstet Gynecol* 1996;174: 288–291.
67. deJong CL, Paarlberg KM, van Geijn HP, et al. Decreased first trimester uric acid production in future preeclamptic patients. *J Perinat Med* 1997;25:347–352.
68. Pitts R. Physiology of the kidney and body fluids, 3rd ed. Chicago: Year Book Medical Publishers, 1974.
69. Kurtzman N, White M, Rogers P, Flynn J. Relationship of sodium reabsorption and glomerular filtration rate to renal glucose reabsorption. *J Clin Invest* 1972;51:127–133.
70. Davison J, Hydden F. The effect of pregnancy on the renal handling of glucose. *Br J Obstet Gynaecol* 1975;82:374–381.
71. Christensen P. Tubular reabsorption of glucose during pregnancy. *Scand J Clin Lab Invest* 1958;10:364–371.
72. Welsh G, Sims E. The mechanisms of renal glucosuria in pregnancy. *Diabetes* 1960;9:363–369.
73. Zarowitz M, Newhouse S. Renal glycosuria in normoglycemic glycosuric pregnancy: a quantitative study. *Metabolism* 1973;11:755–761.
74. Lind J, Hytten F. The excretion of glucose during normal pregnancy. *J Obstet Gynecol Br Commonw* 1972;79:961–965.
75. Lindheimer MD, Katz AI. Renal physiology and disease in pregnancy. In: Seldin DW, Giebisch G, ed. The kidney: physiology and pathophysiology, 2nd ed. New York: Raven Press, 1992:3378.
76. Chugh K, Singhal P, Sharma B, Pal Y, Matthew M, Dhall K, Datta B. Acute renal failure of obstetric origin. *Obstet Gynecol* 1976;48:642–646.
77. Grunfeld JP, Ganeval D, Bournerias F. Acute renal failure in pregnancy. *Kidney Int* 1980;18:179–191.
78. Harkins J, Wilson P, Muggah H. Acute renal failure in obstetrics. *Am J Obstet Gynecol* 1976;118:331–336.
79. Smith K, Browne J, Shackman R, Wrong O. Acute renal failure of obstetric origin. *Lancet* 1965;2:351–354.
80. Stein J, Lifschitz M, Barnes L. Current concepts on the pathophysiology of acute renal failure. *Am J Physiol* 1978;234:F171–F181.
81. Cole E, Bear R, Steinberg W. Acute renal failure at 24 weeks of pregnancy: A case report. *Can Med Assoc J* 1980;122:1161–1162.
82. Fox J, Katz M, Klein S. Young B. Sudden anuria in a pregnant women with a solitary kidney. *Am J Obstet Gynecol* 1978;132:583–585.
83. Goldberg K, Kwart A. Intermittent urinary retention in first trimester of pregnancy. *Urology* 1981;17:270–271.
84. Knapp R, Hellman L. Acute renal failure in pregnancy. *Am J Obstet Gynecol* 1959;78:570–577.
85. O'Shaughnessy R, Weprin S, Zuspan F. Obstructive renal failure by an overdistended uterus. *Obstet Gynecol* 1980;55:247–249.
86. Kleinknecht D, Grunfeld JP, Gomez P, Moreau JF, Garcia-Torres R. Diagnostic procedures and long-term prognosis in bilateral renal cortical necrosis. *Kidney Int* 1973;4:390–400.
87. Stirling Y, Woolf L, North RS, Seghatchian MJ, Meade TW. Haemostasis in Normal Pregnancy. *Thromb Haemostas* 1984;52: 176–182.
88. Kincaid-Smith P. The similarity of lesions and underlying mechanism in preeclampsia toxemia and postpartum renal failure. In: Kincaid-Smith P, Matthew TH, Becker EL, eds. Glomerulonephritis morphology natural history and treatment. New York: John Wiley & Sons, 1972:809.
89. MacDonald M, Clarkson A, Davison M. The role of coagulation in renal disease. In: Kincaid-Smith P, Matthew TH, Becker EL, eds. Glomerulonephritis morphology natural history and treatment. New York: John Wiley & Sons, 1972:809.
90. McKay D. Blood coagulation and toxemia of pregnancy. In: Kincaid-Smith P, Matthew TH, Becker EL, eds. Glomerulonephritis morphology natural history and treatment. New York: John Wiley & Sons, 1972:809.
91. Morris R, Vassalli P, Beller F, McCluskey R. Immunofluorescent studies of renal biopsies in the diagnosis of toxemia in pregnancy. *Obstet Gynecol* 1964;24:32–46.
92. Vassalli P, McCluskey R. The coagulation process and glomerular disease. *Am J Med* 1965;39:175–183.
93. Vassalli P, Morris R, McCluskey R. The pathogenesis role of fibrin deposition in the glomerular lesions of toxemia of pregnancy. *J Exper Med* 1963;118:467–478.
94. Cerneca F, Ricci G, Simeone R, Malisano M, Alberico S, Guaschino S. Coagulation and fibrinolysis changes in normal pregnancy. Increased levels of procoagulants and reduced levels of inhibitors during pregnancy induce a hypercoagulable state, combined with a reactive fibrinolysis. *Eur J Obstet Gynecol Reprod Biol* 1997;73:31–36.
95. Hallak M, Senderowicz J, Cassel A, et al. Activated protein C resistance (factor V Leiden) associated with thrombosis in pregnancy. *Am J Obstet Gynecol* 1997;176:889–893.
96. Raij L. Glomerular thrombosis in pregnancy: Role of the L-argininenitric oxide pathway. *Kidney Int* 1994;45:775–781.
97. McKay D, Merrill S, Weiner A, Herlig A, Reid D. The pathologic anatomy of eclampsia, bilateral renal cortical necrosis, pituitary necrosis and other acute fetal complications of pregnancy and its pos-

sible relationship to the generalized Shwartzman phenomenon. *Am J Obstet Gynecol* 1953;66:507–539.
98. McKay D, DeBacalao E, Sedlis A. Platelet adhesiveness in toxemia of pregnancy. *Am J Obstet Gynecol* 1964;90:1315–1318.
99. McKay D, LaTour J, Lopez A. Production of the generalized Shwartzman reaction by activated Hageman factor and α-adrenergic stimulation. *Thromb Diath Haemorrh* 1971;26:71–76.
100. Pritchard J, Cunningham F, Mason R. Does coagulation have a role in eclampsia? In: Lindheimer M, Katz A, Zuspan F, eds. Hypertension in pregnancy. New York: John Wiley & Sons, 1976:95.
101. Ferris T. Toxemia and hypertension in pregnancy. In: Burrow G, Ferris T, eds. Medical complications during pregnancy. Philadelphia: WB Saunders, 1982:1.
102. Fischer K, Luger A, Spargo B, Lindheimer M. Hypertension in pregnancy: clinical pathological correlations and remote prognosis. *Medicine* 1981;60:267–276.
103. Fisher K, Luger A, Spargo B, Lindheimer MD. Hypertension in pregnancy: clinico-pathological correlations and remote prognosis. *Medicine* 1981;60:267–276.
104. Davey D, MacGillivay I. The classification and definition of the hypertensive disorders of pregnancy. *Am J Obstet Gynecol* 1988; 158:892–898.
105. Apargo R, McCartney CP, Winemiller R. Glomerular capillary endotheliosis in toxemia of pregnancy. *Arch Pathol* 1959;68:593–599.
106. Petrucco O, Thonson N, Lawrence JR, Weldon M. Immunofluorescent studies in renal biopsies in pre-eclampsia. *BMJ* 1974;1:473–476.
107. Gaber LW, Spargo BR. Pregnancy-induced nephropathy: the significance of focal segmental glomerulosclerosis. *Am J Kidney Dis* 1987; 9:317–323.
108. Bucht M, Werko L. Glomerular filtration rate and renal blood flow in hypertensive toxemias of pregnancy. *J Obstet Gynecol Br Commonw* 1953;60:157–164.
109. Pritchard J, Pritchard S. Standardized treatment of 154 consecutive cases of eclampsia. *Am J Obstet Gynecol* 1975;123:543–549.
110. Pritchard J, Stone S. Clinical and laboratory observations on eclampsia. *Am J Obstet Gynecol* 1967;99:754–765.
111. Ober W, Reid D, Romney J, Merrill J. Renal lesions and acute renal failure in pregnancy. *Am J Med* 1956;21:781–810.
112. Kincaid-Smith P, Fairley KF. The differential diagnosis between preeclampsia toxemia and glomerulonephritis in patients with proteinuria during pregnancy. In: Lindheimer MD, Katz AI, Zuspan FP, eds. Hypertension in pregnancy. New York: John Wiley & Sons, 1957:157.
113. Higgins JR, Brennecke SP. Preeclampsia—still a disease of theories? *Curr Opin Obstet Gynecol* 1998;10:129–133.
114. Zemel MB, Zemel PC, Berry S, et al. Altered platelet calcium metabolism as an early predictor of increased peripherl vascular resistance and preeclampsia in urban black women. *N Engl J Med* 1990;323: 434–438.
115. Konijnenberg A, van der Post JAM, Mol BW, et al. Can flow cytometric detection of platelet activation early in pregnancy predict the occurrence of preeclampsia? A prospective study. *Am J Obstet Gynecol* 1997;177:434–442.
116. Churg J, Koffler D, Paronetto F, Rorat E, Barnett R. Hemolytic syndrome as a cause of postpartum renal failure. *Am J Obstet Gynecol* 1970;108:253–261.
117. Finkelstein FO, Kashgarian M, Hayslett JP. Clinical spectrum of postpartum renal failure. *Am J Med* 1974;57:649–654.
118. Robson J, Martin A, Ruckley V, MacDonald M. Irreversible postpartum renal failure. *QJM* 1968;37:423–435.
119. Williams G, Hughes M. Postpartum renal failure. *J Pathol* 1974;114: 149–154.
120. Ford PM, Levison DA, Down PF, McConnell JB. Clinicopathological spectrum of late postpartum: renal failure: two contrasting cases. *J Clin Pathol* 1976;29:101–110.
121. Schoolwerth AC, Sandler RS, Klahr S, Kissane JM. Nephrosclerosis postpartum and in women taking oral contraceptives. *Arch Intern Med* 1976;136:178–185.
122. Zacherle BJ, Richardson JA. Irreversible renal failure secondary to hypertension induced by oral contraceptives. *Ann Intern Med* 1972;77:83–85.
123. Brown CB, Rodson JS, Thompson D, Clarkson AR, Cameron JS, Ogg CS. Haemolytic uraemic syndrome in women taking oral contraceptives. *Lancet* 1973;1:1479–1481.
124. Tobon H. Malignant hypertension, uremia and hemolytic anemia in a patient on oral contraceptives. *Obstet Gynecol* 1972;40:681–685.
125. Ferris T. Renal diseases. In: Burrow G, Ferris T, eds. Medical complications during pregnancy. Philadelphia: WB Saunders, 1982:250.
126. Bronfitt W. The effects of bacteriuria in pregnancy on maternal and fetal health. *Kidney Int* 1975;8:S1113–S119.
127. McFayden IR, Gardner NHN, Bennet AE, Mayo MF, Lloyd-Davis RW. Bacteriuria in pregnancy. *J Obstet Gynaecol Br Commonw* 1973;80: 385–405.
128. Harris RE, Thomas VL, Skelokov A. Asymptomatic bacteriuria in pregnancy: Antibody coated bacteria, renal function and intrauterine growth retardation. *Am J Obstet Gynecol* 1976;126:20–25.
129. Kass EH. Bacteriuria and pyelonephritis of pregnancy. *Arch Int Med* 1960;105:194–198.
130. Kincaid-Smith P, Bullen M. Bacteriuria in pregnancy. *Lancet* 1965;1: 395–399.
131. Whalley P. Bacteriuric of pregnancy. *Am J Obstet Gynecol* 1967;97: 723–738.
132. Charles D. Urinary tract infection in pregnancy. In: Infections in obstetrics and gynecology. Philadelphia: WB Saunders, 1980:351.
133. Milutinovic J, Fialkow PJ, Agoda LY, Phillips LA, Bryant JI. Fertility and pregnancy complications in women with autosomal dominant polycystic kidney disease. *Obstet Gynecol* 1983;61:566–570.
134. Katz AI, Davison J, Hayslett JP, Singson E, Lindheimer MD. Pregnancy in women with kidney disease. *Kidney Int* 1980;18:192–206.
135. Jungers P, Houillier P, Forget D, et al. Influence of pregnancy on the course of primary chornic glomerulonephritis. *Lancet* 1995;346: 1122–1124.
136. Jungers P, Chauveau G, Choukroun G, et al. Pregnancy in women with impaired renal function. *Clin Nephrol* 1997;47:281–288.
137. Lin C, Lindheimer M, River P, Moawad A. Fetal outcome in hypertensive disorders of pregnancy. *Am J Obstet Gynecol* 1982;142: 255–260.
138. Baylis C, Reese K, Wilson CB. Glomerular effects of pregnancy in a model of glomerulonephritis in the rat. *Am J Kidney Dis* 1989;14: 452–456.
139. Hou Sh, Grossman SD, Madias NE. Pregnancy in women with renal disease and moderate renal insufficiency. *Am J Med* 1985;78: 185–194.
140. Strauch BS, Hayslett JP. Kidney disease and pregnancy. *Br Med J* 1974;4:578–582.
141. Hayslett JP. Interaction of renal disease and pregnancy. *Kidney Int* 1984;25:579–587.
142. Haslam AJ, Wallace MR. The transient nephrotic syndrome of pregnancy. *N Z Med J* 1975;81:470–472.
143. Seftel HC, Schewitz LJ. The nephrotic syndrome in pregnancy. *J Obstet Gynecol Br Commonw* 1957;64:862–870.
144. Studd J. The origin and effects of proteinuria in pregnancy. *J Obstet Gynaecol Br Commonw* 1973;80:872–883.
145. Studd JW, Blainey JD. Pregnancy and the nephrotic syndrome. *Br Med J* 1969;1:276–280.
146. Weisman SA, Simon NM, Herdson PB, Frnaklin WA. Nephrotic syndrome in pregnancy. *Am J Obstet Gynecol* 117:867–883, 1973.
147. Lindheimer MD, Spargo B, Katz AI. Renal biopsy in pregnancy-induced hypertension. *J Reprod Med* 1975;15:189–194.
148. Anonymous. Systemic lupus in pregnancy. *Ann Intern Med* 1981;94: 667–677.
149. Hayslett JP, Lynn R. Effect of pregnancy in patients with lupus nephritis. *Kidney Int* 1980;18:207–220.
150. Huser M, Fish A, Tagatz G, Williams P, Michael A. Pregnancy and systemic lupus erythematosus. *Am J Obst Gynecol* 1980;138:409–413.
151. Tozman G, Urowitz M, Gladman D. Systemic lupus erythematosus and pregnancy. *J Rheumatol* 1980;7:624–632.
152. Zulman J, Talal N, Hoffman G, Epstein W. Problems associated with management of pregnancies in patients with systemic lupus erythematosus. *J Rheumatol* 1980;7:37–49.
153. Bear R. Pregnancy and lupus nephritis. *Obstet Gynecol* 1976;47: 715–718.
154. Lindheimer MD, Spargo B, Katz AI. Renal biopsy in pregnancy-induced hypertension. *J Reprod Med* 1975;15:189–194.
155. Lindheimer MD, Davison JM. Renal biopsy during pregnancy: to b...or not to b... *Br J Obstet Gynaecol* 1987;94:932–934.
156. Best RM, Chakravarthy U. Diabetic Retinopathy in pregnancy. *Br J Ophthalmol* 1997;81:249–251.

157. Purdy LP, Hantsch CE, Molitch ME, Metzger BE, Phelps RL, Dooley SL, Hou SH. Effect of pregnancy on renal function in patients with moderate to severe diabetic renal insufficiency. *Diabetes Care* 1996; 19:1067–1074.
158. Kitzmiller JL, Gavin IA, Gin GD, Jovanovic-Peterson L, Main EK, Zigrang WD. Preconception care of diabetes: glycemic control prevents congenital anomalies. *JAMA* 1991;265:731–736.
159. Okundaye I, Abrinko P, Hou S. Registry of pregnancy in dialysis patients. *Am J Kidney Dis* 1998;31:766–773.
160. Souqiyyeh MZ, Huraib SO, Mohd AG, Aswad S. Pregnancy in chronic dialysis patients in the Kingdom of Saudi Arabia. *Am J Kidney Dis* 1992;19:235–238.
161. Bagon J, Vernaeve H, DeMuylder X, Lafontaine J-J, Martens J, Van Roost G. Pregnancy and dialysis. *Am J Kidney Dis* 1998;31:756–765.
162. Schwarz A, Post KG, Keller F, Molzahn M. Value of human chorionic gonadotropin measurements in blood as a pregnancy test in women on maintenance hemodialysis. *Nephron* 1985;39:341–343.
163. Hou S. Pregnancy in women on hemodialysis and peritoneal dialysis. *Ballieres Clin Obstet Gynecol* 1994;8:481–500.
164. Hou S, Firanek C. Management of the pregnant dialysis patient. *Adv Renal Repl Ther* 1998;5:24–30.
165. Redrow M, Cherem L, Elliot J, et al. Dialysis in the management of pregnant patients with renal insufficiency. *Medicine* 1988;67: 199–208.
166. Murray JE, Reid DE, Harrison JH, Merrill JP. Successful pregnancies after human renal transplantation. *N Engl J Med* 1963;269:341–343.
167. Rudolph JE, Schweizer RT, Bartus S. Pregnancy in renal transplant patients. *Transplantation* 1979;27:26–29.
168. Davison JM. Pregnancy in renal allograft recipients: problems, prognosis and practicalities. *Ballieres Clin Obstet Gynaecol* 1994;8:501–525.
169. Sturgiss SN, Davison JM. Effect of pregnancy on the long term function of renal allografts: an update. *Am J Kidney Dis* 1995;26: 54–56.
170. Fist MR, Combs CA, Weiskittel P, Miodovnik M. Lack of effect of pregnancy on renal allograft survival or function. *Transplantation* 1995;59:472–476.
171. Armenti V, Ahlswede KM, Ahlswede BA, et al. Variables affecting birthweight and graft survival in 197 pregnancies in cyclosporine treated kidney transplant recipients. *Transplant* 1995;59:476–478.
172. Lamarque V, Leleu MF, Monka C, Krupp P. Analysis of 629 pregnancy outcomes in transplant recipients treated with Sandimmun. *Transplant Proc* 1997;29:2480.
173. Penn I, Makowski E, Harris P. Parenthood following renal transplantation. *Kidney Int* 1980;18:221–233.
174. Sciarra J, Toledo-Pereyra L, Bendel R, Simmons RL. Pregnancy following renal transplantation. *Am J Obstet Gynecol* 1975;123: 411–422.
175. Waltzer WC, Coulam CB, Zincke H, Sterioff S, Frohnert PP. Pregnancy in renal transplantation. *Transplant Proc* 1980;12:221–226.
176. Davison JM, Lind T, Uldall PR. Planned pregnancy in a renal transplant recipient. *Br J Obstet Gynaecol* 1976;83:518–527.
177. O Connell PJ, Caterson RJ, Stewart JH, Mahoney JF. Proglems associated with pregnancy in renal allograft recipients. *Int J Artif Organs* 1989;12:247–152.
178. Churg J. In: Churg J, Sobin LM, eds. Renal disease classification and atlas of glomerular disease. Tokyo: Igaku-Shoin, 1982.
179. Churg J. In: Trump B, Jones RT, eds. Diagnostic electron microscopy of renal diseases. New York, John Wiley & Sons, 1980.
180. Spargo BH. In: Trump B, Jones RT, eds. Diagnostic electron microscopy of renal diseases. New York: John Wiley & Sons, 1980.

Cherry and Merkatz's Complications of Pregnancy,
Fifth Edition, edited by W. R. Cohen.
Lippincott Williams & Wilkins, Philadelphia © 2000.

CHAPTER 17

Urologic Complications

Gregory T. Bales and Glenn S. Gerber

There are many urologic issues that arise during pregnancy. Many pertain to the dramatic physiologic changes that occur during gestation. An appreciation and understanding of these changes is critical when assessing a pregnant patient. In addition, health care workers must consider both the health and comfort of the mother-to-be as well as the developing fetus. This chapter will review the physiologic alterations of pregnancy germane to the urinary system and describe urologic surgical and anesthetic problems unique to pregnancy. We will also review the latest recommendations regarding antibiotic use during pregnancy for the treatment of upper and lower urinary tract infections, the management of hydronephrosis and urolithiasis during pregnancy, and an overview of urologic trauma and urologic malignancies that occur in the gestational period. Finally, birthing and postpartum complications that are encountered frequently will be reviewed.

PHYSIOLOGIC CHANGES OF PREGNANCY

Most of the major organ systems undergo changes during the gestational period. Physicians need to be aware of these alterations to better diagnose and manage complications in their pregnant patients. Although this review will concentrate mainly on those alterations unique to the genitourinary system, a brief synopsis of several other organ systems (reviewed in more depth in other chapters) is pertinent because they impact on possible urologic interventions.

Pulmonary

The pulmonary system undergoes one of the most profound changes. The functional residual capacity (FRC) is reduced by 20% by the fifth month of pregnancy (1). While the FRC is reduced, oxygen consumption increases by 15%. The combination of these factors causes the pregnant woman to experience hypoxia and exertional dyspnea more easily (2).

It is critical that consideration to these effects be given before performing general and regional anesthesia. Less anesthetic is required for women during all stages of pregnancy. Epidural requirements are diminished because of venous engorgement reducing the volume of the peridural space (3). Local anesthetic requirements are also lessened. It is thought that progesterone enhances membrane sensitivity to local agents (4).

Hematologic

During pregnancy the blood becomes hypercoagulable. This places pregnant women at increased risk of thromboembolism. The hypercoaguable state is caused by an increase in factors VII, VIII, and X and fibrinogen during pregnancy (5). In addition, a reduction in the velocity of venous blood flow in the lower extremities with a concomitant increase in venous pressure compounds the risk. The use of the dorsal lithotomy position for various urologic interventions can also increase the risk of deep venous thrombosis. Therefore, some clinicians feel that low-dosage heparin may be indicated before any surgical procedures (6). Regardless of the deep venous thrombosis prophylaxis used, physicians should have a low threshold for evaluating any pregnant patient with signs or symptoms of a blood clot. In addition, some have maintained that low-dose heparin (which does not cross the placenta) should be used in all pregnant women with a history of thromboembolism (7).

Cardiovascular

Cardiac output increases by 30% to 50% by the third trimester (8). The total blood volume increases by 25% to 40% due principally to a 50% increase in plasma volume. Red cell volume increases appreciably as well to a value about 15% higher than baseline (8). As a result, the cir-

G. T. Bales and G. S. Gerber: Departments of Surgery and Urology, University of Chicago, Chicago, IL 60637.

culating blood hematocrit is reduced. This hemodilution may be associated with an increase in the free fraction of protein-bound drugs, which may alter their effects and toxicity (9,10). Therefore, any addition of medication to the pregnant woman should be carefully assessed.

Surgical considerations need to take into account the gravid uterus filling the pelvis. As pregnancy advances, when women are supine or in the lithotomy position, the great vessels may be compressed with reduced aortic blood flow below the level of obstruction. Venous return also may be impaired from compression of venous channels in the pelvis.

Gastrointestinal

The gastrointestinal tract is also affected during pregnancy. Progesterone slows gastric and intestinal motility and relaxes the gastroesophageal sphincter. In addition, the gravid uterus pushes the abdominal contents toward the diaphragm. This may further compromise the gastroesophageal sphincter competence. Studies have shown that a delay in gastric emptying may begin as early as 8 weeks of gestation (11). Because of these gastrointestinal alterations, the risk of perioperative aspiration in the pregnant patient increases significantly.

Renal

Glomerular filtration rate and renal plasma flow increase by 30% to 50% during pregnancy. As a result, normal ranges of serum creatinine and blood urea nitrogen decrease by about 25% (12). One important clinical consequence of these changes is that medications given in the gestational period undergo a rapid urinary excretion, and dosing modifications may be necessary to maintain therapeutic plasma levels.

Two other effects on the kidneys during gestation are pelvocalyceal dilation and hypercalciuria. The dilation is thought to be both mechanical and hormonal in nature. The hypercalciuric state is related to the increased levels of 1,25-dihydroxyvitamin D during pregnancy. Both intestinal absorption of calcium and increased urinary calcium excretion contribute to the hypercalciuric state.

SURGERY AND PREGNANCY

The incidence of nonobstetric surgery during pregnancy is approximately 1 in 500 deliveries (13). The three most common etiologies of nonobstetric surgery are appendicitis, intestinal obstruction, and cholecystitis (13–15).

When evaluating a pregnant patient, it is important to remember that pregnancy-specific causes of abdominal pain outnumber nonobstetric causes.

An important point regarding the evaluation of a pregnant woman with abdominal pain are the displacement of the appendix and the separation of the viscera from the anterior abdominal wall. Both of these effects contribute to the difficulty in assessing the pregnant woman. In fact, the superior displacement of the appendix toward the right upper quadrant results in the inability to reliably differentiate appendicitis from right pyelonephritis and cholecystitis.

There is controversy surrounding the best time for surgical intervention during pregnancy. The most opportune time appears to be during the second trimester. Surgery performed during the last trimester carries a risk of premature labor, whereas intervention occurring in the first trimester can induce spontaneous abortion.

URINARY TRACT INFECTIONS DURING PREGNANCY

Urinary tract infection (UTI) is one of the most common and potentially serious complications of pregnancy. It is estimated that urinary infections account for five times as many febrile episodes as do viral infections during pregnancy (16). Because urinary tract infections are relatively easy to treat, it is essential that pregnant women are screened throughout pregnancy to diagnose these infections when they occur. Failure to treat lower tract infections adequately during pregnancy often leads to acute pyelonephritis.

Significant bacteriuria is defined as the presence of greater than 10^5 colony-forming units per milliliter (CFU/mL) of a single organism in a mid-stream, clean-catch urine specimen, whether or not symptoms are present (17). In symptomatic patients, however, fewer organisms also may indicate infection. Interestingly, the prevalence of bacteriuria among pregnant women does not differ from that of age-matched, sexually active, non-pregnant women. Prevalence has been reported at approximately 1.1% in school girls, with an increase of 1% to 2% each decade up to 10% by the age of 50 years. This predicts that 4% to 7% of childbearing-aged women will become bacteriuric. Indeed, Sweet determined that a mean of 6% of pregnant women met the criteria for bacteriuria, with a range of 2% to 12% (18).

The majority of pregnant women with bacteriuria are diagnosed at their first prenatal visit. Only 1% to 2% develop symptomatic UTI after an initial negative culture (19). The major concern related to bacteriuria is the increased risk of pyelonephritis, which is a rare outcome of uncomplicated UTI among nonpregnant women. However, among pregnant women, 28% of those with bacteriuria will develop pyelonephritis, compared with 1.4% of those with an initial negative urine culture.

Several changes in maternal anatomy and physiology are believed to contribute to the increased risk of ascending infection. The kidneys increase in length during pregnancy by approximately 1 cm (20). This change is attributed to increased interstitial volume. The bladder itself also becomes congested and is displaced anterosuperiorly from its normal anatomic position. Physiologically, hormonal effects of the elevated progesterone levels during pregnancy may contribute to the dilation of the ureters commonly seen during gestation (Fig. 17-1). The higher progesterone levels may exert a muscle-relaxing effect on the bladder and ureters, resulting in decreased peristalsis and diminished urine flow. As pregnancy continues past the first trimester, mechanical obstruction of the ureters by the enlarging uterus contributes to hydronephroureter, which is usually more exaggerated on the right side. The combined effects result in stasis and ureteral volumes as great as 200 mL, an environment conducive to bacterial growth (21). Also, it has been demonstrated that urine from pregnant women tends to have more rapid bacterial growth, likely secondary to the higher glucose content and more favorable pH (22). In addition, in a study analyzing the urinary mucosal surface, leukocytes of pregnant women with infection did not demonstrate the usual increase in phagocytic activity normally seen in pregnancy (23).

Urinary infections during pregnancy can be subdivided into pyelonephritis, cystitis, and asymptomatic bacteriuria. Acute pyelonephritis is the most severe infection with the most serious consequences to the pregnancy. It is more prevalent during the last two trimesters, with 20% of the diagnoses being made in the immediate postpartum period (21). The greater incidence of cases seen toward

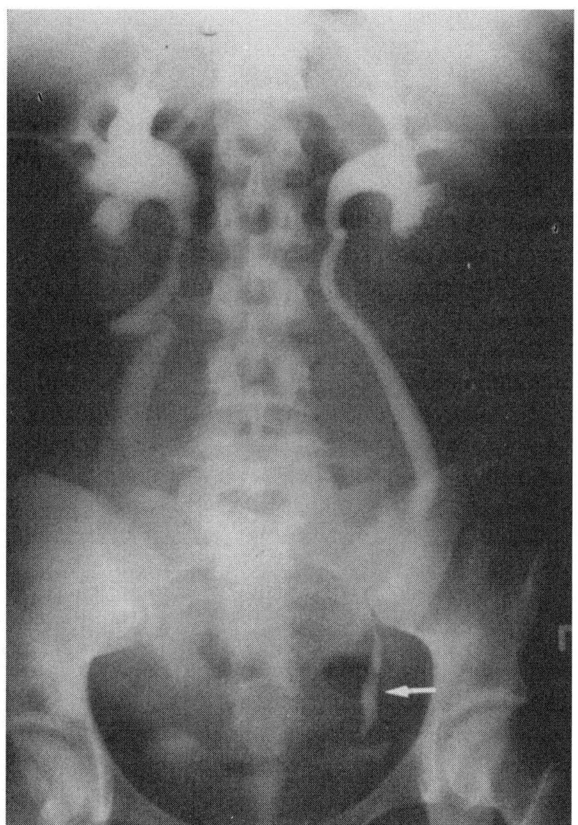

FIG. 17-1. Intravenous urogram in the sixth week of pregnancy demonstrates early dilatation of upper ureters bilaterally. Note that the lower ureter (*arrow*) retains its normal caliber. (From Freed SZ, Herzig N, eds. Urology in pregnancy. Baltimore: Williams & Wilkins, 1982.)

the end of pregnancy is the result of the worsening obstruction of the ureters, with increasing urinary stasis occurring toward term. The mechanism by which bacteria reach the kidney from the bladder is still uncertain. Vesicoureteral reflux may play a role, but bacteria may ascend to the kidney when reflux is not present. The decreased urine flow rate of pregnancy may allow easier passage of bacteria in a retrograde manner.

Some investigators feel that reflux plays a definite contributory role. Hutch and colleagues studied 12 patients whose pregnancies were complicated by pyelonephritis and demonstrated reflux in five cases (24). A different study determined that 23 women with a history of pyelonephritis in pregnancy demonstrated reflux on subsequent voiding cystography (21). Reflux occurring during their pregnancy, along with the upper tract dilation, likely put these women at risk for upper tract infection.

The signs and symptoms of acute pyelonephritis do not differ in the pregnant and nonpregnant states. Women present with fever, chills, flank pain, lower urinary tract symptoms, nausea, and vomiting. It is important not to mistake other complications of pregnancy, such as premature labor or placental abruption, for acute pyelonephritis. A study evaluating 24,000 pregnant women over a 4.5-year period determined that 656 of the women (2.7%) developed acute pyelonephritis (25). The primary feature of the infection was costovertebral angle tenderness, with the right side predominating over the left. This is likely due to the greater degree of right-sided hydronephrosis. Lower urinary tract symptoms were seen in 40% of the affected individuals, with only 24% presenting with lower urinary tract symptoms alone. A urinalysis and urine culture are mandatory whenever pyelonephritis is suspected. Clumps of white cells and white cell casts may be seen in the sediment. Leukocytosis is also frequently seen, with a shift to the left on a peripheral smear.

In the past, a diagnosis of pyelonephritis mandated hospital admission. For pregnant patients with a high fever and elevated white blood cell count, the safest course of action is hospitalization and the use of broad-spectrum parenteral antibiotics such as cephalosporins. The use of fluoroquinolones has facilitated outpatient treatment of nonpregnant patients with pyelonephritis. However, the use of fluoroquinolones in animal studies has been demonstrated to cause cartilaginous changes, including erosions, blisters, and disturbances in limb bud development. Therefore, the use of these drugs in pregnancy or postpartum in nursing mothers is contraindicated.

Antibiotics must be administered judiciously during pregnancy because of the increased maternal glomerular filtration rate and the attendant risks to the fetus associated with certain antibiotics. After treatment of acute pyelonephritis for a 7- to 10-day period, careful follow-up is imperative. The incidence of recurrent pyelonephritis has been estimated to be 18.5% and tends to be caused by the same pathogen that provoked the initial infection. After appropriate intravenous treatment, patients with recurrent pyelonephritis may be maintained on suppressive oral medication. Both nitrofurantoin crystals or sulfamethoxazole have been used effectively for this purpose. These medications are also safe in the postpartum period because only small amounts are found in breast milk.

Acute cystitis occurs in 1.3% of all pregnancies. Two thirds of these patients were reported to have negative urine cultures at their initial office visit. The etiology of cystitis is the same in the gravid and nongravid state. Essentially, the introitus and anterior urethra become colonized by gastrointestinal organisms, which gain entrance into the bladder and establish an infection. Stamey and colleagues have demonstrated that 25% of women have *Escherichia coli, Klebsiella,* and *Proteus* organisms in their vagina and anterior urethra (26).

The symptoms of cystitis in pregnant and nonpregnant women are similar. Urinary urgency, frequency, and suprapubic pain are common. Gross hematuria also occurs frequently. Dysuria, a prominent and common symptom encountered in nonpregnant women with cystitis, is often less pronounced during pregnancy (27). Systemic symptoms such as fever, chills, and flank pain are usually absent. A pregnant woman presenting with some of these signs and symptoms should have an immediate urine culture performed to confirm the clinical suspicion of infection and isolate the responsible pathogen.

The treatment of lower urinary tract infections has traditionally consisted of a week-long course of antibiotics. Recently, however, one dose or 3-day therapy has been shown to yield results equivalent to those of 7 days of therapy, at least in nonpregnant patients (28). Shorter term treatment has the advantage of causing less toxicity and potential for side effects. The incidence of antibiotic-induced vaginal candidiasis is also reduced.

Short-term therapy consists of either a single dose or 3-day course of an oral antibiotic. Three grams of amoxicillin, 3 g of fosfomycin, 1.9 g of cotrimoxazole (trimethoprim-sulfamethoxazole), and 200 mg of nitrofurantoin have all been used successfully as single-dose treatment in nonpregnant women (29,30). Three-day therapy may consist of nitrofurantoin, cotrimoxazole, or amoxicillin. The concomitant intake of copious amounts of fluids is thought to assist with resolution of the infection and help resolve the associated symptoms. Clotrimoxazole and nitrofurantoin have generally given way to oral cephalosporins (e.g., cephalexin) as first-line drugs during pregnancy (see Chapter 7).

A number of women do not manifest signs or symptoms of infection but have bacteriuria on clean-catch urinalysis. Asymptomatic bacteriuria, which is defined as the presence of bacteria in the urine in the absence of urinary symptoms, is not uncommon. It has been estimated that 4% to 6% of pregnant women will develop sequelae of their asymptomatic bacteriuria (21). The treatment of asymptomatic bacteruria is probably best undertaken with single-dose therapy, as outlined above. Repeat urinalysis to confirm adequate therapy is essential. One third of treated patients will develop recurrences, and some will subsequently develop pyelonephritis. When a recurrence of infection occurs, full-dose week-long therapy is mandatory. For patients whose bacteruria continues to recur, diagnostic tests should be undertaken to rule out underlying pathology (such as calculi) or a congenital abnormality that might be responsible for predisposing to the recurrent infections.

HYDRONEPHROSIS

Dilation of the upper urinary system is common during pregnancy, and considered physiologic. As mentioned earlier, both hormonal and mechanical factors cause this to occur. Although hydronephrosis is frequently encountered, this phenomenon is responsible for an array of clinical sequelae (21).

The term "acute hydronephrosis of pregnancy" refers to an abrupt increase in intraurethral and intrapelvic pressure, usually caused by a change in position of the uterus. Stretching of the renal capsule causes a colicky pain, which mimics that of renal colic. Ultrasonography reveals the dilated collecting system. The colicky symptoms may be relieved by having the patient lie on the contralateral side or by assuming the knee-chest position. Sometimes ureteral stenting becomes necessary if pain persists from the obstruction.

Ongoing obstruction may cause a forniceal rupture in the proximal collecting system. This occurs at the junction between the calyceal fornices and the renal parenchyma. Sometimes a ureteric obstruction from a stone may cause this phenomenon. If a forniceal rupture is suspected, then sonography may confirm the diagnosis by revealing a perinephric collection. Drainage of the collecting system becomes necessary in this circumstance.

A less common result of dilation is actual renal rupture. A review of the literature determined that 17 cases of rupture of the collecting system and/or renal parenchyma during pregnancy have been reported. As expected, 14 of the 17 occurred on the right side. Oesterling and colleagues identified three categories of spontaneous renal rupture during pregnancy: rupture secondary to pregnancy alone; rupture secondary to underlying infection or ureteral obstruction; and rupture secondary to a renal tumor, usually an angiomyolipoma (31).

Patients who suffer a renal rupture need prompt evaluation and treatment. One maternal death has been reported. If the patient is stable, then an attempt at conservative management is indicated. Ureteral stenting with or without nephrostomy or percutaneous tube placement into the urinoma should be attempted. If this is unsuccessful, then exploration with open repair or nephrectomy should be performed. If a patient presents with hemorrhage causing shock, immediate open surgical management is necessary.

Renal Failure

The hydronephrosis of pregnancy can rarely be so significant as to cause obstructive renal failure. Several reports have clearly established this as a real clinical entity, which usually occurs with polyhydramnios or the presence of multiple gestation. After delivery, the hydronephrosis resolves, usually with recovery of the renal function. If renal failure occurs at the end of gestation, the treatment of choice is to deliver the baby. When the renal failure is encountered earlier in gestation, placement of ureteral stents is indicated to preserve and protect renal function until the postpartum period.

UROLITHIASIS

Renal calculi are associated with 1 in 1,500 pregnancies. Typically, the stones are diagnosed in the second and third trimesters. As with nongravid patients, the majority of renal calculi will pass spontaneously. It is estimated that 50% to 80% of all stones require no treatment because they will be passed spontaneously in the urinary stream. In pregnant patients, however, additional concerns regarding the pregnancy arise. Acute episodes of renal colic have been associated with the initiation of premature labor. Therefore, clinicians should be aware of the unique mode of intervention used for the gravid patient.

When conservative management fails, and severe pain or fever is present, treatment becomes necessary. First, the exact diagnosis and site of urolithiasis needs to be made. The use of diagnostic studies using radiation should be discouraged, especially in the first trimester, the most significant risk period for increasing the incidence of subsequent birth defects (32). Some investigators feel that a single abdominal film (delivering 0.2 rad to the fetus) or even a two- or three-film intravenous pyelogram can be performed after the first trimester. The total exposure to the developing fetus is less than 1 rad.

A recent report by Harvey and colleagues caused many to rethink any radiation exposure (33). In their study, a retrospective evaluation of twins born in Connecticut over a 40-year period was undertaken to determine if any correlation exists between prenatal x-ray exposure and subsequent childhood cancer. An abdominal plain film had been obtained to confirm the presence of the twin gestation. Their statistical analysis revealed a 1.6 relative risk of leukemia, a 3.2 relative risk of solid childhood cancers, and an overall risk of 2.4 for all childhood malignancies. Because additional studies also have demonstrated a possible relationship between irradiation and malignancy in childhood, it would seem most reasonable to avoid any radiographic exposure during pregnancy unless the potential benefits are felt to outweigh the risks (34,35).

Improvements in technology have allowed less dependence on radiographs. Ultrasonography is a sensitive modality that has demonstrated efficacy in the evaluation of the urinary tract in the pregnant patient (36). Several papers have confirmed the ability to place stents with ultrasonographic guidance. Transvaginal ultrasonography has further enhanced the visualization of distal ureteral calculi, which may not be apparent on abdominal ultrasonography. Endoluminal ultrasonography is another new technology that can be used during pregnancy for evaluation of the collecting system and placement of stents (37).

When ureteral stenting cannot be accomplished, or if the patient shows any signs of sepsis, percutaneous nephrostomy tube placement should be performed. Several papers have confirmed the satisfactory treatment of renal colic with percutaneous nephrostomy, which can be accomplished with minimal anesthesia using ultrasonographic guidance (38,39). Under some circumstances, nephrostomy placement may increase the risk of infection and contribute more discomfort than an internal stent. Open surgical procedures to remove stones also have been reported. However, due to the complexity of such procedures they should generally be left to the postpartum period.

Ureteroscopic extraction of calculi also has been advocated by some clinicians (40,41), but can potentially put the fetus at risk. Therefore, when possible, the ureteroscopic approach should await the postpartum period. Extracorporeal shock wave lithotripsy is contraindicated during pregnancy. Animal studies have demonstrated intrauterine growth retardation. An algorithm reported by Loughlin for the approach to the pregnant patient with stone disease is depicted in Fig. 17-2 (3).

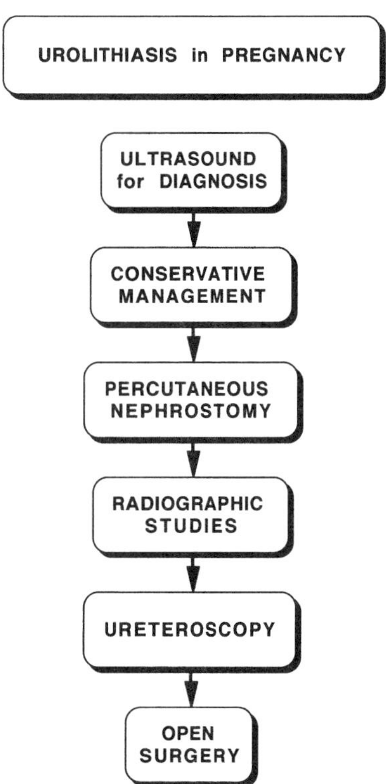

FIG. 17-2. Paradigm for the management of urolithiasis in pregnancy.

PREGNANCY AND URINARY DIVERSION

Urinary diversions are being used more frequently for a variety of disease processes. Advances in reconstructive surgical techniques have allowed many patients to have a continent urinary reservoir or even neobladder constructed, resulting in an improved quality of life. As a result, more pregnant patients are encountered with these various reconstructions. Fortunately, normal vaginal deliveries can usually be performed irrespective of these prior procedures. When a cesarean section is necessary, urologic consultation should be available to assist when necessary with the identification of any urologic reconstruction so it is not affected by the obstetric surgery.

Patients with ileal conduits may develop hematuria during the third trimester. This is thought to be secondary to stretching of the section of ileal reservoir by the gravid uterus. In addition, due to the refluxing nature of the ureteral anastomoses to the conduit, these patients may be at greater risk of developing pyelonephritis. Women with ureterosigmoidostomies need to be concerned with the metabolic complications that can occur from this form of diversion. Hyperchloremic metabolic acidosis is frequently noted secondary to wasting of bicarbonate and to chloride absorption. Pregnancy may exacerbate this condition, so electrolytes need to be monitored carefully in such patients.

Other urinary procedures such as enterocystoplasty also may affect pregnancy. One study evaluated 15 patients after augmentation cystoplasty (42). Infections developed in 9 of the 15 women, and in 4 women premature labor ensued. The conclusion from this work was that vaginal delivery can be attempted. However, cesarean section should be used in those patients with previous bladder neck reconstruction.

RENAL TRANSPLANTATION

Renal transplantation is generally not a major impediment to pregnancy and childbirth. Murray and colleagues first documented a successful pregnancy after transplantation in 1963 (43). Transplantation does increase the fertility rate compared with women with chronic renal failure on dialysis. It is estimated that pregnancy occurs in 1:200 women of reproductive age on dialysis and 1:50 women of childbearing age after successful renal transplantation. There does appear to be a higher incidence of complications in pregnant patients with a renal allograft. Urinary tract infection, preeclampsia, premature delivery, premature rupture of membranes, premature onset of labor, and small-for-gestational-age babies are some of the complications reported to occur with increased frequency in transplanted women. Acute rejection occurs approximately 9% of the time during pregnancy, and this mirrors the rate of rejection in the nonpregnant population (44). Immunosuppressive agents such as prednisone, azathioprine, and cyclosporine A present potential teratogenic risk. These agents should not be discontinued though, because the potential fetal malformation risk is relatively low, and the drugs have obvious importance for the long-term integrity of the transplant.

GENITOURINARY TRAUMA DURING PREGNANCY

In underdeveloped countries, trauma during delivery is a significant cause of urinary complications. Damage to the lower urinary tract typically occurs because of prolonged labor. This causes tissue necrosis of the anterior vaginal wall and damage to the bladder neck and urethra secondary to their impaction against the bony pelvis. Further injury can occur with the injudicious use of forceps during delivery. Fortunately, the use of complex forceps delivery has markedly diminished over recent decades. A laceration also can occur because of a prolonged second stage of labor. Typically, however, a cesarean section is used to reduce this complication and for the safety of both mother and child (45).

Cesarean section can infrequently cause urologic injury, which typically occurs during dissection of the posterior bladder wall off the anterior lower uterine segment. The posterior bladder wall is sometimes adherent to the anterior surface of the uterus, and separating these structures can result in a bladder laceration. When this injury is noted, hemostasis needs to be obtained to identify the extent of the injury clearly. If the tear extends down to the trigone, urologic consultation may be necessary to help visualize and possibly to help place stents in the ureters. The bladder needs to be closed in a watertight fashion using absorbable suture material. A suprapubic cystostomy tube should be left to allow bladder decompression during the healing process. A cystogram should be obtained 7 to 10 days after the repair to be sure there is no extravasation before the drainage tube is removed.

Another infrequent complication with potentially serious ramifications after labor and delivery can be a urinary fistula. Several different types of fistulas may result, and a systematic approach to the postpartum patient with a fistula will allow proper diagnosis and treatment. Vesicovaginal fistulas are the most common and are particularly associated with prolonged labor, laceration by forceps, or direct injury during cesarean section. The common presenting complaint is total urinary incontinence, which is most marked in the upright position.

The initial evaluation of a woman with total incontinence postpartum should include a tampon test. This is performed by placing a vaginal pack or gauze into the vagina and then instilling a dilute methylene blue solution into the bladder. The patient is then asked to move about for a few minutes, and the pack is removed. Evidence of blue discoloration on the pad is indicative of a vaginal communication with the urinary tract. Direct inspection can then be conducted using a vaginal speculum in an attempt to visualize the defect. It is important to exclude involvement of the ureters prior to any surgical intervention. An intravenous pyelogram or bilateral retrograde pyelograms should be performed to ensure that the upper tracts are intact.

The management of fistulas in the acute postpartum period is best tailored to the individual patient. Smaller vesicovaginal fistulas can be managed with a urethral catheter for a period of up to 4 weeks, which may allow for spontaneous closure. In addition, transurethral fulguration may be performed to aid in closure. The resulting inflammatory response can cause scarring to occur and assist in healing. In general, most fistulas will not respond to these conservative means and will require surgical repair.

Surgical correction of vesicovaginal fistulas can be performed via a vaginal or abdominal approach. For low fistulas located away from the ureteral orifices, vaginal repair is indicated. Cystoscopic examination is essential prior to surgery to assist in planning the repair. If the ureteral orifices are close to the site of the fistula, diversionary ureteral catheters should be passed in a retrograde fashion to avoid incorporation of an orifice into the repair. Urinary infection should be ruled out prior to surgery. If infection is present, antibiotic therapy should be given before attempting the repair.

The key to obtaining successful results is careful approximation of bladder mucosa in a watertight, tension-free fashion. Overlapping suture lines should be avoided. It is unclear if the fistulous tract needs to be excised, because this excision can convert a small opening into a much larger defect. Healthy tissue should be interposed to aid further in healing. When the fistula cannot be accessed via the vagina secondary to vaginal scarring, anatomy, or location, then an abdominal approach should be used. The abdominal route also is used when the fistula incorporates the ureteral orifice and a ureteral reimplantation must be performed. Via the abdominal route, omentum is easily available and can be used to separate the bladder and the vagina. In all instances of repair, decompression of the bladder during the healing process is mandatory. A suprapubic tube is best used for urinary diversion, and a urethral catheter can be used concomitantly to enhance drainage. Diversionary ureteral stents that directly drain the kidneys externally will provide complete urinary diversion and also can be used. Bladder spasms, if they occur, should be managed with anticholinergic agents such as oxybutynin.

Ureteral injuries are fortunately much less common than lower urinary tract injuries and usually occur during cesarean section. Typically, bleeding from the uterine vessels in the broad ligament ensues after delivery and suture ligation of the bleeding points incorporates the ureter, which runs immediately posteriorly. Two situations may arise from distal ureteral injury, which may be noted immediately or in a delayed fashion. If the ureteral injury is identified intraoperatively, then hemostasis is achieved and the ureter is inspected. The type of injury may include ligation, laceration, transection, or resection. If the ureter can be isolated and the offending clamp or suture removed, frequently no further treatment is necessary. It is always reasonable to stent the ureter for a week after the injury to assist in healing after this type of contusion. If there is any doubt about the viability of the ureter, ureteral reimplantation should be performed. Similarly, if the ureter has been cut or resected, then reimplantation or reanastamosis is necessary. The various techniques of ureteral reimplantation are best performed by a surgeon who has experience with these procedures.

The timing of intervention is controversial when urinary tract injury is noted in a delayed fashion. The immediate concern is adequate drainage of an obstructed kidney or urinoma secondary to extravasation. Foley catheter placement and drainage of the kidney with a ureteral stent or percutaneous nephrostomy are mandatory. Generally, if a patient is medically stable, then intervention to correct the problem can be performed at any time. Some surgeons prefer to intervene in the first week after cesarean section, with a waiting period of approximately 3 months when the injury is noted after the first week. This interval allows associated inflammation to diminish and may facilitate surgical repair.

PLACENTA PERCRETA

The placenta is adherent to the decidual lining of the uterus during gestation. An uncommon and serious phenomenon occurs when the placental chorionic villi penetrate into or through the uterine wall. Invasion of contiguous organs can then occur. Placenta percreta, in which the trophoblastic tissues penetrate through the uterine serosa, can frequently invade the bladder. It is important to consider this diagnosis in any woman who presents with hematuria during pregnancy. Ultrasonographic examination is the best screening modality because it identifies loss of the subplacental sonolucent area. If cystoscopy reveals a bladder lesion in this situation, biopsy is contraindicated.

The literature suggests that most cases of placenta percreta with bladder invasion are best managed with cesarean section, hysterectomy, and transfusion and replacement of massive amounts of coagulation products. A urologist should be called to evaluate the bladder. Typically, the bladder needs to be widely opened to identify bleeding areas. Proper closure with appropriate hemostasis can then be accomplished.

UNCOMMON UROLOGIC COMPLICATIONS OF PREGNANCY

There are several uncommon conditions that can occur with pregnancy. Although relatively rare, medical personnel should be at least familiar with their occurrence. Aldosteronism is rarely associated with pregnancy, with only 15 cases reported in the literature (46). In the normal pregnant state, both aldosterone production and plasma renin activity are markedly elevated. When primary aldosteronism occurs, a decreased plasma renin level is noted. Hypokalemia and hypertension typically are seen in affected patients. Conservative medical management with antihypertensive medication and potassium supplementation is appropriate in the majority of women, with surgery reserved only for those who do not respond.

Urethral diverticula can occasionally complicate labor. This may be secondary to the diverticulum itself or the accumulation of a large amount of urine within the diverticulum obstructing the bladder and disrupting labor. Usually these diverticula can be left to the postpartum period for appropriate excision. Transurethral bladder inversion has been reported during labor. It is associated with grand parity, marked weakness of the pelvic floor, and uterovaginal prolapse. This is usually not serious, and manual replacement of the bladder can be performed. If manual decompression fails, then open surgical repair may be necessary.

Finally, an unusual form of bladder irritation may be seen secondary to eosinophilic cystitis. Associated with allergic reactions, the common findings include typical lower urinary symptoms such as can be seen with bacterial cystitis. Sterile urine cultures are characteristically noted. The diagnosis is established by transurethral bladder biopsy demonstrating edema, perivascular eosinophilic infiltration, and lymphangiectasia. Antihistamines and intravesical dimethylsulfoxide have been used to provide symptomatic relief.

SUMMARY

Many of the urologic complications of pregnancy manifest themselves in the nongravid state as well. When encountered in the pregnant patient, strict attention to both the mother and fetus during intervention is essential to allow any of the variety of problems to be treated appropriately. By effectively diagnosing and treating the urologic complications in an orderly and systematic manner, both mother and fetus should be well served and pregnancy can usually conclude uneventfully.

REFERENCES

1. Prowse CM, Gaensler EA. Respiratory and acid-base changes during pregnancy. Anesthesiology 1965;26:381–392.
2. Archer GW, Marx GF. Arterial oxygenation during apnea in parturient women. Br J Anaesth 1974;46:358–360.
3. Loughlin KR. Management of urologic problems in the pregnant patient. AUA Update Series, Vol. 16, No. 2, 1997.
4. Datta S, Lambert DH, Gregus J. Differential sensitivities of mammalian nerve fibers during pregnancy. Anesth Analg 1983;62:1070–1072.
5. Barron WM. Medical evaluation of the pregnant patient requiring nonobstetric surgery. Clin Perinatol 1985;12:481–496.
6. Hathaway WE, Bonnar J. Perinatal coagulation. New York: Grune & Stratton, 1978:27–51.
7. Kakkar VV. The current status of low-dose heparin in the prophylaxis of thrombophlebitis and pulmonary embolism. World J Surg 1978; 2:3–13.
8. Letsky E. The haematological system. In: Hytten F, Chamberlain G, eds. Clinical physiology in obstetrics. Oxford, England: Blackwell Scientific Publications. 1980:43–78.
9. Dean M, Stock B, Patterson RJ, Levy G. Serum protein binding of drugs during and after pregnancy in humans. Clin Pharmacol Ther 1980;28:253–261.
10. Santos AC, Pederson H, Harmon TW, et al. Does pregnancy alter the systemic toxicity of local anesthetics? Anesthesiology 1989;70: 991–995.
11. Simpson KH, Stakes AF, Miller M. Pregnancy delays paracetamol absorption and gastric emptying in patients undergoing surgery. Br J Anaesth 1988;60:24– 27.
12. Barron WM. Medical evaluation of the pregnant patient requiring nonobstetric surgery. Clin Perinatol 1985;12:481–496.
13. Kammerer WS. Non-obstetric surgery during pregnancy. Med Clin NA 1979;6:1157–1164.
14. Babaknia A, Parsa H, Woodruff JD. Appendicitis during pregnancy. Obstet Gynecol 1977;50:40–44.
15. Welch JP. Miscellaneous causes of small bowel obstruction. In: Welch JP, ed. Bowel obstruction: differential diagnosis and clinical management. London: WB Saunders, 1990.
16. Schaeffer AJ. Infections of the urinary tract. In: Walsh PC, Retik AB, Stamey TA, et al., eds. Campbell's urology. Philadelphia: WB Saunders, 1992.
17. Maranchie JK, Capelouto CC, Loughlin KR. Urinary tract infections during pregnancy. Infect Urol 1997;10:152–157.
18. Sweet RL. Bacteriuria and pyelonephritis during pregnancy. Semin Perinatol 1977;1:25–40.
19. Andriole VT, Patterson TF. Epidemiology, natural history, and management of urinary tract infections in pregnancy. Med Clin North Am 1991;75:359–373.
20. Maranchie JK, Capelouto CC, Loughlin KR. Urinary tract infections during pregnancy. Infect Urol 1997;10:152–157.
21. Weber HN, Dillon RW, Sotolongo JR. Urologic complications in pregnancy. In: Cherry SH, Merkatz IR, eds. Complications of pregnancy, 4th ed. Baltimore: Williams & Wilkins, 1991:536–559.
22. Roberts JA, Auger M. The effect of a progestational agent on ureteral physiology. Invest Urol 1971;9:206.
23. MacDonald P. Summary of a workshop on maternal genitourinary infections and the outcome of pregnancy. J Infect Dis 1983;147:596–605.
24. Hutch JA, Miller ER, Hinman F Jr. Vesicoureteral reflux-role in pyelonephritis. Am J Obstet Gynecol 1963;87:478.
25. Gilstrap LC, Levenao KJ, Cunningham FG, Whalley PJ, Roark ML. Renal infection and pregnancy outcome. Am J Obstet Gynecol 1981; 141:709.
26. Stamey TA, Timothy M, Millar M, Mihara G. Recurrent urinary infections in adult women. The role of enterobacteria. Calif Med 1971;1:115.
27. Sweet RL, Ledger WJ. Puerperal infections morbidity. Am J Obstet Gynecol 1973;117:1093–1100.
28. Baily RR. Single dose antibacterial treatment for bacteriuria of pregnancy. Drugs 1987;27:183–186.
29. Anderton KJ, Abbas AMA, Davey A, Ancill RJ. High dose short-course amoxicillin in the treatment of bacteriuria in pregnancy. Br J Clin Pract 1983;37:212–214.
30. Ragni N, Pivetta C, Paccagnella F. Urinary tract infections in pregnancy. Fosfomycin trometamol single-dose treatment versus conventional therapy with pipemidic acid. In: Neu HC, Williams JD, eds. New trends in urinary tract infection. Basel, Switzerland: Karger, 1988.
31. Oesterling JE, Besinger RE, Brendler CB. Spontaneous rupture of the renal collecting system during pregnancy: successful management with a temporary ureteral catheter. J Urol 1988;140:588–590.
32. Swartz HM, Reichling BA. Hazards of radiation exposure for pregnant women. JAMA 1978;239:1907–1908.
33. Harvey EB, Boice JD Jr, Honeyman M, Flannery JT. Prenatal x-ray exposure and childhood cancer in twins. N Engl J Med 1985;312: 541–545.
34. MacMahon B. Prenatal x-ray exposure and childhood cancer. J Natl Can Inst 1962;28:1173–1191.

35. Mole RH. Antenatal irradiation and childhood cancer: causation or coincidence? Br J Cancer 1974;30:199–208.
36. Loughlin KR, Bailey RB Jr. Internal ureteral stents for conservative management of ureteral calculi during pregnancy. N Engl J Med 1986; 315:1647–1649.
37. Wolf MC, Hollander JB, Salisz JA, Kearney DJ. A new technique for ureteral stent placement during pregnancy using endoluminal ultrasound. Surg Gynecol Obstet 1992;175:575–576.
38. Denstedt JD, Razvi H. Management of urinary calculi during pregnancy. J Urol 1992;148:1072–1075.
39. Horowitz E, Schmidt JD. Renal calculi in pregnancy. Clin Obstet Gynecol 1985;28:324–338.
40. Vest JM, Warden SS. Ureteroscopic diagnosis and treatment of urinary calculi during pregnancy. Urology 1990;35:250–252.
41. Rittenberg MH, Bagley DH. Ureteroscopic diagnosis and treatment of urinary calculi during pregnancy. Urology 1988;32:427–428.
42. Hill DE, Kramer SA. Management of pregnancy after augmentation cystoplasty. J Urol 1990;144:457–459.
43. Murray JE, Reid DE, Harrson JH, Merrill JP. Successful pregnancies after human renal transplantation. N Engl J Med 1963;269: 341–343.
44. Fine RN. Pregnancy in renal allograft recipients. Am J Nephrol 1982; 2:117–121.
45. McCausland AM, Caillonette JC, Bennallack DA, Holmes F. A comparative study of vesicovaginal fistulas following delivery. Am J Obstet Gynecol 1960;79:1110.
46. Webb JC, Bayliss P. Pregnancy complicated by primary aldosteronism. South Med J 1997;90:243–245.

SECTION VI

Gastrointestinal Disorders

Cherry and Merkatz's Complications of Pregnancy,
Fifth Edition, edited by W. R. Cohen.
Lippincott Williams & Wilkins, Philadelphia © 2000.

CHAPTER 18

Digestive Tract Disorders

Peter H. Rubin and Henry D. Janowitz

Among the more frequent complaints of pregnancy are those related to the gastrointestinal tract. In a large survey of prenatal clinic visits, approximately 20% of pregnant women with symptoms severe enough to seek medical attention related them to the gastrointestinal system (1). This is no wonder, because pregnancy, with its attendant physical, hormonal, and physiologic alterations, significantly affects the functioning of the gut at many levels.

Physically, it displaces the stomach, small intestine, and mobile portions of the colon (including the appendix) from their customary anatomic locations; it alters motility of every portion of the hollow gut and the biliary tree; it impairs appropriate functioning of the lower esophageal sphincter; it decreases gastric acidity; it affects the selective absorptive mechanisms of the small intestine and colon and perhaps pancreatic secretion as well; and, in the setting of such intraabdominal crises as inflammation, perforation, and obstruction, it attenuates the body's response, thus further complicating correct diagnosis.

It follows that history and physical examination of the gravid patient may be misleading, and such laboratory data as leukocyte counts, erythrocyte sedimentation rates, and liver chemistries may be of limited clinical use. Furthermore, the presence of the fetus may restrain the clinician from aggressively pursuing diagnosis with plain and contrast x-rays, scans, and endoscopies. Finally, even if the correct diagnosis is made, concerns for the pregnancy may limit the use of the entire available therapeutic armamentarium.

P.H. Rubin and H.D. Janowitz: Mount Sinai School of Medicine, New York, NY 10029.

NAUSEA AND VOMITING

Nausea in early pregnancy usually is a common, self-limiting, suggestively diagnostic symptom of pregnancy itself. Occasionally, however, vomiting may be a harbinger of life-threatening fluid and electrolyte imbalances or other serious gastrointestinal or systemic disease.

In its most innocuous form, it is the nausea of morning sickness, experienced by as many as 80% of pregnant women (2), or vomiting in 30% of women during their first trimester (3). But when on occasion it persists and disturbs nutritional balance, leading to weight loss and deficiencies of fluids and electrolytes, it is *hyperemesis gravidarum.*

Nausea and vomiting generally occur during the first 14 weeks of pregnancy. Nausea, in fact, may be the first symptom of pregnancy, presenting as early as 3 weeks after the last menstrual period (4). It is experienced usually upon arising, often before any food has been ingested. It may continue at 14 weeks in as many as 40%, at 16 weeks in less than 20%, and at 20 weeks in less than 10% of women (5). It may be more prevalent in multiple than in single gestations (2) and in those who experienced it during previous pregnancies (6).

The designation hyperemesis gravidarum is reserved for those who experience persistent nausea and vomiting, resulting in a reduction of 5% or more in body weight, with disturbed electrolyte levels (3). Specifically, these include reduction in serum sodium, potassium, and chloride, as well as metabolic alkalosis. In the most severe cases, jaundice, hyperpyrexia, peripheral neuritis, gastrointestinal hemorrhage from a Mallory-Weiss tear of the esophagus (7), and a Wernicke-like encephalopathy may develop.

Pathogenesis

In neither morning sickness nor hyperemesis has a specific gastrointestinal lesion been demonstrated. Early pathologic descriptions in hyperemesis of fatty infiltration of liver and kidneys and retinal hemorrhages may have been nonspecific sequelae of malnutrition (3,8). The literature seeking to explain the nausea and vomiting of early pregnancy has centered on four general areas: alteration in gastrointestinal motility; hormonal excesses or deficiencies acting on either the gut directly or the central nervous system; *Helicobacter pylori* gastropathy; and psychosomatic factors.

Gastrointestinal transit in general and gastric emptying in particular are slower as pregnancy progresses (9,10). Abnormalities in gastric myoelectrical rhythms have been documented during pregnancy primarily in women who are experiencing nausea (11).

Progesterone and estrogen have been implicated as mediators in these dysrhythmias (12). In earlier literature, human chorionic gonadotropin (hCG) was implicated circumstantially by the higher incidence of vomiting seen in women with hydatidiform moles and in those carrying more than one fetus. But measurements of the hormone have not correlated with the symptoms of nausea and vomiting (13). Similarly, relative adrenal dysfunction, adrenocorticotropin deficiency, and imbalances in luteinizing hormone and prolactin have been suggested but not substantiated by correlative assays (13–16).

The prevalence of *H. pylori* (as judged by seropositivity to *H. pylori* antibodies) has been found to be significantly higher in women with hyperemesis than in pregnant controls without vomiting (17). This infestation may be facilitated by the relative gastric hypoacidity associated with pregnancy (18).

A psychological basis for the nausea and vomiting of pregnancy has been suggested from observation of dramatic improvement with hospitalization alone and from history of similar symptoms associated with coitus (19). However, no significant correlation has been demonstrated between vomiting in early pregnancy and such factors as patient attitude toward pregnancy, prepregnancy psychopathology, tendency to psychoneurotic symptoms, personality profiles, and marital or socioeconomic status (20).

Other Causes of Nausea and Vomiting in Pregnancy

The occasional patients whose symptoms arise from conditions other than pregnancy *per se* include those with urinary tract infections, gastroenteritis, peptic ulcer, gastric volvulus, pancreatitis, biliary tract disease, early hepatitis, appendicitis, intestinal obstruction, torsion of ovarian cyst, pneumonia, adrenal insufficiency, and increased intracranial pressure. Of these, urinary tract infection, specifically pyelonephritis, is the most common, with peak incidence at 18 to 24 weeks' gestation (21). In later pregnancy, the index of suspicion for one of these conditions is higher because purely pregnancy-related nausea and vomiting are less common. In late pregnancy, additional obstetric considerations are hydramnios, preeclampsia, and onset of labor.

Diagnosis

Persistent nausea and vomiting, especially in the second and third trimesters, necessitates early consideration of etiologies other than the pregnancy. This can be accomplished by thorough physical examination with particular attention to funduscopy, skin turgor, mucus membranes, absent or high-pitched bowel sounds, preservation of hepatic dullness, abdominal or flank tenderness, and extrauterine masses. Laboratory testing includes urine cultures and multiphasic blood tests with amylase. Abdominal sonography is indicated to assess the gallbladder, pancreas, and kidneys, and perhaps to assist in diagnosing acute appendicitis.

If intestinal obstruction or perforation is suggested by the history and physical examination, then supine and standing abdominal x-rays may be considered. The hazards of diagnostic radiation exposure in pregnancy have been studied and considerable reassurance offered (22). No significant increase in congenital malformations or growth retardation has been proved at exposure to the pelvis of less than 5 rad, well above the levels involved in the combined radiation of chest x-ray, abdominal flat plate, intravenous pyelogram, barium enema and gastrointestinal series (22–25). Subsequent development of leukemia and other neoplasms in children exposed to diagnostic radiation *in utero* has been suggested (23), but the risk appears very low (25). The advice of Swartz and Reichling remains cogent: "If there is a valid medical indication to perform a diagnostic study using radiation on a pregnant woman, this will generally outweigh the remote possibility of harm to the patient or her fetus" (25).

Very occasionally, fiberoptic esophagogastroduodenoscopy is needed and can be used safely to evaluate persistent vomiting suspected to arise from the upper gut (26). Strictures can be brushed, examined via biopsy, and dilated. Premedication with meperidine is safe for the fetus, but benzodiazepines and naloxone are best avoided (27).

Treatment

In its milder forms, vomiting can be treated by reassurance and the time-honored dry soda biscuit before arising, and advice to consume small, frequent meals. In more severe cases, restriction of milk and other fats and even a liquid diet may be necessary temporarily. Prenatal vitamins, coffee, and spicy foods should be withheld until symptoms abate, then cautiously reintroduced.

If an antiemetic is necessary, the central-acting phenothiazines such as prochlorperazine appear to be effective and safe, as is the prokinetic agent metoclopramide (28–31). Cisapride, another prokinetic agent, has not been extensively studied in pregnancy, but appears to be safe to the developing infant (29,32).

Other classes of medication that appear useful in treating the nausea and vomiting of pregnancy include mild tranquilizers such as phenobarbitol, antihistamines such as meclizine (33), and vitamins such as pyridoxine (34). Although the safety of these agents to the fetus has been questioned, no strong evidence links them to adverse outcomes of pregnancy (30,35–38). The 5-hydroxytryptamine receptor antagonist ondansetron (Zofran) has been found to be comparable with promethazine in hyperemesis (39) but has not been extensively studied in pregnancy (29). A number of alternative therapies have been reviewed favorably in treating the nausea and vomiting of pregnancy. Among these are acupuncture, ginger root, and hypnosis (40).

For many cases of true hyperemesis, hospitalization is necessary. Intravenous fluid and electrolyte replacement and perhaps antiemetics are administered (41). Total parenteral nutrition (42–44), nasogastric tube feedings (45), or psychotherapeutic intervention (46) may be required. Percutaneous endoscopic gastrostomy has been performed successfully in pregnancy, but in very few cases (47). In obdurate cases, corticosteroid therapy is often helpful.

Prognosis

Outlook for both mother and child is good, even with hyperemesis (29), except when there is advanced malnutrition (48). Some surveys have demonstrated higher perinatal mortality and lower birth weight in mothers who had experienced no first-trimester nausea and vomiting (2). Supporting this are the earlier observations that women likely to abort have less nausea and vomiting than those who do not (36,49,50).

HEARTBURN

Substernal burning discomfort, often with pyrosis, has been reported in 30% to 70% of pregnancies, daily in as many as 25% (51–53). Onset is typically in the second trimester; frequency and intensity often escalate as the pregnancy advances, only to vanish after delivery and not recur in the puerperium (54,55). It occurs more often in women with a prior history of reflux (51,55).

Pathogenesis

Heartburn is the result of refluxing gastric contents. All pregnant women, irrespective of heartburn, tend to exhibit more nonpropulsive motor activity of the esophagus, with decreased wave amplitude and slower peristaltic speed (56). In those who are symptomatic, about half also have significant secondary esophageal peristalsis, suggestive of reflux, a finding observed in neither nonpregnant women nor gravidas without heartburn (56). These secondary waves disappear after pregnancy, suggesting that reflux is prominent in patients with heartburn.

The increase in intragastric pressure that accompanies advancing pregnancy is probably only of secondary importance in causing reflux. The major determinant is (as is the case in the nonpregnant state) the competency of the lower esophageal sphincter (LES). Pregnant women without heartburn have elevated LES pressures sufficient to maintain a gastric-esophageal gradient across the sphincter approximating that in the normal state, whereas gravidas with heartburn do not exhibit this compensatory elevation in LES pressure (57). Some investigators have found LES pressure depressed throughout pregnancy, reaching a nadir at 36 weeks and recovering postpartum (58), whereas others found normal basal LES pressures in early pregnancy but decreased responsiveness of LES to stimulation with pentagastrin, edrophonium, methacholine, and protein meal, suggestive of inhibition (59).

The factors responsible for LES pressure decrease in pregnancy appear to be hormonal (60). It is known that LES pressure is lower in the setting of oral contraceptives (61). Progesterone inhibits gastrin-stimulated LES contraction (59). Other factors contributing to the heartburn may be decreased gastric emptying (9) (perhaps a consequence of the gastric hypoacidity associated with pregnancy) (62) and alkaline reflux of duodenal contents (51).

Diagnosis

Substernal burning discomfort with pyrosis is usually sufficiently suggestive of reflux to allow treatment without further diagnostic measures (63). Dysphagia may be due to stricturing from chronic reflux (64). Odynophagia may indicate infectious esophagitis due to monilia, herpes, or cytomegalovirus. These conditions are more common in diabetic and immunocompromised patients, as well as after antibiotic therapy. Monilial esophagitis may be suspected by inspection for oral thrush. Substernal pain also may be due to esophageal spasm, not necessarily related to reflux.

Nonesophageal causes of substernal chest pain include costochondritis, pericarditis, myocardial ischemia, pleurisy, pulmonary infarction, and pneumonia. These usually can be distinguished from reflux on clinical grounds.

As discussed above in the diagnosis of vomiting, if upper gastrointestinal endoscopy is needed to evaluate chest pain, it can be done safely during pregnancy (20,26, 27,62).

Therapy

Treatment is aimed at reducing reflux or neutralizing the material being refluxed. Relief often can be obtained by avoiding recumbence after meals, elevating the head of the bed, and eliminating the consumption of substances that lower LES pressure, such as alcohol, nicotine, caffeine, chocolate, fatty foods, peppermint, and tomatoes. Ingesting antacids after meals and at bedtime may suffice for pharmacotherapy and is safe during pregnancy (64).

If symptoms persist, histamine type 2 (H_2) blocking agents or proton pump inhibitors may be used. As a group, the H_2 blocking agents appear safe when taken during the first trimester (65). Cimetidine does cross the placenta but has not been found to cause toxicity (66,67). Similarly, ranitidine and famotidine appear safe for mother and fetus (68,69). The proton pump inhibitors omeprazole and lansoprazole have been used widely in treating reflux in the nonpregnant state and are regarded as more effective than the H_2 blockers. Large studies in pregnancy are lacking, however, although they have been used safely throughout pregnancy in women with Zollinger-Ellison syndrome (70). As discussed in the therapy of nausea during pregnancy, the prokinetic agents metoclopramide and cisapride appear to be safe (71), but, like the proton pump inhibitors, they are used reluctantly if at all (63).

PEPTIC ULCER DISEASE

This common condition is distinctly rare in pregnancy (72,73). In a series of 83 upper endoscopies performed in pregnancy, only 7% had peptic ulcer disease (26). Peptic disease antedating pregnancy tends to improve in at least 80% of cases as the pregnancy progresses but recurs in 50% by the third postpartum month and in virtually all by 2 years postpartum (74). In animal studies pregnancy reduced the incidence of steroid-induced ulcers by 50% (75). Those with persistent peptic symptoms during pregnancy may have a coexistent condition such as hyperemesis or albuminuria (74) or a gastric hypersecretion syndrome such as Zollinger-Ellison.

Complications of peptic disease such as hemorrhage and perforation are more likely to occur in pregnancies already complicated by toxemia or by coexistent renal disease (76).

Pathogenesis

The rarity of the condition and its improvement during pregnancy have been linked to alterations in gastric acidity. Hydrochloric acid levels, both basal and after stimulation with histamine, are diminished during most of pregnancy with a tendency to revert to normal levels after 30 weeks (18). The decreased acidity during most of pregnancy has been attributed to increased serum histaminase from placenta (77) and to elevated levels of estrogen. Estrogen has been reported to heal peptic ulcers in men (78). This is supported by the epidemiologic observation that an unduly large proportion of ulcers start, flare up, or undergo complications at or about the time of the menopause (74). Serum gastrin levels remain normal during most of pregnancy but increase markedly late in the third trimester and in the early puerperium, with highest levels immediately after delivery (79). By late pregnancy, gastric pH and basal and stimulated acid output do not differ significantly from those in nonpregnant women (58). This correlates with the clinical observation that peptic symptoms and their complications, if they occur at all during pregnancy, do so in the late third trimester.

Helicobacter pylori infection is now accepted as a major pathogenic factor in peptic ulcer disease. A study in Belgium found about 20% of pregnant women in their late twenties and 30% of those in their late thirties were seropositive, similar to the prevalence in nonpregnant women of these ages (80). Transmission of *Helicobacter* from infected mother to newborn has been documented (81).

Diagnosis

Gnawing upper abdominal pain, often relieved by meals, may lead to empiric treatment without further diagnostic measures. The differential diagnosis includes gastroesophageal reflux, biliary tract disease, pancreatitis, and irritable bowel syndrome. When symptoms do not respond to empiric measures, or in the setting of upper gastrointestinal bleeding, upper tract endoscopy may be indicated. As discussed earlier, diagnostic upper gastrointestinal endoscopy can be used safely in pregnancy (20,27). To maximize safety to the fetus, attention must be directed to assuring hemodynamic stability prior to endoscopy (27,82), and fetal heart rate monitoring should be considered in late pregnancy (27). In the setting of bleeding, endoscopy brings the added advantage of therapy with electrocoagulation or injection of bleeding sites. Esophageal varices, Mallory-Weiss tears, and peptic ulcers have been treated safely endoscopically (7,26,83), but large, controlled studies are lacking. A flatplate and upright x-ray of the abdomen may be indicated in suspected cases of perforation or obstruction without harm to the fetus (22,25).

Therapy

Alcohol, nicotine, salicylates, and nonsteroidal antiinflammatory agents are prohibited. The traditional mainstay of medical management of peptic disease has been antacids, taken 1 and 3 hours after meals and at bedtime. As a group these are safe during pregnancy (64,84), but some caution has been expressed about bicarbonate agents that could produce alkalosis and fluid overload if used in large doses (85).

Specific H_2 antagonists have now supplanted antacids as the most widely prescribed agents in managing peptic disease. These include cimetidine, ranitidine, famotidine, and nizatidine. As discussed earlier, these agents have not been found to have teratogenicity or to affect labor or delivery adversely, despite crossing the placental barrier and the presence of histamine receptors in uterine myometrium (67,69). The proton pump inhibitors omeprazole and lansoprazole have not been found to be teratogenic (86). In fact, the short-term use of H_2 or proton-pump blockers has been advocated in preventing Mendelson syndrome, aspiration of gastric contents by pregnant patients during general anesthesia (67,87).

Synthetic prostaglandins (misoprostol) have been developed for prophylaxis of gastric ulcerations in patients who must take potentially ulcerogenic medication. These agents are contraindicated during pregnancy because they are capable of inducing uterine contractions (66).

No literature has appeared bearing on the treatment of *H. pylori* in the pregnant patient. In view of the side effects and possible teratogenicity of the antibiotics used to eradicate *H. pylori*, it would seem reasonable to defer such treatment until the puerperium.

Therapeutic upper endoscopy has been reported in relatively small numbers of pregnant women (26). Nevertheless, it is reasonable to attempt this approach if the only other course is abdominal surgery (88). Biopsy of gastric ulcer probably adds no morbidity to the procedure, although malignant gastric ulcer is distinctly rare in pregnancy (89).

Mother and child have survived emergency gastric surgery performed for intractable bleeding, perforation, and gastric outlet obstruction (90–93). The fetal death rate in such situations has been reported to be 20% (90). Although some authorities recommend cesarean section prior to ulcer surgery (94), others propose vaginal delivery after early surgical repair (95,96). Subsequent pregnancies are not adversely affected by gastric resection (97).

BOWEL DISORDERS: CONSTIPATION OR DIARRHEA

The functioning of the bowels in pregnancy is variable. Gastrointestinal transit time is delayed in pregnancy and returns to normal in the puerperium (10). Retrospective interviews with 1,000 postpartum women found that 55% experienced no change in prior bowel habits during pregnancy, 34% recalled increased frequency, and 11% reported decreased stooling (98). In the latter group only 1.5% required laxatives. Other surveys have reported constipation in up to 30% of pregnant women, particularly during the first and third trimesters (99). Bowel disturbance may be higher in women with previous irregular bowel habits and habitual laxative use. Possible consequences of constipation in pregnancy are backache, fecal impaction, and hemorrhoids.

Causes of Constipation

The pathophysiology of constipation in pregnancy may be explained in part by prolonged small bowel transit time (10,100). Colonic perfusion and motility studies during pregnancy have not been conducted. Whether constipation is a consequence of hormonal influences (such as aldosterone or progesterone), primary changes in colonic motility, or extrinsic compression on the rectosigmoid by the enlarging uterus, have not been established. Ingestion of prenatal vitamins fortified with iron and calcium also may contribute to constipation. Rarely, constipation in pregnancy can be caused by a coexisting colonic neoplasm (101–103), endometriosis (104), Hirschsprung's disease (105), or a pseudoobstruction syndrome (106).

Diagnosis of Constipation

Usually constipation can be treated without extensive diagnostic evaluation. Sigmoidoscopy should be considered when there is no prior history of bleeding hemorrhoids and the constipation is associated with either frank rectal bleeding or the presence of occult blood. Sigmoidoscopy during pregnancy has been studied carefully and is safe (107).

Treatment of Constipation

The management of constipation consists, as in the nonpregnant state, of a high fiber diet, increased ingestion of liquids, and physical activity. Hydrophilic stool bulking agents such as bran or psyllium and glycerine suppositories may be useful and are considered safe in pregnancy because they are not absorbed (108). Stool softeners such as docusate sodium also have been found safe in pregnancy (99). If laxatives must be used, milk of magnesia, senna concentrate, or bisacodyl suppositories seem safe (25,28) if used occasionally (66). Because phenolphthalein-containing laxatives are excreted in breast milk and may cause colic in breastfeeding infants, these are to be avoided in the puerperium if the woman is planning to breastfeed. Castor oil is to be avoided because of the possibility of uterine stimulation (66).

Causes of Diarrhea

Diarrhea occurring during pregnancy may be attributable to diet, medication, infection, irritable bowel syndrome (IBS), or inflammatory bowel disease (IBD). Dietary considerations include (a) underlying lactase deficiency unmasked by increased ingestion of milk and other dairy products, (b) dietary indiscretion, (c) osmotic diarrhea from liberal ingestion of diet sodas and gums containing nonabsorbable, noncaloric sweeteners, and (d) underlying gluten enteropathy.

Medications implicated in diarrhea include high doses of supplemental vitamins, antacids, and antibiotics. Antibiotic-associated colitis attributable to *Clostridium difficile* is an important diagnosis to make by assaying stools for the toxin. Most of the infectious diarrheas are viral, but other infectious etiologies include *Salmonella, Shigella, Campylobacter, Escherichia coli,* and protozoans such as *Giardia* (28,109).

Although there are no detailed studies on the appearance or relapse of IBS during pregnancy, IBS is known to exacerbate during menses, presumably secondary to fluxes of estrogenic or progestational hormones or prostaglandins (108,110). Preexisting IBD may flare and occasionally appear *de novo* during pregnancy.

Diagnosis and Treatment of Diarrhea

Elimination of any medication or dietary factors that could be causing diarrhea is the first therapy, followed, if necessary, by a short course of antidiarrheal agents such as kaolin-pectin, diphenoxylate, or loperamide (69,108). Bismuth subsalicylate (Pepto-Bismol) is best avoided because its content of salicylate is high (111).

Pathogenic microorganisms such as *Giardia,* ameba, *Salmonella, Shigella, Campylobacter, Yersinia,* and *C. difficile* can be documented by stool analysis or culture, although several specimens may need to be submitted. Sigmoidoscopy is rarely necessary, but, as discussed above, it can be performed safely (107) to document distal colitis.

Although metronidazole, sulfas, tetracyclines, and quinolones are usually avoided during pregnancy (110), erythromycin and ampicillin are safe (108). Severe *C. difficile* could be treated with oral vancomycin, because it is not absorbed, or with metronidazole after the first trimester (69,109). Irritable bowel symptoms are safely managed with a high roughage diet and stool bulking, rather than with antispasmotics or sedatives (69,108,110).

HEMORRHOIDS

In a retrospective survey of their pregnancies, about one third of women recalled symptoms attributable to hemorrhoids and one tenth required treatment (112). Presumably hemorrhoids are a consequence of compromised venous drainage by the enlarging uterus, with heightened pressure within common iliac vein transmitted to inferior and middle hemorrhoidal veins. Constipation and straining at stool would be expected to aggravate this condition.

Symptoms commonly include itching, pain, or bleeding. The diagnosis can be confirmed by gentle proctoscopy or flexible sigmoidoscopy. In experienced hands these procedures are safely tolerated in pregnancy (27). It is recommended that the patient not be placed in the supine position during rectal endoscopy, to minimize compression on the inferior vena cava, and thereby the uterine blood supply, by the enlarged uterus (113).

The goal is to correct any coexisting constipation, using diet, stool softeners, sitz baths, and topical ointments or suppositories of bismuth subgallate. Soaking may facilitate digital reduction of prolapsed hemorrhoids. For severe pain, local injection with phenol or sodium morrhuate (114) or hemorrhoidectomy under local anesthesia (115) may be required.

COLON CANCER

Carcinoma of the colon in pregnancy has been variably estimated to occur in 1 in 10,000 to 1 in 50,000 (103,116). The mean age is 31 years (117). The most common symptoms are rectal bleeding, abdominal pain, distension, and constipation (118), all of which can be, as discussed elsewhere in this chapter, common in uncomplicated pregnancy. Sometimes the patients present with rectal prolapse, intestinal obstruction (with or without intussusception), or colonic perforation with peritonitis. Distribution within the colon has been reported to be the same as in the nonpregnant population (119), although in other series the majority (up to 88%) were located in the rectum or distal colon, that is, within the reach of a sigmoidoscope (102,117).

The pathologic stage of the colon cancers found in pregnancy tends to be more advanced than that in the nonpregnant population. In one series of 39 cases of colonic carcinoma in pregnancy, more than 50% were Dukes C or D (117). This is most likely due in part to delays in diagnosis during pregnancy. The incidence of metastases of colonic carcinoma to ovaries in pregnancy has been reported as high as 25% (120), much higher than in the nonpregnant population.

Diagnosis

The diagnosis is driven by clinical suspicion and confirmed by colonoscopy and biopsy (121). Serum carcinoembryonic antigen (CEA) is normal or slightly elevated during uncomplicated pregnancy (122). Although of low sensitivity and specificity, CEA elevation may be useful in diagnosing colonic carcinoma in pregnancy. Abdominal ultrasonography (123) may demonstrate a bulk lesion or hepatic metastases. Although computed tomography (CT) scan is generally avoided during pregnancy because of concern of radiation exposure to the fetus, these small risks may be outweighed by the benefits of diagnosis. Accumulating experience with magnetic resonance imaging suggests that it is a safe diagnostic alternative in pregnancy (124,125).

Treatment

The therapeutic approach involves first correction of any nutritional deficits from the combined neoplasm and pregnancy. This will enable continued fetal development, maximize the chance of delivering a viable baby (126), and improve the mother's postoperative course and response to chemotherapy or radiotherapy (127,128). Anemia and iron deficiency must be addressed with transfusion and iron supplementation as necessary (129).

In early pregnancy, prompt surgical intervention is recommended, as if the pregnancy did not exist (117,130). In later pregnancy, surgery is delayed, if possible, only long enough for reasonable fetal viability (118). Some investigators (102), but not all (118), have advised cesarean section prior to colonic resection. If cesarean section is not performed, some investigators have advised delaying cancer resection for several days to weeks postdelivery to eliminate the risks associated with uterine size (making surgical exposure difficult) and increased pelvic vascularity and blood flow (102,131). Because of the high coexistence of ovarian metastases, some investigators have advocated simultaneous bilateral salpingoophorectomy (132), but because this is associated with a high rate of spontaneous abortion, especially in the first trimester, others have advocated bilateral ovarian biopsy and removal only if metastasis is documented (118).

Prognosis

Older series emphasized a high fetal loss rate after laparotomy. Recent experience is more optimistic, reporting less than 5% fetal loss after surgery, although there is still an appreciable risk of premature delivery and low birth weight babies (133). Vaginal delivery is feasible after colonic resection, although some investigators have recommended cesarean section if the neoplasm has invaded the anterior rectal wall or compressed the birth canal, so as to avoid obstructed labor and postpartum hemorrhage (102,112). Subsequent successful pregnancy has been reported after prior resection, with or without radiotherapy (134), although radiotherapy can lead to sterility (135).

Primarily because of delay in diagnosis, the prognosis for women developing carcinoma of the rectum or colon during pregnancy is poor, with a 5-year survival rate of 0% to 40% (117,118). The prognosis for the baby depends on the mother's state of nutrition and hemoglobin, but overall has been reported at about 80% (116). The fetus is spared from metastases, although the placenta may be involved (103,136).

INTESTINAL OBSTRUCTION

The incidence has been estimated at 1 in 1,500 to 1 in 66,000 pregnancies (137–140). It is most likely to occur in the third trimester (corresponding to fetal head descent), at 4 to 5 months (as the uterus ascends from pelvis to abdomen), or in the puerperium (141,142). The most common cause is adhesions from prior laparotomy, such as appendectomy (141,143). Less likely causes are volvulus (143–147), intussception, internal hernia, and tumor. Internal hernia is rare, perhaps because the enlarging uterus moves bowel away from the inguinal and femoral rings (142,148). Diaphragmatic hernias have been reported, with incarceration secondary to adjacent pressure by the uterus (149).

Diagnosis

The diagnosis may be difficult to make in pregnancy because abdominal pain, vomiting, and constipation may be ascribed to the pregnancy itself. The most common symptom is pain, followed by nausea, vomiting, and constipation (143). Bilious or feculent vomiting are more likely due to obstruction than to pregnancy (150,151). Beck's warning remains pertinent: "All too often the obstetrician is lulled into a sense of well-being by explaining away symptoms in the belief that they represent acceptable normal variations of pregnancy-induced problems" (141). The correct diagnosis requires a high index of suspicion and often the ordering of abdominal x-rays (143,148).

Treatment

After fluid and electrolyte stabilization and an attempt at tube decompression, early laparotomy is recommended (142,143,152). Volvulus may be decompressed endoscopically (153) but has been reported to carry a high mortality rate (154). Intestinal obstruction in pregnancy carries a high risk of bowel strangulation, with fetal survival of 50% to 80% and maternal survival of 90% (142,152,155).

APPENDICITIS

The most common extrauterine surgical complication of pregnancy is acute appendicitis (156). Its incidence has been estimated at 0.06% to 0.2%, similar to that in the general population (156–159). The second trimester is the most likely but by no means the only time for appendicitis to present (160–163).

Diagnosis

The diagnosis of acute appendicitis is notoriously difficult in pregnancy, especially as the gestation progresses. Accurate preoperative diagnosis is made in less than 70% of cases (156,160,163). The classic location of the pain is increasingly variable in advanced pregnancy, as the cecum becomes displaced toward the iliac crest, bringing the appendix upward, lateral, and posterior, with its long axis no longer downward but upward in as many as 60% by the eighth month (164). The premonitory symptoms of anorexia, nausea, and vomiting are often ascribed to the pregnancy. Fever may be absent or low grade in as many as 90% of cases (159,160,163,165). Elevated white blood count or sedimentation rates are frequently misleading because they may be affected by pregnancy (158,160, 161,165,166). It is no wonder, therefore, that appendicitis in pregnancy is often associated with perforation and peritonitis, particularly in the third trimester (161,164). This may be due not only to delayed diagnosis but also to alterations in omental topography preventing walling off of the perforated viscus.

The considerable differential diagnosis includes pyelonephritis, urolithiasis, threatened abortion, ectopic or heterotopic pregnancy, salpingitis, adnexal torsion, rupture of corpus luteum cyst, infarction of omentum, degenerating leiomyoma, abruptio placentae, chorioamnionitis, and cholecystitis.

Treatment

The therapy is prompt laparotomy, spurred by a high diagnostic index of suspicion (167). Laparoscopic appendectomy can be offered to pregnant women, particularly in the first two trimesters (168,169). It is less useful in the third trimester and in the setting of diffuse peritonitis (151).

As noted, preoperative diagnosis is more often incorrect in pregnant as compared with nonpregnant patients. As summarized by Brant: "The fact that 50% of appendices removed were uninflamed is of little importance since in that case the operation carries a negligible risk to a mother and baby. This additional operation rate is a small price to pay for discovering the undetected case" (158). It remains to be determined whether new diagnostic approaches that include abdominal CT will reduce this false-positive rate.

Prognosis

Both fetal and maternal mortality rates increase with advancing pregnancy (158,160). The reported maternal mortality rate has been as high as 4% in perforated appendicitis (170), and fetal loss can reach 35% (158,160,171). This risk is influenced favorably by early laparotomy (157,172,173). Appendectomy even in the third trimester does not necessarily induce labor or obligate cesarean section (160). Section may be necessary prior to appendectomy, however, during prolonged labor or when appendiceal perforation has occurred (151).

MALABSORPTION SYNDROMES

Absorption of dietary iron across duodenal mucosa is low in early pregnancy but increases as gestation progresses, paralleling but falling short of the 10-fold increase in iron demands (174). Folic acid absorption is the same as that in the nonpregnant state (175), but postpartum serum folic acid concentration is below normal in many pregnant women unless supplemented earlier in the pregnancy (41,116).

Obstetrical sprue has been described, characterized by anemia, sluggish weight gain, and glossitis (176). These patients have folic acid deficiency and intestinal malabsorption of varying combinations of D-xylose, carotene, and fats. Small bowel biopsies demonstrate mild to severe villous atrophy. A childhood history of celiac disease is rare. Cure is achieved in most by administering folic acid at a dosage of 2.5 mg/day.

Patients with even mild classical celiac disease prior to pregnancy may have difficulty conceiving and have abortion rates as high as 20%, low-birth-weight babies, and decreased duration of lactation. All these are apparently improved by restricting gluten and adding appropriate nutritional supplements (177–180). Occasionally patients with iron and folic acid deficiency in pregnancy are found on investigation to have previously undiagnosed celiac disease (179). Celiac disease has been reported to begin or exacerbate in the puerperium (181,182).

INFLAMMATORY BOWEL DISEASE (ULCERATIVE COLITIS AND CROHN DISEASE)

These diseases most often affect women during their reproductive years (183,184) and have been investigated extensively in pregnancy.

Conception

Ulcerative colitis does not alter the ability to conceive (185), but Crohn disease may (186–189), particularly in those with involvement of the colon (190). This may be due to periadnexal adhesions from the adjacent transmural inflammatory disease that characterizes Crohn disease. Rarely there is direct adnexal involvement with granulomatous salpingitis (191). Perineal inflammation may lead to dyspareunia and this, as well as the weakness and malaise of active IBD, may adversely influence conception.

Effect on Pregnancy

Once a woman with either ulcerative colitis or Crohn disease does become pregnant, her gestation is likely to proceed to term with the same success as the normal population (185–188,190,192–199), especially if her IBD is quiescent (116). Duration of pregnancy, maternal weight gain, hemoglobin concentration, hypertension, proteinuria, neonatal hyperbilirubinemia, congenital malformations, prematurity, and spontaneous abortions are not more common than in normal pregnancies (198,

200–202). Normal spontaneous vaginal delivery is the rule, although cesarean section may be indicated, particularly in Crohn with perineal disease (192,103,203).

Mothers with IBD, especially Crohn disease, may be more likely to give birth to low-birth-weight infants (189, 200–202,204) and to deliver preterm (200,205). Certain subsets of Crohn patients may have more fetal wastage. These include Crohn disease appearing for the first time during pregnancy, Crohn disease active at the time of conception, and Crohn disease flaring during pregnancy (192,198,206–210).

Effect of Pregnancy on the Mother's Disease

The extensive literature on this subject is divided into two camps. One asserts that pregnancy exerts no significant influence on the natural course of IBD to exacerbate and remit, with relapse rates of 30% to 50% per year (184,186,187,190,194,198,201,211). The other point of view is that the effect of the pregnancy on the bowel disease depends on how active the disease was at conception: if quiescent at conception, it will tend to remain so throughout the pregnancy; if active at conception, most will continue to flare during the pregnancy and postpartum (185,186,188,190,193,206,212–214).

Most agree that 25% to 40% of patients with Crohn disease may exacerbate within the first 4 postpartum months. This may be due to the marked increase in serum cortisol levels in late pregnancy and its rapid decline in the puerperium (215–217).

Diagnosis

Diarrhea during pregnancy in a woman with a history of ulcerative colitis or Crohn disease first requires evaluation for noninflammatory bowel disease. Thus, review of diet, medication, travel, and consideration of intercurrent viral, bacterial, or protozoan enteritis is indicated. If this search is not fruitful and symptoms persist, the underlying IBD must be implicated.

Bloody diarrhea should be investigated with gentle flexible sigmoidoscopy to differentiate among proctitis, proctosigmoiditis, and more extensive ulcerative colitis. Crohn may be more difficult to prove because it frequently spares the distal colon, has a more protean clinical presentation, and is less likely to present with frankly bloody diarrhea.

Medical Treatment

The medical armamentarium includes the azosalicylates, antibiotics, corticosteroids, immunosuppressives, antidiarrheals, and antispasmotics (218). Sulfasalazine crosses the placenta, achieving levels in cord serum of 50% to 100% of that in maternal serum (219,220). It also may pass into breast milk, with levels up to 30% of that in serum (219). Nevertheless large studies have concluded that sulfasalazine can be used safely throughout gestation and the postpartum period (185,198,201,206, 208,221). As in the nonpregnant state, sulfasalazine may impair absorption of folic acid (222), necessitating supplementation with 1 to 2 mg of folic acid per day.

For those intolerant to sulfasalazine, 5-aminosalicylate is available as suppositories, enemas, and oral preparations (218). These include olsalazine (Dipentum) and mesalamine (Asacol and Pentasa). These agents have been found to be at least as safe in pregnancy as sulfasalazine (223–226), but experience is more limited and the average dose studied relatively low. A case report has appeared of renal insufficiency in an infant exposed *in utero* to 4 g per day of mesalamine (227).

Antibiotics are often used as adjuncts to sulfasalazine, particularly in Crohn disease. Ampicillin and cephalosporins are considered safe in pregnancy (28,228). Ciprofloxacin has been used in pregnancy without documented teratogenicity (229) but is a category C drug. Metronidazole is used for Crohn disease of the colon and perineum, but is often avoided during pregnancy because of controversial reports of teratogenicity (230), yet no convincing teratogenicity has been demonstrated in humans (231–234).

Corticosteroid use in pregnancy has been associated with placental insufficiency, lower birth weight, and fetal distress (235–237), but large studies have not found an increase in congenital abnormalities or other pregnancy complications (198,201,208,238). Although hydrocortisone does cross the placenta, it is largely converted to the less active cortisone, and little enters maternal milk (239). If necessary to control the IBD, corticosteroids can be used safely during pregnancy (240).

Immunomodulating agents have now been generally accepted as effective therapy in both ulcerative colitis and Crohn disease, but their safety in pregnancy remains a concern. Extensive experience reported in both renal transplantation and gastroenterologic literature suggests that azathioprine and 6-mercaptopurine can be continued throughout pregnancy without increased teratogenicity (210,238,241–243) or suppression of fetal immunoglobulin levels (244). A review of 1,200 gestations in 789 women with renal transplants found that more than 80% of pregnancies that continued beyond the first trimester were completed successfully (241). The influence of azathioprine in pregnant women with IBD has been studied and no complications or congenital anomalies detected (245,246).

These immunosuppressives do cross the placenta (247), and there are case reports of pulmonic stenosis, hyaline membrane disease, respiratory distress syndrome, combined immunodeficiency syndrome, myelomeningocele, leukopenia, growth retardation, and chromosomal aberrations in newborns (241,248–251). These reports have left many hesitant to use these agents in pregnancy unless deemed absolutely necessary to control active IBD (240).

Other immunomodulating agents used in IBD are methotrexate and cyclosporine. Methotrexate is considered contraindicated during pregnancy because of demonstrated mutagenicity and teratogenicity (210). In the transplantation literature, cyclosporine has been variably associated with prematurity and low birth weight, but not with immunosuppression in the newborn (252) or with any significant side effect on mother or offspring (253). In IBD patients case reports and a small series have found no undue renal toxicity or congenital anomalies (254–255).

Antidiarrheal agents such as diphenoxylate and codeine can be used in pregnancy, although codeine in high doses may lead to neonatal withdrawal (28). Total parenteral nutrition has been administered throughout pregnancy in advanced Crohn disease and short bowel syndrome (256,257).

All in all, the advice of Crohn et al. is still germane:

> What should be the attitude of the clinician toward the patient in whom pregnancy occurs during a bout of the colitis, or colitis occurs during the pregnancy? Since the life of the patient is rarely threatened by even severe colitis . . . the recommended procedure is to treat . . . in a symptomatic manner and to carry the pregnancy to its natural fruition. Such an approach is usually successful, since the chances of delivery of a viable infant are as good as in the control population . . . . The corticotropins apparently exert no deleterious effect . . . (112).

Surgical Treatment

Surgery is mandated by persistent intestinal obstruction, free perforation, intractable disease activity, toxic megacolon (258–260), or the development of colonic cancer (261). If urgent surgery is needed for ulcerative colitis, the procedure of choice is subtotal colectomy and ileostomy (258,262). Colectomy, even in the third trimester, does not necessarily require coincident cesarean section, although, as is the case with other abdominal surgery during pregnancy, onset of labor may follow laparotomy within several days (263,264).

Fetal and maternal mortality rates after surgery as high as 53% and 29%, respectively, were reported in earlier literature (263), but these rates are probably considerably lower now. More recently, emergent surgery during pregnancy for Crohn disease has been reported, with excellent maternal and infant survival (265).

Patients with ileostomy fare well in subsequent pregnancies, especially if the IBD is quiescent. Ileostomy function throughout pregnancy is usually normal, although prolapse may occur (184,266) and there may be an increased risk of intestinal obstruction (138). Cesarean section may be required, particularly after extensive perineal disease or surgery (138,267,268), although many women can deliver vaginally (266).

Ulcerative colitis patients requiring colectomy now often opt for ileoanal anastomosis with an ileal pelvic pouch. Conception and pregnancy are not impaired significantly after these procedures (269). Increased stooling and temporary incontinence may occur from the enlarged adjacent uterus (270). Obstruction of the pouch has been reported in advanced pregnancy, relieved by delivery (131). Although some have advocated cesarean section in ileoanal anastomoses to avoid damage to anal sphincters (271), vaginal delivery is possible and advised in most cases (270,272).

PANCREATITIS

Acute pancreatitis occurs in 1 of every 1,000 to 10,000 pregnancies, probably more often than in the nonpregnant state (273–276). It may be more common in primigravidas than multiparas (277), although this has been called into question (278–280). During pregnancy it is most likely to occur during the third trimester or within 5 months of delivery (152,275,277).

Pathogenesis

In dogs, pregnancy has been shown to increase pancreatic basal flow, as well as bicarbonate concentration and output, all of which revert to normal in the postpartum period (281). The hormonal alterations of pregnancy have been implicated in acute pancreatitis on the basis of their similarities to the hormonal state induced by oral contraceptives and their putative link to pancreatitis (278), but supporting studies in humans are lacking.

By far the most common etiology is cholelithiasis, found by ultrasonography in as many as 90% of pregnant women with acute pancreatitis (275,282). Less common associations include thiazide ingestion (283), hyperparathyroidism (284,285), prepregnancy hyperlipidemia (286), and physiologic hyperlipidemia of second and third trimesters, a number of viral infections, trauma, and vasculitis (287). Alcohol and drugs are less frequent etiologies than in the nonpregnant population (288).

Diagnosis

As in the nonpregnant state, the diagnosis of acute pancreatitis in pregnancy is made by obtaining a history of abdominal or back pain, often associated with nausea, low-grade fever, decreased or absent bowel sounds, hyperamylasemia, and elevated urinary amylase (152, 277,287). A prior history of recurrent bouts of abdominal pain, gallstones, or hyperlipidemia increases the clinical index of suspicion. Vomiting alone or other upper gastrointestinal symptoms besides pain may be the presenting symptoms (273).

Serum amylase may fluctuate somewhat during pregnancy but not enough to confuse the diagnostic issue

(275,288–290). What can confound, however, is the hyperamylasemia seen with perforated or strangulated intestinal viscus or ruptured tubal pregnancy. Serum lipase remains normal in uneventful pregnancy (289), is not affected by coincident hyperlipidemia, and is therefore helpful in diagnosing acute pancreatitis.

Abdominal sonography is useful in demonstrating edema of the pancreas, pseudocyst, or gallstones. Occasionally the diagnosis is made by cul-de-sac extraction of nonclotting, turbid, wine-colored fluid high in amylase (291).

The differential diagnosis includes acute cholecystitis, penetrating ulcer, splenic infarction or rupture, pyelonephritis or perinephric abscess, pulmonary infarction, appendicitis, ruptured ectopic pregnancy, and preeclampsia.

Treatment

Management of acute pancreatitis includes putting the gut at rest and administering intravenous fluids to prevent or correct hypovolemia. Analgesics are administered as needed. Parenteral hyperalimentation has become a significant addition to the medical management of severe acute pancreatitis (292).

Laparoscopic cholecystectomy is feasible during pregnancy (293). For biliary pancreatitis in the first trimester, cholecystectomy performed in the second trimester has been advocated. This procedure is justified because fetal organogenesis has been completed, the likelihood of spontaneous abortion and premature labor are decreased, the relative smallness of the uterus does not obscure the operative field, and the likelihood of further episodes of biliary colic, cholecystitis, or pancreatitis later in the same pregnancy is decreased (273, 275,282).

Other investigators favor a nonoperative approach, except in cases of bile duct obstruction, empyema, or intractable or repeated attacks of pancreatitis (276). Attacks during the third trimester are managed nonoperatively if possible, postponing cholecystectomy until the postpartum period (282).

Endoscopic retrograde cholangiography, sphincterotomy, and, if necessary, common duct stone extraction are available as adjuncts or alternatives to cholecystectomy. Fetal shielding and minimal x-ray fluoroscopy are mandatory (294,295).

When hyperlipidemia is the cause, a low-fat and low-carbohydrate diet must be instituted (296). If this is unsuccessful in lowering plasma triglyceride levels below 1,000 mg/dL, total parenteral nutrition (297) and even extracorporeal lipid elimination (298) may be required.

Dreaded sequelae of acute pancreatitis, such as hypocalcemia, retroperitoneal hemorrhage, abscess, and pseudocyst, may occur in pregnancy. Pseudocysts have been drained surgically during pregnancy (299).

Prognosis

Subsequent attacks of acute pancreatitis occur in as many as 50% of patients, often antepartum. A maternal mortality rate as great as 37% has been reported by some investigators (204,300) but not all (273). Hypovolemia appears to be a major factor in the mortality figures, underscoring the need for vigorous rehydration (277). With modern management, fetal salvage of 80% to 90% is the rule (273,277).

REFERENCES

1. Peckham CH, King RW. A study of intercurrent conditions observed during pregnancy. Am J Obstet Gynecol 1963;87:909.
2. Brandes JM. First-trimester nausea and vomiting as related to outcome of pregnancy. Obstet Gynecol 1967;30:427–431.
3. Fairweather DV. Nausea and vomiting in pregnancy. Am J Obstet Gynecol 1968;102:135–175.
4. Scher E. Treatment for nausea of pregnancy. Postgrad Med 1965;37: 610.
5. Diggory PLC, Tomkinson JS. Nausea and vomiting in pregnancy: a trial of meclazine dihydrochloride with and without pyridoxine. Lancet 1962;2:370.
6. Weigel MM, Weigel RM. The association of reproductive history, demographic factors, and alcohol and tobacco consumption with the risk of developing nausea and vomiting in early pregnancy. Am J Epidemiol 1988;127:562–570.
7. Macedo G, Carvalho L, Ribeiro T. Endoscopic sclerotherapy for upper gastrointestinal bleeding due to Mallory-Weiss syndrome. Am J Gastroenterol 1995;90:1364–1365.
8. Adams RH, Gordon J, Combes B. Hyperemesis gravidarum: I. Evidence of hepatic dysfunction. Obstet Gynecol 1968;31:659–664.
9. Davison JS, Davison MC, Hay DM. Gastric emptying time in late pregnancy and labour. J Obstet Gynaecol Br Commonw 1970;77:37–41.
10. Lawson M, Kern F, Everson JT. Gastrointestinal transit time in human pregnancy. Prolongation in the second and third trimesters followed by postpartum normalization. Gastroenterology 1985;89:996–999.
11. Koch KL, Stern RM, Vasey M, Botti JJ, Creasy GW, Dwyer A. Gastric dysrhythmias and nausea of pregnancy. Dig Dis Sci 1990;35: 961–986.
12. Walsh JW, Hasler WL, Nugent CE, Owyang C. Progesterone and estrogen are potential mediators of gastric slow-wave dysrhythmias in nausea of pregnancy. Am J Physiol 1996;270:G506.
13. Soules MR, Hughes CL, Garcia JA, Livengood CH, Prystowsky MR, Alexander E. Nausea and vomiting of pregnancy: role of human chorionic gonadotropin and 17-hydroxyprogesterone. Obstet Gynecol 1980; 55:696–700.
14. Jarvinen PA Pesonen S, Vaanaanen P. Fractional determinations of urinary 17-ketosteroids in hyperemesis gravidarum. Acta Endocrinol 1962:41:123.
15. Kauppila A, Ylikorkala O, Jarvinen PA, Haapalahti J. The function of the anterior pituitary-adrenal cortex axis in hyperemesis gravidarum. Br J Obstet Gynaecol 1976;83:11–16.
16. Ylikorkala O, Kauppila A, Haapalaht J. Follicle stimulating hormone, thyrotropin, human growth hormone and prolactin in hyperemesis gravidarum. Br J Obstet Gynaecol 1976;83:529–533.
17. Frigo P, Lang C, ReisenbergerK, Kolbl H, Hirshl AM. Hyperemesis gravidarum associated with *Helicobacter pylori* seropositivity. Obstet Gynecol 1998;91:615–617.
18. Murray FA, Erskine JP, Fielding J. Gastric secretion in pregnancy. J Obstet Gynaecol Br Emp 1957;64:373.
19. Harvey WA, Sherfey MJ. Vomiting in pregnancy: a psychological study. Psychosom Med 1954;6:1.
20. Palmer ED. Upper gastrointestinal hemorrhage during pregnancy. Am J Med Sci 1961;242:223.
21. Midwinter A. Vomiting in pregnancy. Practitioner 1971;206:743–750.
22. Janower ML, Linton OW, eds. Radiation risk: a primer. American College of Radiology, Commission on Physics and Radiation Safety, Committee on Radiologic Units, Standards and Protection, 1996. Reston, Virginia.

23. Brent RL. The effects of embryonic and fetal exposure to x-rays, microwaves, and ultrasound. Clin Obstet Gynecol 1983;26:484–510.
24. Mole RH. Radiation effects on pre-natal development and their radiological significance. Br J Radiol 1979;52:89–101.
25. Swartz HM, Reichling BA. Hazards of radiation exposure for pregnant women. JAMA 1978;239:1907–1908.
26. Cappell MS, Colon V, Sidhom OA. A study of eight medical centers of the safety and clinical efficacy of esophagogastroduodenoscopy in 83 pregnant females with follow-up of fetal outcome and with comparison to control groups. Am J Gastroenterol 1996;91:348–354.
27. Cappell MS. The safety and efficacy of gastrointestinal endoscopy during pregnancy. Gastroenterol Clin North Am 1998;27:37–71.
28. Atlay RD, Weekes AR. The treatment of gastrointestinal disease in pregnancy. Clin Obstet Gynecol 1986;13:335–347.
29. Broussard CN, Richter JE. Nausea and vomiting of pregnancy. Gastroenterol Clin North Am 1998;27:123–151.
30. Leathem AM. Safety and efficacy of antiemetics used to treat nausea and vomiting of pregnancy. Clin Pharmacy 1986;5:660–668.
31. Singh MS, Lean TH. The use of metoclopramide (Maxalon) in hyperemesis gravidarum. Proc Obstet Gynecol Soc Singapore 1970;1:43.
32. Bailey B, Addis A, Lee A, et al. Cisapride use during human pregnancy: a prospective, controlled multicenter study. Dig Dis Sci 1997; 42:1848–1852.
33. Witter FR, King TM, Blake DA. The effects of chronic gastrointestinal medication on the fetus and neonate. Obstet Gynecol 1981;58 (suppl):79–84.
34. Sahakian V, Riuse D, Sipes S, Rose N, Nebyl J. Vitamin B_6 is effective therapy for nausea and vomiting of pregnancy: a randomized, double-blind placebo-controlled study. Obstet Gynecol 1991;78:33–36.
35. Huff PS. Safety of drug therapy for nausea and vomiting of pregnancy. J Fam Pract 1980;11:969–970.
36. Kullander S, Kollen B. A prospective study of drugs and pregnancy: II. Anti-emetic drugs. Acta Obstet Gynecol Scand 1976;55:105–111.
37. Milkovich L, van den Berg BJ. Effects of antenatal exposure to anorectic drugs. Am J Obstet Gynecol 1977;129:637–642.
38. Shapiro S. Kaufman DW, Rosenberg L, et al. Meclizine in pregnancy in relation to congenital malformations. Br Med J 1978;1:483.
39. Sullivan CA, Johnson CA, Roach H, Martin RW, Stewart DK, Morrison JC. A pilot study of intravenous ondansetron for hyperemesis gravidarum. Am J Obstet Gynecol 1996;174:1565–1568.
40. Aikens Murphy P. Alternative therapies for nausea and vomiting of pregnancy. Obstet Gynecol 1998;91:149–155.
41. Hamaoui E, Hamaoui M. Nutritional assessment and support during pregnancy. Gastroenterol Clin North Am 1998;27:89–121.
42. van Stuijvenberg ME, Schabort I, Labadarios D, Nel JT. The nutritional status and treatment of patients with hyperemesis gravidarum. Am J Obstet Gynecol 1995;172:1585–1591.
43. Charlin V, Borghesi L, Hasbun J, Von Mulenbrock R, Moreno MI. Parenteral nurition in hyperemesis gravidarum. Nutrition 1993;9:29–32.
44. Levine MG, Esser D. Total parenteral nutrition for the treatment of severe hyperemesis gravidarum: maternal nutritional effects and fetal outcome. Obstet Gynecol 1988;72:102–107.
45. Hsu JJ, Clark-Glena R, Nelson DK, Kim CH. Nasogastric enteral feeding in the management of hyperemesis gravidarum. Obstet Gynecol 1996;88:343–346.
46. Deuchar N. Nausea and vomiting in pregnancy: a review of the problem with particular regard to psychological and social aspects. Br J Obstet Gynaecol 1995;102:6–8.
47. Shaheen NJ, Crosby MA, Grimm IS, Isaacs K. The use of percutaneous endoscopic gastrostomy in pregnancy. Gastrointest Endosc 1997;46:564–565.
48. Gross S, Librach C, Cecutti A. Maternal weight loss associated with hyperemesis gravidarum: a predictor of fetal outcome. Am J Obstet Gynecol 1989;160:906–909.
49. Medalie JH. Relationship between nausea and/or vomiting in early pregnancy and abortion. Lancet 1957;273:117.
50. Weigel RM, Weigel MM. Nausea and vomiting of early pregnancy and pregnancy outcome: a meta-analytical review. Br J Obstet Gynaecol 1989;96:1312–1318.
51. Atlay RD, Gillison EW, Horton AL. A fresh look at pregnancy heartburn. J Obstet Gynaecol Br Commonw 1973;80:63–66.
52. Baron TH, Richter JE. Gastroesophageal reflux disease in pregnancy. Gastroenterol Clin North Am 1992;21:777–791.
53. Nebel OT, Fornes MF, Castell DO. Symptomatic gastroesophageal reflux: incidence and precipitating factors. Am J Dig Dis 1976:21: 953–956.
54. Feeney JG. Heartburn in pregnancy. Br Med J 1982;284:1138–1139.
55. Marrero JM, Goggin PM, de Caestecker JS, Pearce JM, Maxwell JD. Determinants of pregnancy heartburn. Br J Obstet Gynaecol 1992;99: 731–734.
56. Ulmsten U, Sundstrom G. Esophageal manometry in pregnant and nonpregnant women. Am J Obstet Gynecol 1978;132:260–264.
57. Lind JF, Smith AM, McIver DK, Coopland AT, Crispin JS. Heartburn in pregnancy: a manometric study. Can Med Assoc J 1968;98:571–574.
58. van Thiel DH, Gavaler JS, Joshi SN, Sara RK, Stremple J. Heartburn of pregnancy. Gastroenterology 1977;72:666–668.
59. Fisher RS, Roberts GS, Grabowski C, Cohen S. Altered lower esophageal sphincter function during early pregnancy. Gastroenterology 1978;74:1233–1237.
60. Dodd WJ, Dent J, Hogan WJ. Pregnancy and the lower esophageal sphincter. Gastroenterology 1978;74:1334–1336.
61. van Thiel DH, Gavaler JS, Stremple J. Lower esophageal sphincter pressure in women using sequential oral contraceptives. Gastroenterology 1976;71:232–234.
62. Castro L. Reflux esophagitis as the cause of heartburn in pregnancy. Am J Obstet Gynecol 1967;98:1–10.
63. Katz PO, Castell DO. Gastroesophageal reflux disease during pregnancy. Gastroenterol Clin North Am 1998;27:153–167.
64. Swinhoe JR, Cochrane GW, Wishart R. Oesophageal stricture due to reflux oesophagitis in pregnancy: case report. Br J Obstet Gynaecol 1981;88:1249–1251.
65. Magee LA, Inocencion G, Kamboj L, Rosetti F, Koren G. Safety of first trimester exposure to histamine H_2 blockers: a prospective cohort study. Dig Dis Sci 1996;41:1145–1149.
66. Lewis JH, Weingold AB. The use of gastrointestinal drugs during pregnancy and lactation. Am J Gastroenterol 1985;80:912–923.
67. McGowan WAW. Safety of cimetidine in obstetric patients. J R Soc Med 1979;72:902–902.
68. Beeley L. Does ranitidine have an adverse effect on a pregnant woman or her fetus? Br Med J 1985;290:308.
69. Briggs GG, Freeman RK, Yaffe SJ. In: Drugs in pregnancy and lactation: a reference guide to fetal and neonatal risk, 4th ed. Baltimore: Williams & Wilkins, 1994.
70. Harper MA, McVeigh E, Thompson W, Ardill JE, Buchanan KD. Successful pregnancy in association with Zollinger-Ellison syndrome. Am J Obstet Gynecol 1995;173:863–864.
71. Hey VMF, Ostick DG. Metoclopromide and the gastro-oesophageal sphincter: a study in pregnant women with heartburn. Anesthesia 1978;33:462–465.
72. Baird RM. Peptic ulceration in pregnancy: report of a case with perforation. Can Med Assoc J 1966;94:861–994.
73. Sandweiss DJ, Podolsky HM, Saltzstein HC. Deaths from perforation and hemorrhage of gastroduodenal ulcer during pregnancy and puerperium: review of literature and report of one case. Am J Obstet Gynecol 1943;45:131.
74. Clark DH. Peptic ulcer in women. Br Med J 1953:1:1254.
75. Kelly P, Robert A. Inhibition by pregnancy and lactation of steroid-induced ulcers in the rat. Gastroenterology 1969;56:24–29.
76. Landmade CF. Epigastric pain in pregnancy toxemias. West J Surg 1956;64:540.
77. Barnes LW. Serum histaminase during pregnancy. Obstet Gynecol 1957;9:730.
78. Truelove SC. Stilbesterol, phenobarbitone and diet in chronic duodenal ulcer. Br Med J 1960;2:559.
79. Rooney PJ, Dow TGB, Brooks PM, Dick WC, Buchanan KD. Immunoreactive gastrin and gestation. Am J Obstet Gynecol 1975; 122:834–836.
80. Blecker U, Lanciers S, Hauser B, Vandenplas Y. The prevalence of *Helicobacter pylori* positivity in a symptom-free population, aged 1 to 40 years. J Clin Epidemiol 1994;47:1095–1098.
81. Blecker U, Lanciers S, Keppans E, Vandenplas Y. Evolution of *Helicobacter pylori* positivity in infants born from positive mothers. J Pediatr Gastroenterol Nutr 1994;19:87–90.
82. Esposito TJ. Trauma during pregnancy. Emerg Med Clin North Am 1994;12:167–199.
83. Potzi R, Ferenci P, Gangl A. Endoscopic sclerotherapy of esophageal varices during pregnancy: case report. J Gastroenterol 1991;29: 246–247.

84. Hill LM, Kleinberg F. Effects of drugs and chemicals on fetus and newborn. Mayo Clin Proc 1984;59:707–716.
85. Ching CK, Lam SK. Antacids: indications and limitations. Drugs 1994;47:305–317.
86. Smallwood RA, Berlin RG, Castagnoli N, et al. Safety of acid-suppressing drugs. Dig Dis Sci 1995;40(suppl):63–80.
87. Lin CJ, Huang CL, Hsu HW, Chent L. Prophylaxis against acid aspiration in regional anesthesia for elective cesarean section: a comparison between oral single-dose ranitidine, famotidine and omeprazole assessed with fiberoptic gastric aspiration. Acta Anaesthesiol Sin 1996;34:179–184.
88. Cappell MS, Garcia A. Gastric and duodenal ulcers during pregnancy. Gastroenterol Clin North Am 1998;27:169–195.
89. Maeta M, Yamashiro H, Oka A, Tsujitani S. Ikeguchi M, Kaibara N. Gastric cancer in the young, with special reference to 14 pregnancy-associated cases: analysis based on 2,325 consecutive cases of gastric cancer. J Surg Oncol 1995;58:191–195.
90. Becker-Andersen H, Husfeldt V. Peptic ulcer in pregnancy. Report of two cases of surgically treated bleeding duodenal ulcer. Acta Obstet Gynecol Scand 1971;50:391–395.
91. Grosfeld JL. Massive gastric hemorrhage in late pregnancy: survival of mother and offspring after vagotomy and pyloroplasty. Ann Surg 1968;168:971–973.
92. Honiotes G, Clark PF, Cavanaugh D. Gastric ulcer perforation during pregnancy. Am J Obstet Gynecol 1970;106:619–621.
93. Winchester DP, Bancroft BR. Perforated peptic ulcer in pregnancy. Am J Obstet Gynecol 1966;94:280–281.
94. Jones PF, McEwan AB, Bernard RM. Haemorrrhage and perforation complicating peptic ulcer in pregnancy. Lancet 1969;2:350–352.
95. Paul M, Tew WL, Holliday RL. Perforated peptic ulcer in pregnancy with survival of mother and child: case report and review of the literature. Can J Surg 1976;19:427–429.
96. Tew WL, Holliday RL, Phibbs G. Perforated duodenal ulcer in pregnancy with double survival. Am J Obstet Gynecol 1976;125:1151–1152.
97. Peck DA, Welch JS, Waugh JM, et al. Pregnancy following gastric resection. Am J Obstet Gynecol 1964;90:517.
98. Levy N, Lemberg E, Sharf M. Bowel habit in pregnancy. Digestion 1971;4:216–222.
99. Greenhalf JO, Leonard HS. Laxatives in the treatment of constipation in pregnant and breast-feeding mother. Practitioner 1973;210:259–263.
100. Baron TH, Ramirez B, Richter J. Gastrointestinal motility disorders during pregnancy. Ann Intern Med 1993;118:366–375.
101. Nash AG. Perforated large bowel carcinoma in late pregnancy. Proc R Soc Med 1967;60:504.
102. O'Leary FA, Pratt JH, Symmonds RE. Rectal carcinoma and pregnancy: a review of 17 cases. Obstet Gynecol 1967;30:862–868.
103. Rothman LA, Cohen CJ, Astarloa J. Placental and fetal involvement by maternal malignancy; a report of rectal carcinoma and review of the literature. Am J Obstet Gynecol 1973;116:1023–1034.
104. Clement PB. Perforation of the sigmoid colon during pregnancy: a rare complication of endometriosis. Case report. Br J Obstet Gynaecol 1977;84:548–550.
105. Balfour RP, Burke M. Hirschsprung's disease complicating pregnancy. Br J Clin Pract 1976;30:70.
106. Shaxted EJ, Jukes R. Pseudo-obstruction of the bowel in pregnancy. Case reports. Br J Obstet Gynaecol 1979;86:411–413.
107. Cappell MS, Sidhom O, Colon V. A study at ten medical centers of the safety and efficacy of 48 flexible sigmoidoscopies and 8 colonoscopies during pregnancy with follow-up of fetal outcome and with comparison to control groups. Dig Dis Sci 1996;41:2353–2361.
108. Bonapace ES, Fisher RS. Constipation and diarrhea in pregnancy. Gastroenterol Clin North Am 1998;27:197–211.
109. Grandien M, Sterner G, Kalin M, Engardt L. Management of pregnant women with diarrhoea at term and of healthy carriers of infectious agents in stools at delivery. Scand J Infect Dis 1990;71(suppl): 9–18.
110. West L, Waren J, Cutts T. Diagnosis and management of irritable bowel syndrome, constipation, and diarrhea in pregnancy. Gastroenterol Clin North Am 1992;21:793–802.
111. Collins E. Maternal and fetal effects of acetaminophen and salicylates in pregnancy. Obstet Gynecol 1981;58(suppl):57–62.
112. Medich DS, Fazio VW. Hemorrhoids, anal fissure, and carcinoma of the colon, rectum and anus during pregnancy. Surg Clin North Am 1995;75:77–88.
113. Martin C, Varner MW. Physiologic changes in pregnancy: surgical implications. Clin Obstet Gynecol 1994;37:241–255.
114. Lieberman W. Anus and rectum. Relation to obstetrics and gynecology. Am J Proctol 1971;22:41–43.
115. Saleeby RG, Rosen L, Stasik JJ, Riether RD, Sheets J, Khubchandeni IT. Hemorrhoidectomy during pregnancy: risk or relief? Dis Colon Rectum 1991;34:260–261.
116. Woods JB, Martin JN, Ingram FH, Odom CD, Scott-Conner CE, Rhodes RS. Pregnancy complicated by carcinoma of the colon above the rectum. Am J Perinatol 1992;9:102–110.
117. Bernstein MA, Madoff RD, Caushaj PF. Colon and rectal cancer in pregnancy. Dis Colon Rectum 1993;36:172–178.
118. Nesbitt JC, Moise KJ, Sawyers JL. Colorectal carcinoma in pregnancy. Arch Surg 1985;120:636–640.
119. McGowan L. Cancer and pregnancy. Obstet Gynecol Surv 1964;19: 285.
120. Matsuyama T,Tsukamoto N, Matsukuma K, Kamura T, Kaku T, Saito T. Malignant ovarian tumors associated with pregnancy: report of six cases. Int J Gynecol Obstet 1989;28:61–66.
121. Cappell MS. Colon cancer during pregnancy. Gastroenterol Clinic North Am 1998;27:225–236.
122. Lamerz R, Reider H. Significance of CEA determination in patients with cancer of the colon-rectum and the mammary gland in comparison to physiolgical states in connection with pregnancy. Bull Cancer 1976;63:575–586.
123. Reece EA, Assimakopoulos E, Zheng XZ, Hagay Z, Hobbins JC. The safety of obstetric ultrasonography: concern for the fetus. Obstet Gynecol 1990;76:139–146.
124. Elster AD. Does MR imaging have any known effects on the developing fetus? Am J Roentgenol 1994;162:1493.
125. Seidman DS, Heyman Z, Ben-ari G, Mashiach S, Karkai G. Use of magnetic imaging in pregnancy to diagnose intussusception induced by colon cancer. Obstet Gynecol 1992;79:822–823.
126. Luke B. Nutritional influences on fetal growth. Clin Obstet Gynecol 1994;37:538–549.
127. DeWys WD, Begg C, Lavin PT, et al. Prognostic effect of weight loss prior to chemotherapy in cancer patients. Am J Med 1980;69: 491–497.
128. Donaldson SS. Nutritional support as an adjuvant to radiation therapy. J Parenter Enteral Nutr 1984;8:302–310.
129. Scholl TO, Hediger ML. Anemia and iron-deficiency anemia: compilation of data on pregnancy outcome. Am J Clin Nutr 1994;59(suppl): 492–500.
130. Lea AW. Pregnancy following radical operation for rectal carcinoma. Am J Obstet Gynecol 1972;113:504–510.
131. Walsh C, Fazio VW. Cancer of the colon, rectum, and anus during pregnancy. Gastroenterol Clinic North Am 1998;27:257–267.
132. Pitluk H, Poticha SM. Carcinoma of the colon and rectum in patients less than 40 years of age. Surg Gynecol Obstet 1983;157:335–337.
133. Kort B, Katz VL, Watson WJ. The effect of nonobstetric operation during pregnancy. Surg Gynecol Obstet 1993;177:371–376.
134. Barber HR, Brunschwig A. Carcinoma of the bowel. Radiation and surgical management and pregnancy. Am J Obstet Gynecol 1968;100: 926–933.
135. Mettler FA, Upton AC. Direct effects of radiation. In: Medical effects of ionizing radiation. Philadelphia: WB Saunders, 1995.
136. Dildy GA, Moise KJ, Carpenter RJ, Klima T. Maternal malignancy metastatic to the products of conception: a review. Obstet Gynecol Surv 1989;44:535–540.
137. Hoff WS, D'Amelio LF, Tinkoff GH, et al. Maternal predictors of fetal demise in trauma during pregnancy. Surg Gynecol Obstet 1991;172: 175–180.
138. Hudson CN. Ileostomy in pregnancy. Proc R Soc Med 1972;65: 281–283.
139. Smith JA, Bartlett MK. Acute surgical emergencies of the abdomen in pregnancy. N Engl J Med 1940;223:529.
140. Stewardson RH, Bombeck CT, Nyhus LM. Critical operative management of small bowel obstruction. Ann Surg 1979;187:189–193.
141. Beck WW. Intestinal obstruction in pregnancy. Obstet Gynecol 1974;43:374–378.
142. Meyerson S, Holtz T, Ehrinpreis M, Dhar R. Small bowel obstruction in pregnancy. Am J Gastroenterol 1995;90:299–302.
143. Perdue PW, Johnson HW, Stafford HW. Intestinal obstruction complicating pregnancy. Am J Surg 1992;164:384–388.

144. Brannen EA. Four cases of volvulus of the small bowel complicating early pregnancy. Am J Obstet Gynecol 1962:84:854.
145. Hamlin CH, Palermino DA. Volvulus associated with pregnancy. Am J Obstet Gynecol 1966;94:1147–1148.
146. Lazaro EJ, Das PB, Abraham PV. Volvulus of the sigmoid colon complicating pregnancy. Obstet Gynecol 1969;33:553–557.
147. Lord SA, Boswell WC, Hungerpiller JC. Sigmoid volvulus in pregnancy. Am Surg 1996;62:380–382.
148. Hill LM, Symmonds RE. Small bowel obstruction in pregnancy: a review and report of four cases. Obstet Gynecol 1977;49:170–173.
149. Kurzel RB, Naunheim KS, Schwartz RA. Repair of symptomatic diaphragmatic hernia during pregnancy. Obstet Gynecol 1988;71: 869–871.
150. Connolly MM, Unti JA, Nora PF. Bowel obstruction in pregnancy. Surg Clin North Am 1995;75:101–113.
151. Firstenberg MS, Malangoni MA. Gastrointestinal surgery during pregnancy. Gastroenterol Clin North Am 1998;27:73–88.
152. Nathan L, Huddleston JF. Acute abdominal pain in pregnancy. Obstet Gynecol Clin North Am 1995;22:55–68.
153. Brothers TE, Strodel WE, Eckhauser FE. Endoscopy in colonic volvulus. Ann Surg 1987;206:1–4.
154. Ballantyne GH. Review of sigmoid volvulus: clinical patterns and pathogenesis. Dis Colon Rectum 1982;25:823–830.
155. Davis MR, Bohon CJ. Intestinal obstruction in pregnancy. Clin Obstet Gynecol 1983;26:832–842.
156. Sarason EL, Bauman S. Acute appendicitis in pregnancy: difficulties in diagnosis. Obstet Gynecol 1963;22:382.
157. Al-Mulhim AA. Acute appendicitis in pregnancy: a review of 52 cases. Int Surg 1996;81:295–297.
158. Brant HA. Acute appendicitis in pregnancy. Obstet Gynecol 1967; 29:130–138.
159. Lee RA, Johnson CE, Symmonds G. Appendicitis during pregnancy. JAMA 1965;193:966.
160. Babaknia A, Parsa H, Woodruff JD. Appendicitis during pregnancy. Obstet Gynecol 1977;50:40–44.
161. MacBeth RA. Acute surgical disease of the abdomen complicating pregnancy. Can J Surg 1961;4:419.
162. Mazze RI, Kallen B. Appendectomy during pregnancy: a Swedish registry study of 778 cases. Obstet Gynecol 1991;77:835–840.
163. Tamir IL, Bongard FS, Klein SR. Acute appendicitis in the pregnant patient. Am J Surg 1990;160:571–575.
164. Baer JL, Reis RA, Arens RA. Appendicitis in pregnancy with changes in position and axis of the normal appendix in pregnancy. JAMA 1932;98:1359.
165. Weingold AB. Appendicitis in pregnancy. Clin Obstet Gynecol 1983; 26:801–809.
166. Masters K, Levine BA, Gaskill HV, Sirinek KR. Diagnosing appendicitis during pregnancy. Am J Surg 1984;148:768–771.
167. Thomford NR, Patti RW, Teteris NJ. Appendectomy during pregnancy. Surg Gynecol Obstet 1969;129:489–492.
168. Gurbuz AT, Peetz ME. The acute abdomen in the pregnant patient: is there a role for laparoscopy? Surg Endosc 1997;11:98–102.
169. Schreiber JH. Laparoscopic appendectomy in pregnancy. Surg Endosc 1990;4:100–102.
170. DeVore GR. Acute abdominal pain in the pregnant patient due to pancreatitis, acute appendicitis, cholecystitis, or peptic ulcer disease. Clin Perinatol 1980;7:349–369.
171. McComb P, Laimon H. Appendicitis complicating pregnancy. Can J Surg 1980;23:92–94.
172. Frisenda R, Roty AR, Kilway JB, Brown AL, Peelen M. Acute appendicitis during pregnancy. Am Surg 1979;45:503–506.
173. Zaitoon MM, Mrazek RG. Acute appendicitis associated with pregnancy, labor, and the puerperium. Am Surg 1977;43:395–398.
174. Svanberg B. Absorption of iron in pregnancy. Acta Obstet Gynecol Scand Suppl 1975;48:1108.
175. Iyengar L, Babu S. Folic acid absorption in pregnancy. Br J Obstet Gynaecol 1975;82:20–23.
176. Whitfield CR. Obstetric sprue. J Obstet Gynaecol Br Commonw 1970;77:577–586.
177. Ciacci C, Cirillo M, Auriemma G, DiDato G, Sabbatini F, Mazzacca G. Celiac disease and pregnancy outcome. Am J Gastroenterol 1996; 91:718–722.
178. Collin P, Vilska S, Heinonen PK, Hallstrom O, Pikkarainen P. Infertility and coeliac disease. Gut 1996;39:382–384.
179. Joske RA, Martin JHD. Coeliac disease presenting as recurrent abortion. J Obstet Gynaecol Br Commonw 1971;78:754–758.
180. Ogborn AD. Pregnancy in patients with coeliac disease. Br J Obstet Gynaecol 1975;82:293–296.
181. Erdozain JC, Martin de Argila C, Cerezo E, Lizasoain J, Presa M. Adult celiac disease: reactivation during pregnancy and puerperium. Am J Gastroenterol 1993;88:1139–1140.
182. Pauzner R, Rothman P, Schwartz E, Neuman G, Farfel Z. Acute onset of celiac disease in the puerperium. Am J Gastroenterol 1992;87: 1037–1039.
183. Donaldson RM. Management of medical problems in pregnancy—inflammatory bowel disease. N Engl J Med 1985;312:1616–1619.
184. Vender RJ, Spiro HM. Inflammatory bowel disease and pregnancy. J Clin Gastroenterol 1982;4:231–249.
185. Willoughby CP, Truelove SC. Ulcerative colitis and pregnancy. Gut 1980;21:469–474.
186. DeDombal FT, Burton IL, Goligher JC. Crohn's disease and pregnancy. Br Med J 1972;3:550.
187. Donaldson LB. Crohn's disease: its gynecologic aspect. Am J Obstet Gynecol 1978;131:196–202.
188. Homan WP, Thorbjarmarson B. Crohn disease and pregnancy. Arch Surg 1976;111:545–547.
189. Mayberry JF, Weterman IT. European survey of fertility and pregnancy in women with Crohn's disease: a case control study by European collaborative group. Gut 1986;27:821–825.
190. Fielding JF, Cooke WT. Pregnancy and Crohn's disease. Br Med J 1970;2:76–77.
191. Brooks JJ, Wheeler JE. Granulomatous salpingitis secondary to Crohn's disease. Obstet Gynecol 1977;49:31–33.
192. Baiocco PJ, Korelitz BI. The influence of inflammatory bowel disease and its treatment on pregnancy and fetal outcome. J Clin Gastroenterol 1984;6:211–216.
193. Banks PM, Korelitz BI, Setzel L. The course of nonspecific ulcerative colitis: review of twenty years experience and late results. Gastroenterology 1957;32:983.
194. DeDombal FT, Watt JM, Watkinson G, et al. Ulcerative colitis and pregnancy. Lancet 1965;2:599.
195. Hanan IM, Kirsner JB. Inflammatory bowel disease in pregnant women. Clin Perinatol 1985;12:669–682.
196. Lindhagen T, Bohe M, Ekelund S, Valentin L. Fertility and outcome of pregnancy in patients operated on for Crohn's disease. Int J Colorect Dis 1986;1:25–27.
197. McEwan HP. Ulcerative colitis in pregnancy. Proc R Soc Med 1972;65:279–281.
198. Nielsen OH, Andreasson B, Bondesen S, Jacobson O, Jarnum S. Pregnancy in Crohn's disease. Scand J Gastroenterol 1984;19:724–732.
199. Webb MJ, Sedlack RE. Ulcerative colitis in pregnancy. Med Clin North Am 1974;58:823–827.
200. Fedorkow DM, Persaud D, Nimrod CA. Inflammatory bowel disease: a controlled study of late pregnancy outcome. Am J Obstet Gynecol 1989;160:998–1001.
201. Nielsen OH, Andreasson B, Bondesen S, Jarnum S. Pregnancy in ulcerative colitis. Scand J Gastroenterol 1983;18:735–742.
202. Porter RJ, Stirrat GM. The effects of inflammatory bowel disease on pregnancy: a case-controlled retrospective analysis. Br J Obstet Gynaecol 1986;93:1124–1131.
203. Brandt LJ, Estabrook SG, Reinus JF. Results of a survey to evaluate whether vaginal delivery and episiotomy lead to perirectal involvement in women with Crohn's disease. Am J Gastroenterol 1995;90: 1918–1922.
204. Schade RR, van Thiel DH, Gavaler JS. Chronic idiopathic ulcerative colitis. Pregnancy and fetal outcome. Dig Dis Sci 1984;29:614–619.
205. Baird DD, Naraendranahtan M, Sandler RS. Increased risk of preterm birth for women with inflammatory bowel disease. Gastroenterology 1990;99:987–994.
206. Khosla R, Willoughby CP, Jewell DP. Crohn's disease and pregnancy. Gut 1984;25:52–56.
207. Martinbeau PW, Welch FS, Weiland LH. Crohn's disease and pregnancy. Am J Obstet Gynecol 1975;122:746–749.
208. Mogadam M, Dobbins WO, Korelitz BI, Ahmed SW. Pregnancy in inflammatory bowel disease: effect of sulfasalazine and corticosteroids on fetal outcome. Gastroenterology 1981;80:72–76.
209. Schonfield PF, Turnbull RB, Hawk WA. Crohn's disease and pregnancy. Br Med J 1970;1:364.

210. Weinstein GD. Methotrexate. Ann Intern Med 1977;86:199–204.
211. Levy N, Roisman I, Teodor I. Ulcerative colitis in pregnancy in Israel. Dis Colon Rectum 1981;24:351–354.
212. Abramson D, Jankelson IR, Milner FR. Pregnancy in idiopathic ulcerative colitis. Am J Obstet Gynecol 1951;61:121.
213. Crohn BB, Yarnis H, Crohn EB, Walter RI, et al. Ulcerative colitis and pregnancy. Gastroenterology 1956;30:391.
214. Crohn BB, Yarnis H, Korelitz BI. Regional ileitis complicating pregnancy. Gastroenterology 1956;31:615.
215. Burke CW, Roulet F. Increased exposure of tissues to cortisol in late pregnancy. Br Med J 1970;1:657–659.
216. Jarnerot G. Fertility, sterility, and pregnancy in chronic inflammatory bowel disease. Scan J Gastroenterol 1982;17:1–4.
217. Jolivet A, Blanchier H, Gautray JP, Dhem N. Blood cortisol variations during late pregnancy and labor. Am J Obstet Gynecol 1974;119: 775–783.
218. Peppercorn MA. Advances in drug therapy for inflammatory bowel disease. Ann Intern Med 1990;112:50–60.
219. Khan AK, Truelove SC. Placental and mammary transfer of sulfasalazine. Br Med J 1979;2:1553.
220. Klotz U. Clinical pharmokinetics of suphasalazine, its metabolites and other prodrugs of 5-aminosalicylic acid. Clin Pharmacokinet 1985; 10:285–302.
221. Jarnerot G, Into-Malmberg MB. Sulphasalazine treatment during breast feeding. Scand J Gastroenterol 1979;14:869–871.
222. Franklin JL, Rosenberg HH. Impaired folic acid absorption in inflammatory bowel disease: effects of salicylazasulfapyridine (Azulfidine). Gastroenterology 1973:64:517–525.
223. Bell CM, Habal FM. Safety of topical 5-aminosalicylic acid in pregnancy. Am J Gastroenterol 1997;92:2201–2202.
224. Bell CM, Habal FM. Safety of topical 5-aminosalicylic acid in pregnancy. Am J Gastroenterol 1997;92:2201–2202.
225. Habal FM, Hui G, Greenberg GR. Oral 5-aminosalicylic acid for inflammatory bowel disease in pregnancy: safety and clinical course. Gastroenterology 1993;105:1057–1060.
226. Traillori G, d'Albasio G, Bardazzi G, et al. 5-aminosalicylic acid in pregnancy: clinical report. Ital J Gastroenterol 1994;26:75–78.
227. Colombel JF, Brabant G, Gubler MC, et al. Renal insufficiency in infant: side-effect of prenatal exposure to mesalazine? Lancet 1994;344:620–621.
228. Landers DV, Green JR, Sweet RL. Antibiotic use during pregnancy and the postpartum period. Clin Obstet Gynecol 1983;26:391–406.
229. Bomford JAL, Ledjer JC, O'Keefe BJ. Ciprofloxacin used during pregnancy. Drugs 1993;45:461–462(Suppl. 3).
230. Rustia M, Shubid K. Induction of lung tumors and malignant lymphomas in mice by metronidazole. J Natl Cancer Inst 1972;48:721–729.
231. Morgan IFK. Metronidazole treatment in pregnancy. Int J Gynaecol Obstet 1978;15:501–502.
232. Roe FJ. Safety of nitroimidazoles. Scand J Infect Dis Suppl 1985;46: 72–81.
233. Roe FJ. Toxicologic evaluation of metronidazole with particular reference to carcinogenic, mutagenic and teratogenic potential. Surgery 1983;93:158–164.
234. Rosa FW, Baum C, Shaw M. Pregnancy outcomes after first-trimester vaginitis drug therapy. Obstet Gynecol 1987;69:751–755.
235. Bongiovanni AM, McPadden AJ. Steroids during pregnancy and possible fetal consequences. Fertil Steril 1960;11:181.
236. Reinisch JM, Simon NG, Karow WG, Gandelman R. Prenatal exposure to prednisone in humans and animals retards intrauterine growth. Science 1978;202:436–438.
237. Warrell DW, Taylor R. Outcome for the foetus of mothers receiving prednisolone during pregnancy. Lancet 1968;1:117–118.
238. Golbus MS. Teratology for the obstetrician: current status. Obstet Gynecol 1980;55:269–277.
239. McKenzie SA, Selley JA, Agnew JE. Secretion of prednisolone into breast milk. Arch Dis Child 1975;50:894–896.
240. Korelitz BI. Inflammatory bowel disease and pregnancy. Gastroenterol Clinic North Am 1998;27:213–224.
241. Davison JM, Lindheimer MD. Pregnancy in renal transplant recipients. J Reprod Med 1982;27:613–621.
242. Symington GR, Mackay IR, Lambert RP. Cancer and teratogenesis: infrequent occurrence after medical use of immunosuppressive drugs. Aust N Z J Med 1977;7:368–372.
243. Sharon E, Jones J, Diamond H, Kaplan D. Pregnancy and azathioprine in systemic lupus erythematosus. Am J Obstet Gynecol 1974;118: 25–28.
244. Cederqvist LL, Merkatz IR, Litwin SD. Fetal immunoglobulin synthesis following maternal immunosuppression. Am J Obstet Gynecol 1977;129:687–690.
245. Alstead EM, Ritchie JR, Lennard-Jones JE, Farthing MJ, Clark ML. Safety of azathioprine in pregnancy in inflammatory bowel disease. Gastroenterology 1990;99:443–446.
246. Francella A, Dayan A, Rubin PH, et al. 6-Mercaptopurine (6-MP) is safe therapy for child bearing patients with inflammatory bowel disease (IBD): a case controlled study (abst). Gastroenterology 1996; 110:909.
247. Saarikoski S, Seppala M. Immunosuppression during pregnancy: transmission of azathioprine and its metabolites from the mother to the fetus. Am J Obstet Gynecol 1973;115:1100–1106.
248. Cote CJ, Meuwissen HJ, Pickering RJ. Effects on the neonate of prednisone and azathioprine administered to the mother during pregnancy. J Pediatr 1974;85:324– 328.
249. de Witte DB, Buick MK, Cyran SE, Maisels MJ. Neonatal pancytopenia and severe combined immunodeficiency associated with antenatal administration of azathioprine and prednisone. J Pediatr 1984;105: 625–628.
250. Price HV, Salaman JR, Lawrence KM, Langmaid H. Immunosuppressive drugs and the foetus. Transplantation 1976;21:294–298.
251. Scott JR. Fetal growth retardation associated with maternal administration of immunosuppressive drugs. Am J Obstet Gynecol 1977;128: 668–676.
252. Al-Khader AA, Absy M, Al-Hasani MK. Successful pregnancy in renal transplant recipients treated with cyclosporine. Transplantation 1988;45:987–988.
253. Armenti VT, Ahlswede KM, Ahlswede BA, Jarrell BE, Moritz MJ, Burke JF. National transplantation pregnancy registry: outcomes of 154 pregnancies in cyclosporine-treated female kidney transplant recipients. Transplantation 1994;57:502–506.
254. Bertschinger P, Himmelmann A, Risti B, Follath F. Cyclosporine treatment of severe ulcerative colitis during pregnancy. Am J Gastroenterol 1995;90:330.
255. Marion JF, Rubin PH, Lichtiger S, et al. Cyclosporine is safe for severe colitis complicating pregnancy [Abstract]. Am J Gastroenterol 1996;91:1975.
256. Jacobson LB, Clapp DH. Total parenteral nutrition in pregnancy complicated by Crohn's disease. J Parenter Enteral Nutr 1987;11:93–96.
257. Nugent FW, Rajala M, O'Shea RA, et al. Total parenteral nutrition in pregnancy: conception to delivery. J Parenter Enteral Nutr 1987;11: 424–427.
258. Boulton R, Hamilton M, Lewis A, Walker P, Painder R. Fulminant ulcerative colitis in pregnancy. Am J Gastroenterol 1994;89: 931–933.
259. Cooksey G, Gunn A,Wotherspoon WC. Surgery for acute ulcerative colitis and toxic megacolon during pregnancy. Br J Surg 1985;72:547.
260. Holzbach RT. Toxic megacolon in pregnancy. Am J Dig Dis 1969;14:908–910.
261. Green LK, Harris RE, Massey FM. Cancer of the colon during pregnancy. A review of the literature and report of a case associated with ulcerative colitis. Obstet Gynecol 1975;46:480–483.
262. Bohe MG, Ekelund E, Genell SN, et al. Surgery for fulminating colitis during pregnancy. Dis Colon Rectum 1983;26:119–122.
263. Anderson JB, Turner GM, Williamson RCN. Fulminant ulcerative colitis in late pregnancy and the puerperium. J R Soc Med 1987;80: 492–494.
264. Watson WJ, Gaines TE. Third-trimester colectomy for severe ulcerative colitis. J Reprod Med 1987;32:869–872.
265. Hill J, Clark A, Scott NA. Surgical treatment of acute manifestations of Crohn's disease during pregnancy. J R Soc Med 1997;90:64–66.
266. Priest FO, Gilchrist RV, Long JS. Pregnancy in the patient with ileostomy and colectomy. JAMA 1959;169:213.
267. Barwin BN, Harley JMG, Wilson W. Ileostomy and pregnancy. Br J Clin Pract 1974;28:256–258.
268. Scudmore HH, Rogers AC, Bargen JA, et al. Pregnancy after ileostomy for chronic ulcerative colitis. Gastroenterology 1957;32: 295.
269. Nelson H, Dozois RR, Kelly KA, Malkasian GD, Wolff BG, Ilstrup DM. The effect of pregnancy and delivery on the ileal pouch-anal anastomosis functions. Dis Colon Rectum 1989;32:384–288.

270. Juhasz ES, Fozard B, Dozois RR, Ilstrup DM, Nelson H. Ileal pouch-anal anstomosis function following childbirth. An extended evaluation. Dis Colon Rectum 1995;38:159–165.
271. Pezim ME. Successful childbirth after restorative proctocolectomy with pelvic ileal reservoir. Br J Surg 1984;71;292.
272. Metcalf AM, Dozois RR, Kelly KA. Sexual function in women after proctocolectomy. Ann Surg 1986;204:624–627.
273. Corlett RC, Mishell DR. Pancreatitis in pregnancy. Am J Obstet Gynecol 1972;113:281–290.
274. Joupilla P, Mokka R, Larmi TKI. Acute pancreatitis in pregnancy. Surg Gynecol Obstet 1974;139:879–882.
275. McKay AJ, O'Neill J, Imrie CW. Pancreatitis, pregnancy and gallstones. Br J Obstet Gynaecol 1980;87:47–50.
276. Wilkinson EJ. Acute pancreatitis in pregnancy: a review of 98 cases and a report of 8 new cases. Obstet Gynecol Surv 1973;28:281–303.
277. Montgomery WH, Miller FC. Pancreatitis and pregnancy. Obstet Gynecol 1970;35:658–664.
278. Davidoff F, Tishler S, Rosoff C. Marked hyperlipidemia and pancreatitis associated with oral contraceptive therapy. N Engl J Med 1973; 289:552–555.
279. Scott LD. Gallstone disease and pancreatitis in pregnancy. Gastroenterol Clin North Am 1992;21:803–815.
280. Young KR. Acute pancreatitis in pregnancy: two case reports. Obstet Gynecol 1982;60:653–657.
281. Dreiling DA, Bordalo O, Rosenberg V, Rudick J. Pregnancy and pancreatitis. Am J Gastroenterol 1975;64:23–25.
282. Block P, Kelly TR. Management of gallstone pancreatitis during pregnancy and the postpartum period. Surg Gynecol Obstet 1989;168: 426–428.
283. Minkowitz, S, Soloway HB, Hall JE, et al. Fatal hemorrhagic pancreatitis following chlorothiazide administration in pregnancy. Obstet Gynecol 1964;24:337.
284. Inabnet WB, Baldwin D, Daniel DO, Staren ED. Hyperparathyroidism and pancreatitis during pregnancy. Surgery 1996;119:710–713.
285. Levine G, Tsin D, Risk A. Acute pancreatitis and hyperparathyroidism in pregnancy. Obstet Gynecol 1979;54:246–248.
286. DeChalain TM, Michell WL, Berger GM. Hyperlipidemia, pregnancy and pancreatitis. Surg Gynecol Obstet 1988;167:469–473.
287. Sharp HT. Gastrointestinal surgical conditions during pregnancy. Clin Obstet Gynecol 1994;37:306–315.
288. Epstein FB. Acute abdominal pain in pregnancy. Emerg Med Clin North Am 1994;12:151–165.
289. Ordorica SA, Frieden FJ, Marks F, Hoskins IA, Young BK. Pancreatic enzyme activity in pregnancy. J Reprod Med 1991;36:359–362.
290. Strickland DM, Hauth JC, Widish J, Strickland K, Perez R. Amylase and isoamylase activities in serum of pregnant women. Obstet Gynecol 1984;63:389–391.
291. Walker BE, Diddle AW. Acute pancreatitis in gynecologic and obstetric practice. Am J Obstet Gynecol 1969;105:206–211.
292. Gineston JL, Capron JP, Delcenserie R, Delamarre J, Blot M, Boulanger JC. Prolonged total parenteral nutrition in a pregnant woman with acute pancreatitis. J Clin Gastroenterol 1984;6:249–252.
293. Gouldman JW, Sticca RP, Rippon MB, McAlhany JC. Laparoscopic cholecystectomy in pregnancy. Am Surg 1998;64:93–97.
294. Baillie J, Carins SR, Putnam WS, Cotton PB. Endoscopic management of choledocholithiasis during pregnancy. Surg Gynecol Obstet 1990;171:1–4.
295. Bartell JS, Chowdhury T, Miedema BW. Endoscopic sphincterotomy for the treatment of gallstone pancreatitis during pregnancy. Surg Endosc 1998;12:387–389.
296. Sanderson SL, Iverium PH, Wilson DE. Successful hyperlipemic pregnancy. JAMA 1991;265:1858–1860.
297. Weinberg RB, Sitrin MD, Adkins GM, Lin CC. Treatment of hyperlipidemic pancreatitis in pregnancy with total parenteral nutrition. Gastroenterology 1982;83:1300–1305.
298. Swoboda K, Derfler K, Koppensteiner R, et al. Extracorporeal lipid elimination for treatment of gestational hyperlipidemic pancreatitis. Gastroenterology 1993;104:1527–1531.
299. Strickland N. Acute pancreatitis with pseudocyst formation during pregnancy: report of a case. Obstet Gynecol 1966;27:347.
300. Palmer RL. A psychosomatic study of vomiting of early pregnancy. J Psychosom Res 1973;17:303.

Cherry and Merkatz's Complications of Pregnancy,
Fifth Edition, edited by W. R. Cohen.
Lippincott Williams & Wilkins, Philadelphia © 2000.

CHAPTER 19

Diseases of the Biliary Tract and Liver

David H. Berman and Sonia Friedman

An estimated 10% of the adult population of the Western world has gallstones, resulting in approximately 500,000 cholecystectomies yearly in the United States alone. Cholesterol gallstones account for 75% to 90% of all gallstones (1), and multiple factors are involved in their pathogenesis. There have been numerous reports that cholesterol gallstones are more common in women than in men and that the events that lead to this disparity have their onset during puberty (2). These theories have been confirmed by one prospective study of the prevalence of both symptomatic and asymptomatic stones as determined by ultrasound, in which 14.6% of female subjects had stones compared with 6.7% of male subjects (3). Many of these asymptomatic patients will experience symptoms, at a probable rate of 18% over 20 years (4). There is evidence of an increased incidence of gallstones associated with menarche at a young age, abortions, increased parity, estrogen replacement therapy, and use of oral contraceptives (5) and that pregnancy also increases the risk of gallstones in women (1,6). Although all the mechanisms of action responsible for this increased risk are not known, recent work has given us a better understanding of the problem.

PATHOGENESIS OF GALLSTONE FORMATION

The main types of stones found in the gallbladder are cholesterol stones, pigment stones, and mixed cholesterol and pigment stones, which are probably a variant of cholesterol stones, since they contain more than 50% cholesterol. Pigment stones are insoluble in water and are the consequence of the metabolism of hemoglobin; they contain little cholesterol and are mostly made up of calcium bilirubinate. Pigment stones are associated with hemolytic disease, biliary tract infection, and alcoholic liver disease, although most patients with these stones lack a specific predisposing factor. Bacteria are found at the center of most pigment stones but rarely in cholesterol stones (7). In this chapter, we do not discuss the pigment stone, which was capably reviewed by Soloway et al. (8).

Cholesterol gallstones form when cholesterol precipitates in bile. One of the three major classes of lipids, cholesterol is insoluble in water. It is held in aqueous solution in bile by mixing with bile acids and phospholipids to form complex aggregates known as micelles. These aggregated complexes have their lipophilic portions in the center and their hydrophobic portions peripherally placed, which allows them to be soluble in bile. Bile salt micelles alone are not effective in solubilizing bile, and the incorporation of phospholipid into the hydrophobic core of the micelle is required to enhance the capacity to solubilize cholesterol. The principal type of phospholipid in human bile is lecithin, and the three major species of bile acids present in humans are cholic acid, chenodeoxycholic acid, and deoxycholic acid. Human bile has approximately one lecithin molecule for every four bile acid molecules. Cholesterol is also held in suspension in the form of cholesterol–lecithin vesicles. These mixed lipid vesicles are unstable, and fusion of them is the initial step resulting in cholesterol crystallization (9–11).

Admirand and Small found that the solubility of cholesterol was dependent on the relative molar concentrations of cholesterol, bile acids, and phospholipids (12). The authors graphically plotted the concentrations of bile in these three lipids and found that cholesterol will precipitate if the concentration of bile acids or phospholipids falls below a critical level. Patients with cholesterol gallstones appear to secrete supersaturated bile (13,14).

The formation of supersaturated bile can result from several possible factors: a high rate of cholesterol secretion, a reduced rate of bile acid secretion, a decreased bile acid pool, decreased secretion of phospholipids, or an altered water content of bile. It has been shown that with the same lipid composition, dilute bile is less capable of

D.H. Berman and S. Friedman: Mount Sinai Medical Center, New York, NY 10029.

solubilizing cholesterol than concentrated bile, and this might be a factor leading to stone formation (9).

Prolonged stasis of bile from hypomotility of the gallbladder is another important factor in the pathogenesis of gallstone formation. Van der Linden assessed gallbladder function with oral cholecystography in 21 subjects without gallstones and found weakly contracting gallbladders in 12 subjects. After 14 years it was found that gallstones developed in seven of twelve subjects with weakly contracting gallbladders, but in only one of the subjects with a strongly contracting gallbladder (11). Patients with diabetes mellitus, truncal vagotomy, or spinal cord injuries and those on total parenteral nutrition (TPN) are most affected by gallbladder hypomotility and prone to gallstone formation (15).

More complex physical–chemical changes are being investigated, to clarify the mechanisms of action promoting gallstone formation. These events include more rapid nucleation of cholesterol crystals in lithogenic bile and an interaction between mucin and cholesterol–phospholipid vesicles and proteins that both promote and inhibit nucleation. Mucosal inflammation of the gallbladder, which is common in cholesterol gallstone disease, might be important in producing gallbladder-derived pronucleating agents (16). Increased biliary group II phospholipase A_2, an inflammatory mediator, can potentiate this inflammation and favor cholesterol crystal formation (17).

RISK FACTORS IN GALLSTONE FORMATION

Obesity

A high rate of cholesterol secretion is seen with obesity (18,19). Numerous epidemiologic studies have confirmed that obese patients have gallstones more frequently (6,20–22) and that increased body mass index is one of the principal risk factors for gallstones; this relationship is usually stronger in women than in men. In addition to the effect of obesity itself, the pattern of body fat distribution has emerged as an independent risk factor for clinical gallbladder disease (23). The waist-to-hip ratio was directly associated with gallbladder disease risk even after controlling for relative weight (1). It is agreed that obese people secrete more cholesterol into their bile than people of normal weight, a finding possibly related to increased total body cholesterol synthesis. Other observations concerning mechanisms of action in obese patients include abnormal nucleating factors and gallbladder emptying (24,25).

Diet

A high-calorie diet can also promote gallstone formation as the result of increased secretion of biliary cholesterol mediated via an increase in the rate-limiting enzyme in cholesterol synthesis (hydroxymethyl-glutaryl coenzyme A reductase) and decreased bile salt and phospholipid secretion (26–28). This cholestatic state in obesity likely reflects the accumulation of intracellular microvesicular fat and mitochondrial damage (29). Dietary cholesterol and high levels of fat intake are independent risk factors for increasing biliary cholesterol concentrations, and adverse effects on lipid concentrations in plasma and bile tend to be exacerbated by ingestion of diets rich in fat and cholesterol (30). A high-cholesterol diet is also associated with altered small-intestinal smooth-muscle contractility and prolonged small-intestinal transit in addition to diminished gallbladder contractility (31,32). The resulting sluggish enterohepatic cycling of bile acids, associated with an expanded deoxycholate pool, contributes to cholesterol gallstone formation (33).

Serum Lipids

There is an inverse relationship between total serum cholesterol levels and the risk of gallstones, higher levels being associated with a lower risk of gallstone disease. The risk of gallstones increases with decreasing high-density lipoproteins and increasing triglyceride levels (34).

Rapid Weight Loss

Low-calorie diets that are recurrently undertaken by the obese might favor the formation of stones (24). A low-calorie diet will lower the secretion rate of all biliary lipids, and the bile acid pool will decrease. In some patients, the decrease of bile acids is greater proportionately to that of cholesterol, with a subsequent rise in bile saturation. A study of the effect of dieting in 51 obese people showed the presence of sludge in three and gallstones in 13 (26%) after eight weeks (35). Disappearance of gallstones due to dissolution or evacuation was noted in some patients after they resumed a normal diet. Other reports have indicated that ursodeoxycholic acid and aspirin prevented lithogenic bile and the formation of gallstones in obese dieting patients (23).

Gallbladder stasis may also play a role in the development of stones in the context of weight-reduction diets. In obese subjects randomized to a 520-kcal diet with less than 2 g fat/day or a 900-kcal diet with 30 g fat/day (including one 10-g fat meal to stimulate maximal gallbladder emptying), gallstones developed in four of six patients in the first group and no patients in the second group (36). Gallstones also develop in 23% to 35% of patients receiving TPN, most likely owing to reduced gallbladder contractions and subsequent development of sludge and stones (37,38).

Ileal Disease or Bypass

Bile salts are synthesized from cholesterol in the liver and excreted into the bile. They are stored in the gallbladder and, in response to a meal, empty into the intestine, where they are involved in fat absorption. Bile salts are actively reabsorbed into the terminal ileum, about 98% returning via the portal vein to the liver for resumption of the cycle. The rate of synthesis of bile salts is governed by a feedback mechanism to replenish losses in the stool. Alteration of this cycle can result in increased saturation of bile. For example, excess loss of bile acids can occur in malabsorption states, with subsequent inability of the liver to synthesize adequate new bile acids to compensate for these losses. There is thus a relative deficiency of bile acids (39). Regional enteritis or ileal resection or bypass are examples of conditions associated with an increased prevalence of gallstones, presumably as the result of this mechanism of action (40,41). Gallstones develop in approximately 30% of patients with Crohn's disease who have had the ileum resected. Ileal bypass procedures for obesity increase the incidence of gallstones by tenfold within a few years of surgery compared with obese controls. A large body of information suggests that alterations in the enterohepatic cycle play an important role in stone formation. Alteration of rates of gallbladder emptying and intestinal transit time may enhance stone formation (42)—this is discussed later with regard to pregnant women.

Other Risk Factors

Iron deficiency can enhance cholesterol gallstone formation by altering hepatic enzyme metabolism to increase gallbladder bile cholesterol and promote crystal formation (43). This deficiency may have a role in gallstone formation in multiparous women, who are frequently iron deficient. Physical activity may play an important part in the prevention of symptomatic gallstone disease even beyond its control of body weight. The results of one study indicate that 34% of cases of symptomatic gallstone disease in men could be prevented by increasing exercise to 30 minutes of endurance training five times per week (44).

Diabetes mellitus might be a significant risk factor for gallstone disease (45,46). One study using ultrasonography shows almost twice the prevalence of gallstones in diabetic men and more than three times in diabetic women than in patients without diabetes (47). There are several possible reasons for the greater risk of cholelithiasis among diabetics. Bile from diabetic subjects is frequently supersaturated with cholesterol, gallbladder motility might be impaired, and the hyperinsulinemia associated with diabetes has been linked to gallstone risk (1).

Clofibrate, used to lower serum cholesterol, is associated with a high incidence of gallstones, possibly by increasing biliary cholesterol secretion or by decreasing bile acid synthesis (48,49). Genetic factors might play a role in the formation of gallstones (50). A history of gallstones in first-degree relatives confers a doubled risk of cholelithiasis (1). Pima Indians in the southwestern United States have an unusually high rate of formation of cholesterol stones owing not only to increased secretion of excessive cholesterol but also to decreased secretion of bile acids (51). A higher incidence of stones has been noted in certain northern European countries and other racial groups and also in family aggregations (43,52). This genetic predisposition appears to be related to a secretion of a more highly saturated bile.

Aging alone is a risk factor for gallstone formation, the incidence of which increases with each successive decade. It is probably related to increased cholesterol secretion into bile. Stones are uncommon before age 20, and 40 is a typical age at diagnosis (53).

SPECIAL RISK FACTORS IN WOMEN

As noted in the introduction, there is a higher incidence of gallstones in women compared with men (6,20,54). The onset of this difference in puberty and its decline after menopause suggest that it is mediated by differences in estrogen or progesterone levels, or both (6,55). Many studies have likewise confirmed that oral contraceptives are associated with an increased incidence of gallbladder disease (5). Using a duodenal tube, Bennion et al. (56) found that after an overnight fast, bile is significantly more saturated with cholesterol in women using oral contraceptives than in women not using oral contraceptives. A decrease in the proportion of chenodeoxycholic acid in the bile acid pool in oral contraceptive users has also been documented (57,58). Because chenodeoxycholic acid feedings are used to dissolve gallstones, this decrease could increase biliary cholesterol secretion (59).

A study by Wingrave and Kay (60) showed that the risk of development of stones associated with the use of contraceptives is short term and that their use possibly accelerates gallbladder disease in those women who are already susceptible. This report suggests that the long-term risk is not greatly increased. A study by Scragg et al. (61) suggested that using oral contraceptives raises the risk of gallstone formation among many young subjects but that there is a lowered risk in older women. The authors suggested that there is a subpopulation of women who have a metabolic susceptibility to the formation of gallstones and in whom stones develop soon after exposure to contraceptives. This would explain why earlier studies showed an increased risk of stones soon after starting oral contraceptives that could not be confirmed in subsequent trials. The risk of gallstones declines with increasing age at the first pregnancy. Scragg and colleagues noted that stones develop in this susceptible subpopulation of women in their first rather than in subsequent pregnancies.

There is also a risk of gallbladder disease in users of exogenous estrogens. The Boston Collaborative Drug

Surveillance Program gathered data on hospitalized women aged 45 to 69 years and found that postmenopausal women undergoing cholecystectomy were 2.5 times more likely than controls to use estrogens (62). The Coronary Drug Project (63) examined the effects of estrogen therapy on the incidence of diagnosed gallstones in a placebo-controlled trial of men who had recently suffered myocardial infarctions. Estrogen-treated men had a higher rate of definite gallbladder disease than controls, although no dose–response effect was observed. Similar findings were reported in men treated with estrogens for prostate cancer. Honore reported a relative risk of 3.7 for symptomatic gallbladder disease in women who used estrogen replacement therapy (64), and Petitti et al. found a relative risk of 2.1 for cholecystectomy among women who used supplemental estrogen (65).

Endogenous hormones probably have a similar effect on bile saturation in women as do oral contraceptives and other exogenous estrogens, by inducing increased cholesterol secretion and a contraction of chenodeoxycholic acid with subsequent supersaturation of bile (66). Estrogens could also affect lower-density lipoproteins, leading to gallbladder disease (62,67). In laboratory animals, estrogenic compounds increase expression of low-density lipoprotein receptors on the hepatocyte membrane; similar effects are seen in male subjects treated with exogenous estrogen. Thus, enhanced clearance of plasma low-density lipoprotein cholesterol might be the source of the increased cholesterol secretion in bile induced by estrogens (68).

It may be the progestin in the oral contraceptives that is responsible for the increased cholesterol saturation of bile. Although it has been incompletely studied, progesterone itself increases cholesterol secretion in bile in rats by inhibiting acyl coenzyme A—cholesterol acyltransferase, the enzyme that esterifies cholesterol. This effect is offset by co-administration of ethinyl estradiol, a known cholesterol acyltransferase stimulator (68).

Progesterone's smooth-muscle-relaxing effects might also play a role in stone formation (69,70). The possible mechanism of action is shown in animal studies that suggest that the gallbladder contains progesterone receptors that regulate gallbladder motility (71). Subsequent research has found that decreased gallbladder emptying correlates with the presence of receptors in the wall of the gallbladder (72). Receptors for cholecystokinin in the muscle of the gallbladder wall also represent an important mechanism in gallbladder function, because fewer receptors are found in gallbladders that contract poorly in response to a standard meal (73).

Once saturated bile has been formed, crystals can develop in one of two ways (74). The first is spontaneous (homogeneous) nucleation; it occurs with marked supersaturation. The bile becomes labile, the rate of aggregation exceeds the rate of disaggregation, and bile precipitates spontaneously and rapidly. The second method requires a nucleating agent, a foreign substance, such as calcium bilirubinate, coalesced mucus, or cells desquamated from the gallbladder. The bile in this solution need not be supersaturated, and the precipitation takes place around this foreign particle.

Gallstones can then grow either by aggregation of many small crystals or by addition of further solute molecules. Impaired evacuation of the gallbladder, as seen in pregnancy, might contribute to the subsequent growth of stones. Mucin may play a role, because a mucin glycoprotein gel accumulates on the mucosa of the gallbladder and crystal nucleation and growth likely develop in this gel layer. This accumulation of gel with entrapped cholesterol monohydrate crystals forms biliary "sludge" (75). The significance of sludge in pregnancy is discussed later herein.

EFFECTS OF PREGNANCY ON GALLBLADDER FUNCTION

There is an epidemiologic link between pregnancy and cholesterol gallstone disease, but more research needs to be done to quantify this risk. Alterations of biliary physiology in pregnancy are manifest in both gallbladder function and biliary lipid composition. Until recent years, there had been few studies on bile and pregnancy. In 1935, Riegel et al. found evidence of impaired bile fluid absorption in women at term (76). Radiographic studies at that time suggested impaired emptying of the gallbladder in pregnancy. Studies obviously have been limited because of the reluctance to expose pregnant women to radiation. In a descriptive analysis of his experience as an obstetrician, Potter reported in 1936 that in 75% of women undergoing cesarean section at term, palpation of the gallbladder revealed it to be large, atonic, and often distended, in contrast to what normally would be expected (1). In a more quantitative study published 2 years later, Gerdes and Boyden viewed the gallbladder on radiography by using intravenous contrast (77). By analyzing sequential films taken after a fatty meal, changes in gallbladder volume were estimated. In third-trimester pregnancies, the volume was 48% of baseline at 40 minutes, but in nonpregnant and postpartum controls, the volume was 27% of baseline; a comparison of these results showed a significant increase in residual volume in the pregnant group (77).

Braverman et al. (78) used real-time ultrasonography to evaluate gallbladder kinetics in pregnant women and contrasted these results with those of normal controls and women using contraceptive steroids. Their results showed that in women using contraceptive steroids, measurements of gallbladder function were similar to those seen in controls, so that fasting gallbladder volumes were in the normal range (4–24 mL). Residual volumes after a standard meal were also in the normal range (1.5–9 mL), and the rate of gallbladder emptying was unchanged. By contrast, in women pregnant for 14 or more weeks, all measurements of gallbladder function were altered. Fasting volume (range, 15–30 mL) and residual volume were higher (range, 2.5–16 mL), and the rate of emptying was markedly lower. Pregnancies of less than 14 weeks showed normal fasting and residual volumes, but the rate of emptying was somewhat slower compared with controls (although much less slow than that seen in later pregnancy).

In laboratory studies, the gallbladder of the pregnant guinea pig is also abnormal: the contractile responsiveness of gallbladder smooth muscle to both acetylcholine and cholecystokinin (CCK) octapeptide has been found to be significantly impaired. Thus, pregnancy appears to create an environment in which gallbladder motility is inhibited. The result is bile stasis, currently thought to be an important pathogenetic factor in gallstone formation (79).

Progesterone, which circulates in high concentrations during pregnancy, likely plays a role in altering gallbladder motility. A generalized inhibitor of smooth-muscle function, progesterone has been shown to impair the uterine motility response to oxytocin and blunt the lower esophageal sphincter response to gastrin, with subsequent heartburn (most marked in the last trimester) (80). Gallbladder emptying normally takes place after ingesting a meal, with subsequent CCK release (81). Progesterone might lessen the responsiveness of the gallbladder to CCK in humans by inhibiting CCK-mediated smooth-muscle contraction, as has been shown in guinea pigs (70). In addition, progesterone receptors with high specific binding have been identified in the gallbladder and have been hypothesized to be a regulatory variable in gallbladder contractility (79,82).

Another mechanism of action that might explain the higher fasting gallbladder volume is diminished absorption of water from the gallbladder mucosa. This may be related to high concentrations of estrogens, which have been shown to decrease the activity of the sodium pump in gallbladder epithelium (78). Sludge, a collection of cholesterol crystals, mucus, and calcium bilirubinate, is easily recognized on sonography. In an attempt to define the significance of sludge, Lee et al. (83) prospectively followed patients with gallbladder sludge using ultrasonography and found that sludge disappeared in 18% and did not recur quickly, whereas in 60% it disappeared and returned quickly. Asymptomatic gallstones developed in 8% of the patients, symptomatic gallstones in 6%, and biliary-type pain in 7%. These researchers concluded that in some patients sludge is a precursor form of gallstone disease.

In a series of studies, Maringhini et al. showed that both sludge and gallstones can form very rapidly during pregnancy (84–86). In a cohort of 272 pregnant women recruited during the first trimester and followed by ultrasonography, 67 (24%) were newly diagnosed with biliary sludge and 6 (2%) with gallstones. After delivery, 92 women had sludge, and 23 had stones. Sludge disappeared in 61% of these women after a mean follow-up of 5 months, and stones disappeared in 28% of women after 9.7 months of follow-up. During pregnancy, 28% of women experienced biliary pain, which was associated only with the presence of stones. Thus, sludge was common, generally asymptomatic, and disappeared spontaneously after delivery, whereas gallstones were much less common but more likely to be associated with biliary pain.

EFFECTS OF PREGNANCY ON BILIARY LIPID SECRETION AND COMPOSITION

Intricate studies measuring biliary lipid secretion and composition have provided further evidence for the method of formation of gallstones during pregnancy. Kern and colleagues (87) measured duodenal fluid after fasting and gallbladder stimulation in nonobese, healthy, pregnant and nonpregnant women and evaluated biliary lipid composition and secretion, bile acid composition and kinetics, and gallbladder storage and emptying. They found that the stage of ovulation had no apparent effect on any of these parameters. Other comparable studies in humans, although they have generated conflicting results, tend to confirm these findings (56,88,89).

In further experiments of biliary composition in pregnant women (87), bile was found to be more saturated with cholesterol in the second and third trimesters. Although cholesterol crystals were not found in any patient, this supersaturation suggests that pregnancy increases the risk of formation of gallstones. The mean rate of secretion of biliary lipids was not affected by pregnancy, but there was a higher rate of cholesterol secretion relative to the rate of bile acid and phospholipid secretion in the last two trimesters. This is again suggestive of the secretion of a more lithogenic bile. The increased total bile acid pool size became evident early in the first trimester. There was also a decline in the percentage of chenodeoxycholic acid with an increase in the percentage of cholic acid. Subsequently, chenodeoxycholic acid and deoxycholic acid levels both dropped, in contrast to a rise in the cholic acid synthesis rate. These findings are similar to those changes seen with the use of contraceptive steroids, suggesting that both exogenous and endogenous female sex hormones are associated with a relative increase in cholic acid and a decrease in chenodeoxycholic acid.

There is evidence that the individual primary bile acids have different effects on the coupling of cholesterol and phospholipid to bile acids, and these changes in bile acids could be a factor in making the bile more lithogenic. Kern et al. suggested that the following mechanisms of action are at work in pregnancy: an early increase in serum progesterone, with incomplete and delayed gallbladder emptying as well as slowing of transit time through the small intestine, and a subsequent decrease in bile acid return to the liver, stimulating synthesis of bile acids (enhanced by estrogen-induced liver responsiveness) with an expanded bile acid pool (87). Chenodeoxycholic acid synthesis declines relative to cholic acid, which affects coupling of bile acid to cholesterol and phospholipids. Biliary cholesterol saturation increases with subsequent nucleation and precipitation of cholesterol crystals. Incomplete gallbladder emptying and a high residual volume then enhance sludge or stone formation.

CLINICAL PROBLEMS OF BILIARY TRACT DISEASE IN PREGNANCY

Cholecystitis in Pregnancy

Despite the previously noted evidence that pregnancy predisposes to gallstones, acute cholecystitis infrequently coincides with pregnancy (90,91). The incidence is lower than that of acute appendicitis, and reported figures range from 0.02% to 0.16% (46,92–94). Two-thirds of the patients are multiparous, and more than one-third have a history of gallbladder disease before pregnancy. This does not exceed the rate for nonpregnant women in the same age group; in fact, parity and age do not affect the occurrence of symptoms. The clinical picture is no different from that seen in nonpregnant women. Pain usually manifests in the right-upper quadrant or epigastrium, reaching a peak between 12 and 24 hours. There might be radiation toward the back, and chills and fever are not uncommon.

On physical examination, there might be epigastric or right-upper-quadrant tenderness and a nonpalpable gallbladder, unless obstruction is present. Right-sided tenderness at the tip of the ninth costal cartilage as the patient inspires (Murphy's sign) is much less common in pregnant women—it is seen only 5% of the time (95,96). Involuntary guarding, rebound tenderness, and rigidity suggest the presence of a perforated duodenal ulcer or gallbladder or pancreatitis. In more severe cases, gallbladder empyema can result; a mass might be palpable, or jaundice might be evident. During pregnancy, jaundice due to cholecystitis or choledocholithiasis occurs only 5% of the time (97).

With regard to the differential diagnosis, in more than 50% of patients with stones, a history of fatty food intolerance can be pinpointed. In the pregnant patient, the differential diagnosis is unique and includes acute viral hepatitis, acute alcoholic hepatitis, peptic ulcer disease, acute pancreatitis, right-lower-lobe pneumonia, acute myocardial infarction, pyelonephritis, early herpes zoster, acute fatty liver of pregnancy, preeclampsia, HELLP syndrome (hemolysis, elevated liver injury tests, and a low platelet count), and acute appendicitis. Appendicitis must be considered, because in later pregnancy the appendix might be pushed up into the right-upper quadrant. Appendicitis is four to five times more common than cholecystitis in pregnancy (98). After acute appendicitis, diseases of the biliary tract are the next most common surgical conditions complicating pregnancy (99).

Several other rare causes of cholecystitis or cholelithiasis during pregnancy include hemoglobin SC disease and *Salmonella typhi* infection (100,101). A diagnosis of cholelithiasis should be entertained in the patient with the HELLP syndrome if gallstones are identified during the evaluation (102). Diagnostic evaluation should include routine blood tests (complete blood count with differential, amylase, and sequential multiple analysis of chemistries), urinalysis, and abdominal imaging studies. Laboratory testing is seldom diagnostic, and normal changes of pregnancy might confuse the issue. An elevation of alkaline phosphatase is not a reliable sign in pregnant patients because the level normally is elevated during pregnancy owing to placental production of an isoenzyme (103).

Radiographic diagnostic procedures are rarely performed, for fear of harming the fetus, although the risk of fetal abnormalities associated with routine flat plates or operative cholangiograms is probably minimal. Sonography has greatly enhanced our ability to diagnose biliary tract disease safely and accurately in pregnancy (104). Accuracy rates higher than 90%, with rare false positives, have been reported. A mobile echogenic focus in the gallbladder, producing a distal acoustic shadow, is diagnostic of cholelithiasis (105). The accuracy is increased if the acoustic shadow moves with the gallbladder in the decubitus position. Gallbladder wall thickening and pericholecystic fluid would also indicate cholecystitis. Most errors with sonography are those of the false-negative type.

The bulk of the literature before 1987 favored conservative management of cholecystitis in pregnancy and described symptom resolution with nonoperative treatment. A review of patients at the Massachusetts General Hospital found that in 23 cases, symptoms of cholelithiasis remitted without surgery and that all patients went to term uneventfully (106). On the other hand, an 11-year review found that 58% of 54 patients had recurrent episodes of biliary colic and that 27% required two to three hospitalizations (107). There was significant fetal loss, leading to the recommendation of medical treatment in the first and third trimester but elective surgery during the second trimester in patients with biliary colic or cholecystitis. In a study by Swisher et al., the relapse rate of biliary disease in pregnancy after initially successful medical therapy decreased as the pregnancy progressed; it was 92% in the first trimester, 64% in the second, and 44% in the third (108).

Management should initially be conservative and depends on the severity of the process. If there is significant inflammation, hospitalization and intravenous hydration is indicated. A nasogastric tube may be required on occasion, and the patient should receive adequate analgesia (meperidine) to control pain. If the patient has a fever, antibiotics are indicated. The choice of antibiotics is dictated in part by the trimester: chloramphenicol and tetracycline should be avoided during early pregnancy, whereas sulfa drugs should not be used in the later stages of pregnancy. The current consensus is to initiate broad-spectrum coverage with a β-lactam antibiotic. In more than 90% of cases, the acute process will resolve; however, subsequent attacks may necessitate surgery.

TPN has been used in pregnant patients for several conditions, including chronic cholecystitis (109). Advocates report no significant untoward effects of TPN use during pregnancy, and it can provide an alternative to surgery in patients who fail conservative treatment, especially those in the first and third trimesters of pregnancy. The use of the bile acid ursodeoxycholic acid (ursodiol) in the attempt to dissolve cholesterol gallstones should be avoided in pregnant patients. Although it is not known to cause teratogenic or abortifacient effects in humans, there have been no adequate and well-controlled studies of its use in pregnant women (110,111).

Surgical intervention is required in about 30% to 35% of all patients who have cholecystitis during pregnancy. Indications for surgery include repeated attacks of biliary colic, acute cholecystitis, obstructive jaundice, gallstone pancreatitis, peritonitis, or uncertainty in diagnosis (112). In several reviews, surgical intervention is reported as necessary in 1 in 5,000 to 1 in 15,000 pregnancies (113–116). Laparoscopic cholecystectomy can be performed safely and is probably the procedure of choice for cholecystitis in pregnancy. It should be undertaken in the second trimester because organogenesis is complete, uterine size is not large enough to interfere with trochar placement, and the risk of spontaneous abortion is low.

Low-pressure carbon dioxide pneumoperitoneum and reverse Trendelenberg, in the left-side-down position should be used. Perioperative monitoring of the fetal heart rate and uterine contractions should be available. Some investigators have advocated the use of indomethacin as a prophylactic tocolytic. Positioning of the ports is no different from that in nonpregnant patients. No significant increase in abnormal fetal heart rate patterns was seen in response to positioning on the operating table, induction of anesthetic, insufflation of pneumoperitoneum, or sustained pneumoperitoneum for the duration of the surgery or during recovery (114). Most surgeons perform cholangiography on a selective basis only when there is a suspicion or risk of common duct stones. They place a lead shield over the lower abdomen to protect the fetus from radiation exposure (114,115).

Several studies have documented the successful use of laparoscopic cholecystectomy in pregnancy. Lanzafame reviewed 20 reports of such treatment and another three reports of 14 patients who underwent laparoscopic cholecystectomy during pregnancy without any fetal or maternal morbidity (117). Glasgow et al. reported the cases of 14 patients who underwent laparoscopic cholecystectomy, also without any fetal or maternal complication or morbidity (114). Usually, it is the severity of the surgical disease itself and not the surgery per se that appears to be the more important factor in determining prematurity, spontaneous abortion, perinatal mortality, and maternal morbidity and mortality.

Open cholecystectomy has also been shown to be safe during pregnancy. McKellar et al. reported nine open cholecystectomies performed during pregnancy, with no fetal deaths (55). Swisher et al. reviewed 16 open cholecystectomies and found no higher rates of perioperative fetal or maternal morbidity (108). Patients who had surgery spent fewer days in the hospital than patients treated medically. The morbidity is no greater for pregnant patients undergoing uncomplicated cholecystectomy than it is for nonpregnant patients. The increased risk, if any, is due to possible delays in diagnosis and resulting complications, especially pancreatitis. Following uncomplicated cholecystectomy, there is no increase in maternal mortality, and the rate of fetal loss is approximately 5% (118). For cholecystectomy with common bile duct exploration, particularly in patients with pancreatitis, there is a 15% maternal mortality rate and a 60% fetal loss rate. These rates will likely be reduced with the advent of laparoscopic cholecystectomy, endoscopic sphincterotomy, or placement of common bile duct stents in pregnant patients (68). In summary, if it is indicated, cholecystectomy can be performed in the second trimester with only minimal risk to both fetus and mother in a stable pregnancy. Laparoscopic cholecystectomy is safe and effective and is emerging as the procedure of choice.

Endoscopic Management of Choledocholithiasis

Choledocholithiasis develops in one of approximately 1,200 births and can cause acute cholangitis and pancreatitis. The traditional approach is to perform cholecystectomy and common bile duct exploration (119). During the past two decades, the role of endoscopy in treating nonpregnant patients has expanded exponentially. The success rate for endoscopic sphincterotomy and removal of common bile duct stones approaches 90% (120). The complication rate remains constant in most published articles at approximately 6.5% to 10%, with a mortality rate of 1.5%. These are roughly one-third the expected mortality and complication rates for surgical intervention in such patients (121).

Several case reports have described the success of endoscopic retrograde cholangiopancreatography (ERCP) with endoscopic sphincterotomy or stenting of the common bile duct during all trimesters of pregnancy

(122). Nesbitt et al. treated three women with cholelithiasis, acute cholecystitis, or gallstone pancreatitis with sphincterotomy and stone extraction (123). Fluoroscopy was kept to a minimum with a lead shield over the abdomen, and all patients experienced rapid resolution of symptoms and successful pregnancy outcomes. Uomo and associates treated two pregnant patients with acute gallstone pancreatitis and obvious common bile duct stones on ultrasound with sphincterotomy and stone extraction. No fluoroscopy was used, and both women had uneventful pregnancies with cholecystectomies after delivery (124). Baillie et al. successfully treated five pregnant women with choledocholithiasis with endoscopic sphincterotomy (125). A lead shield was placed over the abdomen, and fetal irradiation was monitored with a dosimeter placed over the uterine fundus. No exposure was detected. Elective cholecystectomies were performed after completion of pregnancy.

Farca et al. used biliary stents to promote temporary drainage in 10 pregnant women with choledocholithiasis, acute gallstone pancreatitis, or residual common bile duct stones after emergency cholecystectomy (119). All 10 women had uneventful pregnancies and had definitive endoscopic sphincterotomies after delivery. The authors claim that stent placement is associated with a lower complication rate than sphincterotomy and that radiation exposure is minimized. This has yet to be proved in a prospective clinical trial.

Gallstone Pancreatitis and Pregnancy

Schmidt (126) described the first association of pregnancy and acute pancreatitis in 1919. The first significant review of acute pancreatitis and pregnancy was generated in 1951 by Langmade and Edmondson (127), who defined pancreatitis as arising at any stage of pregnancy and in the first six weeks postpartum. The incidence of pancreatitis ranges from 1 in 2,000 to 1 in 10,000 pregnancies. (128–130). Gallstones play a major role in the development of pancreatitis; they are probably the most common etiologic factor (131). Gallstones can be pinpointed as the source in 25% to 90% of pregnant patients with pancreatitis, compared with 37% of nonpregnant patients (129,131,132).

The clinical picture is not different from that of nongravid patients: nausea, vomiting, mild abdominal distension, diminished bowel sounds, upper-abdominal tenderness that might be poorly localized and radiates to the flanks or shoulders, and minimal temperature elevation with, at times, biliary colic. Symptoms can resemble those of other conditions found in pregnancy, including hyperemesis gravidarum, ectopic pregnancy, salpingitis, and pyelonephritis.

Laboratory studies include complete blood count, sequential multiple analysis of blood chemistries, and determinations of serum amylase and lipase. Serum amylase levels are normal or only slightly raised during normal pregnancy, peaking at 21 to 25 weeks' gestation and then gradually decreasing. Toxemia of pregnancy usually lowers serum amylase levels. A rise in the serum amylase of more than 300 Somogyi units or a urine amylase level of more than 300 U/ml is considered diagnostic of pancreatitis. No correlation between fetal or maternal mortality and amylase levels has ever been established. Other conditions that can elevate serum amylase levels include renal failure, perforated viscus, ruptured ectopic pregnancy, cholecystitis, mumps, or small-bowel obstruction. The use of amylase clearance and creatinine clearance ratios in diagnosing pancreatitis has been explored (133). These ratios must be interpreted carefully because an elevated ratio can be caused not only by pancreatitis but also by severe preeclampsia and severe hyperemesis gravidarum. During pregnancy the creatinine clearance is greater than normal, thus lowering the clearance ratio.

The differential diagnosis from other acute conditions that can require interventional therapy includes mesenteric infarction, acute cholangitis or cholecystitis, and perforated peptic ulceration. The use of diagnostic imaging methods is different in the pregnant patient. In an attempt to avoid radiation, abdominal ultrasonography should be performed; it is 73% accurate in the diagnosis of gallstone pancreatitis (134). Although there are additional biochemical parameters used to entertain the diagnosis of pancreatitis, the clinical picture and a raised serum amylase level are sufficient to confirm the diagnosis (135).

Episodes of gallstone pancreatitis can develop during any trimester of pregnancy, but the incidence is greatest during the third trimester and in the immediate postpartum period (131). A review by Ramin and co-workers of the cases of acute pancreatitis at Parkland Hospital over a 10-year period describes pancreatitis as more common with increasing gestational age (136). Nineteen percent of women were diagnosed in the first trimester, 26% in the second, and 53% after 28 weeks' gestation. Parity does not alter the incidence of the disease. Treatment of these patients does not differ from that of the nonpregnant patient. Conservative treatment includes nasogastric suction if the patient has nausea or vomiting, fluid and electrolyte replacement, analgesia, and monitoring for signs and symptoms of complications related to the disease process.

Complications of pancreatitis include disseminated intravascular coagulation, jaundice, preeclampsia, fetal growth restriction, and premature labor, which occurs in 60% of patients affected in late pregnancy (137). Other complications include sepsis, embolic phenomena, pleural effusion, and electrolyte disturbances. Complications that can lead to surgery are pseudocyst formation (138), biliary obstruction, gastrointestinal hemorrhage, and splenic rupture. The majority of patients will experience spontaneous passage of their gallstones (139).

In patients with gallstone pancreatitis, it is best to wait until the episode of pancreatitis has subsided before proceeding with definitive treatment of the biliary tract (128,131,140). The ultimate mode of therapy depends on the patient's condition and the stage of the patient's pregnancy. Indications for cholecystectomy in pregnant patients should not be significantly different from those of nonpregnant patients; in uncomplicated cases, conservative therapy during the first trimester is best followed by surgical intervention in the second trimester (139). During the second trimester, uncomplicated cases should be operated on during the initial hospital stay, after pancreatitis has subsided. Surgery is safest when performed in the second trimester of pregnancy because organogenesis is complete, premature labor and spontaneous abortion are less likely, and the uterus does not obstruct the operative field (96). Patients in the third trimester should be treated conservatively and should be operated on during the early part of the postpartum period.

Parenteral nutrition has been employed by Stowell et al. (138) in the treatment of pseudocysts complicating pregnancy. These researchers concluded from a review of the literature that TPN is a safe and reliable method for nutritional support of mother and fetus and that this conservative management should be followed because of the technical difficulties of surgical intervention during the third trimester. The role of ERCP and sphincterotomy with stone removal or destruction or of stenting of the common bile duct in gallstone pancreatitis is now expanding in pregnant patients. Successful procedures have been performed with minimal fluoroscopy time and no morbidity in the mother or fetus. Laparoscopic cholecystectomy can then often be delayed until after delivery.

In past studies, maternal mortality rates from pancreatitis have been reported as ranging from 15% to 60%, but recent reviews document lower maternal morbidity rates. Ramin and co-workers reported no maternal deaths among 43 pregnant women with acute pancreatitis (136), Legro and Laifer had no maternal deaths in 11 patients (141), and Swisher and colleagues described no deaths in 30 patients (140). However, most patients had fairly mild courses, and there would likely have been higher mortality rates with severe disease. Treatment should initially be conservative. With the increased understanding of the course of acute pancreatitis in pregnancy and with modern methods of therapy, maternal mortality rates should continue to improve.

In summary, we have presented the evidence for increased pathogenesis of gallstones in pregnancy. Although cholecystitis is not a common clinical problem during pregnancy, newer techniques, such as ERCP with sphincterotomy or stent and/or laparoscopic cholecystectomy, are safe and effective when medical therapy fails. Pancreatitis and its severe complications are becoming amenable to newer forms of therapy as well as surgical or endoscopic intervention when required.

THE LIVER*

Most of the liver's functions are not affected in a clinically significant way by pregnancy. Commonly used measures of hepatocellular function, alanine aminotransferase and aspartate aminotransferase serum levels, remain unchanged, as does that of bilirubin. Serum alkaline phosphatase levels increase during pregnancy, primarily the consequence of a placental heat-stable isoenzyme. Some synthetic functions of the liver are altered during gestation. Serum albumin levels fall, mainly as the result of hemodilution. Ceruloplasmin concentrations are increased twofold, and plasma fibrinogen rises by at least 50%. Serum levels of vitamin K–dependent clotting factors rise, as do those of cholesterol. Neither the gross nor the histologic appearance of the liver changes in normal pregnancy. Pregnant women are susceptible to any hepatic disease or dysfunction that can arise in nonpregnant women. In addition, however, there are several liver disorders that are unique to pregnancy. These include intrahepatic cholestasis of pregnancy (discussed previously in this chapter), acute fatty liver of pregnancy, and preeclamptic liver disease.

Acute Fatty Liver of Pregnancy

Acute fatty liver of pregnancy is a rare disorder that can produce acute hepatic failure and death. It develops in about 1 in 10,000 pregnancies as an acute illness with nausea, vomiting, and abdominal pain. Symptoms usually begin in the 35th week of gestation, but they can occur as early as the 13th week (142,143). It can also develop in the immediate puerperium. Jaundice follows shortly after the onset of symptoms and becomes intense in most patients. The course can be fulminant, with gastrointestinal bleeding, hepatic coma, and renal failure; this makes differentiating it from severe and rapidly progressive hepatitis difficult. Pancreatitis, hypoglycemia, and disseminated intravascular coagulation frequently complicate the clinical course (144). Maternal mortality can reach 75% and fetal loss 85%; however, earlier recognition is associated with an improved prognosis (145). Resolution generally occurs with delivery, and recovery is usually complete.

When hepatic failure occurs, cerebral edema and hepatic encephalopathy ensue. The syndrome develops more frequently in nulliparas and can accompany preeclampsia, sometimes in association with hemolysis and thrombocytopenia. The cause is uncertain, and the rarity of the disease has made study difficult. Recent evidence has emerged that women who have acute fatty liver of pregnancy might be heterozygous for a mutant gene that results in a defect in fatty acid oxidation (146,147). Children with a deficiency of long-chain 3-hydroxyacyl

*Portions of this section were contributed to the fourth edition by Franklin M. Klion, M.D.

coenzyme A dehydrogenase have been born to mothers with acute fatty liver. Whether the fetus or the mother produces abnormal fatty acid metabolites that are toxic to the maternal liver is uncertain, but acute fatty liver of pregnancy is remarkably similar to a group of hepatic microvesicular steatoses (e.g., Reye's syndrome, valproic acid hepatotoxicity, and acyl CoA dehydrogenase deficiency) in which hepatotoxic free fatty acids are produced.

Jaundice that accompanies signs of renal failure should suggest the diagnosis. The white blood cell count is frequently elevated; aspartate aminotransferase and alanine aminotransferase levels are only modestly high early in the disease. Once a coagulopathy develops, prolongation of the prothrombin time and partial thromboplastin time and depression of fibrinogen levels will occur. Neutrophilia, thrombocytopenia, and normoblasts in the periphery are seen (148). Enzyme levels are occasionally quite high; serum bilirubin is increased to varying degrees.

The diagnosis is made on the basis of these clinical and laboratory findings. The disease must be distinguished from acute viral hepatitis and preeclamptic liver disease. Although liver biopsy could be extremely helpful in making the diagnosis, because fat staining can identify microvesicular steatosis, coagulation problems often develop rapidly and preclude the use of biopsy (Fig. 19–1). Computerized tomography or magnetic resonance imaging may show reduced attenuation in the liver (149). On electron microscopy, which can sometimes be necessary to confirm the diagnosis, one sees honeycombing of the smooth endoplasmic reticulum (150).

Many treatments have been attempted, including corticosteroid therapy and hemodialysis; none has been shown to be clearly successful. If the patient survives, the disease usually resolves spontaneously after delivery. Although it has not been proved that prompt delivery will cure the disease, it is generally recommended. Most of the treatment should be aggressively directed to support and maintain blood volume and normal glucose and electrolyte levels and to correct the disseminated intravascular coagulation. With good supportive care and timely delivery, it is likely that many lives can be saved. Under any circumstances, however, this disorder will continue to take a significant maternal and fetal toll.

Preeclamptic Liver Disease

Most patients with preeclampsia have normal liver function test results and no histologic abnormalities, but elevations of transferase activity are present in at least 20% of patients. Jaundice is uncommon, except when it is a consequence of hemolysis and intravascular coagulation (151). Histologic lesions are characterized by sinusoidal fibrin deposition in the periportal areas, with surrounding hemorrhage (152). Inflammation is absent, but centrilobular necrosis can occur, perhaps as a conse-

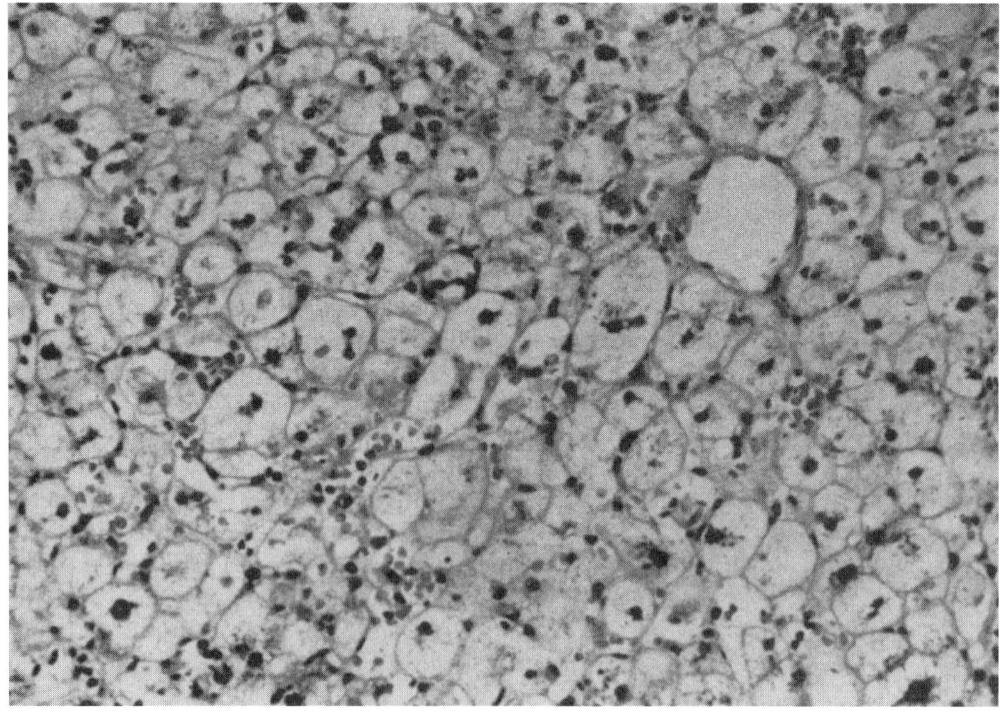

FIG. 19-1. Fatty liver of pregnancy shows enlargement and rarefaction of the cytoplasm of the hepatocyte, stemming from a small droplet of fat. (Courtesy of Dr. S.N. Thung.)

quence of systemic or local reductions in perfusion (Fig. 19–2). Thrombi develop in portal capillaries.

It should not be difficult to distinguish preeclamptic liver disease from other causes of jaundice in pregnancy when preeclamptic liver disease is associated with hypertension, renal dysfunction, and other typical manifestations. On occasion, however, hepatic dysfunction is one of the earliest signs of the preeclamptic process. Sometimes intrahepatic hematomas develop, usually in the context of severe liver necrosis and disseminated intravascular coagulation. Rupture of the liver, which is usually fatal, can occur in this situation (see later discussion). Smaller subcapsular hematomas can also arise and are frequently associated with the HELLP syndrome. This constellation of findings is a manifestation of severe preeclampsia. Advancing liver involvement is often associated with the clinical manifestation of right-upper-quadrant or epigastric pain. If a tender mass is palpated, one should be concerned about the possibility of a large subcapsular hematoma and impending rupture. Computed tomography scan is usually useful in establishing a diagnosis in such circumstances. There is no available specific treatment for the hepatic dysfunction produced by preeclampsia. In general, when the disease is seen in association with significant hepatic dysfunction, delivery should be considered. The early manifestations of preeclamptic liver disease are completely reversible.

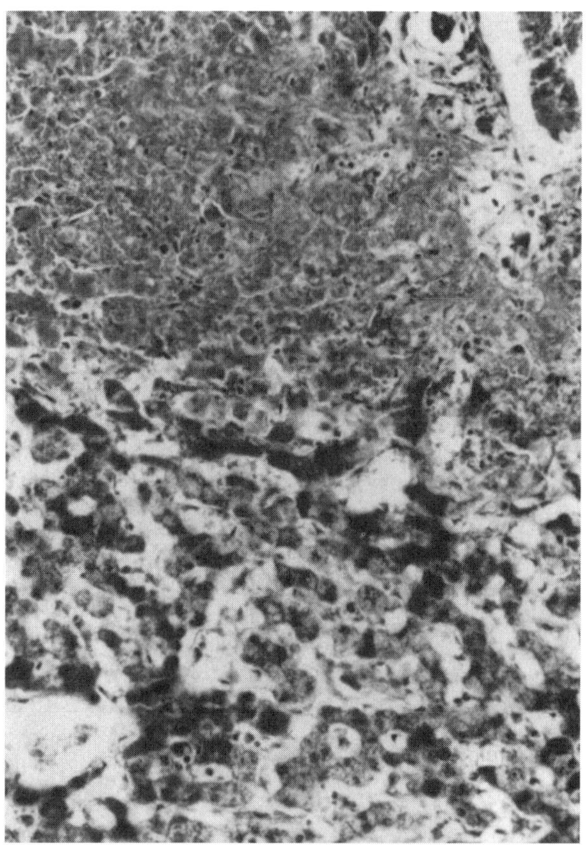

FIG. 19-2. The liver in preeclampsia. There is severe periportal necrosis with fibrin deposits in the sinusoids and minimal portal and parenchymal inflammation. (Courtesy of Dr. M. Gerber.)

Hyperemesis Gravidarum

When hyperemesis occurs in early pregnancy and is associated with prolonged fasting and dehydration, hepatic manifestations can arise. These are generally mild and are sometimes associated with elevations in hepatic enzymes and cholestasis. The pathophysiologic basis for these changes is uncertain. They are reversible once nutrition returns to normal.

Hepatic Rupture

Spontaneous rupture of the liver is an unusual but serious complication of pregnancy and the puerperium. Severe preeclampsia or eclampsia is the major predisposing factor (153). Vascular abnormalities (e.g., arteriovenous malformations, aneurysms, fibromuscular dysplasia) cause a few cases. In most cases the associated preeclampsia is accompanied by significant coagulopathy. Onset can be acute, but antecedent right-upper-quadrant or epigastric pain may be present for some time. Once rupture occurs, hypovolemic shock ensues rapidly. Maternal mortality will exceed 50% unless the diagnosis is made promptly and surgical intervention is undertaken. Ultrasound imaging, as well as computed tomography or magnetic resonance imaging, might help establish a diagnosis. In hemodynamically stable patients, selective angiography and embolization might be helpful.

Liver Disease Independent of Pregnancy

Acute Viral Hepatitis

Acute viral hepatitis is the most common cause of jaundice in pregnancy. Several viruses have been implicated. Hepatitis viruses A, B, C, and D appear to have no adverse effect on pregnancy in well-nourished women who receive good medical care. Hepatitis E, which is rare in industrialized countries, seems to be associated with a high risk of maternal mortality (154). Other viruses (see Chapter 45) also can cause hepatitis in pregnancy, including cytomegalovirus, herpes simplex virus, and Epstein-Barr virus.

The incidence of hepatitis varies around the world. In North America and northern Europe, an incidence as low as 0.03% to 0.1% (143) has been reported, whereas Africa, India, and the Middle East have reported a 3% to 20% or higher rate (155). Studies from Europe and North America have shown no differences in the course of hepatitis in pregnant and nonpregnant women (156,157). Studies from less developed areas of the world have found a higher incidence of fulminant hepatitis and infant mortality (158,159). This variance might reflect different population studies, nutritional status, and prenatal care.

Hepatitis A, an RNA enterovirus, has an incubation time of 15 to 50 days and is transmitted by the fecal–oral route or through contaminated food or water. It occurs sporadically or epidemically. Pregnant women in close contact with excreta of children are at high risk of contracting hepatitis A. About 2 to 6 weeks after exposure, flulike symptoms develop, characterized by weakness, fatigue, fever, anorexia, arthralgias, and headaches, followed by jaundice, dark urine, light stools, and right-upper-quadrant tenderness. It is most contagious during the week before the onset of jaundice. Death occurs in less than 1% of patients with acute hepatitis A. The usual course of the disease is 2 to 3 weeks. There is no chronic form, and recovery confers immunity against reinfection.

Before the onset of symptoms, hepatitis A antigen is present in the stool, but it can be identified only by specialized laboratories. At the onset of symptoms, the liver enzymes alanine aminotransferase and aspartate aminotransferase are elevated, and the IgM antibody is detectable in the serum. This antibody persists for 3 to 6 months and is followed by the appearance of IgG antibodies, which persist for life. Thus, the IgM antibody is a marker of acute disease, and the IgG antibody is a marker of previous exposure.

The disease is self-limited and is treated symptomatically. It is important to carefully isolate infected women to prevent spread. Symptomatic treatment requires prevention of maternal dehydration and maintenance of adequate nutrition. Pregnant women who have been exposed to infection may be given immune globulin (0.02 mg/kg) to protect against infection. Immune globulin therapy is effective only if given within 2 weeks of exposure. Hepatitis A vaccine can be given with immune globulin. The vaccine produces protective levels of antibody in 10 to 14 days.

There is no clear evidence of vertical transmission of acute hepatitis A, and if IgM antibody is present in the mother during the third trimester, prophylactic treatment of the newborn is probably not necessary. However, if hepatitis A antigen is present in the stool at the time of delivery or, alternatively, when the illness has occurred in the last 2 to 3 weeks of pregnancy, newborns should receive immunoglobulin prophylaxis because they can be infected by their mothers. Pregnancy does not confer an increased risk of mortality in women with hepatitis A (160).

Hepatitis B virus (HBV) is a doubled-stranded DNA virus that is the most common cause of acute viral hepatitis in pregnancy. The disease can appear in an acute, a subclinical, or a chronic form. The acute form is similar in clinical symptoms to those of hepatitis A, although extrahepatic symptoms, such as serum sickness (161), nephritis (162), essential mixed cryoglobulinemia (163), and aplastic anemia (164), are more common. HBV is found in whole blood, semen, saliva, breast milk, amniotic fluid, and cord blood. The disease can be transmitted sexually, by intravenous drug use with a contaminated needle, acupuncture, tattooing, and administration of blood products. Most offspring who become infected do so in the neonatal period.

The serologic characteristics of hepatitis B are complex but well understood. Viral surface antigen (HBsAg) is detectable shortly after onset of infection, peaks in the serum early in the illness, and is undetectable in the majority of cases during the few weeks after clinical recovery. If HbsAg persists after 6 months, patients are considered to be chronic carriers of the antigen.

Shortly after surface antigen is detectable, antibodies to the viral core protein emerge (HBcAb) and generally persist for life. Antibodies to surface antigen (HBsAb) are not detectable until several weeks after resolution of HbsAg. The e antigen (HbeAg) appears in the serum shortly after HbsAg and, after about 2 weeks, disappears, with the emergence of its corresponding antibody (HBeAb). This antibody is strongly correlated with DNA polymerase activity in the viral core and indicates a high risk of infectivity. The presence of maternal HbeAb is associated with an approximately 90% risk of perinatal transmission.

The overall risk of neonatal infection is about 75% if maternal infection occurs in the third trimester or the puerperium; it is much less (5%–10%) if maternal disease develops early in pregnancy (160). Most newborn infection probably takes place during labor and delivery or through maternal–newborn contact, rather than transplacentally. Although most babies show signs of mild anicteric infections, they tend to become chronic antigen carriers. These carriers have a considerable lifetime risk of hepatic cirrhosis and carcinoma. Newborns of infected mothers (including chronic HbsAg carriers) should be protected with a combination of passive antibodies (hepatitis B immune globulin) and active immunization with hepatitis B vaccine. Universal screening of pregnant women for HBV is a cost-effective strategy.

Hepatitis C (HCV), previously known as non-A non-B hepatitis, is caused by an RNA flavivirus and is the most common blood-borne infection in the United States. More than 220,000 infections occur worldwide each year. Many patients are chronically infected, the consequence in 70% to 90% of cases. Of these patients, 15% to 20% ultimately develop cirrhosis, which contributes to 40% of deaths from chronic liver disease (165). Most cases result from percutaneous routes of infection, primarily illicit drug use. Donated blood is screened for HCV. Sexual transmission is very uncommon, and the likelihood of vertical transmission from an infected mother is less than 10% (166). The risk of neonatal HCV infection is considerably higher if the mother is infected with the human immunodeficiency virus (HIV) (168). Transmission risks are related to the HCV RNA titer, which tends to be high in HIV-infected individuals. Immune serum globulin provides no postexposure protection.

Time from exposure to illness (which is often mild or even subclinical) is 6 to 9 weeks. Enzyme immunoassay techniques can detect HCV antibodies 3 to 5 months after infection but cannot distinguish among cases of acute, chronic, or resolved infection. HCV RNA analyses by polymerase chain reaction, now in development, should allow detection of virus 1 to 3 weeks after onset of disease. At present, all positive enzyme immunoassay tests should be confirmed by a recombinant immunoblot assay (169). Chronic HCV infection should be treated with parenteral interferon alpha in patients at high risk of cirrhosis, that is, those with persistently elevated serum alanine aminotransferase levels, detectable HCV RNA, or evidence of progression on biopsy. Interferon can be used during pregnancy (FDA category C), but ribavirin, which is sometimes used as an adjunct in the treatment of nonpregnant women, is teratogenic in most species. Children born to HCV-positive women should be tested for infection. Antibody testing should be postponed for 1 year, but RNA analysis can be used to confirm infection sooner, if necessary.

Hepatitis D virus is a parenterally transmitted agent that develops as a co-infection or superinfection with hepatitis B, on which it depends to replicate. Vertical transmission of HDV happens considerably less frequently than vertical transmission of HBV. Co-infection with HBV and HDV often leads to severe hepatitis, and where it is endemic, it is a common cause of hepatic failure.

REFERENCES

1. Diehl AK. Epidemiology and natural history of gallstone disease. Gastroenterol Clin North Am 1991;20:1–17.
2. Bennion LJ, Grundy SM. Risk factors for the development of cholelithiasis in man. N Engl J Med 1978;299:1161–1167.
3. Barbara L, Sama C, Morselli Labate AM, et al. A population study on the prevalence of gallstone disease: the Sirmione study. Hepatology 1987;7:913–917.
4. Ransahoff DF, Gracie WA, Wolfenson LB, Neuhauser D. Prophylactic cholecystectomy or expectant management for silent gallstones: a decision analysis to assess survival. Ann Intern Med 1983;99: 199–204.
5. Boston Collaborative Drug Surveillance Program. Oral contraceptives and venous thromboembolic disease, surgically confirmed gallbladder disease and breast tumors. Lancet 1973;1:1399–1404.
6. Friedman GD, Kannel WB, Dawber TR. The epidemiology of gallbladder disease: observations in the Framingham study. J Chronic Dis 1966;19:273–292.
7. Stewart L, Smith AL, Pellegrini CA, Motson RW, Way LW. Pigment gallstones form as a composite of bacterial microcolonies and pigment solids. Ann Surg 1987;206:242–250.
8. Soloway RD, Trotman BW, Osman JD. Pigment gallstones. Gastroenterology 1977;72:167–182.
9. Cooper AD. Metabolic basis of cholesterol gallstone disease. Gastroenterol Clin North Am 1991;20:21–46.
10. Donovan JM, Carey MC. Physical-chemical basis of gallstone formation. Gastroenterol Clin North Am 1991;20:47–67.
11. Holzbach RT. Newer pathogenetic concepts in cholesterol gallstone formation: a unitary hypothesis. Digestion 1997;58[Suppl 1]:29–32.
12. Admirand WH, Small DM. The physicochemical basis of cholesterol gallstone formation in man. J Clin Invest 1968;47:1043–1051.
13. Small DM, Rapo S. The source of abnormal bile in patients with cholesterol gallstones. N Engl J Med 1970;283:53–57.
14. Vlahcevic ZR, Bell CC Jr, Swell L. Significance of the liver in the production of lithogenic bile in man. Gastroenterology 1970;59: 62–69.
15. Portincasa P, Stolk MFJ, Van Erpectum KJ, Palasciano G, vanBerge-Henegouwen GP. Cholesterol gallstone formation in man and potential treatments of the gallbladder motility defect. Scand J Gastroenterol 1995;30[Suppl 212]:63–78.
16. Afdhal NH, Smith BF. Cholesterol crystal nucleation: a decade long search for the missing link in gallstone pathogenesis [Editorial]. Hepatology 1990;19:699–702.
17. Shoda J, Ueda T, Ikegami T, et al. Increased biliary group II phospholipase A2 and altered gallbladder bile in patients with multiple cholesterol stones. Gastroenterology 1997;112:2036–2047.
18. Bennion LJ, Grundy SM. Effects of obesity and caloric intake on biliary lipid metabolism in man. J Clin Invest 1975;56:996–1011.
19. Mabee TM, Meyer P, Denbesten L, et al. The mechanism of increased gallstone formation in obese human subjects. Surgery 1976;79: 460–468.
20. Gross DMB. A statistical study of cholelithiasis. J Pathol Bacteriol 1929;32:503–526.
21. Kono S, Shinchi K, Todoroki I. Gallstone disease among Japanese men in relation to obesity, glucose intolerance, exercise, alcohol use, and smoking. Scand J Gastroenterol 1995;30:372–376.
22. Van Der Linden W. Some biological traits in female gallstone patients: a study of body build, parity and serum cholesterol levels. Acta Chir Scand 1961;269[Suppl]:1–94.
23. Broomfield PH, Chopra R, Sheinbaum RC, et al. The effects of ursodeoxycholic acid and aspirin on the formation of lithogenic bile and gallstones during loss of weight. N Engl J Med 1988;319: 1567–1572.
24. Schreibman PH, Pertsemlidis D, Liu GCK, et al. Lithogenic bile: a consequence of weight reduction. Presented at the 66th Annual Meeting of the American Society for Clinical Investigation, Atlantic City, 1974.
25. Whiting MJ, Watts JM. Supersaturated bile formation from obese patients without gallstones supports cholesterol crystal growth but not nucleation. Gastroenterology 1984;86:243–248.
26. Kratzer W, Kachele V, Mason RA, et al. Gallstone prevalence in relation to smoking, alcohol, coffee consumption, and nutrition: the Ulm gallstone study. Scand J Gastroenterol 1997;32:953–958.
27. Moerman CJ, Smeets FW, Kromhouit D. Dietary risk factors for clinically diagnosed gallstones in middle-aged men. Ann Epidemiol 1994; 4:248–254.
28. Sarles H, Hauton J, Planche NE, Lafont H, Gerolami A. Diet cholesterol gallstone composition of the bile. Am J Dig Dis 1970;15: 251–260.
29. St. George CM, Russel JC, Shaffer EA. Effects of obesity on bile formation and biliary lipid secretion in the genetically obese JCR:LA-corpulent rat. Hepatology 1994;20:1541–1547.
30. Booker ML, LaMorte WW, Beer ER, Hopkins SR. Effects of dietary cholesterol and triglycerides on lipid concentrations in liver, plasma, and bile. Lipids 1997;32:163–172.
31. Denbesten L, Connor WE, Bell S. The effect of dietary cholesterol on the composition of human bile. Surgery 1973;73:266–273.
32. Sarles H, Cruite C, Gerolami A, Mule A, Domingo N, Hauton J. Influence of cholestyramine, bile salt and cholesterol feeding on the lipid composition of hepatic bile in man. Scand J Gastroenterol 1970;5: 603–608.
33. Xu Q, Mantle M, Pauletzki JG, Shaffer EA. Sustained gallbladder stasis promotes cholesterol gallstone formation in the ground squirrel. Hepatology 1997;26:831.
34. Atilli AF, Capocaccia R, Carulli N, et al. Factors associated with gallstone disease in the MICOL experience. Hepatology 1997;26: 809–818.
35. Liddle RA, Goldstein RB, Saxton J. Gallstone formation during weight-reduction dieting. Arch Intern Med 1989;149:1750–1753.
36. Gebhard RL, Prigge WF, Ansel HJ, et al. The role of gallbladder emptying in gallstone formation during diet-induced rapid weight loss. Hepatology 1996;24:544–548.
37. Klein S, Nealon WH. Hepatobiliary abnormalities associated with total parenteral nutrition. Semin Liver Dis 1988;8:237–246.

38. Messing B, Bories C, Kunstlinger F, Bernier JJ. Does total parenteral nutrition induce gallbladder sludge formation and lithiasis? Gastroenterology 1983;84:1012–1019.
39. Rovsing H, Sloth R. Microgallbladders and biliary calculi in mucoviscidosis. Acta Radiol 1973;14:588—592.
40. Cohen S, Kaplan M, Gottlieb J, Patterson J. Liver disease and gallstones in regional enteritis. Gastroenterology 1971;60:237–245.
41. Miehoff WE, Kern F Jr. Bile salt malabsorption in regional ileitis, ileal resection and mannitol-induced diarrhea. J Clin Invest 1978;47: 261–267.
42. Xu Q, Scott B, Tan DMT, Shaffer EA. Slow intestinal transit: a motor disorder contributing to cholesterol gallstone formation in the ground squirrel. Hepatology 1996;23:1664–1672.
43. Johnston SM, Murray KP, Martin S, et al. Iron deficiency enhances cholesterol gallstone formation. Surgery 1997;122:354–362.
44. Leitzman MF, Giovanucci EL, Rimm EB, et al. The relation of physical activity to risk for symptomatic gallstone disease in men. Ann Intern Med 1998;128:417–425.
45. Hahm JS, Park JY, Park KG, Ahn YH, Lee MH, Park KN. Gallbladder motility in diabetes mellitus using real time ultrasonography. Am J Gastroenterol 996;91:2391–2394.
46. Patankar R, Ozmen MM, Bailey IS, Johnson CD. Gallbladder motility, gallstones, and the surgeon. Dig Dis Sci 1995;40:2323–2335.
47. De Santis A, Attili AF, Corradini G, et al. Gallstones and diabetes: a case-control study in a free-living population sample. Hepatology 1997;25:787–790.
48. Cooper J, Geizerova H, Oliver MF. Clofibrate and gallstones. Lancet 1975;1:1083.
49. Pertsemlidis D, Panveliwalla D, Ahrens EH Jr. Effects of clofibrate and of an estrogen–progestin combination on fasting biliary lipids and cholic acid kinetics in man. Gastroenterology 1974;66:565–573.
50. Durst RY, Burvin R, Eitan A, Barzilay A. A familial risk factor in cholesterol gallstone disease. J Clin Gastroenterol 1996;23(4):289–291.
51. Grundy SM, Metzger AL, Adler RD. Mechanisms of lithogenic bile formation in American Indian women with cholesterol gallstones. J Clin Invest 1972;51:3026–3043.
52. Zahor Z, Sternby NH, Kagan A, Uemura K, Vanecek R, Vichert AM. Frequency of cholelithiasis in Prague and Malmo: an autopsy study. Scand J Gastroenterol 1974;9:3–7.
53. GREPCO. The Rome Group for Epidemiology and Prevention of Cholelithiasis: the epidemiology of gallstone disease in Rome, Italy, part 1. Hepatology 1988;8:904–906.
54. Heaton KW. The epidemiology of gallstones and suggested aetiology. Clin Gastroenterol 1973;2:67–83.
55. McKellar DP, Anderson CT, Boynton CJ, Peoples JB. Cholecystectomy during pregnancy without fetal loss. Surg Gynecol Obstet 1992; 174:465–468.
56. Bennion LJ, Ginzberg RL, Garnick MB. Effects of oral contraceptives on the gallbladder bile of normal women. N Engl J Med 1976;294: 189–192.
57. Bennion LJ. Changes in bile lipids accompanying oophorectomy in a premenopausal woman. N Engl J Med 1977;297:709–711.
58. Bennion LJ, Ginzberg RL, Garnick JB, Bennett PH. Effects of the normal menstrual cycle on human gallbladder bile. N Engl J Med 1976;294:1187.
59. Thistle JL, Hofmann AF, Yu PYS, Ott B. Effect of varying doses of chenodeoxycholic acid on bile lipid and biliary acid composition in gallstone patients: a dose-response study. Am J Dig Dis 1977;22:1–6.
60. Wingrave SJ, Kay CR. Oral contraceptives and gallbladder disease. Lancet 1982;2:957–959.
61. Scragg RKR, McMichel AJ, Seamark RF. Oral contraceptives and endogenous oestrogens in gallstone disease: a case controlled study. Br Med J 1984;288:1795–1799.
62. Bradley DD, Wingerd J, Petitti DB, et al. Serum high-density lipoprotein cholesterol in women using oral contraceptives, estrogens and progestins. N Engl J Med 1978;299:17–20.
63. Coronary Drug Project Research Group. Gallbladder disease as a side effect of drugs influencing lipid metabolism: experience in the Coronary Drug Project. N Engl J Med 1977;296:1185–1190.
64. Honore LH. Increased incidence of symptomatic cholesterol cholelithiasis in perimenopausal women receiving estrogen replacement therapy: a retrospective study. J Reprod Med 1980;25:187–190.
65. Petitti DB, Sidney S, Perlman JA. Increased risk of cholecystectomy in users of supplemental estrogen. Gastroenterology 1988;94:91–95.
66. Bennion LJ, Drabny E, Knowler WC, et al. Sex differences in the size of bile acid pools. Metabolism 1978;27:961–969.
67. Thornton JR, Heaton KW, Macfarlane DG. A relation between high-density lipoprotein cholesterol and bile cholesterol saturation. Br Med J 1951;283:1352–1354.
68. Scott LD. Gallstone disease and pancreatitis in pregnancy. Gastroenterol Clin North Am 1992;21:803–815.
69. Cohen S. The sluggish gallbladder of pregnancy [Editorial]. N Engl J Med 1980;302:397–399.
70. Smith JJ, Pomaranc MM, Ivy AC. The influence of pregnancy and sex hormones on gallbladder motility in the guinea pig. Am J Physiol 1941;132:129–140.
71. Hould FS, Fried GM, Fazekas AG, Tremblay S, Mersereau WA. Progesterone receptors regulate gallbladder motility. J Surg Res 1988;45: 505–514.
72. Daignault PG, Fazekas AG, Rosenthall L, Fried GM. Relationship between gallbladder contraction and progesterone receptors in patients with gallstones. Am J Surg 1988;155:147–151.
73. Upp JR, Nealon WH, Singh P, et al. Correlation of cholecystokinin receptors with gallbladder contractility in patients with gallstones. Ann Surg 1987;205:641–648.
74. Small DM. Cholesterol nucleation and growth in gallstone formation [Editorial]. N Engl J Med 1980;302:1305–1307.
75. Carey MC, Cahalane MJ. Whither biliary sludge? Gastroenterology 1988;95:508–523.
76. Riegel C, Raudin IS, Morrison PJ, et al. Studies of gallbladder function. XI. The composition of the gallbladder bile in pregnancy. JAMA 1935;105:1343–1344.
77. Gerdes MM, Boyden EA. The rate of emptying of the human gallbladder in pregnancy. Surg Gynecol Obstet 1938;66:145–156.
78. Braverman DZ, Johnson ML, Kern F Jr. Effects of pregnancy and contraceptive steroids on gallbladder function. N Engl J Med 1980;302: 362–364.
79. Radberg G, Friman S, Svanvik J. The influence of pregnancy and contraceptive steroids on the biliary tract and its reference to cholesterol gallstone formation. Scand J Gastroenterol 1989;25:97–102.
80. Fisher RS, Roberts GS, Grabowski CJ, Cohen S. Inhibition of lower esophageal sphincter circular muscle by female sex hormones. Am J Physiol 1978;234:E243–E247.
81. Northfield TC, Kuffer RM, Maudgal DP, et al. Gallbladder sensitivity to cholecystokinin in patients with gallstones. Br Med J 1980;280: 143–145.
82. Basso L, McCollum PT, Darling MR, Tocchi A, Tanner WA. A study of cholelithiasis during pregnancy and its relationship with age, parity, menarche, breast-feeding, dysmenorrhea, oral contraception, and a maternal history of cholelithiasis. Surg Gynecol Obstet 1992;175: 41–46.
83. Lee SP, Maher K, Nicholls JF. Origin and fate of biliary sludge. Gastroenterology 1988;94:170–176.
84. Maringhini A, Marceno MP, Lanzarone F, et al. Sludge and stones in gallbladder after pregnancy: prevalence and risk factors. J Hepatol 1987;5:218–223.
85. Maringhini A, Ciambra M, Baccelliere P, Raimondo M, Pagliaro L. Sludge, stones and pregnancy. Gastroenterology 1988;95:1160–1161.
86. Maringhini A, Ciambra, M, Baccelliere P, et al. Biliary sludge and gallstones in pregnancy: incidence, risk factors, and natural history. Ann Intern Med 1993;119:116–120.
87. Kern F Jr, Everson GT, Demark B, et al. Biliary lipids, bile acids and gallbladder function in the human female: effects of pregnancy and the ovulatory cycle. J Clin Invest 1981;68:1229–1242.
88. Low-Beer TS, Wicks ACB, Heaton KW, Durrington P, Yeates J. Fluctuations of serum and bile lipid concentration during the menstrual cycle. Br Med J 1977;1:1568–1570.
89. Whiting MJ, Down RHL, Watts JMCK. Precision and accuracy in the measurement of the cholesterol saturation index of duodenal bile. Gastroenterology 1981;80:533–538.
90. Friley MD, Douglas G. Acute cholecystitis in pregnancy and the puerperium. Am Surg 1972;38:314–317.
91. Valdivieso V, Covarrubias C, Siegel F, Cruz F. Pregnancy and cholelithiasis: pathogenesis and natural course of gallstones diagnosed in early puerperium. Hepatology 1993;17:1–4.
92. Aufses AH Jr. Biliary tract disease. In: Rovinsky JJ, Guttmacher AF, eds. Medical, surgical and gynecologic complications of pregnancy, 2nd ed. Baltimore: Williams & Wilkins, 1965:251–253.

93. Landers D, Carmona R, Crombleholme W, Lim R. Acute cholecystitis in pregnancy. Obstet Gynecol 1987;69:131–133.
94. Sali A, Oats JN, Acton CM, Elzarka A, Vitetta L. Effect of pregnancy on gallstone formation. Aust N Z J Obstet Gynaecol 1989;29: 386–389.
95. Hiatt JR, Hiatt JG, Williams RA, Klein SR. Biliary disease in pregnancy and strategy for surgical management. Am J Surg 1986;151: 263–265.
96. Hill LM, Johnson CE, Lee RA. Cholecystectomy in pregnancy. Obstet Gynecol 1975;46:291–293.
97. Haemmerli UP. Jaundice during pregnancy with special reference to recurrent jaundice during pregnancy and its differential diagnosis. Acta Med Scand 966;444[Suppl]:1.
98. Printen KJ, Ott RA. Cholecystectomy during pregnancy. Am Surg 1978;44:432–434.
99. O'Neill JP. Surgical conditions complicating pregnancy: diseases of the gallbladder and pancreas. Aust N Z J Obstet Gynaecol 1969;9: 249–252.
100. Lewis GJ. A rare cause of cholecystitis in pregnancy. Int J Gynecol Obstet 1983;21:175–177.
101. Spinapolice RX, Colmorgen GHC, Spisso K. Hemoglobin SC disease associated with cholecystitis and cholelithiasis in pregnancy. Obstet Gynecol 1982;60:388–390.
102. Duffy BL, Watson RI. The HELLP syndrome mimics cholecystitis. Med J Aust 1988;148:473–475.
103. Pritchard JA, MacDonald PC, eds. Williams Obstetrics, 6th ed. New York: Appleton-Century-Crofts, 1980:248.
104. DeGraaf CS, Grade M. Gallstones, pregnancy and ultrasound. Conn Med 1979;43:424–425.
105. Worthen NJ, Uszler JM, Funamura JL. Cholecystitis: prospective evaluation of sonography and ^{99m}Tc Hida cholescintigraphy. AJR 1981; 137:973–978.
106. Hamlin E, Bartlett MK, Smith JA. Acute surgical emergencies of the abdomen in pregnancy. N Engl J Med 1951;244:128–131.
107. Dixon DP, Faddis DM, Silberman H. Aggressive management of cholecystitis during pregnancy. Am J Surg 1987;154:292–294.
108. Swisher SG, Schmit PJ, Hunt KK, et al. Biliary disease during pregnancy. Am J Surg 1994;168:576–581.
109. Lockwood C, Stiller RJ, Bolognese RJ. Maternal total parenteral nutrition in chronic cholecystitis. J Reprod Med 1987;32:785–788.
110. Fromm H. Gallstone dissolution therapy with ursodiol. Dig Dis Sci 1989;34:365–385.
111. Palmer AK, Heywood R. Pathological changes in the rhesus fetus associated with oral administration of chenodeoxycholic acid. Toxicology 1974;2:239–246.
112. Vincent CR. Jaundice in pregnancy: a review from the Charity Hospital, New Orleans, 1941–1956. Obstet Gynecol 1957;9:595–598.
113. Ghumman E, Barry M, Grace PA. Management of gallstones in pregnancy. Br J Surg 1997;84:1646–1650.
114. Glasgow RE, Visser BC, Harris HW, Patti MG, Kilpatrick SJ, Mulvihill SJ. Changing management of gallstone disease during pregnancy. Surg Endosc 1998;12:241–246.
115. Gouldman JW, Sticca RP, Rippon MB, McAlhany JC. Laparoscopic cholecystectomy in pregnancy. Am Surg 1998;64:93–97.
116. McCorriston CC. Nonobstetrical abdominal surgery during pregnancy. Am J Obstet Gynecol 1963;86:593–599.
117. Lanzafame RJ. Laparoscopic cholecystectomy. Surgery 1995;118: 627–631.
118. Greene J, Rogers A, Rubin L. Fetal loss after cholecystectomy during pregnancy. Can Med Assoc J 1963;88:576–577.
119. Farca A, Aguilar ME, Rodriguez G, delaMora G, Arango L. Biliary stents as temporary treatment for choledocholithiasis in pregnant patients. Gastrointest Endosc 1997;46:99–101.
120. Cotton PB. Endoscopic management of bile duct stones (apples and oranges). Gut 1984;25:587–597.
121. McSherry CK, Glenn F. The incidence and causes of death following surgery for non-malignant biliary tract disease. Ann Surg 1980;191: 271.
122. Friedman RL, Friedman IH. Acute cholecystitis with calculous biliary duct obstruction in the gravid patient. Surg Endosc 1995;9:910–913.
123. Nesbitt TH, Kay HH, McCoy MC, Herbert WN. Endoscopic management of biliary disease during pregnancy. Obstet Gynecol 1996;87: 806–809.
124. Uomo G, Manes G, Picciotto FP, Rabitti PG. Endoscopic treatment of acute biliary pancreatitis in pregnancy. J Clin Gastroenterol 1994;18: 250–252.
125. Baillie J, Cairns SR, Cotton PB. Endoscopic management of choledocholithiasis during pregnancy. Surg Gynecol Obstet 1990;171:1–4.
126. Schmidt WJ. Sammlung-Zweifelhafter schwangerschaft Faille nebst einer kritischen Einleitung. Vienna: F. Wimmer, 1918:172–180.
127. Langmade CF, Edmondson HA. Acute pancreatitis in pregnancy and the postpartum period. Surg Gynecol Obstet 1951;92:43.
128. Corlett RC, Mishell DR. Pancreatitis in pregnancy. Am J Obstet Gynecol 1972;113:281–290.
129. Jouppila P, Mokka R, Larmi TKI. Acute pancreatitis in pregnancy. Surg Gynecol Obstet 1974;139:879–882.
130. Walker BE, Diddle A. Acute pancreatitis in a gynecologic and obstetric practice. Am J Obstet Gynecol 1969;105:206–211.
131. McKay AJ, O'Neill J, Imbrie CW. Pancreatitis, pregnancy and gallstones. Br J Obstet Gynaecol 1980;87:47–50.
132. Wilkinson EJ. Acute pancreatitis in pregnancy: a review of 98 cases and a report of 9 new cases. Obstet Gynecol Surv 1973;28:281–303.
133. DeVore GR, Bracken M, Berkowitz RL. The amylase/creatinine clearance ratio in normal pregnancy and pregnancies complicated by pancreatitis, hyperemesis and toxemia. Am J Obstet Gynecol 1980;136: 747.
134. McKay AJ, Duncan JG, Imre CW, Joffe SN, Blumgart LH. A prospective study of the clinical value and accuracy of grey scale ultrasound in detecting gallstones. Br J Surg 1978;5:330–333.
135. Young KR. Acute pancreatitis in pregnancy: two case reports. Obstet Gynecol 1982;60:653–657.
136. Ramin KD, Ramin SM, Richey SD, Cunningham FG. Acute pancreatitis in pregnancy. Am J Obstet Gynecol 1995;173:187–191.
137. Ranson JHC, Rifkind KM, Turner JW. Prognostic signs and nonoperative peritoneal lavage in acute pancreatitis. Surg Gynecol Obstet 1976;143:209–219.
138. Stowell JC, Bottsford JE, Rubel HR. Pancreatitis with pseudocyst and cholelithiasis in the third trimester of pregnancy: management with total parenteral nutrition. South Med J 1984;77:502–504.
139. Block P, Kelly T. Management of gallstone pancreatitis during pregnancy and the postpartum period. Surg Gynecol Obstet 1989;168: 426–428.
140. Swisher SG, Hunt KK, Schmit PJ, Hiyama DT, Bennion RS, Thompson JE. Management of pancreatitis complicating pregnancy. Am Surg 1994;60:759–762.
141. Legro RS, Laifer SA, First-trimester pancreatitis: maternal and fetal outcome. J Reprod Med 1995;40:689–695.
142. Sheehan HL. Jaundice in pregnancy. Am J Obstet Gynecol 1961;81: 427–432.
143. Haemmerli UP. Jaundice during pregnancy. Acta Med Scand 1966; 179[Suppl]:9–21.
144. Hatfield AK, Stein JH, Greenberger NJ, Abernathy RW, Ferris TF. Idiopathic acute fatty liver of pregnancy: death from extrahepatic manifestations. J Dig Dis 1972;17:167–178.
145. Riely CA. Acute hepatic failure at term: diagnostic problems posed by broad clinical spectrum. Postgrad Med 1980;68:118–122, 125–127.
146. Schoeman MN, Batey RG, Wilcken B. Recurrent acute fatty liver of pregnancy associated with a fatty-acid oxidation defect in the offspring. Gastroenterology 1991;100:544–548.
147. Isaacs JD, Sims HF, Powell CK, et al. Maternal acute fatty liver of pregnancy associated with fetal trifunctional protein deficiency: molecular characterization of a novel maternal mutant allele. Pediatr Res 1996;40:393.
148. Burroughs AK, Seong NGH, Dojcinov M, Scheuer PJ, Sherlock SV. Idiopathic acute fatty liver of pregnancy in 12 patients. Q J Med 1982;51:481–497.
149. Castro MA, Ouyounian JG, Colletti PM, et al. Radiologic studies in acute fatty liver of pregnancy: a review of the literature and 19 new cases. J Reprod Med 1996;41:839–843.
150. Weber FL, Snodgrass PJ, Powell DE, Rao P, Huffman SL, Brady PG. Abnormalities of hepatic mitochrondrial urea-cycle enzyme activities and hepatic ultrastructure in acute fatty liver of pregnancy. J Lab Clin Med 1979;94:27–41.
151. Long RG, Scheuer PJ, Sherlock S. Preeclampsia presenting with deep jaundice. J Clin Pathol 1977;30:212–215.
152. Killiam AP, Dillard SH, Patton RC, Pederson PR. Pregnancy-induced hypertension complicated by acute liver disease and disseminated intravascular coagulation. Am J Obstet Gynecol 1975;123:823–828.

153. Pereira SP, O'Donouhue J, Wendon J, Williams R. Maternal and perinatal outcome in severe pregnancy-related liver disease. Hepatology 1997;26:1258–1262.
154. Rab MA, Bile MK, Mubarik MM, et al. Water-borne hepatitis E virus epidemic in Islamabad, Pakistan: a common source outbreak traced to the malfunction of a modern water treatment plant. Am J Trop Med Hyg 1997;57:151–157.
155. Stevens CE, Palmer-Beasley R, Tsui J, Wy-Chon L. Vertical transmission of hepatitis B antigen in Taiwan. J Med Virol 1979;3:237–241.
156. Adams RN, Conkes R. Viral hepatitis during pregnancy. JAMA 1965; 192:195–199.
157. Cahill KM. Hepatitis in pregnancy. Surg Gynecol Obstet 1962;114: 545–548.
158. Borhanmanesh F, Haghigh P, Hekmat K, Reziazadeh K, Ghavami AG. Viral hepatitis during pregnancy: severity and effect on gestation. Gastroenterology 1973;64:304–312.
159. Malkani PK, Greuval AK. Observations on infectious hepatitis in pregnancy. Indian J Med Res 1957;45[Suppl]:77–87.
160. Ton MJ, Thursby M, Rakela J, McPeak C, Edwards VM, Mosley JW. Maternal-infant transmission of the viruses which cause acute hepatitis. Gastroenterology 1981;80:999–1004.
161. Wands JR, Alpert E, Isselbacher KJ. Arthritis associated with chronic active hepatitis: complement activations and characterization of circulating immune complexes. Gastroenterology 1975;69: 1286–1291.
162. Brzosko WJ, Krawczynski K, Nazarewicz T, Morzycka M, Nowoslawski A. Glomerulonephritis associated with hepatitis B surface antigen immune complexes in children. Lancet 1974;2:477–482.
163. Levo Y, Gorevic PD, Kassab HJ, Zucker-Franklin D, Franklin EC. Association between hepatitis B virus and essential mixed cryoglobulinemia. N Engl J Med 1977;296:1501–1504.
164. Hagler L, Pastore RA, Bergin JJ, Wrensch MR. Aplastic anemia following viral hepatitis. Medicine 1975;54:139–164.
165. Alter MJ. Transmission of hepatitis C virus: route, dose and titer. N Engl J Med 1994;330:784–786.
166. Chang MH. Mother-to-infant transmission of hepatitis C virus. Clin Invest Med 1996;19:368–372.
167. Hunt CM, Carson KL, Sharara AI. Hepatitis C in pregnancy. Obstet Gynecol 1997;89:883–890.
168. Thomas DL, Villano SA, Riester KA, et al. Perinatal transmission of hepatitis C virus from human immunodeficiency virus type 1–infected mothers. Women and Infants Transmission Study. J Infect Dis 1998;177:1480–1488.
169. Centers for Disease Control. Recommendations for prevention and control of hepatitis C virus (HCV) infection and HCV-related chronic disease. MMWR 1998;47:RR-19.

SECTION VII

Hematopoietic Disorders

Cherry and Merkatz's Complications of Pregnancy,
Fifth Edition, edited by W. R. Cohen.
Lippincott Williams & Wilkins, Philadelphia © 2000.

CHAPTER 20

Disorders of Hemostasis

Wayne B. Kramer and Carl P. Weiner

In the past few years, dramatic progress has been made in the understanding, diagnosis, and treatment of clotting disorders. A working knowledge of coagulation physiology and pathology is necessary to select the optimal evaluation path to establish a timely diagnosis and to direct therapy. Although hemorrhage remains a leading cause of maternal death, timely administration of the correct therapy improves the likelihood of the patient's survival.

PHYSIOLOGY OF COAGULATION

Hemostasis involves a complex interrelationship between the ability of the circulatory system to respond to injury and the ability of the vessel wall to protect against thrombosis. A complex series of interactions ultimately leads to the formation of thrombin and fibrin clot. Hypocoagulability or hypercoagulability is produced by any acquired or inherited abnormality affecting any of these interactions.

Hemostasis is divided into two phases: formation of platelet plug and deposition of a fibrin cap over the platelet plug, thus strengthening and stabilizing it. Clot extension is prevented by multiple regulatory systems.

W. B. Kramer and C. P. Weiner: Department of Obstetrics and Gynecology, University of Maryland Medical Systems, Baltimore, MD 21201.

THE PLATELET

Disruption of the vascular endothelium results in exposure of the subendothelial collagen layer, which leads to a complicated chain of events resulting in platelet adherence to this exposed layer. Actual deposition of platelets is controlled by flow factors governing their transport to the surface and by the kinetics of their interaction with the surface (1). Contact is initiated by the platelet membrane glycoprotein complex Ib–IX binding to the von Willebrand factor (VWF) present on subendothelial collagen and noncollagen microfibrillar material; this material activates the platelets and exposes activated glycoprotein IIb–IIIa on the platelet, to which VWF can bind irreversibly and promote platelet aggregation. The binding of VWF to glycoprotein complex Ib–IX causes a transmembrane flux of calcium ions. This influx of calcium ions, which is required for platelet aggregation, can be provoked in a number of ways. Thromboxane A_2 (TxA_2), thrombin, platelet-activating factor, and adenosine diphosphate are all able to promote the influx of calcium ions; and TxA_2 has ionophoric activity, which enables it to transport calcium ions across intracellular membranes (2). At first, the platelet plug is loose, allowing blood to flow continuously over and through it. With additional platelet aggregation and adherence, the plug becomes progressively more dense, and within minutes a fibrin cap is formed over the platelet plug and blood flow through the defect is no longer possible. This event is followed by clot retraction, which is mediated by the platelet fibrinogen. In this process, the platelet is attached firmly to fibrin strands (3,4). The adjacent normal vascular endothelium limits the size of the forming thrombus by releasing endothelium-derived relaxing factors and prostacyclin in response to the adenosine diphosphate (ADP), TxA_2, and serotonin released by the platelets.

SOLUBLE COMPONENTS

The end stage of the coagulation pathway is thrombin production. Coagulation can be divided into two stages: (a) an initiation stage and (b) an augmentation stage (Fig. 20-1) (5). The initiation stage, referred to as the *extrinsic pathway*, is dependent on the tissue factor (TF)-dependent pathway. The augmentation stage is handled by components of the formerly termed *intrinsic pathway*. In both pathways, thrombin is generated. The initiation stage of the pathway, which is dependent on tissue factor, is shut off soon after initiation by tissue factor pathway inhibitor (TFPI). Usually, enough thrombin is generated to activate factors V, VIII, and XI before this occurrs.

Tissue factor is the initiating molecule in these complex interactions (Fig. 20-2). It catalyzes the activation of VII to VIIa. The TF–VIIa complex then activates coagulation factors IX and X. The activation of IX and X is limited by the binding of the TF-VIIa complex to the TFPI. A limited amount of Xa provides sufficient thrombin to induce local aggregation of platelets and activation of critical cofactors V, VIII, and XI. The amount of Xa produced by the TF–VIIa complex and dampened by TFPI is insufficient to sustain hemostasis and must be amplified by the actions of cofactors IXa, VIIIa, and XIa for ultimate and persistent hemostasis.

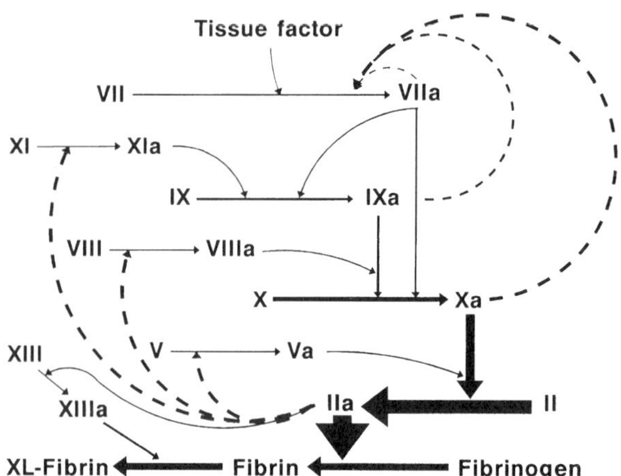

FIG. 20-2. Activation of coagulation by tissue factor. *Stippled lines* are positive feed-back mechanisms. XL-fibrin, cross-linked fibrin. (From Nielson JD. Thromogenesis. Ann Chir Gynaecol 1995;84:327–334.)

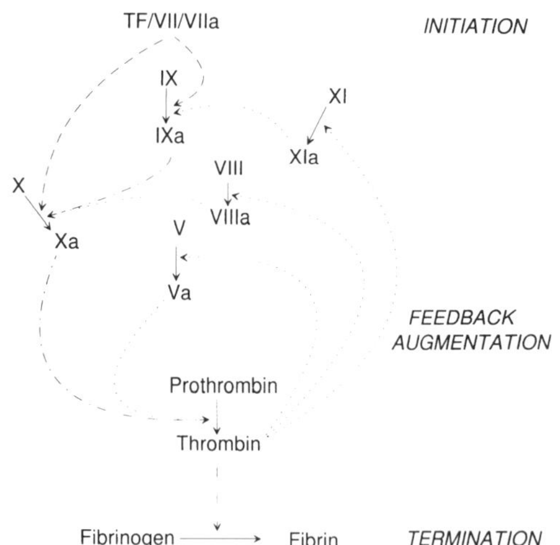

FIG. 20-1. The tissue factor-dependent pathway of blood coagulation. A simplified version of the blood coagulation cascade demonstrating how TF initiates the cascade and how feedback inhibition by thrombin takes over when TF/VIIa is inhibited by TFPI-1. (From Camerer E, Kolsto AB, Prydz H. Cell biology of tissue factor, the principal initiator of blood coagulation. Thromb Res 1996;81:1–41.)

Tissue factor can be found in most tissues, with high levels in the brain, lung, and kidney (6). Cells express it based on the degree of cellular differentiation (7). It is expressed constitutively, is prohibited, or is induced. It is expressed constitutively by epithelial and glial cells. The lymphocytes are examples of the prohibited phenotype. Neither the T cells nor the B class of cells express TF in resting form or after activation. The endothelial cells and cells of monocytic lineage are examples of the induced form. The cellular immune response induces TF production in monocytes by antigen-driven T-helper cell signaling (8). TF production in monocytes is also induced by endotoxin and anaphylotoxin C5a (9). Interleukin 1, tumor necrosis factor, endotoxins, virus infections, thrombin, insulin, and various mitogens can induce TF production in both endothelial cells and monocytes (10).

The binding of TF to VII enhances the ability of trace factors of VIIa, IXa, Xa, or thrombin to activate VII (11–15). Calcium and phospholipid enhances activity, although neither is absolutely required for interaction (16,17). The small picomolar concentrations of factor VIIa in circulating blood trigger the initial TF–VIIa catalyzed generation of factors IX and X when blood is exposed to extravascular blood (18,19). A newly discovered serine protease hepsin, which is present in many tissues, activates VII in a calcium action independent of TF and may play a significant role in the initial activation of VII (20,21). Once Xa is made available to the prothrombinase complex, enough thrombin is generated to back-activate the cascade through VIII and IX (*augmentation*). The thrombin that is formed also enhances platelet aggregation; catalyzes the formation of the proteases XIa, Xa, and VIIa; and activates cofactor V. In the final step of coagulation, thrombin splits off the fibrinopeptides A and B from fibrinogen and finally enables the cross-linking of fibrin by activation of factor XIII.

COAGULATION MODULATORS

The coagulation process is downregulated by several proteases that slow fibrin generation. TF–VIIa complex activity is regulated by both TFPI and antithrombin III (AT III) (22,23). The *TFPI* gene has been cloned and sequenced (24) and contains three inhibitory domains that act as slow, tight-binding, competitive, and reversible inhibitors (25). It inhibits Xa directly and in a Xa-dependent fashion produces feedback inhibition of the TF–VIIa complex (26,27). Factor VIIa of the TF–VIIa complex binds to the first domain (28). Factor Xa binds to and is inhibited by the second domain, but other regions of the molecule assist in formation of the Xa/TFPI complex (29,30). The function of the third domain is unknown. Inhibition of the factor VIIa/tissue factor complex at normal concentrations of TFPI involves the formation of a quaternary complex containing factor Xa/TFPI/VIIa/TF, which is dependent on the presence of factor Xa (31). This inhibitory ability is not influenced by free VIIa concentration, whereas that of AT III is. Fiftyfold greater concentrations of TFPI are required to inhibit factor VIIa/TF in the absence of factor Xa (28). TFPI also inhibits activation of IX. Most of the TFPI in plasma is bound to lipoproteins, with platelets carrying about 10% (32). Thrombin and other agents stimulate the platelets to release TFPI at sites of coagulation, which increases the local concentration of TFPI at the site of a wound (33). TFPI is also thought to be bound to surface glycosaminoglycans in the endothelium and is released with heparin infusion (34).

Antithrombin III is a thrombin inhibitor that also irreversibly inhibits Xa, IXa, VIIa, and XIa. It inhibits the TF–VIIa complex before the generation of Xa. TF is released from the TF–VIIa complex, which then is free to bind with free VIIa. Heparin enhances the inhibitory effect of AT III from the tissue factor VIIa complex and thus may be ineffective in the absence of AT III (35). The variable response of patients with disseminated intravascular coagulopathy (DIC) to heparin may result from the variable AT III concentration. The interaction between AT III and thrombin also is facilitated by PAPP-A, a pregnancy-specific protein that functions like heparin; however, it does not aid in the interaction of AT III and factor Xa (36). AT III has a half-life of 2 to 3 days, but this is reduced to a few hours in DIC patients (37).

Two types of AT III deficiency have been delineated (38). Type I deficiency is the result of reduced synthesis of normal protease inhibitor molecules. Type II deficiency is secondary to a particular molecular defect within the inhibitor, which now has been further subdivided. AT III deficiency is inherited as an autosomal dominant condition, with homozygous AT III deficiency being incompatible with life. The prevalence of AT III deficiency in patients with venous thromboembolism is estimated to be 2% to 3% (39,40). In the normal population, AT III deficiency is estimated to affect 1 in 2,000 to 1 in 5,000 persons (41). Patients are predisposed to venous thrombosis when the AT III level is below 50% (42).

Thrombin also is inhibited by heparin cofactor II (HC-II), whose full role in hemostasis has not been determined. One percent of patients with venous thrombosis will have a heparin HC-II deficiency (43). A 50% decrease in plasma HC-II levels has been associated with an increased risk of thrombosis (44). The fibrin-bound thrombin is still active, but both AT III and HC-II are unable to access this molecule. Breakdown of the fibrin network releases the active thrombin, which then can stimulate the coagulation cascade (45). Direct thrombin inhibitors such as hirudin have been developed to access the fibrin-bound thrombin that neither AT III nor HC-II can access (46). About 1% of patients presenting with venous thrombosis may have some sort of dysfibrinogenemia.

Excess thrombin generated at the wound site interacts with thrombomodulin, and this complex activates protein C. Thrombin bound to thrombomodulin no longer can clot fibrinogen or activate platelets. The binding of thrombomodulin to thrombin also accelerates thrombin inhibition by thrombomodulin. Thrombomodulin is detectable on endothelial cells, platelets, synovial cells, neutrophils, and mononuclear phagocytes (47). The activated protein C complex (APC) interacts with protein S on endothelial cells or platelet membranes and then proteolytically inactivates Va (a necessary cofactor for catalyzing thrombin formation). APC also can inactivate VIIIa (involved in formation of Xa). Factors Va and VIIIa in complex with Xa and IXa are relatively resistant to inactivation by APC. Protein S renders these enzymes susceptible to inactivation by APC (48,49). APC has a relatively long half-life of 15 minutes, which allows APC to inhibit coagulation complexes on cell surfaces and inactivate them before a coagulation response occurs. APC is inhibited by α_2-macroglobulin, α_1-antitrypsin, and protein C inhibitor (50,51). The concentration of protein C is stable during normal pregnancy, whereas the concentration of protein S is markedly decreased (52,53). Increased protein C and protein S levels are found in women with mild to moderate preeclampsia (52). Recently, resistance to APC has been described. This abnormality, which causes Va to be resistant to inhibition by APC (54–58), is present in 30% to 40% of patients presenting with venous thrombosis (59). In most cases, the substitution of glutamine for arginine at amino acid 506 in V (a variation termed *factor V Leiden*) is responsible for this disorder (56,58).

FIBRINOLYSIS

As soon as the hemostatic task of fibrin has been completed, the plasmin system begins the process of fibrinolysis. (The fibrinolytic system, however, appears to play a less important role in preventing thrombosis than do inhibitors of procoagulant pathways.) Reduced fibrinolytic activity in the plasma may predispose to both venous thromboembolism and arterial thrombosis (59–61). Activation of plasminogen to plasmin is a major function of this system. Plasminogen activators such as tissue plasminogen activator (t-PA), urokinase, and kallikrein are responsible for this reaction; t-PA, which is released from the endothelial cell in response to stresses such as exercise and venous occlusion, is one of the most important plasminogen activators. The secretion of t-PA from endothelial cells also is stimulated by thrombin (62). It has a half-life in plasma of about 4 minutes (63). Several inhibitors of t-PA have been identified, of which plasminogen activator inhibitor 1 (PAI-1) is the most significant. It is released from endothelial cells and platelets. PAI-1 levels have a diurnal variation with 90% of the total blood PAI-1 being of platelet origin (64). The plasma levels of PAI-1 are difficult to interpret, as they are influenced by a wide variety of factors including age, sex, pregnancy, recent trauma, infection, fat distribution, blood pressure, and triglyceride level and are raised in obese patients with type II diabetes. It is suggested that PAI-1 levels may be related to insulin precursor molecules (61). High levels of plasma PAI-1 and depressed levels of t-PA have been shown to cause recurrent venous thromboembolism (59,60). The major plasma inhibitor of plasmin is α_2-plasmin inhibitor. It rapidly inactivates free plasmin, whereas fibrin-bound plasmin is protected from inactivation (65).

THE VASCULATURE

The fluid state of blood within vessels is maintained by the antithrombotic inner surface of the vasculature. Blood flow remains the most important modulator of this fluid state. It removes activated coagulants, thus limiting clot extension. Other local modulators include endothelium-derived factors, endothelial cell receptors, and fibrin.

TABLE 20-1. *Vasomotor products secreted by the endothelial cell*

Vasodilating agents
Nitric oxide
Prostacyclin
Endothelium-derived hyperpolarizing factor
Vasoconstricting agents
Thromboxane
Angiotensin-converting enzyme
Endothelin

TABLE 20-2. *Endothelial cell regulation of coagulation*

Procoagulant	Anticoagulant
Platelet-activating factor	Tissue factor pathway inhibitor
von Willebrand factor	Activated protein C Complex
Tissue factor	Thromboxane
Plasminogen activator inhibitor-1	Thrombomodulin
Thromboxane	Heparin sulfate
	Urokinase
	Tissue plasminogen activator

Together, the fibrin and the platelet plug limit enzyme activation by blocking access to the initiating stimuli. Fibrin also neutralizes large quantities of thrombin by reversibly absorbing it (66).

The endothelial cells are responsible for maintaining vasomotor tone (Table 20-1), but they also play an important role in coagulation (Table 20-2). Normal intact endothelium is responsible for binding and synthesis of VWF (67,68). The secretion and expression of the various procoagulants and anticoagulants by the endothelium are continuously modified by cytokines, which are released in disease states such as the development of DIC in septic shock. The endothelium is also the primary source of t-PA, prostacyclin, and nitric oxide. Both nitric oxide and prostacyclin are also potent inhibitors of platelet adhesion and aggregation (69). The production and release of each increase during pregnancy. A deficiency of prostacyclin has been reported in obstetric conditions such as preeclampsia (70,71). Elevated hematocrit and levels of plasma fibrinogen also are associated with an increased risk of thrombotic disease (72,73). Hyperviscosity syndromes result in increased risk of thrombotic events (72). Patients with vasculitis or other diseases resulting in endothelial damage also have elevated levels of VWF and thrombomodulin (74). The vascular smooth muscle aids hemostasis only by retraction and spasm.

PREGNANCY-ASSOCIATED CHANGES IN COAGULATION

Pregnancy probably exerts its impact on the clotting system through enhanced hormonal synthesis. Pregnancy is thought to be a state of chronic compensated DIC in which component synthesis equals or exceeds consumption. Fibrinopeptide A (FPA), which is increased before the end of the first trimester, supports this theory (75), reflects increased thrombin generation, and is the earliest documented pregnancy-mediated alteration in coagulation. AT III activity is not significantly altered by pregnancy; however, a minor illness during pregnancy, such as a viral upper respiratory infection, can cause a dramatic decline in plasma AT III activity (76). There is minimal fibrin deposition in the maternal microvasculature during normal pregnancy, because fibrinolytic activity increases

TABLE 20-3. *Changes in coagulation during pregnancy*

Increased	Unchanged	Decreased
Fibrinogen	II	XI
VII	V	XIII
VWF:C (function)	IX	Platelets
VWF:Ag (antigen)	Protein C	Protein S
VWF:ROc (ristocetin cofactor activity)	TFPI	
X	Antithrombin III	
XII	Plasminogen	
Fibrinopeptide A	Prekallikrein	
PAI-I		
PAI-II		
α2-macroglobulin		

VWF, von Willebrand factor; PAI, plasminogen activator inhibitor; TFPI, tissue factor plasma inhibitor.

during the first and second trimester (although it decreases in the early third trimester) (77). The concentrations of other coagulation factors also change during pregnancy (Table 20-3).

Later in pregnancy, it can be considered to be a "hypercoagulable state," which is confirmed by the elevation of FPA and thrombin–AT complexes in late gestation. Together with the venous stasis present in the dependent limbs throughout pregnancy and the vascular damage that occurs during delivery, they would account for the high incidence of thromboembolic disease in the peripartum period.

CLINICAL EVALUATION OF A BLEEDING DISORDER

History and Physical Examination

Any routine prenatal evaluation should include a complete bleeding history and physical examination. All suspicious findings should be pursued actively. Bleeding disorders often are missed unless specific inquiries are made in addition to the standard questions concerning a family history of bleeding or past transfusions. For example, patients with hereditary bleeding disorders rarely have problems shedding deciduous teeth; however, it must be ascertained whether the patient bled briskly for more than 1 hour after a dental extraction or oozed for more than 2 days. This finding may indicate VWD or the fact that the patient was a symptomatic carrier of factor VIII deficiency. It is also important to inquire about recent medications, because numerous drugs are associated with either qualitative or quantitative platelet disorders. A history of when bleeding occurred is also very important. Bleeding of immediate onset often is associated with platelet abnormalities. A delayed-onset bleed often is associated with a soluble component disorder.

The first step in the evaluation of any bleeding disorder is to determine whether it results from local pathology, a generalized defect in the clotting system, or a combination of both. Information about signs and symptoms associated with the bleeding can be virtually diagnostic and may prevent costly laboratory evaluation. For example, petechiae that appear in crops and are common on the dependent parts of the body are characteristic of either a platelet or vascular disorder. Deep dissecting hematomas and hemarthroses are more characteristic of a soluble component disorder.

Vascular abnormalities often are associated with unexplained easy bruising. These disorders are important because the frequency of hemorrhage and thrombosis is increased after operative or traumatic stress. These defects often are associated with collagen disorders, Cushing syndrome, diabetes, and infections. Evaluation of the kinin and autoimmune systems and tissue biopsy is often necessary to make this diagnosis.

Basic Laboratory Evaluation

The basic components of a clotting screen should include the prothrombin time (PT), the partial thromboplastin time (PTT), the platelet count, and fibrinogen level. The PTT evaluates the intrinsic (augmentation) and common pathways. It is often used to monitor heparin therapy; however, it correlates poorly with the plasma heparin level and is not so important as the fact that the therapeutic level of heparin remains poorly defined and clinical experience confirms that a 50% increase in the PTT is associated with a marked reduction in subsequent thrombotic events. A prolonged PTT can be taken to imply an intact heparin–AT III pathway. A reduction in AT III, as seen in DIC, increases the heparin requirement.

The PT evaluates the initiation and common pathways. It is most sensitive to deficiencies of factors V, VII, and X. The PT is a useful monitor of warfarin therapy, because factor VII has the shortest half-life of the vitamin K-dependent factors (i.e., II, VII, IX, and X). Hypofibrinogenemia will not alter the PT unless the fibrinogen concentration is below 100 mg/dL. Eventually, automated tests for specific components of the extrinsic and intrinsic pathways will replace the PT and PTT.

The platelet contribution to hemostasis is evaluated by doing a platelet count. The incidence of thrombocytopenia has been demonstrated to increase during pregnancy (78). Thrombocytopenia is not a diagnosis but rather a symptom of an underlying disease. Generally, whereas most laboratories use a platelet cutoff of 150,000/mm^3, a count below 120,000/mm^3 is clearly atypical. When the platelet count exceeds 50,000/mm^3, excessive bleeding is rare. If bleeding occurs when the count is above this level, a functional platelet disorder should be considered. Spontaneous bleeding may be seen when the platelet count is below 50,000/mm^3. It is rarely severe if the count is above 10,000/mm^3. A low count always should be confirmed by a manual count, because the anticoagulant EDTA does not always prevent platelet clumping. These clumps are not recognized by the automated counters, which then erroneously report a low count.

The bleeding time is measured from a series of standardized stab wounds and reflects both platelet number and function. The bleeding time can be prolonged by a qualitative platelet disorder such as that which occurs in association with VWD, Glanzmann thromboasthenia, the ingestion of antiprostaglandin drugs (e.g., aspirin, ibuprofen), and preeclampsia. It also may be associated with a vascular abnormality, but this possibility is much less common and should be pursued last. Platelet function also can be evaluated by the *in vitro* response of platelets to aggregating agents as measured by the change in optical density of a light beam passed through platelet-rich plasma. The aggregating agents most commonly used include ADP, serotonin, epinephrine, collagen, arachidonic acid, and ristocetin. Diseases associated with acquired platelet dysfunction include autoimmune disorders, preeclampsia, anemia, drug-induced disorders, uremia, and myeloproliferative syndromes.

In the absence of overwhelming liver disease, a decline in fibrinogen level suggests that consumption is exceeding production and the cause should be determined. In the emergency situation, a bedside clotting test should be performed. Five milliliters of blood should be placed in a silicone-coated vacuum blood collection tube (red top). The absence of clot after 10 minutes indicates a fibrinogen concentration below 50 mg/dL. Should a clot occur and then rapidly break down, this may demonstrate the presence of excess circulating FSP.

Interpretations of the various screening tests are listed in Table 20-4. An isolated prolongation of the PTT is quite common. In an asymptomatic patient, this may be due to an acquired inhibitor (most often an antibody) or to a deficiency of either prekallikrein, factor XII, or high-molecular-weight kinogen. If the abnormality is due to an antibody, the PTT will not correct when the patient's plasma is mixed 1:1 with normal plasma. Inhibitors usually are not associated with hemorrhage, except when directed against factor VIII or IX.

Commonly, both the PT and PTT are prolonged, often because of DIC with fibrin-fibrinogenolysis, which also is caused by isolated deficiencies or inhibitors of the common pathway clotting factors, hypofibrinogenemia, liver disease, massive transfusion of banked blood, and vitamin K deficiency. Often, ingestion of a prolonged broad-spectrum antibiotic may lead to vitamin K deficiency. A woman with a clinical bleeding disorder characterized by a normal coagulation screen has either a factor XIII deficiency or a vascular abnormality.

Specialized Tests

Fibrin degradation products or *fibrin split products* (FSP) are the result of plasmin catabolism of fibrinogen and fibrin resulting in X, Y, D, and E fragments. These fragments are cleared by the reticuloendothelial system

TABLE 20-4. *Laboratory tests in bleeding disorders*

Clinical bleeding	PTT	PT	Bleeding time	Platelet count	Fibrinogen	Common causes	
						Acquired	Hereditary
–	P	N	N	N	N	Lupus anticoagulant	High-molecular—weight kinogen; prekallikrein, factor XII deficiencies
+	P	N	N	N	N	Heparin, factor VIII inhibitors	Hemophilia A and B, factor XI deficiency
+	P	P	N	N	N	Heparin, warfarin, vitamin K deficiency, antibiotics	Deficiency in factors V, X, and II and dysfibrinogenemia
+	N	P	N	N	N		Factor VII deficiency
+	P	N	P	N	N	Lupuslike anticoagulant, factor VIII complex inhibitor	von Willebrand syndrome
+	P	P	P	N			Afibrinogenemia
+	N	N	P		N	Thrombocytopenia secondary to ITP, drugs, etc.	Aldrich syndrome
+	N	N	P	N	N	Aspirin, uremia, etc.	Thrombasthenia, deficient platelet release, Bernard-Soulier syndrome
+	N	N	N	N	N		Factor XIII deficiency
+	P	P				DIC, liver disease	

+, present; DIC, disseminated intravascular coagulation; ITP, immune thrombotic thrombocytopenia; N, normal; P, prolonged; –, absent; PT, prothrombin time; PTT, partial prothrombin time.

From Colman RW, Hirsh J, Marder VJ, Salzman EW. Approach to the bleeding patient. In: Colman RW, Hirsh J, Marder VJ, Salzman EW, eds. Hemostasis and thrombosis. Philadelphia: JB Lippincott, 1982:700.

and have a half-life of approximately 9 hours. The Y and D fragments are especially potent antithrombins and impair platelet aggregation (79). Although fibrinolysis occurs slowly within large blood vessels, it is rapid within the microvasculature (80). The FSP can be measured by several techniques. Fibrin is finally degraded into the D-dimer. The measurement of D-dimer is thus specific for fibrin degradation products.

Fibrinopeptide A (FPA) is the first peptide cleaved from fibrinogen during thrombin-mediated fibrin generation. The concentration of FPA directly reflects fibrin generation, which has a short half-life of 3 minutes and is measured by radioimmunoassay and is elevated during normal pregnancy. Significantly higher concentrations are found during pregnancies complicated by preeclampsia, sepsis, and thromboembolic disease (76,81,82). A normal FPA during pregnancy is inconsistent with an acute thrombosis of any size.

AT III inhibits most active soluble clotting components. It has become one of the most useful laboratory parameters for monitoring the effect of therapy on DIC (83). When AT III consumption is limited or has ceased, it may be assumed that the causative process has been either eliminated or blunted. Reduction in AT III activity during pregnancy is seen with infection, preeclampsia, and thromboembolic disease, suggesting a low reserve (76). The finding of a normal AT III value during pregnancy would be inconsistent with the diagnosis of DIC.

Euglobulin lysis time is a crude but practical measure of plasminogen activator and plasmin activity.

DIAGNOSIS AND MANAGEMENT OF COAGULATION DISORDERS

Disseminated Intravascular Coagulation

Thrombin generation at the site of tissue injury results in coagulation of blood and stops blood loss from damaged microvessels. In patients with DIC, the excess thrombin production results in the release of free thrombin into the circulation, which leads to widespread microvascular thrombosis resulting in tissue ischemia and organ damage. To maintain vascular patency, excess plasmin is generated so that local fibrinolysis and systemic fibrinogenolysis occur. It is the excess of free thrombin and plasmin in the circulation that results in the clinical features of DIC. A number of diseases unique to pregnancy or complications of pregnancy are associated with intravascular clotting abnormalities: the preeclampsia/eclampsia syndrome, abruptio placentae, saline abortion, the dead fetus syndrome, amniotic fluid embolus, and septic abortion and shock. DIC is not a unique disease entity but an intermediate mechanism of many well-defined diseases (Table 20-5) (84). It is a continuum in which a variety of symptoms may appear. Understanding the disorders that promote DIC and recognizing the syndrome are paramount in making the diagnosis and directing management.

TABLE 20-5. *Conditions that may be associated with disseminated intravascular coagulation*

Obstetric conditions
Amniotic fluid embolism
Placental abruption
Retained fetus syndrome
Preeclampsia/eclampsia
Abortion
Viremias
HIV
Varicella
Cytomegalovirus
Hepatitis
Intravascular hemolysis
Massive transfusion
Hemolytic transfusion reaction
Septicemia
Gram-negative (endotoxin)
Gram positive (mucopolysaccharides)
Metastatic malignancy
Burns, trauma
Acid-base imbalance
Vascular disorders
Prosthetic devices
Acute liver disease

HIV, human immunodeficiency virus.

Pathophysiology

The release of TF into the circulation triggers DIC, which activates the coagulation system and the production of both thrombin and plasmin (Fig. 20-3) (85). Intact endothelium concentrates both AT III molecules on its surface and expresses thrombomodulin molecules. If thrombin is generated close to intact endothelium, it is inactivated by the AT III or bound by thrombomodulin in such a way as to alter its substrate specificity and prevent

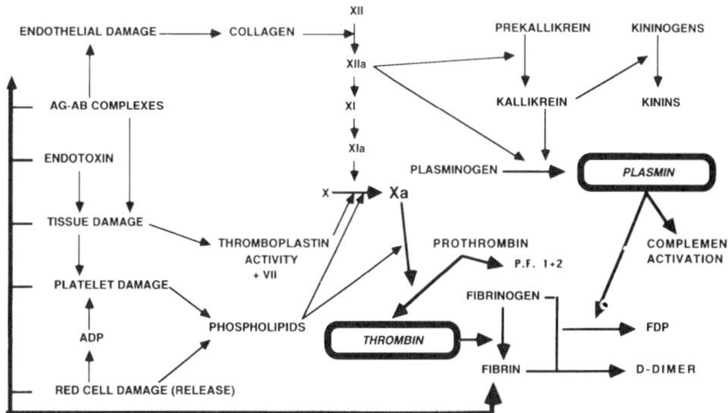

FIG. 20-3. Triggering mechanisms for DIC. (Reproduced with permission from Bick RL. Disseminated intravascular coagulation: objective clinical and laboratory diagnosis, treatment, and assessment of therapeutic response. Semin Thromb Hemostas 1996;22:69.)

it from converting fibrinogen to fibrin. Without an intact endothelium, the thrombin is allowed to circulate systemically, resulting in fibrinopeptides A and B being cleaved from fibrinogen and leaving behind fibrin monomers that polymerize into fibrin in the circulation. These fibrin monomers then lead to microvascular and macrovascular thrombosis and interference with blood flow, peripheral ischemia, and end-organ damage (86–89). Fibrin deposits occur within the microcirculation, platelets are trapped, and thrombocytopenia ensues (86–88). In response to stresses such as tissue ischemia and venous occlusion, plasminogen activators such as t-PA are released from the endothelial cell. This release of t-PA from the endothelial cells also is stimulated by thrombin. The plasmin circulating systemically cleaves the carboxy end of fibrinogen into FSPs, which interfere with fibrin monomer polymerization. This interference impairs hemostasis and leads to hemorrhage (86). Further platelet dysfunction and hemorrhage are induced by fragments D and E. Plasmin also degrades factors V, VIIIc, IX, XI, and other plasma proteins such as adrenocorticotropic hormone, insulin, and growth hormone (86–91). It also activates the common pathway leading to activation of C8-9 and both platelet and red cell lysis (92). Platelet entrapment in the fibrin-webbed microvasculature results in thrombocytopenia. Complement-induced platelet lysis produces further platelet destruction and more platelet procoagulant material. The fibrin in contact with red blood cells produces hemolysis, releasing components capable of propagating the DIC cycle. With generation of factor XIIa, there is activation of the kinin system with production of circulating kinins (93,94). Excess bradykinin produces several common clinical manifestations of DIC, such as systemic hypotension and increased vascular permeability (95,96). Thus, once begun, the cycle of DIC is self-propagating.

Diagnosis

Essentially, DIC is a clinical diagnosis (Table 20-6). Confirmatory laboratory tests are required because the signs and symptoms are so variable (Table 20-7). The most common presentation of DIC is hemorrhage, which usually occurs when secondary fibrinogenolysis dominates and FSPs are present in a high concentration (e.g., abruptio placentae) (39). Spontaneous bruising, prolonged bleeding from venipuncture sites or intraarterial lines, oozing from traumatic or surgical wounds, and petechiae are common (86,88,95). When DIC occurs acutely, hemorrhage is associated with hypovolemia, hypotension, and shock. Low-grade DIC, however, presents with subacute bleeding and diffuse thrombosis (86,88,95). When the intravascular clotting process dominates and secondary fibrinogenolysis is minimal, diffuse thrombosis is a common presentation (e.g., malignancy) (39). Both microvascular and large vessel thrombosis occurs, which may not be clinically apparent (86,88,95). Similarly, microvascular thrombosis in the kidneys leads to acute renal failure, and acute tubular necrosis is common. Microvascular thrombosis also may lead to generalized cortical and brainstem dysfunction with impaired consciousness and coma. The combination of hemorrhage and thrombosis in the lungs leads to progressive respiratory failure. In the obstetric patient, DIC can occur as a chronic disorder without clinical signs and may manifest only by laboratory abnormalities.

The clinical diagnosis always should be confirmed by laboratory diagnosis (Table 20-8). The characteristic findings include prolongation of the PT and PTT, an abnormal platelet count (low and high), abnormal clotting factor concentrations, elevated FSP, abnormal clot retraction, reduced AT III activity, a positive protamine sulfate test, leukocytosis, and schistocytosis on a smear of peripheral blood. All parameters may be abnormal in an acute DIC, whereas in chronic DIC only individual factor consumption rates may be elevated.

The key event in the coagulation of blood is the conversion of prothrombin to thrombin. Thrombin then com-

TABLE 20-6. *Clinical presentation of disseminated intravascular coagulation*

Evidence of hemorrhage	Petechiae and purpura Wound bleeding Spontaneous bruising Bleeding venipuncture sites or intraarterial lines Intracranial hemorrhage Gastrointestinal hemorrhage Respiratory tract hemorrhage
Evidence of thrombosis	Organ failure Skin necrosis Gangrene Venous thromboembolism Coma
Evidence of cytokine and kinin generation	Fever Tachycardia Hypotension Edema

TABLE 20-7. *Laboratory tests used for diagnosing DIC*

Most reliable	Often abnormal
D-Dimer	PT
AT III	PTT
FPA	Platelet count
FSP	Fibrinogen

AT III, antithrombin factor III; DIC, disseminated intravascular coagulation; FPA, fibrinopeptide A; FSP, fibrin split product; PT, prothrombin time; PTT, partial thromboplastin time.

TABLE 20-8. *Therapy for acute disseminated intravascular coagulation*

Treatment of triggering event
Evacuation of uterus
Antibiotics
Volume expansion and replacement
Component therapy
Packaged red cells
Platelets
Fresh-frozen plasma
Prothrombin complex
Anticoagulant therapy
Low-dose heparin
Heparin
Antiplatelet drugs
Antithrombin concentrates
Inhibition of residual fibrinolysis
Epsilon-amino caproic acid or tranexamic acid

bines with its antagonist AT III to form the thrombin-AT III (TAT) complex or proteolyses fibrinogen with the release of FPA (96). The FPA levels are abnormal in about 88% of patients with DIC (97). The FPA levels increase as a function of age and may be involved in many other types of thrombotic events (98). AT III is a major *in vivo* inhibitor of thrombin production, and it usually declines as consumption exceeds production. It is abnormal in 89% of patients with DIC. In patients with malignancy and diabetes, it can behave as an acute-phase reactant and may be normal or slightly increased despite rapid consumption. Thus, the sensitivity of the test is reduced. In contrast, the sensitivity of AT III measurement to excess clotting activity seems to increase. During normal pregnancy, plasma AT III activity is essentially unchanged (95); however, it declines in the presence of systemic illnesses such as pyelonephritis, viral infection, and bacterial pneumonia (84). The most sensitive test in diagnosing DIC is measurement of the D-dimer, which is abnormal in 93% of patients with confirmed DIC (97). Fifty percent of patients with acute DIC have both a prolonged PT and PTT, although these times may be shortened in patients with chronic DIC. The FSP will be abnormal in 85% of patients with DIC (88). Ten percent of patients with acute DIC will have negative paracoagulation tests (84). It is possible that the FSPs are degraded past the point of detection for commercially available assays. As a result of variations in renal clearance, the actual FSP titer may have little clinical relevance.

Treatment

The primary therapeutic goal is to treat the underlying disorder and thus remove the triggering event (see Table 20-8) (99). Because DIC is complicated by hemorrhage, treatment must include aggressive support of blood volume (washed packed red cells, crystalloids, and colloids), blood pressure (pressor medications), and antibiotics as needed. Underreplacement of volume is a common error, as hypotension and hypoperfusion may lead to hypoxic ischemia, which in turn damages the microvascular endothelium, thus providing a new trigger for the DIC cycle. In most obstetric-related DIC cases, these steps constitute adequate therapy. Component replacement [platelets, cryoprecipitate, or fresh frozen plasma (FFP)] occasionally may be helpful to aid in controlling bleeding. FFP and cryoprecipitate contain fibrinogen, which may lead to higher levels of FSP, which impairs hemostasis. When the underlying cause of DIC has been treated and the cycle is broken, replacement does not add fuel to the fire (100).

Anticoagulation should be initiated only when the aforementioned measures fail to correct a clinically significant DIC. This situation is exceedingly rare in the obstetric patient. If the hemorrhage is not severe, the patient should be observed for 4 hours after treatment of the underlying disease before starting anticoagulants to allow adequate time for laboratory evaluation to identify the precise clotting defect. In the past, heparin has been given for anticoagulation, but its efficacy was unpredictable, partially because of the variable AT III concentration at the time of anticoagulation (101,102). If the use of heparain is being considered, the AT III activity should be determined.

In many circumstances, low-dose heparin appears to be as effective as larger doses. It also minimizes the possibility of exacerbating the hemorrhage. Heparin is given subcutaneously (5,000 U every 8 to 12 hours). The PTT should normalize with treatment. Acute DIC secondary to obstetric complications also has been treated successfully with the use of concentrated AT III (103,104). The dose of AT III concentrate is calculated as follows (105):

$$\text{Total units needed} = (\text{desired} - \text{initial level}) \times 0.6 \times \text{total body weight (kg)}$$

One should attempt to obtain a level of 125% of normal or greater. This calculated dose can be delivered every 8 hours. Newer agents with potential therapeutic benefit being tested at this time include recombinant hirudin, defibrotide, and gabexate (106,107). After this therapy, a rare patient may continue to bleed secondary to residual fibrinogenolysis. This is one of two instances in obstetrics when antifibrinolytic agents such as epsilon-amino caproic acid or tranexamic acid may be of value for the treatment of DIC.

Obstetric Causes

Pregnancy is, as noted, a hypercoagulable condition (75). There is good clinical and experimental evidence that pregnancy predisposes young women to develop DIC

(108,109). Five major pregnancy-related entities can be associated with DIC: preeclampsia, placental abruption, dead fetus syndrome, septic abortion, and amniotic fluid embolism.

Preeclampsia/Eclampsia Syndrome

Overt DIC is uncommon in women with preeclampsia. Although thrombocytopenia is present in some 10% of women with severe preeclampsia or eclampsia, only a small percentage develop symptomatic bleeding.

There is overwhelming evidence that a subclinical, consumptive coagulopathy occurs in women with the clinical diagnosis of preeclampsia. The earliest laboratory sign of preeclampsia is a decrease in the number of platelets (110). Platelet factor 4 and β-thromboglobulin are elevated (111). These changes often occur before the clinical onset of disease (112). Fibrinlike material often is identified in renal and liver biopsy specimens from preeclamptic women (40,112,113). A decrease in AT III occurs in preeclampsia, which is in proportion to severity and secondary to increased consumption (76,114,115). Factor VIII consumption increases in amounts that also correlate with disease severity. These changes occur before the clinical manifestations of the disease appearing (116–118). The FPA concentration also is elevated significantly in women who have preeclampsia (82,119). Other laboratory findings include a reduction in plasma protein C antigenicity and activity (120), elevation of the D-dimer (121), elevation of the TAT complex (122), and elevation of plasminogen activator inhibitor (123). Between 30 and 32 weeks' gestation, the fibrinolytic activity of whole blood decreases and is decreased additionally in women who have preeclampsia (77). This is often the time in which preeclampsia manifests itself clinically. These coagulation abnormalities are not seen in women who have chronic hypertension but no other evidence of preeclampsia. The observation that some women with the clinical diagnosis of preeclampsia do not show these changes is consistent with the reported 15% to 65% error in the clinical diagnosis of preeclampsia (definitive diagnosis based on renal biopsies) (124). The clinical diagnosis of preeclampsia is frequently wrong if a renal biopsy is taken as the ultimate test. This situation may lead to a preterm delivery being performed on the assumption that pharmacologic therapy of hypertension is inappropriate. The measurement of plasma AT III activity may be helpful because normal activity is uncommon in women who have significant preeclampsia (125). In a patient whose AT III activity is normal, a trial of oral antihypertensive therapy is a reasonable approach in the absence of maternal or fetal distress.

All hypertensive women in labor should have a platelet count because the degree of thrombocytopenia does not necessarily correlate with disease severity. No other tests are needed for vaginal delivery. PT and PTT also can be justified based on an increased likelihood of cesarean delivery, especially in patients remote from term. In the absence of significant hemorrhage, measurement of the FSP is unnecessary. In the presence of DIC, AT III concentrate reportedly normalizes consumption (104). If AT III concentrate is not available, FFP should be used because of its high concentration of AT III. No other anticoagulation is needed. A bleeding diathesis can develop in a preeclamptic woman based on component depletion; however, this is a rare occurrence. The effect of preeclampsia on the fetal and neonatal clotting system is unclear.

Abruptio Placentae

Placental abruption is the most common obstetric cause of an acute DIC. In about 20% of women with abruptio placentae, there is a gross defect in clotting (126). Of these, one fourth will have a postpartum hemorrhage. This number excludes women whose clotting disorder is based on massive blood loss and tissue hypoxia.

Massive extravascular clot formation with secondary component consumption does not explain the alterations in coagulation in women with placental abruption. The consumption of the soluble components and activation of the fibrinolytic system are out of proportion to the blood loss. Hypofibrinogenemia often precedes postpartum hemorrhage, with FSP concentration having the greatest correlation with postpartum hemorrhage of any laboratory parameter (127). The source of FSP in patients with abruption is unclear. Fibrinolytic activity is similar in both uterine artery and vein when both placenta and fetus are healthy (127,128); however, the FSP and presumably plasminogen activator increase significantly in the uterine vein effluent after normal delivery. This occurs after an abruption, even if the fetus and placenta remain *in utero* (127). Thus, placental separation itself contributes to the FSP elevation. The concentration of FSP continues to increase during labor if the placenta has separated only partially and peaks shortly after complete placental separation. After delivery, it is cleared from the circulation within 12 to 24 hours (129). The FSP concentration in the lochia of women with abruptio placentae is also significantly higher than that in the lochia of normal women after delivery (127). High doses of FSP inhibit myometrial contractility (127), and intravenous infusion of an antifibrinogenolytic agent reverses uterine inertia secondary to placental abruption (129).

The management of acute abruptio placentae follows general guidelines for management of DIC. The uterus should be emptied and blood volume supported with crystalloid, colloid, or blood products as necessary. Coagulation components may be required if surgical intervention is contemplated. Once emptied, the uterus responds well to oxytocin (and antifibrinolytic agents, primarily used for experimental purposes).

A chronic placental abruption is as difficult to manage as it is to diagnose. A suspected small abruption remote from term may be managed expectantly if symptoms resolve, laboratory abnormalities do not exist, and fetal testing remains normal.

The perinatal morbidity and mortality from abruptio placentae increase with delay in diagnosis and management. If the fetus is alive when the mother is admitted but subsequently died *in utero*, 75% of these deaths occurred more than 90 minutes after admission. Seventy percent of the perinatal mortality occurred 2 hours or longer after the diagnosis of placental abruption was entered into the record (130). In a patient with abruptio placentae, if labor progresses appropriately with normal coagulation parameters, the fetus is not in distress, and an emergency cesarean section can be performed, a closely observed labor is preferred. If any of these abnormalities are observed, delivery should be effected immediately.

Fetal Death Syndrome

This syndrome may occur following the death of a singleton fetus or of one fetus in a multiple gestation. Onset of FDS is gradual, with most standard laboratory test abnormalities not detected until 3 to 4 weeks after the death (131). The concentration of fibrinopeptide A has been shown to increase within days. Manifestations of the coagulopathy include a varying degree of hypofibrinogenemia, decreased plasminogen, decreased AT III activity, increased generation of both FPA and FSP, and thrombocytopenia (132). The laboratory picture is consistent with a true chronic DIC condition (133). The cause of the syndrome is unknown. Theories have been proposed that include a leak of tissue thromboplastin from a decaying fetus into the maternal circulation. Anitfibrinolytics have little benefit, suggesting that fibrinolysis does not contribute to the syndrome significantly (132).

About 80% of women with an intrauterine fetal demise (IUFD) have labor spontaneously within 2 to 3 weeks. Of the undelivered patients, one third will develop a progressive hemostatic defect within 4 to 5 weeks after the death. The incidence of coagulopathy increases with the duration of the delay, but only 1% to 2% of these women suffer a significant hemorrhagic complication. The treatment of a medically stable patient with a singleton IUFD is delivery.

A dilemma arises when a fetus who has died is part of a preterm multiple gestation. Recent reports document a limited duration of the coagulopathy secondary to the death of one fetus, suggesting that delivery need not be effected immediately (134–136).

There are also fetal implications in multiple gestations with FDS. In monozygotic gestations with vascular anastomoses, thromboplastic material theoretically might embolize to the surviving fetus, producing fetal DIC, multicystic encephalomalacia, or other structural anomalies. Whether this occurs or not is unclear (137–140). Heparin does not cross the placenta; therefore, it would not protect the fetus in this scenario.

Heparin is the treatment of choice when the mother's coagulopathy is associated with FDS. Most women require 5,000 to 10,000 U subcutaneously twice a day. There are case reports in which heparin was inadequate to reverse laboratory anomalies, even in large doses (136). This resistance to heparin may reflect a decreased concentration of AT III. Theoretically, it should be possible to titrate the heparin dose based on normalization of the fibrinopeptide A level. A prompt increase in plasma fibrinogen should follow.

Septic Abortion

All patients with septic shock and septic abortion can be demonstrated to have an altered coagulation profile if tested thoroughly (141). The resultant coagulopathy is consistent with a true DIC accompanied by various degrees of fibrinolysis (142). The degree of coagulopathy correlates with the severity of the disease. Bacterial endotoxin is usually the initiating mechanism. Increased sensitivity to bacterial endotoxin has been demonstrated during pregnancy (143–146). The shock syndrome results from a complex interaction between endotoxin, the vascular endothelium, platelets, and complement, ultimately generating histamines, kinins, and serotonin. This situation results in hypotension, hypoxia, and acidosis, which then perpetuate the cycle of kinin activation.

The main clinical findings of septic shock are secondary to DIC. Kinin activation occurs early in the clotting cascade; the amount of kallikrein generated correlates directly with the severity of the shock (95). Fibrin emboli within the microvasculature create massive perfusion disturbances that affect blood stasis and cause hypotension. Death most often results from pulmonary complications (147,148).

Aggressive antibiotic therapy and evacuation of the uterus in the absence of shock are the foundations of treatment. If septic shock is present, fluid replacement should be guided by pulmonary artery catheter measurements. Ringer's lactate solution should be avoided because it may potentiate a metabolic acidosis (149). Red blood cells should be used to maintain the hematocrit above 36%. High-dose corticosteroids (30 mg/kg) may be useful in stabilizing biomembranes, exerting a positive inotropic effect upon the heart, dilating the vasculature, and preventing beta-endorphin release by the pituitary (150–152). In reference to the latter, pretreatment with naloxone may reduce the severity of septic shock (153,154). Mortality from septic shock in an otherwise healthy patient is 20% compared with 80% in cancer patients (150).

Rapid resolution of the coagulopathy in septic shock depends on eradication of the septic source. The use of anticoagulation is controversial. Because sepsis is associated with widespread activation of the clotting cascade and microvascular fibrin thrombi would disrupt flow even further, administration of heparin would seem logical to prevent further fibrin generation; however, it neither prevents kinin activation nor eliminates platelet aggregation.

The published clinical experience with septic shock does not resolve this controversy. Reports have demonstrated both no difference and increased survival in patients receiving heparin therapy (155,156). Heterogeneity of both AT III and underlying disease may be responsible for the differences in patient response to heparin. Heparin administration is suggested in a patient with a profound hypofibrinogenemia and thrombocytopenia in conjunction with factor coagulation replacement. In this instance, the therapeutic goal is a PTT 1.5 to 2.0 times baseline. Coagulation factor replacement is done best with FFP. Prophylactic heparin seems to be indicated in women with septic abortions because it decreases the incidence of subsequent septic shock and reduces the level of soluble fibrin monomer to normal. Subcutaneous heparin 5,000 U given two or three times daily is sufficient (141,157).

Amniotic Fluid Embolus

The incidence of amniotic fluid embolism (AFE) ranges between 1 in 8,000 and 1 in 800,000 deliveries. It is also responsible for 10% of the maternal mortality in industrialized countries. The associated mortality rate approximates 80% in most series. As a result of its rarity, no large therapeutic trials have been done to guide the treatment of AFE.

Diagnosis

An AFE may occur anytime during the peripartal period. The initial phase (phase 1) is that of profound cardiovascular collapse, which is of short duration. Phase 2 begins shortly afterward but may occur up to 4 hours after phase 1. Phase 2 is associated with the onset of uterine bleeding refractory to oxytocin, bleeding from old puncture sites, and easy bruisability (158).

Diagnostically, it is difficult to document an AFE without a postmortem examination. The presence of fetal debris in a blood sample drawn from a right-sided cardiac catheter is thought to be diagnostic of AFE (159). This conclusion was based on a unique and unrepeated study of the transfer of radiolabeled red blood cells from the amniotic cavity into the maternal circulation (160). Fetal debris, however, can be found in samples obtained from the right heart of asymptomatic women (161). Therefore, the finding of fetal squames in a right-sided cardiac blood sample is consistent with but not diagnostic of AFE.

Pathophysiology

The pathophysiology of AFE is not completely understood. Phase 1 is associated with intense pulmonary vasospasm and interstitial edema, which results in myocardial necrosis with characteristic electrocardiographic changes (162). It was thought that the pulmonary arterial pressure increases with cardiac output decreasing secondary to increased afterload; however, recent studies reveal that left ventricular failure occurs without pulmonary hypertension (163). Phase 1 has been difficult to document because few patients have had a Swan Ganz catheter in place at time of AFE. Animal model studies have demonstrated that pulmonary artery pressure does increase; however, it returns to normal within 30 minutes and usually presents as a mixed respiratory-metabolic acidosis. The appearance of pulmonary edema and shock is evidence of worsening clinical status.

About 50% of patients survive phase 1. Patients who survive phase 1 are at risk of developing severe coagulopathy and uterine atony during phase 2. Few hematologically well-studied cases of AFE are reported in the literature. Each reports a profound excess of fibrinolytic activity as demonstrated by decreased plasminogen levels, increased plasmin activator, or a high concentration of FSPs (164–166). Laboratory abnormalities precede the clinical manifestations by 30 to 60 minutes (162,164). Numerous soluble clotting factors are decreased, and in most cases there is hypofibrinogenemia. The excess plasmin activation results in nonspecific proteolysis of various proenzymes. It is difficult to predict how much of the reduced clotting component concentration represents proenzyme degradation rather than thrombin-mediated consumption, because FPA has yet to be studied during an AFE. Potentially, this information would affect therapy.

The amniotic fluid volume necessary to cause the syndrome is unknown; however, it may not be the volume of intravascular amniotic fluid per se but rather the result of an abnormal substance(s) in the amniotic fluid (167). The cause of the coagulopathy is also controversial. When amniotic fluid is added to human plasma, it accelerates the clotting pathway through factor X (168). This procoagulant effect persists even after filtering the amniotic fluid and correlates with both gestational age and phospholipid content (169,170). Parenteral administration of unfiltered but not of filtered amniotic fluid evokes the syndrome in dogs, showing that there are species differences (171). Human amniotic fluid collected during labor is far more toxic to the cat than amniotic fluid collected from nonlaboring women (172). Some hemodynamic and procoagulant effects of the AFE syndrome can be mimicked by prostaglandins and leukotrienes, which are increased during labor (173), and pretreatment with an inhibitor of the lipoxygenase system (including leukotrienes) prevents death after intravascular injection of amniotic fluid in the rabbit (174).

Controversy exists over the cause of hypofibrinogenemia in the AFE syndrome. Some investigators favor primary fibrinogenolysis as the mechanism rather than a consumptive coagulopathy with secondary fibrinolysis (165,166). The finding of fibrin thrombi scattered throughout the pulmonary vascular bed argues against primary fibrinogenolysis as the sole explanation. Endothelial abrasion from particulate emboli coupled with cardiovascular collapse may produce sufficient damage to initiate fibrin generation, resulting in elevated FPA. Thrombin-mediated fibrin generation secondary to pulmonary endothelial damage would activate both plasmin and kinin which, in the absence of antiplasmin, would perpetuate their own generation. If thrombin generation occurred in the setting of excess plasmin proactivator, a coagulopathy dominated by fibrin fibrinogenolysis could result (175), which would lead to lysis of recent fibrin thrombi within the uterine spiral arteries and at previous puncture sites and result in bleeding. The high level of FSP could inhibit uterine contractility, leading to frank hemorrhage.

Treatment

There is no successful therapeutic protocol. Phase 1 therapy should be directed toward cardiovascular and ventilatory support. A pulmonary artery catheter should be placed. A clotting profile and heparinized sample for histologic study, as well as extra tubes of citrated blood for later study, next should be drawn from the catheter. Resuscitation with colloids and the use of pressor agents should be dictated by the information obtained from the pulmonary artery catheter. Fluid overload must be carefully avoided. Rapid digitalization may help.

Patients should be intubated immediately to provide ventilatory support. Use of positive end-expiratory pressure (PEEP) should be guided by parameters obtained from the pulmonary artery catheter (150). If, for example, the contributions of interstitial edema and capillary permeability abnormalities to pulmonary edema are minimal, the lungs may remain compliant. With compliant lungs, PEEP could increase right ventricular afterload, produce bulging of the interventricular septum into the left ventricle, and decrease stroke volume and cardiac output. Such an event would more than offset any ventilatory gain from PEEP (150). Both corticosteroids and aminophylline have been used to treat coexistent bronchospasm.

Whether the AFE-associated coagulopathy can be prevented is unclear. Survival after administration of a small dose of heparin has been documented in one patient (176). This patient had evidence of a clotting abnormality without evidence of hemorrhage. Heparin would be the logical choice to blunt cascade activation and the resulting plasmin generation; however, the quantity of heparin necessary to do this is unknown. Knowledge of the FPA level would be helpful in this situation. If the FPA concentration is high, it would indicate massive thrombin generation and the need for large quantities of heparin. A single intravenous heparin bolus of 3,000 to 5,000 U on diagnosis would be an option (174).

Once fibrin fibrinogenolysis is well established, component therapy alone may be adequate (164,177). Should the patient fail to respond to this plan, administration of an antifibrinolytic agent (epsilon-amino caproic acid or aprotinin) should be considered. The dose of epsilon-amino caproic acid is 4 to 6 g every 4 to 6 hours.

Other Obstetrically Related Causes

DIC has been demonstrated to occur in patients with placenta previa, placenta accreta, degenerating leiomyomas, and hydatidiform mole (178–181). Some data are consistent with DIC and secondary fibrinolysis, whereas other reports merely reflect extravascular consumption with associated intravascular depletion.

Nonobstetric Causes

Antibiotics

Many broad-spectrum antibiotics are associated with hypoprothrombinemia. Malnourished patients seem to be those at highest risk. Different mechanisms have been proposed (182,183). The first is depletion of the bowel flora that synthesize vitamin K. Methyltetrazolethiol, a cephalosporin metabolite that directly inhibits hepatic prothrombin synthesis, suggests another possible mechanism. A PT should be obtained periodically on patients at risk, such as before surgery. The parental administration of vitamin K reverses these abnormalities. These same antibiotics augment warfarin anticoagulation by depleting bowel flora and by displacing warfarin from albumin (182).

Some antibiotics inhibit platelet function directly. The mechanism of action is due to a decreased ADP-mediated platelet aggregation (184,185). One metabolite of penicillin is thought to bind to the platelet membrane ADP receptor. Effects are dose related and are detectable 12 to 24 hours after first administration of the drug. The effects may last for up to 12 days and usually are seen in the setting of high-dose penicillin or of cephalosporin administration for severe gram-negative infections.

Acquired Inhibitors

Specific inhibitors of individual clotting factors have been identified in previously healthy women during pregnancy. Often they are antibodies. Inhibitors of factors V, VIII:C, VIII:RCo, IX, XI, and XIII all have been reported in previously healthy women (186–192). The most common inhibitors are antiphospolipid antibodies and antifactor VIII antibodies.

A factor deficit is most easily differentiated from an inhibitor by performing a 1:1 mix of the patient's plasma with normal plasma. If the clotting time remains prolonged, an inhibitor is present; however, a low-titer inhibitor may become apparent only after incubating the plasma mix. An antibody inhibitor usually shows progressive, time-dependent prolongation of the clotting time.

The antiphospholipid antibodies are a group of autoantibodies that include the lupus anticoagulant (LA) and anticardiolipin antibodies (ACA) and antibodies found in serologic tests for syphilis. They have been identified in association with a wide variety of diseases and drugs, including chlorpromazine and penicillin (192–194). ACAs block the binding of phospholipids and interfere with the action of the preformed prothrombinase complex, prolonging both the PT and PTT (195,196). The addition of phospholipid corrects the abnormality. Incubation of LA with normal plasma does not decrease clotting time further. This anticoagulant has been associated with recurrent fetal demise, congenital heart block, and intrauterine growth restriction (187,197–199). The fetal heart block is secondary to an associated antibody, anti-SS-A (Ro), which binds RNA in the right atrial wall (200). Women with lupus and an inhibitor have a worse perinatal outcome with the presence of lupus and no inhibitor. Any combination of an inhibitor with prior fetal demise has a high incidence of perinatal death (201). Factor VIII is not decreased and bleeding is uncommon. Rather, these women are at highest risk for thrombosis.

Treatment has been demonstrated to be beneficial during pregnancy, although the optimal regimen is unclear. Several regimens have been tried with outcomes judged on the basis of prepregnancy and postpregnancy loss rates (202,203). See Chapter 37 for management guidelines.

Factor VIII inhibitors are associated with hemorrhage indistinguishable clinically from hemophilia (190). These inhibitors are autoantibodies in the nonhemophilic population, or they may be alloinhibitors (complication of treatment with factor VIII infusates in patients with classic hemophilia). The severity of disease and number of treatments are risk factors for the development of alloinhibitors (204,205). Autoantibodies to factor VIII are time and temperature dependent and are usually an IgG class antibody that therefore may cross the placenta. Only the PTT is prolonged. This syndrome often presents as a catastrophic, delayed postpartum hemorrhage (186, 188–190). Factor VIII inhibitor usually is missed or identified after surgical intervention for presumed uterine atony. Autoinhibitors may disappear within 18 months of delivery and, once gone, there are no reports of recurrences during a subsequent pregnancy.

Treatment regimens available for patients with factor VIII inhibitor are most unsatisfactory (206). These regimens include factor VIII replacement, which actually may increase the antibody titer. Treatment options include bovine or porcine factor VIII concentrate; continuous slow infusion of the concentrate, which may be more effective than bolus administration; or administration of prothrombin complex concentrate (PCC) or activated prothrombin concentrates (APC) (205,206). Corticosteroids, immunosuppressants, exchange transfusion, and plasmapheresis are ineffective. Antifactor IX antibodies are predominantly immunoglobulin G (IgG) and not temperature or time dependent. They are more common in hemophilia B than in hemophilia A and usually are treated with high-purity concentrates PCC and APC.

Inhibitors to coagulation factors V, VII, IX, X, and XI are rare. A reasonable approach to treat them is to treat the underlying disease. Therapeutic measures include IgG, plasma exchange, immunoabsorption procedures, and immunosuppressant agents.

HEREDITARY COAGULOPATHIES

A genetically determined defect has been identified at most points in the coagulation cascade. These defects are found in the smallest group of patients with a clotting abnormality seen by the practicing obstetrician. The discussion that follows focuses on the more common of these defects.

Von Willebrand Disease

von Willebrand disease (VWD), a disorder of hemostasis, is caused by a reduction in or abnormality of VWF, which is a glycoprotein normally found in plasma, endothelial cells, the subendothelial space, megakaryocytes, and platelets (208). VWF is synthesized in megakaryoctes and endothelial cells (209,210). Adhesion of platelets to the injured subendothelium is mediated by VWF. It also participates in platelet aggregation, carries factor VIII, and provides a protective role for factor VIII. Defects in VWF can cause bleeding by impairing platelet adhesion or blood clotting (211).

VWD is a heterogeneous group of disorders with different phenotypes that are inherited as an autosomal dominant trait. There are three major categories based on the type of factor VIII deficiency (Table 20-9) (212). Type 1 is a partial qualitative deficiency, type 2 is a qualitative deficiency that is subdivided into four variants (2A, 2B, 2M, 2N), and type 3 is a total deficiency. Patients with VWD have mucocutaneous, posttraumatic, and postoperative bleeding. Occasionally, VWD presents as menorrhagia or postpartum hemorrhage. It can be difficult to diagnose, because only moderate to severe forms are characterized by a prolonged bleeding time. Inconsistently abnormal bleeding times are common in patients who have milder forms. A single normal factor VIII level or bleeding time therefore does not exclude the diagnosis of VWD.

TABLE 20-9. *Classification, diagnosis and treatment of von Willebrand disease*

Type	Frequency	Clinical features	Diagnosis	Treatment
1	1/10,000 Autosomal dominant	Mild to moderate bleeding	VWF:Ag and VWF:RCo in the range of 20%–50%, VIII:C activity reduced	DDAVP FVIII concentrates (Hemate P)
2A	10%–15% of cases General autosomal dominant	Mild to moderate bleeding	Variably decreased VWF:Ag, VWF:RCo and VIII:C; absent high and intermediate size VWF multimers with prominent satellite bands	FVIII concentrates (Hemate P)
2B	<5% of cases Autosomal dominant	Mild to moderate bleeding	Variably decreased VWF:Ag, VWF:RCo and VIII:C; loss of large VWF multimers; thrombocytopenia	FVIII concentrates (Hemate P); platelet transfusion
2M	Rare Autosomal dominant	Variable bleeding	Variably decreased VWF:Ag, and VIII:C, VWF:RCo decreased	FVIII concentrates (Hemate P)
2N	Rare Autosomal dominant	Variable bleeding	Variably decreased VWF:Ag and VWF:RCo; disproportionately low VIII:C	DDAVP
3	1–5/1,000,000 Autosomal recessive	Severe bleeding	Markedly decreased or undetectable VWF:Ag, VWF:RCo and VIII:C	FVIII concentrates (Hemate P), DDAVP, recombinant factor VIII

Ag, antigen; DDAVP, 1-deamino-8-D-arginine vasopressin; FVIII, factor VIII; RCo, ristocein cofactor; VWF, von Willebrand factor.

Diagnosis

Laboratory evaluation from VWD includes ristocetin cofactor activity (VWF:RCo), which measures the VWF binding to platelet glycoprotein Ib in the presence of ristocetin and measures VWF functional activity. Normal VWF:RCo results are expressed as a percentage of the activity of a normal pooled plasma standard. Ristocetin-induced platelet aggregation (RIPA) is similar to VWF:RCo, except the patient's own platelets are used and the ristocetin is varied. An enhanced RIPA is necessary for the diagnosis of VWD type 2B and platelet-type pseudo-VWD. The VWF antigen (VWF:Ag), factor VIII function (VIII:C), and VWF multimer structure should be obtained (see Table 20-9).

Patients with VWD have been monitored during pregnancy (213–221). Labor and delivery are often uneventful, because VIII:C, VWF:AG, and VWF:RCo usually increase to hemostatic levels during pregnancy. This gradual increase (if it occurs) is seen after 11 to 12 weeks of gestation. This increase is not uniform in occurrence or degree; therefore, it should not be assumed that factor VIII complex is increasing (217,220). Individual components may decrease at varying rates, which could account for the 20% incidence of postpartum hemorrhage (213,217,219,220). A baseline VWF:AG and VWF:RCo should be obtained early in pregnancy; if the initial value is abnormal, the test should be repeated once or twice in the third trimester. Individual levels may be altered by blood type (persons with type O blood have lower levels than type AB), collagen vascular diseases, hyperthyroidism, DIC, and stress (221).

Treatment

A 50% level of VWF:RCo is sufficient for most hemostatic stresses (217). Thus, women with clinically mild disease whose indices normalize antepartum will not need prophylaxis for vaginal delivery. Episiotomy, deep injection of a local anesthetic, and conduction anesthesia should be avoided. Treatment of choice for mild type 1 VWD is DDAVP (1-deamino-8-D-arginine vasopressin, or desmopressin). Its mode of action is unknown. It is administered intravenously at a rate of 0.2 to 0.4 mg/kg over 15 to 30 minutes (222). The intranasal dose is as effective as the intravenous form (223). DDAVP elevates the VWF:AG and VWF:RCo activity to three to five times that of basal level within 30 minutes, lasting for 6 to 12 hours (224). A trial infusion of DDAVP should be attempted before its therapeutic use. Up to 20% of type 1 patients will not respond to this therapy. This group is known as the *platelet low group* based on plasma and platelet VWF levels (225). In patients with type 2 and 3 VWD, DDAVP is of limited usefulness. It may even be contraindicated in type 2B (226). Factor replacement should be given to patients who are unresponsive to DDAVP or in whom it is contraindicated (227). Preparations containing large quantities of VWF are used for replacement therapy. The most frequently used concentrate in the United States is Hemate P. Therapy with Hemate P is empiric, often determined by prior response to treatment. There are no clear guidelines for monitoring therapy. If factor replacement in unavailable, cryoprecipitate can be used. Cryoprecipitate should also be available in case of emergency. Patients with thrombocytopenia may need platelet transfusions in addition to factor replacement.

Prophylactic DDAVP is indicated for vaginal delivery if the VIII:RCo level fails to reach 80% by term. Postpartum, serial VIII:RCo levels or bleeding times are obtained and DDAVP therapy is given for 7 days to prevent delayed hemorrhage. Postpartum hemorrhage may occur for up to a month after delivery; therefore, it may be advisable to monitor serial VIII:RCo levels or bleeding times weekly after discontinuation of therapy. DDAVP or factor replacement should be given regardless of the laboratory parameters to all but the mildest cases of VWD if cesarean section is contemplated. Therapy is given to raise the VIII:RCo level above 100%. Postoperatively, the VIII:RCo level is maintained at 100% until the abdominal sutures are removed (217). Antiplatelet drugs and intramuscular injections should be avoided.

The fetus is assumed to be affected unless proven otherwise. The use of a scalp electrode is precluded. Fetal hemorrhage during labor resulting from VWD is rare, although intracranial hemorrhage (ICH) during labor has been reported. Circumcision should be avoided until the diagnosis is ruled out. Prenatal diagnosis is possible from fetal blood. Fetal factor VIII:RCo can be measured by the technique of Weiss and co-workers (228). Type 1 is usually a mild condition; so cordocentesis usually can be performed without significant risk of maternal hemorrhage. Types 2 and 3, however, can be severe, and maternal transfusion of factor replacement may be necessary before cordocentesis.

Hemophilia A and B

Hemophilia A and B are characterized, respectively, by low levels of either factor VIII coagulant (VIII:C) or factor IX coagulant (IX:C) activity and a normal to increased level of the factor-related antigen (VIII:Ag, IX:Ag). Both are X-linked and cannot be distinguished clinically. Hemophilia affects 20 in 100,000 males; thus, an estimated 1 in 5,000 women are carriers (229,230). Eighty-five percent of hemophilia cases are of hemophilia A. One third of men with hemophilia have no family history of a bleeding disorder, suggesting that their illness is the result of a spontaneous mutation (231).

The smallest unit in the factor VIII complex is the factor VIII protein (VIII). It contains the locus responsible for the coagulation activity of factor VIII. Coagulant activity also can be determined immunologically using an antibody directed against this section of the multimer (VIII:C) (232). Its immunologic presence can be measured (VIII:Ag). Factor IX also may be measured by both its coagulant activity (IX:C) and its immunologic presence (IX:Ag).

The task of the obstetrician includes carrier identification, treatment of the symptomatic pregnant women, and prenatal diagnosis. Because one X chromosome is randomly inactivated in each cell (lyonization), the average ratio of the related antigen to coagulant activity is 2:1. Measurement of this ratio allows the diagnosis of 80% to 90% of nonpregnant carrier women (233–237). In 10% to 20% of carriers, extreme lyonization occurs, resulting in significantly lower levels of VIII and IX (<40%) and an increase in hemorrhagic problems (238). Pregnancy induces an increase in VIII levels in carriers of hemophilia A but not in IX levels in carriers of hemophilia B (239). Although the ratio of antigen-to-coagulant activity increases with increasing gestational age to a variable degree, pregnant women should not be denied carrier analysis before 20 weeks' gestation. For reasons unknown, a higher percentage of carrier identification has been reported in the second trimester than in the nonpregnant state (240).

Rarely are carriers of hemophilia symptomatic. Levels of VIII:C and VIII:Ag should be determined at the patient's first visit and again at 28 and 34 weeks' gestation (239). Women whose VIII:C is less than 50% at delivery and who undergo cesarean section should be given DDAVP adequate to elevate the VIII:C level above 80% before surgery and to keep it above 30% to 40% for 3 to 4 days postoperatively. If the VIII:C level is less than 30% DDAVP, high-purity factor concentrates or recombinant FVIII should be given before delivery regardless of the type. High-purity factor concentrate is given to women who have hemophilia B. Similarly, women undergoing invasive prenatal diagnostic procedures, spontaneous abortion, and termination of pregnancy whose level is less than 30% should receive prophylaxis. Cryoprecipitate can be used if first-line agents are not available. Cryoprecipitate contains little active factor IX. Therefore, FFP can be used in women with hemophilia B. Prothrombin complex concentrates are given only to patients who have severe disease because of the risk of thrombosis.

Hemophilia A and B may be diagnosed prenatally by either DNA analysis or direct study of fetal blood. A database of mutations in the factor VIII gene has been published and is updated constantly (242). The method depends on the gestational age at which the patient is first seen and the degree to which the patient's family has been studied. The first step is to determine the karyotype. Before 10 weeks' gestation, chorionic villus sampling may be done, and amniocentesis may be done thereafter. Because there seems to be a variety of possible deletions and point mutations involved, family members should be investigated. If the restriction fragment length polymorphism linkage studies of the family are informative, they can be applied for a definitive diagnosis. All normal results should be confirmed later by coagulation studies of fetal blood (241). By the midsecond trimester, definitive diagnosis of fetal hemophilia A is possible by measuring the ratio of VIII:Ag to VIII:C in a blood sample obtained by cordocentesis (230,243). Cord blood should be collected at birth for confirmation or diagnosis if prenatal testing is refused. Prenatal diagnosis of an affected fetus changes intrapartum and early postnatal management. Intrapartum use of scalp electrodes, the vacuum extractor, forceps, and prolonged labor should be avoided (239,241,244). Six to ten percent of hemophiliac neonates suffer a perinatal hemorrhagic complication. Intramuscular injections should be avoided in affected male infants or when the coagulation status is not known (239).

Antibodies directed against factor VIII have been identified in the puerperium. They are acquired and may lead to severe hemorrhage, especially in the postpartum period (245,246). Administering prothrombin complex concentrates or porcine factor VIII to these patients may result in a therapeutic response (247).

Antithrombin III Deficiency

AT III is a major *in vivo* inhibitor of thrombin activity. The risk of thrombosis in women with AT III deficiency is increased exponentially in pregnancy (248–251). The activity of AT III is not significantly altered by pregnancy. Approximately two thirds of pregnant women with congenital AT III deficiency experience thrombosis; 75% of these occur antepartum (251). If the patient has a history of thromboembolism, the risk of thrombosis increases. Thrombosis occurs even after a first-trimester abortion. AT III deficiency also places a women at increased risk for abortion and stillbirth (252).

Treatment

The ideal regimen for thrombosis prophylaxis during pregnancy in women with an AT III deficiency until recently was somewhat controversial. The regimen of choice presently is to administer subcutaneous heparin throughout the pregnancy (252,253). Prophylactic AT III administration reduces thrombin hyperactivity in pregnancy (254), although large studies have not addressed this issue. Concentrates of AT III can be given during labor or if a thrombosis develops. FFP is less helpful than AT III in this situation (248,251,255–257). Low-molecular-weight heparins and thrombin inhibitors such as hirudin and argatroban are being evaluated for prophylaxis of medical and surgical deep venous thrombosis and in the treatment of patients with preexisting thrombosis (258).

Patients with AT III deficiency are resistant to heparin; so the quantity of heparin required for a given effect is usually larger than in the nondeficient patient. Effective prophylaxis requires enough heparin administered subcutaneously to prolong the activated PTT five to ten times above the patient's baseline throughout the pregnancy and puerperium (251). AT III deficiency also requires a higher dose of heparin secondary to heparin resistance. The PTT should be measured just before the next dose. When functional AT III activity is 40% to 50% of normal, the daily requirement is 20,000 to 45,000 IU of heparin. During an acute thrombotic episode, the daily requirement is 40,000 to 80,000 IU of heparin to prolong the PTT to 1.5 to 2 times above baseline (251). The patient continues to take heparin for 4 weeks postpartum or until conversion to chronic warfarin anticoagulation can be done successfully (259). AT III concentrate also may be of benefit. In a congenitally deficient person with a baseline level of 50%, the infusion of 50 U per kilogram of body weight of AT III concentrate will raise the plasma AT III level to 120% (260,261). Plasma levels should be monitored so that they are always higher than 80% (260). Warfarin, which is not known to affect AT III concentrations, may be used with danazol to provide anticoagulation postpartum; however, the dose of warfarin may need to be reduced to prevent excessive anticoagulation (262).

The newborn delivered to a woman with AT III deficiency should have plasma AT III activity measured, and if it is less than 10%, FFP should be administered. Possible neonatal complications include fatal thrombosis.

Protein C and Protein S Deficiencies

A number of other inherited coagulation disorders have implications for management in pregnancy. In general, small patient numbers preclude prospective trials of the recommended interventions, although some observations may be made.

Protein C deficiency is a heterozygous disorder associated with a propensity for venous thrombosis in early adulthood (263). It is an autosomal dominant trait with incomplete penetrance. The homozygous disorder can result in massive thrombosis during the neonatal period (264). Intrauterine central nervous system infarction has been described in homozygous fetuses (265). Pregnant patients may exhibit manifestations of protein C deficiency, usually presenting with thromboembolism (266, 267). Prophylaxis of thromboembolism during pregnancy with full anticoagulation with heparin is advised (267). Protein S, a protein C cofactor, as discussed previously, is associated with outcomes similar to protein C deficiency (268). For both disorders, prenatal diagnosis is possible using cordocentesis (269).

The result of APC resistance is a hypercoagulable state. Factor V Leiden (factor V Leiden mutation) occurs in 80% of patients with this disorder (56–58). It may be the most important hereditary cause of venous thrombosis, affecting up to 8% of the general population (270, 271). Persons who are heterozygous for this condition have an estimated fivefold to tenfold increased risk for venous thrombosis. Homozygosity for this condition has a 50- to 100-fold increased risk of venous thrombosis, and this risk increases with age. Factor V Leiden mutation is an important risk factor for the development of venous thromboembolism in pregnancy (272); 60% of women with this mutation who had a deep venous thrombosis or pulmonary embolism in pregnancy had evidence of venous thromboembolism in the first trimester (272). Patients known to have factor V Leiden mutation should have early prophylaxis with subcutaneous heparin therapy. Other causes of APC resistance in pregnancy should be managed in a similar way.

Other Inherited Coagulation Disorders

Factor V deficiency is an autosomal recessive disorder. It is commonly associated with menorrhagia and easy bruisability but rarely with hemarthrosis and intramuscular bleeding. Factor V increases to nearly normal concentrations during pregnancy. The major risk to the pregnant patient is postpartum hemorrhage (273–275). Treatment of choice is FFP. A report of severe fetal central nervous system hemorrhage at birth and *in utero* exists (276).

Factor X deficiency is an autosomal recessive disorder that appears to be well tolerated during pregnancy (277). Favorable pregnancy outcomes have been obtained using prophylactic clotting factor replacement with FFP (278). Clotting factor replacement only during labor has also been shown to be effective (277).

Factor XI deficiency is most common among Ashkenazi Jewish families and is an autosomal recessive disorder. Severity of the effect varies in a manner unrelated to the degree of factor XI deficiency. There is a slight decline in factor XI during pregnancy; however, these women tend to have pregnancies marked only by increased bleeding from delivery lacerations (279,280). It is recommended that levels of greater than 30% during labor, delivery, and postpartum be maintained with FFP (281).

Factor XII deficiency is an autosomal recessive trait in which affected women tolerate pregnancy well (282,283). Usually, it is not associated with clinically significant hemostatic abnormalities.

Factor XIII deficiency is also autosomal recessive. Levels of factor XIII decline during normal pregnancy. The deficiency is generally well tolerated in patients; however, the risk of postpartum hemorrhage seems to be increased (280). Factor XIII levels from 3% to 10% have been suggested to be sufficient to prevent spontaneous hemorrhages (284). Occasional patients with activity levels between 30% and 50% have prolonged secondary hemorrhages after an abortion or delivery (285). These cases require therapy during surgery and acute bleeding episodes. Long-term therapy is recommended to maintain the patient's factor XIII activity above 1% to 2% (286), achieved by either intermittent infusion of 300 to 450 mL of fresh-frozen plasma every 14 days or 30 IU per kilogram of body weight of concentrate every 4 weeks. Classically, the deficiency presents in the neonate as delayed bleeding from the umbilical cord stump. This disorder also has been associated with increased fetal wastage.

PLATELET DISORDERS

Quantitative or qualitative platelet disorders are common causes of abnormal coagulation in a pregnant woman. They often manifest as bleeding from mucous membranes or into the skin. Associated findings include easy bruising, epistaxis, gastrointestinal or gingival bleeding, hematuria, menorrhagia, and petechiae. The most serious complication is maternal or fetal central nervous system hemorrhage. A thorough understanding of these platelet disorders is essential because the implications are serious.

Thrombocytopenia

Thrombocytopenia is defined as a platelet count of less than 150,000 platelets/mm^3. Primary bone marrow disorders such as leukemias, lymphomas, megaloblastic anemia, and metastatic malignancies can cause thrombocytopenia. This review concentrates on the most likely and significant causes of isolated thrombocytopenia during pregnancy.

A combination of either decreased platelet production or increased consumption or destruction itself may lead to thrombocytopenia. We can make this distinction by measuring mean platelet volume and by doing a bone marrow evaluation. When production is down, megakaryocytes are decreased; when production is up, megakaryocytic hyperplasia is found. A relative but not an absolute thrombocytopenia may be caused by platelets pooling in the spleen. A bone marrow biopsy is also helpful in ruling out a primary marrow dyscrasia.

There are numerous causes of thrombocytopenia, including primary bone marrow disorders such as leukemia, lymphoma, regular aplastic anemia and metastatic malignancies, which will not be covered in this review. Environmental causes include drugs, chemicals, and ionizing radiation. Virtually all medications have been implicated in one or more cases of thrombocytopenia; because this is a common cause of thrombocytopenia, a careful search for drug exposure should be made. All implicated medications should be changed or stopped completely if possible. In a previously sensitized person with drug-related, immune-mediated thrombocytopenia, even a small amount of a drug can cause profound thrombocytopenia. A good example is heparin-induced thrombocytopenia, which is associated with heparin resistance, thromboembolism, heparin-related platelet aggregation, and even DIC. If this condition develops, the heparin should be discontinued. Heparin is not a single substance, and its molecular makeup varies with each preparation; thus, another manufacturer's lot of heparin or low-molecular-weight heparin often can be substituted (287, 288). The small amounts of quinine in some soft drinks can trigger a similar response (289). Once the medication has been discontinued, drug-induced thrombocytopenia usually resolves.

Immune Thrombocytopenic Purpura

The diagnosis of immune thrombocytopenic purpura (ITP) is made after all other causes of thrombocytopenia have been excluded and a platelet-associated antibody has been demonstrated. Megakaryocyte hyperplasia is seen on bone marrow, and there is an increase in the mean platelet volume. Similar to other autoimmune diseases, ITP is common in young patients. It occurs in about 1 in 300 to 600 pregnancies (290). Of these cases, 82% to 100% have IgG antibody directed against the platelet (291). The coated platelets then are removed from the circulation by the reticuloendothelial cells. Autologous platelets transfused to ITP patients have a survival span of a few minutes to 3 days compared with the normal platelet lifespan of 9 to 12 days (289). When the platelet count declines to less than 100,000 cells/mm^3, abnormal skin and mucous bleeding may appear. Spontaneous bleeding commonly occurs with counts below 20,000 cells/mm^3. Specific complications and bleeding severity vary greatly among patients.

An increased incidence of mild thrombocytopenia (platelet count between 100,000 and 150,000 cells/mm^3) has been recognized during pregnancy. This is called *gestational thrombocytopenia*, and it occurs in up to 7% to 9% of pregnant patients (290,292,293). Many of these women have been treated, perhaps unnecessarily, as though they have ITP. This disorder differs from ITP in that C3, rather than IgG, binds to the platelets (294). The outcome is good in patients with gestational thrombocytopenia once an underlying medical disorder has been ruled out. The risk of fetal thrombocytopenia in this condition seems no more than that of a normal pregnancy (295). The risk of maternal or neonatal complications associated with the thrombocytopenia is extremely small (296,297). It is not associated with any other abnormalities and requires no treatment. A recommendation for cesarean delivery or even a routine fetal scalp platelet count in labor for all thrombocytopenic women would expose these pregnancies to unnecessary interventions (296).

When a platelet count is at least 100,000 cells/mm^3, epidural anesthesia is considered safe. The maternal bleeding time is neither a necessary nor useful test in this setting. Patients with a platelet count between 50,000 and 100,000 cell/mm^3 have had epidural anesthesia without evidence of an epidural hematoma (298). Experience with severely thrombocytopenic patients is limited, and the safety of epidural anesthesia in this circumstance is unknown.

Treatment

When the platelet count declines to below 100,000/mm^3 secondary to an immune mechanism, corticosteroid therapy should be considered. Oral prednisone is given at a dose of 0.5 to 1 mg/kg daily in divided doses. Corticosteroids increase platelet production without any change in the platelet life span (299). If the platelet count is below 50,000/mm^3, patient activity should be restricted to avoid hemorrhage secondary to trauma. Once therapy has been initiated, the platelet count should begin to improve within 3 to 10 days. The steroid dose is tapered to maintain a minimum platelet count that exceeds 100,000/mm^3. An initial course of therapy will induce remission in up to 60% of patients, but there is a high rate of treatment failure and relapse. Other immunosuppressive medications, such as azathioprine, vincristine, and cyclophosphamide, have been used successfully for the treatment of ITP, but they should be avoided during pregnancy if possible (289). Corticoteroids usually can be discontinued in drug-related cases. In immune-mediated cases, 5 to 40 mg of prednisone per day may be necessary over the long term to prevent relapse. In some patients, corticosteroid treatment may be necessary only during periods of high risk, such as near term. During pregnancy, splenectomy may precipitate abortion and has been virtually replaced by corticosteroids and other medical treatments (300). Postpartum, splenectomy may be preferable to chronic corticosteroid therapy. Splenectomy induces remission in 60% to 70% of patients, including those who failed first-line therapy. Antibody production may persist, but the patient may go into a serologic remission. In immune-mediated disorders, platelet transfusion is only transiently effective because the antiplatelet IgG binds to donor platelets as well and is recommended only to treat life-threatening bleeding during pregnancy.

Intravenous infusion of gamma globulin (IVIG, 400 mg/kg daily for 5 days) has been used to treat immune thrombocytopenia during pregnancy. Most patients respond to therapy with an increased platelet count within a few days. This improvement may last for a few days to a few weeks (287,299). The neonatal response is more variable, however; some reports describe severe neonatal thrombocytopenia despite the recommended IVIG regimen (301,302). This problem may be overcome by increasing the dose and frequency of IVIG. Therapeutic fetal blood levels of gamma globulin have been demonstrated after repeated semiweekly maternal intravenous infusions (302). This therapy is expensive and effective. Normally, therapy should be directed toward raising the platelet count to an acceptable level for delivery (>50,000/mm^3). If satisfactory counts are not obtained using prednisone, IVIG started 7 days before delivery is often successful.

Fetal Considerations

Maternal treatment has no effect on circulating IgG antibodies, which cross the placenta to the fetus. In fact, splenectomy may enhance the fetal risk. The currently recommended steroids and IVIG also have not been shown to cross the placenta well (301). Neither the maternal platelet count nor platelet-associated IgG levels are useful in predicting neonatal thrombocytopenia (303, 304). Some have demonstrated that the presence of free antiplatelet antibody may be a significant risk factor for developing fetal thrombocytopenia (297,305).

Cesarean section in patients with thrombocytopenia is unnecessary for most pregnancies (306). With a fetal platelet count above 50,000/mm^3 vaginal delivery is thought to be safe. For lower fetal platelet counts, the best route of delivery is debatable. Two intracranial bleeds in 17 vaginally delivered infants of mothers with ITP were documented in one study (305). Other studies have documented none (297). It is also not known whether cesarean section protects against fetal hemorrhage, and it was recently suggested that cesarean section be reserved for obstetric indications only (306).

Fetal scalp blood sampling permits measurement of fetal platelet count early in labor. It is associated with a low incidence of false-negative results and is a safe technique (307). A modest false-positive rate exists secondary to platelet aggregation in the sample, especially if it is contaminated by amniotic fluid or vernix (241,290,308).

Cordocentesis also has been used to diagnose fetal thrombocytopenia in patients with ITP. The risk of cordocentesis is fairly low, at 0.1% to 2%; however, the likelihood of antenatal hemorrhage is even lower, suggesting that there is no benefit from cordocentesis. A scalp platelet count is preferred if necessary. All infants should be watched closely after birth, as thrombocytopenia may become evident only after the first few days of life.

Alloimmune Thrombocytopenia in the Fetus

Alloimmune thrombocytopenia (AITP) is the platelet equivalent of Rh sensitization. Most often, the diagnosis is made after birth of an affected sibling. Of all affected women, 50% will have an affected fetus during their first pregnancy, with 83% to 97% of fetuses in subsequent pregnancies being affected (309). It is more severe and occurs earlier in gestation in fetuses with an older sibling who had an ICH (310).

The sensitized mother produces IgG antibodies to a foreign platelet antigen. There are seven studied platelet antigen systems: HPA (Human Platelet Antigen)-1 to HPA-7, with HPA-1a being the most potent of the isoantigens. In the white population, most cases of AITP are caused by antibodies to HPA-1a (311,312), which is inherited as an autosomal dominant trait (313). HPA-4 is the most frequently implicated system in the Japanese population (314). There are several leukoplatelet antigens, including HLA-5, HLA-9, PLGrLyC1, and PLGrLyB1 (315). Various human leukocyte antigen (HLA) subtypes are high-risk groups for alloimmunization and include types B8, DR3, and Drw52 (316,317). HPA-1a occurs in 98% of the population. One would thus expect 2% of all pregnancies to be incompatible and at risk for alloimmunization. Prospective follow-up shows that 6% of HPA-1a-negative women become alloimmunized, an incidence of 1 in 1,666 pregnancies (318). The incidence of AITP is 1 in 5,000 in the population overall, suggesting that alloimmunization is not an inevitable consequence in all incompatible pregnancies. There is also no correlation between the maternal antiplatelet antibody titers and the severity of the disease by present laboratory methods (313). In cases with a heterozygous or unknown father, antigenic status can be determined by amniocentesis or chorionic villus sampling.

The neonate may present with varying symptoms, such as hematemesis, melena, hematochezia, hematuria, cephalohematoma, and petechial rash. The most severe complication is an ICH. Most children (90%) present with only mild bleeding, which resolves without residual deficits within 1 to 4 weeks after birth (75). There is a high rate of perinatal morbidity and a 10% incidence of perinatal mortality, usually due to ICH. About a third of ICHs occur *in utero* (319–322). Fetuses at greatest risk are those in the last trimester because the longer the platelet count is depressed, the greater the risk of ICH. The risk of early neonatal bleeding is about 20% (241).

Treatment

All pregnancies at risk for AITP should have fetal blood sampling (FBS) performed. Diagnostic FBS is best performed at 21 to 22 weeks' gestation (323,324) and should be repeated at 28 to 32 weeks because a normal fetal platelet count does not preclude an affected fetus. Treatment options include one or more of the following: fetal platelet transfusions, maternal or fetal administration of IVIG, or maternal steroids.

Fetal platelet transfusion can be used to prevent bleeding at the time of FBS, prophylactically during pregnancy, or before delivery. The platelets should be used as soon as possible after harvesting to maximize platelet lifespan after transfusion. The volume of platelet concentrate to be transfused can be calculated from the following equation (325,326):

$$\text{Volume} = \frac{\text{fetal placental blood volume} \times 2 \times \text{desired increment}}{\text{concentrate platelet count}}$$

A posttransfusion platelet level of 400 to 500 × 10^9/L should be aimed for, especially if repeated transfusions are planned (327). Platelets survive only 4 to 5 days in the fetal circulation; therefore, fetal platelet transfusions need to be repeated every 7 to 10 days. Prophylactic transfusion programs have been used successfully (327, 328); however, the loss rate with the repeated procedures may be as great as in untreated cases, and frequent fetal transfusions are extremely arduous for the mother (329). A fetal platelet transfusion immediately before delivery is an effective method for raising the fetal platelet count for delivery (88). If the fetal platelet count at the end of this final transfusion is 100×10^9 cells per liter, several authors believe a vaginal delivery can be attempted without risk to the fetus (241,308).

High-dose IVIG administered antenatally has been demonstrated to increase the fetal platelet count and prevent ICH (330,331). The IVIG is infused at 1 g per kilogram weekly starting within 1 week of documentation of fetal thrombocytopenia (331). Daily dexamethasone added to the IVIG regimen resulted in no better effect, but 50% of those who did not respond to IVIG plus dexamethasone responded to IVIG plus prednisone (60 mg/day) (331). Direct administration of IVIG to the fetus has had no effect on severe AITP (328,329).

Corticosteroid therapy has no effect on the fetal platelet count (332). The role of maternal steroid treatment alone or in combination with IVIG needs to be further explored.

Recognizing these treatment options, the following strategies are proposed: (a) conservative management with frequent ultrasounds until delivery or lung maturity is reached (before delivery the platelet count is determined and a platelet transfusion administered if necessary); (b) high-dose IVIG with or without steroids (cases of treatment failure will need to have repeated platelet transfusions); (c) repeated platelet transfusions until fetal maturity is reached.

A combination of these approaches seems prudent. When an affected fetus is documented, IVIG therapy should be initiated. If the fetus is unresponsive to medical therapy, fetal platelet transfusions are necessary. This sequence would reduce the number of fetal platelet transfusions needed. Preimplantation selection of a HPA-compatible embryo also may become a practical possibility soon (333).

Thrombotic Thrombocytopenic Purpura

Thrombotic thrombocytopenic purpura (TTP) is characterized by a diagnostic pentad of fever, microangiopathic hemolytic anemia, thrombocytopenia, central nervous system symptoms, and renal impairment (334). It occurs with increased frequency in pregnancy, constituting up to 10% of all cases of TTP (335). The presentation and management of this disorder during pregnancy have been reviewed (336,337). Few women present with the classic pentad, making the diagnosis of TTP in the third trimester or postpartum extremely difficult because most women will present with thrombocytopenia, microangiopathic hemolytic anemia, and subtle neurologic findings, all of which may not occur together (337,338).

The primary event in this syndrome is platelet aggregation, which leads to the characteristic microvascular thrombotic lesions seen throughout the body. This results in generalized endothelial injury and the release of ultra-large multimeric forms of VWF and thrombomodulin into the circulation (334–336). In TTP the distinctive clotting abnormalities found enable easier and earlier diagnosis of this disorder (339–341), which is distinct from DIC in that fibrinogen turnover is normal in TTP (342). In contrast to preeclampsia, the serum fibronectin concentration is usually normal and not elevated (343). The PT/PTT, AT III, protein C, fibrinogen, the ratio of factor VIII antigen to activity, and FSP are almost always normal in patients with TTP (344).

In a compilation of 40 published cases, 58% of the patients initially presented with TTP at or before 24 weeks' gestation. In 89% of patients, TTP preceded delivery (336). The clinical definition of preeclampsia was fulfilled in 38% of women who developed TTP after 24 weeks; however, clear-cut preeclampsia occurred simultaneously only three times. TTP places both mother and fetus in extreme jeopardy. When TTP was present antepartum, only 25% of mother–infant pairs survived (336). Eighty percent of the infants died directly or indirectly as a result of maternal disease (336). In a recent series (11 cases), the maternal mortality was 18%, with a fetal loss rate of 30% (341).

Treatment

Corticosteroids, aspirin, dextran, dipyridamole, plasma infusion, and plasmapheresis have shown some therapeutic efficacy (336,345,346). Plasmapheresis has increased survival up to 90% and is the treatment of choice (347, 348). Because the disease is rapidly progressive, therapy should be initiated promptly (349). A delay in initiating therapy can result in treatment failure. In a review of published cases associated with pregnancy, the overall maternal mortality rate was 44% (336). When divided by the mode of treatment, the mortality rate was 68% (19/28) if plasma therapy was not used and 0% (0/17) if it was used (336). Plasmapheresis with FFP should be initiated with a single exchange (40 mL/kg body mass) on a daily basis. It is continued until a few days after the thrombocytopenia has resolved, the hemoglobin is stable, neurologic abnormalities are gone, and the lactate dehydrogenase level has normalized. Then it is tapered over 1 to 2 weeks. If there is no response to initial therapy, plasmapheresis can be done twice daily or increased to 80 mL per kilogram of body mass. Relapses often occur within 1 week to 1 month of completing therapy (346).

If plasmapheresis cannot be done immediately, plasma infusion may be beneficial. Infusion of packed red blood cells is used to treat life-threatening anemia, and renal failure is treated by dialysis. Patients who have a relapse after plasmapheresis or who did not respond to the initial plasmapheresis protocol occasionally respond to a splenectomy (350,351). It usually is performed as salvage therapy in patients refractory to plasmapheresis or to reduce the recurrence rate in patients with relapsing TTP (352,353). Splenectomy is rarely of use during pregnancy. Heparin and immunosuppressive agents have not improved on response rates achieved by plasmapheresis alone. Platelet transfusions have disastrous results, actually increasing intravascular thrombus formation and exacerbating the disease (345).

Based on literature review and the largest compilation of published cases, the following treatment protocol for TTP in pregnancy is suggested (336). Plasma exchange with donor plasma should be initiated promptly, exchanging one plasma volume during the first 24 hours. The concentration of lactic dehydrogenase (LDH) levels is monitored as an indicator of ongoing hemolysis and ischemic tissue damage. If there is an inadequate response to plasmapheresis, glucocorticoids (1 to 2 mg/kg daily of prednisone) and antiplatelet agents are added. Splenectomy during pregnancy should be considered the last resort.

Fetal Considerations

When TTP presents in the first trimester, the fetus typically does not survive. Successful treatment of TTP presenting in the second or third trimester allows the pregnancy to be lengthened by 4 weeks or more (336). As a result, fetal survival has been reported when TTP develops in the late second and third trimester (336,341,347, 348). Maternal TTP does not improve with delivery (336).

TABLE 20-10. *Differentiating causes of thrombocytopenia in pregnancy*

	TTP	HUS	Preeclampsia	ITP
Clinical features				
CNS	+	–	+	–
Fever	+	–	–	–
Hypertension	–	–	+	–
Petechiae	+	–	+	+
Laboratory findings				
Hemolytic anemia	+	+	+	–
Lactate dehydrogenase	↑	↑	↑	N
AST/ALT	N	N	↑	N
Antithrombin III activity	N	N	↓	N
Autoantibodies	–	–	–	+
Proteinuria	+	+	+	–
Serum creatinine	↑	↑	↑	N
Blood urea nitrogen	↑	↑	↑	N

+, Present; ALT, alanine aminotransferase; AST, aspartate aminotransferase; CNS, central nervous system symptoms; HUS, hemolytic uremic syndrome; ITP, idiopathic thrombocytopenic purpura; N, normal; ↓ decreased; TTP, thrombotic thrombocytopenia purpura; ↑, increased; –, absent.

From Sipes SL, Weiner CP. Coagulation disorders in pregnancy. In: Reece EA, Hobbins JC, Mahoney MJ, Petrie RH, eds. Medicine of the fetus and mother. Philadelphia: JB Lippincott, 1992:1131.

Other Disorders

Pregnancy-associated disorders may present similarly to TTP (Table 20-10).

Preeclampsia

Thrombocytopenia occurs in 10% of women with severe preeclampsia. Occasionally, it precedes the clinical manifestations of preeclampsia itself (354). The preeclampsia-associated thrombocytopenia is due to accelerated platelet destruction and results in bone marrow compensation, which accelerates platelet production, resulting in younger, larger platelets on the peripheral smear with an increased platelet distribution width (355). Platelet aggregation is probably secondary to the damaged vascular endothelium (355). In most preeclamptic patients, there is no correlation between the maternal or fetal platelet counts and an abnormal antiplatelet IgG, IgM, or C3 titers (356). Antiplatelet IgG is found most often; however, the significance of the increased antiglobulin titers in preeclampsia is unclear (306,356,357).

There is significant overlap in the presentation of severe preeclampsia and TTP. Both may present with thrombocytopenia, microangiopathic hemolysis, and renal failure. Measurements of AT III activity may help to separate the two syndromes. The activity AT III is decreased in women with severe preeclampsia but remains stable in TTP and hemolytic uremic syndrome.

The following management protocol is suggested when the differential diagnosis is TTP versus severe atypical preeclampsia. At 34 weeks' gestation or beyond, the AT III activity should be measured and the patient delivered. If the patient has preeclampsia, the AT III activity level is decreased and the patient will recover soon after delivery. If the AT III level was normal and the patient does not recover, the correct diagnosis is TTP, and plasmapheresis should be initiated. Before 28 weeks' gestation, the AT III activity level should be measured. If the fetal condition is satisfactory, a trial of plasmapheresis is recommended. If the patient improves after plasmapheresis, a presumptive diagnosis of TTP is made. If there is no improvement with treatment, the diagnosis is most likely preeclampsia. There is little evidence that preeclampsia is altered by plasmapheresis in the absence of confounding variables such as delivery. Between 28 and 34 weeks' gestation, treatment should be individualized. Again, if the AT III activity level is normal, without a compromised fetus, a trial of plasmapheresis should be initiated. Once plasmapheresis has begun, it should be continued into the postpartum period until remission has been achieved. Once initiated, plasmapheresis should not be discontinued during pregnancy because the likelihood of relapse increases during pregnancy. A patient with atypical severe preeclampsia who does not respond to plasmapharesis should be delivered.

Postpartum Hemolytic Uremic Syndrome.

Hemolytic uremic syndrome (HUS), often confused with TTP, presents with microangiopathic anemia, thrombocytopenia, and renal failure. It is rarely associated with neurologic changes, and the seizures associated with it are usually due to renal failure or hypertension. Other distinguishing features of HUS include the following: onset 48 hours after a normal delivery (289); a history of a prodromal gastrointestinal disorder with diarrhea; milder bleeding and thrombocytopenia than in TTP; early, severe renal failure with anuria and hypertension.

The primary coagulation defect in HUS involves the platelet, with thrombocytopenia present most of the time. AT III activity is also usually normal in HUS (336). FSPs are frequently increased, possibly as a result of fibrinogen rather than fibrin degradation, in contrast to TTP, in which FSPs are normal. Urinary free hemoglobin is common secondary to hemolysis (336).

Treatment

Treatment recommendations for HUS are similar to those for TTP, with the addition of dialysis. Heparin has not been shown to be effective. Compared with TTP in pregnancy, the outcome for patients with HUS was worse (336). The overall maternal mortality rate was 55% (34/66), with half of the survivors requiring long-term dialysis (13/28). Five patients underwent kidney transplantation, and one died after organ rejection. Again, plasmapheresis is apparently beneficial, although the numbers of reported cases are small.

Systemic lupus erythematosus and variant VWD (type 2B) can cause thrombocytopenia in pregnancy. In VWD (type 2D), the abnormal VWF binds to the patient's platelets, producing thrombocytopenia. This results in platelet aggregate formation and clearance (358). Variant VWF synthesis increases in pregnancy (359,360).

Functional Platelet Defects

Acquired disorders of platelet function can occur in conjunction with numerous medical illnesses, including myeloproliferative disorders, congestive heart failure, and uremia. Drug-induced platelet dysfunction is, however, more common in pregnancy.

The most important drugs affecting platelet function in pregnancy are aspirin and other nonsteroidal antiinflammatory agents. Aspirin is the longest acting of these drugs. It inhibits thromboxane synthesis by irreversibly acetylating platelet cyclooxygenase. This results in decreased platelet aggregation in the presence of collagen and prolongation of bleeding time. This may result in mild bruising or bleeding in someone who has recently taken aspirin. Pregnant women who ingest aspirin within 10 days of delivery rarely have any clinically significant effects; however, they have been reported to have increased blood loss both intrapartum and postpartum. Their infants also have an increased incidence of abnormal coagulation (361). Other nonsteroidal antiinflammatory agents have similar effects on platelet function, although most are of shorter duration and less potent. These medications are not recommended during pregnancy. Numerous other drugs have been associated with thrombocytopenia. A review of all the drugs involved would be beyond the scope of this chapter.

Congenital disorders of platelet function are extremely rare, and there is little experience with them in pregnancy. A discussion of these disorders is beyond the scope of this chapter. Good reviews exist in the hematology and pathology literature (362).

REFERENCES

1. Weiss HJ. Flow-related platelet deposition on subendothelium. Thromb Haemost 1995;74:117–122.
2. Moncada S, Vane JR. Pharmacology and endogenous roles of prostaglandin endoperoxides, thromboxane A_2 and prostacyclin. Pharmacol Rev 1978;30:293–331.
3. Bettex-Galland M, Trescher EF. Thrombosthenin, the contractile protein from blood platelets and its relation to other contractile proteins. Adv Protein Chem 1965;20:1–35.
4. Erichson RB, Katz AJ, Cintron JR. Ultrastructural observations on platelet adhesion reactions: platelet fibrin interaction. Blood 1967;29: 385–400.
5. Camerer E, Kolsto AB, Prydz H. Cell biology of tissue factor, the principal initator of blood coagulation. Thromb Res 1996;81:1–41.
6. Astrup T. Assay and content of tissue thromboplastin in different organs. Thromb Diath Haemorrh 1965;14:401–416.
7. Drake TA, Morrissey JH, Edgington TS. Selective cellular expression of tissue factor in human tissues: implications for disorders of hemostasis and thrombosis. Am J Pathol 1989;134:1087–1097.
8. Gregory SA, Morrissey JH, Edgington TS. Regulation of tissue factor gene expression in the monocyte procoagulant response to endotoxin. Mol Cell Biol 1989;9:2752–2755.
9. Gregory SA, Kornbluth RS, Helin H, Remold HG, Edgington TS. Monocyte procoagulant inducing factor: a lymphokine involved in the T cell-instructed monocyte procoagulant response to antigen. J Immunol 1986;137:3231–3239.
10. Edgington TS, Mackman N, Brand K, Ruf W. The structural biology of expression and function of tissue factor. Thromb Haemost 1991; 66:67–79.
11. Rao LVM, Rapaport SI, Bajaj SP. Activation of human factor VII in the initiation of tissue of factor-dependent coagulation. Blood 1986; 68:685–691.
12. Rao LVM, Rapaport SI. Activation of factor VII bound to tissue factor: a key early step in the tissue factor pathway of blood coagulation. Proc Natl Acad Sci USA 1988;85:6687–6691.
13. Broze GJ Jr, Majerus PW. Purification and properties of human coagulation factor VII. J Biol Chem 1980;255:1242–1247.
14. Bajaj SP, Rapaport SI, Brown SF. Isolation and characterization of human factor VII: activation of factor VII by factor Xa. J Biol Chem 1981;256:253–259.
15. Davie EW, Fujikawa K, Kisiel W. The coagulation cascade: initiation, maintenance, and regulation [Review]. Biochemistry 1991;30: 10363–10370.
16. Bach R, Gentry R, Nemerson Y. Factor VII binding to tissue factor in reconstituted phospholipid vesicles: induction of cooperativity by phosphatidylserine. Biochemistry 1986;25:4007–4020.
17. Sabharwal AK, Birktoft JJ, Gorka J, Wildgoose P, Petersen LC, Bajaj SP. High affinity Ca(2-)binding site in the serine protease domain of human factor VIIa and its role in tissue factor binding and development of catalytic activity. J Biol Chem 1995;270:15523–15530.
18. Wildgoose P, Nemerson Y, Hansen LL, Neilsen FE, Glazer S, Hedner

U. Measurement of basal levels of factor pathway blood coagulation. Proc Natl Acad Sci USA 1988;85:6687.
19. Morrissey JH, Macik BG, Neuenschwander PF, Comp PC. Quantitation of activated factor VII levels in plasma using a tissue factor mutant selectively deficient in promoting factor VII activation. Blood 1993;81:734–744.
20. Tsuji A, Torres-Rosado A, Arai T, et al. Hepsin, a cell membrane-associated protease: characterization, tissue distribution, and gene localization. J Biol Chem 1991;266:16948–16953.
21. Kazama Y, Hamaamoto T, Foster DC, Kisiel W. Hepsin, a putative membrane-associated serine protease, activates human factor VII and initiates a pathway of blood coagulation on the cell surface leading to thrombin. J Biol Chem 1995;270:66–72.
22. Broze GJ, Likert K, Higuchi D. Inhibition of factor VIIa/tissue factor by antithrombin III and tissue factor pathway inhibitor. Blood 1993; 82:1679–1681.
23. Lawson JH, Butenas S, Ribarik N, Mann KG. Complex-dependent inhibition of factor VIIa by antithrombin II and heparin. J Biol Chem 1993;268:767–770.
24. Wun TC, Kretzmer KK, Girard TJ, Miletich JP, Broze GJ Jr. Cloning and characterization of a cDNA coding for the lipoprotein-associated coagulation inhibitor shows that it consists of three tandem Kunitz-type inhibitory domains. J Biol Chem 1988;263:6001–6004.
25. Laskowski M Jr, Kato I. Protein inhibitors of proteinases. Annu Rev Biochem 1980;49:593–626.
26. Rapaport SI, Rao LV. Initiation and regulation of tissue factor-dependent blood coagulation. Arterioscler Thromb Vasc Biol 1992;12: 1111–1121.
27. Broze GJ Jr. The role of tissue factor pathway inhibitor in a revised coagulation cascade. Semin Hematol 1992;29:159–169.
28. Girard TJ, Warren LA, Novotny WF, et al. Functional significance of the Kunitz-type inhibitory domains of lipo-protein-associated coagulation inhibitor. Nature 1989;338:518–520.
29. Wesselschmidt RL, Girard TJ, Likert KM, Wun TC, Broze GJ Jr. Tissue factor pathway inhibitor: the carboxy-terminus is required for optimal inhibition of factor Xa. Blood 1992;79:2004–2010.
30. Higuchi D, Wun TC, Likert KM, Broze GJ Jr. The effect of leukocyte elastase on tissue factor pathway inhibitor. Blood 1992;79: 1712–1719.
31. Broze GJ Jr, Warren LA, Novotny WF, Higuchi DA, Girard TJ, Miletich JP. The lipoprotein-associated coagulation inhibitor that inhibits the factor VII-tissue factor complex also inhibits factor Xa: insight into its possible mechanism of action. Blood 1988;71: 335–343.
32. Novotny WF, Girard TJ, Miletich JP, Broze GJ Jr. Purification and characterization of the lipoprotein-associated coagulation inhibitor from human plasma. J Biol Chem 1989;264:18832–18837.
33. Novotny WF, Girard TJ, Miletich JP, Broze GJ Jr. Platelets secrete a coagulation inhibitor functionally and antigenically similar to the lipoprotein-associated coagulation inhibitor. Blood 1988;72: 2020–2025.
34. Sandset PM, Abildgaard U, Larsen ML. Heparin induces release of extrinsic coagulation pathway inhibitor (EPI). Thromb Res 1988;50: 803–813.
35. Gruenberg JC, Smallridge RC, Rosenberg RD. Inherited antithrombin III deficiency causing mesenteric thrombosis: a new clinical enity. Ann Surg 1975;181:791–794.
36. Bischof P, Meisser A. Sizonenko PC, Herrmann WL. Pregnancy-associated plasma protein A inhibits thrombin-induced coagulation. Washington DC: Proceedings of the Society for Gynecologic Investigation, 1984 (abst. 321).
37. Blauhut B, Necek S, Vinazzer H, Bergmann H. Substitution therapy with an antithrombin III concentrate in shock and DIC. Thromb Res 1982;27:271–278.
38. Lane DA, Ireland H, Olds RJ, Thein SL, Perry DJ, Aiach M. Antithrombin III: a database of mutations. Thromb Haemost 1991; 66:657–661.
39. Mersky C. Defibrination syndrome. In: Biggs R, ed. Human blood coagulation, hemostasis and thrombosis. London: Blackwell Scientific, 1976:492.
40. Morris RH, Vassalli P, Beller FK, McCluskey RT. Immunofluorescent studies of renal biopsies in the diagnosis of toxemia of pregnancy. Obstet Gynecol 1964;24:32.
41. Meade T, Syer S, Howarth DJ, Imeson JD, Stirling Y. Antithrombin III and procoagulant activity: sex differences and effects of the menopause. Br J Haematol 1990;74:77–81.
42. Fourrier F, Chopin C, Goudemand J, et al. Septic shock, multiple organ failure, and disseminated intravascular coagulation. Compared patterns of anthithrombin III, protein C, and protein S deficiencies. Chest 1992;101:816–823.
43. Bertina RM, van der Linden IK, Engesser L, Muller HP, Brommer EJ. Hereditary heparin cofactor II deficiency and the risk of development of thrombosis. Thromb Haemost 1987;57:196–200.
44. Weisdorf DJ, Edson JR. Recurrent venous thrombosis associated with inherited deficiency of heparin cofactor II. Br J Haematol 1990;77: 125–126.
45. Jorgensen B, Neilsen JD. Intra-arterial thrombin activity produced by percutaneous transluminal angioplasty eliminated by segmentally enclosed thrombolysis. Eur J Vasc Surg 1992;6:153–157.
46. Weitz JI, Hudoba M, Massel D, Maraganore J, Hirsh J. Clot-bound thrombin is protected from inhibition of heparin-an-tithrombin III but is susceptible to inactivation by antithrombin III-independent inhibitors. J Clin Invest 1990;86:385–391.
47. Dittman WA, Majerus PW. Structure and function of thrombomodulin: a natural anticoagulant. Blood 1990;75:329–336.
48. Solymoss S, Tucker MM, Tracy PB. Kinetics of inactivation of membrane-bound factor Va by activated protein C. J Biol Chem 1988;263: 14884–14890.
49. Regan LM, Lamphear BJ, Huggins CF, Walker FJ, Fay PJ. Factor Ixa protects factor VIIIa from activated protein C. J Biol Chem 1994;269: 9445–9452.
50. Scully MF, Toh CH, Hoogendoorn H, et al. Activation of protein C and its distribution between its inhibitors, protein C inhibitor, 1-antitrypsin and 2-macroglobulin, in patients with disseminated intravascular coagulation. Thromb Haemostas 1993;69:448–453.
51. Heeb MJ, Gruber A, Griffin JH. Identification of divalent metal ion-dependent inhibition of activated protein C by alpha$_2$macroglobulin and alpha$_2$antiplasmin in blood and comparisons to inhibition of factor Xa, thrombin, and plasmin. J Biol Chem 1991;266:17606–17612.
52. Comp PC, Esmon CT, Evidence for multiple roles of activated protein C in fibrinolysis. In: Mann KG, Taylor FB Jr, eds. The regulation of coagulation. New York: Elsevier/North-Holland, 1980:583
53. Hopmeier P, Halbmayer M, Schwarz HP, Heuss F, Fischer M. Protein C and protein S in mild and moderate preeclampsia. Thromb Haemost 1987;58:794–795.
54. Dahlback B, Carlsson M, Svensson PJ. Familial thrombophilia due to a previously unrecognized mechanism characterized by poor anticoagulant response to activated protein C. Proc Natl Acad Sci USA 1993;90:1004–1008.
55. Greengard JS, Eichinger S, Griffin JH, Bauer KA. Brief report: variability of thrombosis among homozygous siblings with resistance to activated protein C due to an Arg Gln mutation in the gene for factor V. N Engl J Med 1994;331:1559–1562.
56. Bertina RM, Koeleman BPC, Koster T, et al. Mutation in blood coagulation factor V associated with resistance to activated protein C. Nature 1994;369:64–67.
57. Greengard JS, Sun X, Xu X, Fernandez JA, Griffin JH, Evatt B. Activated protein C resistance caused by Arg506Gln mutation in factor VA. Lancet 1994;343:1361–1362.
58. Zoller B, Dahlback B. Linkage between inherited resistance to activated protein C and factor V gene mutation in venous thrombosis. Lancet 1994;343:1536–1538.
59. Dahlback B. Inherited thrombophilia: resistance to activiated protein C as a pathogenic factor of venous thromboembolism. Blood 1995;85: 607–614.
60. Juhan-Vague I, Valadier J, Alessi MC, et al. Deficient t-PA release and elevated PA inhibitor levels in patients with spontaneous or recurrent deep vein thrombosis. Thromb Haemost 1987;57:67–72.
61. Nagi DK, Hendra TJ, Ryle AJ, et al. The relationships of concentration of insulin, intact proinsulin and 32-33 split proinsulin to cardiovascular risk factors in type 2 diabetic subjects. Diabetologia 1990;33: 532–537.
62. Dichek D, Quertemous T. Thrombin regulation of mRNA levels of tissue plasminogen activator inhibitor-1 in cultured human umbilical vein endothelial cells. Blood 1989;74:222–228.
63. Collen D. Molecular mechanisms of fibrinolysis and their application to fibrin-specific thrombolytic therapy. J Cell Biochem 1987;33: 77–86.

64. Booth NA, Simpson AJ, Croll A. Plasminogen activator inhibitor (PAI-1) in plasma and platelets. Br J Haematol 1988;70:327–333.
65. Collen D, Lijnen HR, Todd PA, Goa KL. Tissue-type plasminogen activator: a review of its pharmacology and therapeutic use as thrombolytic agent. Drugs 1989;38:346–388.
66. Ogston D, Bennett B. Naturally occurring inhibitors of coagulation. In: Ogston B, Bennett B, eds. Haemostasis: biochemistry, physiology and pathology. London: John Wiley & Sons, 1977:230.
67. Jaffe EA, Hoyer LW, Nachman RL. Synthesis of antihemophilic factor antigen by cultured human endothelial cells. J Clin Invest 1973;52: 2757–2764.
68. Tschopp TB, Weiss JH, Baumgartner HR. Decreased adhesion of platelets to subendothelium in von Willebrand's disease. J Lab Clin Med 1974;83:296–300.
69. Moncada S, Vane JR. The role of prostacyclin in vascular tissue. Fed Proc 1979;38:66–71.
70. Goodman RP, Killam AP, Brash AR, Branch RA. Prostacyclin production during pregnancy: comparison of production during normal pregnancy and pregnancy complicated by hypertension. Am J Obstet Gynecol 1982;142:817–822.
71. Dadak C, Kefalides A, Sinzinger H, Weber G. Reduced umbilical artery prostacyclin formation in complicated pregnancies. Am J Obstet Gynecol 1982;144:792–795.
72. Elwood PC, Benjamin IT, Waters WE, Sweetnam PM. Mortality and anaemia in women. Lancet 1974;1:891–894.
73. Koster R, Rosendaal FR, Briet E. Risk factors for deep vein thrombosis: LETS interim analysis. Thromb Haemost 1993;69:764.
74. Takahashi H, Ito S, Hanano M, et al. Circulating thromboglobulin as a novel endothelial cell marker: comparison of its behavior with von Willebrand factor and tissue-type plasminogen activator. Am J Hematol 1992;41:32–39.
75. Weiner CP, Kwaan H, Hauck WW, Duboe FJ, Paul M, Wallemark CB. Fibrin generation in normal pregnancy. Obstet Gynecol 1984;64: 46–48.
76. Weiner CP, Brandt J. Plasma antithrombin III activity: an aid in the diagnosis of preeclampsia-eclampsia. Am J Obstet Gynecol 1982;142: 275–281.
77. Arias F, Andrenopoulos G, Zamora J. Whole blood fibrinolytic activity in normal and hypertensive pregnancies and its relation to placental concentration of urokinase inhibitor. Am J Obstet Gynecol 1979; 133:624–629.
78. Bertina RM, van der Linden IK, Engesser L, Muller HP, Brommer EJ. Hereditary heparin cofactor II deficiency and the risk of development of thrombosis. Thromb Haemost 1987;57:196–200.
79. Larrieu MJ, Rigollot C, Marder VJ. Comparative effects of fibrinogen degradation fragments D & E on coagulation. Br J Haematol 1972;22: 719–733.
80. Ogston D, Ogston CM, Fullerton HW. The plasminogen content of thrombi. Thromb Haemost 1966;15:220–230.
81. Weiner CP, Kwaan H, Duboe F. Diagnosis of septic pelvic vein thrombophlebitis by measurement of fibrinopeptide A. Am J Perinatol 1985; 2:93–95.
82. Weiner CP, Sabbagha RE, Vaisrub N. Distinguishing preeclampsia from chronic hypertension using antithrombin III. Washington, DC: Proceedings of the Society for Gynecologic Investigation, 1983 (abst. 29).
83. Bick RL. Disseminated intravascular coagulation: clinical and laboratory characteristics in 48 patients. Ann NY Acad Sci 1981;370: 843–850.
84. Bick RL. Disseminated intravascular coagulation and related syndromes: etiology, pathophysiology, diagnosis, and management. Am J Hematol 1978;5:265–282.
85. Bick RL. Disseminated intravascular coagulation: objective clinical and laboratory diagnosis, treatment, and assessment of therapeutic response. Semin Thromb Hemost 1996;22:69–88.
86. Bick RL. Disseminated intravascular coagulation and related syndromes: a clinical review. Semin Thromb Hemost 1988;14:299–338.
87. Bick RL. Disseminated intravascular coagulation. In: Bick RL, ed. Disorders of thrombosis and hemostasis: clinical and laboratory practice. Chicago: ASCP Press, 1992:137.
88. Bick RL, WF Baker. Disseminated intravascular coagulation. Hematol Pathol 1992;6:1–24.
89. Mullo-Berghaus G. Pathophysiologic and biochemical events, in disseminated intravascular coagulation: dysregulation of procoagulant and anticoagulant pathways. Semin Thromb Hemost 1989;15:58.
90. Nilsson IM. Local fibrinolysis as a mechanism for haemorrhage. Thromb Diath Haemorrh 1975;34:623–633.
91. Stormorken H. Relation of the fibrinolytic to other biological systems. Thromb Diath Haemorrh 1975;34:378–385.
92. Schreiber AD, Austen KF. Interrelationships of the fibrinolytic, coagulation, kinin generation, and complement systems. Semin Hematol 1973:6:593–600.
93. Kaplan A, Meier H, Mandel R. The Hageman factor dependent pathways of coagulation, fibrinolysis, and kinin generation. Semin Thromb Hemost 1976;3:1–26.
94. van Iwaarden F, Bouma B. Role of high molecular weight kininogen in contact activation. Semin Thromb Hemost 1987;13:15–24.
95. Baker WF. Clinical aspects of disseminated intravascular coagulation: a clinician's point of view. Semin Thromb Hemost 1989;15:1–57.
96. Rosenberg JS, Beeler DL, Rosenberg RD. Activation of Human prothrombin by highly purified human factors V and Xa in the presence of human antithrombin. J Biol Chem 1975;250:1607–1617.
97. Bick RL, Baker W. Diagnostic efficacy of the D-dimer assay in DIC and related disorders. Thromb Res 1992;65:785–790.
98. Bauer KA, Weiss LM, Sparrow D, Vokonas PS, Rosenberg RD. Aging-associated changes in indices of thrombin generation and protein C activation in humans: normative aging study. J Clin Invest 1987;80:1527–1534.
99. Weiner CP, Brandt J. Plasma antithrombin III activity in normal pregnancy. Obstet Gynecol 1980;56:601–603.
100. Wintrobe WM, Lee GR, Boggs DR, et al, eds. Clinical hematology. 8th ed. Philadelphia: Lea & Febiger, 1981:1223–1226.
101. Turpie AGG, Hirsh J. When and how to use heparin prophylaxis and treatment. Geriatrics 1979;34:59–70.
102. Yin ET. Effect of heparin on neutralization of factor X and thrombin by the plasma alpha-2 globulin inhibitor. Thromb Haemost 1974;33: 43–50.
103. Brandt P, Jespersen J, Gregersen G. Postpartum hemolytic-uremic syndrome successfully treated with antithrombin III. BMJ 1980; 280:449.
104. Buller HR, Weenink AH, Treffers PE, Kahle LH, Otten HA, TenCate JW. Severe antithrombin III deficiency in a patient with preeclampsia: observations on the effect of human AT III concentrate transfusion. Scand J Haematol 1980;25:81–86.
105. Bick RL. Disseminated intravascular coagulation. Hematol Oncol Clin North Am 1992;6:1259–1285.
106. Vinazzer HA. Antithrombin III in shock and disseminated intravascular coagulation. Clin Appl Thromb Hemost 1995;1:62–68.
107. Niada R, Prota R, Pescador R, Mantovani M, Prino G. Thrombolytic activity of defibrotide against old venous thrombi. Semin Thromb Hemost 1989;15:474–479.
108. Mueller-Eckhardt C, Heene D, Muller-Berghaus G, Lasch HG. Hamolytische Transfusion-szwischenfalle mit Verbrauschkoagulopathie durch seltene Blutgruppenatikorper. Thromb Haemost 1969; 22:336–343.
109. Woodfield DG, Cole SK, Allan AG, Cash JD. Systemic fibrinolysis during and following elective cesarean section and gynecologic operations. J Obstet Gynaecol Br Commonw 1972;79:538–543.
110. Redman CWG, Bonnar J, Berlin L. Early platelet consumption in preeclampsia. BMJ 1978;1:467–469.
111. Socol ML, Weiner CP, Louis G, Rehnberg K, Ross EC. Platelet activation in preeclampsia. Am J Obstet Gynecol 1985;151:494–497.
112. Romero R, Snyder E, Rickles F, et al. The clinical significance and mechanism of thrombocytopenia in pregnancy-induced hypertension. Dallas: Proceedings, Society for Gynecologic Investigation, 1982 (abst. 69).
113. Arias F, Mancilla-Jimenez R. Hepatic fibrinogen deposits in preeclampsia: immunofluorescent evidence. N Engl J Med 1976;295: 578–582.
114. Weenink GH, Borm JJ, TenCate JW, Treffers PE. Antithrombin III levels in normotensive and hypertensive pregnancy. Gynecol Obstet Invest 1983;16:230–242.
115. Elyan A, Abdelhady M, Halim HA, Altohamy S, Goubran F. Antithrombin III levels in normal pregnancy and preeclampsia. Proceedings, 4th World Congress of the International Society for the Study of Hypertension in Pregnancy. Nottingham, England, 1984:211.
116. Redman CW, Denson KW, Berlin LJ, Bolton FG, Stirrat GM. Factor VIII consumption in preeclampsia. Lancet 1977;2:1249–1252.
117. Howie PW, Begg CB, Purdie DW, Prentice CR. The use of coagulation

tests to predict the clinical progress of preeclampsia. Lancet 1976; 2:323–325.
118. Fournie A, Monrozies M, Pontonnier T, Boneu B, Bierme R. Factor VIII complex in normal pregnancy, preeclampsia and fetal growth retardation. Br J Obstet Gynecol 1981;88:250–254.
119. Douglas JT, Shah M, Lowe GD, Belch JJ, Forbes CD. Plasma fibrinopeptide A and beta-thromboglobulin levels in preeclampsia and hypertensive pregnancy. Thromb Haemost 1982;47:54–55.
120. Aznar J, Gilabert J, Estelles A, Espana F. Fibrinolytic acitivity and protein C in preeclampsia. Thromb Haemost 1986;55:314–317.
121. Trofatter KF Jr, Trofatter MO, Caudle MR, Offutt DQ. Detection of fibrin d-dimer in plasma and urine of pregnant women using Dimertest latex assay. South Med J 1993;86:1017–1021.
122. Kobayashi T, Terao T. Preeclampsia as chronic disseminated intravascular coagulation: study of two parameters: thrombin-antithrombin complex and D-dimers. Gyneco Obstet Invest 1987;24:170–178.
123. Halligan A, Bonnar J, Sheppard B, Darling M, Walshe J. Haemostatic, fibrinolytic and endothelial variables in normal pregnancies and preeclampsia. Br J Obstet Gynaecol 1994;101:488–492.
124. Fisher KA, Luger A, Spango BH, Linheimer MD. Hypertension in pregnancy: clinical-pathological correlations and late prognosis. Medicine 1981;60:267–276.
125. Weiner CP, Kwaan HC, Xu C, Paul M, Burmeister L, Hauck W. Antithrombin III activity in women with hypertension during pregnancy. Obstet Gynecol 1985;65:301–306.
126. Douglas RG, Buckman MI, MacDonald PF. Premature separation of the normally implanted placenta. J Obstet Gynaecol Br Emp 1955; 62:710.
127. Basu HK. Fibrinolysis and abruptio placentae. Br J Obstet Gynaecol 1969;76:481–496.
128. Sutton DMC, Hauser R, Kulapongs P, Bachmann F. Intravascular coagulation in abruptio placentae. Am J Obstet Gynecol 1971;109: 604–614.
129. Sher G. Pathogenesis and management of uterine inertia complicating abruptio placentae with consumption coagulopathy. Am J Obstet Gynecol 1977;129:164–170.
130. Knab DR. Abruptio placentae: an assessment of the time and method of delivery. Am J Obstet Gynecol 1978;52:625–629.
131. Pritchard JA. Fetal death in utero. Obstet Gynecol 1959;14:573.
132. Jimenez JM, Pritchard JA. Pathogenesis and treatment of coagulation defects resulting from fetal death. Obstet Gynecol 1968;32:449–459.
133. Waxman B, Gambrill R. Use of heparin in disseminated intravascular coagulation. Am J Obstet Gynecol 1972;112:434–438.
134. Levine W, Rosengart M, Siegler A. Spontaneous correction of hypofibrinogenemia with fetal death *in utero*. Obstet Gynecol 1962; 19:551.
135. Romero R, Duffy TP, Berkowitz RL, Chang E, Hobbins JC. Prolongation of a preterm pregnancy complicated by death of a single twin *in utero* and disseminated intravascular coagulation. Effects of treatment with heparin. N Engl J Med 1984;310:772–774.
136. Skelly H, Marivate M, Norman R, Kenoyer G, Martin R. Consumptive coagulopathy following fetal death in a triplet pregnancy. Am J Obstet Gynecol 1982;142:595–596.
137. Moore CM, McAdams AJ, Southerland J. Intrauterine disseminated intravascular coagulation: a syndrome of multiple pregnancy with a dead twin fetus. J Pediatr 1969;74:523–528.
138. Benirschke K. Twin placenta and perinatal mortality. NY J Med 1961; 61:1499.
139. Reisman LE, Pathak A. Bilateral renal cortical necrosis in the newborn. Am J Dis Child 1966;111:541.
140. Yoshioka H, Kadomoto Y, Mino M, Morikawa Y, Kasubuchi Y, Kusunoki T. Multicystic encephalomalacia in live-born twin with a stillborn macerated co-twin. J Pediatr 1979;95:798–800.
141. Graeff H, Ernst E, Bocaz R, von Hugo R, Hafter R. Evaluation of hypercoagulability in septic abortion. Hemostasis 1976;5:285–294.
142. Phillips LL, Margaretten W, McKay DG. Changes in the fibrinolytic enzyme system following intravascular coagulation induced by thrombin and endotoxin. Am J Obstet Gynecol 1968;100:319.
143. Kuhn W, Graeff H. Prophylaktische massnahmen beim septischen abort. In Zander J, ed. Septischer Abort und Bakterieller Schock. Heidelburg: Springer, 1968:74.
144. McKay DG. Disseminated intravascular coagulation. New York: Harper & Row, 1965.
145. McKay DG, Jewett JF, Reid DE. Endotoxin shock and the generalized Shwartzman reaction in pregnancy. Am J Obstet Gynecol 1959; 78:546.
146. Beller FK, Schoendorf T. Augmentation of endotoxin-induced fibrin deposits by pregnancy and estrogen-progesterone treatment. Gynecol Obstet Invest 1972;3:176–183.
147. Beller FK, Uszynski M. Disseminated intravascular coagulation in pregnancy. Clin Obstet Gynecol 1974;17:250–278.
148. Duff P. Pathophysiology and management of septic shock. J Reprod Med 1980;24:109–117.
149. Margulis RR, Dustin RW, Lovell JR, Robb H, Jabs C. Heparin for septic abortion and the prevention of endotoxic shock. Obstet Gynecol 1971;37:474–483.
150. McLees BD. Critical care medicine. In: Wyngaarden JB, Smith LH, eds. Cecil textbook of medicine. Philadelphia: WB Saunders, 1982:2186.
151. Schumer W. Steroids in the treatment of clinical septic shock. Ann Surg 1976;184:333–341.
152. Glenn TM, Leffer AM. Role of lysosomes in the pathogenesis of splanchnic ischemic shock in cats. Circ Res 1970;27:783–797.
153. Gahhos FN, Chiu RC, Hinchey EJ, Richards GK. Endorphins in septic shock: hemodynamic and endocrine effects of an opiate receptor antagonist and agonist. Arch Surg 1982;117:1053–1057.
154. Peters WP, Johnson MW, Friedman PA, Mitch WE. Pressor effect of naloxone in septic shock. Lancet 1981;1:529-532.
155. Colman RW, Robboy SJ, Minna JD. Disseminated intravascular coagulation: a reappraisal. Annu Rev Med 1979;30:359–374.
156. Corrigan JJ Jr. Heparin therapy in bacterial septicemia. J Pediatr 1977; 91:695–700.
157. Kuhn W, Graeff H. Gerinnungsstorungen in der Geburtshilfe. Stuttgart: Thieme, 1970:848–852.
158. Steiner PE, Lushbaugh CC. Maternal pulmonary embolism by amniotic fluid as a cause of obstetrical shock and unexpected deaths in obstetrics. JAMA 1941;117:1245–1255.
159. Resnik R, Swartz WH, Plumer MH, Benirschke K, Stratthaus ME. Amniotic fluid embolism with survival. Obstet Gynecol 1976;47: 295–298.
160. Sparr RA, Pritchard JA. Studies to detect the escape of amniotic fluid into the maternal circulation during parturition. Surg Gynecol Obstet 1958;107:560–564.
161. Kuhlman K, Hidvegi D, Tamura RK, Deep R. Is amniotic fluid material in the central circulation of peripartum patients pathologic? Am J Perinatol 1985;2:295–299.
162. Graeff J, Kuhn W. Coagulation disorders in obstetrics—pathobiochemistry, pathophysiology, diagnosis, treatment. Philadelphia: WB Saunders, 1980.
163. Clark SL, Montz FJ, Phelan JP. Hemodynamic alterations associated with amniotic fluid embolism: a reappraisal. Am J Obstet Gynecol 1985;151:617–621.
164. Skjodt P. Amniotic fluid embolism: a case investigated by coagulation and fibrinolysis studies. Acta Obstet Gynecol Scand 1965;44:437–457.
165. Beller FK, Douglas GW, Debrovner CH, Robinson R. The fibrinolytic system in amniotic fluid embolism. Am J Obstet Gynecol 1963;87: 48–55.
166. Albrechtsen OK, Storm O, Trolle D. Fibrinolytic activity in circulating blood following amniotic fluid infusion. Acta Haematol 1955; 14:309.
167. Clark SL, Pavlova Z, Greenspoon J, Horenstein J, Phelan JP. Squamous cells in the maternal pulmonary circulation. Am J Obstet Gynecol 1986;154:104–106.
168. Phillips LL, Davidson EC. Procoagulant properties of amniotic fluid. Am J Obstet Gynecol 1972;113:911–919.
169. Yaffe H, Bar-On H, Eldor A, Ron M, Sadovsky E. Correlation between thromboplastin activity and lecithin/sphingomyelin ratio in amniotic fluid: preliminary report. Br J Obstet Gynecol 1977;84: 354–356.
170. Weiner CP, Brandt J. A modified activated partial thromboplastin time with the use of amniotic fluid. Am J Obstet Gynecol 1982;144: 234–240.
171. Attwood HD, Downing SE. Experimental amniotic fluid in meconium embolism. Surg Gynecol Obstet 1965;120:255–262.
172. Kitzmiller JL, Lucas WE. Studies on a model of amniotic fluid embolism. Obstet Gynecol 1972;39:626.
173. Karim SMM, Devlin J. Prostaglandin content of amniotic fluid during pregnancy and labor. J Obstet Gynecol Br Commonw 1979;74:230.

174. Azegami M, Mori N. Amniotic fluid embolism and leukotrienes. Am J Obstet Gynecol 1986;155:1119–1124.
175. Albrechtsen OK, Trolle D. A fibrinolytic system in human amniotic fluid. Acta Haematol 1955;14:376–382.
176. Maki M, Tachita K, Kawasaki Y, Nagasawa K. Heparin treatment of amniotic fluid embolism. Tohoku J Exp Med 1969;97:155–160.
177. Lalos O, von Schoultz B. Amniotic fluid embolism: a review of the literature with two case reports. Int J Gynaecol Obstet 1977;15:48–53.
178. Henderson SR, Lund CJ. Severe preeclampsia, disseminated intravascular coagulopathy and hydatiform mole complicating a 20 week pregnancy with a fetus. Obstet Gynecol 1971;37:722–729.
179. Talbert LM, Easterling WE, Flowers CE, Graham JB. Acquired coagulation defects of pregnancy—including a case of a patient with hydatiform mole. Obstet Gynecol 1961;18:69–76.
180. Glueck HI, Burket RL, Sutherland JM, Garber ST. Afibrinogenemia in pregnancy apparently due to a degenerating leiomyoma. Obstet Gynecol 1961;18:285–290.
181. Koren Z, Zuckerman H, Brzezinski A. Placenta previa accreta with afibrinogenemia: report of three cases. Obstet Gynecol 1961;18:138–145.
182. Antimicrobials and haemostasis [Editorial]. Lancet 1983;1:510.
183. Neu HC. The *in vitro* activity, human pharmacology and clinical effectiveness of new beta-lactam antibiotics. Annu Rev Pharmacol Toxicol 1982;22:599–642
184. Brown CH, Natelson EA, Bradshaw MW, Williams TW Jr, Alfrey CP Jr. The hemostatic defect produced by carbenicillin. N Engl J Med 1974;291:265–270.
185. Ikeda Y, Kikuchi M, Matsuda S, et al. Inhibition of platelet function by sulbenicillin and its metabolite. Antimicrob Agents Chemother 1978;5:881–883.
186. Margolius A, Jackson DP, Ratnoff OD. Circulating anticoagulants: a study of 40 cases and a review of the literature. Medicine 1961; 40:145.
187. Carreras LO, Defreyn G, Machin SJ, et al. Arterial thrombosis, intrauterine death and "lupus" anticoagulant: detection of immunoglobulin interfering with prostacyclin formation. Lancet 1981;1:244–246.
188. Marengo-Rowe AJ, Murff G, Leveson JE, Cook J. Hemophilia-like disease associated with pregnancy. Obstet Gynecol 1972;40:56–64.
189. Greenwood RJ, Rabin SC. Hemophilia-like postpartum bleeding. Obstet Gynecol 1967;30:362–366.
190. Voke J, Letsky E. Pregnancy and antibody to factor VIII. J Clin Pathol 1977;30:928–932.
191. Fischer DS, Clyne LP. Circulating factor XI antibody and disseminated intravascular coagulation. Arch Intern Med 1981;141:515–517.
192. Lechner K. Acquired inhibitors in nonhemophiliac patients. Hemostasis 1974;3:65.
193. Boxer M, Elleman L, Carvalho A. The lupus anticoagulant. Arthritis Rheum 1976;19:1244–1248.
194. Canoso RT, Hutton RA. A chlorpromazine-induced inhibitor of blood coagulation. Am J Hematol 1977;2:183–191.
195. Feinstein DI, Rapaport SI. Acquired inhibitors of blood coagulation. Prog Hemost Thromb 1972;1:75–95.
196. Feinstein DI, Rapaport SI. Anticoagulants in systemic lupus erythematosus. In: Dubois EL, ed. Lupus erythematosus. Supplement 2. Los Angeles: University of Southern California Press, 1974:438.
197. De Wolf F, Carreras LO, Moerman P, Vermylen J, Van-Assche A, Renaer M. Decidual vasculopathy and extensive placental infarction in a patient with repeated thromboembolic accidents, recurrent fetal loss, and a lupus anticoagulant. Am J Obstet Gynecol 1982;142: 829–834.
198. Stephensen O, Cleland WP, Hallidie-Smith K. Congenital complete heart block and persistent ductus arteriosus associated with maternal systemic lupus erythematosus. Br Heart J 1981;46:104–106.
199. Chameides L, Truex R, Vetter V, Rashkind WJ, Galioto FM, Jr, Noonan JA. Association of maternal systemic lupus erythematosus with congenital complete heart block. N Engl J Med 1977;297:1204–1207.
200. Scott JS, Maddison PJ, Taylor PV, Esscher E, Scott O, Skinner RP. Connective tissue disease, antibodies to ribonucleoprotein, and congenital heart block. N Engl J Med 1983;309:209–212.
201. Lockshin MD, Druzin ML, Qamar T. Prednisone does not prevent recurrent fetal death in women with antiphospholipid antibody. Am J Obstet Gynecol 1989;160:439–443.
202. Lubbe WF, Butler WS, Palmer SJ, Wiggins GC. Fetal survival after prednisone suppression of maternal lupus-anticoagulant. Lancet 1983; 1:1361–1363.
203. Prednisone and maternal lupus anticoagulant blood;cb. Lancet 1983;2:576–577.
204. McMillan CW, Shapiro SS, Whitehurst D, Hoyer LW, Rao AV, Lazerson J. The natural history of factor VIII inhibitors in patients with hemophilia A: a national cooperative study. II. Observations on the initial development of factor VIII C inhibitors. Blood 1988;71: 344–348.
205. Hoyer LW. Factor VIII inhibitors. Curr Opin Hematol 1995;2: 365–371.
206. Feinstein DI. Acquired inhibitors against factor VIII and other clotting proteins. In: Coleman RW, Hirsch J, Marder VJ, Salzman EW, eds. Hemostasis and thrombosis. Philadelphia: JB Lippincott, 1982: 567–570.
207. Holmberg L, Nilsson IM. von Willebrand's disease. Eur J Haematol 1992;48:127–141.
208. Sporn LA, Chavin SI, Marder VJ, Wagner DD. Biosynthesis of von Willebrand protein by heman megakaryocytes. J Clin Invest 1985; 76:1102–1106.
209. Wagner DD, Marder VJ. Biosynthesis of von Willebrand protein by human endothelial cells. J Bio Chem 1983;258:2065–2067.
210. Ginsburg D, Sadler JE. von Willebrand disease: a database of point mutations, insertions, and deletions. Thromb Haemost 1993;69: 177–184.
211. Sadler JE. A revised classification of von Willebrand disease. Thromb Haemost 1994;71:520–525.
212. Hanna W, McCarroll D, McDonald T, et al. Variant von Willebrand's disease and pregnancy. Blood 1981;58:873–879.
213. Punnonen R, Nyman D, Gronroos M, Wallen O. Von Willebrand's disease in pregnancy. Acta Obstet Gynecol Scand 1981;60:507–509.
214. Evans PC. Obstetric and gynecologic patients with von Willebrand's disease. Obstet Gynecol 1971;38:37–43.
215. Sorosky J, Klatsky A, Nobert GF, Burchell RC. Von Willebrand's disease complicating second trimester abortion. Obstet Gynecol 1980; 55:253–254.
216. Lipton RA, Ayromlooi J, Coller BS. Severe von Willebrand's disease during labor and delivery. JAMA 1982;248:1355–1357.
217. Krishnamurthy M, Miotti AB. Von Willebrand's disease in pregnancy. Obstet Gynecol 1977;49:244–247.
218. Noller KL, Bowie EJW, Kempers RD, Owen CA Jr. Von Willebrand's disease in pregnancy. Obstet Gynecol 1973;41:865–872.
219. Adashi EY. Lack of improvement in von Willebrand's disease during pregnancy. N Engl J Med 1980;303:1178.
220. Lusher JM. Screening and diagnosis of coagulation disorders. Am J Obstet Gynecol 1996;175:778–783.
221. Lusher JM. Response to 1-deamino-8-D-arginine vasopressin in von Willebrand disease. Haemostasis 1994;24:276–284.
222. Rose EH, Aledort LM. Nasal spray desmopressin (DDAVP) for mild hemophilia A and von Willebrand disease. Ann Intern Med 1991; 114:563–568.
223. Aledort LM. Treatment of von Willebrand's disease. Mayo Clin Proc 1991;66:841–846.
224. Mannucci PM, Lombardi R, Bader R, et al. Heterogeneity of Type I von Willebrand disease: evidence for a subgroup with an abnormal von Willebrand factor. Blood 1985;66:796–802.
225. Casonato A, Sartori MT, De Marco L, Girolami A. 1-Desamino-8-D-arginine vasopressin (DDAVP) infusion in type IIB von Willebrand's disease: shortening of bleeding time and induction of a variable pseudothrombocytopenia. Thromb Haemost 1990;64:117–120.
226. Foster PA. A perspective on the use of FVIII concentrates and cryoprecipitate prophylactically in surgery or therapeutically in severe bleeds in patients with von Willebrand disease unresponsive to DDAVP: results of an international survey. Thromb Haemost 1995; 74:1370–1378.
227. Weiss HJ, Rogers J, Brand H. Defective ristocetin-induced aggregation in von Willebrand's disease: its correction by factor VIII. J Clin Invest 1973;52:2697–2707.
228. Ramgren O. A clinical and medical social study of hemophilia in Sweden. Acta Med Scand 1962;171:759.
229. Department of Health, Education and Welfare. National Heart, Lung and Blood Institute study to evaluate the supply–demand relationships for AHF and PTC through 1980. Washington, DC: US Government Printing Office, 1977.
230. Barrai I, Cann HM, Cavalli-Sforza LL, DeNicola P. The effect of parental age on rates of mutation for hemophilia and evidence for dif-

fering mutation rates for hemophilia A and B. Am J Hum Genet 1968;20:175–196.

231. Firshein SI, Hoyer LW, Lazarchick J, et al. Prenatal diagnosis of classic hemophilia. N Engl J Med 1979;300:937–941.
232. Elston RC, Graham JB, Miller CH, Reisner HM, Bouma BN. Probabilistic classification of hemophilia A carriers by discriminant analysis. Thromb Res 1976;8:683–695.
233. Seligsohn U, Zivelin A, Perez C, Modan M. Detection of hemophilia A carriers by replicate factor VIII activity and factor VIII antigenicity determinations. Br J Haematol 1979;42:433–439
234. Ratnoff OD, Steinberg AG. Detection of the carrier state of classic hemophilia. NY Acad Sci 1975;240:95–96.
235. Klein HG, Aledort LM, Bouma BN, Hoyer LW, Zimmerman TS, DeMets DL. Cooperative study for detection of the carrier state of classic hemophilia. N Engl J Med 1977;296:959–962.
236. Orstavik KH, Veltkamp JJ, Bertina RM, Hermans J. Detection of carriers of hemophilia B. Br J Haematol 1979;42:293–301.
237. Lusher JM, McMillan CW. Severe factor VIII and factor IX deficiency in females. Am J Med 1978;65:637–648.
238. Kadir RA, Economides DL, Braithwaite J, Goldman E, Lee CA. The obstetric experience of carriers of haemophilia. Br J Obstet Gynecol 1997;104:803–810.
239. Hoyer LW, Carta CA, Mahoney MJ. Detection of hemophilia carriers during pregnancy. Blood 1982;60:1407.
240. Daffos F, Forestier F, Kaplan C, Cox W. Prenatal diagnosis and management of bleeding disorders with fetal blood sampling. Am J Obstet Gynecol 1988;158:939–946.
241. Tuddenham EGD, Schwaab R, Seehafer J, et al. Haemophilia A: database of nucleotide substitutions, deletions, insertions and rearrangements of the factor VIII gene. Nucleic Acids Res 1994;22:3511.
242. Mibashan RS, Peake IR, Rodeck CH, et al. Dual diagnosis of prenatal haemophilia A by measurement of fetal factor VIII C and VIII C antigen (VIII C Ag). Lancet 1980;2:994–997.
243. Ljung R, Lindgren AC, Petrini P, Tengborn L. Normal vaginal delivery is to recommended for haemophilia carrier gravidae. Acta Paediatr 1994;83:609–611.
244. Kadir RA, Koh MB, Lee CA, Pasi KJ. Acquired haemophilia, an unusual cause of severe postpartum haemorrhage. Br J Obstet Gynaecol 1997;104:854–856.
245. Vicente V, Alberca I, Gonzalez R, Alegre A. Normal pregnancy in a patient with a postpartum factor VIII inhibitor. Am J Hematol 1987; 24:107–109.
246. Aledort LM. Hemophilia: yesterday, today, and tomorrow. Mt Sinai J Med 1996;63:225–235.
247. Brandt P, Stemberg S. Subcutaneous heparin for thrombosis in pregnant women with hereditary antithrombin deficiency. BMJ 1980; 1:449.
248. Egeberg O. Inherited antithrombin deficiency causing thrombophilia. Thromb Haemost 1965;13:516.
249. Johansson L. Hedner U, Nilsson IM. Familial antithrombin III deficiency as pathogenesis of deep venous thrombin. Acta Med Scand 1978;204:491–495.
250. Hellgren M, Tengborn L, Abildgaard U. Pregnancy in women with congenital antithrombin III deficiency: experience of treatment with heparin and antithrombin. Gynecol Obstet Invest 1982;14:127–141.
251. Sanson BJ, Friederich PW, Simioni P, et al. The risk of abortion and stillbirth in antithrombin-, protein C-, and protein S-deficient women. Thromb Haemost 1996;75:387–388.
252. Weiner CP. Thromboembolic disease in the obstetric patient: evaluation, diagnosis, and treatment. In: Kwaan HC, ed. Clinical thrombosis, vol 2. Boca Raton, FL: CRC Press, 1989:291.
253. Kazuomi K, Matsuo T, Kodama K, Matsuo M. Prophylactic antithrombin III administration during pregnancy immediately reduces the thrombin hyperactivity of cogenital antithrombin III deficiency by forming thrombin-antithrombin III complexes. Thromb Res 1992; 66:509.
254. Vellenga E, Van Imhoff GW, Aarnoudse JG. Effect of prophylaxis with oral anticoagulants and low dose heparin during pregnancy in an antithrombin III deficient woman. Lancet 1983;2:224.
255. Samson D, Stirling Y, Woolf L, Howarth D, Seghatehian MJ. Management of planned pregnancy in a patient with congenital antithrombin III deficiency. Br J Haematol 1984;56:243–249.
256. LeClerc JR, Geerts W, Panju A, Nguyen P, Hirsh J. Management of antithrombin III deficiency during pregnancy without administration of anti-thrombin III. Thromb Res 1986;41:567–573.
257. Walenga JM, Fareed J. Current status on new anticoagulant and antithrombotic drugs and devices. Curr Opin Pulm Med 1997;3:291–302.
258. Gallus AS. Familial venous thromboembolism and inherited abnormalities of the blood clotting system. Aust NZ J Med 1984;14: 807–810.
259. Bauer-Menache D, O'Malley JP, Schorr JB, Wagner B, Williams C, the Cooperative Study Group. Evaluation of the safety, recovery, half-life, and clinical efficacy of antithrombin III (human) in patients with hereditary antithrombin III deficiency. Blood 1990;75:33–39.
260. Bauer-Schwartz RS, Bauer KA, Rosenberg RD, Kavanaugh EJ, Davies DC, Bogdanoff DA. Clinical experience with antithrombin III concentrate in treatment to congenital and acquired deficiency of antithrombin. Am J Med 1989;87:53S,605.
261. Fairfax AJ, Ibbotson RM. Effect of danazol on the biochemical abnormality of inherited antithrombin III deficiency. Thorax 1985;40: 646–650.
262. Malm J, Laurell M, Dahlback B. Changes in the plasma levels of vitamin K-dependent proteins C and S and C4b-binding protein during pregnancy and oral contraception. Br J Haematol 1988;68:437–443.
263. Griffin JH, Evatt B, Zimmerman TS, Kleiss AJ, Wideman C. Deficiency of protein C in congenital thrombotic disease. J Clin Invest 1981;68:1370–1373.
264. Manco-Johnson MJ, Marlar RA, Jacobson CJ, Hays T, Warody BA. Severe protein C deficiency in newborn infants. J Pediatr 1988; 113:359.
265. Morrison AE, Walker ID, Black WP. Protein C deficiency presenting as deep venous thrombosis in pregnancy: case report. Br J Obstet Gynaecol 1988;95:1077–1080.
266. Vogel JJ, de Moerloose A, Bounameaux H. Protein C deficiency and pregnancy: a case report. Obstet Gynecol 1989;73:455–456.
267. Comp PC, Esmon CT. Recurrent venous thromboembolism in patients with a partial deficiency of protein S. N Engl J Med 1984;311: 1525–1528.
268. Melissari E, Nicolaides KH, Scully MF, Kakkar VV. Protein S and C4b-binding protein in fetal and neonatal blood. Br J Haematol 1988; 70:199–203.
269. Koster T, Rosendaal FR, de Ronde H, Briet E, Vandenbroucke JP, Bertina RM. Venous thrombosis due to poor anticoagulant response to activated protein C: Leiden Thrombophilia Study. Lancet 1993;342: 1503–1506.
270. Legnani C, Palareti G, Giagi R, Coccheri S. Activated protein C resistance in deep-vein-thrombosis. Lancet 1994;343:541–542.
271. Hirsch DR, Mikkola KM, Marks PW, et al. Pulmonary embolism and deep venous thrombosis during pregnancy or oral contraceptive use: prevalence of factor V Leiden. Am Heart J 1996;131:1145–1148.
272. Stahlman F, Herrington WJ, Maloney WC. Parahemophilia: report of a case in a woman with studies on other members of her family. J Lab Clin Med 1951;38:842.
273. Field JB, Ware AG. Studies on parahemophilia. J Clin Invest 1954; 33:932.
274. Philips LL, Little WA. Factor V deficiency in obstetrics. Obstet Gynecol 1962;19:507–512.
275. Whitelaw A, Haines ME, Bolsover W, Harris E. Factor V deficiency and antenatal intraventricular haemorrhage. Arch Dis Child 1984;59: 997–999.
276. Bofill JA, Young RA, Perry KG Jr. Successful pregnancy in a woman with severe factor X deficiency. Obstet Gynecol 1996;88:723.
277. Kumar M, Mehta P. Cogenitial coagulopathies and pregnancy: report of four pregnancies in factor X deficient patient. Am J Hematol 1994; 46:241–244.
278. Purcell G, Nossel HL. Factor XI (PTA) deficiency: surgical and obstetric aspects. Obstet Gynecol 1970;35:69–74.
279. Czapek EE. Coagulation problems. Int Anesthesiol Clin 1973;11: 175–201.
280. Steinberg MH, Saletan S, Funt M, Baker D, Coller BS. Management of factor XI deficiency in gynecologic and obstetric patients. Obstet Gynecol 1986;68:130–133.
281. Saidi P, Siegelman M, Mitchell VB. Effect of factor XII deficiency on pregnancy and parturition. Thromb Haemost 1979;41:523–528.
282. Lao TT, Lewinsky RM, Ohlsson A, Cohen H. Factor XII deficiency and pregnancy. Obstet Gynecol 1991;78:491–493.
283. Duckert F, Jung E, Shmerling. A hitherto undescribed congential haemorrhagic diathesis probably due to fibrin stabilizing factor deficiency. Thromb Diath Haemorrh 1961;5:179.
284. Egbring R, Kroniger A, Seitz R. Factor XIII deficiency: pathogenic

mechanisms and clinical significance. Semin Thromb Hemost 1996; 22:419–425.

285. Trobisch H, Egbring R. Substitution mit einem neuen Faktor XIII-Konzentrat bei kongenitalelm Faktor XIII-Mangel. Dtsch Med Wochenschr 1972;97:499–502.
286. Coppleston A. Oscier DG. Heparin-induced thrombocytopenia in pregnancy [Letter]. Br J Haematol 1987;65:248.
287. Meytes D, Ayalon H, Virag I, Weisbort Y, Zakut H. Heparin-induced thrombocytopenia and recurrent thrombosis in pregnancy: a case report. J Reprod Med 1986;31:993–996.
288. Anderson HM. Maternal hematologic disorders. In: Creasy RK, Resnick R, eds. Maternal–fetal medicine: principles and practice. Philadelphia: WB Saunders, 1989:890.
289. Burrows RF, Kelton JG. Thrombocytopenia at delivery: a prospective survey of 6715 deliveries. Am J Obstet Gynecol 1990;163:731–734.
290. von dem Borne AEG, Vos JJ, van der Lelie E, Bossers B, van Dalen CM. Clinical significance of a positive platelet immunofluorscence test in thrombocytopenia. Br Jr Haematol 1986;64:767–776.
291. Burrows RF, Kelton, JG. Fetal thrombocytopenia and its relation to maternal thrombocytopenia. N Engl J Med 1993;329:1463–1466.
292. Kaplan C, Daffos F, Forestier F, Tertian G. Fetal platelet counts in thrombocytopenic pregnancy. Lancet 1990;336:979–982.
293. Freedman J, Musclow E, Garvey B, Abott D. Unexplained perparturient thrombocytopenia. Am J Hematol 1986;21:397–407.
294. Burrows RF, Kelton JG. Incidentally detected thrombocytopenia in healthy mothers and their infants. N Engl J Med 1988;319:142–145.
295. Burrows RF, Kelton JG. Low fetal risks in pregnancies associated with idiopathic thrombocytopenic purpura. Am J Obstet Gynecol 1990; 163:1147–1150.
296. Rolbin SH, Abbott D, Musclow E, Papsin F, Lie LM, Freedman J. Epidural anesthesia in pregnant patients with low platelet counts. Obstet Gynecol 1988;71:918–920.
297. Bofill JA, Young RA, Perry KG Jr. Successful pregnancy in a woman with severe factor X deficiency. Obstet Gynecol 1996;88:723.
298. Tancer LM. Idiopathic thrombocytopenic purpura and pregnancy. Am J Obstet Gynecol 1960;79:148.
299. Davies SV, Murray JA, Gee H, Giles HM. Transplacental effect of high-dose immunoglobulin in idiopathic thrombocytopenia (ITP). Lancet 1986;1:1098–1099.
300. Hammarstrom L, Smith CI. Placental transfer of intravenous immunoglobulin. Lancet 1986;1:681.
301. Kelton JG. Management of the pregnant patient with idiopathic thrombocytopenic purpura. Ann Intern Med 1983;99:796–800.
302. Kelton JG, Inwood MJ, Barr RM. The prenatal prediction of thrombocytopenia in infants of mothers with clinically diagnosed immune thrombocytopenia. Am J Obstet Gynecol 1982;144:449–454.
303. Samuels P, Bussel JB, Braitman LE, et al. Estimation of the risk of thrombocytopenia in the offspring of pregnant women with presumed immune thrombocytopenic purpura. N Engl J Med 1990;323:229–235.
304. Payne SD, Resnik R, Moore TR, Hedriana HL, Kelly TF. Maternal characteristics and risk of severe neonatal thrombocytopenia and intracranial hemorrhage in pregnancies complicated by autoimmune thrombocytopenia. Am J Obstet Gynecol 1997;177:149–155.
305. Christiaens GCML, Helmerhorst FM. Validity of intrapartum diagnosis of fetal thrombocytopenia. Am J Obstet Gynecol 1987;157: 864–865.
306. Weiner CP. Cordocentesis. Obstet Gynecol Clin North Am 1988;15: 283–301.
307. Bussel JB and the Neonatal Immune Thrombocytopenia Study Group. Neonatal alloimmune thrombocytopenia (NAIT): information derived from a prospective international registry. Paediatr Res 1988b;23:337A (abst).
308. Bussel JB, Zabusky MR, Berkowitz RL, McFarland JG. Fetal alloimmune thrombocytopenia. N Engl J Med 1997;337:22–26.
309. Schulman NR, Marder VJ, Hiller MC, Collier EM. Platelet and leukocyte antigens and their antibodies: serologic, physiologic, and clinical studies. Prog Hematol 1964;4:222.
310. Mueller-Eckhardt C, Kiefel V, Grubert A, et al. 348 cases of suspected neonatal alloimmune thrombocytopenia. Lancet 1989a;1:363–366.
311. Patriarco M, Yeh SY. Immunologic thrombocytopenia in pregnancy. Obstet Gynecol Surv 1986;41:661–671.
312. Shibata Y, Matsuda I, Miyaji T, Ichikawa Y. Yuk[a], a new platelet antigen involved in two cases of neonatal alloimmune thrombocytopenia. Vox Sang 1986;50:177–180.
313. Pearson HA, Schulman N, Marder V, Cone T. Immune neonatal thrombocytopenic purpura: clinical and therapeutic considerations. Blood 1964;23:154–177.
314. Kaplan C, Daffos F, Forestier F, et al. Management of alloimmune thrombocytopenia: antenatal diagnosis and in utero transfusion of maternal platelets. Blood 1988;72:340–343.
315. de Waal LP, van Dalen CM, Engelfreit CD, von dem Borne AEG. Alloimmunization against the platelet-specific Zwa antigen, resulting in neonatal alloimmune thrombocytopenia or post transfusion purpura, is associated with the supertypic DRw52 antigen including DR3 and DRw6. Hum Immunol 1986;17:45–53.
316. Blanchette VS, Chen L, Salomon de Freidberg S, Hoghan VA, Trudel E, Decary F. Alloimmunization to the Pl^{A1} antigen: results of a prospective study. Br J Haematol 1990;74:209–215.
317. Zalneraitis EL, Young RS, Krischnamoorthy KS. Intracranial hemorrhage in utero, a complication of isoimmune thrombocytopenia. J Pediatr 1979;95:611–614.
318. de Vries LS, Connell J, Bydder GM, et al. Recurrent intracranial haemorrhages *in utero* in an infant with alloimmune thrombocytopenia. Case report. Br J Obstet Gynaecol 1988;95:299–302.
319. Burrows RF, Caco CC, Kelton JG. Neonatal alloimmune thrombocytopenia: spontaneous in utero intracranial hemorrhage. Am J Hematol 1988;28:98–102.
320. Herman JH, Jumbelic MI, Ancona RJ, Kickler TS. *In utero* cerebral hemorrhage in alloimmune thrombocytopenia. Am J Pediatr Hematol Oncol 1986;8:312–317.
321. Bussel JB, McFarland JG, Berkowitz RL. Antenatal management of fetal alloimmune and autoimmune thrombocytopenia. Transfusion Medicine Reviews 1990;4:149–162.
322. Kaplan C, Daffos F, Forestier F, et al. Management of alloimmune thrombocytopenia: antenatal diagnosis and *in utero* transfusion of maternal platelets. Blood 1988;72:340–343.
323. Murphy MF, Pullon HWH, Metcalfe P, et al. Management of fetal alloimmune thrombocytopenia by weekly *in utero* platelet transfusions. Vox Sang 1990;58:45–49.
324. Nicholaides KH, Clewell W, Rodeck CH. Measurement of human fetoplacental blood volume in erythroblastosis fetalis. Am J Obstet Gynecol 1987;157:50–53.
325. Nicolini U, Rodeck CH, Kochenur NK, Greco P, Fisk NM, Letsky E. *In utero* platelet transfusion for alloimmune thrombocytopenia. Lancet 1988;2;506.
326. Murphy MF, Metcalfe P, Waters AH, Ord J, Hambley H, Nicolaides K. Antenatal management of severe feto-maternal alloimmune thrombocytopenia: HLA incompatibility may affect responses to fetal platelet transfusions. Blood 1993;81:2174–2179.
327. Weiner E, Zosmer N, Bajoria R, et al. Direct fetal administration of immunoglobulins: another disappointing therapy in alloimmune thrombocytopenia. Fetal Diagn Ther 1994;9:159–164.
328. Lynch L, Bussel JB, McFarland JG, Chitkara U, Berkowitz RL. Antenatal treatment of alloimmune thrombocytopenia. Obstet Gynecol 1992;62:67–71.
329. Bussel JB, Berkowitz RL, Lynch L, et al. Antenatal management of alloimmune thrombocytopenia with intravenous γ-globulin: a randomized trial of the addition of low-dose steroid to intravenous γ-globulin. Am J Obstet Gynecol 1996;174:1414–1423.
330. Donner M, Aronsson S, Holmberg L, Olofsson P. Corticosteroid treatment of maternal ITP and risk of neonatal thrombocytopenia. Acta Paediatr Scand 1987;76:369–371.
331. Van den Veyer IB, Chong SS, Kristjansson K, Snabes MC, Moise KJ Jr, Hughes MR. Molecular analysis of human platelet antigen system 1 antigen on single cells can be applied to preimplantation genetic diagnosis for prevention of alloimmune thrombocytopenia. Am J Obstet Gynecol 1994;170:807–812.
332. Moschowitz E. An acute febrile pleiochromic anemia with hyaline thrombosis of terminal arterioles and capillaries: an undescribed disease. Thromb Haemost 1978;40:4–8.
333. Ezra Y, Rose M, Eldor A. Therapy and prevention of thrombotic thrombocytopenic purpura during pregnancy: a clinical study of 16 pregnancies. Am J Hematol 1996;51:1–6.
334. Weiner CP. Thrombotic microangiopathy in pregnancy and the postpartum period. Semin Hematol 1987;24:119–129.
335. Egerman RS, Witlin AG, Friedman SA, Sibai BM. Thrombotic thrombocytopenic purpura and hemolytic uremic syndrome in pregnancy: review of 11 cases. Am J Obstet Gynecol 1996;175:950–956.
336. Ridofi RL, Bell WR. Thrombotic thrombocytopenic purpura: report of 25 cases and review of the literature. Medicine 1981;60:413–428.

337. Moake JL, Byrnes JJ, Troll JH, et al. Effects of fresh-frozen plasma and its cryosupernatant fraction on von Willebrand factor multimeric forms in chronic thrombotic thrombocytopenic purpura. Blood 1985; 65:1232–1236.
338. Moake JL, Rudy CK, Troll JH, et al. Unusually large plasma factor VIII: von Willebrand factor multimers in chronic relapsing thrombotic thrombocytopenic purpura. N Engl J Med 1982;307:1432–1435.
339. Takahashi H, Hanano M, Wada K, et al. Circulating thrombomodulin in thrombotic thrombocytopenic purpura. Am J Hematol 1991;38: 174–177.
340. Harker LA, Slichter SJ. Platelet and fibrinogen consumption in man. N Engl J Med 1972;287:999–1005.
341. Byrnes JJ, Moake JL. Thrombotic thrombocytopenic purpura and the haemolytic–uraemic syndrome: evolving concepts of pathogenesis and therapy. Clin Haematol 1986;15:413–442.
342. Jaffe EA, Nachman RL, Herskey C. Thrombotic thrombocytopenic purpura: coagulation parameters in twelve patients. Blood 1973;42: 499–507.
343. Pinette MG, Vintzileos AM, Ingardia CJ. Thrombotic thrombocytopenic purpura as a cause of thrombocytopenia in pregnancy: literature review. Am J Perinatol 1989;6:55–57.
344. Rock GA, Shumak KH, Buskard NA, et al. Comparison of plasma exchange with plasma infusion in the treatment of thrombotic thrombocytopenic purpura. Canadian Apheresis Study Group. N Engl J Med 1991;325:393–397.
345. Ambrose A, Welham RT, Cefalo RC. Thrombotic thrombocytopenic purpura in early pregnancy. Obstet Gynecol 1985;66:267–272.
346. Vandekerchove F. Thrombotic thrombocytopenic purpura mimicking toxemia. Am J Obstet Gynecol 1984;150:320–322.
347. Pereira A, Mazzara R, Monteagudo J, et al. Thrombotic thrombocytopenic purpura/hemolytic uremic syndrome: a multivariate analysis of factors predicting the response to plasma exchange. Ann Hematol 1995;70:319–323.
348. Schneider PA, Rayner AA, Linker CA, Schuman MA, Liu ET, Hohn DC. The role of splenectomy in multimodality treatment of thrombotic thrombocytopenic purpura. Ann Surg 1985;202:318–322.
349. Thompson CE, Damon LE, Reis CA, Linker CA. Thrombotic microangiopathies in the 1980's: clinical features, response to treatment, and the impact of the human immunodeficiency virus epidemic. Blood 1992;80:1890–1895.
350. Veltman GA, Brand A, Leeksma OC, ten Bosch GJ, van Krieken JH, Briet E. The role of splenectomy in the treatment of relapsing thrombotic thrombocytopenic purpura. Ann Hematol 1995;70:231–236.
351. Winslow GA, Nelson EW. Thrombotic thrombocytopenic purpura: indications for and results of splenectomy. Am J Surg 1995;170: 558–561.
352. Romero R, Mazor M, Lockwood CJ, et al. Clinical significance, prevalence, and natural history of thrombocytopenia in pregnancy-induced hypertension. Am J Perinatol 1989;6:32–38.
353. Stubbs TM, Lazarchick J, Van Dorsten P, Cox J, Loadholt CB. Evidence of accelerated platelet production and consumption in nonthrombocytopenic preeclampsia. Am J Obstet Gynecol 1986;155: 263–265.
354. Samuels P, Main EK, Tomaski A, Mennuti MT, Gabbe SG, Cines D. Abnormalities in platelet antiglobulin tests in preeclamptic mothers and their neonates. Am J Obstet Gynecol 1987;157:109–113.
355. Hart D, Dunetz C, Nardi M, Porges RF, Weiss A, Karpatkin M. An epidemic of maternal thrombocytopenia associated with elevated antiplatelet antibody: platelet count and antiplatelet antibody in 116 consecutive pregnancies. Relationship to neonatal platelet count. Am J Obstet Gynecol 1986;154:878–883.
356. Rick ME, Williams SB, Sacher RA, McKeown LP. Thrombocytopenia associated with pregnancy in a patient with type IIB von Willebrand's disease. Blood 1987;69:786–789.
357. Giles AR, Hoogendoorn H, Benford K. Type IIB von Willebrand's disease presenting as thrombocytopenia during pregnancy. Br J Haematol 1987;67:349–353.
358. Conti M, Mari D, Conti E, Muggiasca ML, Mannucci PM. Pregnancy in women with different types of von Willebrand disease. Obstet Gynecol 1986;68:282–285.
359. Stuart MJ, Gross SJ, Elred H, Graeber JE. Effects of acetylsalicylic-acid ingestion on maternal and neonatal hemostasis. N Engl J Med 1982;307:909–912.
360. White JG. Inherited abnormalities of the platelet membrane and secretory granules. Hum Pathol 1987;18:123–139.
361. Stuart MJ, Gross SJ, Elred H, Graeber JE. Effects of acetylsalicylic acid in gestation on maternal and neonatal homeostasis. N Engl J Med 1982;307:909–912.
362. White JG. Inherited abnormalities of the platelet membrane and secretory granules. Hum Path 1987;18:123–139.

Cherry and Merkatz's Complications of Pregnancy,
Fifth Edition, edited by W. R. Cohen.
Lippincott Williams & Wilkins, Philadelphia © 2000.

CHAPTER 21

Anemia

Christopher O'Reilly-Green

Anemia is defined as a reduction below normal in the number of erythrocytes per cubic millimeter, in the quantity of hemoglobin, or in the volume of packed red cells. The detection of symptomatic anemia is based initially on history and physical examination. The diagnosis is confirmed by evaluating the complete blood count (CBC), which might also have been obtained from an asymptomatic person as a screening test. Morphologic classification of anemia begins with an evaluation of red cell indexes, followed by a microscopic evaluation of the peripheral blood smear. Measurement of the reticulocyte count provides information regarding the individual's capacity to respond to and correct the anemia and, in the context of the morphologic data, allows for a preliminary etiologic classification of the anemia. The clinician uses this classification for guidance in selecting further tests that will specify the cause of the anemia.

DEFINITION IN WOMEN

The normal ranges of hemoglobin and hematocrit change with age and during pregnancy and are lower for women than for men (1–3). The Second National Health and Nutrition Examination Survey provided population-based information that gave a definition of norms for hemoglobin and hematocrit (1). These norms were determined after excluding from a cross-sectional population-based survey those women who were pregnant, who had known hemoglobinopathies, or who had an iron-to-iron binding capacity ratio <16%, a mean cell volume (MCV) <80 fL, or an erythrocyte protoporphyrin level >75 μg/dL, values usually associated with anemia. Using this subpopulation, the median venous hemoglobin for all "normal" women aged 18 to 44 was 13.5 g/dL (Table 21-1). For all normal women aged 18 to 44, the 95th percentile range for venous hemoglobin was 11.7 to 15.5 g/dL. For black normal women aged 18 to 44, the 95th percentile range for venous hemoglobin was 10.7 to 15.3 g/dL. For normal men it was 13.2 to 17.3 g/dL.

TABLE 21-1. *Sex and race differences in hemoglobin values*

NHANES II values for ages 18–44	Median venous hemoglobin (g/dL)	95% Confidence limits around the median venous hemoglobin (g/dL)
All normal women	13.5	11.7–15.5
Black normal women	12.8	10.7–15.3
All normal men	15.3	13.2–17.3

NHANES II, Second National Health and Nutrition Examination Survey.

[a]Median venous hemoglobin values and 95% confidence limits derived from a "normal" subset of the NHANES II study population (from ref. 2).

DEFINITION IN PREGNANCY

Based on pooled data from four European surveys of healthy pregnant women taking iron supplements, the fifth percentile for hemoglobin fell from 11.0 g/dL at 12 weeks' gestation to a nadir of 10.5 at 24 weeks' gestation and rose to 11.9 at 40 weeks (Table 21-2) (2). The normal values are higher at every gestational age in women subject to chronic hypoxic stress, such as smoking tobacco or living at high altitude.

When low-income women attending prenatal clinics in the United States were studied, blacks had lower hemoglobin levels than whites at every week of gestation (4). Hemoglobin levels among these women were lowest for teenagers and for women who first enrolled in the third trimester. Thalassemia and sickle cell disease, sickle cell trait, hemoglobin C disease, and hemoglobin C trait are

C. O'Reilly-Green: Lenox Hill Hospital, New York, NY.

TABLE 21-2. *Fifth percentile values for hemoglobin by week of pregnancy*[a]

Gestation (wk)	12	16	20	24	28	32	36	40
Mean hemoglobin (g/dL)	12.2	11.8	11.6	11.6	11.8	12.1	12.5	12.9
Fifth percentile hemoglobin (g/dL)	11.0	10.6	10.5	10.5	10.7	11.0	11.4	11.9
Fifth percentile hematocrit (%)	33.0	32.0	32.0	32.0	32.0	33.0	34.0	36.0

[a]Fifth percentile values for hemoglobin by week of pregnancy from four European surveys of healthy women taking iron supplements (from ref. 1).

more common among blacks and might account for a part of the mean difference (5). However, these subgroups may have worse nutritional status or an additional factor that causes anemia.

In 1980, the Public Health Service published nutrition objectives for the nation to achieve by 1990. Among them was a stated goal that the proportion of pregnant women with iron-deficiency anemia should be reduced to 3.5% (6). In 1992, the Centers for Disease Control reported that the prevalence of anemia at each trimester among low-income pregnant women participating in public health programs in the United States had remained stable since 1979 (7). In 1990, 9.8%, 13.8%, and 33% of the women reported by the Centers for Disease Control pregnancy nutrition surveillance system were anemic in the first, second, and third trimesters, respectively. Anemia in the first trimester was associated with a high risk of low birth weight.

EPIDEMIOLOGY

Mortality and Morbidity Among Women

The American College of Obstetricians and Gynecologists recommends screening women for asymptomatic anemia and correcting it before considering pregnancy or at least as early in pregnancy as possible (8). A significant effort is spent in prenatal care to diagnose and treat asymptomatic anemia. The reason for this is the perception that anemia contributes to pregnancy morbidity and mortality. The magnitude of this problem is difficult to assess, because these outcomes are not common and their association with anemia is usually made through connecting databases in which the sources and causes of anemia are not well defined. Some systemic diseases that cause maternal and fetal morbidity and mortality are associated with anemia, but it is likely that the risk is related to the global manifestations of the systemic disease itself rather than simply the anemia.

In the United States, iron deficiency is the most common cause of anemia among women (2). Such deficiency results from acute and chronic loss of iron through bleeding without adequate dietary replacement. Iron-deficiency anemia can contribute to maternal and fetal mortality if the hemoglobin level falls low enough to cause tissue hypoxia. This can occur in the asymptomatic iron-deficient woman who experiences acute blood loss during pregnancy. Correction of the iron-deficient state before the onset of hemorrhage might lessen the risk of mortality. These risks account for the reluctance of surgeons to undertake elective surgery when the hemoglobin level is less than 10 g/dL.

The prevalence of iron-deficiency anemia worldwide in 1990 was 36,715 per 100,000 women (9). Disability-adjusted life years (DALYs) measure disease burden by adjusting the absolute measured life span according to the number of years of disability preceding death and report the number of productive years of life lost because of a disease (10). In 1990, iron-deficiency anemia was ranked 12th worldwide among causes of diminished DALYs in women. It is projected to drop to a rank of 39th by the year 2020, replaced by newly rising causes, such as war, human immunodeficiency virus infection, violence, self-inflicted injuries, and tobacco-related cancers. Iron-deficiency anemia ranks second among leading causes of disability worldwide, behind unipolar major depression.

There is a conviction among obstetricians, patients, and public health authorities that maternal anemia contributes to poor perinatal outcome. This belief is based on research associating the two. Data from the U.S. Pregnancy Nutrition Surveillance System showed that anemia in the first trimester was strongly associated with a risk of low birth weight (7). This association was attenuated in later trimesters. These investigators concluded that their findings indicated a need to improve iron nutrition among low-income women. These sentiments echo those expressed by numerous others. The analyses of epidemiologic data, however, did not control sufficiently for confounding variables. Thus, whether anemia is a cause of poor outcome or a consequence of other factors that are themselves the underlying causes of poor fetal and neonatal outcomes cannot be determined from these data.

PHYSIOLOGY OF ERYTHROCYTE HOMEOSTASIS

Most women show hematologic changes during pregnancy that could be attributed to iron deficiency (11). Hemoglobin and serum iron concentrations fall, and total iron-binding capacity rises; the mean corpuscular hemoglobin concentration can remain constant or fall. Much of this change cannot be considered anemia if it is defined as total oxygen-carrying capacity or sufficient oxygen-carrying capacity to meet physiologic needs. In the well-nourished patient, the red cell mass actually increases during pregnancy. Hemoglobin and hematocrit fall because the increase in plasma volume exceeds the increase in red cell mass. The circulating red cells have a greater percentage of reticulocytes, which are larger and younger than mature red cells, and have a lower concentration of hemoglobin. There is no evidence that this physiologic response in well-nourished, healthy women is inadequate. The increased demands for iron are offset in part by amenorrhea and the increased absorption of iron during pregnancy.

Physiology of Erythropoiesis in Pregnancy

Anemia can be considered a breakdown in the mechanism responsible for maintaining homeostasis in the red cell compartment. The feedback loop for this mechanism involves oxygen delivery. Red cells are nonreplicating, differentiated cells with an average life span of 120 days. They contain hemoglobin, which, in turn, carries molecular oxygen bound to the heme moiety in a reversible fashion described by the sigmoid-shaped oxygen–hemoglobin dissociation curve. Red cells carry oxygen bound to hemoglobin to the kidneys, which contain cells that synthesize erythropoietin. A decline in oxygen delivery to these cells results in an increase in the synthesis and release of erythropoietin, which is transported out of the kidney in blood and exerts its effect in the erythroid marrow, enhancing multiplication and differentiation of erythroid cell precursors. This process requires the supply of iron stored in reticuloendothelial cells as well as important cofactors in DNA synthesis, including cobalamin (vitamin B_{12}) and folate.

Various hematopoietic growth factors derived from other members of the marrow compartment influence the development of erythroid cells. Interleukin-3 (IL-3), derived from T-lymphocytes, and granulocyte–macrophage colony–stimulating factor (GM-CSF), derived from T-lymphocytes, monocytes, fibroblasts, and endothelial cells, interact with erythropoietin. The result is stimulation of erythroid burst-forming units (BFU-E) to differentiate into erythroid colony-forming units and then into pro-erythroblasts and erythroblasts (10).

Beguin and colleagues investigated serum immunoreactive erythropoietin in 74 nonpregnant women, including 33 normal subjects and 41 women with hypoplastic, hemolytic, dyserythropoietic, or iron-deficiency anemia (11). The mean value for erythropoietin in normal women was 16.4 mU/mL. An inverse linear relationship between the log of the erythropoietin concentration and hematocrit was observed. Serum erythropoietin levels were significantly higher during pregnancy (30 mU/mL), at delivery (31 mU/mL), and on day 7 postpartum (37 mU/mL) than in normal nonpregnant women. Erythropoietin levels increased steadily from 18 mU/mL in the first trimester to 26 mU/mL in the second trimester and to 35 mU/mL in the third trimester. The negative correlation between the log of the erythropoietin concentration and hematocrit was not present in the first two trimesters. It was present during the third trimester and at delivery, but it had a reduced slope. The previously observed negative correlation was reestablished postpartum. The authors concluded that the erythropoietin response to anemia was impaired in early pregnancy, recovered in late pregnancy, and normalized rapidly in the postpartum period.

A randomized, double-blind, placebo-controlled study of iron supplementation showed that from 27 weeks of gestation to 8 weeks postpartum, the placebo-treated group had significantly lower hemoglobin levels than the iron-treated group. The placebo group had significantly higher values for erythropoietin than the iron-treated group from the 27th week of gestation to 1 week postpartum (12). Harstad et al. found that the mean hematocrit level in normal pregnancy reached a nadir late in the second trimester and the serum erythropoietin level reached a plateau at a 50% increase (13). Those pregnancies complicated by anemia, defined by a hematocrit less than 30 vol%, showed a statistically significant increase in serum erythropoietin above the levels of those pregnancies not complicated by anemia.

In a trial of iron supplementation, Milman et al. found that in the placebo-treated women, median serum erythropoietin rose from 22.5 mU/mL at inclusion to 35.0 mU/mL at delivery (14). In the iron-treated women, median serum erythropoietin rose from 23.9 to 29.9 mU/mL. Serum erythropoietin showed a steeper increase in the placebo-treated women than in the iron-treated women. After delivery, serum erythropoietin became normal in both groups. Most studies found a steady rise in erythropoietin as gestation progressed and a negative correlation between the log of erythropoietin and indexes of iron depletion, as in nonpregnant patients. Iron supplementation of pregnant women results in suppression of erythropoietin production.

ETIOLOGY, CLASSIFICATION, AND DIAGNOSIS OF ANEMIAS

Anemias can be classified in terms of clinical, morphologic, or etiological factors and characteristics. There are advantages to each system, and they mesh with each other. Clinical classification allows the physician to adjust the pace of diagnosis and treatment according to the severity of the patient's condition. Morphologic classification, based on examination of the peripheral smear, is the most common way to arrive at a specific diagnosis and a good way to proceed in a cost-effective search for the source of anemia. The most common cause of anemia is iron deficiency, and when the history, physical examination, and evaluation of the CBC, the red cell indexes, and the peripheral smear lead to no other diagnosis, a cost-effective approach to confirming the diagnosis is to initiate therapy and reevaluate the results in 1 month. If anemia fails to improve with this regimen, a more intensive clinical and laboratory evaluation is justified.

Clinical Classification of Anemias

Anemias can be classified as either symptomatic or asymptomatic. Symptomatic anemia manifests as pallor of the skin and mucous membranes, shortness of breath, palpitations, soft systolic murmurs, lethargy, and fatigability. Some women will enter pregnancy with a diagnosis of anemia that was made before pregnancy on the basis of symptoms. These patients are at high risk not only because they have more severe anemias but also because they might have an underlying systemic disease that itself imparts risks to pregnancy. Other women will be discovered to have anemia during pregnancy as a result of screening tests. These anemias will generally be of a milder sort, but the interaction with pregnancy can result in an unexpectedly severe outcome. One example is a previously undiagnosed heterozygous hemoglobinopathy for hemoglobin S and hemoglobin C. This condition might have been asymptomatic before pregnancy, yet it can lead to a fatal outcome in gestation. Stages of iron deficiency (more fully discussed later) are presented in Fig. 21-1.

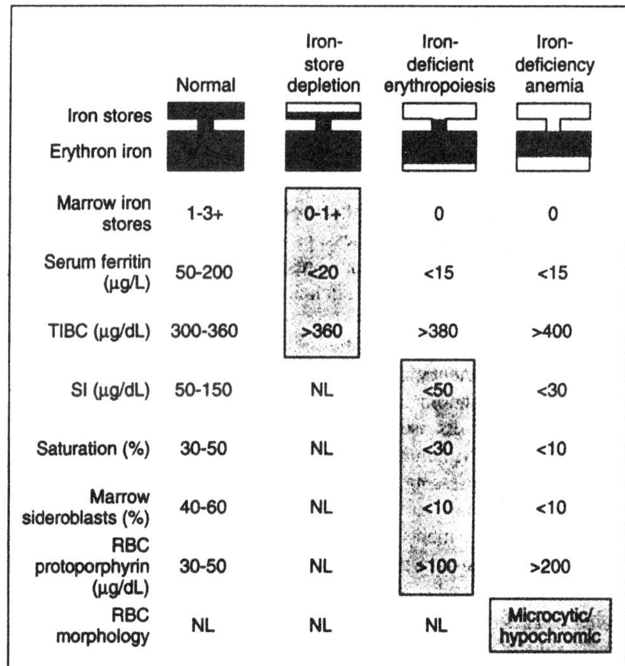

	Normal	Iron-store depletion	Iron-deficient erythropoiesis	Iron-deficiency anemia
Iron stores				
Erythron iron				
Marrow iron stores	1-3+	0-1+	0	0
Serum ferritin (μg/L)	50-200	<20	<15	<15
TIBC (μg/dL)	300-360	>360	>380	>400
SI (μg/dL)	50-150	NL	<50	<30
Saturation (%)	30-50	NL	<30	<10
Marrow sideroblasts (%)	40-60	NL	<10	<10
RBC protoporphyrin (μg/dL)	30-50	NL	>100	>200
RBC morphology	NL	NL	NL	Microcytic/hypochromic

FIG. 21-1. Stages of iron deficiency. From Hillman RS, Finch CA. Red Cell Manual, 7th ed. Philadelphia, F.A. Davis, 1996.

History

Rapidly developing anemia is symptomatic, and the patient's chief complaint can be hemorrhage or such dramatic symptoms as syncope or cardiac arrest. Anemia that develops slowly is initially asymptomatic. Increased intracellular 2,3-diphosphoglycerate (2,3-DPG) is generated, which shifts the oxyhemoglobin dissociation curve to the right, decreasing the affinity of hemoglobin for oxygen and allowing increased extraction by tissues (15). Atrial volume receptors and the carotid sinus stimulate aldosterone- and cortisol-mediated water and salt retention by the kidneys to increase plasma volume and thus maintain the total blood volume and cardiac preload.

Some symptoms of anemia are caused directly by the resulting tissue hypoxia; most, however, are a consequence of compensatory mechanisms. Vasoconstriction and oxygen deprivation in the subcutaneous tissue are in part responsible for the characteristic pallor of the skin and mucous membranes. This allows selectively increased perfusion to more vital areas and is tolerated well. Increased cardiac output generates the increased perfusion necessary to maintain oxygen delivery. The patient might notice palpitations as the signs of cardiac hyperactivity emerge. Increased blood flow might cause a roaring in the ears. Shortness of breath, exertional dyspnea, and orthopnea are characteristic clinical manifestations of anemia. They are rarely related to incipient congestive heart failure. Increased bone marrow activity in response to exponential increases of erythropoietin can result in sternal tenderness and diffuse bone aches and pains.

If tissue hypoxia persists in spite of compensatory mechanisms, disturbing or disabling symptoms can emerge, including headache, light-headedness and faintness, loss of stamina, lethargy and fatigability, night cramps, and, in those with vascular disease, intermittent claudication or angina pectoris. The medical history should include information about pregnancies, menstrual characteristics, operations, trauma, transfusions, allergies, medications, drugs, cigarette smoking, ingestion of alcohol and other toxins, infections, hospitalizations, and other medical problems.

Physical Examination

The physical examination of the anemic patient can reveal signs of uncompensated hypovolemia, including resting or postural tachycardia or hypotension. The compensated patient might show signs only of pallor of the mucous membranes, nail beds, and palmar creases; mild tachycardia; and increased arterial and capillary pulsation with wide pulse pressures. The apical impulse will be forceful, and soft systolic murmurs and bruits due to increased flow and turbulence will be apparent. Atrophy of the papillae of the tongue might indicate cobalamin, folate, or iron deficiency. Angular stomatitis develops in iron deficiency, abnormal gait or impaired vibration or other sensory changes in cobalamin deficiency, and scleral icterus, splenomegaly, and leg ulcers in hemolytic conditions.

Morphologic Classification of Anemia

Red Blood Cell Indexes of the Complete Blood Count

After the history and physical examination, the next step in evaluating anemia is review of the CBC. The severity of the reduction in hemoglobin or hematocrit in conjunction with the patient's symptoms will indicate the chronic nature of the condition. The asymptomatic patient might come to attention because of an abnormal screening test for anemia. If this test is not a CBC, obtain a CBC and a reticulocyte count and look at the peripheral smear. Significant progress can be made toward diagnosis with just this information. The MCV, the mean cell hemoglobin (MCH), and the peripheral smear will allow for a morphologic classification of the anemia.

The normal MCV is 90 ± 9 fL. An MCV level of >99 fL represents macrocytosis, whereas an MCV <81 fL indicates microcytosis. If the onset of anemia is recent or a response to therapy is in progress, two populations of cells will be present, and the MCV level may not be abnormal, since it represents the mean of a distribution of cell sizes. However, two distinct populations will be found on the peripheral smear. In this case, another index of the CBC is useful, the red cell distribution width (RDW). The RDW-CV is the width of the distribution at one standard deviation divided by the MCV, while the RDW-SD is the width of the distribution curve at the 20% frequency level. Since it is a ratio, the RDW-CV tends to magnify variations in cell size in patients with microcytosis. The RDW-SD is very sensitive to the appearance of small populations of macrocytes or microcytes. The normal MCH is 32 ± 2 pg. A reduction in this level represents hypochromia. Changes in red cell population morphologic characteristics suspected by evaluating the indexes should be confirmed by microscopic examination of the peripheral smear.

Peripheral Smear

The peripheral blood smear is invaluable in establishing the cause of anemia. Macrocytes are associated with dyserythropoiesis or premature release from the marrow. They might indicate megaloblastic erythropoiesis or release of reticulocytes in response to hemolysis. With macrocytosis, polymorphonuclear white blood cells should be evaluated for increased nuclear segmentation or lobulation (more than five clumps of chromatin per nucleus). In addition, in the context of anemia, the white blood cell differential morphology counts should be evaluated, since anemia can be a manifestation of marrow replacement by leukemic cells. Macrocytes are found in liver disease, cobalamin or folate deficiency, and reticulocytosis.

Polychromasia is a grayish-blue color found in the polychromatic macrocytes, which are called reticulocytes when they are stained for reticulin or RNA. Anisochromia represents variability of hemoglobinization or the presence of a young red cell population, as seen in hemolysis with the release of an increased number of reticulocytes. Hypochromic microcytes are the product of defective hemoglobin synthesis, such as occurs in iron deficiency or thalassemia. Anisocytosis describes variability in the observed cell size and correlates with RDW. Poikilocytosis refers to variability in cell shape. Abnormal cell shapes include burr cells, with a characteristic evenly spaced scalloped border, which are seen in uremia, and helmet cells, schistocytes, and cell fragments, which are seen in cases of trauma to red cells, such as occurs with microvascular hemolysis or severe oxidant damage.

Microspherocytes are red cells that lack the pale central biconcavity typical of red blood cells and are shaped like spheres. Their shape is a consequence of antibody-mediated damage to the cell membrane, damage due to other agents, the presence of homozygous hemoglobin C, or hereditary spherocytosis. Elliptocytes have an oval or elliptical shape and can be found in a variety of conditions, including iron deficiency, or be caused by a genetic defect in the red cell membrane. Irregularly shaped spur cells with multiple spicules and bizarrely spiculated acanthocytes manifest in severe hepatocellular disease, starvation, and some genetic disorders of lipid metabolism. Sickle cells have a flattened, curved shape and look like a sickle or the waning moon seen end-on. They occur in the sickling disorders, hemoglobin S-S, hemoglobin S-C, or hemoglobin S-A/thalassemia.

Reticulocyte Count

Reticulocytes are red blood cells that contain a substance called reticulin that can be recognized using light microscopy when stained with a specific dye. They also can be recognized with some difficulty in a Wright's stain preparation as slightly larger and slightly blue-tinged red blood cells. Reticulin has residual RNA, and these cells are thus immature red blood cells. They are counted and reported as a percentage of the total number of red blood cells. Normally 1% to 2% of red blood cells are reticulocytes. Increases in the reticulocyte count in response to anemia provide a measure of the bone marrow's ability to increase production. In a normal patient, reticulocyte production can increase two to three times in response to a drop in hematocrit to 30%, and production can rise five to six times normal in patients with chronic hemolytic anemias. Thus, a reticulocyte response to anemia shows appropriate erythropoietin release, a marrow capable of producing red cell precursors, and sufficient iron to increase production. An inadequate reticulocyte response indicates a defect in production of red blood cells, identifying the anemia as hypoplastic, at least in part.

To confirm an inadequate response, two modifications of the reticulocyte count must be calculated. The first is a correction for the early release of reticulocytes into the circulation in response to the anemic stress. These reticulocytes will remain in the circulation 3 to 4 days instead of the normal 1 to 2 days. Thus, they will cause the immediate reticulocyte count to be an overestimate of the daily production of red blood cells. A second correction must be made to convert the reticulocyte count into an absolute number rather than a percentage of total red blood cells. This calculation must be made because as the number of red cells declines, the same percentage of reticulocytes represents less and less of a marrow response.

A reassuring marrow response should produce a 100% increase in reticulocytes over the normal amount, given the potential error present in the assumptions on which these calculations are based. However, any increase over normal values probably represents a response. If the number calculated falls below the normal replacement value, a defective marrow response is likely. In this way, the reticulocyte count can help the clinician decide if a hypoplastic response is part of the picture of the anemia under investigation. This is important, because among the most treatable causes of anemia are the hypoplastic responses to cobalamin, folic acid, and iron deficiency.

Iron Studies

Because of the common occurrence of iron deficiency, iron studies are frequently recommended as part of the initial workup. These include evaluations of serum ferritin and serum iron and iron-binding capacity.

MAKING THE DIAGNOSIS

The information obtained from these preliminary investigations and pathophysiologic considerations is used to diagnose the specific cause of anemia. One approach to narrow the differential diagnosis is as follows.

Step 1: Does the history lead to a previous diagnosis?
Yes: Do the physical examination and laboratory tests confirm this diagnosis? If so, obtain copies of old records and initiate or maintain appropriate therapy.
No: Step 2

Step 2: Does the physical examination suggest the diagnosis?
Yes: Do the laboratory tests confirm this diagnosis? If so, complete the testing pathway leading to this diagnosis. If diagnosis is assured, initiate appropriate therapy.
No: Step 3

Step 3: Is the peripheral smear compatible with the MCV, the MCH, and the RDW-CV and RDW-SD?
Yes: Step 3a
No: Repeat the CBC, prepare the peripheral smear yourself, and repeat step 3.

Step 3a: Does the peripheral smear suggest a hemolytic diagnosis?
Yes: Proceed to an etiologic diagnosis based on specific morphologic criteria.
No: Step 4

Step 4: Is the MCV low, normal, or high?
MCV 81–99: Step 4a
MCV >99: Step 4b
MCV <81: Step 4c

Step 4a: Draw blood for another CBC, reticulocyte count, and sedimentation rate. Start the patient on iron supplements, review the sedimentation rate and evaluate the response to a month of therapy, and follow the pathway given below for normal MCV.

Step 4b: Obtain further history regarding alcohol use; repeat physical examination, focusing on the liver, venous spiders, and varicosities; examine the peripheral smear; and draw blood for CBC, reticulocyte count, liver enzymes, and cobalamin and folic acid levels. Follow the pathway given below for high MCV.

Step 4c: Is Mentzer's index (see below) <14?
Yes: Step 5a
No: Step 5b

Step 5a: Draw blood for another CBC, reticulocyte count, serum iron, total iron-binding capacity, ferritin, and hemoglobin electrophoresis and follow the pathway given below for low MCV.

Step 5b: Is the patient at more than 12 weeks' gestation?
Yes: Step 6a
No: Step 6b

Step 6a: Does the patient wish to have prenatal diagnosis?
Yes: Step 5a
No: Step 6b

Step 6b: Draw blood for another CBC and reticulocyte count. Start the patient on iron supplements and confirm the diagnosis by evaluating the response to a month of therapy. If the diagnosis of iron deficiency is not confirmed (failure of microcytic hypochromic anemia to resolve after iron studies have become normal), go to step 5a.

Normal MCV

The most common causes of anemia associated with a normal MCV are iron-deficiency anemia and anemia of chronic disease. The latter is more likely to be present as the sedimentation rate rises. If the sedimentation rate is high, search for acute or chronic infection or inflammation.

High MCV

If the test results indicate liver disease, consultation should be obtained from a maternal–fetal medicine specialist. If the source is alcohol ingestion, the patient should be withdrawn from alcohol in a supervised setting.

Low MCV

The most common causes of a low MCV are iron deficiency anemia, thalassemia, sideroblastic anemia, and the anemia of chronic disease. Iron deficiency is by far the most common cause of microcytosis. In addition, up to 25% of patients with the anemia of chronic disease have microcytosis, but the MCV is seldom less than 70 fl. The next most common cause of severe microcytosis is thalassemia. In areas of the world where parasitism is endemic, these three conditions commonly coexist. Sideroblastic anemia is rare.

High Reticulocyte Count

A high absolute reticulocyte count indicates a responding bone marrow and anemia due to either acute blood loss or hemolysis. The history and physical examination should be reviewed for signs and symptoms of bleeding, severe preeclampsia, hemolytic–uremic syndrome, thrombotic thrombocytopenic purpura, or systemic lupus erythematosus. The spleen should be reexamined for enlargement or tenderness. The peripheral smear should be inspected for abnormal forms indicating intravascular hemolysis, sickle cells, elliptocytes, microspherocytes, or inclusion bodies. A hemoglobin electrophoresis should be obtained if no other cause of hemolysis or bleeding can be found. The presence of microspherocytes should prompt the measurement of anti-red-blood-cell immunoglobulins with both the direct and the indirect Coombs' tests.

Low Reticulocyte Count

If the reticulocyte count is abnormally low, the marrow response is inadequate. The most common causes are nutritional—lack of iron, folate, or cobalamin. A low reticulocyte count, however, does not indicate that hypoplastic marrow is the only cause of anemia. Hemorrhage or hemolysis normally bring about an elevated reticulocyte count. But if nutrients were borderline to begin with, they might soon be exhausted; the reticulocyte count will then not indicate the initial cause of anemia until the nutrients have been replaced. In this case, the peripheral smear can be a powerful indicator that another process is taking place.

Abnormal Hemoglobin Electrophoresis

Finding that the hemoglobin has abnormal electrophoretic mobility suggests that hemoglobinopathy is the explanation for hemolysis. This condition might produce only anemia or might be associated with systemic disease, as with hemoglobins S-S and S-C and hemoglobin S-A in conjunction with thalassemia. Often the latter two conditions are unrecognized until pregnancy, which can elicit symptoms for the first time, occasionally with fatal results. Abnormal amounts of normal hemoglobins are occasionally encountered. An elevated hemoglobin A_2 level might indicate β-thalassemia. An elevated fetal hemoglobin (hemoglobin F) level is occasionally encountered in an asymptomatic individual.

EXTRINSIC ANEMIAS

Extrinsic anemias are caused by acute or chronic blood loss as the result of escape of blood from the circulation due to loss of mechanical integrity of the blood vessels. Acute blood loss comes to immediate attention because of dramatic symptoms. Anemia resulting from acute blood loss is usually symptomatic. Its source is apparent from the history. Chronic blood loss is blood loss that is either asymptomatic or has subtle symptoms. Its cause is not immediately apparent and must be discerned through investigation. Chronic blood loss might not cause symptoms until enough loss has taken place that an essential precursor, such as iron, is depleted. The reticulocytosis will not be apparent, and the picture will be one of iron-deficiency anemia. Thus, the workup of iron-deficiency anemia always includes a search for a route of chronic blood loss. A primary nutritional deficiency of iron is a diagnosis of exclusion.

Anemia of Chronic Blood Loss

This anemia stems from blood loss that is slow enough to make the hemodynamic effects subtle and allow for compensation. In the pregnant woman it usually occurs as a consequence of disease in the pulmonary tree, the gastrointestinal tract, or the genitourinary tract. The symptoms of anemia gradually become apparent, especially loss of stamina, lethargy, and fatigability. There may also be such symptoms as hematochezia or melena owing to the underlying disease. The reticulocyte count is appropriately elevated until the level of some critical (usually iron) nutrient declines and the marrow response becomes hypoplastic.

Radiographic imaging studies, especially barium enema and barium swallow with upper-gastrointestinal follow-through, are relatively contraindicated during pregnancy. Computerized tomography or magnetic resonance imaging delivers less radiation; endoscopy might be best suited to gastrointestinal diagnosis. Treatment is based on identifying and managing the underlying disease.

HEMOLYTIC ANEMIAS

Hemolytic anemias result from an increased rate of red cell destruction. They are classified as inherited or acquired: in general, the former are due to intrinsic red cell defects in the erythrocyte membrane, glycolytic pathway, glutathione metabolism, or hemoglobin molecule, and the latter are due to actions of such extrinsic factors as infectious agents, poisons, physical trauma, or antibodies. They usually cause an increase in the reticulocyte count. However, if the process is chronic and nutrients such as iron, cobalamin, or folate are depleted, appropriate reticulocytosis might not occur. Nevertheless, the peripheral smear will generally indicate the nature of the process.

Autoimmune Hemolytic Anemia

This anemia results from autoantibodies against red cell antigens. The cold-antibody types are caused by hemagglutinating antibody (usually IgM) maximally active at 4°C. These anemias include cold agglutinin syndrome and paroxysmal cold hemoglobinuria, and usually involve complement-dependent intravascular hemolysis or sequestration of erythrocytes by the liver. The warm-antibody type is caused by serum autoantibodies (usually IgG) maximally active at 37°C, which react with the patient's red blood cells.

Autoimmune hemolytic anemias can be idiopathic or can stem from hematologic neoplasms, autoimmune diseases, viral infections, or immunodeficiency diseases. Coombs' test is positive for IgG or complement. The antibodies might be a manifestation of an underlying disorder, such as systemic autoimmune diseases, lymphoproliferative disorders, nonlymphoid neoplasms (e.g., ovarian tumors), chronic inflammatory diseases (e.g., ulcerative colitis), drug ingestion (e.g., α-methyldopa), and infections (e.g., mononucleosis, mycoplasma pneumonia, and paroxysmal cold hemoglobinuria associated with syphilis) (16). The antibodies are directed against components of the red cell membrane and attach to the patient's red cells. These are then subject to hemolysis by complement or, more commonly, to removal from the circulation by the reticuloendothelial system, especially in the spleen.

The smear shows polychromasia, reticulocytosis, spherocytosis, red cell fragments, nucleated red cells, and erythrophagocytosis; reticulocytopenia has also been observed. There is erythroid marrow hyperplasia, hyperbilirubinemia, and hemoglobinuria. The diagnosis is made by the presence of spherocytosis and associated red cell autoantibodies bound to the patient's red cells, measured by the direct (Coombs') antiglobulin test. Transfusion, glucocorticosteroids, splenectomy, immunosuppressive drugs, plasmapheresis, intravenous Swiss immunoglobulin, and other therapies are used. Fetal well-being in pregnancies complicated by autoimmune hemolytic anemia should be monitored by biophysical testing and sonographic evaluation for hydrops.

α-Thalassemia

This congenital hypoplastic anemia is related to a disturbance of hemoglobin synthesis: a congenital defect in the number or regulation of expression of one or more of the genes for the α-globin chain leads to decreased synthesis of the α-chain. It occurs with a high frequency in selected ethnic groups. A double gene deletion is common among Asian patients; a single gene deletion is native to West Africa; and both are common in Mediterranean, Indian, and mixed populations. Clinical problems occur because an excess of γ- and β-chains accumulate as the result of diminished synthesis of the α-globin chain, with normal or near normal synthesis of the γ- and β-chains (Table 21-3).

The excess unpaired γ- and β-chains form tetramers (Bart's hemoglobin and hemoglobin H); these tetramers aggregate in the presence of oxidative stress, such as infection; accumulate to toxic levels in the erythroid precursor cells; and have destructive effects on developing erythrocytic normoblasts. The cells may die in the marrow, and, for this reason, erythropoiesis is ineffective. In addition, affected cell membranes are rigid, and cell removal is accelerated in the reticuloendothelial system; thus, anemia is caused by a variable combination of ineffective erythropoiesis and premature destruction of red cells. With chronic hypoxia, there is expansion of the marrow cavity, osteopenia, and enlargement of the reticuloendothelial organs. Because there are no variants of the α-globin chain to form complexes with the excess γ- and β-globin chains, the untreated homozygous state is fatal in the perinatal period.

TABLE 21-3. *The α-thalassemias*

Condition	Hemoglobin A (%)	Hemoglobin H (β^4) (%)	Hemoglobin level (g/dL)	Mean cell volume (fL)
Normal	97	0	15	90
Silent thalassemia: –α/αα	98–100	0	15	90
Thalassemia trait –α/–α homozygous α-thal-2[a] or – –/αα heterozygous α-thal-1[a]	85–95	Red blood cell inclusions	12–13	70–80
Hemoglobin H disease -/-α heterozygous α-thal-2	70–95	5–306	6–10	60–70
Hemoglobin Bart's disease – –/– – homozygous α-thal-1	0	5–10[b]	0 (fatal in utero or at birth)	—

[a]When both α-alleles on one chromosome are deleted, the locus is called α-thal-1; when only a single α-allele on one chromosome is deleted, the locus is called α-thal-2.
[b]90–95% of the hemoglobin is Bart's hemoglobin [tetramers of γ (fetal) globin chain].
From ref. 17.

Clinical Manifestations

In Bart's hemoglobin, the consequence is fetal hydrops and intrauterine or neonatal death. In hemoglobin H disease, splenomegaly is common, and cholelithiasis and jaundice occur. Anemia is variable. Heterozygous α-thalassemia-1 and homozygous α-thalassemia-2 have mild clinical symptoms. Heterozygous α-thalassemia-2 is clinically undetectable. There are no fetal, neonatal, or adult substitutes for the α-gene; since there are two α-genes on each chromosome 16, there are two haplotypes. One is the α-thalassemia-1 variant, or α^0, which is common among Asian patients and has a deletion of two α-genes. The second is the α-thalassemia-2 variant, or α^+, with one α-gene deleted; this type is common among blacks but is also found among Asian and Mediterranean populations. Five clinically distinct syndromes are distinguished among the various genotypes for α-chain deletions.

Homozygous α-thalassemia-1, or Bart's hemoglobin, arises when there are no functioning α-genes. In Bart's hemoglobin, γ-tetramers predominate, with a few β-tetramers. Neither can release oxygen. Doubly heterozygous α-thalassemia, the combination of the α-thalassemia-1 and α-thalassemia-2 gene defects, is also called hemoglobin H disease. It is associated with the presence of a single functioning α-gene. The others might be deleted, have defective regulation, or produce an abnormal gene product. Hemolysis is brisk, and reticulocytosis is inadequate. In splenectomized patients, large single red cell inclusions are present, whereas in patients with intact spleens, several smaller punctate inclusions are evident. Bart's hemoglobin can be detected at birth. Hemoglobin H can be identified by precipitation on staining with brilliant cresyl blue. The severity of the condition varies with the cause of the reduction in α-globin chains. Nondeletional mutations usually are more severe than deletions.

Heterozygous α-thalassemia-1 is associated with no functioning α-globin genes on one of the chromosomes in the pair and two on the other. Anemia is mild or absent except during aplastic events, such as parvovirus infection. Red cells are hypochromic and microcytic. Homozygous α-thalassemia-2 is associated with one functional and one nonfunctional α-gene on each chromosome 16. It is similar to heterozygous α-thalassemia-1, with mild anemia or no anemia at all except during aplastic events, such as parvovirus infection. Red cells are hypochromic and microcytic. Both of these conditions must be differentiated from, or can be associated with, iron-deficiency anemia. In the silent carrier state, or heterozygous α-thalassemia-2, one chromosome contains one nonfunctional and one functional α-gene, and the other chromosome is normal.

Diagnosis is made by a suggestive clinical history in a patient with microcytic, hypochromic anemia; normal iron study results; and normal hemoglobin electrophoresis. The hemoglobin electrophoresis shows γ-tetramers (Bart's hemoglobin) and β-tetramers (hemoglobin H) in homozygous α-thalassemia and β-tetramers (hemoglobin H) in hemoglobin H disease. If iron deficiency coexists, the diagnosis can be made if microcytosis and reticulocytosis persist after iron has been repleted. Confirmation of the diagnosis can be obtained using specific gene probes.

Treatment

There is no practical treatment for Bart's hemoglobin. In hemoglobin H disease, regular transfusions are not usually required, but they can be necessary in the context of an aplastic crisis or if infection or other oxidative stress leads to increased precipitation of hemoglobin H and increased hemolysis. In heterozygous α-thalassemia, there is no transfusion requirement.

Effect of α-Thalassemia on Pregnancy

Homozygous α-Thalassemia

Bart's hemoglobin releases oxygen poorly to the periphery, resulting in hydrops and fetal death. Since this condition has previously been lethal in the perinatal period, there are no reported pregnancies affected by the condition. However, one fetus has been rescued from hydrops due to homozygous α-thalassemia (17). The outcome of this newborn is uncertain, since it had minor malformations, possibly owing to hypoxia (18–20), and is awaiting bone marrow transplant. Nevertheless, we can expect to see pregnancies in patients with homozygous α-thalassemia in the future.

At present, the condition is important in obstetrics principally as a target for prenatal diagnosis and as a concomitant of early preeclampsia (21-24). Patients of Southeast Asian or Mediterranean extraction are at risk for homozygous α-thalassemia (25). The condition has not been reported in blacks (26). Early sonographic diagnosis of homozygous α-thalassemia is suggested by unusual placental thickening in the first trimester (27). Cure of the condition by establishing hematochimerism using fetal stem-cell transplantation is a compelling approach in theory, but results are disappointing so far (28).

Hemoglobin H disease

In hemoglobin H disease, the patient has one functional α-globin gene, leading to a deficiency of α-globin chains and moderately severe hemolytic anemia. The excess β-chains form tetramers (hemoglobin H) that precipitate as inclusion bodies that are removed by the reticuloendothelial system, thus decreasing the life span of the affected red cell. Hemoglobin H disease is common among patients from Asia or the Mediterranean who have α-thalassemia, but it is rare among patients of African or East Indian origin.

Pregnancy outcome is reported to be normal in hemoglobin H disease (29,30); however, too few pregnancies among patients with hemoglobin H disease have been reported to allow for definite conclusions. Anemia can become severe enough to require transfusions, and the folic acid requirement, as in all forms of hemolytic anemia, is higher. Iron deficiency is rare, but it should be ruled out definitively as a cause of worsening anemia. Oxidant drugs, such as nitrofurantoin and the sulfonamides, should be avoided because they increase the precipitation of hemoglobin H (31). Hydrops fetalis has also been reported as a cause of perinatal death in fetuses affected by hemoglobin H disease (32–34). These reports might represent the coincident occurrence of intrauterine parvovirus infection or another undetected cause of hydrops fetalis. Otherwise, pregnancy outcome has been reported to be benign, except for neonatal anemia in newborns with hemoglobin H disease.

α-Thalassemia Trait

The α-thalassemia trait is a heterogeneous group of conditions. In heterozygous α-thalassemia-1 and homozygous α-thalassemia-2, only two functioning α-genes are present, leading to a shortage of normal hemoglobin molecules and microcytic, hypochromic anemia. Rarely, there is an imbalance in globin chain synthesis, resulting in an excess of β-chains. However, hemoglobin electrophoresis is usually normal. The absence of an imbalance in globin chain synthesis in these conditions can be explained by a compensatory increase in α_1-globin gene expression in individuals with either α-globin gene deletion (35). Pregnancy does not seem to be specifically affected by any of these deletional diseases except to target the individual for prenatal diagnosis, unless an additional condition results in increased severity of anemia (36–38). Detection of coexisting iron-deficiency anemia is mandatory, and prevention of folic acid deficiency is usually accomplished by giving 1 mg of folic acid daily.

Prenatal Diagnosis of α-Thalassemia

The early detection of a fetus with a lethal genotype—Bart's hemoglobin—is a goal of prenatal diagnosis. A patient with homozygous α-thalassemia-2 might be targeted for prenatal diagnosis, since the patient's fetus is at risk for homozygous α-thalassemia-2 and doubly heterozygous α-thalassemia-1 and -2 (hemoglobin H disease). In heterozygous α-thalassemia-2, three functioning α-globin genes are present and no defect in hemoglobin production is detectable. The individual is phenotypically normal, and there is no demonstrable effect on pregnancy. A patient with heterozygous α-thalassemia-2 might be also targeted for prenatal diagnosis, since the patient's fetus is at risk for homozygous α-thalassemia-2 and doubly heterozygous α-thalassemia-1 and -2 (hemoglobin H disease).

Methods using gene probes are available for prenatal detection of α-thalassemia (39–45). Detection of α-thalassemia-2 heterozygotes and homozygotes and compound heterozygotes is now possible by the polymerase chain reaction (PCR) technique. Specific oligonucleotides have been developed that selectively amplify appropriate segments of both the abnormal chromosome (which contains the area of deletion) and the normal chromosome. PCR can potentially provide a way to screen populations where α-gene defects are prevalent. For patients who want more than a predicted probability before subjecting their fetus to the risk of prenatal diagnosis, sonographic methods for early detection of hydrops are being developed (46–50).

β-Thalassemia

The condition of β-thalassemia results from a congenital defect in the number or regulation of expression of one or more of the genes for the β-globin chain, leading to its diminished synthesis. An excess of unpaired α-chains accumulates. They aggregate and precipitate in the erythroid precursor cell, causing some of these cells to die; thus, erythropoiesis is ineffective. Overall, there is less hemoglobin per cell, accounting for hypochromia and target cell formation. The affected erythrocytes are misshapen and relatively rigid, and cell removal is accelerated in the reticuloendothelial system; thus, anemia is caused by a combination of ineffective erythropoiesis and premature destruction of red cells. With the resulting chronic hypoxia, there is expansion of the marrow cavity, osteopenia, and enlargement of the reticuloendothelial organs. Tumors can arise at these sites, and transfusions predispose to iron-overload illnesses. The presence of more δ- and/or τ-globin chains to pair with the excess α-chains ameliorates the illness. Multiple mutations exist, with marked variability in the degree to which production of the β-globin messenger RNA is reduced.

Variants of β-thalassemia cause three clinical syndromes (17). Beta-thalassemia major (Cooley's anemia) is an illness with severe manifestations that appears in the first year of life with symptoms of jaundice, hepatosplenomegaly, expansion of erythroid marrow, growth restriction, and susceptibility to infection. Chronic transfusions are needed, leading to iron overload and death in adolescence if cardiac hemochromatosis is left untreated. In β-thalassemia minor, symptoms are rare unless the defect is found in combination with the sickle trait; in this case, symptoms are intermittently those of sickling. Occasionally, there is splenomegaly. In β-thalassemia intermedia, there are clinical manifestations of moderate severity, intermediate between those of thalassemia major and minor, and there are variable degrees of hepatosplenomegaly.

The peripheral smear in β-thalassemia major, the homozygous or doubly heterozygous condition, shows nucleated red cells, distorted hypochromic erythrocytes, and basophilic stippling. There are three variants: in β^0-thalassemia, no β-globin chains are synthesized, and only hemoglobin F and A_2 are found; in β^+-thalassemia, small amounts of β-chain and consequently hemoglobin A are made; in δ-β-thalassemia, due to deletion of δ-globin and β-globin genes, only hemoglobin F is made.

Beta-thalassemia minor, or β-thalassemia trait, takes the form of mild anemia that might emerge only with an aplastic crisis. The peripheral smear shows hypochromia and microcytosis with basophilic stippling. The hemoglobin A_2 level is elevated in most individuals to above 5%, and in half of patients the amount of hemoglobin F is raised above 2%. The hemoglobin F concentration varies from one red cell to another; the higher the hemoglobin F, the less severe the anemia. In heterozygotes for the δ-β variant, increased amounts of hemoglobin F are made, but there are normal amounts of hemoglobin A_2. Iron deficiency must be ruled out in the differential diagnosis of hypochromic, microcytic anemia. In iron deficiency, there is hypoproliferation of red cells, whereas in thalassemia trait, red cell numbers are only minimally depressed, and a hemoglobin level of 9 g/dL will be associated with a red cell count of five million cells per microliter. This provides the basis for such indexes as the Mentzer index in distinguishing the two conditions. However, the thalassemia trait and iron deficiency can coexist as a consequence of vaginal or gastrointestinal bleeding.

In β-thalassemia intermedia, the hemoglobin level can be as low as 6 or 7 g/dL. This low level is caused by mild variants of β^+- or δ-β-thalassemia major (homozygous) or by interactions between α- and β-thalassemia. In this case, the diminished synthesis of α-chains lessens cell damage due to an excess of α-globin chains. In hemoglobin Lepore, the genes for the δ- and β-chains are fused, and synthesis of the resulting chain is impaired. Homozygous patients might have a clinical picture of Cooley's anemia or thalassemia intermedia; their red cells contain only hemoglobin Lepore and hemoglobin F. In hemoglobin E disease, synthesis of the abnormal β-chain E is impaired, and heterozygotes have clinical symptoms of thalassemia minor. In the case of hereditary persistence of fetal hemoglobin, homozygotes have 100% hemoglobin F, and heterozygotes have about 50% hemoglobin F. These individuals can have mild to moderate anemia.

Beta-thalassemia is diagnosed when microcytic, hypochromic anemia exists in the context of normal or high iron stores, relatively normal red cell numbers, more numerous reticulocytes, and increased amounts of hemoglobin A_2 (over 4%). The three syndromes are usually distinguishable in terms of clinical symptoms. Beta-thalassemia major is diagnosed when the patient is transfusion dependent; the intermedia form is diagnosed when the patient has severe anemia but is not normally transfusion dependent. In the minor form, the patient has relatively mild and clinically insignificant anemia. There are ways to make these diagnoses more specifically by using gene probes and measuring messenger RNA, but these methods are not needed for clinical treatment.

In β-thalassemia major, aggressive transfusion therapy is used to keep the hemoglobin above 12 g/dL. Deferoxamine chelation therapy and, occasionally, splenectomy is necessary. The application of these therapies has allowed women with this disease to survive to childbearing age. Bone marrow transplantation is an experimental therapy, as is treatment with such chemotherapeutic agents as azacitidine or hydroxyurea to raise hemoglobin F levels. Beta-thalassemia minor usually requires no treatment. In β-thalassemia intermedia, regular transfusions are typically not required but might be needed during an aplastic crisis.

Effect of β-Thalassemia on Pregnancy

Homozygous β-Thalassemia

Homozygous β-thalassemia (major) was fatal before the advent of transfusion therapy, but patients now live to reproductive age (51); many are infertile as the result of end-organ damage from progressive iron deposition in endocrine tissues. Pregnancy in patients with homozygous β-thalassemia major is unusual. Fifteen pregnancies were reported between 1969 and 1994 (52,53). In fact, many previously reported pregnancies might have been in doubly heterozygous women (54). With current therapy, the incidence of true homozygotes is rising: 58 pregnancies have been reported since 1995 (53,55,56). The improvement in endocrine function in these patients is attributed to iron chelation therapy. Thirty-one of these pregnancies were spontaneous; ovulation induction or in vitro fertilization was necessary in the others (53,56,57).

Cephalopelvic disproportion is common and results from normal fetal growth in patients with short stature due to previous growth problems associated with their disease. Although intrauterine growth retardation might be expected in patients with chronic fetal hypoxia due to severe maternal anemia, this effect was not seen in these series, in which maternal hemoglobin levels were kept over 10 g/dL. Transfusion therapy was continued throughout pregnancy, while withholding chelation. Nevertheless, serum ferritin levels rose no more than 10% in any patient. The fetus actively takes up iron, and the placenta can accumulate iron (58). The functional significance of the latter is uncertain.

Counseling before conception is of great value for women with homozygous β-thalassemia—it allows the mother's medical status to be evaluated and optimized before conception. Several serious medical disorders can exist in these patients. Iron deposition in the pancreas and thyroid can cause type I diabetes and hypothyroidism, respectively. Congestive heart failure from iron deposition cardiomyopathy can be precipitated by transfusion in the context of the increased cardiac work of pregnancy; consequently, myocardial function must be assessed before pregnancy. Cardiomyopathy is associated with a maternal mortality rate of up to 50%. In addition, the mother can be expected to have a shortened life span, and she needs to consider the consequences of leaving young children behind.

The fetus is at risk for homozygous β-thalassemia as well, and knowledge of the fetal genotype is necessary if the mother is willing to consider pregnancy termination for an affected fetus. Knowledge of the paternal genotype is sufficient if he is not a carrier of the β-thalassemia gene. Although chelation therapy with deferoxamine causes skeletal anomalies in laboratory animals, none were reported in the offspring of nine women who took deferoxamine at various times during pregnancy, including three who took it throughout pregnancy (53,59).

Isoimmunization of the mother from multiple blood transfusions is common in homozygous β-thalassemia. Passively transferred antibodies might affect the fetus, causing hemolytic anemia progressing to hydrops fetalis. Amniotic fluid bilirubin might not reflect fetal disease because of passively transferred maternal bilirubin, as reported for sickle cell disease (60–62). Fetal blood sampled for the effects of isoimmunization can be used for genetic testing for β-thalassemia as well. Hepatitis C is the most common transfusion-acquired hepatitis in β-thalassemia patients (63), and screening in pregnancy for hepatitis C is appropriate. Patients with homozygous β-thalassemia have received bone marrow transplantation for attempted cure of their disease, and pregnancy has been reported in a patient who underwent transplant for β-thalassemia major (64).

Doubly Heterozygous β-Thalassemia/Thalassemia Intermedia

There are few reports of doubly heterozygous β-thalassemia or thalassemia intermedia in pregnancy (54). Chronic anemia among patients with these diseases might predispose to a poor fetal outcome. The disorder is probably underdiagnosed, since diagnosis requires specialized gene probes for specific alleles not generally available. The stress of pregnancy is unlikely to affect women with doubly heterozygous β-thalassemia unless some other cause of anemia compounds their problems. Thus, iron deficiency must be ruled out in every case, and folic acid deficiency must be avoided. Prenatal diagnosis should be considered (65).

Heterozygous β-Thalassemia

There is little effect of this mild anemia on pregnancy (66,67). In one study, patients with the β-thalassemia trait had normal reticulocyte counts and higher mean serum ferritin values, less iron deficiency, and similar folate and cobalamin concentrations compared with normal patients (67). Multiple genetic variants of β-thalassemia exist (68). Considerations for prenatal diagnosis of the heterozygous patient are similar to those for doubly heterozygous and homozygous patients.

Prenatal Diagnosis of β-Thalassemia

Successful use of enzymatically amplified DNA and nonradioactive allele-specific oligonucleotide probes for the prenatal diagnosis of β-thalassemia was reported in 1988 (69), and there have been many reports since that time on the rapid prenatal diagnosis of β-thalassemia using DNA amplification and specific gene probes (70–80). Fetal DNA is obtained using amniocentesis, chorionic villus sampling, and fetal blood sampling. Anion-exchange high-performance liquid chromatography has been used for the prenatal diagnosis of thalassemias from fetal blood samples. This method may be useful where PCR methods are not available but high-performance liquid chromatography is available.

Less-invasive techniques for obtaining fetal DNA are under investigation. Cheung and associates reported successful prenatal diagnosis in two patients at risk for β-thalassemia, using fetal cells found in maternal blood (81). Prenatal diagnosis using cells aspirated from transcervical mucus might also be possible (82). Further development of less invasive techniques for prenatal diagnosis is anticipated. *In utero* fetal transplantation to correct β-thalassemia following prenatal diagnosis is a goal of maternal–fetal medicine. Work is under way to solve technical problems surrounding this procedure (83,84).

Screening for Thalassemia in the United States

The first step to select patients for screening is to assess the MCV, as determined from the patient's CBC. When the MCV is below 80 fL, the significant differential diagnoses are thalassemia, anemia of chronic disease, and iron deficiency (66,85,86). Further evaluation uses hemoglobin electrophoresis and serum iron studies. The yield of such a program is dependent, however, on the ethnic mixture in the population. For example, in an African-American population, the overwhelming majority of patients will prove to have iron deficiency or anemia of chronic disease, while the form of thalassemia detected will likely be α-thalassemia of the African type, which is unlikely to cause fetal disease and may even be genetically advantageous.

If the patient is first seen for prenatal care at or before 12 weeks of gestation, a trial of 4 weeks of iron therapy can be implemented. This therapy will result in confirmation of iron-deficiency anemia in most cases, evidenced by elevation of the MCV into the normal range; an increase in total red blood cells, hemoglobin and hematocrit; and a rise in the number of reticulocytes. If iron deficiency is not confirmed, the opportunity for prenatal diagnosis is not compromised.

If the MCV is less than 75 fL and the red cell count is more than five million, there is an 85% chance that the patient has a thalassemia syndrome (87–90). Although this discriminant has excellent sensitivity and specificity, its predictive value would be limited in a population where the prevalence of iron deficiency far outweighs that of the thalassemia trait. Mentzer developed a simplified index using patients with hemoglobins above 9 g/dL (91). This population is expected to comprise patients with only mild iron deficiency. Mentzer's index can be used to evaluate a low MCV and guide the decision regarding the next step in the diagnosis of microcytic anemia. The MCV is divided by the total number of red blood cells per million to produce Mentzer's index. If it is <11.5, thalassemia is likely. If it is >14, iron deficiency is probable. This is based on the biological difference between iron deficiency and thalassemia, namely, that for a given reduction of MCV, there are many more red blood cells in thalassemia than in iron deficiency.

Sickle Cell Anemia

This form of hemolytic anemia is characterized by red cells with sicklelike morphologic characteristics and multi-organ system disease, the consequence of the presence of hemoglobin S or another sickling hemoglobin (Table 21-4). The gene that codes for hemoglobin S is present in 10% of all black people in the United States; the homozygous condition exists in 0.2% (92). The disease results from a defect in a single DNA base pair that results in a defect in the globin molecule that induces sickling, owing to the presence of the S β-globin chain. Deoxyhemoglobin S has reduced solubility and polymerizes into long, tubelike fibers, which cause red blood cells to assume a sickle shape. The sickle shape and the hemoglobin S polymers enhance reticuloendothelial clearance of the abnormal cells.

In addition, when the percentage of sickle cells in the microcirculation passes a threshold, the sickle cells obstruct capillary beds, causing a vaso-occlusive crisis that can lead to ischemic damage in widespread capillary beds, organ failure, and sometimes death. The pain of the vaso-occlusive crisis is usually caused by avascular necrosis of the bone marrow. In addition to episodic bone and joint pain, multiple organ compromise occurs, including hepatic necrosis, renal insufficiency, pulmonary sequestration and failure, gallstones, splenic infarction, neurologic disorders, susceptibility to infection, and aplastic episodes.

If the patient is heterozygous for β-globin S (sickle cell disease), disease expression is different compared with its expression in patients who are heterozygous for the β-globin S gene in conjunction with the β-globin C gene (sickle S-C disease) or heterozygous in conjunction with a β-globin A gene affected by a production defect (sickle cell/β-thalassemia disease). Disease expression may be affected in these individuals, depending on whether α-thalassemia is present. If the heterozygote is also heterozygous for hemoglobin C (sickle S-C disease) or has β-thalassemia (sickle/thalassemia disease), reducing the synthesis of the β-globin A chain, a disease similar to sickle cell disease is produced, with variable forms of expression. It can first become symptomatic during surgery or pregnancy.

Patients heterozygous for hemoglobin S can experience sickling under extreme conditions of nonadapted stress, temperature, or altitude. In addition, their cells routinely sickle in the hypertonic renal medulla, leading to destruction of the vasa recta, inability to concentrate (isosthenuria), papillary necrosis, and hematuria. Laboratory studies show reticulocytosis except during an aplastic crisis. The peripheral smear can show sickle cells, holly-leaf cells, and Howell-Jolly bodies. Hemoglobin electrophoresis shows varying amounts of hemoglobin S and hemoglobin F; the higher the hemoglobin F, the less severe the anemia. Other varieties of sickling hemoglobin are rare.

TABLE 21-4. *Clinical features of sickle hemoglobinopathies*

Condition	Clinical abnormalities	Hemoglobin level (g/dL)	Mean corpuscular volume (fL)	Hemoglobin electrophoresis
Sickle cell trait	None: rare painless hematuria	Normal	Normal	Hb S/A: 40/60%
Sickle cell anemia	Vaso-occlusive crises with infarction of spleen, brain, marrow, kidney, lung; aseptic necrosis of bone; gallstones; priapism; ankle ulcers	7–10	80–100	Hb S/A: 100/0% Hb F: 2%–25%
S/β^0 thalassemia	Vaso-occlusive crises, aseptic necrosis of bone	7–10	60–80	Hb S/A: 100/0% Hb F: 1%–10%
S/β$^+$/thalassemia	Rare crises and aseptic necrosis	10–14	70–80	Hb S/A:60/40%
Hemoglobin S-C	Rare crises and aseptic necrosis, painless hematuria	10–14	80–100	Hb S/A: 50/0% Hb C: 50%

Hb, hemoglobin.
From ref. 17.

Therapy for Sickle Cell Disease

The mutational event responsible for altering the β-globin gene to produce hemoglobin S occurred more than once. There are five variants with different disease expressions, ranging from mild to severe (93). Treatment is primarily supportive during a vaso-occlusive crisis, with analgesia to relieve pain and oxygen therapy to attempt to reduce sickling. Several new treatments hold promise. The level of hemoglobin F among these variants correlates partly with their severity. The higher the hemoglobin F level, the less severe the disease. Increases in hemoglobin F might lessen the intracellular polymerization of hemoglobin S. These observations have led to attempts to increase the level of hemoglobin F in sickle cell patients.

Nagel and co-workers (94) reported that recombinant human erythropoietin can stimulate the F-reticulocyte responses in some patients with sickle cell anemia. Administration of recombinant human erythropoietin to patients with heterozygous hemoglobin S β-thalassemia during pregnancy (95) resulted in a 1.5- to twofold increase in the hemoglobin F levels, a dramatic reduction in pain episodes and transfusion requirements, and better pregnancy outcomes in the five patients studied.

In a randomized trial, Charache and colleagues reported that hydroxyurea therapy ameliorated the clinical course of sickle cell anemia in some adults with three or more painful crises per year. The long-term safety of hydroxyurea in patients with sickle cell anemia was considered uncertain (96). This therapy should be avoided in pregnancy because of its potential effects on fetal DNA synthesis and function.

Perrine and colleagues reported the response of sickle cell patients to infusions of arginine butyrate (97). Fetal globin synthesis increased from 6% to 45% above pretreatment levels. The authors concluded that further trials of this class of compounds were warranted, to determine long-term tolerance and efficacy in patients with sickle cell anemia or β-thalassemia. The minimal side effects and the natural origin of the compound suggest the likelihood of safety in pregnancy.

A remarkable trial (98) of zinc supplementation in the prevention of vaso-occlusive episodes showed that the number of painful episodes over 1.5 years was 2.46 in the intervention group and 5.29 in the control group ($p < 0.025$). There was a significant reduction in the mean number of infective episodes and associated morbidity in treated patients. Tschumi and co-workers had previously shown that such doses (220 mg three times a day) were well tolerated and did not cause hematologic, renal, or hepatic toxicity (99). If similar doses can be tolerated by pregnant women without untoward side effects, this might be a promising prophylactic therapy for complications of sickling hemoglobinopathies. Bone marrow transplantation is the only currently available cure for sickle cell disease. Its complications and expense are too great to warrant its widespread use. Attempts to engraft nonsickling stem cells *in utero* have been disappointing. Specific gene therapy is a future goal of research.

Pregnancy Outcome in Sickling Hemoglobinopathies

Women with sickle cell disease were once often counseled against pregnancy (100–101). These opinions reflected the grave outcomes for mother and fetus at the time, with maternal mortality rates of 14% and perinatal mortality rates of 55%. In 1973, Pritchard and associates reported their experience with sickle cell disease in pregnancy (102). Although maternal and fetal morbidity and mortality were still significant, improvement over past experience was noted and attributed to the introduction of prophylactic exchange transfusion throughout pregnancy. In this procedure, pregnant women with sickling hemoglobinopathy were given transfusions to keep their hematocrit levels over 25% and their sickle hemoglobin level no higher than 60%. Experiments with this policy (103) showed a reduction in maternal mortality to zero and improvement in perinatal mortality. However, there was an increased incidence of growth-restricted fetuses, meconium staining of amniotic fluid, and ominous decelerations of the fetal heart rate compared to the general obstetric population. Morbidity from the transfusions was troublesome.

In 1976, Morrison and Wiser reported perinatal outcomes in 35 patients prophylactically transfused during pregnancy (104,105). The results were similar in the group receiving transfusions to those in a control group. Moreover, when compared with historical controls, there was a decrease in perinatal wastage and prematurity and in the incidence of low-birth-weight infants in the prophylactic transfusion group. These results led to a National Institutes of Health consensus development conference recommending prophylactic exchange transfusion for pregnant women with sickle cell disease (106).

In 1981, Miller et al. reviewed their experience in sickle cell patients treated over a 7-year period (107). Prophylactic exchange transfusion was not associated with improved pregnancy outcomes and was associated with significant antibody formation. The authors concluded that exchange transfusion might best be reserved as a treatment for infection, crisis, or symptomatic anemia in patients with sickle hemoglobinopathy. Tuck and associates later assessed the benefits of prophylactic blood transfusion in 51 pregnancies among women with hemoglobin S-S, hemoglobin S-C, and hemoglobin S β-thalassaemia in a retrospective study (108). Their data showed no significant difference in fetal or maternal outcomes between those patients who were transfused prophylactically and those who were not.

In 1988, Koshy et al. randomly assigned 72 pregnant patients with sickle cell anemia to treatment groups: 36 received prophylactic transfusions, and 36 received red cell transfusions only for medical or obstetric emergencies (109). Perinatal mortality rates were not significantly different between the patients who were given prophylactic transfusions and those who received transfusion for cause (15% vs. 5%). Prophylactic transfusions significantly lowered the incidence of painful episodes of sickle cell disease (14% vs. 50%) but did not significantly reduce the cumulative incidence of other complications of this disorder. The authors concluded that the omission of prophylactic red cell transfusion would not harm pregnant patients with sickle cell disease or their offspring, but the study lacked sufficient power to address the issues of perinatal and maternal mortality for which prophylactic transfusion was initiated (110).

Morrison et al. studied the role of partial prophylactic red cell exchange transfusion using continuous flow erythrocytapheresis in the treatment of pregnant patients with major sickle hemoglobinopathies (111). Among 131 pregnant patients with major hemoglobinopathies (hemoglobin S, hemoglobin S-C), 103 received partial prophylactic exchange transfusion early during prenatal care, whereas 28 received blood only when serious complications developed. Patients treated with exchange transfusion underwent outpatient continuous flow erythrocytapheresis with buffy-coat-poor blood. Directed donations from family members were used whenever possible. One maternal death occurred in the group of patients transfused for indications only. There were significantly fewer painful episodes, a significant reduction in other serious medical complications, and a significant decrease in maternal hospital days in women given prophylactic transfusions compared with women in the control group. The number of preterm deliveries, the prevalence of low-birth-weight infants, and the perinatal death rate were significantly lower among those who were routinely transfused. Among those receiving prophylactic transfusions, 1.9% had hepatitis, 4.9% had transfusion reactions, and 11% had alloantibodies versus 3.6%, 7.1%, and 17.9%, respectively, in the control group.

In 1995, Koshy reviewed the subject of prophylactic transfusion in pregnancy and concluded that there is no proof that prophylactic transfusion alters the outcome of pregnancy (112). She recommended that transfusion therapy be reserved for those patients who have already undergone a pregnancy that ended in the death of the fetus or for those with preeclampsia, acute chest syndrome, neurologic events of recent onset, and severe anemia and in preparation for surgical intervention. This approach is reasonable in terms of our current state of knowledge.

A review (113) of the outcomes of pregnancies complicated by sickle cell disease in the United Kingdom from 1991 to 1993 documented two maternal deaths among 81 pregnancies (2.5% maternal mortality rate); the perinatal mortality rate was 60/1,000. Sickling complications developed antenatally in 46.2% of pregnancies and postnatally in 7.7% of pregnancies. Pregnancies complicated by sickle cell disease were significantly more likely to be associated with anemia, preterm delivery, proteinuric hypertension, birth weights below the 10th percentile, and cesarean section as an emergency procedure than pregnancies in the control group. Severe sickling complications occurred more commonly in the third trimester; prophylactic transfusions reduced this risk but did not improve obstetric outcome.

In homozygous sickle cell disease (hemoglobin S-S), maternal mortality declined from an average of 3.2% before 1972 to 0.67% from 1972 to 1982 and to 0.59% in a prospective multicenter study from 1979 to 1986 (114,115). Live births rose from 68.1% before 1972 to 76.5% from 1972 to 1982. A similar trend in improved maternal and fetal outcomes has been seen in patients with hemoglobin S-C and hemoglobin S β-thalassemia diseases (114,115).

In summary, pregnancy outcomes in sickling syndromes are still highly variable around the world. Prophylactic partial exchange transfusion has been advocated as a means of preventing maternal death in several centers with extensive experience and excellent outcomes. Using current techniques, transfusion reactions and alloimmunization can be kept at a low level. A randomized trial to study the effects of prophylactic partial exchange transfusion did not have enough power to address the primary outcome variable of interest, the maternal mortality rate. Thus, prophylactic partial exchange transfusion remains the subject of controversy. The American College of Obstetricians and Gynecologists suggests that either plan of management could be considered appropriate and that care should be individualized (116). Mahomed (117) came to similar conclusions on reviewing the subject for the pregnancy and childbirth module of the Cochrane database of systematic reviews.

Transfusion for Complications of Sickling Hemoglobinopathies During Pregnancy

While the relationship between prophylactic partial exchange transfusion and pregnancy outcome in sickling syndromes remains contentious, there are agreed-on indications for therapeutic red blood cell transfusion. They include symptomatic splenic sequestration episodes, symptomatic aplastic events, severe symptomatic anemia, prevention of stroke recurrence, and severe acute chest episodes with hypoxia (118). Transfusion might also be useful in complicated forms of surgery, such as cardiovascular or thoracic surgery, or with complicated obstetric problems, severe right-upper-quadrant syndromes, extreme hyperbilirubinemia, refractory leg ulcers, refractory and protracted pain episodes, acute and severe priapism, and multi-organ failure syndrome.

Exchange transfusion has been recommended for selected patients with acute chest syndrome and priapism. A chronic transfusion regimen is under investigation for preoperative preparation and might have a benefit in the context of retinal–arterial vaso-occlusion, hepatic failure, septic shock, and cerebral angiography (119). Simple long-term transfusion might be indicated for cerebrovascular disease and for selected patients with debilitating vaso-occlusive symptoms, pulmonary disease, cardiac disease, and complicated pregnancy. In addition to severe sickle-related complications, transfusions for pregnant women are recommended for multiple gestation or a history of recurrent fetal loss. Indications for simple transfusion are symptomatic anemia, including that associated with splenic sequestration episodes, aplastic episodes, accelerated hemolysis, and blood loss. Koshy et al. (112,119) recommended simple transfusion during pregnancy if the hemoglobin level is less than 5 g, the hematocrit level is less than 15%, or the reticulocyte count is less than 3%. Otherwise, partial exchange transfusion using manual methods was suggested, removing 500 mL of the patient's blood and transfusing 2 units of packed red blood cells.

Two studies (120,121) indicated that preoperative transfusion to bring hemoglobin levels over 10 g/dL and hemoglobin S levels below 60% works as well as a more aggressive regimen to lessen mortality and morbidity rates associated with surgery. Pregnant sickle cell patients stand at least a 25% risk of cesarean section; their hemoglobin levels should be raised above 10 g/dL by partial exchange transfusion with buffy-coat-poor, extensively cross-matched red cells before cesarean section.

Complications of simple transfusions in sickle cell patients include hyperviscosity, which can precipitate or worsen a vaso-occlusive episode; hypersplenism, with decreased red cell half-life; iron overload; viral transmission; non-hemolytic transfusion reactions; red cell alloimmunization; and complications of central venous catheters in patients with poor venous access. Exchange transfusions avoid hyperviscosity, hypersplenism, and iron overload. Additional complications of exchange transfusion include anticoagulant effects of acid citrate buffer, rare neurologic complications of uncertain origin, risks of unmonitored volume shifts, and 2,3-DPG deficiency.

Management of Specific Complications of Sickling Hemoglobinopathies During Pregnancy

Anemia

Sickling hemoglobinopathies result in mild to moderate chronic hemolytic anemia. In addition, many patients with sickle cell anemia have inappropriately low erythropoietin production. Anemia is most severe in patients with homozygous hemoglobin S-S disease or heterozygous hemoglobin S β^0-thalassemia disease. It is milder in patients with heterozygous hemoglobin S β^+-thalassemia or heterozygous hemoglobin S-C disease. In patients with homozygous hemoglobin S-S disease, the anemia might be less severe with coexisting α-thalassemia (93).

There are several specific circumstances in which anemia can become more severe. There may be acute sequestration of red blood cells in an organ with a large vascular bed, such as the spleen, liver, or lung. Such episodes are usually caused by obstruction of flow through the organ and are accompanied or immediately followed by ischemia and necrosis. Treatment for sequestration is correction of the inciting factors responsible for increased sickling and capillary bed obstruction, restoration of blood volume with intravenous fluids, and oxygen delivery with red cell transfusion. Splenic sequestration occurs in children and adults with hemoglobin S-C disease or sickle thalassemia syndromes. Adults with hemoglobin S-S disease usually have infarcted spleens from previous sequestration events or have undergone splenectomy.

Another cause of worsening anemia can be a nutritional deficit of key building blocks. If the patient has undergone multiple transfusions, she might have an iron overload, but if the patient has not had many transfusions or has had excessive blood loss, iron deficiency is possible. Similarly, a high rate of DNA synthesis requires a high rate of folic acid turnover, which a diet deficient in vegetables might not provide. It is prudent to supplement the patient's diet with folic acid, 1 mg orally per day. More rarely, nutritional cobalamin deficiency can occur with high-protein cobalamin-deficient lacto-ovo vegetarian diets. The possibility of nutrient deficiencies should be evaluated when worsening anemia in a patient with hemoglobinopathy (or any hemolytic anemia) is being investigated.

Decreased bone marrow production of precursors due to an acute bacterial or viral infection can also worsen anemia in sickle cell disease. Parvovirus B19 has been specifically implicated in this form of reversible aplastic anemia. Impaired bone marrow production of precursors due to widespread bone marrow necrosis during a vaso-occlusive event can also exacerbate anemia. Transfusion is necessary, as is intensive supportive therapy for the associated bone marrow or fat embolization that frequently accompanies bone marrow necrosis. Bone marrow/fat embolism is one of the common fatal events in sickle cell disease, leading to hypoxemia and cardiac ischemia. As with all acute anemias, an external source of blood loss must be considered. Specific pregnancy-related causes of external blood loss should come to mind, particularly concealed placental abruption and uterine rupture.

Transfusions are indicated for symptomatic anemia, which usually is associated with an acute event. Oxygen delivery in such cases does not approach normal levels until very low levels of hemoglobin S are achieved (122).

The optimal hematocrit for patients with sickle cell disease has been found to be 26% using this perspective. A rule of thumb for transfusion is to restore the hematocrit to the level the patient had during a period of health free of complications.

Pain

Pain in a pregnant sickle cell patient must be evaluated first as a possible pregnancy-related complication. The pain associated with abruptio placentae, ectopic pregnancy, pyelonephritis, uterine rupture, and pulmonary embolism all have the potential to be misdiagnosed as vaso-occlusive events. Simultaneous evaluation of fetal health must run in parallel with evaluation of the cause of pain. Pain specific to sickling hemoglobinopathies is caused by tissue hypoxemia and inflammatory responses to necrosis of ischemic tissues. It therefore signals the presence or previous occurrence of a vaso-occlusive event at the location identified by the pain.

Vaso-occlusion can be precipitated by cold, dehydration, a sickle hemoglobin level greater than 8.5 g/dL, transfusion, infection, hypoxemia, metabolic or respiratory acidosis, stress, alcohol consumption, or preexisting microvascular disease, such as that associated with preeclampsia or other causes of disseminated intravascular coagulation. Common locations for pain include the back, chest, extremities (especially the tibial and periarticular areas) and abdomen; but any area of the body can be affected.

Management of pain begins with a thorough history and physical examination, searching for a precipitating cause of vaso-occlusion, particularly infection. Laboratory tests of the functional status of each organ system are evaluated, including CBC, reticulocyte count, erythrocyte sedimentation rate, urinalysis, arterial blood gas analysis, blood urea nitrogen, serum creatinine, serum electrolytes, bicarbonate, lactate dehydrogenase, total bilirubin, aspartate aminotransferase, alanine aminotransferase, alkaline phosphatase, and creatine kinase. A chest radiograph is indicated in the case of pulmonary findings or hypoxemia. Nonspecific therapy is concurrently initiated, including rehydration with intravenous fluids, oxygen (123), and narcotics. Specific therapy is instituted when a precipitating cause has been identified (for example, infection). Transfusion is not recommended for treatment of pain, because the tissue damage that has already occurred will not be relieved by therapy for vaso-occlusion; however, evidence of ongoing vaso-occlusion not relieved by conservative measures might be an indication for transfusion.

Neurologic Complications

Neurologic complications, which are seen in 25% of patients with sickle cell disease, include hemorrhagic and ischemic stroke, subarachnoid hemorrhage, isolated functional losses that suggest focal occlusion, seizures, and coma. Since the neurologic complications that accompany sickle cell disease also develop in conjunction with severe preeclampsia or eclampsia, the presence of one of these complications in pregnancy should prompt investigation for other signs of preeclampsia.

Ophthalmologic Complications

Vaso-occlusive episodes can result in retinal artery occlusion, retinal and anterior chamber ischemia, proliferative retinopathy, and retinal detachment and hemorrhage. Retinal examinations in pregnancy are indicated. The ophthalmic complications of sickle cell disease mimic those of preeclampsia and can be confused with them.

Acute Chest Syndrome

Acute chest syndrome is a nonspecific designation for acute, severe pulmonary disease in a patient with a sickling hemoglobinopathy. Symptoms and signs include dyspnea, chest pain, fever, tachypnea, leukocytosis, and a pulmonary infiltrate on chest radiography. It can be caused by viral or bacterial infection, acute pulmonary sequestration, or fat/bone marrow embolization resulting from infarction elsewhere or embolization from a venous thrombus. These conditions may be difficult to distinguish, and one may precipitate the other. Sputum macrophages that stain positively for fat suggest the presence of pulmonary fat embolism.

Pregnant patients should be monitored in an intensive care unit. Antibiotics to cover possible pathogens are indicated until definitive microbiological results are returned. Acute chest syndrome in pregnancy is an indication for a partial exchange transfusion, to bring the hemoglobin S concentration to 30% to 40% (124). Incentive spirometry is useful in decreasing atelectasis and pulmonary infiltrates (125).

Chronic Lung Disease

The patient who has recovered from acute chest syndrome will frequently manifest evidence of chronic pulmonary compromise, with pulmonary infarcts leading to restrictive lung disease, hypoxemia, pulmonary hypertension, and cor pulmonale. With diminished reserve, subsequent pulmonary events are more likely to be fatal. Baseline blood gases and pulmonary function testing should be obtained in all sickle cell patients.

Cardiac Complications

The anemia of sickle cell disease leads to a demand for expanded cardiac output and consequent left-ventricular hypertrophy, with chronic chamber enlargement and cardiomegaly. Vaso-occlusive events in the heart lead to loss of cardiac reserve and diminished exercise capacity. Myocardial infarction can arise even in the context of normal coronary arteries. Pulmonary infarction leads to pulmonary hypertension and right-ventricular failure. Congestive heart failure can result from exacerbations of anemia, hypertension, and volume overload, all of which can be associated with pregnancy.

Splenic Complications

Vaso-occlusive episodes in the spleen can lead to acute splenic sequestration, splenic ischemia, and infarction. The adult patient with sickle disease frequently is hyposplenic and more susceptible to bacterial infections. Pregnancy can exacerbate previously asymptomatic heterozygous sickle hemoglobin C disease and heterozygous sickle β^{+}-thalassemia disease, resulting in acute splenic sequestration and infarction in adulthood. Acute splenic sequestration is an indication for blood transfusion, which can usually reverse the process.

Hepatobiliary Complications

Acute hepatic vaso-occlusion can lead to sequestration, hepatomegaly, and ischemic necrosis with fever, pain, elevation of liver enzymes, and possibly hepatic failure. The abnormalities of liver function associated with vaso-occlusion can be difficult to distinguish from similar abnormalities associated with severe preeclampsia. Patients with known biliary tract disease should ideally undergo cholecystectomy before pregnancy, to avoid life-threatening episodes of cholecystitis and ascending cholangitis.

Renal Complications

Owing to the hypertonicity of the renal medulla, sickling frequently develops in the vasa recta, with consequent ischemia and infarction resulting in isosthenuria, incomplete renal tubular acidosis, abnormal potassium excretion, hematuria, and papillary necrosis. Hyperuricemia can result from proximal tubular dysfunction. Vaso-occlusive events can affect the glomeruli, leading to hypertension, proteinuria, and chronic renal insufficiency. In pregnancy, hyperuricemia, elevated creatinine, hypertension, and proteinuria are also manifestations of preeclampsia, which can be confused with the sickle renal disease or complicate it.

Infectious Complications

The sickle cell patient is susceptible to bacterial infections, including meningitis, pneumonia, osteomyelitis, and pyelonephritis. This predisposition can be a consequence of complement system abnormalities, reticuloendothelial system dysfunction, or infarction and consequent decreased opsonizing activity. Sickle cell patients might be more susceptible to salmonella osteomyelitis owing to defective opsonizing activity.

Dermatologic Complications

Vaso-occlusive events in the skin lead to myofascial syndromes with soft-tissue swelling and subcutaneous edema. Chronic ulcers can appear at sites of trauma, especially at the medial and lateral malleoli. Infected ulcers can be the site of origin for bacteremia or osteomyelitis. They resist healing as the result of the local ischemia of vaso-occlusion, and they frequently recur.

Placental Complications

Sickling in the uteroplacental circulation causes ischemia and infarction, with decreased placental perfusion. Early in pregnancy, this can provoke spontaneous abortion. A history of recurrent fetal loss in sickle cell disease is an obstetric indication for exchange transfusion.

Late fetal heart rate decelerations that develop during a vaso-occlusive crisis can disappear with maternal therapy. If the fetus recovers from an acute placental vaso-occlusive event, it is faced with decreased placental reserve and nutrient flow. The result may be intrauterine growth retardation. The identification of intrauterine growth restriction in pregnancy complicated by sickle cell disease is an indication for exchange transfusion. Sickle cell patients with multiple gestations are at extremely high risk for stillbirth, and prophylactic partial exchange transfusions are also indicated for these patients (119). Evidence of uteroplacental insufficiency using techniques of antepartum fetal biophysical monitoring is an indication for exchange transfusion, followed by delivery as soon as fetal lung maturity is established.

Preeclampsia

The pregnant patient with sickle cell disease is at high risk for preeclampsia. This predisposition may be due to placental events caused by sickling or to the presence of chronic renal disease and hypertension or both. Vaso-occlusive events in various organ systems can be difficult to distinguish from preeclampsia, as noted earlier. In addition, preeclampsia and vaso-occlusive events can coexist and exacerbate one another (126). Preeclampsia is associated with many of the fatal outcomes of sickle cell disease in pregnancy (127) and is an indication for exchange transfusion followed by delivery as soon as is obstetrically appropriate (112).

Isoimmunization

Isoimmunization from multiple previous blood transfusions is common in pregnant sickle hemoglobinopathy patients. Passively transferred antibodies might affect the fetus, causing hemolytic anemia progressing to hydrops fetalis. Sickle cell patients frequently have elevated serum bilirubin levels because of excessive hemolysis and impaired hepatic function. This bilirubin diffuses into the amniotic fluid and can make an amniotic fluid bilirubin reading uninterpretable in terms of the contribution of fetal hemolysis to the reading (128,129). If amniotic fluid analysis suggests severe fetal compromise, fetal cord blood sampling is the most direct way to assess the extent of fetal hemolysis and anemia. Isoimmunization can make cross-matching and further transfusion difficult. The most advanced methods for preventing this complication must be used in every transfusion.

Labor, Delivery, and the Puerperium

A sickle cell patient with an uncomplicated pregnancy can be observed for spontaneous labor at term, although most clinicians would intervene by 41 weeks. Oxytocin should be used at low doses because of the concern that it might diminish blood flow to bone. Postpartum anemia and endometritis must be treated aggressively. If any sign of preeclampsia or a vaso-occlusive episode appears during labor, partial exchange transfusion is indicated.

Hemoglobin C Disease

This hemolytic anemia is related to the presence of hemoglobin C. In the homozygous condition, relatively insoluble hemoglobin C crystallizes in the oxyhemoglobin state, causing the red cells to become rigid and thus subject to fragmentation and loss of membrane material, leading to the presence of microspherocytes on the peripheral smear. Hemoglobin C crystals dissolve in the deoxyhemoglobin state, probably explaining the absence of vaso-occlusive episodes in these patients. In the heterozygous state, illness is rare unless the patient is also heterozygous for hemoglobin S, in which case the pathophysiologic characteristics of sickling due to hemoglobin S might predominate.

Patients with hemoglobin C disease have few symptoms or physical findings. Laboratory studies indicate mild hemolytic anemia with microcytosis and target cells. The outcome of 72 pregnancies in 20 women with heterozygous hemoglobin C or doubly heterozygous hemoglobin C β-thalassemia were reported (130). Maternal complications attributable to hemoglobinopathy were rare, and perinatal outcomes were good. There is an enhanced requirement for folic acid because of increased synthetic activity in the marrow, reticulocytosis, and splenic destructive activity. Splenomegaly and hypersplenism can complicate pregnancy. Otherwise, a normal outcome can be expected. Prenatal diagnosis is important for parents who would like to know if their fetus is at risk for doubly heterozygous hemoglobin S-C disease. These genetic considerations should be sorted out by first identifying hemoglobinopathies in the patient as well as in her partner.

Hemoglobin E Disease

This hemolytic anemia is related to the presence of hemoglobin E. Beta-globin is normally derived from three separate DNA exons, which are transcribed; the resulting messenger RNA is then processed to splice these separate exons, removing the intervening intron sequences. A specific gene defect in the DNA for hemoglobin E leads to abnormal splicing, resulting in a decrease in chain synthesis—a "thalassemic" effect. In addition, the β-globin chain produced is structurally abnormal. Heterozygotes have no splenomegaly, and their clinical symptoms are similar to those of patients who are heterozygotes for β-thalassemia. Homozygotes have mild anemia, an elevated red cell count but no reticulocytosis, a low MCV, microcytes, and target cells. Chronic hemolysis does not develop. Heterozygotes have microcytosis with normal hemoglobin values, except during an aplastic crisis.

Hemoglobin E trait occurs in as many as 25% of Southeast Asian women (131) and has been reported in 50% of an isolated population in India (132). Growth restriction and fetal wastage can occur in homozygotes for hemoglobin E (133,134), but there is no difference in mortality rates among live-born infants. Thus, hemoglobin E disease appears to affect pregnancy in a manner similar to thalassemia intermedia, which hemoglobin E disease resembles.

ENZYME-DEFICIENCY ANEMIAS

Forms of congenital nonspherocytic hemolytic anemia can be caused by deficiencies of many enzymes necessary for red cell metabolism. These include glucose-6-phosphate dehydrogenase (G6PD) deficiency, pyruvate kinase (PK) deficiency, and glucose-6-phosphate isomerase (G6PI) deficiency. Others are quite rare. For G6PD deficiency, an X-linked recessive trait, the prevalence is high: 10% of black men in the United States are affected. Two defects of the glycolytic pathway enzymes account for most of the remaining enzyme deficiencies: 95% are due to PK deficiency, and 4% are due to G6PI deficiency.

G6PD is a key enzyme in the hexose–monophosphate shunt. Lack of G6PD lessens the reducing power of the erythrocyte. Oxidative stress caused by exogenous oxidants, including certain drugs (Table 21-5), leads to oxidative degradation and membrane binding of hemo-

TABLE 21-5. *Drugs causing hemolysis in subjects deficient in G6PD*

Antimalarials: primaquine, pamaquine, dapsone
Sulfonamides: sulfamethoxazole
Nitrofurantoin
Analgesics: acetanilid
Miscellaneous: vitamin K (water-soluble form), doxorubicin, methylene blue, nalidixic acid, furazolidone, niridazole, phenazopyridine

G6PD, glucose-6-phosphate dehydrogenase.
From ref. 135.

globin, producing Heinz bodies. These membranes are rigid and rapidly removed from the circulation. Favism is the name given to the clinical syndrome of hemolysis and profound anemia that arises in patients with G6PD deficiency when they eat fava beans, a staple food in the Mediterranean area, where G6PD deficiency is endemic.

There are three clinical classes of G6PD deficiency. Class I is a chronic, congenital, nonspherocytic, hemolytic anemia that resembles thalassemia and can be transfusion dependent. In class II, characterized by severe enzyme deficiency, there is episodic hemolysis. Class III is the most common; the enzyme deficiency is moderate, and hemolysis is precipitated by oxidant drugs or substances. Hepatitis, diabetes, and renal failure can also trigger hemolysis. Patients with deficiencies of glycolytic enzymes (PK and G6PI) show symptoms of anemia, jaundice, and splenomegaly in childhood (135–142).

Tests for G6PD or autohemolysis are abnormal after the reticulocytes have aged following an acute episode; any type of congenital nonspherocytic anemia not caused by hemoglobinopathy or membrane abnormality is probably due to an enzyme deficiency, even if the defect is unknown. Treatment includes vitamin E supplements and folic acid. Most patients do not require therapy except during a hemolytic or aplastic event, when blood transfusions might become necessary. The prognosis is generally good if oxidative stress is avoided.

In spite of its prevalence, reports of G6PD deficiency in pregnancy are rare, perhaps because it is usually a benign condition in women (143–147). One study documented increased anemia during pregnancy in patients with G6PD deficiency compared with controls selected from a consecutive cohort of patients who were screened for the enzyme deficiency (145). The implication made in several articles that pregnancy facilitates hemolysis is unsubstantiated because the studies lack appropriate controls (136,144). Two studies reported an increased rate of spontaneous abortions in mothers with G6PD deficiency compared with controls (143,145). The explanation for this is uncertain, but the rare association of fetal hydrops warrants antepartum surveillance and consideration of amniocentesis.

IRON-DEFICIENCY ANEMIA

This hypoplastic anemia is caused by lack of iron for synthesis of the heme molecule (Table 21-6) (148). It is caused by blood loss, including idiopathic pulmonary hemosiderosis, dietary iron deficiency, or congenital atransferrinemia. About 3% of American women of reproductive age have iron-deficiency anemia. This rate is much lower than the worldwide estimate of 15%. The anemia related to a disturbance of hemoglobin synthesis—absent mobilizable marrow iron stores—is the proximate cause. Dietary iron deficiency is a diagnosis of exclusion. Anemia in pregnancy is a major public health problem in developing countries because malaria and helminthic infections, in addition to inadequate dietary iron, contribute to the burden of anemia and increased rates of maternal and perinatal morbidity and mortality.

Iron deficiency proceeds in stages (Fig. 21-1). At first, only the serum ferritin and iron-binding capacity give clues to the deficient iron stores. When the deficiency becomes moderate, the iron saturation declines, and the marrow and heme precursors show evidence of diminished production of red cells. Only when the deficiency is severe do the cells take on the typical microcytic morphologic characteristics (Fig. 21-1). Laboratory abnormalities include anemia, normal or microcytic MCV, increased RDW-CV and RDW-SD, a low reticulocyte count, microcytes and target cells, low serum iron, high iron-binding capacity, low saturation of transferrin, low levels of ferritin, and absent bone marrow iron stores. Bone marrow biopsy is not usually needed.

TABLE 21-6. *Causes of iron depletion and deficiency*

Iron-store depletion	Iron-deficient erythropoiesis	Iron-deficiency anemia
Rapid growth	Blood loss	Blood loss
Infancy	Excessive menses or donation	GI hemorrhage
Adolescence	Hemodialysis	Intravascular hemolysis
Menstrual blood loss	GI hemorrhage	Surgical blood loss
Inadequate diet	Pregnancy	Hookworm infestation
Blood donation	Malabsorption	Severe malabsorption
	Polycythemia vera treated with phlebotomy	Gastrectomy
		Sprue
		Inflammatory bowel disease

GI, gastrointestinal.
From ref. 148.

TABLE 21-7. *Oral iron preparations*

Generic name	Tablet weight (iron content) mg
Ferrous sulfate	325 (65)
	195 (39)
Extended release	525 (105)
Ferrous fumarate	325 (107)
	195 (64)
Ferrous gluconate	325 (39)
Polysaccharide iron	150 (150)
	50 (50)

From ref. 148.

Diagnosed iron deficiency is easily corrected with iron supplements. Absorption of iron is increased in proportion to the severity of the deficiency. Asorbic acid enhances the absorption of inorganic iron. Lower doses of iron to correct iron deficiency have been advocated. The Centers for Disease Control have suggested a 60- to 120-mg iron supplement for all pregnant women with proven iron deficiency (3,149). Alternative preparations to ferrous sulfate have been introduced, to minimize the gastrointestinal toxicity of iron therapy (Table 21-7).

Iron Deficiency in Pregnancy

In spite of the fact that in developed countries the decline in hematocrit during pregnancy is unlikely to represent a pathologic process in women receiving an adequate diet, it has been almost universal practice to recommend routine iron supplementation during pregnancy. The value of this approach is uncertain. It is theoretically possible that iron supplementation in these women will increase blood viscosity and thus impair placental circulation and fetal growth. In addition, higher amounts of serum iron can negatively influence the absorption of other minerals.

There has been considerable research on iron deficiency in pregnancy and a body of randomized control trials (150). In most trials, diets were supplemented orally with 100 mg of elemental iron. The control groups received a placebo tablet or no iron. Mahomed reviewed the quality and content of the world literature on iron supplementation in pregnancy (150). Based on trials of acceptable methodologic quality, it appeared that routine iron supplementation raised or maintained the serum ferritin above 10 μg/L. This resulted in a substantial reduction in the proportion of women with a hemoglobin level below 10 or 10.5 g/dL in late pregnancy. Thus, iron supplementation was effective in controlling severe degrees of anemia associated with iron deficiency.

Surprisingly little information exists regarding the effect of iron supplementation on measures of either maternal or fetal outcome The only possible statistically significant effects of routine supplementation, suggested by the largest trial, were a reduced likelihood of cesarean section and postpartum blood transfusion (151). However, this same investigation showed an increase in dead infants and in those diagnosed as having hyperviscosity. These associations were not predicted before the analysis. The investigators speculated that some of the apparently worse outcomes in the selectively supplemented group were due to reactions of midwives and physicians to low hematocrit values. This trial had 2,912 participants, which exceeds the numbers in other studies by tenfold. No other methodologically sound trial showed a beneficial effect of supplementation on pregnancy outcome, even in areas with a greater burden of anemia, disease, and poverty than is seen in the developed countries where most research was conducted.

In spite of an abundance of published information on this subject, there is a dearth of well-constructed trials, and we continue to be ignorant of the potential benefits of this widespread practice of iron supplementation (152). The finding of a significant adverse outcome in one large, well-conducted trial suggests that iron supplementation should be given cautiously and selectively. In addition, the literature suggests a need for other large, properly designed trials to investigate fetal and neonatal death as endpoints in both developed and underdeveloped areas.

Heme iron is more easily absorbed than inorganic supplements; however, since heme iron is present in high quantities only in blood, muscle, spleen, and liver, consumption of heme iron from food results in consumption of increased amounts of cholesterol, saturated fats, and animal protein along with salt, all of which have deleterious effects, probably more so than modest iron deficiency. Heme iron is available as a pharmaceutical supplement and provides slight advantages over inorganic iron in pregnancy. For example, 27 mg of elemental iron in a product containing both heme and non-heme iron prevented anemia and increased iron stores during pregnancy and was safe and well tolerated (149). The same dose of completely inorganic iron had the same hematologic effect but did not maintain iron stores in all patients. The clinical usefulness of heme iron compared with inorganic iron is uncertain, but it is reasonable to try heme iron before resorting to more dangerous and untested methods, such as parenteral iron or erythropoietin supplements. Anemia in association with pregnancy that is resistant to iron supplementation might have a different origin or several sources. The anemia of chronic disease must be considered, as well as other hypoplastic conditions.

MEGALOBLASTIC ANEMIA

These hypoplastic anemias are the consequence of a disturbance in DNA synthesis that results from cobalamin deficiency, folic acid deficiency, and acquired and congenital defects of purine or pyrimidine metabolism (153,154). Cobalamin is released from microbial sources in food by acid-pepsin attack and transported by gastric intrinsic factor or salivary R proteins. It is absorbed in the terminal ileum. Alcohol addiction, phenytoin use, and absence of microbial sources of cobalamin from the diet thus lead to dietary deficiencies of folate and cobalamin. Various genetic defects can impair the absorption and utilization of cobalamin. In addition, there are genetic defects of purine and pyrimidine metabolism that impair DNA synthesis, but RNA and protein synthesis continue, and larger cells are produced. Pregnancy normally causes a relative folate deficiency, as do hemolytic disorders with a high turnover of cells and DNA synthesis.

Clinical Manifestations

Symptoms of anemia as well as progressive neuropathy occur (paresthesias are an early sign) in cobalamin deficiency, as do atrophy of lingual papillae and glossitis. Neuropsychiatric disorders, hallucinations, and personality and mood changes sometimes develop without obvious megaloblastosis. Symptoms of anemia without neuropathy or glossitis occur in folate deficiency. Affective disorders are common.

Laboratory abnormalities include macrocytosis, or elevation of the MCV. Macrocytosis might not be readily apparent from the peripheral smear, but a slight elevation of the MCV together with an elevated RDW indicates the presence of a small population of enlarged cells. Fish-tailed red blood cells and hypersegmented neutrophils are seen and, in severe cases, there are nucleated red blood cells, granulocytopenia, and thrombocytopenia. Concurrent iron deficiency will block full morphologic expression of megaloblastosis, as will thalassemia, but hypersegmentation of neutrophils will persist. Serum cobalamin levels of 250 pg/mL or less are suggestive; levels are falsely low in pregnancy and folate deficiency and after administration of radioisotopes. Serum folate and red blood cell folate can be depressed primarily or concurrently with cobalamin deficiency. Anti-intrinsic-factor antibodies may be present, and serum levels of homocysteine and methylmalonic acid increase. Treatment requires a supply of the missing nutrient.

While folic acid is a vitamin and cannot be manufactured in the body, normal requirements can usually be met from dietary intake, except when cooking methods destroy the folic acid available in food or when starvation occurs. Fetal growth increases the total number of rapidly dividing cells, leading to higher requirements for folic acid (154). Without folate supplementation, more than a third of pregnant women show signs of subnormal postpartum serum folate levels, and up to 3.4% have megaloblastic anemia (155). Folic acid demands can be further amplified in women with sickle cell disease, thalassemia, and other hemolytic anemias and in women with anemias with ineffective erythropoiesis where precursors fail to mature properly, such as the dyserythropoietic, sideroblastic, and myelodysplastic anemias. Folic acid demand may also be higher in areas where malaria is endemic (156). Routine folate supplementation raises or maintains serum and red cell folate levels and substantially cuts down the proportion of women with low hemoglobin levels in late pregnancy (157). It has been shown that some neural tube defects can be prevented by supplementation of the maternal diet with folic acid (see Chapter 2).

Anemia due to cobalamin deficiency generally stems from an inability to absorb the vitamin from food, a condition known as pernicious anemia, rather than to dietary deficiency (158,159). Cobalamin deficiency is uncommon in pregnancy, partly because of the rarity of pernicious anemia and partly because of the infertility that often accompanies it (160). Nevertheless, there have been isolated reports of newborn infants with dietary cobalamin deficiency due to maternal pernicious anemia (161) or to maternal dietary deficiency associated with a vegan diet (162). Folic acid supplementation of a mother with pernicious anemia could theoretically mask the symptoms of anemia and allow the neuropathy of cobalamin deficiency to progress. The presence of megaloblastic anemia therefore requires careful evaluation and specific replacement therapy.

REFERENCES

1. Centers for Disease Control. CDC criteria for anemia in children and childbearing-aged women. MMWR 1989;38:400–404.
2. Dallman PR, Yip R, Johnson C. Prevalence and causes of anemia in the United States, 1976 to 1980. Am J Clin Nutr 1984;39:437–445.
3. Centers for Disease Control. Recommendations to prevent and control iron deficiency in the United States. Centers for Disease Control and Prevention MMWR 1998;47(RR-3):1–29.
4. Centers for Disease Control. Anemia during pregnancy in low-income women—United States, 1987. MMWR 1990;39:73–76 and 81.
5. Fleming AF. Hematologic diseases. In: Strickland GT, ed. Hunter's tropical medicine, 7th ed. Philadelphia: WB Saunders, 1991.
6. Public Health Service. Promoting health/preventing disease: Public Health Service implementation plans for attaining the objectives for the nation. Public Health Rep 1983;Sept–Oct[Suppl]:132–155.
7. Kim I, Hungeford DW, Yip R, Kuester SA, Zyrkowski C, Trowbridge FL. Pregnancy nutrition surveillance system—United States, 1979–1990. MMWR CDL Surveillance Summaries 1992;41:25–41.
8. Hauth JC, Merenstein GB. Antepartum care. In: Guidelines for prenatal care, fourth edition. Elk Grove Village, The American Academy of Pediatrics, and Washington D.C., The American College of Obstetrics and Gynecologists, 1997:65–92.
9. Murray CJL, Lopez AD. Global health statistics: a compendium of prevalence and mortality estimates for over 200 conditions. Cambridge: Harvard University Press, 1996.
10. Murray CJL, Lopez AD. The global burden of disease: a comprehensive assessment of mortality and disability from diseases, injuries and risk factors in 1990 and projected to 2020. Cambridge: Harvard University Press, 1996.
11. Letsky EA. Erythropoiesis in pregnancy. J Perinat Med 1995;23: 39–45.
12. Schrier SL. Hematopoiesis and red blood cell function. In: Rubenstin E., Federman DD (eds.), Scientific American Medicine. New York, Scientific American, 1994.
13. Harstad TW, Mason RA, Cox SM. Serum erythropoietin quantitation in pregnancy using an enzyme-linked immunoassay. Am J Perinatol 1992:9:233–235.
14. Milman N, Graudal N, Nielsen OJ, Agger AO. Serum erythropoietin during normal pregnancy: relationship to hemoglobin and iron status

markers and impact of iron supplementation in a longitudinal placebo-controlled study on 18 women. Int J Hematol 1997;66:159–168.
15. Beutler E. Disorders of hemoglobin. In: Fauci AS, Braunwald E, Isselbacher KJ, et al. (eds.) Harrison's Principles of internal medicine, 14th edition, New York, McGraw-Hill, 1998:645–652.
16. Packman CH, Leffy JP. Acquired hemolytic anemia due to warm-reacting autoantibodies. In: Beutler E, Lichtman MA, Coller BS, Kipps TJ, eds. Williams hematology, 5th ed. New York: McGraw Hill, 1995.
17. Carr S, Rubin L, Dixon D, Star J, Dailey J. Intrauterine therapy for homozygous alpha-thalassemia. Obstet Gynecol 1995;85:876–879.
18. Chitayat D, Silver MM, O'Brien K, et al. Limb defects in homozygous alpha-thalassemia: report of three cases. Am J Med Genet 1997;68: 162, 167.
19. Abuelo DN, Forman EN, Rubin LP. Limb defects and congenital anomalies of the genitalia in an infant with homozygous alpha-thalassemia. Am J Med Genet 1997;68:158–161.
20. Harmon JV Jr, Osathanondh R, Holmes LB. Symmetrical terminal transverse limb defects: report of a twenty-week fetus. Teratology 1995;51:237–242
21. Tongsong T, Wanapirak C, Srisomboon J, Piyamongkol W, Sirichotiyakul S. Antenatal sonographic features of 100 alpha-thalassemia hydrops fetalis fetuses. J Clin Ultrasound 1996;24:73–77.
22. Guy G, Coady DJ, Jansen V, Snyder J, Zinberg S. Alpha-thalassemia hydrops fetalis: clinical and ultrasonographic considerations. Am J Obstet Gynecol 1985;153:500–504.
23. Kurtz AB, Foy PM, Wapner RJ, Rubin CS, Dubbins PA, Cole-Beuglet C. Fetal ultrasound findings in alpha-thalassemia major. J Clin Ultrasound 1981;9:257–259.
24. Lie-Injo LE, Lopez CG, Dutt AK. Pathological findings in hydrops foetalis due to alpha-thalassemia: a review of 32 cases. Trans R Soc Trop Med Hyg 1968;62:874–879.
25. Petrou M, Brugiatelli M, Old J, et al. Alpha thalassemia hydrops foetalis in the UK: the importance of screening pregnant women of Chinese, other South East Asian and Mediterranean extraction for alpha thalassaemia trait. Br J Obstet Gynaecol 1992;99:985–989.
26. Stein J, Berg C, Jones JA, Detter JC. A screening protocol for a prenatal population at risk for inherited hemoglobin disorders: results of its application to a group of Southeast Asians and blacks. Am J Obstet Gynecol 1984;150:333–341.
27. Lam YH, Ghosh A, Tang MH, Lee CP, Sin SY. Early ultrasound prediction of pregnancies affected by homozygous alpha thalassemia-1. Prenat Diagn 1997;17:327–332.
28. Westgren M, Ringden O, Eik-Nes S, et al. Lack of evidence of permanent engraftment after in utero fetal stem cell transplantation in congenital hemoglobinopathies. Transplantation 1996;61:1176–1179.
29. Ong HC, White JC, Sinnathuray TA. Haemoglobin H disease and pregnancy in a Malaysian woman. Acta Haematol 1977;58:229–233.
30. Laros RK. Blood disorders in pregnancy. Philadelphia: Lea & Febiger, 1986.
31. Horger EO III. Hemoglobinopathies in pregnancy. Clin Obstet Gynecol 1974;17:127–162.
32. Chan V, Chan TK, Liang ST, Ghosh A, Kan YW, Todd D. Hydrops fetalis due to an unusual form of Hb H disease. Blood 1985;66:224–228.
33. Gadoth N, Kornmehl P, Gueron M, Moses SW. Haemorrhagic infarction of the myocardium in a newborn with haemoglobin H disease and erythroblastosis. Acta Paediatr Scand 1978;67:245–247.
34. Halbrecht I, Shabtai F. An unusual case of hemoglobin Bart's hydrops fetalis. Acta Genet Med Gemellol (Roma) 1975;24:97–103.
35. Liebhaber SA, Cash FE, Main DM. Compensatory increase in alpha 1-globin gene expression in individuals heterozygous for the alpha-thalassemia-2 deletion. J Clin Invest 1985;76:1057–1064.
36. White JM, Richards R, Byrne M, Buchanan T, White YS, Jelenski G. Thalassemia trait and pregnancy. J Clin Pathol 1985;38:810–817.
37. Miller JM Jr. Alpha thalassemia minor in pregnancy. J Reprod Med 1982;27:207–209.
38. Alger LS, Golbus MS, Laros RK Jr. Thalassemia and pregnancy: results of an antenatal screening program. Am J Obstet Gynecol 1979;134:662–673.
39. Lam YH, Tang MH. Prenatal diagnosis of haemoglobin Bart's disease by cordocentesis at 12–14 weeks gestation. Prenat Diagn 1997;17:501–504.
40. George E, Mokhtar AB, Azman ZA, Hasnida K, Saripah S, Hwang CM. Prenatal diagnosis of Hb Bart's hydrops fetalis in West Malaysia: the identification of the alpha and 1 defect by PCR based strategies. Singapore Med J 1996;37:501–504.
41. Chang MY, Soong YK, Wang ML. Preimplantation diagnosis of alpha-thalassemia by blastomere aspiration and polymerase chain reaction: preliminary experience. J Formos Med Assoc 1996;95:203–208.
42. Torcharus K, Sriphaisal T, Krutvecho T, et al. Prenatal diagnosis of Hb Bart's hydrops fetalis by PCR technique: Pramongkutklao experience. Southeast Asian J Trop Med Public Health 1995;26[Suppl 1]:287–290.
43. Winichagoon P, Fucharoen S, Kanokpongsakdi S, Fukumaki Y. Detection of alpha-thalassemia 1 (Southeast Asian type) and its application for prenatal diagnosis. Clin Genet 1995;47:318–320.
44. Kuo PL, Lin TM, Huang KF, et al. Carrier screening and prenatal diagnosis for alpha-thalassemia with biphasic polymerase chain reaction. J Formos Med Assoc 1994;93:765–769.
45. Hofstaetter C, Gonser M, Goelz R. Perinatal case report of unexpected thalassemia Hb Bart. Fetal Diagn Ther 1993;8:418–422.
46. Lam YH, Ghosh A, Tang MH, Lee CP, Sincerely SY. Second-trimester hydrops fetalis in pregnancies affected by homozygous alpha-thalassaemia-1. Prenat Diagn 1997;17:267–269.
47. Lam YH, Ghosh A, Tang MH, Lee CP, Sincerely SY. Early ultrasound prediction of pregnancies affected by homozygous alpha-thalassemia-1. Prenat Diagn 1997;17:327–332.
48. Tongsong T, Wanapirak C, Srisomboon J, Piyamongkol W, Sirichotiyakul S. Antenatal sonographic features of 100 alpha-thalassemia hydrops fetalis fetuses. J Clin Ultrasound 1996;24:73–77.
49. Ko TM, Tseng LH, Hsu PM, Hwa HL, Lee TY, Chuang SM. Ultrasonographic scanning of placental thickness and the prenatal diagnosis of homozygous alpha-thalassemia 1 in the second trimester. Prenat Diagn 1995;15:7–10.
50. Ghosh A, Tang MH, Lam YH, Fung E, Chan VTI. Ultrasound measurement of placental thickness to detect pregnancies affected by homozygous alpha-thalassemia 1. Lancet 1994;344:988–989.
51. Pearson HA, O'Brien RT. The management of thalassemia major. Semin Hematol 1975;12:255–265.
52. Mordel N, Birkenfeld A, Goldfarb AN, Rachmilewitz EA. Successful full-term pregnancy in homozygous beta-thalassemia major: case report and review of the literature. Obstet Gynecol 1989;73:837–840.
53. Jensen CE, Tuck SM, Wonke B. Fertility in beta thalassaemia major: a report of 16 pregnancies, preconceptual evaluation and a review of the literature. Br J Obstet Gynaecol 1995;102:625–629.
54. Savona-Ventura C, Bonello F. Beta-thalassemia syndromes and pregnancy. Obstet Gynecol Surv 1994;49:129–137.
55. Kumar RM, Rizk DE, Khuranna A. Beta-thalassemia major and successful pregnancy. J Reprod Med 1997;42:294–298.
56. Seracchioli R, Porcu E, Colombi C, et al. Transfusion-dependent homozygous beta-thalassaemia major: successful twin pregnancy following in-vitro fertilization and tubal embryo transfer. Hum Reprod 1994;9:1964–1965.
57. Surbek D, Koller A, Pavic N. Successful twin pregnancy in homozygous beta-thalassemia after ovulation induction with growth hormone and gonadotropins. Fertil Steril 1996;65:670–672.
58. Birkenfeld A, Mordel N, Okon E. Direct demonstration of iron in a term placenta in a case of beta-thalassemia major. Am J Obstet Gynecol 1989;160:562–563.
59. Vaskaridou E, Konstantopoulos K, Kyriakou D, Loukipoulos D. Deferoxamine treatment during early pregnancy: absence of teratogenicity in two cases. Haematologica 1993;78:183–184.
60. Fort AT, Morrison JC, Ragland JB, Morgan BS, Fish SA. Correlation of maternal serum and amniotic fluid bilirubin in gravid patients with sickle cell anemia who were actively hemolyzing. Am J Obstet Gynecol 1972;112:227–232.
61. Lindsay MK, Kupo VR. Nonpredictive value of measurements of delta optical density at 450 mm in SS disease. Am J Obstet Gynecol 1985;152:75–76.
62. Hadi HA, Fadel HE, Nelson GH, Hill J. The unreliability of amniotic fluid bilirubin measurements in isoimmunized pregnancies in sickle cell disease patients. Obstet Gynecol 1985;65:758–760.
63. Rund D, Rachmilewitz E. Thalassemia major 1995: older patients, new therapies. Blood Rev 1995;9:25–32.
64. Borgna-Pignatti C, Marradi P, Rugolotto S, Marcolongo A. Successful pregnancy after bone marrow transplantation for thalassaemia. Bone Marrow Transplant 1996;18:235–236.
65. Ratip S, Skuse D, Porter J, Wonke B, Yardumian A, Modell B. Psychosocial and clinical burden of thalassaemia intermedia and its implications for prenatal diagnosis. Arch Dis Child 1995;72:408–412.
66. Alger LS, Golbus MS, Laros RK Jr. Thalassemia and pregnancy:

results of an antenatal screening program. Am J Obstet Gynecol 1979;134:662–673.
67. White JM, Richards R, Byrne M, Buchanan T, White YS, Jelenski G. Thalassaemia trait and pregnancy. J Clin Pathol 1985;38:810–817.
68. Xu X, Liao C, Liu Z, et al. Antenatal screening and fetal diagnosis of beta-thalassemia in a Chinese population: prevalence of the beta-thalassemia trait in the Guangzhou area of China. Hum Genet 1996;98: 199–202.
69. Saliki RK, Chang CA, Levenson CH, et al. Diagnosis of sickle cell anemia and beta-thalassemia with enzymatically amplified DNA and nonradioactive allele-specific oligonucleotide probes. N Engl J Med 1988;319:537–541.
70. Cai SP, Chang CA, Zhang JZ, Saiki RK, Erlich HA, Kan YW. Rapid prenatal diagnosis of beta thalassemia using DNA amplification and nonradioactive probes. Blood 1989;73:372–374.
71. Maggio A, Giambona A, Cai SP, Wall J, Kan YW, Chehab FF. Rapid and simultaneous typing of hemoglobin S, hemoglobin C, and seven Mediterranean beta-thalassemia mutations by covalent reverse dot-blot analysis: application to prenatal diagnosis in Sicily. Blood 1993; 81:239–242.
72. Hatcher SL, Lambert QT, Teplitz RL, Carlson JR. Heteroduplex formation: a potential source of genotyping error from PCR products. Prenat Diagn 1993;13:171–177.
73. Chan V, Chan TP, Lau K, Todd D, Chan TK. False non-paternity in a family for prenatal diagnosis of beta-thalassaemia. Prenat Diagn 1993;13:977–982.
74. Tan JA, Tay SH, Kham KY, Wong HB. BamH1 polymorphism in the Chinese, Malays, and Indians in Singapore and its application in the prenatal diagnosis of beta-thalassemia. Jpn J Hum Genet 1993;38: 315–318.
75. Chandran R, Ainoon O, Anson I, Anne J, Cheong SK. First trimester prenatal diagnosis of beta-thalassaemia following chorionic villus sampling. Med J Malaysia 1993;48:341–344.
76. Lee HH, Chang JG, Chen RT, Yang ML, Choo KB. Prenatal diagnosis of beta-thalassemic mutations in Chinese by multiple restriction fragment–single strand conformation polymorphism analysis. Proceedings of the National Science Council, Republic of China–Part B. Life Sci 1994;18:112–117.
77. Fucharoen S, Fucharoen G, Ratanasiri T, Jetsrisuparb A, Fukumaki Y. A simple nonradioactive method for detecting beta-thalassemia/HbE disease: application to prenatal diagnosis. Southeast Asian J Trop Med Public Health 1995;26[Suppl 1]:278–281.
78. Winichagoon P, Fucharoen S, Siritanaratkul N, et al. Prenatal diagnosis for beta-thalassemia syndromes using HRP-labeled oligonucleotide probes at Siriraj Hospital. Southeast Asian J Trop Med Public Health 1995;26[Suppl 1]:282–286.
79. Tuzmen S, Tadmouri GO, Ozer A, et al. Prenatal diagnosis of beta-thalassaemia and sickle cell anaemia in Turkey. Prenat Diagn 1996;16: 252–258.
80. Muralitharan S, Srivastava A, Shaji RV, et al. Prenatal diagnosis of beta-thalassaemia mutations using the reverse dot blot technique. Natl Med J India 1996;9:70–71.
81. Cheung MC, Goldberg JD, Kan YW. Prenatal diagnosis of sickle cell anaemia and thalassaemia by analysis of fetal cells in maternal blood. Nature Genet 1996;14:264–268.
82. Adinolfi M, el-Hashemite N, Sherlock J, Ward RH, Petrou M, Rodeck C. Prenatal detection of Hb mutations using transcervical cells. Prenat Diagn 1997;17:539–543.
83. Touraine JL. In utero transplantation of fetal liver stem cells into human fetuses. J Hematother 1996;5:195–199.
84. Westgren M, Ringden O, Eik-Nes S, et al. Lack of evidence of permanent engraftment after in utero fetal stem cell transplantation in congenital hemoglobinopathies. Transplantation 1996;61:1176–1179.
85. Gehlbach DL, Morgenstern LL. Antenatal screening for thalassemia minor. Obstet Gynecol 1988;71:801–803.
86. Yeo GS, Tan KH, Liu TC. Screening for beta thalassaemia and HbE traits with the mean red cell volume in pregnant women. Ann Acad Med Singapore 1994;23:363–366.
87. Schrier SL. Anemia: blood loss and disorders of iron metabolism. In: Rubenstein E, Federman DD, eds. Scientific American medicine. New York: Scientific American, 1991.
88. Hansen RM, Hanson G, Anderson T. Failure to suspect and diagnose thalassemic syndromes: interpretation of RBC indices by the non-hematologist. Arch Intern Med 1985;145:93–94.
89. Fairbanks VV, Beutler E. Iron deficiency. In Williams WJ, Beutler E, Erslev AJ, Lichtman MA, eds. Hematology, 3rd ed. New York: McGraw-Hill, 1983.
90. England JM, Fraser PM. Differentiation of iron deficiency from thalassaemia trait by routine blood count. Lancet 1973;1:449.
91. Mentzer WC Jr. Differentiation of iron deficiency from thalassaemia trait. Lancet 1973;1:882.
92. Motulsky AG. Frequency of sickling disorders in U.S. blacks. N Engl J Med 1973;288:31–33.
93. Powars D, Hiti A. Sickle cell anemia. Beta S gene cluster haplotypes as genetic markers for severe disease expression. Am J Dis Child 1993;147:1197–1202.
94. Nagel RL, Vichinsky E, Shah M, et al. F reticulocyte response in sickle cell anemia treated with recombinant human erythropoietin: a double-blind study. Blood 1993;81:9–14.
95. Bourantas K, Makrydimas G, Georgiou J, Tsiara S, Lolis D. Preliminary results with administration of recombinant human erythropoietin in sickle cell/beta-thalassemia patients during pregnancy. Eur J Haematol 1996;56:326–328.
96. Charache S, Terrin ML, Moore RD, et al. Effect of hydroxyurea on the frequency of painful crises in sickle cell anemia. N Engl J Med 1995;332:1317–1322.
97. Perrine SP, Ginder GD, Faller DV, et al. A short-term trial of butyrate to stimulate fetal-globin-gene expression in the beta-globin disorders. N Engl J Med 1993;328:81–86.
98. Gupa VA, Chaubey SB. Efficacy of zinc therapy in prevention of crisis in sickle cell anemia: a double blind, randomized controlled clinical trial. J Assoc Physicians India 1995;43:467–469.
99. Tschumi P, Gloersheim GL. Zur Vertraglichkeit von hochdosiertem peroralem Zinksulfat. Schweiz Med Wochenschr 1981;111:1573–1577.
100. Bopp JR, Hall DG III. Indications for surgical sterilization. Obstet Gynecol 1970;35:760–764.
101. Fort AT, Morrison JC, Diggs LW, Fish SA, Berreras L. Counseling the patient with sickle cell disease about reproduction: pregnancy outcome does not justify the maternal risk. Am J Obstet Gynecol 1971; 111:324–327.
102. Pritchard JA, Scott DE, Whalley PH, Cunningham FG, Mason RA. The effects of maternal sickle cell hemoglobinopathies and sickle cell trait on reproductive performance. Am J Obstet Gynecol 1973;117: 662–670.
103. Cunningham FG, Pritchard JA, Mason R, Chase G. Prophylactic transfusions of normal red blood cells during pregnancies complicated by sickle cell hemoglobinopathies. Am J Obstet Gynecol 1979;135: 994–1003.
104. Morrison JC, Wiser WL. The effect of maternal partial exchange transfusion on the infants of patients with sickle cell anemia. J Pediatr 1976;89:286–289.
105. Morrison JC, Wiser WL. The use of prophylactic partial exchange tranfusion in pregnancies associated with sickle cell hemoglobinopathies. Obstet Gynecol 1976;48:516–520.
106. Transfusion therapy in pregnancy sickle cell disease patients. National Institutes of Health Consensus Development Conference Summaries 1979;1:17–20.
107. Miller JM Jr, Horger EO III, Key TC, Walker-EM Jr. Management of sickle hemoglobinopathies in pregnant patients. Am J Obstet Gynecol 1981;141:237–241.
108. Tuck SM, James CE, Brewster EM, Pearson TC, Studd JW. Prophylactic blood transfusion in maternal sickle cell syndromes. Br J Obstet Gynaecol 1987;94:121–125.
109. Koshy M, Burd L, Wallace D, Moawad A, Baron J. Prophylactic red-cell transfusions in pregnant patients with sickle cell. N Engl J Med 1988;319:1447–1452.
110. Koshy M. Prophylactic transfusions in pregnant patients with sickle cell disease. N Engl J Med 1989;320:1286–1287.
111. Morrison JC, Morrison FS, Floyd RC, Roberts WE, Hess LW, Wiser WL. Use of continuous flow erythrocytapheresis in pregnant patients with sickle cell disease. J Clin Apheresis 1991;6:224–229.
112. Koshy M. Sickle cell disease and pregnancy. Blood Rev 1995;9: 157–164.
113. Howard RJ. Tuck SM. Pearson TC.: Pregnancy in sickle cell disease in the UK: results of a multicentre survey of the effect of prophylactic blood transfusion on maternal and fetal outcome. British J Obstet Gynaecol 1995;102:947–951.
114. Smith JA, Espeland M, Bellevue R, Bonds D, Brown AK, Koshy M.

Pregnancy in sickle cell disease: experience of the Cooperative Study of Sickle Cell Disease. Obstet Gynecol 1996;87:199–204.
115. Powars DR, Sandhu M, Niland-Weiss J, Johnson C, Bruce S, Manning PR. Pregnancy in sickle cell disease. Obstet Gynecol 1986;67:217–228.
116. Hemoglobinopathies in pregnancy. Technical Bulletin number 220. Washington, D.C.: American College of Obstetricians and Gynecologists, 1996.
117. Mahomed K. Prophylactic vs. selective blood transfusion in sickle cell anaemia. In: Neilson JP, Crowther CA, Hodnett ED, Hofmeyr GJ, eds. Pregnancy and childbirth module of the Cochrane database of systematic reviews [updated 01 September 1997]. The Cochrane Library database on disk and CD ROM. The Cochrane Collaboration, Issue 4. Oxford: Update Software, 1997.
118. Wayne AS, Kevy SV, Nathan DG. Transfusion management of sickle cell disease. Blood 1993;81:1109–1123.
119. Koshy M, Chisum D, Burd L, Orlina A, How H. Management of sickle cell anemia and pregnancy. J Clin Apheresis 1991;6:230–233.
120. Vichinsky EP, Haberkern CM, Neumayr L, et al. A comparison of conservative and aggressive transfusion regimens in the perioperative management of sickle cell disease. The Preoperative Transfusion in Sickle Cell Disease Study Group. N Engl J Med 1995;333:206–213.
121. Haberkern CM, Neumayr LD, Orringer EP, et al. Cholecystectomy in sickle cell anemia patients: perioperative outcome of 364 cases from the National Preoperative Transfusion Study. Preoperative Transfusion in Sickle Cell Disease Study Group. Blood 1997;89:1533–1542.
122. Howard RJ, Tuck SM, Pearson TC. Optimal haematocrit and haemoglobin S levels in pregnant women with sickle cell disease. Clin Lab Haematol 1995;17:157–161.
123. Zipursky A, Robieux IC, Brown EJ, et al. Oxygen therapy in sickle cell disease. Am J Pediatr Hematol Oncol 1992;14:222–228.
124. Koshy M, Burd L. Management of pregnancy in sickle cell syndromes. Hematol Oncol Clin North Am 1991;5:585–596.
125. Bellet PS, Kalinyak KA, Shukla R, Gelfand MJ, Rucknagel DL. Incentive spirometry to prevent acute pulmonary complications in sickle cell diseases. N Engl J Med 1995;333:699–703.
126. Chmel H, Bertles JF. Hemoglobin S/C disease in a pregnant woman with crisis and fat embolization syndrome. Am J Med 1975;58: 563–566.
127. Perkins RP. Inherited disorders of hemoglobin synthesis and pregnancy. Am J Obstet Gynecol 1971;111:120–159.
128. Hadi HA, Fadel HE, Nelson GH, Hill J. The unreliability of amniotic fluid bilirubin measurements in isoimmunized pregnancies in sickle cell disease patients. Obstet Gynecol 1985;65:758–760.
129. Lindsay MK, Lupo VR. Nonpredictive value of measurements of delta optical density at 450 nm in SS disease. Am J Obstet Gynecol 1985; 153:75–76.
130. Mayberry MC, Mason RA, Cunningham FG, Pritchard JA. Pregnancy complicated by hemoglobin CC and C-beta-thalassemia disease. Obstet Gynecol 1990;76:324–327.
131. Pravatmuang P, Tilokhus M, Suannum M, Chaipat C. Phitsanulok population: the highest incidence of hemoglobin E in the northern provinces of Thailand and PND counseling. Southeast Asian J Trop Med Public Health 1995;26[Suppl 1]:266–270.
132. Deka R. Fertility and haemoglobin genotypes: a population study in Upper Assam. Hum Genet 1981;59:172–174.
133. Ong HC. Maternal and fetal outcome associated with hemoglobin E trait and hemoglobin E disease. Obstet Gynecol 1975;45:672–674.
134. Belgir RS. Reproductive profile of mothers in relation to hemoglobin E genotypes. Indian J Pediatr 1992;59:449–454.
135. Rosse W, Bunn HF. Hemolytic anemias and acute blood loss. In: Fauci AS, Braunwald E, Isselbacher KJ, et al. (eds). Harrison's Principles of internal medicine, 14th edition. New York, McGraw-Hill, 1998: 659–671.
136. Vives Corrons JL, Garcia AM, Sosa AM, Pujades A, Colomer D, Linares M. Heterozygous pyruvate kinase de deficiency and severe hemolytic anemia in a pregnant woman with concomitant, glucose-6-phosphate dehydrogenase deficiency. Ann Hematol 1991;62:190–193.
137. Fanning J, Hinkle RS. Pyruvate kinase deficiency hemolytic anemia: two successful pregnancy outcomes. Am J Obstet Gynecol 1985;153: 313–314.
138. Amankwah KS, Dick BW, Dodge S. Hemolytic anemia and pyruvate kinase deficiency in pregnancy. Obstet Gynecol 1980;55:42S–44S.
139. Nieling C, Pottgen W. Hamolytische Anamie durch Pyruvatkinase-Mangel und Schwangerschaft. Verh Dtsch Ges Inn Med 1974;80: 1517–1520.
140. Gilsanz F, Vega MA, Gomez-Castillo E, Ruiz-Balda JA, Omenaca F. Fetal anaemia due to pyruvate kinase deficiency. Arch Dis Child 1993; 69:523–524.
141. Ghindini A, Sirtori M, Romero R, Yarkoni S, Solomon L, Hobbins JC. Hepatosplenomegaly as the only prenatal finding in a fetus with pyruvate kinase deficiency anemia. Am J Perinatol 1991;8:44–46.
142. Volpato S, Vigi V, Cattarozzi G. Nonspherocytic haemolytic anaemia and severe jaundice in a newborn with partial pyruvate kinase deficiency. Acta Paediatr Scand 1968;57:59–64.
143. Toncheva D, Tzoneva M. Prenatal selection and fetal development disturbances occurring in carriers of G6PD deficiency. Hum Genet 1985; 69:88.
144. Horanyi M, Szelenyi J, Rona G, Lang A, Lehmann H, Hollan SR. Haemoglobin O Arab, beta-thalassaemia and glucose-6-phosphate dehydrogenase deficiency in a Hungarian family. Folia Haematol 1980;107:654–660.
145. Perkins RP. The significance of glucose-6-phosphate dehydrogenase deficiency in pregnancy. Am J Obstet Gynecol 1976;125:215–223.
146. Silverstein E, Roadman C, Byers RH, Kitay DZ. Hematologic problems in pregnancy. III. Glucose-6-phosphate dehydrogenase deficiency. J Reprod Med 1974;12:153–158.
147. Bernard EE. Glucose-6-phosphate dehydrogenase deficiency in pregnancy. J Obstet Gynaecol Br Commonw 1969;76:370–372.
148. Hillman RS. Iron deficiency and other hyproliferative anemias. In: Fauci AS, Braunwald E, Isselbacher KJ, et al. (eds). Harrison's Principles of internal medicine, 14th edition. New York, McGraw-Hill, 1998:638–644.
149. Eskeland B, Malterud K, Ulvik RJ, Hunskaar S. Iron supplementation in pregnancy: Is less enough? A randomized, placebo controlled trial of low dose iron supplementation with and without heme iron. Acta Obstet Gynecol Scand 1997;76:822–828.
150. Mahomed K. Routine iron supplementation during pregnancy. In: Neilson JP, Crowther CA, Hodnett ED, Hofmeyr GJ, eds. Pregnancy and childbirth module of the Cochrane database of systematic reviews in the Cochrane Library. The Cochrane Collaboration, issue 4. Oxford: Update Software, 1997.
151. Hemminki E, Rimpela U. A randomized comparison of routine versus selective iron supplementation during pregnancy. J Am Coll Nutr 1991;10:3–10.
152. Hollan S, Johansen KS. Adequate iron stores and the nil nocere principle. Haematologia 1993;25:69–84.
153. Louis-Ferdinand RT. Myelotoxic, neurotoxic and reproductive adverse effects of nitrous oxide. Adverse Drug React Toxicol Rev 1994;13: 193–206.
154. Campbell BA. Megaloblastic anemia in pregnancy. Clin Obstet Gynecol 1995;38:455–462.
155. Willoughby ML, Jewell FG. Folate status throughout pregnancy and in postpartum period. Br Med J 1968;4:356–360.
156. Fleming AF, Ghatoura GB, Harrison KA, Briggs ND, Dunn DT. The prevention of anaemia in pregnancy in primigravidae in the guinea savanna of Nigeria. Ann Trop Med Parasitol 1986;80:211–233.
157. Mahomed K. Routine folate supplementation in pregnancy. In: Neilson JP, Crowther CA, Hodnett ED, Hofmeyr GJ, eds. Pregnancy and childbirth module of the Cochrane database of systematic reviews, September 1997.
158. Schilling RF, Williams WJ. Vitamin B_{12} deficiency: underdiagnosed, overtreated?. Hosp Pract (Off Ed) 1995;30:47–52.
159. Pruthi RK, Tefferi A. Pernicious anemia revisited. Mayo Clin Proc 1994;69:144–150.
160. Marty H. Perniziose Anamie als Ursache einer sekundaren Sterilitat. Schweiz Med Wochenschr 1984;114:178–179.
161. Heaton D. Another case of megaloblastic anemia of infancy due to maternal pernicious anemia. N Engl J Med 1979;300:202–203.
162. Sklar R. Nutritional vitamin B_{12} deficiency in a breast-fed infant of a vegan-diet mother. Clin Pediatr (Phila) 1986;25:219–221.

SECTION VIII

Endocrine Disorders

Cherry and Merkatz's Complications of Pregnancy,
Fifth Edition, edited by W. R. Cohen.
Lippincott Williams & Wilkins, Philadelphia © 2000.

CHAPTER 22

Thyroid Disease in Pregnancy and the Postpartum Period

Terry F. Davies and Rhoda H. Cobin

The evaluation and management of thyroid function and dysfunction in pregnancy poses a challenge to the combined efforts of the thyroidologist and obstetrician. Thyroid disease is so prevalent in the population that the combination of pregnancy and thyroid disease is commonplace. Furthermore, the fact that postpartum thyroid dysfunction occurs in 8% to 10% of pregnant women has aroused great interest in the relationship between thyroid function and pregnancy. In one of the earliest descriptions of hyperthyroidism [by Parry in 1825 (1)], a large swollen thyroid gland was described some three months "after lying in." To quote Parry, "The carotid arteries on each side were greatly distended; the eyes were protruded from their sockets, and the countenance exhibited an appearance of agitation and distress . . . which I have rarely seen equaled." Treatment of such thyroid disorders requires an awareness of many fundamental concepts in thyroid pathophysiology because they accurately predict the effect of disease and therapy on both the mother and child.

T. F. Davies and R. H. Cobin: Departments of Endocrinology and Medicine, Mount Sinai School of Medicine, New York, NY 10029.

NORMAL THYROID PHYSIOLOGY

Control of Thyroid Function

The thyroid gland accumulates iodine from the circulation in an active, energy-requiring process against a concentration gradient via the iodine transporters present in the thyroid cell membrane (2). The transport of iodine is regulated primarily by thyroid-stimulating hormone (TSH) and the plasma iodine concentration (Fig. 22-1). Iodine is then organified by a thyroid peroxidase (TPO) enzyme system (TPO used to be referred to as the microsomal antigen). Tyrosine rings within thyroglobulin (Tg) molecules are progressively iodinated and coupled to form the thyroid hormones triiodothyronine (T_3) and thyroxine (T_4) (Fig. 22-1). T_3 and T_4 generally exist within the thyroid gland in a ratio of 1:10 to 1:20. These molecules are hydrolyzed off the Tg molecule and released concomitantly into the circulation. All steps are accelerated by pituitary TSH. This glycoprotein hormone binds to specific thyroid cell surface receptors (TSHR) and induces the generation of cyclic adenosine monophosphate (cAMP) and phosphoinositol as second messengers (Fig. 22-2) (3). As well as serving as an accelerator of thyroid hormone synthesis, TSH is a trophic factor for the thyroid gland. The release of TSH is guided by a pituitary set-point, which is influ-

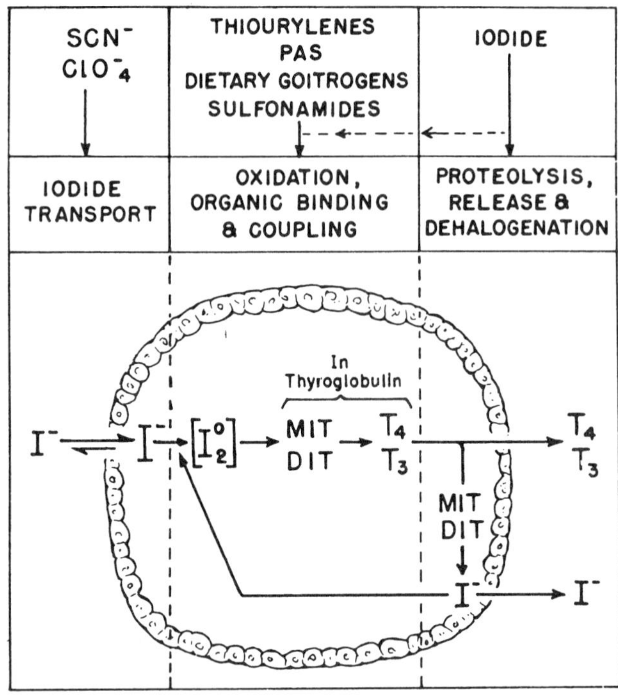

FIG. 22-1. Thyroid hormone synthesis. The intrafollicular lumen represents the interstitial compartment rather than the true follicle lumen. Also shown are the major inhibitors of the several steps in hormone biosynthesis. In addition, lithium acts like iodide as an inhibitor of proteolysis and release. (From Ingbar S, Woeber S. In: Williams RH, ed. Textbook of endocrinology, 6th ed. Philadelphia: WB Saunders, 1981.)

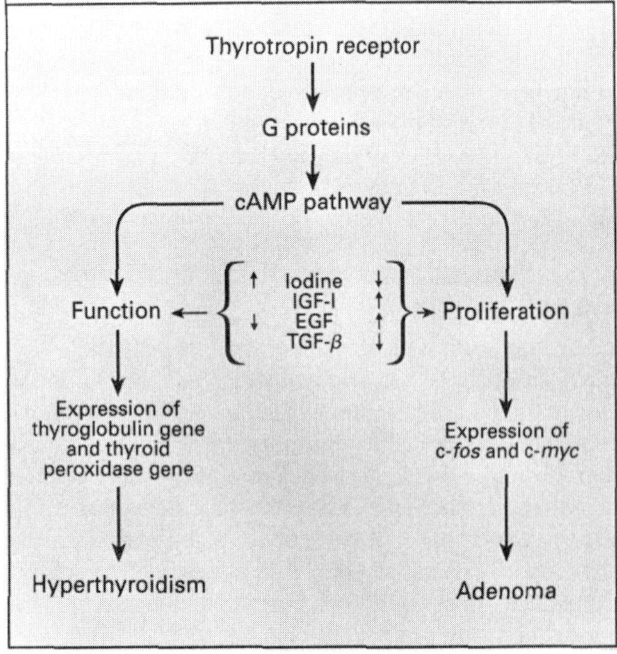

FIG. 22-2. Signal transduction at the TSH receptor.

enced by hypothalamic TSH-releasing hormone (TRH) and thyroid hormone feedback. TRH increases TSH release and synthesis. Conversely, T_3 exerts negative feedback directly on the pituitary by binding to thyroid hormone receptors, which act as negative transcription factors and inhibit TSH β gene transcription. Thyroid hormones also inhibit TRH release at the level of the hypothalamus. Hence, a classic negative feedback loop occurs (Fig. 22-3).

Thyroid Hormones

Once released into the circulation, T_4 is 99.5% bound to carrier proteins; only 0.5% is in the free and active state. Thyroid binding globulin (TBG) binds 60% to 70% of the circulating T_4 at a high affinity and relatively low capacity, whereas thyroid binding prealbumin (transthyretin) binds 20% to 30% of the circulating hormone with a lower affinity but greater capacity. The remaining 10% of bound circulating thyroid hormone is associated with serum albumin. Occasionally individuals have aberrant binding proteins that require careful evaluation. There is 60-fold more T_4 than T_3 in the peripheral circulation, but the free T_4:T_3 ratio is only about 3:1. This is because the affinity of T_3 for TBG is one tenth that of T_4, and the circulating free T_3 level is therefore less affected by alterations in the thyroid binding proteins. A small amount of T_3 is secreted directly from the thyroid gland, especially in situations of iodine deficiency. However, 80% of circulating T_3 is derived from peripheral deiodination of T_4 by 5′-mono-deiodination occurring in liver, muscle, and a variety of other tissues, including the pituitary gland. Thus, T_4 may be thought of as a secretory product that serves as a precursor or prohormone for biologically active T_3. The nature of the three deiodinase enzymes that accomplish this task has now been clarified (4). These enzymes contain the rare amino acid selenocysteine. Their properties are summarized in Table 22-1. Of particular importance has been the recognition that these enzymes have differing specific activities and, because they are critical for conversion of T_4 to T_3, the effects in the pituitary and brain may be different from muscle and liver, depending on the presence of the different enzyme subtypes. Brain tissue, for example, possesses deiodinase enzymes that, in circumstances of low iodine or low T_3, may preferentially shunt T_4 to T_3 to preserve metabolically active cerebral T_3. Placental type II deiodinase activity may serve to regulate intraplacental concentrations of T_3 necessary for local placental function, whereas type III deiodinase activity may be regulated by circulating T_3 levels and serves to regulate fetal thyroid hormone economy (5). T_4 also can be monodeiodinated to an inactive 3,3′,5′-reverse T_3. Metabolic disturbances frequently result in preferential deiodination to reverse T_3 which, together with its decreased clearance, contributes to the low-T_3 syndromes seen commonly in hospitalized sick patients.

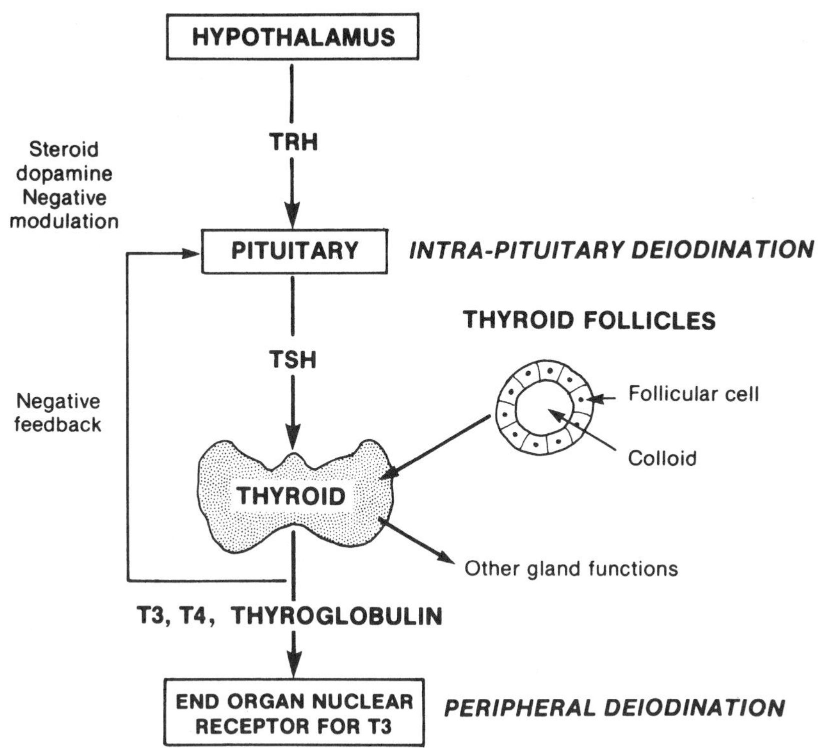

FIG. 22-3. Outline of hypothalamic-pituitary-thyroid axis with its classic feedback network.

TABLE 22-1. *A simple comparison of properties of the human iodothyronine selenodeiodinases*

	Type 1	Type 2	Type 3
Tissue location	Liver, kidney, thyroid, central nervous system	Central nervous system, pituitary, brown fat, placenta, thyroid, skeletal muscle, heart	Central nervous system, placenta, skin
Substrate preference	r $T_3 > T_4 > T_3$	$T_4 >$ r T_3	$T_3 > T_4$
Deiodination site	Outer and inner ring	Outer ring	Inner ring
Inhibition by propylthiouracil	Sensitive	Resistant	Resistant

Thyroid hormones diffuse through cell membranes by a poorly characterized mechanism and are then transferred to the cell nucleus bound to a family of thyroid hormone alpha and beta receptors. These complexes in turn bind to thyroid response elements (TREs) on the DNA and may activate or repress mRNA transcription and protein synthesis depending on the gene engaged and the presence of a variety of cooperative factors (6,7). Thyroid hormone receptors belong to the same family as the steroid hormone receptors and have been characterized thoroughly. The different subtypes are expressed to different degrees in different tissues, and the effect of thyroid hormone on cell function is therefore determined by which receptors and cofactors are expressed in that particular cell.

THYROID FUNCTION IN PREGNANCY

The Thyroid Gland

In the pregnant woman the thyroid gland responds to a number of physiologic alterations:

1. Iodine turnover is increased as a consequence of a higher glomerular filtration rate and renal iodine clearance. In theory this would cause a decrease in the proportion of iodine accumulated by the thyroid gland and a decrease in thyroid hormone released, and it may be responsible for some degree of organ hypertrophy induced by excess TSH (8).
2. Estrogen increases the half-life of TBG by altering its degree of sialylation as it is synthesized in the liver, and more T_4 is then bound to circulating protein. Total circulating thyroid hormone is increased as TBG increases, but the free and biologically active T_4 is normally maintained within the eumetabolic range (Table 22-2). Metabolic clearance of T_4 and T_3 during pregnancy reaches a new steady state, the metabolic clearance rate (MCR) of T_4 having been measured at 97 μg/day, similar to the nonpregnant rate of 90 μg/day (9).
3. The TSH response to TRH has been reported to be increased during the 16th to 20th week of pregnancy (10), presumably as a function of both estrogen

TABLE 22-2. *Thyroid function tests in normal pregnancy*[a]

Variables	Female controls	2nd trimester	3rd trimester
Number	100	21	80
T_4 (μg/100 mL)	9.0 ± 2.5	13.1 ± 2.6	13.5 ± 2.6
TBG (μg/mL)	22.8 ± 4.9	41.8 ± 6.0	41.7 ± 5.6
T_4:TBG ratio	4.2 ± 0.7	3.2 ± 0.6	3.2 ± 0.6
T_3 (μg/100 mL)	120 ± 12	188 ± 42	210 ± 25

[a]Normal range varies for every laboratory depending on assays used.

effects on the pituitary gland and possibly elevated endogenous TRH.

4. Human chorionic gonadotropin (hCG) has intrinsic thyroid-stimulating activity due to its low-affinity interaction with the TSH receptor (11–13). Studies have indicated small elevations of free thyroid hormone (still within the normal range) corresponding to the time of peak hCG levels early in pregnancy (14,15), along with lower TSH levels. Physiologically, this may be of little consequence, but in hydatidiform mole or choriocarcinoma, hyperthyroidism secondary to hCG stimulation may result (12,16,17).

Placental Transfer

The placental barrier in pregnancy effectively screens the fetus from many alterations in maternal thyroid status because neither TSH nor TBG penetrate significantly. Placental transfer of thyroid hormone is variable at different times during pregnancy (18). Although previously the placental membrane was felt to be relatively impermeable to T_4 and T_3, investigators have demonstrated the presence of T_3 in the brain of human fetuses before the presence of a fetal thyroid (19). Human fetuses with severe iodide organification defects or thyroid agenesis have been noted to have sufficient T_4 in cord blood, implying maternal transfer (20). In Dutch goats carrying a mutation for thyroglobulin synthesis, affected fetuses with unaffected mothers had normal T_4 and brain weights (21). Rat studies have also revealed T_4 and T_3 maternal-fetal transfer in early pregnancy (22). In areas of severe iodine deficiency with a high prevalence of endemic cretinism, supplementation of maternal iodine in the first and second trimester reduced the frequency of fetal neurologic abnormalities from 9% to 2% (23). This maternal-fetal transfer mechanism may be of great import in areas of endemic goiter and in congenital hypothyroidism (24).

Under pathologic conditions, the fetus may be exposed to alterations in thyroid function by the passage of nonphysiologic molecules across the placental barrier. Immunoglobulin G (IgG) antibodies, including the TSH receptor antibodies with thyroid-stimulating or blocking activity (TSHR-Ab) found in Graves disease and Hashimoto's disease (25–27), traverse the placenta, as do iodine, TRH, antithyroid drugs, and β blockers, including propranolol (28–30).

Immune Function

Much of thyroid disease seen during the childbearing years is autoimmune in etiology. The fact that normal immune surveillance is diminished in pregnancy has been well documented (see Chapter 37). Depressed cellular immunity has been characterized by decreased skin graft rejection, reduced phytohemagglutinin-induced immunocyte stimulation, and a lower response to PPD and dinitrochlorobenzene in skin testing. More recently, the observations of a decrease in the Th1 T-cell subsets in pregnancy is also reflective of a shift from cell-mediated immunity (31). Such diminished immune function may be partially related to changes in estrogen and cortisol levels, hCG, or circulating placental cytokines in pregnancy and to the transfer of immune suppressor factors from the fetus to the maternal circulation.

Diminished thyroid immunosurveillance may be associated clinically with declining goiter size, decreased thyroid antibody titers, reduced circulating peripheral lymphocyte function, and with partial or complete autoimmune thyroid disease remission in pregnancy (32–34). The practical implications of this concept are clear:

1. If thyroid autoimmune disease severity is altered, medical therapy may require adjustments during pregnancy.
2. Rebound of autoimmune disease with elevated cytotoxic Th1 cells and antibody titers in the postpartum period may lead to either transient or permanent abnormalities in thyroid function.

Fetal Considerations

Fetal maturation of the hypothalamic-pituitary-thyroid axis must be considered in the management of maternal thyroid disease (Fig. 22-4). After development as an outpouching of gut endoderm and migration from the buccal area into the neck, at 12 weeks the fetal thyroid gland has developed a normal histologic appearance and can organify iodine and secrete thyroid hormone. Near mid-gestation, pituitary TSH has increased into the physiologic range and may exceed maternal levels. Other parameters of pituitary function also appear by this time, as evidenced by growth hormone and prolactin levels (35), both of which are measurable during the first trimester and increase progressively toward term. There is a con-

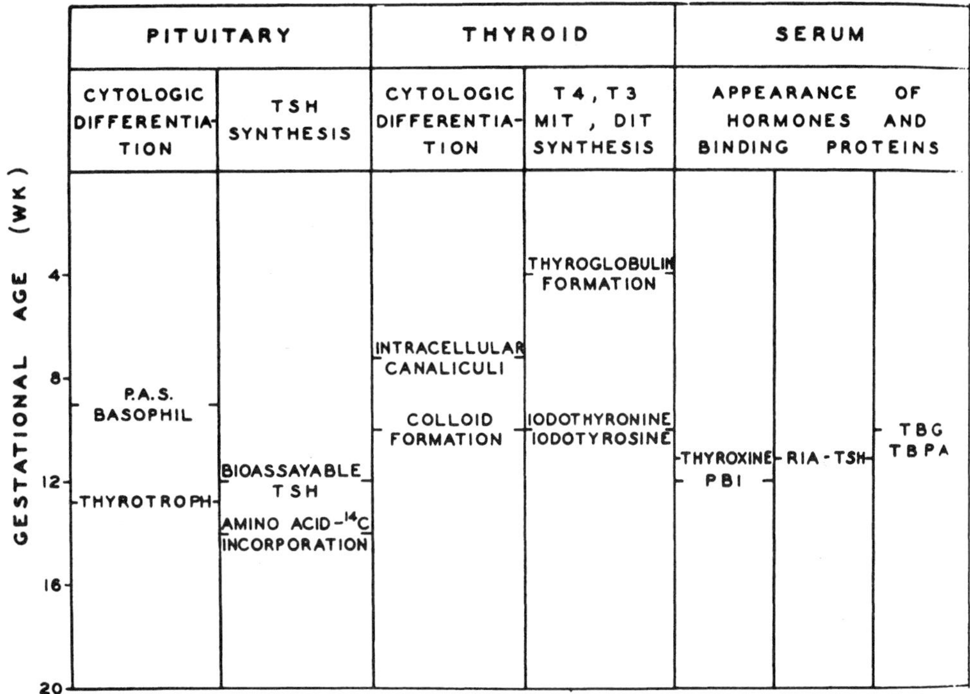

FIG. 22-4. Histologic and functional differentiation of the human thyroid. (From Greenberg AH, Czernichow P, Reba RC, Tyson J, Blizzard RM, et al. Observations on the maturation of thyroid function in early fetal life. J Clin Invest 1970;49:1790–1803.)

comitant increase in fetal TBG production, but free T_4 values may be higher than expected, suggesting either increased biological activity of TSH or an immature set-point mechanism. Near-term values of free T_4 may exceed the maternal range (Table 22-2). By contrast, total T_3 is consistently low, with elevated reverse T_3. Metabolic clearance studies of fetal sheep T_4, T_3, and reverse T_3 suggest that immaturity of the 5′-deiodinase enzymes may be responsible for this phenomenon. Despite the reduced T_3, the fetus is eumetabolic by clinical assessment. After delivery, there is a rapid transient surge in TRH, TSH, T_4, and T_3, all of which return to the normal adult range within 3 to 4 days (Table 22-3) (36).

Clinical Aspects

The normal thyroid gland has been said both to enlarge and to remain unchanged (37–39) in healthy pregnant females. The incidence of goiter in pregnancy varies geographically, perhaps in relation to ambient iodine supply. However, the presence of thyromegaly may imply a primary thyroid disorder rather than the result of pregnancy alone. Postmortem studies of unfortunate pregnant women demonstrated increased cellular hypertrophy and vascularity of the thyroid (40), but the presence of gross glandular hypertrophy in iodine-suficient areas most often implies disease, however subtle. The presence of estrogen receptors in thyroid tissue also suggests the possibility of a direct impact on the thyroid follicular cell (41).

Normal pregnant subjects often mimic the hyperthyroid state by appearing nervous, having a resting tachycardia, having smooth, moist, slightly diaphoretic skin, with warm, soft erythematous palms, and clinically apparent systolic cardiac murmurs. There is cutaneous vasodilatation, and the basal metabolic rate is elevated because of increased oxidative metabolism in pregnancy. Careful biochemical evaluation of thyroid function is therefore often more decisive than clinical evaluation, especially in the presence of a goiter.

TABLE 22-3. *Thyroid function tests in the neonatal period*

	Approximation values for thyroid function tests in infants (range)		
Tests	Newborn cord blood	3–5 days	2 weeks to 3 months
T_4 (μg/100 mL)	12 (6–17)	15 (9–20)	11 (7–15)
T_3 (ng/100 mL)	50 (10–90)	130 (50–210)	160 (160–240)
TSH (μg/mL)	9.5 (1–20)	6 (U–20)	4 (U–10)

Values are means and 95% ranges.
U, undetectable.

Thyroid Function Testing in Pregnancy

The availability of accurate measurements for total T_4, total T_3, TBG (or T_3 resin uptake), and TSH by radioimmunoassay (RIA) makes the calculation of thyroid function status precise. Indirect measurements of free T_4 and free T_3, relying on resin binding, may be compromised by increasing TBG levels (10,18). However, the chemical diagnoses of hyper- and hypothyroidism are now made with little difficulty, even when clinical signs are conflicting. The ratio of T_4 to TBG (or a resin binding test) correlates well with free T_4 measurements (Table 22-4), but should always be combined with serum TSH assessment. It is important to note that the T_4:TBG ratio decreases during pregnancy for uncertain reasons, perhaps because of inhibition of T_4 binding to the carrier protein. Free thyroid hormone analysis by equilibrium dialysis is expensive, time consuming, and unnecessary. Other ancillary measures of thyroid function are unwise in pregnancy, for example, thyroid scanning and measurement of radioactive iodine uptake. A T_3 RIA still remains a helpful, widely available, additional investigation in the presence of a suppressed TSH. TRH testing, which used to be performed under such circumstances, is no longer recommended and should never be performed in pregnancy because TRH crosses the placenta and also may be associated with smooth muscle (including uterine) contractions. Furthermore, the new third-generation TSH assays are highly reliable and precise. A suppressed TSH (usually less than 0.1 μU/mL) is almost always indicative of thyroid overactivity (42). Mild hyperthyroidism has not been demonstrated to be dangerous in pregnancy, and repeat testing and clinical observation before the institution of therapy is most advisable when thyroid function tests are borderline.

Hypothyroidism is straightforward to diagnose because of the great efficacy of TSH levels as a monitor of thyroid hormone deficiency. In hypothyroidism secondary to thyroidal disease, the TSH level is always raised, and further stimulation with TRH is never indicated even in borderline situations. Total T_4 or a derived T_4 index is generally low or in the low normal range. Free hormone levels by equilibrium dialysis are poor indicators of reduced thyroid function and are not indicated (43). Similarly, total T_3 levels are of little help in detecting thyroid failure and should not be requested.

TABLE 22-4. *Appropriate thyroid function tests in relation to suspected diagnosis*

	Thyroid function test strategy		
Suspected disorder	Primary test	Secondary test	Antibody confirmation
Hyperthyroidism	TSH	T_3 or free T3	TSHR-Ab
Hypothyroidism	TSH	T_4 : TBG ratio or free T4	Anti-Tg Anti-TPO

Gestational Thyrotoxicosis

During the second trimester, when hCG production reaches its peak, there is enhanced stimulation of the TSH receptor by crossover specificity with hCG, manifested in normal pregnancy by slight elevation of free T_4 and lowering of TSH. These changes are both within the normal range and only seen clearly in group comparisons. This is a clinically silent phenomenon, but an increase in thyroid size, tachycardia, and failure to gain weight may occur, sometimes in association with hyperemesis gravidarum (44). The more pronounced syndrome has been linked to the presence of an asialo hCG with greater thyroid-stimulating activity (45) and seems to be more common in Asian women (46). Because it is self-limited, the importance of the disorder is primarily to distinguish it from true Graves disease requiring treatment. TSHR-Abs are not detectable in gestational thyrotoxicosis and Graves ophthalmopathy is absent. Among all patients with hyperemesis, thyrotoxicosis is often sought but rarely found (47).

Fundamentals of Autoimmune Thyroid Disease

Because the majority of pregnant patients with thyroid disease have Graves or Hashimoto disease, it is important to understand what we know of the etiology of these common diseases. Two principal forms of immunologic influence on thyroid function are known: stimulation by stimulating antibodies to the TSH receptor aided by helper-inducer T cells in Graves disease and destruction of thyroid epithelial cells by antibodies capable of destroying cells, cytotoxic T cells, and thyroid cell apoptosis in Hashimoto's thyroiditis. Hence, there is a spectrum of disease from hyperthyroid Graves patients to those in gross thyroid failure due to autoimmune thyroiditis (Hashimoto's disease) (Fig. 22-5). The presentation of disease in patients appears to depend on the balance between these influences.

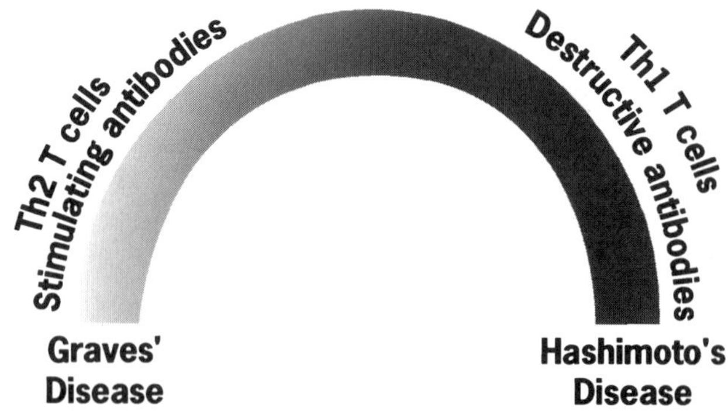

FIG. 22-5. The contrasting causes of Graves disease and Hashimoto disease. Graves disease is associated with stimulating antibodies and T-helper cells with primarily Th2-type cytokine secretion. In contrast, Hashimoto disease is associated with destructive antibodies and T-helper cells with primarily Th1-type cytokine secretion.

Evidence for the association of disordered immunity and thyroid disease is based on the pathologic nature of the thyroid lesions, the presence of a variety of thyroid autoantibodies and thyroid-specific T cells in the circulation and within the thyroid tissue itself, and the association of thyroid disease with other autoimmune abnormalities. It is important to be aware of the data indicating the primary nature of the immune abnormalities rather than their being secondary to some other thyroid abnormality. In certain situations, for example, subacute (granulomatous) thyroiditis, thyroid autoantibodies are detected only in transiently increased titers and usually fade with decline of the disease. In contrast, in autoimmune thyroid disease, autoantibodies and T cells may predate obvious tissue changes, and both destructive and stimulating antibodies are capable of tissue effects *in vitro* (48,49) and *in vivo* (50,51). Furthermore, the development of immunization-induced animal models of thyroiditis and Graves disease that closely resemble human disease further supports the autoimmune nature of the disorders (52,53).

Immunogenetics of Thyroid Disease

Both Graves disease and autoimmune thyroiditis are familial diseases in the sense that both may occur, and indeed often do, within the same extended family. Thyroid disease is also found in families with other autoimmune diseases such as diabetes, pernicious anemia, Sjögren syndrome, rheumatoid arthritis, and Addison's disease. In keeping with these observations has been the increased frequency of HLA-DR3 in such patients, but with a risk ratio of only threefold. Moreover, this increased frequency has been shown to be an association and not true linkage (54). This implies that HLA makes only a small contribution to genetic susceptibility to autoimmune thyroid disease. This is shown most clearly by the fact that HLA-identical siblings have only a 7% to 10% concordance for disease (55). This indicates that non-HLA genes contribute significantly to susceptibility in patients with Graves disease and Hashimoto's disease. A search is therefore underway in many laboratories to identify such genes.

THYROID AUTOANTIBODIES

Thyroid-Stimulating Hormone Receptor Antibodies

Sera from patients with hyperthyroid Graves disease contain thyroid-stimulating antibodies discovered by Adams and Purves (49) in 1956 in the form of long-acting thyroid stimulator (LATS). Such antibodies are now measured by *in vitro* thyroid cell or TSH receptor–transfected cell techniques that rely on antibody-induced stimulation of cAMP, thyroglobulin, iodine uptake, or even thyroid hormone release (56–58). These autoantibodies are known to be directed toward an epitope on the TSH receptor and are generically referred to as TSH receptor antibodies (TSHR-Abs). Of untreated patients, about 90% demonstrate easily measurable TSHR-Ab levels, and administration of Graves immunoglobulins intravenously induced thyroid stimulation in human volunteers (50). Thus, TSHR-Abs are the primary causative agent of Graves disease hyperthyroidism, and their presence is diagnostic of the disease when they are biologically acting as TSH agonists (Fig. 22-6). IgG preparations from patients with TSHR-Ab inhibit the binding of radiolabeled TSH to thyroid cells or isolated TSH receptors (59–62). This forms the basis of a widely available radioreceptor assay for TSHR-Ab, which is much cheaper to perform as a clinical investigation than thyroid cell bioassays.

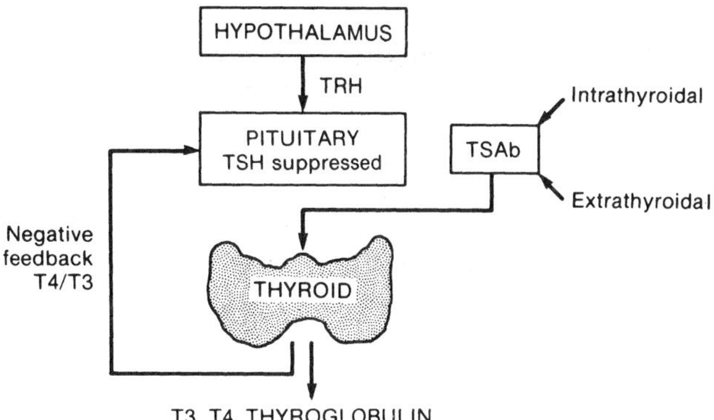

FIG. 22-6. Action of thyroid-stimulating antibodies (TSAbs). Compare with Fig. 22-3.

It is now clear, however, that not all TSH receptor antibodies measured by TSH radioreceptor competition assay are necessarily able to stimulate the TSH receptor sites. Some are able to block TSH action at the receptor, acting therefore as TSH antagonists or partial agonists (63,64). However, in hyperthyroid patients, the receptor assay is the measurement of choice because the patient acts as the real bioassay. However, if the patient is not hyperthyroid, some assessment of TSH-like bioactivity may be helpful, particularly in pregnancy.

Thyroglobulin Antibodies

The pathogenic role of autoantibodies to human thyroglobulin (hTg-Ab) has been inferred by their correlation with lymphocytic infiltration and their high titer in autoimmune thyroiditis (Hashimoto disease) (65,66). Antibody to hTg would clearly have access to antigen on the surface of the thyroid cell and has the potential to initiate thyroiditis, as demonstrated in animal models (67). The mechanism of such damage may include complement fixation and antibody-dependent cytotoxicity (ADCC). hTg-Abs are best measured by radioassay or enzyme-linked immunosorbent assay (ELISA) systems (68), which have replaced the less sensitive hemagglutination tests. Of the general population, up to 20% may have hTg-Ab by sensitive assay, but titers are much higher and more common in patients with either Graves or Hashimoto disease (30%–80%, respectively). The polyclonality of hTg-Ab strongly suggests that hTg-Abs are a secondary phenomenon in these diseases.

Thyroid Peroxidase Antibodies

Many patients with autoimmune thyroid disease demonstrate high titers of antibody to a sonicated 80,000-g fraction of thyroid homogenate, especially patients with Hashimoto thyroiditis. The antigen in question, formerly called microsomal antigen, is now known to be the enzyme thyroid peroxidase (TPO) (69). Such antibodies to TPO are readily measured using sensitive radioassay and ELISA techniques (68,70). Of people with TPO-Ab, 70% to 80% have evidence of thyroid disease (71), and such antibodies show a better correlation with thyroiditis and elevated TSH in the general population than hTg-Ab (66). Up to 20% of the normal population also have TPO-Abs, and that prevalence increases with age (72). More than 90% of patients with Hashimoto and 50% with Graves disease have easily detectable TPO-Ab, the titers often being extremely high in Hashimoto thyroiditis.

Antibodies to the Iodine Transporter

The transporter for iodine has recently been characterized and has been suggested as another important thyroid cell autoantigen (73). Although autoantibodies to this structure have been demonstrated in patients with autoimmune thyroid disease, their importance in disease etiology is uncertain. Nevertheless, the fact that such antibodies may inhibit iodine transport suggests that they may well have a pathologic role.

T-Cell Meditated Immunity in Thyroid Disease

The role of cell-meditated, rather than humoral, immunity in the etiology of thyroid disease has become much clearer in recent years (74). The demonstration of intrathyroidal T-cell clonal expansion and a bias in the use of particular T-cell receptor V genes has indicated the primary nature of T cells in disease etiology (75). The helper ($CD4^+$) and cytotoxic ($CD8^+$) T cells have been more precisely defined and thyroid antigen-specific T-cells have been identified in both Graves and Hashimoto's diseases. Of particular help has been the concept of $CD4^+$ T cells being divided into Th1 cells (cytotoxic and secreting IL-2 and γIF) and Th2 cells (antibody-enhancing by IL-4 secretion) (76). Shifts in such T-cell populations could move a disease from antibody secreting to cell destruction, not unlike the progression from Graves to Hashimoto disease seen in a significant proportion of patients. However, the evidence to date suggests that both types of T cells are plentiful in both these diseases. Although mild nonspecific suppressor T-cell abnormalities have been described, the role of a thyroid-specific suppressor T-cell defect as the primary cause of such diseases is not widely accepted (77). The concepts of T-cell deletion (apoptosis) and anergy (desensitization), in which cells are destroyed or inhibited by direct contact with antigen, are more important modulators of immune function but are outside the scope of this review.

THYROID DYSFUNCTION IN PREGNANCY

Prevalence of Thyroid Dysfunction

Autoimmune thyroid disease is found in about 1% to 2% of the general population but has a marked preference for women in the reproductive age range, in which 5% to 15% may be affected (72). There have been relatively few direct studies on the prevalence of thyroid disease in pregnancy. It appears that significant thyroid disease complicates about 0.8% of all pregnancies, approximately 0.2% hyperthyroid and 0.6% hyperthyroid, much less than expected from an age-matched population, probably a reflection of the problem of decreased fertility in thyroid dysfunction (Table 22-5). Pregnant patients make up about 1% of patients with thyroid disease. In addition, about 10% of women have detectable thyroid dysfunction in the postpartum period (PPTD), much of which appears to be transient in nature.

Fertility and Thyroid Disease

Prevalence studies indicate a marked reduction in fertility associated with thyroid dysfunction. On a clinical basis, this is reflected in menstrual irregularity and anovulation in both hyper- and hypothyroidism (78–80) and a marked rebound in fertility during the early stages of treatment of the disorder. It is imperative, therefore, that patients be warned of the increased risk of pregnancy at the initiation of treatment. Up to 70% of hypothyroid females have ovulatory failure, inadequate corpus luteum formation, and menorrhagia. Hyperthyroid women have oligomenorrhea or scant menstrual flow in up to 90% of cases, and half such patients fail to ovulate. The physiologic mechanisms for these disturbances in normal ovarian function lie at a number of levels.

1. The hyperthyroid pituitary demonstrates exaggerated responses to gonadotropin-releasing hormone (GnRH), which interrupt the finely tuned control of gonadotropin pulsatility necessary for ovulation. (Fig. 22-7) (81,82).

TABLE 22-5. *Prevalence of thyroid dysfunction in pregnancy and the postpartum period*

Status	Prevalence (%)		
	Nonpregnant	Pregnant	Postpartum
Hyperthyroid	1.9	0.2	—
Hypothyroid	1.4	0.6	—
PPYD	—	—	7.0–10.0

PPTD, postpartum thyroid dysfunction.

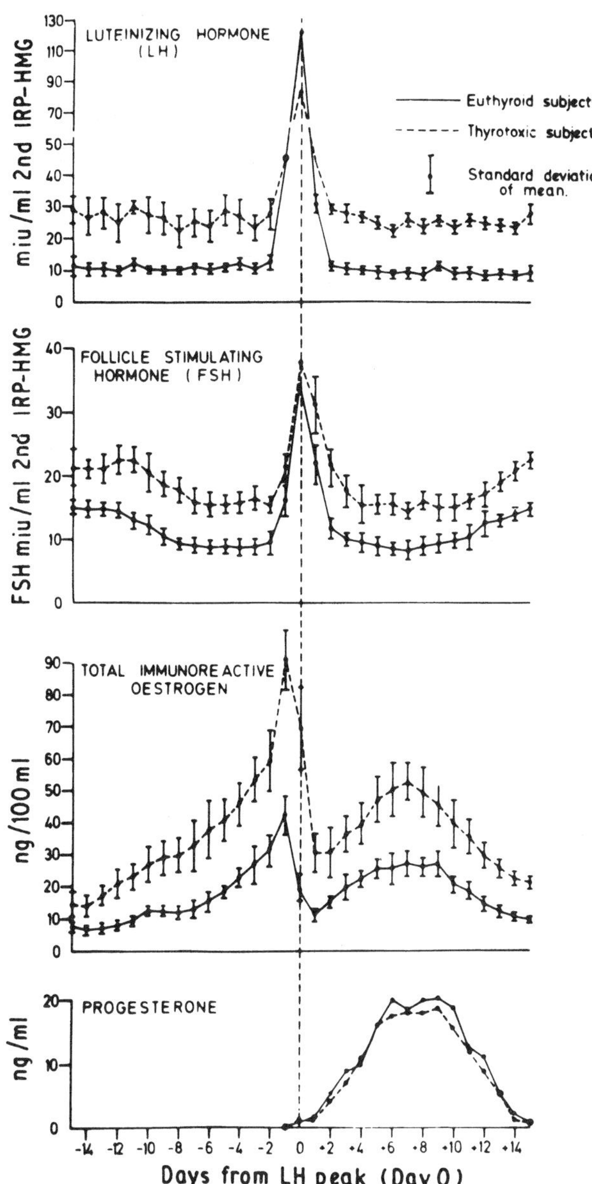

FIG. 22-7. Gonadotropin levels in hyperthyroid women through the menstrual cycle. The graphs were constructed around the day of the luteinizing hormone peak (day 0). (From Akande EO, Hockaday TDR. Plasma concentration of gonadotropins, estrogens and progesterone in thyrotoxic women. Br J Obstet Gynaecol 1975:82:541–551.)

2. Levels of sex hormone–binding globulin (SHBG) are elevated in hyperthyroidism, and estrogen, both bound and free, is also increased. This results from both an increased production rate, via excessive conversion of testosterone to estradiol and androstenedione to estrone, together with decreased clearance, perhaps related to increased SHBG levels (83–85). The opposite occurs in thyroid failure, although SHBG levels may remain unchanged.
3. The ovary is also known to accumulate iodine and to be dependent on thyroid hormone for normal function (86–87). However, ovarian iodine transporters have not been demonstrated (88).

The impact of thyroid hormone deficiency or excess on the reproductive process is therefore complex, and many areas of normal physiology may be interrupted. We have no reliable data on the influence of thyroid hormone status on female sexuality, although it is well known to affect male potency and fertility (89).

Who Should Treat Thyroid Disease in Pregnancy?

Physicians who are expert in dealing with pregnancy and physicians who have extensive experience in treating thyroid disease should work together to manage the complex and unique problems of pregnancy complicated by thyroid dysfunction. It is common sense, supported by mortality and morbidity changes, that thyroid disease in pregnancy requires dual care by both obstetricians and endocrinologists, working as a team with the common goal of caring for both mother and fetus in the short and long term. This approach allows a few interested individuals to share their expertise for the general good of the community. Furthermore, an experienced pediatrician should also be on hand for those unusual situations in which the newborn is at risk.

HYPERTHYROID GRAVES DISEASE IN PREGNANCY

The syndrome of Graves disease has three facets: thyroid dysfunction, ophthalmic involvement, and the dermatologic manifestation usually referred to as pretibial myxedema. As discussed earlier, some signs and symptoms of normal pregnancy may mimic hyperthyroidism. Systemic symptoms such as fatigue, heat intolerance, emotional lability, and hyperhidrosis are often part of normal pregnancy, as are tachycardia and hyperdynamic systolic murmurs. Warm, moist skin and palmar erythema may be observed. These nonspecific findings, therefore, cannot be a guide to the diagnosis of hyperthyroidism. Failure to gain weight adequately may be one of the more helpful clinical signs. Although the size of the thyroid in pregnancy may increase (see section on Thyroid Function Testing), a visible goiter is most likely to be an indication of thyroid dysfunction. The presence of classical signs of Graves disease, such as ophthalmic and skin changes, although uncommon, make the diagnosis straightforward (Table 22-6), and a family history should always alert the clinician. However, in all patients, bio-

TABLE 22-6. *Diagnostic signs in Graves disease*

System	Sign
Thyroid	Visible, soft, diffusely enlarged gland
Eyes	Periorbital edema
	Conjunctival injection
	Exophthalmos
	Muscle dysfunction
Skin	Pretibial myxedema

chemical parameters with reference to the normal pregnant ranges have to be evaluated carefully before a therapeutic decision can be made.

Morbidity and Mortality

Because many patients with severe thyrotoxicosis are amenorrheic or anovulatory, fertility is impaired, and often hyperthyroidism is observed in the setting of a partially treated woman who has been on antithyroid drugs and has subsequently become pregnant. Careful management with consideration of physiologic principles is essential for avoiding maternal and fetal morbidity and mortality. Maternal complications of untreated hyperthyroidism now occur rarely, but may still be life threatening in the severe case with accelerating hyperthyroidism. Even recent reports emphasize that untreated hyperthyroidism, particularly of relatively long duration in pregnancy, may result in an increased risk of preeclampsia and heart failure (90). It has been estimated that in untreated hyperthyroidism, early fetal loss of 5% is similar to the general population, but late fetal loss may be as much as four times greater (6.6% versus 1.6%) if the mother is untreated (10,18,91). Stillbirths and prematurity are both significantly increased. Nonimmune fetal hydrops may occur (92,93). In a 1994 study, there was an increase in the incidence of low-birth-weight babies and the risk of severe preeclampsia was increased fivefold (94). In most series, however, congenital anomalies were not found to be increased.

TREATMENT OF HYPERTHYROIDISM

The General Approach

An antithyroid drug regimen is the appropriate treatment for most women with hyperthyroidism in pregnancy. Radioactive iodine is contraindicated. In the past, surgery during the mid-trimester of pregnancy after preparation with antithyroid drugs was considered the most advisable therapy. Subsequently, however, many series have been published with favorable results from the use of antithyroid drugs alone, thus avoiding the risks of anesthesia and surgery (95). This is our standard therapy for hyperthyroidism in pregnancy. Surgical intervention is reserved for those patients with significant drug intolerance or extremely poor compliance and has proven safe and effective in the mid-trimester.

Our aim in the therapy of pregnant hyperthyroid patients is to reduce the circulating free T_4 concentration into the high normal or just elevated range. Earlier poor results from medically treated patients were a direct consequence of difficulty in measuring the free hormone indices or failure to perform frequent thyroid function monitoring. A TSH and a free hormone assessment (e.g., T_4:TBG, free thyroxine index) must be measured frequently to prevent decreasing levels and avoid excessive fetal thyroid blockade by antithyroid drugs. Often the drug dosage requires relatively rapid tapering because we prefer to act when the T_4 is decreasing rather than waiting until below normal levels are achieved and TSH is increasing. Once the TSH is elevated, the fetus must have been exposed to excessive antithyroid drug. We believe that maternal levels are a reliable indication of clinical fetal thyroid status and have found no fetal hypothyroidism with meticulous maternal control. Amniotic fluid measurements of thyroid hormones are unreliable and unnecessary.

Antithyroid Drugs

When the diagnosis of hyperthyroidism has been established by appropriate thyroid function tests, including TSHR-Ab titers, antithyroid drugs can be introduced. Propylthiouracil (PTU) and methimazole are thionamide drugs that act by blocking thyroid hormone synthesis at the start of organification and iodotyrosine coupling (see Fig. 22-2). Inhibition of peripheral deiodination by PTU has been much discussed but appears to be unimportant at normal therapeutic doses. Because of the strange occurrence of fetal aplasia cutis reported with methimazole (96), PTU has become the standard antithyroid drug for use during pregnancy in the United States, but methimazole has remained the first drug used in many parts of the world without any apparent ill effects. There is no compelling evidence that this disorder is a consequence of the therapy itself (97). In one of the few studies directly comparing the use of methimazole to PTU during pregnancy, there was no aplasia cutis with either drug and no difference in the efficacy of the two drugs or their side effects (98). The suggestion that PTU accumulates less than methimazole in breast milk and crosses the placenta with less ease has also been disproven. What is important is that maternal thyroid function must be carefully monitored throughout pregnancy.

Therapy should begin with as low a dose as possible (e.g. 50 mg PTU three times daily), a dose lower than normally prescribed in nonpregnant patients. Because the drug interrupts organification, its action is not reflected in circulating hormone reduction for 7 to 10 days, depending on the level of preformed hormone left in storage within the gland. In many patients a therapeutic effect may not be seen for 3 or 4 weeks. As the free T_4 index decreases, the dose is reduced as rapidly as possible. Generally the amount of drug necessary to control hyperthyroidism decreases as TSHR-Ab levels decrease during pregnancy. A dose of as little as 25 to 50 mg may provide adequate control by late pregnancy. Each patient must be treated individually, however, with the goal of therapy being adequate control of maternal hyperthyroidism without excess drug crossing the placenta.

The commonly used block and replace regimen is not appropriate in pregnancy. Because of the unpredictable transplacental passage of thyroid hormone, supplementation with either T_4 or T_3 provides a false sense of security, making the mother euthyroid while continuing fetal exposure to higher doses of antithyroid drugs than would be necessary without thyroid hormone supplementation.

Adjunctive therapy with stable iodine is not justified in pregnancy because it crosses the placenta easily and may be responsible for large goiters leading to dystocia, fetal hypothyroidism, and fetal death (30). Propranolol and other β-adrenergic blocking drugs are used to control the sympathomimetic symptoms of hyperthyroidism in nonpregnant patients but have been associated with placental insufficiency, intrauterine growth retardation, excessive uterine irritability, and fetal bradycardia (99). However, reports of fetal hypoglycemia, hyperbilirubinemia, and polycythemia have not been substantiated. There has been controversy regarding the use of propranolol in hypertensive pregnant patients, and its occasional uneventful use in hyperthyroid pregnancies has been reported (100). At present we do not recommend propranolol during pregnancy, except preoperatively, when antithyroid drugs are contraindicated, and in the rare cases of severe hyperthyroidism precipitated by the onset of delivery in an untreated or inadequately treated patient.

Fetal Impact of Antithyroid Drugs

Logic emphasizes the need for the smallest dose of antithyroid drug possible. Even with low doses of PTU (100–200 mg daily), the mean cord serum T_4 may be lower than in controls (101–103). An exaggerated newborn TSH response on day 1 may be a reflection of such mild hypothyroidism (104). Thus, assurance of maternal euthyroidism does not guarantee freedom from neonatal hypothyroidism. We therefore taper antithyroid drugs rapidly and find that in most patients minimal doses in the range of 50 to 100 mg or less of PTU are all that is necessary to achieve euthyroidism in the third trimester. Attempts at providing the fetus with thyroid hormone by the use of intraamniotic or placental delivery and placental-passing analogues also have been reported. The clinical relevance of excessive transient neonatal TSH evaluations, described above, is uncertain. Although subsequent growth and development of such children is thought to be normal (105,106), two additional issues warrant consideration. The first is that maternal thyroid autoantibodies have themselves been related to impaired child development (107); and second, neonatal hypothyroxinemia in preterm infants has been related to neurologic and mental retardation (108). Using a regimen of antithyroid drug therapy similar to ours, studies have indicated no fetal goiters and no obvious hypothyroidism (102), but other investigations have suggested continuing hypothyroidism in some newborn infants, and careful monitoring is mandatory.

Subtotal Thyroidectomy in a Pregnant Patient

In the case of a pregnant hyperthyroid patient who sustains major drug toxicity (marked leukopenia, significant liver disease), surgery may be the only means of successfully effecting euthyroidism. Subtotal thyroidectomy in the nonpregnant patient cures most such patients, with hypothyroidism occurring in about 15% to 50% and recurrent disease in approximately 5%, depending on the experience of the surgical teams involved. Recurrent laryngeal nerve injury and permanent hypoparathyroidism are unusual, with a subtotal procedure but remain a significant risk outside major centers (109). Anesthetic complications in pregnancy are apparently no greater than in the general population, and fetal losses are not increased in euthyroid patients. However, untreated pregnant thyrotoxic patients in their second trimester have been reported to have increased rates of abortion, intrauterine death, and stillbirth rates affecting 10% to 25% of cases (110). The use of propranolol before, during, and after such surgical intervention has helped greatly in the management of these patients, and the brief exposure time to which the fetus is subjected to the drug is perfectly justifiable (111). With proper preparation and surgical intervention in the second trimester, complication rates are comparable with those in nonpregnant patients (112).

Management of Labor with Graves Disease

Most pregnant hyperthyroid women will have been reasonably well controlled with antithyroid drugs by the time labor ensues. Such euthyroid patients seem to sustain no increased risk of complications of labor or of exacerbated hyperthyroidism. In the case of a patient who has previously escaped medical therapy and arrives at the hospital in labor or close to term with untreated hyperthyroidism, more drastic measures are necessary to avoid the risk of severe accelerated hyperthyroidism precipitated by the stress of labor and delivery. The poorly prepared patient should be started on blocking doses of antithyroid drugs at the start of labor and begin sodium iodide therapy to block the release of preformed thyroid hormone from the thyroid gland. Then, beta blockers such as propranolol may be used cautiously in the event of tachycardia and circulatory distress. Oral or parenteral corticosteroids (e.g., dexamethasone 2 mg four times daily for 24 hours) should be added because there is evidence that they rapidly decrease circulating T_3 levels (113) and may reduce the morbidity of what is often termed thyroid storm. Steroids may affect thyroid hormones by decreasing thyroid cell prostaglandin action at the level of the thyroid and reducing hormone release. In addition, they may inhibit peripheral deiodination of T_4 to T_3. This combination drug regimen reduces maternal morbidity without undue danger to the fetus. However, complications in the presence of such an accelerating degree of hyperthyroidism remain significant. Thankfully, such acceleration is unusual in the pregnant thyrotoxic patient, so gestation-specific mortality and morbidity figures are not available.

THE NEONATAL PERIOD AND PREDICTION OF NEONATAL GRAVES DISEASE

Munro and Major (114,115) first suggested in 1960 that neonatal hyperthyroidism may be caused by transplacental passage of TSHR-Abs. We now know that neonatal thyrotoxicosis, occurring as a result of transplacental passage of TSHR-Abs is rare, occurring in less than 1% of mothers with Graves disease (25,26). It also may be seen in babies whose mothers are euthyroid on T_4 during pregnancy after previous thyroid destruction for Graves disease but who have persistently high TSHR-Ab levels. Knowing the bioactivity of circulating TSHR-Abs in pregnancy is therefore most helpful.

Because of the placental passage of antithyroid drugs, neonates who have been exposed to high titers of TSHR-Abs may not demonstrate symptoms of neonatal thyrotoxicosis until they have been discharged from the nursery. This is because the half-life of antithyroid drug action is approximately 10 days, whereas that for the action of TSHR-Abs may be more than 3 weeks. Maternal TSH receptor–blocking antibodies with a shorter effective half-life than stimulating antibodies also have been suggested to be a cause of delayed neonatal hyperthyroidism in mothers who have coincidental stimulating TSHR-Abs (116). Much depends on the maternal antithyroid drug regimen in the last week of pregnancy. Babies of mothers with high titers of TSHR-Abs and no antithyroid drugs may have obvious neonatal hyperthyroidism soon after birth.

Neonatal Graves disease persists for as long as the TSHR-Ab is present at a sufficient concentration in the circulation. The disease is therefore transient and must be distinguished from the rare familial hyperthyroidism caused by activating mutations of the TSH receptor (117) and early onset of true Graves disease in the infant or young child. This latter situation is unusual in early childhood and can best be recognized by persistent or newly developed TSHR-Ab levels.

The pediatrician caring for an infant at risk should be alert for tachycardia, fever, congestive heart failure, failure to gain weight, and failure to thrive in the first weeks of life, rather than awaiting the customary 1-month well baby examination. The use of TSHR-Ab assays in the prediction of neonatal hyperthyroidism has received considerable attention and has found its place in routine clinical care in most centers. The transplacental passage of TSHR-Abs is responsible for the development of the neonatal thyrotoxicosis, but studies have indicated that only those patients with markedly elevated titers during pregnancy deliver babies who are at risk for the development of neonatal thyrotoxicosis (118). It is logical, therefore, to screen all women at risk antenatally, reserving neonatal screening for those newborns at risk whose mothers have not been tested. Hence, quantitative and qualitative assays of TSHR-Abs should be available to all pregnant patients with a history of autoimmune thyroid disease as a means of predicting which infants will be at greater risk. A mother may have undergone a subtotal thyroidectomy or radioiodine ablation for Graves disease and may be maintained on thyroxine replacement. Such patients may have persistent TSHR-Abs in high titer, and treatment with antithyroid drugs may be initiated to treat the fetus itself. Careful monitoring of the fetus for hyperthyroidism under such conditions (e.g., by the presence of a constant tachycardia) is difficult, and sampling of fetal blood for thyroid function may be necessary, as may careful fetal sonography for goiter development.

OPHTHALMIC GRAVES DISEASE

The retroorbital accumulation of inflammatory cells and the induction of connective tissue and muscle swelling, followed by fibrosis of orbital muscles, is evidence of autoimmune involvement in Graves orbitopathy (119). However, the disease course does not parallel the thyroid dysfunction. It may even be seen without any detectable thyroid involvement, so-called euthyroid ophthalmic Graves disease. Treatment of the hyperthyroidism does not usually influence the ophthalmic abnormality, apart from reducing thyrotoxic stare, unless hypothyroidism ensues, which worsens the retroorbital swelling. The disease was thought to be a separate but closely linked inherited abnormality, with the genes for Graves thyroid and ophthalmic disease occurring close together. However, recent suggestions that the TSH receptor may be a common antigen to both clinical phenotypes, because the receptor is found expressed in both retroorbitol fibroblasts and adipose cells, may indicate that they are manifestations of the same disease. Eye disease is clinically apparent in about 15% of cases of Graves disease, but exacerbations during pregnancy are very uncommon. Indeed, such disease is usually clinically quiescent during pregnancy.

AUTOIMMUNE THYROIDITIS AND HYPOTHYROIDISM IN PREGNANCY

Presentation and Diagnosis

Because significant thyroid insufficiency may be associated with ovulatory failure, pregnant patients are usually known to have established thyroid disease and may have discontinued their medications. In addition, previous thyroid surgery and radioactive iodine treatment must be excluded. The clinical presentation in such cases remains typical of the nonpregnant woman, with marked lack of energy, excessive weight gain, general malaise, cold intolerance, dry skin, constipation, myalgia, and early fatigue. Hence, there is often a marked contrast to the usual metabolically hyperkinetic state of a normal pregnancy. Typically, however, the pregnancy is progressing normally despite the maternal thyroid failure.

Diagnosis is confirmed by the measurement of serum TSH and T_4 and a binding assessment (TBG or T_3 resin uptake). Autoimmune thyroiditis is suggested by significant thyroglobulin and TPO antibody titers and perhaps by a family history of autoimmune endocrine disease. Any significant increase in TSH levels during pregnancy indicates thyroid insufficiency and requires therapy.

Morbidity and Mortality

In untreated patients the rate of first trimester fetal loss may approach 50%, with a 20% rate of stillbirths and neonatal deaths (120,121). Study results suggest that good obstetric practice is as important as treating the hypothyroid mother with replacement therapy (122,123), but also indicate that the developing fetal brain may be affected by maternal hypothyroidism. Every effort therefore should be made to keep mothers adequately replaced. When the fetal thyroid is normal and there is no iodine deficiency, maternal hypothyroidism may not adversely affect subsequent mental development of the offspring (124). With only mild elevations of TSH, the fetus is at less risk from mild maternal thyroid failure and TSH does not cross the placenta.

TREATMENT OF HYPOTHYROIDISM

The New Patient

Appropriate therapy is replacement with T_4 itself, adequate to bring the maternal calculated free T_4 index into the normal pregnant range with concomitant reduction in TSH. T_3 is provided via peripheral deiodination of administered T_4. There is no evidence to suggest that additional T_3 therapy is necessary in most patients. Persistent elevations in TSH, indicating inadequate replacement, probably have no effect on the fetus because TSH does not cross the placenta, but such elevations should nevertheless not be accepted. During a normal pregnancy, the metabolic clearance rate of T_4 does not change, so in theory, the dose of T_4 required to achieve euthyroidism should not differ from the normal nonpregnant woman and, most importantly, from the same patient before pregnancy. Using a highly sensitive assay for TSH, however, studies have found an increase in the replacement dose of thyroxine necessary during many pregnancies. This may represent slight underreplacement prior to pregnancy or a true increase in need because of the increased clearance of T_4 or secondary to TBG increases and changes in the distribution space for free T_4 (104,125).

The use of thyroid extract for thyroid hormone replacement is no longer acceptable, and such preparations have already been withdrawn from some European markets. Their problem is one of unpredictability, particularly in the high serum T_3 levels that patients may develop.

Treated Hypothyroidism

Because the clearance rate for T_4 remains unchanged during pregnancy, many patients who are already on long-term replacement therapy will not need their dosage adjusted. Nevertheless, it is essential to monitor T_4 and TSH during the pregnancy. Some patients require increased T_4 doses; but apparently inadequate doses may be secondary to the patient not adhering to the prescribed regimen for a variety of reasons, including the fear of harming the baby by taking a drug. Careful explanation to all patients of the safety and benefits of T_4 will help to avoid such problems.

The Maternal Impact of Thyroid Autoantibodies

Patients with euthyroid autoimmune thyroid disease manifested by high levels of thyroid autoantibodies—particularly anti-TPO—are at increased risk for the development of subclinical hypothyroidism during pregnancy (103) and increased risk of first trimester fetal loss (126,127). Up to 30% develop postpartum thyroiditis (128). Abnormal thyroid echogenicity, possibly as a result of autoimmune thyroiditis, has been associated with pregnancy-induced hypertension (129). It is our policy, therefore, to screen all newly pregnant women for the presence of thyroid autoantibodies in addition to TSH. An increased TSH must be corrected and then monitored in each trimester. The fetal loss associated with anti-TPO is considered to be a reflection of an abnormal immune response to pregnancy, not abnormal thyroid function.

Fetal Impact of Maternal Thyroid Antibodies

There appears to be no fetal thyroid impact by placental passage of maternal thyroglobulin and TPO autoantibodies (130). Presumably an abnormal immune system, including appropriate T cells, is necessary for thyroidal destruction. Alternatively, the fetal thyroid may be particularly resistant to destruction. It is important to remember that titers of such antibodies in the maternal serum are depressed by the end of pregnancy, and passage of suppressive cells to the fetus also may be protective (131). One recent report has suggested that later childhood development may be impaired in children with mothers who have anti-TPO (107,132). This notion requires further confirmation, but may reflect the existence of subtle fetal hypothyroidism that has been missed. One antibody in women with autoimmune thyroiditis that is reportedly associated with neonatal hypothyroidism, the TSH receptor blocking antibody, is discussed under the section on TSH Receptor Antibodies. Familial neonatal hypothyroidism is associated with maternal and fetal TSHR-Abs, which do not stimulate but block TSH action (63,64,133). Such antibodies may be one cause of neonatal hypothyroidism, and the results of one large study indicated that this occurs in 1 in 180,000 births and makes up 2% of congenital hypothyroidism (134). Although one mother with receptor-blocking antibodies was reported to have had three children, each with a different congenital abnormality (135), most series indicate that if the transient neonatal hypothyroidism is corrected appropriately, such children are neurodevelopmentally normal and remain euthyroid later in childhood (136). Hence, mothers with autoimmune thyroid disease may have variable titers of TSH receptor stimulators and blockers that may be independent of their current thyroid status. Bioassay of the circulatory TSHR-Abs allows the prediction of their effects on the fetus.

THE POSTPARTUM THYROID SYNDROMES

Nature and Prevalence of the Diseases

The onset of autoimmune thyroid disease in the postpartum period has been known since the earliest description of the disease (1). Pregnancy induces dramatic suppression of both humoral and cell-medicated immunity. In the postpartum state, reversal of this phenomenon may induce rebound activation of autoimmune disease, with marked increases in thyroid antibody titers and reversal of helper/suppressor T-cell ratios (Fig. 22-8) (137). Robertson (138) in 1948 recognized the increased frequency of postpartum thyroid failure in patients with goiter, and it was Amino and Miya who reawakened interest in the autoimmune nature of the postpartum syndromes (139). During the 1990's, postpartum thyroiditis has been recognized with increasing frequency, with an incidence of 5.5% in Japan (140) and up to 10% in the United States and Europe (44,107,137,141). The varied presentation and course of the disorders indicates that multiple factors influence the thyroid dysfunction, but the greatest risk factor appears to be the mother's susceptibility to autoimmune thyroid disease (Fig. 22-9). Patients with anti-TPO in their first trimester have an increased risk of developing postpartum thyroid disease (25% compared with 8%), as do women with type I IDDM (25%), particularly if they have anti-TPO (50%) (142–144). About 75% of women with postpartum hyperthyroid disease will have transient destruction-induced disease, whereas the remainder will have postpartum Graves disease or its recurrence. This distinction is important because the transient variety may resolve quickly.

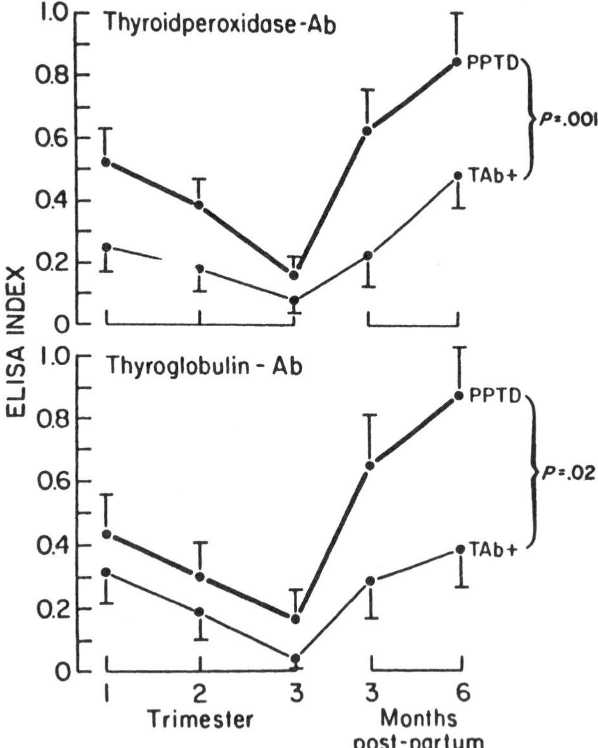

FIG. 22-8. Thyroid autoantibody titers for patients with postpartum thyroid disease (PPTD+) and thyroid autoantibodies without disease (TAb+), expressed as the mean and SEM at different time points. (From Stagnaro-Green A, Roman SH, Cobin RH, el-Harazy E, Wallenstein S, Davies TF, et al. A prospective study of lymphocyte-initiated immunosuppression in normal pregnancy: evidence of a T-cell etiology for postpartum thyroid dysfunction. J Clin Endocrinol Metab 1992;74:645–653.)

Transient Postpartum Thyroiditis

Patients who develop thyroiditis in the postpartum period may present in either a hyper- or hypothyroid phase, the former usually preceding the latter (139). A painless thyroid enlargement may be seen, and occasionally tenderness may occur. Patients may have a history of previous autoimmune thyroid disease, but typically this is not the case and thyroiditis is not expected unless anti-TPO has been measured.

Patients seen in the hyperthyroid phase of thyroiditis have destruction-induced hyperthyroidism similar to that seen in subacute thyroiditis and occasionally seen at the

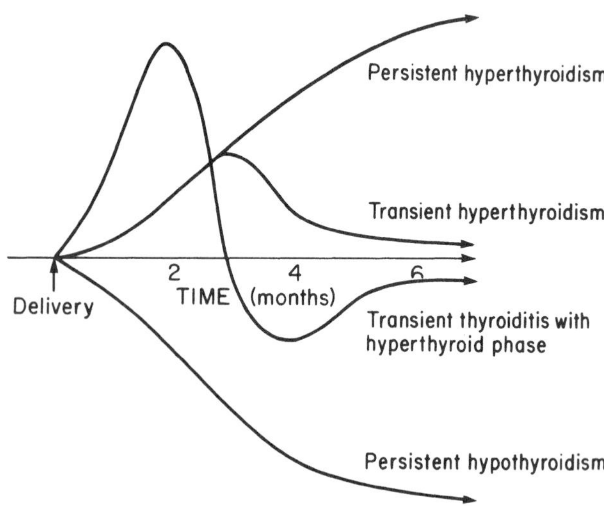

FIG. 22-9. Representation of the natural history of postpartum thyroid syndromes. (Adapted from Amino N, Miyai K. In: Davies TF, ed. Autoimmune endocrine disease. New York: Wiley, 1983.)

onset of a more classical Hashimoto thyroiditis (145). Radioiodine uptake is low, sedimentation rate may be normal or only mildly elevated, and the T_3:T_4 ratio may be low due to excessive T_4 release. The disease is generally brief in duration, occurring 3 to 6 months postpartum, and is often followed by a transient hypothyroid phase as described below. Titers of thyroid antibodies, particularly anti-TPO, are characteristically high (33). Antithyroid drugs are best avoided because they are not likely to be helpful in a thyroid undergoing inflammatory destruction, they may cloud the onset of thyroid failure, and they may introduce complications for mothers who are breastfeeding.

Patients who present initially with transient hypothyroidism may have had a preexistent hyperthyroid phase with glandular destruction that was not diagnosed. Recovery to the euthyroid state may take 3 to 5 months. Diagnosis is made on the basis of thyroid function tests, particularly an elevated TSH level and high antibody titers. If the results of a thyroid biopsy were available, they would show a marked lymphocytic component with widespread thyroid follicle destruction. Treatment with thyroxine may be required to alleviate symptoms of fatigue and weight gain and may need to be continued for 6 months. Attempts should then be made to withdraw therapy and to determine if the disease is permanent or transient. Generally, by 1 year postpartum, the gland has recovered, but some patients remain permanently hypothyroid. Fifty percent of patients with postpartum thyroiditis will have a recurrence in subsequent pregnancies, and 17% to 25% will develop permanent hypothyroidism within 5 years (146). Some studies have reported an increase in postpartum depression in women with anti-TPO independent of thyroid function (132). No clear mechanism exists to explain this relationship other than anti-TPO being an innocent marker for a genetic predisposition to depression.

Transient Postpartum Graves Disease

Some patients present with thyroid enlargement and hyperthyroid function tests but with increased rather than decreased radioiodine uptake excluding the presence of destructive thyroiditis. This syndrome may have a slightly later onset than classical thyroiditis and may persist for 4 to 6 months. Our interpretation of this disorder has been that it represents a transient form of Graves disease (147), and the failure to demonstrate TSHR-Ab in some such cases could be explained by assay insensitivity.

Permanent Postpartum Thyroid Disease

Both Graves and Hashimoto diseases are known to present for the first time in the postpartum period. This was often assumed to be just coincidence, but our understanding of the immune changes in the postpartum period indicates that such patients decompensate for understandable reasons. Often they have had a previous history, especially Graves disease patients, and recurrence is diagnosed in the postpartum period (148,149). Treatment of these conditions is the same as for the nonpregnant patient with particular attention to issues surrounding breastfeeding.

Why Do Patients Recover So Often from Postpartum Thyroid Disease?

The ability of a patient with marked thyroiditis and high thyroid antibody titers in the postpartum period to ultimately regain control of her immune system and suppress destructive T cells, apoptosis, and autoantibody secretion is one of the great enigmas of thyroid immunology. Such individuals obviously have the inherited clones of thyroid-specific T cells and thyroid antibody-secreting cells that, during a particular interlude, are allowed to expand and cause thyroid cell destruction or stimulation. The factors that allow such expansion and their ultimate suppression most likely lie in pregnancy- and postpregnancy–induced swings in T-cell subsets and in the release and induction of T-cell and B-cell desensitization (the concept of anergy) (150). It is the families of specific helper T cells that ultimately control T- and B-cell differentiation. Understanding this sequence of events may allow us to help patients with chronic thyroid disease unrelated to pregnancy also regain control of their immune repertoire.

BREASTFEEDING AND THYROID DISEASE

Most women with thyroid dysfunction come successfully to term and deliver normal infants. Many are concerned about the risks and benefits of nursing in this special situation. T_4 is present in breast milk and may be beneficial to the congenitally hypothyroid baby (151). No evidence has linked postpartum hyperthyroidism with excessive T_4 passage via breastfeeding; indeed the mother's metabolic status appears to be irrelevant to the infant.

Antithyroid Drugs

Antithyroid drugs enter breast milk, and many physicians persuade mothers not to breastfeed under such circumstances. Early studies suggested that the concentration of antithyroid drugs in breast milk may be significant enough to influence the child's thyroid function. More recent investigators with improved analytic techniques have shown that drug levels are much lower than originally thought (152,153). For example, maternal ingestion of methimazole in doses of 5 to 20 mg daily did not cause abnormal thyroid function in 35 infants nursing from 1 to 4 months (154). Hence, antithyroid drugs are not an absolute contraindication to breastfeeding, assuming the mother is taking a low dose and that infant thyroid hormone levels can be monitored if necessary.

Other Concerns

Little is known of the immediate consequences of lymphocyte and thyroid antibody transfer to the neonate via breast milk. Obviously the nursing mother must not be given radioiodine for either diagnostic purposes or treatment in the postpartum period because iodine is also secreted by the breast. Indeed, the iodine transporter has recently been identified in mammary tissue.

NON-AUTOIMMUNE THYROID DISEASES IN PREGNANCY

Multinodular Goiter

We know a great deal about the causes of multiple nodule formation in the thyroid gland. Activating mutations of the TSH receptor have been found in many hot nodules, both single and within multinodular goiters (117), and activating mutations of g proteins have also been reported (155). In cold nodules, defective iodine transporter molecules have been identified. Furthermore, the follicular heterogeneity of the normal thyroid has been well documented (156), indicating the potential for nodule development in all thyroid tissue, particularly in the presence of iodine deficiency and increased TSH secretion.

If a pregnant patient has previously been on thyroid hormone suppression therapy with the aim of suppressing further enlargement, this should be continued throughout the pregnancy without change. Desuppression may be associated with enlargement of a goiter or nodule in as many as 20% of cases (157). Withdrawal also may reveal permanent hypothyroidism due to an associated autoimmune thyroiditis and is not recommended during pregnancy. In the euthyroid patient, observation is all that is required.

Thyroid Nodules

About 5% of the population has one or more palpable nodules in the thyroid, and this rate increases with age. The development of a single thyroid nodule during pregnancy is unusual, but the great concern is the possibility of a rare thyroid carcinoma. Pregnancy does not, however, increase the frequency of thyroid cancer or exacerbate its growth or metastasis (158,159). Thyroid biopsy is the investigation of choice, along with routine thyroid function tests (160). Thyroid scanning is contraindicated, but this is a time when ultrasonography may be very helpful. A diagnosis of definite or suspicious malignancy should lead directly to surgical therapy. This may be safely performed in the second trimester (161). If the diagnosis is made later, then surgery can reasonably be delayed until after delivery. When the biopsy is benign and the nodule is enlarging, then an attempt at thyroid hormone suppression can be introduced without any risk to the fetus, or the nodule may just be observed until after delivery.

Subacute (DeQuervain's) Thyroiditis

Subacute thyroiditis is a viral-like inflammation of the thyroid gland, which may present with a painful or painless enlargement associated initially with release of thyroid hormone from damaged tissue, followed by thyroid failure when widespread cell death occurs (162). It may be associated with the transient appearance of thyroid antibodies in low titers in susceptible individuals (163). Most patients then have total recovery of normal thyroid function. The onset of painful subacute thyroiditis in pregnancy is rare. Should it become apparent, then thyroid hormone supplementation may be needed for the hypothyroid phase. Low-dose steroids are effective for extreme pain, but their potential influence on the fetus must be balanced against the benefits of use in pregnancy. The painless variety has to be distinguished from autoimmune thyroiditis (Hashimoto disease) by the absence of thyroid antibodies or their transient presence in low titer. Similarly, in the postpartum period, the two syndromes must be distinguished by thyroid antibody titers because both will exhibit low radioiodine uptakes.

ACKNOWLEDGMENTS

We thank Nathan Kase, M.D., for his continuing support and encouragement of our interest in thyroid disease in pregnancy. T.F.D. is supported in part by Grants DK 45011, DK 35764, and DK 52464 from the National Institute of Diabetes, Digestive and Kidney Diseases.

REFERENCES

1. Parry CH. Disease of the heart. In: Collections from the unpublished writings, 1st ed., Vol. 2. London: Underwoods, 1825:111–125.
2. Dai G, Levy O, Carrasco N. Cloning and characterization of the thyroid iodide transporter. Nature 1996;379:458–460.
3. Vassart G, Dumont JE. The thyrotropin receptor and the regulation of thyrocyte function and growth. Endocr Rev 1992;13:596–611.
4. Larsen PR. Update on the human iodothyronine selenodeiodinases, the enzymes regulating the activation and inactivation of thyroid hormone. Biochem Soc Trans 1997;25:588–592.
5. Kooperdonk-Kool J, De Vijldar J, Veenboer GJM. Type II and type III deiodinase activity in human placenta as a function of gestational age. J Clin Endocrinol Metab 1996;81:2154–2158.
6. Hodin RA, Lazar MA, Chin WW. Differential and tissue-specific regulation of multiple rat c-erbA messenger RNA species by thyroid hormone. J Clin Invest 1990;85:101–106.
7. Lazar MA. Recent progress in understanding thyroid hormone action. Thyroid Today 1997;20:1–9.
8. Dowling JT, Appleton WG, Nicoloff JT. Thyroxine turnover during human pregnancy. J Clin Endocrinol Metab 1967;27:1749–1750.
9. Fisher DA, Klein HH. Thyroid development and disorders of thyroid function in newborn. N Engl J Med 1981;304:702–702.

10. Burrow GN. Thyroid function and hyperfunction during gestation. Endocrinol Rev 1993;14:194–202.
11. Nisula BC, Ketelslegers J. Thyroid-stimulating activity and chorionic gonadotropin. J Clin Invest 1974;54:494–501.
12. Davies TF, Taliadouros GS, Catt KJ, Nisula BC. Assessment of urinary thyrotropin-competing activity in choriocarcinoma and thyroid disease: further evidence for human chorionic gonadotropin interacting at the thyroid cell membrane. J Clin Endocrinol Metab 1979;49:353–357.
13. Tomer Y, Huber GK, Davies TF. Human chorionic gonadotropin (hCG) interacts directly with recombinant human TSH receptors. J Clin Endocrinol Metab 1992;74:1477–1479.
14. Glinoer D, De Nayer P, Bourdoux P, et al. Regulation of maternal thyroid during pregnancy. J Clin Endocrinol Metab 1990;71:276–287.
15. Ballabio M, Poshyachinda M, Ekins RP. Pregnancy induced changes in thyroid function: role of hCG as putative regulator of maternal function. J Clin Endocrinol Metab 1991;73:824–831.
16. Kenimer JG, Hershman JM, Higgins HP. The thyrotropin in hydatidiform mole is human chorionic gonadotropin. J Clin Endocrinol Metab 1975;40:482–491.
17. Nisula B, Taliadouros G. Thyroid function in gestational trophoblastic neoplasia: evidence that the thyrotropic activity of chorionic gonadotropin mediates the thyrotoxicosis of choriocarcinoma. Am J Obstet Gynecol 1979;138:77–85.
18. Burrows GN. Mothers are important! Endocrinology 1997;138:3–4.
19. Bernal J, Pekonen F. Ontogenesis of the nuclear 3,5,3′ triodothyronine receptor in the human fetal brain. Endocrinology 1984;114:677–677.
20. Vulsma T, Gons MH, DeVilder JJM. Maternal-fetal transfer of thyroxine in congenital hypothyroidism due to a total organification defect or thyroid agenesis. N Engl J Med 1989;321:13–16.
21. Piosik PA, van Groenigen M, van Doorn J, Bass F, deVijlder JJ. Effects of maternal thyroid status on thyroid hormones and growth in congenitally hypothyroid goat fetuses during the second half of gestation. Endocrinology 1997;138:5–11.
22. Obregon MJ, Mallol J, Pastor R, Morreale de Escobar G, Escobar del Rey F. L-thyroxine and 3,5,3, triiodo-L-thyronine in rat embryos before onset of fetal thyroid function. Endocrinology 1984;114:305–307.
23. Xui-Yi C, Xin-Min JZ-HD, Cao XY, et al. Timing of vulnerability of the brain to iodine deficiency in endemic cretinism. N Engl J Med 1994;331:1739–1744.
24. Morreale de Escobar G, Calvo R, Obregon MJ, Escobar del Rey F. Contribution of maternal thyroxine to fetal thyroxine pools in normal rats near term. Endocrinology 1990;126:2765–2767.
25. Munro DS, Dirmikis SM, Humphries H, Smith T, Broadhead GD. The role of thyroid-stimulating immunoglobulins of Graves' disease in neonatal thyrotoxicosis. Br J Obstet Gynaecol 1978;85:837–843.
26. McKenzie JM. Neonatal Graves' disease. J Clin Endocrinol Metab 1964;24:660–664.
27. Zakarija M, McKenzie JM, Eidson MS. Transient neonatal hypothyroidism: characterization of maternal antibodies to the thyrotropin receptor. J Clin Endocrinol Metab 1990;70:1239–1246.
28. Burrow GN. Neonatal goiter after maternal propylthiouracil therapy. J Clin Endocrinol 1975;24:403–408.
29. Cottrill CM, McAllister RG Jr, Gettes L, Noonan J. Propranolol therapy during pregnancy, labor and delivery: evidence for transplacental drug transfer and impaired neonatal drug disposition. J Pediatr 1977; 91:812–814.
30. Galina MP, Arnet ML, Einhorn A. Iodides during pregnancy. N Engl J Med 1962;267:1124–1127.
31. Russell AS, Johnston C, Chew C, Maksymowych WP. Evidence for reduced TH1 function in normal pregnancy: a hypothesis for the remission of rheumatoid arthritis. J Rheumatol 1997;24:1045–1050.
32. Selenkow HA, Birnbaum MD, Hollander CS. Thyroid function and dysfunction during pregnancy. Clin Obstet Gynaecol 1973;16:66–108.
33. Amino N, Kuro R, Tanizawa O, et al. Changes of serum anti-thyroid antibodies during and after pregnancy in autoimmune thyroid diseases. Clin Exp Immunol 1978;31:30–37.
34. Buyon JP, Nelson JL, Lockshin MD. The effects of pregnancy on autoimmune thyroid diseases. Clin Immunol Immunopathol 1996;78: 99–104.
35. Grumbach MM, Kaplan SL. Ontogenesis of growth hormone, insulin, prolactin and gonadotropin secretion in the human fetus. In: Anonymous, foetal and neonatal physiology. Cambridge: Cambridge University Press, 1973:467–487.
36. Fisher DA. Thyroid physiology in the perinatal period and during childhood. In: Braverman LE, Utiger RD, eds. Werner and Ingbar's the thyroid, 7th ed. Philadelphia: JB Lippincott, 1996:974–983.
37. Crooks J, Tullock MI, Turnbull AC, Davidson D, Skulason G, Snaedel G. Comparative incidence of goiter in pregnancy in Iceland and Scotland. Lancet 1967;2:225–229.
38. Levy RP, Newman DM, Rejeal LS, Barford D. The myth of goiter in pregnancy. Am J Obstet Gynecol 1980;137:701–703.
39. Berghout A, Endert E, Ross A, Hogerzeil HV, Smits NJ, Wiersinga WM. Thyroid function and thyroid size in normal pregnant women living in an iodine replete area. Clin Endocrinol 1994;41:375–379.
40. Stoffer RP, Koeneke IA, Chesky VE, Helling CA. The thyroid in pregnancy. Am J Obstet Gynecol 1957;74:300–306.
41. Clark OH, Gerend PL, Davis M, Goretzki PE, Hoffman PG. Estrogen and TSH receptors in neoplastic and non-neoplastic thyroid tissue. J Surg Res 1985;85:89–96.
42. Spencer CA, Eigan A, Shen D, Nicoloff JT. Specificity of sensitive assays for TSH used to screen for thyroid disease in hospitalized patients. Clin Chem 1987;33:1391–1396.
43. Yeo PPB, Lewis M, Evered DC. Radioimmunoassay of free thyroid hormone concentrations in the investigation of thyroid disease. Clin Endocrinol 1977;6:159–165.
44. Lazarus JH, Othman. Thyroid disease in relation to pregnancy. Clin Endocrinol (Oxf) 1991;34:91–98.
45. Tsuruta E, Tada H, Tamaki H, et al. Pathogenic role of asialo human chorionic gonadotropin in gestational thyrotoxicosis. J Clin Endocrinol Metab 1995;80:350–355.
46. Price A, Davies R, Heller SR. Asian women are at increased risk of gestational thyrotoxicosis. J Clin Endocrinol Metab 1996;81:1160–1163.
47. Wilson R, McKillop JH, MacLean M, et al. Thyroid function tests are rarely abnormal in patients with severe hyperemesis gravidarum. Clin Endocrinol 1992;37:331–334.
48. Irvine WJ. Studies on the cytotoxic factor in thyroid disease. Br Med J 1962;1444–1449.
49. Adams DD, Purves HD. Abnormal responses in the assay of thyrotropin. Proc Univ Otago Med School 1956;34:11–12.
50. Adams DD, Fastier FN, Howie JB, Kennedy TH, Kilpatrick JA, Stewart RDH. Stimulation of the human thyroid by infusions of plasma containing LATS protector. J Clin Endocrinol Metab 1974;39:826–832.
51. Clagett JA, Wilson CB, Weigle WO. Interstitial immune complex thyroiditis in mice: the role of autoantibody to thyroglobulin. J Exp Med 1974;140:1439–1456.
52. Rose NR, Kong YM. T cell regulation of experimental autoimmune thyroiditis in the mouse. Life Sci 1983;32:85–95.
53. Shimojo N, Kohno Y, Kikioka S-I, et al. Induction of Graves'-like disease in mice by immunization with fibroblasts transfected with thyrotropin receptor and a class II molecule. Proc Natl Acad Sci U S A 1996;93:11074–11079.
54. Tomer Y, Barbesino G, Greenberg D, Davies TF. The immunogenetics of autoimmune diabetes and autoimmune thyroid disease. Trends Endocrinol 1997;8:63–70.
55. Stenszky V, Kozma L, Balazs C, Rochkitz S, Bear JC, Farid NR. The genetics of Graves' disease: HLA and disease susceptibility. J Clin Endocrinol Metab 1985;61:735–740.
56. Davies TF, Platzer M, Schwartz A, Friedman E. Functionality of thyroid-stimulating antibodies assessed by cryopreserved human thyroid cell bioassay. J Clin Endocrinol Metab 1983;57:1021–1027.
57. Vitti PV, Valente WA, Ambesi-Impiombato FS, et al. Graves' IgG stimulation of continuously cultured rat thyroid cells: a sensitive and potentially useful clinical assay. J Endocrinol Invest 1982;5:179–185.
58. Ludgate M, Perret J, Parmentier M, et al. Use of recombinant human thyrotropin receptor (TSH-R) expressed in mamalian cell lines to assay TSH-R autoantibodies. Mol Cell Endocrinol 1990;73:R13–R18
59. Fayet G, Vernier B, Girand A, et al. Effect of LATS on the reorganization into follicles of isolated thyroid cells and on the binding of radioiodine TSH to reassociated cells. FEBS Lett 1973;32:299–301.
60. Manley SW, Bourke JR, Hawker RW. The thyrotrophin receptor in guinea pig thyroid homogenate: interaction with the long-acting thyroid stimulator. J Endocrinol 1974;61:437–445.
61. Smith BR, Hall R. Thyroid-stimulating immunoglobulins in Graves' disease. Lancet 1974;2:427–429.
62. Shewring G, Rees Smith B. An improved radioreceptor assay for TSH receptor antibodies. Clin Endocrinol 1982;17:409–411.
63. Endo K, Kasagi K, Konish J, et al. Detection and properties of TSH-binding inhibitory immunoglobulins in patients with Graves' disease

and Hashimoto's thyroiditis. J Clin Endocrinol Metab 1978;46: 734–739.

64. Kraiem Z, Lahat N, Glaser B, Baron E, Sadeh O, Sheinfeld M. Thyrotropin receptor blocking antibodies: incidence, characterization and in-vitro synthesis. Clin Endocrinol 1987;27:409–421.
65. Roitt IM, Doniach D, Campbell PN, Vaughan-Hudson R. Autoantibodies in Hashimoto's disease (lymphadenoid goitre). Lancet 1956;2: 820–822.
66. Yoshida H, Amino N, Yagawa K, et al. Association of serum antithyroid antibodies with lymphocytic infiltration of the thryoid gland: studies of seventy autopsied cases. J Clin Endocrinol Metab 1978;46: 859–862.
67. Witebsky E, Rose NR, Terplan K, Paine JR, Egan RW. Chronic thyroiditis and autoimmunization. JAMA 1957;164:1439–1447.
68. Roman SH, Korn F, Davies TF. Enzyme-linked immunosorbent microassay and hemagglutination compared for detection of thyroglobulin and thyroid microsomal autoantibodies. Clin Chem 1984; 30:246–251.
69. Magnusson RP, Chazenbalk GD, Gestautas J, et al. Molecular cloning of the complementary deoxyribonucleic acid for human thyroid peroxidase. Mol Endocrinol 1987;1:856–861.
70. Mori T, Kriss JP. Measurement by competitive binding radioassay of serum antimicrosmal and antithyroglobulin antibodies in Graves' disease and other thyroid disorders. J Clin Endocrinol 1971;33:688–698.
71. Vanderpump MPJ, Tunbridge WMG, French JM, et al. The incidence of thyroid disorders in the community: a twenty-year follow-up of the Whickham survey. Clin Endocrinol 1995;43:55–68.
72. Tunbridge WMG, Evered DC, Hall R, et al. The spectrum of thyroid disease in a community. Clin Endocrinol 1977;7:483–493.
73. Endo T, Kaneshige M, Nakazato M, Kogai T, Saito T, Onaya T. Autoantibody against thyroid iodide transporter in the sera from patients with Hashimoto's thyroiditis possesses iodide transport inhibitory activity. Biochem Biophys Res Commun 1996;228:199–202.
74. Martin A, Davies TF. T cells and human autoimmune thyroid disease: Emerging data show lack of need to invoke suppressor T-cell problems. Thyroid 1992;2:247–261.
75. Davies TF. The Pathogenesis of Graves' disease. In: Braverman LE, Utiger RD, eds. The Thyroid: a fundamental text, 7th ed. Philadelphia: JB Lippincott, 1996:525–536.
76. Romagnani S. An update on human Th1 and Th2 cells. Int Arch Allergy Appl Immunol 1997;113:153–156.
77. Davies TF, Martin A, Graves P. Human autoimmune thyroid disease: cellular and molecular aspects. Bailliere's Clin Endocrinol Metab 1988;2:911–939.
78. Benson RC, Dailey ME. The menstrual pattern in hyperthyroidism and subsequent post-therapy hypothyroidism. Surg Gynecol Obstet 1955;100:19–24.
79. Goldsmith RE, Somers H, Sturgis JL, Stanbury JB. The menstrual pattern in thyroid disease. J Clin Endocrinol Metab 1952;42:853–855.
80. Russell PMG, Dean EM. Influence of thyrotoxicosis on menstruation. Lancet 1942;2:66–69.
81. Akande EO, Hockaday TDR. Plasma concentration of gonadotrophins, estrogen and progesterone thyrotoxic women. Br J Obstet Gynaecol 1975;82:541–551.
82. Chopra IJ. Gonadotropins in hyperthyroidism. Med Clin North Am 1975;59:1109–1121.
83. Akande EO, Anderson DC. Role of SHBG in hormonal changes and amenorrhea in thyroxic women. Br J Obstet Gynaecol 1975;82:557–561.
84. Ridgeway EC, Longcope C, Maloof F. Metabolic clearance and blood production rates of estradiol in hyperthyroidism. J Clin Endocrinol Metab 1975;41:491–497.
85. Southern AL, Olivo J, Gordon GG. The conversion of androgen to estrogens in hyperthyroidism. J Clin Endocrinol Metab 1974;38:207–214.
86. Robinson GA, Wasridge DC, Floto F, Downie SE. Excess iodide and the accumulation of ^{125}I by the thyroid plasma and developing oocytes of the Japanese quail. Br Poult Sci 1977;18:151–157.
87. Karlsen AE, Hagopian WA, Grubin CE, et al. Cloning and primary structure of a human islet isoform of glutamic acid decarboxylase from chromosome-10. Proc Natl Acad Sci U S A 1991;88:8337–8341.
88. Ajjan RA, Kamaruddin NA, Crisp M, Watson PF, Ludgate M, Weetman AP. Reguation and tissue distribution of the human sodium iodide symparter gene. Clin Endocrinol 1993;49:517–523.
89. Kidd GS, Glass AR, Vigersky RA. The hypothalamic-pituitary-testicular axis in thyroxicosis. J Clin Endocrinol Metab 19979;48:798–802.
90. Davies LE, Lucas MJ, Hawkens GDV, Micki L, Roalk B, Cunningham FG. Thyrotoxicosis complicating pregnancy. Am J Obstet Gynecol 1989;160:63–70.
91. Gardner Hill H. Pregnancy complications, simple goiter and Graves' disease. Lancet 1929;1:120–124.
92. Watson WJ, Fiegen MM. Fetal thyrotoxicosis associated with nonimmune hydrops. Am J Obstet Gynecol 1995;172:1039–1040.
93. Treadwell MC, Sherer DM, Sacks AJ. Successful treatment of recurrent non-immune hydrops secondary to fetal hypothyroidism. Obstet Gynecol 1996;87:838–840.
94. Millar LK, Wing DA, Leung AS. Low birth weight and preeclampsia in pregnancies complicated by hyperthyroidism. Obstet Gynecol 1994;84:946–949.
95. Momotani N, Noh J, Oyanaji H, Ishikawa N, Ito K. Antithyroid drug therapy for Graves' disease during pregnancy: optimal regimen for fetal thyroid status. N Engl J Med 1986;315:24–24.
96. Mujitaba Q, Burrow GN. Treatment of hyperthyroidism in pregnancy with propylthiouracil and methimazole. Obstet Gynecol 1975;46: 282–286.
97. Roti E, Minelli R, Salvi M. Management of hyperthyroidism and hypothyroidism in the pregnant woman. J Clin Endocrinol Metab 1996;81:1679–1682.
98. Wing D, Millar LK, Koonings PP, Montoro MN, Mestman JH. A comparison of propylthiouracil versus methimazole in the treatment of hyperthyroidism in pregnancy. Am J Obstet Gynecol 1994;170:90–95.
99. Pruyn SC, Phelan JP, Buchanan GC. Long-term propranolol therapy in pregnancy: maternal and fetal outcome. Am J Obstet Gynecol 1979; 135:485–489.
100. Langer A, Hung CT, McNulty JA, Harrington T, Washington E. Adrenergic blockade, a new approach to hyperthyroidism during pregnancy. Obstet Gynecol 1974;44:181–186.
101. Cheron RG, Kaplan M, Larsen PR, Selenkow H, Crigler JF Jr. Neonatal thyroid function after propylthiouracil therapy for maternal Graves' disease. N Engl J Med 1981;304:525–528.
102. Lamberg BA, Konen EI, Teramo K, et al. Treatment of maternal hyperthyroidism with antithyroid agents and changes in thyrotropin and thyroxine in the newborn. Acta Endocrinol 1981;97:186–195.
103. Glinoer D, Riahi M, Grun JP. Risk of subclinical hypothyroidism in pregnant women with asymptomatic thyroid disorders. J Clin Endocrinol Metab 1994;79:197–204.
104. Mandel SJ, Larsen PR, Seely EW, Brent GA. Increased need for thyroxine during pregnancy in women with primary hypothyroidism. N Engl J Med 1990;323:91–95.
105. Burrow GN, Bartsocas C, Klatsin E, Grunt J. The subsequent intellectual and physical development of children exposed in-vitro to propylthiouracil. Am J Dis Child 1968;116:161–166.
106. McCarroll AM, Hutchinson M, McAuley R, Montgomery D. Long-term assessment of children exposed in-vitro to cabizamole. Arch Dis Child 1976;51:532–536.
107. Pop VJ, DeVries E, VanBaar E, et al. Maternal thyroid peroxidase antibodies during pregnancy: a marker of impaired child development. J Clin Endocrinol Metab 1995;60:3561–3566.
108. Reuss ML, Paneth N, Pinto-Martin JA, Lorenz JM, Susser M. The relation of transient hypothyroxinemia in preterm infants to neurologic development at two years of age. N Engl J Med 1996;334:821–827.
109. Toft AD, Irvine WJ, Sinclair I, McIntosh D, Seth J, Cameron E. Thyroid function after surgical treatment of thyrotoxicosis. A report of 100 cases treated with propranolol before operation. N Engl J Med 1978;298:643–647.
110. Holt WA, Talbert LM, Thomas CG, Rankin P. Hyperthyroidism during pregnancy. Obstet Gynecol 1970;36:779–785.
111. Levy C, Waite J, Dickey R. Thyrotoxicosis and pregnancy. Use of preoperative propranolol for thyroidectomy. Am J Surg 1977;133:319–321.
112. Roben IB, Walfry PS, Nikore U. Pregnancy and surgical thyroid disease. Surgery 1985;98:1135–1140.
113. Mechanick JI, Davies TF. Medical management of hyperthyroidism: theoretical and practical aspects. In: Falk SA, ed. Thyroid disease: endocrinolgy, surgery, nuclear medicine and radiotherapy. New York: Raven Press, 1990:197–232.
114. Munro DS, Dirmikis SM, Humphrey H, Smith T, Broadhead SD. The role of thyroid-stimulating immunoglobulins of Graves' disease in neonatal thyrotoxicosis. Br J Obstet Gynecol 1978;85:837–843.
115. Munro DS, Major PW. Thyroid stimulating activity in human sera. J Endocrinol 1960;2:xix–xx.

116. Fort P, Lifshitz F, Pugliese M, Klein I. Neonatal thyroid disease: differential expression in three successive offspring. J Clin Endocrinol Metab 1987;66:645–647.
117. Van Sande J, Parma J, Tonacchera M, Swillens S, Dumont J, Vassart G. Somatic and germline mutations of the TSH receptor gene in thyroid diseases. J Clin Endocrinol Metab 1995;80:2577–2585.
118. Mejias-Heredia A, Litchfield WR, Zurakowski D. Assessing the risk of neonatal Graves' disease using TSI measurements [Abstract]. 77th Meeting of the Endocrine Society 1995;P3:460.
119. Bahn RS, Heufelder AE. Pathogenesis of Graves' ophthalmopathy. N Engl J Med 1993;329:1468–1475.
120. Hodges RE, Hamilton HE, Keetel WC. Pregnancy in myxedema. Arch Intern Med 1952;90:863–870.
121. Greenman GW, Gabrielson MA, Flanders H, Wessel MA. Thyroid dysfunction in pregnancy, fetal loss and follow-up: evaluation of surviving infants. N Engl J Med 1962;267:426–430.
122. Wasserstrum N, Anania CA. Perinatal consequences of maternal hypothyroidism in early pregnancy and inadequate replacement. Clin Endocrinol 1995;42:353–358.
123. Montoro M, Lollea J, Frasier D, Mestman J. Successful outcome of pregnancy in women with hypothyroidism. Ann Intern Med 1981; 94:31–33.
124. Liu H, Momotani N, Yoshimura J. Maternal hypothyroidism during early pregnancy and intellectual development of the progeny. Arch Intern Med 1994;154:785–787.
125. McDougall IR, Maclin N. Hypothyroid women need more thyroxine when pregnant. J Fam Pract 1995;41:238–240.
126. Stagnaro-Green A, Roman SH, Cobin RH, El-Harazy E, Alverez-Marfany M, Davies TF. Detection of at-risk pregnancy by means of highly sensitive assays for thyroid autoantibodies. JAMA 1990;264: 1422–1426.
127. Glinoer D, Fernandez-Soto M, Bourdoux P, et al. Pregnancy in patients with mild thyroid abnormalities: maternal and neonatal repercussions. J Clin Endocrinol Metab 1991;73:421–427.
128. Stagnaro-Green A. Pregnancy and thyroid disease. Immunol Allergy Clin North Am 1994;14:865–878.
129. Lejeune B, Grun, DeNayer P. Antithyroid antibodies underlying thyroid abnormalities and miscarriage or pregnancy induced hypertension. Br J Obstet Gynaecol 1991;100:669–672.
130. Parker RH, Beirwaltes WH. Thyroid antibodies during pregnancy and in the newborn. J Clin Endocrinol Metab 1961;21:792–798.
131. Haw J, Thompson AW, Scott RM, Gerrie LM, Khir B, Bewsher P. Autoimmune thyroid disease and pregnancy. Br Med J 1984;289: 253–254.
132. Pop VJ, DeRoy HA, Vader HL, et al. Postpartum thyroid dysfunction and depression in an unselected population. N Engl J Med 1991;325: 1815–1816.
133. Matsoura N, Yamada Y, Nohara Y, et al. Familial neonatal transient hypothyroidism due to maternal TSH-binding inhibitor immunoglobulins. N Engl J Med 1980;303:738–742.
134. Brown RS, Bellisario RL, Botero D, et al. Incidence of transient congenital hypothyroidism due to maternal thyrotropin receptor antibodies in over one million babies. J Clin Endocrinol Metab 1996;81: 1147–1151.
135. Pacaud D, Huot C, Gattereau A, et al. Outcome in three siblings with antibody-mediated transient congenital hypothyroidism. J Pediatr 1995;127:275–277.
136. Kohler B, Schnabel, Biebermann H, Gruters A. Transient congenital hypothyroidism and hyperthyrotropinemia: normal thyroid function and physical development at the ages of 6–14 years. J Clin Endo Metab 1996;81:1563–1567.
137. Stagnaro-Green A, Roman SH, Cobin RH, El-Harazy E, Wallenstein S, Davies TF. A prospective study of lymphocyte-initiated immunosuppression in normal pregnancy: evidence of a T-cell etiology for postpartum thyroid dysfunction. J Clin Endocrinol Metab 1992;74:645–653.
138. Robertson HEW. Lassitude, coldness and hair changes following pregnancy and their response to tratment with thyroid extract. Br Med J 1948;2(suppl):2275–2276.
139. Amino N, Miyai K. Postpartum autoimmune endocrine syndromes. In: Davies TF, ed. Autoimmune endocrine disease. New York: Wiley, 1983:247–272.
140. Amino N, Mur H, Iwatani Y, et al. High prevalence of transient post partum thyrotoxicosis and hypothyroidism. N Engl J Med 1982;306: 851–855.
141. Gerstein HC. How common is postpartum thyroiditis? A methodologic overview of the literature. Arch Intern Med 1990;150: 1397–1400.
142. Gerstein HC. Incidence of post partum thyroid dysfunction in patients with type 1 diabetes mellitus. Ann Intern Med 1993;118:419–423.
143. Weetman AP. Insulin dependent diabetes mellitus and postpartum thyroiditis: an important association. J Clin Endocrinol Metab 1994;79: 7–9.
144. Alverez-Marfany M, Roman SH, Drexler A, Robertson C, Stagnaro-Green A. Long-term prospective study of postpartum thyroid dysfunction in women with insulin dependent diabetes mellitus. J Clin Endo Metab 1997;79:10–16.
145. Ginsberg J, Walfish PG. Postpartum transient thyrotoxicosis with painless thyroiditis. Lancet 1977;1:1125–1128.
146. Tachi J, Amino N, Tamaki H, Aozasa M, Iwatani Y, Miyai K. Long term followup and HLA association in patients with postpartum hyperthyroidism. J Clin Endocrinol Metab 1988;66:480–484.
147. Tamaki H, Amino N, Aozasa M, Mori M, Tanizawa O, Miyai K. Serial changes in thyroid-stimulating antibody and thyroid binding inhibitor immunoglobublin at the time of postpartum occurrence of thyrotoxicosis in Graves' disease. J Clin Endocrinol Metab 1987;65: 324–330.
148. Amino N, Miyai K, Yamamoto T, Kuro R, Tanaka F, Tanizawa O, Kumahara Y. Transient recurrence of hyperthyroidism after delivery in Graves' disease. J Clin Endocrinol Metab 1977;44:130–136.
149. Eckel RH, Green WI. Postpartum thyrotoxicosis in a patient with Graves' disease. JAMA 1980;243:1454–1458.
150. Schwartz RH. T cell anergy. Sci Am 1993;269:66–71.
151. Bode HH, Vanjonack WJ, Crawford JD. Mitigation of cretinism by breast feeding. Pediatrics 1978;62:13–16.
152. Kampmann JP, Johansen K, Hansen JM, Helweg J. Propylthiouracil in human milk. Lancet 1980;1:736–738.
153. Tegler L, Lindstrom B. Antithyroid drugs in milk. Lancet 1980;2: 591–591.
154. Azizi F. Effect of methimazole treatment of maternal thyrotoxicosis on thyroid function in breast-feeding infants. J Pediatr 1996;128: 855–858.
155. Tonacchera M, Van Sande J, Parma J, et al. TSH receptor and disease. Clin Endocrinol 1996;44:621–633.
156. Peter H.J., Struder H, Forster R, Gerber H. The pathogenesis of hot and cold follicles in multinodular goiters. J Clin Endocrinol Metab 1982;55:941–946.
157. Koroscil T, Glowienka PR. Effect of desuppression on nodular thyroid disease. Endocrinol Pract 1997;3:222–224.
158. Herzon FS, Morris DM, Segal MN, Rauch G, Parnell T. Coexistent thyroid cancer and pregnancy. Arch Otolaryngol Head Neck Surg 1994;120:1191–1193.
159. Walker RP, Lawrence AM, Paloyan E. Nodular disease during pregnancy. Surg Clin North Am 1995;75:53–58.
160. Schwartz AE, Nieburgs HE, Davies TF, Gilbert PG, Friedman EW. The place of fine needle biopsy in the diagnosis of nodules of the thyroid. Surg Gynecol Obstet 1982;155:54–58.
161. Tan GH, Gharib H, Goellner JR. Management of thyroid nodules in pregnancy. Arch Intern Med 1996;156:2317–2320.
162. Davies TF. Thyroiditis. In: Rakel RE, ed. Conn's currrent therapy. Philadelphia: WB Saunders, 1998:662–665.
163. Volpe R, Row VV, Ezrin V. Circulating viral and thyroid antibodies in subacute thyroiditis. J Clin Endocrinol Metab 1967;27:1275–1284.

Cherry and Merkatz's Complications of Pregnancy,
Fifth Edition, edited by W. R. Cohen.
Lippincott Williams & Wilkins, Philadelphia © 2000.

CHAPTER 23

Diabetes

Oded Langer

Diabetes during pregnancy continues to be a significant public health problem that affects more than 200,000 pregnancies annually in the United States. The National Diabetes Data Group (NDDG) has estimated that women with pregestational diabetes (type I or type II) account for 4 to 15 in 1,000 pregnancies; 25 to 50 in 1,000 pregnancies are complicated by gestational diabetes (diagnosed for the first time in pregnancy and resolved upon delivery) (1). These conditions contribute disproportionately to maternal and fetal morbidity and mortality.

Among diabetic women in the preinsulin era, the maternal mortality rate was 27%, the stillbirth rate 30%, and the spontaneous abortion rate 12% to 30%. Macrosomia and metabolic complications occurred in 20% to 40% of pregnant diabetic women. Although today maternal and fetal mortality have become rare in well-treated pregnant diabetic women, the combination of diabetes and pregnancy still presents a special challenge to the obstetrician to minimize adverse maternal and fetal morbidity. The major acute complications of diabetes during pregnancy include hypoglycemia, ketoacidosis, and pregnancy-induced hypertension. Chronic maternal complications include diabetic retinopathy, nephropathy, coronary artery disease, and unstable metabolic control, which, in turn, may lead to further exacerbation of the acute complications. Neonatal macrosomia, respiratory distress syndrome, hypoglycemia, hypocalcemia, hyperbilirubinemia, congenital malformation, and intrauterine death of the fetus have been associated with diabetes in pregnancy. Overall, diabetes in pregnancy results in a 10% risk of fetal morbidity and a 4% risk of fetal mortality (2).

This chapter focuses on the approach used for the detection and management of diabetes during pregnancy at The University of Texas Health Science Center at San Antonio and Bexar County Hospital District's Medical Center Hospital (a regional tertiary care center). In general, the population served in the Bexar County Medical Center comprises inner city women who have been referred from various health care facilities. The goal of therapy for these patients is to supply state-of-the-art diabetes care and fetal surveillance testing to minimize adverse outcome of pregnancy.

CLASSIFICATION OF DIABETES

The classification of the different types of diabetes mellitus is shown in Table 23-1. Patients are divided into two main categories: those in whom the disease exists prior to pregnancy, and those in whom the disease will be exposed or developed during pregnancy (i.e., gestational diabetes).

Gestational diabetes mellitus (GDM) is defined as glucose intolerance first recognized during pregnancy that resolves following delivery. Pregestational diabetes mellitus (PGDM) is characterized by chronic hyperglycemia and other disturbances of carbohydrate and lipid metabolism. PGDM is often associated with the development of specific microvascular complications, especially affecting the eye and kidney. There may be increased frequency of macrovascular disease, such as peripheral vascular and coronary heart disease unrelated to pregnancy.

For patients with pregestational diabetes mellitus, there are two main categories, type 1 and type 2. Type 1 diabetes (previously termed insulin-dependent or juvenile diabetes) is characterized by a patient profile with insulin deficiency, insulinopenia, dependency on exogenous insulin, propensity to ketoacidosis, lean body habitus, and abrupt onset of symptoms, usually before age 30, although it may occur in the elderly. Type 1 patients are further stratified by the White classification system, originally published in 1949, based on the patient's condition before pregnancy, type of therapy required (insulin or diet), duration of the diabetes, and presence

O. Langer: Department of Obstetrics and Gynecology, Health Sciences Center at San Antonio, University of Texas, San Antonio, Texas 78284.

TABLE 23-1. *Classification of diabetes mellitus*

I. Insulin dependent—type 1
II. Noninsulin dependent—type 2
   A. Nonobese
   B. Obese
III. Secondary diabetes
IV. Impaired glucose tolerance
   A. Nonobese
   B. Obese
   C. Secondary
V. Gestational diabetes
   A. Diet control
   B. Insulin required

of vascular disease (Table 23-2). In PGDM patients, fetal mortality and morbidity are increased in classes D, F, and RF, whereas pregnancy threatens maternal survival in class H.

Women with type 2 diabetes (formerly termed non–insulin-dependent diabetes mellitus or adult-onset diabetes) may be free of classic symptoms, may require exogenous insulin, and are not prone to ketoacidosis. They usually have a family history of diabetes mellitus, are obese or have a history of obesity, and are usually diagnosed after age 30.

The National Diabetes Data Group has recommended that type 2 diabetes be diagnosed according to the following criteria: the patient must have either (a) diabetic symptoms (polyuria, polydipsia, and unexplained weight loss) and a casual plasma glucose concentration (defined as any time of day without regard to time since last meal) equal to or greater than 200 mg/dL (11.1 mmol/L) or a fasting plasma glucose (fasting defined as no caloric intake for at least 8 hours) greater than or equal to 126 mg/dL (7.0 mmol/L), or (b) a 2-hour plasma glucose level at or above 200 mg/dL during an oral glucose tolerance test (OGTT) in a nonpregnant individual. The OGTT is not recommended for routine clinical use. When done, it should be performed as described by the World Health Organization (WHO), using a glucose load containing the equivalent of 75 g of anhydrous glucose dissolved in water. The results should be confirmed by repeat testing on a different day.

TABLE 23-2. *White's classification*

Gestational diabetes:	Maintained by diet alone (A_1)
	Insulin required (A_2)
Pregestational class	
A	Euglycemia by diet alone, any duration, onset at any age
B	Onset age 20 or older, duration <10 yr
C	Onset during age 10–19 yr, or duration of 10–19 yr
D	Onset at age <10 yr, duration of >20 yr, background retinopathy or hypertension (not PIH)
R	Proliferative retinopathy or vitreous hemorrhage
F	Nephropathy with proteinuria >500 mg/day
RF	Criteria for Classes R and F
H	Arteriosclerotic heart disease clinically evident
T	Prior renal transplantation

Modified from Shade DS, Santiago JV, Skyler JS, Rizza RA. Intensive insulin therapy. Princeton, NJ: Medical Examination Publishing, 1983.

The Data Group further classified normality (the nondiabetic state) as a fasting plasma glucose concentration less than 111 mg/dL and 2-hour postglucose load value of less than 141 mg/dL. Impaired glucose tolerance results reflect a fasting range between 111 and 125 mg/dL and 2-hour postprandial levels greater than 140 mg/dL but less than 200 mg/dL. This change in criteria doubled the incidence of diabetes in the general population, recategorizing many women previously thought to have GDM instead as type 2 (PGDM) patients. Moreover, in the Fourth Diabetes Workshop for gestational diabetes, it was recommended to decrease the diagnostic limits for the OGTT to 95 mg/dL for fasting; 180 mg/dL for 1 hour; 160 mg/dL for 2 hours; and 140 mg/dL for 3 hours regardless of whether the glucose load was 75 or 100 g. This change in criteria will probably double the rate of diagnosed GDM from 3% to 6%.

PREGNANCY-INDUCED METABOLIC CHANGES AND THEIR EFFECT ON THE DIABETIC WOMAN

Pregnancy is accompanied by extensive hormonal and physiologic readjustment by the mother. Almost every endocrine tissue and system participates in adaptive changes that maintain metabolic hemostasis during normal pregnancy. The placenta, anterior pituitary, and adrenal cortex all perform key functions in the endocrine adaptation to pregnancy. When the body is unable to adjust completely to the physiologic stress of gestation, latent pathology such as gestational diabetes may be expressed.

In normal pregnancy, glucose metabolism is characterized by lower fasting and elevated postprandial plasma glucose values. These changes occur as early as the 10th week of gestation. They continue to evolve, and only in the third trimester does the carbohydrate level stabilize. Insulin concentrations are increased in response to the high OGTT glucose changes. In contrast, fasting insulin concentration is significantly elevated in the third trimester of pregnancy in comparison with the nonpregnant state. In general, the rate of glucose disappearance after glucose ingestion is enhanced beginning in the first trimester and then declines toward the normal range in late pregnancy. Thus, there is scant evidence that the first few months of pregnancy are accompanied by diabetogenic stress or insulin resistance. On the contrary, insulin action on carbohydrate metabolism is enhanced during the first 20 weeks of gestation. Estrogen and progesterone may have a positive effect on the pancreatic beta cell, resulting in increased insulin sensitivity and release.

In summary, during the first 20 weeks of gestation, the increase in glycogen storage, the decrease in fasting plasma glucose, and the increase in glucose disappearance rate are affected by the sex steroid hormones, which cause reduction of hepatic glucose production and increased peripheral glucose utilization. In the second half of pregnancy, the counterinsulin hormones, especially human placental lactogen (HPL) and prolactin, as well as growth hormone and cortisol in a lesser capacity, affect glucose metabolism. These hormones augment glycogen storage with prolonged excursion of plasma glucose during the fed state, with emphasis on glycogen mobilization and gluconeogenesis during the fasting state (3).

Pregnancy-related metabolic changes in the second half of pregnancy coincide with the increasing elaboration of metabolically active steroids and peptides by the placenta. At this time, the fasting state is characterized by a more rapid, profound diversion to the metabolism of fat (accelerated starvation) (4). This physiologic finding is traditionally attributed to the growing fetus siphoning nutrients from the maternal to the fetal compartment. Thus, concentrations of circulating free fatty acids and ketones ascend to higher levels than under nongravid conditions whenever food is withheld, and plasma glucose and amino acid levels decrease more rapidly. The temporal relationships vary for individual fuels, but all aspects of accelerated starvation may be achieved by such mild dietary deprivations as that involved in skipping breakfast after an overnight fast (5).

The fed state is also altered. The ingestion of glucose results in greater, more prolonged elevations of the plasma glucose level and a tendency toward carbohydrate-induced triglyceridemia; the increases in plasma levels of amino acids after mixed meals are smaller and of a shorter duration (6). As a result of the changes in the fed and fasting states, an overall decrease of plasma glucose and amino acid levels and a sustained elevation of plasma triglyceride and cholesterol levels (particularly in the very-low-density lipoprotein fraction) occur. These changes in the levels of fuels during normal pregnancy are accompanied by modifications in circulating insulin. Basal insulin levels are higher than nongravid levels, especially in late pregnancy, and alimentation effects a two- to threefold greater outpouring of insulin compared with the nonpregnant state (3). The chronic and acute increases in plasma insulin are accompanied by diminished responsiveness to insulin action in the periphery. The resistance appears to be mediated at the postreceptor level (7–9).

It may be too simplistic to assume that these changes alone cause gestational diabetes. A more reasonable concept is that an underlying carbohydrate metabolism abnormality is exposed by pregnancy-induced changes. In fact, some evidence suggests that gestational diabetes is characterized by impairment of insulin secretion as well as increases in insulin resistance. This segment of the pregnant population cannot withstand the physiologic stresses accompanying pregnancy, resulting in abnormal glucose tolerance with elevated postprandial and, under more severe conditions, fasting plasma glucose levels. An insulin secretion abnormality is frequently but not categorically present in pregnant women with elevated fasting glucose levels. Insulin secretion, however, would not be expected to be affected in normal and milder forms of glucose tolerance (fasting plasma less than 95 mg/dL). Insulin resistance, however, is present uniformly in women with any degree of clinically detectable glucose intolerance. This insulin resistance is located both in the liver and the peripheral tissues, especially skeletal muscle. Hepatic resistance results in inappropriately high glucose production in the fasting state and deficient glucose uptake following food intake.

Peripheral insulin resistance manifests itself as reduced glucose uptake (mainly in muscle) after exposure to endogenous or exogenous insulin, and reduced clearance of plasma glucose in the fasting state (10–12). We can thus hypothesize that the pathogenesis of gestational diabetes mellitus resides in a defect in the secretory activity of the beta cells and in the interaction among the gastrointestinal tract, the liver, and peripheral tissues manifested as insulin resistance.

PROBLEMS RELATED TO PREGESTATIONAL DIABETES

The estimated 10,000 to 14,000 infants born yearly in the United States to women with overt diabetes are at high risk for mortality, prematurity, congenital defects, macrosomia, neonatal hypoglycemia or brain damage, respiratory distress syndrome, and newborn hyperbilirubinemia. All these conditions are especially common with poor maternal glycemic control, and their occurrence can be diminished by maintenance of euglycemia (13). When a center for disease control in California conducted a study of preexisting diabetes in women, it reported high rates of major congenital anomalies (8%), respiratory distress syndrome (7%), and stillbirth (2%) (14).

A direct relationship has been demonstrated between the degree of maternal hyperglycemia and the perinatal mortality rate (15). In most cases, maintenance of euglycemia in the pregnant diabetic woman has been associated with perinatal mortality rates equal to those in the nondiabetic population when deaths from major congenital anomalies are excluded (4,15). This normalization in fetal mortality rates, however, is contingent on intensive therapy for controlling glycemia and achieving near-normal glucose levels. This is not the case when significant maternal vascular involvement is evident (5). Fetal surveillance testing during pregnancy is especially indicated in these patients because the underlying vasculopathy can by itself place the fetus at risk for stillbirth. Thus, to maximize pregnancy outcome (16), these patients must undergo an intensive testing scheme even in the presence of normal glycemia.

White's classification (17) has withstood the test of time, enabling patients with vasculopathy to be identified and, in turn, allowing more intensive care of this subgroup of patients. What is not yet clear is the net contribution of glycemic control in perinatal mortality versus the aggregate effect of modern aspects of perinatal care. Contemporary care includes modern techniques of fetal surveillance testing (ultrasonographic examination, biophysical fetal testing), prenatal determination of lung maturation, and genetic counseling and testing. Thus, there is early identification of the fetus with defects not compatible with life and the ability to prepare for prompt neonatal treatment of some anomalies. Modern care offers the pregnant diabetic mother alternatives and control over the outcome and course of her pregnancy (including induced abortion). The prevention of congenital malformations through good glycemic control, dietary supplements, and early pregnancy termination has assumed a major role in further reduction of the perinatal mortality rate among diabetic women.

The pregnant pregestational diabetic patient is confronted with major health risks. Research has confirmed the presence of severe acute and chronic maternal consequences. Among the acute maternal complications are ketoacidosis, hypoglycemia, and conditions complicated by hypertension, urinary tract infections, toxemia, and hydramnios (13). Acceleration of microvascular, renal, ocular, and neural complications may result, especially when women do not receive optimal care in pregnancy. Serious maternal and fetal complications can result in extended hospitalization in pregnancy. Contemporary health economic trends toward stringent adherence to cost-effective strategies has highlighted the need for strategies to provide intensive diabetic care in nonhospitalized women.

Congenital Anomalies

Preconceptional Counseling: Primary Prevention

The concept of community-based prevention to reduce risks in diabetes and pregnancy is important to ensure further gains are realized in reduction of maternal and perinatal morbidity and mortality. In pregestational diabetes, attention is focused on primary prevention by initiation of tight metabolic control regimens in the preconceptional period and throughout pregnancy to prevent fetal anomalies.

Congenital anomalies are major contributors to perinatal morbidity and mortality in infants of diabetic mothers. Furthermore, the types of malformations most commonly seen in these infants (e.g., congenital heart disease, caudal regression syndrome) occur embryologically before 7 weeks of gestation, indicating that prevention strategies must begin very early in or, preferably, before pregnancy (18).

The identification and diagnosis of diabetes in pregnancy present the primary opportunity for medical interventions to prevent adverse outcome. Prepregnancy counseling and implementation of strategies that contribute to tight glycemic control for women with type I or type II diabetes provides the best mode of prevention of stillbirth and fetal anomalies.

The rate of birth defects over recent decades has not diminished significantly in major perinatal centers. This raises two key questions: What are the causes of birth defects? and when should intervention occur to reduce effectively the rate of fetal malformation? Most congenital malformations occur early in the first trimester, emphasizing the significance of preconceptional counseling and glycemic control. Unfortunately, only a small segment of the PGDM mothers are enrolled in care programs prior to conception (fewer than 15%). The majority of PGDM mothers enroll after the 7th week. This fact alone explains the lack of significant reduction in the rate of anomalies. It is therefore an important public health objective to enhance primary prevention in the form of education and counseling prior to pregnancy rather than to resort belatedly to secondary prevention in the form of pregnancy termination.

Congenital malformations continue to occur among diabetic individuals at least three times more frequently than the 2% to 3% background incidence in the general population. The most widely accepted theory to explain the cause of these malformations in diabetic individuals is that hyperglycemia, prior to and early in conception, plays the major causative role. Several groups noted higher levels of glycosylated hemoglobin during the first trimester in diabetic women who delivered infants with major congenital anomalies than in those with normal offspring. Many studies on animals have reinforced the link between birth defects and elevated maternal blood glucose during early gestation. Studies of whole-embryo tissue cultures in animals have shown that disturbances in levels of glucose, as well as of other energy sources, were associated with various anomalies (19,20).

Increased concentrations of glucose, ketones, somatomedin inhibitors, and factors linked to abnormal glucose and lipid fuel disposition have been suggested so far. Introduction of these materials to media during culture of intact rodent embryos has produced profound dysmorphogenesis. In addition, synergistic interactions among these factors were described. For example, the addition of subteratogenic amounts of glucose in combination with subteratogenic amounts of ketones to the medium can produce debilitating congenital anomalies in cultured embryos. Therefore, a multifactorial metabolic foundation may explain the diabetic embryopathy. Additionally, genetic predisposition may be an important contributor to risks.

Research has shown in the rat *in vivo* that brief intervals of hypoglycemia can impair embryogenesis during the postimplantation period, which is particularly dependent on consistent glycolysis for metabolic substrate. This finding raises the question of whether achievement of stringent glycemic control during preconception and early gestation may be dangerous because attempts at strict control may result in episodes of hypoglycemia. It should be remembered, however, that poorly controlled diabetes is also associated with frequent hypoglycemic episodes. Thus, near normalization of the plasma glucose profile (minimizing hypoglycemic episodes) is the most appropriate goal for insulin therapy during the first 8 weeks of gestation in the pregnant diabetic woman.

In a retrospective study, Miller and colleagues (21) confirmed earlier evidence that the incidence of malformations was higher among pregestational diabetic mothers with an abnormally high hemoglobin A1c value detected in early pregnancy. The overlap between individual values of mothers bearing normal and abnormal infants suggested that blood glucose concentration was not the only factor in the occurrence of fetal anomalies. The results of a study of 2,041 diabetic pregnancies conducted in Copenhagen (22) and of the United Kingdom National Inquiry into Diabetic Pregnancy (unpublished observations) have supported the concept that the greater the severity of maternal diabetes, the higher the incidence of fetal anomalies. In the Copenhagen study, patients with class A diabetes treated with diet alone had an anomaly rate of 4.1% compared with a rate of 2.6% in the control group.

The association between class of diabetes, presence of vasculopathy, and risk of major malformations was studied by Miodovnik and colleagues (23), who suggested that the significant variables associated with malformations were maternal vasculopathy and high HbA1c at 9 weeks' gestation. They concluded that congenital malformations were associated with poor first-trimester glycemic control and maternal vasculopathy as reflected in the White classification.

The Diabetes in Early Pregnancy project was a multicenter prospective study that enrolled diabetic and nondiabetic women prior to or within three weeks of conception. The investigators found that the diabetic women who entered the study early had a moderate degree of glycemic control. A mean glucose value of 140 to 234 mg/dL was recorded for 90% of the women. A malformation rate of 4.9% was found in these women, compared with 9% for those who enrolled after 3 weeks' gestation and 2.1% in the nondiabetic subjects. The research demonstrated that intervention in early pregnancy can reduce dramatically the incidence of congenital anomalies. Preconceptional glycemic control did not occur in women enrolled early in pregnancy, who consequently suffered a twofold higher rate of malformations compared with the control group. This reconfirms the importance of tight metabolic control and preconceptional intervention (24). In Germany, Fuhrmann and colleagues (25) initiated strict blood glucose control before conception, resulting in a malformation rate of 0.8% compared with 7.5% in subjects in whom intensive treatment was started 8 weeks or more after conception.

Available data are sufficient to support the concept that the risk of congenital anomalies in pregestational diabetes is associated closely with the level of glycemic control. Thus, preconceptional enrollment into educational and clinical programs that will help improve patient compliance and level of glycemic control will decrease the rate of malformations.

In contrast to PGDM, evidence is insufficient to support the concept that there is increased risk of congenital anomalies in gestational diabetes. It appears likely, however, that the notion of a metabolic teratogen induced by diabetes, as proposed by Freinkel (26), is a distinct possibility and that normalization of glycemia among the few gestational diabetic mothers who are detected very early in pregnancy is a sensible and desirable goal.

Diabetes, Ketoacidosis, and Hypoglycemia

Diabetic ketoacidosis (DKA) is a medical emergency that continues to result in substantial morbidity and mortality, despite advances in therapy, such as low-dose insulin therapy (27) and intensive insulin therapy (28). The current low-dose insulin approach (5–10 U/h) produces plasma insulin concentrations that are in the high physiologic to pharmacologic range (75–200 μU/mL). DKA is a severe metabolic decompensation characterized by uncontrolled hyperglycemia (generally more than 300 mg/dL), metabolic acidosis (arterial blood pH usually less than 7.30), and an increase in circulating total blood ketone (beta-hydroxybutyric and acetoacetic acid) concentrations (more than 5 mmol/L). The key diagnostic feature is the elevation in total blood ketone body concentration, which is reflected in an increase in the anion gap.

From the epidemiologic point of view, the annual incidence of DKA among type 1 diabetic individuals ranges from 8% to 13%, with ketoacidosis accounting for 2% to 8% of all diabetic hospital admissions. The most common cause of DKA is infection, which accounts for 30% to 40% of all hospital admissions for DKA. Interruption of insulin therapy accounts for only 15% to 20% of episodes of DKA. Medications such as glucocorticoids and diuretics precipitate 10% to 15% of cases. Previously undiagnosed diabetic patients account for 20% to 25% of all hospital admissions for DKA, whereas in about 25% of cases of DKA no obvious event can be defined. Approximately 20% of all cases of DKA are recurrent and are especially common in women under 20 years of age.

Blood glucose concentration is a reflection of the equilibrium between the processes that control the entry and exit of glucose from the body. Glucose entry is achieved by the ingestion of glucose and/or hepatic glucose production (HGP); glucose exit is the consequence of tissue metabolism or urinary excretion. A study of persons with DKA prior to treatment revealed that hepatic glucose production increased by 150% to 200% and glucose disposal was reduced by 20%. This demonstrates that glucose production is the main cause of the hyperglycemia (29). The mean blood glucose level in these patients is less than 800 mg/dL (range 500–600 mg/dL).

At the opposite end of the continuum are subjects with severe DKA but mild to modest hyperglycemia. Approximately 15% of individuals with DKA have glucose concentrations below 350 mg/dL (30), which is defined as euglycemic DKA. Pregnant women with diabetes mellitus may have severe DKA with minimal hyperglycemia, owing to the volume expansion that occurs during pregnancy and increased glomerular filtration, or the continued use of glucose by the fetoplacental unit in the presence of maternal insulin deficiency. This represents a nonhepatic mechanism, which can be characterized by lack of association between plasma glucose and bicarbonate levels.

Correction of fluid deficits is especially important in these patients because it promotes glucosuria and decreases the release of insulin counterregulatory hormones that produce insulin resistance. Thus, in diabetes in pregnancy, glucose-containing fluid must be initially administered even when glucose concentrations are approximating 300 to 350 mg/dL (31).

The pathogenesis of DKA may be characterized by insulin resistance or insulin deficiency. Almost all patients who present with DKA have either an absolute or relative deficiency of insulin. Therefore, in all pregnant diabetic patients who present with ketoacidosis, both insulin deficiency and insulin resistance contribute simultaneously to the metabolic decompensated state. Most diabetic patients who are admitted in ketoacidosis maintain or even increase their daily dose of insulin, and circulating insulin levels are increased. In these patients, there is relative insulin deficiency due to the increase in the circulating counterregulatory hormones and an altered metabolic environment represented by an increase in free fatty and amino acids as well as metabolic acidosis. Both epinephrine and glucagon cause insulin resistance by inhibiting insulin-mediated glucose uptake in muscle and by stimulating hepatic glucose production (HGP) through an augmentation of both glycogenolysis and gluconeogenesis. Cortisol and growth hormone block insulin action in peripheral tissues.

The therapeutic approach to DKA is based on the pathophysiology described above. All components are treated with insulin in addition to free water for the hyperglycemia and hypertonicity; sodium bicarbonate for the ketoacidosis; and potassium and sodium chloride for the fluid and electrolyte losses.

Insulin management in conjunction with fluid and electrolyte replacement remains the foundation of DKA therapy. Insulin will correct the hyperglycemia and inhibit ketogenesis, reversing the metabolic acidosis. Regular insulin given intravenously remains the drug of choice. Unless the insulin resistance is extremely severe, 5 to 10 U/h, after a 5- to 10-U intravenous bolus, usually is sufficient to break up the ketoacidosis and to correct all of the metabolic disturbances. Whether one uses low-dose or conventional insulin therapy, the rate of decline in plasma glucose concentration is approximately 75 to 100 mg/dL per hour. However, because higher doses of insulin are associated with more hypokalemia, as well as hypophosphatemia, a conservative approach is to start with an insulin infusion rate of 5 to 10 U/h. The insulin dose should be increased in the 10% of DKA patients who fail to demonstrate the expected decline in plasma glucose concentration after the first 60 minutes of insulin therapy. Finally, it should be noted that plasma glucose concentration will decrease much more rapidly than the serum ketones. Therefore, the insulin infusion should be continued until the ketoacidosis is under control.

The metabolic acidosis is characterized by a decrease in the serum bicarbonate concentration. DKA patients who are most likely to benefit from bicarbonate therapy are those with severe hypobicarbonatemia (less than 5–6 mEq/L) and a blood pH below 7.15. These patients present a major risk for the development of fulminant acidemia and cardiovascular collapse. When deciding to treat with bicarbonate, it is important to give amounts of alkali only sufficient to raise the serum bicarbonate level to 10 to 12 mEq/L.

Replenishing salt and water losses in addition to insulin replacement is the next foundation of DKA therapy. For most patients with DKA, insulin and sodium chloride fluid replacement are begun simultaneously.

Because plasma sodium concentration is normal or increased in the majority of patients with DKA, the presence of severe hyponatremia (less than 125–130 mEq/L) should alert the physician to the presence of marked sodium deficits. The best predictor for diagnosis of fluid deficit and hyponatremia is plasma osmolality.

In evaluating potassium replacement, several factors need to be considered. If the initial plasma potassium concentration is increased (more than 5.0 mEq/L), no additional potassium should be added to the first liter of normal saline replacement. If the initial plasma potassium is normal (3.6–4.5 mEq/L), 20 to 40 mEq/L of potassium should be added to the first liter of normal saline. If the initial potassium is very low (less than 2.5–3.0 mEq/L), insulin should be withheld for 30 to 60 minutes until sufficient intravenous potassium can be administered to increase the plasma potassium concentration into the normal range.

Hypoglycemia

Hypoglycemia is an intrusive event that deteriorates the life-style of the patient. Severe hypoglycemia results in cerebral impairment (coma, severe confusion, and seizures) before the development of warning symptoms of hypoglycemia (excessive sweating, tremors, etc.). It is important to educate patients about the warning signs, which characteristically are tingling of the tongue, numbness, sweating, and loss of level of concentration. Patients should be educated to respond immediately by measuring blood glucose and consuming carbohydrates or milk.

Hypoglycemia is classified into mild, moderate, and severe. Mild hypoglycemia can be self-treated. Mild or chemical hypoglycemia can accompany pregnancy because of the continuous glucose consumption by the fetus. The classic symptoms are shaking, nervousness, sweating, and extreme hunger. It can accompany the sudden improvement in glycemic control from a previously poorly controlled stage. Although the blood glucose level will be within the near normoglycemic range, the patient may complain of these symptoms. The self-treatment of mild hypoglycemia is 10 to 15 g of carbohydrate followed by a protein such as a cup of milk and crackers.

Moderate hypoglycemia may require assistance in treatment. Symptoms may include headache, mood or behavior swings, confusion, and maternal tachycardia. Treatment often involves a large dose of carbohydrate (total of 20–30 g). This should be followed with a protein snack such as a cup of milk.

Severe hypoglycemia usually requires emergency measures. Unresponsiveness, unconsciousness, or convulsions are the usual symptoms. Patients should be injected with glucagon or given intravenous hydration with a glucose solution.

In general, pregnant women are more prone to prolonged hypoglycemic episodes than are nonpregnant women. We have observed that hypoglycemia in levels ranging from 50 to 30 mg/dL may accompany even gestational diabetic women (6%–10% rate) regardless of treatment modality (diet or insulin).

PROBLEMS RELATED TO GESTATIONAL DIABETES

Between 25 and 50 per 1,000 pregnancies are complicated by gestational diabetes (diagnosed for the first time in pregnancy and resolved immediately following delivery). It has been reported that up to 50% of those women diagnosed with gestational diabetes will go on to develop overt (type II) diabetes (32,33). This tendency for later development of diabetes may be the most compelling reason for screening. Gestational diabetes occurs in 2% to 5% of the total pregnant population (1,34,35), the incidence depending on the demographic characteristics found in a specific geographic location. For example, in areas with a mean maternal population age of 30 or older, or in populations with large proportions of high-risk groups (such as the higher incidence of Mexican Americans in San Antonio, Texas), or populations in which a chronic health problem such as obesity is prevalent, the gestational diabetes rate can increase dramatically to as high as 7% to 9% of the population. Thus, results of pregnancy outcome and prevalence of disease are not always comparable for different geographic areas.

Approximately 60,000 to 100,000 women with gestational diabetes give birth each year in the United States. The disease usually develops during the second or third trimester of pregnancy, when levels of insulin-antagonist hormones are high and insulin resistance normally occurs. The main effects on offspring and mother can include large birth weight [macrosomia and large for gestational age (LGA)], premature delivery with respiratory distress syndrome, difficult delivery associated with maternal or fetal trauma, and increased incidence of delivery by cesarean section. The neonatal metabolic complications include hypoglycemia, polycythemia, hyperbilirubinemia, and hypocalcemia. In addition, there is an increased risk for fetal and neonatal mortality. As noted, gestational diabetes also is associated with a tendency for later development of overt (type II) diabetes in the mother 5 to 10 years after parturition (32).

The significant public health problems associated with diabetes in pregnancy and the possible preventive interventions that may reduce overall morbidity and mortality are presently well known.

IDENTIFICATION AND DIAGNOSIS OF GESTATIONAL DIABETES

Identification of women with gestational diabetes through the use of a universal screening approach provides the best opportunity for prevention of both maternal and fetal complications. It is important to identify the pregnant woman with GDM because it is associated with significantly elevated perinatal mortality. For example, a fourfold increase in perinatal mortality was shown to exist between untreated gestational diabetic women and a control group with normal OGTT results, 6.4% versus 1.5% (36). In another study, a linear relationship was shown to exist between the 2-hour OGTT plasma glucose determination and perinatal mortality, especially when the values were greater than 160 mg/dL (37). Today it would be unethical to conduct studies to reconfirm the relationship between perinatal mortality and gestational diabetes. Efforts and resources could be better directed toward management and prevention.

Until recently, it was believed that only women with risk factors (obesity, previous stillbirth of an LGA infant, family history of diabetes, or age over 35 years) needed to be screened for gestational diabetes. Evidence from several sources now suggests that if only these women were screened, as many as 50% of the women with gestational diabetes would be missed. It is still not certain what the relative costs (in dollars and morbidity) are of universal versus selective screening. Because there is an increase in perinatal mortality (threefold) when GDM subjects are not identified as well as a substantial increase in perinatal morbidity, mainly macrosomia (30% to 50%) and its related complications, it is reasonable to assume that establishment of universal screening, early identification, and proper treatment will result in lower overall cost than the social and financial burdens of managing the results of untreated diabetes. It is recommended (38) that all pregnant patients regardless of age, family history, ethnicity, or other risk factors for diabetes be screened between the 24th and 28th gestational weeks. If the results of screening are normal, some investigators recommend repeating the test at 32 weeks if the patient is obese or over 33 years of age. It also is recommended that women with positive screening and normal glucose tolerance test (GTT) results be retested using an OGTT by the 32nd week. Finally, women with risk factors (previous GDM, obesity, and previous macrosomia) are recommended to be screened at the first prenatal visit and, if screening is negative, rescreened at 24 to 28 weeks' gestation. Recently, the controversy over selective versus universal screening has resurfaced because of economic rather than medical considerations. The screening protocol at the Health Science Center at San Antonio is shown in Fig. 23-1.

Lack of uniformity exists in the method of screening. Different studies have used different gestational ages and different concentrations of glucose, have varied the time of the test during the day, and have used different means to verify the sensitivity and specificity of the screening test. Therefore, the true incidence of GDM remains unknown. The recommended screening method today is the 1-hour blood glucose determination after a 50-g oral glucose load regardless of time of day. Screening results are considered abnormal when they are less than or equal to 140 mg/dL. At the University of Texas at San Antonio, we have chosen to use a lower threshold for abnormality of 130 mg/dL because the rate of abnormal GTT results in women in our community with screening outcomes of 130 to 140 mg/dL is about 10%. In contrast, when screening results are less than 130 mg/dL, only 1% of the women will have an abnormal GTT result.

Similar problems arise in consideration of the diagnostic GTT. Although the OGTT has been the accepted gold standard for detection of GDM, variations in methodology and interpretation are a source of misunderstanding among clinicians. O'Sullivan and Mahan (33) established carefully derived limits of carbohydrate tolerance based on a 100-g OGTT outcome. The test result is abnormal if two or more blood glucose levels meet or exceed specified values. The collected evidence regarding the long-term prognosis for the mother drawn from the studies of O'Sullivan presents a strong argument for using his method (39,40).

Despite the existence of some consensus on the diagnostic criteria established by the national Diabetes Data Group (any two values must be greater than or equal to fasting 105, 1-hour 190, 2-hour 165, 3-hour 145 mg/dL) (Table 23-3), researchers have questioned the ability of the OGTT to identify women who are at high risk for LGA infants. Because the appropriate identification of all women at risk for adverse fetal outcome is critical, several studies have examined the patients who, although not meeting the criteria of two abnormal values during an OGTT, appear to have impaired glucose tolerance by virtue of either high normal values or the presence of one abnormal value during the OGTT. These women who remain untreated are at a threefold higher risk for LGA infants and macrosomia (41).

In a prospective randomized study the hypothesis was tested that treatment of women with one abnormal OGTT value will yield a reduced adverse outcome. One hundred twenty-six women with one abnormal OGTT value and 146 women in the control group (normal OGTT values) participated in a clinical trial during the third trimester of pregnancy. The subjects with one abnormal test result were randomized into treated and untreated groups. Treated subjects were managed with a strict diabetic protocol to maintain tight glycemic control by means of diet and insulin therapy. Untreated subjects tested their capillary blood glucose for a baseline period but had no diet or insulin intervention. The study revealed that the level of glycemic control was similar before initiation of therapy between the treated and untreated groups. The overall incidence of neonatal metabolic complications was 4% in the treated group and 14% in the untreated group. Macrosomia was present in 7% of the treated women and 24% in the untreated women (42). Thus, women with one abnormal value are similar to patients with gestational diabetes (i.e., those with two abnormal values) in their glycemic control prior to therapy and rate of macrosomia (30%). Treatment of these women also will result in perinatal outcome comparable with that of nondiabetic subjects.

The OGTT has many potential uses in evaluating patients with glucose homeostatic disorders and can be used in several clinical situations. It was shown that a relatively "flat" OGTT curve is associated with small-for-gestational-age (SGA) infants (43). This suggests a subgroup within the intrauterine growth restriction (IUGR) population whose growth problems may be metabolic in origin.

Treatment

For all types of diabetes in pregnancy, current approaches call for intensive treatment to manage glucose levels with the target of achieving and maintaining

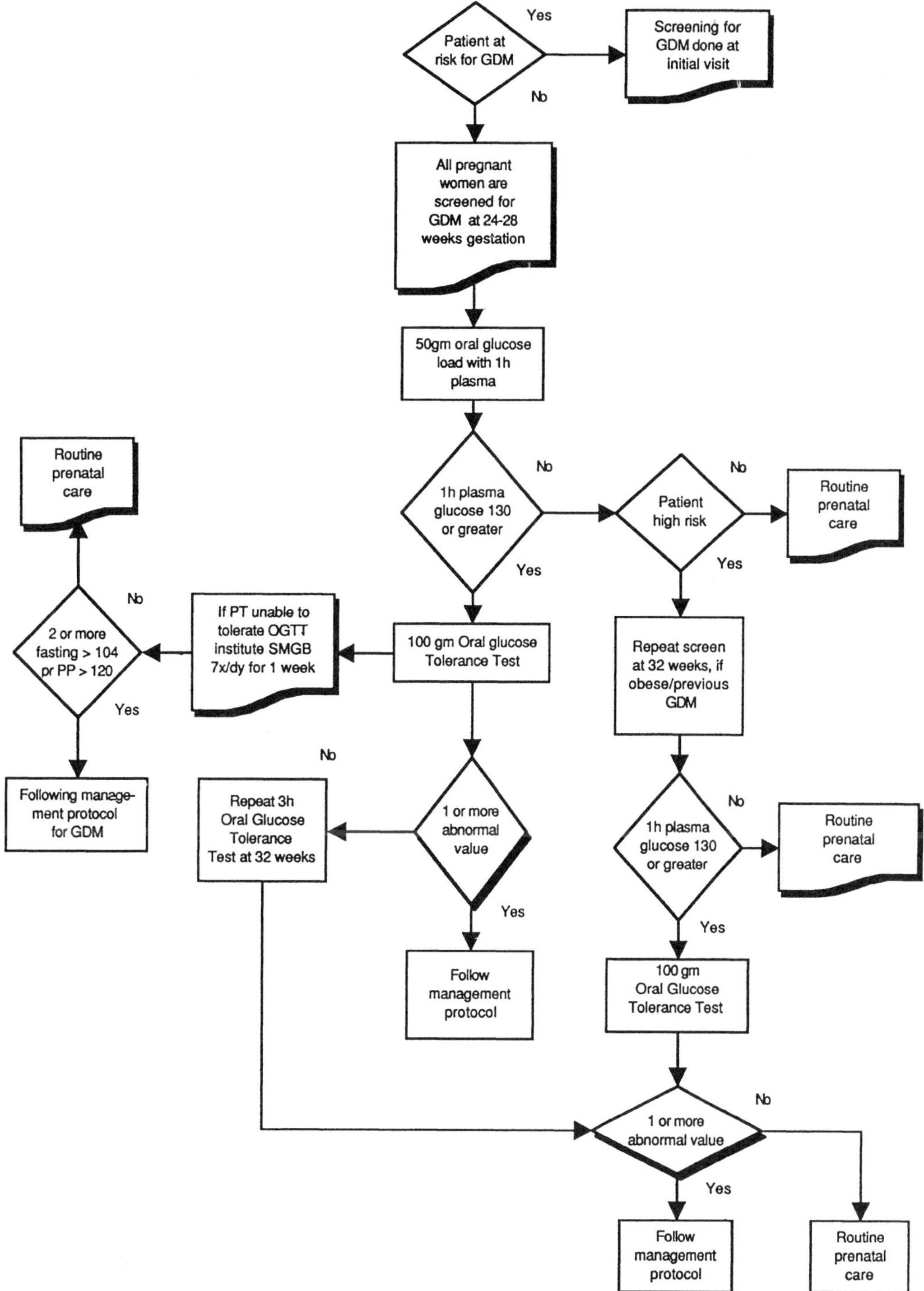

FIG. 23-1. Screening protocol for gestational diabetes.

near-normal glycemia throughout pregnancy. To accomplish this, the decision whether to administer insulin or diet-only regimens must be made.

The cornerstone of treatment for the pregnant diabetic is diet and administration of short- and intermediate-acting insulin when required. Dietary therapy for the pregnant diabetic requires attention to appropriate maternal weight gain, nutrient needs, and meal planning. The current recommendations call for a 10- to 12-kg weight gain to occur during the second and third trimesters in a linear rate of 350 to 400 g per week. There is little doubt that caloric restriction and weight reduction improve insulin

TABLE 23-3. *Criteria for OGTT in pregnancy*

	Glucose concentration (MG%)			
Clinical status	Fasting	1 hr	2 hr	3 hr
Whole blood	90	165	145	125
Plasma/Serum	105	190	165	145
Coustan	95	180	160	140

Diagnostic if elevated fasting or two or more values equal or exceed the stated levels (National Diabetes Data Group Criteria)(1).

sensitivity and insulin binding in obese and gestational diabetic women. Diet can appreciably enhance *in vivo* insulin sensitivity in healthy women after only 2 weeks, a result of influence on postreceptor steps of insulin action. The question remains, however, whether we should allow a 2- to 3-week hiatus in treatment to await results from diet alone when the entire period available for intervention is only 8 to 12 weeks. Although it is generally important for weight gain in pregnancy to meet expected norms, our group found that well-controlled diabetic women gained approximately 2 kg throughout the third trimester from initiation of therapy to delivery (12 weeks) without any observable adverse effect on the fetus. This finding alerts us to the need for further evaluation of the weight gain criteria in the pregnant diabetic. Caloric requirements are increased to about 300 kcal per day above basal requirements during pregnancy. In general, obese patients should receive 25 kcal/kg body weight and nonobese 30 to 35 kcal/kg body weight daily. Carbohydrates should constitute 40% to 60% of calories and no fewer than 200 g per day. Protein should make up 20% to 30% of the total diet with the remainder (25%–40%) provided as fat. The goal of meal planning is to individualize the meal to the patient's eating habits, thus maximizing compliance and limiting the extent of hyperglycemia. Because pregnancy is characterized by accelerated starvation, multiple meals are recommended. This is achieved by three meals and four snacks, with the last snack at bedtime to minimize overnight hypoglycemia and starvation ketosis.

Urine should be tested frequently for ketones as a reflection of the success of the diet therapy, but not as an indicator of glycemic control (Fig. 23-2). It should be further noted that a positive test result for ketones in the urine can be misleading and can be caused by the normal metabolic

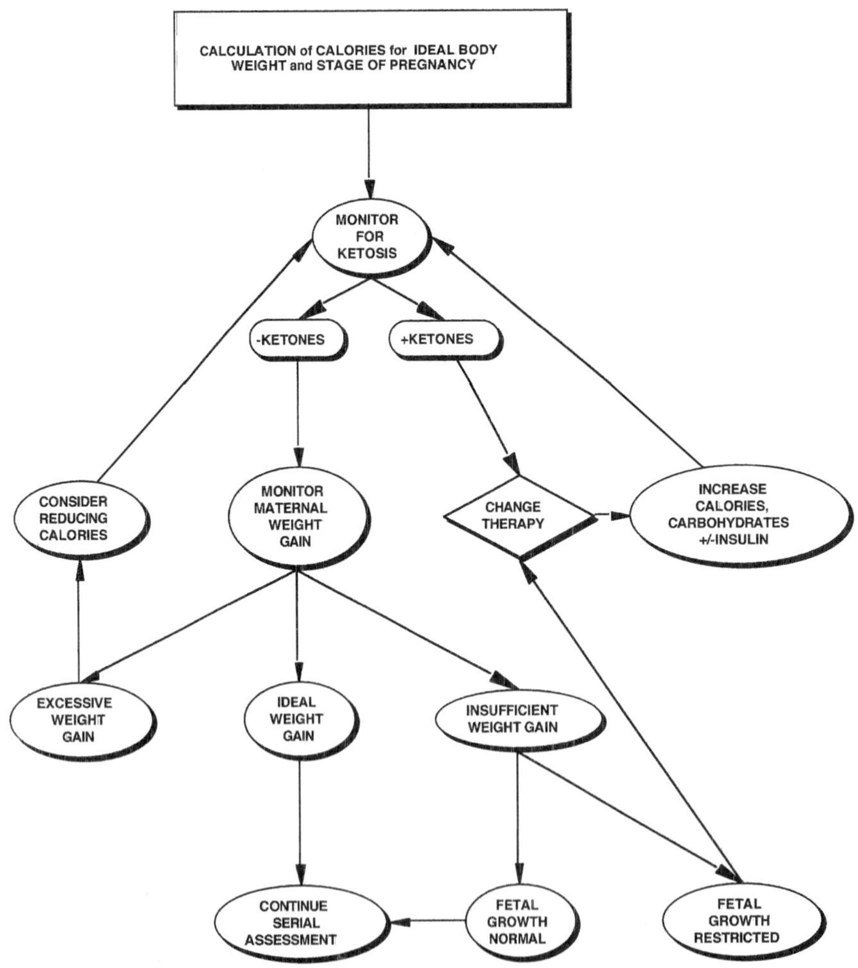

FIG. 23-2. Calculation of calories for ideal body weight and stage of pregnancy.

changes of pregnancy (i.e., accelerated starvation). Therefore, when ketones are present in the urine, blood analysis for ketones also should be performed prior to establishing diagnosis of ketonemia and initiating intervention.

Few studies have reported the use of diet alone to reverse metabolic dysfunction and lessen perinatal morbidities in patients with gestational diabetes. Although caloric restrictions have been advocated and implemented without detrimental effects (44), maternal and fetal outcomes for these patients have not been adequately analyzed. Presently, the use of diet control is usually restricted to patients with normal values of fasting glucose in the OGTT (less than 95 mg/dL) (39,40), or patients who are able to maintain fasting plasma levels of less than 105 mg/dL and postprandial values of less than 120 mg/dL.

Effective control of gestational diabetes by insulin administered at or before 32 weeks' gestation has been reported since the 1970's (45). In women at least 25 years of age, a decreased incidence of both macrosomia and perinatal mortality has been documented (46,47). The approach of "maximally tolerated" doses of insulin for treating gestational and insulin-dependent pregestational diabetes also has been reported (48). The results of this work indicate a decrease in the incidence of neonatal hypoglycemia, prevention of macrosomia, and no increase in perinatal mortality.

These results, however, reflect inconsistent stratification in the analyses by either type of diabetes (gestational or pregestational) or by severity of metabolic derangements. Consequently, the recommendation that all gestational diabetic patients receive insulin, made without defining criteria for treatment or endpoints to assess outcome, must be carefully examined (49).

Although tight control for pregestational insulin-dependent diabetic women is advocated by several groups (50,51), the data cannot be extrapolated to gestational diabetic patients. The fasting blood glucose level at which insulin should be initiated is controversial: some clinicians consider 130 mg/dL the threshold (52); others have proposed either 105 or 110 mg/dL (53,54). It is important to correlate perinatal outcomes with the gray zone of daily fasting blood glucose levels of 90 to 150 mg/dL. Published data support little improvement in perinatal outcome when control is changed from poor to fair (55). In most of the studies cited, however, small sample sizes with heterogeneous groups and inadequate stratification or control of important factors such as gestational age, birth weight, maternal age, and severity of maternal metabolic derangements introduce bias into the analyses that influences interpretation of the results and generalization of the conclusions.

It is now generally agreed that perinatal morbidity and mortality are increased when gestational diabetes is undetected or treated casually (47). It also is apparent that when gestational diabetes is identified early in pregnancy and patients are enrolled in programs for "high risk" obstetric monitoring, excessive perinatal mortality is eliminated (55–57). Perinatal morbidity, however, despite intensive obstetric care, appears unaffected (58).

We attempted to answer the question of whether a large-scale program based on verified blood glucose data, uniform criteria for insulin initiation (fasting plasma of less than 95 mg/dL), appropriate insulin dosage, and frequent glycemic assessment would result in improved perinatal outcome that was also cost effective. In a prospective large-scale study of over 2,500 GDM patients and approximately 5,000 nondiabetic control individuals, we demonstrated that intensified therapy significantly improved perinatal outcome when compared with the conventional approach. In addition, the perinatal outcome was similar for both the intensified and nondiabetic subjects. Moreover, the cost effectiveness of the intensified therapy showed a four- to seven-fold higher benefit/cost ratio when compared with the conventional approach (59).

The paucity of existing information precludes definitive, informed therapeutic recommendations despite the enormity of the population for which such recommendations might be indicated. Although there are no current universal guides to help decide between insulin- and diet-only regimens, several investigators have suggested useful algorithms that rapidly produce near-normal levels of control. Insulin treatment for pregnant women with type I diabetes generally consists of multiple injections of mixed insulins or initiating pump (continuous subcutaneous infusion of insulin) therapy. To ensure optimization of therapy, self-monitoring of blood glucose also is considered to be a part of the treatment approach. This permits the patient to determine as accurately as possible the level of glucose control achieved through different amounts of insulin. It also permits synchronization with diet. The same treatment approach (insulin and self-monitoring) may be used with type II diabetic women and gestational diabetic women. Here, again, achievement of control is the goal. The type II diabetic woman should be treated with insulin during pregnancy.

For the gestational diabetic woman, the initiation of insulin versus diet only is based on the level of control desired (usually normoglycemia), the ability to achieve tight control rapidly, and the willingness of the patient to accept the insulin modality.

Three major issues need to be considered regarding insulin therapy: who should get it; how much insulin should be given; and does this treatment improve perinatal outcome? As mentioned before, gestational diabetes is characterized by a combination of diminished insulin secretion accompanied by insulin resistance. The diminished secretion in pregnancy is reflected in fasting plasma glucose levels of greater than 95 mg/dL. Thus, these patients will probably need additional exogenous insulin to meet their requirements (11). In earlier work, we described the insulin requirements in gestational and pregestational diabetic women using memory reflectance meters to obtain accurate, reliable data. We found that in type II and gestational diabetes the total daily dose ranged from 60 to 90 units per day and that the time of greatest instability in glucose metabolism was at 20 to 32 weeks' gestation, when frequent adjustments of insulin were required. In contrast, a lower dose of about 40 to 50 units per day was necessary in insulin-dependent diabetic individuals (type I), who had a three-phase insulin requirement during pregnancy (27,28). We can conclude from this that in gestational diabetes, insulin requirements are dependent on fasting plasma glucose level and gestational age, and that type I and type II diabetes have characteristically increased insulin requirements throughout pregnancy. Using this approach, we also managed to achieve pregnancy outcomes comparable with those of nondiabetic women. For a detailed scheme of insulin initiation, see Fig. 23-3.

At what level should maternal glucose be maintained to prevent perinatal morbidity and mortality in pregnancies complicated by diabetes mellitus? Can so-called "tight" control limit fetal growth? In a large study of patients with gestational diabetes, the relationship between optimal levels of glycemic control and perinatal outcome was examined (60). Three groups were identified on the basis of mean blood glucose level throughout pregnancy. The low group (86 mg/dL) had a significantly higher incidence of IUGR infants (20%). In contrast, the incidence of LGA infants was 21-fold higher in the high mean blood glucose category (≥105mg/dL). No significant difference was found between the control and the mean blood glucose category of 87 to 104 mg/dL in the incidence of SGA or LGA infants. Thus, a relationship exists between the level of glycemic control and neonatal weight. This information is useful in targeting the level of glycemic control to optimize pregnancy outcome (60). Here, again, self-monitoring plays a major role in the assurance of maintenance of metabolic control. For these patients poor control presents a higher risk of developing large infants, who in turn may require cesarean section and premature delivery.

Because constant evaluation of glycemia in pregnancy is the best gauge of the efficacy of the treatment, the use of self-monitoring of blood glucose has become a principal component of management. However, self-monitoring blood glucose presents a dilemma in actual compliance and reliability of reporting. We found that to obtain reliable data, it is necessary to use memory reflectance meters (61). Data collected without this technique based solely on patient reporting are of dubious value.

The introduction of reflectance meters to measure capillary blood glucose more than a decade ago provided the first opportunity to gauge glucose levels accurately on an ambulatory basis. Recent advances in self-monitoring blood glucose have made it possible to gather significant amounts of glucose data, interpret these data rapidly, and make alterations in treatment to optimize control. The addition to this device of a memory that permits the storage of 2 weeks to 3 months of glucose data (up to 400 readings), helps to assure accurate and reliable data. More importantly, the data can be rapidly analyzed by computer to assess control by hour, day, week, and month.

An alternative method for analysis of capillary blood glucose, the ambulatory glucose profile (62), was used to demonstrate the difference in patterns of metabolic control in different types of diabetes in pregnancy. This new approach to representation of metabolic control in pregnancy also provided an innovative computer-based system for interpretation and analysis. This, in turn, may facilitate a rapid, efficient evaluation of control, enable easy interpretation, and lead to an overall improved method for characterization of metabolic control in pregnancy.

Blood glucose level is an important indicator of overall maternal and fetal well-being in pregnancy, but other approaches also are necessary to detect complications. Examination of the fetus by ultrasonography provides the best avenue for assessment of fetal growth (16,63). Fetal measurements at the 28th, 32nd, and 37th gestational weeks are a means of detecting both macrosomia and intrauterine growth retardation. Based on these measurements, alterations in management and decisions concerning early delivery can be made. Again, the focus is prevention of complications, assurance of normal fetal development, and normal delivery.

Delivery

Because diabetes in pregnancy has been associated so closely with macrosomia, the question of when cesarean section is appropriate is often raised. The LGA infant of a diabetic mother is at higher risk for shoulder dystocia, even in weight categories of less than 4,000 g, when compared with babies of nondiabetic women. This risk is even greater when the macrosomic infant weighs more than 4,250 g. Thus, in weight estimation of this number or greater, delivery by elective cesarean section is preferred. It should be noted that fetal weight estimation by ultrasonographic methods carries a 15% to 20% absolute error (mean ± 2 standard deviations). Normal delivery is usually achievable in the well-controlled diabetic woman, provided that evidence of normal fetal development exists. Indications for early delivery, therefore, should include large fetal size relative to gestational age, poor compliance to the prescribed insulin regimen, maternal vasculopathy, and history of previous stillbirth.

During labor, careful attention to insulin needs is necessary. A variety of regimens have been proposed for intravenous insulin delivery and glucose administration. I prefer the approach of a mixed solution of 5% to 10% dextrose in water with insulin added to the dextrose solution. An initial loading dose of 0.1 U/kg is used, and the rate is adjusted to maintain plasma glucose in the range of 80 to 100 mg/dL. Gestational diabetic women will be

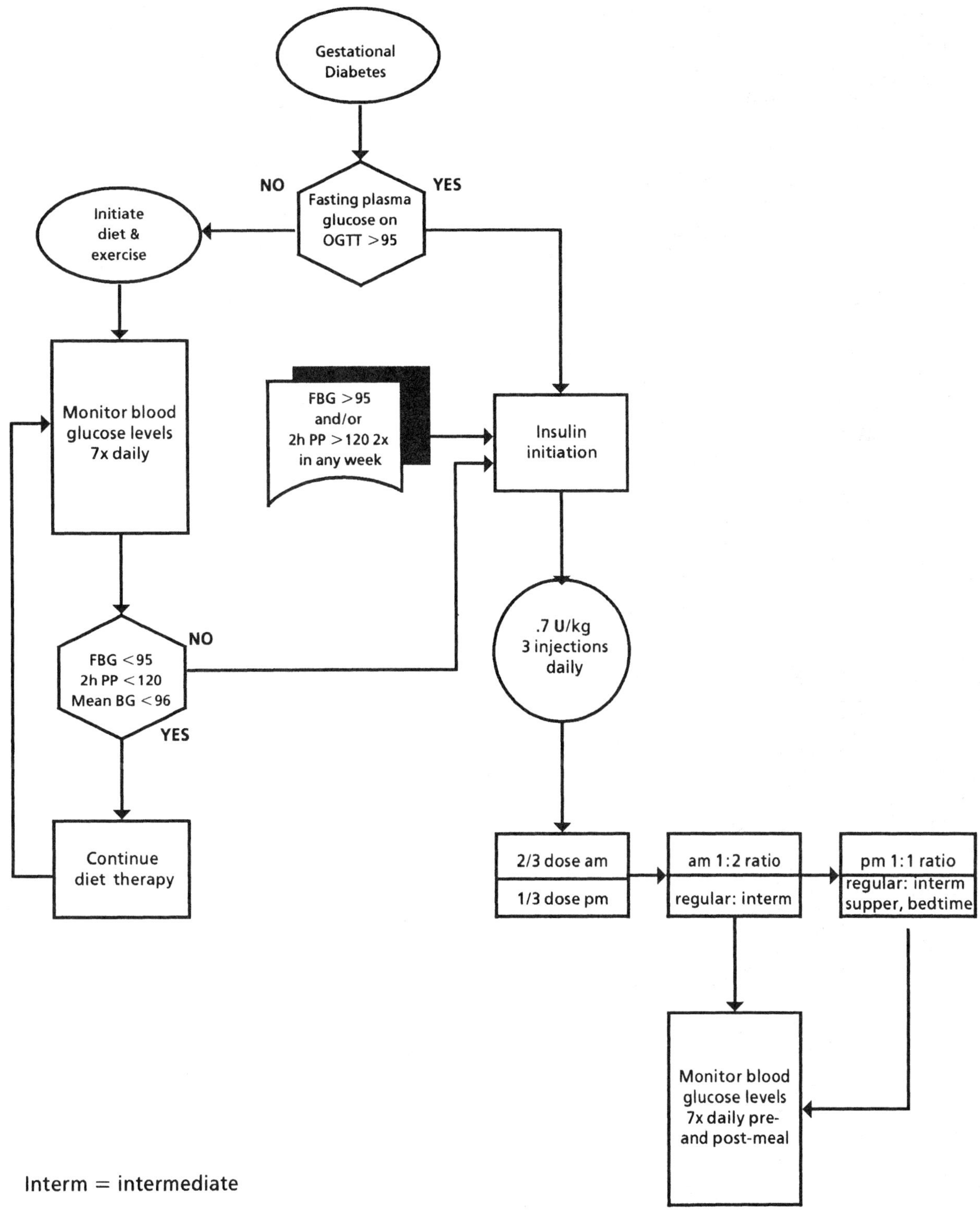

FIG. 23-3. Scheme of insulin initiation.

in normal glycemia without insulin administration soon after delivery. In pregestational diabetes, one third of the dose used during late pregnancy should be given to the patient during the immediate postpartum period, with subsequent adjustments made according to the level of control desired.

Postpartum

For the pregestational diabetic woman, maintenance of glycemic control and counseling for future pregnancies are the best means to minimize complications in pregnancy. Careful attention to issues prior to pregnancy prepares the diabetic for the intensive care needed to ensure normal outcome. Patient education, introduction to the concept of long-term commitment to tight control, planned pregnancies, counseling regarding the risk of fetal anomalies, and the risk of maternal complications are part of the recommended comprehensive program of care and education prior to pregnancy. The significant psychological and social stress experienced by diabetic women prior to and in pregnancy also must be addressed. These factors may, in the long run, have a greater influence on outcome than metabolic control per se.

For the gestational diabetic woman the key issue is to address those risk factors that can be altered prior to future pregnancies. Obesity is the principal factor that needs to be resolved soon after delivery and well in advance of the next pregnancy. Nutritional counseling with follow-up provides the best opportunity to intervene to regain ideal body weight. Detection of type II diabetes through periodic reassessment by OGTT (13) also provides early identification and implementation of appropriate therapy.

REFERENCES

1. National Diabetes Data Group. Diabetes in America. Washington, DC: USDHHS, 1985.
2. Mazze RS, Langer O. Primary, secondary, and tertiary prevention. Program for diabetes in pregnancy. Diabetes Care 1988;11:263–268.
3. Fuhrmann K. Diabetic control and outcome in the pregnant patient. In: Peterson CM, ed. Diabetes management in the 80's. New York: Praeger, 1982:66–81.
4. Fuhrmann K. Effect of the conceptus on maternal metabolism during pregnancy. In: Leibel BS, Wrenshall GA, eds. On the nature and treatment of diabetes. Amsterdam: Excerpta Medica, 1965:679–691.
5. Metzger BE, Ravnikar V, Vileisis RA, Freinkel N. "Accelerated starvation" and the skipped breakfast in late normal pregnancy. Lancet 1982; 1:588–592.
6. Freinkel N, Metzger BE, Nitzan M, Daniel R, Surmaczynska BZ, Nagel TC. Facilitated anabolism in late pregnancy: some novel maternal compensations for accelerated starvation. In Malaisse WJ, Pirart J, eds. Proceedings of the VIIth Congress of the International Diabetes Federation. International Congress Series No. 312. Amsterdam: Excerpta Medica, 1974:474–488.
7. Tsibris JCM, Raynor LO, Buhi WC, Buggie J, Spellacy WN. Insulin receptors in circulating erythrocytes and monocytes from women on oral contraceptives or pregnant women near term. J Clin Endocrinol Metab 1980;51:711–717.
8. Moore P, Kolterman O, Weyant J, Olefsky JM. Insulin binding in human pregnancy: comparisons to the postpartum, luteal, and follicular states. J Clin Endocrinol Metab 1981;52:937–941.
9. Puavilai G, Drobny EC, Domont LA, Baumann G. Insulin receptors and insulin resistance in human pregnancy: evidence for a postreceptor defect in insulin action. J Clin Endocrinol Metab 1982;54:247–253.
10. DeFronzo RA. The triumvirate: β-cell, muscle, liver: a collusion responsible for NIDDM. Diabetes 1988;37:667–687.
11. DeFronzo RA, Ferrannini E. The pathogenesis of non-insulin-dependent diabetes: an update. Medicine 1982;61:125–140.
12. Langer O, Berkus M, Brustman L, Anyaegbunam A, Gonzales D, Mazze R. The rationale for insulin management in gestational diabetes mellitus. Diabetes 1991;40(suppl 2):186–190.
13. Lowy C. Management of diabetes in pregnancy. Diabetes Rev 1993;9: 147–160.
14. Kitzmiller J. A regional perinatal program to prevent congenital anomalies in infants of diabetic mothers. Proceedings of the Society for Gynecological Investigation, Toronto, 1986.
15. Karlson K, Kjellmer I. The outcome of diabetic pregnancies in relation to the mother's blood sugar level. Am J Obstet Gynecol 1972;112:213–220.
16. Landon MB, Langer O, Gabbe SG, Schick C, Brustman L. Fetal surveillance in pregnancies complicated by insulin-dependent diabetes mellitus. Am J Obstet Gynecol 1992;167:617–621.
17. White P. Diabetes mellitus in pregnancy. Clin Perinatol 1974;1:331–347.
18. Mills JL, Baker L, Goldman AS. Malformations in infants of diabetic mothers occur before the seventh gestational week. Diabetes 1979;28: 292–293.
19. Salder TW. Effects of maternal diabetes on embryogenesis, II. Hyperglycemia-induced exencephaly. Teratology 1980;21:349–356.
20. Reece EA, Pinter EA, Leranth CZ, et al. Ultrastructural analysis of malformations of the embryonic neural axis induced by in vitro hyperglycemia conditions. Teratology 1985;32:363–373.
21. Miller E, Hare JW, Cloherty JP, et al. Elevated maternal hemoglobin A1c in early pregnancy and major congenital anomalies in infants of diabetic mothers. N Engl J Med 1981;304:1331–1334.
22. Pedersen LM. Pregnancy and diabetes. A survey. Acta Endocrinol 1980;94:(suppl 238):13–19.
23. Miodovnik M, Mimouni F, Dignan PS, et al. Major malformations in infants of IDDM women: vasculopathy and early first-trimester poor glycemic control. Diabetes Care 1988;11:713–718.
24. Mills JL, Knopp RH, Simpson JL, et al. Lack of relation of increased malformation rates in infants of diabetic mothers to glycemic control during organogenesis. N Engl J Med 1988;318:671–676.
25. Fuhrmann K, Reiher H, Semmler K, Fischer FF, Fischer M, Glockner E. Prevention of congenital malformation in infants of insulin-dependent diabetic mothers. Diabetes Care 1983;6:219–223.
26. Freinkel N. Of pregnancy and progeny. Diabetes 1980;20:1023–1025.
27. Page MM, Alberti KG, Greenwood R, et al. Treatment of diabetic coma with continuous low-dose infusion of insulin. Br Med J 1974;2:687–690.
28. Schade DS, Santiago JV, Skyler JS, Rizza RA. Intensive insulin therapy. Amsterdam: Excerpta Medica, 1983.
29. Fisher JN, Kitabchi AE. A randomized study of phosphate therapy in the treatment of diabetic ketoacidosis. J Clin Endocrinol Metab 1983;57: 177–180.
30. Defronzo R, ed. Ketoacidosis and lactic acidosis. Diabetes Rev 1994;2: 131–254.
31. Kreisberg RA. Diabetic ketoacidosis: revisited again. Mayo Clin Proc 1988;63:1144–1146.
32. Report of the Expert Committee on the Diagnosis and Classification of Diabetes Mellitus. Diabetes Care 1997;20:1183–1197.
33. O'Sullivan JB, Mahan CM. Criteria for the oral glucose tolerance test in pregnancy. Diabetes 1964;13:278–285.
34. Carpenter MW, Coustan DR. Criteria for screening tests for gestational diabetes. Am J Obstet Gynecol 1982;144:768–772.
35. Langer O. Management of gestational diabetes. Clin Perinatol 1993;30: 603–617.
36. Olofsson P, Liedholm H, Sartor G, Sjoberg NO, Svenningsen NW, Ursing D. Diabetes and pregnancy. A 21-year Swedish material. Acta Obstet Gynecol Scand 1984;122(suppl):3–62.
37. Pedersen J, Molsted-Pedersen L. Prognosis of the outcome of pregnancy in diabetics. Acta Endocrinol 1965;50:70–75.
38. White P. Pregnancy complicating diabetes. Am J Med 1949;7:609.
39. Freinkel N, Josimovich J. Report of workshop chairman: summary and recommendations. Diabetes Care 1980;3:499–501.
40. Proceedings of the Second International Workshop-Conference on Gestational Diabetes Mellitus, October 25–27, 1984, Chicago, Illinois. Diabetes 1985;34(suppl 2):123–126.
41. Langer O, Brustman L, Anyaegbunam A, Mazze RS. The significance of one abnormal OGTT value on adverse outcome in pregnancy. Am J Obstet Gynecol 1987;157:758–763.
42. Langer O, Anyaegbunam A, Brustman L, Divon M. A prospective randomized study: management of women with one abnormal oral glucose tolerance test value reduces adverse outcome in pregnancy. Am J Obstet Gynecol 1989;161:593–599.
43. Langer O, Damus K, Maiman M, Divon M, Levy J, Bauman W. A link between relative hypoglycemia-hypoinsulinemia during oral glucose tolerance tests and intrauterine growth retardation. Am J Obstet Gynecol 1986;155:711–716.
44. Wilkerson HLC, Remein QR. Studies of abnormal carbohydrate metabolism in pregnancy: the significance of impaired glucose tolerance. Diabetes 1957;6:324–329.
45. Langer O, Anyaegbunam A, Brustman L, Guidetti D, Mazze RS. Gestational diabetes: insulin requirements throughout pregnancy. Am J Obstet Gynecol 1988;159:544–547.

46. Langer O. Maternal glycemic criteria for insulin therapy in GDM. Diabetes Care. In press.
47. Merkatz IR, Adam PAJ, eds. The diabetic pregnancy: a perinatal perspective. New York: Grune & Stratton, 1979.
48. Roversi GD, Gargiulo M, Nicolini U, et al. A new approach to the treatment of pregnant diabetic women. Report of 479 cases seen from 1963–1975. Am J Obstet Gynecol 1979;135:567–576.
49. Coustan DR, Imarah J. Prophylactic insulin treatment of gestational diabetes reduces the incidence of macrosomia, operative delivery, and birth trauma. Am J Obstet Gynecol 1984;150:836–842.
50. Jovanovic L. Effect of euglycemia on the outcome of pregnancy in insulin-dependent diabetic women as compared with normal control subjects. Am J Med 1981;71:921–927.
51. Jovanovic L. Management of the pregnant, insulin-dependent diabetic woman. Diabetes Care 1980;3:63–68.
52. Frienkel N. In: Ellenberg M, Rifkin H, eds. Diabetes mellitus: theory and practice, 3rd ed. New York: Medical Examination Publishers, 1983: 689–714.
53. Gabbe S. Management and outcome of class A diabetes mellitus. Am J Obstet Gynecol 1977;127:465–469.
54. Oakley NW. The management of diabetes in pregnancy. In: Bratt RG, ed. Perinatal medicine, 2nd ed. Stockholm: Almguist & Wiksell, 1976:92–97.
55. Ogata ES, Sabbagha R, Metzger BE, Phelps RL, Depp R, Frienkel N. Serial ultrasonography to assess evolving fetal macrosomia: studies in 23 pregnant diabetic women. JAMA 1980;243:2405–2408.
56. Garn SM, Clark DC. Trends in fatness and the origins of obesity. Pediatrics 1976;57:443–456.
57. Goldberg JD, Franklin B, Lasser D, et al. Gestational diabetes: impact of home glucose monitoring on neonatal birth weight. Am J Obstet Gynecol 1986;154:546–550.
58. Gyves MT, Schulman PK, Merkatz IR. Results of individualized intervention in gestational diabetes. Diabetes Care 1980;3:495–496.
59. Langer O, Rodriguez DA, Xenakis EMJ, McFarland MB, Berkus MD, Arredondo F. Intensified vs. conventional management of gestational diabetes. Am J Obstet Gynecol 1994;170:1036–1047.
60. Langer O, Levy J, Brustman L, Anyaegbunam A, Merkatz R, Divon M. Glycemic control in gestational diabetes mellitus—how tight is tight enough: small for gestational age versus large for gestational age? Am J Obstet Gynecol 1989;161:646–653.
61. Brustman, Langer O, Engel S, Anyaegbunam A. Verified self-monitored blood glucose data versus glycosylated hemoglobin and glycosylated serum protein as a means of predicting short- and long-term metabolic control in gestational diabetes. Am J Obstet Gynecol 1987;157: 699–703.
62. Mazze RS, Lucido D, Langer O, Hartmann K, Rodbard D. Ambulatory glucose profile: representation of verified self-monitored blood glucose data. Diabetes Care 1987;10:111–117.
63. Langer O, Kozlowski S, Brustman L. Abnormal growth patterns in diabetes in pregnancy: longitudinal study. Isr J Med Sci 1991;27: 516–523.

Cherry and Merkatz's Complications of Pregnancy,
Fifth Edition, edited by W. R. Cohen.
Lippincott Williams & Wilkins, Philadelphia © 2000.

CHAPTER 24

Pituitary and Adrenal Cortical Disorders

Brian L. Cohen and Charmaine D. Cohen

PITUITARY AND ADRENAL CORTICAL DISORDERS

The pituitary, thyroid, and adrenal glands have important and pivotal roles in conception, pregnancy, and parturition. Disorders of these endocrine systems during pregnancy may exert profound effects on both maternal and fetal physiology. Patients with any of these conditions may suffer significant abnormal clinical courses of which physicians need to be aware. This chapter outlines the more important facets of management of pituitary and adrenocortical complications associated with pregnancy.

THE PITUITARY GLAND

Alterations in anterior and posterior pituitary function are uncommon in pregnancy. Many disorders result in infertility, but after these disorders are treated, successful pregnancy can occur. Surveillance during pregnancy is indicated, particularly with anterior pituitary adenomas.

Anterior Pituitary Gland

The cells of the anterior pituitary gland undergo differential changes during pregnancy. Pituitary enlargement is recognized to be a normal and expected occurrence in pregnancy (1). Marked hyperplasia of the lactotrophs occurs throughout the various stages of pregnancy and is sustained for a significant period in the postpartum months (2). The corticotroph and thyrotroph cell populations are unchanged throughout pregnancy (3), whereas the numbers of follicle-stimulating hormone and luteinizing hormone cells are considerably reduced. The consequences of these cytologic changes are readily seen by magnetic resonance imaging studies (MRI) (4,5) accompanied by nonvisualization of the posterior pituitary gland.

B. L. Cohen and C. D. Cohen: Albert Einstein College of Medicine, Bronx, NY 10461-1602.

Pituitary Adenomas

Prolactin-secreting pituitary adenomas are the most common anterior pituitary lesions. They are benign neoplasms composed mainly of lactotroph cells. Malignant tumors almost never are encountered, and few have been reported in the literature (6,7).

Normal prolactin secretion by the anterior pituitary gland is under tonic inhibitory control by dopamine. In pituitary adenomas, hypersecretion of prolactin occurs with variable clinical manifestations, including anovulatory infertility. Prolactinomas are diagnosed by radiologic imaging in the presence of hyperprolactinemic states. They are classified by size: *microadenomas*, smaller than 10 mm in diameter; *macroadenomas*, larger than 10 mm in diameter; and *macroadenomas*, with *extrasellar extension* (8). Compression of the optic chiasm with consequent visual field defects is a potentially serious complication of pituitary gland enlargement.

Management of Prolactinomas during Pregnancy

Anovulatory patients with prolactin-secreting pituitary adenomas who wish to become pregnant usually are treated with the dopamine agonist bromocriptine. Other therapeutic options include surgery, radiotherapy, or a combination of these treatments. The major issues to be considered in a pregnant woman with a prolactinoma are the effect of pregnancy on the prolactinoma and the effect of treatment, in particular bromocriptine, on the pregnancy and fetus.

Effect of Pregnancy on the Prolactinoma

Microadenoma

Symptomatic enlargement of pituitary tumors during pregnancy is possible as a result of the stimulating effects of estrogen on lactotroph growth (9). Molitch (7) reported that, of 246 patients with microadenomas from

16 series, 4 (1.6%) had symptoms compatible with tumor enlargement (i.e., headaches or visual disturbance). In the same report, 11 (4.5%) patients had asymptomatic tumor expansion as evidenced by radiologic assessment. In the group of 45 patients with macroadenomas without any treatment before pregnancy, 7 (15.5%) had symptomatic growth and 4 (9.8%) had asymptomatic enlargement. Molitch also reported on 46 patients with macroadenomas with treatment (i.e., surgery or radiotherapy) before pregnancy. Only 2 (4.3%) developed symptomatic tumor growth (8). There were no patients with asymptomatic tumor growth (8). Spontaneous regression of a prolactinoma during pregnancy also has been reported (9).

For the hyperprolactinemic woman with a microadenoma or a macroadenoma that is confined to the sella turcica, bromocriptine alone is recommended because of its efficacy in restoring ovulation and the relatively low risk of tumor enlargement (8). After this type of medical therapy, 80% to 85% of patients will become pregnant (10). When pregnancy has been achieved, these patients should have careful follow-up for the duration of gestation. Bromocriptine therapy should be discontinued. Prolactin levels may increase for the first 6 to 10 weeks of gestation and then do not increase further. Divers and Yen have reported an absence of increasing prolactin levels in the presence of continuing tumor enlargement (11). Because of these observations, the periodic estimation of prolactin levels in pregnancy is of no benefit. Visual field testing and radiologic evaluation are recommended only for patients who become symptomatic (7). The option of surgical treatment is exercised in situations in which patients have not responded to bromocriptine treatment.

Macroadenoma

If suprasellar extension was present, Molitch reported a 15% to 35% risk of clinically serious tumor enlargement during pregnancy when only bromocriptine was used and then discontinued once the pregnancy was diagnosed (8). These patients must undergo intense surveillance with monthly Goldman perimetric visual field testing (12). MRI is indicated for patients with developing visual field deficiencies.

An alternative form of therapy involves prepregnancy transphenoidal debulking of the tumor followed by medical therapy to restore normal prolactin levels and ovulation, which greatly reduces the risk of subsequent pregnancy-related tumor enlargement (8).

With either of these management strategies, tumor enlargement may occur. Under these circumstances, the best management is the reinstitution of bromocriptine therapy. Surgery has a 1.5-fold risk of fetal loss in the first trimester and a fivefold risk in the second trimester (13). In patients with little or no response to medical therapy and in whom symptoms are developing, consideration must be given to the option of surgery or delivery if fetal maturity is sufficiently advanced.

Radiotherapy is viewed primarily as effective for the prepregnancy treatment of large adenomas when the patient is an unsuitable candidate for surgery, or as secondary treatment when surgical removal has been incomplete. Complications associated with radiotherapy include hypopituitarism and optic nerve atrophy.

Effect of Bromocriptine on the Pregnancy

Bromocriptine is a dopamine receptor agonist and a potent inhibitor of prolactin secretion. It is effective in inducing ovulation in hyperprolactinemic women. Treatment should be discontinued as soon as pregnancy is diagnosed. Although complications of pregnancy or birth defects in children of women treated with bromocriptine either before or during pregnancy are not increased (14), fetal exposure should be limited to the shortest possible period. Long-term follow-up of children exposed to bromocriptine during pregnancy has revealed normal growth and development (15). The use of bromocriptine throughout gestation has been reported, and no abnormalities were noted in the infants except for one who had an undescended testicle and one who had a talipes deformity (16).

Lactation

Prolactin is an important hormone for the initiation of lactation, but its importance is short-lived. In hyperprolactinemic states with or without radiologic evidence of an adenoma, breastfeeding is not contraindicated. In patients who have prolactinomas, breastfeeding does not stimulate tumor growth (17). Once breastfeeding is complete, bromocriptine therapy should be reinstituted if necessary. Occasionally, this therapy is unnecessary, because some women may resume normal spontaneous ovulatory cycles postpartum because of tumor infarction occurring as a result of expansion and shrinkage of pituitary blood flow during and after pregnancy (17).

Summary

Medical therapy (bromocriptine) can induce normal ovulatory cycles and permit pregnancy in up to 80% of women with prolactinonas (8). Transphenoidal surgery is an option for patients who do not respond to medical treatment. Only 50% to 60% of patients with microadenoma and a much smaller percentage with macroadenoma achieve long-term cure (8). When pregnancy is achieved, bromocriptine should be discontinued. A small percentage of patients with microadenomas will experience tumor expansion during pregnancy. This risk is higher for macroadenomas. Symptoms of headache and impairment of visual fields with radiologic evidence of tumor expansion generally regress promptly with bromocriptine treatment (18).

POSTERIOR PITUITARY GLAND

Diabetes Insipidus

Vasopression, like oxytocin, is a polypeptide hormone consisting of nine amino acids. Both hormones are synthesized in the hypothalamus and are transported to the posterior pituitary gland along neural tracts emanating from the supraoptic and paraventricular nuclei. After descending through the median eminence, they terminate in the posterior lobe of the pituitary gland.

The major functions of vasopressin are regulation of osmolality and blood volume. Vasopressin is a potent vasoconstrictor and has powerful antidiuretic properties. Oxytocin is a stimulant of muscular contractions in the uterus and myoepithelial activity in the breast.

Diabetes insipidus occurs as a result of a deficiency of vasopressin action in the tubules of the kidney, resulting in inadequate renal tubular reabsorption and a marked loss of water. The vasopressin deficiency is secondary to a defect in its synthesis or secretion and may be primary or idiopathic (30% of cases) or acquired secondary to a variety of conditions such as cranial injuries (16%), sellar and suprasellar tumors (25%), and vascular lesions (19). The condition is characterized by polydypsia, polyuria, and a low urinary specific gravity. The diagnosis is confirmed by using a water-deprivation test during which the patient is unable to concentrate urine in the presence of dehydration. Treatment is by means of L-deamino-8-D-arginine vasopressin (DDAVP or desmopressin acetate), a synthetic analog of vasopressin administered by the intranasal route.

Women who have a prior diagnosis of diabetes insipidus do not have any contraindication to achieving pregnancy (20). If pregnancy occurs, there appears to be no alteration in its clinical course, and labor is normal (21). This finding is of particular interest considering the common origin of vasopressin and oxytocin.

Pregnancy has an unpredictable effect on diabetes insipidus. In more than half of the cases (58%) described in one report, the patients' condition deteriorated in pregnancy (22). One explanation offered is the deactivation of vasopressin that can occur in placental tissue (23).

Most women who have diabetes insipidus require increasing doses of DDAVP during pregnancy in part because of increased metabolic clearance, probably mediated through placental vasopressinase (24). No adequate, well-controlled studies concerning any effects of DDAVP on the fetus have been reported. Available evidence has not suggested a causal relationship between DDAVP and congenital anomalies.

Sheehan Syndrome

Ischemic necrosis of the anterior pituitary gland following postpartum hemorrhage and shock is a well-known complication of pregnancy. The original description was in 1937 by Sheehan (25). Most cases have panhypopituitarism, with destruction of 95% to 99% of the anterior pituitary (26). The classic presentation is one of failure of lactation in the puerperium followed by amenorrhea, loss of axillary and pubic hair, infertility, hypothyroidism, and adrenocortical insufficiency (26). Less extensive destruction of the anterior pituitary gland is associated with variable degrees of hypopituitarism. Clinical features range from total hypopituitarism to insufficiency of just a single anterior pituitary hormone. Growth hormone is most commonly deficient and is an early signal of anterior pituitary failure. Gonodal function may be preserved. It is therefore possible for patients to become pregnant spontaneously; under these circumstances, if the condition is not recognized and treated appropriately, serious consequences to the mother and fetus may occur (27,28).

In the complete and classic case, both the basal and stress levels of the anterior pituitary hormones are low. If the pituitary necrosis is incomplete and partial, the basal hormone levels can be normal, but severely attenuated in response to stress, stimuli, or pregnancy (29). Patients with Sheehan syndrome can develop an empty fossa of normal size, which occurs secondary to a reduction in gland mass following the pituitary necrosis (30) and can be demonstrated clearly by radiologic imaging.

Posterior pituitary necrosis is an extremely rare association (31). Plasma oxytocin levels increase in normal pregnancy, and these patients have been reported to have normal labor (31).

In the classic and complete case of Sheehan syndrome, induction of ovulation followed by successful pregnancy has been achieved with human menopausal gonadotropins (32). During pregnancy, no abnormal placental function attributable to maternal anterior pituitary insufficiency has been reported, and pregnancy-specific placental hormones all have been noted to be normal (30,33). During pregnancy, full replacement for thyroid and adrenal function is indicated, especially if prepregnancy insufficiency of these systems is present (32).

The occurrence of spontaneous pregnancy does not exclude the possibility of the existence of Sheehan syndrome. The condition should be considered in all patients with a prior history of severe postpartum hemorrhage and circulatory collapse. Patients may not provide a clear history of these obstetric events, and laboratory testing always should be performed if suspicion exists. Laboratory testing for diagnosis in pregnancy requires careful interpretation.

Lymphocytic Hypophysitis

This is a rare complication with an autoimmune basis associated with pregnancy. Most cases occur during or shortly after delivery, and affected women manifest with varying degrees of panhypopituitarism or a mass lesion in the pituitary, leading to headaches and visual disturbances. Lymphocytic hypophysitis may be indistinguishable from a pituitary adenoma and is characterized by massive infiltration of the pituitary gland by lymphocytes and plasma cells with accompanying destruction of the normal parenchyma. Hyperprolactinemia and diabetes insipidus are often present, and radiologic studies mimic an anterior pituitary adenoma (34). This uncommon diagnosis should be considered in any patient who has features suggestive of pituitary insufficiency in the absence of obstetric hemorrhage. Evaluation of pituitary function is indicated, and appropriate hormone replacement therapy should be promptly instituted if hypopituitarism is confirmed. Spontaneous regression of the mass with return of normal pituitary function may occur (35,36). Emergent surgical intervention is warranted if radiologic evidence is found of progressive sellar enlargement with encroachment of the optic chiasm and visual field symptoms.

ADRENAL CORTEX

Both the adrenal cortex and the adrenal medulla exert important roles in the maintenance of normal pregnancy. Abnormalities of the adrenal glands can lead to potentially hazardous conditions in pregnancy with adverse consequences to both the mother and the fetus.

Glucocorticoids are synthesized in the adrenal cortex. Cortisol synthesis and release are under the control of pituitary adrenocorticotropin-releasing hormone (ACTH). Plasma ACTH levels increase throughout pregnancy, and significantly greater levels are present in laboring women than in nonpregnant women at rest (37). The weight of the maternal adrenal glands does not change during pregnancy, although there is a morphological increase in width of the zona fasciculata. In pregnancy, total serum concentrations of cortisol increase between 12 weeks and term, with levels reaching three to five times the nonpregnant state. The increase is largely related to the estrogen-induced increase in corticosteroid-binding globulin by the liver (37). Free cortisol levels in pregnancy are higher than in the nongravid woman (38). Although diurnal circadian variations are preserved during pregnancy, they have been reported to be blunted (38,39). The adrenal cortex also secretes mineralocorticoids, of which aldosterone is the most significant. Its role is to maintain electrolyte balance by retaining sodium and excreting potassium, therefore having a major influence on the regulation of blood pressure and the extracellular fluid compartment.

Cushing Syndrome in Pregnancy

Pregnancy in patients with untreated Cushing syndrome is rare because the endocrine consequences of hypercortisolemia often include anovulation and infertility. The diagnosis may be difficult because, in some women, pregnancy itself produces clinical signs suggestive of cortisol excess, such as central obesity, abdominal striae, and glucose intolerance (40). When the two conditions coexist, the physical features are enhanced and the diagnosis of Cushing syndrome may be suspected with greater confidence. Greater maternal morbidity is present because of the hypertension and diabetes that are features of Cushing syndrome and can be exacerbated by pregnancy.

The etiology of Cushing syndrome can be divided into exogenous (i.e., produced by iatrogenic administration of corticosteroids) and endogenous causes. The causes in a series of 108 patients over 17 years were reported by Orth and Liddle (41). The most common etiology was pituitary-dependent adrenal hyperplasia, followed by adrenal adenoma, adrenal carcinoma, and the syndrome caused by the ectopic secretion of ACTH. Most pituitary ACTH-secreting tumors are microadenomas. Most cases found in association with pregnancy are caused by an adrenal adenoma (42). Ectopic ACTH production as a cause of Cushing syndrome in pregnancy is rare; most reported cases occur in older people, with a male-to-female ratio of 10:1 (43).

The clinical features of Cushing syndrome are consequent to the catabolic state induced by the hypercortisolemia. There is muscle weakness, atrophy of the skin, striae, delayed wound healing, osteoporosis, blood vessel weakness leading to ecchymoses, and insulin antagonism causing glucose intolerance. Weight gain is centripetal, and hypertension and hirsutism may be severe. In pregnancy, maternal complications include hypertension, preeclampsia, diabetes, congestive heart failure, wound breakdown, and death (42) (Table 24-1). Affective changes of depression and overt psychosis may occur in up to two thirds of all patients with Cushing syndrome (42,44).

Table 24-2 describes the perinatal complications of patients with Cushing syndrome (42). There is a high perinatal mortality and morbidity, with premature labor and birth occurring in two thirds of the pregnancies. The overall perinatal mortality rate is 15% of reported cases, half of which were stillbirths. Intrauterine growth restriction, as evidenced by a birth weight less than the tenth percentile for gestational age, is reported in at least 25% of cases. Uteroplacental insufficiency resulting from the hypercortisolemia and hypertension is the underlying cause (42,45). Infants born to mothers with Cushing syndrome do not appear to suffer from any congenital malformation or virilization (42). An infant born with a cleft palate has been reported (46).

Laboratory confirmation of the diagnosis and interpretation of endocrine studies are complicated by the presence of the high estrogen levels found in pregnancy. The biochemical evaluation relies on the measurement of urinary free cortisol, the plasma cortisol response to low- and high-dose dexamethasone suppression tests, and the plasma ACTH levels. Radiologic localization of pituitary, adrenal, and ectopic ACTH-producing tumors depends mainly on MRI. Interpretation of pituitary imaging stud-

TABLE 24-1. *Cushing syndrome and maternal complications in 65 pregnancies*

		Etiology				
Complication	No. of patients	Adrenal hyperplasia	Adrenal adenoma	Adrenal carcinoma	Ectopic ACTH	Unknown
Hypertension	42 (64.6%)	7	27	4	1	3
Preeclampsia						
Simple	2 (3.1%)	1	1	0	0	0
Superimposed	4 (6.2%)	0	3	1	0	0
Diabetes	21 (32.3%)	2	15	3	0	1
Congestive heart failure	7 (10.8%)	0	7	0	0	0
Death	3 (4.6%)	0	1	1	1	0
Wound breakdown	5 (7.7%)	1	4	0	0	0

From Briescher MA, McClamrock HD, Adashi EY. Cushing syndrome in pregnancy. Obstet Gynecol 1992;79:130.

ies may be limited as the pituitary normally increases in size during pregnancy.

Treatment objectives focus on the elimination of hypercortisolemia. During pregnancy, this is accomplished by unilateral or bilateral adrenalectomy in cases of adrenal adenoma. Subsequent steroid replacement for the remainder of pregnancy and long-term replacement after delivery are mandatory. In Cushing syndrome resulting from a pituitary microadenoma (Cushing disease), transphenoidal adenectomy can be contemplated in pregnancy (47). Treatment must be individualized to the patient and the gestational age. Broad recommendations have appeared in the literature (48); definitive surgical treatment is suggested in early pregnancy. In late pregnancy, consideration may be given to delaying such definitive treatment until after delivery. Under these circumstances, specific medical treatment can be considered. Metyrapone, an inhibitor of 11-hydroxylase, can be administered. This drug has not been associated with any identifiable fetal effects (49), but the role of medical therapy remains limited to patients with mild hypercortisolemia. Other clinically useful medical therapies include aminoglutethimide, a 3β-ol-hydroxysteroid dehydrogenase inhibitor, and cyproheptadine, a serotonin antagonist. Adrenal surgery performed during pregnancy has not been associated with any adverse perinatal effects, and premature labor has not been a significant event (42).

In summary, although rare in pregnancy, the diagnosis of Cushing syndrome should be considered in certain clinical presentations. Unrecognized or untreated, maternal and fetal mortality and morbidity are high. A high index of clinical suspicion must be maintained and, when Cushing syndrome is diagnosed, treatment must be individualized between a definitive surgical approach and temporary medical intervention.

Addison Disease

Adrenal insufficiency is classified into *primary* (Addison disease), caused by adrenal gland hypofunction, and

TABLE 24-2. *Cushing syndrome and perinatal complications in 65 pregnancies*

		Etiology				
Complication	No. of patients	Adrenal hyperplasia	Adrenal adenoma	Adrenal carcinoma	Ectopic ACTH	Unknown
Spontaneous abortion[a]	2 (3.1%)	1	0	1	0	0
Perinatal death						
Neonatal death	5 (7.7%)	2	2	1	0	0
Stillbirth	5 (7.7%)	1	3	0	0	1
Premature birth[b]	42 (64.6%)	13	24	3	1	1
Intrauterine growth retardation[c]	7 (10.8%)	0	7	0	0	0
Death	3 (4.6%)	0	1	1	1	0
Wound breakdown	5 (7.7%)	1	4	0	0	0

ACTH, adrenocorticotropic hormone.
[a]Pregnancies terminating before 20 weeks' gestation.
[b]Pregnancies terminating between 20 and 38 weeks' gestation.
[c]Birth weight less than the tenth percentile for gestational age.
From Briescher MA, McClamrock HD, Adashi EY. Cushing syndrome in pregnancy. Obstet Gynecol 1992;79:130.

secondary, resulting from disorders of the hypothalamic–pituitary axis. Primary adrenocortical insufficiency is much less common than Cushing syndrome and has two main causes: autoimmune adrenal destruction and tuberculosis. The former may be part of a broader autoimmune polyendocrine deficiency syndrome of other endocrine glands (e.g., thyroid involvement resulting in thyroiditis and ovarian failure with subsequent amenorrhea and infertility).

Adrenal insufficiency in pregnancy is not associated with any problems specific to fetal development and health, because the fetoplacental unit initiates and controls its own intrauterine steroid environment. The pregnant woman, however, may exhibit marked clinical manifestations related to cardiovascular function with decreased cardiac output, loss of vascular tone, and profound hypovolemia, all of which can affect fetal oxygenation and nutrition adversely. If mineralocorticoid output also is compromised, electrolyte imbalance with hyponatremia and hypercalemia can cause death (50,51).

Adrenocortical insufficiency may present in a chronic or acute form. In the chronic syndrome, weakness, fatigue, abdominal pain and weight loss are the predominant symptoms, which may be accompanied by nausea, anorexia, increased pigmentation, and orthostatic hypotension. The acute syndrome or crisis may occur during the course of the chronic illness, or it may be the initial presentation of new-onset disease. More commonly, the acute crisis is consequent on the sudden withdrawal of exogenously administered adrenocortical hormones. It is an endocrine emergency and is characterized by abdominal, muscle, and joint pain, hypotension, and confusion.

Mild cases of previously unrecognized adrenocortical deficiency may first present with adrenal crisis in labor or the postpartum period (51). In less severe cases, glucocorticoids of fetal origin can cross the placenta and maintain maternal homeostasis (52).

In the primary form, laboratory findings confirm the clinical diagnosis and include hyponatremia, hyperkalemia, high blood urea nitrogen, and, in some instances, hypoglycemia and metabolic acidosis. Secondary adrenal insufficiency may be accompanied by normal electrolyte balance (53). Because the mineralocorticoid-producing component of the adrenal is not under pituitary ACTH control, the diagnosis is confirmed by a low cortisol level and a blunted or absent adrenal response to ACTH stimulation in the secondary variety.

Patients with Addison disease should be treated with specific hormone replacement to correct both glucocorticoid and mineralocorticoid deficiencies. Cortisol in divided doses is the mainstay of treatment, with a higher dose in the morning to mimic normal diurnal variation. The mineralocorticoid replacement is provided by the administration of fluorocortisone, the dose of which is adjusted according to postural blood pressure and measurement of serum electrolytes. All patients require continued education regarding their disease. During physiologically stressful situations, such as surgery or intercurrent illness, the dose of the replacement drugs should be increased to reflect the normally increased output of cortisol in normal persons exposed to such stress.

Exogenous Glucocorticoid Administration in Pregnancy

Numerous medical conditions are treated with exogenously administered steroids. When used in high doses, as in severe asthma or status asthmatics, appropriate therapies have not been teratogenic, nor have they exerted any other adverse effects on pregnancy (54). Initial indications from animal experiments suggesting an increased risk of cleft lip and palate have not been confirmed in humans. The pharmacologic effect of the active steroid in the fetus appears to be reduced by the placental enzyme 11β-OH dehydrogenase, which probably inactivates certain glucocorticoids (54). In asthma and autoimmune disorders, corticosteroids are known to be safe therapeutic agents in the pregnant state. If the underlying disease undergoes exacerbations during pregnancy, appropriate higher doses of steroids are indicated and can be used (55,56).

Caution must be exercised when prolonged glucocorticoid therapy is anticipated. Chronic infections may be exacerbated, and diabetes mellitus can be unmasked. All patients who receive long-term steroid therapy must be considered at high risk for the development of osteoporosis. High doses can predispose patients to peptic ulceration or esophagitis, and existing hypertension may be exacerbated.

When glucocorticoids are used in pregnancy on a long-term basis, it is critically important to administer stress doses of steroids at the time of delivery because of their effects of adrenal suppression. Equally important is that the complete withdrawal of steroids, when indicated, should be implemented on a gradual transition schedule. Normal pituitary–adrenal function will resume as the dose of exogenous steroids is gradually reduced to an alternate-day dosage schedule (or stopped completely) over a few weeks.

REFERENCES

1. Scheithauer BW, Sano T, Kovacs KT, Young WF, Ryan N, Randall RV. The pituitary gland in pregnancy: a clinico-pathologic and immunohistochemical study of 69 cases. Mayo Clin Proc 1990;65:461–474.
2. Stephaneau L, Kovacs K, Lloyd RV, et al. Pituitary lactotrophs and aomatotrophs in pregnancy: a correlative in situ hybridization and immunohistochemical study. Virchows Arch B Cell Pathol 1992;62: 291–296.
3. Gonzalez JG, Elizondo G, Saldivar D, Nanez H, Todd LE, Villarreal JZ. Pituitary gland growth during normal pregnancy: an in vivo study using magnetic resonance imaging. Am J Med 1988;85:217–220.
4. Hinshaw DB, Hasso AN, Thompson JR, Davidson BJ. High resolution computed tomography of the postpartum pituitary gland. Neuroradiology 1986;26:299–301.
5. Schelthauer BW, Randall RV, Laws ER Jr, Kovacs KT, Horvath E, Whitaker MD. Prolactin cell carcinoma of the pituitary. Cancer 1985; 55:598–604.

6. Walker JD, Grossman A, Anderson JV, et al. Malignant prolactinoma with extracranial metastases: a report of three cases. Clin Endocrinol 1993;38:411–419.
7. Molitch ME. Pathologic hyperprolactinemia. Endocrinol Metab Clin North Am 1992;21:887–901.
8. Molitch ME. Pregnancy and the hyperprolactinemic woman. N Engl J Med 1985;312:1364–1370.
9. Comtois R, Bertrand S, Beauregard H, Leger JL, Serri O. Spontaneous regression of a prolactin producing pituitary adenoma during pregnancy. Am J Med 1987;83:1105–1106.
10. Samaan NA, Schultz PN, Leavens TA, Leavens ME, Lee YY. Pregnancy after treatment in patients with prolactinoma: Operation versus bromocriptine. Am J Obstet Gynecol 1986;155:1300–1305.
11. Divers WA Jr, Yen SS. Prolactin-producing microadenomas in pregnancy. Obstet Gynecol 1983;61:425–429.
12. Prager D, Braunstein GD. Pituitary disorders during pregnancy. Endocrinol Metab Clin North Am 1995;24:1–14.
13. Brodsky JB, Cohen EN, Brown BW Jr, Wu ML, Whitcher C. Surgery during pregnancy and fetal outcome. Am J Obstet Gynecol 1980;138: 1165–1167.
14. Weil C. The safety of bromocriptine in long term use: a review of the literature. Curr Med Res Opin 1986;10:25–51.
15. Turkalj I, Braun P, Krupp P. Surveillance of bromocriptine in pregnancy. JAMA 1982;247:1589–1591.
16. Konopka P, Raymond JP, Merceron RE, Seneze J. Continuous administration of bromocriptine in the prevention of neurological complications in pregnant women with prolactinomas. Am J Obstet Gynecol 1983;146:935–938.
17. Speroff L, Olass RH, Kase NG, eds. Amenorrhea. In: Clinical gynecologic endocrinology and infertility, 5th ed, Baltimore: Williams & Wilkins:1994:401A56.
18. Bevan JS, Webster J, Burke CW, Scanton MF. Dopamine agonists and pituitary tumor shrinkage. Endocr Rev 1992;13:220–240.
19. Moses AM, Notman DD. Diabetes insipidus and syndrome of inappropriate antidiuretic hormone secretion (ADH). In: Stillerman GH, ed. Advances in internal medicine, vol 27. Chicago: Year Book Medical, 1982:73–100.
20. Hendricks CH. The neurohypophysis in pregnancy. Obstet Gynecol Surv 1954:9:323.
21. Gordon G, Bradford WP. Pregnancy in a patient with diabetes insipidus following induction of ovulation with clomiphene. J Obstet Gynaecol Br Commonw 1970;77:467–469.
22. Hime MC, Richardson JA. Diabetes insipidus and pregnancy: case report, incidence and review of literature. Obstet Gynecol Surv 1978;3: 375–379.
23. Campbell JW. Diabetes insipidus and complicated pregnancy. JAMA 1980;243:1744–1765.
24. Durr JA. Diabetes insipidus in pregnancy. Am J Kidney Dis 1987;9: 276–283.
25. Sheehan HL. Post-partum necrosis of the anterior pituitary. J Pathol Bacteriol 1937;45:189.
26. Haddock L, Vega LA, Aguilo F, Rodriquez O. Adrenocortical, thyroidal and human growth hormone reserve in Sheehan's syndrome. J Hopkins Med J 1972;131:80–99.
27. Israel S, Conston A. Unrecognized pituitary necrosis (Sheehan's syndrome): a cause of sudden death. JAMA 1952;148:189.
28. Moszkowski EF. Postpartum pituitary insufficiency: report of five unusual cases with long term follow-up. South Med J 1973;66: 878–882.
29. Grimes HG, Brooks MH. Pregnancy in Sheehan's syndrome: report of a case and review. Obstet Gynecol Surv 1980;35:451–458.
30. Fleckman AM, Schubart VK, Danziger A, Fleischer N. Empty sella of normal size in Sheehan's syndrome. Am J Med 1983;75:585–591.
31. Corral J, Calderon J, Goldzieher JW. Induction of ovulation and term pregnancy in a hypophysectomized woman. Obstet Gynecol 1972;39: 397–400.
32. Cohen BL, Baillie P. Sheehan's syndrome followed by successful pregnancy. S Afr Med J 1980;57:838–840.
33. Polishuk WZ, Palti Z, Rabau E, Lunenfield B, David A. Pregnancy in a case of Sheehan's syndrome following treatment with human gonadotropins. J Obstet Gynaecol Br Commonw 1965;72:778–780.
34. Pressman EK, Zeidman SM, Reddy UM, Epstein JL, Brem H. Differentiating lymphocytic adenohypophysitis from pituitary adenoma in the peripartum patient. J Reprod Med 1995;40:251–259.
35. McGrail KM, Beyerl BD, Black PM, Klibanski A, Zervas NT. Lymphocytic adenohypophysitis of pregnancy with complete recovery. Neurosurgery 1987;20:791–793.
36. Leiba S, Schindel B, Weinstein R, Lidor I, Friedman S, Matz S. Spontaneous postpartum regression of pituitary mass with return of function. JAMA 1986;255:230–232.
37. Carr BR, Parker CR Jr, Madden JD, MacDonald PC, Porter JC. Maternal plasma adrenocorticotrophin and cortisol relationships throughout human pregnancy. Am J Obstet Gynecol 1981;139:416–422.
38. Petersen RE. Cortisol. In: Fuchs F, Klopper A, eds. Endocrinology of pregnancy. 2nd ed, Hagerstown, MD: Harper and Row, 1977:157.
39. Nolten W, Lindheimer M, Rueckert P, Oparil S, Ehrlich EN. Diurnal patterns and regulation of cortisol secretion in pregnancy. J Clin Endocrinol Metab 1980;51:466–471.
40. Montgomery DA, Harley JM. Endocrine disorders [Review]. Clin Obstet Gynecol 1977;4:339–470.
41. Orth DN, Liddle GW. Results of treatment in 108 patients with Cushing syndrome. N Engl J Med 1971;285:243–247.
42. Buescher MA, McClamrock HD, Adashi EY. Cushing syndrome in pregnancy. Obstet Gynecol 1992;79:130–137.
43. Bandy PK. Disorders of the adrenal cortex. In: Wilson JD, Foster DW, eds. Williams textbook of endocrinology. 7th ed. Philadelphia: WB Saunders, 1985:816..
44. Plotz CM, Knowlton AI, Raga C. The natural history of Cushing syndrome. Am J Med 1952;13:597.
45. Warrell DW, Taylor R. Outcome for the fetus of mothers receiving prednisolone during pregnancy. Lancet 1968;1:117–118.
46. Khakoo H, Schwartz E, Pillari V, Peterson RE. Cushing syndrome in pregnancy. Int J Gynecol Obstet 1982;20:49–55.
47. Casson IF, Davis JC, Jeffreys RV, Silas JH, Williams SJ, Belchetz PE. Successful management of Cushing disease during pregnancy by transphenoidal adenectomy. Clin Endocrinol 1987;27:423–428.
48. Van der Spuy ZM, Jacobs HS. Management of endocrine disorders in pregnancy. Part II. Pituitary, ovarian and adrenal disease. Postgrad Med J 1984;60:312–320.
49. Gormley MJ, Hadden DR, Kennedy TL, Montgomery DA, Murnaghan GA, Sheridan B. Cushing syndrome in pregnancy-treatment with metyrapone. Clin Endocrinol 1982;16:283–293.
50. Vita JA, Silverberg SJ, Goland RS, Austin JH, Knowlton AI. Clinical clues to the cause of Addison's disease. Am J Med 1985;78:461–466.
51. O'Shaughnessy RW, Hackett KJ. Maternal Addison's disease and fetal growth retardation. J Reprod Med 1984;29:752–756.
52. Druker D, Shumak S, Angel A. Schmidt's syndrome presenting with intrauterine growth retardation and postpartum addisonian crisis. Am J Obstet Gynecol 1984;149:229–230.
53. Sipes SL, Malee MP. Endocrine disorders in pregnancy. Obstet Gynecol Clin North Am 1992;19:666–677.
54. Greenberger PA. Asthma in pregnancy. Clin Chest Med 1992;13:597–605.
55. Fitzsimons R, Greenberger PA, Patterson R. Outcome of pregnancy in women requiring corticosteroids for severe asthma. J Allergy Clin Immunol 1986;78:349–353.
56. Friedman SA, Bernstein MS, Kitzmiller JL. Pregnancy complicated by collagen vascular disease. Obstet Gynecol Clin North Am 1991;18: 213–236.

Cherry and Merkatz's Complications of Pregnancy,
Fifth Edition, edited by W. R. Cohen.
Lippincott Williams & Wilkins, Philadelphia © 2000.

CHAPTER 25

Pheochromocytoma

Wayne R. Cohen and James B. Young

THE SYMPATHOADRENAL SYSTEM

Chromaffin cells and postganglionic sympathetic neurons derive from a common embryonic cell type. Primitive neuroectodermal cells differentiate into sympathoadrenal system anlage. These sympathogonia become ganglion and chromaffin cells, the latter named for their propensity to stain with chromium salts. Whereas sympathetic nerves persist into adult life and are distributed widely, most chromaffin cells present in fetal life degenerate. Those that persist are found primarily in the adrenal medullae.

In addition to the adrenal, extensive chromaffin tissue is found in the fetus and newborn, from the neck to the pelvis along the sympathetic chain (1–4). In humans, the largest concentration of these cells is found in the preaortic retroperitoneal area near the origin of the inferior mesenteric artery; it is referred to as the organ of Zuckerkandl. This tissue involutes rapidly and becomes nonfunctional within weeks of birth. The paired adrenal medullae, together with the peripheral sympathetic nerves and ganglia and small clusters of persistent extraadrenal chromaffin cells, make up the sympathoadrenal system of the adult. This system influences a broad range of physiologic processes and is a major factor in the maintenance of cardiovascular and metabolic homeostasis.

The adrenal medullae synthesize, store, and release catecholamines. Epinephrine is the primary adrenal catecholamine secretory product in adult life; norepinephrine is also released, as is dopamine, to a lesser extent. Epinephrine and norepinephrine are probably secreted differentially in response to specific stresses (5). The medullae also release several physiologically active peptides, including substance P.

W.R. Cohen: Sinai Hospital of Baltimore, Baltimore, MD 21215; J.B. Young: Northwestern University Medical School, Chicago, IL 60611.

EPIDEMIOLOGY AND PATHOLOGY

Other than hypertension, the disease of the sympathoadrenal system that is of greatest significance during pregnancy is pheochromocytoma, a catecholamine-secreting tumor of chromaffin cells. Almost all of these neoplasms originate in the adrenal; about 5% to 10% are bilateral. Of the approximately 15% to 20% of pheochromocytomas that are of extraadrenal origin, most are found in remnants of the major abdominal para-aortic chromaffin bodies (6). The remainder arise along the sympathetic chain, anywhere from the cervical region to the lower pelvis. They have been found in the bladder, broad ligament, vagina, and sacrococcygeal area. Extraadrenal pheochromocytomas are sometimes referred to as paraganglionomas.

Pheochromocytomas are rare tumors. Their exact prevalence is impossible to determine. Somewhat more than 200 pregnancy-associated cases have been reported. They cause perhaps 1 in 1,000 cases of adult hypertension (7) and complicate approximately 1 in 30,000 pregnancies. Autopsy series suggest that these tumors are more common than is usually assumed, and many go undetected clinically (8,9). They are, nevertheless, well-known neoplasms, because their symptoms are often distinctive and dramatic, their removal promptly cures the hypertension and metabolic disturbances that accompany them, and their diagnosis and treatment are immensely gratifying to doctor and patient. Moreover, our understanding of pheochromocytoma has contributed to our knowledge of many aspects of sympathoadrenal physiology.

Untreated pheochromocytomas are often fatal, a risk that seems to be magnified during pregnancy, and for that reason prompt identification and treatment during gestation are especially important (10,11). If these tumors remain undiagnosed during pregnancy, maternal and fetal mortality can be as high as 50%. Diagnosis and proper treatment should lower the maternal mortality risk to near

1% and the fetal mortality rate to less than 25%. In a review of 35 cases of pheochromocytoma in pregnancy, Oishi and Sato (10) reported an 11% maternal mortality rate. Of the cases treated since 1981, in which modern techniques were used, the death rate was only 6%; all these maternal deaths were among women who were not diagnosed with pheochromocytoma before death. Their results, and those of many others (12–22), emphasize two principles: (a) failure to diagnose pheochromocytoma markedly increases the risks of morbidity and mortality for mother and fetus, and (b) diagnosis, if followed by scrupulous medical and surgical therapy, results in a good outcome in the great majority of cases.

In addition to the dangers of the associated hypertension and metabolic effects of catecholamines released by these tumors, about 10% to 15% are malignant, another motivation for prompt diagnosis. Malignancy seems to be more common at extraadrenal sites. Long-term follow-up of these cancers (as well as of benign pheochromocytomas) is particularly important, because metastases have been known to develop years after removal of the primary lesion (23).

Pheochromocytomas are encapsulated, highly vascular tumors that contain two cell types (Fig. 25-1a,b). The neurosecretory chief cell predominates, with a small number of spindle-shaped sustentacular cells. The chief cells are large and usually pleomorphic. The cytoplasm has many fine granules, which stain brown with chromium salts. Sometimes the cells assume a trabecular or areolar pattern. Central necrosis and hemorrhage are not unusual, especially in large tumors. Histologic examination is not helpful in determining whether a pheochromocytoma is malignant, because even benign tumors can have considerable cellular pleomorphism, atypia, and mitotic activity. Even those tumors with gross or microscopic invasion of the capsule can act in a benign fashion. The ability to identify malignant pheochromocytomas is further confounded by the fact that even benign cases are sometimes of multicentric origin, and distinguishing a remote second benign lesion from a metastasis is not possible. Benign pheochromocytomas may persist or recur, or a second benign tumor may arise at a distant site years after the first was excised (24).

The potential for malignancy must therefore be judged by the activity of the disease rather than its histologic or biochemical features. When they are cancerous, pheochromocytomas tend to spread slowly. However, there are cases of distant metastases, which can be hormonally functional. In fact, even in the case of malignant tumors it is usually the difficulty in controlling their catecholamine production that causes the majority of morbidity and mortality. Unfortunately, the tumors are not particularly sensitive to radiation or chemotherapy in most cases, and the 5-year survival rate is about 50%. Some tumors have responded to combination chemotherapy with cyclophosphamide, vincristine, and dicarbazine

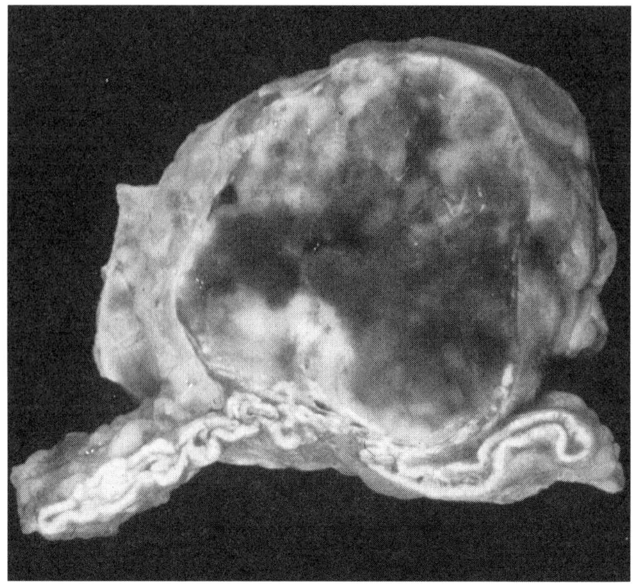

A

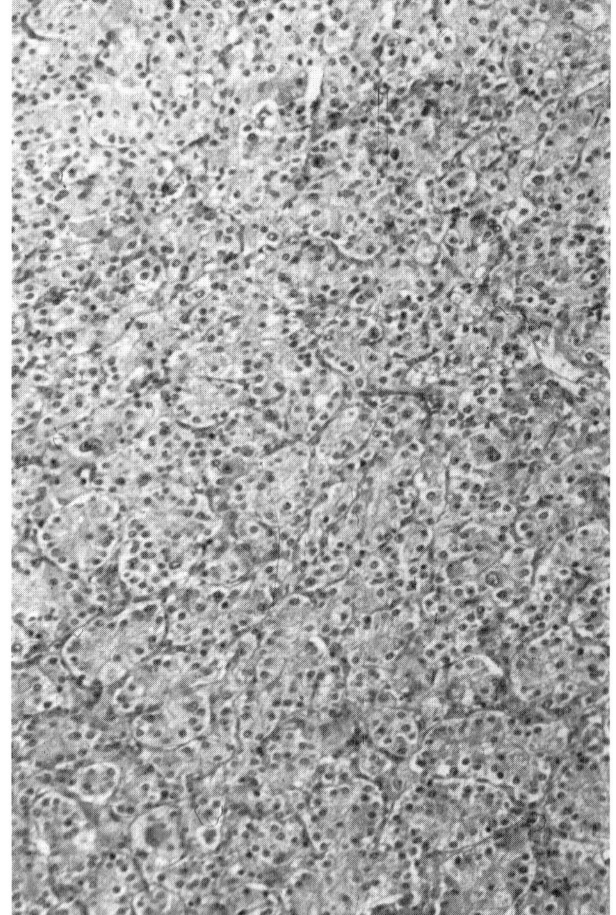

B

FIG. 25-1. a: Gross appearance of a small, bisected pheochromocytoma and adjacent adrenal. **b:** Histologic features of the same tumor. Large, pleomorphic chief cells predominate in a trabecular pattern. (Courtesy of Belur Bhagavan, M.D., Sinai Hospital of Baltimore.)

(25). Malignant pheochromocytomas have been reported in pregnancy (26–29).

Although the great majority of pheochromocytomas arise sporadically, at least 10% to 15% develop as part of multiple endocrine neoplasia (MEN) syndromes (30). If precise screening techniques were widely employed, a larger proportion would likely be identified. In addition, pheochromocytomas may be found in families as isolated autosomal dominantly inherited tumors. They are also found with increased frequency in patients with various heritable neuroectodermal dysplasias, including von Hippel–Lindau disease, von Recklinghausen neurofibromatosis, Stürge-Weber syndrome, and tuberous sclerosis (31). Whereas sporadic cases are generally unilateral, familial cases are more likely to be bilateral in the adrenals or even at multiple sites. Indeed, one of the virtues of accurate chromaffin tumor diagnosis, aside from the potentially life-saving benefit to mother and fetus, is the possibility of recognizing the presence of a familial syndrome. This has potential benefits not only for the patient but for her family members as well.

Two MEN syndromes are identified. MEN 1 is an autosomal dominant trait with high penetrance. Its gene has been identified (32) and found to encode for a nucleoprotein the function of which is uncertain. The ability to identify affected individuals should be available soon. MEN 1 patients have one or more of parathyroid, islet cell, and pituitary tumors, but not pheochromocytoma. Patients with MEN 2 may have parathyroid hyperplasia or adenoma (15%–30%), medullary carcinoma of the thyroid (95%), and pheochromocytoma, which occurs in more than half the patients. Some individuals with a subtype of this syndrome also have multiple mucosal neuromas. There are, in fact, several MEN 2 clinical subtypes with different phenotypic expression. Mutations in the *RET* proto-oncogene, which codes for a tyrosine kinase receptor, have been found in more than 90% of families with MEN 2. This finding allows testing of family members to identify at-risk individuals. The fact that the gene has now been identified has important implications for management and even preventive therapy (33,34).

The von Hippel–Lindau syndrome, also an autosomal dominant disease, has a number of manifestations, including pheochromocytoma, renal cell carcinoma, cerebellar hemangioblastomas, and renal, pancreatic, and epididymal cysts. Most patients with von Hippel–Lindau disease have deletional mutations in the *VHL* gene (35). *VHL* mutations also have been found in two-thirds of families with heritable pheochromocytoma. In such families, occult von Hippel–Lindau disease should be considered, and a search should be undertaken for the *VHL* mutation (35,36). With regard to heredity, it is important to note that as many as 10% of inherited isolated pheochromocytomas are malignant, as may be nearly 25% of those that occur in MEN 2 (37,38).

CLINICAL PRESENTATION

Pheochromocytoma is a remarkably protean disease, a characteristic that makes it both difficult and challenging to recognize (38,39). It is often emphasized that the first key to diagnosis is to have a high index of clinical suspicion. Like most rare diseases, pheochromocytoma is often not identified simply because the clinician does not consider it in a differential diagnosis. The consequence of failing to recognize the presence of this tumor is often fatal for mother and fetus. The differential diagnosis is broad and requires a thorough diagnostic analysis (Table 25-1).

The classically described triad of symptoms includes episodic attacks of palpitations, headaches, and profuse sweating. Anxiety and tremors often accompany these attacks, which may last from minutes to several days; over the long term the patient may experience weakness, constipation, and general wasting. The latter is a consequence of the marked increase in metabolic rate caused by catecholamine excess. Other symptoms can include pallor and, more rarely, facial flushing and episodes of collapse, sometimes accompanied by focal neurologic findings. It must be emphasized that patients sometimes will have normal blood pressure, and, occasionally, they will experience long symptom-free periods. The increased metabolic rate, as noted, can result in weight loss and complaints of heat intolerance, but some patients with pheochromocytomas are obese. Many of the complications caused by pheochromocytomas are quite serious (Table 25-2).

TABLE 25-1. *Pheochromocytoma: differential diagnosis*

Cardiovascular
Preeclampsia/eclampsia
Essential hypertension
Coronary insufficiency
Paroxysmal tachycardias
Cardiovascular collapse
Dissecting aneurysms
Dilated cardiomyopathy
Neuropsychiatric
Hypertensive encephalopathy
Intracranial lesions
Anxiety, panic attacks
Migraine
Endocrine
Thyrotoxicosis
Diabetes mellitus
Carcinoid
Drugs
Amphetamine intoxication
Cocaine intoxication
Opiate withdrawal
Clonidine withdrawal
Miscellaneous
Septic shock
Malignant hyperthermia

TABLE 25-2. *Pheochromocytoma: associated medical complications*

Severe hypertension
Pulmonary edema
Coronary artery spasm
Cardiomyopathy
Arrhythmias
Stroke
Orthostatic hypotension
Hypercalcemia
Polycythemia

Headaches are a symptom in at least 60% of patients (3,39). They are most often occipital, but they may be frontal, and often wake the patient from sleep. Sometimes the headaches of pheochromocytoma improve when the patient stands. At least a third of these headaches are accompanied by nausea or vomiting, and they are often mistaken for migraine. When a patient shows classic symptoms, the diagnosis is often entertained early in the evaluation. Table 25-1 provides a partial list of conditions that pheochromocytoma can masquerade as. Unusual signs and symptoms are common, and sometimes these tumors are remarkably effective mimics of other diseases (39–44). For example, patients can experience diarrhea or hypokalemic alkalosis (from ectopic tumor production of vasoactive intestinal peptide or corticotropic hormone, respectively), hypercalcemia (from ectopic calcitonin production or as part of MEN with primary parathyroid disease), diabetes mellitus (because adrenergic stimulation can antagonize insulin release and epinephrine stimulates glycogen breakdown) or acute pulmonary edema (from effects on myocardial performance or from pulmonary vasconstriction, which raises pulmonary capillary hydrostatic pressure).

Patients with pheochromocytoma can succumb to sudden cardiac death from arrhythmias or from sudden and profound hypotension, which can occur when catecholamine support of blood pressure during a paroxysm is suddenly withdrawn; they may also have frank myocardial infarction (45). Acute neurologic symptoms (39,46,47), including transient loss of consciousness and temporary hemiparesis, have been reported in pregnancy (47,48), as have psychiatric symptoms, including severe depression and delusion (48). Some women show signs of emesis, abdominal pain, or unexplained fever.

Renovascular hypertension may be confused with or even accompany pheochromocytomas as a secondary phenomenon if the tumor compresses the renal artery or, theoretically, in the context of reduced renal blood flow from α-adrenergic stimulation. Some acute medical conditions can mimic pheochromocytoma's symptoms and are also associated with increased catecholamine release. Examples are sepsis and stroke. Cocaine or amphetamine intoxication may produce symptoms similar to those elicited by the catecholamine release of pheochromocytoma.

Hyperemesis can develop in women with pheochromocytomas, who sometimes develop marked hypotension when a phenothiazine is administered (49). Drug reactions out of proportion to what is expected should raise the clinician's suspicions. Several drugs can induce the release of catecholamines from pheochromocytomas and provoke a paroxysm of hypertension and other symptoms. These drugs include glucagon, opiates, corticotropin, saralasin, histamine, and metoclopramide.

Whereas most pheochromocytomas, as noted, release predominantly norepinephrine, a few release primarily epinephrine (39). Patients with such tumors may have a different spectrum of symptoms than is seen ordinarily. Vasodilation predominates, and women may experience episodic syncope or a feeling of weakness or faintness. Such symptoms are not uncommon in normal pregnancy, which can lead to potential diagnostic confusion.

Some epinephrine-predominant pheochromocytomas may be associated with symptoms related to β-adrenergic stimulation, such as hyperglycemia (owing to the potent effect of epinephrine on glycogenolysis and gluconeogenesis), hyperpyrexia (from cutaneous vasoconstriction), and marked leukocytosis. These signs, especially in combination with syncope or other manifestations of reduced central perfusion, can be confused with sepsis. In most cases, however, the clinical picture does not predict the catecholamine profile of the tumor. This may be because symptoms are also related to the panoply of neuropeptides elaborated by pheochromocytomas.

Under most circumstances, the initial pharmacologic approach to any pheochromocytoma should be α-adrenergic blockade. Beta-antagonist drugs given before alpha blockers are potentially hazardous. Patients with epinephrine-predominant pheochromocytoma must be differentiated clinically and pharmacologically from those with predominantly norepinephrine release, because α-adrenergic blockade, the standard and sometimes life-saving approach to managing most pheochromocytomas, can worsen symptoms and signs in women with tumors that secrete primarily epinephrine. Such patients benefit from early beta blockade, which, if initiated as first-line therapy, would not help and could even worsen the clinical situation in most cases of pheochromocytoma.

Many of the symptoms of pheochromocytoma are not specific, and the diagnosis in pregnancy is further confounded by the fact that some symptoms can be mistaken for those that can occur in normal pregnancies or for those that accompany far more common pregnancy-related disorders. Heat intolerance, flushing, fainting episodes, headaches, palpitations, nausea and vomiting, fatigue, dyspnea, and constipation all are common in otherwise uncomplicated pregnancies, but they can also be manifestations of pheochromocytoma. Some of the signs and symptoms that accompany pheochromocytomas or their medical complications can develop during the course of pregnancy and be attributed to other diseases. For example, hypertension, anxiety or tremulousness, nausea, heart murmurs, stroke, shock, or chest pain can all arise during pregnancy as the result of various medical disorders unrelated to pheochromocytoma. They can all also be caused by that tumor. Rarely, a tumor may be present but not suspected or diagnosed until after a successful delivery (4). Some patients who harbor a pheochromocytoma may have symptoms that manifest only when they are pregnant, and symptoms may recur in subsequent pregnancies (39).

By far the most common error is to diagnose preeclampsia or some other form of pregnancy-induced or pregnancy-aggravated hypertension in a patient with pheochromocytoma (50). While the error is understandable because of the rarity of adrenal tumors and the prevalence of preeclampsia, failure to consider pheochromocytoma can result in maternal and fetal death, and has in many instances. The two conditions are not always easy to distinguish, and, to make the matter more challenging, preeclampsia can be superimposed on the hypertension of pheochromocytoma. In general, thrombocytopenia and marked proteinuria would not be expected in the context of pheochromocytoma, nor would hyperuricemia or azotemia. Hyperglycemia is not caused by preeclampsia. When present, those findings can help guide diagnostic decision making.

Fetal risks from pheochromocytoma are related to the high maternal catecholamine levels and their consequences. Hypertension of any origin can be associated with reduced uterine perfusion, and α-adrenergic stimulation can reduce uterine blood flow. Other complications of the tumor that potentially interfere with maternal or fetal oxygenation (e.g., hypotension, cardiac arrhythmias, heart failure, etc.) will also create an unfavorable environment for the fetus. The consequence of all these potential problems is an increased likelihood of intrauterine fetal growth restriction (26,51,52). Maternal catecholamines probably have little direct effect on the fetus. They do not cross the placenta well, because of considerable metabolism by placental monoamine *oxidase* (MAO) and catechol-*O*-methyltransferase (COMT) and perhaps also because by reducing uterine blood flow, they inhibit their own transfer potential (53).

Some hemodynamic data have been obtained in pregnant women with pheochromocytomas (54,55). These data show that, as expected, during a paroxysm of symptoms there is a marked increase in systemic vascular resistance accompanied by a rise in blood pressure and a fall in cardiac output, the latter presumably related to a sudden increase in afterload. This physiologic situation would be expected to be associated with a significant drop in uterine blood flow (perhaps superimposed on a chronically low flow from alpha stimulation) and would explain both acute and chronic fetal oxygen and nutritional deprivation in patients with pheochromocytoma.

Another specific area of confusion deserves mention. Pheochromocytoma can cause hypertrophic or dilated cardiomyopathy (56). The patient may show signs of acute congestive heart failure, sometimes with severe impairment of ventricular function. The cause is probably related to chronically increased afterload and lessened coronary flow from α-adrenergic stimulation. Catecholamine-induced cardiomyopathy is associated with histologic evidence of myocarditis. In many cases, the disorder appears to be reversible after the pheochromocytoma is removed (57). It is important not to misinterpret catecholamine cardiomyopathy as peripartum cardiomyopathy or the heart failure that can accompany severe preeclampsia.

DIAGNOSIS

Once the diagnosis of pheochromocytoma is suspected by the clinical picture, its identification depends on two diagnostic approaches—confirmation of increased catecholamine secretion and imaging techniques to localize the tumor. Most often, imaging is delayed until the presence of pheochromocytoma is suggested by the clinical or laboratory findings. Physical examination is most likely to be revealing if it is performed during a paroxysmal attack. During intervals between paroxysms, hypertension may still be present and, if it has been long-standing, there may be evidence of hypertensive retinopathy. Many patients with pheochromocytomas have postural hypotension. There may also be symptoms related to cardiomyopathy or arrhythmias, and some patients appear tired and thin. Fever may be present, and a fine tremor is common. The pupils may be dilated, and Raynaud's phenomenon develops. Occasionally, a large tumor may be palpable in the abdomen or flank. Indeed, if pheochromocytoma is suspected, extensive abdominal palpation is not wise, because it may provoke a severe paroxysm. Conversely, if abdominal probing of a patient unexpectedly causes an acute attack of typical symptoms, pheochromocytoma should be suspected.

Biochemical Techniques

Biochemical techniques involve measurements of catecholamines or their metabolites in plasma or urine (1,58,59). In addition, chromogranin A, a protein stored and released with catecholamines from the adrenal medulla and from pheochromocytoma cells, can be measured in the plasma (60). This is sometimes used as a complementary technique to help establish the diagnosis, but it is rarely necessary. Screening all hypertensive pregnant women for pheochromocytoma would not be cost effective, and the sensitivity and specificity of diagnostic testing would be low. Testing should obviously be done in patients with suggestive symptoms, but given the propensity of pheochromocytomas to masquerade as various disorders, some other patients should be considered for testing. Pregnant women with hypertension that is severe or is not readily controlled with standard therapy, especially in the first half of gestation; those with unusual and otherwise unexplainable symptoms (e.g., anxiety, fainting episodes, rapid glycemic fluctuations, etc.); or those with hypertension and glucose intolerance deserve testing (61).

Whichever approach is chosen, it is important that the laboratory be experienced in the measurement of catecholamines and that it uses refined analytic techniques. Assays with high precision and sensitivity include radioenzymatic assay, gas chromatography/mass spectroscopy, and, most commonly, high-performance liquid chromatography with electrochemical detection. As an initial screening tool in patients suspected of harboring pheochromocytoma, measurement of catecholamines or their metabolites in a 24-hour urine sample is preferred (Table 25-3). According to some studies, this approach has better specificity than does measurement of plasma catecholamines (62). The latter are more likely to give false-positive or negative results, especially if the samples are collected improperly. Regardless of the fluid used, scrupulous care in the collection of samples is vital if the results are to be meaningfully interpreted.

Collection of 24-hour urine samples is inconvenient and cumbersome for patients and subject to collection error. Nevertheless, there are several advantages to urine analysis, described below. The samples should be collected in acid and, ideally, under oil, to minimize oxidation. Adding 10 mL of 5N hydrochloric acid to the collection container is usually sufficient to maintain the pH of the total sample below 3. The use of 10 to 20 mL of mineral oil is optional, but it may serve as further protection. During the course of the collection day, the container should be kept refrigerated.

TABLE 25-3. *Biochemical assays for diagnosis of pheochromocytoma*

Assay	Normal limit[a]
Urine assays	
Norepinephrine	80 μg/day
Epinephrine	50 μg/day
Metanephrines	1.3 mg/day
Vanillylmandelic acid	8.0 mg/day
Plasma assays	
Norepinephrine	750 pg/mL
Epinephrine	110 pg/mL

[a]Values represent the upper 95% confidence interval for measurements among hypertensive patients without pheochromocytoma. Measured levels vary somewhat according to laboratory technique. Altering the limit will influence the specificity and sensitivity of the assay.

When plasma measurements are used, samples should be obtained only after the pregnant patient has been in lateral recumbency for at least 20 minutes in a quiet environment. Ideally, an indwelling needle should be put in place before the resting period, to avoid any effect of anxiety or pain from the venipuncture on catecholamine levels. Blood samples should be placed immediately in ice and the plasma separated at 4°C and frozen promptly at −70°C until assayed. Samples obtained by acute venipuncture are not useful.

Naturally occurring catecholamines are norepinephrine, epinephrine, and dopamine. Each can be measured in peripheral plasma, urine, and tissue samples. Catecholamines are synthesized from the amino acid tyrosine through a series of enzymatic steps (Fig. 25-2). These enzymes can be present in pheochromocytomas and often show very high levels of activity. Phenylethanolamine-*N*-methyltransferase, normally found in significant concentrations in the adrenal and, to a much lesser degree, in myocardium and brain, is necessary for the formation of epinephrine by methylation of norepinephrine. Phenylethanolamine-*N*-methyltransferase can be identified in adrenal and in some extraadrenal pheochromocytomas (63). The spectrum of pathologic symptoms in patients with pheochromocytomas depends to an extent on the relative amount of synthetic enzyme activity in the tumor as well as that of metabolizing enzymes and the receptor status of target organs. Severity of symptoms does not always correlate with the size of the tumor or the observed plasma or urinary catecholamine levels.

Virtually all circulating epinephrine in healthy individuals derives from the adrenal medulla. Various forms of stress (e.g., hypoglycemia, hypoxemia, anxiety) cause increased adrenal secretion of epinephrine, which can be observed in plasma measurements. Using modern assay techniques, basal levels of plasma epinephrine are also usually measurable. Norepinephrine is also secreted by the adrenal medulla and is the primary neurotransmitter in the peripheral postganglionic sympathetic nerves. Plasma norepinephrine derives partly from the adrenal and mostly from norepinephrine released from sympathetic nerve endings that escapes reuptake into the proximal neuron and is released into the circulation. Dopamine, a precursor of norepinephrine and epinephrine, is also secreted by the adrenal in measurable quantities and has physiologic effects.

Catecholamines are enzymatically metabolized by deamination (MAO), *O*-methylation (COMT), and sulfoconjugation (phenolsulfotransferase) (64). Catecholamines released into the circulation are excreted predominantly via the kidney by filtration and tubular secretion. Those measured in clinical plasma and urinary assays are free (unconjugated). Epinephrine and norepinephrine from the circulation appear in the urine primarily through glomerular filtration, but a substantial proportion of these two catecholamines undergoes

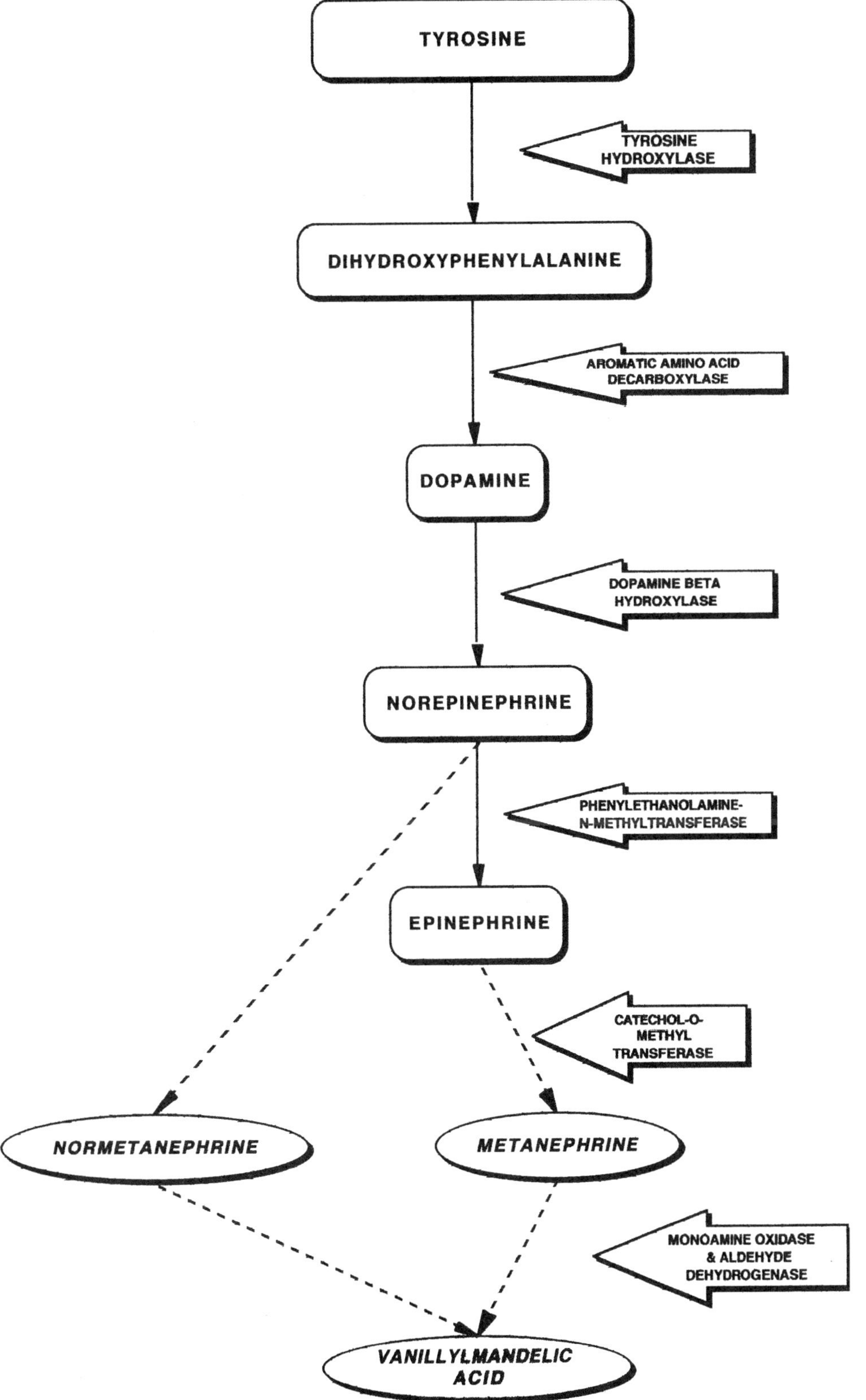

FIG. 25-2. Summary of catecholamine biosynthesis and metabolism. Critical enzymes are denoted by horizontal arrows. Broken lines show the pathways to metabolites used in diagnostic testing.

O-methylation, and these metabolites arrive in urine via tubular secretion. Urinary metabolites commonly measured in the diagnosis of pheochromocytoma are metanephrines and vanillylmandelic acid (VMA). Metanephrine and normetanephrine are the *O*-methylated derivatives of epinephrine and norepinephrine, respectively. They are reported individually or sometimes as total metanephrines in 24-hour urine samples. VMA derives primarily from the action of MAO and aldehyde dehydrogenase on metanephrines. Most VMA found in the urine derives from norepinephrine.

Twenty-four-hour urine collections are better reflections of the aggregate of sympathoadrenal or pheochromocytoma catecholamine release over the course of the day, and they may identify periodic release overlooked by a plasma sample, which reflects catecholamine secretion only around the time it is obtained. However, if symptomatic paroxysms are infrequent, catecholamine elevations may also be missed in urine samples, because they are diluted by normal release for most of the day. Normal plasma norepinephrine levels are sometimes found in women with pheochromocytoma, especially during normotensive (interparoxysmal) periods of time. Similarly, patients with MEN who are asymptomatic and are being screened because they are at risk not uncommonly have normal levels as well. Obviously, as with all laboratory results, interpretation must be tempered by the clinical presentation. In addition, false-positive results can be caused by some antihypertensive agents (e.g., hydralazine, calcium channel blockers), as well as by cigarette smoking, caffeine, emotional stress, and physical exertion. Drugs of various kinds can interfere with assay specificity, especially for metabolites; this is less true of the measurement of catecholamines (65).

Graham et al., who assessed various diagnostic 24-hour urine analyses, showed that using either norepinephrine and epinephrine or normetanephrine and metanephrine yielded specificity and sensitivity results above 95% in the identification of pheochromocytomas (66). Although some pheochromocytomas do secrete dopamine, it is rare for them to do so exclusively. For this reason, dopamine measurements generally do not add to the diagnostic sensitivity of the other two catecholamines.

The sensitivity (about 80%) and specificity (at least 95%) of the three most commonly used urine assays are high and quite similar (59). Those of VMA are somewhat lower than those of metanephrines or catecholamines. When the values from any of the tests are extraordinarily elevated and the clinical situation is suggestive, the diagnosis is highly likely. When results are less certain, the predictive value of testing can be increased considerably if all three tests are done. In a given patient with pheochromocytoma, one or more of the standard tests can be normal. In general, when two of these tests are positive, the probability of a pheochromocytoma is very strong (59). Serially obtained urine samples may reveal abnormalities that are not seen in a single day's specimen, especially in a tumor that is not very active or that secretes high amounts of catecholamines only intermittently.

Choosing the threshold for diagnosis requires accepting a suitable balance between sensitivity and specificity. The use of upper limits of normal from patients with essential hypertension has been recommended by Graham and others (66,67). Using upper limits of normal from the normotensive population to diagnose pheochromocytomas would lead to an unacceptably high number of false-positive results.

Another approach that can be helpful, but which has never been tested in pregnancy, is the clonidine suppression test. Clonidine inhibits catecholamine release from sympathetic nerves by stimulation of α_2-adrenergic receptors in the brain stem. An oral dose of 300 μg is given, which results in a fall in blood pressure in normal patients as well as in those with pheochromocytoma; however, the drug will cause a drop in plasma epinephrine and norepineprhine levels in normal patients but not in those with catecholamine-secreting tumors. This test is not recommended during pregnancy unless the information to be obtained is sufficiently important to justify the risks. Clonidine can cause a considerable decline in blood pressure in some patients, leading to a reduction in uterine blood flow and potential fetal jeopardy. Other provocative tests that rely on histamine, tyramine, or glucagon to stimulate catecholamine release should also not be used in pregnancy.

Imaging Techniques

A variety of approaches to localize pheochromocytomas were used in the past, including intravenous pyelography, presacral gas insufflation, and vena caval catheterization with blood sampling for catecholamines at various levels. These approaches have given way to three techniques in current use: scintigraphic localization, computerized tomography (CT), and magnetic resonance imaging (MRI) (Fig. 25-3a,b) (68,69). Exact preoperative localization is vital, to avoid the need for extensive abdominal exploration and inadvertent pressure on the tumor. It must be borne in mind that in searching for a pheochromocytoma, both adrenal glands should always be imaged, as should the para-aortic areas in the abdomen, since bilateral tumors in the adrenals or multifocal tumors can occur (51,65,70).

MRI is now the procedure of choice under most circumstances, particularly during pregnancy. Both T_1- and T_2-weighted images are helpful. T_2-weighted images are sometimes sufficient, particularly if the tumor is large. T_1-weighted pictures may be useful, especially if one is looking for small or extraadrenal tumors, because T_1 imaging allows for clearer demarcation of the tumor–fat

A

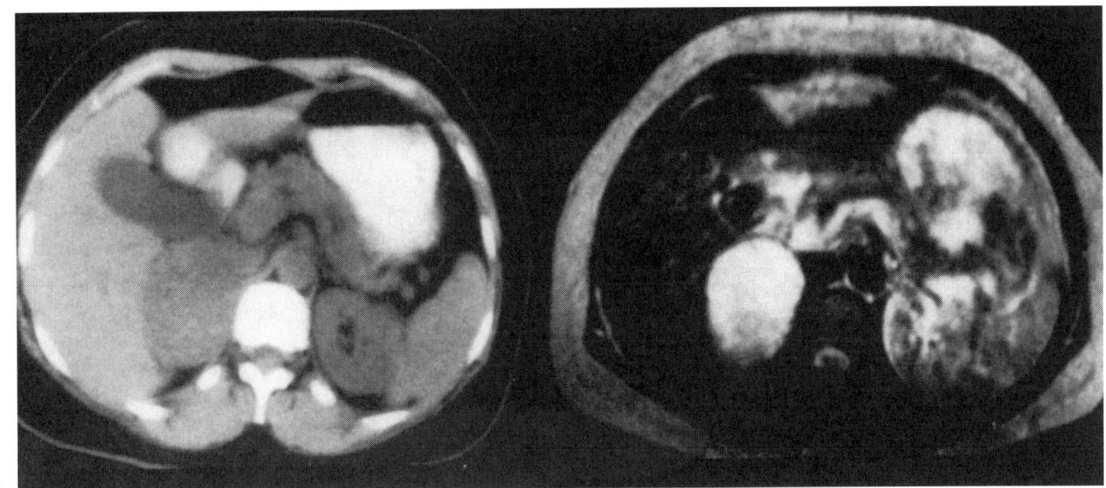

B

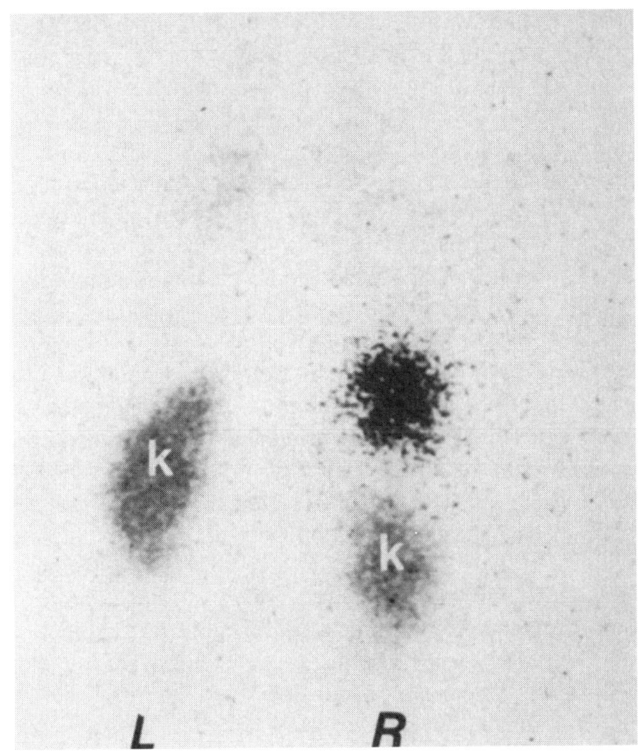

FIG. 25-3. Imaging techniques. The same tumor of the right adrenal is imaged with computerized tomography (**a**, left), T_2-weighted magnetic resonance (**a**, right), and iodine 123–meta-iodobenzylguanidine scintigraphy k, kidney (**b**). (From Bravo E. Pheochromocytoma: new concepts and future trends. Kidney Int 1991;40:544–556.)

interface. Coronal scanning may be particularly appropriate in evaluating the sympathetic chain. In general, pheochromocytomas appear as homogeneous low-intensity masses on T_1-weighted images and as higher-intensity signals with T_2 weighting. The pregnant uterus does not interfere with image quality, even in retroperitoneal areas (71). As noted previously, necrosis and hemorrhage within the tumor mass are not uncommon and can result in a more atypical heterogeneous image. MRI is also helpful in searching for metastases or for persistent or recurrent benign tumors in patients who have previously undergone resection of a pheochromocytoma and who have symptomatic or biochemical evidence of excess catecholamine secretion.

MR images are highly sensitive and as a rule should be used initially during pregnancy. No fetal risks of exposure to the magnetic field of the MRI machine have been noted. The best images are obtained with turbo spin-echo T_2-weighted imaging and with fat-suppressed imaging. These fast spin-echo techniques allow for shorter examination times and therefore reduce artifact from fetal motion and provide more comfort for the patient (71).

CT scanning usually shows a pheochromocytoma as a solid inhomogeneous mass (72). If it is necessary to use CT for localization of a pheochromocytoma during pregnancy, the scan should begin in the adrenal area. Only if no tumor is identified should imaging of the remainder of the abdomen and pelvis be done. This approach means there would be a very small risk of overlooking a second or metastatic nonadrenal lesion, but this is countervailed by the need to minimize fetal radiation exposure. If abdominal scans do not show the pheochromocytoma, the chest and neck should then be imaged. With CT, the use of oral contrast to opacify bowel helps clarify the tumor image. Intravenous contrast may also be helpful in distinguishing adrenal from renal masses. The fetal radiation dose consequent to CT scanning is, in fact, relatively low, especially if only the upper abdomen is imaged, and should be well below the generally accepted 0.05 Gy threshold for teratogenicity. There may be small potential carcinogenic effects of low-level fetal radiation, but they would be justified by the importance of identifying and localizing the neoplasm in preparation for surgical removal.

Ultrasound can also be used to detect these tumors, especially using recently marketed high-resolution scanners. It is sometimes difficult, however, to image both the adrenals and the para-aortic area clearly by this technique, especially in late pregnancy. Although ultrasound can be used as a screening technique, the failure to identify a suspected pheochromocytoma using this method should lead to further evaluation by MRI or CT imaging. Moreover, the latter approaches would usually be necessary to confirm an ultrasound finding.

Nuclear medicine techniques can also be used to localize pheochromocytomas (73). MIBG (meta-iodobenzylguanidine) labeled with iodine 123 or iodine 131 is a norepinephrine analog that is taken up into pheochromocytoma tissue and stored. The approach has the disadvantage that it usually takes 2 days to obtain the necessary images. Although maternal and fetal thyroids can be blocked with iodine before the study, there is still a risk of fetal radiation. MIBG scintigraphy is thus not recommended during pregnancy. However, its use during gestation can sometimes be justified when there is a strong clinical and biochemical suspicion of a functioning chromaffin tumor and MRI is inconclusive. While the sensitivity of MIBG is lower than that of MRI (about 80% versus 90%), the scintigraphic technique is more specific (73). Furthermore, MIBG may help differentiate pheochromocytomas from other adrenal lesions, such as adrenal adenomas or adrenal cortical carcinoma. It must be remembered that some other neural crest tumors, including carcinoid, neuroblastoma, and oat cell carcinoma, among others, can concentrate MIBG.

Although MRI is the procedure of choice, it may be contraindicated in some patients. Women with metal heart valves or intracranial surgical clips should not be placed in the MRI machine. Moreover, extreme obesity or even a large pregnant abdomen can make scanning technically challenging or even dangerous. For some severely claustrophobic patients, even anxiolytics may not sufficiently allay their fear of being placed in the MRI tube. In these situations, ultrasound complemented by CT scanning becomes the method of choice. When CT or MRI, in particular, is used, the radiologist must be reminded of the importance of left-lateral displacement during the study so as to avoid aortacaval compression in third-trimester pregnancies. A new approach that holds promise for the future uses positron emission tomography scanning after administration of fluorodeoxyglucose. This has proved effective in pinpointing pheochromocytomas that could not be imaged with MIBG (74).

THERAPY

In virtually all circumstances, adrenergic blockade is instituted after the diagnosis is confirmed. After stabilization of symptoms, prompt surgical extirpation is the most appropriate therapy. In preparation for surgery or in patients for whom definitive treatment must be delayed, proper medical therapy is critically important (75). The general approach is to use adrenergic-blocking drugs to mitigate the end-organ effects of excess catecholamines.

Phenoxybenzamine is usually the initial drug of choice. It is a noncompetitive long-acting alpha blocker that is relatively selective for α_1-adrenergic receptors. When necessary, it can be administered intravenously to achieve significant alpha blockade within an hour. The half-life of the block is about 24 hours. Typically, beta blockers are used as well and may have important antiarrhythmic effects, especially in perioperative or intraoperative situations. Initiating beta blockade alone in the case of a pheochromocytoma that releases mostly norepinephrine, as do the vast majority, is dangerous and can precipitate worsening of hypertension and even cause angina or myocardial infarction from unopposed α-agonist effects. When beta blockade is appropriate, propranolol is the agent used most frequently; esmolol, a newer parenteral β-adrenergic blocker with rapid onset and a short half-life, is most useful for close control during surgery.

There is now considerable experience in the management of hypertensive disorders in pregnancy using labetelol. It would seem that this drug could be used to advantage in the context of pheochromocytoma because of its combined α- and β-receptor antagonism. Dose requirements, however, are quite high, and other drugs are usually needed as well. Prazosin, a highly selective postsynaptic α_1-antagonist is sometimes used in patients with pheochromocytoma (10), but it is not usually sufficient by itself. Angiotensin-converting enzyme inhibitors and angiotensin receptor antagonists can sometimes be useful in the medical management of pheochromocytoma, because some of the hypertension associated with these tumors is probably related to adrenergic stimulation of renin release. These drugs are generally contraindicated in pregnancy because of adverse effects on fetal development and well-being. Most recently, calcium channel blockers have been used to advantage in controlling blood pressure in these patients, and such agents can be used during pregnancy. Although various antihypertensives are potentially useful, none has been shown to be superior to alpha blockade with phenoxybenzamine. For this reason and in light of the considerable experience with this drug, its use as an initial agent is recommended. For the acute control of very high blood pressure when parenteral drugs are needed (e.g., during surgery) sodium nitroprusside is effective (70). Arfonad should be avoided in patients with pheochromocytoma.

Because all of the drugs used to control blood pressure and other pathologic manifestations of excess catecholamine release have the potential to diminish uterine blood flow, frequent fetal evaluation by nonstress testing and biophysical profile scoring is mandatory. This is especially true when a new drug is added or a dose is altered. Although its use has never been subject to critical evaluation, Doppler flow-velocity study of the uterine arteries might be helpful in adjusting and planning therapy. In addition, all antihypertensives cross the placenta, and large doses can cause fetal and newborn hypotension or interfere with fetal and neonatal blood pressure regulation. Phenoxybenzamine, for example, accumulates in the fetus after maternal administration and can result in neonatal hypotension (76). For these reasons, close fetal surveillance is mandatory, and even term newborns should be observed carefully for several days for lingering effects of antihypertensives.

It has generally been advocated that once the tumor is diagnosed, alpha and then beta blockade be instituted during pregnancy. In most reported cases, phenoxybenzamine has been used in doses of 10 mg b.i.d. increasing to 10 mg t.i.d. over 7 to 10 days, until symptomatic paroxysms are eliminated. Orthostatic hypotension often worsens or first develops in patients on phenoxybenzamine. Pregnant women should scrupulously avoid the supine position when taking this drug, and they should sit up or stand up gradually and cautiously. During the last few days before surgery, propanolol can be added at doses of 10 to 20 mg q.i.d. In the first trimester, surgery with adrenalectomy can often be accomplished without disturbing the pregnancy; during the third trimester, when there is a high likelihood of fetal survival, combined cesarean delivery and removal of the pheochromocytoma is usually advised.

In mid-pregnancy, when surgical exposure to the adrenals may be severely compromised by the large uterus and when delivery would impose unacceptable risks from prematurity, most patients can be treated with medical therapy until neonatal viability is likely and the chromaffin tumor can be resected at surgery after cesarean delivery. Although vaginal delivery has been accomplished safely in patients with pheochromocytoma (77), it is not generally advisable. Paroxysmal symptoms, including severe hypertension, can be provoked by uterine contractions, by changes in the patient's position (presumably putting direct pressure on the tumor), or by the events of delivery (78). Although emergency surgery is possible, it is less hazardous if patients are treated for 10 to 14 days before operation. This permits the cardiovascular system to adapt to diminished adrenergic receptor stimulation, resulting in less vascular lability during and after surgery.

In preparation for surgery, the patient should be sedated and the necessary intravascular lines inserted. Intravenous access that will allow rapid volume replacement is vital, and an intraarterial line for continuous monitoring of blood pressure is very important. Central venous pressure should be measured; a Swan-Ganz pulmonary artery catheter to assess left ventricular function more precisely is preferred by some physicians. The latter technique should always be used if there is evidence of heart failure or cardiomyopathy or if there is an extant or anticipated problem with fluid management. Significant lactic acidosis, which is present in some patients, should be corrected preoperatively (79).

Before surgery there is some virtue in maximizing circulatory volume with crystalloid (or, if appropriate, blood) infusions. Patients with persistently elevated norepinephrine levels are often quite volume restricted. When the pheochromocytoma is removed and vasoconstriction is released, they may become suddenly hypotensive. Pharmacologic alpha blockade and good preoperative hydration can help minimize this effect. Nevertheless, failure to see a decline in blood pressure after the tumor is resected strongly suggests that there is a second tumor.

Various anesthetic techniques have been used with success in the operative management of pheochromocytoma. The overriding principle is to achieve adequate adrenergic blockade and avoid stimuli for catecholamine release (80). More important than the drugs chosen is that the anesthesiologist be alert to the need for controlling wide fluctuations in blood pressure, to the potential for serious cardiac arrhythmias, and to the importance of scrupulous attention to volume repletion. As noted previously, a period of preoperative alpha blockade is important in this regard. It allows volume expansion and lowers the incidence and severity of broad postextirpation shifts in blood pressure.

General anesthesia is most often used because it affords the best opportunity to control hemodynamics. Sodium thiopental is favored for induction of anesthesia. Vercuronium is probably the best muscle relaxant because, unlike most alternatives, it does not cause histamine or catecholamine release. Before endotracheal intubation is attempted, the larynx and trachea should be sprayed with a 4% lidocaine solution, because intubation frequently provokes paroxysms of hypertension in these patients. Obviously, drugs should be prepared and immediately available to counteract cardiac arrhythmias, hypertension, and hypotension. The use of magnesium sulfate as an adjunct to anesthesia has been recommended because it can inhibit the release of catecholamines (80,81). Moreover, some patients with pheochromocytomas may be magnesium deficient. If magnesium is used, the fact that it can potentiate the effects of neuromuscular blocking drugs must be considered.

Some drugs have theoretical risks when used in women with pheochromocytoma. Although adrenergic blockade can obviate many of these concerns, these drugs should not be used unless a suitable alternative is not appropriate. For example, halothane should be avoided because it sensitizes the myocardium to the effects of catecholamines. Enflurane or influorane may be preferable as inhalational agents. Parasympatholytics (atropine, scopolomine) can worsen tachycardias, and drugs that release histamine (curare, morphine) can potentiate catecholamine release from pheochromocytomas. Pancuronium can have sympathomimetic effects, and Innovar (a combination of fentanyl citrate and droperidol) can occasionally cause hypertension.

The surgical approach in late pregnancy is usually to make a subumbilical midline skin incision and perform a cesarean section through a low transverse uterine incision. This minimizes disturbing the tumor in the upper abdomen. Surgical packs should not be used, and upper-abdominal exploration should be delayed. The uterus should be displaced (to whichever side causes no increase in blood pressure) until the fetus is delivered. In addition to its obvious benefits for uterine blood flow, avoiding aortocaval compression can serve to minimize sudden swings in blood pressure. Once the hysterotomy is closed, the abdominal incision is extended to the level of the xiphoid process and the pheochromocytoma is removed. If it is in the adrenal, adrenalectomy is performed.

Although it is unusual with modern imaging techniques to overlook a second pheochromocytoma, there is some virtue in thorough abdominal exploration, emphasizing the adrenals, pre-aortic abdominal areas, and renal hila. Squeezing a pheochromocytoma will usually cause a sudden rise in blood pressure. It should be remembered that compensatory adrenocortical hypertrophy can occur on the side opposite an adrenal pheochromocytoma if compression from the tumor markedly impedes ipsilateral cortical function. The hypertrophied gland should not be mistaken for a second tumor.

Other surgical approaches are possible. Bilateral flank or subcostal incisions can be made and could be considered in early pregnancy when hysterotomy is not planned. These approaches sometimes provide better exposure in very obese patients. They do not, however, allow thorough exploration of the abdomen. The same is true of laparoscopic adrenalectomy. The latter form of surgery can be treacherous because some pheochromocytomas are extensively vascular and require a formidable amount of dissection. Nevertheless, skilled laparoscopic surgeons often recommend this approach for tumors <5cm in diameter if coincident cesarean is not planned.

Postsurgical care is critically important, and the early postoperative period is particularly hazardous for these patients. They are best treated in a critical care unit until they are completely stabilized. In addition to marked hypotension, severe hypoglycemia can sometimes arise as the catecholamine-induced inhibition of insulin release is removed and the counterregulatory benefit of epinephrine from the tumor disappears. About 2 weeks after surgery, catecholamine excretion should be remeasured in a search for residual tumor. If patients remain asymptomatic, retesting should be done at least yearly because of the propensity of pheochromocytomas to recur or arise at another site. Long-term follow-up is especially important in women with familial syndromes, in which pheochromocytomas are more likely to be multicentric or malignant.

REFERENCES

1. Young JB, Landsberg L. Catecholamines and the adrenal medulla. In: Williams textbook of endocrinology, 9th ed. Philadelphia: WB Saunders, 1998:665–728.
2. Fawcett FJ, Kimbell NKB. Phaeochromocytoma of the ovary. J Obstet Gynaecol Br Commonw 1971;78:458–459.
3. Lance JW, Hinterberger H. The headaches of phaeochromocytoma. Proc Aust Assoc Neurol 1975;12:49–53.
4. Bouziani A, Zidi B, Kamoun N, et al. Phéochromocytome vésical et grossesse: une observation. Rev Fr Gynecol Obstet 1993;88:385–389.
5. Cohen WR, Piasecki GJ, Cohn HE, Susa JB, Jackson BT. Sympathoadrenal responses during hypoglycemia, hyperinsulinemia and hypoxemia in the ovine fetus. Am J Physiol 1991;261:E95–E102.
6. Whalen RK, Althausen AF, Daniels GH. Extra-adrenal pheochromocytoma. J Urol 1992;147:1–10.
7. Kaplan NM. Clinical hypertension, 5th ed. Baltimore: Williams & Wilkins, 1990:1–25.
8. Sutton MG, Sheps SG, Lie JT. Prevalence of clinically unsuspected pheochromocytoma. Mayo Clin Proc 1981;56:354–360.
9. Krane NK. Clinically unsuspected pheochromocytomas. Arch Intern Med 1986;146:54–57.
10. Oishi S, Sato T. Pheochromocytoma in pregnancy: a review of the Japanese literature. Endocr J 1994;41:219–225.
11. Graham JB. Pheochromocytoma and hypertension: an analysis of 207 cases. Int Abst Surg 1951;92:105–115.
12. Leak D, Carroll JJ, Robinson DC, Ashworth EJ. Management of pheochromocytoma during pregnancy. Can Med Assoc J 1977;116: 371–375.
13. Landsberg L. Pheochromocytoma complicating pregnancy. Eur J Endocrinol 1994;130:215–216.
14. Venuto R, Burstein P, Schneider R. Pheochromocytoma: antepartum diagnosis and management with tumor resection in the puerperium. Am J Obstet Gynecol 1984;150:431–432.
15. Burgess GE. Alpha blockade and surgical intervention of pheochromocytoma in pregnancy. Obstet Gynecol 1979;53:266–270.
16. Botchan A, Hauser R, Kupperminc M, Grisaru D, Peyser MR, Lessing JB. Pheochromocytoma in pregnancy: case report and review of the literature. Obstet Gynecol Surv 1995;50:321–327.
17. Shroff CP, Deodhar KP. Bilateral adrenal phaeochromocytoma with pregnancy. Aust N Z J Obstet Gynaecol 1980;20:185–186.
18. Oliver MD, Brownjohn AM, Vinall PS. Medical management of phaeochromocytoma in pregnancy. Aust N Z J Obstet Gynaecol 1990;30:268.
19. Sprague AD, Thelin TJ, Dilts PV Jr. Pheochromocytoma associated with pregnancy. Obstet Gynecol 1972;39:887–891.
20. Lyons CN, Colmorgen GHC. Medical management of pheochromocytoma in pregnancy. Obstet Gynecol 1988;72:450–451.
21. Kleiner GJ, Greston WM, Yang PT, Levy JL, Newman AD. Paraganglioma complicating pregnancy and the puerperium. Obstet Gynecol 1982;59:25–65.
22. Proyce C, Cecat P, Delahousse G, Le Monies De Sagaza H, Vansey-

mortier L, Lagacue G. Phéochromocytome et grossesse: bloquage alpha-adrénergique; césarienne et surrénalectomie simultanées. Chirurgie 1982;108:397–401.

23. van Heerden JA, Roland CF, Carney JA, Sheps SG, Grant CS. Long-term evaluation following resection of apparently benign pheochromocytoma(s) paraganglioma(s). World J Surg 1990;14:325–329.
24. Sweeney WJ, Katz VL. Recurrent pheochromocytoma during pregnancy. Obstet Gynecol 1994;83:820–822.
25. Averbuch SD, Steakley CS, Young RC, et al. Malignant pheochromocytoma: effective treatment with a combination of cyclophosphamide, vincristine, and dicarbazine. Ann Intern Med 1988;109: 267–273.
26. Devoe LD, O'Dell BE, Castillo RA, Hadi HA, Searle N. Metastatic pheochromocytoma in pregnancy and fetal biophysical assessment after maternal administration of alpha-adrenergic, beta-adrenergic, and dopamine agonists. Obstet Gynecol 1986;68:155–185.
27. Jaffe RB, Harrison TS, Cerny JC. Localization of metastatic pheochromocytoma in pregnancy by caval catheterization: including urinary catecholamine values in uncomplicated pregnancies. Am J Obstet Gynecol 1969;104:939–944.
28. Simanis J, Amerson JR, Hendee AE, Anton AH. Unresectable pheochromocytoma in pregnancy: pharmacology and biochemistry. Am J Med 1972;53:381–385.
29. Stenström G, Swolin K. Pheochromocytoma in pregnancy: experience of treatment with phenoxybenzamine in three patients. Acta Obstet Gynecol Scand 1985;64:357–361.
30. Epstein H, Morehouse M, Cowles T, King CR. MEA III presenting as pheochromocytoma and complicating pregnancy and the puerperium. J Reprod Med 1985;30:501–504.
31. Glowniak JV, Shapiro B, Sisson JC, et al. Familial extra-adrenal pheochromocytoma: a new syndrome. Arch Intern Med 1985;145: 257–261.
32. Chandrosekharappa SC, Guru SC, Manickam P, et al. Positional cloning of the gene for multiple endocrine neoplasia-type 1. Science 1997;276:404–407.
33. Chodankar CM, Abhyankar SC, Deddhar KP, Shanbhag AM. Sipple's syndrome (multiple endocrine neoplasia) in pregnancy: case report. Aust N Z J Obstet Gynaecol 1982;22:243–244.
34. Eng C. The RET proto-oncogene in multiple endocrine neoplasia type 2 and Hirschsprung's disease. N Engl J Med 1996;335:943–951.
35. Richards FM, Webster AR, McMahon R, Woodward ER, Rose S, Maher ER. Molecular genetic analysis of von Hippel–Lindau disease. J Intern Med 1998;243:527–533.
36. Gross DJ, Arishai N, Meiner V, Filon D, Zbar B, Abeliovich D. Familial pheochromocytoma associated with a novel mutation in the von Hippel–Lindau gene. J Clin Endocrinol Metab 1996;81:147–149.
37. Carney JA, Sizemore GW, Sheps SG. Adrenal medullary disease in multiple endocrine neoplasia, type 2: pheochromocytoma and its precursors. Am J Clin Pathol 1976;66:279–290.
38. Monkelban JF, Cats HA, Beerenhout CH, Dullaart RPF, van Haeften TN. Phaeochromocytoma in various disguises. Neth J Med 1995;47:70–75.
39. Ross EJ, Griffith DNW. The clinical presentation of phaeochromocytoma. Q J Med 1989;71:485–496.
40. Potts JM, Larrimer J. Pheochromocytoma in a pregnant patient. J Fam Pract 1994;38:289–293.
41. Raue F, Bayer JM, Rahn KH, Herfarth C, Minne H, Ziegler R. Hypercalcitoninaemia in patients with pheochromocytoma. Klin Wochenschr 1978;56:697–701.
42. Bravo E. Pheochromocytoma: new concepts and future trends. Kidney Int 1991;40:544–556.
43. Ober KP. Hyperthyroidism or pheochromocytoma? N Carol Med J 1983;44:285-286.
44. Feldman JM. Adult respiratory distress syndrome in a pregnant patient with a pheochromocytoma. J Surg Oncol 1985;29:5–7.
45. Jessurun CR, Adam K, Moise K, Wilansky S. Pheochromocytoma-induced myocardial infarction in pregnancy. Tex Heart Inst J 1993;20: 120–122.
46. Weintraub MI, Manning EJ, Kinkel WR. Neurological complications in pheochromocytoma of pregnancy: report of a case and review of the literature. Am J Obstet Gynecol 1970;107:423–428.
47. Juimo AG, Doh AS, Gaggni J. Phéochromocytome et grossesse: àpropos d'un cas. J Radiol 1987;68:643–646.
48. El Matri A, Slim R, Zmerli S, Ben Ayed H. Phéochromocytome avec troubles psychiatrique. Nouv Presse Med 1978;7:1467–1470.
49. Montminy M, Teres D. Shock after phenothiazine administration in a pregnant patient with a pheochromocytoma. J Reprod Med 1983;28: 159–162.
50. El-Minawi MF, Paulino E, Cuesta M, Ceballos J. Pheochromocytoma masquerading as preeclamptic toxemia. Am J Obstet Gynecol 1971; 109:389–395.
51. Pinaud M, Michel J, Arnould F, et al. Association phéochromocytome surrénalien bilatérel et grossesse: césarienne et surrénalectomies simultanées. Cah Anesthesiol 1985;33:321–324.
52. Verstraeten PR, deBoer R. Pregnancy and functional paraganglionoma. Eur J Obstet Gynecol Reprod Biol 1987;26:157–164.
53. Dahia PLM, Hayashida CY, Strunz C, Abelin N, Toledo SPA. Low cord blood levels of catecholamine from a newborn of a pheochromocytoma patient. Eur J Endocrinol 1994;130:217–219.
54. Combs CA, Easterling TR, Schmucker BC, Benedetti TJ. Hemodynamic observations during paroxysmal hypertension in a pregnancy with pheochromocytoma. Obstet Gynecol 1989;74:439–441.
55. Easterling TR, Carlson K, Benedetti TJ, Mancuso JJ. Hemodynamics associated with the diagnosis and treatment of pheochromocytoma in pregnancy. Am J Perinatol 1992;9:464–466.
56. Nanda AS, Feldman A, Liang C. Acute reversal of pheochromocytoma-induced catecholamine cardiomyopathy. Clin Cardiol 1995;18: 421–423.
57. Simons M, Downing SE. Coronary vasoconstriction and catecholamine cardiomyopathy. Am Heart J 1985;109:297–304.
58. Ratge D, Knoll E, Wisser H. Plasma free and conjugated catecholamines in clinical disorders. Life Sci 1986;39:557–564.
59. Pauker SG, Kopelman RI. Interpreting hoofbeats: can Bayes help clear the haze? N Engl J Med 1992;327:1009–1013.
60. Hsiao RJ, Parmer RJ, Takiyyuddin MA, O'Connor DT. Chromogranin A storage and secretion: sensitivity and specificity for the diagnosis of pheochromocytoma. Medicine 1991;70:33–45.
61. Harper MA, Murnaghan GA, Kennedy L, Hadden DR, Atkinson AB. Phaeochromocytoma in pregnancy: five cases and a review of the literature. Br J Obstet Gynaecol 1989;96:594–606.
62. Greene JP, Guay AT. New perspectives in pheochromocytoma. Urol Clin North Am 1989;16:487–502.
63. Funahashi H, Imai T, Tanaka Y, et al. Discrepancy between PNMT presence and relative lack of adrenaline production in extra-adrenal pheochromocytoma. J Surg Oncol 1994;57:196–200.
64. Kopin IJ. Catecholamine metabolism: basic aspects and clinical significance. Pharmacol Rev 1985;37:333–364.
65. Levine SN, McDonald JC. The evaluation and management of pheochromocytomas. Adv Surg 1984;18:281–313.
66. Graham PE, Smythe GA, Edwards GA, Lazarus L. Laboratory diagnosis of phaeochromocytoma: Which analytes should we measure? Clin Biochem 1993;30:129–134.
67. Bravo EL, Gifford RW Jr. Pheochromocytoma: diagnosis, localization and management. N Engl J Med 1984;311:1298–1303.
68. Chatal J. Can we agree on the best imaging procedure(s) for localization of pheochromocytomas? J Nucl Med 1993;34:180–181.
69. Puvaneswary M, Beckhouse M. Phaeochromocytoma during pregnancy: ultrasound and MRI appearances. Med J Malaysia 1992;47: 81–85.
70. Greenberg M, Moawad AH, Wieties BM, et al. Extraadrenal pheochromocytoma detection during pregnancy using MR imaging. Radiology 1986;161:475–476.
71. Carson BJW, Johnson MA, Iwaniuk G. Extra-adrenal pheochromocytoma in pregnancy: ultrasonography and magnetic resonance imaging findings. Can Assoc Radiol J 1995;46:122–124.
72. Stanley JH, Sanchez F, Frey GD, Schabel SI. Computed tomography evaluation of pheochromocytoma in pregnancy. J Comput Tomogr 1985;9:369–372.
73. van Gils APG, Falke THM, van Erkel AR, et al. MR imaging and MIBG scintigraphy of pheochromocytomas and extraadrenal functioning paragangliomas. Radiographics 1991;11:37–57.
74. Shulkin BL, Loeppe RA, Francis IR, Deeb GM, Lloyd RV, Thompson NW. Pheochromocytomas that do not accumulate metaiodo-benzyl guanidine: localization with PET and administration of FDG. Radiology 1993;186:711–715.
75. Rogaly E. Pelvic phaeochromocytoma. S Afr Med J 1977;15:55–56.

76. Santeiro ML, Stromquist C, Wyble L. Pheoxybenzamine placental transfer during the third trimester. Ann Pharmacother 1996;30:1249–1251.
77. Davies AE, Navaratnarajah M. Vaginal delivery in a patient with a phaeochromocytoma. Br J Anaesth 1984;56:913–916.
78. Bakri YN, Ingemansson SE, Ali A, Parikh S. Pheochromocytoma and pregnancy: report of three cases. Acta Obstet Gynecol Scand 1992;71: 301–304.
79. Bornemann M, Hill SC, Kidd GS. Lactic acidosis in pheochromocytoma. Ann Intern Med 1986;105:880.
80. James MFM, Huddle KRL, Owen AD, van der Veen BW. Use of magnesium sulphate in the anaesthetic management of phaeochromocytoma in pregnnacy. Can J Anaesth 1988;35:178–182.
81. James MFM. Magnesium sulfate in pheochromocytoma. Anesthesiology 1985;62:188–189.

Cherry and Merkatz's Complications of Pregnancy,
Fifth Edition, edited by W. R. Cohen.
Lippincott Williams & Wilkins, Philadelphia © 2000.

CHAPTER 26

Calcium and Parathyroid Disorders

Richard Eastell and Kim Naylor

CALCIUM HOMEOSTASIS IN PREGNANCY

During pregnancy, maternal calcium homeostasis adapts to meet the calcium demands of the growing fetus (Fig. 26-1). It is important for maternal adaptation to occur with no detrimental effect on the mother's own skeleton. Loss of bone mineral content from the maternal skeleton can result in osteoporosis and fracture during pregnancy or postpartum. The mother can adapt to meet the calcium requirements of the fetus by increased dietary intake of calcium, amplified calcium absorption from the gut, decreased urinary calcium excretion, or increased bone resorption, resulting in loss of mineral from the maternal skeleton.

The fetus requires approximately 30 g of calcium, 80% of which is acquired during the third trimester (1). This represents about 3% of the total maternal body calcium of approximately 1,000 g. The skeleton has about 99% of the body calcium, and the remaining 1% is in the soft tissues and extracellular fluid (2). Although the maximal fetal demand for calcium is during the third trimester (approximately 200 mg/day) (3), adjustments to maternal calcium homeostasis begin in early pregnancy.

Physiologic responses to the demand for calcium include an increase in the fractional absorption of calcium, which is doubled by the second trimester (4) and is most likely a consequence of elevated serum calcitriol (1,25-dehydroxyvitamin D3) (5). Based on an average daily intake of calcium of 1,000 mg per day, approximately 200 mg per day is absorbed by the intestine; by 24 weeks of pregnancy this absorption has doubled to 400 mg per day and remains elevated throughout the rest of gestation. An increase in dietary calcium may not affect the fractional absorption of calcium.

R. Eastell and Kim Naylor: Bone Metabolism Group, Section of Medicine, Clinical Sciences Centre (NGHT), University of Sheffield, Sheffield, England.

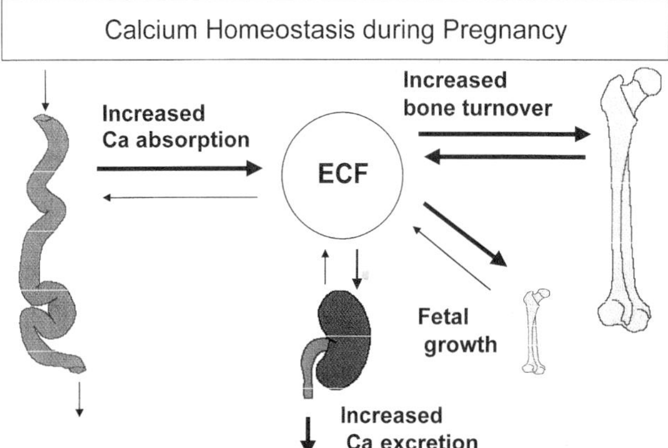

FIG. 26-1. Changes in calcium homeostasis during pregnancy. The most important adaptation in the mother is the increase in calcium absorption. This allows mineralization of the fetal skeleton. ECF, maternal extracellular fluid space.

The adaptations to calcium metabolism during pregnancy occur without elevations of parathyroid hormone (PTH) or calcifediol (25-hydroxyvitamin D3) (6). The increase in calcitriol could be due to increased renal calcifediol hydroxylase activity or increased production of this enzyme from nonrenal sources, such as the fetal kidney and the placenta (Fig. 26-2). Levels of calcifediol hydroxylase have been found to be higher in the kidney during pregnancy compared with levels among nonpregnant controls (7). During pregnancy, there is placental production of calcitriol and an increase in vitamin D–binding protein (8). Other factors, including prolactin, growth hormone, and estrogen, can also regulate calcitriol synthesis during pregnancy (9).

Parathyroid hormone is an important factor in calcium homeostasis. PTH secretion is regulated by serum calcium, with low serum calcium stimulating secretion of PTH. PTH acts on the bone and kidney to increase serum calcium levels. Bone resorption is amplified, and the

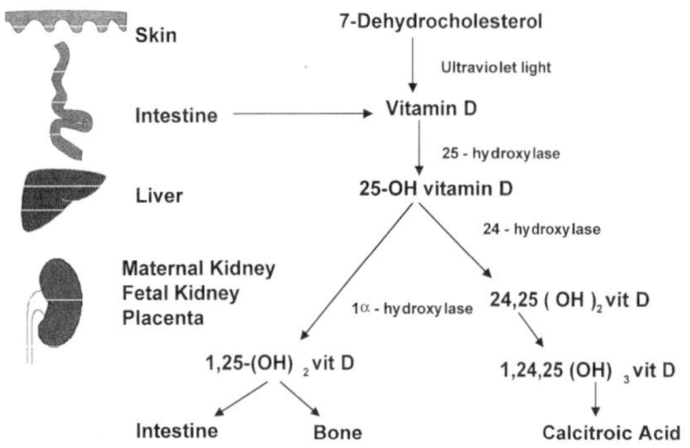

FIG. 26-2. Vitamin D biosynthesis during pregnancy. The increase in the active form of vitamin D (calcitriol) in pregnancy is due to 1-α hydroxylase enzyme activity in the placenta.

renal reabsorption of calcium is enhanced in the kidney in response to PTH. In addition, PTH enhances the production of calcitriol, which in turn increases intestinal absorption of calcium. Immunoreactive PTH levels decline early in pregnancy and subsequently rise (Fig. 26-3). PTH bioactivity, however, is unchanged during pregnancy, possibly as a result of PTH-related protein (PTHrP) production (10). Nephrogenous cyclic AMP, a sensitive marker of PTH activity, is reported to be unchanged during pregnancy (11). PTHrP levels have been shown to rise significantly during pregnancy (12). This protein is produced by the fetal parathyroid glands and the placenta.

The placental transfer of calcium is an active process, with bidirectional fluxes of calcium through the placenta (13). It might involve a calcium-binding protein and ATPase. Placental calcium transport is possibly regulated by uteroplacental blood flow, and chronic placental energy deprivation might impair the mechanism (9). The maternal serum calcium concentration affects fetal calcium, since hypercalcemia during pregnancy can result in neonatal hypocalcemia owing to transient fetal and neonatal hypoparathyroidism (14). Hypocalcemic mothers can have infants with neonatal hyperparathyroidism who are hypercalcemic and who may show signs of parathyroid bone disease (see later discussion). Placental calcium transport can be influenced by such hormones as calcitriol and calcitonin. PTHrP can also increase placental calcium transfer.

Serum calcium levels fall during pregnancy (Fig. 26-3) (15,16). The decrease in serum calcium is probably due to hemodilution and the consequent drop in the protein-bound fraction (17). The ionized calcium fraction remains unchanged during pregnancy. Urinary calcium excretion increases during pregnancy, probably as a result of increased calcium absorption (Fig. 26-3).

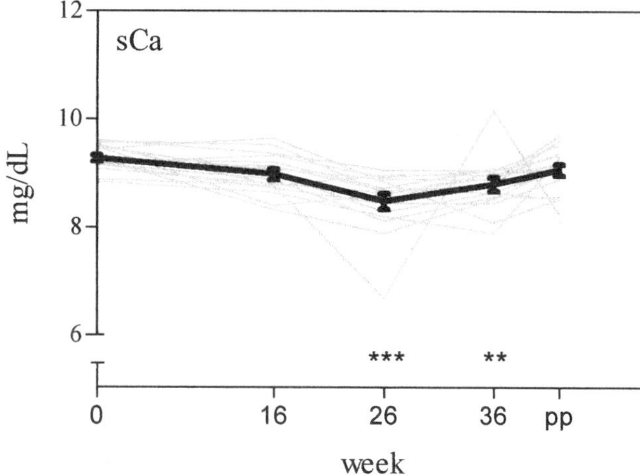

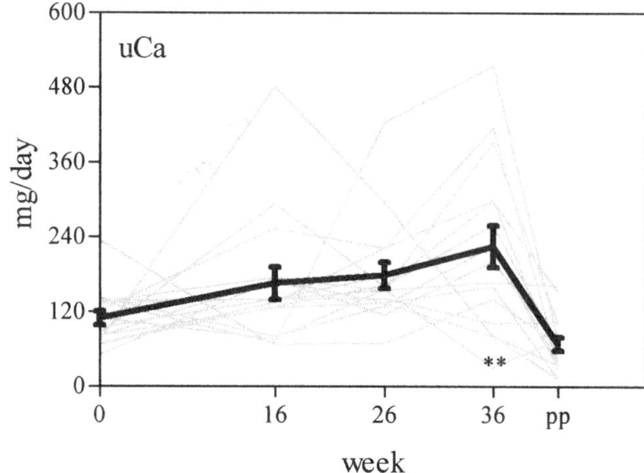

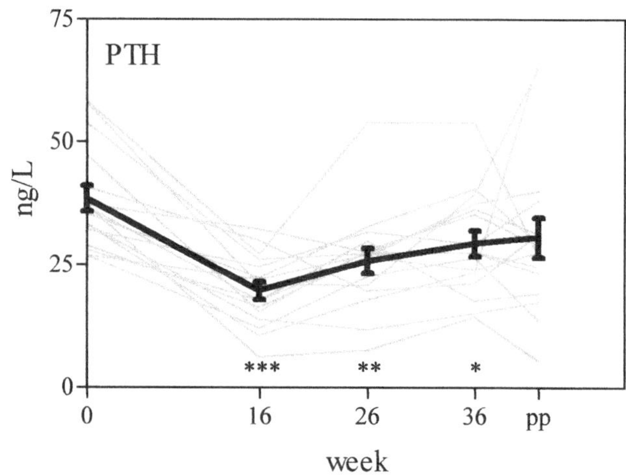

FIG. 26-3. Changes in calcium homeostasis during pregnancy: serum calcium (sCa) decreases, and urinary calcium (uCa) increases. Parathyroid hormone (PTH) decreases and then increases. Solid lines represent the mean (SE); asterisks represent the level of significance (*$p < 0.05$, **$p < 0.01$, ***$p < 0.001$) compared with levels before pregnancy. (From Naylor KE. Biochemical markers of bone turnover: evaluation of high bone turnover states, including pregnancy [Ph.D. thesis]. Sheffield, England: University of Sheffield, 1998.)

BONE DENSITY AND BONE TURNOVER

Lamke et al. measured two sites of the radius and reported loss in cancellous but not cortical bone during pregnancy (18). Other researchers have reported decreased bone mineral density (BMD) at the radial shaft (19) or no change in BMD of the radius (20,21). Lumbar spine BMD has been shown to decline during pregnancy by 3.3% (19), which is in agreement with our findings of diminished BMD of the total spine. In a prospective study, Sowers et al. (22) reported no significant change in proximal femur BMD with pregnancy .

Bone turnover increases in the mother during pregnancy. The increase in bone resorption occurs by the second trimester. Results in the postpartum period can show false elevations because of a contribution from the involuting uterus to the excretion of collagen cross-links (Fig. 26-4a). Bone formation markers increase in the mother, particularly in the third trimester (Fig. 26-4b). This high turnover state might be a consequence of enhanced secretion of insulin-like growth factor type I (by the placenta) and might help explain the higher perinatal risk of vertebral fractures in women with preexisting low bone density (see later discussion).

OSTEOPOROSIS ASSOCIATED WITH PREGNANCY

There are two distinct syndromes of osteoporosis that are related to pregnancy (Table 26-1). Postpregnancy spinal osteoporosis usually is seen a few weeks after delivery, with initial signs of vertebral fracture. Transient osteoporosis of the hip of pregnancy occurs after week 20 and takes the form of hip pain. Useful reviews are available (23,24). The largest group of cases was reported by Smith and associates (25). The spinal syndrome was first described by Nordin and Roper (26) and the hip syndrome by Curtis and Kincaid (27).

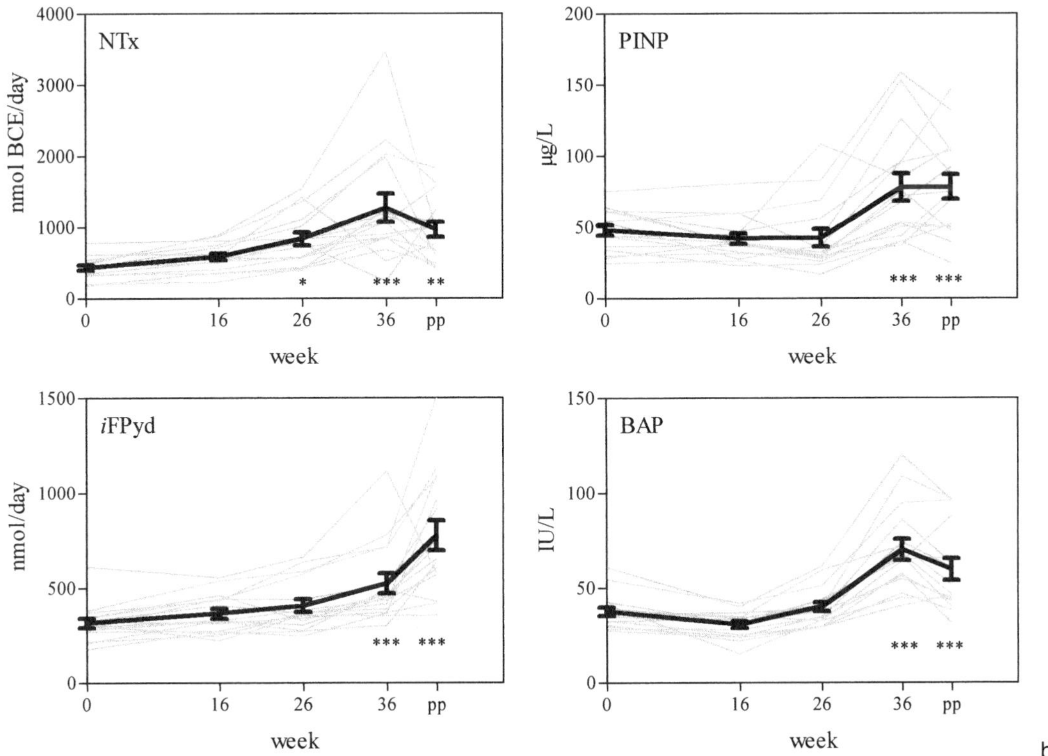

FIG. 26-4. Changes in bone turnover during and after pregnancy. **a:** Bone resorption increases early, reaching a peak at term. There is a decline in the postpartum period in markers specific to bone (N-telopeptide, NTx) but not in markers influenced by degradation of collagen in the involuting uterus (free pyridinoline, iFPyd). **b:** Bone formation increases during pregnancy, especially in the third trimester (serum procollagen type I C-propeptide, or PINP, and bone alkaline phosphatase, or BAP). Solid lines represent the mean (SE); asterisks represent the level of significance (*$p < 0.05$, **$p < 0.01$, ***$p < 0.001$) compared with levels before pregnancy. (From Naylor KE. Biochemical markers of bone turnover: evaluation of high bone turnover states, including pregnancy [Ph.D. thesis]. Sheffield, England: University of Sheffield, 1998.)

TABLE 26-1. *Comparison of post-pregnancy spinal osteoporosis and transient osteoporosis of the hip in pregnancy*

Clinical Features	Spinal osteoporosis	Transient osteoporosis of the hip
Usual onset	Within 3 months of delivery of first child	Third trimester
Symptoms	Back pain, height loss	Hip and groin pain, restricted hip motion
Prognosis	Usually self-limited, spontaneous recovery of bone mass	Usually self-limited; spontaneous recovery of bone mass, but hip pain may persist
Recurrence in later pregnancy	No	Rare
Proposed origin	↑Cytokines ↑Parathyroid hormone–related protein	↓ calcitriol Reflex sympathetic dystrophy

Modified from Kohlmeier L, Marcus R. Osteoporosis associated with pregnancy. In Marcus R, Feldman D, Kelsey JL, eds. Osteoporosis. San Diego: Academic Press, 1996: 959–967.

Postpregnancy Spinal Osteoporosis

Postpregnancy spinal osteoporosis develops as acute-onset back pain that can be associated with height loss and kyphosis. The affected woman may attribute the pain to lifting her infant, and the fracture might become apparent only many years later. Spinal radiographs generally indicate one or several vertebral fractures (Fig. 26-5). An isotope bone scan shows increased uptake only in the fractured vertebrae. Bone density of the spine is usually low (50%–75% of the expected value) (28), but forearm bone density is typically normal. Biochemical findings are generally normal, although a case with increased serum calcium, PTHrP, and urinary hydroxyproline has been reported (28). One patient with high cytokine levels (interleukin-1 bioactivity 80 times the expected level) has also been reported (29). This syndrome has been described in a series of case reports (25,29–31). Bone biopsies have been taken in order to understand the mechanism of bone loss. They have shown increased bone resorption (31) and decreased bone formation (25), but they are difficult to interpret because the biopsies were often taken well after the fracture event.

It is likely that this disorder is caused by a preexisting low spinal BMD, and with the high bone turnover and spinal bone loss of pregnancy there is increased fragility of the vertebrae. In the series of Smith and co-workers (25), four of 24 patients had preexisting risk factors (Table 26–2) for osteoporosis (anorexia nervosa, corticosteroid therapy, heparin therapy, or osteogenesis imperfecta). Kohlmeier and Marcus (23) reported the case of a patient who had vertebral fractures likely related to thyrotoxicosis that developed during pregnancy. Fractures are not inevitable; most patients do not have fractures in subsequent pregnancies (25), and one patient with juvenile osteoporosis had a pregnancy without fractures (32). Bone density has been measured after fracture, and usually there is an increase (Fig. 26–5) (33,34). As noted, it is unusual to experience fractures in a subsequent pregnancy.

In our treatment of patients with postpregnancy spinal osteoporosis, we confirm the fractures by obtaining radiographs of the thoracic and lumbar spine. We measure BMD of the spine and hip and carry out a thorough clinical examination and biochemical workup for secondary forms of osteoporosis. This assessment includes serum calcium, alkaline phosphatase, thyroid-stimulating hormone, complete blood count, protein electrophoresis, and 24-hour urinary calcium and creatinine. We ensure an adequate intake of calcium and vitamin D and then observe the results by measuring BMD every 6 months. If there is no increase in BMD, we consider bisphosphonate therapy.

Transient Osteoporosis of the Hip in Pregnancy

This disorder has also been referred to as idiopathic osteoporosis or algodystrophy. The latter term is appropriate, because the syndrome has many features in common with reflex sympathetic dystrophy. The initial signs are pain in the hip and groin region after the 20th week of pregnancy. The condition is usually unilateral, but it can be bilateral (35) and can extend to affect the knee (35) or sacroiliac region (36). It is occasionally associated with fracture of the rib, wrist, and spine (37). There is usually no preceding trauma. There might have been a similar event in a previous pregnancy. Movement of the hip can be limited by the pain.

Radiographs show indistinct subchondral cortical bone in the femoral head. The bone is generally osteopenic, and there might be a proximal femur fracture or pelvic insufficiency fracture. The magnetic resonance imaging (MRI) scan shows marrow edema (low signal on T_1, high signal on T_2) (Fig. 26-6) and joint fluid. The isotope bone scan shows increased uptake, usually in the femoral head, and the distribution of isotope is even. This picture contrasts with that of avascular necrosis, in which there is diminished uptake initially and patchy uptake later. These symptoms and radiographic findings are similar to those of reflex sympathetic dystrophy. Biopsy of the synovium

The Osteoporosis Centre, NGH, Sheffield

k = 1.148 d0 = 44.9(1.000H) 6.206

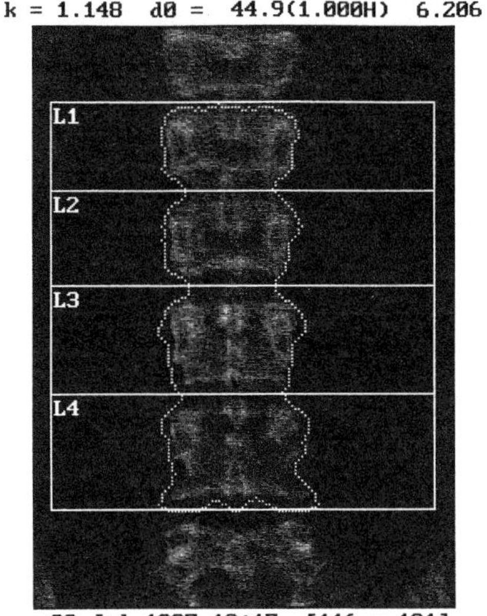

·02.Jul.1997 10:17 [116 x 121]
Hologic QDR-4500A (S/N 45045)
Lumbar Spine V8.17a:3

S0702970C Wed 02.Jul.1997 10:15
Name:
Comment:
I.D.: 832056 Sex: F
S.S.#: - - Ethnic: W
ZIPCode: 1/52 Height: 149.10 cm
Operator: AJ Weight: 48.00 kg
BirthDate: 06.Apr.71 Age: 26
Physician: BAX
Image not for diagnostic use

TOTAL BMD CV FOR L1 - L4 1.0%

C.F. 1.022 1.014 1.000

Region	Est.Area (cm^2)	Est.BMC (grams)	BMD (gms/cm^2)
L1	9.33	6.51	0.697
L2	10.26	7.85	0.765
L3	12.07	9.83	0.815
L4	14.19	11.21	0.790
TOTAL	45.86	35.40	0.772

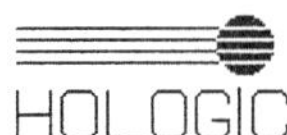

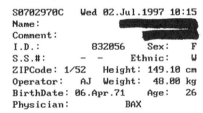

The Osteoporosis Centre, NGH, Sheffield

a Lumbar Spine
Reference Database •

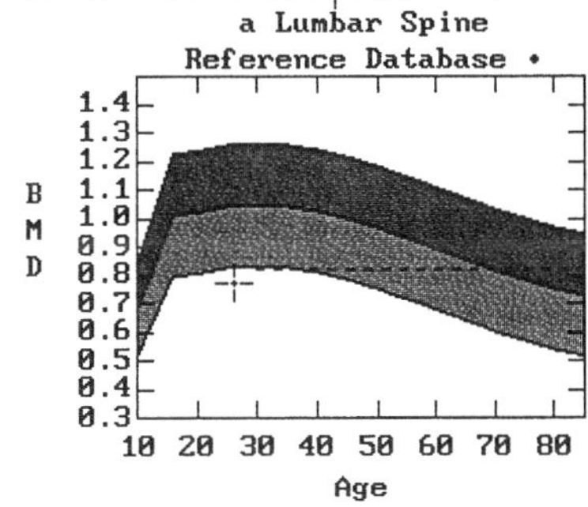

BMD(L1-L4) = 0.772 g/cm^2

Region	BMD	T(30.0)		Z	
L1	0.697	-2.07	75%	-2.03	76%
L2	0.765	-2.39	74%	-2.34	75%
L3	0.815	-2.45	75%	-2.40	76%
L4	0.790	-2.97	71%	-2.92	71%
L1-L4	0.772	-2.50	74%	-2.45	74%

• Age and sex matched
T = peak BMD matched
Z = age matched TK 04 Nov 91

S0702970C Wed 02.Jul.1997 10:15
Name:
Comment:
I.D.: 832056 Sex: F
S.S.#: - - Ethnic: W
ZIPCode: 1/52 Height: 149.10 cm
Operator: AJ Weight: 48.00 kg
BirthDate: 06.Apr.71 Age: 26
Physician: BAX

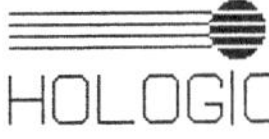

a

FIG. 26-5. Postpregnancy spinal osteoporosis. This 26-year-old woman experienced back pain during the last 2 weeks of her first pregnancy, which became more severe 4 days postpartum. **a:** Bone mineral density at the lumbar spine was 74% of the expected value.

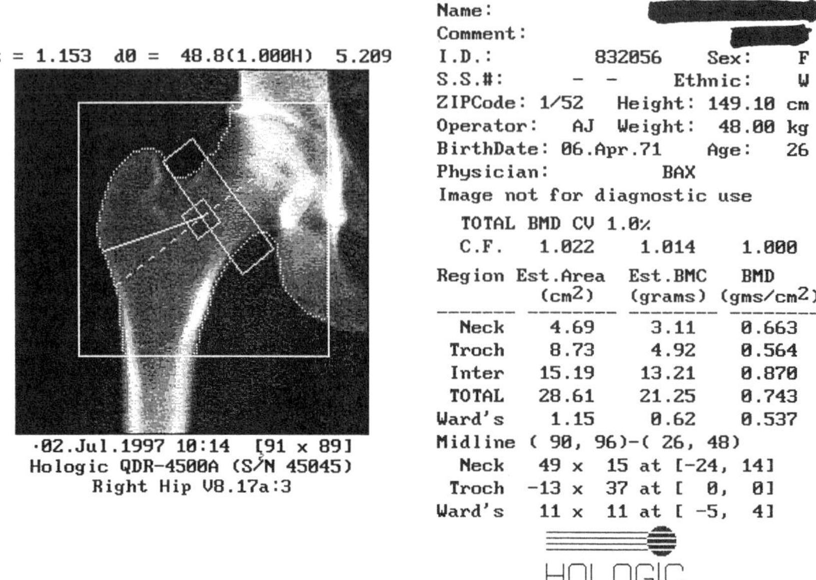

The Osteoporosis Centre, NGH, Sheffield
k = 1.153 d0 = 48.8(1.000H) 5.209
·02.Jul.1997 10:14 [91 x 89]
Hologic QDR-4500A (S/N 45045)
Right Hip V8.17a:3
S0702970B Wed 02.Jul.1997 10:12
Name:
Comment:
I.D.: 832056 Sex: F
S.S.#: - - Ethnic: W
ZIPCode: 1/52 Height: 149.10 cm
Operator: AJ Weight: 48.00 kg
BirthDate: 06.Apr.71 Age: 26
Physician: BAX
Image not for diagnostic use
TOTAL BMD CV 1.0%
C.F. 1.022 1.014 1.000
Region Est.Area (cm2) Est.BMC (grams) BMD (gms/cm2)
Neck 4.69 3.11 0.663
Troch 8.73 4.92 0.564
Inter 15.19 13.21 0.870
TOTAL 28.61 21.25 0.743
Ward's 1.15 0.62 0.537
Midline (90, 96)-(26, 48)
Neck 49 x 15 at [-24, 14]
Troch -13 x 37 at [0, 0]
Ward's 11 x 11 at [-5, 4]
HOLOGIC

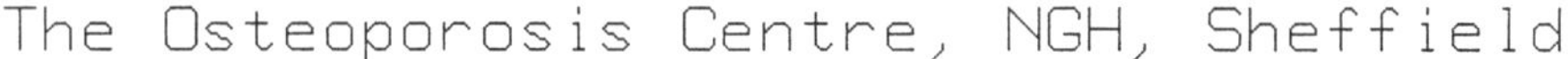

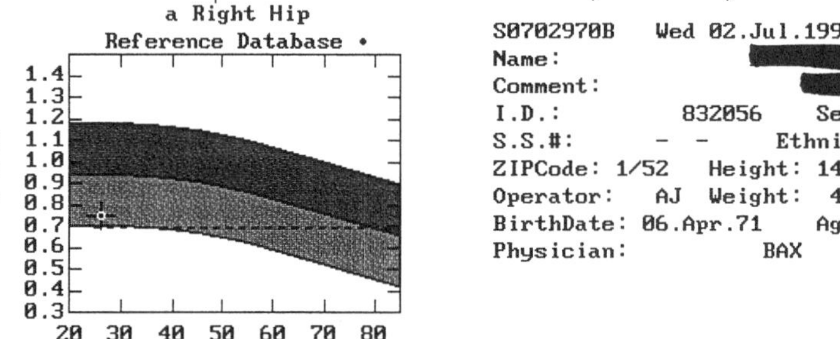

BMD(Total[R]) = 0.743 g/cm²

Region	BMD	T		Z	
Neck	0.663	-1.67 (25.0)	78%	-1.65	78%
Troch	0.564	-1.38 (25.0)	80%	-1.38	80%
Inter	0.870	-1.49 (35.0)	79%	-1.41	80%
TOTAL	0.743	-1.63 (25.0)	79%	-1.63	79%
Ward's	0.537	-1.68 (25.0)	73%	-1.64	74%

• Age and sex matched
T = peak BMD matched
Z = age matched NHA 01 Feb 97

HOLOGIC

b

FIG. 26-5. *Continued.* **b:** Total hip bone mineral density was 79% of the density expected for her age.

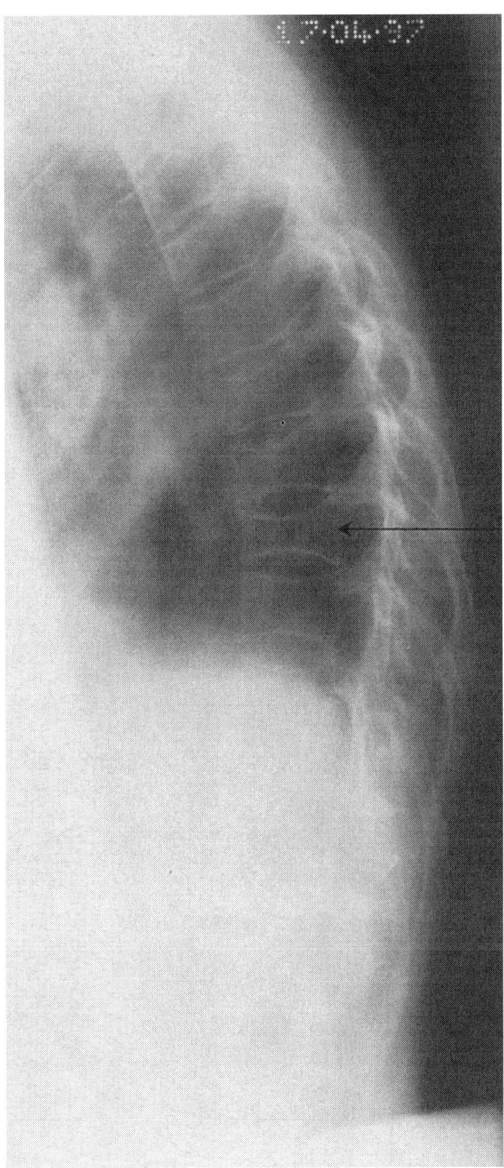

C

FIG. 26-5. *Continued.* **c:** Radiographs of the spine showing fractures at vertebrae T-6, T-7, T-8, T-9, T-12 and L-1 (arrow indicates vertebra T-9). The patient had predisposing factors for osteoporosis (an episode of amenorrhea for a year at age 24 and long-standing low calcium intake). She become hypercalcemic postpartum (serum calcium level of 10.9 mg/dL, serum phosphate level of 1.6 mg/dL), but the condition subsequently resolved, and bone density at the spine increased by 6% over 12 months. Hypercalcemia has been reported previously (28) in postpartum osteoporosis.

shows nonspecific inflammation (38) and is sterile (39). The bone biopsy indicates decreased trabecular bone volume (39).

The biochemical findings have been inconsistent. Serum levels of calcitriol are usually elevated two- to threefold in pregnancy but are relatively low in these patients (37,40). This low level could be the result of increased bone resorption (and suppressed PTH). There is no clear evidence of a humoral mechanism. The

TABLE 26-2. *Risk factors for osteoporosis*

Genetic factor
First-degree relative with low-trauma fracture
Environmental factors
Cigarette smoking
Alcohol abuse
Physical inactivity
Thin habitus
Diet low in calcium
Little exposure to sunlight
Menstrual status
Early menopause (before the age of 45 years)
Previous amenorrhea (e.g., due to anorexia nervosa, hyperprolactinemia)
Drug therapy
Glucocorticoids (7.5 mg/day or more of prednisone for more than 6 months)
Antiepileptic drugs (e.g., phenytoin)
Excessive substitution therapy (e.g., thyroxine, hydrocortisone)
Anticoagulant drugs (e.g., heparin, warfarin)
Endocrine diseases
Primary hyperparathyroidism
Thyrotoxicosis
Cushing syndrome
Addison disease
Hematologic diseases
Multiple myeloma
Systematic mastocytosis
Lymphoma, leukemia
Pernicious anemia
Rheumatologic diseases
Rheumatoid arthritis
Ankylosing spondylitis
Gastrointestinal diseases
Malabsorption syndromes (e.g., celiac disease, Crohn's disease, surgery for peptic ulcer)
Chronic liver diseases (e.g., primary biliary cirrhosis)

From Eastell R. Treatment of postmenopausal osteoporosis. N Engl J Med 1998;338:736–746.

women usually have low bone density, particularly at the hips. Their mothers were more likely to have fractures than expected (41), and their daughters might have low bone density. [The latter finding has been reported for only two women, whose daughters were in puberty (42)]. The groin pain usually improves 2 to 9 months after delivery (43), and bone density of the spine and hip increases (43). The MRI appearance resolves (44). One patient with persistent pain was treated with alendronate, and the pain rapidly resolved (35).

We evaluate these patients by carrying out MRI of the hips to confirm the diagnosis. Because the women are pregnant, we prefer not to make a radiographic absorptiometry measurement until the early postpartum period. We rule out any form of secondary osteoporosis (as noted earlier), and recommend bed rest (the patient might insist on it if the pain is very severe) but arrange for physiotherapy to avoid contractures. We have used calcitonin therapy (50 IU given subcutaneously at bedtime) for its

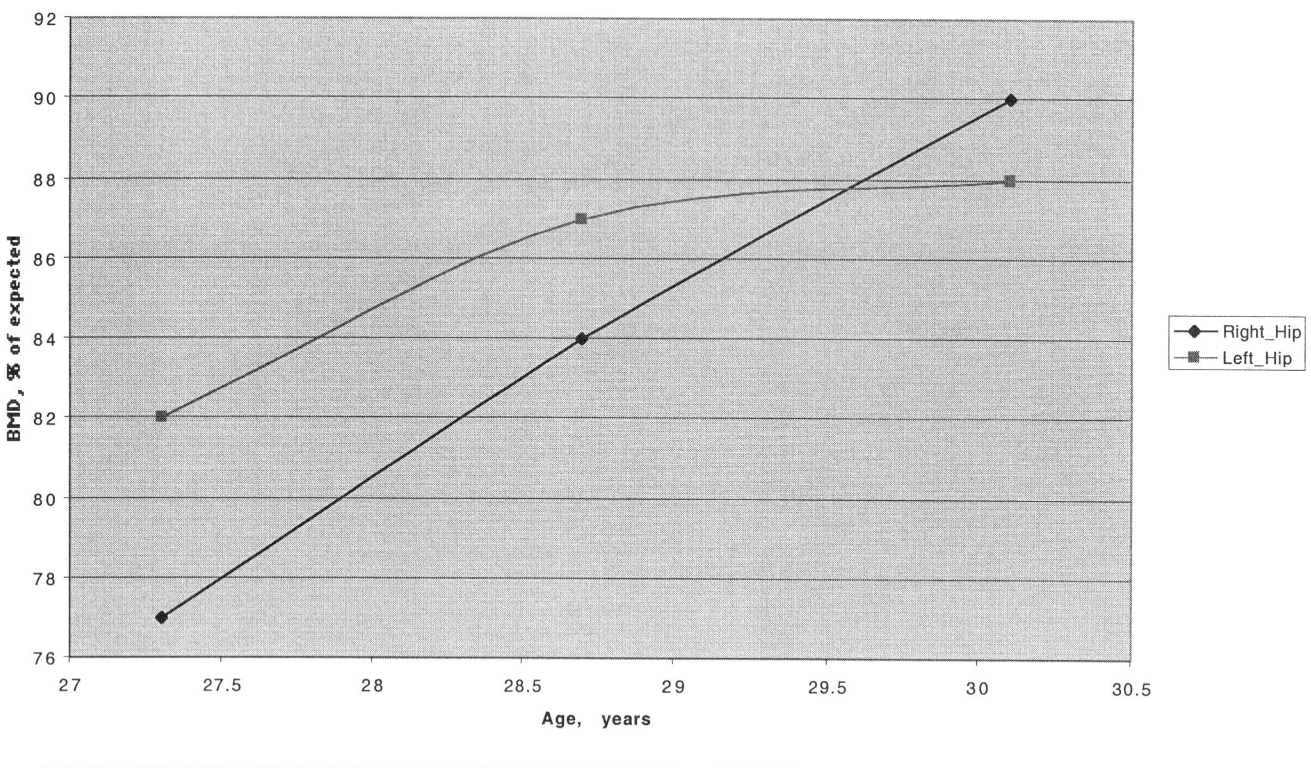

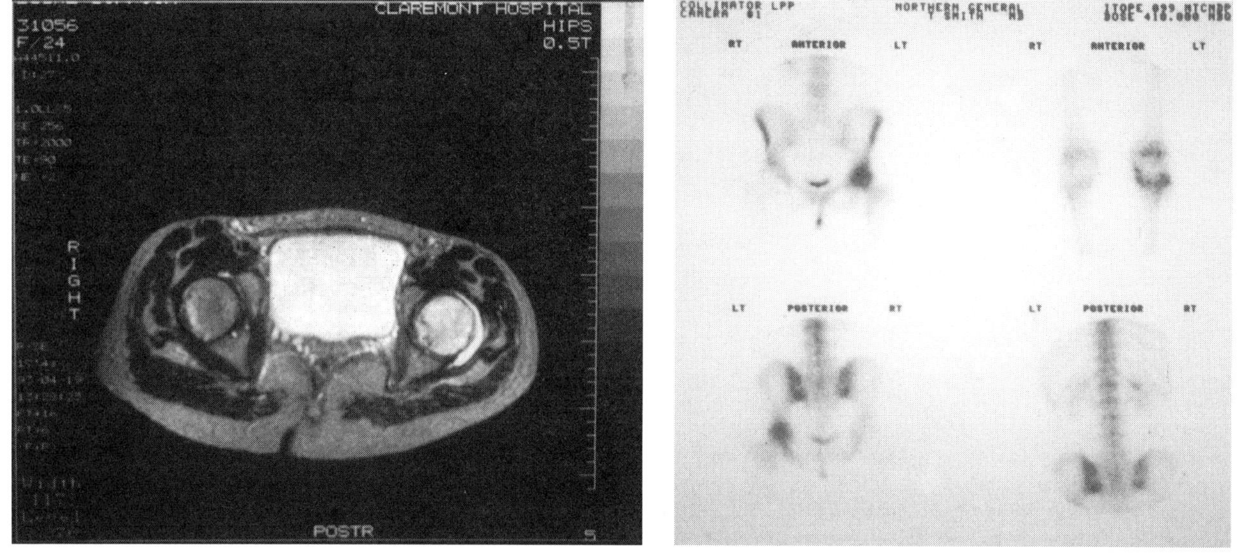

FIG. 26-6. Transient osteoporosis of the hip in pregnancy. This 28-year-old woman had had pain in her right hip in her first and second pregnancies at 16 and 24 weeks of gestation, respectively. In her second pregnancy she was found to have tenderness over the pubic bone and limited movement of the hip. She was unable to walk without crutches. She was treated with periods of bed rest and subcutaneous calcitonin therapy. **a:** Bone mineral density (BMD) was measured shortly after the first and second pregnancies and then 17 months after the second pregnancy. The calcitonin therapy might account for the higher bone density after the second pregnancy than after the first; note how BMD improved after pregnancy. **b:** The magnetic resonance image (T_2-weighted sequence) from another woman with left hip pain showed increased signal, indicating marrow edema. **c:** The isotope bone scan taken showed even uptake over the proximal femur. Pain resolved shortly after delivery.

analgesic and antiresorptive properties. The bone pain usually improves quickly postpartum, and we monitor bone density to ensure it recovers fully. If the pain is persistent postpartum, we would consider bisphosphonate therapy. This therapy can be dangerous, however, if the woman were to become pregnant again (because bisphosphonates impair the skeletal development of the fetus).

Other Forms of Osteoporosis

Heparin therapy can be administered during pregnancy to prevent recurrence of venous thromboembolic disease or for other reasons. Heparin is known to be a direct stimulant of bone resorption *in vitro*. Its administration for 6 months or more would be expected to result in bone loss. Vertebral fractures were observed in 2% of 184 women who were treated with heparin (45). A progressive decrease in BMD was observed in one prospective study (46). Hip BMD declined by more than 10% in a third of women, and this effect was not dose dependent. Even short courses of heparin have been associated with fracture (47), which might indicate variability in individual susceptibility. In another prospective, controlled study there was significant bone loss from the spine (about 8%) (48).

It is unclear how to prevent the bone loss from heparin therapy. Ringe and Keller (47) treated nine women with calcium hydroxyapatite with some success. It has been suggested that low-molecular-weight heparin be used in the first trimester and warfarin in the second trimester (49) in patients at particularly high risk of osteoporosis. It may be too risky to use warfarin, however, because of the embryopathy and devastating hemorrhage that can result from its use (50).

Magnesium sulfate is used for prevention of preterm labor (tocolytic therapy). It has been associated with abnormalities of calcium homeostasis (increased levels of urinary calcium and decreased levels of serum calcium) and low forearm BMD (51). In one patient, bilateral stress fractures of the calcaneus developed postpartum (52), but she had other risk factors for fracture (treatment with betamethasone and heparin). Corticosteroid therapy for the prevention of neonatal respiratory distress syndrome can diminish bone formation in the mother, which can predispose her to osteoporosis (53). These osteoporosis syndromes in pregnancy are rare. It is of interest that the bone loss of pregnancy and lactation has no long-term consequences. Indeed, nulliparous women are more likely to be at risk of postmenopausal osteoporosis (54).

DISORDERS OF MINERAL HOMEOSTASIS

Hypocalcemia

The most common forms of chronic hypocalcemia are hypoparathyroidism, pseudohypoparathyroidism, and osteomalacia (Table 26-3) (55). Hypocalcemia manifests as neuromuscular irritability with carpopedal spasms (cramps in the hands and feet), depression, and worsening of epilepsy. There may be cataracts, basal ganglion calcification, and enamel hypoplasia (if hypocalcemia was present before age 8 years). The signs of latent tetany—the Chvostek test and Trousseau sign—are present. These signs are useful for monitoring the clinical response to therapy.

Hypocalcemia during pregnancy can result in midtrimester abortion or preterm labor. Such complications are more likely if the serum calcium is below 1.7 mmol/L (6.8 mg/dL) (Table 26-4). As an illustration, a 27-year-old woman came to us for spontaneous abortion at 15 weeks of pregnancy. Her serum calcium level was 1.7 mmol/L (6.8 mg/dL), and she had a positive Trousseau sign. She had hypoparathyroidism as result of subtotal thyroidectomy for hyperthyroidism. She had had three full-term pregnancies before the thyroidectomy. Thus, hypocalcemia during pregnancy can result in

TABLE 26-3. *Causes of chronic hypocalcemia*

Hypoparathyroidism
Surgically induced
Idiopathic
Early
DiGeorge syndrome (with thymic aplasia)
MEDAC/HAM
Isolated persistent neonatal
Isolated late onset
Functional
Hypomagnesemia
Neonatal (e.g., maternal hyperparathyroidism)
Infiltrative
Hemosiderosis
Wilson disease
Secondary neoplasia
Pseudohypoparathyroidism
Osteomalacia
Decreased bioavailability of vitamin D
Decreased ultraviolet light exposure
Nutritional
Nephrosis
Malabsorption
Abnormal metabolism of vitamin D
Chronic renal failure
Vitamin D–dependent rickets type 1 (autosomal recessive)
Anticonvulsants
Abnormal response to vitamin D
Vitamin D–dependent rickets type 2
Malabsorption (celiac/Crohn/short bowel)

MEDAC, multiple endocrine deficiency–autoimmune candidiasis; HAM juvenile familial endocrinopathy–hypoparathyroidism/Addison disease/moniliasis.

From Eastell R, Heath H III. The hypocalcemic states: Their differential diagnosis and management. In: Coe FL, Favus MJ, eds. Disorders of bone and mineral metabolism. New York: Raven Press, 1992: 571–586.

TABLE 26-4. *Hypoparathyroidism in pregnancy: outcome of pregnancy*

Case report	Serum calcium, (mg/dL)	Pregnancy duration (wk)
Bronsky et al. (72), case 1	5.6	26
Eastell et al. (73)	6.4	18, 27
Salle et al. (74)	6.8	27
Case described in text	6.8	15
Gradus et al. (75)	7.6	36
Glass and Barr (76)	7.6	Term
Sadeghi-Nejad and Wolfsdorf (77)	8.0	Term
Bronsky et al. (72), 2 case	8.4	Term
Sann et al. (78)	8.4	Term

enhanced uterine irritability. This finding would agree with the results of *in vitro* experiments, which found that a decrease in the media concentration of calcium bathing rat uterine muscle results in a decline in resting potential and alters spike frequency (56).

Hypoparathyroidism

This is most commonly a consequence of neck surgery, but it can be idiopathic (probably autoimmune) or a result of hypomagnesemia. In the mildest form, treatment with calcium alone is sufficient. In more severe cases, vitamin D supplementation is required. Vitamin D is inexpensive, but intoxication can result in long-standing hypercalcemia and renal failure. Treatment with an active form of vitamin D—calcitriol or alphacalcidol—is easier to control (57–59). The requirements for the active form of vitamin D can increase during pregnancy, and it is best to monitor serum calcium at 2- to 4-week intervals over the course of pregnancy. Some investigators find that the addition of thiazide diuretics can improve control of hypocalcemia. If hypocalcemia is not controlled, the neonate can suffer from hypercalcemia as a result of stimulation of the fetal parathyroid glands by chronic hypocalcemia. This hypercalcemia usually lasts a few weeks (60–63).

Pseudohypoparathyroidism

There have been few case reports of pseudohypoparathyroidism in pregnancy. This disorder is inherited and results from a mutation in the gene coding for G-protein. In two women (who had four pregnancies), the serum calcium levels remained normal throughout pregnancy, with the usual two- to threefold increase in serum calcitriol (18). During pregnancy, the placenta is an important site of the 1-α hydroxylation of vitamin D. This enzyme is present in the mitochondria of fetal trophoblasts and is not under the control of PTH (in contrast to the usual form of the enzyme in the kidney). In the uterine tissue from three patients with pseudohypoparathyroidism, 1-α hydroxylase activity was normal (64).

There are several types of this inherited disorder. In the rare type II form (normal cyclic AMP but subnormal phosphaturic response to PTH), hypocalcemia is worse during pregnancy (4.8–6.4 mg/dL) than before pregnancy (7.7–8.4 mg/dL) (65). Transient hyperparathyroidism can develop in the neonate (66). One neonate with normocalcemic hyperparathyroidism had parathyroid bone disease; the hyperparathyroidism resolved after 4 weeks and the bone disease after 5 months. The mother had previously undiagnosed pseudohypoparathyroidism (67).

Osteomalacia

Contracted pelvis is a complication of osteomalacia if it is complicated by pseudofractures (Looser's zones) of the pelvis. One of the earliest cases requiring cesarean section was described in 1820 by Dr. Hamilton of Perth, Scotland (68). This condition is considered rare today, but the cases of three Bedouin women who experienced contracted pelvis after having two to three normal vaginal deliveries have been described (69). In these women, the consumption of high phytate diets (unleavened bread) was thought to be a cause of the osteomalacia. Phytate forms insoluble salts with calcium and prevents its absorption.

In Europe, osteomalacia is typically found in young women from Asia, especially the Indian subcontinent. This condition might relate to their dress (poor ultraviolet exposure of the skin) and their consumption of phytates (also in unleavened bread). It might also relate to the use of anticonvulsants and antituberculosis drugs (70). Asian women attending antenatal clinics have lower calcifediol levels than white women, and their neonates suffer from rickets and hypocalcemia more often (70).

Hypercalcemia

The most common causes of hypercalcemia in women of childbearing age are primary hyperparathyroidism (PHPT) and familial benign hypercalcemia (FBH). Less common sources include vitamin D intoxication, sarcoidosis, and humoral hypercalcemia of malignancy. The only forms of hypercalcemia that have been reported in pregnancy are PHPT and FBH. The differential diagnosis of hypercalcemia is straightforward using assays for intact PTH. An elevated serum calcium level with a raised (or high normal) PTH level indicates PHPT. The only difficulty is in distinguishing between PHPT and FBH. The latter condition is characterized by an autosomal dominant pattern of inheritance. Moreover, the serum calcium level is usually less than 12 mg/dL, and the urinary calcium level is typically low (or low normal).

It is wise to carry out a family study because 50% of first-degree relatives are affected in FBH.

Primary Hyperparathyroidism

Primary hyperparathyroidism (63,71) is usually caused by a single adenoma (about 85%), although it can be caused by hyperplasia (or adenoma) of several parathyroid glands or, rarely, by carcinoma. PTH secretion causes hypercalcemia as the result of increased calcium absorption (indirectly by increased calcitriol synthesis in the kidney, enhanced net bone resorption, and amplified renal calcium reabsorption). The diagnosis is made based on raised serum calcium and PTH levels. The serum calcium level can be misleading, in that serum albumin declines during pregnancy (Fig. 26-3). This problem can be avoided by calculating a calcium value corrected for albumin or by measuring serum ionized calcium. The reference range for PTH changes throughout pregnancy (Fig. 26-3), with lower levels in the first trimester and higher levels in the third trimester.

Primary hyperparathyroidism is usually asymptomatic. In the mother it can be associated with nonspecific symptoms (fatigue, weakness), hyperemesis gravidarum, renal calculi, pancreatitis (72), and psychiatric disturbances (73). In the neonate, it can result in neonatal hypocalcemia (in about half of cases) and in spontaneous abortion or fetal death. Neonatal hypocalcemia may be the first identified manifestation of maternal hyperparathyroidism (74).

Kelly (75) reviewed 109 cases reported in the literature of patients with PHPT in pregnancy. Of these women, 70 had medical treatment, and 53% suffered neonatal complications, including neonatal death. Of the 39 who underwent surgical treatment, only 10% had neonatal complications. The best time for surgery is in the second trimester. In the first trimester, the risks of teratogenesis from medications is greatest. Of the seven cases of patients who underwent surgery in the third trimester, four were complicated by premature labor and neonatal death (76). The neonatal hypocalcemia associated with PHPT is usually temporary, but it can result in seizures. FBH is usually asymptomatic in the mother. There has been one described case of FBH with hypocalcemia in a neonate (77). Thus, PHPT can result in complications for both the mother and the neonate. The optimal approach is surgical resection in the second trimester. There is no successful medical treatment for PHPT in pregnancy, other than ensuring adequate hydration.

Case Report of PHPT

A 28-year-old Asian woman had vomiting and abdominal pain in her 13th week of pregnancy. She had had one normal term pregnancy, and her father had suffered from renal calculi. She was found to have a raised serum calcium level of 3.11 mmol/L and a low serum phosphate level of 0.66 mmol/L. The urinary calcium was low, at 2 mmol/day, and the calcifediol was 3.9 ng/mL, indicating vitamin D insufficiency. Serum PTH was increased at 165 pg/mL (reference range <120). At 27 weeks, her adenomatous right superior parathyroid (24 × 18 mm) was removed. She became hypocalcemic in the postoperative period (serum calcium 7.7 mg/dL), and this value returned to normal (9.2 mg/dL) with 2,400 mg elementary calcium given daily. She had a full-term pregnancy, and the neonate had a normal serum calcium level.

This case illustrates several points:

1. The initial signs of PHPT are often nonspecific, for example, vomiting.
2. The family history of renal calculi illustrates the importance of a family survey of serum calcium to identify FBH or familial parathyroid states, for example, multiple endocrine neoplasia.
3. The low urinary calcium level in this Asian woman was likely caused by vitamin D deficiency, and this was confirmed by measuring calcifediol. The vitamin D should be replaced.
4. A serum calcium level greater than 3 mmol/L would be rare in FBH. With the elevated PTH value, it most likely represents PHPT. Also, this level of hypercalcemia would be an indication for surgery even in nonpregnant adults.
5. Surgery was done at the correct time, that is, during the second trimester.
6. It was important to correct the hypocalcemia. If it had persisted, the neonate might have had hyperparathyroidism.

REFERENCES

1. Givens MH, Mach IG. The chemical composition of the human fetus. J Biol Chem 1933;102:7–17.
2. Broadus AE. Mineral balance and homeostasis. In: Favus MJ, ed. Primer on the metabolic bone diseases and disorders of mineral metabolism. Philadelphia: Lippincott–Raven Publishers, 1996:57–63.
3. Prentice A. Maternal calcium requirements during pregnancy and lactation. Am J Clin Nutr 1994;59:477S–483S.
4. Heaney RP, Skillman TG. Calcium metabolism in normal human pregnancy. J Clin Endocrinol 1971;33:661–670.
5. Kumar R, Cohen WR, Silva P, Epstein FH. Elevated 1,25 dihydroxyvitamin D plasma levels in normal human pregnancy and lactation. J Clin Invest 1979;63:342–344.
6. Whitehead M, Lane G, Young O, et al. Interrelations of calcium-regulating hormones during normal pregnancy. Br Med J 1981;283:10–12.
7. Fenton E, Brillon HG. 25-Hydroxycholecalciferol 1 alpha-hydroxylase activity in the kidney of the fetal, neonatal and adult guinea pig. Biol Neonate 1980;37:254–261.
8. Bouillon R, Van Baelen H, DeMoor P. 25-Hydroxyvitamin D and its binding protein in maternal cord serum. J Clin Endocrinol Metab 1977;45:679–684.
9. Chesney RW, Specker BL, Mimouni F, McKay CP. Mineral metabolism during pregnancy and lactation. In: Coe FL, Favus MJ, eds. Disorders of bone and mineral metabolism. New York: Raven Press, 1992: 383–393.
10. Hosking DJ. Calcium homeostasis in pregnancy. Clin Endocrinol 1996; 45:1–6.
11. Gallacher SJ, Fraser WD, Owens OJ, et al. Changes in calciotrophic

hormones and biochemical markers of bone turnover in normal human pregnancy. Eur J Endocrinol 1994;131:369–374.
12. Bertelloni S, Baroncelli GI, Pelletti A, Battini R, Saggese G. Parathyroid hormone–related protein in healthy pregnant women. Calcif Tissue Int 1994;54:195–197.
13. Ramberg CF, Delivoria-Papadopoulos M, Crandall ED, Kronfield DS. Kinetic analysis of calcium transport across the placenta. J Appl Physiol 1973;35:662–688.
14. Croom RD, Thomas CG. Primary hyperparathyroidism in pregnancy. Surgery 1984;96:1109–1116.
15. Pitkin RM, Reynolds WA, Williams GA, Hargis GK. Calcium metabolism in normal pregnancy: a longitudinal study. Am J Obstet Gynecol 1979;133:781–790.
16. Pitkin RM. Calcium metabolism in pregnancy: a review. Am J Obstet Gynecol 1975;121:724–737.
17. Reeve J. Calcium metabolism. In: Hytten F, Chamberlain G, eds. Clinical physiology in obstetrics, 2nd ed. Oxford: Blackwell Science, 1991.
18. Lamke B, Brundin J, Moberg P. Changes of bone mineral content during pregnancy and lactation. Acta Obstet Gynecol Scand 1977;56: 217–219.
19. Drinkwater BL, Chesnut CH III. Bone density changes during pregnancy and lactation in active women: a longitudinal study. Bone Miner 1991;14:153–160.
20. Cross NA, Hillman LS, Allen SH, Krause GF, Vieira NE. Calcium homeostasis and bone metabolism during pregnancy, lactation and postweaning: a longitudinal study. Am J Clin Nutr 1995;61:514–523.
21. Kent GN, Price RI, Gutteridge DH, et al. Effect of pregnancy and lactation on maternal bone mass and calcium metabolism. Osteoporos Int 1993;[Suppl 1]:S44–S47.
22. Sowers M, Crutchfield M, Jannausch M, Updike S, Corton G. A prospective evaluation of bone mineral changes in pregnancy. Obstet Gynecol 1991;77:841–845.
23. Kohlmeier L, Marcus R. Osteoporosis associated with pregnancy. In: Marcus R, Feldman D, Kelsey JL, eds. Osteoporosis. San Diego: Academic Press, 1996:959–967.
24. Rizzoli R, Bonjour JP. Pregnancy-associated osteoporosis. Lancet 1996;347:1274–1276.
25. Smith R, Athanasou NA, Ostlere SJ, et al. Pregnancy-associated osteoporosis. Q J Med 1995;88:865–878.
26. Nordin BEC, Roper A. Post pregnancy osteoporosis: a syndrome? Lancet 1955;1:431–434.
27. Curtis PH, Kincaid W. Transient demineralization of the hip in pregnancy: a report of three cases. J Bone Joint Surg 1959;41:1327(abst).
28. Reid IR, Wattie DJ, Evans MC, et al. Case report and review: post-pregnancy osteoporosis associated with hypercalcemia. Clin Endocrinol 1992;37:298–303.
29. Blanch J, Pacifici R, Chines A. Pregnancy-associated osteoporosis: report of two cases with long-term bone density follow-up. Br J Rheumatol 1994;33:269–272.
30. Chung HC, Lim SK, Lee MK, et al. Osteoporosis of pregnancy. Lancet 1985;1:1178–1180.
31. Yamamoto N, Takahashi HE, Tanizawa T, et al. Bone mineral density and bone histomorphometric assessments of postpregnancy osteoporosis: a report of five patients. Calcif Tissue Int 1994;54:20–25.
32. Koo WW, Chesney RW, Mitchell N. Case report: effect of pregnancy on idiopathic juvenile osteoporosis. Am J Med Sci 1995;309:223–225.
33. Rillo OL, Di Stefano CA, Bermudez J, et al. Pregnancy-associated osteoporosis: report of two cases with long-term bone density follow-up. Br J Rheumatol 1994;33:269 272.
34. Liel Y, Atar D, Ohana N. Pregnancy-associated osteoporosis: preliminary densitometric evidence of extremely rapid recovery of bone mineral density. South Med J 1998;91:33–35.
35. Samdani A, Lachmann E, Nagler W. Transient osteoporosis of the hip during pregnancy: a case report. Am J Phys Med Rehabil 1998;77: 153–156.
36. Breuil V, Brocq O, Euller-Ziegler L, et al. Displaced subcapital fracture of the hip in transient osteoporosis of pregnancy: a case report. Int Orthop 1997;21:201–203.
37. Gruber HE, Gutteridge DH, Baylink DJ. Osteoporosis associated with pregnancy and lactation: bone biopsies and skeletal features in three patients. Metab Bone Dis Rel Res 1984;5:159–165(abst).
38. Lequesne M, Kerboull M, Bensasson M, et al. Transient osteoporosis of the hip: magnetic resonance imaging. Clin Orthop 1991;190–194.
39. Bramlett KW, Killian JT, Nasca RJ, et al. Pregnancy associated osteoporosis. Clin Endocrinol (Oxf) 1993;39:487–490.
40. Smith R, Stevenson JC, Winearls CG, et al. Osteoporosis of pregnancy. Lancet 1985;1:1178–1180.
41. Dunne F, Walters B, Marshall T, et al. Pregnancy associated osteoporosis. Clin Endocrinol (Oxf) 1993;39:487–490.
42. Carbone LD, Palmieri GM, Graves SC, et al. Osteoporosis of pregnancy: long-term follow-up of patients and their offspring. Obstet Gynecol 1995;86:664–666.
43. Funk JL, Shoback DM, Genant HK. Transient osteoporosis of the hip in pregnancy: natural history of changes in bone mineral density. Clin Endocrinol (Oxf) 1995;43:373–382.
44. Takatori Y, Kokubo T, Ninomiya S, et al. Transient osteoporosis of the hip: magnetic resonance imaging. Clin Orthop 1991;271:190–194.
45. Dahlman TC. Osteoporotic fractures and the recurrence of thromboembolism during pregnancy and the puerperium in 184 women undergoing thromboprophylaxis with heparin. Am J Obstet Gynecol 1993;168: 1265–1270.
46. Barbour LA, Kick SD, Steiner JF, et al. A prospective study of heparin-induced osteoporosis in pregnancy using bone densitometry. Am J Obstet Gynecol 1994;170:862–869.
47. Ringe JD, Keller A. Calcium homeostasis in pregnant women receiving long-term magnesium sulfate therapy for preterm labor. Am J Obstet Gynecol 1992;167:45–51.
48. Douketis JD, Ginsberg JS, Burrows RF, et al. The effects of long-term heparin therapy during pregnancy on bone density: a prospective matched cohort study. Thromb Haemost 1996;75:254–257.
49. Kyei-Mensah A, Machin SJ, Jacobs HS. Balancing the risk of recurrent thromboembolism and pre-existing osteoporosis in pregnancy. Curr Opin Obstet Gynecol 1995;7:77–81.
50. Ginsberg JS, Hirsh J. Osteoporotic fractures and the recurrence of thromboembolism during pregnancy and the puerperium in 184 women undergoing thromboprophylaxis with heparin. Am J Obstet Gynecol 1993;168:1265–1270.
51. Smith LG, Burns PA, Schanler RJ. Calcium homeostasis in pregnant women receiving long-term magnesium sulfate therapy for preterm labor. Am J Obstet Gynecol 1992;167:45–51.
52. Levav AL, Chan L, Wapner RJ. Long-term magnesium sulfate tocolysis and maternal osteoporosis in a triplet pregnancy: a case report. Am J Perinatol 1998;15:43–46.
53. Ogueh O, Khastgir G, Studd JW, et al. Antenatal corticosteroid therapy and risk of osteoporosis. Br J Obstet Gynaecol 1998;105:551–555.
54. Sowers M. Changes in bone density and biochemical markers of bone turnover in pregnancy-associated osteoporosis. Br J Obstet Gynaecol 1996;103:716–718.
55. Eastell R, Heath H III. The hypocalcemic states: their differential diagnosis and management. In: Coe FL, Favus MJ, eds. Disorders of bone and mineral metabolism. New York: Raven Press, 1992:571–586.
56. Abe Y. Effects of changing the ionic environment on passive and active membrane properties of pregnant rat uterus. J Physiol 1971;214: 173–190.
57. Callies F, Arlt W, Scholz HJ, et al. Management of hypoparathyroidism during pregnancy: report of twelve cases. Eur J Endocrinol 1998;139: 284–289.
58. Salle BL, Berthezene F, Glorieux FH, et al. Hypoparathyroidism during pregnancy: treatment with calcitriol. J Clin Endocrinol Metab 1981;52: 810–813(abst).
59. Sadeghi-Nejad A, Wolfsdorf JI. Hypoparathyroidism and pregnancy: treatment with calcitriol. JAMA 1980;243:254–255.
60. Bronsky D, Kiamko RT, Moncada R, et al. Intra-uterine hyperparathyroidism secondary to maternal hypoparathyroidism. Paediatrics 1968; 42:606–613.
61. Eastell R, Edmonds CJ, de Chayal RC, et al. Prolonged hypoparathyroidism presenting eventually as second trimester abortion. Br Med J (Clin Res Ed) 1985;291:955–956.
62. Gradus D, LeRoith D, Karplus M, et al. Congenital hyperparathyroidism and rickets: secondary to maternal hypoparathyroidism and vitamin D deficiency. Isr J Med Sci 1981;17:705–708.
63. Sann L, David L, Thomas A, et al. Congenital hyperparathyroidism and vitamin D deficiency secondary to maternal hypoparathyroidism. Acta Paediatr Scand 1976;65:381–385.
64. Zerwekh JE, Breslau NA. Human placental production of 1-alpha,25-dihydroxyvitamin D3: biochemical characterization and production in

normal subjects and patients with pseudohypoparathyroidism. J Clin Endocrinol Metab 1986;62:192–196.

65. Saito H, Saito M, Saito K, et al. Subclinical pseudohypoparathyroidism type II: evidence for failure of physiologic adjustment in calcium metabolism during pregnancy. Am J Med Sci 1989;297:247–250.
66. Glass EJ, Barr DGD. Transient neonatal hyperparathyroidism secondary to maternal pseudohypoparathyroidism. Arch Dis Child 1981;56:565–568.
67. Ozsoylu S. Management of pseudohypoparathyroidism in pregnancy: case report. Br J Obstet Gynaecol 1985;92:639–641.
68. Kaufman MH. Reflections on Dr Henderson of Perth's case of impracticable labour: an early case (1820) in which the caesarean operation was performed. Scott Med J 1993;38:85–88.
69. Chaim W, Alroi A, Leiberman JR, et al. Severe contracted pelvis appearing after normal deliveries. Acta Obstet Gynecol Scand 1981;60: 131–134.
70. Peacock M. Osteomalacia and rickets. In: Nordin BEC, Need AG, Morris HA, eds. Metabolic bone and stone disease. Edinburgh: Churchill Livingstone, 1993:83–118.
71. Murray JA, Newman WA III, Dacus JV. Hyperparathyroidism in pregnancy: diagnostic dilemma? Obstet Gynecol Surv 1997;52: 202–205.
72. Kondo Y, Nagai H, Kasahara K, et al. Primary hyperparathyroidism and acute pancreatitis during pregnancy: report of a case and review of the English and Japanese literature. Int J Pancreatol 1998;24: 43–47.
73. Pitkin RM. Calcium metabolism in pregnancy and the perinatal period: a review. Am J Obstet Gynecol 1985;151:99–109.
74. Better OS, Levi J, Grief E, et al. Prolonged neonatal parathyroid suppression. A sequel to asymptomatic maternal hyperparathyroidism. Arch Surg 1973;106:722–724.
75. Kelly TR. Primary hyperparathyroidism during pregnancy. Surgery 1991;110:1028–1034.
76. Carella MJ, Gossain W. Hyperparathyroidism and pregnancy: case report and review. J Gen Intern Med 1992;7:448–453(abst).
77. Thomas BR, Bennett JD. Symptomatic hypocalcemia and hypoparathyroidism in two infants of mothers with hyperparathyroidism and familial benign hypercalcemia. J Perinatol 1996;16:513–514.

SECTION IX

Neurologic Disorders

Cherry and Merkatz's Complications of Pregnancy,
Fifth Edition, edited by W. R. Cohen.
Lippincott Williams & Wilkins, Philadelphia © 2000.

CHAPTER 27

Cerebrovascular Disorders

Efraim P. David and Robert J. Wityk

Although stroke is commonly thought of as a disease of the elderly, approximately 5% to 10% of stroke victims are children or young adults aged under 45 years (1). A discussion of the diagnosis and management of stroke patients can be found in a number of current textbooks (2,3), and texts dealing with stroke in young patients are particularly germane to women of childbearing age (1,4,5). This chapter focuses primarily on cerebrovascular disorders that are either unique to pregnancy or can be seen in young women of childbearing age.

Stroke is a general term encompassing ischemic stroke, intracerebral hemorrhage (ICH), subarachnoid hemorrhage (SAH), and cerebral venous thrombosis (CVT). Although the initial clinical presentation may be similar in these subtypes of stroke, prognosis and management are often quite different. The goal of evaluation of the stroke patient is to distinguish quickly between ischemic and hemorrhagic stroke and to determine expeditiously the underlying mechanism of stroke to plan appropriate therapy (6).

EPIDEMIOLOGY

A number of studies have estimated the incidence of stroke during pregnancy and the postpartum period, but many of these studies involve only small numbers of stroke patients or are potentially subject to referral bias (Table 27-1) (7–13). One large, prospective study at Parkland Memorial Hospital reviewed 89,913 deliveries over a 6-year period and found nine patients with ischemic stroke and six patients with ICH, giving an incidence rate of 1 in 6,000 pregnancies (16.7/100,000) (10). A population-based study in central France surveyed more than 350,000 deliveries at 63 community and academic hospitals and found a lower incidence of 4.3 per 100,000 for ischemic stroke and 4.6 per 100,000 for intraparenchymal hemorrhage (11). The most common cause of both ischemic and hemorrhagic stroke in this study was eclampsia. Ischemic strokes occurred most often in the postpartum period, followed by the third trimester. Hemorrhagic strokes, however, presented most often in the third trimester (not including the period of labor).

A more recent population-based study (the Baltimore–Washington Young Stroke Study) was derived from a registry of stroke patients aged under 45 years in the central Maryland and Washington D.C. area during the years 1988 and 1991 (13). All area hospitals participated, and cases were ascertained from the International Classification of Diseases (ICD)-9 discharge codes and referral from community neurologists. The puerperium was defined as up to 6 weeks postpartum, and pregnancies terminated by spontaneous or induced abortion were included. The pregnancy- and puerperium-associated

E. P. David and R. J. Wityk: Department of Neurology, Johns Hopkins University School of Medicine, Johns Hopkins Hospital, Baltimore, MD 21287.

TABLE 27-1. *Epidemiologic studies of stroke in pregnancy*

Year	First author	Location	Period	Pregnancies	Number of strokes	Incidence per 10^5	Comments
1962	Lorincz (124)	Chicago, IL	1955–1959	15,198	6	40	Puerperal cases only; abortions not included; all cases had excellent recovery
1964	Goldman (123)	Israel	1950–1963	25,000	15	60	Abortions not included; seven autopsies performed; all CVT
1968	Cross (7)	Glasgow	1956–1967	600,000	31	5	Referral center
1983	Srinivasan (14)	India	1974–1983	65,000?	135	208	Puerperal cases only; total number of population at risk not clear
1985	Wiebers (9)	Rochester, MN	1955–1979	26,099	1	4	Puerperium and abortion-related cases not included; homogenous sample
1991	Simolke (10)	Dallas, TX	1984–1990	89,913	15	17	Abortions not included
1995	Sharshar (11)	France	1989–1992	348,295	31	9	Puerperal period is 2 wk; TIA, CVT, pure SAH excluded; population based
1996	Kittner (13)	Baltimore, MD	1988–1991	234,023	31	13	SAH not included; population based
1997	Witlin (105)	Memphis, TN	1985–1995	79,301	20	25	Abortions not included
1997	Lanska (125)	USA	1979–1991	50,110,949	9938	18	Abortions not included; only strokes during hospitalization

CVT, cerebral venous thrombosis; SAH, subarachnoid hemorrhage; TIA, transient ischemic attack.

stroke rate was 1 in 7,500 pregnancies (13.3/100,000). The relative risk for pregnant women compared with nonpregnant women of the same age was calculated using state vital statistics and estimated at risk years for all women of childbearing age during the study period (Table 27-2). Interestingly, the relative risk (RR) for ischemic stroke was not elevated during pregnancy [RR, 0.7; 95% confidence interval (CI), 0.3–1.6] but was significantly elevated in the puerperium (RR, 5.4; 95% CI, 2.9–10.0). For hemorrhagic stroke, the relative risk was 2.5 (95% CI, 1.0–6.4) during pregnancy and 28.3 (95% CI, 13.0–61.4) during the puerperium. The temporal distribution during pregnancy of ischemic and hemorrhagic strokes from this study is shown in Figs. 27-1 and 27-2. Unlike the French study, the Baltimore–Washington study considered the puerperal period to be up to 6 weeks postpartum (rather than 2 weeks) and included patients with CVT. These differences may explain the higher incidence rates. In both studies, however, a substantial proportion of ischemic strokes and hemorrhages were attributed to eclampsia (Fig. 27-3).

In developing countries, the incidence of maternal stroke may be much higher. Srinivasan reported an incidence rate of 208/100,000 in India, with most strokes attributed to venous thrombosis (14). In the early literature from the United States and Europe, CVT appeared to

TABLE 27-2. *Relative risk of stroke during pregnancy*

Period	RR of infarction	RR of ICH	Total RR
Pregnancy	0.7 (0.3–1.6)	2.5 (1.0–6.4)	1.1 (0.6–2.0)
Puerperium	5.4 (2.9–10.0)	18.2 (8.7–38.1)	7.9 (5.0–12.7)
Puerperium (delivered)	8.7 (4.6–16.7)	28.3 (13.0–61.4)	12.7 (7.8–20.7)
Puerperium (induced abortion)	1.1 (0.2–7.9)	4.5 (0.6–33.1)	1.8 (0.4–7.2)
Entire pregnancy and puerperium	1.6 (1.0–2.7)	5.6 (3.0–10.5)	2.4 (1.6–3.6)

RR, relative risk; ICH, intracerebral hemorrhage.

From Kittner SJ, Stern BJ, Feeser BR, et al. Pregnancy and the risk of stroke. N Engl J Med 1996;335:768–774, with permission.

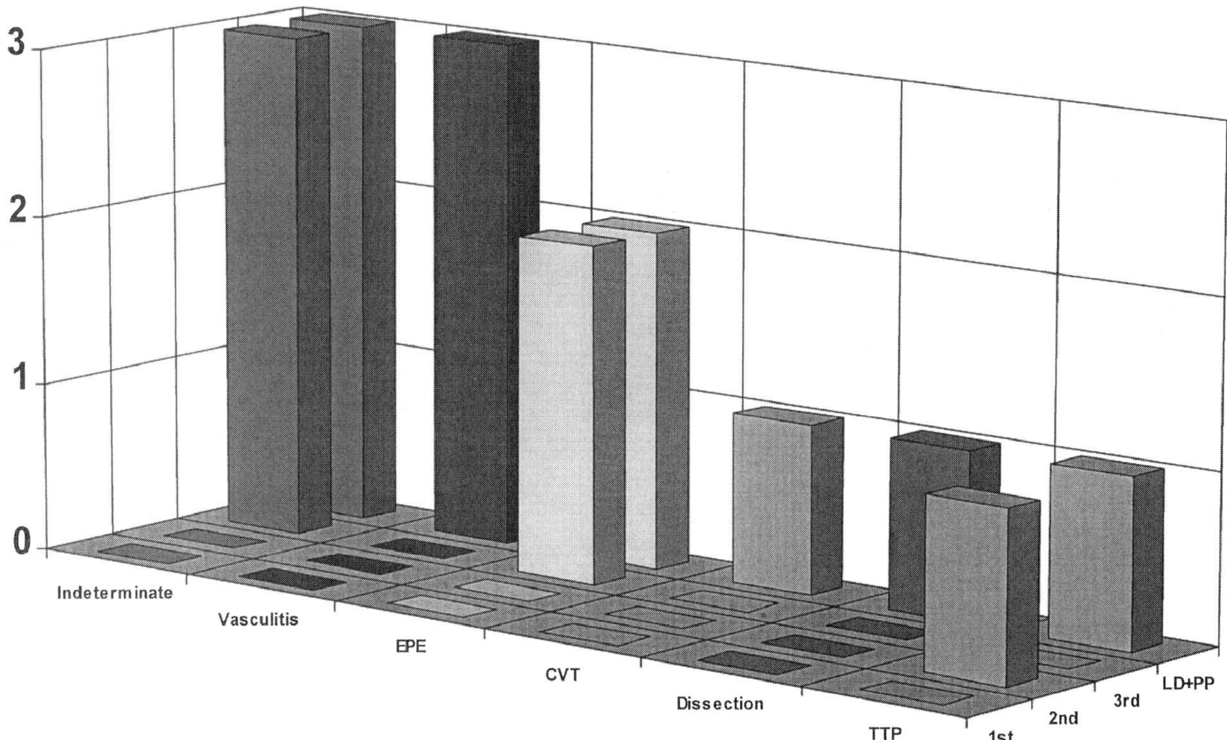

FIG. 27-1. Ischemic stroke in pregnancy. (Adapted from Sharshar T, Lamy C, Mas JL. Incidence and causes of strokes associated with pregnancy and puerperium: a study in public hospitals of Ile de France. Stroke in Pregnancy Study Group. Stroke 1995;26:930–936. Kittner SJ, Stern BJ, Feeser BR, et al. Pregnancy and the risk of stroke. N Engl J. Med 1996;335:768–774.)

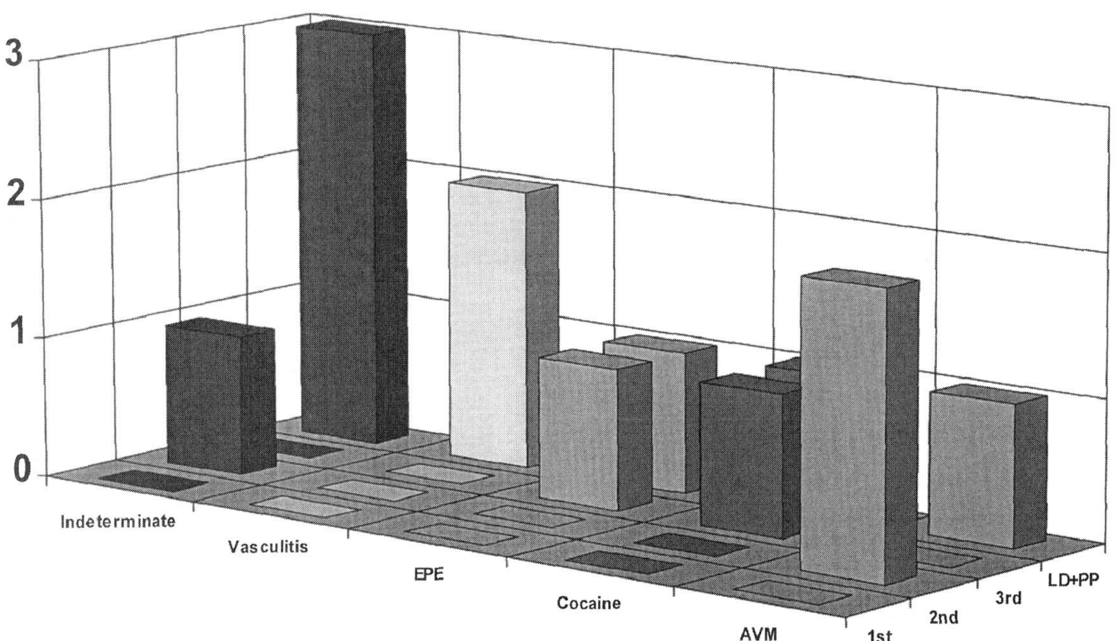

FIG. 27-2. Intracerebral hemorrhage in pregnancy. (Adapted from ref. Sharshar T, Lamy C, Mas JL. Incidence and causes of strokes associated with pregnancy and puerperium: a study in public hospitals of Ile de France. Stroke in Pregnancy Study Group. Stroke 1995;26:930–936. Kittner SJ, Stern BJ, Feeser BR, et al. Pregnancy and the risk of stroke. N Engl J. Med 1996;335:768–774.)

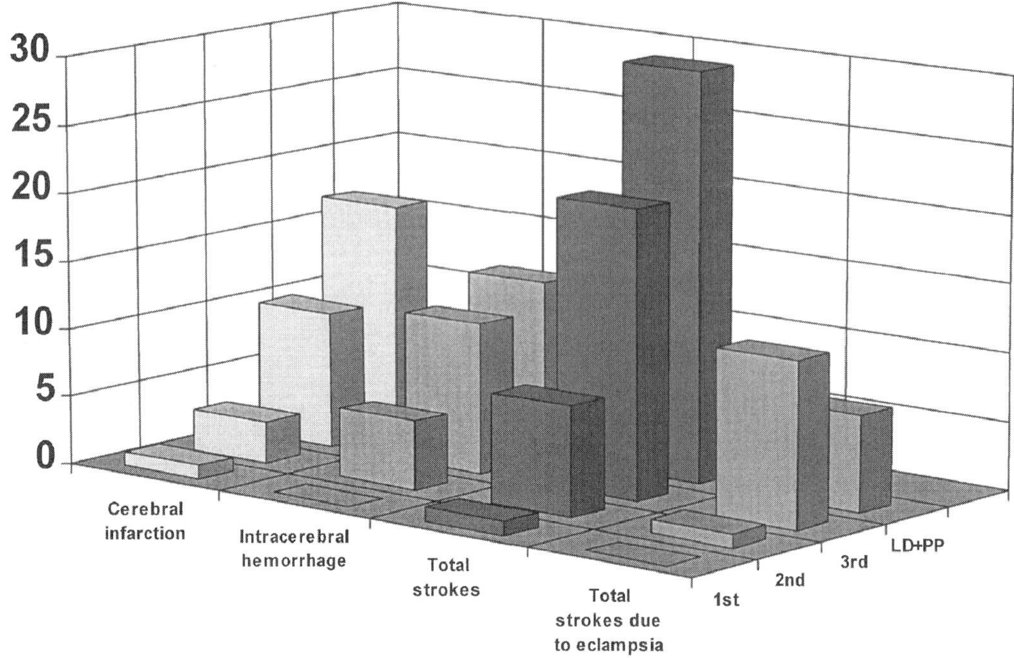

FIG. 27-3. Stroke and eclampsia in pregnancy. (Adapted from refs. Sharshar T, Lamy C, Mas JL. Incidence and causes of strokes associated with pregnancy and puerperium: a study in public hospitals of Ile de France. Stroke in Pregnancy Study Group. Stroke 1995;26:930–936. Kittner SJ, Stern BJ, Feeser BR, et al. Pregnancy and the risk of stroke. N Engl J. Med 1996;335:768–774.)

be a common cause of maternal stroke, but it has become distinctly less frequent in more recent series. Venous thrombosis is considered related to dehydration and a hypercoagulable state during the postpartum period. Better hydration and general medical care in developed countries may explain the currently reduced incidence of venous thrombosis.

Despite its relative infrequency (0.01% of pregnancies), stroke nevertheless contributes an estimated 4.3% to 8.5% of maternal mortality (15,16). These figures probably underestimate the actual contribution of stroke to maternal mortality. The leading cause of maternal mortality is systemic embolism (which includes intracranial embolism as well) followed by hypertensive disease of pregnancy (15,16), and both these causes of maternal death are proven risk factors for stroke (Fig. 27-4). In cases when the stroke was secondary to hypertensive disease of pregnancy, for example, the cause of death was not attributed to stroke but to the hypertensive disorder (15). It is important to point out that the concomitant occurrence of stroke increases disease morbidity and complicates medical management; overall mortality may

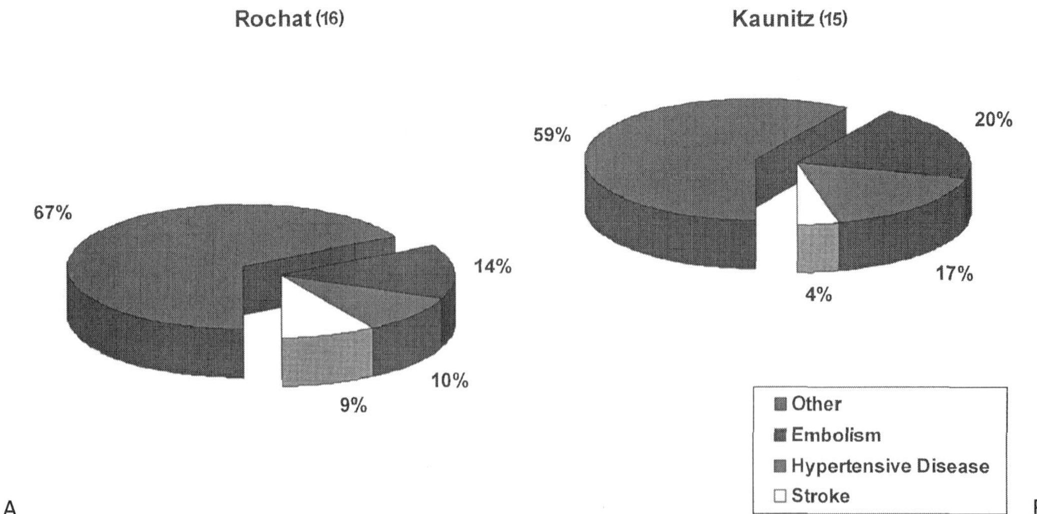

FIG. 27-4 A and **B.** Stroke and maternal mortality.

be worsened. In a smaller but more detailed study (17), Barnes and Abbott reported that ICH and SAH contributed to 9% of maternal fatalities. Interestingly, no deaths were attributed to cerebral infarction. A similar study (18) by Barno and Freeman showed ICH and SAH as contributing to 9% of maternal deaths; again, no figure was mentioned for ischemic strokes.

ISCHEMIC STROKE

Ischemic stroke results from a critical loss of blood flow to a particular region of the brain. If the degree and length of hypoperfusion are limited, the ischemic neurons may recover, and the neurologic deficit can resolve completely, resulting in a transient ischemic attack (TIA). Although TIAs are defined as a neurologic deficit resulting from ischemia that resolves within 24 hours, most TIAs last only 5 to 15 minutes and rarely last more than a few hours. More severe and prolonged hypoperfusion triggers a cascade of neurochemical changes in neural tissue, which eventually leads to cellular necrosis and a permanent neurologic deficit. The molecular details of these events are the focus of intense interest in stroke research at this time. Development of pharmacologic agents that interfere with neuronal death has resulted in clinical trials of a number of potential neuroprotective agents (19). Glutamate, for example, is an excitatory amino acid neurotransmitter with wide distribution in the cerebral cortex (20). In experimental animal models of ischemic stroke, excessive amounts of glutamate are released and are felt to cause secondary neuronal injury (the excitotoxic theory) through a nitric oxide-dependent mechanism (19,21,22) Administration of glutamate antagonists either before or shortly after the ischemic insult in animal models results in a substantial reduction in cerebral infarct size. Whereas this type of experimental data has generated much interest in the clinical application of these pharmacologic agents, none has yet been proven effective in clinical trials in humans (19,23).

Ischemic stroke can be classified by presumed cause or mechanism of stroke (Table 27-3), with the realization that some patients may have more than one potential cause. In older patients, large-artery atherosclerosis, cardioembolism, and lacunar (small vessel) stroke are the three most common etiologies. In young stroke patients, cardioembolism is the most common etiology, followed by hematologic causes, with large-artery atherosclerosis and lacunes less common, except for patients in the 40- to 50-year age range who have premature atherosclerosis

TABLE 27-3. *Etiology and predisposing factors of ischemic stroke*

- Cardiac-embolic
  - Wall-motion abnormality predisposing to intracardiac thrombus
    - Atrial fibrillation
    - Atrial septal aneurysm
    - Peripartum cardiomyopathy
  - Valvular abnormality
    - Rheumatic heart disease
    - Subacute bacterial endocarditis
    - Marantic endocarditis
    - Mitral valve prolapse
  - Paradoxical embolism through right-to-left shunt
    - Patent foramen ovale
    - Atrial septal defect
    - Ventricular septal defect
    - *Other embolic material* (foreign body embolism such as amniotic fluid, fat, and air)
- Vascular-thrombotic
  - Premature atherosclerosis
  - Arterial dissection
  - Fibromuscular dysplasia
  - Vasculitis
    - Systemic lupus erythematosis
    - Takayasu's arteritis
    - Syphilitic arteritis
    - Primary central nervous system vasculitis
  - Moyamoya disease
  - Postpartum angiopathy
  - Lacunar stroke
- Hematologic
  - Primary hypercoagulable state
    - Antithrombin disorders
      - Antithrombin III deficiency
      - Heparin cofactor II deficiency
    - Protein C and protein S disorders
      - Protein S deficiency
      - Protein C deficiency
      - Activated protein C resistance
    - Fibrinolytic disorders
      - Hypoplasminogenemia
      - Plasminogen activator deficiency
      - Dysfibrinogenemia
  - Secondary hypercoagulable state
    - Activation of coagulation system
      - Systemic malignancy
      - Estrogen use
      - Nephrotic syndrome
      - Lupus anticoagulant
    - Platelet activation and vascular disorders
      - Myeloproliferative disorders, e.g., leukemias, polycythemia vera
      - Sickle cell disease
      - Heparin associated thrombosis
      - Thrombocytopenic purpura
      - Homocystenuria
      - Paroxysmal nocturnal hemoglobinuria
    - Venous stasis
      - Immobilization
      - Obesity
      - Congestive heart failure
      - Postoperative state
- Eclampsia/preeclampsia
- Cerebral venous thrombosis
- Miscellaneous
  - Substance abuse
  - Migraine
  - Chronic meningitis

(5,24–26). Hematologic disorders, unusual vasculopathies, and vasculitis must be considered in young patients. Despite increasing sophistication in diagnostic evaluation, up to 30% of young patients still have no clearly defined cause of their stroke (5,24,25).

Cardioembolic strokes are responsible for one fifth of ischemic strokes, and in the case of stroke in young patients, about a third (27). The classic presentation is maximal neurologic deficit at onset. Findings on physical examination may include cardiac rhythm irregularities, murmurs, and cardiomegaly. Isolated aphasias and hemianopias are suggestive of embolic infarction. Neuroimaging typically shows a wedge-shaped infarct or several such infarcts in multiple vascular territories. Transesophageal echocardiography detects most potential cardiac sources of emboli, such as mural thrombi, left atrial appendage thrombi, left atrial spontaneous echo contrast, atrial septal aneurysm, right-left shunts (e.g., patent foramen ovale), aortic arch atheroma, and cardiac-wall motion abnormalities such as dyskineasia, akinesia, and hypokinesia (28–30). An electrocardiogram (ECG) can identify cardiac arrhythmias, and 24-hour Holter monitoring can pick up intermittent arrhythmias that the routine electrocardiogram may miss. Anticoagulation is generally recommended for secondary prevention of further embolic events. Contraindications to anticoagulation include massive acute infarction, severe hypertension, infective endocarditis, or ICH. The duration of the anticoagulation depends on the underlying pathology. Global and severe left ventricular dysfunction and atrial fibrillation may require lifetime anticoagulation (31).

Peripartum cardiomyopathy (PPC) is a form of dilated congestive cardiomyopathy of unknown etiology occurring predominantly in the last trimester of pregnancy or up to 6 months postpartum (32). The incidence is about 1 in 10,000 (33), and there may be a familial component (34). Patients present with signs and symptoms of congestive heart failure. Multiparity, twin gestation, age over 30, and black race appear to be risk factors. Echocardiography shows dilatation of all cardiac chambers and reduced ejection fraction. Endomyocardial biopsy may reveal evidence of myocarditis (35). The diagnosis is established by exclusion of other causes of heart failure. Maternal cocaine abuse is an important differential of PPC (36). About half of patients recover without sequelae, whereas the other half deteriorate and die (33). There is a risk of recurrence in subsequent pregnancies (37). Treatment is supportive and symptomatic with judicious use of digitalis (as a result of enhanced digitalis sensitivity and a risk of toxicity), afterload and preload reduction, and anticoagulation because of the high risk of embolization (38). Immunosuppressive therapy may play a role, especially in those with inflammatory changes on biopsy (39). Heart transplant is an option for those who do not respond to conventional treament (33,40–42). PPC is a state of high risk for cardioembolism. Postmortem dissection of affected hearts frequently shows mural thrombi in the left ventricle and left atrial appendage (35,38). Stroke is not an infrequent complication of PPC (38,43–45) and even may be the presenting sign (45). Prophylactic anticoagulation is indicated (32,33,38), especially in patients with low ejection fraction and evidence of mural thrombi (37), or as long as cardiomegaly persists (46).

Amniotic fluid embolism (AFE) is a rare complication of pregnancy occurring in about 1 in 8,000 to 1 in 80,000 deliveries and accounts for as much as 10% of maternal deaths. It is usually secondary to a tear in the membranes as may occur in placenta accreta, cesarean section, ruptured uterus, or through small tears in the endocervical veins during normal labor (47). Possible predisposing factors include preeclampsia, twins, hydramnios, low placental insertion, postterm pregnancy, hypertonic contractions, abruptio placentae, uterine rupture, shoulder dystocia, and umbilical cord prolapse (48). The classic clinical presentation is sudden dyspnea and hypotension, leading to cardiopulmonary collapse. Seizure is also a presenting symptom in a third of cases (49). There is a greater than 50% mortality within the first hour and only a 15% survival rate with intact neurologic function (50). Neurologic deficits are attributed to hypoxic–ischemic injury secondary to respiratory failure, although cerebral embolism may occur through pulmonary or cardiac right-to-left shunts. Because the emboli are small, the radiologic picture may mimic global ischemia (51). Disseminated intravascular coagulation occurs early in the disorder. Diagnosis often is established at autopsy by identification of fetal squames in the maternal pulmonary vascular bed; however, fetal squames also have been recovered in pulmonary circulation of mothers otherwise asymptomatic for AFE (47). Management is aimed to maintain left ventricular output and may consist of cardiopulmonary resuscitation, oxygen, and mechanical ventilation.

Large-artery atherosclerosis is a common cause of stroke in the general population, but it is a relatively uncommon cause of stroke in women of childbearing age. Risk factors for the development of large-artery atherosclerosis include advancing age, hypertension, diabetes mellitus, smoking, and hypercholesterolemia. Relative elevation of the amino acid homocysteine in the blood is a recently described risk factor for premature atherosclerosis. Treatment of large-artery atherosclerosis requires optimal management of risk factors, such as control of blood pressure and diabetes, smoking cessation, and use of cholesterol-lowering agents. Vitamins B_6 and B_{12} and folate supplements may be beneficial in patients with homocystenemia. Aspirin in daily doses of 80 to 1,300 mg reduces the recurrence of stroke. When the arterial lumen diameter is significantly reduced by atherosclerotic plaque (more than 70% diameter stenosis), blood flow is compromised. When this occurs in surgically accessible locations (for example, in the extracranial segment of the internal carotid artery) operative interventions such as carotid endarterectomy have proved beneficial in symptomatic patients. In nonsurgically accessible locations such as the intracranial blood vessels, treatment options include medical management with aspirin or anticoagulation with warfarin. Endovascular interventions such as angioplasty or stenting are investigational procedures that hold promise.

Arterial dissection is a tearing of a cerebral vessel with hematoma formation in the wall of the vessel between the intima and the media (52). Although dissections may penetrate the vessel wall (resulting in a pseudoaneurysm), the more common complication is narrowing of the vascular lumen by the hematoma or development of an intraluminal clot that can embolize distally. As a consequence, patients have ischemic rather than hemorrhagic stroke from arterial dissection of cerebral vessels. Patients with dissection who present with minor symptoms have a good prognosis. Generally, anticoagulation with heparin and warfarin is recommended. With time, there is reabsorption of the hematoma and often complete resolution of the vascular lesion. Disorders of the vessel wall, such as fibromuscular dysplasia, cystic medial necrosis, and other connective tissue disorders, may predispose to dissection, but in most cases no associated cause can be found (52,53). The peak age for arterial dissection is in the 40's, with most cases occurring between 30 and 50 years of age. No data linking pregnancy or labor with an increased risk of dissection have been found.

Fibromuscular dysplasia (FMD) is a vasculopathy of unknown etiology in which fibrous thickening of the vessel wall may result in hemodynamically significant stenosis of large vessels (commonly the extracranial carotid or vertebral arteries) (54). Patients often present with TIAs, but sometimes the stenosis may become so severe as to cause occlusion and results in a stroke. FMD is associated with arterial dissection 12% of the time, which may lead to cerebral infarction, and it is associated with saccular aneurysms 20% of the time, which may lead to subarachnoid hemorrhage. Diagnosis is established by conventional angiography and increasingly by magnetic resonance angiography (MRA) showing the classic "string-of-beads" appearance. Management consists of surgical excision of severely affected segments or endovascular interventions. Most patients with less severe disease are treated with antiplatelet agents.

Vasculitis should be suspected in a young stroke patient with fever, headache, and inflammatory changes in the cerebrospinal fluid (CSF). Vasculitis can result from a systemic vasculitis [e.g., systemic lupus erythematosus (SLE), polyarteritis nodosa, sarcoid], hypersensitivity reaction (e.g., intravenous drug abuse), or primary central nervous system (CNS) angiitis (55). Cerebral angiography shows findings of multiple and diffuse segmental narrowing and dilatation, occlusion, and sluggish blood flow in the arteries (56). The vascular changes may result from inflammation and vasospasm initially and from scarring later. The diagnosis is confirmed by brain biopsy showing vascular inflammatory changes, although this is done infrequently, and treatment with immunosuppressive agents, such as steroids, is often used on a presumptive basis.

Systemic lupus erythematosus is the most frequent type of symptomatic vasculitis during pregnancy (57). Neurologic symptoms include encephalopathy, seizures, cranial nerve palsies, chorea gravidarum, and stroke. There are a few reported cases of stroke during pregnancy in a patient with SLE (58–60). The management of the pregnant patient with SLE is complex, requiring a multidisciplinary approach and close prenatal follow-up to monitor disease exacerbation during pregnancy.

Primary CNS vasculitis is an uncommon disorder of unknown etiology. It occurs rarely during pregnancy and the puerperium, with only two reported cases (61,62). The diagnosis is one of exclusion and is confirmed by brain biopsy showing vascular inflammatory changes. Treatment consists of corticosteroids and cyclophosphamide. The prognosis is unpredictable.

Takayasu disease ("pulseless disease") is an inflammatory arteriopathy with preferential involvement of large vessels arising from the aorta (63). The condition is more common in Asians, but it is seen in a variety of ethnic groups. The consequence of arterial inflammation is an occlusive fibrous thickening of involved vessels. Progressive stenosis or occlusion of the carotid arteries can result in stroke, TIA, or chronic ocular ischemia. Narrowing of the aorta often results in secondary hypertension, which may be difficult to detect because of falsely low blood pressure readings in the arms, which is caused by subclavian stenosis. The diagnosis is suspected from finding asymmetric radial pulses or hearing bruits over the supraclavicular fossa. Involvement of the proximal aorta can result in aortic insufficiency and aortic root dilatation. During pregnancy, the inflammatory component of the disease appears unaffected, and the primary concern relates to cardiac decompensation in patients with aortic arch involvement and labile hypertension (64,65). The most common cerebrovascular complication described in one review was ICH associated with accelerated hypertension at the time of labor (65). Patients with extensive occlusive disease are at higher risk for obstetric complications, and measurement of blood pressure in the arms may be inaccurate. Cesarean section has been recommended for patients with extensive disease who develop severe hypertension during the first stage of labor (65).

Moyamoya is a vasculopathy of unknown etiology in which there is gradual occlusion of the distal intracranial carotid arteries (66). An extensive collateral circulation develops deep within the base of the brain in the form of a mesh of fine, fragile vessels that appear as a puff of smoke on cerebral angiography. Moyamoya has an incidence of about 1 per one million in Japan, where the disease is most common. The male-to-female ratio is about 2:3. The age distribution is bimodal, with the first peak in children presenting with ischemia from progressive arterial stenosis and a second peak in adults, presenting most often as ICH from rupture of the fragile collateral vessels (66–68). Hemorrhages in young adults are in the basal ganglia and deep white matter in two thirds and intraventricular or subependymal in one third (69,70). In one prospective series of 210 young adults with stroke, eight patients had moyamoya disease; in one patient, the stroke occurred in the peripartum period (71). The diagnosis is established by cerebral angiography, although the condition can be recognized by magnetic resonance imaging (MRI) and MRA. Many treatment options are available, mainly surgical, such as superior cervical ganglionectomy, perivascular sympathectomy, encephaloduroarteriosynangiosis, and superior temporal artery to middle cerebral artery anastomosis (66).

Postpartum angiopathy is a poorly defined syndrome in which neurologic symptoms in the puerperium are associated with sometimes transient changes in the caliber of intracranial vessels. The patients typically present with headache, vomiting, seizures, and occasionally focal neurologic findings. The computed tomography (CT) scan may show areas of infarct. Angiography in reported cases usually reveals segmental narrowing in multiple cerebral vessels that is suggestive of either focal vasospasm or possibly vasculitis. In some cases, the clinical and angiographic findings normalize over time.

In many of the reported cases, there is a history of use of vasoconstrictive agents, such as bromocriptine (72–75), ergonovine (74,76), ergometrine (77), and phenylephrine (75). Bromocriptine increases the risk of postpartum hypertension in women with antepartum pregnancy-induced hypertension (78). Some of these patients have a history of antepartum (79–83) or immediate postpartum preeclampsia.

An acute hypertensive state could trigger vasospasm and explain the angiographic findings. This mechanism is believed to underlie the same process in pheochromocytoma, eclampsia, and other acute hypertensive states (74). The remaining cases without an inciting event may represent true postpartum eclampsia (79,84,85) in which the clinical presentation and angiographic findings are similar.

Delayed postpartum eclampsia represents about a sixth of all cases of eclampsia (86). It is believed that retained placental tissue may play a role in its pathogenesis (80, 84,87). Dilatation and curretage after delivery may play a role (88) in prevention, but this is not proven.

Lacunar stroke is a stroke in the territory of the small, deep-penetrating branches of the large arteries, primarily the middle cerebral arteries and the basilar artery. These branches arise perpendicularly from the parent artery and supply a small portion of brain tissue, usually an area no larger than 15 mm in diameter. These small infarcts can be seen on CT but are better visualized by MRI. Damage to penetrating arteries is associated strongly with a history of hypertension, and histopathology usually reveals lipohyalinosis of the artery. Clinically, lacunar stroke has been described by syndromes, such as pure-motor hemiparesis, pure sensory stroke, ataxic-hemiparesis, and clumsy-hand dysarthria. One must bear in mind, however, that these clinical syndromes do not always equate with small deep hemispheric infarcts. Furthermore, even radiologically proven lacunar infarcts may be caused by large-artery atheroslerosis occluding the penetrating artery at its origin or by cardiac or arterial emboli that propagate along the parent artery and occlude the branches or lodge in the penetrating artery itself. Patients with lacunar stroke should therefore be evaluated for large-artery disease and potential sources of emboli; this is particularly important for young or pregnant stroke patients, who often do not have a long history of hypertension.

Hematologic abnormalities are reported to contribute approximately 4% (89) to 17% (90) of strokes in young patients. The actual numbers are probably higher, because these percentages were derived before the discovery of activated protein C (APC) resistance, now considered the most common underlying abnormality in patients with deep venous thrombosis (DVT). The actual percentage may increase even more as new inherited coagulation abnormalities are discovered. The percentage of hematologic abnormalities in stroke during pregnancy has not been defined but most likely parallels that of stroke in other young persons.

Hematologic abnormalities can be subdivided into primary and secondary hypercoagulable states (see Table 27-3), which include intrinsic hematologic abnormalities such as antithrombin deficiency, protein C deficiency, protein S deficiency (91), APC resistance (92), lupus anticoagulant, and the presence of anticardiolipin antibody. The diagnosis is made by the identification and measurement in the serum of the specific protein deficiency. Secondary hypercoagulable states are due to systemic diseases that produce a procoagulable state and include malignancy, estrogen use, thrombotic thrombocytopenic purpura (TTP), immobilization, postoperative state, and even pregnancy. These hypercoagulable states may be clinically silent by themselves but become symptomatic when two or more states interact (93), such as in the postoperative patient with underlying APC resistance.

APC resistance is primarily a genetic disorder secondary to a point mutation in the factor V Leiden gene. In patients with DVT, APC resistance is present in 20% to 60%. In patients with CVT, APC resistance is present in about 20% (94,95).

When a hypercoagulable state becomes clinically symptomatic, the treatment of choice is systemic anticoagulation. The duration of anticoagulation may range from a few weeks to lifelong, depending on the underlying coagulation abnormality.

GENERAL DIAGNOSIS AND MANAGEMENT OF STROKE

Rapid diagnosis of a pregnant patient with focal neurologic deficits is essential because of the potentially

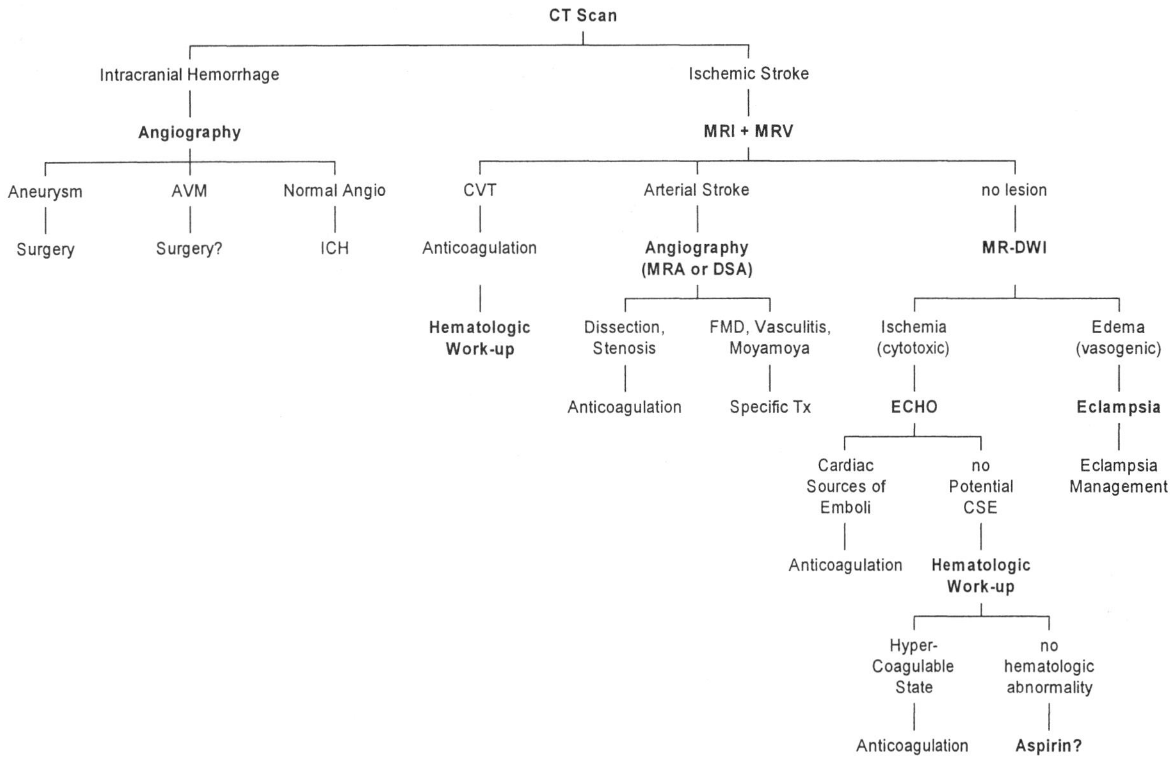

FIG. 27-5. Diagnostic workup of stroke in pregnancy.

high morbidity and mortality of patients with ischemic and hemorrhagic stroke (Fig. 27-5). CT scan should be performed as soon as possible, because it is sensitive to the presence of ICH and can detect more than 90% of subarachnoid bleeds. In patients in whom the clinical picture is suggestive of SAH (e.g., the patient complains of the worst headache of her life) and the CT is negative, then a spinal tap is needed to assess for red blood cells or xanthochromia in the CSF.

The CT may be negative, or it may show a hypodense area within the first 24 hours in a patient with an ischemic stroke (Fig. 27-6). A patient with ischemic stroke is evaluated for large-vessel disease, potential cardiac sources of emboli, hematologic disorders, and an inflammatory processes, such as vasculitis and infection. A carotid ultrasound is the quickest way to evaluate the extracranial internal carotid arteries. MRA can screen for both extracranial and intracranial large-artery disease such as the circle of Willis and its major branches. Cerebral angiography is still the gold standard for diagnosis, but it carries a small risk of complications, such as local hematoma, dye toxicity, and stroke.

An echocardiogram is used to evaluate for potential embolic sources from the heart and is best accomplished by using transesophageal echocardiography, looking for left atrial or left ventricular thrombi, left atrial smoke, segmental akinesia or hypokinesia, atrial septal aneurysm, or right-to-left shunts (e.g., patent foramen ovale, atrial septal defect, ventricular septal defect). A Holter monitor may

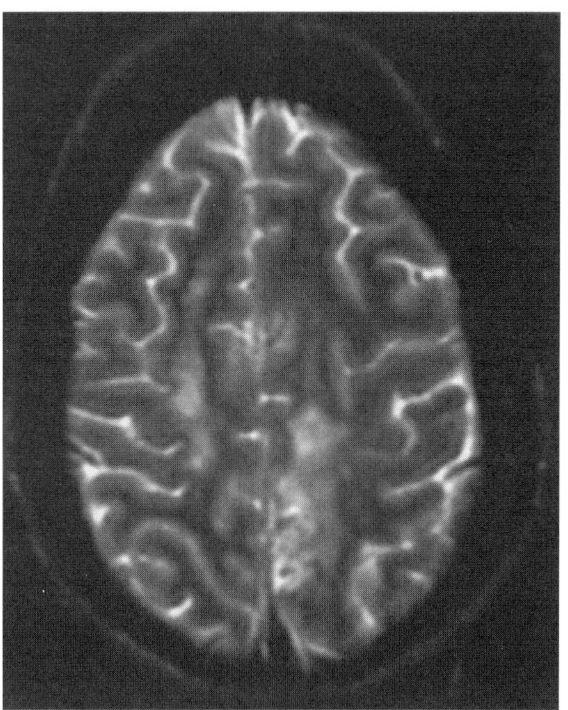

FIG. 27-6. MRI of a patient who developed multifocal neurologic deficits 2 weeks postpartum demonstrating multiple infarcts. In addition, the patient had diffuse vasospasm and a patent foramen ovale. The MRI appearance is similar in appearance to that found in some patients with eclampsia.

identify intermittent arrhythmias, such as atrial fibrillation or sick sinus syndrome, that predispose to embolization.

Workup for hematologic disorders includes a standard complete blood count, prothrombin time, partial thromboplastin time, protein C, protein S, antithrombin, antiphospholipid or anticardiolipin antibody, and lupus anticoagulant screen (e.g., Russel viper venom titer). Many young stroke patients have a remarkably good recovery so that a thorough evaluation is necessary to prevent future events.

Because cerebral autoregulation may be impaired during ischemia, cerebral perfusion pressures must be maintained. Mild to moderate blood pressure elevations are seen acutely, and these need not be treated. Patients who have low blood pressure may benefit from volume expansion using intravenous fluids, and sometimes even pharmacologic blood pressure elevation is indicated. In patients with stroke and hypertensive encephalopathy or hypertensive crises, blood pressure should be reduced cautiously by no more than 25% of the mean arterial pressure within 24 hours.

Thrombolytic therapy has been effective for ischemic stroke when it is given within 3 hours of onset of symptoms; however, experience in the use of thrombolytics during pregnancy is limited to a few cases of myocardial infarction, thrombosed mitral valve prosthesis and massive pulmonary embolism, and DVT (96–104). No experience has been reported of using thrombolytic therapy for stroke during pregnancy or the puerperium. Because of the risks of placental and fetal hemorrhage during pregnancy and maternal hemorrhage during pregnancy and the puerperium, thrombolysis for stroke during pregnancy cannot be recommended at this time.

Anticoagulation is indicated when either a potential source of emboli or a hypercoagulable state is identified. Intravenous heparin can be used in the acute setting. Warfarin should be avoided during weeks 6 to 12 of gestation, when teratogenic risk is high, and close to term, when delivery is imminent, to avoid excessive bleeding during delivery or cesarean section (see Chapters 7 and 15).

Supportive therapies must not be overlooked. These consist of low-flow oxygen by nasal cannula, correction of any underlying metabolic derangements, treatment of concommitant infections, gastrointestinal prophylaxis for peptic ulcer disease, and DVT prophylaxis with sequential compression devices or subcutaneous heparin (except in patients with ICH) or both. Once the stroke is established or completed, rehabilitation is the treatment for attempting to restore function. Physical therapy and occupational therapy may begin as soon as the patient is hemodynamically stable.

ECLAMPSIA–PREECLAMPSIA AND STROKE

Preeclampsia is the occurrence of hypertension and proteinuria during pregnancy. Severe preeclampsia occurs when there is the additional presence of oliguria (output less than 400 mL per 24 hours); pulmonary edema; hepatic dysfunction or right upper quadrant pain; thrombocytopenia; and cerebral disturbances manifested as headache, stupor, scotomata, and visual blurring (see Chapter 13).

Eclampsia is the occurrence of seizures or convulsions in the setting of preeclampsia. The seizures may be focal or multifocal in onset with generalization. Differentiation between early preeclampsia, severe preeclampsia, and eclampsia is not always clear-cut. Eclampsia implies CNS involvement, although CNS abnormalities such as alteration of level of consciousness, subclinical seizures, and cortical blindness may occur before or without clinically identifiable seizures. These probably represent different stages in the spectrum of the pathogenesis of a single disease. For the rest of the discussion, they will be considered under one rubric of eclampsia–preeclampsia (EPE).

Once the diagnosis of EPE is made, the determination of cerebral involvement, particularly stroke, is not easily established or excluded. A presumptive diagnosis of eclampsia actually may delay identification of stroke (105). The differential diagnosis of neurologic symptoms in a patient with EPE should include CVT, ICH, ischemic stroke, meningitis, and cerebral neoplasm.

A CT scan of the head is the preferred initial diagnostic imaging test. The CT scan in eclampsia may show hypodense areas, most commonly in the parietooccipital region, which may represent areas of edema (106–109) or ischemia (110). These two types of lesions are difficult to distinguish by CT. Focal neurologic deficits such as visual loss or weakness may resolve over time (107,111, 112) along with the CT findings (106–108,112), confirming that the lesions are not infarcts.

MRI may show changes that are not seen on CT or more extensive changes than those revealed by CT (112). Magentic resonance venography (MRV) can rule out CVT. One case report highlights the potential value of new MRI techniques, namely diffusion-weghted imaging (DWI) to distinguish areas of edema from infarction (113). With DWI, areas of vasogenic edema have increased diffusion coefficients and areas of ischemia (cytotoxic edema) have decreased diffusion coefficients. The distinction is important because edema responds favorably to blood pressure reduction, and ischemia does not.

The behavior of intracranial blood vessels in eclampsia is not well documented. Some angiographic (110,111, 114) and transcranial Doppler (115,116) studies have documented diffuse narrowing of both proximal and distal vessels. In some cases, these are associated with SAH (80,114) or ischemic stroke (110,111). Although the exact chronology of these neurovascular changes is not well delineated, the ischemic strokes appear to be secondary to the vasospasm (see Fig. 27-6). There are nevertheless reports of normal angiographic (117) and transcranial Doppler (116) findings.

CEREBRAL VENOUS THROMBOSIS

The cerebral venous system consists of small cortical veins on the surface of the brain. These veins drain into the large dural sinuses (sagittal sinus, transverse and sigmoid sinuses), which in turn empty into the jugular veins and a deep venous system draining the ventricles and base of the brain. Thrombosis of a cerebral vein impairs circulation of a region of the brain as a result of passive congestion, resulting in venous infarction. Because of high venous pressure, these infarcts often become hemorrhagic. Thrombosis of large sinuses can cause sufficient impairment of venous drainage to lead to increased intracranial pressure (ICP), even in the absence of cerebral infarction or mass effect.

The cause of CVT has been attributed to factors such as infection (obvious or occult), a hypercoagulable state during pregnancy, a relative dehydration in the puerperium, and the unique anatomy of cerebral venous drainage (118–120). Before the antibiotic era, most cerebral venous thrombosis was secondary to infection, such as otitis or mastoiditis, with spread of inflammation to the lateral venous sinus (121). The higher incidence of CVT in developing countries may reflect a higher rate of infection. Martin and Sheehan proposed the possibility of a symptomless infection and noted that positive blood cultures are found in a high percentage of normal women within 2 hours of a normal delivery (118).

A hypercoagulable state is responsible for some of the CVT in the general population. In particular, recent studies suggest that up to a fifth of patients with CVT have resistance to activated protein C because of an inherited mutation in the factor V gene (94,95). In the postpartum period, a hypercoagulable state, relative dehydration, and infection (122) are believed to account for most cases of pregnancy-related CVT, and older theories of extension of extracranial venous thrombosis into the cerebral veins have lost credibility (118,120).

Early estimates of the incidence of CVT range from 1 in 1,666 (123) to 1 in 2,500 (124) deliveries. A recent review of the National Hospital Discharge Survey for the period of 1979 to 1991 yielded an estimated 4,454 cases of intracranial venous thrombosis among 50 million deliveries, or about 1 in 11,000 deliveries (125). CVT usually occurs in the postpartum period (126–128). In a review by Biback and colleagues, 23% (9 of 37) occurred within the first 24 hours and nearly half within the first week (127) (Fig. 27-7). CVT has been reported to occur up to week 20 postpartum (127).

The most common presenting signs and symptoms are headache, seizures, and hemiparesis (123,127,129). Other signs include vomiting, depression of level of consciousness, fever, aphasia, hypertension, and psychosis (123). Headaches are usually generalized and throbbing and are probably secondary to elevated ICP. Papilledema may not be seen in the acute stage, but it is present in patients with chronic venous thrombosis. Hemorrhagic venous infarcts are typically cortical and high in the convexity of the brain, causing hemiparesis and cortical sensory loss (57,130). The presence of blood in the cortex is believed to irritate the brain and to cause the relatively high incidence of seizures. Frequently, the seizures are focal, causing motor twitching involving the hand or face, but then may spread to become generalized convulsions (57).

The pregnant or postpartum patient with CVT tends to differ from other patients with CVT. Patients with CVT associated with pregnancy tend to be younger, the disease onset is more acute, the resolution is faster, and the prognosis is better. In addition, there appears to be a higher prevalence of anemia. The reason for these differences is not clear, although the anemia may be secondary to blood loss during delivery or poor nutrition during pregnancy (128).

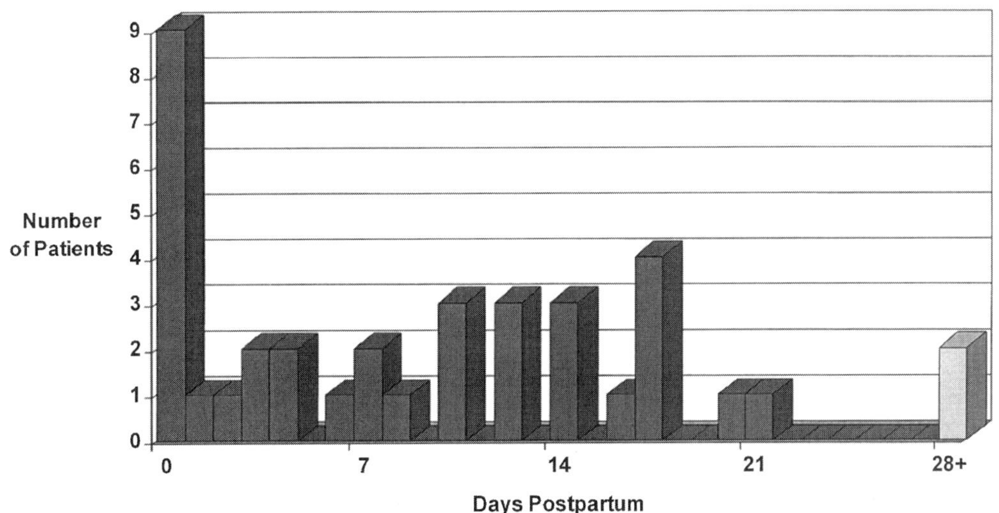

FIG. 27-7. CVT frequency in the postpartum period. (Adapted from Biback SM, Franklin A, Sata WK. Puerperal hemiplegia. Am J Obstet Gynecol 1962;83:45–53.)

CT scan may show a cortical hemorrhagic infarction, which often does not follow arterial territories. Contrast-enhanced CT can show the empty delta sign of thrombus in the sagittal sinus, but MRI has much better sensitivity and has become the imaging procedure of choice. The sinuses can be visualized both on MRI (particularly sagittal T1- and T2-weighted images) and ideally by MRV, which shows noninvasively both major sinuses and many smaller veins. MRI has the advantage of being able to date and follow the evolution of the thrombus (131). Conventional venography using a late-phase intraarterial contrast injection may reveal smaller isolated cortical venous occlusions that are harder to see on MRV (130). If a spinal tap is performed, the results may show elevated opening pressure and a higher protein concentration in one third of cases and increased red blood cells in one fourth of cases (129).

The treatment of choice is anticoagulation with heparin unless extensive ICH is present (57,118,120,132, 133). Some authors recommend anticoagulation despite the presence of ICH (133), whereas some are more conservative (132). Anticoagulation in the face of cortical hemorrhage may seem risky, but the bleeding is due to venous occlusion and is not from an arterial source. Anticoagulation to prevent propagation of thrombosis reduces the risk of further intracerebral bleeding and mortality. Hydration is also an important aspect in the management of these patients. The blood pressure must be followed carefully, because hypotension may exacerbate venous thrombosis. Direct endovascular thrombolysis of the CVT has been reported (134–136) but has not been tried during pregnancy.

The mortality rate varies between 0% (124–125) and 50% (129), depending on the study. In patients who survive, recovery tends to be almost complete. In one series, nine patients died, giving a 23% mortality rate; 24 (62%) had complete recovery (127).

INTRACRANIAL HEMORRHAGE

Intracranial bleeding can be divided into intracerebral (parenchymal) hemorrhage or SAH. The causes of ICH include intracranial vascular anomalies [aneurysm, arteriovenous malformation (AVM), cavernous angioma, moyamoya disease], hypertension, preeclampsia–eclampsia, CVT, hemorrhagic transformation of an ischemic stroke, coagulation disorders, and intracranial neoplasm (primary and metastatic) (1,137,138). The most frequent cause for pure ICH during pregnancy is preeclampsia–eclampsia (13).

SAH can be due to ruptured aneurysms (berry aneurysms, mycotic aneurysm, fusiform aneurysm of intracranial vessels) or extension of ICH into the subarachnoid space, which is often the case with arteriovenous malformations. The most frequent cause for SAH during pregnancy is ruptured aneurysm, followed by AVM. SAH contributes to most intracranial hemorrhages during pregnancy. Although symptomatic aneurysms and AVMs during pregnancy are rare (139), the mortality rate ranges from 40% to 80% (140) and contributes to 10% of maternal deaths (17).

INTRACEREBRAL HEMORRHAGE

The most common cause of nontraumatic ICH in patients aged younger than 45 years is AVM and in patients aged older than 45 years is hypertension (137,141). Hypertensive ICH is believed to result from rupture of the small penetrating arteries possibly secondary to fibrinoid necrosis, medial degeneration, lipohyalinosis, or microaneurysms (142). Hypertensive ICH frequently arises in the basal ganglia, especially the putamen, the lobar white matter, thalamus, pons, and cerebellum. Nonhypertensive ICH (e.g., resulting from AVM or tumor) frequently arises in the lobar white matter. ICH expands by tearing through adjacent brain tissue and occasionally ruptures into the ventricular system and causes intraventricular hemorrhage.

The incidence of ICH during pregnancy is about 1 in 10,000. When the etiology can be determined, AVMs and preeclampsia–eclampsia are the most common causes (13).

The symptoms at the onset of ICH are sudden, with evolution of neurologic deficits over the ensuing minutes to hours. Patients have headache, nausea, meningismus, and focal neurologic deficits. Signs suggestive of cerebral herniation include decreasing level of consciousness, pupillary dilatation (usually on the side of the herniation), hemiplegia with decorticate posturing, and a change in respiratory pattern. Patients with ICH in the temporal lobe or frontal pole may have minimal objective deficits early but complain of headache and drowsiness.

CT scan of the head is sensitive for the detection of acute intracranial hemorrhage. MRI is also adequate in the visualization of acute hemorrhage if appropriate sequences are done, but it is less reliable for subarachnoid and intraventricular hemorrhage (Figs. 27-8 and 27-9). Imaging studies usually obviate the need for lumbar puncture; withdrawal of spinal fluid in a patient with an intracerebral mass may result in neurologic deterioration.

The etiology of ICH in young patients is heterogeneous (Table 27-4), and a rigorous search for a cause should be undertaken even if the patient has known hypertension. Testing includes routine hematologic and coagulation profiles and a urine toxicology screen (for illicit drugs and sympathomimetic agents). Bromocriptine use for suppression of lactation has been associated with hemorrhagic infarction (143). Vasculitis should be considered in patients with known connective tissue disorders or in patients with unexplained fever, headache, elevated sedimentation rate, and multifocal strokes (Fig. 27-9). In a patient with fever or heart murmur, bacterial endocarditis must be considered, prompting blood cultures and an echocardiogram.

MRI of the brain may reveal an underlying neoplasm or vascular anomaly. A repeat MRI imaging 6 weeks later, when the hemorrhage has started to resolve, may better visualize an underlying lesion. Most young patients with unexplained ICH should have cerebral angiography at some point to looking for an AVM or other vascular abnormality (Fig. 27-10).

The management of patients with ICH is mainly supportive, with particular attention to management of ICP. Elevated blood pressure may increase ICP, but excessive blood pressure reduction can precipitate cerebral ischemia by lowering cerebral perfusion pressure. Fever, hypoxia, seizures, positive end-expiratory pressure (PEEP), endotrachial suctioning, and coughing contribute to ele-

TABLE 27-4. *Etiology and predisposing factors of nontraumatic intracerebral hemorrhage*

- Hypertension
  - Chronic hypertension
  - Preeclampsia-eclampsia
  - Pregnancy-induced hypertension
  - Sympathomimetic agents
    - Amphetamine, phenylpropanolamine, ephedrine, pseudoephedrine, cocaine
- Hematologic abnormalities
  - Hemostatic disorders
    - Platelet adhesion disorder, e.g., von Willebrand disease, uremia
    - Platelet aggregation disorder, e.g., antiplatelet drugs such as Ticlid, Reopro
    - Platelet granule release disorder, e.g., drugs such as aspirin and nonsteroidal antiinflammatory drugs
  - Vessel wall disorders
    - TTP, hemolytic-uremic syndrome, Henoch-Schönlein purpura
  - Coagulation disorders
    - Factor deficiency, e.g., factor VIII, IX, XI
    - Afribrogenemia, dysfibrogenemia
    - Vitamin K deficiency
    - Disseminated intravascular coagulation
    - Thrombolytic drugs, e.g., tPA, urokinase, streptokinase
- Intracranial tumors
  - Primary intracranial neoplasm, e.g., glioblastoma multiforme
  - Metastatic carcinoma
    - Choriocarcinoma, melanoma, bronchogenic carcinoma, renal cell carcinoma
- Hemorrhagic transformation of ischemic infarct
  - Septic embolic infarct, e.g., subacute bacterial endocarditis
  - Nonseptic embolic infarcts
  - Venous infarct, e.g., sinus thrombosis
- Vascular anomalies
  - Aneurysms
  - Vascular malformations
    - Arteriovenous malformations, cavernous angiomas, venous angiomas
  - Moyamoya disease
  - Vasculitis

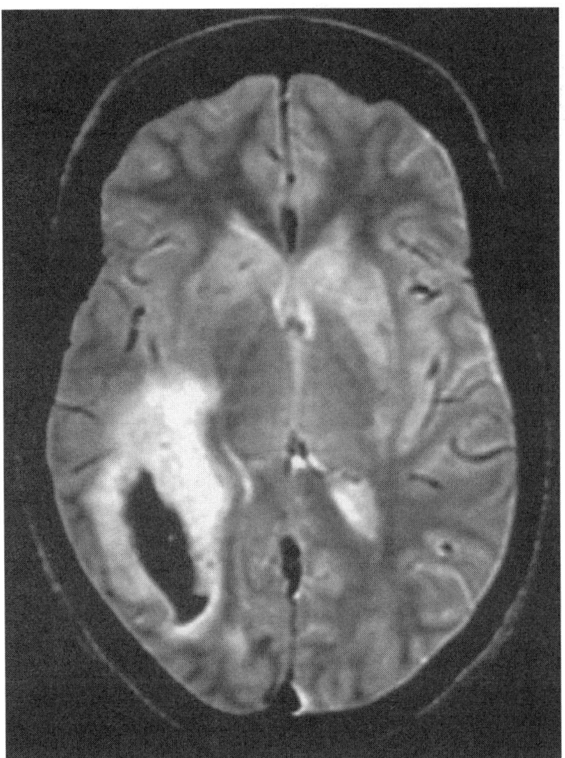

FIG. 27-8. MRI of a patient who developed a right parietal intracerebral hemorrhage postpartum.

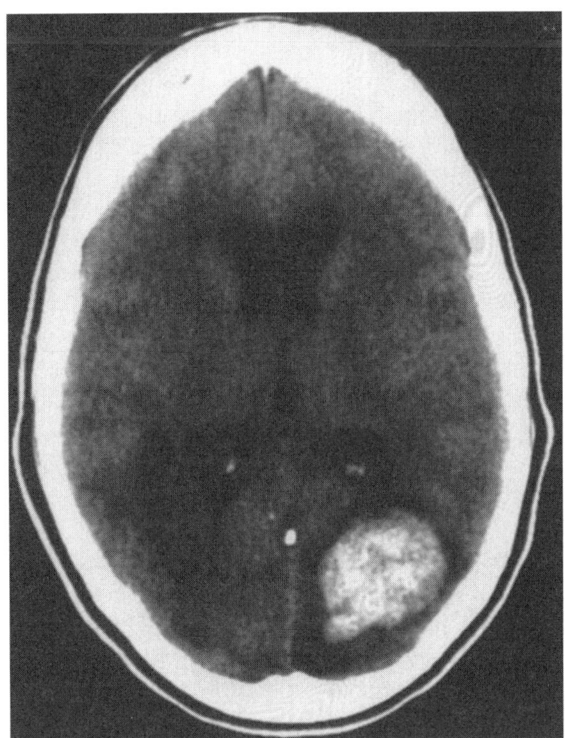

FIG. 27-9. Follow-up CT scan a few weeks later of the patient in Fig. 27-8. Note the development of a new intracerebral hemorrhage in the contralateral hemisphere, and the resolving hemorrhage in the right parietal region appearing as a hypodense area.

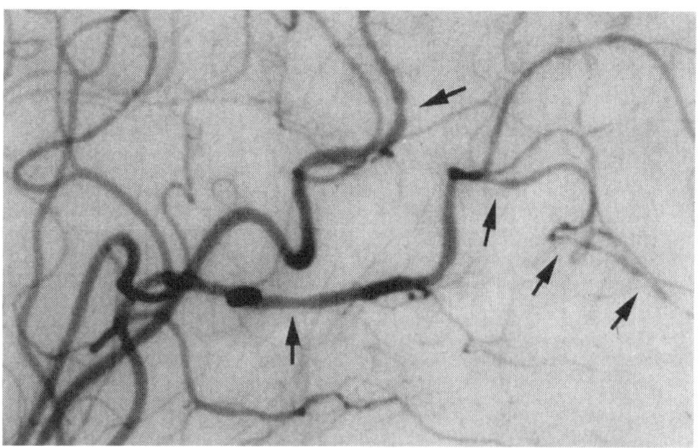

FIG. 27-10. Cerebral angiogram of the patient in Fig. 27-9 demonstrating multiple focal areas of narrowing *(arrows)*. These areas represent either vasculitis or vasospasm.

vated ICP. Hyperventilation, aiming for a partial pressure of carbon dioxide (pCO_2) of 25 to 35 mm Hg, acutely lowers ICP but is only a temporizing maneuver. Osmotic diuretics are also useful, although their use in pregnancy may lead to fetal dehydration (57). The usefulness of corticosteroids in the treatment of ICH is unproven.

The role of acute surgery in ICH is still debated. Some authors recommend surgical removal of a hematoma when it threatens life, especially in a young person with clinical deterioration (144). Furthermore, exploratory surgery may help to establish etiology and pathogenesis in cases in which the diagnosis is uncertain. Patients with superficial lobar hematomas tend to do better with surgery than do patients with deep basal ganglia bleeds. Cerebellar ICH is a notable exception. Cerebellar hematomas have the potential to cause rapid clinical deterioration secondary to brainstem compression, hydrocephalus, and upward transtentorial herniation. Hematomas larger than 3 cm in diameter usually are evacuated surgically by a suboccipital craniotomy approach, significantly improving outcome. Smaller lesions are monitored closely for clinical deterioration and potential surgical evacuation.

The acute mortality within the first 24 to 48 hours is about one fourth (145,146) and the in-hospital mortality about 40% (147). The 30-day mortality rate ranges from one third to one half (145,146,148–152). The size of the hematoma, the presence of intraventricular extension, and the clinical severity as measured by the Glasgow Coma Scale correlate with mortality (145,147,149,150,153, 154). Pontine hematomas larger than 3 cm in diameter are usually fatal, and supratentorial hematomas with a volume greater than 60 to 80 mL have a poor prognosis. When there is intraventricular extension, hydrocephalus may develop later. Prognosis is good for survivors, most of whom are ambulatory or functional on follow-up (144).

Choriocarcinoma is an extremely vascular and invasive form of gestational trophoblastic neoplasm (155). The incidence is about 1 in 20,000 pregnancies. There is a history of hydatidiform mole in about half of the cases, term pregnancy in a fourth, abortion in the other fourth, and ectopic pregnancy in a small portion (156,157). There are also reports of choriocarcinoma in recipients of organs from donors at high risk for the cancer (158). Younger women appear to be at higher risk, as are certain ethnic groups, such as the Ibadan in Nigeria (159). In postpartum women who develop choriocarcinoma, the offspring is free of metastatic cancer; when the offspring has metastatic choriocarcinoma, the mother is free of the cancer (160). Thus, the spread of cancer depends on which side of the placenta it originates. It appears not to cross the maternofetal barrier.

The clinical presentation is usually irregular bleeding in the puerperium, although symptoms related to metastasis may be the initial presentation (155,161,162). The cancer is highly metastatic (155) and appears to propagate by arterial embolization (159,163). The metastatic lesions have a tendency to bleed as a result of invasion and erosion of vascular structures. Cerebral metastasis occurs in about 20% of cases (164,165). Sometimes the primary tumor is never demonstrated (162). In the CNS, it frequently causes intracranial hemorrhage, although bland infarction (166), aneurysms (157,163,165,167), and carotid–cavernous fistulas (167) have been reported. A noncontrast CT scan of the head identifies the presence of intracranial hemorrhage immediately, although the presence of an underlying neoplasm is best demonstrated by MRI, preferably with gadolinium contrast. Cerebral angiography may demonstrate occlusion of distal branches of the major cerebral arteries (157,165,166, 168), neoplastic aneurysms (resembling mycotic aneurysms) (163,165,169–172), or even findings suggestive of vasculitis (157). Diagnosis is confirmed by elevated beta-human chorionic gonadotrophic (HCG) titers. Treatment consists of aggressive chemotherapy centered on etoposide, and radiotherapy, with or without hysterectomy (164). Advances in treatment have significantly increased remission rates in patients with evidence of metastasis from practically zero to about 70% (173). The associated intracranial aneurysms (170) and carotid–cavernous fistulas (167) may resolve spontaneously with successful medical treatment of the underlying cancer, although some authors use surgical intervention for the aneurysms (163,167,169,171,172). Cerebral metastasis, especially if associated with ICH, carries a relatively poor prognosis (161). Intracranial hemorrhage is the leading cause of death in all patients with choriocarcinoma (161,165).

ANEURYSMAL SUBARACHNOID HEMORRHAGE

Aneurysms may be classified morphologically into saccular, fusiform, mycotic, and dissecting aneurysms (174). Saccular aneurysms are the most important clinically and, based on autopsy series, occur in at least 5% of the general population (174). Saccular aneurysms form most often in the circle of Willis at arterial bifurcations where a discontinuity or defect of the medial smooth muscle is believed to exist and hemodynamic stress is maximal. Most intracranial aneurysms are found in the anterior circulation (175), and about 20% of patients have multiple aneurysms (176).

In the general population, unruptured asymptomatic aneurysms rupture at the rate of about 1% per year (177,178). The rate appears higher during pregnancy, especially in the second and third trimester (126,140) and the puerperium (140). The increased rate is thought to be secondary to the hemodynamic and hormonal changes of gestation. Aneurysmal growth has been documented during pregnancy (179), with return to baseline after delivery. Even after surgical clipping, the residual aneurysmal neck may exhibit rapid growth (180).

The classic presentation is that of a sudden, severe headache usually described as the worst headache of one's life (181,182). Other symptoms include nuchal rigidity, loss of consciousness, and nausea and vomiting (139,175). Seizures, diplopia, and focal neurologic signs referable to the site of aneurysm rupture, such as cranial nerve III palsy, also may be present (175,176,181). A warning hemorrhage manifested by so-called *sentinel headaches* precedes the major hemorrhage by 7 to 10 days in about half of cases (183).

A noncontrast CT scan of the head is the diagnostic procedure of choice in suspected cases of SAH (Fig. 27-11). CT scans still will miss about 10% of cases, depending on the amount of hemorrhage and the timing of the scan in relation to the onset of the SAH. A lumbar puncture is indicated in patients with suspected SAH and a negative CT scan. The CSF is analyzed for blood and spun down to evaluate for xanthochromia, a yellowish color caused by the presence of hemoglobin breakdown products.

Cerebral angiography should be considered in patients who are awake and with mild or moderate deficits (Fig. 27-12). A complete four-vessel angiogram is essential so as not to miss multiple aneurysms (175,176). Because radiation is potentially teratogenic, the fetus must be protected by abdominal shielding. Iodinated contrast agents can lead to fetal dehydration; so the mother must be adequately hydrated before the procedure.

The management of aneurysmal SAH in the pregnant patient is based on neurosurgical principles (1,139,140, 175,181,182,184–186). Patients who are good surgical candidates should have the aneurysm surgically clipped as expeditiously as possible before it has a chance to rebleed. Surgical intervention decreases maternal and fetal mortality by as much as 80% as shown by a retrospective review of multiple series (140). In patients with profound alteration of consciousness where prognosis is poor and operative mortality high, medical management

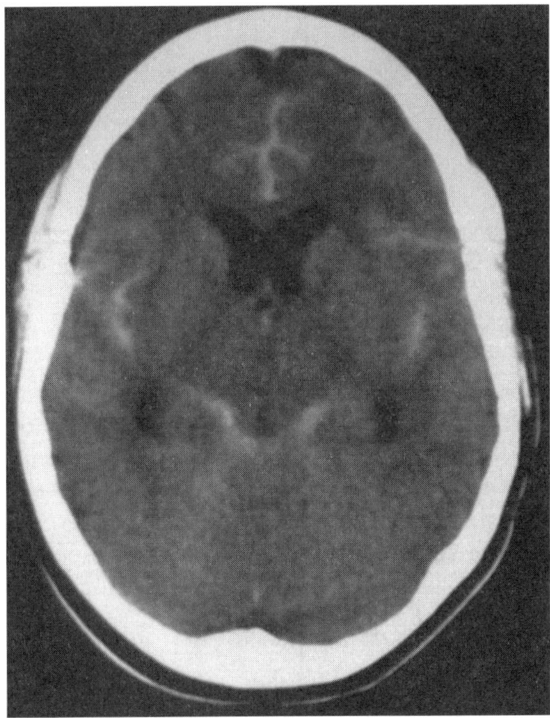

FIG. 27-11. CT scan of a patient who developed subarachnoid hemorrhage in the postpartum period.

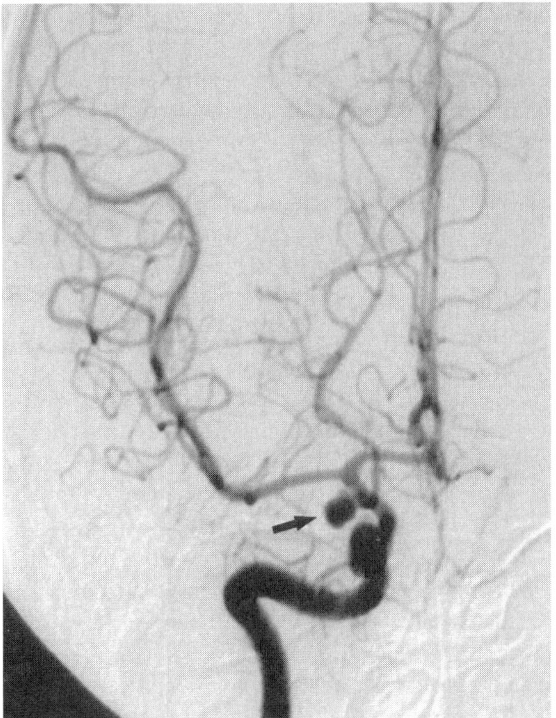

FIG. 27-12. Cerebral angiogram of the patient in Fig. 27-11 showing a posterior communicating artery aneurysm *(arrow)*.

is the main recourse (122). In the postpartum patient with aneurysmal SAH, management is the same as in the nonpregnant patient. Endovascular interventions such as coiling and balloon occlusion have been playing an increasing role, especially in surgically inaccessible lesions or in patients who are not surgical candidates (187,188). It appears to be a safe alternative (187), although no studies comparing the efficacy and safety of surgical versus endovascular therapy have been reported, nor has its use during pregnancy been reported. Pregnancy does not appear to be a contraindication as long as proper abdominal shielding is maintained during fluoroscopy.

The mode of delivery of the fetus depends on whether the aneurysm has been successfully clipped. Once the aneurysm is clipped, it becomes irrelevant to the choice of the mode of delivery. Delivery proceeds according to obstetric indications (140). In the conservatively managed aneurysm (meaning there is still the risk of rerupture), the mode of delivery is controversial. Most authors recommend low-forceps delivery to shorten the second stage of labor under epidural anesthesia (1,140,184). Others recommend cesarean section if aneurysmal rupture occurred in the third trimester (122) and vaginal delivery if rupture occurred in the first two trimesters. When aneurysmal rupture occurs at term, simultaneous cesarean section and aneurysmal clipping under the same general anesthesia have been reported (189).

SAH can be complicated by the potential occurrence of aneurysmal rebleeding, cerebral vasospasm, increased ICP, communicating and noncommunicating hydrocephalus, cardiac arrhythmia, seizures, and syndrome of inappropriate antidiuretic hormone secretion (SIAHS). Vasospasm is the most feared complication of aneurysmal SAH and results in cerebral ischemic complications in about a quarter of cases. Vasospasm starts to occur on the third day after hemorrhage and may continue for up to 2 weeks thereafter. Transcranial Doppler (TCD) ultrasonography indirectly measures vessel caliber by measuring blood flow velocity. The intracranial arteries are insonated through the temporal window of the skull or the foramen magnum. Serial TCD measurements monitor for the development of vasospasm, which is manifested by an upward trend in blood-flow velocities.

The management of vasospasm includes expansion of intravascular volume, augmentation of cardiac index, and induction of systemic hypertension (183). Calcium channel blockers such as nimodipine may be used prophylactically when the benefit outweighs the potential risk to the fetus (1). The effect of nimodipine on the fetus and the uteroplacental circulation is unknown. It has the potential to cause heart block in the mother when used in combination with magnesium sulfate (190). There are no reports of its use in pregnant women. Successful endovascular treatment of vasospasm also has been reported (191). This has not been tried during pregnancy, although there appears to be no major contraindication to attempt its use.

SAH contributes to about 4% of maternal mortality (17–18). Most fatal cases occur in the postpartum period (17,18). In more than half of patients, death ensues within the first 24 hours of symptom onset (17–18). The maternal mortality rate from aneurysmal SAH is about a third and the fetal mortality rate about a sixth (140,181,192). Mortality depends on the initial clinical severity. In their review, Dias and Sekhar reported that maternal and fetal mortality was about five and a half times higher in the nonsurgically treated patients compared with the surgically managed patients (140). Outcome may have been biased by patient selection because the moribund patients were treated nonsurgically. Recurrent hemorrhage complicates a third of cases within 3 days to 6 weeks, and mortality increases to 60% with a recurrent hemorrhage (175).

ARTERIOVENOUS MALFORMATIONS

AVMs are tangles of abnormal blood vessels in the brain or spinal cord that result from the formation of aberrant primitive channels between arteries and veins. The histologic characteristics of the blood vessels are intermediate between arteries and veins. Roughly two thirds are located superficially in the cerebrum (193). AVMs typically bleed in patients between the ages of 10 and 30. In a tenth of the patients, the bleeding is solely intraparenchymal; in a fourth, it is subarachnoid, and in the remaining majority it is mixed parenchymal and subarachnoid (194).

The natural history of unruptured, unoperated AVMs is not clearly defined. There is controversy about whether they are congenital or develop later in life. Most AVMs come to the attention of the medical establishment because of symptoms related to hemorrhage, seizures, or as an incidental finding in the management of an unrelated medical condition. It is difficult to define the actual incidence of AVMs in the general population and, therefore, it is hard to estimate the bleeding rate of unruptured asymptomatic AVMs. Unruptured symptomatic AVMs have a hemorrhage rate of about 3% per year (195). Once AVMs bleed, the rebleeding rate for the first year thereafter is 6% and about 3% yearly afterward (195).

The risk of bleeding from AVMs during pregnancy is generally believed to be increased (140,184,192), although some authors suggest that it is not increased (181,196,197). The prepartum history of the AVM is not predictive of its behavior during pregnancy (198). AVMs do not present evenly during the course of pregnancy (Fig. 27-13). There is a clustering of cases in the second (184,198) and third (192) trimesters and at the time of labor and delivery (184).

AVMs manifest with hemorrhage about three times more often in pregnant women compared with nonpregnant women (184,199,200). AVMs also contribute a larger proportion to SAH during pregnancy of up to 50%

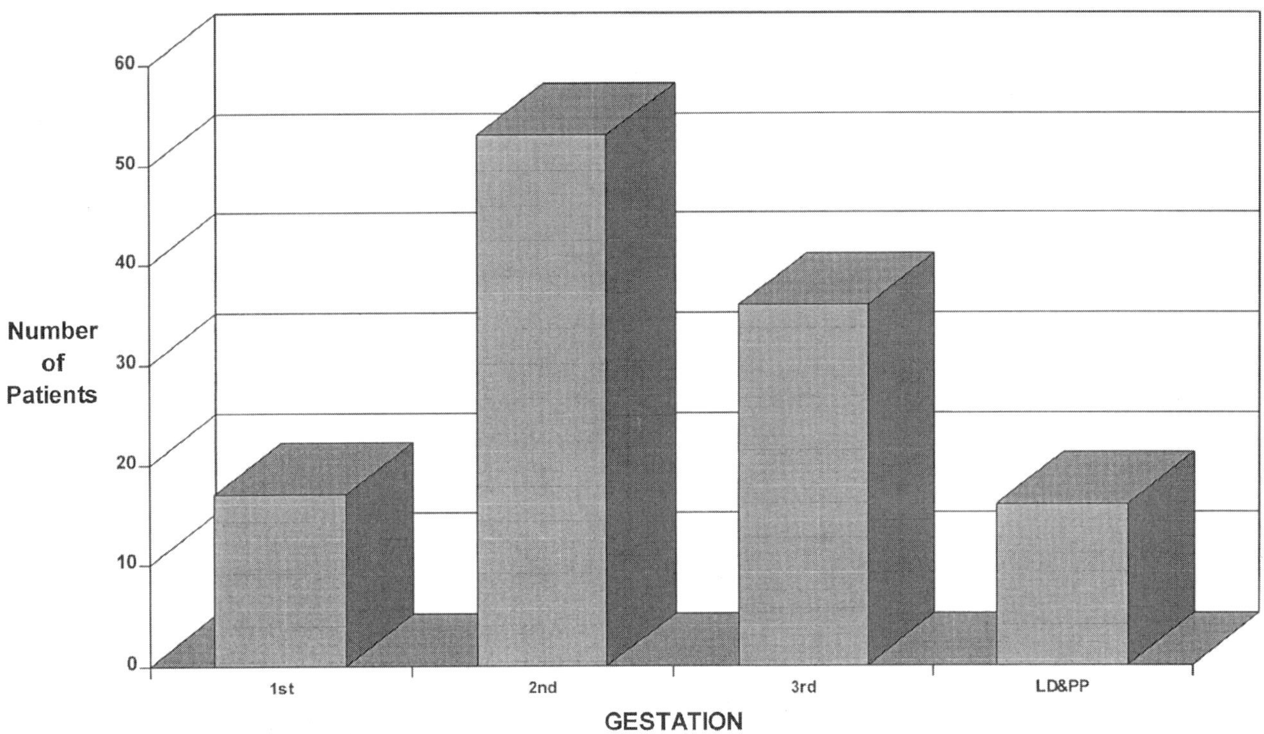

FIG. 27-13. Gestation and AVM hemorrhage.

(126,184,199) compared with about 10% in nonpregnant women and 6% in the general population. The exact reason for the relatively higher incidence of AVM hemorrhage compared with aneurysm hemorrhage in pregnancy is not known.

AVMs commonly present with headache, seizures, and focal neurologic signs caused by either rupture or vascular steal. Headaches in patients with AVMs may be similar to migraine. Seizures occur in at least a third as the presenting symptom and are usually focal with secondary generalization. Clues to an AVM on physical examination include a bruit over the eye or cranium. A noncontrast CT scan of the brain may show a hemorrhage or calcification within the AVM and a contrast-enhanced CT scan or MRI may show the serpentine appearance of the vascular channels in the AVM. A four-vessel angiogram with external carotid injections is necessary to identify the feeding and draining vessels and the presence of any associated aneurysms (which are present in 10% of cases of AVMs).

Surgery is the definitive treatment when the AVM is operable. An AVM grading system such as proposed by Spetzlar and Martin, based on size, venous drainage, and eloquence of adjacent cerebral cortex, may help to determine surgical risk and outcome (201,202). Grades I through III are definite surgical candidates, whereas grades IV or V are assessed on a case-by-case basis, depending on symptoms (recurrent hemorrhage or progressing neurologic disability) and surgical risk. When surgery is incomplete, difficult, or is nonfeasible, endovascular interventions such as coiling and embolization or stereotactic radiosurgery are complementary or alternative methods (203).

During pregnancy, the decision to operate on ruptured and unruptured AVMs is based on neurosurgical rather than obstetric criteria (122,140,192,204). According to Robinson et al., once AVMs bleed during pregnancy, the risk of rebleeding during the same pregnancy is as high as 27% (192), which may be an overestimate, because pregnancy was defined in that study as 2 years before and after the actual period that the patient was gravid. Spreading the 27% risk over that whole interval would result in a rebleeding rate close to the 6% of the general population. Nonetheless, there are advocates for early surgical intervention (122,184) and there are advocates for deferring the surgery until after pregnancy (205), specifically 2 months after delivery (199), when maternal hemodynamics have returned to normal. Patients who are deteriorating neurologically often require emergent surgical intervention (199).

The optimal mode of delivery in patients with unoperated AVMs is unclear. In Dias and Sekhar's review (140), among the nonsurgically treated AVMs, three maternal deaths occurred in the ten women who were delivered vaginally and one maternal death occurred in the eight women delivered by cesarean section. The numbers are too small to draw firm conclusions. Parturients with unoperated AVMs have been successfully delivered vaginally as well as by elective cesarean section at term (126,

140,192,199,204,206,207). Some authors recommend cesarean section for hemorrhage occurring in the advanced stages of pregnancy (207). Women with successfully operated AVMs are delivered according to obstetric indications (140).

Vaginal or cesarean delivery is done under lumbar epidural anesthesia (140,192,206,208). Epidural anesthesia offers advantages over general anesthesia such as avoidance of elevation of blood pressure and ICP associated with laryngoscopy and endotracheal incubation and the ability to assess the patient neurologically during surgery (206,208). Epidural anesthesia carries a risk of dural puncture in inexperienced hands, however, and may be contraindicated when there is evidence of increased ICP (206). If labor occurs during neurosurgical intervention, the operation may have to be interrupted momentarily while forceps delivery or cesarean section is done (192).

Anticonvulsants are given when there is an associated seizure. The role of prohylactic anticonvulsants must be weighed against potential teratogenic risk to the fetus. Oxytoctic agents may be given, although excessive use should be avoided (192,204).

The mortality from untreated symptomatic AVMs is about 1.5 % per year and the morbidity about 3.5% per year (209,210), although these numbers may be higher for the at-risk segment of 20- to 40-year-old women (193). For each episode of bleeding, there is an approximate 10% mortality rate and a 20% morbidity rate (211).

In mothers with untreated AVMs, subsequent pregnancies carry a higher likelihood of hemorrhage (204), with a 33% maternal morbidity and mortality risk and 26% fetal mortality (184) for each hemorrhage. Thus, treatment of AVMs is advisable in patients who plan to become pregnant again.

REFERENCES

1. Stern BJ, Wityk RJ. Stroke in the young. In: Gilman S, Goldstein GW, Waxman SG, eds. Neurobase, 2nd ed. San Diego: Arbor Publishing; 1998 (CD-ROM).
2. Caplan LR. Stroke: a clinical approach. 2nd ed. Boston: Butterworth, 1993:1–562.
3. Barnett HJM, Stein BM, Mohr JP, Yatsu FM. Stroke: pathophysiology, diagnosis and management, 2nd ed. New York: Churchill-Livingstone, 1992:1–1270.
4. Biller J, Mathews KD, Love BB. Stroke in children and young adults. Boston: Butterworth-Heinemann, 1994.
5. Stern BJ, Wityk RJ. Stroke in the young. In: Goldstein PJ, Stern BJ, eds. Neurological disorders of pregnancy, 2nd ed. Mount Kisco, NY: Futura Publishing, 1992:51–84.
6. Wityk RJ. Early recognition and treatment of acute ischemic stroke. Heart Dis Stroke 1993;2:397–406.
7. Cross JN, Castro PO, Jennett WB. Cerebral strokes associated with pregnancy and the puerperium. BMJ 1968;3:214–218.
8. Wiebers DO, Whisnant JP. The incidence of stroke among pregnant women in Rochester, Minn, 1955 through 1979. JAMA 1985;254: 3055–3057.
9. Wiebers DO. Ischemic cerebrovascular complications of pregnancy. Arch Neurol 1985;42:1106–1113.
10. Simolke GA, Cox SM, Cunningham FG. Cerebrovascular accidents complicating pregnancy and the puerperium. Obstet Gynecol 1991; 78:37–42.
11. Sharshar T, Lamy C, Mas JL. Incidence and causes of strokes associated with pregnancy and puerperium: a study in public hospitals of Ile de France. Stroke in Pregnancy Study Group. Stroke 1995;26: 930–936.
12. Grosset DG, Ebrahim S, Bone I, Warlow C. Stroke in pregnancy and the puerperium: what magnitude of risk? [editorial]. J Neurol Neurosurg Psychiatry 1995;58:129–131.
13. Kittner SJ, Stern BJ, Feeser BR, et al. Pregnancy and the risk of stroke. N Engl J Med 1996;335:768–774.
14. Srinivasan K. Cerebral venous and arterial thrombosis in pregnancy and puerperium: a study of 135 patients. Angiology 1983;34:731–746.
15. Kaunitz AM, Hughes JM, Grimes DA, Smith JC, Rochat RW, Kafrissen ME. Causes of maternal mortality in the United States. Obstet Gynecol 1985;65:605–612.
16. Rochat RW, Koonin LM, Atrash HK, Jewett JF. Maternal mortality in the United States: report from the Maternal Mortality Collaborative. Obstet Gynecol 1988;72:91–97.
17. Barnes JE, Abbott KE. Cerebral complications incurred during pregnancy and the puerperium. Am J Obstet Gynecol 1961;82:192–207.
18. Barno A, Freeman DW. Maternal deaths due to spontaneous subarachnoid hemorrhage. Am J Obstet Gynecol 1976;125:384–392.
19. Wityk RJ, Stern BJ. Ischemic stroke: today and tomorrow. Crit Care Med 1994;22:1278–1293.
20. Lipton SA, Rosenberg PA. Excitatory amino acids as a final common pathway for neurologic disorders. N Engl J Med 1994;330:613–622.
21. Zhang J, Benveniste H, Klitzman B, Piantadosi CA. Nitric oxide synthase inhibition and extracellular glutamate concentration after cerebral ischemia/reperfusion. Stroke 1995;26:298–304.
22. Nanri K, Takizawa S, Fujita H, Ogawa S, Shinohara Y. Modulation of extracellular glutamate concentration by nitric oxide synthase inhibitor in rat transient forebrain ischemia. Brain Res 1996;738: 243–248.
23. Goldszmidt A, Wityk RJ. Recent advances in stroke therapy. Curr Opin Neurol 1998;11:57–64.
24. Kittner SJ, Stern BJ, Wozniak M, et al. Cerebral infarction in young adults: the Baltimore–Washington Cooperative Young Stroke Study. Neurology 1998;50:890–894.
25. Stern BJ, Kittner S, Sloan M, et al. Stroke in the young. Md Med J 1991;40:453–571.
26. Rohr J, Kittner S, Feeser B, et al. Traditional risk factors and ischemic stroke in young adults: the Baltimore–Washington Cooperative Young Stroke. Arch Neurol 1996;53:603–607.
27. Poole RM, Chimowitz MI. Cardiac sources of embolism: diagnosis, management and prevention. In: Batjer HH, ed. Cerebrovascular disease. Philadelphia: Lippincott-Raven,1997:377–383.
28. DeRook FA, Pearlman AS. Transesophageal echocardiographic assessment of embolic sources: intracardiac and extracardiac masses and aortic degenerative disease. Crit Care Clin 1996;12:273–294.
29. Manning WJ. Role of transesophageal echocardiography in the management of thromboembolic stroke. Am J Cardiol 1997;80:19D–39D.
30. Meacham RR, Headley AS, Bronze MS, Lewis JB, Rester MM. Impending paradoxical embolism. Arch Intern Med 1998;158: 438–448.
31. Oppenheimer SM, Hachinski VC. The cardiac consequences of stroke. Neurologic Clinics 1992;10:167–176.
32. Elkayam U, Ostrzega EL, Shotan A. Peripartum cardiomyopathy. In: Gleicher N, ed. Principles and practice of medical therapy in pregnancy. 2nd ed. Norwalk: Appleton & Lange, 1992:812–814.
33. Elkayam U. Peripartum cardiomyopathy. In: Braunwald E, ed. Heart disease. Philadelphia: WB Saunders, 1997:1843–1864.
34. Pearl W. Familial occurrence of peripartum cardiomyopathy. Am Heart J 1995;129:421–422.
35. Ferrans VJ. Pathologic anatomy of the dilated cardiomyopathies. Am J Cardiol 1989;64:9c–11c.
36. Mendelson MA, Chandler J. Postpartum cardiomyopathy associated with maternal cocaine abuse. Am J Cardiol 1992;70:1092–1094.
37. Homans DC. Peripartum cardiomyopathy. N Engl J Med 1985;312: 1432–1437.
38. Ribner HS, Silverman RI. Peripartal cariomyopathy. In: Elkayam U, Gleicher N, eds. Cardiac problems in pregnancy: diagnosis and management of maternal and fetal disease, 2nd ed. New York: Alan R. Liss, 1990:115–127.

39. Midei MG, DeMent SH, Feldman AM, Hutchins GM, Baughman KL. Peripartum myocarditis and cardiomyopathy. Circulation 1990;81: 922–928.
40. Rickenbacher PR, Rizeq MN, Hunt SA, Billingham ME, Fowler MB. Long-term outcome after heart transplantation for peripartum cardiomyopathy. Am Heart J 1994;127:1318–1323.
41. Keogh AM, Freund J, Baron DW, Hickie JB. Timing of cardiac transplantation in idiopathic dilated cardiomyopathy. Am J Cardiol 1988; 61:418–422.
42. Keogh A, Macdonald P, Spratt P, Marshman D, Larbalestier R, Kaan A. Outcome in peripartum cardiomyopathy after heart transplantation. J Heart Lung Transplant 1994;13:202–207.
43. McAdams SA, Maguire FE. Unusual manifestations of peripartal cardiac disease. Crit Care Med 1986;14:910–912.
44. Ladwig P, Fischer E. Peripartum cardiomyopathy. Aust N Z J Obstet Gynaecol 1997;37:156–160.
45. Hodgman MT, Pessin MS, Homans DC, et al. Cerebral embolism as the initial manifestation of peripartum cardiomyopathy. Neurology 1982;32:668–671.
46. Demakis JG, Rahimtoola SH. Peripartum cardiomyopathy. Circulation 1971;44:964–968.
47. Martin RW. Amniotic fluid embolism. Clin Obstet Gynecol 1996;39: 101–106.
48. Joelsson UHI. Amniotic fluid embolism in Sweden, 1951–1980. Gynecol Obstet Invest 1985;20:130–137.
49. Clark SL. New concepts of amniotic fluid embolism: a review. Obstet Gynecol Surv 1990;45:360–368.
50. Clark SL, Hankins GD, Dudley DA, Dildy GA, Porter TF. Amniotic fluid embolism: analysis of the national registry. Am J Obstet Gynecol 1995;172(4 Pt 1):1158–1169.
51. Noble WH, St-Amand J. Amniotic fluid embolus. Can J Anaesth 1993;40:971–980.
52. Leys D, Lucas C, Gobert M, Deklunder G, Pruvo JP. Cervical artery dissections. Eur Neurol 1997;37:3–12.
53. Stahmer SA, Raps EC, Mines DI. Carotid and vertebral artery dissections. Emerg Med Clin North Am 1997;15:677–698.
54. Kalimo H, Kaste M, Haltia M. Fibromuscular dysplasia. In: Graham DI, Lantos PL, eds. Greenfield's neuropathology, 6th ed. New York: Oxford University Press, 1996:315–396.
55. Nadeau SE, Watson RT. Neurologic manifestations of vasculitis and collagen vascular disease. In: Joynt RE, ed. Neurology, vol 4. Philadelphia: JB Lippincott, 1994:1–133.
56. Alhalabi M, Moore PM. Serial angiography in isolated angiitis of the central nervous system. Neurology 1994;44:1221–1226.
57. Donaldson JO. Cerebrovascular disease. In: Donaldson JO, ed. Neurology of pregnancy. Philadelphia: WB Saunders, 1989:347.
58. Suzuki Y, Kitagawa Y, Matsuoka Y, Fukuda J, Mizushima Y. Severe cerebral and systemic necrotizing vasculitis developing during pregnancy in a case of systemic lupus erythematosus. J Rheumatol 1990; 17:1408–1411.
59. Pryse-Phillips W, Yorkston NJ. Hysterical contracture complicating hemiplegia in a patient with systemic lupus erythematosus, activated in pregnancy. Guys Hosp Rep 1965;114:239–247.
60. Traboulsi EI, Mansour AM, Aswad MI, Gharzuddin W, Frayha RA. Homonymous hemianopia and systemic lupus erythematosus. J Clin Neuroophthalmol 1985;5:63–66.
61. Farine D, Andreyko J, Lysikiewicz A, Simha S, Addison A. Isolated angiitis of brain in pregnancy and puerperium. Obstet Gynecol 1984; 63:586–588.
62. Yasuda Y, Matsuda I, Kang Y, Saiga T, Kameyama M. Isolated angiitis of the central nervous system first presenting as intracranial hemorrhage during cesarean section. Intern Med 1993;32:745–748.
63. Ishikawa K. Natural history and classification of occlusive thromboaortopathy (Takayasu's disease). Circulation 1978;57:27–35.
64. Wong VW, Wang RYC, Tse TF. Pregnancy and Takayasu's arteritis. Am J Med 1983;75:597–601.
65. Ishikawa K, Matsuura S. Occlusive thromboaortopathy (Takayasu's disease) and pregnancy: clinical course and management of 33 pregnancies and deliveries. Am J Cardiol 1982;50:1293–1300.
66. Suzuki J. Moyamoya disease. Berlin: Springer-Verlag, 1986:1–143.
67. Suzuki J, Kodama N. Moyamoya disease—a review. Stroke 1983;14: 104–109.
68. Fukui M. Current state of study on moyamoya disease in Japan. Surg Neurol 1997;47:138–143.
69. Yonekawa Y, Ogata N. Spontaneous occlusion of the circle of Willis: with special reference to its disease entity and etiological controversy. Brain Dev 1992;14:253–254.
70. Yonekawa Y, Goto Y, Ogata N. Moyamoya disease. In: Barnett HJM, Stein BM, Mohr JP, Yatsu FM, eds. Stroke: pathophysiology, diagnosis and management, 2nd ed. New York: Churchill-Livingstone, 1992: 721–747.
71. Bruno A, Adams HP Jr, Biller J, Rezai K, Cornell S, Aschenbrener CA. Cerebral infarction due to moyamoya disease in young adults. Stroke 1988;19:826–833.
72. Janssens E, Hommel M, Mounier-Vehier F, Leclerc X, Guerin du Masgenet B, Leys D. Postpartum cerebral angiopathy possibly due to bromocriptine therapy. Stroke 1995;26:128–130.
73. Comabella M, Alvarez-Sabin J, Rovira A, Codina A. Bromocriptine and postpartum cerebral angiopathy: a causal relationship? Neurology 1996;46:1754–1756.
74. Bogousslavsky J, Despland PA, Regli F, Dubuis PY. Postpartum cerebral angiopathy: reversible vasoconstriction assessed by transcranial Doppler ultrasounds. Eur Neurol 1989;29:102–105.
75. Chartier JP, Bousigue JY, Teisseyre A, Morel C, Delpuech-Formosa F. [Postpartum cerebral angiopathy of iatrogenic origin]. Rev Neurol (Paris) 1997;153:212–214.
76. Barinagarrementeria F, Cantu C, Balderrama J. Postpartum cerebral angiopathy with cerebral infarction due to ergonovine use. Stroke 1992;23:1364–1366.
77. Dua JA. Postpartum eclampsia associated with ergometrine maleate administration. Br J Obstet Gynaecol 1994;101:72–73.
78. Watson DL, Bhatia RK, Norman GS, Brindley BA, Sokol RJ. Bromocriptine mesylate for lactation suppression: a risk for postpartum hypertension? Obstet Gynecol 1989;74:573–576.
79. Raps EC, Galetta SL, Broderick M, Atlas SW. Delayed peripartum vasculopathy: cerebral eclampsia revisited. Ann Neurol 1993;33: 222–225.
80. Chapman K, Karimi R. A case of postpartum eclampsia of late onset confirmed by autopsy. Am J Obstet Gynecol 1973;117:858–861.
81. Brady WJ, DeBehnke DJ, Carter CT. Postpartum toxemia: hypertension, edema, proteinuria and unresponsiveness in an unknown female. J Emerg Med 1995;13:643–648.
82. Tso E, Reid RP, Barish RA, Browne BJ. Late postpartum eclampsia. Ann Emerg Med 1987;16:907–909.
83. D'Addesio JP. Postpartum eclampsia. Ann Emerg Med 1989;18: 1105–1106.
84. Sibai BM, Schneider JM, Morrison JC, et al. The late postpartum eclampsia controversy. Obstet Gynecol 1980;55:74–78.
85. Amon E, Sibai BM.The late appearance of postpartum eclampsia [letter]. JAMA 1986;255:2292.
86. Lubarsky SL, Barton JR, Friedman SA, Nasreddine S, Ramadan MK, Sibai BM. Late postpartum eclampsia revisited. Obstet Gynecol 1994; 83:502–505.
87. Lopez-Llera M. Personal communication through Sibai, B.M. ; 1979.
88. Hunter CA, Howard WF, McCormick COJ. Amelioration of the hypertension of toxemia by postpartum curettage. Am J Obstet Gynecol 1961;81:884–889.
89. Hart RG, Kanter MC. Hematologic disorders and ischemic stroke. Stroke 1990;21:1111–1121.
90. Martinez HR, Rangel-Guerra RA, Marfil LJ. Ischemic stroke due to deficiency of coagulation inhibitors: report of 10 young adults. Stroke 1993;24:19–25.
91. Barinagarrementeria F, Cantu-Brito C, De La Pena A, Izaguirre R. Prothrombotic states in young people with idiopathic stroke. A prospective study. Stroke 1994;25:287–290.
92. Martinelli I, Landi G, Merati G, Cella R, Tosetto A, Mannucci PM. Factor V gene mutation is a risk factor for cerebral venous thrombosis. Thromb Haemost 1996;75:393–394.
93. Schafer AI. Hypercoagulable states: molecular genetics to clinical practice. Lancet 1994;344:1739–1742.
94. Brey RL, Coull BM. Cerebral venous thrombosis: role of activated protein C resistance and factor V gene mutation [editorial; comment]. Stroke 1996;27:1719–1720.
95. Zuber M, Toulon P, Marnet L, Mas JL. Factor V Leiden mutation in cerebral venous thrombosis. Stroke 1996;27:1721–1723.
96. Webber MD, Halligan RE, Schumacher JA. Acute infarction, intracoronary thrombolysis, and primary PTCA in pregnancy. Cathet Cardiovasc Diagn 1997;42:38–43.

97. Schumacher M, Schmidt D, Wakhloo AK. Intra-arterial fibrinolytic therapy in central retinal artery occlusion. Neuroradiology 1993;35: 600–605.
98. Fleyfel M, Bourzoufi K, Huin G, Subtil D, Puech F. Recombinant tissue type plasminogen activator treatment of thrombosed mitral valve prosthesis during pregnancy. Can J Anaesth 1997;44:735–738.
99. Ramamurthy S, Talwar KK, Saxena A, Juneja R, Takkar D. Prosthetic mitral valve thrombosis in pregnancy successfully treated with streptokinase. Am Heart J 1994;127:446–448.
100. Onoyama Y, Minamitani M, Takeuchi H, Sakai S, Eguchi H. Use of recombinant tissue-type plasminogen activator to treat massive pulmonary embolism after cesarean section: a case report. J Obstet Gynaecol Res 1996;22:201–208.
101. Mazeika PK, Oakley CM. Massive pulmonary embolism in pregnancy treated with streptokinase and percutaneous catheter fragmentation. Eur Heart J 1994;15:1281–1283.
102. Fagher B, Ahlgren M, Astedt B. Acute massive pulmonary embolism treated with streptokinase during labor and the early puerperium. Acta Obstet Gynecol Scand 1990;69:659–661.
103. Patterson DE, Raviola CA, Ea DO, et al. Thrombolytic and endovascular treatment of peripartum iliac vein thrombosis: a case report. J Vasc Surg 1996;24:1030–1033.
104. La Valleur J, Molina E, Williams PP, Rolnick SJ. Use of urokinase in pregnancy: two success stories. Postgrad Med 1996;99:269–273.
105. Witlin AG, Friedman SA, Egerman RS, Frangieh AY, Sibai BM. Cerebrovascular disorders complicating pregnancy—beyond eclampsia. Am J Obstet Gynecol 1997;176:1139–1148.
106. Beeson JH, Duda EE. Computed axial tomography scan demonstration of cerebral edema in eclampsia preceded by blindness. Obstet Gynecol 1982;60:529–532.
107. Naheedy MH, Biller J, Schiffer M, Azar-Kia B, Gianopoulous J, Zarandy S. Toxemia of pregnancy: cerebral CT findings. *J Comput Assist Tomogr* 1985;9:497–501.
108. Colosimo JC, Fileni A, Guerrini P. CT findings in eclampsia. Neuroradiology 1985;27:313–317.
109. Coughlin WF, McMurdo KS, Reeves T. MR imaging of postpartum cortical blindness. J Comput Assist Tomogr 1989;13:572–576.
110. Lewis LK, Hinshaw DB Jr, Will AD, Hasso AN, Thompson JR. CT and angiographic correlation of severe neurological disease in toxemia of pregnancy. Neuroradiology 1988;30:59–64.
111. Trommer BL, Homer D, Mikhael MA. Cerebral vasospasm and eclampsia. Stroke 1988;19:326–329.
112. Raroque HG, Jr. Cerebral vasospasm in eclampsia [Letter]. Stroke 1989;20:826.
113. Schaefer PW, Buonanno FS, Gonzalez RG, Schwamm LH. Diffusion-weighted imaging discriminates between cytotoxic and vasogenic edema in a patient with eclampsia. Stroke 1997;28:1082–1085.
114. Finelli PF. Postpartum eclampsia and subarachnoid hemorrhage. J Stroke Cerebrovasc Dis 1992;2:151–153.
115. Williams K, McLean C. Maternal cerebral vasospasm in eclampsia assessed by transcranial Doppler. Am J Perinatol 1993;10:243–244.
116. Demarin V, Rundek T, Hodek B. Maternal cerebral circulation in normal and abnormal pregnancies. Acta Obstet Gynecol Scand 1997;76: 619–624.
117. Klingler D, Necek S. Eclampsia—monitoring of intraventricular CSF pressure. J Neurol 1980;223:147–150.
118. Martin JP, Sheehan HL. Primary thrombosis of cerebral veins (following childbirth). BMJ 1941;1:349–353.
119. Sinclair MAM, Glasg MD, Cantab DPH. Puerperal aphasia: analysis of 18 cases. Lancet 1902;2:204–205.
120. Kendall D. Thrombosis of intracranial veins. Brain 1948;71:386–402.
121. Stevens H. Puerperal hemiplegia. Neurology 1954;4:723–738.
122. Wiebers DO. Subarachnoid hemorrhage in pregnancy. Semin Neurol 1988;8:226–229.
123. Goldman JA, Eckerling B, Gans B. Intracranial venous sinus thrombosis in pregnancy and puerperium: report of 15 cases. J Obstet Gynecol Br Commonw 1964;71:791–796.
124. Lorincz AB, Moore RY. Puerperal cerebral venous thrombosis. Am J Obstet Gynecol 1962;83:311–318.
125. Lanska DJ, Kryscio RJ. Peripartum stroke and intracranial venous thrombosis in the National Hospital Discharge Survey. Obstet Gynecol 1997;89:413–418.
126. Amias AG. Cerebral vascular disease in pregnancy. J Obstet Gynaecol Br Commonw 1970;77:100–120, 312–315.
127. Biback SM, Franklin A, Sata WK. Puerperal hemiplegia. Am J Obstet Gynecol 1962;83:45–53.
128. Cantu C, Barinagarrementeria F. Cerebral venous thrombosis associated with pregnancy and puerperium: review of 67 cases. Stroke 1993; 24:1880–1884.
129. Carroll JD, Leak D, Lee HA. Cerebral thrombophlebitis in pregnancy and the puerperium. QJM 1966;35:347–368.
130. Jacobs K, Moulin T, Bogousslavsky J, et al. The stroke syndrome of cortical vein thrombosis. Neurology 1996;47:376–382.
131. Macchi PJ, Grossman RI, Gomori JM, Goldberg HI, Zimmerman RA, Bilaniuk LT. High field MR imaging of cerebral venous thrombosis. J Comput Assist Tomogr 1986;10:10–15.
132. Levine SR, Twyman RE, Gilman S. The role of anticoagulation in cavernous sinus thrombosis. Neurology 1988;38:517–522.
133. Einhaupl KM, Villringer A, Meister W, et al. Heparin treatment in sinus venous thrombosis [published erratum appears in Lancet 1991 Oct 12;338:958] Lancet 1991;338:597–600.
134. Horowitz M, Purdy P, Unwin H, et al. Treatment of dural sinus thrombosis using selective catheterization and urokinase. Ann Neurol 1995; 38:58–67.
135. Barnwell SL, Higashida RT, Halbach VV, Dowd CF. Direct endovascular thrombolytic therapy for dural sinus thrombosis. Neurosurgery 1991;28:135–142.
136. Gerszten PC, Welch WC, Spearman MP, Jungreis CA, Redner RL. Isolated deep cerebral venous thrombosis treated by direct endovascular thrombolysis. Surg Neurol 1997;48:261–266.
137. Wityk RJ, Caplan LR. Hypertensive intracerebral hemorrhage. Epidemiology and clinical pathology. Neurosurg Clin N Am 1992;3:521–532.
138. Wilterdink JL, Feldmann E. Cerebral hemorrhage. Adv Neurol 1994; 64:13–23.
139. Pedowitz P, Perell A. Aneurysms complicated by pregnancy. Part II. Aneurysms of the cerebral vessels. Am J Obstet Gynecol 1957;73: 736–749.
140. Dias MS, Sekhar LN. Intracranial hemorrhage from aneurysms and arteriovenous malformations during pregnancy and the puerperium. Neurosurgery 1990;27:855–866.
141. Hamilton MG, Zabramski JM. Spontaneous brain hemorrhage. In: Tindall GT, Cooper PR, Barrow DL, eds. The practice of neurosurgery, vol 2. Baltimore: Williams & Wilkins, 1996:2295–2312.
142. Caplan LR. Hypertensive intracerebral hemorrhage. In: Kase CS, Caplan LR, eds. Intracerebral hemorrhage. Boston: Butterworth-Heinemann, 1994:99–116.
143. Iffy L, Lindenthal J, McArdle JJ, Ganesh V. Severe cerebral accidents postpartum in patients taking bromocriptine for milk suppression. Isr J Med Sci 1996;32:309–312.
144. Kase CS, Cromwell RM. Prognosis and treatment of patients with intracerebral hemorrhage. In: Kase CS, Caplan LR, eds. Intracerebral hemorrhage. Boston: Butterworth-Heinemann, 1994:467–489.
145. Fogelholm R, Nuutila M, Vuorela AL. Primary intracerebral haemorrhage in the Jyvaskyla region, central Finland, 1985–89: incidence, case fatality rate, and functional outcome. J Neurol Neurosurg Psychiatry 1992;55:546–552.
146. Franke CL, van SJ, Algra A, van GJ. Prognostic factors in patients with intracerebral haematoma. J Neurol Neurosurg Psychiatry 1992; 55:653–657.
147. Douglas MA, Haerer AF. Long-term prognosis of hypertensive intracerebral hemorrhage. Stroke 1982;13:488–491.
148. Daverat P, Castel JP, Dartigues JF, Orgogozo JM. Death and functional outcome after spontaneous intracerebral hemorrhage: a prospective study of 166 cases using multivariate analysis. Stroke 1991;22:1–6.
149. Fieschi C, Carolei A, Fiorelli M, et al. Changing prognosis of primary intracerebral hemorrhage: results of a clinical and computed tomographic follow-up study of 104 patients. Stroke 1988;19:192–195.
150. Tuhrim S, Dambrosia JM, Price TR, et al. Prediction of intracerebral hemorrhage survival. Ann Neurol 1988;24:258–263.
151. Bamford J, Dennis M, Sandercock P, Burn J, Warlow C. The frequency, causes and timing of death within 30 days of a first stroke: the Oxfordshire Community Stroke Project. J Neurol Neurosurg Psychiatry 1990;53:824–829.
152. Silver FL, Norris JW, Lewis AJ, Hachinski VC. Early mortality following stroke: a prospective review. Stroke 1984;15:492–496.
153. Dixon AA, Holness RO, Howes WJ, Garner JB. Spontaneous intracerebral haemorrhage: an analysis of factors affecting prognosis. Can J Neurol Sci 1985;12:267–271.
154. Portenoy RK, Lipton RB, Berger AR, Lesser ML, Lantos G. Intracerebral haemorrhage: a model for the prediction of outcome. J Neurol Neurosurg Psychiatry 1987;50:976–979.
155. Cunningham FG, MacDonald PC, Leveno KJ, Gilstrap LCI, Hankins

GDV, Clark SL. Diseases and abnormalities of the placenta. Williams obsetetrics, 20th ed. Stamford, CT: Appleton & Lange, 1997:669–691.
156. Gurwitt LJ, Long JM, Clark RE. Cerebral metastatic choriocarcinoma: a postpartum cause of "stroke." Obstet Gynecol 1975;45:583–588.
157. Watanabe AS, Smoker WR. Computed tomography and angiographic findings in metastatic choriocarcinoma. J Comput Assist Tomogr 1989;13:319–322.
158. Baquero A, Penn I, Bannett A, Werner DJ, Kim P. Misdiagnosis of metastatic cerebral choriocarcinoma in female cadaver donors. Transplant Proc 1988;20:776–777.
159. Adeloye A, Osuntokun BO, Hendrickse JP, Odeku EL. The neurology of metastatic chorion carcinoma of the uterus. J Neurol Sci 1972;16: 315–329.
160. Kelly DL Jr, Kushner J, McLean WT. Neonatal intracranial choriocarcinoma. Case report. J Neurosurg 1971;35:465–471.
161. Wilkinson AG, Sellar RJ. Case report: cerebral metastases from choriocarcinoma in the absence of detectable extracranial disease. Clin Radiol 1991;43:278–279.
162. van den Doel EM, van Merrienboer FJ, Tulleken CA. Cerebral hemorrhage from unsuspected choriocarcinoma. Clin Neurol Neurosurg 1985;87:287–290.
163. Giannakopoulos G, Nair S, Snider C, Amenta PS. Implications for the pathogenesis of aneurysm formation: metastatic choriocarcinoma with spontaneous splenic rupture. Case report and a review. Surg Neurol 1992;38:236–240.
164. Weed JC Jr, Hammond CB. Cerebral metastatic choriocarcinoma: intensive therapy and prognosis. Obstet Gynecol 1980;55:89–94.
165. Seigle JM, Caputy AJ, Manz HJ, Wheeler C, Fox JL. Multiple oncotic intracranial aneurysms and cardiac metastasis from choriocarcinoma: case report and review of the literature. Neurosurgery 1987;20:39–42.
166. Rose PG. Cerebrovascular embolization of choriocarcinoma. Obstet Gynecol 1996;88:738.
167. Weir B, MacDonald N, Mielke B. Intracranial vascular complications of choriocarcinoma. Neurosurgery 1978;2:138–142.
168. Nakagawa Y, Tashiro K, Isu T, Tsuru M. Occlusion of cerebral artery due to metastasis of chorioepithelioma: case report. J Neurosurg 1979;51:247–250.
169. Momma F, Beck H, Miyamoto T, Nagao S. Intracranial aneurysm due to metastatic choriocarcinoma. Surg Neurol 1986;25:74–76.
170. Hove B, Andersen BB, Christiansen TM. Intracranial oncotic aneurysms from choriocarcinoma: case report and review of the literature. Neuroradiology 1990;32:526–528.
171. Fujiwara T, Mino S, Nagao S, Ohmoto T. Metastatic choriocarcinoma with neoplastic aneurysms cured by aneurysm resection and chemotherapy: case report. J Neurosurg 1992;76:148–151.
172. Pullar M, Blumbergs PC, Phillips GE, Carney PG. Neoplastic cerebral aneurysm from metastatic gestational choriocarcinoma: case report. J Neurosurg 1985;63:644–647.
173. Hammond CB, Weed JC Jr, Currie JL. The role of operation in the current therapy of gestational trophoblastic disease. Am J Obstet Gynecol 1980;136:844–858.
174. Sekhar LN, Heros RC. Origin, growth, and rupture of saccular aneurysms: a review. Neurosurgery 1981;8:248–260.
175. Pool JL. Treatment of intracranial aneurysms during pregnancy. JAMA 1965;192:209–214.
176. Locksley HB. Natural history of subarachnoid hemorrhage, intracranial aneurysms, and arteriovenous malformations. Neurosurgery 1966;25:219.
177. Heiskanen O. Risk of bleeding from unruptured aneurysm in cases with multiple intracranial aneurysms. J Neurosurg 1981;55:524–526.
178. Winn HR, Almaani WS, Berga SL, Jane JA, Richardson AE. The long-term outcome in patients with multiple aneurysms: incidence of late hemorrhage and implications for treatment of incidental aneurysms. J Neurosurg 1983;59:642–651.
179. Ortiz O, Voelker J, Eneorji F. Transient enlargement of an intracranial aneurysm during pregnancy: case report. Surg Neurol 1997;47:527–531.
180. Weir BK, Drake CG. Rapid growth of residual aneurysmal neck during pregnancy: case report. J Neurosurg 1991;75:780–782.
181. Cannell DE, Botterell EH. Subarachnoid hemorrhage and pregnancy. Am J Obstet Gynecol 1956;72:844–855.
182. Donaldson JO, Lee NS. Arterial and venous stroke associated with pregnancy. Neurol Clin 1994;12:583–599.
183. Selman WR, Ratcheson RA. Intracranial aneurysms. In: Bradley WG, Daroff RB, Fenichel GM, Marsden CD, eds. Neurology in clinical practice. Boston: Butterworth-Heinemann, 1996:1048–1062.
184. Robinson JL, Hall CS, Sedzimir CB. Arteriovenous malformations, aneurysms, and pregnancy. J Neurosurg 1974;41:63–70.
185. Barrett JM, Van Hooydonk JE, Boehm FH. Pregnancy-related rupture of arterial aneurysms. Obstet Gynecol Surv 1982;37:557–566.
186. Hunt HB, Schifrin BS, Suzuki K. Ruptured berry aneurysms and pregnancy. Obstet Gynecol 1974;43:827–837.
187. Casasco AE, Aymard A, Gobin P, et al. Selective endovascular treatment of 71 intracranial aneurysms with platinum coils. J Neurosurg 1993;79:3–10.
188. Taki W, Nishi S, Yamashita K, et al. Selection and combination of various endovascular techniques in the treatment of giant aneurysms. J Neurosurg 1992;77:37–42.
189. Whitburn RH, Laishley RS, Jewkes DA. Anaesthesia for simultaneous caesarean section and clipping of intracerebral aneurysm. Br J Anaesth 1990;64:642–645.
190. Briggs GG, Freeman RK, Yaffe SJ. Drugs in pregnancy and lactation: a reference guide to fetal and neonatal risk, 4th ed. Baltimore: Williams & Wilkins, 1994:624–625.
191. Higashida RT, Halbach VV, Dowd CF, Dormandy B, Bell J, Hieshima GB. Intravascular balloon dilatation therapy for intracranial arterial vasospasm: patient selection, technique, and clinical results. Neurosurg Rev 1992;15:89–95.
192. Robinson JL, Hall CJ, Sedzimir CB. Subarachnoid hemorrhage in pregnancy. J Neurosurg 1972;36:27–33.
193. Selman WR, Ratcheson RA. Arteriovenous malformations. In: Bradley WG, Daroff RB, Fenichel GM, Marsden CD, eds. Neurology in clinical practice. Boston: Butterworth-Heinemann, 1996:1063–1070.
194. Robbins SL, Cotran RS, Kumar V. Pathologic basis of disease, 5th ed. Philadelphia: WB Saunders, 1994:1408.
195. Graf CJ, Perret GE, Torner JC. Bleeding from cerebral arteriovenous malformations as part of their natural history. J Neurosurg 1983;58: 331–337.
196. Horton JC, Chambers WA, Lyons SL, Adams RD, Kjellberg RN. Pregnancy and the risk of hemorrhage from cerebral arteriovenous malformations. Neurosurgery 1990;27:867–872.
197. Walton JN. Subarachnoid hemorrhage in pregnancy. BMJ 1953; 2:869–871.
198. Forster DM, Kunkler IH, Hartland P. Risk of cerebral bleeding from arteriovenous malformations in pregnancy: the Sheffield experience. Stereotact Funct Neurosurg 1993;61:20–22.
199. Sadasivan B, Malik GM, Lee C, Ausman JI. Vascular malformations and pregnancy. Surg Neurol 1990;33:305–313.
200. Pelletierri L, Carlsson CA, Grevsten S. Surgical versus conservative treatment of intracranial vascular malformations: a study in surgical decision-making. Acta Neurochir Suppl 1989;29:1–86.
201. Spetzler RF, Martin NA. A proposed grading system for arteriovenous malformations. J Neurosurg 1986;65:476–483.
202. Hamilton MG, Spetzler RF. The prospective application of a grading system for arteriovenous malformations. Neurosurgery 1994;34:2–7.
203. Lawton MT, Hamilton MG, Spetzler RF. Multimodality treatment of deep arteriovenous malformations: thalamus, basal ganglia, and brain stem. Neurosurgery 1995;37:29–36.
204. Tuttelman RM, Gleicher N. Central nervous system hemorrhage complicating pregnancy. Obstet Gynecol 1981;58:651–657.
205. Aminoff MJ. Pregnancy and disorders of the nervous system. In: Aminoff MJ, ed. Neurology and general medicine. New York: Churchill Livingstone, 1995:571–574.
206. Sharma SK, Herrera ER, Sidawi JE, Leveno KJ. The pregnant patient with an intracranial arteriovenous malformation: cesarean or vaginal delivery using regional or general anesthesia? Reg Anesth 1995;20: 455–458.
207. Laidler JA, Jackson IJ, Redfern N. The management of caesarean section in a patient with an intracranial arteriovenous malformation. Anaesthesia 1989;44:490–491.
208. Viscomi CM, Wilson J, Bernstein I. Anesthetic management of a parturient with an incompletely resected cerebral arteriovenous malformation. Reg Anesth 1997;22:192–197.
209. Ondra SL, Troupp H, George ED, Schwab K. The natural history of symptomatic arteriovenous malformations of the brain: a 24-year follow-up assessment. J Neurosurg 1990;73:387–391.
210. Troupp H. Arteriovenous malformations of the brain: what are the indications for operation? In: Morley TP, ed. Current controversies in neurosurgery. Philadelphia: WB Saunders, 1976:210–216.
211. Wilkins RH. Natural history of intracranial vascular malformations. Neurosurgery 1985;16:421–430.

Cherry and Merkatz's Complications of Pregnancy,
Fifth Edition, edited by W. R. Cohen.
Lippincott Williams & Wilkins, Philadelphia © 2000.

CHAPTER 28

Epilepsy

Page B. Pennell

DEFINITION AND CLINICAL MANIFESTATIONS

A *seizure* is caused by paroxysmal abnormal cerebral neuronal discharges. It is clinically characterized by an episodic alteration in behavior or perception, which is stereotyped. *Epilepsy* is a chronic brain disorder of various etiologies characterized by recurrent unprovoked seizures. Seizures that occur only once or in a single cluster are not sufficient evidence to diagnose epilepsy, particularly if there is a probable exogenous cause, such as eclampsia or a toxic or metabolic disturbance (e.g., hypoglycemia, alcohol withdrawal).

The International League Against Epilepsy has provided a classification scheme for both seizures and epilepsy syndromes, and this classification is accepted worldwide (1,2). Seizures are classified according to clinical *semiology* (behavior), *interictal* (between seizures) electroencephalography (EEG), and *ictal* (during seizures) EEG. Seizures are divided into either generalized seizures or partial seizures. *Generalized seizures* have a bilateral, diffuse onset and can be nonconvulsive (e.g., absence, atonic) or convulsive [e.g., generalized tonic–clonic seizures (GTCS)]. Partial seizures are focal at onset. *Simple partial seizures* (SPS) do not involve any alteration in level of awareness or responsiveness and can have many different clinical symptoms and signs. *Complex partial seizures* (CPS) begin focally and have some alteration in level of awareness or responsiveness. Partial seizures may evolve and spread to involve the entire brain and are classified as partial seizures that have secondarily generalized.

An *epilepsy syndrome* is classified according to type of seizure, etiology, anatomy, precipitating factors, age of onset, family history, severity, chronicity, circadian cycling, and prognosis. Patients may have one type of epilepsy syndrome but more than one type of seizure. *Primary epilepsies* are idiopathic and occur in patients who have no identifiable underlying cerebral pathology, a normal developmental history, often a genetic predisposition; these patients tend to be controlled easily with medication and may have spontaneous remission as the patient enters adulthood. *Secondary epilepsies* are symptomatic of underlying focal or diffuse cerebral injury and occur in patients with neurologic abnormalities. Seizures usually occur frequently and are often difficult to control, with little abatement throughout life.

Status epilepticus is defined as a seizure that persists for a sufficient time or repeated frequently enough that the patient does not regain consciousness within 30 minutes. Status epilepticus can be partial and involve repetitive or prolonged focal seizures, or it can be generalized with convulsive or nonconvulsive seizures. Postictal weakness is common after isolated partial epileptic seizures but tends to increase in severity and duration with the length and number of seizures and is termed Todd's paralysis.

ETIOLOGY

Two thirds of incident cases of epilepsy are idiopathic (3). The most common identifiable etiologies of epilepsy vary with the age of onset. Between birth and age 2 years, the most common etiologies are perinatal injury, metabolic defect, and congenital malformation. Between the ages of 2 and 5 years, the most common causes are infection and postnatal trauma. Between the ages of 5 and 30 years, the most common etiologies are postnatal trauma and genetic predisposition, with infection still providing a major contribution. After the age of 30 years, brain tumor and vascular disease are the most common identifiable etiologies.

P. B. Pennell: Department of Neurology, Emory University School of Medicine, Emory University Hospital, Atlanta, GA 30322.

INCIDENCE AND PREVALENCE

Epilepsy is the most common neurologic disorder after stroke. The prevalence of active epilepsy is about 0.64% in the United States (3) and slightly higher for men than for women. About a million women of childbearing age in the United States have epilepsy and give birth to some 20,000 infants each year (4).

PATHOGENESIS

A seizure is caused by transient, hypersynchronous, excessive discharges of cerebral neurons. The excessive discharges are likely to result at least in part from increased excitatory neurotransmission via glutamate receptors or decreased activity of γ-aminobutyric acid $(GABA)_A$-benzodiazepine receptor complexes. Many antiepileptic drugs (AEDs) target these specific mechanisms; for example, tiagabine blocks GABA uptake from the synaptic cleft.

Sex steroid hormones likely also contribute to seizure frequency. In animal studies, estrogen exhibits a seizure-activating effect (5), whereas progesterone provides a seizure-protective effect (6), possibly by enhancement of GABA-mediated neuronal inhibition and lowering glutamate excitation (7). Many women with epilepsy report an increase in their seizures just before and during the menstrual flow and during ovulation (8–11). Bäckström (10) demonstrated a positive correlation between seizure frequency and the serum estrogen-to-progesterone ratio; seizure frequency was highest at the beginning of menstruation and just before ovulation when the concentration of estrogen was relatively higher than that of progesterone.

NEW-ONSET SEIZURES DURING PREGNANCY

New-onset seizures during pregnancy demand quick and efficient evaluation and treatment. Adequate maternal oxygenation should be provided, and secondary effects on the fetus should be monitored. A careful and detailed history and physical examination are essential for the correct diagnosis. The history should determine whether the event was a seizure and, if so, what type. Questions should be asked about the presence of aura, loss of awareness, body movements and their type, urinary incontinence, oral trauma, postictal phase, and duration. The actual cause of some seizures may be identified by history alone (e.g., hypoglycemia resulting from insulin, meningitis, medications). The number of disorders that can cause secondary seizures is extensive (Table 28-1); a general rule is that any disorder that can be associated with an agitated encephalopathy also can be associated with seizures. During pregnancy, it is imperative to rule out eclampsia, because management of the patient would be considerably different. It is important to rule out concurrent neurologic symptoms and signs. Occasionally, physical examination will suggest other possibilities (e.g., hypertension resulting from eclampsia, cardiac emboli, metastatic tumor). Laboratory tests should be performed to rule out metabolic causes. History and a toxicology screen should be obtained to rule out recreational and prescription drug use or withdrawal from barbiturates, benzodiazepines, and alcohol. Some prescription drugs more likely to be encountered in the obstetric setting are narcotic analgesics, inhalation anesthetics such as enflurane and isoflurane, and oxytocin. Oxytocin-induced seizures could be secondary to its antidiuretic effect producing hyponatremia (12). If no precipitant can be identified, if the patient is immunocompromised, if any signs of infection (elevated temperature, stiff neck, headache) are present, or if the patient does not recover normal mentation in a timely manner, a lumbar puncture should be performed to rule out meningitis or encephalitis once signs of increased intracranial pressure are excluded. Precipitating factors such as sleep deprivation and stress should be documented because these factors would favor withholding initiation of chronic anticonvulsant treatment. A computed tomography (CT) scan of the head will help to rule out hemorrhage or large tumor, but ultimately the patient should undergo magnetic resonance imaging (MRI) to identify more subtle, commonly asso-

TABLE 28-1. *Differential diagnosis of peripartum seizures*

Eclampsia
Cerebrovascular disorders
Cerebral venous thrombosis
Cerebral arterial occlusion
Intracerebral hemorrhage
Subarachnoid hemorrhage
Mass lesions
Brain tumor
Brain abscess
Vascular malformations
Infectious diseases
Viral
Bacterial
Parasitic
HIV
Toxic/metabolic disorders
Hypoglycemia
Hypocalcemia
Hyponatremia
Hypomagnesemia
Hypophosphatemia
Nonketotic hyperglycemia
Hypoxia
Hypothyroidism or hyperthyroidism
Uremia
Hepatic failure
Drug effects
Epilepsy

HIV, human immunodeficiency virus.

ciated abnormalities, such as mesial temporal sclerosis, cavernous angioma, low-grade glioma, or heterotopias. An EEG should also be obtained to aid in decisions about the need for long-term treatment. Recurrence of seizures will occur in 30% to 70% of patients presenting with a single unprovoked seizure; half of these patients will have a recurrence in the first year and most by the end of the second year. The general rule is that chronic anticonvulsant treatment is not started until a second seizure occurs. If, however, the first seizure was unprecipitated, focal signs are present, the patient has a significant underlying neurologic abnormality or risk factor for epilepsy, or the EEG demonstrates epileptiform activity, then the risk of seizure recurrence is substantially higher and warrants treatment. After the first trimester, the risk to the fetus of another convulsive seizure probably outweighs the risk attributed to AEDs.

PRECONCEPTIONAL PLANNING FOR WOMEN WITH EPILEPSY

Both neurologists and obstetricians treating women with epilepsy are often not appropriately knowledgeable about issues of pregnancy and epilepsy (13), and current recommended guidelines (14–16) regarding preconceptional counseling often are not followed (17). Rarely, some women still are advised to undergo sterilization because of their epilepsy, and rather commonly epileptic women are discouraged, even by physicians, from childbearing. Other patients are told that they have to stop all AEDs before becoming pregnant, regardless of their current seizure control. More than 90% of pregnancies in women with epilepsy occur without complications. Because there are potential increased complications to both the mother and the fetus during pregnancy, careful planning and management of any pregnancy in a woman with epilepsy are essential.

Careful planning necessitates effective birth control. Many of the AEDs enhance the activity of the hepatic microsomal oxidative enzymes and share the same cytochrome P-450 system with the sex steroid hormones. The resulting increased enzymatic activity can lead to rapid clearance of steroid hormones, which may allow ovulation, especially in women taking low-dose oral contraceptives (18). An estradiol dose of 50 μg or its equivalent needs to be prescribed when using oral contraceptive agents with the enzyme-inducing AEDs. The effects of five common AEDs on hormonal contraceptives are listed in Table 28-2 (13,19).

TABLE 28-2. *Effects of antiepileptic drugs on plasma levels of hormonal contraceptive agents*

Enzyme-inducing AEDs	Estradiol	Norgestrel/ norethindrone
Phenobarbital	–38%	–19%
Phenytoin	–49%	–42%
Carbamazepine	–42%	–40%
Topiramate	–21%	–4%
Oxcarbazepine	–47%	–36%

MANAGEMENT OF WOMEN WITH EPILEPSY DURING PREGNANCY

Seizures During Pregnancy

The effect of pregnancy on seizure frequency is variable and unpredictable. Approximately 20% of patients will have an increase in their seizures, 5% to 25% of patients will have a decline, and 60% to 83% will have no significant change in seizure frequency during pregnancy (20–23). Unfortunately, which route a person's course will take is impossible to know and cannot be predicted based on factors such as age, ethnic origin, number of pregnancies, seizure type(s), AED(s), and seizure frequency during a previous pregnancy (4,24).

Pregnancy is associated with several physiologic and psychologic changes that can alter seizure frequency, including changes in sex hormone concentrations, changes in metabolism, sleep deprivation, and new stresses. Plasma levels of estrogen and progesterone increase gradually throughout pregnancy and peak during the last trimester. It may be that during pregnancy women who have a relatively greater increase in estrogen than progesterone are more likely to have a worsening of their seizures, whereas those with a higher progesterone-to-estrogen ratio have improvement in their seizures (10,25). No studies have addressed this question adequately. Also, plasma chorionic gonadotropin levels rise during the first trimester before falling again, and animal studies suggest that this may contribute to increases in seizures during the first trimester (26). Metabolic changes include increased weight, fluid and sodium retention, compensated respiratory alkalosis, and hypomagnesemia. No convincing evidence has been found, however, that links these factors to seizure control (4).

Sleep deprivation and noncompliance are two of the most frequent factors that lead to worsening of seizures during pregnancy but yet are largely modifiable. Studies showed that sleep deprivation or noncompliance played a clear role in 40% to 90% of women in whom seizures increased during pregnancy (27). It is important to inquire about both sleep patterns and compliance in pregnant patients with epilepsy. Sleep deprivation can be due to physical discomforts, such as nausea, back pain, entrapment neuropathies (carpal tunnel syndrome), pressure and movements of the fetus, and nocturia. Marital and financial stress and personal doubts and concerns can contribute to sleep deprivation as well as cause a more direct increase in the likelihood of seizure occurrence. Noncompliance with medications is common during pregnancy and is due in large part to the strong message that any drugs during pregnancy are harmful to the fetus. Teratogenic effects of AEDs are well described, but risks to the fetus are often exaggerated or misrepresented. Proper education about the risks of AEDs versus the risks of seizures can be helpful in ensuring compliance during pregnancy.

For women with epilepsy who have seizures during pregnancy, the risk of seizures to the fetus is important and should be discussed thoroughly with the patient and other family members. Maternal seizures of all types in the first trimester have been associated with a higher malformation rate of 12.3% compared with a malformation rate of 4% for infants of epileptic mothers (IEMs) not exposed to seizures during the first trimester (28). No significant differences in malformation rates have been observed between the offspring of women with different types of epilepsy (28,29). Trauma that is the consequence of a seizure can result in ruptured fetal membranes, which increases the risk of infection, premature labor, and even fetal death (27). Abruptio placentae will occur after 1% to 5% of minor and 20% to 50% of major blunt injuries (30). Restrictions from driving and climbing heights should be reinforced with each patient, and the substantial risk to the fetus of a seemingly minor injury should be discussed.

Generalized tonic–clonic seizures (GTCS) can cause maternal and fetal hypoxia and acidosis. After a single GTCS, miscarriages and stillbirths have been reported. Status epilepticus is an uncommon complication of pregnancy, but when it does occur it carries a high maternal and fetal mortality rate. One series of 29 cases reported nine maternal deaths and 14 infant deaths (31). A single brief tonic–clonic seizure has been shown to cause depression of fetal heart rate for more than 20 minutes (32), and longer or repetitive tonic–clonic seizures are incrementally more hazardous to the fetus as well as to the mother.

Antiepileptic Drugs during Pregnancy

Management of AEDs during pregnancy can be complex, and ideally the patient's obstetrician and neurologist should work closely together. The ideal AED level needs to be established for each patient, preferably before conception, and should be the level at which seizure control is the best possible for that patient without debilitating side effects (Table 28-3). AED levels need to be monitored regularly during pregnancy and the first 1 to 2 months postpartum. Plasma AED concentrations decrease during pregnancy despite steady or increasing doses (Table 28-4) (33). Lamotrigine appears to behave in the same fashion during pregnancy (34). The total AED levels generally decline more than the free levels (33). Several factors contribute to the decline in AED levels during pregnancy (27). Impaired absorption is one cause, although it is relatively uncommon. The volume of distribution increases throughout pregnancy, but this would not account for the relatively lesser reduction in free levels compared with total levels. The most important contributing mechanisms are thought to be decreased albumin concentration, reduced plasma protein binding, and increased drug clearance. The decline in albumin concentration and plasma protein binding creates an increased percentage of unbound AED, which in turn provides an increased proportion of the drug available for metabolic degradation. Additionally, the increased sex steroid hormone levels may cause an induction of the hepatic microsomal enzymes and may contribute to the increased clearance of AEDs (35).

TABLE 28-3. *Antiepileptic drugs: indications and dose-related side effects*

Drug	Seizure type	Dose-related side effects
Carbamazepine	Partial or GTCS	Nausea, sedation, diplopia, dizziness, hyponatremia, neutropenia, dyskinesias
Phenytoin	Partial or GTCS	Nytagmus, ataxia, nausea, gum hypertrophy, drowsiness, megaloblastic anemia, increased seizures, lymphadenopathy
Valproic acid	All generalized or partial seizures	Tremor, weight gain, nausea, alopecia, peripheral edema, platelet dysfunction
Phenobarbital	Partial or GTCS, MC, clonic or tonic seizures	Sedation, depression, fatigue
Primidone	Partial or GTCS	Above plus psychosis, impotence
Clonazepam	MC or GTCS	Sedation, dizziness
Gabapentin	Partial seizures	Sedation, fatigue, dizziness, weight gain
Lamotrigine	Partial or Generalized seizures	Drowsiness, diplopia, dizziness, nausea, HA
Ethosuximide	Abence seizures	Nausea, anorexia, drowsiness, HA, agitation
Topiramate	Partial seizures	Confusion, ataxia, abnormal thinking, anorexia
Tiagabine	Partial seizures	Dizziness, tremor, HA, depression somnolence

GTCS, generalized tonic-clonic seizures; HA, headache; MC, myoclonic.

TABLE 28-4. *Pharmacokinetics of antiepileptic drugs during pregnancy*

AED	Decline in total level by 3rd trimester (%)	Percentage free fraction		
		Normal	Maternal	Neonatal
Carbamazepine	40	22	25	35
Phenytoin	56	9	11	13
Valproic acid	50	9	15	19
Phenobarbital	55	51	58	66
Primidone	55			
Derived PB	70	75	80	?
Ethosuximide	90	?	?	

AED, antiepileptic drug; PB, phenobarbital.

The optimal approach to monitoring AED levels during pregnancy is one that measures free levels of the AED on a monthly basis. Although the ratio of free to bound drug increases during pregnancy, the amount of free AED still declines for all major AEDs (33). The changes in total and free AEDs during pregnancy can vary widely and are not predictable for the individual patient based on reported group changes or total levels only. The frequency of monitoring levels often will need to be tailored to each situation, including the availability of tests, affordability, seizure control, and adverse effects. Unfortunately, many health facilities are not able to obtain free AED levels promptly enough to allow for timely AED adjustments, and the total AED levels may be the only possible guide. When the physician adjusts AEDs according to levels, he or she should take into consideration that it takes four to five half-lives for a medication to reach steady state (Table 28-5), and levels should be obtained as trough measurements for accurate comparisons.

Obstetric Complications

Women with epilepsy do have a slightly increased risk of certain obstetric complications. There is an approximate twofold increased risk of vaginal bleeding, anemia, hyperemesis gravidarum, abruptio placentae, eclampsia, and premature labor associated with epilepsy (36,37). Weak uterine contractions have been described in women taking AEDs, which may account for the twofold increased use of interventions during labor and delivery, including induction, mechanical rupture of membranes, forceps or vacuum assistance, and cesarean section (36,37).

Fetal death (fetal loss at greater than 20 weeks' gestational age) is another increased risk for pregnancies of epileptic mothers. Reported stillbirth rates vary between 1.3% to 14.0% for women with epilepsy compared with rates of 1.2% to 7.8% for women without epilepsy (38). Neonatal death rates also appear to be slightly increased for women who have epilepsy (1.3%–7.8%) compared with controls (1.0–3.9%). In contrast, spontaneous abortions before 20 weeks' gestational age do not appear to occur more frequently in epileptics (38).

Adverse Outcomes of Infants of Epileptic Mothers

IEMs are at increased risk for minor anomalies, major congenital malformations, and developmental disability (27,39–41). *Minor anomalies* are defined as structural

TABLE 28-5. *Pharmacologic properties of the common antiepileptic drugs*

Medication	Starting dose (mg)	Maintenance dose (mg/kg/d)	Therapeutic plasma conc. (µg/mL)	Serum half-life (hr)	Route of elimination	Serum protein binding (%)
Carbamazepine	200	10–20	6–12	8–24	Hepatic	70–80
Phenytoin	200	5–7	10–20	10–50	Hepatic	90–93
Valproic acid[a]	500	20–50	50–100	7–17	Hepatic	88–92
Phenobarbital	60	3–5	15–45	72–144	Hepatic	48–54
Primidone	250	20	5–15	4–12	Hepatic	20–30
Clonazepam	1	0.05–0.1	None	30–40	Hepatic	80–90
Gabapentin	600	20–70	None	5–7	Renal	0
Lamotrigine	100	4–9	?0.5–3.0	21–50	Hepatic	55
Ethosuximide	500	15–30	40–100	20–60	Hepatic	0
Topiramate	50	5–6	None	19–25	Renal	15
Tiagabine	8	0.3–1	None	5–8	Hepatic	96

[a]The therapeutic effects of valproic acid do not directly follow the plasma levels and suggest a longer therapeutic half-life.

deviations from the norm that do not constitute a threat to health and occur in fewer than 4% of the population. *Major malformations* are defined as an abnormality of an essential anatomic structure present at birth that interferes significantly with function or requires major intervention. Minor anomalies affect 6% to 20% of IEMs. Major malformations affect 4% to 8% of IEMs compared with 2% of the general population. Some component may be due to traits carried by mothers with epilepsy, but there is also a definite contribution from AEDs. The fetal anticonvulsant syndrome includes the minor anomalies, major malformations, mental deficiency, microcephaly, and intrauterine growth retardation, in various combinations. The fetal anticonvulsant syndrome has been described for phenytoin (PHT), carbamazepine (CBZ), phenobarbital (PB), and valproic acid (VPA). Consensus guidelines from a workshop and symposium in 1990 concluded that based on available data each of these four AEDs carried a similar teratogenic risk (14). Trimethadione (Tridione) is considered contraindicated during pregnancy because of the high prevalence of severe birth defects (14). As yet, no convincing evidence has been found for teratogenicity for gabapentin (GBP), tiagabine (TGB), or vigabatrin (VGB), but experience with these agents during pregnancy has been exceptionally limited. Information from the lamotrigine pregnancy registry (42) indicates that congenital defects have occurred at similar frequencies to older AEDs (about 5% of live births) in the 81 prospectively collected cases thus far. Although many of these women were on additional AEDs, some of the cases with major malformations did involve infants of epileptic mothers on LTG monotherapy. Animal studies suggest that topiramate (TPM) does have teratogenic effects at clinically relevant doses (43). It is clear that the risk increases with the number of AEDs to which the fetus is exposed during pregnancy, especially during the first trimester. Previous studies have reported major malformations in 25% of IEMs using four or more AEDs (39). Recent studies indicate that if a patient is on monotherapy, the risk of major malformations is probably as low as 4% to 6% (38).

Children of women who have epilepsy, including those born to mothers who are not taking AEDs, tend to have slightly more minor anomalies than controls or children of men with epilepsy (28). The minor anomalies may be outgrown in the first several years of life. They include distal digital and nail hypoplasia and the craniofacial anomalies, including ocular hypertelorism, broad nasal bridge, short upturned nose, altered lips, epicanthal folds, abnormal ears, and low hairline (27,39–41).

Major congenital malformations (Table 28-6) associated with AEDs include congenital heart disease, cleft lip/palate, neural tube defects, and urogenital defects (27,39–41). Urogenital defects commonly involve glandular hypospadias. The congenital heart defects include atrial septal defect, ventricular septal defect, tetralogy of Fallot, coarctation of the aorta, patent ductus arteriosus,

TABLE 28-6. *Major malformations in infants of epileptic mothers compared to the general population*

	General population	IEMs
Congenital heart	0.5%	1.5–2%
Cleft lip/palate	0.15%	1.4%
Neural tube defect	0.1%	1–2% (VPA) 0.5–1% (CBZ)
Urogenital defects		1.7%

CBZ, carbamazepine; IEM, infants of epileptic mothers; VPA, valproic acid.

and pulmonary stenosis. The neural tube defects usually consist of spina bifida and not anencephaly, but they tend to be severe open abnormalities that are frequently complicated by hydrocephaly and other midline defects (44). CBZ and VPA are associated with neural tube defects at a rate of about 10 and 20 times the general population, respectively (45,46). A recent paper pooling data from five prospective studies suggested that the absolute risk of malformations in children of women treated with VPA monotherapy may be as high as 3.8% and that offspring of women who received more than 1,000 mg per day of VPA during pregnancy were at particularly increased risk (29). PB monotherapy also showed a trend for increased risk of major malformations with increasing dose, but the differences were not significant.

Prenatal screening should be offered to all women with epilepsy to detect any major fetal malformations. Screening for neural tube defects should be done using a combination of maternal serum alpha-fetoprotein at 16 weeks and expert, targeted ultrasonography at 18 weeks, which can identify at least 95% of fetuses with open neural tube defects (47). Early transvaginal ultrasonography at 11 to 13 weeks to screen for neural tube defects is possible. Amniocentesis (with measurements of amniotic fluid alpha-fetoprotein and acetylcholinesterase) should be offered if these tests are equivocal. Detailed sonographic imaging of the fetal heart should be performed at 18 to 20 weeks' gestation, followed by fetal echocardiography if visualization is suboptimal. This approach can detect up to 85% of prenatally diagnosable cardiac abnormalities (47). Careful imaging of the fetal face for cleft lip and palate also can be performed at 18 to 20 weeks' gestational age, although the accuracy of prenatal diagnosis is less well established (47). If the patient's weight gain and fundal growth do not appear appropriate, serial sonography should be performed to assess fetal size and amniotic fluid volume (16).

Results of studies investigating psychomotor retardation in IEMs have been as varied as the protocols used, but most studies report a twofold to sevenfold increased risk of mental deficiency, affecting 1.2% to 6.2% of IEMs (48). Verbal scores on neuropsychometric measures may be selectively more involved (38). An association has been found between cognitive impairment in IEMs and *in utero* AED exposure, seizures, a high number of minor anomalies, major malformations, decreased maternal education, impaired maternal–child relations, and maternal partial-seizure disorder (49). Microcephaly also is associated with all AEDs (38).

Low birth weight (<2,500 g) and prematurity have been reported in IEMs at rates of 7% to 10% and 4% to 11%, respectively (38). The risk of epilepsy in children of women who have epilepsy is higher (relative risk of 3.2) compared with controls. Children of fathers with epilepsy do not demonstrate this same degree of increased risk. This may be related to the finding that the occurrence of maternal seizures during pregnancy, but not AED use, confers an increased risk of seizures in offspring (50).

Teratogenecity of AEDs is thought to be mediated by several mechanisms, including folate deficiency, AED free radical intermediates, and oxidative metabolites. Antifolate effects are well established for PHT, PB, and primidone, whereas VPA and CBZ also have been implicated (51,52). LTG and GBP do not have any obvious antifolate properties. Low serum and red blood cell folate levels are associated with an increased incidence of spontaneous abortions and malformations in animal and human epilepsy studies (51). Folate supplementation provides a 72% protective effect for offspring of nonepileptic women at high risk for neural tube defects (53) and probably reduces the incidence of other major malformations (54). The maximal benefit of folate is achieved with supplementation beginning before and continuing after conception. Therefore, all women of childbearing potential who have epilepsy should be placed on folate supplementation, regardless of family plans and birth control use.

Oxidative metabolites also may play a role in AED teratogenesis (55). The enzyme epoxide hydrolase normally eliminates these epoxide metabolites. Fetuses who are homozygous for the recessive allele have low enzyme activity and are probably at greater risk for developing features of the fetal anticonvulsant syndrome. AED polytherapy may promote epoxide production and inhibit epoxide metabolism. Fetuses who are at risk may benefit from AEDs that lack epoxide intermediates (such as the investigational AED oxcarbazepine) and from avoidance of polytherapy.

A hemorrhagic disorder can occur during the neonatal period as a result of a deficiency of vitamin K-dependent clotting factors (56). It has been reported in association with CBZ, PHT, PB, ethosuximide (ESX), primidone (PRM), diazepam, mephobarbital, and amobarbital (38,57). Infant mortality from this bleeding disorder is greater than 30% and is usually due to bleeding in the abdominal and pleural cavities leading to shock. At least part of this newborn disorder is due to inhibition by AEDs of the transport of vitamin K across the placenta. These effects can be overcome by large concentrations of vitamin K. Prophylactic treatment consists of vitamin K administered orally as 20 mg daily to the mother during the last month of pregnancy and 1 mg administered intramuscularly or intraveneously to the newborn at birth (58). If two of the coagulation factors fall below 5% of the normal values, intraveneous fresh frozen plasma needs to be administered (38).

Vitamin D levels can be lowered by PHT, PB, and PRM, probably by increasing metabolism. Epileptic women should be encouraged to take prenatal vitamins that include an adequate amount of vitamin D (59).

Labor and Delivery

A generalized tonic–clonic seizure occurs during labor in only 1% to 2% of women with epilepsy and in another 1% to 2% of women with epilepsy during the first 24 hours after delivery (14). The length of sleep deprivation should be monitored, and obstetric anesthesia may be used to allow for some rest before delivery if sleep deprivation has been prolonged. Although there is an approximately twofold increased use of interventions during labor and delivery in women with seizure disorders (37), most will have a safe vaginal delivery. During a prolonged labor, oral absorption of AEDs may be erratic, and any emesis will confound the problem. PHT, PB, and VPA may be given intravenously at the same maintenance dosage as is used orally. Convulsive seizures and repeated seizures during labor should be treated promptly with intravenous lorazepam (14). Benzodiazepines in large doses can cause neonatal depression, decreased heart rate, and maternal apnea, and it is important to watch closely for these potential side effects. Administration of other, longer-acting AEDs is controversial because of the potential inhibitory effects on myometrial contractions (14). Boluses of PHT or PB will need to be accompanied by cardiac and blood pressure monitoring because dysrhythmias and hypotension can occur, although rarely. The use of fosphenytoin instead of intravenous phenytoin can minimize this risk. Status epilepticus, or even a single GTCS, needs to be treated aggressively because of the high risk to the mother and fetus. Oxygen should be administered to the patient, who should be placed on her left side to increase uterine blood flow and decrease the risk of maternal aspiration (16). Prompt cesarean section should be performed when repeated GTCS cannot be controlled during labor or when the mother is unable to cooperate during labor because of impaired awareness during repetitive absence or complex partial seizures (14).

Postpartum Care

Serum levels of AEDs rise again after delivery and plateau after 8 to 10 weeks. AED levels need to be followed closely during this postpartum period.

Perinatal lethargy, irritability, and feeding difficulties have been attributed to intrauterine exposure to AEDs, especially the barbiturates and the benzodiazepines. IEMs who are breastfed may continue to demonstrate these behavioral patterns and even potentially develop

TABLE 28-7. *Concentration of antiepileptic drugs in breast milk and neonatal elimination*

AED	Breast milk/plasma concentration ratio	Adult $t_{1/2}$ (hr)	Neonate $t_{1/2}$ (hr)
Carbamazepine	0.4–0.6	8–25	8–28
Phenytoin	0.2–0.4	12–50	15–105
Phenobarbital	0.4–0.6	75–126	45–500
Ethosuximide	0.9	40–60	40
Primidone	0.7–0.9	4–12	7–60
Valproic acid	0.01	6–18	30–60
Lamotrigine	0.6	–	–

AED, antiepileptic drug; $t_{1/2}$, half-life.

failure to thrive. In addition, prenatal or neonatal exposure to PB can produce withdrawal symptoms beginning approximately 7 days after last exposure and lasting 2 to 6 weeks (60). Most IEMs, however, can breastfeed successfully without complications if the mother is not taking a barbiturate or benzodiazepine. The amount of AED excreted into the breast milk is based in part on the portion that is not protein bound in plasma (Table 28-7). The infant's serum concentration is determined by this factor as well as by the AED elimination half-life in neonates, which is usually more prolonged than that in adults (see Table 28-7) (35,38).

Appropriate individualized safety issues must consider the mother's ictal semiology. If she is likely to drop objects she is holding, then she should use a harness when carrying the infant. If she is likely to fall, a stroller in the house is an even better option. Changing diapers and clothes is best performed on the floor rather than on an elevated changing table. Bathing should never be performed alone, as a brief lapse in attention can result in a fatal drowning. The important role of sleep deprivation in exacerbation of seizures must be emphasized. Especially if the mother is breastfeeding, sleep deprivation may be unavoidable. The possibility of other family members sharing the burden of nighttime feedings through the use of formula or harvested breastmilk should be considered, and the mother should attempt to make up any missed sleep during the infant's daytime naps.

SUMMARY OF MANAGEMENT OF EPILEPSY AND PREGNANCY

The initial visit between the physician and a woman with epilepsy of childbearing age should include a discussion about family planning. Topics should include effective birth control, the importance of planned pregnancies with AED optimization and folate supplementation before conception, the risks of AEDs, and the risks of seizures during pregnancy. The goal is effective control of maternal seizures with the least risk to the fetus. Because each of the major AEDs is teratogenic, the medication that is most effective for that woman's epilepsy and seizure type should be prescribed. The one exception is in the case of neural tube defects. If a woman is at high risk for bearing a child with a neural tube defect because of her family history, then VPA and CBZ should be chosen only if other AEDs are ineffective.

Seizure control remains an important goal during pregnancy in epileptic women. Convulsive seizures in particular place the mother and fetus at risk. Nonconvulsive seizures are also harmful, especially if they may involve falling or other forms of potential trauma. Any decision to withdraw medications before a planned pregnancy should be based on the same principles used for AED withdrawal in any person with epilepsy.

Monotherapy is an important goal in women with seizure disorders of childbearing potential, and AEDs should be used at the lowest effective doses. The risk of teratogenicity may increase with higher doses of all AEDs, as has been shown for VPA and spina bifida (61). If high daily doses are needed, frequent small doses may be helpful to avoid high peak levels.

Folate supplementation should begin before conception and is crucial during the first 30 days of gestation to protect against neural tube defects. The optimal dosage has not been established for women with epilepsy, and recommendations vary between 0.4 and 5 mg per day.

A common but usually erroneous reason to change medications is the woman who presents to her physician after she has discovered she is pregnant. In many cases, she is already in or past the critical period of organogenesis (Table 28-8). It is important to try to achieve optimal monotherapy before conception. Stopping or abruptly modifying AEDs during weeks 6 to 8 of pregnancy does little to lower the risk of major congenital defects and only increases the risk of seizures, which are potentially harmful to both the mother and the fetus. If a woman with epilepsy presents after conception and she is taking a single drug that is effective, her medication usually should not be changed. The teratogenic risk is increased only by exposing the fetus to a second agent during a crossover of AEDs, and seizures are more likely to occur with any medication changes. If a woman is receiving polytherapy and is seizure free, it may be possible to switch safely to monotherapy.

Prenatal screening can detect major malformations in the first and second trimesters. Vitamin K is given as 20 mg per

TABLE 28-8. *Relative timing and developmental pathology of certain malformations*

Tissues	Malformations	Time after LMP
CNS	Meningomyelocele	28 d
Heart	Ventricular septal defect	6 wk
Face	Cleft lip	36 d
	Cleft maxillary palate	10 wk

CNS, central nervous system. LMP, first day of last menstrual period.

day orally during the last month of pregnancy, followed by 1 mg intramuscularly or intravenously to the newborn.

With the above information and guidelines, most women with epilepsy will have healthy pregnancies without major maternal or fetal complications. The most effective tool in achieving this goal is thorough education and careful planning before conception.

REFERENCES

1. Commission on Classification and Terminology of the International League Against Epilepsy. Proposal for revised classification of epilepsies and epileptic syndromes. Epilepsia 1989;30:389–399.
2. Commission on Classification and Terminology of the International League Against Epilepsy. Proposal for revised clinical and electroencephalographic classification of epileptic seizures. Epilepsia 1981;22: 489–501.
3. Hauser WA, Hersdorffer DC. Epilepsy: frequency, causes and consequences. New York: Demos Publications, 1990:1–51.
4. Devinsky O, Yerby M. Women with epilepsy. Neurol Clin 1994;12: 479–495.
5. Logothetis J, Harner R, Morell F, Torres F. The role of oestrogen in catamenial exacerbation of epilepsy. Neurology 1959;9:352–360.
6. Woolley D, Timiras P. The gonad-brain relationship: effects of female sex hormones and electroshock convulsions in the rat. Endocrinology 1962;70:169–209.
7. Morrell MJ. Hormones and epilepsy through the lifetime. Epilepsia 1992;33:S49–S61.
8. Laidlaw J. Catamenial epilepsy. Lancet 1956;2:1235–1237.
9. Mattson RH, Cramer JA. Epilepsy, sex hormones and antiepileptic drugs. Epilepsia 1985;26(Suppl 1):S40–51.
10. Bäckström T. Epileptic seizures in women related to plasma estrogen and progesterone during the menstrual cycle. Acta Neurol Scand 1976; 54:321–347.
11. Herzog AG, Klein P, Ransil BJ. Three patterns of catamenial epilepsy. Epilepsia 1997;38:1082–1088.
12. Schacter SC. Iatrogenic seizures. Neurol Clin 1998;16:157–170.
13. Krauss GL, Brandt J, Campbell M, Plate C, Summerfield M. Antiepileptic medication and oral contraceptive interactions: a national survey of neurologists and obstetricians. Neurology 1996;46:1534–1539.
14. Delgado-Escueta A, Janz D. Consensus guidelines: preconception counseling, management, and care of the pregnant woman with epilepsy. Neurology 1992;42:149–160.
15. Commission on Genetics, Pregnancy, and the Child, International League Against Epilepsy. Guidelines for the care of women of childbearing age with epilepsy. Epilepsia 1993;34:588–589.
16. Committee on Educational Bulletins of the American College of Obstetricians and Gynecologists. Seizure disorders in pregnancy. Int J Gynecol Obstet 1997;56:279–286.
17. Seale C, Morrell MJ, Nelson L, Druzin MI. Analysis of the prenatal and gestational care given to women with epilepsy. Epilepsia 1997;38 (Suppl 8):231.
18. Janz D, Schmidt D. Anti-epileptic drugs and failure of oral contraceptives. Lancet 1974;1:1113.
19. Rosenfeld WE, Doose DR, Walker SA, Nayak RK. Effect of topiramate on the pharmacokinetics of an oral contraceptive containing norethindrone and ethinyl estradiol in patients with epilepsy. Epilepsia 1997;38: 317–323.
20. Gjerde IO, Strandjord RE, Ulstein M. The course of epilepsy during pregnancy: a study of 78 cases. Acta Neurol Scand 1988;78:198–205.
21. Otani K. Risk factors for the increased seizure frequency during pregnancy and the puerperium. Folia Psych Neurol Jap 1985;39:33–42.
22. Svigos JM. Epilepsy and pregnancy. Aust N Z J Obstet Gynaecol 1984; 24:182–185.
23. Tanganelli P, Regesta G. Epilepsy, pregnancy, and major birth anomalies: an Italian prospective, controlled study. Neurology 1992;42:89–93.
24. Cantrell DC, Riela SJ, Ramus R, Riela AR. Epilepsy and pregnancy: a study of seizure frequency and patient demographics. Epilepsia 1997; 38(Suppl 8):231.
25. Ramsay RE. Effect of hormones on seizure activity during pregnancy. J Clin Neurophys 1987;4:23–25.
26. Loiseau P, Legroux M, Henry PO. Epilepsies et grossesses. Bordeaux Medicine 1974;7:1157–1164.
27. Yerby MS, Devinsky O. Epilepsy and pregnancy. In: Devinsky O, Feldmann E, Hainline B, eds. Neurological complications of pregnancy. New York: Raven Press, 1994:45–63.
28. Lindhout D, Meinardi H, Meijer JWA, Nau H. Antiepileptic drugs and teratogenesis in two consecutive cohorts: changes in prescription policy paralleled by changes in pattern of malformations. Neurology 1992; 42(Suppl 5):94–110.
29. Samrén EB, van Duijn CM, Koch S, et al. Maternal use of antiepileptic drugs and the risk of major congenital malformations: a joint European prospective study of human teratogenesis asssociated with maternal epilepsy. Epilepsia 1997;38:981–990.
30. Pearlman MD, Tintinalli JE, Lorenz RP. Blunt trauma during pregnancy. N Engl J Med 1990;323:1609–1613.
31. Teramo K, Hiilesmaa VK. Pregnancy and fetal complications in epileptic pregnancies: review of the literature. In: Janz D, Bossi L, Dam M, et al., eds. Epilepsy, pregnancy and the child. New York: Raven Press, 1982:53–59.
32. Teramo K, Hiilesmaa V, Bardy A, Saarikoski S. Fetal heart rate during a maternal grand mal epileptic seizure. J Perinat Med 1979;7:3–6.
33. Yerby MS, Collins SD. Pregnancy and the mother. In: Engel J, Pedley TA, eds. Epilepsy, a comprehensive textbook. Philadelphia: Lippincott-Raven Publishers, 1997:2030.
34. Tomson T, Ohman I, Vitols S. Lamotrigine in pregnancy and lactation: a case report. Epilepsia 1997;48:1039–1041.
35. Krauer B, Krauer F. Drug kinetics in pregnancy. Clin Pharmacokinet 1977;2:167–181.
36. Yerby M. Risks of pregnancy in women with epilepsy. Epilepsia 1992; 33:S23–S27.
37. Yerby MS, Koepsell T, Daling J. Pregnancy complications and outcomes in a cohort of women with epilepsy. Epilepsia 1985;26:631–635.
38. Yerby MS, Collins SD. Teratogenicity of antiepileptic drugs. In: Engel J, Pedley TA, eds. Epilepsy, a comprehensive textbook. Philadelphia: Lippincott-Raven Publishers, 1997:1195–1203.
39. Lindhout D, Omtzigt J. Pregnancy and the risk of teratogenicity. Epilepsia 1992;33:S41–S48.
40. Lindhout D, Omtzigt J. Teratogenic effects of antiepileptic drugs: implications for the management of epilepsy in women of childbearing age. Epilepsia 1994;35:S19–S28.
41. Yerby M. Pregnancy, teratogenesis and epilepsy. Neurol Clin 1994;12: 749–771.
42. Glaxo-Wellcome. International lamotrigine pregnancy registry, interim report, 9/1/92–3/31/97.
43. Topiramate prescribing information package insert. McNeil Pharmaceutical, Ortho Pharmaceutical Corporation, 1996.
44. Lindhout D, Omtzigt JGC, Cornel MT. Spectrum of neural-tube defects in 34 infants pernatally exposed to antiepileptic drugs. Neurology 1992;42(Suppl 5):111–118.
45. Rosa FW. Spina bifida in infants of women treated with carbamazepine during pregnancy. N Engl J Med 1991;324:674–677.
46. Lindhout D, Schmidt D. In-utero exposure to valproate and neural tube defects. Lancet 1986;2:1392–1393.
47. Malone FD, D'Alton ME. Drugs in pregnancy: anticonvulsants. Semin Perinatol 1997;21:114–123.
48. Ganström ML, Gaily E. Psychomotor development in children of mothers with epilepsy. Neurology 1992;42(Suppl 5):144–148.
49. Meador KJ. Cognitive effects of epilepsy and of antiepileptic medications. In: Wyllie E, ed. The treatment of epilepsy: principles and practice, 2nd ed. Baltimore: Williams & Wilkins, 1996:1121–1130.
50. Ottman R, Annegers JF, Hauser WA, Kurland LT. Higher risk of seizures in offspring of mothers than fathers with epilepsy. Am J Hum Genet 1988;43:357–364.
51. Dansky L, Rosenblatt D, Andermann E. Mechanisms of teratogenesis: folic acid and antiepileptic therapy. Neurology 1992;42:32–42.
52. Wegner C, Nau H. Alteration of embryonic folate metabolism by valproic acid during organogenesis: implications for mechanisms of teratogenesis. Neurology 1992;42(Suppl 5):17–24.
53. MRC Vitamin Study Research Group. Prevention of neural-tube defects: results of the Medical Research Council Vitamin Study. Lancet 1991;338:131–137.
54. Ogawa Y, Kaneko S, Otani K, Fukushima Y. Serum folic acid in epileptic mothers and their relationship to congenital malformations. Epilepsy Res 1991;8:75–78.

55. Buehler BA, Rao V, Finnell RH. Biochemical and molecular teratology of fetal hydantoin syndrome. Pediatric Neurogenetics 1994;12: 741–748.
56. Srinivasan G, Seeler RA, Tiruvury A, Pildes RS. Maternal anticonvulsant therapy and hemorrhagic disease of the newborn. Obstet Gynecol 1982;59:250–252.
57. Nelson KB, Ellenber JH. Maternal seizure disorder, outcomes of pregnancy, and neurologic abnormalities in the children. Neurology 1982; 32:1247–1254.
58. Krumholz A. Epilepsy in pregnancy. In: Goldstein PJ, Stern BJ, eds. Neurological disorders of pregnancy, 2nd ed. Mount Kisco, NY: Futura Publishing, 1992:25–50.
59. Friis B, Sardemann H. Neonatal hypocalcaemia after intrauterine exposure to anticonvulsant drugs. Arch Dis Child 1977;52:239–247.
60. Desmond MM, Schwanecke RP, Wilson GS, Yasunaga S, Burgdorff I. Maternal barbiturate utilization and neonatal withdrawal symptomatology. J Pediatr 1972;80:190–197.
61. Omtzigt JGC, Los FJ, Grobee DE, et al. The risk of spina bifida aperta after first-trimester exposure to valproate in a prenatal cohort. Neurology 1992;42(Suppl 5):119–125.

Cherry and Merkatz's Complications of Pregnancy,
Fifth Edition, edited by W. R. Cohen.
Lippincott Williams & Wilkins, Philadelphia © 2000.

CHAPTER 29

Peripheral Nerve Disorders

Bruce A. Rabin

Disorders of the peripheral nervous system occur with an increased frequency during pregnancy. This increase may be due to many causes, including anatomic changes, hormonal changes, fluid and electrolyte imbalance, inflammatory diseases, and other as yet unidentified causes. Most of the pregnancy-related peripheral nervous system disorders discussed in this chapter resolve following delivery.

MONONEUROPATHIES

Mononeuropathies are disorders that affect a single nerve. The causes of mononeuropathies are varied and range from compression of a single nerve to focal inflammation. If several different nerves are selectively and discretely involved, the term *mononeuritis multiplex* is used. These syndromes are named to contrast with polyneuropathies, in which the disorders are less selective and tend to affect many nerves. Symptoms of peripheral neuropathies allow identification of affected nerves and nerve roots (Table 29-1).

Bell's Palsy

Since Bell described a woman who developed idiopathic facial weakness during gestation (1), idiopathic facial nerve palsy (Bell's palsy) has been noted to occur with an increased frequency in pregnancy (2,3).

The incidence in nonpregnant women is about 15 to 20 per 100,000. The incidence doubles in pregnancy, to approximately 40 to 45 per 100,000, with most cases occurring in the third trimester and in the puerperium (2). The reason for this increase is uncertain. There is no apparent association with preeclampsia or eclampsia. Most affected women have normal glycemic control (4). Although Bell's palsy in both pregnant and nonpregnant women is usually unilateral, there are rare cases (3%) of bilateral Bell's palsy in both groups (5). Some women have a recurrence with subsequent pregnancies (3). The cause of Bell's palsy in pregnant women is not known. Treatable causes of isolated cranial neuropathies should be excluded, including Lyme disease and sarcoidosis. Idiopathic Bell's palsy has not been associated with an increased risk to the fetus or the mother.

The diagnosis of Bell's palsy is based on the clinical observation of acute paralysis of the facial muscles on one half of the face. Weakness of the forehead and lower face localizes the lesion to the facial nerve (cranial nerve VII). Sensation over the anterior two thirds of the tongue on the affected side may be reduced, and there may be hyperacusis. Nerve conduction studies and electromyography may provide additional information related to prognosis, because recovery appears to be directly related to the severity of denervation, with partial lesions having the best prognosis. Recovery in most patients with Bell's palsy is good and occurs within the first 3 months postpartum; however, patients with complete lesions demonstrated by electromyography (EMG) will likely have only a partial recovery.

Treatment of Bell's palsy is controversial. Acute therapy with a 10-day course of corticosteroids beginning in the first 24 hours (e.g., 60 mg of prednisone a day for 10 days with a rapid taper) is believed to decrease the duration and severity of symptoms (2,6). Initiation of treatment after the first 24 hours has not been shown to be of benefit. Attention to ophthalmologic care is critical to prevent corneal abrasions if there is weakness of the orbicularis oculi muscles.

Median Neuropathy at the Wrist (Carpal Tunnel Syndrome)

The median nerve contains nerve fibers arising from the C5–T1 spinal roots. It is formed by the union of fibers

B. A. Rabin: Department of Neurology, Johns Hopkins School of Medicine, Division of Neurology; Sinai Hospital of Baltimore, Baltimore, MD 21215.

TABLE 29-1. *Localization of common peripheral nerve symptoms in pregnancy*

Symptom	Affected nerve	Root
Numb hand and thumb	Median	C-6, C-7
Numb hand and digit 5	Ulnar	C-8, T-1
Foot drop	Peroneal or sciatic	L-4, L-5
Quadriceps weakness	Femoral	L-2, L-3, L-4
Lateral thigh numbness	Lateral femoral cutaneous nerve of the thigh	L-2, L-3
Thigh adductor weakness	Obturator	L-2, L-3, L-4
Severe shoulder pain and weakness	Brachial plexus	variable, often C5-T1

of the medial and lateral cords of the brachial plexus. It crosses the elbow in the antecubital fossa and courses through the carpal tunnel to terminate in the hand (Fig. 29-1). In the hand, the motor fibers innervate the abductor pollicis brevis, opponens pollicis, and the first two lumbricals. Sensory fibers innervate the palmar surface of the thumb, second, third, and half of the fourth digit.

Carpal tunnel syndrome is the most common entrapment syndrome of pregnancy, although it was not recognized as such until the late 1950's (7,8). As many as 20% to 30% of pregnant women experience typical symptoms (9), although only 2% to 5% of pregnant women will have clinical or electrophysiologic abnormalities (10). Symptoms are more prominent in the second and third trimesters and usually resolve within 2 weeks of delivery. Recurrence during subsequent pregnancies is common. Lactation-related carpal tunnel syndrome occurs near the end of the first postpartum month in women who are breastfeeding their infants and resolves when the infants are weaned. The cause is unknown but may be the positioning of the infant during feeding.

Symptoms begin with intermittent paresthesias over the palmar surface of the hand, although many patients have difficulty localizing the symptoms. Typically, patients awaken with tingling, burning, or numb hands and complain of poor circulation in their hands or that they feel swollen. Gestational carpal tunnel syndrome is frequently bilateral. The patient often shakes or flicks her hands (*flick sign*), with symptoms usually relieved by repositioning. Examination may reveal numbness over the palmar aspect of the first three and a half digits. In severe cases, atrophy of the thenar eminence and weakness of thumb abduction are present. Provocative maneuvers include tapping over the wrist to elicit Tinel's sign and hyperflexion of the wrist for 30 to 60 seconds to produce Phalen's sign. Hyperextension of the wrist may produce a reverse Phalen's sign. Unfortunately, the sensitivity and specificity of all these clinical tests are low.

Carpal tunnel syndrome is caused by compression or inflammation of the median nerve within the carpal tunnel. There is progressive injury to the nerve, ranging from mild focal demyelination to frank axonal injury and denervation. In pregnancy, pressure on the median nerve is likely to result from the reduction of free space within the carpal tunnel as a result of tissue swelling.

Prognosis of gestational carpal tunnel syndrome is usually excellent, although patients with axonal injury may have persistent or progressive symptoms. These patients should undergo electrodiagnostic testing to ensure correct diagnosis and to assess the severity of disease.

The differential diagnosis of carpal tunnel syndrome includes C6 or C7 radiculopathy, thoracic outlet syndrome, and de Quervain's tenosynovitis. The latter also has a predilection for pregnancy and the postpartum period. C6–7 root disease results in numbness of the median-innervated fingers, and, unlike carpal tunnel syndrome, often involves the dorsal surface. When weakness is present, the hand muscles are spared, whereas the triceps and pronator teres muscles are affected. Thoracic outlet syndrome results in weakness and atrophy of the abductor pollicis brevis muscle and numbness in the ulnar nerve distribution (median motor and ulnar sensory involvement). De Quervain's tenosynovitis results in dorsolateral wrist pain and tenderness in the absence of paresthesias. Thus, carpal tunnel syndrome usually can be distinguished from these three processes by clinical criteria alone.

Because prognosis of gestational carpal tunnel syndrome is so good, conservative management is usually sufficient. Wrist splints are effective, especially if worn at

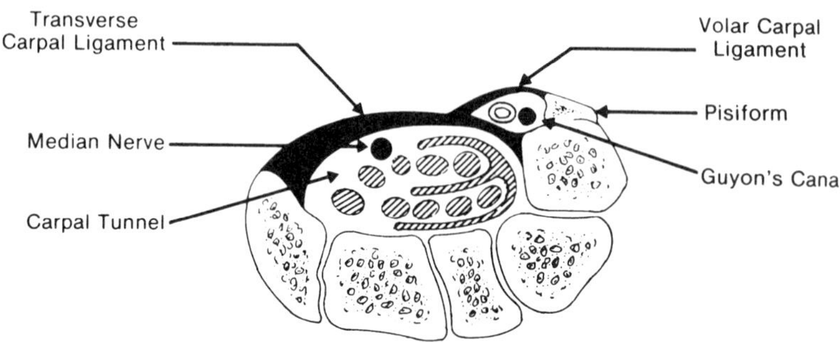

FIG. 29-1. Diagram of a cross section through the wrist illustrating the relationship of the median and ulnar nerves to the transverse carpal ligament, carpal bones, and intrinsic hand muscle ligaments. (From Stewart JD. Focal peripheral neuropathies, 2nd ed. New York: Raven Press, 1993.)

night. At least 80% of patients receive full relief from nocturnal splinting of the wrist.

Thiazide diuretics also may be of some benefit in patients for whom splinting fails. For those with severe carpal tunnel syndrome (i.e., those with weakness, atrophy, or denervation of the abductor pollicis brevis on electrophysiologic testing), surgical release of the transverse carpal ligament (flexor retinaculum) is usually effective in relieving symptoms and halting any further injury to the median nerve.

Ulnar Neuropathy

The ulnar nerve is formed from the C8 and T1 spinal nerves as they pass through the lower trunk and medial cord of the brachial plexus. The nerve runs posterior to the medial epicondyle in the ulnar groove, under the aponeurosis of the flexor carpi ulnaris, and through the cubital tunnel (Fig 29-2). The ulnar nerve passes through Guyon's canal in the wrist (see Fig. 29-1).

Compression at the elbow is the most common cause of ulnar neuropathy, although compression in Guyon's canal also occurs. Patients typically have paresthesias along the ulnar side of the hand involving the little finger, although many have difficulty localizing the sensory symptoms. Weakness is rare in pregnancy but, when present, usually involves the interossei. Sensory loss typically is seen in the fifth digit, over the palmar surface of the ulnar side of the fourth digit, and over the ulnar side of the hand.

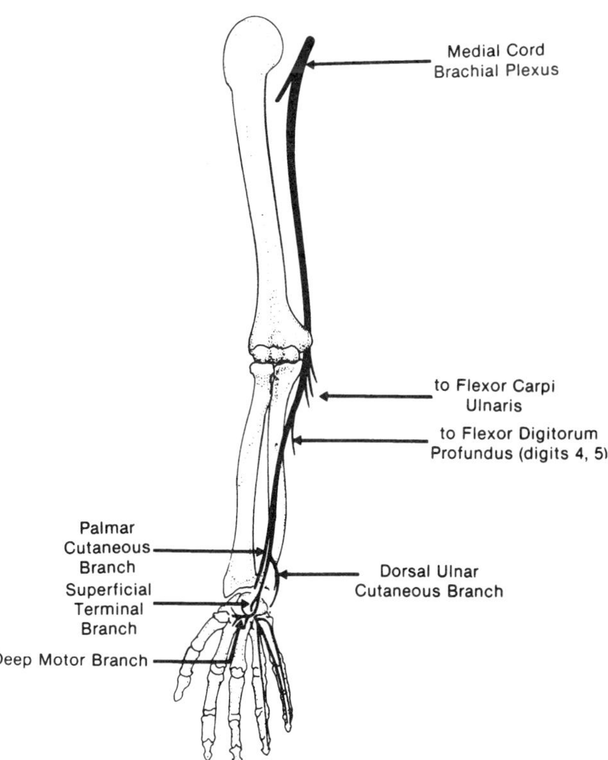

FIG. 29-2. Diagram of the ulnar nerve and its branches. Note how the ulnar nerve runs posterior to the medial epicondyle in the ulnar groove at the elbow. (From Stewart JD. Focal peripheral neuropathies, 2nd ed. New York: Raven Press, 1993.)

Electrodiagnostic studies are useful in differentiating ulnar neuropathy from carpal tunnel syndrome and to assess severity of disease. Protection of the elbow with an elbow pad, particularly at night, is usually adequate to relieve symptoms. In most affected patients, recovery is complete following delivery. For severe cases with atrophy or weakness, or for those whose EMG studies demonstrate denervation, surgical transposition of the ulnar nerve is necessary to prevent further nerve injury.

Meralgia Paresthetica

Meralgia paresthetica results from injury to the lateral femoral cutaneous nerve of the thigh. This purely sensory nerve arises from the L2 and L3 spinal nerves and passes under or through the lateral portion of the inguinal ligament to innervate the skin over the anterolateral thigh (Fig 29-3). In pregnancy, symptoms usually occur in the third trimester and may be unilateral or bilateral (11). Symptoms may reappear with subsequent pregnancies (12). The cause of gestational meralgia paresthetica is likely to be due to entrapment of the lateral femoral cutaneous nerve of the thigh as it traverses the inguinal ligament (13). Women who have had rapid weight gain or who are obese appear to be more susceptible to this focal neuropathy (14).

Characteristic symptoms are numbness, burning, and tingling in the lateral thigh, often worsened by walking or standing. Many patients report allodynia. Some patients experience improvement after prolonged sitting, whereas others report increased symptoms. If numbness is present, it occupies a relatively small area (usually a few centimeters in diameter) of the midlateral thigh. The remainder of the neurologic examination is normal, with preserved power and deep tendon reflexes.

Differential diagnosis of lateral thigh numbness includes radiculopathy at the L2 level, lumbar plexopathy, and femoral neuropathy. All three of these entities would be expected to result in more extensive sensory changes as well as weakness and abnormal deep tendon reflexes. Nerve conduction and EMG studies may be useful to exclude these other disorders but rarely are needed or helpful for a diagnosis of meralgia paresthetica.

Although symptoms typically improve spontaneously several months postpartum, if they are particularly bothersome, they can be managed with either anticonvulsant (e.g., gabapentin or carbamazepene) or tricyclic antidepressant (e.g., amitriptyline) medications in the postpartum period. More severe symptoms may require the combined use of analgesic and neuropathic pain medications.

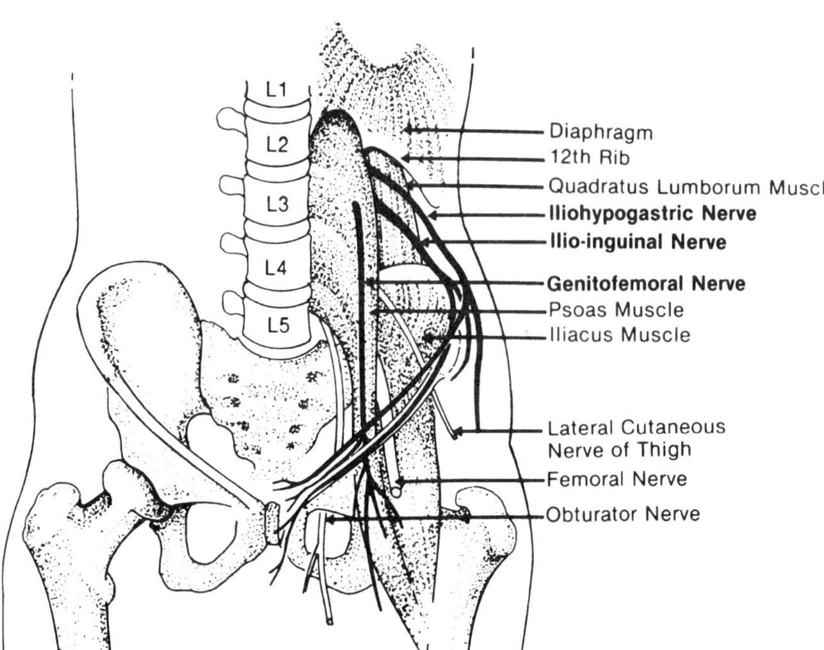

FIG. 29-3. Diagram demonstrating the relationship of the iliohypogastric, ilioinguinal, genitofemoral, femoral, and obturator nerves within the pelvis. (From Stewart JD. Focal peripheral neuropathies, 2nd ed. New York: Raven Press, 1993.)

Femoral Nerve Injury

The femoral nerve arises from the L2–4 spinal nerve roots and passes under the inguinal ligament lateral to the femoral artery and nerve (Fig. 29-3). Femoral neuropathy may occur after vaginal delivery. The most common symptom is painless knee extension weakness, with hip flexion weakness encountered less frequently. There also may be associated thigh numbness. On examination, the patellar reflex is reduced or absent on the affected side. Most cases resolve spontaneously 1 to 2 months postpartum. The cause of femoral neuropathy is unknown but is believed to be due to positioning of the leg with hip flexion and external rotation during childbirth with subsequent compression of the femoral nerve at or near the inguinal canal (15–17). If hip flexion weakness is present, the lesion must be proximal to the branch to the iliopsoas and may be due to compression from the fetal head, instrumentation, or leg positioning. Femoral neuropathies that result from cesarean section may be due to prolonged positioning in the lithotomy position or the presence of self-retaining retractors causing pressure on the iliopsoas muscle and the femoral nerve as it courses through this muscle (18,19).

Obturator Nerve Palsy

The obturator nerve arises from the L2–L4 spinal nerves. It runs through the psoas muscle to its medial border, around the pelvic side wall, and descends through the obturator canal to innervate the thigh adductors and skin of the upper thigh (Fig. 29-3). Obturator nerve palsy, a rare syndrome in pregnancy and the postpartum period (20), may occur during pelvic surgery as a result of stretch or compression or during delivery as a result of compression of the nerve against the bony pelvis by the fetal head (21). Obturator nerve lesions result in thigh adductor weakness and numbness over the medial thigh; however, more common causes of thigh adductor weakness include lumbar radiculopathy at the L3 or L4 level and lumbar plexopathy. Prognosis is good for recovery, usually in the first month after delivery.

Peroneal Nerve Injury

The common peroneal nerve arises in the popliteal fossa as a branch of the sciatic nerve. It runs posteriorly over the fibular head and divides into the superficial and deep peroneal nerves. Footdrop may result from direct compression of the common peroneal nerve as it crosses the fibular head. This usually occurs in pregnancy as a result of prolonged positioning of the legs in the lithotomy position during labor, although forceps delivery also may cause injury (22). There are case reports of footdrop resulting from compression of the nerves during natural childbirth, either from prolonged pushing or squatting (23,24). Patients on prolonged bed rest are also at increased risk.

Footdrop that results from compression of the peroneal nerve needs to be differentiated from that caused by an L5 radiculopathy, sciatic neuropathy, or lumbar plexopathy. Peroneal nerve injuries cause ankle dorsiflexion and eversion weakness, whereas an L5 radiculopathy has the additional sign of ankle inversion weakness. Electrodiagnostic studies are useful in more severe cases to localize the lesion and guide therapy.

Treatment is usually conservative, with measures taken to prevent compression of the peroneal nerve. Ankle orthoses are used to prevent slapping of the foot and dragging of the toes. Physical therapy helps to maintain residual strength and prevents contractures. Only rarely is surgical decompression of the nerve necessary.

DISORDERS OF THE BRACHIAL PLEXUS

The brachial plexus is formed from spinal roots C5–T1 (Fig. 29-4). Acute brachial plexus neuropathy, also known as neuralgic amyotrophy, brachial plexus neuritis, and Parsonage-Turner syndrome, is characterized by severe pain in the shoulder girdle lasting from days to weeks, followed by muscle weakness and wasting (25). As the weakness appears, the pain tends to dissipate. Weakness is usually proximal, resulting from focal involvement of the upper trunk of the brachial plexus. Patients with acute brachial plexus neuropathy tend to have asymmetric, bilateral involvement of both plexi. Sensory symptoms other than pain are present in only one third of patients. Rarely, patients may develop shortness of breath as a result of involvement of the phrenic nerve in the cervical plexus.

The cause of acute brachial plexus neuropathy is unknown. There has been an association with immunizations, suggesting the possibility that there is an inflammatory component, but immunosuppressive treatments have not been of much benefit. Recurrent brachial plexus neuropathy may be inherited as an autosomal dominant trait, with acute attacks occurring in pregnancy or immediately postpartum (26–28).

Many patients have evidence of moderate to severe axonal injury in affected muscles on EMG testing. Recovery may require a year or longer, with full recovery seen in most patients by 3 years; however, patients with severe axonal injury, with denervation seen by EMG, are less likely to make a complete recovery.

DISORDERS OF THE LUMBOSACRAL PLEXUS

The lumbosacral plexus is formed from the L4–S4 spinal nerve roots. Vaginal delivery may result in injury to the lumbosacral plexus by direct compression from the fetal head or from obstetric forceps. The usual presenting complaint is postpartum pain referable to the sciatic nerve, with the peroneal fibers affected more often than the tibial fibers (29). The incidence of obstetric lumbosacral plexopathies originally was estimated to be between 1 in 2,600 and 1 in 6,400 (30,31); however, a more recent review of obstetric plexopathies did not find any association (32), possibly reflecting the fact that fewer forceps deliveries are done in modern obstetrics.

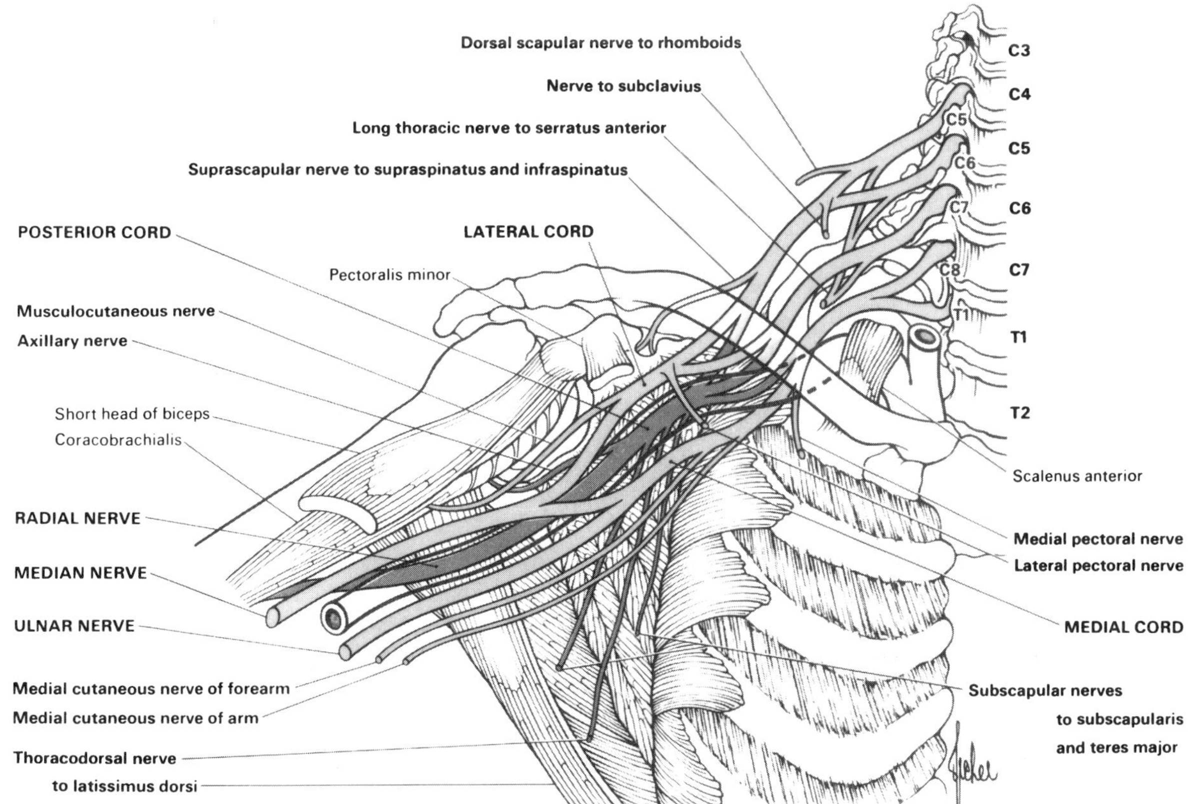

FIG. 29-4. Diagram of the brachial plexus. (The Guarantors of *Brain*: From AIDS to the examination of the peripheral nervous system. Oxford, England: Baillière-Tindall, The Alden Press, 1986, p. 4.)

Risk factors for developing lumbosacral plexopathy are thought to include nulliparity, cephalopelvic disproportion, use of instrumentation for delivery, and prolonged labor (21). The anatomic features predisposing to lumbosacral plexus injury are short ilium, flat sacral promontory, and shallow sacral alae (31). As in brachial plexus lesions, prognosis is usually good but depends on the severity of axonal injury (32,33).

DISORDERS OF THE LUMBOSACRAL ROOTS

Lumbosacral Radiculopathy

About 50% of all pregnant women develop significant low back pain during pregnancy, usually during the second or third trimester (34). Most of these patients suffer because of laxity of the sacroiliac joint(s) rather than nerve or root injury; however, relaxation of the spinal joints as well as exaggerated lumbar lordosis may alter facet articulation enough to cause nerve irritation, which results in pain radiating into the leg.

Treatment is usually conservative with home exercise, heat, and massage. Elevating one foot on a low stool; sitting and standing may help to alleviate discomfort by reversing the lumbar lordosis. More aggressive treatments are reserved for women with acute lumbar disc herniation. These patients develop severe, sudden pain that radiates into the ankle or foot. Symptoms are worsened by coughing, sneezing, or Valsalva maneuver. The distribution of observed weakness and numbness depends on the particular root involved (Table 29-2). Focal neurologic deficits, including bladder and bowel dysfunction, may indicate the need for neuroradiologic evaluation, preferably with magnetic resonance imaging (MRI) and possible surgery. Strict bed rest, heat, and analgesics may make the patient more comfortable, allowing a more accurate assessment of actual neurologic deficits when the pain is better controlled.

TABLE 29-2. *Lumbosacral root innervation*

Root	Muscle	Deep tendon reflex
L-2	Adductors, quadriceps, iliopsoas	Patella, L2-4
L-3	Adductors, quadriceps, iliopsoas	Patella, L2-4
L-4	Adductors, quadriceps, tibialis anterior, tibialis posterior, gluteus medius	Patella, L2-4
L-5	Peroneus longus, tibialis anterior, tibialis posterior, extensor hallucis longus, extensor digitorum brevis, hamstrings, gluteus maximus, gluteus medius	
S-1	Peroneus longus, extensor hallucis longus, extensor digitorum brevis, hamstrings, gluteus maximus, gluteus medius, gastrocnemius, soleus	Ankle, S1-2
S-2	Gluteus maximus, gastrocnemius, soleus, hamstrings, gluteus maximus	Ankle, S1-2

POLYNEUROPATHIES

Guillain-Barré Syndrome

The clinical syndrome of Guillain-Barré is characterized by transient back pain and progressive weakness. Sensory symptoms are usually much less prominent. Early symptoms may be mild but can progress rapidly to quadriplegia with respiratory and bulbar muscle weakness requiring mechanical ventilation. On examination, there is muscle weakness, areflexia, and sensory loss. Occasionally, autonomic instability resulting from involvement of the peripheral autonomic nervous system can be life threatening.

Spinal fluid examination shows a cytoalbuminemic dissociation with elevated spinal fluid protein and normal or mildly elevated white blood count. Electrodiagnostic studies typically show prolonged distal and F-wave latencies early in the course of the disease. Later they show reduced conduction velocities with or without conduction block, reduced compound motor action potentials, and evidence of acute denervation on EMG testing in severe cases. Pathologic examination of affected nerves shows segmental demyelination.

The cause of the Guillain-Barré syndrome is unknown, although there has been an association with immunizations and various infections occurring several weeks before the appearance of symptoms (35). Although many believe an association exists with respiratory and gastrointestinal viruses, recent evidence suggests that infection with *Campylobacter jejuni* is a predisposing factor for the development of the disease (36).

Guillain-Barré syndrome occurs with equal frequency in pregnant and nonpregnant women (37). It occurs throughout pregnancy and appears to have no direct effect on the fetus (38). Although uterine contractions are normal, if the patient is weak at delivery, pushing may be difficult and forceps may be necessary to complete the delivery. If there is evidence of autonomic dysfunction, tocolytic agents should be not be used.

Treatment for Guillain-Barré syndrome is through a combination of supportive measures and either plasmapheresis or intravenous immunoglobulin (IVIg). Typically, plasmapheresis is given for five treatments on an every-other-day basis (39). If the treatments are provided over a shorter time course, recurrence is more likely. Plasmapheresis is generally safe in pregnancy. A large number of pregnant women have been treated for diseases as varied as Guillain-Barré syndrome, myasthenia gravis, and Rhesus antibody incompatibility. Experience with IVIg for Guillain-Barré syndrome in pregnancy is limited, but generally is believed to be safe for mother and fetus. If IVIg is used, the usual dose is 2 g per kilogram given over 3 to 5 days (40).

Chronic Inflammatory Demyelinating Neuropathy

In contrast with the Guillain-Barré syndrome, the incidence of chronic inflammatory demyelinating polyneuropathy (CIDP) in pregnancy is almost three times that seen in the general population (41). CIDP is a chronic neuropathy characterized by progressive muscle weakness and atrophy as well as large fiber sensory loss. In addition to weakness and atrophy of the limbs, examination may show decreased vibration and position sense, cranial nerve involvement, and hyporeflexia or areflexia.

Spinal fluid examination shows an elevated protein level and normal white cell count. Electrodiagnostic studies demonstrate the presence of a neuropathy with demyelinating features of prolonged distal and F-wave latencies as well as reduced nerve conduction velocities.

Most exacerbations occur in the third trimester (42), although symptoms may worsen throughout pregnancy and the postpartum period (43,44). Some women who have had pregnancy-related worsening of their symptoms may later have episodes unrelated to pregnancy. Therapeutic regimens have been developed with IVIg, plasmapheresis, or steroids (40). CIDP does not appear to have any effect on the developing fetus, and infants born to women with CIDP are normal.

Nutritional Polyneuropathies

Wernicke's encephalopathy is characterized by the acute onset of confusion, ophthalmoplegia, nystagmus, and ataxia. It is usually associated with chronic alcohol use, although malnutrition from any cause (e.g., starvation, anorexia nervosa, malabsorption, and hyperemesis) can lead to symptoms. In all cases, the underlying cause of Wernicke encephalopathy is thiamine deficiency, and the characteristic neuropathologic lesion is petechial hemorrhages in the mammillary bodies. In pregnancy, hyperemesis gravidarum may lead to thiamine deficiency and subsequent development of Wernicke encephalopathy alone or in combination with a distal symmetric polyneuropathy (45,46). This type of neuropathy, also referred to as gestational distal polyneuropathy, also may occur in the absence of Wernicke encephalopathy.

The neuropathy is usually mild but may be severe enough to lead to gait ataxia and inability to walk. Patients complain of paresthesias, dysesthesias, and numbness. On examination, there is weakness, hyporeflexia or areflexia, and distal sensory loss. If the autonomic nervous system is involved, there may be orthostatic hypotension and fluctuations of heart rate and blood pressure. On electrodiagnostic testing, distal axonal loss is found.

Treatment with thiamine and multivitamins usually results in improvement. Untreated, prognosis is poor and the disease often leads to death. If recognition of the condition is delayed and treatment with thiamine is initiated late, recovery may require many months, and residual deficits are not uncommon.

NEUROLOGIC COMPLICATIONS RELATED TO REGIONAL ANESTHESIA

Regional anesthesia is a safe and effective mode of administration of anesthetic agents. Although neurologic deficits are among the most feared complications, they rarely occur. Estimates indicate one neurologic complication for every 10,000 to 20,000 epidural blocks (47,48). Typical symptoms related to epidural anesthesia include headache and persistent numbness. Spinal headaches are usually due to a leak of spinal fluid through a hole in the dura and can be differentiated from other headaches by the fact that symptoms are usually positional in nature. Bed rest, fluids, and caffeine have been advocated as treatments. If the headache is persistent, autologous blood patches are helpful (49). Leg weakness, sphincter dysfunction, Horner syndrome, and cranial neuropathies are the most common complications (50).

Among the most serious complications of regional anesthesia are those related to central nervous system bleeding such as epidural hematoma. Epidural hematomas present with severe back pain and myelopathic symptoms including sphincter dysfunction, leg weakness, and a sensory loss level. Immediate neurosurgical evaluation must be obtained for consideration of surgical decompression.

Serious complications also may arise from direct injection of anesthetic agent into the subarachnoid or subdural space as a result of hypotension, apnea, or paralysis. Injection into epidural fat may cause persistent numbness resulting from slow leaching out of the anesthetic agent from the fat.

Infections also have been reported. Epidural abscess may occur as a result of spinal anesthesia, although spontaneous epidural abscess is a more frequent occurrence. Bacterial meningitis is an obvious risk and can be avoided by good technique and declining to perform epidural injections in bacteremic patients. Aseptic meningitis also may occur, usually as a toxic reaction to the anesthetic agent or the carrier. Arachnoiditis, a chronic inflammation of the cauda equina, has been reported (51).

DISORDERS OF THE NEUROMUSCULAR JUNCTION

Mysathenia Gravis

Myasthenia gravis (see Chapter 30) is an autoimmune disease characterized by fluctuating weakness. The cause of the disease is usually the production of antibodies directed against acetylcholine receptors located on the postsynaptic membrane of the neuromuscular junction. These antibodies block the action of acetylcholine and inhibit muscle contraction. Diagnosis is made by the appropriate clinical history and examination as well as the finding of acetylcholine receptor antibodies in the serum. Repetitive nerve stimulation is another useful diagnostic test and often shows a decrimental response with repeated stimulation at 2 to 3 Hz.

Weakness may be generalized or restricted to the eyes (ocular myasthenia). When generalized, bulbar and respiratory muscle weaknesses are ominous signs. The course of myasthenia is changed little by pregnancy. One third of pregnant women with myasthenia worsen, one third remain stable, and one third improve (52). Delivery or termination of pregnancy does not alter the severity of the symptoms. Increased weakness often is found in the first postpartum month, and close follow-up is advised.

Treatment of myasthenia gravis usually requires some form of immunosuppressive therapy, which may be combined with an acetylcholinesterase inhibitor, such as pyridostigmine. Thymectomy reduces the severity of the disease and occasionally results in complete remission. In young women, thymectomy should be considered before pregnancy, although pregnancy is not an absolute contraindication for surgery, particularly for those with thymoma, because these tumors may become quite aggressive during pregnancy. For acute exacerbations during pregnancy (myasthenic crisis), treatment is identical to that of a nonpregnant woman. Severe weakness requires either plasmaphoresis or intravenous immunoglobulin therapy. Immunosuppression with corticosteroids is the usual mode of treatment of young women, as most of the other immunosuppressants may result in sterility and are teratogenic; however, corticosteroids must be used cautiously, because they may exacerbate hyperglycemia, emotional instability, and weight gain.

Labor and delivery are usually unaffected by myasthenia, although tocolytic agents such as magnesium sulfate may lead to increased weakness or myasthenic crisis as a result of decreased neuromuscular junction transmission and therefore should be avoided. Anesthesiologists should avoid the use of curare-like drugs, as this class of drugs may lead to severe respiratory compromise. In addition, chloroprocaine metabolism is blocked by acetylcholinesterase inhibitors, and its use may lead to toxicity and seizures; therefore, lidocaine is the preferred medication for regional anesthesia.

REFERENCES

1. Bell C. Appendix. In: Taylor J, ed. The nervous system of the human body. iv-v. London: Longman, Rees, Orme, Brown, and Greene, 1830: iv–v.
2. Hilsinger RL, Adour KK, Doty HE. Idiopathic facial paralysis, pregnancy, and the menstrual cycle. Ann Otol 1975;84:433–442.
3. McGregor JA, Guberman A, Amer J, Goodlin R. Idiopathic facial nerve paralysis (Bell's palsy) in late pregnancy and the early puerperium. Obstet Gynecol 1987;69:435–438.
4. Korczyn AD. Bell's palsy and pregnancy. Acta Neurol Scand 1971;47: 603–607.
5. Matthews WB. The treatment of Bell's palsy. In: Matthews WB GG, ed. Recent advances in clinical neurology, vol 3. Edinburgh: Churchill Livingstone, 1982:239–248.
6. Adour KK, Winegerd J, Bell DN. Prednisone treatment for idiopathic facial nerve paralysis (Bell's palsy). N Engl J Med 1972;287: 1268–1272.
7. Wallace JT, Cook AW. Carpal tunnel syndrome in pregnancy: a report of two cases. Am J Obstet Gynecol 1957;73:1333–1336.
8. Tobin SM. Carpal tunnel syndrome in pregnancy. Am J Obstet Gynecol 1967;97:493–498.
9. Voitk AJ, Mueller JC, Farlinger DE, Johnston RU. Carpal tunnel syndrome in pregnancy. Can Med Assoc J 1983;128:277–281.
10. Ekman-Ordeberg G, Salgeback S, Ordeberg G. Carpal tunnel syndrome in pregnancy. Acta Obstet Gynecol Scand 1987;66:233–235.
11. Rhodes P. Meralgia paresthetica in pregnancy. Lancet 1957;2:831.
12. Price GE. Meralgia paresthetica, recurring with repeated pregnancies. Am Med 1909;4:210–212.
13. Keegan JJ, Holyoke EJ. Meralgia paresthetica: an anatomical and surgical study. J Neurosurg 1962;19:341–345.
14. Ecker AD, Woltman HW. Meralgia paresthetica: a report of one hundred and fifty cases. JAMA 1938;110:1650–1652.
15. Al-Hakim M, Katirji MB. Femoral mononeuropathy induced by the lithotomy position: a report of 5 cases with a review of the literature. Muscle Nerve 1993;16:891–895.
16. Vargo MM, Robinson LR, Nicholas JJ, Rubin MC. Postpartum femoral neuropathy: relic of an earlier era. Arch Phys Med Rehabil 1990;71: 591–596.
17. Donaldson JO, Wirz D, Mashman J. Bilateral postpartum femoral neuropathy. Conn Med 1985;49:496–498.
18. Rosenbaum J, Schwarz GA, Bendler E. Femoral neuropathy: a neurological complication of hysterectomy. JAMA 1966;195:409–414.
19. Adelman JU, Goldberg GS, Puckett JD. Postpartum bilateral femoral neuropathy. Obstet Gynecol 1973;42:845–850.
20. Warfield CA. Obturator neuropathy after forceps delivery. Obstet Gynecol 1984;64:47S–48S.
21. Graham JG. Neurological complications of pregnancy and anesthesia. Clin Obstet Gynecol 1982;9:333–350.
22. Goldstein PJ. The lithotomy position: surgical aspects: obstetrics and gynecology. In: Martin I, ed. Positioning in anesthesia and surgery, 2nd ed. Philadelphia: WB Saunders, 1987:1–50.
23. Adornato BT, Carlini WG. Pushing palsy: a case of self-induced bilateral peroneal palsy during natural childbirth. Neurology 1992;42: 936–937.
24. Reif ME. Bilateral common peroneal nerve palsy secondary to prolonged squatting in natural childbirth. Birth 1988;15:100–102.
25. Tsairis PDP, Mulder DW. Natural history of brachial plexus neuropathy. Arch Neurol 1972;27:109–117.
26. Redmond JMT, Cros D, Martin JB, Shahani BT. Relapsing bilateral brachial plexopathy during pregnancy. Arch Neurol 1989;46:462–464.
27. Geiger LR, Mancall EL, Penn AS, Tucker SH. Familial neuralgic amyotrophy: a report of three families with review of the literature. Brain 1974;97:87–102.
28. Dumitru D, Liles RA. Postpartum idiopathic brachial neuritis. Obstet Gynecol 1989;73:473–475.
29. Feasby TE, Burton SR, Hahn AF. Obstetrical lumbosacral plexus injury. Muscle Nerve 1992;15:937–940.
30. Hill EC. Maternal obstetric paralysis. Am J Obstet Gynecol 1962;83: 1452–1460.
31. Cole JT. Maternal obstetric paralysis. Am J Obstet Gynecol 1946;52: 372–385.
32. Sabra A, Dawson D. Peripheral nerve injuries during labor and delivery. Neurology 1989;9:S292.
33. Gibbs MA, Beydoun SR. Obstetrical lumbosacral plexus injury. Muscle Nerve 1993;16:801.
34. Fast A, Shapiro D, Ducommun EJ, Friedmann LW, Bouklas T, Floman Y. Low back pain in pregnancy. Spine 1987;12:368–371.
35. Hughes RA, Rees JH. Clinical and epidemiologic features of Guillain-Barré syndrome. J Infect Dis 1997;176:S92–S98.
36. Allo BM. *Campylobacter jejuni* infection as a cause of the Guillain-Barré syndrome. Infect Dis Clin North Am 1998;12:173–184.

37. Rodin A, Ferner R, Russell R. Guillain-Barré syndrome in pregnancy and puerperium. J Obstet Gynaecol 1988;9:39–42.
38. Sudo N, Weingold AB. Obstetric aspects of the Guillain-Barré syndrome. Obstet Gynecol 1975;45:39–43.
39. Guillain-Barré Study Group. Plasmaphoresis and acute Guillain-Barré syndrome. Neurology 1985;35:1096–1104.
40. Dalakas MC. Intravenous immune globulin therapy for neurologic disease. Ann Intern Med 1997;126:721–730.
41. Jones MW, Berry K. Chronic relapsing polyneuritis associated with pregnancy. Ann Neurol 1981;9:413.
42. McCombe PA, McManis PG, Frith JA, Pollard JD, McLeod JG. Chronic inflammatory demyelinating polyradiculoneuropathy associated with pregnancy. Ann Neurol 1987;21:102–104.
43. Calderon-Gonzalez R, Gonzalez-Canter N, Rizzo-Hernandez H. Recurrent polyneuropathy with pregnancy and oral contraceptives. N Engl J Med 1970;282:1307–1308.
44. Novak DJ, Johnson KP. Relapsing idiopathic polyneuritis during pregnancy. Immunologic aspects and literature review. Arch Neurol 1973; 28:219–223.
45. Lavin PJM, Smith D, Kori SH, Ellenberger C. Wernicke's encephalopathy: a predictable complication of hyperemesis gravidarum. Obstet Gynecol 1983;62:13S–15S.
46. McGoogan LS. Severe polyneuritis due to vitamin B deficiency in pregnancy. Am J Obstet Gynecol 1942;43:752–762.
47. Bromage PR. Neurologic complications of regional anaesthesia. In: Schnider SM LG, ed. Anaesthesia for obstetrics. Baltimore: Williams & Wilkins, 1987:316–324.
48. Crawford J. Some maternal complications of epidural analgesia for labour. Anaesthesia 1985;40:1219–1225.
49. DiGiovanni AJ, Dunbar BS. Epidural injections of autologous blood for postlumbar puncture headache. Anesth Analg 1970;49:268–271.
50. Tubridy N, Redmond JMT. Neurological symptoms attributed to epidural analgesia in labour: an observational study in seven cases. Br J Obstet Gynaecol 1996;103:832–833.
51. Greene NM. Neurologic sequelae of spinal anesthesia. Anesthesiology 1961;22:682–698.
52. Fennell D, Ringel SP. Myasthenia gravis and pregnancy. Obstet Gynecol Surv 1987;41:414–421.

Cherry and Merkatz's Complications of Pregnancy,
Fifth Edition, edited by W. R. Cohen.
Lippincott Williams & Wilkins, Philadelphia © 2000.

CHAPTER 30

Muscle Disease

James M. Gilchrist

Muscle disease is a nonspecific term meant to include primary disorders of muscle and the neuromuscular junction. This chapter discusses those diseases in which pregnancy confers a risk to either mother or fetus and also includes a few muscle diseases that do not directly affect pregnancy if prenatal genetic counseling and testing are important. A comprehensive view of the latter diseases was published in 1997 (1). Advances in molecular genetics have profoundly changed the field of inherited neuromuscular disease, and advances continue. Therefore, specific mention of genetic localizations and counseling are limited to those diseases considered of paramount importance. All patients with a presumption of genetic muscle disease should be seen by a physician or genetic counselor who is conversant in the latest in genetic diagnosis and screening techniques. This chapter also presents a brief explication of maternal inheritance as it pertains to mitochondrial encephalomyopathies.

MYASTHENIA GRAVIS

Myasthenia gravis is an autoimmune disorder in which polyclonal antibodies are directed against the nicotinic acetylcholine receptor of skeletal muscle (2,3), which results in degradation of the neuromuscular junction and failure of neuromuscular transmission (2). The clinical hallmark of the disease is fatigable weakness, causing intermittent symptoms, usually following repetitive action, such as ptosis, diplopia, dysphagia, dysarthria, and facial and limb muscle weakness. Respiratory compromise can occur in severe cases.

The disease has a bimodal peak incidence, affecting older men and young women of childbearing age (4). Although the clinical history and examination are often typical and highly suggestive, confirmation of the diagnosis rests on pharmacologic, immunologic, and electrodiagnostic grounds. Edrophonium (Tensilon) given intravenously quickly but briefly reverses the signs of myasthenia gravis and serves as a good bedside test (5). Assay for the presence of serum acetylcholine receptor antibodies is specific for myasthenia gravis, and is abnormal in 70% to 90% of cases (6,7). Sensitivity is lower in patients who show only ocular signs. Electrodiagnostic tests of neuromuscular transmission include repetitive nerve stimulation (abnormal in 50%–75% of cases) (8,9) and single-fiber electromyography (abnormal in 98%) (8).

Treatment may be curative or only address symptoms. Anticholinesterase drugs can be used to abate for a short time or improve symptoms attributable to myasthenia gravis, but will not affect the underlying immunologic dysfunction. These drugs work by inhibiting the breakdown of acetylcholine, the neurotransmitter released by terminal motor nerve fibers. Edrophonium, neostigmine, and pyridostigmine (Mestinon) are all anticholinesterases, the last being most commonly used given its longer duration of action (2–4 hours) and lesser muscarinic side effects. Mestinon is used commonly by itself in mild cases and in conjunction with immune suppression in more severe cases. Side effects include diaphoresis, hypersalivation, diarrhea, nausea, abdominal cramping, bradycardia, and fasciculations. The above-mentioned anticholinesterases are all quaternary ammonium compounds, and placental transfer is minimal (10). Parenteral formulations of neostigmine and pyridostigmine are available when needed before or after surgery, during labor, or early in pregnancy if emesis gravidarum is severe. Intravenous dosages are one thirtieth the oral dose for both drugs.

Suppression of the immune system attack on the acetylcholine receptor is indicated when the disease is generalized, involves vital functions such as ventilation or swallowing, or is not amenable to symptomatic treatment alone. Various treatments can be used, including corticosteroids, immune suppressants such as azathio-

J. M. Gilchrist: Department of Clinical Neuroscience, Brown University School of Medicine, Department of Neurology, Rhode Island Hospital, Providence, RI 02903.

prine and cyclosporine, plasmapheresis, intravenous human immune globulin, and thymectomy. In the pregnant patient, corticosteroids are preferred over other immune suppressants. Corticosteroids can cause dramatic worsening of symptoms at initiation of therapy, and patients must be watched carefully early in treatment, preferably as inpatients (11,12). This worsening can be lessened by starting patients on low doses with a slow titration upward, although this approach delays clinical benefit (13). Plasmapheresis is indicated in the severely compromised patient, in the patient refractory to other treatment modalities, and in the patient in whom an immediate response is required. Plasmapheresis rapidly lowers acetylcholine antibody titers and may be indicated when high maternal titers threaten fetal development (14) or predict development of neonatal myasthenia. The technique has been used to treat fulminant myasthenia gravis successfully in a pregnant patient (15), and the low rate of complications does not differ from that in nonpregnant patients (16).

Thymomas are present in 10% to 15% of patients with myasthenia gravis, and myasthenia gravis occurs in 30% of patients with thymomas (17). Malignant thymoma is uncommon in the pregnant patient but carries a poor prognosis when associated with pregnancy (18). The relationship between myasthenia gravis and thymic tissue remains unknown, but removal of thymic tissue increases the remission rate from 15% to 30% and results in significant clinical improvement in two thirds of patients, although the improvement may take up to 5 years (19). Thymectomy favorably influences the incidence of neonatal myasthenia gravis (discussed later) (20). Thymectomy has been performed in pregnant women who have refractory disease (21) and, if done before pregnancy, can decrease the incidence of disease exacerbation during pregnancy (22). If possible, it is advisable for a woman with generalized myasthenia gravis who is considering pregnancy to have thymectomy before becoming pregnant (23). Generally, thymectomy may be recommended in all patients aged between 18 and 55 years with generalized myasthenia gravis.

Drug Interactions

Many drugs can cause worsening of myasthenia gravis (Table 30-1) (24,25). Iodinated contrast dye also has been noted to cause transient worsening of myasthenic symptoms (26).

Effect of Pregnancy on Myasthenia Gravis

Review of the literature revealed that 31% of pregnancies in myasthenic women caused no change in the status of the myasthenia, 28% had improvement, and 40% had worsening of symptoms during the pregnancy or, most commonly, in the puerperium (27). Mortality of mothers was 10%, most commonly from myasthenic crisis but also from cholinergic crisis and postpartum hemorrhage (27). These numbers probably reflect a reporting bias toward more severe disease, but they indicate that pregnancy often may have an adverse effect on the myasthenic patient. Exacerbations tend to be most sudden and dangerous in the postpartum period and frequently are accompanied by respiratory failure (27). Therapeutic abortion is of little benefit in the treatment of myasthenia gravis (28,29).

Alpha-fetoprotein (AFP) effectively inhibits binding of acetylcholine antibodies to the acetylcholine receptor (30). The presence of AFP in maternal serum during pregnancy may explain the symptomatic improvement often seen in the third trimester (20), and its absence may

TABLE 30-1. *Drugs potentially harmful in myasthenia gravis*

Antibiotics	Cardiovascular	Anticonvulsants	Antirheumatics	Neuromuscular blocking agents[a]	Psychotropics	Others
Aminoglycosides	Lidocaine	Dilantin	Chloroquine	Curare	Lithium carbonate	Magnesium sulfate
Neomycin	Quinidine	Trimethadione	D-penicillamine	Pancuronium	Chlorpromazine	Corticosteroids
Streptomycin	Quinine			Succinylcholine	Phenelzine	Thyroid replacement
Kanamycin	Procaineamide				Promazine	ACTH
Gentamycin	Beta-blockers	-				Anticholinesterases
Tobramycin	Ca^{++} channel blockers					
Amikacin	Trimethaphan					
Polymyxin A						
Polymyxin B						
Colistin						
Lincomycin						
Clindamycin						
Tetracyclines						

ACTH, adrenocorticotrophic hormone.
[a]Partial list.

account for the frequent postpartum exacerbation of myasthenia gravis when AFP levels fall precipitously.

Effects of Myasthenia Gravis on Pregnancy

Myasthenia gravis increases the risk of premature delivery (27,31) slightly, but it does not affect the incidence of preeclampsia (31,32). Magnesium sulfate is contraindicated in the myasthenic patient because it interferes with neuromuscular transmission and muscle fiber excitability (33) and may lead to increased weakness.

Myasthenia gravis does not affect the smooth muscles but may weaken the voluntary muscles used during the second stage of labor; parenteral anticholinesterases (e.g., intravenous pyridostigmine, 2 mg) may be useful at this point. Care must be taken not to push the myasthenic patient beyond her physical capabilities during labor, and in some situations, the criteria for cesarean section should be broadened. Myasthenia gravis does not appear to affect the overall length of labor (34,35). Women on corticosteroid therapy for myasthemia during pregnancy should have stress doses given during labor and delivery.

Regional anesthesia is preferred over other anesthetic methods. Myasthenic patients are particularly sensitive to even small doses of neuromuscular blocking agents, especially of the nondepolarizing type, such as curare, and these drugs should be avoided. Lidocaine is the recommended local anesthetic because it is an aminoacyl amide and is not affected by the decreased cholinesterase activity seen in patients receiving anticholinesterase drugs (36,37).

There is an increased perinatal death rate in myasthenia gravis (34) secondary to antenatal and neonatal myasthenia gravis. Both conditions are presumed secondary to transplacental transfer of maternal acetylcholine receptor antibodies (38). Antenatal effects derive from inhibited skeletal muscle movement and development resulting in pulmonary hypoplasia, arthrogryposis multiplex, and polyhydramnios (14), which is consistent with the fetal akinesia deformation sequence (39). Mothers with previously affected infants or especially high titers of acetylcholine receptor antibodies are at higher risk of having such children, who have a very high perinatal mortality rate. Measurement of the fetal/adult antiacetylcholine receptor antibody ratio may be predictive of risk for neonatal myasthenia gravis (40). Ultrasound monitoring of total fetal and diaphragmatic movement and assessment of acetylcholine receptor antibody titers also may indicate the at-risk women in whom aggressive lowering of antibody load to the placenta, such as with plasmapheresis, could prevent congenital anomalies (14,41). The syndrome may occur in asymptomatic women (42).

A less severe but more common occurrence is *neonatal myasthenia gravis*, characterized by transient weakness in the newborn infant (43). The disease affects up to 19% of children born to mothers with myasthenia gravis; it becomes symptomatic within the first 3 days of life and can persist for weeks before improving (43). Symptoms include poor feeding, weak suck, feeble cry, floppiness, generalized weakness, and respiratory distress. Treatment is supportive but can be supplemented by cholinesterase inhibitors. Neostigmine 0.1 mg administered intramuscularly (i.m.) or subcutaneously or pyridostigmine 0.15 mg i.m. will be effective (43); however, these drugs must be used sparingly because they may increase oral secretions. Further therapeutic interventions, for example, plasmapheresis, are rarely needed. The disease is self-limited and does not represent a risk to the infant for later myasthenia gravis. Subsequent infants born to mothers with affected newborns are at higher risk for neonatal myasthenia gravis (43).

The etiology of neonatal myasthenia gravis is not entirely clear. Nearly all infants born to myasthenic mothers were exposed to maternal acetylcholine receptor antibodies *in utero* (44); yet only a minority develop symptoms. Conversely, neonatal myasthenia has occurred in infants born to mothers in remission (45), although there is a positive correlation between maternal acetylcholine receptor antibody titers and the occurrence of neonatal myasthenia gravis (44). Because AFP binds acetylcholine receptor antibody (30), its decline after birth may result in the emergence of symptoms (27,31).

MUSCULAR DYSTROPHY

There are several forms of muscular dystrophy, all of which are progressive, inherited muscular diseases. Most are inherited as autosomal dominant traits (myotonic dystrophy, facioscapulohumeral dystrophy, oculopharyngeal dystrophy), some as autosomal recessive (e.g., limb–girdle muscular dystrophy, congenital muscular dystrophy), and several as X-linked (e.g., Duchenne's muscular dystrophy, Becker muscular dystrophy, Emery-Driefuss muscular dystrophy). All have had chromosomal localization, many have had genes localized, and some have had the affected genetic product elucidated. The discussion on genetic counseling issues herein is limited to those dystrophies with a known gene product and accurate, easily available gene testing (i.e., Duchenne's and Becker dystrophy, and myotonic dystrophy). In the near future, such testing probably will be available for other dystrophies. Emery-Driefuss and oculopharyngeal muscular dystrophy are not discussed here, because there is no known effect either of or on pregnancy.

Myotonic Dystrophy

Myotonic dystrophy is a multisystem disorder characterized by variable expression of progressive, predominantly distal, skeletal muscle weakness; cataracts; frontal balding; cardiac conduction defects; clinical and electrical myotonia; smooth-muscle weakness of the esophagus, stomach, bowel, and uterus; and endocrine disturbances (46). Onset can be as early as birth but is more likely in the second to third decade of life (47,48).

Myotonic dystrophy is inherited as an autosomal dominant trait, and the abnormal gene has been localized to chromosome 19 (49–51). It encodes for myotonin, a member of the protein kinase family (49), whose function remains poorly understood. A triplet repeat expansion (CTG) of the gene, present in essentially all patients with myotonic dystrophy (52), can increase in size in succeeding generations, explaining the clinical phenomenon of *anticipation*, in which subsequent generations manifest the disease more severely and at an earlier age (52).

To begin with, myotonic dystrophy has an effect on fertility. Large sibships are not uncommon in families with myotonic dystrophy, and fertility is not drastically reduced; however, testicular atrophy occurs in about 80% of affected men (53). This atrophy is of primary gonadal origin, as shown by elevated follicle-stimulating hormone (FSH) and luteinizing hormone (LH) levels (54–56), normal secondary sexual characteristics, and low testosterone levels (54), abnormalities that can be seen prepubertally (57). Seminiferous tubule destruction is seen histologically and constitutes the bulk of the gonadal pathology; Leydig cells are normal until total tubular fibrosis is present (55,58). Despite these findings, men with testicular atrophy have been reported to father children (59). Women with myotonic dystrophy have few clinical or hormonal gonadal abnormalities (57,60). In two studies of six women each, no abnormalities of estrogen, gonadotrophin, or testosterone levels were found (60,61). In a group of 33 women studied by Thomasen, menstrual irregularities correlated with the severity of myotonic dystrophy (62), although other authors have expressed uncertainty about the significance of this finding (57). Harper studied 44 affected women and compared them with unaffected siblings and spouses. He found a tendency toward irregular and painful menses and an earlier onset of menopause (57). A case with amenorrhea from hypothalamic hypogonadism reported normal gonadal hormone levels (55). Fertility seems to be reduced to 75% of normal in both sexes. Because this includes severely affected members who are unlikely to conceive, the fertility of less affected women may well be normal or even increased (63).

Effect of Pregnancy on Myotonic Dystrophy

Pregnancy uncommonly has an ill effect on the woman with myotonic dystrophy (64), and there is no evidence to suggest that pregnancy has a beneficial effect on the disease. Several case reports indicate that myotonia, muscle wasting, and weakness can become symptomatic or dramatically worsen during pregnancy (65–69). Usually, but not exclusively, this occurs during the third trimester (66,70), corresponding to the time of maximal progesterone levels and leading some to speculate progesterone is involved in the increased symptoms (66). The worsened clinical state is temporary, and return to baseline is usual after delivery. Because progressive loss of muscle function in the mother is expected regardless of pregnancy, the question of whether pregnancy accelerates permanent disability is difficult to answer but rarely may occur (64).

Fall et al. (71) reported a pregnant myotonic woman who developed heart failure at 32 weeks' gestation, with an endomyocardial biopsy consistent with myotonic dystrophy. She improved after delivery but died suddenly of cardiac arrhythmia 8 weeks later.

Effect of Myotonic Dystrophy on Pregnancy and Delivery

Myotonic dystrophy has a potentially devastating impact on pregnancy and delivery (Table 30-2) for both the mother (64,65,68,70,72–77) and the fetus (64,70,72, 73,77,78). Postpartum hemorrhage related to failure of uterine contraction after delivery is particularly worrisome (73,76). Labor can be prolonged in both the first (66) and second stages because of poor uterine contraction from myometrial involvement (65,70) and an inability to "bear down" because of voluntary muscle weakness (67,69). Nonetheless, labor is not prolonged for most women with myotonic dystrophy (64). Extended bed rest should be avoided because disuse of muscles will further weaken any patient with myotonic dystrophy.

Anesthesia carries special risks as well. Depolarizing neuromuscular blockade, such as with succinylcholine, in patients with myotonic dystrophy has been reported to cause myotonic spasm (79,80) in which muscles diffusely contract and cannot be relaxed. This is temporary and without permanent sequelae; however, it may be impossible to ventilate the patient during the spasm. Nondepolarizing agents (e.g., curare) do not cause this reaction and can be used. Thiopental has been noted to cause marked respiratory depression in patients with myotonic dystrophy (76). All things considered, local anesthesia is preferable to general anesthesia (76).

TABLE 30-2. *Effects of myotonic dystrophy on the pregnant mother and her fetus*

Maternal effects	Fetal effects
Prolonged labor	Hydramnios
Premature labor	Increased neonatal mortality
Uterine atony	Reduced fetal movements
Retained placenta	
Placenta previa	
Spontaneous abortion	
Postpartum hemorrhage	
Variable response to oxytocin	

Congenital Myotonic Dystrophy

Myotonic dystrophy can present *in utero,* at birth, or in early childhood. For reasons still unexplained (81,82), this congenital myotonic dystrophy occurs only when the mother is the affected parent (83). The risk of an affected woman having a congenitally affected child is 10%, but this risk increases to about 40% if she has already had congenitally affected offspring (81). Women with multisystem disease at the time of pregnancy and delivery are at highest risk for a child with congenital myotonic dystrophy (81), but even asymptomatic women have borne congenitally affected children (84). The mother's age at birth may have an effect on the severity of her offspring's disease, suggesting that the older the woman, the more severely affected are her children (85).

The disease can manifest *in utero* as polyhydramnios and reduced fetal movements, resulting in arthrogryposis multiplex congenita at birth (70,72,78,86). Vanier first described congenital myotonic dystrophy in 1960 (87), and Dyken and Harper later described 38 patients from 24 families who had symptoms attributable to myotonic dystrophy from birth (48). Symptoms varied from severe respiratory involvement at birth to clumsiness and mental retardation evident in early childhood. Neonatal onset of myotonic dystrophy is frequently fatal as a result of respiratory failure (72,86). Survivors are impaired, with hypotonia, diffuse weakness, developmental delay, poor feeding, mental retardation (88), and arthrogryposis (86). Fetal muscle in these cases exhibits maturational arrest most severely involving limb, pharyngeal, and diaphragmatic muscles (89). Rutherford and colleagues reported that respiratory function at birth determined the likelihood of survival in congenital myotonic dystrophy and that the duration of mechanical ventilation was the best guide to prognosis (90). Electrodiagnostic studies sometimes can confirm the diagnosis (91) but often do not show myotonia and may be more informative when done on the mother than on the infant. A high index of suspicion for congenital myotonic dystrophy is important in the infant with respiratory failure and failure to feed, because the mother commonly has not been previously diagnosed. Affected children without the fetal or neonatal presentation exhibit talipes, facial diplegia, mental retardation, developmental delay, weakness, clumsiness, strabismus, and dysarthria (47,48).

Genetic Counseling

In the absence of a foreseeable cure for myotonic dystrophy, genetic counseling offers an opportunity to help develop a patient's understanding of the disease, establish individual risk for symptoms, determine the risk for myotonic dystrophy, and offer advice for dealing with these risks. Carrier and prenatal detection now can be done with near 100% accuracy by measuring fetal trinucleotide repeat length (92), allowing better genetic counseling and the option of elective abortion of affected fetuses. For prenatal detection, chorionic villus sampling at about 11 weeks or amniocentesis at about 16 weeks is required to establish fetal genotype. Trophoblast cells obtained from endocervical canal flushing between 7 and 9 weeks' gestation also can provide fetal DNA for this purpose (93).

Accurate genetic testing for myotonic dystrophy has revealed families without either a triplet repeat expansion or linkage to DNA markers on chromosome 19. These patients are clinically similar to myotonic dystrophy except for proximal rather than distal weakness, thus the newly coined diagnosis of *proximal myotonic myopathy* (PROMM) (94). This entity affects genetic counseling because asymptomatic patients with a family history of myotonic dystrophy and normal triplet repeat numbers cannot be excluded definitely as carriers until an affected family member has been shown to have an expanded triplet repeat region.

Duchenne's and Becker Muscular Dystrophy

Duchenne's and *Becker muscular dystrophy* are allelic X-linked recessive disorders arising from defects in a gene coding for a large structural protein called *dystrophin* (95,96). Boys become symptomatic for Duchenne's dystrophy at around 5 years of age, become wheelchair bound by about age 10 to 12, and die by their early 20's. Becker dystrophy is milder; the symptoms, although similar, reach the same milestones about a decade later (97). Females, by nature of the chromosomal location, are at risk for being carriers but not for the dystrophy (infrequently, carrier females can manifest a milder form of the disease) (98,99).

Prenatal Diagnosis and Counseling

Because of the devastating effect on both parent and child, and the lack of a cure, it is important to provide prepregnancy genetic counseling regarding the risk of being a carrier to women with affected offspring, siblings, or other relatives. Unfortunately, the dystrophin gene region is quite large, and up to one third of cases of Duchenne's and Becker dystrophy are new mutations (97). In families with known dystrophinopathies, carrier detection and prenatal diagnosis of affected fetuses are nevertheless available (100). The calculated risk of being a carrier depends on the pedigree (i.e., the number of affected males and their relationship to the female patient). Bayesian analysis enables calculation of the genetic risk for being a carrier (97). For a known carrier, each of her offspring, whether male or female, carries a 50% chance of inheriting the abnormal gene. The situation is often more complex (97), and the risk calculation may be improved by DNA analysis (100).

Abnormal dystrophin quantity and quality are the *sine qua non* of Duchenne's and Becker muscular dystrophy, and this can be determined by muscle assay (101); however, female carriers are not diagnosed reliably by quantitation of dystrophin (99). Immunostaining of muscle for dystrophin may be useful (99), but a normal examination does not exclude being a carrier and DNA analysis is essential (102). About 60% of Duchenne cases arise from a deletion of the dystrophin gene, and another 7% arise from duplications (103). If either is present in the affected male(s) of a family, the presence or absence of the deletion or duplication can be determined in at-risk females by a blood test for DNA analysis. Absence of the DNA abnormality can exclude the risk, although germline mosaicism also must be considered. Presence of the DNA defect indicates that the female is a carrier. If a deletion or duplication is not found in the affected male, then DNA analysis is indicated (100,104), which necessitates obtaining blood from members of the family and, most especially, from affected males, if they are alive. If the fetus is male, DNA linkage using polymerase chain reaction (PCR) techniques can be done to determine whether the fetus carries the defective gene and may be accomplished on cells obtained by chorionic villus sampling or amniocentesis. Other approaches include fetal muscle biopsy for dystrophin analysis (105), cleavage cell embryo biopsy (106), and dystrophin deletion analysis of nucleated maternal erythrocytes (107). These tests are helpful only if therapeutic abortion is being considered.

Limb-Girdle Muscular Dystrophy

In the past, a diagnosis of limb-girdle muscular dystrophy (LGMD) was given to patients with muscle disease not otherwise explained. In the past 5 years, the molecular genetics of LGMD have been much clarified, with localization of seven autosomal recessive forms and one autosomal dominant form (108,109). Several of the genes code for proteins of the dystrophin-associated glycoprotein complex, which, with dystrophin, constitute the major underlying structural support of the muscle fiber membrane (110). This has enabled a genetic classification of the LGMD syndromes and foretells the eventual ability to predict carrier and prenatal status (108,110).

Typically, LGMD appears in the second and third decade of life, with proximal legs, then arms affected over a prolonged course. Ambulation may be lost, but this does not occur until about 20 years after onset. LGMD is sporadic or inherited as an autosomal recessive trait in 95% of patients, with the remaining cases inherited in an autosomal dominant pattern.

Less commonly, a severe childhood form of the disease is seen, which looks very much like Duchenne's muscular dystrophy but is distinguishable by an autosomal recessive pattern of inheritance (severe childhood autosomal recessive muscular dystrophy, or SCARMD).

LGMD and Pregnancy

Delivery can be difficult when a patient with LGMD is severely affected and wheelchair bound (111). In an unpublished study, Lauren Donald and I did a retrospective survey of 38 women with autosomal recessive LGMD from 31 families. There were 59 pregnancies in 22 women with 38 children, a known spontaneous abortion rate of 31%, and one perinatal death. Difficulty with labor and delivery was reported in 29% of births without other complications. Seven women suffered significant permanent decline in function while pregnant, most frequently in the more severely affected women and usually in the first two trimesters.

Similar findings were reported from a retrospective review of nine women with LGMD who had 15 pregnancies (112). Therapeutic abortion occurred in three women (20%); no miscarriages were noted. Operative delivery was necessary in five of the remaining 12 pregnancies, of which two were emergencies. Five of the nine women experienced worsening weakness during pregnancy, one of whom improved after delivery. Five of the women required assistance in child care after delivery because of physical limitations. Therefore, women with LGMD should be counseled that pregnancy may increase spontaneous abortion and also may significantly and permanently increase weakness, the risk being greater with increasing disease severity.

Genetic Counseling

Most LGMD patients have an autosomal recessively inherited trait. Therefore, the risk of their offspring inheriting the disease is only marginally increased over the general population as long as the mating is not consanguinous. The real question arises in families who would like to have another child and who already have one child with SCARMD. The risk of any additional children having the disease is 25% if there is no consanguinity. Prenatal screening is possible but requires either linkage analysis or fetal muscle biopsy at a center able to do the testing, which is not widely available (113). In autosomal dominant LGMD families, a large, multigeneration family was linked to chromosome 5q(109), and conceivably linkage analysis could be done in members of that family if they wished to clarify the odds of transmitting the disease beyond 50%. At present, no other dominant LGMD family has been linked to the same or any other locus.

Facioscapulohumeral Dystrophy

Facioscapulohumeral muscular dystrophy (FSHD) is inherited as an autosomal dominant trait. About 90% to 95% of families have been linked to chromosome 4q35, near the telomere (114). FSHD is a muscular dystrophy of characteristic and defining weakness involving the face and scapular muscles. The age of onset is variable, from childhood (these patients are frequently more severely affected) to the early third decade. The weakness is slowly progressive and may arrest for several years or more; however, the disease may also progress in sudden accelerations.

Despite the relative frequency of FSHD, there is but one report, which describes 26 pregnancies in 11 patients (112). There were three miscarriages (12%), two preterm births, and six operative deliveries. Three women had symptomatic worsening during gestation, but all recovered after delivery, and there were no long-term sequelae.

Genetic Counseling

As with any autosomal dominantly inherited trait, the risk of intergenerational transmission is 50% for each child. The gene for FSH has not been found, nor is the gene product known. Therefore, prenatal genetic testing requires linkage analysis using DNA markers, which is available at only a few research laboratories (115).

Congenital Muscular Dystrophy

Congenital muscular dystrophy (CMD) comprises a group of inherited disorders with progressive muscular weakness and variable amounts of central nervous system (CNS) involvement. CMD has been classified into the *classic form*, without CNS involvement, and *Fukuyama muscular dystrophy*. The classic form has been further divided by the presence or absence of merosin, which connects the dystrophin-associated glycoprotein complex to the extracellular matrix. Merosin-deficient CMD has been linked to the locus of the laminin alpha-2 chain of merosin, which is located on chromosome 6q2 (116). It and merosin-positive CMD share similar characteristics of hypotonia, muscle weakness, and developmental delay, with onset in early infancy (117). Imaging studies of the brain reveal white matter changes but no malformations. Mental retardation occurs in a minority of patients with classic CMD. The progressive weakness and mental retardation may be milder in the merosin-positive patients (117). Fukuyama CMD has early infantile onset of severe weakness, brain malformation, severe mental retardation, and early death. It has been linked to a locus on chromosome 9q31(118).

The finding of a genetic locus for merosin-negative CMD and for Fukuyama CMD has made possible prenatal genetic determination in families at risk. Trophoblast tissue immunocytochemistry and DNA linkage analysis have been used to identify affected and unaffected merosin-negative CMD fetuses (119). Linkage analysis using PCR markers has been used in Fukuyama CMD for the same purpose(120).

OTHER MUSCLE DISEASES

Channelopathies

Channelopathy refers to a group of inherited muscle disorders caused by genetic defects of muscle membrane channels. These include the *SCN4A* gene on chromosome 17q23 coding for the adult sodium channel α-subunit (121), the *CLCN1* gene on chromosome 7q35 encoding the chloride channel (121), and the *CACNL1A3* gene on 1q31-32 coding for the dihydropyridine receptor of the calcium channel (121). Mutations of the *SCN4A* gene result in several autosomal dominant phenotypes, including hyperkalemic periodic paralysis, normokalemic periodic paralysis, and paramyotonia congenita (121). These diseases cause transient paralysis of muscles, beginning in the legs and progressing to involve arm and even facial muscles, and, rarely, muscles of respiration. Each attack lasts hours to days, and onset is in childhood. All have electric, and to a lesser extent, clinical myotonia. Mutations of the *CLCN1* gene cause either autosomal dominant (Thomsen disease) or autosomal recessive (Becker-type myotonia) myotonia congenita (121); the former is more common. Both are characterized by electric and clinical myotonia of skeletal muscles, with normal muscle strength. Patients complain of stiffness, which abates with continued use of the muscle (i.e., after "warming up"). Sudden movement, however, may result in such stiffness as to cause falls. The multisystem involvement of myotonic dystrophy is not present in any of the channelopathies. Mutations of the calcium channel gene result in hypokalemic periodic paralysis in which patients suffer transient weakness of limbs, as in the hyperkalemic form, but have no myotonia. These mutations are associated with low serum potassium.

The effect of pregnancy on myotonia congenita in two women was temporary worsening in the second half of the pregnancy (122,123). As with myotonic dystrophy, increased symptoms in the pregnant mother occur but are probably uncommon. Obstetric problems have not been described.

Anesthetics pose some risks to pregnant women with myotonia congenita. "Myotonic spasms" may occur with depolarizing neuromuscular blockers such as succinylcholine (79). Malignant hyperthermia has been reported in two cases of myotonia congenita (124,125), although a connection between the two disorders remains unproved (126).

There are no reports of pregnancy in periodic paralysis. In a multigeneration family with hyperkalemic periodic paralysis, affected women have had multiple uneventful pregnancies. It is uncertain whether certain anesthetics precipitate attacks of paralysis (126). Paralytic attacks with surgery may be related more to the stress of the operation, long periods of fasting, or overeating the night before surgery than to any anesthetic agent.

Polymyositis and Dermatomyositis

Polymyositis and *dermatomyositis* are inflammatory disorders that affect striated and cardiac muscle (see Chapter 37). Dermatomyositis differs clinically from polymyositis primarily by the presence of skin involvement and is thought to be a vasculopathy. The etiology of polymyositis and dermatomyositis is unknown. Both diseases can be seen in isolation or in conjunction with a variety of connective diseases. Both are characterized by proximal weakness, elevated creatine phosphokinase (CPK) levels, myopathic electromyography, and inflammatory myonecrosis on muscle biopsy.

Polymyositis and dermatomyositis are encountered rarely in the pregnant patient. Alhough women are affected twice as often as men, the bimodal age of onset largely spares the childbearing years, and the average age of onset of the inflammatory myopathies is 47 years (127). A review of the literature reveals 24 patients with 36 examined pregnancies, about evenly split between polymyositis or dermatomyositis antedating pregnancy or starting during pregnancy (128–144). Preexisting inflammatory myopathy generally does not result in gestational exacerbation (possibly because pregnancy is avoided in patients with poorly controlled disease); but when it does, it occurs in later pregnancy (128). This is in contrast to *de novo* disease, which usually occurs during the first trimester (128) but can appear as late as the postpartum period (134). In preexisting polymyositis or dermatomyositis, the inflammatory myopathy is rarely fulminant or difficult to control. *De novo* inflammatory myopathy is often active throughout gestation, even on treatment, but remission follows close on the heels of delivery (128).

Several complications of pregnancy have been reported in patients with polymyositis or dermatomyositis, including postpartum microangiopathic hemolytic anemia (132), placental abruption, uterine atony, and postpartum maternal death (138). More frequently encountered is intrauterine growth retardation, spontaneous abortion, and preterm labor, the latter of which is common (128).

Fetal wastage is increased in pregnancies complicated by inflammatory myopathies, with a rate of 50% to 60% found by Gutierrez and colleagues (134). My review is not quite so gloomy: In *de novo* disease, 36% fetal deaths occurred; and in preexisting disease, the rate was 21%.

Treatment of gestational polymyositis and dermatomyositis is determined by the clinical condition of the patient and the length of gestation. Mild disease may not need to be treated. For patients who require treatment, corticosteroids are the drug of choice, in doses of about 1 mg per kilogram daily. Although the effect of corticosteroids on fetal development is not clear, these agents are a much better choice than the antimetabolites, which in the first trimester may result in spontaneous abortion or fetal malformation (see Chapter 7) (145,146). Unfortunately, even with corticosteroids, no controlled studies of efficacy are available.

In general, women with either mildly active inflammatory myopathy or women who are in remission should have a relatively uneventful pregnancy, using corticosteroids to manage any exacerbations. Pregnancy should not be undertaken electively in severe disease or in any patient requiring antimetabolite therapy. In patients with onset in pregnancy, attempts to manage the disease early with corticosteroids can be made, but if these attempts are unsuccessful therapeutic abortion should be considered (147). Tapering of corticosteroids postpartum should be done conservatively to avoid exacerbations.

Metabolic Myopathies

Myophosphorylase Deficiency

Metabolic myopathies can be loosely defined as inborn errors of metabolism affecting muscle. *Myophosphorylase deficiency*, or *McArdle's disease*, is caused by lack of an enzyme in the muscle glycolytic pathway manifesting as exercise-induced muscle contracture and myoglobinuria. There are several glycogen storage disorders, all of which are rare, and little is known of their effect on pregnancy. A single report documents an uneventful pregnancy and delivery in a woman with McArdle's disease (148). Dawson and colleagues (149) mention one multiparous woman with McArdle's disease who suffered leg "cramps" and myoglobinuria after her last delivery. Smooth-muscle phosphorylase is normal in McArdle's patients (150), and uterine activity should be unimpaired. Neither deterioration nor exacerbation is expected during pregnancy.

Myoglobinuria

Myoglobinuria is a sign of rhabdomyolysis rather than a disease. Dramatically elevated levels of CPK in the serum and the presence of myoglobin in the urine are the biochemical hallmarks of the syndrome. Idiopathic and polymyositis-associated myoglobinuria have been reported during pregnancy (129,151). Increased estrogens will cause a decrease in muscle enzyme efflux and are proposed to have some stabilizing effect on muscle (152), including lowering baseline CPK levels during pregnancy. Oral contraceptives have no effect on serum levels of CPK (153).

Malignant Hyperthermia

Malignant hyperthermia is a syndrome of hyperpyrexia, muscle rigidity, rhabdomyolysis, and death, triggered by certain anesthetic agents (e.g., depolarizing muscle relaxants, inhalation anesthetics) and, in susceptible patients, stress and infection. The incidence in adults is 1:50,000 operative cases, and the question relating to pregnancy and malignant hyperthermia is why more cases are not encountered (154). Thus far, familial malignant hyperthermia has been linked to three different chromosomal loci (1). Only three cases of malignant hyperthermia during pregnancy have been reported, all during cesarean section (155–157) and all managed successfully with dantrolene. Malignant hyperthermia-susceptible patients can be managed uneventfully through labor and delivery, including cesarean section, by using agents not associated with malignant hyperthermia, careful monitoring (154), and prophylactic dantrolene if needed (158–160). Dantrolene crosses the placenta (160) and although its effects on the newborn have not been well studied, one report of 20 exposed pregnancies found no adverse effect on fetus or newborn (158).

Mitochondrial Myopathy

Mitochondrial myopathies are a heterogeneous group of diseases in which mitochondrial metabolism is defective. The disorders are best grouped into four categories (161): defects of mitochondrial substrate transport, defects of the respiratory chain, defects of substrate utilization, and defects of energy conservation and transduction. In the context of the pregnant woman, only the first two categories are discussed herein.

Intramitochondrial fatty acid oxidation is largely dependent on the transport of long-chain fatty acids across the mitochondrial membrane by attachment to carnitine. Deficiency of carnitine can be purely myopathic, in which case pregnancy is unlikely to be a factor, or systemic. Primary systemic carnitine deficiency is rare, with most deficiencies secondary to other metabolic disorders (161). Weakness, predominantly of proximal muscles, is frequent, and muscle biopsy shows abnormal lipid storage. Rapid progression of weakness has been reported during pregnancy (162) and in the postpartum period (163,164) in three cases, two of which were fatal (162, 164). The one patient treated with carnitine replacement, 2 g daily, improved (163). A fourth patient with systemic carnitine deficiency and a defect in the respiratory chain had rapidly progressive worsening of her weakness in the last trimester. She improved following treatment with 6 g of carnitine daily (161). The dramatic worsening of disease probably is related to already low carnitine stores experienced normally by pregnant women (163), which are further depleted by lactation (163) and increased fetal demand. Carnitine is actively transported placentally to the fetus (165), which has a relatively poor ability to produce carnitine (166). Untreated, systemic carnitine deficiency in pregnancy can be fatal; treated, patients do well.

A relatively common cause of myoglobinuria, but a rare disease nonetheless, is *carnitine palmitoyltransferase deficiency* (CPT). This enzyme attaches and detaches long-chain fatty acids to carnitine for transport across the mitochondrial membrane, where they will undergo oxidation, providing a major source of muscle energy, especially during aerobic exercise lasting more than 20 minutes (glycolysis is the main source of anaerobic energy production). The prolonged exertion required during labor would seem to make patients with CPT deficiency susceptible to rhabdomyolysis and myoglobinuria, but no reports of this exist. I have personal experience of one woman with an uneventful pregnancy before her diagnosis, when she was mildly symptomatic. Although the disease is inherited as an autosomal recessive trait, only 20% of documented cases are women (167), and some of those patients were diagnosed as siblings of affected males. A hormonal protective effect has been postulated (167).

Two case reports detail the pregnancies of women with defects in the respiratory chain (168,169). Other than mild exercise intolerance, pregnancy and labor (cesarean section in one) were unremarkable and the infants were healthy. Neither had postpartum progression of symptoms.

Mitochondrial Maternal Inheritance

About 85% of the proteins constituting the mitochondrial respiratory chain are encoded by nuclear DNA, with 15% (in total, 13 proteins) encoded on DNA within the mitochondrion itself (161). All human mitochondria arise from maternal sources (i.e., the ova), because there are no mitochondria in spermatozoa. This results in maternal (nonmendelian) inheritance of many mitochondrial encephalomyopathies (170). Mitochondrial diseases do not all arise from mitochondrial genomic defects; some follow mendelian inheritance patterns. Because mitochondria replicate autonomously, a range of mitochondrial genomes exists in any ovum. The presence and percentage of mutated mitochondria determine the expression of a particular mitochondrial defect, which explains the variable expression of mitochondrial encephalomyopathies. The disease is passed between generations by females only, although all offspring of a carrier mother may carry the genetic defect and may be affected.

Congenital Myopathy

There are a number of congenital myopathies, often requiring muscle biopsy for diagnosis. These disorders reflect a developmental arrest of muscle, with the pathologic and clinical manifestations dependent on the timing of insult or the nature of the genetic defect. These diseases do not progress, but the patient may be severely affected and may die. Myotubular myopathy has been linked to the X-chromosome, and prenatal diagnosis is possible by linkage analysis of DNA markers in the Xq28 region (171).

Congenital nemaline myopathy is a static muscle disease of variable severity and usually is diagnosed in childhood. Antenatal onset may occur, with severe consequences characteristic of the fetal akinesia sequence (39, 172), including arthrygryposis, polyhydramnios, lung hypoplasia, and neonatal demise (172). Hypotonia, weakness, jaw and palatal abnormalities, and scoliosis are frequent findings in milder cases. It is inherited as either an autosomal dominant or recessive trait. Four cases of pregnant women with congenital nemaline myopathy have ben reported: Pregnancy was uneventful in all, and vaginal or cesarean deliveries were normal, except when micrognathia, prognathia, and high arched palate made intubation difficult and scoliosis inhibited epidural anesthesia (173,174). All infants were unaffected.

A retrospective report (112) detailed the 12 pregnancies of five women with central-core congenital myopathy and the two pregnancies of a woman with cytoplasmic body congenital myopathy. For the most part, all the women had mild weakness that was not progressive before pregnancy. Three patients with central-core myopathy had worsening of weakness during pregnancy, with no improvement after delivery. No miscarriages, three preterm deliveries, and two assisted deliveries (prolonged labor in one, threatened fetal asphyxia in another), and no adverse fetal outcomes occurred. Two children inherited central-core myopathy. The chromosomal locus for central-core myopathy is 19q13.1, and the gene product is the ryanodine receptor, the same as for one of the familial malignant hyperthermia types (175).

Cramps

Cramps are uncommonly a sign of muscle disease but rather suggest neuronal or metabolic disturbance. The word *cramp* often is misused to cover any type of muscle pain, or *myalgia*. In fact, a muscle cramp is a specific clinical and electrophysiologic syndrome that must be differentiated from muscle contracture, myalgia, tetany, stiffness, spasticity, myotonia, neuromyotonia, and dystonia.

A cramp is a "sudden, forceful, painful, involuntary contraction of one muscle or part of a muscle, lasting anywhere from a few seconds to several minutes" (176). EMG during a cramp reveals a full interference pattern indistinguishable from a maximal voluntary contraction of the muscle. Cramps often begin and end with fasciculations, in contrast with muscle contractures, as in McArdle's disease, which are electrically silent.

Cramps can occur in normal persons, at night or related to exercise. Several metabolic disorders also may cause cramps, including uremia, hypothyroidism, and hypoadrenalism. Acute extracellular volume depletion (e.g., from perspiration, diarrhea, vomiting, diuresis, hemodialysis) also is associated with cramps (176). Pregnant women suffer an increased frequency of cramping, probably secondary to changes in metabolic and extracellular volume parameters. Cramps are seen most seriously in disorders of the motor neuron (e.g., amyotrophic lateral sclerosis, radiculopathy, neuropathy, old polio). Layzer (176) hypothesized the pathophysiology to be ectopic nerve excitation in the distal, intramuscular portion of the motor axon. Stretching the affected muscle is the best immediate treatment for cramping. If no correctable cause is present, recurrent cramps can be treated with quinine, oral magnesium (177), phenytoin, or carbamazepine for prophylaxis, although the latter two drugs carry some risk for teratogenesis.

REFERENCES

1. Gene location table. *Neuromuscul Disord* 1997;7:III.
2. Fambrough DM, Drachman DB, Satyamurti S. Neuromuscular junction in myasthenia gravis: decreased acetylcholine receptors. *Science* 1973;182:293–295.
3. Lindstrom JM, Seybold ME, Lennon VA, Whittingham S, Duane DD. Antibody to acetylcholine receptor in myasthenia gravis: prevalence, clinical correlates, and diagnostic value. *Neurology* 1976;26:1054–1059.
4. Schwab RS, Leland CC. Sex and age in myasthenia gravis as critical factors in incidence and remission. *JAMA* 1953;153:1270–1273.
5. Daroff RB. The office Tensilon test for ocular myasthenia gravis. *Arch Neurol* 1986;43:843–844.
6. Lindstrom J, Shelton D, Fujii Y. Myasthenia gravis. *Adv Immunol* 1988;42:233–284.
7. Appel SH, Almon RR, Levy NR. Acetylcholine receptor antibodies in myasthenia gravis. *N Engl J Med* 1975;293:760–761.
8. Sanders DB, Howard JF, Johns TR. Single-fiber electromyography in myasthenia gravis. *Neurology* 1979;29:68–76.
9. Oh SJ, Eslami N, Nishihira T, et al. Electrophysiological and clinical correlation in myasthenia gravis. *Ann Neurol* 1982;12:348–354.
10. Edery H, Porath G, Zahavy J. Passage of 2-hydroxyiminomethyl-*N*-methyl-pyridium methanesulfate to the fetus and cerebral spaces. *Toxicol Appl Pharmacol* 1966;9:341–346.
11. Pascuzzi RM, Coslett HB, Johns TR. Long-term corticosteroid treatment of myasthenia gravis: report of 116 patients. *Ann Neurol* 1984;15:291–298.
12. Miller RG, Milner-Brown HS, Mirka A. Prednisone-induced worsening of neuromuscular function in myasthenia gravis. *Neurology* 1986;36:729–732.
13. Seybold ME, Drachman DB. Gradually increasing doses of prednisone in myasthenia gravis. *N Engl J Med* 1974;290:81–84.
14. Carr SC, Gilchrist JM, Abuelo D, Clark D. Antenatal treatment of myasthenia gravis. *Obstet Gynecol* 1991;78:485–489.
15. Levine SE, Keesey JC. Successful plasmapheresis for fulminant myasthenia gravis during pregnancy. *Arch Neurol* 1986;43:197–198.
16. Watson WJ, Katz VL, Bowes WA. Plasmapheresis during pregnancy. *Obstet Gynecol* 1990;76:451–457.
17. Castleman B. The pathology of the thymus gland in myasthenia gravis. *Ann NY Acad Sci* 1966;135:496–503.
18. Goldman KP. Malignant thymomas in pregnancy. *Br J Dis Chest* 1974;68:279–283.
19. Perlo VP, Arnason B, Poskanzer D, et al. The role of thymectomy in treatment of myasthenia gravis. *Ann NY Acad Sci* 1971;183:308–315.
20. Genkins G, Kornfeld P, Papatestas AE, Bender AN, Matta RJ. Clinical experience in more than 2000 patients with myasthenia gravis. *Ann NY Acad Sci* 1987;505:500–513.
21. Ip MSM, So SY, Lam WK, Tang LCH, Mok CK. Thymectomy in myasthenia gravis during pregnancy. *Postgrad Med J* 1986;62:473–474.
22. Eden RD, Gall SA. Myasthenia gravis and pregnancy: a reappraisal of thymectomy. *Obstet Gynecol* 1983;62:328.
23. Donaldson JO. Neurologic emergencies in pregnancy. *Obstet Gynecol Clin North Am* 1991;18:199–212.
24. Kaeser HE. Drug-induced myasthenic syndromes. *Acta Neurol Scand* 1984;70(Suppl):39–47.
25. Argov Z, Mastaglia FL. Disorders of neuromuscular transmission caused by drugs. *N Engl J Med* 1979;301:409–413.
26. Chagnac Y, Hadani M, Goldhammer Y. Myasthenic crisis after intravenous administration of iodinated contrast agent. *Neurology* 1985;35:1219–1220.
27. Plauche WC. Myasthenia gravis in mothers and their newborn. *Clin Obstet Gynecol* 1991;34:82–99.

28. Hay DM. Myasthenia gravis and pregnancy. *J Obstet Gynaecol* 1969; 76:323–329.
29. Viets HR, Schwab RS, Brazier MAB. The effect of pregnancy on the course of Myasthenia gravis. *JAMA* 1942;119:236–242.
30. Brenner T, Beyth Y, Abramsky O. Inhibitory effect of alpha fetoprotein on the binding of myasthenia gravis antibody to acetylcholine receptor. *Proc Natl Acad Sci U S A* 1977;77:3635–3639.
31. Fennell DF, Ringel SP. Myasthenia gravis and pregnancy. *Obstet Gynecol Surv* 1987;41:414–421.
32. Duff GB. Preeclampsia and the patient with myasthenia gravis. *Obstet Gynecol* 1979;54:355–358.
33. Bashuk RG, Krendel DA. Myasthenia gravis presenting as weakness after magnesium administration. *Muscle Nerve* 1990;13:708–712.
34. Frenkel M, Ehrlich EN. The influence of progesterone and mineral-corticoids upon myasthenia gravis. *Ann Intern Med* 1964;60:971–981.
35. Giwa-Osagie OF, Newton JR, Larcher V. Obstetric performance of patients with myasthenia gravis. *Int J Gynecol Obstet* 1981;19:267.
36. Kalow W. Hydrolysis of local anesthetics by human serum cholinesterase. *J Pharm Exp Ther* 1952;104:122–134.
37. Rolbin SH, Levinson G, Shnider SM, Wright RG. Anesthetic consideration for myasthenia gravis and pregnancy. *Anesth Analg* 1978;57: 441–447.
38. Keesey J, Lindstrom J, Cokely H. Anti-acetylcholine receptor antibody in neonatal myasthenia gravis. *N Engl J Med* 1977;296:55.
39. Moessinger AC. Fetal akinesia deformation sequence: an animal model. *Pediatrics* 1983;72:857–863.
40. Gardnerova M, Eymard B, Morel E, et al. The fetal/adult acetylcholine receptor antibody ratio in mothers with myasthenia gravis as a marker for transfer of the disease to the newborn. *Neurology* 1997; 48:50–54.
41. Stoll C, Ehret-Mentre MC, Treisser A, Tranchant C. Prenatal diagnosis of congenital myasthenia with arthrogryposis in a myasthenic mother. *Prenat Diagn* 1991;11:17–22.
42. Barnes PR, Kanabar DJ, Brueton L, et al. Recurrent congenital arthrogryposis leading to a diagnosis of myasthenia gravis in an initially asymptomatic mother. *Neuromuscul Disord* 1995;5:59–65.
43. Namba T, Brown SB, Grob D. Neonatal myasthenia gravis: report of two cases and review of the literature. *Pediatrics* 1970;45:488–504.
44. Eymard B, Morel E, Dulac O, et al. Myasthenie et grossesse: une étude clinique et immunologique de 42 cas (21 myasthenies neonatales). *Rev Neurol* 1989;145:696–701.
45. Elias SB, Butler I, Appel S. Neonatal myasthenia gravis in an infant of a myasthenic mother in remission. *Ann Neurol* 1979;6:72.
46. Harper PS. Myotonic dystrophy, 2nd ed. Philadelphia: WB Saunders, 1989;13–36.
47. Harper PS. Myotonic dystophy, 2nd ed. Philadelphia: WB Saunders, 1989:187–214.
48. Dyken PR, Harper PS. Congenital dystrophica myotonica. *Neurology* 1973;23:465–473.
49. Brook JD, McCurrach ME, Harley HG, et al. Molecular basis of myotonic dystrophy: expansion of a trinucleotide (CTG) repeat at the 3' end of a transcript encoding a protein kinase family member. *Cell* 1992;68:799–808.
50. Fu Y-H, Pizzuti A, Fenwick RG, et al. An unstable triplet repeat in a gene related to myotonic muscular dystrophy. *Science* 1992;255: 1256–1258.
51. Mahadevan M, Tsilfidis C, Sabourin L, et al. Myotonic dystrophy mutation: an unstable CTG repeat in the 3′translated region of the gene. *Science* 1992;255:1253–1255.
52. Redman JB, Fenwick RG, Fu Y-H, Pizzuti A, Caskey CT. Relationship between parental trinucleotide GCT repeat length and severity of myotonic dystrophy in offspring. *JAMA* 1993;269:1960–1965.
53. Drucker WD, Rowland LP, Sterling K, Christy NP. On the function of the endocrine glands in myotonic muscular dystrophy. *Am J Med* 1961;31:941–950.
54. Harper P, Penny R, Foley TP, Migeon CJ, Blizzard RM. Gonadal function in males with myotonic dystrophy. *J Clin Endocrinol* 1972;35: 852–856.
55. Febres F, Scaglia H, Lisker R, et al. Hypothalamic-pituitary-gonadal function in patients with myotonic dystrophy. *J Clin Endocrinol* 1975; 41:833–840.
56. Sagel J, Distiller LA, Morley JE, Issacs H. Myotonia dystrophica: studies on gonadal function using luteinizing hormone-releasing hormone. *J Clin Endocrinol Metab* 1975;40:1110–1113.
57. Harper PS. Myotonic dystrophy, 2nd ed. Philadelphia: WB Saunders, 1989:127–132.
58. Drucker WD, Blanc WA, Rowland LP, Grumbach MM, Christy NP. *J Clin Endocrinol Metab* 1963;23:59.
59. Caughey JE, Myrianthopoulos NC. Dystrophica Myotonica and related disorders. Springfield, IL: Charles C Thomas, 1963.
60. Sagel J, Distiller LA, Morley JE, Issacs H. Myotonia dystrophica: studies on gonadal function using luteinizing hormone-releasing hormone. *J Clin Endocrinol Metab* 1975;40:1110–1113.
61. Marshall J. Observations on endocrine function in dystrophica myotonica. *Brain* 1959;82:221–231.
62. Thomasen E. Myotonia: Thomsen's disease (myotonic congenita), paramyotonia, and dystrophica myotonica: a clinical and heredobiologic investigation. London: MK Lewis, 1948.
63. Harper PS. Myotonic Dystrophy, 2nd ed. Philadelphia:W.B. Saunders, 1989:320.
64. O'Brien TA, Harper PS. Reproductive problems and neonatal loss in women with myotonic dystrophy. *J Obstet Gynecol* 1984;4:170–173.
65. Sciarra JJ, Steer CM. Uterine contractions during labor in myotonic muscular dystrophy. *Am J Obstet Gynecol* 1961;82:612–615.
66. Hopkins A, Wray S. The effect of pregnancy on dystrophica myotonica. *Neurology* 1967;17166–17168.
67. Gardy HH. Dystrophica myotonica in pregnancy. *Obstet Gynecol* 1963;21:441–445.
68. Jaffe R, Mock M, Abramowitz J, Ben-Aderet N. Myotonic dystrophy and pregnancy: a review. *Obstet Gynecol Surv* 1986;41:272–278.
69. Davis HA. Pregnancy in myotonica dystrophica. *J Obstet Gynaecol Br Emp* 1958;65:479–480.
70. Shore RN, MacLachlan TB. Pregnancy with myotonic dystrophy: course, complications and management. *Obstet Gynecol* 1971;38: 448–454.
71. Fall LH, Young WW, Power JA, Faulkner CS, Hettleman BD. Severe congestive heart failure and cardiomyopathy as a complication of myotonic dystrophy in pregnancy. *Obstet Gynecol* 1990;76:481–485.
72. Broekhuizen FF, Elejalde de M, Elejalde R, Hamilton PR. Neonatal myotonic dystrophy as a cause of hydramnios and neonatal death. *J Reprod Med* 1983;28:595–599.
73. Webb D, Muir I, Faulker J, Johnson G. Myotonia dystrophica: obstetric complications. *Am J Obstet Gynecol* 1978;132:265–270.
74. Maas O. Observations on dystrophica myotonica. *Brain* 1937;60: 498–524.
75. Watters GV, Williams TV. Early onset myotonic dystrophy. Clinical and laboratory findings in five families and a review of the literature. *Arch Neurol* 1967;17:137–152.
76. Hook R, Anderson EF, Noto P. Anesthetic management of a parturient with myotonia atrophia. *Anesthesiology* 1975;43:689–692.
77. Risseeuw JJ, Oudsboorn JH, van der Straaten PJ, Kuypers JC. Myotonic dystrophy in pregnancy: a report of two cases within one family. *Eur J Obstet Gynecol Reprod Biol* 1997;73:145–148.
78. Sarnat HB, O'Connor T, Byrne PA. Clinical effects of myotonic dystrophy on pregnancy and the neonate. *Arch Neurol* 1976;33:459–465.
79. Thiel RE. The myotonic response to suxamethonium. *Br J Anaesth* 1967;39:815–820.
80. Mitchell MM, Ali HH, Savarese JJ. Myotonia and neuromuscular blocking agents. *Anesthiology* 1978;49:44–48.
81. Koch MC, Grimm T, Harley HG, Harper PS. Genetic risks for children of women with myotonic dystrophy. *Am J Hum Genet* 1991;48: 1084–1091.
82. Poulton J. Congenital myotonic dystrophy and mtDNA. *Am J Hum Genet* 1992;50:651–652.
83. Harper PS, Dyken PR. Early onset dystrophica myotonica: evidence supporting a maternal environmental factor. *Lancet* 1972;2:53–55.
84. Howeler CJ, Bush HTM. An asymptomatic mother of children with congenital myotonic dystrophy. *J Neurol Sci* 1990;98(Suppl):197.
85. Andrews PI, Wilson J. Relative disease severity in siblings with myotonic dystrophy. *J Child Neurol* 1992;7:161–167.
86. Pearse RG, Howeler CJ. Neonatal form of dystrophica myotonica. *Arch Dis Child* 1979;54:331–338.
87. Vanier TM. Dystrophica myotonica in childhood. *BMJ* 1960;2: 1284–1288.
88. Calderon R. Myotonic dystrophy: a neglected cause of mental retardation. *J Pediatr* 1966;68:423–431.
89. Sarnat HB, Silbert SW. Maturational arrest of fetal muscle in neonatal myotonic dystrophy. *Arch Neurol* 1976;33:466–474.

90. Rutherford MA, Heckmatt JZ, Dubowitz V. Congenital myotonic dystrophy: respiratory function at birth determines survival. *Arch Dis Child* 1989;64:191–195.
91. Swift TR, Ignacio OJ, Dyken PR. Neonatal dystrophica myotonica: electrophysiological studies. *Am J Dis Child* 1975;29:734–737.
92. Caskey CT, Pizzuti A, Fu Y-H, Fenwick RG, Nelson DL. Triplet repeat mutations in human disease. *Science* 1992;256:784–789.
93. Massari A, Novelli G, Colosimo AG, et al. Non-invasive early prenatal molecular diagnosis using retrieved transcervical trophoblast cells. *Hum Genet* 1996;97:150–155.
94. Moxley RT. Proximal myotonic myopathy: mini-review of a recently delineated clinical disorder. *Neuromuscul Disord* 1996;6:87–93.
95. Hoffman EP, Brown RH, Kunkel LM. Dystrophin: the protein product of the Duchenne muscular dystrophy locus. *Cell* 1987;51:919–928.
96. Multicenter Study Group. Diagnosis of Duchenne's and Becker muscular dystrophies by polymerase chain reaction. *JAMA* 1992;267: 2609–2615.
97. Emery AEH. Duchenne muscular dystrophy. New York: Oxford University Press, 1987:73–77.
98. Barkhaus PB, Gilchrist JM. Duchenne muscular dystrophy manifesting carriers. *Arch Neurol* 1989;46:673–675.
99. Hoffman EP, Arahata K, Minetti C, Bonilla E, Rowland LP. Dystrophinopathy in isolated cases of myopathy in females. *Neurology* 1992;42:967–975.
100. Clemens PR, Fenwick RG, Chamberlain JS, et al. Carrier detection and prenatal diagnosis in Duchenne's and Becker muscular dystrophy families, using dinucleotide repeat polymorphisms. *Am J Hum Genet* 1991;49:951–960.
101. Hoffman EP, Fischbeck KH, Brown RH, et al. Characterization of dystrophin in muscle-biopsy specimens from patients with Duchenne's or Becker's muscular dystrophy. *N Engl J Med* 1988;318:1363–1368.
102. Hoffman EP, Pegoraro E, Scacheri P, et al. Genetic counseling of isolated carriers of Duchenne muscular dystrophy. *Am J Med Genet* 1996;63:573–580.
103. Den Duneen JT, Grootscholten PM, Bakker E, et al. Topography of the Duchenne muscular dystrophy (DMD) gene: FIGE and cDNA analysis of 194 cases reveals 115 deletions and 13 duplications. *Am J Hum Genet* 1989;45:835–847.
104. Abbs S. Prenatal diagnosis of Duchenne's and Becker muscular dystrophy. *Prenat Diagn* 1996;16:1187–1198.
105. Evans MI, Krivchenia EL, Johnson MP, et al. *In utero* fetal muscle biopsy alters diagnosis and carrier risks in Duchenne's and Becker muscular dystrophy. *Fetal Diagn Ther* 1995;10:71–75.
106. Liu J, Lissens W, Devroey P, Liebaers I, Van Steirteghem A. Cystic fibrosis, Duchenne muscular dystrophy and preimplantation genetic diagnosis. *Hum Reprod Update* 1996;2:531–539.
107. Sekizawa A, Kimura T, Sasaki M, Nakamura S, Kobayashi R, Sato T. Prenatal diagnosis of Duchenne muscular dystrophy using a single fetal nucleated erythrocyte in maternal blood. *Neurology* 1996;46: 1350–1353
108. Bushby K. Towards the classification of the autosomal recessive limb-girdle muscular dystrophies. *Neuromuscul Disord* 1996;6:439–441.
109. Speer MC, Yamaoka LH, Gilchrist JH, et al. Confirmation of genetic heterogeneity in limb-girdle muscular dystrophy: linkage of an autosomal dominant form to chromosome 5q. *Am J Hum Genet* 1992;50: 1211–1217.
110. Anderson LVB. Optimized protein diagnosis in the autosomal recessive limb-girdle muscular dsytrophies. *Neuromusc Disord* 1996;6: 443–446.
111. Pash MP, Balaton J, Eagle C. Anesthetic management of a parturient with severe muscular dystrophy, lumbar lordosis and a difficult airway. *Can J Anaesth* 1996;43:959–963.
112. Rudnick-Schoneborn S, Glauner B, Rohrig D, Zerres K. Obstetric aspects in women with facioscapulohumeral muscular dystrophy, limb-girdle muscular dystrophy, and congenital myopathies. *Arch Neurol* 1997;54:888–894.
113. Restagno G, Romero N, Richard I, et al. Prenatal diagnosis of limb-girdle muscular dystrophy type 2A. *Neuromuscul Disord* 1996;6:173–176.
114. Fisher J, Upadhyaya M. Molecular genetics of facioscapulohumeral muscular dystrophy (FSH). *Neuromuscul Disord* 1997;7:55–62.
115. Bakker E, van der Wielen MJ, Voorhoeve E, et al. Diagnostic, predictive, and prenatal testing for facioscapulohumeral muscular dystrophy: diagnostic approach for sporadic and familial cases. *J Med Genet* 1996;33:29–35.
116. Helbling-Leclerc A, Zhang X, Topaloglu H, et al. Mutations in the laminin alpha 2-chain gene (LAMA 2) cause merosin-deficient congenital muscular dystrophy. *Nat Genet* 1995;11:216–218.
117. Kobayashi O, Hayashi Y, Arahata K, Ozawa E, Nonaka I. Congenital muscular dystrophy: clinical and pathologic study of 50 patients with classical (Occidental) merosin-positive form. *Neurology* 1996;46: 815–818.
118. Toda T, Segawa M, Nomura Y, et al. Localization of a gene for Fukuyama type congenital muscular dystrophy to chromosome 9q31-33. *Nat Genet* 1993;5:283–286.
119. Naom I, Sewry C, D'Alessandro M, et al. Prenatal diagnosis of merosin-deficient congenital muscular dystrophy. *Neuromuscul Disord* 1997;7:176–179.
120. Kondo E, Saito K, Toda T, et al. Prenatal diagnosis of Fukuyama type congenital muscular dystrophy by polymorphism analsysis. *Am J Med Genet* 1996;66:169–174.
121. Lehmann-Horn F, Rudel R. Hereditary nondystrophic myotonias and periodic paralyses. *Curr Opin Neurol* 1995;8:402–410.
122. Gardiner CF. A case of myotonia congenita. *Arch Pediatr* 1901;18: 925–928.
123. Hakim CA, Thomlinson J. Myotonia congenita in pregnancy. *J Obstet Gynaecol Br Commonw* 1969;76:561–562.
124. Morley JB, Lambert TF, Kakulas BA. *Excerpta Medica International Congress Series* 1973;295:543.
125. Saidman LJ, Havard ES, Eger EI. Hyperthermia during anesthesia. *JAMA* 1964;190:1029–1032.
126. Miller JD, Lee C. Muscle diseases. In: Katz J, Benumof JL, Kadis LB, eds. Anesthesia and uncommon diseases, 3rd ed. Philadelphia: WB Saunders, 1990;622–626.
127. Bohan AJ, Peter JB, Pearson CM. A computer-assisted analysis of 150 patients with polymyositis and dermatomyositis. *Medicine* 1977; 56:255.
128. Rosenzweig BA, Rotmensch S, Binnette SP, Phillippe M. Primary idiopathic polymyositis and dermatomyositis complicating pregnancy: diagnosis and management. *Obstet Gynecol Surv* 1989;44:162–170.
129. Ditzian-Kadanoff R, Reinhard JD, Thomas C, Segal AS. Polymyositis with myoglobinuria in pregnancy: a report and review of the literature. *J Rheumatol* 1988;15:513–514.
130. Ishii N, Ono H, Kawaguchi T, Nakajima H. Dermatomyositis and pregnancy: case report and review of the literature. *Dermatologica* 1991;183:146–149.
131. Glickman FS. Dermatomyositis associated with pregnancy. *United States Armed Forces Medical Journal* 1958;9:417–425.
132. Tsai A, Lindheimer MD, Lamberg SI. Dermatomyositis complicating pregnancy. *Obstet Gynecol* 1973;41:570–573.
133. Katz AL. Another case of polymyositis in pregnancy. *Arch Intern Med* 1980;140:1123.
134. Gutierrez G, Dagnino R, Mintz G. Polymyositis/dermatomyositis and pregnancy. *Arthritis Rheum* 1984;27:291–294.
135. Barnes AB, Lisak DA. Childhood dermatomyositis and pregnancy. *Am J Obstet Gynecol* 1983;146:335–336.
136. Bauer KA, Siegler M, Lindheimer MA. Polymyositis complicating pregnancy. *Arch Intern Med* 1979;139:449.
137. Houck W, Melnyk C, Gast MJ. Polymyositis in pregnancy. *J Reprod Med* 1987;32:208–210.
138. England MJ, Perlmann T, Veriava Y. Dermatomyositis in pregnancy. *J Reprod Med* 1986;31:633–636.
139. King CR, Chow S. Dermatomyositis and pregnancy. *Obstet Gynecol* 1985;66:589–592.
140. Emy PH, Lenormand V, Maitre F, et al. Polymyosites, dermatomyosites et grossesse: grossesse a haut risk, nouvelle observation et revue de la literature. *J Gynecol Obstet Biol Reprod* 1986;15:785.
141. Masse MR. Grossesses et dermatomyosite. *Bull Soc Franc Derm Syph* 1962;69:921.
142. Satoh M, Ajmani AK, Hirakata M, Suwa A, Winfield JB, Reeves WH. Onset of polymyositis with autoantibodies to threonyl-tRNA synthetase during pregnancy. *J Rheumatol* 1994;21:1564–1566.
143. Harris A, Webley M, Usherwood M, Burge S. Dermatomyositis presenting in pregnancy. *Br J Dermatol* 1995;133:783–785.
144. Boggess KA, Easterling TR, Raghu G. Management and outcome of pregnant women with interstitial and restrictive lung disease. *Am J Obstet Gynecol* 1995;173:1007–1014.
145. Nicholson HO. Cytotoxic drugs in pregnancy. *J Obstet Gynaecol Br Commonw* 1968;75:307–312.

146. Hausknect RU. Methotrexate and misoprostol to terminate early pregnancy. *N Engl J Med* 1995;333:537–540.
147. Mintz G. Dermatomyositis. *Rheum Dis Clin North Am* 1989;15: 375–382.
148. Cochrane P, Alderman B. Normal pregnancy and succesful delivery in myophosphorylase deficiency (McArdle's disease). *J Neuro Neurosurg Psychiat* 1973;36:225–227.
149. Dawson DM, Spong FL, Harrington JF. McArdle's disease: lack of muscle phosphorylase. *Ann Intern Med* 1968;69:229–235.
150. Engel WK, Eyerman EL, Williams HE. Late-onset type of skeletal-muscle phosphorylase deficiency: a new familial variety with completely and partially affected members. *N Engl J Med* 1962;268:135–137.
151. Owens OJ, Macdonald R. Idiopathic myoglobinuria in the early puerperium. *Scott Med J* 1989;34:564–565.
152. Thomsen WHS, Smith I. Effects of oestrogen on erythrocyte enzyme efflux in normal men and women. *Clin Chim Acta* 1980;103: 203–208.
153. Simpson J, Zellweger H, Burmeister LF, Christee R, Nielsen MK. Effect of oral contraceptive pills on the level of creatine phosphokinase with regard to carrier detection in Duchenne muscular dystrophy. *Clin Chim Acta* 1974;52:219–223.
154. Kaplan RF, Kellner KR. More on malignant hyperthermia during delivery. *Am J Obstet Gynecol* 1985;152:608–609.
155. Liebenschutz F, Mai C, Pickerodt VWA. Increased carbon dioxide production in two patients with malignant hyperthermia and its control by dantrolene. *Br J Anaesth* 1979;51:899–903.
156. Lips FJ, Newland M, Dutton G. Malignant hyperthermia triggered by cyclopropane during cesarean section. *Anesthesiology* 1982;56: 144–146.
157. Cupryn JP, Kennedy A, Byrick RJ. Malignant hyperthermia in pregnancy. *Am J Obstet Gynecol* 1984;150:327–328.
158. Sorosky JI, Ingardia CJ, Botti JJ. Diagnosis and management of susceptibility to malignant hyperthermia in pregnancy. *Am J Perinatol* 1989;6:46–48.
159. Shime J, Gare D, Andrews J, Britt B. Dantrolene in pregnancy: lack of adverse effects on the fetus and newborn infant. *Am J Obstet Gynecol* 1988;159:831–834.
160. Morison DH. Placental transfer of dantrolene. *Anesthesiology* 1983; 59:265.
161. Morgan-Hughes JA. The mitochondrial myopathies. In: Engel AG, Franzini-Armstrong C, eds. Myology, 2nd ed. New York: McGraw-Hill 1994;1610–1660.
162. Cornelio F, DiDonato S, Peluchetti D, et al. Fatal cases of lipid storage myopathy with carnitine deficiency. *J Neurol Neurosurg Psychiatry* 1977;40:170–178.
163. Angelini C, Govoni E, Bragaglia M, Vergani L. Carnitine deficiency: acute postpartum crisis. *Ann Neurol* 1978;4:558–561.
164. Boudin G, Mikol J, Guillard A, Engel AG. Fatal systemic carnitine deficiency with lipid storage in skeletal muscle, heart, liver and kidney. *J Neurol Sci* 1976;30:313–325.
165. Hahn P, Skala JP, Secombe DW, et al. Carnitine content of blood and amniotic fluid. *Pediatr Res* 1977;11:878–880.
166. Warshaw JB, Terry ML. Cellular energy metabolism during fetal development, Part 2. *J Cell Biol* 1970;44:354–360.
167. Zierz S, Papadimitriou A. Carnitine palmitoyltransferase deficiency. In: Engel AG, Franzini-Armstrong C, ed. Myology, 2nd ed. New York: McGraw-Hill, 1994;1577.
168. Berkowitz K, Monteagudo A, Marks F, Jackson U, Baxi L. Mitochondrial myopathy and preeclampsia associated with pregnancy. *Am J Obstet Gynecol* 1990;162:146–147.
169. Rosaeg OP, Morrison S, MacLeod JP. Anaesthetic management of labour and delivery in the parturient with mitochondrial myopathy. *Can J Anaesth* 1996;43:403–407.
170. Giles RE, Blanc H, Cann HM, Wallace DC. Maternal inheritance of human mitochondrial DNA. *Proc Natl Acad Sci U S A* 1980;77:6715.
171. Hu LJ, Laporte J, Kress W, Dahl N. Prenatal diagnosis of X-linked myotubular myopathy: strategies using new and tightly linked DNA markers. *Prenat Diagn* 1996;16:231–237.
172. Lammens M, Moerman P, Fryns JP, Lemmens F, ran de Kamp GM, Goemans N, Dom R. Fetal akinesia sequence caused by nemaline myopathy. *Neuropediatrics* 1997;28:116–119.
173. Stackhouse R, Chwlmow D, Dattel BJ. Anesthetic complications in a pregnant patient with nemaline myopathy. *Anesth Analg* 1994;79: 1195–1197.
174. Wallgren-Pettersson C, Hilesmaa VK, Paatero H. Pregnancy and delivery in congenital nemaline myopathy. *Acta Obstet Gynecol Scand* 1995;74:659–661.
175. Quane KA, Healey JMS, Keating KE, Manning BM, Couch FJ, Palmacci LM, Doriguzzi C, Fagerland TH, Berg K, Ording H, et al. Mutations in the ryanodine receptor gene in central core disease and malignant hyperthermia. *Nature Genet* 1993;5:51–55.
176. Layzer RB. Neuromuscular manifestations of systemic disease. Philadelphia: FA Davis 1985:19–22.
177. Dahle LO, Berg G, Hammar M, Hurtig M, Larsson L. The effect of oral magnesium substitution on pregnancy-induced leg cramps. *Am J Obstet Gynecol* 1995;173:175–180.

Cherry and Merkatz's Complications of Pregnancy,
Fifth Edition, edited by W. R. Cohen
Lippincott Williams & Wilkins, Philadelphia © 2000.

CHAPTER 31

Multiple Sclerosis

Rene Elkin

Multiple sclerosis (MS) is a common disease of the central nervous system (CNS) that primarily affects young adults and is more common in women. It is an acquired inflammatory disease that has a variable and unpredictable clinical course, with protean manifestations. Despite extensive research, the etiology and pathogenesis of the disease remain unproved, and to date there is no treatment available that effects a cure. Because the disease affects young persons in the prime of their lives, the resultant physical disability may have profound psychosocial and economic implications for the patient, the patient's family, and society.

DEFINITION

MS is an immune-mediated inflammatory disease of the CNS that involves myelin and the myelin-producing cells, oligodendrocytes. In contrast to other immune-mediated diseases such as systemic lupus erythematosus, the process of inflammation is confined to the CNS. Several hypotheses to explain the etiology and pathogenesis of this disease have been presented, but to date no single etiologic factor has been implicated. Because the disease occurs in young persons, the impact on the quality of life is enormous. In many cases, progressive physical disability renders the individual with MS incapable of living an independent life.

ETIOLOGY

Three main factors appear to be involved in the etiology of MS: an abnormal immune response to an unidentified self-antigen within the CNS, a genetic predisposition, and an environmental trigger, which is presumed to be a virus.

R. Elkin: Department of Neurology, Albert Einstein College of Medicine, Bronx, NY 10461.

Evidence for Immunopathogenesis

Although the clinical and pathologic features of MS were described by Charcot as early as 1868, the precise etiology of this primary demyelinating disease of the CNS remains an enigma. In recent years, development of sophisticated laboratory techniques has greatly facilitated our knowledge and understanding of the complex mechanisms that are responsible for lesion formation in MS. The currently accepted hypothesis for the pathogenesis of MS is that in a genetically susceptible person, viral infections can trigger a white-matter–specific, cell-mediated immune response that results in selective destruction of myelin and oligodendrocytes. There is a combination of both exogenous and endogenous factors that play a role in the pathogenesis of autoimmune diseases, involving both humoral and cell-mediated immune reactions (1,2). Prevailing immunologic tolerance may be overcome when normally anergic autoreactive T cells are activated by myelin-antigen cross-reactive pathogens, resulting in the production of high-affinity–binding pathologic autoreactive T cells with consequent tissue damage. Furthermore, T cells may be activated polyclonally by proinflammatory cytokines that are produced by unrelated immune

TABLE 31-1. *Detection of immune dysfunction in the blood in multiple sclerosis*

Increased in serum
IFN-α
TNF
IL-2
IL-2 receptor
INF-α intermittently
Decreased in serum
CD-8+ suppressor cell function
PGE_2 release by macrophages

IFN, interferon; TNF, tumor necrosis factor; IL-2, interleukin 2; PGE_2, prostaglandin E_2. Created from (1, 9–14).

TABLE 31-2. *Detection of Immune dysfunction in the cerebrospinal fluid in multiple sclerosis*

Increased IgG, IgG index, oligoclonal bands
Increased INF-α-secreting cells
Increased tumor necrosis factor
Increased activated CD4+ T-cells

From refs. 1, 9–14, with permission.

responses, resulting in activation of physiologic autoreactive T cells. These cytokines facilitate extravasation of leucocytes and the development of inflammatory lesions in target organs by upregulating adhesion molecules and vascular addressins and by inducing aberrant class II major histocompatibility complex (MHC) expression on endothelial and glial elements (3–5). The increase in the exacerbation rate following intercurrent viral illnesses (6), systemic administration of interferon gamma (IFN-γ) (7), and the observed close association between optic neuritis and vaccinations in children (8) lend strong clinical support for the hypothesis of disease activation by cytokines. The specificity of the disease process for myelin and oligodendrocytes, the type IV delayed hypersensitivity-like features of the inflammatory lesions, the wide spectrum of the immunologic abnormalities in both the blood and the cerebrospinal fluid (CSF), and the similarities of these changes with those observed in human autoimmune diseases and in the animal model experimental allergic encephalomyelitis (EAE) have provided strong support for the conclusion that MS is an immune-mediated disease. A number of quantitative and qualitative abnormalities of both the humoral and cellular immune system and activation of bone marrow cells have been described in MS. Because enhancement of the immune response by cytokines is random, most of these observed changes in the blood and CSF are not specific for MS but also are observed in other immune-mediated diseases. These abnormalities are believed to reflect mainly immunoregulatory defects in T-cell function that are associated with hyperactivity of T and B cells (9). These abnormalities are summarized in Tables 31-1 through 31-3 (1,9–14).

TABLE 31-3. *Detection of immune dysfunction in active multiple sclerosis plaques*

IFN-γ on astrocytes
Class II MHC on astrocytes
TNF on astrocytes and macrophages
Lymphotoxin on T-cells and macrophages
IFN-α on macrophages
IFN-γ on astrocytes, lymphocytes, and macrophages

TNF, tumor necrosis factor; IL, interleukin; PGE, prostoglandin; MHC, major histocompatibility class; IFN, interferon. From refs. 11, 12, 14, with permission.

TABLE 31-4. *Pattern of inheritance in multiple sclerosis (MS)*

MS does not fit a mendelian inheritance pattern, but rather a polygenic model
Up to 20% of MS subjects have at least one relative with MS
In monozygotic twins with MS the risk for development of MS in the co-twin is 26%–36%
In a parent with MS, the risk for a child is 4%
In an MS subject the risk for a sibling is 4%–5%

From ref. 20, with permission.

GENETICS

The prevailing hypothesis in the 1990's is that MS is a polygenic disease. It has long been known that a gene located on the short arm of chromosome 6 in the HLA class II region is associated with a predisposition to the development of MS. Other HLA haplotypes that are associated with MS include HLA-DR-DQ, HLA-DW2, and HLA-DR3,DQ2. Bearing a certain HLA type is neither sufficient nor essential for the development of MS, however (15). Family studies and twin studies have shed further light on the genetic basis for this disease. The combined data from a population-based study of MS included 27 monozygotic and 43 dizygotic pairs (16). A 7.5-year follow-up showed a concordance rate for MS of 28% for monozygotic pairs compared with 4% for dizygotic pairs, which is not significantly different from the 5% concordance rate for nontwin siblings. Because the concordance rate for monozygotic twins significantly exceeds those of the other two groups, there is clearly a major genetic component in susceptibility to MS. Furthermore, the 7:1 monozygotic–dizygotic concordance ratio indicates the operation of at least two or more genes, because this ratio would approximate only 2:1 or 4:1, respectively, if only a single dominant or recessive susceptibility locus were implicated. Of note, most of the monozygotic twins pairs were discordant, demonstrating the powerful effect of environmental and other noninheritable factors (17).

Studies by Sandovnick and Baird in 1988 (18) and Ebers and Sandovnick in 1994 (19) report a family history in 20% of persons with MS, which not only invokes a genetic basis for the disease, but it also implicates the environment and lifestyle that are shared by family members. The risks of developing MS were calculated from data collected over 7 years at an MS clinic in Vancouver that serves a white population in a region at high risk for MS (Table 31-4) (20).

EVIDENCE FOR A VIRAL ETIOLOGY

Although a single environmental trigger for the development of MS has not been identified, there is a high suspicion that one or more infectious agents is involved.

Indirect evidence that viruses may play a role includes similarities to acute disseminated encephalomyelitis, a primarily demyelinating condition that may occur following infection with measles, EBV, varicella, and other pathogens. Canine distemper virus can induce demyelination in dogs, as can Theiler's murine encephalomyelitis virus in mice. Although there is an increased level of antibody titers to the measles virus in the serum and CSF of patients with MS, this increase appears to be caused by a nonspecific generalized B-cell hyperactivity. To date, no virus has been identified consistently or specifically in MS tissues. Herpes type 6 virus was recently reported in MS brain tissue (22), but the relevance of this finding in MS remains to be ascertained.

EPIDEMIOLOGY

In the United States, an estimated 250,000 to 300,000 persons had physician-diagnosed MS in 1990. Most of the patients are female, and peak age of onset is between 15 and 50 years (mean, 33 years). Most patients are diagnosed in the third and fourth decades of life (21,24).

There is a strong relation between geographic latitude and the risk of developing MS. Prevalence varies from 5 to 10 per 100,000 in tropical zones to 50 to 100 per 100,000 in temperate zones (21). A further observation from migration studies (21,23) is that the location where one spends the first 15 years of life determines to a greater or lesser extent the risk for subsequent development of MS. A person who is born in the north and migrates to the south after the age of 15 is more likely to develop MS than one who moves from south to north. Prevalence also varies by race: It is highest among northern Europeans and those of northern European descent. The disease is rare among Asians and in the black population of Africa. The incidence among black Americans is much greater than in Africa and represents 40% of all Americans with MS (25).

The high incidence of MS in certain regions is known as *clustering*, but even evaluation of such groups has failed to identify a single cause for the disease. MS is a complex trait that appears to be determined by both genetic and environmental factors.

PATHOLOGY

The pathognomonic pathologic findings in MS are (a) the focal nature of the lesions; (b) the relatively large size of the lesions; (c) the perivenous location; and (d) the histologic findings within the lesions of extensive demyelination and destruction of oligodendrocytes, the myelin-producing cells within the CNS, with relative sparing of nerve cells and axons.

On gross inspection of a brain of a person with MS, mild or severe cortical atrophy and depressed gray areas of scarring, firm to the touch in unfixed tissue, may be present. On the cut surface, there is usually ventricular enlargement, and plaques are seen in the periventricular grey matter. Some areas of the brain are more susceptible to plaque formation. These areas include the tissue around the lateral and fourth ventricles, the periaqueductal tissue, corpus callosum, the optic nerves, chiasm and tracts, the corticomedullary junction, and the subpial brainstem (26).

At autopsy it is usual to find lesions of different ages (i.e., old, inactive lesions and evidence of recent activity). In cases of long standing, there may be only old, inactive lesions. It is these inactive lesions that are responsible for the neurologic manifestations of the disease. They consist of demyelinated axons embedded in a mesh of astroglial processes, with few macrophages and few inflammatory cells. This finding is in contrast to the acute lesions, which reveal macrophages at the periphery of the lesion that frequently contain phagocytosed myelin fragments and a mononuclear leukocyte infiltration. Plaques may be discovered incidentally at autopsy in older persons with no history of neurologic dysfunction in life. At the other extreme, MS on rare occasions may present as a fulminant disease with a rapid downhill course and early death. Tissue damage in MS is highly selective, resulting in the permanent loss of oligodendrocytes and myelin from circumscribed areas of the CNS. Ultrastructurally, there is evidence of myelin destruction by macrophages that contain fragments of ingested myelin. At present, why remyelination fails to occur in long-standing MS lesions is a subject of controversy. Hypotheses include the presence of myelin-inhibiting antibodies (27) or T cells or antibodies reactive against oligodendrocyte differentiation antigens (28), among others.

CLINICAL PRESENTATION

The hallmark of the clinical presentation of MS is the waxing and waning of symptoms and signs that are variable and unpredictable in both their frequency and severity. The clinical picture reflects the site(s) of disease activity. The course of MS is variable and recently was classified into four categories, depending on the clinical manifestations of the disease (29), including (a) relapsing remitting, (b) primary progressive, (c) secondary progressive, and (d) progressive relapsing (Figs. 31.1 through 31.4). The clinical signs and symptoms include the following:

Motor Symptoms

Involvement of the corticospinal tracts may be the first manifestation of MS in 30% to 40% patients. In patients with chronic disease, the frequency increases to almost 62% (30). The lower extremities are involved more frequently than the upper extremities, and when all four limbs are affected, the legs usually are involved first. The

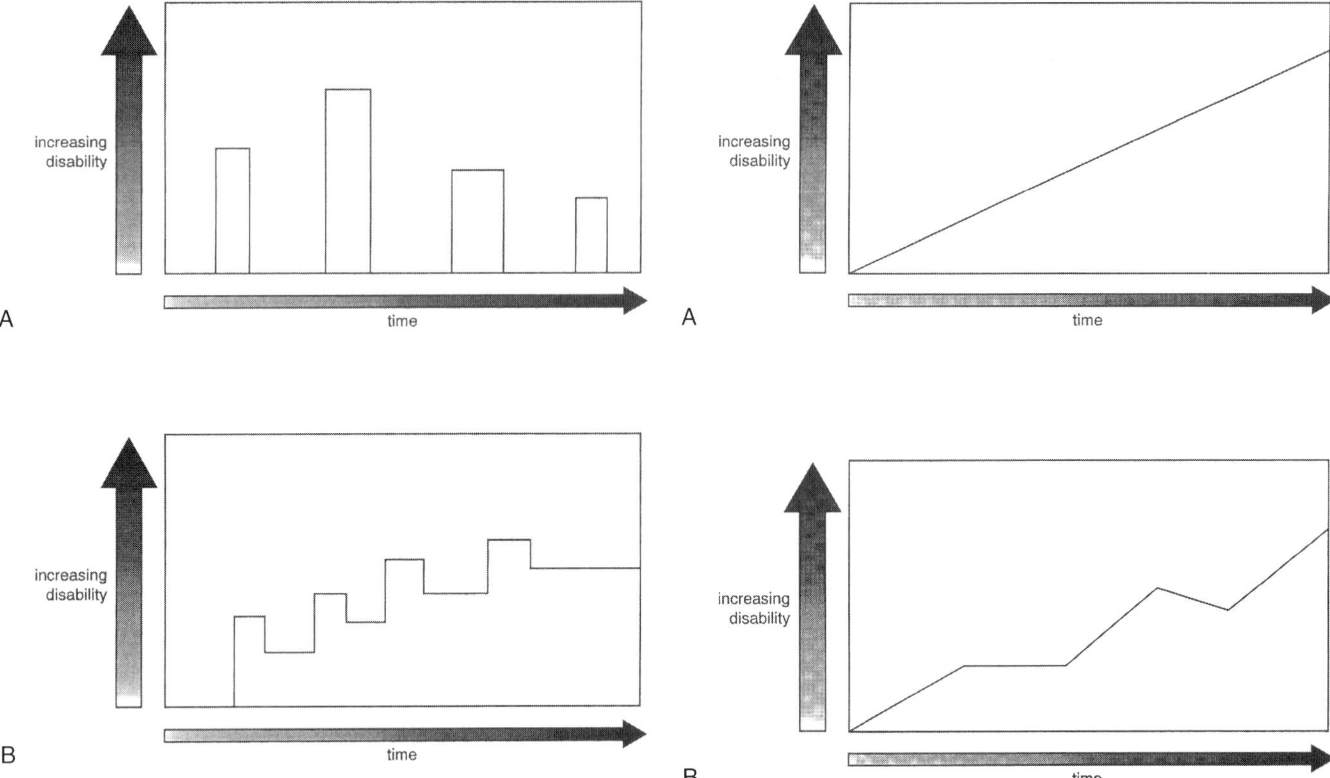

FIG. 31-1. Relapsing-remitting *(RR)* MS is characterized by clearly defined acute attacks with full recovery (**A**) or with sequelae and residual deficit on recovery (**B**). Periods between disease relapses are characterized by lack of disease progression. (From ref. 29, with permission.)

FIG. 31-2. Primary progressive *(PP)* MS is characterized by disease showing progression of disability from onset, without plateaus or remissions (**A**) or with occasional plateaus and temporary minor improvements (**B**). (From ref. 29, with permission.)

clinical findings are those of upper motor neuron dysfunction, with hyperreflexia, hypertonia, clonus, and Babinski responses. There is commonly demyelination of the corticospinal tracts in the spinal cord, but there may be involvement of the brainstem or deep cerebral white matter to account for these findings. The weakness may be asymmetric and on occasion may be mistaken for a stroke.

Sensory Symptoms

Aberrant sensation is extremely common in MS. It may be the presenting symptom in 20% to 55% of patients and is present in up to 70% of patients during the course of their disease (30). Sensory complaints include tingling, burning, or tightness. These may be patchy and fail to conform to any known dermatomal peripheral nerve distribution. The most frequent site of demyelinating lesions is in the posterior columns. Hence, vibratory sense is almost always reduced in the distal lower extremities; less frequently, joint position sense is impaired. Reduced pain and temperature sensation is sometimes detected (36).

L'hermitte's symptom is a sudden electric sensation that runs down the spine, usually when flexing the neck. Although not confined to MS, it is a well-recognized association that occurs in about 15% of cases (31). Another well-known but infrequent symptom in MS is trigeminal neuralgia, which is indistinguishable from that due to non-MS causes (32,33). It usually responds to carbamazepine. Headache is a rare symptom in MS, although it has been described in the literature in association with a lesion in the periaqueductal grey region (34).

Brainstem Symptoms

These symptoms include abnormalities in external ocular movements most frequently, including nystagmus and oscillopsia. Internuclear ophthalmoplegias, when present in a young person, are most characteristic of MS and should alert the clinician to this diagnosis. The pathologic lesion is in the medial longitudinal fasciculus.

Dysarthria, cranial nerve involvement, and myokymia are well-described brainstem findings in MS. Auditory dysfunction is rare, but on occasion it may be the presenting symptom of MS (35). Vertigo usually occurs as part of an exacerbation.

Dysphagia is not infrequent in MS, although it is usually associated with more severe, long-standing cases of

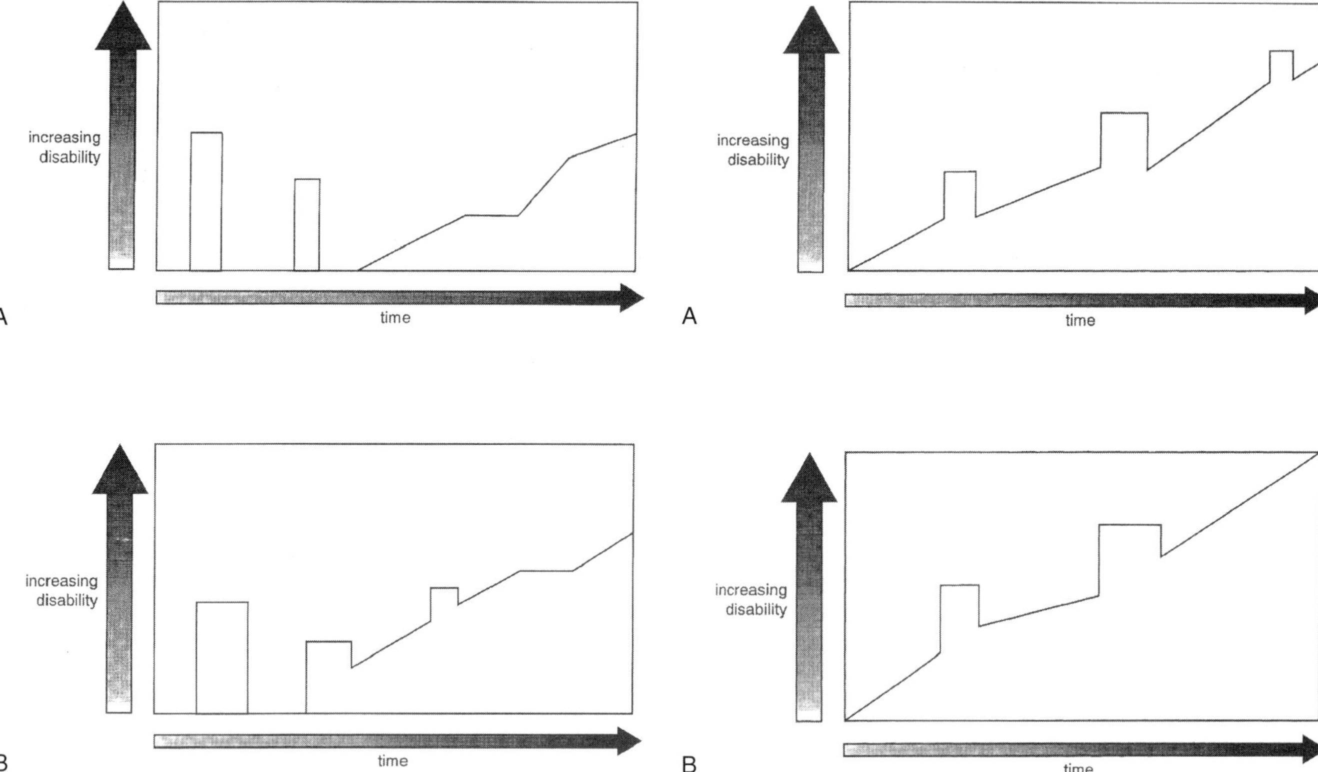

FIG. 31-3. Secondary progressive *(SP)* MS begins with an initial RR course, followed by progression of variable rate (**A**) that may also include occasional relapses and minor remissions (**B**). (From Ref. 29, with permission.)

FIG. 31-4. Progressive-relapsing *(PR)* MS shows progression from onset but with clear acute relapses with (**A**) or without (**B**) full recovery. (From ref. 29, with permission.)

the disease. Choking and coughing indicate aspiration into the airway. The only reliable way to determine the cause of aspiration is through a modified barium swallow, during which the swallowing process is observed and analyzed fluoroscopically. On the basis of the test, appropriate dietary interventions can be made. There may be no alternative to a feeding gastrostomy in patients who are at high risk for aspiration.

Visual Symptoms

Optic neuritis, which occurs frequently in MS, is one of the most characteristic symptoms. Visual acuity is decreased, often accompanied by ocular pain. Testing the visual fields may reveal a central scotoma or a variety of visual field abnormalities (37). The fundal examination may show a swollen disc, or it may appear quite normal. Frequently, an episode of optic neuritis may go undetected by the patient, but the clinical examination may reveal an afferent pupillary defect on the swinging light test. Visual evoked responses will detect asymptomatic involvement of the optic nerve.

Patients who are sensitive to the ambient temperature and who complain of heat sensitivity may experience transient visual, motor, or sensory deterioration when the core body temperature is increased. This is known as Uthoff's phenomenon. It is not associated with heightened disease activity, but rather it reflects slowed conduction in a demyelinated nerve in a warm environment. Cooling results in return of function to baseline (36).

The presence of cerebellar dysfunction is determined by the presence of dysmetria, intention tremor, dysdiadokokinesia, and gait ataxia. These result from both vermian and cerebellar hemispheral involvement. Cerebellar disease often is associated with a poor long-term outcome.

Cognitive and Psychiatric Symptoms

It was recognized recently that cognitive dysfunction in MS is common. The reported incidence varies, but it may be present in up to 90% of cases. Not all patients demonstrate profound dementia, but subtle abnormalities of cognition are common. Frequent reports include memory disturbance, poor concentration, and poor processing and acquisition of new information (38). Both euphoria and depression are common, and the incidence of suicide among persons with MS is significantly higher than in the general population (39).

Fatigue and Sleep

Fatigue, a common and disabling symptom, occurs in as many as 78% of patients. This problem can be differentiated from depression, side effects of medication, and the increased physical demands placed on a compromised neuromuscular system. Patients with MS also complain of disturbed sleep, which is more common than in the normal population, and may be associated with lesions at specific sites in the CNS. The cause of MS fatigue is unknown.

Treatment with pemoline or amantadine may be useful. In addition, the patient should be encouraged to arrange the day's activities to be able to rest whenever needed and to plan most activities for a time when fatigue is least (40,41).

Bowel, Bladder, and Sexual Dysfuntion

These common symptoms are among the most common and most disabling features of MS. There may be urinary frequency, urgency, or incontinence. These symptoms may result from a bladder that is irritable and fails to store urine or from a bladder that fails to empty properly. Measurement of a post-void residual volume will provide information as to the nature of the problem, whereafter appropriate treatment can be instituted. This would include an anticholinergic agent when the bladder is irritable and fails to store urine or having the patient learn the technique of intermittent straight catheterization when there is failure to empty the bladder. Sometimes there is a condition of a combination of failure to store and failure to empty, a condition known as *detrusor-sphinter-dyssynergia*, which requires a combination of anticholinergic medication together with intermittent catheterization. In patients who are catheterizing or who have an element of urinary retention, use of a urinary antiseptic such as HiprexR, one tablet twice a day, together with high doses of vitamin C (1 g, four times daily) may reduce the likelihood of urinary tract infection (42). When infection occurs, appropriate antibiotic treatment must be instituted.

Constipation is attributed to reduced bowel motility and possibly nonneuronal factors, such as lack of exercise, lack of fiber and adequate hydration, and the effects of medications, particularly the anticholinergic agents used for bladder dysfunction. Treatment includes high-fiber diets, adequate intake of water by mouth, and judicious use of bulking agents and laxatives. Diarrhea is uncommon in MS and, when present, should alert the physician to the possibility of spurious diarrhea secondary to constipation. A rectal examination should be performed, and regular bowel movements should be induced with suppositories or enemas.

Impotence in men is now amenable to effective intervention with intracavernous papavarine or prostaglandin E_1. A recent and exciting treatment of men with erectile dysfunction with prostaglandin E_1 delivered transurethrally has been described as having good clinical results (43,44). Women regularly complain of anorgasmia or decreased libido. These symptoms may reflect the primary disease or psychologic complications, and frequently both. The psychologic dysfunction is best managed by individual, couples, or group counseling.

CLINICAL COURSE

The course of MS is unpredictable. Typically, the early years are characterized by attacks and remissions. After about 10 years, almost 50% of patients will enter into a progressive phase of the disease, known as secondary progressive MS. Although this progression is insidious, the disease may remain stable for many years. In other cases, the disease may remain benign, with little or no disability. The factors that predispose to deterioration are not known. The role of stress and trauma have not been proved. In a prospective study by Bamford and colleagues, no association was found between trauma and the exacerbation of MS (45). Viral infections appear to trigger attacks, which may be due to the presence of high levels of γ-IFN associated with these events.

Because the course of the disease is difficult to predict clinically, attempts have been made to quantify impairment and disability in an attempt to prognosticate, to select patients for experimental protocols, and to determine their future needs. The most widely used of these scales is the Minimal Record of Disability (MRD), which addresses impairment, disability, and handicap. The Kurtzke system (46) is a two-part evaluation that assesses neurologic impairment. The Expanded Disability Status Scale (EDSS), originally constructed by Kurtzke and Granger, is a 20-step ordinal scale based on the neurologic examination that measures overall function of the patient through assignment of a numeric score selected from this scale. It relies heavily on the functional systems (FS), a series of eight functional groupings based on objective deficits elicited on the neurologic examination (Tables 31-5 and 31-6). Disability is measured by the Incapacity Status Scale, and handicap is measured by the Environmental Status Scale of Mellerup and Fog (47), which addresses the individual's social dysfunction as defined in different cultural settings. Another commonly used assessment scale is the Ambulation Index (AI), a 10-point ordinal scale that, similar to the EDSS, which is heavily weighted to gait. The timed 25-foot walk often is used by clinicians for evaluation of lower extremity function, and the 9-hole peg test is used to quantitatively evaluate upper extremity function (Table 31-7).

LABORATORY ABNORMALITIES

The diagnosis of MS is a clinical one, despite the development of new and sophisticated tests. The exami-

TABLE 31-5. *Kurtzke Expanded Disability Status Scale[a] and Functional Systems (FS) Scores*

Score	Definition
0.0	Normal neurologic examination (all grade 0 in FS)
1.0	No disability, minimal signs in one FS (i.e., grade 1).
1.5	No disability, minimal signs in more than one FS (more than one grade 1).
2.0	Minimal disability in one FS (one FS grade 2, others 0 or 1).
2.5	Minimal disability in two FS (two FS grade 2, others 0 or 1).
3.0	Moderate disability if one FS (one FS grade 3, others 0 or 1) or mild disability in three or four FS (three or four FS grade 2, others 0 or 1) though fully ambulatory.
3.5	Fully ambulatory, but with moderate disability in one FS (one grade 3) and one or two FS grade 2; or two grade 3 (others 0 or 1); or five grade 2 (others 0 or 1).
4.0	Fully ambulatory without aid, self-sufficient, up and about some 12 h/day, despite relatively severe disability consisting of one FS grade 4 (others 0 or 1), or combination of lesser grades exceeding limits of previous steps and the patient can walk ≥ 500 m without assist or rest.
4.5	Fully ambulatory without aid, up and about much of the day, may otherwise require minimal assistance; characterized by relatively severe disability, usually consisting of one FS grade 4 (others or 1) or combinations of lesser grades exceeding limits of previous steps and the patient can walk ≥ 300 m without assist or rest.
5.0	Ambulatory without aid or rest for at least 200 m; disability severe enough to impair full daily activities (e.g., to work a full day without special provision). (Usual FS equivalents are one grade 5 alone, others 0 or 1; combinations of lesser grades.)
5.5	Ambulatory without aid for at least 100 m; disability severe enough to preclude full daily activities. (Usual FS equivalents are one grade 5 alone, others 0 or 1; or combinations of lesser grades). Enough to preclude full daily activities.
6.0	Intermittent or unilateral constant assistance (cane, crutch, brace) required to walk at least 100 m with or without resting. (Usual FS equivalents are combinations with more than one FS grade 3.)
6.5	Constant bilateral assistance (canes, crutches, braces) required to walk at least 20 m. (Usual FS equivalents are combinations with more than one FS grade 3.)
7.0	Unable to walk at least 5 m even with aid, essentially restricted to wheelchair; wheels self and transfers alone; up and about in wheelchair some 12 h/day. (Usual FS equivalents are combinations with more than one FS grade 4+; very rarely pyramidal grade 5 alone.)
7.5	Unable to take more than a few steps; restricted to wheelchair; may need aid in transfer; wheels self but cannot carry on in wheelchair a full day. (Usual FS equivalents are combinations with more than one FS grade 4+.)
8.0	Essentially restricted to chair or perambulated in wheelchair, but out of bed most of day; retains many self-care functions; generally has effective use of arms. (Usual FS equivalents are combinations generally 4+ in several systems.)
8.5	Essentially restricted to bed most of day; has some effective use of arm(s); retains some self-care functions. (Usual FS equivalents are combinations generally 4+ in several systems.)
9.0	Helpless bed patient; can communicate and eat. (Usual FS equivalents are combinations, mostly grade 4+.)
9.5	Totally helpless bed patient; unable to communicate effectively or eat or swallow. (Usual FS equivalents are combinations almost all grade 4+.)
10.0	Death due to MS.

[a]EDSS steps below 5 refer to patients who are fully ambulatory, and the precise step is defined by the Functional System (FS) score(s). EDSS steps from 5 up are defined by ability to ambulate, and usual equivalents in FS score are provided.

nation of cerebrospinal fluid (CSF) was the first test to provide laboratory confirmation of MS. The typical profile is fewer than 50 mononuclear white blood cells, a mildly elevated protein concentration (<100 mg/mL), a normal glucose level, and an increase in immunoglobulin G (IgG) and oligoclonal bands. During an exacerbation, there may be myelin-basic protein detectable in the CSF. Since the advent of magnetic resonance imaging (MRI), there is seldom a need to perform a spinal tap when the clinical picture supports the diagnosis.

MRI has provided a useful adjunct for demonstrating periventricular, subcortical, callosal, brainstem, and spinal-cord white-matter abnormalities, which are present in about 90% of cases. The multifocal white matter lesions are seen on the T2-weighted images. The Fazekas criteria (48) for T2-weighted images consistent with MS require at least two of three findings to be present: a lesion next to the body of the lateral ventricles, an infratentorial lesion, and a lesion larger than 5 mm in diameter. Another set of criteria (49) requires at least four hyperintense lesions or three lesions larger than or equal to 3 mm, with at least one periventricular in location to be strongly suggestive of MS. Several other conditions may reveal white-matter abnormalities on MRI. These include normal aging, cerebrovascular disease, human T-cell lymphotrophic virus (HTLV)-I-associated myelopoathy, the collagen vascular disorders, human immunodeficiency virus (HIV) encephalitis, progressive multifocal leukoen-

TABLE 31-6. *Kurtzke Functional Systems (FS)*

Pyramidal functions
- 0 Normal
- 1 Abnormal signs without disability
- 2 Minimal disability
- 3 Mild to moderate paraparesis or hemiparesis; or severe monoparesis
- 4 Marked paraparesis or hemiparesis; moderate quadriparesis; or monoplegia
- 5 Paraplegia, hemiplegia, or marked quadriparesis
- 6 Quadriplegia
- 9 Unknown

Cerebellar functions
- 0 Normal
- 1 Abnormal signs without disability
- 2 Mild ataxia
- 3 Moderate truncal or limb ataxia
- 4 Severe ataxia in all limbs
- 5 Unable to perform coordinated movements because of ataxia
- 9 Unknown

Brain stem functions
- 0 Normal
- 1 Signs only
- 2 Moderate nystagmus or some other mild disability
- 3 Severe nystagmus, marked extraocular weakness, or moderate disability of other cranial nerves
- 4 Marked dysarthria or other marked disability
- 5 Inability to swallow or speak
- 9 Unknown

Sensory function
- 0 Normal
- 1 Vibration or figure-writing decrease only in one or two limbs
- 2 Mild decrease in touch or pain or position sense, and/or moderate decrease in vibration in one or two limbs; or vibratory decrease alone in three or four limbs
- 3 Moderate decrease in touch or pain or position sense, and/or essentially lost vibration in one or two limbs; or mild decrease in touch or pain and/or moderate decrease in all proprioceptive tests in three of four limbs
- 4 Marked decrease in touch or pain or loss of proprioception, alone or combined, in one or two limbs; or moderate decrease in touch or pain and/or severe proprioceptive decrease in more than two limbs
- 5 Loss (essentially) of sensation in one or two limbs; or moderate decrease in touch or pain and/or loss of proprioception for most of the body below the head
- 6 Sensation essentially lost below the head
- 9 Unknown

Bowel and bladder function: (rate on the basis of worse function, either bowel or bladder)
- 0 Normal
- 1 Mild urinary hesitancy, urgency, or retention
- 2 Moderate hesitancy, urgency, retention of bowel or bladder or rare urinary incontinence (intermittent self-catheterization, manual compression to evacuate bladder, or finger evacuation of stool)
- 3 Frequent urinary incontinence
- 4 In need of almost constant catheterization (and constant measures to evacuate stool)
- 5 Loss of bladder function
- 6 Loss of bladder and bowel function
- 9 Unknown

Visual (or optic) functions
- 0 Normal
- 1 Scotoma with visual acuity (corrected) better than or equal to 20/30
- 2 Worse eye with scotoma with maximal visual acuity (corrected) of 20/30 or 20/59
- 3 Worse eye with large scotoma, or moderate decrease in fields, but with maximal visual acuity (corrected) of 20/60 to 20/99
- 4 Worse eye with marked decrease of fields and maximal visual acuity (corrected) of 20/100 or 20/200; grade 3 plus maximal acuity of better eye of 20/60 or less
- 5 Worse eye with maximal visual acuity (corrected) less than 20/200; grade 4 plus maximal acuity of better eye of 20/60 or less
- 6 Grade 5 plus maximal visual acuity of better eye of 20/60 or less
- 9 Unknown

Cerebral (or mental) function
- 0 Normal
- 1 Mood alteration only (does not affect DSS score)
- 2 Mild decrease in mentation
- 3 Moderate decrease in mentation
- 4 Marked decrease in mentation (chronic brain syndrome—moderate)
- 5 Dementia or chronic brain syndrome—severe or incompetent
- 9 Unknown

Other functions (any other neurological findings attributable to MS)
- Spasticity
  - 0 None
  - 1 Mild (detectable only)
  - 2 Moderate (minor interference with function)
  - 3 Severe (major interference with function)
  - 9 Unknown
- Other
  - 0 None
  - 1 Any neurological findings attributed to MS: specify__________
  - 9 Unknown

cephalopathy, and migraine, among others. Although still a controversial topic, there is increasing evidence that there is a substantial relation between the MRI parameters and the clinical manifestations of the disease. The MRI is widely used and is an invaluable tool in clinical trials in MS. Magnetic resonance spectroscopic imaging may yield further information on the natural history and response to therapeutic interventions.

Evoked potential tests (EPs) have been used for the past 20 years to aid in the diagnosis of MS. They are sensitive, reproducible, objective, and can be quantified easily to two or three significant figures. They represent electric potentials that are evoked by brief sensory stimuli. At a site of demyelination, the signals are either delayed or blocked. Visual EPs can be elicited with a checkerboard-patterned reversal device or a strobe flash;

TABLE 31-7. *Ambulation Index (AI)*

Score	Definition
0	Asymptomatic; fully active; no gait abnormality reported or observed.
1	Walks normally but reports fatigue or difficulty running which interferes with athletic or other demanding activities.
2	Abnormal gait or episodic imbalance; gait disorder is noticeable to family and friends, and evident to examiner. Able to walk 25 ft in 10 sec or less.
3	Walks independently; requires ≥ 10 sec, but able to walk 25 ft in 20 sec or less.
4	Requires unilateral support (cane, single crutch) to walk; uses support more than 80% of the time. Walks 25 ft in 20 sec or less.
5	Requires bilateral support (canes, crutches, walker) and walks 25 ft in 20 sec or less; or requires unilateral support, but walks 25 feet in greater than 20 sec.
6	Requires bilateral support and walks 25 ft in greater than 20 secs. May use wheelchair on occasion.
7	Walking limited to several steps with bilateral support; unable to walk 25 ft. May use wheelchair for most activities.
8	Restricted to wheelchair; able to transfer independently.
9	Restricted to wheelchair; unable to transfer independently.

Reprinted with permission from Hauser, Dawson, Lehrich et al. Immunosuppression in progressive multiple sclerosis and randomized high dose intravenous cyclophosphamide plasma and ACTH. N Engl Med 1983;308;173–180.

the former is more sensitive. The large positive polarity seen at 100 ms after each stimulus is called the P100. This is delayed in the optic nerve that has been demyelinated. It is abnormal in virtually all patients who have had an episode of optic neuritis and is more sensitive than the MRI in detecting demyelinating lesions in the optic nerves, chiasm, and optic tracts. In the absence of a history of optic neuritis, the visual EPs are abnormal in about 50% of patients (50).

Brainstem auditory EPs detect lesions in the pons and midbrain (51). The typical abnormalities that occur in MS include a prolongation of waves II–V, as determined by the I–V interpeak latencies, and a loss of amplitude of wave V, determined by V/I amplitude ratio, and disappearance of V.

Neither brainstem nor visual EPs are pathognomonic of MS. Brainstem auditory EPs are more sensitive than MRI in the diagnosis of pontine lesions, but they are not more sensitive than MRI in making an initial diagnosis of MS. Somatosensory EPs may detect clinically silent lesions in sensory pathways in MS. They may be useful in the assessment of spinal cord pathways and may complement the MRI in atypical MS cases.

In summary, several laboratory tests are available to aid in the diagnosis of MS. In typical cases, these tests may be redundant, but they are useful tools in the not infrequent atypical case that may pose a diagnostic dilemma.

DIAGNOSIS

The most common presenting symptom of MS is numbness in the extremities. Weakness, fatigue, visual loss (optic neuritis), ataxia, sphincteric disturbances, and acute brainstem dysfunction (e.g.,vertigo, diplopia, facial weakness) are also frequent initial symptoms. By definition, these symptoms must be present for at least 24 hours. The diagnosis is made on clinical grounds. A solid history of at least two separate episodes of dysfunction involving the cerebral white matter (e.g., visual loss, weakness, ataxia, brainstem dysfunction) in addition to support on the clinical examination for at least two lesions in anatomically separate sites is required. The MRI may be a useful adjunct in making the diagnosis. As mentioned, evoked potentials and examination of the spinal fluid may be necessary in atypical cases.

The prognosis is uncertain and cannot be stated with certainty. There are known clinical associations with both benign and poor outcomes. These are outlined in the list below:

Type of course	Characteristics
Benign	None or few exacerbations No or little disability noted Identified incidentally on MRI or autopsy
Relapsing-progressive	Random attacks over a number of years, may be more frequent in the first years Variable recovery, may be incomplete Permanent residual deficits may result with each attack
Chronic progressive	Slow decline in neurologic function, primarily with spinal cord involvement, in patients with onset of disease after age 40 years

Most patients with relapsing remitting MS eventually develop chronic disease. By 10 years after the diagnosis, as many as 58% of patients have entered into a chronic progressive phase of the disease, with rare or no exacerbations but rather a slow and steady decline. The older the age of onset, the more progressive the nature of the disease. Men tend to have poorer outcomes compared with women (52).

TREATMENT

Recent exciting developments in the treatment of MS afford hope that finally there may be a treatment intervention that may alter the natural history of the disease. The drug treatments for MS recently were reviewed (92), and three treatments were approved for use in treating remitting-relapsing MS. These include two synthetically produced beta-interferons: Betaseron (53,54,55) and Avonex (56,57). A third agent, called Copaxone, a glatirimer acetate, is now available (58,59). These treatments are all injectable compounds known to cause allergic side effects that vary in severity and duration in individual users. These agents reduce the frequency of MS exacerbations and, in the case of Avonex, slow disease progression and reduce the number of lesions on serial MRIs. It is important to realize that none of these treatments is complete and that only a third of patients respond to any one treatment. There is no available study concerning use of these agents in pregnancy; they are therefore not recommended in women who are actively planning a pregnancy. If a patient becomes pregnant while taking any of these treatments, discontinuation is advised until after delivery.

Other therapies that have been tried in MS include oral azothiaprine (60,61,62), cyclophosphamide (60,63,64), total lymphoid irradiation (60,65), and plasma exchange (68,69,70). These treatments are not considered useful based on currently availabe information. Weekly treatment with oral methotrexate has been demonstrated to be of benefit in patients with progressive MS, particularly with regard to upper-extremity function (66). Recent studies with cladribine (2Cd-A, Leustatin) in progressive MS have been disappointing (67). Oral myelin was not effective in a recently performed study (72,74,75). T-cell vaccination and T-cell receptor therapy are not clinically applicable at this time (71). Linomide, a promising anticancer compound, was discontinued in clinical trials when it was shown to have cardiotoxicity (73). Monoclonal antibodies may prove effective in slowing the course of the disease (71,72).

Many treatments are available for the symptomatic treatment of MS and include oral or intravenous corticosteroid treatment for acute exacerbations. Treatment usually is indicated for disabling symptoms that are accompanied by objective neurologic dysfunction (77–80). There is no need to treat sensory symptoms with corticosteroids. A special circumstance is that of acute optic neuritis. The results of a recent multicenter study suggest that intravenous corticosteroid treatment is superior to oral prednisone (81,82).

Spasticity, a sign of upper-motor neuron pathology, is treated with baclofen, and sometimes with additional small doses of diazepam. Because both of these agents act on γ-amino butyric acid receptors in the spinal cord, they are synergistic in their effect in reducing spasticity. A new agent called tizanidine (Zanaflex) was recently approved by the U.S. Food and Drug Administration (FDA) for treatment of spasticity (83). In cases refractory to oral agents, placement of a pump to deliver baclofen intrathecally has been most successful (84). Management of the bladder, bowel, and sexual dysfunction already has been alluded to in an earlier section of this chapter.

PREGNANCY

MS does not appear to affect fertility and is not associated with an increased incidence of birth defects, spontaneous abortions, or stillbirths among women with MS. Uncomplicated MS has no effect on the pregnancy, labor, or delivery. The effect of pregnancy on MS has been studied (85). There is no evidence that the relapse rate is increased during pregnancy. In fact, some data suggest that there may be a reduction in the number of relapses during gestation (86–88). The relapse rate appears to increase during the first 3 months postpartum, and about 30% to 40% of women will experience an exacerbation at this time. This period may extend 6 months into the postpartum period. The reasons are unclear. There is evidence that other autoimmune diseases are improved during pregnancy and worsen during the postpartum period. It is possible that proteins secreted by the placenta and fetus, together with the high glucocorticoid environment caused during pregnancy, may suppress the disease, as shown in the experimental animal model of MS, EAE, whereby there is a decline in the susceptibility of pregnant animals to induction of EAE, and they experience a more benign course (90).

Retrospective studies have shown that there is no difference in the long-term outcome of disability in MS patients who have had children compared with those who have not. Poser and Poser, in a study of 512 women with MS, concluded that pregnancy was not linked to an increased rate of disease progression (89).

Before becoming pregnant, patients should discontinue use of all immunosuppressant drugs and all nonessential medications. These precautions should have been discussed with the patient before the initiation of potentially teratogenic therapies.

Patients should be aware of the increased risk for urinary tract infections, and appropriate treatment should be initiated if infection does occur. There may be worsening of both bladder and bowel function as a result of the mechanical effects of the pregnancy.

No special provisions are necessary for delivery. In patients with myelopathy, outlet forceps may be needed to assist delivery, because the mother may be unable to exert bearing-down efforts or may be too exhausted to do so. Whereas epidural anesthesia is preferred, there is no evidence that general, spinal, or epidural anesthesia may predispose to disease exacerbations.

The patient may require extra temporary help at home, or more disabled patients may need permanent assistance. A study investigating the use of immune globulin in the postpartum period to prevent exacerbations suggests that this may be useful, but the numbers are too small to draw definitive conclusions (91). Some physicians recommend prophylactic treatment with corticosteroids following delivery in an attempt to diminish the possibility of an exacerbation, but there is no documentation that this is beneficial or even wise. There is no evidence for the use of β-IFN to prevent a disease exacerbation at this time (86). Although only a theoretic concern, the medication is precluded in nursing mothers, because the effects of β-IFN on breastfeeding infants are unknown.

Preconceptional Counseling

There is no reason to advise an abortion in a pregnant MS patient. The patient should be warned of the potential for a flareup of the disease in the first 6 months postpartum. There is no evidence that pregnancy affects the long-term disability outcome in a woman who has given birth to a child. The only difference appears to be when the patient becomes a mother. The risk of her offspring developing MS was discussed earlier in this chapter. Patients need to be aware of the potential for physical deterioration over time and the need to ensure that the child will be cared for adequately, if not by the mother, then by another reliable and caring person. In many cases, this person turns out to be a family member. Because the course of the disease is not altered by pregnancy over the long term, there is a good chance that the mother may remain well without experiencing increasing disability. There is little information regarding the effect of MS on offspring whose parents have MS. A study by Kalb and colleagues (unpublished) involving parents and children in 20 families revealed that children, in many ways, cope better than their parents. The children's primary concerns were with their parents' emotional distress and the emotional climate within the household. Parents who were clearly in need of help and support were reluctant to seek this help in the belief that their children were not being affected by the MS. Education of families from the time of diagnosis and inclusion of children in the comprehensive care model from the outset may allow families to communicate more effectively, enable them to address the needs of a parent with MS more effectively, and alleviate for the parent with the disease the anxiety and guilt associated with having to ask for help with family issues.

SUMMARY AND CONCLUSIONS

MS remains an enigmatic and incurable disease of the CNS. There are many facets to the disease that impact on all aspects of the life of the affected individual. The challenge to develop and treat the disease continues, and research in the field remains extremely active. The mere fact that in the last 5 years there are three FDA-approved treatments for MS gives hope and encouragement to the patient, treating physicians, and the families of affected persons.

REFERENCES

1. Traugott U. Evidence for immunopathogenesis. In: Cook S, ed. Handbook of multiple sclerosis. New York: Marcel Dekker, 1990.
2. Abbas AK, Lichtman AH, Poser JS. Cellular and molecular immunology. In: Diseases caused by humoral and cell-mediated immune reactions. Philadelphia: WB Saunders, 1991.
3. Traugott U. Alterations of the blood-brain barrier by components of the immune system. In: Regulatory mechanisms of neuron to vessel communication in the brain (NATO ASI series H33). Heidelberg: Springer Verlag, 1989.
4. Traugott U, Frohman E, Scheinberg LC. Role of adhesion molecules in the immunopathogenesis of multiple sclerosis lesions. Neurology 1989; 39(Suupl):171.
5. Washington R, Burton J, Todd RF, Newman W, Dragovic L, Dore-Duffy P. Expression of immunologically relevant endothelial cell activation antigens on isolated central nervous system microvessels from patients with multiple sclerosis. Ann Neurol 1994;35:89–97.
6. Sibley WA, Bamford CR, Clark K. Clinical viral infections and multiple sclerosis. Lancet 1985;1313:13–15.
7. Panitch HS, Hirsch RL, Haley AS, Johnson KP. Exacerbations of multiple sclerosis in patients treated with gamma-interferon. Lancet 1987; 8538:893–895.
8. Riikonen R. The role of infection and vaccination in the genesis of optic neuritis and multiple sclerosis in children. Acta Neurol Scand 1989; 80:425–431.
9. Lu C-Z, Jensen MA, Arnason BGW. Interferon gamma and interleukin-4-secreting cells in multiple sclerosis. J Neuroimmunol 1993;46: 123–128.
10. Haffler DA, Weiner HL. Multiple sclerosis: a CNS and systemic autoimmune disease. Immunol Today 1989;10:104–107.
11. Hofman FM, Hinton DR, Johnson K, Merrill JE. Tumor necrosis factor identified in multiple sclerosis brain. J Exp Med 1989;170:607–612.
12. Traugott U, Lebon P. Multiple sclerosis: involvement of interferons in lesion pathogenesis. Ann Neurol 1988;24:243–251.
13. Selmag K, Raine CS, Cannella B, Brosnan CF. Identification of lymphotoxin and tumor necrosis factor in multiple sclerosis lesions. J Clin Invest 1991;87:949–954.
14. Trotter JL, Collins KG, VanderVeen RC. Serum cytokine levels in chronic progressive multiple sclerosis: interleukin-2 levels parallel tumor necrosis factor-alpha levels. J Neuroimmunol 1991;33:29–36.
15. Ebers GC, Paty DW, Stiller CR, Nelson RF, Seland TP, Larsen B. HLA typing in multiple sclerosis sibling pairs. Lancet 1982;2:88–90.
16. Ebers GC, Bulman DE, Sandovnick AD, Paty DW, et al. A population based study of multiple sclerosis in twins. N Engl J Med 1986;315: 1638–1642.
17. Sadovnick AD, Armstrong H, Rice GPA, et al. A population-based study of multiple sclerosis in twins: update. Ann Neurol 1993;33: 281–285.
18. Sandovnick AD, Baird PA, Ward RH. Multiple sclerosis: updated risks for relatives . Am J Med Genet 1988;29:533–541.
19. Ebers GC, Sandovnick AD. The role of genetic factors in multiple sclerosis susceptibility. J Neuroimmunol 1994;54:1–17.
20. Sandovnick AD, Baird PA. The familial nature of multiple sclerosis: age corrected empiric recurrence risks for children and siblings of patients. Neurology 1988;38:990–991.
21. Sandovnick AD, Ebers GC. Epidemiology of multiple sclerosis: a critical overview. Can J Neurol Sci 1993;20:17–29.
22. Challoner PB, Smith KT, Parker JD, et al. Plaque-associated expression of human herpesvirus 6 in multiple sclerosis. Proc Natl Academy Sci U S A 1995;92:7440–7444.
23. Pryse-Phillips W. Epidemiology of multiple sclerosis. In: Cook SD, ed. Handbook of multiple sclerosis. New York: Marcel Dekker, 1996:1–17.
24. Anderson DW, Ellenberg JH, Leventhal CM, Reingold SC, Rodriquez M, Silberberg DH. Revised estimate of the prevalence of multiple sclerosis in the United States. Ann Neurol 1992;31:333–336.
25. Martyn CN. The epidemiolgy of multiple sclerosis. In: Matthews WB ed. McAlpine's multiple sclerosis, 2nd ed. New York: Churchill Livingstone, 1991.
26. Prineas J. Pathology of multiple sclerosis. In: Cook SD. Handbook of multiple sclerosis. New York: Marcel Dekker, 1996.
27. Bornstein MB,Raine CS. Experimental allergic encephalomyelitis. Antiserum inhibition of myelination in vitro. Lab Invest 1970;23: 536–542.

28. Prineas JW, Kwon EE, Goldenberg PL, Cho ES, Sharer LR. Interaction of astrocytes and newly formed oligodendrocytes in resolving multiple sclerosis lesions. Lab Invest 1990;63:624–636.
29. Lublin FD, Reingold SC. Defining the clinical course of multiple sclerosis: results of an international survey. National Multiple Sclerosis Society (USA) Advisory Committee on Clinical Trials of New Agents in Multiple Sclerosis. Neurology 1996;46:907–911.
30. Kurtzke JF. Clinical manifestations of multiple sclerosis. In: Vinken PJ, Bruyn GW, eds. Handbook of clinical neurology, vol 9. Multiple sclerosis and other demyelinating diseases. Amsterdam: North Holland, 1970:161–216.
31. Kunchandi R, Howe JG. Lhermitte's sign in multiple sclerosis: a clinical survey and review of the literature. J Neurol Neurosurg Psychiatry 1982;45:308–312.
32. Clifford DB, Trotter JL. Pain in multiple sclerosis. Arch Neurol 1984; 41:1270–1272.
33. Moulin De, Foley KM, Ebers GC. Pain syndromes in multiple sclerosis. Neurology 1988;38:1830–1834.
34. Haas DC, Kent PR, Friedman DL. Headache caused by a single lesion of multiple sclerosis in peiaqueductal grey area. Headache 1993;33: 452–455.
35. Drulovic B, Riberic-Jankes K, Kostic V, Sternic N. Sudden hearing loss as the initial monosymptom of multiple sclerosis. Neurology 1993;43: 2703–2705.
36. Miller AE. Clinical features. In: Cook SD, ed. Handbook of multiple sclerosis. New York: Marcel Dekker, 1996.
37. Frederiksen JL, Larsson HB, Nordeno AM, Seedorff HH. Plaques causing hemianopsia or quadrantanopsia in multiple sclerosis identified by MRI and VEP. Acta Ophthalmol 1991;69:169–177.
38. Peyser JM.Edwards KR, Poser CM, Filsov SB. Cognitive function in patients with multiple sclerosis. Arch Neurol 1980;37:577–579.
39. Schiffer RB. The spectrum of depression in multiple sclerosis: an approach for clinical management. Arch Neurol 1987;44:596–599.
40. Krupp LB, Alvarez LA, Larocca NG, Scheinberg LC. Fatigue in multiple sclerosis. Arch Neurol 1988;45:435–437.
41. Krupp LB, Coyle PK, Doscher C, et al. Fatigue therapy in multiple sclerosis: results of a double-blind, randomized, parallel trial of amantadine, pemoline and placebo. Neurology 1995;45:1956–1961.
42. Boyarsky S, Labay P, Nanick P, et al. Care of the patient with neurogenic bladder. Boston: Little Brown and Company, 1979.
43. Kirkeby HJ, Poulsen ZV, Petersen T, Dorup J. Erectile dysfunction in multiple sclerosis. Neurology 1988;38:1366–1371.
44. Padma-Nathan H, Hellstrom WJ, Kaiser FE, et al. Treatment of men with erectile dysfunction with tsansurethral alprostadil: medicated urethral system for erection (MUSE) Study Group. N Engl J Med 1997; 336:1–7.
45. Bamford CR, Sibley WA, Thies C, Laguna JF, Smith MS, Clark K. Trauma as an etiologic and aggravating factor in multiple sclerosis. Neurology 1981;31:1229–1234.
46. Kurtzke JF. Rating neurologic impairment in multiple sclerosis: an expanded disability status scale (EDSS). Neurology 1983;33: 1114–1452.
47. Mellerup E, Fog T. The socioeconomic scale. Acta Neurol Scand 1981; 64(Suppl)89:130–138.
48. Fazekas F, Offenbacker H, Fuchs S, Schmidt R, Niederkom K, Horner S, Lechner H. Criteria for an increased specificity of MRI interpretation in elderly subjects with suspected multiple sclerosis. Neurology 1988;38:1822–1825.
49. Paty DW, Oger JJF, Kastrukoff LF, Hashimoto SA, Hooge JP, Eisen AA, Eisen KA, Purves SJ, Low MD, Brandies V, et al. MRI in the diagnosis of MS: a prospective study with comparison of clinical evaluation, evoked potential, oligoclonal banding and CT. Neurology 1988;38: 180–185.
50. Richey ET, Kooi KA, Tourtellotte WW. Visually evoked responses in multiple sclerosis. J Neurol Neurosurg Psychiatry 1971;34:275–280.
51. Purves SJ, Low MD, Galloway J, Reeves B. A comparison of visual, brainstem auditory, and somatosensory evoked potentials in multiple sclerosis. Can J Neurol Sci 1981;8:15–19.
52. Weinshenker BG, Bass B, Rice GPB, Noseworthy JH, Carriere W, Bakersville J, Ebers GC. The natural history of multiple sclerosis: a geographically-based study 1. Clinical course and disability. Brain 1989; 112:133–146.
53. The IFNB Multiple Sclerosis Study Group. Interferon beta-1b is effective in relapsing-remitting multiple sclerosis I. Clinical results of a multicenter, randomized, double-blind, placebo-controlled trial. Neurology 1993;43:655–661.
54. Paty DW, Li DK. Interferon beta- 1b is effective in relapsing- remitting multiple sclerosis: MRI results of a multicenter randomized, double-blind placebo-controlled trial. Neurology 1993;43:662–667.
55. Arnason BGW. Interferon beta in multiple sclerosis. Neurology 1993; 43:641–643.
56. Jacobs L. Results of a phase III trial of intramuscular recombinant beta interferon as treatment for multiple sclerosis. 119th Meeting of the American Neurological Association, San Francisco, CA, 1994.
57. Jacobs LD, Cookfair DL, Rudick RA, et al. Intramuscular interferon beta-1b for disease progression in relapsing multiple sclerosis. Annal Neurol 1996;39:285–294.
58. Bornstein MB, Miller A, Slagel S, et al. A pilot trial of Cop I in exacerbating-remitting multiple sclerosis. N Engl J Med 1987;317:408–414.
59. Johnson KP, Brooks BR, Cohen JA, et al. Copolymer I reduces relapse rate and improves disability in relapsing-remitting multiple sclerosis: results of a phase III multicenter, double-blind, placebo-controlled trial. Neurology 1995;45:1268–1276.
60. Ellison GW. Immunosuppressive drugs in multiple sclerosis. In: Cook SD, ed. Handbook of multiple sclerosis. New York: Marcel Dekker, 1996:465–488.
61. Goodkin DE, Bailly RC, Teetzen ML, Hertsgaard D, Beatty WW . The efficacy of azothiaprine in relapsing-remitting multiple sclerosis. Neurology 1991;41:20–25.
62. Yudkin PL, Ellison GW, Ghezzi A, et al. Overview of azothiaprine treatment in multiple sclerosis. Lancet 1991;338:1051–1055.
63. The Canadian Cooperative Multiple Sclerosis Study Group. The Canadian cooperative trial of cyclphosphamide and plasma exchange in progressive multiple sclerosis. Lancet 1991;337:441–446.
64. Weiner HL, Mackin GA, Orav EJ, et al. Intermittent cyclophosphamide pulse therapy in progressive multiple sclerosis: final report of the Northeast Cooperative Multiple Sclerosis Treatment Group. Neurology 1993;43:910–918.
65. Cook SD, Troiano R, Rohowsky-Kochan C, et al. Treatment of patients with progressive multiple sclerosis with total lymphoid irradiation. In: Cook SD, ed. Handbook of multiple sclerosis. New York: Marcel Dekker, 1996.
66. Goodkin DE, Rudick RA, VanderBrug Medendorp S, Daughty MM, Schwetz KM, Fischer J, VanDyke C. Low dose (7.5 mg) oral methotrexate reduces rate of progression in chronic progressive multiple sclerosis. Ann Neurol 1995;37:30–40.
67. Sipe JC, Romine JS, Koziol JA, McMillan R, Zyroff J, Beutler E. Cladribine in treatment of chronic progressive multiple sclerosis. Lancet 1994;344:9–13.
68. Khatri BO. Plasma exchange and lymphocytopharesis therapy in multiple sclerosis. In: SD Cook, ed. Handbook of multiple sclerosis. New York: Marcel Dekker, 1996.
69. Weiner HL, Dawson DM. Plasmapharesis in multiple sclerosis: preliminary study. Neurology 1980;30:1029–1033.
70. Dau PC, Petajan JM, Johnson KP, Panitch HS, Bornstein MB. Plasmapheresis in multiple sclerosis: preliminary findings. Neurology 1980; 30:1023–1028.
71. Lindsey JW, Hodgkinson S, Mehta R, et al. Phase I clinical trial of chimeric monoclonal anti-CD4 antibody in multiple sclerosis. Neurology 1994;44:413–419.
72. Weiner HL, Hohol MJ, Khoury SJ, Dawson DM, Hafler DA. Therapy for multiple sclerosis. Neurol Clin 1995;13:173–196.
73. Karussis DM, Lehmann D, Slavin S, et al. Inhibition of acute experimental autoimmune encephalomyelitis by the synthetic immunomodulator linomide. Ann Neurol 1993;34:654.
74. Weiner HL, Friedman A, Miller A, et al. Oral tolerance: immunologic mechanisms and treatment of animal murine and human organ specific autoimmune diseases by oral administration of autoantigens. Annu Rev Immunol l994;12:809–837.
75. Weiner HL, Mackin GA, Matsui M, et al. Double-blind pilot trial of oral tolerization with myelin antigens in multiple sclerosis. Science 1993;259:1321–1324.
76. Dowling PC, Bosch VV, Cook SD. Possible beneficial effect of high dose intravenous steroid therapy in acute demyelinating disease and transverse myelitis. Neurology 1980;30:33–36.
77. Goas JY, Marion JL, Missoum A. High dose intravenous methylpred-

nisolone in acute exacerbations of multiple sclerosis. J Neurol Neurosurg Psychiatry 1983;46:99.

78. La Mantia L, Eoli M, Milanese C, Salmaggi A, Dufour A, Torri V. Double blind trial of dexamethasone versus methylprednisolone in multiple sclerosis acute relapses. Eur Neurol 1994;34:194–203.
79. Miller DH, Thompson AJ, Morrissey SP, et al. High dose steroids in acute relapses of multiple sclerosis: MRI evidence for a possible mechanism of therapeutic effect. J Neurol Neurosurg Psychiatry 1992;55: 450–453.
80. Trotter JL, Garvey WF. Prolonged effects of large-dose methylprednisolone infusion in multiple sclerosis. Neurology 1980;30:702–708.
81. Beck RW, Cleary PA, Anderson MM, et al. A randomised controlled trial of corticosteroids in the treatment of acute optic neuritis. N Engl J Med 1992;326:581–588.
82. Beck RW, Cleary PA, Trobe JD, et al. The effect of corticosteroids for acute optic neuritis on the subsequent development of multiple sclerosis. N Engl J Med 1993;329:1764–1769.
83. Smith CR, Birnbaum G, Carter JL, Greenstein J, Lublin FD. Tizanidine treatment of spasticity caused by multiple sclerosis: results of a double-blind placebo-controlled trial. Neurology 1994;44:(Suppl 9):S34–S43.
84. Penn RD, Savoy SM, Corcos D, et al. Intrathecal baclofen for severe spinal spasticity. N Engl J Med 1989;320:1517–1521.
85. Cook SD, Troiano R, Bansil S, Dowling PC. Multiple sclerosis and pregnancy. Adv Neurol 1994;64:83–95.
86. Weinreb HJ. Demyelinating and neoplastic diseases in pregnancy. Neurol Clin 1994;12:509–526.
87. Frith, JA, McLeod JG. Pregnancy and multiple sclerosis. J Neurol Neurosurg Psychiatry 1988;51:495–498.
88. Roullet E, Verdier-Taillefer MH, Amaremco P, Gharbi G, Alperovitch A, Marteau R. Pregnancy and multiple sclerosis: a longitudinal study of 125 remittent patients. J Neurol Neurosurg Psychiatry 1993;56: 1062–1065.
89. Poser S, Poser W. Multiple sclerosis and gestation. Neurology 1983;33: 1422–1427.
90. Abramsky O, Lubetzki-Korn I, Evron S, Brenner T. Suppressive effect on pregnancy on multiple sclerosis and EAE. Prog Clin Biol Res 1984; 146:399.
91. Achiron A, Rotstein Z, Noy S, Mashiach S, Dulitzky M, Achiron R. Intravenous immunoglobulin treatment in the prevention of childbirth-associated acute exacerbations in multiple sclerosis: a pilot study. J Neurol 1996;243:25–28.
92. Rudick RA, Cohen JA, Weinstock-Guttman B, Kinkel RP, Ransohoff RM. Management of multiple sclerosis. N Engl J Med 1997;337: 1604–1611.

Cherry and Merkatz's Complications of Pregnancy,
Fifth Edition, edited by W. R. Cohen.
Lippincott Williams & Wilkins, Philadelphia © 2000.

CHAPTER 32

Headaches

Stephen D. Silberstein

This chapter discusses the diagnosis, differential diagnosis, and prevalence of migraine and other headache disorders that occur during pregnancy and the necessity and safety of diagnostic testing for headache. This is followed by a summary of the adverse effects of drugs on the fetus and recommendations for headache treatment based on a review of the literature and personal experience. The International Headache Society (IHS) divides headaches into two broad categories: *primary* and *secondary* headache disorders. Secondary headaches are symptoms of another disease and can be caused by intracranial or extracranial structural abnormalities or by systemic or metabolic conditions. In the primary headache disorders, the headache itself is the illness (Table 32-1). The primary headache disorders include migraine, tension-type headache (TTH), and cluster headache. Chronic daily headaches (CDH), a term in common use but not recognized by the IHS, may be due to chronic TTH, prolonged or transformed migraine, or hemicrania continua and is often associated with abortive medication overuse (1).

Headache prevalence is age dependent. Migraine prevalence peaks near age 40 and declines afterward (Fig. 32-1). With aging not only is there a change in prevalence of the primary headache disorder, but a shift to new or organic causes of headache (2).

The first step in establishing a diagnosis is a complete history, which should include the patient's age at headache onset; location, severity, and type of pain; attack frequency (including any change in frequency); associated symptoms; precipitating and relieving factors; patient's sleep habits; and family history. A complete medication history should be taken to evaluate the doses, duration of use, and effectiveness of previous headache medications as well as to determine if any medications that could exacerbate headaches are being used or overused (3). This will not only serve as a baseline but will help with preconceptional counseling.

Having patients keep a diary will alert the physician to any changes that occur between office visits, especially if medication was modified. Patients should bring their medications with them periodically in order for the physician to check for compliance, to be sure they are using the medications appropriately, and to see if other physicians have prescribed additional medications.

Headache diagnosis is primarily clinical, based mainly on the history and on the physical and neurologic examinations, and sometimes on diagnostic testing. Primary headache disorders occur during pregnancy; however, conditions that mimic them also may occur at this time (4,5). For example, a new-onset migraine with aura can be due to a symptomatic disorder such as vasculitis, brain tumor, or occipital arteriovenous malformation (AVM)

TABLE 32-1. *International Headache Society classification*

1. Migraine
2. Tension-type headache
3. Cluster headache and chronic paroxysmal hemicrania
4. Miscellaneous headaches unassociated with structural lesion
5. Headache associated with head trauma
6. Headache associated with vascular disorders
7. Headache associated with nonvascular intracranial disorder
8. Headache associated with substances or their withdrawal
9. Headache associated with noncephalic infection
10. Headache associated with metabolic disorder
11. Headache or facial pain associated with disorder of cranium, neck, eyes, ears, nose, sinuses, teeth, mouth, or other facial or cranial structures
12. Cranial neuralgias, nerve trunk pain and deafferentation pain

S. D. Silberstein: Department of Neurology, Thomas Jefferson University, Jefferson Headache Center, Thomas Jefferson University Hospital, Philadelphia, PA 19107.

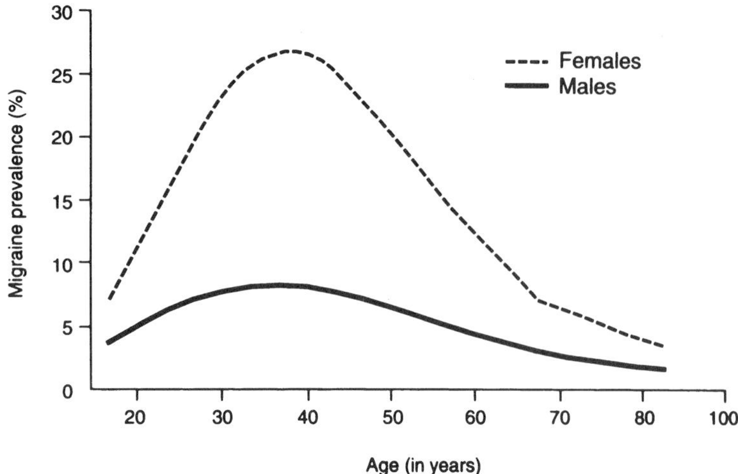

FIG. 32-1. Migraine prevalence by age. Prevalence increased from 12 to 38 years of age in both women and men; the peak was considerably higher among women. (From Silberstein SD, Lipton RB. Headache epidemiology: emphasis on migraine. Neurol Clin 1996;14:421–434.)

(6). Sinusitis, meningitis, and idiopathic intracranial hypertension can present as intractable headache (6). Subarachnoid hemorrhage (SAH) can present as a severe episode of acute-onset headache. These symptomatic conditions require neuroimaging or a lumbar puncture (LP) for diagnosis. Some disorders are more common or occur exclusively during pregnancy and produce headache. These include stroke, cerebral venous thrombosis, eclampsia, SAH, pituitary tumor, and choriocarcinoma (7,8). Idiopathic intracranial hypertension does not occur more frequently than expected during pregnancy (5).

Investigation of headache, and migraine in particular, is controversial, and few guidelines exist. In fact, in a typical healthy migraineur, laboratory tests may not be necessary for diagnosis; however, some laboratory tests are usually recommended prior to treatment. Even less is known about the need to investigate other types of headache. Systemic secondary causes of headache often cannot be diagnosed by physical examination; therefore, laboratory studies are performed to rule them out (6).

Diagnostic testing serves to (a) confirm the clinical diagnosis; (b) exclude other causes of headache; (c) rule out comorbid diseases that could complicate headache and its treatment; (d) establish a baseline for and exclude contraindications to drug treatment; and (e) measure drug levels to determine absorption, patient compliance, or medication overuse (5).

Lumbar Puncture

Lumbar puncture is crucial in four distinct clinical situations: (a) a "first or worst" headache, with the suspicion of an intracranial infection or SAH; (b) a severe, rapid-onset, recurrent headache; (c) a progressive headache; and (d) a chronic intractable or atypical headache disorder (9). If increased intracranial pressure is suspected, LP should be performed after neuroimaging, except when meningitis is suspected, in which case it should not be delayed.

Neuroimaging

Head computerized tomography (CT) is relatively safe during pregnancy and is the study of choice for head trauma and possible nontraumatic subarachnoid, subdural, or intraparenchymal hemorrhage. For all other nontraumatic or nonhemorrhagic craniospinal pathology, magnetic resonance imaging (MRI) is preferred. Magnetic resonance angiography (MRA) should be used first to evaluate any suspected vascular pathology; but when necessary, standard angiography is reasonably safe in the pregnant patient (Table 32-2).

Indications for CT or MRI in headache investigation during pregnancy include the first or worst headache of the patient's life, particularly if it is of abrupt onset (thunderclap headache); a change in the frequency, severity, or

TABLE 32-2. *Guidelines for neuroimaging the patient who is or may be pregnant*

Determine the necessity and the potential risks of the procedure.
If possible, perform the examination during the first 10 days postmenses, or if the patient is pregnant, delay the examination until the third trimester or preferably postpartum.
Pick the procedure with the highest accuracy balanced by the lowest radiation.
Use MRI if possible.
Avoid direct exposure to the abdomen and pelvis.
Avoid contrast agents.
Do not avoid radiologic testing purely for the sake of the pregnancy.
If significant exposure is incurred by a pregnant patient, consult a radiation biologist.
Consent forms are neither required nor recommended.

MRI; magnetic resonance imaging.
Adapted from Schwartz RB. Neurodiagnostic imaging of the pregnant patient. In: Neurologic complications of pregnancy. Devinsky O, Feldman E, Hainline B, eds. New York: Raven Press, 1994.

clinical features of the headache attack; an abnormal neurologic examination; a progressive or new daily persistent headache; neurologic symptoms that do not meet the criteria of migraine with typical aura; persistent neurologic defects; definite electroencephalographic evidence of a focal cerebral lesion; an orbital or skull bruit suggestive of arteriovenous malformation; and new comorbid partial (focal) seizures (6).

MIGRAINE

Prevalence

Migraine is an episodic headache disorder that may be preceded by a prodrome and initiated by an aura. Migraine occurs in 4% of children, 6% of men, and 18% of women. Sixty-two percent of migraineurs also have TTH (10). Migraine usually begins in the first three decades of life, and prevalence peaks in the fifth decade (11). The prognosis for migraine sufferers is good because migraine prevalence decreases with increasing age (10). Migraine in women is influenced by hormonal changes throughout the life cycle: menarche, menstruation, oral contraceptive use, pregnancy, menopause, and hormonal replacement therapy may all influence the presence and nature of migraine. Migraine can occur for the first time during pregnancy; preexisting migraine may worsen, particularly during the first trimester; or the patient may become headache free in later pregnancy. Some women with migraine have no change in their headache pattern during pregnancy (12). The true incidence of migraine in pregnancy is uncertain, and most reported cases have been of migraine with aura or prolonged aura. Migraine prevalence decreases with menopause, although the prevalence does not fall to premenarchal levels.

In the past, migraine headaches were known as either classic migraine or common migraine, based on the presence or absence of an aura (4). Common migraine is now called *migraine without aura;* classic migraine is now called *migraine with aura.* Either type may be associated with premonitory phenomena that develop hours to days before the headache attack. Examples include hyper- or hypoactivity, depression, irritability, difficulty concentrating, or food cravings, especially for chocolate (4).

Clinical Features

Migraine diagnosis depends on the characteristics of the pain and associated features. To diagnose for migraine without aura using the IHS criteria (Table 32-3) requires the patient to have had at least five headache attacks (1). A diagnosis of migraine with aura (classic migraine) requires the patient to have had at least two attacks with at least three of the characteristics listed in Table 32-4. If the aura lasts longer than 1 hour but less than 1 week, the condition is called migraine with prolonged aura (1). The migraine aura may occur without the headache, and migraine may remit or become transformed into chronic daily headache (with or without medication overuse).

Migraine aura occurs in about 20% of patients. It usually develops over 5 to 20 minutes, lasts 20 to 30 minutes, and consists of focal neurologic symptoms (visual, sensory, motor, or speech) that accompany the headache or occur up to an hour before it begins (13). Visual symptoms are the most common and include scintillations (fluorescent flashes of light in the visual field), fortification spectra or teichopsia (alternating light and dark lines in the visual field), photopsia (flashing lights), positive scotomata (bright geometric lights in the visual field), and negative scotomata (blind spots

TABLE 32-3. *Migraine without aura: diagnostic criteria*

A. At least five attacks fulfilling B–D
B. Headache lasting 4–72 h (untreated or unsuccessfully treated)
C. Headache has at least two of the following characteristics:
   1. Unilateral location
   2. Pulsating quality
   3. Moderate or severe intensity (inhibits or prohibits daily activities)
   4. Aggravation by walking stairs or similar routine physical activity
D. During headache at least one of the following:
   1. Nausea and/or vomiting
   2. Photophobia and phonophobia
E. No evidence of organic disease

Adapted from Headache Classification Committee of the International Headache Society. Classification and diagnostic criteria for headache disorders, cranial neuralgia, and facial pain. Cephalalgia 1988;8(suppl 7):1–96.

TABLE 32-4. *Migraine with aura: diagnostic criteria*

A. At least two attacks fulfilling B
B. At least three of the following four characteristics:
   1. One or more fully reversible aura symptoms indicating focal cerebral cortical, brain stem dysfunction, or both
   2 At least one aura symptom develops gradually over more than 4 minutes, or two or more symptoms occur in succession
   3. No aura symptom lasts more than 60 min; if more than one aura symptom is present, accepted duration is proportionally increased
   4. Headache follows aura with a free interval of less than 60 min (it may also begin before or simultaneously with the aura)
C. No evidence of organic disease

Adapted from Headache Classification Committee of the International Headache Society. Classification and diagnostic criteria for headache disorders, cranial neuralgia, and facial pain. Cephalalgia 1988;8(suppl 7):1–96.

that may move across the visual field). Sensory symptoms are less common and include numbness, tingling, or paresthesias of the face or hand. Motor symptoms are usually hemiparetic, whereas language disturbances consist of difficulty speaking (aphasia) or understanding (14,15).

The headache of migraine can begin at any time during the day, usually developing gradually and subsiding after 4 to 72 hours (16). A headache lasting longer than 72 hours defines status migrainosus. The pain is moderate to severe in intensity and usually described as throbbing or pulsating. Pain is usually unilateral, but may begin as, or become, bilateral (16). Strictly unilateral headaches are not of concern because they occur in 20% of migraineurs. Accompanying symptoms are common: most patients are anorectic and have nausea; some vomit or have diarrhea. Photophobia and phonophobia cause patients to seek relief in a dark, quiet room to decrease sensory stimulation. Most patients have one to four attacks a month (15).

After the headache phase, some patients experience a postdrome, or recovery, phase that may last up to 24 hours. Some patients feel tired, others feel alert; some feel depressed, others feel euphoric; some feel worn out, whereas others feel refreshed. Some may complain of poor concentration, food intolerance, or scalp tenderness (13).

Tension-Type Headache

Tension-type headache is the most common headache type, with a lifetime prevalence of 69% in men and 88% in women. TTH can begin at any age, but onset during adolescence or young adulthood is most common. The IHS criteria for TTH are listed in Table 32-5. The headache may be shorter or longer in duration than migraine.

Tension-type headache is mild or moderate in intensity and has no accompanying autonomic symptoms. The cause of this common disorder is unknown, but it is not related to muscular tension (patients with migraine have more muscle tension than patients with TTH).

Acute TTH often responds to nonpharmacologic treatment. If the headache does not respond to this approach and medication is needed, many patients self-medicate with over-the-counter analgesics (aspirin, acetaminophen, ibuprofen, naproxen), with or without caffeine. Combination analgesics contain sedatives or caffeine, and their use should be limited because overuse may cause dependence. Narcotic analgesics and benzodiazepines should be avoided due to their abuse potential. Overusing symptomatic medications, including tranquilizers and analgesics, can cause episodic TTH to convert to chronic TTH (17). In women who are attempting to become or who are pregnant, the drugs should be used with the precautions outlined in the treatment section later in this chapter.

Chronic Daily Headache

Chronic daily headache may be due to chronic TTH or transformed migraine and is often associated with medication overuse (Table 32-6). It is important to determine the cause of CDH so that the appropriate treatment can be chosen. When concurrent depression and medication dependence accompany CDH, treatment is difficult and detoxification may be required. This is particularly

TABLE 32-5. *Tension-type headache (IHS)*

Episodic tension-type headache: diagnostic criteria

- A. At least 10 previous headache episodes fulfilling criteria B–D listed below. Number of days with such headache <180/yr (<15/mo)
- B. Headache lasting from 30 min to 7 days
- C. At least two of the following pain characteristics
  1. Pressing/tightening (nonpulsating) quality
  2. Mild or moderate intensity (may inhibit, but does not prohibit activities)
  3. Bilateral location
  4. No aggravation by walking stairs or similar routine physical activity
- D. Both of the following:
  1. No nausea or vomiting (anorexia may occur)
  2. Photophobia and phonophobia are absent, or one but not the other is present

Chronic tension-type headache: diagnostic criteria

- A. Average headache frequency >15 days/mo (180 days/yr) for >6 months fulfilling criteria B–D
- B. At least two of the following pain characteristics:
  1. Pressing/tightening quality
  2. Mild or moderate severity (may inhibit but does not prohibit activities)
  3. Bilateral location
  4. No aggravation by walking stairs or similar routine physical activity
- C. Both of the following:
  1. No vomiting
  2. No more than one of the following: nausea, photophobia, or phonophobia

Adapted from Headache Classification Committee of the International Headache Society. Classification and diagnostic criteria for headache disorders, cranial neuralgia, and facial pain. Cephalalgia 1988;8 (suppl 7):1–96.

TABLE 32-6. *Chronic daily headache*

Primary
- Headache duration greater than 4 h
  - Transformed migraine
  - Chronic tension-type headache
  - New daily persistent headache
  - Hemicrania continua
- Headache duration less than 4 h
  - Cluster headache
  - Chronic paroxysmal hemicrania
  - Hypnic headache
  - Idiopathic stabbing headache

Secondary
- Posttraumatic headache
- Cervical spine disorders
- Headache associated with vascular disorders [arteriovenous malformation, arteritis (including giant cell arteritis), dissection, subdural hematoma]
- Headache associated with nonvascular intracranial disorders [intracranial hypertension; infection (EBV, HIV), neoplasm]
- Other (temporomandibular joint disorder; sinus infection)

Adapted from Headache Classification Committee of the International Headache Society. Classification and diagnostic criteria for headache disorders, cranial neuralgia, and facial pain. Cephalalgia 1988;8(suppl 7):1–96.

important in women who want to become pregnant. Under these circumstances both the amounts and the types of medicine used must be limited. Refractory rebound headaches may occur when aspirin, acetaminophen, or opiate-containing analgesics are overused or when analgesics are taken more frequently than 3 days a week or ergotamine tartrate more often than 2 days a week. To avoid this situation, headache medication must be used within defined limits (17).

Cluster Headache

Cluster headache prevalence is lower than that of migraine or TTH, with a rate of 0.01% to 0.24% in various populations. In contrast to migraine, prevalence is higher in men (70%–90%) than in women (Table 32-7). Cluster headache can begin at any age: it most commonly begins in the late twenties, rarely in childhood, and occasionally (10%) in patients in their sixties (2,18). The prognosis of cluster headaches is guarded; it is a chronic headache disorder that may last for the patient's entire life.

Episodic cluster headache features symptoms that last 1 week to 1 year, with remission periods lasting at least 14 days. Chronic cluster headache has either no remission periods or remissions that last less than 14 days. Cluster attacks may begin with slight discomfort that rapidly increases (within 15 minutes) to excruciating pain. The attacks often occur at the same time each day and frequently awaken patients from sleep. Attacks generally last for 30 to 90 minutes, but may last up to 180 minutes and often occur once or twice a day. Patients may say, "It's like driving a hot poker in my eye." Tearing occurs in most patients. Patients with cluster headaches should avoid alcohol and nitroglycerin.

TABLE 32-7. *Cluster headache*

A. At least five attacks fulfilling B–D
B. Severe unilateral orbital, supraorbital and/or temporal pain lasting 15–180 min untreated
C. Headache is associated with at least one of the following signs which have to be present on the pain side:
   1. Conjunctival injection
   2. Lacrimation
   3. Nasal congestion
   4. Rhinorrhea
   5. Forehead and facial sweating
   6. Miosis
   7. Ptosis
   8. Eyelid edema
D. Frequency of attacks: from one every other day to eight per day.
E. No evidence of organic disease.

Adapted from Headache Classification Committee of the International Headache Society. Classification and diagnostic criteria for headache disorders, cranial neuralgia, and facial pain. Cephalalgia 1988;8(suppl 7):1–96.

DIFFERENTIAL DIAGNOSIS

Headache of sudden onset and extended duration may result from a subarachnoid hemorrhage or an unruptured aneurysm. More benign causes of this condition include crash migraine and coital cephalgia (6).

Thunderclap Headache

Thunderclap headache is defined as the sudden onset of a severe headache that reaches maximum intensity within 1 minute. Some further define it by the absence of an SAH. An acute neurologic event must be ruled out in all patients who present with severe, acute-onset headache, even though migraine can present in this manner as well.

Exertional and Cough Headaches

Transient, severe head pain upon coughing, sneezing, weight-lifting, bending, straining at stool, or stooping defines exertional headache. MRI must be performed at the appropriate time to rule out hind-brain abnormalities, such as brain tumor (most commonly meningioma), Arnold-Chiari malformation, pineal cyst, basilar impression, and acoustic neurinoma. If no abnormality is found, the diagnosis of benign cough headache may be made.

Other Serious Organic Causes of Headache

Several structural brain abnormalities can cause intense, bilateral headaches that last minutes. Colloid cysts and other third ventricle masses may produce intermittent headaches with dizziness, blurred or double vision (some due to sixth nerve palsy), drop attacks, and, rarely, sudden death.

Headache Associated with Mass Lesions

Headache occurs at presentation in up to half of patients with brain tumors and develops in the course of the disease in 60% (see Chapter 33). Headache is partly dependent on tumor location: it is a rare initial symptom in patients with pituitary tumors, craniopharyngiomas, or cerebellopontine angle tumors (19).

The postulated mechanisms of headache development include traction on pain-sensitive intracerebral vessels, transient herniation of hippocampal gyri, traction on cranial or cervical nerves, or elevation of intracranial pressure. Although increased cerebrospinal fluid (CSF) pressure is not necessary for headache development, it clearly plays a role in a group of patients with central nervous system neoplasms (19).

In a modern series, 111 consecutive patients with primary (34%) or metastatic (66%) brain tumor were diagnosed by neuroimaging procedures (1). Increased intracranial pressure was defined by the presence of papilledema, obstructive hydrocephalus, communicating hydrocephalus from leptomeningeal metastasis, or a CSF opening pressure at lumbar puncture of more than 250 mm. Headache, present in 48% of both primary and metastatic tumor, was similar to TTH in 77% and to migraine in 9% of patients. Unlike true TTH, brain tumor headaches were worsened by bending in 32%, and nausea or vomiting was present in 40% (20).

Most patients with increased intracranial pressure had a bilateral, frontal, aching headache; only 1% had a unilateral headache. The headache was constant in 61%. The pain was often severe, associated with nausea and vomiting, and resistant to common analgesics. Ataxia was present in 61%. In contrast, only 36% of patients with a supratentorial tumor without increased intracranial pressure had headache. These headaches were milder and more likely to be intermittent (however, they were constant in 20% of patients). Nausea, vomiting, and ataxia were much less common (20).

There is a significant overlap between brain tumor headache and migraine and TTH. A headache of recent onset or one that has changed in character, particularly if the headache is severe or occurs with nausea or vomiting, or any headache accompanied by a neurologic sign or symptom that cannot be easily explained by the aura of migraine requires a thorough evaluation. Morning or nocturnal headache associated with vomiting and increased headache frequency may be seen with both migraine and brain tumor. Brain tumor headache is more common in patients with a history of prior headache, increased intracranial pressure, and large tumors with a midline shift (19).

Patients with brain abscesses, in contrast, often have a progressively severe, intractable headache. In published clinical series, headache was present in 70% to 90% of such patients (21). The higher headache prevalence in abscess, as compared with tumor, may be due to the rapid evolution, the associated meningeal reaction, and the occasional low-grade fever that may accompany abscess.

PREGNANCY AND MIGRAINE

Mechanisms

The relationship between migraine and sex hormones is well-known. Menarche, menstruation, oral contraceptive use, pregnancy, menopause, and hormone replacement therapy affect migraine, in part by changing a woman's estrogen levels. Estrogen levels do not differ in nonpregnant women with or without menstrual migraine. Rising or sustained high estrogen levels have been proposed as the mechanism of migraine relief that often occurs during pregnancy; this mechanism, however, cannot explain the worsening or new appearance of migraine that sometimes occurs (22). The rapid decrease of estrogen levels may be responsible for menstrual and postpartum migraine. Women with a prior history of migraine are more likely to develop postpartum migraine (23).

Migraine relief during pregnancy is not dependent on adequate protective levels of progesterone. No statistical differences in progesterone levels, measured near term, are found between women who did not have migraine relief during pregnancy and those who did, suggesting that migraine relief does not depend on the absolute blood level of progesterone (24).

The key to the genesis of migraine may be the intrinsic estrogen receptor sensitivity of the hypothalamic neurons. In most women, increasing or sustained estrogen levels decrease headache. In some women, these same changes could induce headache (25).

Course of Migraine During Pregnancy

Most migraineurs improve during pregnancy, whereas some women without prior migraine will experience their first migraine headache (Table 32-8). Case reports (12, 22,26,27) emphasize the presence of focal neurologic symptoms in new-onset migraine because patients with these dramatic presentations are more likely to be referred to a neurologist.

In reported series of migraineurs, most women improved during pregnancy. Lance (28) found migraine improved in 58% of 120 pregnant women, whereas 42% worsened or had no change. Sixty-four percent of women with menstrual migraine had relief during pregnancy, com-

TABLE 32-8. *Migraine and pregnancy*

	Lance (28)	Callaghan (29)	Somerville (24)	Bousser (30)	Granella et al. (31)	Rasmussen (32)	Chen and Leviton (33)	Maggioni et al. (35)
Women studied		200	200	703	1300	975	55,000	430
History of migraine and pregnancies	120	41	38	116	943	80	484	80
Number of pregnancies	252	200	200	147	943		484	173
New migraine during pregnancy	0	33/41 (80%)	7/38 (18%)	16/147 (11%)	12 (1.3%)	?	0	1/428
New migraine postpartum			?	42 (4.5%)	?	0	?	
Prior migraine	252	8	31	131	571	80	484	93
Prior migraine improved	145/252 (58%)	4 (50%)	24/31 (77%)	102/131 (78%)	384/571 (67.3%)	48%	382/484 (79%)	88%
Prior migraine unchanged or worsened	107/252 (42%)	3 (38%)	7/31 (23%)	29/131 (22%)	187/571 (32.7%)	52%	102/484 (21%)	80/93 86
Type series	R,H	R,H	R,H	R,O	R,H	R,POP	P,O	R,H

H, headache or neurologic; P, prospective; R, retrospective; POP, population based; O, obstetrical.

pared with 48% of those without menstrual migraine. Lance did not look at migraine incidence during pregnancy.

Callaghan (29) found that only eight women of 200 in his study had migraine before their pregnancy; of these, 4 improved. In contrast to all other series, 33 of the 200 patients developed migraine during pregnancy, with new attacks occurring during each trimester (16 during the first, 9 during the second, and 8 during the third trimester).

Callaghan's (29) unusual finding that migraine prevalence during pregnancy is much higher than migraine prevalence prior to pregnancy prompted Somerville (24) to study an antenatal population of 200 women in Australia in the early 1970's. Thirty-eight had migraine; 31 of these had a prior history of migraine, and 7 first developed migraine while pregnant (5 women in the first trimester, 1 in the second trimester, and 1 in the third trimester). Seventy-seven percent of women with preexisting migraine improved during their pregnancy. Somerville did not distinguish between migraine with and without aura.

Bousser (30) interviewed 703 patients postnatally and found that 116 women (147 pregnancies) had IHS migraine. Preexisting migraine improved or disappeared in 102 of 131 pregnancies (77.9%), worsened in 10 (7.6%), was unchanged in 11 (8.4%), and was variable in 8 (6.1%). Migraine appeared for the first time in 16 women. Disappearance or improvement did not differ significantly in migraine with or without aura, but worsening was much more common in migraine with aura. Improvement was more frequent in women with menstrual migraine. No significant difference was found in any of the three trimesters of pregnancy.

Granella and colleagues (31) analyzed retrospectively 1,300 migraineurs attending a headache clinic in Italy. During pregnancy complete remission occurred in 17.4%; 49.2% had significant improvement and only 3.5% worsened. Women whose migraine started with menarche had a higher remission rate than did women whose headaches began at other times (36.4% versus 13.9%). Migraine began during pregnancy in 1.3% of the patients and postpartum in 4.5%.

Rasmussen (32) evaluated 1,000 women in a cross-sectional epidemiologic study. Eighty migraineurs in the group had been pregnant. Of these, 48% had no change, 49% had disappearance or significant improvement in their headache, and only 4% worsened.

Chen and Leviton (33) analyzed the data from the prospective Collaborative Perinatal Project of 55,000 pregnant women in the United States. Only 2% of these women had self-reported migraine, an underascertainment of true migraine prevalence, perhaps because only severe cases were identified. Of those analyzable (n = 484), 17% had a complete remission and another 62% showed some improvement with pregnancy. No correlation to menstrual migraine was attempted. In a much smaller series, Scharff and colleagues (34) recruited 30 women who were more than 10 weeks pregnant. They reported a nonsignificant decrease in all headache types including migraine and TTH, more so for the primiparous women. The general trend toward improvement was supported by Maggioni and colleagues (35), who evaluated 428 women 3 days postpartum. Eighty-one had migraine without aura and 12 had migraine with aura. One new case of migraine without aura began during pregnancy. Of the migraineurs, 86% had at least a 50% decrease in attack frequency, usually after the first trimester.

Outcome of Pregnancy in Migraineurs

The incidence of miscarriage, toxemia, congenital anomalies, and stillbirth was not increased in a sample of 777 migraine sufferers compared with the national averages or controls (36). However, in Chancellor's small series, four of nine patients developed complications, including preeclampsia in two (22). This may be due to selection artifact in a very small sample.

Postpartum Migraine

Stein (23) prospectively followed 71 randomly selected women during their first postpartum week. Postnatal headache (PNH) occurred in 39%. It was most frequent on days 3 to 6 postpartum and was associated with a past history or a family history of migraine. PNH, although less severe than the patients' typical migraine, was bifrontal, prolonged, and associated with photophobia, nausea, and anorexia. MacArthur and colleagues (37) investigated 11,701 women by a postal questionnaire. By 3 months postpartum, newly occurring frequent headache occurred in 3.6% of the women and migraine in 1.4%. The definition of migraine was not stated.

Summary

We can conclude from available data that, although some women have their first attack during pregnancy, most women with migraine improve during pregnancy. Migraine often recurs postpartum and can begin for the first time during that interval. Despite drug use, migraineurs do not differ from nonmigraineurs in the frequency of miscarriages, preeclampsia, congenital anomalies, or stillbirths.

HEADACHE TREATMENT

Risk of Drug Treatment

Although studies have not absolutely established the safety of any medication during pregnancy, some are thought to be relatively safe (38–42). Most drugs cross the placenta and have the potential to affect the fetus adversely. Drugs are routinely tested in animals to uncover any teratogenic effects, but these findings cannot always be extrapolated to humans (39,43–45). Consequently, caution must be exercised to be sure that potential benefits outweigh possible risks of any headache drug given during pregnancy (see Chapter 7).

Drug Risk Categories

The U.S. Food and Drug Administration (FDA) lists five categories of labeling for drug use in pregnancy (Table 32-9) (40,46). These categories are intended to provide therapeutic guidance, weighing the risks as well as the benefits of the drug. An alternative rating system is TERIS, an automated teratogen information resource wherein ratings for each drug or agent are based on a consensus of expert opinion and the literature (Table 32-10) (47). It was designed to assess the teratogenic risk to the fetus from a drug exposure. The FDA categories often have little correlation to the TERIS teratogenic risk assessment. This discrepancy results in part from the fact that the FDA categories were designed to provide therapeutic guidance, and the TERIS ratings are useful for estimating the teratogenic risks of a drug and not vice versa (48).

TABLE 32-9. *FDA risk categories*

Category A:	Controlled human studies show no risk
Category B:	No evidence of risk in humans, but there are no controlled human studies
Category C:	Risk to humans has not been ruled out
Category D:	Positive evidence of risk to humans from human and/or animal studies
Category X:	Contraindicated in pregnancy

Headache Treatment

The major concern in the management of pregnant patients is the effect of both medication and the disease on the fetus. Because of the possible risk of injury to the fetus, medication use should be limited; however, it is not contraindicated during pregnancy (49). Because migraine usually improves after the first trimester, many women can manage their headaches with this reassurance and nonpharmacologic treatment. Some women, however, will continue to have severe, intractable headaches, sometimes associated with nausea, vomiting, and possible dehydration. Not only are these conditions disruptive to the patient, they may pose a risk to the fetus that is greater than the potential risk of the medications used to treat the pregnant patient (44,49).

Symptomatic treatment, designed to reduce the severity and duration of symptoms, is used to treat an acute headache attack (Tables 32-11 and 32-12). Individual attacks should be treated with rest, reassurance, and ice packs. For headaches that do not respond to those measures, symptomatic drugs are indicated. The nonsteroidal antiinflammatory drugs (NSAIDs), acetaminophen (alone or with codeine), codeine alone, or other opiods

TABLE 32-10. *TERIS risk rating*

Undetermined (C)
None (A)
None-minimal (A)
Minimal (B)
Minimal-small (D)
High (X)

Equivalent FDA ratings in parenthesis.

TABLE 32-11. *Some therapeutic medications*

	Fetal risk	
	FDA	TERIS
Simple analgesics		
Aspirin	C^a (D)	None-minimal
Acetaminophen	B^a	None
Caffeine	B^a	None-minimal
NSAIDs		
Ibuprofen	B^a (D)	None-minimal
Indomethacin	B^a (D)	None
Naproxyn	B^a (D)	Undetermined
Narcotics		
Butorphanol	C_M (D)	
Codeine	C_M (D)	None-minimal
Meperidine	B^a (D)	None-minimal
Methadone	B^a (D)	None-minimal
Morphine	B^a (D)	None-minimal
Ergots and serotonin agonists		
Ergotamine	X_M	Minimal
Dihydroergotamine	X_M	Undetermined
Sumatriptan	C_M	Undetermined
Corticosteroids		
Dexamethasone	C^a	None-minimal
Prednisone	B^a	None-minimal
Barbiturates		
Butalbital	C^a (D)	None-minimal
Phenobarbital	D^a	None-minimal
Benzodiazepam		
Chlordiazepoxide	D^a	None-minimal
Diazepam	D^a	None-minimal

Elements within parentheses indicate risk factor if used at the end of the third trimester.
M, manufacturer's; NSAIDs, nonsteroidal antiinflammatory drugs.
[a]Briggs', not manufacturer's list.
Risk factor used at end of third trimester

can be used during pregnancy. Aspirin in low intermittent doses is not a significant teratogenic risk, although large doses, especially if given near term, may be associated with maternal and fetal bleeding. Aspirin should probably be avoided unless there is a definite therapeutic need for it (other than headache). NSAIDs have the potential to close or narrow the ductus arteriosus, especially in late pregnancy. Although there are probably no significant consequences of short-term ductus closure in healthy fetuses, more long-term effects could be considerable. Barbiturate and benzodiazepine use should be limited. Ergotamine, dihydroergotamine, and sumatriptan should be avoided (44).

The associated symptoms of migraine, such as nausea and vomiting, can be as disabling as the headache pain itself. In addition, some medications that are used to treat migraine can produce nausea. Metoclopramide, which decreases the gastric atony seen with migraine and enhances the absorption of coadministered medications, is extremely useful in migraine treatment. Mild nausea can be treated with phosphorylated carbohydrate solution (emetrol) or doxylamine succinate and vitamin B_6 (pyridoxine). More severe nausea may require the use of injections or suppositories. Trimethobenzamide, chlorpromazine, prochlorperazine, and promethazine are available orally, parenterally, and by suppository and can all be used with relative safety. We frequently use promethazine and prochlorperazine suppositories. Corticosteroids can be used occasionally. Some use prednisone in preference to dexamethasone (which crosses the placenta more readily).

TABLE 32-12. *Neuroleptics/antiemetics*

	Fetal risk	
	FDA	TERIS
Antihistamines		
Cyclizine (Marezine)	B^a	
Cyproheptadine	B_M	Undetermined
Dimenhydrinate (Dramamine)	B_M	None-minimal
Meclizine (Antivert)	B_M	None-minimal
Neuroleptics		
Phenothiazines		
Chlorpromazine (Thorazine)	C^a	None-minimal
Prochlorperazine (Compazine)	C^a	None
Metoclopramide (Reglan)	B_M	Minimal
Other		
Emetrol	B	
Doxylamine succinate	—	None
Vitamin B_6 (Pyridoxine)	B	None

M, manufacturers.
[a]Briggs', not manufacturer's list.

Severe acute attacks of migraine should be treated aggressively (42,49). We start intravenous (i.v.) fluids for hydration and then use prochlorperazine 10 mg i.v. to control both nausea and head pain. This can be supplemented by parenteral narcotics or corticosteroids. This is an extremely effective way of handling status migrainosus during pregnancy.

Preventive Treatment

Increased frequency and severity of migraine associated with nausea and vomiting may justify the use of daily preventive medication. This treatment option should be a last resort and used only with the consent of the patient and her partner after the risks have been explained completely. Preventive therapy is designed to reduce the frequency and severity of headache attacks. Prophylaxis should be considered when patients experience at least three or four prolonged, severe attacks a month that are particularly incapacitating or unresponsive to symptomatic therapy and may result in dehydration and fetal distress (44). Beta-adrenergic blockers such as propranolol have been used in these circumstances, although possible adverse effects, including intrauterine growth retardation, have been reported. If the migraine is so severe that drug treatment is essential, the patient should be told of the risks posed by all the drugs that are used (Table 32-13) (44). If the patient has a coexistent illness that requires treatment, an attempt

TABLE 32-13. *Guidelines for prophylactic treatment of headache*

	Dose	Fetal Risk	
		FDA	TERIS
Beta-blockers			
Propranolol (Inderal, Inderal LA)	40–320 mg/day	C_M	Undetermined
Nadolol (Corgard)	40–240 mg/day	C_M	Undetermined
Atenolol (Tenormin)	50–120 mg/day	C_M	Undetermined
Timolol (Blocadren)	10–30 mg/day	C_M	Undetermined
Antidepressants			
Nortriptyline Hcl (Pamelor, Aventyl)	10–100 mg/day	D[a]	Undetermined
Amitriptyline (Elavil, Endep)	10–250 mg/day	D[a]	None-minimal
Doxepin (Sinequan, Adapin)	10–150 mg/day	C[a]	Undetermined
Fluoxetine (Prozac)	10–80 mg/day	B_M	None
Calcium channel blockers			
Verapamil (Calan)	240–720 mg/day	C_M	Undetermined
Nifedipine (Procardia)	30–180 mg/day	C_M	Undetermined
Diltiazem (Cardizem)	120–360 mg/day	C_M	Undetermined
Serotonin antagonists			
Methysergide (Sansert)	2–8 mg/day in divided doses up to 14 mg/day	D	Undetermined
Methylergonovine maleate (Methergine)	0.2–0.4 mg four times daily	C_M	Undetermined
Anticonvulsants			
Phenytoin (Dilantin)	200–400 mg/day	D[a]	Small-moderate
Valproic acid [Depakene and Depakote (enteric coated)]	500–3,000 mg/day	D[a]	Small-moderate

M, manufacturers.
[a]Briggs', not manufacturer's list.

should be made to prescribe one drug that will treat both disorders. For example, propranolol can be used to treat hypertension and migraine, whereas fluoxetine can be used to treat comorbid depression. Patients with intractable CDH and cluster may require treatment. This can be difficult and will require consultation between the treating physician and the obstetrician.

Drug Exposure

The physician should work with the obstetrician to manage the pregnant patient's headaches. If a woman inadvertently takes a drug while she is pregnant or becomes pregnant while taking a drug, determine the dose, timing, and duration of the exposure(s). The patient's past and present state of health and the presence of congenital malformations, mental retardation or chromosomal abnormalities in the family should be ascertained. Using a reliable source of information (such as TERIS), the drug should be identified as a known teratogen (although for many drugs this is not possible) (38–40,47,50).

If the drug is teratogenic or the risk is unknown, gestational age should be confirmed by ultrasonography and the patient should be informed of all potential risks and alternatives.

SUMMARY

Migraine and TTH are primary headache disorders that occur commonly during pregnancy. Migraine sometimes occurs for the first time with pregnancy. The majority of migraineurs improve while pregnant; however, migraine often recurs postpartum. Some disorders that produce headache, such as stroke, cerebral venous thrombosis, eclampsia, and subarachnoid hemorrhage, occur more frequently during pregnancy. Diagnostic testing serves to exclude organic causes of headache, to confirm the diagnosis, and to establish a baseline before treatment. If neurodiagnostic testing is indicated, the study that will provide the most information with the least fetal risk is the study of choice (5).

Although medication use should be limited, it is not absolutely contraindicated in pregnancy. In migraine, the risk of status migrainosus may be greater than the potential risk of the medication used to treat the pregnant patient. Nonpharmacologic treatment is the ideal solution; however, analgesics such as acetaminophen and narcotics can be used on a limited basis. Preventive therapy is the least desirable approach, but may be necessary in some patients (5).

REFERENCES

1. Headache Classification Committee of the International Headache Soceity. Classification and diagnostic criteria for headache disorders, cranial neuralgia, and facial pain. Cephalalgia 1988;8(suppl 7):1–96.
2. Lipton RB, Pfeffer D, Newman L, Solomon S. Headaches in the elderly. J Pain Symptom Manage 1993;8:87–97.
3. Dalessio DJ, Silberstein SD. Diagnosis and classification of headache. In: Dalessio DJ, Silberstein SD, eds. Wolff's headache and other head pain, 6th ed. New York: Oxford University Press, 1993:3–18.
4. Silberstein SD, Saper J. Migraine: diagnosis and treatment. In: Dalessio D, Silberstein SD, eds. Wolff's headache and other head pain, 6th ed. New York: Oxford University Press, 1993:96–170.

5. Silberstein SD. Migraine and pregnancy. Neurol Clin 1997;15: 209–231.
6. Silberstein SD. Evaluation and emergency treatment of headache. Headache 1992;32:396–407.
7. Fox MW, Harms RW, Davis DH. Selected neurologic complications of pregnancy. Mayo Clin Proc 1990;65:1595–1618.
8. Hainline B. Headache. Headache 1994;12:443–460.
9. Silberstein SD, Corbett JJ. The forgotten lumbar puncture. Cephalalgia 1993:13:212–213.
10. Lipton RB, Silberstein SD, Stewart WF. An update on the epidemiology of migraine. Headache 1994;34:319–328.
11. Stewart WF, Lipton RB, Celentano DD, Reed ML. Prevalence of migraine headache in the United States. JAMA 1992;267:64–69.
12. Uknis A, Silberstein SD. Review article: migraine and pregnancy. Headache 1991;31:372–374.
13. Silberstein SD, Lipton RB. Overview of diagnosis and treatment of migraine. Neurology 1994;44(suppl 7):6–16.
14. Silberstein SD, Young WB. Migraine aura and prodrome. Semin Neurol 1995;45:175–182.
15. Silberstein SD. Migraine symptoms: results of a survey of self-reported migraineurs. Headache 1995;35:387–396.
16. Selby G, Lance JW. Observations on 500 cases of migraine and allied vascular headache. J Neurol Neurosurg Psychiatry 1960;23:23–32.
17. Silberstein SD, Lipton RB. Chronic daily headache. In: Silberstein SD, Goadsby P, eds. Headache. Newton, MA: Butterworth Heinemann, 1997:201–225.
18. Silberstein SD. Pharmacological management of cluster headache. CNS Drugs 1994;2:199–207.
19. Silberstein SD, Marcelis J. Headache associated with abnormalities in intracranial structures or pressure including brain tumor and post-LP headache. In: Dalessio D, Silberstein SD, eds. Wolff's headache and other head pain, 6th ed. New York: Oxford University Press, 1993: 438–461.
20. Forsyth PA, Posner JB. Headache in patients with brain tumors. A study of 111 patients. Neurology 1993;43:1678–1683.
21. Britt RH. Brain abscess. In: Wilkins RH, Rengachary SS, eds. Neurosurgery. New York: McGraw-Hill, 1985:1928–1956.
22. Chancellor MD, Wroe SH. Migraine occuring for the first time in pregnancy. Headache 1990;30:224–227.
23. Stein GS. Headaches in the first postpartum week and their relationship to migraine. Headache 1981;21:201–205.
24. Somerville BS. A study of migraine in pregnancy. Neurology 1972; 22:824–828.
25. Silberstein SD, Merriam GR. Estrogens, progestins, and headache. Neurology 1991;41:786–793.
26. Wright DS. Patel MK. Focal migraine and pregnancy. Br Med J 1986; 293:1557–1558.
27. Massey EW. Migraine during pregnancy. Obstet Gynecol Surv 1977; 32:693–696.
28. Lance JW, Anthony M. Some clinical spects of migraine. Arch Neurol 1966;15:356–361.
29. Callaghan N. The migraine syndrome in pregnancy. Neurology 1968; 18:197–201.
30. Bousser MG. Ratinahirana H, Darbois X. Migraine and pregnancy: a prospective study in 703 women after delivery. Abstr Neurol 1990;40: 437.
31. Granella F, Sances G, Zanferrari C, Cosca A, Martignoni E, Manzoni GC. Migraine without aura and reproductive life events: a clinical epidemiologic study in 1300 women. Headache 1993;385–389.
32. Rasmussen BK. Migraine and tension-type headache in a general population: precipitating factors, female hormones, sleep pattern, and relation to lifestyle. Pain 1993;53:65–72.
33. Chen TC, Leviton A. Headache recurrence in pregnant women with migraine. Headache 1994;107–110.
34. Scharff L, Marcus DA, Turk DC. Headache during pregnancy and in the postpartum: a prospective study. Headache 1997;37:203–210.
35. Maggioni F, Alessi C, Maggino T. Primary headaches and pregnancy [Abstract]. Cephalalgia 1995;17:54.
36. Wainscott G, Volans GN. The outcome of pregnancy in women suffering from migraine. Postgrad Med J 1978;54:98–102.
37. MacArthur C, Lewis M, Knox EG. Health after childbirth. Br J Obstet Gynecol 1991;98:1193–1204.
38. Gilstrap LC III, Little BB, eds. Drugs and pregnancy. New York: Elsevier, 1992:23–29.
39. Blake DA, Niebyl JR. Requirements and limitations in reproductive and teratognic risk assessment. In: Niebyl JR, ed. Drug use in pregnancy, 2nd ed. Philadelphia: Lea & Febiger, 1988:1–9.
40. Briggs GG, Freeman RK, Yaffe SJ. Drugs in pregnancy and lactation, 4th ed. Baltimore: Williams & Wilkins, 1994.
41. Niebyl JR. Teratology and drugs in pregnancy and lactation. In: Winters R, ed. Danforth's obstetrics and gynecology, 6th ed. New York: JB Lippincott, 1990.
42. Rayburn WF, Lavin JP. Drug prescribing for chronic medical disorders during pregnancy: an overview. Am J Obstet Gynecol 1986;155: 565–569.
43. Cavagnaro JA. Traditional reproductive toxicology studies and their predictive value. FDA conference on regulated products and pregnant women. Virginia: November 1994.
44. Silberstein SD. Headaches and women: treatment of the pregnant and lactating migraineur. Headache 1993;33:533–540.
45. Heinonen OP, Slone S, Shapiro S. Birth defects and drugs in pregnancy. Littleton, MA: Publishing Sciences Group, 1977.
46. Barnhart ER, ed. Physicians desk reference, 45th ed. Oradell JN: Medical Economics Inc., 1991.
47. Friedman JM, Polifka JE, eds. Teratogenic effects of drugs: a resource for clinicians (TERIS). Baltimore: Johns Hopkins University Press, 1994.
48. Friedman JM, Little BB, Brent RL, Cordero JF, Hanson JW, Shepard TH. Potential human teratogenicity of frequently prescribed drugs. Obstet Gynecol 1990;75:594–599.
49. Raskin NH. Migraine treatment. In: Raskin NH, ed. Headache, 2nd ed. New York: Churchill-Livingstone, 1988.
50. Shepard TH. Catalog of teratogenic agents, 8th ed. Baltimore: Johns Hopkins University Press, 1973.
51. Silberstein SD, Lipton RB. Headache epidemiology: emphasis on migraine. Neurol Clin 1996;14:421–434.

Cherry and Merkatz's Complications of Pregnancy,
Fifth Edition, edited by W. R. Cohen.
Lippincott Williams & Wilkins, Philadelphia © 2000.

CHAPTER 33

Brain Tumors

Robert F. Keating

Although brain tumors are rare in the pregnant patient, their manifestations may easily be missed in this setting of increased cerebral perfusion and the frequently accompanying headaches. The preeclamptic patient presenting with seizures may cause even greater confusion. Nevertheless, certain characteristics provide diagnostic insight to differentiate a cerebral mass from generalized cerebral swelling seen in the later stages of gestation. The overall objective of this chapter is to highlight the signs and symptoms of brain tumors in the pregnant patient as well as to review the diagnosis and treatment of the most common types of tumors presenting during this period. In addition, correlation between hormone levels and tumor growth will be examined.

Fortunately, brain tumors during pregnancy are rare. Isla and colleagues (1) reviewed their experience with 126,413 pregnancies over 12 years and found 7 patients who developed primary brain tumors during their gestation. Three patients had gliomas (one parietal, one brain stem, and one with multiple gliomas), two developed meningiomas, and two had ependymomas. Three patients presented with seizures, two with cranial nerve findings, one with increased intracranial pressure, and one with sudden lethal intracranial hemorrhage during labor. In a report by Haas (2) based on a population-based epidemiologic study from the German Democratic Republic tumor registry from 1961 to 1979, the frequency of all types of cancer was reviewed in the pregnant patient and was seen to be 62% less than expected in the general population. This was felt to be related to the greater likelihood of early interruption of the pregnancy or perhaps to an overall decreased libido in the setting of subclinical cancer. Roelvink and colleagues (3) reviewed 86 literature reports of 223 cases of pregnancy-related primary brain and spinal cord tumors and found that the incidence of brain tumors that became symptomatic during pregnancies seemed to be decreased compared with the incidence in nonpregnant women of the same age. They also found that gliomas manifested themselves more often in the first trimester and that the incidence of brain tumors decreased with increase in parity. Haas and colleagues (4), however, found a higher prevalence for both glioma and meningioma in the pregnant patient. Although some degree of sample bias may have been present, similar findings have been observed elsewhere (5,6). The number of spontaneous abortions in patients with brain tumors also has been reported to be higher in the period before the tumor was clinically apparent (3,4). Whether this was mediated by tumor-induced alterations in the hypothalamic axis remains unclear.

Cushing and Eisenhardt (7) were, in 1938, the first to detail the relationship between meningiomas and pregnancy. Subsequently, the association between meningiomas and estrogen as well as progesterone receptors also was recognized (8–11). In general, a majority of meningiomas (>70%) demonstrate progesterone receptors, whereas only a third will manifest estrogen receptors. In addition, androgen and glucocorticoid receptors have been demonstrated in both meningiomas and gliomas (12–14), as has epidermal growth factor (15).

Although apparent increases in the growth rate of meningiomas during pregnancy would suggest a relationship between high progesterone levels and the growth of the meningioma, this has not been demonstrated in the laboratory. *In vitro* cultured meningiomas manifest only minimal effects of progesterone. However, the presence of epidermal growth factor and progesterone receptors in meningioma tumor growth is modulated by progesterone and can be inhibited by the progesterone receptor blocking agent mifepristone (RU486) (15). It would thus appear that the presence of progesterone may increase the meningioma cell's sensitivity to specific mitogenic agents (e.g., epidermal growth factor). It is likely that

R.F. Keating: Departments of Neurosurgery and Pediatrics, George Washington University School of Medicine, Children's National Medical Center, Washington, DC 20010.

there are different manifestations of various cytokines during the course of pregnancy, and to date the definitive causal relationship between progesterone and brain tumors has yet to be established.

PRESENTATION

Pregnant women with brain tumors may present with localized signs and symptoms secondary to focal brain involvement or may manifest changes due to an overall increase in intracranial pressure (Table 33-1). Focal findings may include seizures, weakness, numbness, aphasia, cranial neuropathies, or even hormonal imbalances. These changes are related to direct neurologic invasion or discrete focal pressure from the neoplasm. This is distinct from the generalized findings seen when concomitant cerebral edema or hydrocephalus promotes a diffuse increase in the intracranial pressure. Patients with increased intracranial pressure may complain of headaches, visual changes (blurred vision, diplopia), nausea, vomiting, lethargy, difficulty with balance, or memory and personality changes. It is not difficult to envision the confusion that may originate in the pregnant patient. Headache undoubtedly is the most common presenting symptom of tumors and is frequently confused with headaches related to hormone-directed changes in the overall cerebral blood volume. Headaches associated with increased intracranial pressure are often pronounced in the morning secondary to nocturnal hypercapnia as a result of a decreased respiratory drive during sleep. In addition, vomiting often provides temporary relief of the headache due to the transient hyperventilation which in turn decreases the pCO_2. A lower pCO_2 will promote cerebral vasoconstriction and eventually lead to a reduction in intracranial pressure. Although the generalized symptoms of increased intracranial pressure may be ascribed to numerous etiologies, including a brain tumor, hydrocephalus, or pregnancy, it is difficult to confuse the cause of a pregnant patient presenting with headache and focal findings. In general, it is common for patients who have only generalized symptoms to present after the tumor has achieved considerable size, whereas patients with focal findings often present at an earlier stage of the neoplasm's growth.

TABLE 33-1. *Clinical manifestation of brain tumors*

Localized (focal tumor involvement)	Generalized (increased intracranial pressure)
Weakness	Headache
Numbness	Visual changes
Aphasia	Nausea/vomiting
Seizures	Lethargy
Cranial nerve palsies	Balance difficulties
Hormonal changes	Memory/personality changes

RADIOLOGIC WORKUP

Although no longer routinely used, the venerable skull X-ray in the past would occasionally provide a diagnostic clue in the clinical evaluation of a pregnant patient with atypical headaches. Erosion of the inner calvarial table due to long-standing increased intracranial pressure may produce skull x-rays with the classic "beaten copper pot" appearance, otherwise known as *Lukenschadel.* The presence of digital markings, while suggestive of increased intracranial pressure, may not always be pathognomonic for elevated pressure. Patients with pituitary lesions frequently manifest an enlarged sella turcica. However, the majority of individuals fail to demonstrate any significant abnormality and thus illustrate the low sensitivity of this diagnostic test in this setting.

Consequently, the role of the accurate and easily obtained computed tomogram (CT) grew in importance during the late 1970's and early 1980's to help diagnose those individuals with brain tumors (Fig. 33-1). If care is taken to shield the abdomen, CT studies may be used safely in the pregnant patient with a suspected intracranial process.

Commercial magnetic resonance imaging (MRI) scanners have nevertheless become the modality of choice in the pregnant patient (Fig. 33-2). At present, there are no data interdicting its use in the pregnant patient. In addition, the sensitivity and overall detail are often superior to that of a corresponding CT.

Contrast materials (iodinated) are considered safe in the pregnant patient with little risk to the fetus. However, it remains important to ensure adequate hydration for both the mother and fetus and be vigilant for any allergic reaction.

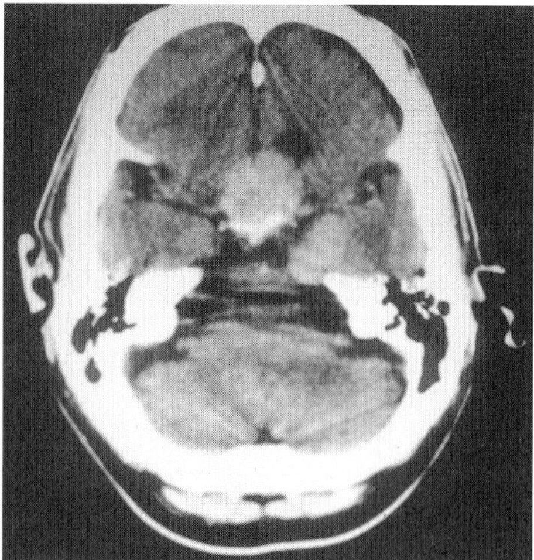

FIG. 33-1. A CT scan of a 34-year-old pregnant woman with a large sellar meningioma with petrous ridge extension. The patient presented initially with visual changes and eventual left sixth nerve palsy in the third trimester of pregnancy. The differential diagnosis included a pituitary adenoma, meningioma, and other sellar lesions.

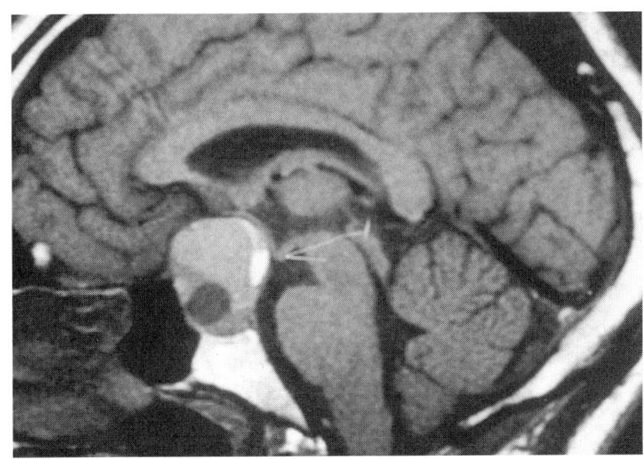
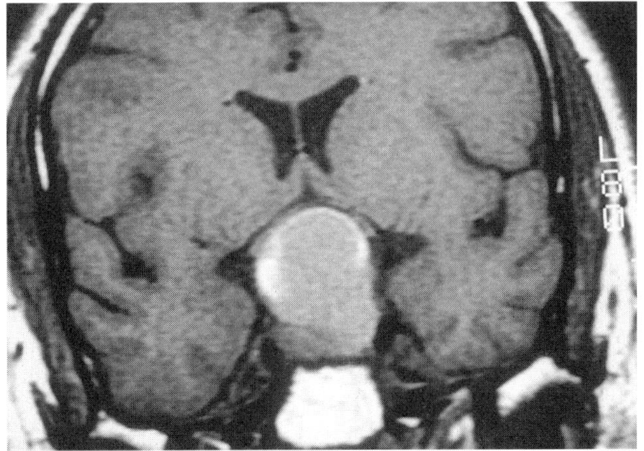

A B

FIG. 33-2. A: A sagittal MRI demonstrating a large sellar mass with suprasellar extension. The patient had a known history of a pituitary adenoma and became noncompliant with her bromocriptine therapy during her pregnancy. The tumor has a heterogeneous composition with cystic and hemorrhagic components. **B:** A coronal view of the pituitary mass demonstrates a thinned optic chiasm draped over the posterosuperior portion of the mass.

At this time, the safety of gadolinium in the pregnant patient has not been investigated.

TUMOR TYPE

The most common type of primary brain tumor encountered in the pregnant patient is the glioma, with meningiomas being close in overall frequency (3). Although the incidence of meningiomas may represent a significantly higher percentage than seen in the general population, it remains unclear whether pregnancy-related hormones contribute to accelerated tumor growth and thus earlier manifestations. In their review of the literature, Roelvink and colleagues (3) noted that gliomas more often made their clinical appearance in the first trimester, whereas meningiomas more commonly had onset of symptoms in the second and third trimesters.

Although less common, pituitary adenomas have long been associated with menstrual irregularities as well as complicating the course of pregnancy (16–22). As expected, a secreting pituitary adenoma may influence any pregnancy as well as the pregnancy causing its own effects upon the tumor. Nevertheless, in the immunohistochemical study by Scheithauer and colleagues (23), a postmortem review of women with pituitary tumors who had died during pregnancy, prolactin-producing adenomas were no more numerous nor larger than were similar tumors in nonpregnant women and in men. They thus concluded that pregnancy neither initiated formation nor accelerated the growth of pituitary adenomas. In another study (20), a review of pregnant women with previously untreated pituitary tumors demonstrated that ovulation had occurred spontaneously in 9%, and visual disturbances in 25%, whereas 61% remained asymptomatic. Within this group, 30% ultimately required surgery or radiation therapy. It also was felt that treatment of the tumor during pregnancy significantly increased prematurity rates but did not affect abortion or perinatal mortality rates. There are numerous examples of pregnant patients who demonstrated symptomatic enlargement of their tumors during pregnancy (24–28). Patients not infrequently manifest visual changes (i.e., bitemporal hemianopia), which is related to an accelerated growth in the size of the tumor during the pregnancy and eventual midline compression of the optic chiasm (24,25). Hormonal changes also may be seen and may result from hemorrhage into the tumor (26), compression of the normal pituitary-hypothalamic axis by an expanding mass, infiltrative lymphocytic hypophysitis, or secondary to pituitary necrosis (29). This in turn may lead to diabetes insipidus (26,27) or other hormonal deficiencies, including panhypopituitarism. Thus, it is imperative to follow closely patients with known tumors for any endocrinologic or visual changes over the course of the pregnancy.

The most common type of pituitary adenoma remains by far the prolactinoma. In prolactin-secreting adenomas, the elevation of serum prolactin witnessed during pregnancy significantly decreases after delivery. Advances in the diagnosis of pituitary microadenomas with accurate anatomical localization initially led to the adoption of surgical management as a mainstay in the treatment of infertile women (16), as well as for patients who discovered a tumor during their pregnancy. The coupling of an old surgical exposure (transphenoidal route) with the microscope as well as petrosal sinus sampling allowed safe, accurate, and often complete surgical excisions of the microadenoma. Before the universal utilization of bromocriptine, surgical excision of the adenoma was often undertaken to prevent any increase in the size of the tumor and potential mass effect upon the optic chiasm or hypothalmus, or obstruction of cerebral spinal fluid pathways leading to hydrocephalus. With U.S. Food and Drug Administration approval of bromocriptine in 1978, the treatment of pituitary prolactinomas was revolutionized. Since then, countless women harboring prolactinomas have had successful conceptions as well as term pregnancies while being maintained on bromocriptine (27,18,30). To date, there has not been any significant association with birth defects in these patients. A combination therapy of bromocriptine in smaller doses in conjunction with tamoxifen (estrogen inhibitor) has been used successfully in the pregnant patient who is unable to tolerate the usual bromocriptine dose (19). There has also been a report of a patient who was initially responsive to bromocriptine but became refractory to treatment despite prior surgical excision, with residual tumor becoming sensitive to bromocriptine after delivery (31). Although management of pituitary adenomas during pregnancy today remains predominantly a conservative choice, advocates for a surgical course nevertheless remain visible (28).

Choriocarcinoma presenting with brain metastases during pregnancy is an uncommon event. Nevertheless, the presence of cerebral metastases has been demonstrated in 66.7% of patients with choriocarcinoma during autopsy study (32). They most often present as solitary lesions with a propensity to bleed. In a reported case by Dana and colleagues (33), a patient who presented at 31 weeks' gestation with a grand mal seizure was subsequently seen to have metastatic choriocarcinoma with diffuse cerebral edema. The mother was treated with chemotherapy, and both the mother and child survived.

The occurrence of distant metastases from primary brain tumors is rare. There is, however, a case report of medulloblastoma metastatic to the placenta complicating a pregnancy at 20 weeks (34). The pregnancy was prolonged to 29 weeks for a delivery by cesarean section. The postoperative course was complicated by coagulopathy, pneumonia, and eventual death.

MANAGEMENT

Clinical management of the pregnant patient with a brain tumor is dependent on presenting symptoms, type and location of the tumor, and stage of pregnancy. When patients clinically manifest early with modest-sized tumors and minimal mass effect, the clinical approach can often take a conservative route. Although tumor diagnosis can never be definitive without a tissue biopsy, advances in the radiologic workup have significantly increased the likelihood of an accurate preoperative diagnosis. Lesions that appear benign may be followed with serial MRIs and will often permit the pregnancy to proceed to term. Should a lesion increase significantly in size or begin to cause mass effect on the brain, one may need to consider a more expeditious extirpative biopsy. Malignant lesions in the early course of a pregnancy generally demonstrate the poorest prognosis (35), and because of the need for aggressive adjuvant therapy, they may raise the issue of elective termination of the pregnancy. Nevertheless, today's surgical armamentarium will permit a safer and more accurate biopsy and resection of tumors in a variety of locations.

Once a diagnosis has been made, the inevitable question involves the next step. This will be dependent on the patient's current neurologic status and presumed tumor diagnosis as well as the stage of gestation. Carmel (35) reviewed this issue in 1974 and stratified patients into benign versus malignant disease, early gestation in contrast to later pregnancy, as well as the ease of medical management. The pregnancies of patients with presumed malignant disease were commonly chosen to be terminated because of the dismal overall prognosis. At that time, radiologic studies lacked today's level of sophistication, often making prognostic predictions less than accurate. In addition, today's approach to malignant disease is more aggressive, with safer and improved means of tumor resection being readily available. Frameless stereotactic resection (Fig. 33-3), improved anesthesia using local and improved agents, and an ever-widening array of adjuvant therapy (gene therapy, immune approaches) have all led to a decreased surgical morbidity. The long-term benefit in improved survival nevertheless is still unclear. Consequently, it is no longer uncommon for patients with malignant disease to have resection of their tumor while maintaining the pregnancy.

There has been significant controversy over the years with respect to the mode of delivery for the patient with a brain tumor. Soutoul and colleagues (36) in 1971 outlined a number of indications for cesarean section, which included the characterization of a malignant tumor, deteriorating clinical course, or whether forceps delivery under general anesthesia would be necessary. Over time the clinical necessity for cesarean section has been reevaluated. During the initial phase of labor, uterine contractions do not appear to increase intracranial pressure. However, during active bearing-down efforts, intracranial pressure may be significantly increased. Thus, for patients with large tumors or those who have significant mass effect and pressure, a cesarean section is generally advised. Whereas for patients with small tumors or without significant cerebral swelling, a vaginal delivery is often acceptable. Other considerations need to include the stage of gestation and whether the mother is multiparous. The pregnant patient with a deteriorating medical or neurologic condition in the third trimester may be best served by an early cesarean delivery for the health of both the mother and child. In a situation in which it is considered safe from a neurosurgical viewpoint to allow a vaginal delivery, this should be considered the preferential route. This decision will obviously be made on an individual basis and will require close coordination between the obstetrician and neurosurgeon (Table 33-2).

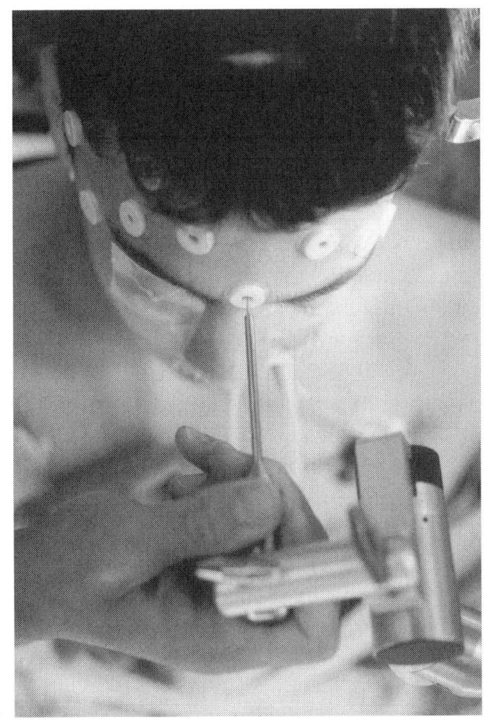

A

FIG. 33-3. **A:** The frameless stereotactic arm is used to register external landmarks (fiducials) in conjunction with a concurrent MRI. The skin markings serve as a reference point when using the same localizing arm within the brain. Current systems now use a camera array and LEDs for three-dimensional localization, which has replaced the need for the fixed and frequently awkward localizing arm. **B:** A current MRI is used with three-dimensional views of the brain for stereotactic localization of the lesion. The position of the probe (or any other instrument) is correlated with real-time updated MRI views of the brain. The cross-hairs on all views are the location of the probe at that instant. Thus, the surgeon knows the intracranial location (within 2–3 mm) at any time, which in turn provides a greater accuracy in removal of such lesions as well as decreased intraoperative morbidity.

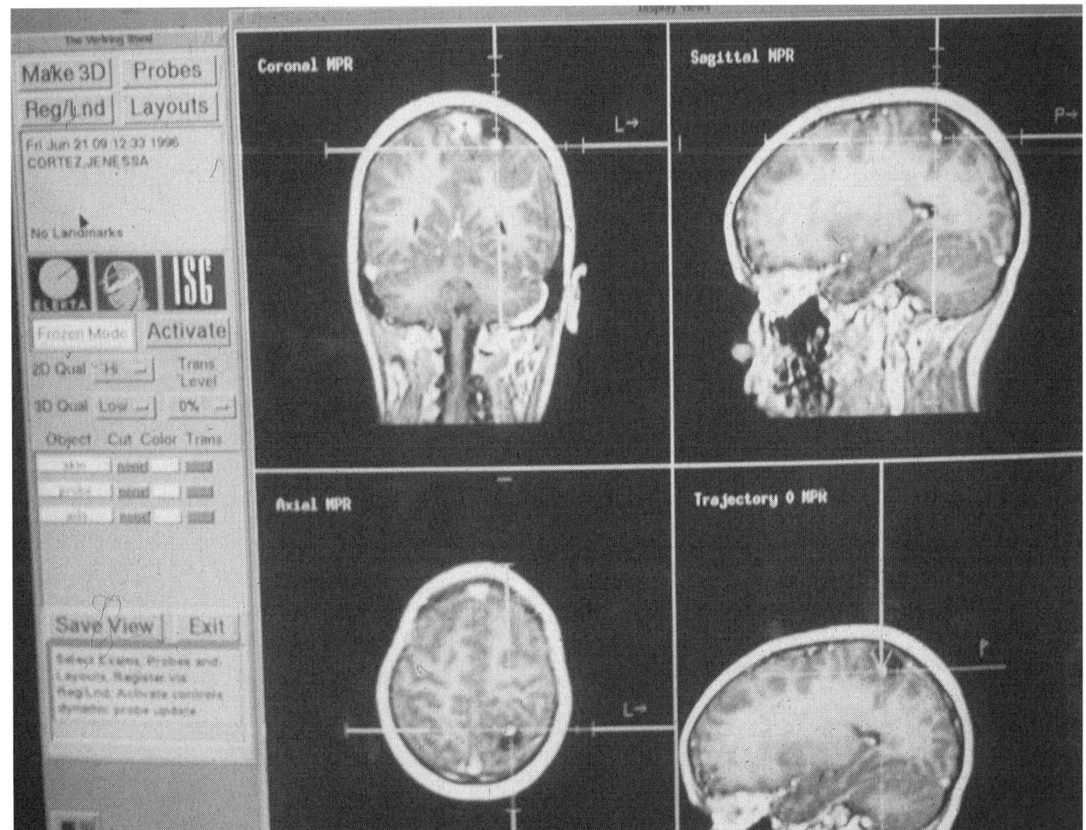

B

TABLE 33-2. *Neurosurgical indications for cesarean section*

Large tumor with significant mass effect
Malignant tumor during late gestation, requiring extirpation/subsequent adjuvant therapy
Moderate sized tumors in primigravid mother with prolonged labor
Deteriorating neurologic condition in 3rd trimester

The treatment of a pregnant patient with a brain tumor parallels that of the nonpregnant patient in the majority of circumstances. The patients are placed on steroids and anticonvulsants in a typical fashion. Patients with cortical lesions demonstrating mass effect or symptoms are started on 2 to 4 mg dexamethasone (orally or intravenously) every 6 hours. This will be tapered to a minimal maintenance level that will in turn provide symptomatic relief for the patient. The patients without significant mass effect generally do not require corticosteroids. Long-term administration of steroids, especially in the last trimester, may potentially lead to adrenal suppression in the fetus and newborn (37).

The benefit of anticonvulsant therapy is considered to outweigh the potential long-term adverse effects to both the mother and fetus. Any seizure experienced by the mother would place both the patient and fetus at risk. Any increase in intracranial pressure in the setting of preexisting swelling may promote cerebral herniation with its potential dire neurologic consequences. The fetus would also be at considerable risk from periictal hypoxia and acidosis. There are no teratogenic issues that commend the use of one anticonvulsant over another (38) in this situation. It is important to monitor serum anticonvulsant levels closely because changes in the mother's serum albumin may increase the unbound fraction of an anticonvulsant, and some agents are cleared more rapidly by the liver during pregnancy.

CONCLUSION

Brain tumors in the pregnant patient are rare. Nevertheless, it remains critical to be able to recognize the signs and symptoms of increased intracranial pressure or other symptoms secondary to a brain tumor and to be able to differentiate these from similar clinical effects caused by pregnancy or preeclampsia.

Over the past few decades significant strides have been made in the diagnosis and treatment of brain tumors. This has benefited the pregnant patient as well. The MRI scan has removed the threat of radiation to the developing fetus and now allows an unparalleled view of the brain and its coverings. Its sensitivity also permits a more accurate preoperative diagnosis, which in turn may help to direct the choice of treatment options. It is now common to allow a pregnancy to continue to term if the radiologic diagnosis is consistent with a benign etiology and the patient's neurologic status permits. For the patient with an aggressive tumor or deteriorating neurologic condition, surgical techniques are more advanced and offer decreased morbidity in the present setting. Nevertheless, the current prognosis for such patients will be dependent on the primary tumor pathology. Patients harboring benign lesions, even in difficult locations, generally do well, whereas malignant disease continues to carry a guarded overall prognosis.

As neurosurgical techniques continue to evolve in a minimalistic direction with the universal incorporation of frameless stereotactic surgery, endoscopically assisted approaches, and robotic and virtual real-time adjuncts, perioperative morbidity and mortality should continue to improve. This will also have a profound impact on the pregnant patient and will benefit both the mother and baby. Nevertheless, today's neurosurgical armamentarium still offers a significant improvement for the pregnant patient with an intracranial mass and often permits the pregnancy to proceed to term. Future advances will be delivered by molecular biologists and perinatologists as we gain a better understanding of hormonal interactions and tumor growth.

REFERENCES

1. Isla A, Alvarez A, Gonzalez A, Garcia-Grande A, Perez-Alvarez M, Garcia-Blazquez M. Brain tumor and pregnancy. Obstet Gynecol 1997;89:19–23.
2. Haas JF, Pregnancy in association with newly diagnosed cancer: a population-based epidemiologic assessment. Int J Cancer 1984;34:229–235.
3. Roelvink CA, Kamphorst W, van Alphen HAM, Rao BR. Pregnancy-related primary brain and spinal tumors. Arch Neurol 1987;44:209–215.
4. Haas JF, Janisch W, Staneczek W. Newly diagnosed primary intracranial neoplasms in pregnant women: a population-based assessment. J Neurol Neurosurg Psychiatry 1986;49:874–880.
5. Chaudhuri P, Wallenburg HCS. Brain tumors and pregnancy. Presentation of a case and a review of the literature. Eur J Obstet Gynecol Reprod Biol 1980;11:109–114.
6. Michelsen JJ, New PFJ. Brain tumour and pregnancy. J Neurol Neurosurg Psychiatry 1969;32:305–307.
7. Cushing H, Eisenhardt L. Meningiomas: their classification, regional behavior, life history, and surgical end result. Springfield, IL: Charles C Thomas, 1938.
8. Glick RP, Molteni A, Fors EM. Hormone binding in brain tumors. Neurosurgery 1983;13:513–519.
9. Tilzer LL, Plapp FV, Evans JP, Stone D, Alward K. Steroid receptor proteins in human meningiomas. Cancer 1982;49:633–636.
10. Cahill DW, Bashirelahi N, Solomon LWE, Dalton T, Salcman M, Ducker TB. Estrogen and progesterone receptors in meningiomas. J Neurosurg 1984;60:985–993.
11. Markwalder TM, Zava DT, Goldhirsch A, Markwalder RV. Estrogen and progesterone receptors in meningiomas in relation to clinical and pathologic features. Surg Neurol 1983;20:42–47.
12. Yu ZY, Wrange O, Boethius J, Hatam A. A study of glucocorticoid receptors in intracranial tumors. J Neurosurg 1981;55:757–760.
13. Brentani MM, Lopes MTP, Martins VR, Plese JP. Steroid receptors in intracranial tumors. Clin Neuropharmacol 1984;7:347–350.
14. Courriere P, Tremoulet M, Eche N, Armand JP. Hormone steroid receptors in intracranial tumours and their relevance in hormone therapy. Eur J Clin Oncol 1985;21:711–714.

15. Koper JW, Lamberts SWJ. Meningiomas, epidermal growth factor and progesterone. Hum Reprod 1994;9:190–194.
16. Laws ER Jr, Fode NC, Randall RV, Abboud CF, Coulam CB. Pregnancy following transphenoidal resection of prolactin-secreting pituitary tumors. J Neurosurg 1983;58:685–688.
17. Bergh T, Nillius SJ,Enoksson P, Larsson SG, Wide L. Bromocriptine-induced pregnancies in women with large prolactinomas. Clin Endocrinol (Oxf) 1982;17:625–631.
18. De Witt W, Coelingh Bennink HJT, Gerrads LJ. Prophylatic bromocriptine treatment during pregnancy in women with macroprolactinomas: report of 13 pregnancies. Br J Obstet Gynaecol 1984;91:1059–1069.
19. Koizumi K, Aono T. Pregnancies after combined treatment with bromocriptine in two patients with pituitary prolactinomas. Fertil Steril 1986;46:312–314.
20. Magyar DM, Marshall JR, Pituitary tumors and pregnancy. Am J Obstet Gynecol 1978;132:739–751.
21. Weinstein D, Yarkoni S, Schenker JG, Sahar A, Siew FP, Ben-David M, Polishuk WZ. Conservative management of suspected prolactinsecreting in pituitary adenoma during pregnancy. Eur J Obstet Gynecol Reprod Biol 1981;11:305–312.
22. Divers WA Jr, Yen SS. Prolactin-producing microadenomas in pregnancy. Obstet Gynecol 1983;62:425–429.
23. Scheithauer BW, Sano T, Kovacs KT, Young WF Jr, Ryan N, Randall RV. The pituitary gland in pregnancy: a clinicopathologic and immunohistochemical study of 69 cases. Mayo Clin Proc 1990;65:461–474.
24. Nelson PB, Robinson AG, Archer DF, Maroon JC. Symptomatic pituitary tumor enlargement after induced pregnancy. J Neurosurg 1978;49: 283–287.
25. Mills RP, Harris AB, Heinrichs L, Burry KA. Pituitary tumor made symptomatic during hormone therapy and induced pregnancy. Ann Ophthalmol 1979;11:1672–1676.
26. Freeman R, Wezenter B, Silverstein M, et al. Pregnancy-associated subacute hemorrhage into a prolactinoma resulting in diabetes insipidus. Fertil Steril 1992;58:427–429.
27. Nader S. Pituitary disorders and pregnancy. Semin Perinatol 1990;14: 24–33.
28. Samaan NA, Leavens ME, Sacca R, Smith K, Schultz PN. The effects of pregnancy on patients with hyperprolactinemia. Am J Obstet Gynecol 1984;148:466–473.
29. Prager D, Braunstein GD. Pituitary disorders during pregnancy. Endocrinol Metab Clin North Am 1995;24:1–14.
30. Tan SL, Jacobs HS. Rapid regression through bromocriptine therapy of a suprasellar prolactinoma during pregnancy. Int J Gynaecol Obstet 1986;24:209–215.
31. Shanis BS, Check JH. Relative resistance of a macroprolactinoma to bromocriptine therapy during pregnancy. Gynecol Endocrinol 1996; 10:91–94.
32. Kobayashi T, Kida Y, Yoshida J, Shibuya N, Kageyama N. Brain metastasis of choricarcinoma. Surg Neurol 1982;17:395–403.
33. Dana A, Saldanha GJ, Doshi R, Rustin GJ. Metastatic cerebral choriocarcinoma coexistent with a viable pregnancy. Gynecol Oncol 1996; 61:147–149.
34. Pollack RN, Pollack M, Rochon L. Pregnancy complicated by medulloblastoma with metastases to the placenta. Obstet Gynecol 1993;81: 858–859.
35. Carmel PW. Neurologic surgery in pregnancy. In: Barber HR, Graber EA, eds. Surgical disease in pregnancy. Philadelphia: WB Saunders, 1974:203–224.
36. Soutoul JH, Gouaze A, Gallier J, Santini JJ. Neurochirugie et grossesse. Rev Fr Gynecol 1971;66:603–618.
37. Biggs JSC, Allan JA. Medication and pregnancy. Drugs 1981; 2169–2175.
38. Kochenour N, Emery MG, Sawchuk RJ. Phenytoin metabolism in pregnancy. Obstet Gynecol 1980;56:577–582.

SECTION X

Sense Organ Disorders

Cherry and Merkatz's Complications of Pregnancy,
Fifth Edition, edited by W. R. Cohen.
Lippincott Williams & Wilkins, Philadelphia © 2000.

CHAPTER 34

Ocular Complications

Laurey G. Mogil and Alan H. Friedman

NORMAL ANATOMY

A transverse section through the eyeball is shown in Fig. 34-1. The diagram illustrates most of the structural features of the eye and provides orientation for the discussion that follows.

The wall of the eyeball is composed of three concentric layers: the retina, the uvea, and the sclera. These layers enclose the transparent media that light rays traverse in their path from the cornea to the retina. The outermost fibrous covering is composed of the sclera and cornea; these serve a refractive as well as a protective function. The middle coat, or uvea, is the vascular and nutritive layer and is composed of the choroid, the ciliary body, and the iris. The inner layer is the retina, the neurosensory layer of the eye. The retina is composed of several layers of cells and a pigment epithelium. The fibers that form the optic nerve originate in the retina. The site at which the optic nerve exits the eyeball, the optic disc, is an area that is not sensitive to light stimulation and is referred to as the blind spot.

The contents of the eyeball consist of the refractive media: the aqueous humor, the lens, and the vitreous body. The area about the lens and its suspensory ligaments is divided into two chambers. In front of the iris is the anterior chamber and behind it is the posterior chamber. Posterior to the lens is the vitreous body.

Figure 34-2 shows the posterior pole of the eye, or the fundus, as seen with an ophthalmoscope. The red background of the fundus results from blood in the choroid and the color of the retinal pigment epithelium. The amount of pigment in the choroidal layer and the retinal pigment epithelium varies and usually parallels the race of the person. The optic disc is about 1.5 mm in diameter and appears pink because of the presence of many capillaries. Slightly temporal or lateral to the center of the disc is the physiologic cup, which appears white. The margins of the disc are usually flat and sharp, but not uncommonly, the nasal margin is slightly less distinct than the temporal margin. Retinal arteries and veins are branches of the central retinal artery and vein. A broad bright streak is reflected from the surface of the arteries. All vessels bifurcate. They do not anastomose; therefore, blockage of the vessels obliterates vision in that part of the retina.

The area lying between the two major vascular arcades temporal to the disc is the macula. It is devoid of blood vessels, is a deeper color red than the rest of the fundus, and often is stippled with pigment. In the center of the macula is the fovea centralis, in which a pinpoint light reflex can be seen. The fovea centralis is the area of the retina responsible for best visual acuity.

L. G. Mogil: Department of Opthalmology, Mount Sinai School of Medicine, New York, NY 10029.

A. H. Friedman: Departments of Ophthalmology and Pathology, Mount Sinai School of Medicine, New York, NY 10029.

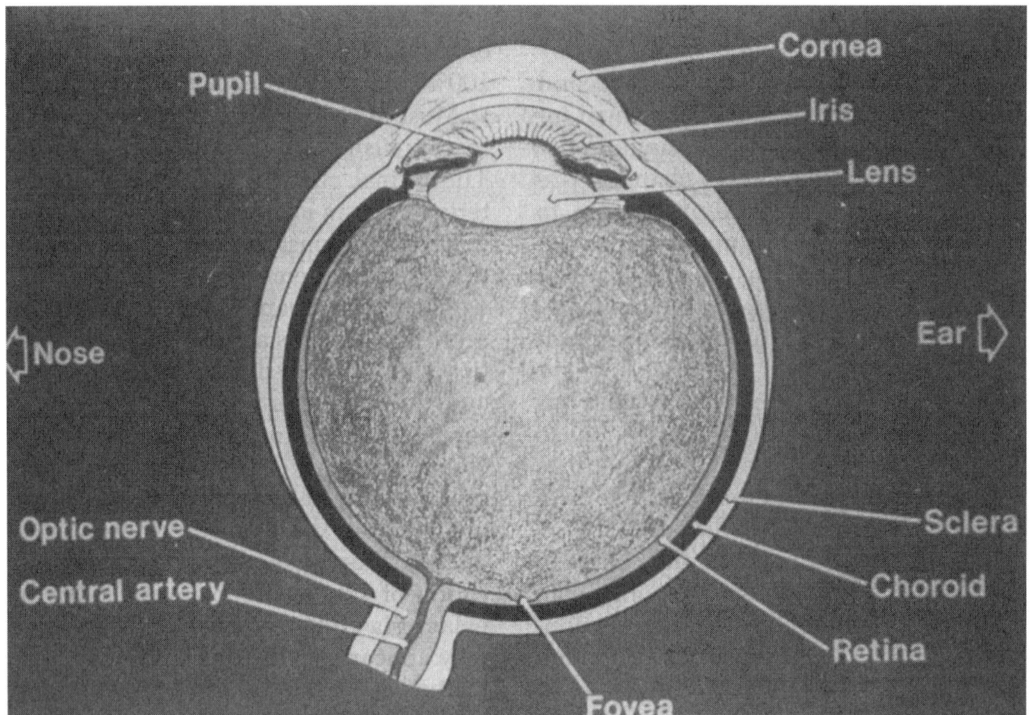

FIG. 34-1. Transverse section through right eyeball.

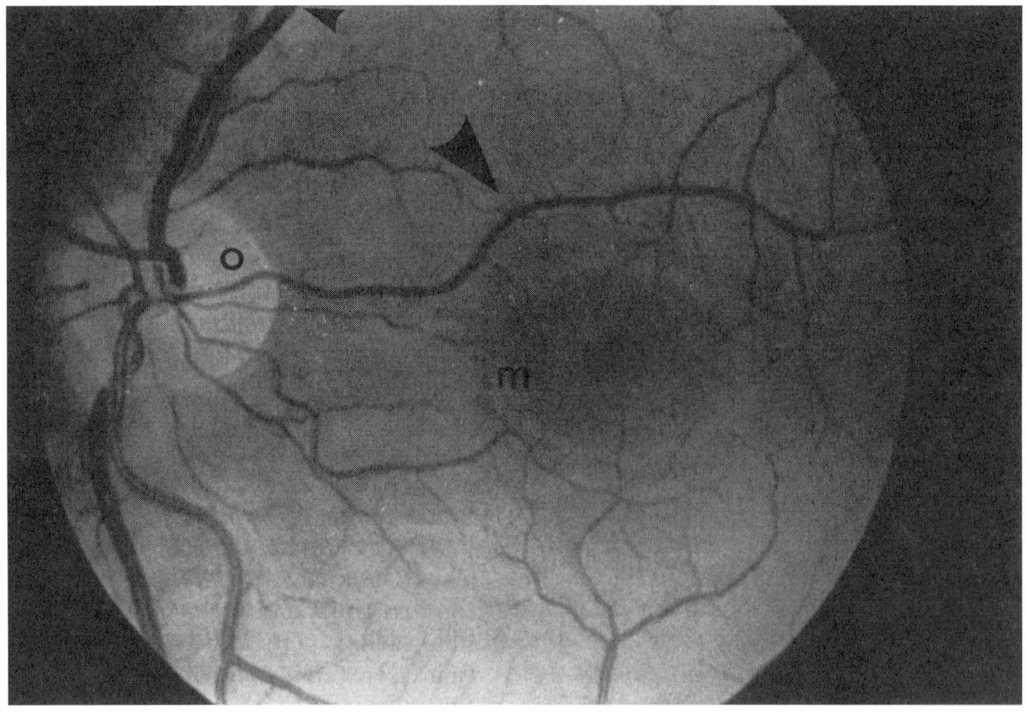

FIG. 34-2. Ophthalmoscopic view of normal left fundus: o, optic nerve head; m, macula; small arrowhead, retinal vein; large arrowhead, retinal artery.

PHYSIOLOGIC CHANGES IN THE MATERNAL EYE DURING PREGNANCY

During the course of normal pregnancy variations in ocular physiology occur. Changes in corneal sensitivity and topography have been associated with intermittent, mild corneal edema occurring during the third trimester of pregnancy. This may account for complaints of discomfort and difficulty in wearing contact lenses. An alteration in the composition of tears, thought due to an increased secretion of lysozyme, may cause contact lenses to become greasy shortly after insertion, with concomitant blurring of vision. The alteration in corneal thickness can result in a change in the refractive index and, therefore, the refractive power of the eye (1–3). A transient insufficiency of accommodation also has been reported (4). For these reasons, it is not advisable to prescribe a new optical correction (spectacles or contact lenses) until a few weeks after delivery.

Intraocular pressure decreases during the second half of pregnancy. This may be secondary to an increased facility of aqueous outflow or change in the episcleral venous pressure. These changes are thought to be hormonally mediated and return to prepartum levels approximately 2 months after delivery (5,6). The ocular hypotensive effect of late pregnancy was found to be similar in systemically hypertensive and nonhypertensive pregnant women (7). The management of a pregnant woman who has preexisting glaucoma can be facilitated by these physiologic hypotensive changes and sometimes can allow the ophthalmologist to reduce the topical medications needed to control the disease.

Blepharoptosis may develop during the course of a normal pregnancy (8). The pregnant woman can complain of this drooped eyelid as a cosmetic concern or as a functional loss of visual field. Although the exact cause is unknown, it has been proposed that the ptosis occurring in mid to late pregnancy may be related to increased levels of estrogen and resultant infiltration of water into the collagen matrix, subsequently stretching the levator muscle and its tendon (9). In most cases the ptosis resolves completely (8), but if it remains for several months postpartum it also can be surgically corrected.

Increased pigmentation around the eyelids may be seen. Commonly called chloasma, or the mask of pregnancy, it may be the result of increased circulating melanocytic-stimulating hormone (10). Pigment deposition on the inner layer of the cornea (Krukenberg spindles), as seen only on slit-lamp biomicroscopy, is noted in increased frequency in pregnant women. Similar to chloasma, it is thought to be caused by increased circulating hormones (11).

Spider angiomas commonly seen during pregnancy can occur on the face and around the eyelids. These telangiectasias are thought to be caused by increased estrogen levels (12).

OCULAR COMPLICATIONS OF PREGNANCY

During normal and complicated pregnancies a variety of changes occur in maternal physiology that can initiate or aggravate eye disease.

Retinopathy of Preeclampsia

A well-known ocular complication of pregnancy is the retinopathy of preeclampsia. It is associated with hypertension, edema, and proteinuria and, in more severe cases, convulsions and coma may occur. Funduscopic changes have been reported in 30% to 100% of cases of preeclampsia (13).

Most of the ocular complications in preeclampsia are readily visible in the posterior pole of the fundus. The retinal changes (Fig. 34-3) include severe arteriolar spasm, characterized by either segmental or generalized constriction of the retinal vessels. Multiple retinal hemorrhages, retinal edema, cotton wool spots and papilledema (Fig. 34-4) also may be seen. These signs are more common in preeclamptics with other systemic diseases such as diabetes and chronic hypertension (12,14). Spasm and narrowing of the retinal vessels is the earliest and most common sign of retinopathy of preeclampsia. The progression of focal spasm to generalized constriction may parallel the worsening of the disease (12,14,15). Exudative retinal detachment is a complication of severe preeclampsia (20% of cases) and eclampsia (10% of cases) (16). Retinal detachments may appear as large bullous areas of cryptlike elevations in the fundus and may be bilateral. The clinical use of intravenous fluorescein angiography has demonstrated that these retinal detachments may be caused by an increased pressure in the

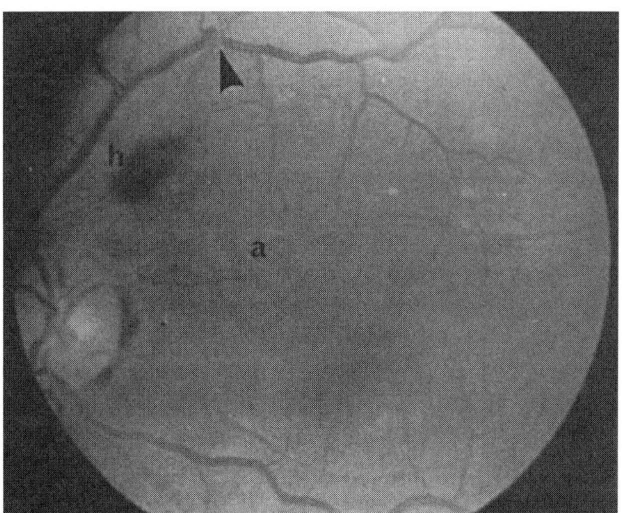

FIG. 34-3. The fundus in toxemia: arrowhead, arteriovenous crossing change; a, copper wiring of retinal artery; h, superficial retinal hemorrhage.

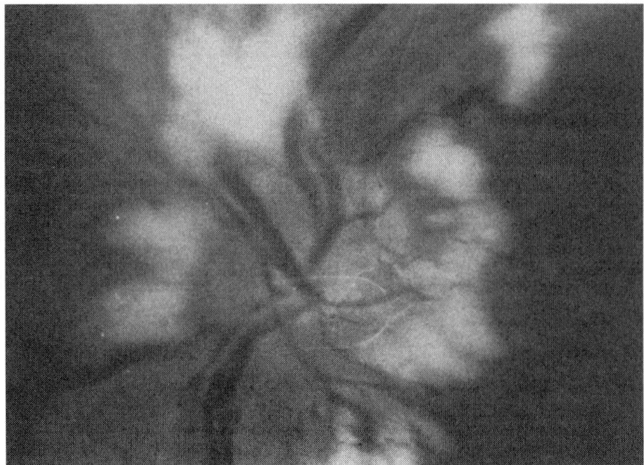

FIG. 34-4. The fundus in toxemia showing many cotton-wool spots.

choroidal vessels with subsequent damage to the retinal pigment epithelium and leakage of fluid into the subretinal space. The accumulation of this fluid causes the detachment. Focal areas of damaged retinal pigment epithelium can be recognized ophthalmoscopically as white-yellow patches in the outer layers of the retina (17).

The fundal changes in preeclampsia may be readily observed using a direct ophthalmoscope. Although obstetricians and ophthalmologists alike are obliged to examine a toxemic patient who presents with visual complaints, they should be aware that convulsions may be precipitated by photic stimulation (18). If a retinal detachment is suspected, indirect ophthalmoscopy should be performed. Fluorescein angiography should not be performed routinely on preeclampsia patients who have visual symptoms because fluorescein crosses the placenta (18). If the diagnosis is not apparent after funduscopic examination, additional noninvasive tests, including electrophysiologic tests of retinal function, may be obtained. These tests may help distinguish retinopathy from the less common causes of blindness seen in toxemia, such as cortical blindness caused by occipital infarct or vasospasm, ischemic optic neuropathy, papillophlebitis, thrombosis of the central retinal artery, or conversion reactions (19).

With the termination of pregnancy, there is usually prompt resolution of the systemic signs of preeclampsia. Concurrently, the previously observed retinal changes are usually reversible. Although the prognosis of retinal detachments is generally good, permanent visual loss can occur in the event of protracted detachments.

Diabetic Retinopathy

Diabetic retinopathy is a complication of type I diabetes mellitus. The prevalence of retinopathy is best correlated with the duration of the disease, and visual symptoms generally appear approximately 15 years after onset. Diabetic retinopathy is usually seen in women of childbearing age who developed diabetes when they were 5 to 15 years of age and is reported in about 25% of diabetic women during their pregnancy. It is not certain whether the incidence of retinopathy is coincidental with age (20 to 30 years, the peak childbearing years) or whether the metabolic and endocrinologic changes of pregnancy influence its onset and progression (20,21). A pregnant woman who acquires gestational diabetes is not at risk for diabetic retinopathy (22).

Diabetic retinopathy can be divided into two types: background and proliferative. Background retinopathy (Fig. 34-5) is manifested by microaneurysms, dot hemorrhages, large hemorrhages, hard exudates, soft exudates (cotton-wool spots), venous dilatation and tortuosity, and areas of retinal edema. Proliferative retinopathy (Fig. 34-6), in addition to background changes, displays areas of new vessel formation. These vessels are small and fragile and are seen on the optic disc or elsewhere in the posterior pole. The new vessels may or may not be accompanied by fibrous tissue proliferation.

Diabetic retinopathy invariably involves the posterior pole of the eye in the area bordered by the superior and inferior temporal arcades. Visual acuity is often not a good indication of the severity of the retinopathy. If the fovea centralis is not affected, there may be excellent vision despite advanced retinopathy (23). Only a careful ophthalmologic evaluation will determine the extent of disease. All pregnant diabetics have a baseline ophthalmologic examination in the first trimester, and follow-up should be judged according to ophthalmic findings and the obstetric course.

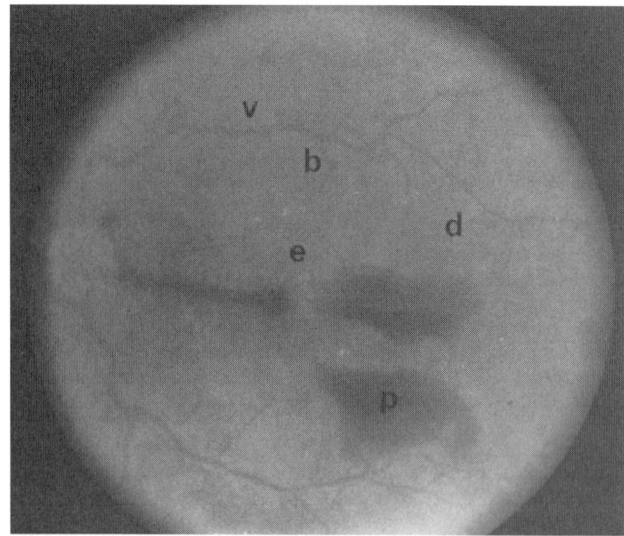

FIG. 34-5. Nonproliferative diabetic retinopathy: d, dot hemorrhages; b, blot hemorrhages; e, hard exudates; v, venous dilatation; p, preretinal hemorrhages.

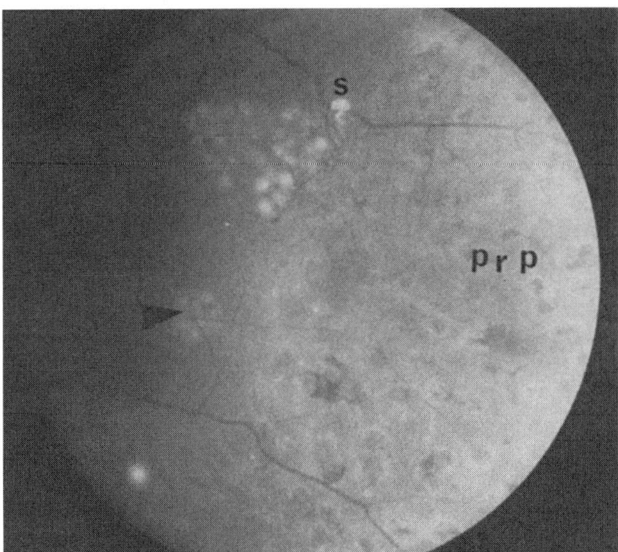

FIG. 34-6. Proliferative diabetic retinopathy: prp, an area of panretinal laser photocoagulation; arrowhead, area of retinal neovascularization following laser treatment; s, a sclerosed vein-vessel tuft.

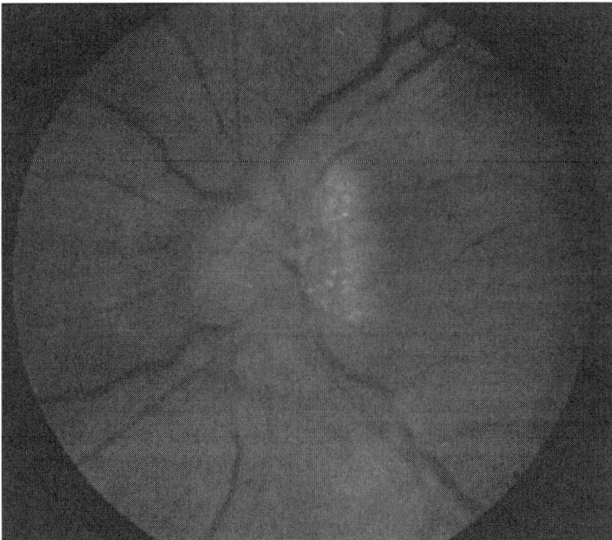

FIG. 34-7. Full-blown papilledema.

Diabetic retinopathy, especially progressive proliferative disease, is a risk to vision and, in the past, had been considered an indication for termination of pregnancy. Treatment and prognosis of diabetic retinopathy during pregnancy have changed dramatically in the last decade. Intravenous fluorescein angiography (IVFA), although helpful, is often not crucial in decision making. In cases of diabetic retinopathy associated with retinal ischemia, however, IVFA is definitely indicated. With the advent of argon laser photocoagulation (panretinal photocoagulation), diabetic retinopathy may be arrested and the pregnancy may be allowed to continue (24,25).

Intracranial Problems

Visual field changes in pregnancy can vary from complaints of transient obscurations in vision to loss of bitemporal fields. Numerous conditions can produce changes in the visual field by exerting pressure on the neural pathways of the visual system or by increasing intracranial pressure. It is often difficult to determine whether pregnancy is responsible for the disease or merely accelerates its development (26).

Pseudotumor cerebri (benign intracranial hypertension) is a rare complication of pregnancy but may occur during any trimester. The ocular danger to patients with pseudotumor cerebri is permanent impairment of vision caused by chronic papilledema. The pregnant woman may complain of headache, blurring of vision, transient obscuration in vision, double vision, or dizziness. On examination she may have bilateral papilledema (Fig. 34-7) and sixth nerve palsy without other focal neurologic deficits. The diagnosis is established by excluding other causes of increased intracranial pressure such as mass lesions, hydrocephalus, and hypertensive encephalopathy. The treatment of pseudotumor during pregnancy includes observation, repeated lumbar puncture with removal of cerebrospinal fluid, diuretics with salt and water restriction, corticosteroids, ventricular shunt procedures, and decompression of the perioptic meninges. If treatment is ineffective, termination of pregnancy may be considered. When medical management has enabled the pregnancy to continue without damage to vision, cesarean delivery may be preferred to avoid an increase in maternal intracranial pressure during the second stage of labor (27).

With advances and treatment of amenorrhea and infertility problems, women who have unrecognized pituitary microadenomas and adenomas may become pregnant. Hormonal changes during pregnancy may stimulate enlargement of pituitary tumors (12,28). The pregnant woman with a pituitary tumor may complain of headaches and visual disturbances, including blurred vision, double vision, and visual field changes. On examination, the optic discs may appear pale and the visual field may demonstrate bitemporal abnormalities. Management of these patients with high-dose corticosteroids and bromocriptine, and careful monitoring of the visual acuity and visual fields may obviate the need for surgical intervention. If progression of visual changes is demonstrated, tumor removal or termination of pregnancy is indicated (29–31) (see Chapter 24).

Vascular tumors have been noted to increase in size during pregnancy. This may be secondary to a change in hemodynamics and endocrinologic systems. Unilateral proptosis (exophthalmos) during pregnancy has been seen with orbital cavernous hemangiomas and spontaneous carotid-cavernous fistulas (32). Cases of rapidly growing craniopharyngioma occurring during pregnancy have also been reported (33).

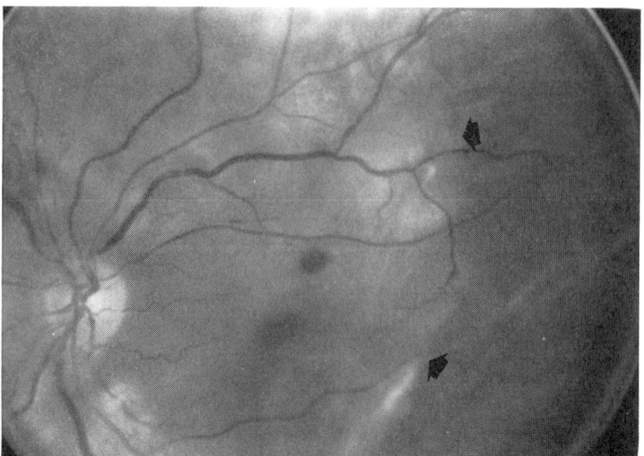

FIG. 34-8. Fundus photograph shows numerous focal retinal detachments in a woman who developed DIC postpartum and died.

Visual disturbances and visual field defects have occurred in the puerperium as a result of cerebral vein thrombosis. This has resulted in cortical blindness or homonymous hemianopsia (34).

Disseminated Intravascular Coagulation

Disseminated intravascular coagulation (DIC) is an acquired coagulopathy characterized by an intravascular consumption of clotting factors and platelets resulting in widespread deposition of fibrin thrombi in the peripheral blood system. Obstetric problems such as abruptio placentae, toxemia, amniotic fluid embolus, retained dead fetus, and postpartum sepsis are factors associated with DIC.

In the eye, DIC affects the choroidal vessel layer, particularly the region below the macula and optic disc (Fig. 34-8). The fibrin clots in the choroidal vessels cause marked vascular congestion and hemorrhage of the posterior pole, which can result in a retinal detachment (Fig. 34-9) (35).

Visual symptoms may be an early manifestation of DIC, presenting as complaints of decreased vision, postural xanthopsia (shimmering of vision), or a visual field cut secondary to a retinal detachment. The findings are often present in both eyes (36,37).

Graves Disease

Ocular findings such as lid lag, thyroid stare, and exophthalmos (Fig. 34-10) may be the initial manifestations of thyrotoxicosis and may be seen in early pregnancy or after delivery. These ocular changes are specific to Graves disease and are not seen in Hashimoto disease (38–40) (see Chapter 22).

Autoimmune Disease

Pregnancy can alter the course of an autoimmune disease. The relationship may vary, causing either a remission or exacerbation of the condition (see Chapter 37). Autoimmune disease may be influenced by various hormones secreted by the ovaries, placenta, and adrenal glands. Several reports have documented the ocular findings as the initial manifestation of the disease and the first clue to the diagnosis.

One such example is Vogt-Koyangi-Harada syndrome, an uncommon condition that has occurred during pregnancy. It is characterized by bilateral anterior and posterior uveitis, retinal detachment, papilledema, vitiligo, alopecia, hearing problems, and central nervous system (CSN) involvement. When this disease occurs during pregnancy, treatment with steroids may be beneficial, but complete remission is thought to occur only after delivery (41).

Other diseases may be suppressed during pregnancy. Uveitis secondary to sarcoidosis may remain dormant throughout pregnancy and may exacerbate in the puerperium. The suppression may be based on the high level of circulating free cortisol during pregnancy. After deliv-

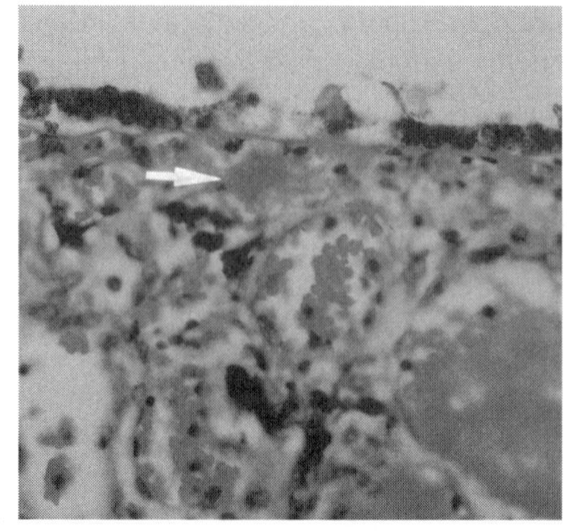

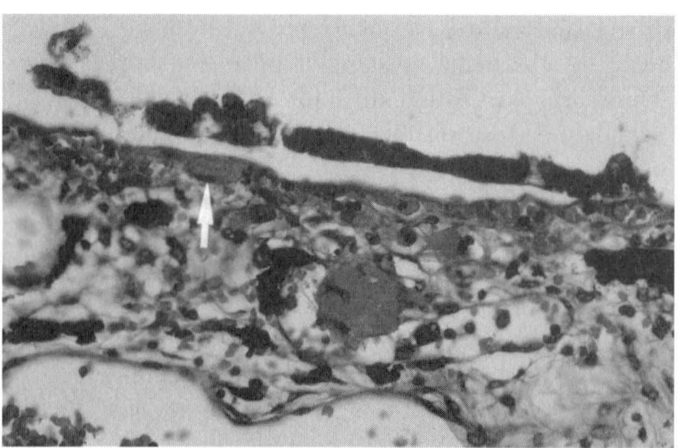

FIG. 34-9. Photomicrograph of eye postmortem shows fibrin thrombi in choroidal blood vessels. **A:** Hematoxylin and eosin. **B:** Trichrome.

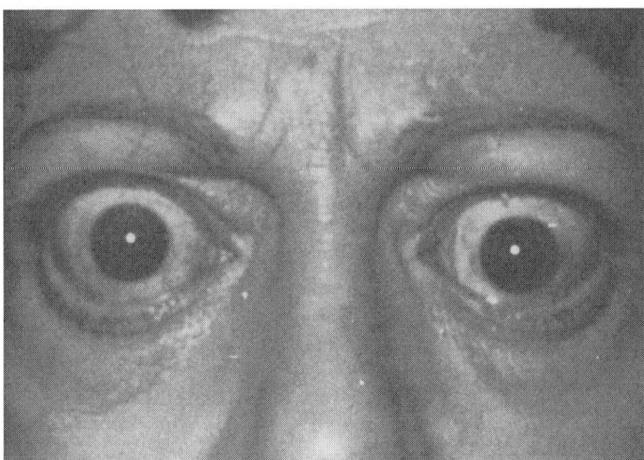

FIG. 34-10. Graves disease with prominent stare and exophthalmos.

ery, there is a rapid reduction of serum cortisol that may exacerbate the uveitis and retinopathy (42).

Systemic lupus erythematosus (SLE) is associated with a variety of ocular problems, including cotton-wool spots (soft exudates) (Fig. 34-11), retinal hemorrhages, retinal edema, retinal vein engorgement, papilledema, conjunctivitis, and episcleritis (Fig. 34-12). Retinal vascular occlusions and retinal neovascularization may develop during pregnancy. The presence and progression of these manifestations of SLE in the absence of a favorable response to medical therapy may necessitate termination of the pregnancy in order to preserve vision (43).

Uveitis associated with rheumatoid arthritis and ulcerative colitis also can occur in the postpregnant state (44).

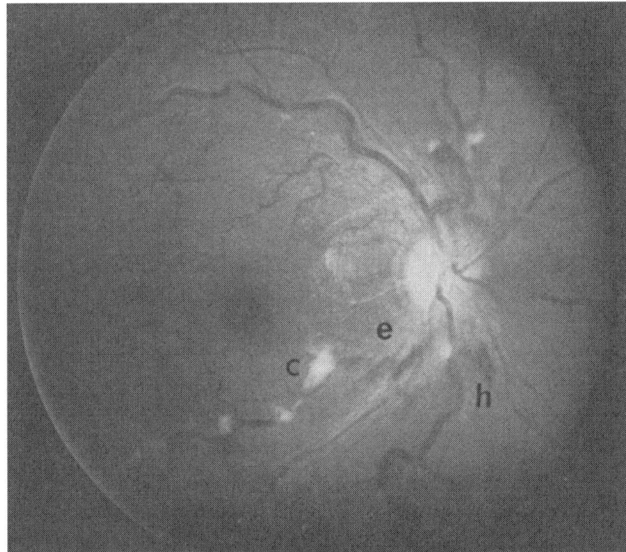

FIG. 34-11. Fundus in systemic lupus erythematosus: h, hemorrhages; c, cotton-wool spots; e, retinal edema.

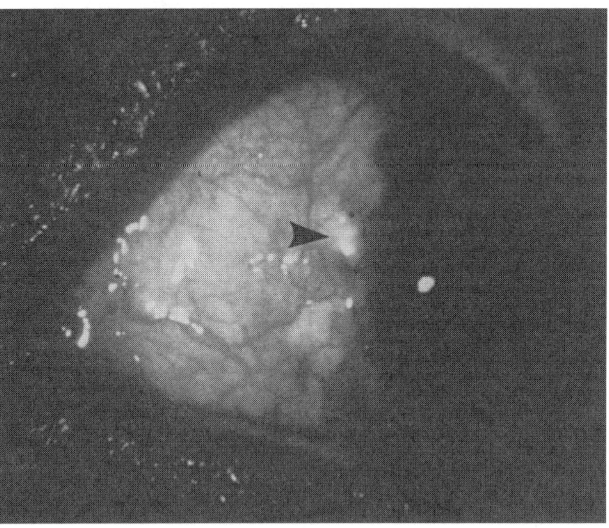

FIG. 34-12. Episcleritis in a patient with SLE. Arrowhead delineates lesion.

Central Serous Choroidopathy

Central serous choroidopathy is a spontaneous condition caused by focal leakage from the choriocapillaris that results in the accumulation of fluid between the retina and the pigment epithelium (Fig. 34-13). The subsequent detachment of the sensory retina causes symptoms of diminished visual acuity, central scotoma, and metamorphopsia. This disease usually affects men but has been seen with increased prevalence among pregnant woman. The visual disturbances that will occur during pregnancy spontaneously resolve after delivery. Pregnancy is otherwise normal, without signs of preeclampsia. Laboratory testing is not beneficial in establishing the cause of this disorder (45).

The visual disturbances in central serous choroidopathy should not be confused with complaints associated with pregnancy-related optic neuritis or expanding intracranial lesions. These various clinical entities can always be distinguished by careful fundus examination.

Migraines

Migraine headaches are a common occurrence, affecting nearly 5% of the general population. There is a greater prevalence of migraine headaches among women, suggesting that hormone levels, especially estrogen, influence the occurrence, frequency, and severity of migraine attacks (16) (see Chapter 32).

Generally, pregnancy is felt to have a beneficial influence on migraine headaches. Many reports show an improvement in the common migraine sufferer during the end of the first and last two trimesters of pregnancy (46). This is not necessarily true in the classical migraine headache, in which some women complain of new onset or increased frequency of their classical migraine attacks (47).

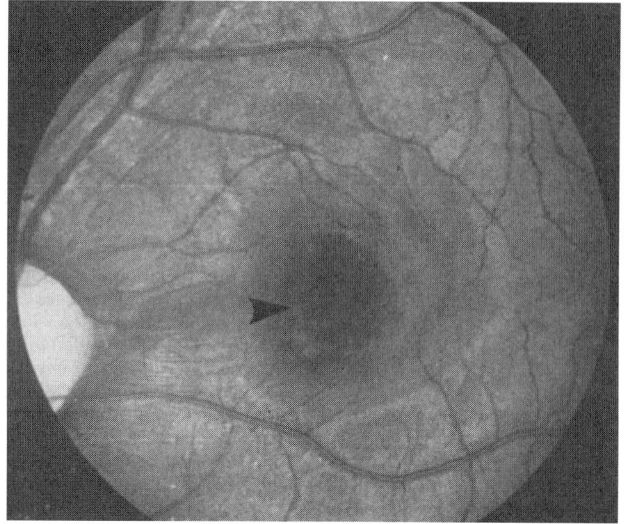
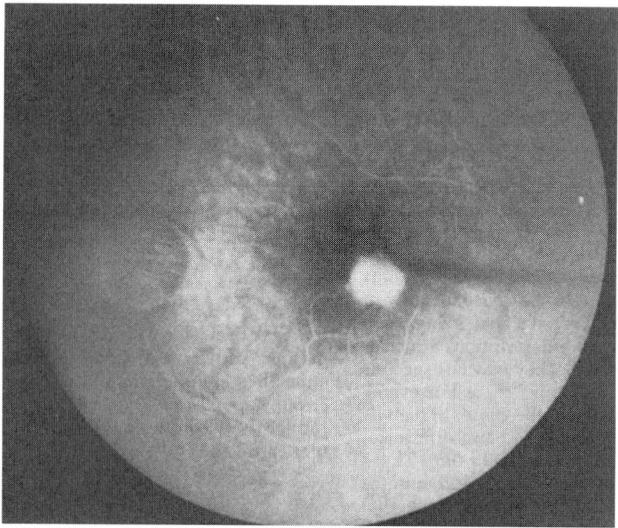

FIG. 34-13. Fundus photograph of left eye in central serous retinopathy. **A:** Arrowhead shows area of macular edema. **B:** Intravenous fluorescein angiogram shows the area of leakage in the arteriovenous phase of the study.

Classic migraine headaches have several characteristic visual symptoms that may alarm pregnant women. These visual experiences (scintillating scotomas or visual field defects) are not painful and precede the actual headache (48). They often are described as waving zig-zag lines, heat-wave flashes, and colored or neon lights. These patients may describe an alteration in their visual acuity or complain that, while reading or looking at a face or an object, a fragment is missing. These descriptions are characteristic of visual scotomas. They may last seconds to minutes, and then luminous C-shaped or horseshoe-shaped zig-zag lines appear in the center of the visual field. These lines may expand and diffuse toward the periphery of the visual field (49). These visual complaints usually last from 20 to 25 minutes and may or may not be followed by a headache that often is contralateral to the involved visual field (48).

OCULAR EMBRYOPATHIES

Embryotoxicities

The extent of ocular maldevelopment caused by teratogens depends on the period in which the embryotoxic agent acts during gestation. The teratogen may be drugs, environmental chemicals, radiation, or infectious agents (see Chapters 6 and 7).

Many factors can play a role in the presence or extent of ocular damage, including teratogenic potential of the agent, dosage, mode of transmission, predilection for a particular tissue, maternal and fetal susceptibility, and, last, the laws of random distribution (8,49).

Drugs

Ethanol. Significant ethanol ingestion during pregnancy may result in a spectrum of fetal malformations known as the "fetal alcohol syndrome." The syndrome includes reduced growth, facial anomalies, and mental retardation. The affected infants may continue to show decreased growth rates after birth (50).

A high percentage (up to 90%) of children who have fetal alcohol syndrome also have eye abnormalities. The classic ophthalmic findings include short horizontal palpebral fissures, ptosis, myopia, and cataracts. The two malformations that are the most typical are hypoplasia of the optic nerve head and increased tortuosity of the retinal vessels. Visual acuity is often seriously reduced (51). There may be a close relationship between the quantity of ethanol consumption and the full expression of the disease (50).

Also noted is the increased occurrence of strabismus in infants born to drug-dependent women. A study indicates that exposure to psychoactive drugs and increased methadone dosages during pregnancy may predispose infants more to the development of strabismus compared with the general population (52).

Lysergic Acid Diethylamide. Lysergic acid diethylamide (LSD) ingestion during the first trimester of pregnancy may result in numerous ocular and CNS abnormalities. Ocular anomalies include microphthalmia, cataracts, optic atrophy, persistent hyperplastic primary vitreous, retinal dysplasia, retinal detachment, and intraocular cartilage (53).

Thalidomide. Thalidomide ingestion during the first trimester of pregnancy can cause a condition called phocomelia, as well as multiple ocular abnormalities. Studies have shown that ocular involvement occurs in 25% of fetuses exposed to the drug between the fifth and seventh weeks of gestation. Ocular findings include colobomas of the uvea and optic nerve, microphthalmos, and paresis of ocular muscles, causing strabismus (53).

Ethambutol. Ethambutol in therapeutic doses is known to damage the optic nerve and ocular tissue in the susceptible person. Although ethambutol has no proven teratogenic effects during the first trimester of pregnancy, it is unclear whether later damage to the myelinization process of the optic nerve is affected by continuance of the drug into late pregnancy. Because the drug possesses an affinity for optic nerve tissue, signs of impaired development would be expected to occur, yet functional impairment may go undetected until the infant is older and full visual function is established. As a precaution, it is advisable that ethambutol not be used in the treatment of tuberculosis during pregnancy (54).

Folic Acid Antagonists. Folic acid antagonists (including methotrexate, pyrimethamine, and other anticancer and antimicrobials) have the potential for human teratogenicity. Ocular abnormalities such as proptosis and hypertelorism have been reported (55).

Phenothiazines and Chloroquine. In utero exposure to phenothiazines such as chlorpromazine and thioridazine and to antimalarial and antirheumatic agents such as chloroquine can cause retinotoxic effects in animals. These observations may reflect a potential toxic effect in humans. Visual impairment and the appearance of retinal damage may appear at a later stage in the infant.

Hydantoins. Seizures occur in 0.3% of pregnant women and require anticonvulsant therapy. Recent data suggest that 11% of infants exposed to hydantoin in utero share a common set of dysmorphic features. These findings include limb, craniofacial, ocular, and growth abnormalities. Ocular defects include ptosis, strabismus, wide epicanthal folds, hypertelorism, and colobomas of the uvea. Animal studies have shown a dose-related teratogenic effect; therefore, monitoring of serum phenytoin levels in women of childbearing age may be warranted (56). Another anticonvulsant, trimethadione, has been associated with epicanthus and V-shaped eyebrows, myopia, and strabismus (57). Thorough counseling of women who take anticonvulsant drugs is necessary to balance risks and benefits in each patient so that informed decisions can be made (see Chapters 7 and 28) (8).

Environmental Agents

Organic mercurials are industrial waste products found in fungicides. They may contaminate water sources and food products. Toxic doses may produce a visual field constriction, decreased visual acuity, tremors, dementia, and death. *In utero* exposure is known to cause a similar condition in the fetus (58).

Radiation

Doses of radiation (500 rad or more in the first trimester of pregnancy) are associated with microphthalmia, pigment degeneration of the retina, and cataracts. The association of human teratogenicity because of radiation is well documented (59,60) and is discussed in detail in Chapter 6.

Ophthalmic Medications and Pregnancy

Limited information exists on the use of topical ophthalmic medications during pregnancy and lactation. Topical eye medications are absorbed systemically via the nasopharyngeal mucosa and must therefore be considered for their potential adverse effects as well as their teratogenicity. Two general principles should be observed in the use of any topical eye medication during pregnancy or lactation:

1. Therapy should be administered in a minimal effective dose for as short a time as is consistent with good eye care.
2. Nasolacrimal occlusion should be performed after instillation of eye medications to minimize systemic absorption.

Nasolacrimal occlusion is accomplished by placement of the index finger between the medial canthus and nose to compress the nasolacrimal sac for 3 to 5 minutes.

Antiglaucoma therapy during pregnancy presents a particular problem because of the chronic nature of the disease requiring ongoing therapy. Topical beta-adrenergic antagonists are thought to be relatively safe during pregnancy (61), but without definitive evidence it is cautioned that beta blockers should be avoided in the first trimester and only the lowest doses needed should be used in the other trimesters. It is also advised to discontinue therapy 2 to 3 days prior to delivery in order to decrease the potential effect of beta blockade on uterine contractility and to prevent neonatal complications such as bradycardia and apnea (61). Beta blockers also have been found in the breast milk of lactating mothers. Infants should be observed for signs of beta blockade (such as bradycardia and apnea). It is best advised that women on beta blockers not breastfeed (12,61,62).

There is limited information regarding miotic therapy, and many of the reports are anecdotal. Transient muscle weakness in the newborn when the mother has received systemic cholinesterase inhibitors has been reported (62). There also is a report of a pregnant woman treated with pilocarpine throughout pregnancy who delivered a healthy baby (62). Pilocarpine given to a pregnant woman near term has been associated with neonatal hyperthermia, seizures, restlessness, and diaphoresis (61).

There are multiple reports in humans and animals of the teratogenic effects of carbonic anhydrase inhibitors taken orally, and this class of antiglaucoma medications should be avoided during pregnancy (61,62). Epinephrine crosses the placenta, can interfere with uterine contractility, and can cause hypoxia in the fetus in doses sufficient to cause deceased uterine blood flow. No data are available on the effects of dipivefirin.

Other dilating agents, such as atropine, homatropine, and scopolamine, have been associated with minor fetal malformations when given systemically. Scopolamine also has been associated with neonatal tachycardia, fever, and lethargy. No data are available regarding the untoward effects of shorter acting anticholinergics such as tropicanide and cyclopentolate (12,61).

It has not been established whether topical corticosteroids cause teratogenic effects in humans. Corticosteroids taken systemically have been associated with teratogenic effects in experimental animals, but data from humans have not proved teratogenesis. Bilateral cataracts have been reported in a child whose mother received systemic corticosteroids throughout her pregnancy (61). Systemic corticosteroids appear in breast milk and can cause growth problems and suppression of endogenous corticosteroid production in the neonate. Nursing is relatively contraindicated in patients who take corticosteroids (61).

Use of topical antibiotics during pregnancy may be needed to treat vision-threatening infections. Topical erythromycin and polymixin B are thought to be the safest antibiotics for this purpose because there are no reports of congenital defects associated with these drugs (61).

The aminoglycosides—gentamicin, neomycin, and tobramycin—have been associated with ototoxicity in the fetus (61), but systemic levels of significance are unlikely if the usual ophthalmic doses are given. Sulfonamides given systemically in the third trimester can lead theoretically to hyperbilirubinemia in infants; tetracycline produces discoloration of the primary teeth after the first trimester and should not be used during lactation (61).

Antivirals are potentially teratogenic and should generally not be used in pregnant or nursing mothers (12,61). To date, no data exist regarding any harmful effects of fluorescein, which is known to cross the placenta.

Ocular Complications Associated with Intrauterine Infections

Ocular disease can be produced by various infectious agents that affect the fetus during pregnancy. Transplacental transmission is the usual route of *in utero* infection, but ocular disease also can be contracted through retrograde infection from the genital tract to the fetus, secondary to premature rupture of membranes. Ophthalmic disease can be acquired as well during delivery of the infant through an infected birth canal.

The ensuing sections address several clinically significant diseases, including the TORCH group (toxoplasmosis/rubella/cytomegalovirus/herpes simplex) and the common causes of ophthalmia neonatorum.

Rubella

When a nonimmune pregnant woman is infected with the rubella virus during the first trimester and a viremia occurs, there is a 30% to 60% chance of ocular defects occurring in the fetus. The mechanism for the development of ocular malformations is thought to be death of infected cells or a change in the rate of growth of these cells, or a contribution of both mechanisms. The diagnosis of congenital rubella is established by rubella titers in the mother and infant and, if needed, titers of the aqueous fluid of the eye (63).

One of the common ocular anomalies associated with the congenital rubella syndrome is cataracts (Fig. 34-14), unilateral or bilateral, which are frequently associated with microphthalmia. The cataracts usually are present at birth but may be too small to be detected without special instrumentation. When the cataract is fully developed, within several weeks the cloudy lens fills the pupillary aperture and is easily detectable on gross examination. Cataract formation is caused by direct viral infection of the lens and is unique with regard to the speed at which it progresses (63,64). Microphthalmic eyes associated with cataracts always have poor vision; therefore, cataract surgery may be of questionable value.

Rubella retinitis (Fig. 34-15) is the most frequent ocular abnormality seen in this syndrome. It is present in 25% to 50% of infants who have congenital rubella. It can be unilateral or bilateral and appears characteristically as pigment deposits in a granular or clumped distribution. The pigmentation is usually limited to the posterior pole, most

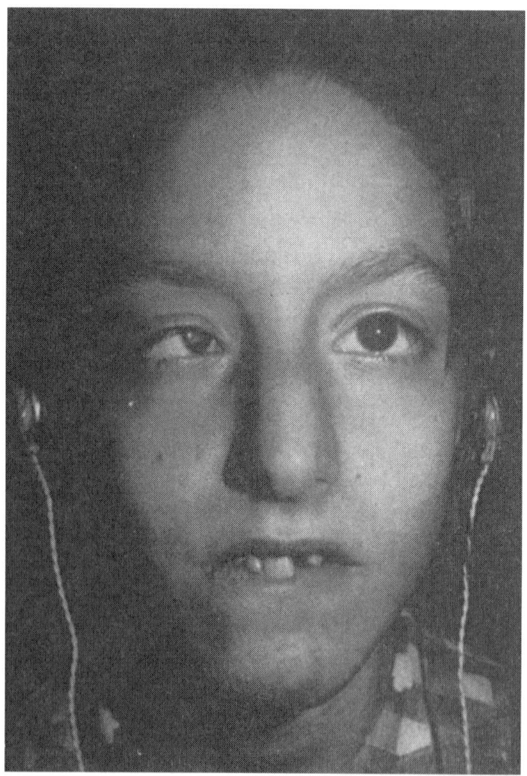

FIG. 34-14. A girl with congenital rubella syndrome. She is deaf, has a cataract in the right eye, and strabismus. The right eye, in addition, is microphthalmic.

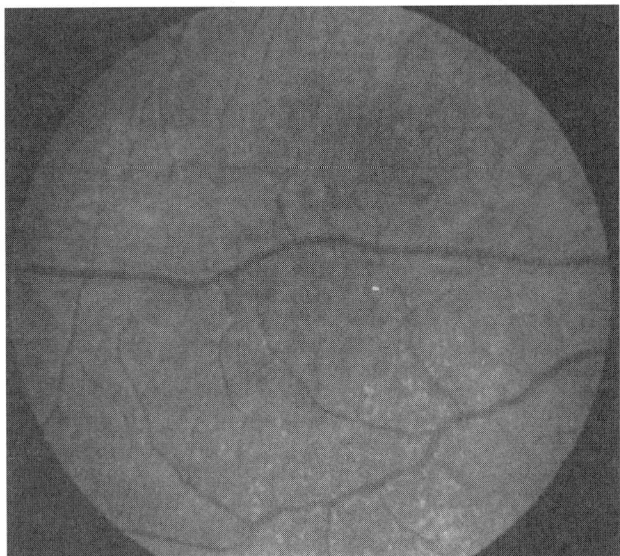

FIG. 34-15. The fundus of a child with rubella retinopathy. Note salt and pepper appearance of retina.

prominently in the macular area. The retinopathy of congenital rubella, commonly called "salt and pepper" fundus, is benign and nonprogressive. It does not interfere with vision unless a network of new blood vessels develops in the macular area beneath the retina (65).

Congenital glaucoma is another complication of the rubella syndrome. If the viral infection occurs during the first trimester, cataracts and glaucoma may develop. If the viremia occurs during the second trimester, only glaucoma may exist because the lens has already completed its embryonic capsular development. The glaucoma is usually caused by maldevelopment of the anterior chamber angle. Although the incidence of cataracts in the rubella syndrome is about tenfold more prevalent than is glaucoma, glaucoma has been reported in approximately 10% to 20% of infants (63,64,66,67). Transient corneal clouding may be seen in congenital rubella. This must be distinguished from the corneal clouding seen in congenital glaucoma. Other ocular defects of the rubella syndrome include strabismus, nystagmus, and inflammation of the lacrimal gland and uvea (63,68).

Congenital Toxoplasmosis

Toxoplasma gondii is usually transmitted to the fetus from a mother who has acquired the infection during pregnancy, and rarely from a mother infected before pregnancy (69). The fetus is infected by transplacental transmission of the parasite (Fig. 34-16). Ocular involvement is thought to be a result of congenital infection only.

Approximately 40% of the infants of actively infected mothers contract this disease. Of that 40%, about 80% have ocular involvement. Signs of ocular involvement may appear acutely or may manifest later in life (69).

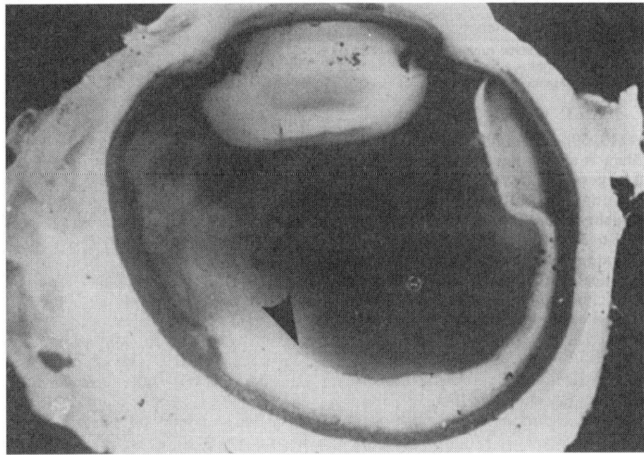

FIG. 34-16. Toxoplasmosis. Gross photograph of the left eye of an aborted fetus showing severe retinal necrosis. (Courtesy of W. Richard Green, M.D.)

Retinochoroiditis is the most common finding in ocular toxoplasmosis and may appear as an acute inflammation at birth or up to 18 months after delivery. An acute retinochoroiditis presents as a white-to-yellow exudative lesion and is commonly seen in the macular region of the fundus. An overlying inflammation of vitreous may give a hazy appearance to the retina. Active retinal lesions usually subside, resulting in chorioretinal scarring within one to several months regardless of treatment (70).

The presence of a focal, pigmented, atrophic chorioretinal scar from toxoplasmosis is evidence of an inactive *in utero* infection. Reactivation (Fig. 34-17) of retinochoroiditis in life is thought to be caused by *T. gondii* cysts dormant in the retina or by a hypersensitivity reaction (71).

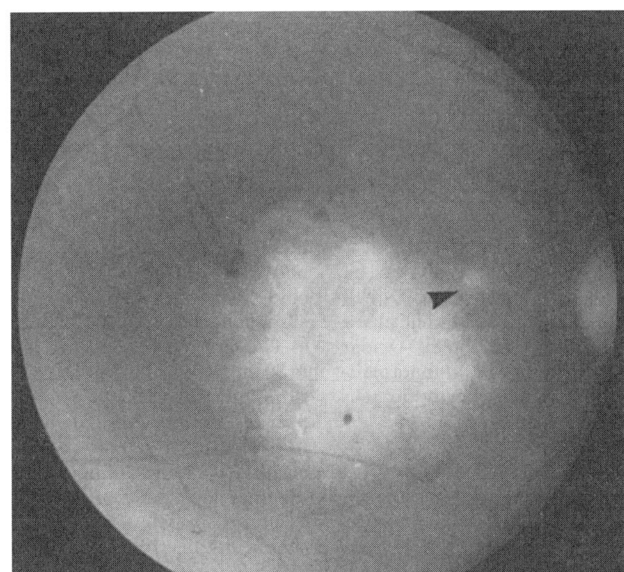

FIG. 34-17. Reactivation of congenital toxoplasmosis produces an acute retinochoroiditis *(arrowhead)*.

Microphthalmia is a severe complication of congenital toxoplasmosis. It may occur in about 20% of infants who have ocular abnormalities and may be associated with retinochoroiditis and secondary cataracts (70).

Mothers who have given birth to toxoplasmic infants rarely infect subsequent offspring because the maternal immunity is important in preventing the disease. A patient who has active ocular toxoplasmosis should be treated if the inflammatory process is severe or threatens the macula. Combined use of various antibiotics (including sulfadiazine and clindamycin) as well as corticosteroids may be used. Pregnant women who have active toxoplasmosis should be treated (see Chapter 44). Pyrimethamine has been reported to cause limb defects in animals (72), but is probably safe in humans. In one recent study it was observed that of 18 pregnancies in 10 women, clinical evidence of active toxoplasmic retinochoroiditis (three patients) was not associated with fetal infection.

Congenital Syphilis

Congenital syphilis is caused by transplacental transmission of the obligate human pathogen *Treponema pallidum.* The fetus is most commonly infected after the third gestational month and, as a result of the late involvement *in utero,* the ocular abnormalities are more inflammatory than developmental. Although the diagnosis and treatment of syphilis has been more effective in recent years, there are still over 20,000 reported cases in the United States each year. In an untreated pregnant woman, there is only a small chance that her fetus will not be involved (70).

Various stages of ocular abnormalities are associated with congenital syphilis, including early inflammatory conditions such as eyelid chancres, uveitis, vitritis, chorioretinitis, and retinal vasculitis. The anterior inflammatory reaction can result in secondary glaucoma and cataracts. The most common ocular manifestation is interstitial keratitis. It occurs in 10% to 15% of infants who have congenital syphilis, and it characteristically occurs later in life, between the age of 5 and 16 years. It is usually bilateral and is thought to be a result of a local immunologic reaction (70,73). An acute infection is characterized by complaints of photophobia, blepharospasm, and lacrimation. The eyes appear to be injected. The cornea is edematous with infiltrates and vessel ingrowth. Untreated, the acute reaction may be prolonged and result in scarring of the cornea with a poor visual prognosis. Of importance is that interstitial keratitis can be prevented if the congenital syphilis is recognized and treated prior to 3 months of age (70).

The fundus of an involved infant can display chorioretinal lesions that may have a focal atrophic or a diffuse granular appearance of the retinal pigment epithelium. This is another example of "salt and pepper" retinopathy. There may be areas of pigment deposition in a distribution resembling retinitis pigmentosa. This retinal picture in congenital syphilis is called pseudoretinitis pigmentosa and can be readily differentiated from true retinitis pigmentosa if the results of electroretinography are normal (71,73,74).

The very late stage of congenital syphilis can be compared with the tertiary stage in the adult. Development of neurosyphilis may follow a latent phase of congenital syphilis during childhood. Ocular findings at this stage include pupillary abnormalities, classically a light-near dissociation, optic neuritis, and optic atrophy (75).

Herpes

A genital infection of increasing clinical importance is herpes simplex virus (HSV), particularly type 2. The virus can be transmitted to the neonate from the infected genital tissues during passage through the birth canal or secondary to an ascending infection because of premature rupture of membranes.

The eye can be the only site of infection in neonatal herpes or it can be seen in conjunction with local or disseminated forms of the disease. Commonly, conjunctivitis is noted. It may be unilateral or bilateral and may be associated with herpetic vesicles on the eyelids. The onset of symptoms varies from 3 days to 2 weeks postpartum. Symptoms are associated with injection of the bulbar conjunctiva and a serosanguinous conjunctival discharge. In approximately 10% of cases, a keratitis may coexist with the conjunctivitis. Corneal herpetic involvement can have the characteristic findings of a dendritic or geographic ulcer. Conjunctivitis in the absence of corneal involvement, therefore, suggests other causes of neonatal ophthalmia (70,76,77).

Numerous reports exist that describe chorioretinitis as a manifestation of neonatal herpetic infection. The inflammation may be detected 1 to 3 months after delivery and may have been preceded by keratoconjunctivitis. The inflammation is characteristically manifested by extensive retinal necrosis with vitreous reaction. Cataracts, intraocular calcification, optic atrophy, and poor vision may be expected (77,78).

Cytomegalovirus

In the differential diagnosis of intrauterine infections, cytomegalic inclusion disease must be considered. Cytomegalovirus (CMV) is frequently cultured from the cervix of pregnant women. Fifty to eighty percent of patients over age 35 have complement fixation antibodies to CMV. Congenital infections therefore may be the result of primary infection of the antibody-deficient pregnant woman (79).

Infection with CMV *in utero* can result in either fetal death or the clinical syndrome of cytomegalic inclusion disease. Contrary to prior reports, CMV is not invariably fatal, although the complex may include hepatosplenomegaly, pneumonitis, CNS disease, chorioretinitis, and optic atrophy (70,79).

The most common ocular lesion, occurring in up to 30% of infected infants, is chorioretinitis. The chorioretinitis present at or shortly after birth may appear as scattered white patches with irregular sheathing of adjacent retinal vessels. The patches may coalesce with areas of hemorrhage around them. In the final stage, the chorioretinitis may be visualized as a posterior pole scar with very little pigment and should not be confused with the scar of toxoplasmosis (70).

Congenital Varicella

Congenital defects following maternal varicella infection are rare compared with congenital rubella anomalies. Nevertheless, there are consistent clinical findings associated with a history of maternal varicella infection during the first trimester of pregnancy. One of these ocular abnormalities includes chorioretinitis, either active inflammation or a chorioretinal scar seen in the posterior pole. Microphthalmia with cataracts, nystagmus, abnormal pupil, and Horner syndrome also have been described in the congenital varicella syndrome. Offspring born to mothers known to have contracted varicella or who have a typical herpes zoster (varicella-zoster virus) rash should have eye examinations for chorioretinal lesions and other ocular anomalies (52).

One report described an acute retinal necrosis (ARN) syndrome following chicken pox in a pregnant woman (80). Acute retinal necrosis is a clinical entity that involves acute inflammation of the retina, vitreous, and anterior segment. This has been associated with a varicella skin eruption in a pregnant woman who had elevated antibody titers to the varicella-zoster virus in the aqueous humor of both eyes (80).

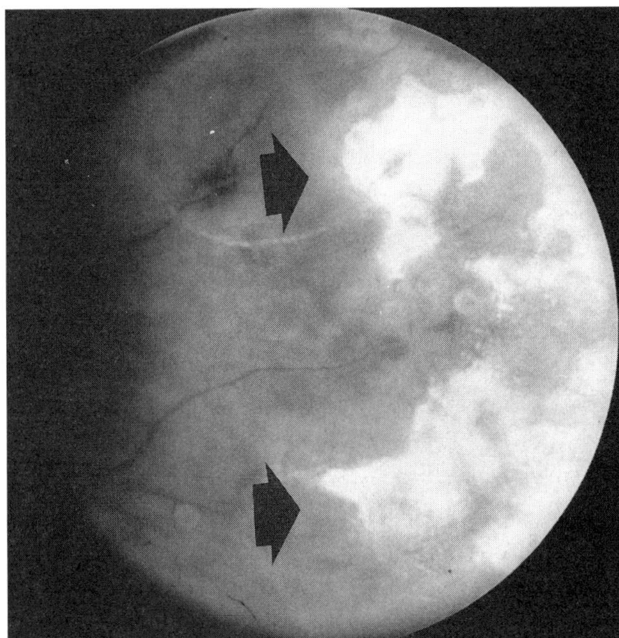

FIG. 34-18. Retinal photograph of left eye in a term pregnant patient with acute retinal necrosis syndrome. Arrows delineate white areas of retinal necrosis.

Another case of ARN was seen by one of the authors (A.H.F.) in the ninth month of pregnancy, caused by herpes virus with no other evidence of systemic herpes infection (Fig. 34-18). The healthy baby was delivered by cesarean section.

Lyme disease is an illness caused by the tick-borne spirochete *Borrelia burgdorferi.* Transplacental transmission of this spirochete has been documented in a pregnant woman who had Lyme disease but who did not receive antimicrobial therapy (81). Adverse outcomes to the fetus have included congenital heart defect, developmental delay, and cortical blindness (81–83). The relationship between the intrauterine infection and these adverse outcomes has not yet been documented (82).

There are many ocular manifestations of Lyme disease that can be recognized in the pregnant women. These include conjunctivitis, keratitis, uveitis, choroiditis with exudative retinal detachment, optic nerve edema or atrophy, pupil abnormalities, and motility problems (84). A pregnant woman with any of these eye findings that cannot otherwise be explained should have serologic testing for Lyme disease.

Acquired Immunodeficiency Syndrome

The human immunodeficiency virus type I is widespread in certain high-risk women of childbearing age and is transmissible to infants. It is well established that maternofetal contamination usually occurs via the transplacental route. Infection is also possible during delivery through the maternal genital tract (85,86). Identification of young women in high-risk groups, risks to the mother, and disease in the infant are addressed elsewhere in this text (see Chapter 43). This discussion focuses on the ocular involvement seen in AIDS patients, such as might occur in women in their childbearing years).

Ocular involvement occurs in approximately 75% of patients who have AIDS. Ocular manifestations are secondary to the opportunistic infections and neoplasias seen in the AIDS syndrome. The most common ocular infections present in the retina, and they include CMV retinitis and toxoplasmosis retinochoroiditis. CMV retinitis manifests as white lesions associated with hemorrhages, most often seen in the posterior pole. The involvement can follow the distribution of the vascular tree seen in the retina. Toxoplasmosis may present as a posterior uveitis with complaints of pain, photophobia, and vitreous floaters. On ophthalmoscopy vitreous opacities and white-yellow intraretinal lesions with irregular borders can be seen. Among AIDS patients, toxoplasmosis often produces bilateral and multifocal retinal lesions, in contradistinction to the involvement seen in the healthy host (86). Significant permanent visual loss can accompany both infections.

Herpes zoster ophthalmicus may occur in AIDS patients and is characterized by a vesicular eruption and neuralgic pain in the distribution of the ophthalmic branch of the trigeminal nerve. Ocular involvement can include blepharitis, conjunctivitis, keratitis, and uveitis (86). A sign of ocular involvement may be a vesicle on the tip of the nose, an area innervated by the nasociliary nerve that also serves the cornea.

Other eye findings seen in AIDS patients include herpes simplex disease, fungal infections (including *Candida* and *Cryptococcus*), and neoplasms (such as Kaposi's sarcoma seen on the eyelid, conjunctiva, and orbit). Cranial nerve palsies can result in extraocular muscle problems with complaints of double vision. Also noted are pupillary abnormalities, optic neuritis, and papilledema.

Ophthalmia Neonatorum

Gonococcal Ophthalmia Neonatorum. The incidence of genital gonorrhea in the obstetric population ranges from 4% to 7.5% (87). Three quarters of these infections are asymptomatic. Gonococcal ophthalmia is acquired during the passage of the infant through an infected cervical and vaginal canal. Conjunctivitis is the most common manifestation of a neonate who has gonorrhea that develops within 4 days of birth. Clinically, the conjunctivitis begins as a serous discharge of both eyes, but a purulent reaction rapidly becomes evident (Fig. 34-19). Untreated gonococcal ophthalmia can progress to an overwhelming ocular infection with corneal ulceration, intraocular spread, and blindness (87).

Diagnosis is suggested by clinical examination and confirmation by laboratory demonstration of gram-negative diplococci seen within polymorphonuclear leukocytes in a Gram stain of the conjunctival exudate. Treatment should not be deferred until culture results are available.

Differential diagnosis of ophthalmia neonatorum includes chlamydial infection, which typically is a less purulent discharge and occurs 5 or more days after birth. Other nongonococcal bacterial pathogens that may be implicated are *Pseudomonas, Pneumococcus, Staphylococcus,* and *Streptococcus.* Identification of the causal agent can be made on Gram stain and culture.

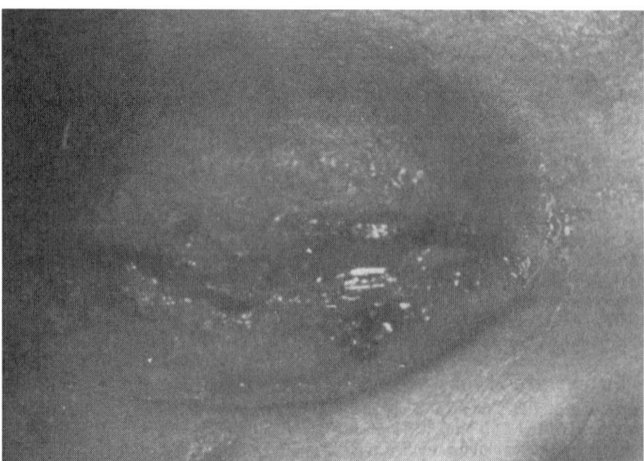

FIG. 34-19. The typical purulent discharge in a case of gonococcal ophthalmia neonatorum. (Courtesy of Drs. Michael Newton and Susan Stenson.)

Recommended treatment of gonococcal conjunctivitis consists of ophthalmic ointment or drops containing 0.5% erythromycin or 1% tetracycline. Systemic therapy is indicated using intravenous aqueous crystalline penicillin G, 50,000 units/kg/day for 7 days. In addition, the parents should be cultured and treated for gonorrhea and the infant should be tested for syphilis (76,87).

Reducing the incidence of gonococcal ophthalmia neonatorum is directed at ocular prophylaxis and screening and treatment of infected mothers before delivery. Since 1880, when Credé discovered that silver nitrate solution was effective in decreasing the rate of ophthalmia from 10% to less than 1%, it has been the basis of ocular prophylaxis (88). Topical antibiotics such as erythromycin and tetracycline are also effective in prevention and may cause less chemical irritation than silver nitrate. Despite the widespread use of ocular prophylaxis, gonococcal conjunctivitis continues to occur. The fetus may be infected prior to delivery, as in premature rupture of membranes, or when the instillation of a prophylactic agent is delayed. In the past, saline irrigation was used in conjunction with antibiotic prophylaxis. Improper or excessive use of saline irrigation may inactivate otherwise effective prophylaxis (88).

Chlamydia. The incidence of *Chlamydia trachomatis* infection of the cervix has been reported as 2% to 16% of pregnant women. The frequency of transmission of infection from an infected birth canal to the infant has been estimated to be 23% to 70% (89).

The conjunctiva are reported to be the portal of entry for this organism, and the infection is thought to spread from this site through the nasolacrimal duct to the nasopharynx. The infants exposed can manifest the infection in the conjunctiva as early as the fifth day of life. By 2 weeks, approximately 90% have the infection in this site. The delay in detection is likely related to the time required for replication of the organism in the conjunctival tissue (87,89).

Genital strains of *C. trachomatis* have been recognized as the cause of many cases of neonatal conjunctivitis. It has been reported that chlamydial infections are the most frequent cause of ophthalmia neonatorum in the United States, except for the transient chemical conjunctivitis associated with silver nitrate instillation. Statistics indicate that *C. trachomatis* causes ophthalmia neonatorum six to ten times more frequently than gonococcus, and that silver nitrate prophylaxis at birth is inactive against chlamydia (8,90).

Clinical signs include a rapid succession of conjunctival hyperemia and a mucopurulent discharge. Diagnosis is confirmed by demonstration of basophilic, intracytoplasmic inclusion bodies in epithelial cells as seen on a Giemsa stain of conjunctival scrapings. Cultures are not a practical diagnostic tool because several weeks of incubation are necessary.

Infants do not routinely experience visual loss because of infection if treated properly. If untreated, however, conjunctival scarring and superficial corneal vascularization can occur. Neonatal chlamydial pneumonia may result from a conjunctivitis (87,89–91).

Treatment of infants who have ophthalmia neonatorum caused by *C. trachomatis* consists of topical sulfacetamide or 1% tetracycline ointment four times daily for 3 weeks. Other topical antibiotics such as penicillin, neomycin-polymyxin combinations, chloramphenicol, and gentamycin are all ineffective.

OCULAR TRAUMA ASSOCIATED WITH LABOR AND DELIVERY

Fetal ocular injury occurring during labor and vaginal delivery results from compression of the fetal head against the bony pelvic outlet, use of forceps, or vacuum extraction. Less commonly, trauma to the globe or ocular adnexae may be caused by instrumentation during elective cesarean section or lacerations by monitoring electrodes or amniocentesis needles (92,93).

Intraocular hemorrhage, predominantly retinal hemorrhage, is one of the most frequent injuries, occurring in approximately 15% of all newborns regardless of the type of delivery (93). Factors contributing to the occurrence of such hemorrhages include compression of the fetal head and neck during a long second stage of labor, particularly in nulliparas; precipitate delivery; nuchal cords; and large-birth-weight fetuses. These may all result in increased venous pressure and congestion leading to subconjunctival, intravitreal, and, most commonly, retinal hemorrhage and anterior chamber hemorrhage (hyphema). Such hemorrhages are uncommon after cesarean section or breech deliveries (93).

Funduscopically, the retinal hemorrhage may appear small or large, flame shaped, and round in configuration. These may be seen readily in the posterior pole and most often surrounding the optic disc. Neonatal retinal hemorrhages are absorbed within 3 weeks in 90% of cases (92,93). There is no treatment for these hemorrhages and there are no long-term sequelae. Visual prognosis therefore is excellent, even if the hemorrhages are in the macular area. An interesting consideration is that epidural analgesia, although potentially increasing the length of the second stage of labor, reduces the intensity of pelvic muscular resistance and pushing. This may relieve the compression of the fetal head and neck and offer some protection against retinal hemorrhage during a spontaneous vaginal delivery.

Unilateral corneal opacification may be seen from birth trauma. The corneal clouding may be caused by direct instrumentation injury to the corneal epithelium and the underlying stroma and may be associated with lacerations or ecchymosis of the eyelids. These usually resolve in 1 week without sequelae. Rupture of Descemet's membrane can result from forceps injuries as well. This is more common when mid-cavity forceps are used and pressure is transmitted to the globe. The ruptures appear as double contoured, linear, scroll-like striae in the posterior layer of the cornea. Corneal edema evidenced as clouding may be present at birth but will resolve in a few months pending regeneration of the endothelial cells and duplication of Descemet's membrane. The injury may result in unilateral high corneal astigmatism and myopia and, if unrecognized and uncorrected, may result in amblyopia (8,94).

Ocular trauma during delivery may produce a transient increase in intraocular pressure, depending on the extent of damage. It is difficult to distinguish between traumatic and developmental forms of congenital glaucoma. Clues such as the forceps bruises on the forehead or cheeks of the neonate may help differentiate the cause of increased intraocular pressure. If birth injury is suspected, improvement of the intraocular pressure as well as the associated corneal clouding will resolve in a few months.

Neurologic injury of ophthalmologic importance has been reported as a consequence of birth trauma. Cranial nerves II, III, VI, and VII, as well as peripheral nerves, are involved. When presented with a neurologic injury, a history of difficult labor, forceps delivery, or breech delivery with shoulder stretching can help differentiate the injury from other causes of neurologic disease (8,95). Compression of the fetal skull, intracranial contusions, and hemorrhage can cause field defects, cortical blindness, or optic nerve injury (96).

Ptosis may result from direct injury to the levator muscle or the third nerve. If a peripheral branch of the seventh nerve is affected, it may result in an inability to close the ipsilateral eyelid. Congenital sixth nerve palsies can cause a strabismus and may be secondary to an increase in intracranial pressure during the second stage of labor (8).

Brachial plexus palsies may cause, among other things, sympathetic denervation resulting in the findings associated with Horner's syndrome, ptosis, miosis, anhydrosis, and heterochromia (97). In all of the conditions reported, the findings may be transient, and supportive therapy should be instituted prior to surgical intervention.

Ocular complications of epidural analgesia have been reported in the mother during delivery. Horner syndrome during epidural analgesia is uncommon but is more likely to occur in the parturient than in the nonpregnant woman. It is a result of chemical interruption of the sympathetic nerve supply to the pupil, levator palpebrae muscle, and the vessels of the conjunctiva caused by the spread of local anesthetic in the epidural space toward the first four thoracic nerve roots. The findings associated with this syndrome include unilateral or bilateral ptosis, miosis, anhydrosis, conjunctival facial vasodilation, and relative enophthalmos. The findings usually resolve within 5 hours after the final dose of local anesthetic is given. In all cases reported there has been complete recovery. The clinical significance of Horner syndrome during epidural analgesia is that it indicates a high level of sympathetic denervation that may precipitate maternal hypotension (98).

The management of labor in a pregnant woman who has a history of high myopia has been a concern in the past. The stresses of the second stage of labor with repeated Valsalva maneuvers were felt to increase ocular pressure with the risk of retinal tears and detachments, especially in patients who have a history of high myopia with peripheral retinal degenerations. In some medical centers it was routine to terminate delivery in such a patient with forceps or vacuum extraction, despite no direct evidence that deterioration occurred. A study involving 50 women who had high myopia with predisposition to retinal detachment showed no change in their fundus after spontaneous vaginal delivery (99). Increased intraocular pressure caused by the Valsalva mechanism is spread equally in all directions in a closed eyeball. This pressure should not be responsible for vitreous traction in a particular direction, thereby precipitating a retinal tear or detachment. The main finding of this study, that a highly myopic patient may be allowed to deliver spontaneously, is thus consistent with physical principles.

During the physical stresses of labor subconjunctival hemorrhages may appear in the mother (Fig. 34-20). They can appear as small or large areas of extravasated blood over the surface of the sclera. The hemorrhage is not associated with pain, change in vision, or any permanent visual sequelae but may be of concern to the patient because of its sudden and dramatic appearance (11).

Two women reportedly demonstrated orbital hematomas that occurred during labor. The development was sudden, evidenced by proptosis and complaints of double vision with orbital pain. Neither patient developed compressive optic neuropathy. The patients were observed clinically and echographically. The hemotomas resolved in approximately 2 weeks (100).

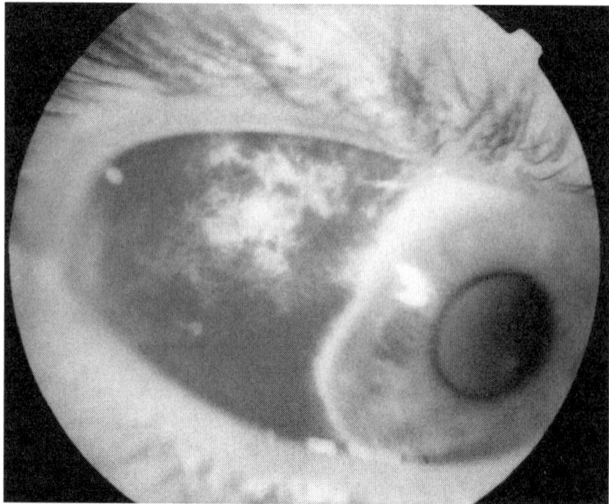

FIG. 34-20. External photograph of right eye showing a subconjunctival hemorrhage temporal to limbus.

REFERENCES

1. Millodot M. The influence of pregnancy on the sensitivity of the cornea. Br J Ophthalmol 1977;61:646–649.
2. Riss B, Riss P. Corneal sensitivity in pregnancy. Ophthalmologica 1981;183:57–62.
3. Sarwar M. Contact lenses and oral contraceptives. Br Med J 1966; 5497:1235.
4. Duke-Elder S, Cook C. In: Duke-Elder S, ed. System of ophthalmology. St. Louis: CV Mosby, 1963.
5. Avasthi P, Sethi P, Mithal S. Effect of pregnancy and labor on intraocular pressure. Int Surg 1976;61:82–84.
6. Horven I, Gjonnaess H. Corneal identation pulse and intraocular pressure in pregnancy. Arch Ophthalmol 1974;91:92–98.
7. Philips I, Gore SM. Ocular hypotensive effect of late pregnancy with and without high blood pressure. Br J Ophthalmol 1985;69: 117–119.
8. Wang FM. Perinatal ophthalmology. In: Duane T, ed. Clinical ophthalmology. New York: Harper & Row, 1982.
9. Sanke RF. Blepharoptosis as a complication of pregnancy. Ann Ophthalmol 1984;8:420–422.
10. Wynn RM. Obstetrics and gynecology. Unit II. Philadelphia: Lea & Febiger, 1974.
11. Weinreb R, Lu A, Key T. Maternal ocular adaptations during pregnancy. Obstet Gynecol Surv 1987;42:471–483.
12. Sunness JS. The pregnant woman's eyes. Surv Ophthalmol 1988;32: 219–238.
13. Kline LB. Retinopathy in toxemia of pregnancy. South Med J 1981; 74:34–36.
14. Jaffe G, Schatz H. Ocular manifestations of preeclampsia. Am J Ophthalmol 1987;103:309–315.
15. Handesman R. Retinal and conjunctival vascular changes in normal and toxemic pregnancy. Bull NY Acad Med 1955;31:376.
16. Mabie WC, Ober RR. Fluorescein angiographyin toxemia of pregnancy. Br J Ophthalmol 1980;64:666–671.
17. Fastenberg DM, Fetkenhour CL, Choromokos E, Shoch DE. Choroidal vascular changes in toxemia of pregnancy. Am J Ophthalmol 1980;89:362–368.
18. Folk JC, Weingeist TA. Fundus changes in toxemia. Ophthalmology 1981;88:1173–1174.
19. Grimes DA, Eklradh LE, McCartney WH. Cortical blindness in preeclampsia. Int J Gynaecol Obstet 1980;17:601–603.
20. Dibble CM, Kochenour NK, Worley RJ, Tyler FH, Swartz M. Effect of pregnancy on diabetic retinopathy. Obstet Gynecol 1982;59:699–704.
21. Johnston GP. Pregnancy and diabetic retinopathy. Am J Ophthalmol 1980;90:519–524.
22. Horvat M, MacLean H, Goldbert L, Crock GW. Diabetic retrinopathy in pregnancy: a 12-year prospective survey. Br J Ophthalmol 1980;64: 398–403.
23. Newell F. Ophthalmology, principles and concepts, 4th ed. St. Louis: CV Mosby, 1978.
24. Cassar J, Kohner EM, Hamilton AM, Gordon H, Joplin GF. Diabetic retinopathy and pregnancy. Diabetologia 1978;15:105–111.
25. Laatikainen L, Larinkari J, Teramo K, Raivio KO. Occurrence and prognostic significance of retinopathy in diabetic pregnancy. Metab Pediatr Ophthalmol 1980;4:191–195.
26. Elian M, Ben-Tovim N, Bechar M, Bornstein B. Recurrent benign intracranial hypertension during pregnancy. Obstet Gynecol 1968; 31:685–688.
27. Shekleton P, Fidler J, Grimwade J. A case of benign intracranial hypertension in pregnancy. Br J Obstet Gynaecol 1980;87:345–347.
28. Carlson DC. Ocular manifestations of pregnancy. J Am Optom Assn 1988;59:49–57.
29. Jewelewicz R, Zimmerman EA, Carmel PW. Conservative management of a pituitary tumor during pregnancy following induction of ovulation with gonadotropins. Fertil Steril 1977;28:35–40.
30. Nelson PB, Robinson AG, Archer DF, Maroon JC. Symptomatic pituitary tumor enlargement after induced pregnancy. J Neurosurg 1978; 44:283–287.
31. Swyer GI, Little V, Harries BJ. Visual disturbance in pregnancy after induction of ovulation. Br Med J 1971;4:90–91.
32. Zauberman H, Feinsod M. Orbital hemangioma growth during pregnancy. Acta Ophthalmol 1970;48:929–933.
33. Sachs BP, Smith SK, Cassar J, Van Iddekinge B. Rapid enlargement of craniopharyngioma in pregnancy. Br J Obstet Gynaecol 1978;85: 557–558.

34. Beal MF, Chapman PH. Cortical blindness and homonymous hemianopia in the post partum period. JAMA 1980;244:2085–2087.
35. Ortiz J, Yanoff M, Cameron D, Schaffer D. Disseminated intravascular coagulation in infancy and in the neonate. Arch Ophthalmol 1982; 100:1413–1415.
36. Azar P, Smith RS, Greenberg MH. Ocular findings in disseminated intravascular coagulation. Am J Ophthalmol 1974;78:493–496.
37. Cogan D. Ocular involvement in disseminated intravascular coagulopathy. Arch Ophthalmol 1975;93:1–8.
38. Amino N, Tanazawa O, Mori H, et al. Aggravation of thyrotoxicosis in early pregnancy and after delivery in Grave's disease. J Clin Endocrinol Metab 1982;55:108–112.
39. Amino N, Miyan K, Yamamoto T, Kuro R, Tanaka F. Transient recurrence of hyperthyroidism after delivery in Grave's disease. J Clin Endocrinol Metab 1977;44:130–136.
40. Innerfield F, Hollander CS. Thyroidal complications of pregnancy. Med Clin North Am 1977;61:67–87.
41. Friedman Z, Granat M, Neumann E. The syndrome of Vogt-Koyanagi-Harada and pregnancy. Metab Pediatr Ophthalmol 1980;4:147–149.
42. Hyman BN. Postpartum uveitis. Ann Ophthalmol 1976;8:677–688.
43. Henkind P, Gold DH. Ocular manifestations of rheumatic disorders, natural and iatrogenic. Oculotaneous manifestation of rheumatid diseases. In: Rheumatology. Basel, Switzerland: Karger, 1973.
44. Scott JS. Immunological diseases in pregnancy. Prog Allergy 1977;23: 321–366.
45. Cruysberg JR, Deutman AF. Visual disturbances during pregnancy caused by central serous choroidopathy. Br J Ophthalmol 1982;66: 240–241.
46. Sjaastad O. Headache and the ameliorating effect of pregnancy: an editorial. Cephalalgia 1984;4:211–212.
47. Callaghan N. The migraine syndrome in pregnancy. Neurology 1968; 18:197–201.
48. Spector RH. Migraine. Surv Ophthal 1984;29:193–207.
49. Duke-Elder S, Cook C. Normal development, Part 1. Embryology. In: Duke-Elder S, ed. System of ophthalmology. St. Louis: CV Mosby, 1963.
50. Miller M, Israel J, Cuttone J. Fetal alcohol syndrome. J Pediatr Ophthalmol Strabismus 1981;18:6–15.
51. Stromland K. Ocular involvement in fetal alcohol syndrome. Surv Ophthalmol 1987;31:277–283.
52. Charles N, Bennett T, Margolis S. Ocular pathology of the congenital varicella syndrome. Arch Ophthalmol 1977;95:2034–2037.
53. Yanoff M, Fine B. Drug embryopathy. In: Ocular pathology, 2nd ed. New York: Harper & Row, 1982.
54. Levit T, Nebell, Terracina S, Karman S. Ethambutol in pregnancy: observations on embryogenesis. Chest 1974;66:25–26.
55. Emerson DJ. Congenital malformations due to attempted abortion with aminopterin. Am J Obstet Gynecol 1962;84:356.
56. Hampton GR, Krepostman JI. Ocular manifestation of the fetal hydantoin syndrome. Clin Pediatr 1981;20:475–478.
57. Zackai EH, Mellman WJ, Neiderer B, Hanson JW. The fetal trimethadione syndrome. J Pediatr 1975;87:280–284.
58. Koos BJ, Longo LD. Mercury toxicity in the pregnant woman, fetus and newborn infant. A review. Am J Obstet Gynecol 1976;126: 390–409.
59. DeKaban AS. Abnormalities in children exposed to X-radiation during various stages of gestation: Tentative timetable of radiation injury to the human fetus. Part 1. J Nucl Med 1968;9:471–477.
60. Rugh R, Sharedoff L. X-rays and the monkey fetal retina. Invest Ophthalmol 1969;8:31–40.
61. Samples JR, Meyer M. Use of ophthalmic medications in pregnant and nursing women. Am J Ophthalmol 1988;106:616–622.
62. Kooner KS, Zimmerman TJ. Antiglaucoma therapy during pregnancy: Part I. Ann Ophthalmol 1988;20:166–169.
63. Rudolph AJ, Desmond MM. Clinical manifestations of the congenital rubella syndrome. Int Ophthalmol Clin 1972;12:3–19.
64. Cooper LZ, Krugman S. Clinical manifestations of postnatal and congenital rubella. Arch Ophthamol 1967;77:434–439.
65. Krill A. Retinopathy secondary to rubella. Int Ophthalmol Clin 1972; 12:89–103.
66. Boniuk M. Glaucoma in the congenital rubella syndrome. Int Ophthalmol Clin 1972;12:121–136.
67. Layden WE. Cataracts and glaucoma. In: Duane T, ed. Clinical ophthalmology. New York: Harper & Row, 1981.
68. O'Neill JF. Strabismus in the rubella syndrome. Int Ophthalmol Clin 1972;12:111–20.
69. Schlaegel TJ Jr. Toxoplasmosis. In: Duane T, ed. Clinical ophthalmology. Philadelphia: Harper & Row, 1981.
70. Schaffer DB. Eye findings in intrauterine infections. Clin Perinatol 1977;83:415–443.
71. O'Connor GR. Protozoan diseases of the uvea. Int Ophthalmol Clin 1977;17:163–176.
72. Sullivan GE, Takacs E. Comparative teratogenicity of pyrimethamine in rats and hamsters. Teratology 1971;4:205–210.
73. Chandler SH. Ocular abnormalities associated with intrauterine infections. Perspect Ophthalmol 1979;3:249.
74. Schaffer DB. Congenital infections. In: Scheie HG, Alert DM, eds. Textbook of Ophthalmology, 9th ed. Philadelphia: WB Saunders, 1977.
75. Rogell G. Congenital syphilis. In: Duane T, ed. Clinical ophthalmology. New York: Harper & Row, 1981.
76. McCormack W. Genital infections of perinatal importance. Clin Obstet Gynecol 1979;22:313–319.
77. Nahmias AJ, Hagler WM. Ocular manifestations of herpes simplex in the newborn (neonatal ocular herpes). Int Ophthalmol 1972;12: 191–213.
78. Hanshaw JB, Dudgeon JA. Herpes simplex infection of the fetus and newborn. Major Probl Clin Pediatr 1978;17:153–181.
79. Boniuk I. The cytomegaloviruses and the eye. Int Ophthalmol Clin 1972;12:169–190.
80. Matsuo T, Ohno A, Matsuo N. Acute retinal neurosis syndrome following chicken pox in pregnant women. Jpn J Ophthalmol 1988; 32:70–74.
81. Leads from MMWR. Update: Lyme disease and cases occurring during pregnancy. JAMA 1985;254:736–737, 741.
82. Smith LG Jr, Pearlmen M, Smith LG, Faro S. Lyme disease: a review with emphasis on the pregnant woman. Obstet Gynecol Surv 1991;46: 125–130.
83. Markowitz LE, Steeve AC, Benach JL, Slade JD, Broome CV. Lyme disease during pregnancy. JAMA 1986;255:3394–3396.
84. Gross J, Gross F, Friedman A. Systemic infectious diseases affecting the eye. In: Duane T, ed. Clinical ophthalmology. New York: Harper & Row, 1990.
85. Henrio R. Pregnancy and AIDS. Hum Reprod 1988;3:257–262.
86. Schuman JS, Orellana J, Friedman AH, Terch SA. Acquired immunodeficiency syndrome (AIDS). Surv Ophthalmol 1987;31:384–410.
87. Eschenbach D. Significance for the fetus of sexually acquired maternal infections with myoplasma, chlamydia and neisseria gonorrhea. Semin Perinatal 1977;1:11–24.
88. Snowe RJ, Wilfert CM. Epidemic reappearance of gonococcal ophthalmia neonatorum. Pediatrics 1973;51:110–114.
89. Heggie AD, Lumicao GG, Stuart LA, Gyves MT. Chlamydia trachomatis infection in mothers and infants. A prospective study. Am J Dis Child 1981;135:507–511.
90. Chandler JW, Alexander ER, Pheiffer TA, Wang SP, Holmes KK, English M. Ophthalmia neonatorum associated with maternal chlamydial infections. Trans Am Acad Ophthalmol Otolaryngol 1977;83: 302–308.
91. Fransen L, Nsanze H, D'Costa L, Brunham R, Piot P. Parents of infants with ophthalmia neonatorum: a high risk group for sexually transmitted diseases. Sexual Transm Dis 1985;12:130–134.
92. Maltau JM, Egge K. Epidural analgesia and perinatal retinal hemorrhages. Acta Anaesthesiol Scand 1980;24:99–101.
93. Sarin L, Reinart C. Retinopathy in ocular trauma. In: Duane T, ed. Clinical ophthalmology. New York: Harper & Row, 1981.
94. Doughman D. Corneal edema. In: Duane T, ed. Clinical ophthalmology. Philadelphia: Harper & Row, 1981.
95. Rubin A. Birth injuries: incidence, mechanisms and end results. Obstet Gynecol 1964;23:218.
96. Walsh TJ, Smith JL, Shipley T. Blindness in infants. Am J Ophthalmol 1966;62:546–556.
97. Eng GD. Neuromuscular diseases. In: Avery GB, ed. Neonatology. Pathophysiology and management of the newborn, 2nd ed. Philadelphia: JB Lippincott, 1981.
98. Schachner SM, Reynolds AC. Horner syndrome during lumbar epidural analgesia for obstetrics. Obstet Gynecol 1982;59:315–325.
99. Neri A, Grausbord R, Kremer I, Ovadia J, Treister G. The management of labor in high myopic patients. Eur J Obstet Gynecol Reprod Biol 1985;19:277–279.
100. Jacobsen DM, Itani K, Digre KB, Ossoinig KC, Varner MW. Maternal orbital hematoma associated with labor. Am J Ophthalmol 1988;105: 547–553.

Cherry and Merkatz's Complications of Pregnancy,
Fifth Edition, edited by W. R. Cohen.
Lippincott Williams & Wilkins, Philadelphia © 2000.

CHAPTER 35

Ear, Nose, and Throat Disorders

William Lawson, Anthony J. Reino, and Hugh F. Biller

The effects of pregnancy on head and neck structures are diverse. Relevant signs and symptoms that are encountered include nasal congestion and rhinorrhea, aural fullness and hearing loss, facial paralysis, hoarseness, neck swelling, and the production of tumors in the nose, oral cavity, and jaws. The pathogenesis of these clinical findings involves disturbances in fluid dynamics, increased protein synthesis and loss, and altered vascular proliferation and permeability induced by hormonal changes. The various head and neck disorders encountered are discussed according to the anatomic site involved.

EAR

Otosclerosis

Otosclerosis is a localized form of osteodystrophy involving the otic capsule of the temporal bone. Clinically, it is characterized by a hearing loss that is generally conductive in nature, secondary to fixation of the stapes footplate. Pregnancy has been traditionally considered to stimulate activity in otosclerosis, presumably by the increased concentration of circulating estrogens. These hormones act as stimulators of osteocytic activity and may play a dominant role during ossification of an otospongeotic bone lesion. This may explain the onset of a conductive hearing loss due to otosclerosis during pregnancy (1). In the premicrosurgical era it often was recommended that abortion be performed in otosclerotic women who became pregnant, in an attempt to preserve their hearing (2).

The concept that pregnancy activates otosclerosis and accelerates the hearing loss from the disease was based primarily on the subjective complaints of affected women. Nager (3) reported that 48% of 164 pregnant women surveyed claimed increased deafness with childbearing. In another survey of 194 otosclerotic women who became pregnant, House (4) found that 87 (45%) claimed increased loss of hearing. This occurred during the first pregnancy in 41 cases, during the second pregnancy in 23 cases, in the third pregnancy in 10 cases, and during one of several pregnancies in 10 other women. Walsh (5) surveyed 243 similar cases and found that 43% of the women stated that pregnancy worsened their hearing. Gristwood and Venables (6) conducted a retrospective study of 479 women who had otosclerosis to determine the effect of pregnancy on their hearing loss. They reported that the risk of a subjective sense of hearing loss was 33% in women who had bilateral otosclerosis after one pregnancy, which increased to 63% after six pregnancies. In women who had unilateral disease, the complaint of increased hearing loss was much less.

When the effect of pregnancy on otosclerosis was documented by audiometric testing, it became apparent that the actual incidence of hearing loss was much lower than subjectively reported by the patients. Day (7) tested 47 women undergoing 75 pregnancies and observed hearing loss in only three women. Sullivan (8) studied 25 otosclerotics who had undergone fenestration surgery and later became pregnant and noted hearing loss in the unoperated ear in three cases; however, this hearing loss occurred 3 to 5 years after the pregnancies. Walsh (5) similarly reviewed patients who became pregnant following fenestration surgery and found two who had hearing loss in the operated ear. Hearing loss was also observed in seven other patients; this also occurred 3 to 5 years following surgery. Walsh concluded that pregnancy had no significant effect on otosclerosis.

Lindsay (9) similarly doubted whether pregnancy had an adverse effect on otosclerosis. He considered the observed onset and increased severity of symptoms in pregnant women represented the coincidental peak incidence of this disorder during the childbearing years.

W. Lawson, A.J. Reino, and H.F. Biller: Department of Otolaryngology, Mt. Sinai School of Medicine, New York, NY 10029.

Meuniere Disease

Meuniere syndrome is characterized by vertigo, tinnitus, hearing loss, and aural fullness believed to be induced by endolymphatic hydrops. Although Lederer and Tardy (10) suggested that the retention of sodium and water occurring during pregnancy may aggravate labyrinthine dysfunction and result in the clinical manifestation of latent Meuniere disease, there are few reports on its course during pregnancy. Uchide and colleagues (11) noted a correlation between the patient's serum osmolality and the frequency of Meuniere symptoms. Interestingly, they found that when the serum osmolality was significantly below normal (<270 mosm/kg) the attacks increased to 10 per month. However, as the pregnancy proceeded and the serum osmolality normalized, the attacks decreased in frequency. The vertigo in this study was treated with oral isosorbide and intramuscular injections of diazepam.

Eustachian Tube Dysfunction

Edema of the nose and upper aerodigestive tract during pregnancy may result in malfunction of the eustachian tube, with failure of equilibration of the pressure within the middle ear and mastoid and nasopharynx. Loss of patency of the eustachian tube produces the troublesome sensation of fullness in the ear that is unrelieved by swallowing. Persistent closure of the eustachian tube may result in the formation of a negative pressure in the middle ear space, secondary to resorption of air by the blood vessels of the lining mucosa. If this is sustained, a serous effusion results. The presence of fluid in the middle ear space produces a conductive hearing loss and carries the potential risk of secondary bacterial infection.

In a prospective study by Derkay (12) using tympanometry and anterior rhinomanometry, objective evidence of eustachian tube dysfunction and nasal obstruction was found in 80% of symptomatic third-trimester patients, compared with 45% of asymptomatic matched pregnant patients and with 30% of nonpregnant controls. Cigarette smoking was found to predispose women to this condition.

On otoscopy, the tympanic membrane may appear to be normal or slightly retracted and does not move on Valsalva's maneuver. Impedance audiometry may reveal normal compliance, a persistent negative pressure in the middle ear, or evidence of fluid. If the condition progresses to serous otitis, a myringotomy and the insertion of a ventilating tube may be necessary. As in all adults with unilateral serous otitis, examination of the nasopharynx is mandatory in order to eliminate the possibility of a lesion obstructing the eustachian tube ostium. A limited trial of topical nasal decongestants (e.g., Neosynephrine) may be used. The symptoms usually subside spontaneously postpartum.

Facial Paralysis

The prevalence of Bell's palsy appears to be greater in pregnant women than in the general population. Robinson and Pou (13) calculated an incidence of 1 case per 2,000 pregnancies over a 10-year period studied. Suggested causative factors include hormonal alterations, hypercoagulability, autoimmune disease, viral infection, vascular injury, and fluid retention (2), with the latter being generally favored, for although interstitial edema occurs in many body areas during pregnancy, swelling of the facial nerve within its bony canal causes direct mechanical injury to the nerve or obstruction to its blood supply. Powers (2) reviewed 46 reported cases of facial paralysis occurring in pregnancy. The mean age of the patients was 26 years. The right and left sides of the face were involved with equal frequency, with bilateral paralysis developing in only one case. There was a peak incidence in the third trimester (79% of the cases), with a small number of cases occurring in the second trimester (8%) and immediately postpartum (13%). Approximately half of the cases were associated with preeclampsia (13,14). The paralysis spontaneously resolved immediately after delivery in the majority of the patients, but persisted for 1 to 2 months in several cases (15). The loss of nerve excitability on electrical testing may be considered an indication for surgical decompression.

In 1995, Ben-David and colleagues (16) studied the effects of ovarian steroids on the brainstem during changes of estrogen and progesterone blood levels. They found, through the use of brainstem evoked response audiometry, that a significant delay in peak III occurred with an increased stimulus rate in the cohort with the highest estrogen level. They concluded that estrogen may cause a brainstem synaptic impairment, presumably because of ischemic changes, and therefore may also be responsible for a higher incidence of Bell's palsy during pregnancy.

Drug Ototoxicity

Numerous chemical agents, including various antibiotics, diuretics, analgesics, and antineoplastic drugs, may produce sensorineural hearing loss, tinnitus, and vertigo from their deleterious effects on the inner ear. Prominent among these substances are the aminoglycoside antiobiotics (e.g., streptomycin, gentamicin, kanamycin, tobramycin, and amikacin), which are markedly cochleotoxic. The degree of placental transportation of these agents is unclear. Streptomycin is said to cross the placenta, whereas kanamycin was found to achieve only very low levels in the fetus (17). Consequently, these drugs should be administered with great caution to pregnant mothers to prevent the occurrence of ototoxicity in newborn infants.

Otitis

The development of serous otitis from the increased tendency toward eustachian tube dysfunction during pregnancy may be complicated by secondary bacterial infection. Pain then supervenes on ear fullness and decreased hearing, with otoscopy revealing a reddened tympanic membrane with loss of landmarks. Antibiotic therapy is directed against *Streptoccus pneumoniae* and *Hemophilus influenzae* (including beta-lactamase–producing strains), which are the most commonly encountered pathogens. Presently, the drugs of choice are amoxicillin-clavulanic acid and the newer cephalosporins (e.g., cefuroxamine).

Naranbhai and colleagues (18) described the development of congenital tuberculous otis in two infants from two mothers who had miliary tuberculosis by infection *in utero* or at birth.

NOSE

Nasal obstruction is a well-recognized accompaniment of pregnancy in some women. The experimental injection of estrogenic hormones has been shown to produce perivascular edema of the nasal mucosa in monkeys (19,20). Mabry (21) suggested that estrogen may produce nasal mucosal congestion through a cholinergic mechanism. Pooling of blood in the nasal tissues secondary to the increased circulating volume and a progesterone-induced smooth-muscle relaxation of blood vessels are other proposed causes of the observed nasal congestion (22,23).

The observation of nasal congestion in pregnancy, swelling of the nasal mucosa during menstruation, and the erectile property of the turbinates and septal mucosa led to the concept of a reciprocal nasogenital relationship in which there was postulated a physiologic association between the nose and the reproductive tract (24). MacKenzie (25) is credited with being the first to report the occurrence of nasal congestion and turbinate enlargement in pregnancy. Proetz (26) reported recurrent polyposis and nasal edema with successive pregnancies. The congested nasal mucosa manifests itself clinically by nasal stuffiness and obstruction, often with serous rhinorrhea or postnasal discharge.

During pregnancy, aggravation of nasal allergic symptoms is occasionally observed in patients with nasal allergy. Hamano and colleagues observed an increase in the expression of histamine (H_1) receptor mRNA in patients with nasal allergy (27). Moreover, this study demonstrated that the female hormones beta-estradiol and progesterone significantly increased the expression of H_1 receptor mRNA on human nasal epithelial cells and human mucosal microvascular endothelial cells. Because of this, they concluded that these sex hormones were related, at least partially, to symptoms of nasal hyperactivity during pregnancy.

Mabry (21) concluded in a study of 66 randomly selected pregnant women and 16 pregnant women under treatment for pregnancy rhinitis that rhinitis gravidarum may not be an isolated entity. Other causes of chronic nasal congestion in pregnant women also include allergic and bacterial rhinosinusitis and rhinitis medicamentosa (22,23).

Pharmacologic treatment of allergic diseases is often necessary during pregnancy. Drugs used should be safe and without serious side effects for either mother or fetus. Topical mucosal agents seem to be safest, due to their minimal or absent absorption. Preferred agents are topical anthihistamines and steroids (for rhinitis and conjunctivitis) and cromolyn with topical steroids (for asthma) because they are both safe and effective (28).

The congested and hyperemic mucosa may result in epistaxis from rupture of a superficial blood vessel. This is generally controlled by the application of a topical vasoconstrictor and chemical or electrocautery. Occasionally anterior nasal packing is required. The nasal edema of pregnancy is self-limiting and disappears after delivery. Derkay (12) noted that the rhinitis of pregnancy resolved spontaneously within 4 to 10 weeks following delivery on objective measuring with anterior rhinomanometry.

The prolonged use of topical nasal sprays containing sympathomimetic substances is to be avoided because of the rebound congestion they produce. In a long-term study by Settipane and colleagues (29) comparing mothers receiving allergy immunotherapy during pregnancy and untreated controls, no statistically significant difference was detectable in the offspring regarding the development of asthma, rhinitis, or positive skin tests.

The nasal hemangioma of pregnancy is a rare lesion. Ash and Old (30) on review of 3,000 benign nasal tumors, found only 23 nasal hemangiomas, one of which arose during pregnancy. Fu and Perzin (31) and Shalit and colleagues (32) each mentioned an additional case. The exact pathogenesis of these tumors is unknown, with suggested causes including hormonal alterations (especially during placentation), changes in blood volume, vessel growth in a preexisting vascular anomaly, or a combination of factors (33). Histologically, the majority of these lesions are of the capillary type. Clinically, these tumors generally arise on the anterior nasal septum and present with epistaxis. They tend to regress after delivery, and those that fail to involute should be excised.

It should be noted that hemangiomas arise at various cutaneous and mucosal sites during pregnancy. Barter and colleagues (33) reported such lesions appearing on the lips, tongue, cheek, and eyelid. They may require excision if they cause bleeding or produce deformity.

Nasal granuloma gravidarum is another rare entity occurring in pregnancy in which the patient rapidly develops an intranasal mass that produces obstruction and bleeding. It generally develops in multiparous women. Whereas McShane and Walsh (34) were able to remove the lesions readily in their cases under local anesthesia, severe bleeding and recurrences were noted by other researchers (35).

Nasopharynx

The congestion of the nasal cavity commonly present during pregnancy may extend to the nasopharynx, producing the previously cited eustachian tube dysfunction. No distinct pathologic entity exists in the nasopharynx that is produced by or aggravated during pregnancy; however, Yan and colleagues (36) found that pregnant women who developed and underwent radiotherapy for nasopharyngeal carcinoma had a much poorer prognosis (5-year survival of 11%) than did women who became pregnant following completion of therapy.

ORAL CAVITY

Gingiva

In response to the hormonal influence of pregnancy and the local irritative effect of subgingival dental plaque or calculus, gingival hypertrophy occurs. It may progress to the development of a reddish-purple, friable, sessile, or pedunculated lobular mass involving one or several teeth. Lindhe and colleagues (37) demonstrated the ability of pregnancy hormones to cause increased vascular permeability and proliferation in the buccal mucosa of the hamster. Gridly (38) reported an incidence of gingivitis of 23% and of pregnancy tumor formation of 2.7% among 1,002 women studied.

The pregnancy tumor may arise anywhere in the oral cavity but has a predilection for the anterior teeth. The lesion is painless and may bleed spontaneously or from minimal trauma on mastication. It generally appears between the third and fifth months of pregnancy and progressively increases in size with gestation (39). Histologically, the lesion is composed of a vascular stroma containing infiltrates of acute and chronic inflammatory cells and is covered by a hyperplastic squamous epithelium. Consequently, these lesions frequently have been diagnosed microscopically as pyogenic granulomas or angiofibromas. Although some small tumors may regress postpartum, most persist and enlarge during subsequent pregnancies. Treatment is local excision; however, recurrence is not uncommon later in the pregnancy (40).

Maxilla and Mandible

McGowan (41) reported a patient who developed a central giant cell tumor of the mandible during pregnancy that reappeared during a subsequent pregnancy. On survey of the literature, he collected four other cases of giant cell tumors of the jaws that had enlarged during pregnancy. Based on review of the clinical histories of these cases, he proposed that a hormonal influence occurred during pregnancy that influenced the growth of these lesions. Additional reports of active enlargement of giant cell tumors were made in the mandible and the maxilla during pregnancy (42,43). Littler (43) reported reactivation of such a mandibular tumor in pregnancy after a quiescent period of 6 years. Fechner and colleagues (44) reported an unusual case of such a lesion of the maxilla that, in the last trimester of pregnancy, rapidly grew and extended intracranially, requiring a craniofacial resection for control.

Histologically these lesions consist of scattered multinucleated giant cells within a fibrous stroma containing focal areas of hemorrhage and osteoid formation. These lesions are considered reparative granulomas rather than true neoplasms, and they are treated by curettage. As with all giant cell lesions of the skeleton, hyperparathyroidism must be ruled out by appropriate biochemical tests.

Larynx

Laryngopathia gravidarum is a temporary condition arising in some pregnant women in which edema, dryness, and crusting of the laryngeal mucosa produce hoarseness (45). The condition is innocuous, but probably has the potential to hinder endotracheal intubation.

Laryngeal edema is occasionally encountered in late pregnancy, which may complicate obstetric anesthesia. The congestion of the mucous membranes of the upper respiratory tract also may involve the false vocal cords (46). This can be aggravated by the increased venous pressure resulting from the strenuous bearing-down efforts of the second stage of labor (47). Jouppila and colleagues (48) reported difficult intubation in a patient requiring early postpartum anesthesia for a vaginal hematoma, and MacKenzie (47) described laryngeal edema complicating intubation in two patients with prolonged labor.

In patients who have preeclampsia with facial edema but no respiratory obstruction, unrecognized laryngeal edema may be present, which may render laryngeal intubation difficult. Several such cases have been reported (47–49). The presumed mechanism for this interstitial edema of the larynx is a decreased serum protein level secondary to the albuminuria of preeclampsia. Why it has a predilection for the larynx in some people is unknown.

Other unusual causes of airway obstruction in pregnancy are the occurrence of hereditary angioedema (50) and the development of necrotizing epiglottitis complicating infectious mononucleosis (51).

Supraglottic hemangiomas of the larynx that enlarged with pregnancy causing airway obstruction were reported by Brandwein and colleagues (52) and Mugliston and Sanewan (53). In the case of Brandwein and colleagues

(52) the lesion spontaneously involuted at 36 weeks of gestation; however, the patient in the study of Mugliston and Sangwan (53) required a tracheostomy because of the severe dyspnea.

Thyroid

Enlargement and increased vascularity of the thyroid gland is noted in more than 50% of normal pregnant patients (see Chapter 22) (54). Although a small amount of diffuse enlargement of the thyroid gland may be considered a normal physiologic response to pregnancy, the presence of a solitary nodule is a matter of greater concern. The reported incidence of autoimmune disease of the thyroid approaches 10% in women. This autoimmune state, which predisposes to the development of thyroid neoplasia, especially in patients with subclinical hypothyroidism, combined with tumor growth and immunologic factors that occur in pregnancy, account for the significant incidence of nodular thyroid disease in the pregnant state (52). Thyroid nodules that produce suspicious aspirates on cytologic examination should be managed with a certain degree of urgency (55). In a series of 30 patients with thyroid neoplasia arising during pregnancy, 43% were carcinoma and 37% adenoma. Given the results, surgical management of thyroid mass during pregnancy should be performed either in the second trimester or immediately after delivery (56).

Doherty and colleagues (56) retrospectively reviewed the records of 23 patients with thyroid nodules that were first detected during pregnancy. The incidence of malignancy in the series was 39%. Because of the apparent increased potential for malignancy in thyroid nodules during pregnancy, the author recommended the following management guidelines: fine-needle aspiration and biopsy to be performed for rapidly enlarging thyroid nodules before 20 weeks' gestation; for nodules associated with palpable cervical adenopathy; for solid nodules larger than 2 cm; and for cystic nodules larger than 4 cm.

In contrast, Cunningham and Slaughter (57) studied 26 patients who underwent surgery for a solitary nodule that had arisen during, or was affected by, pregnancy. The majority were colloid nodules, with nine true adenomas found. Obstetrical parity did not influence the formation of the nodule. The nodules generally appeared in the first and second trimesters, or postpartum, and occurred infrequently during the last trimester. Medical management generally produced no effect. There were eight patients who had thyroid carcinoma, five of whom underwent surgery during pregnancy. Among these operated cases, there were three fetal deaths. In a comparative study of the incidence of carcinoma and adenoma in pregnant and nonpregnant women, the same relative frequency of both lesions was found in the two groups. Also, the number of pregnancies did not influence the development of carcinoma or alter its prognosis.

Rosvoll and Winship (58) studied 60 patients who had thyroid carcinoma: 38 had been treated for carcinoma 2 to 15 years before becoming pregnant and were clinically free of disease; 22 patients had residual and metastatic carcinoma and subsequently became pregnant. In the first group, pregnancy did not reactivate the carcinoma. In the second group it did not appear to accelerate tumor growth. Hill and colleagues (59) analyzed two groups of patients who had thyroid carcinoma: 70 patients had one or more pregnancies after the diagnosis of carcinoma was established, and 109 who had carcinoma did not subsequently become pregnant after it was diagnosed. They found no significant difference in the recurrence rate in both groups and no apparent effect on the clinical course of the disease by one or several pregnancies. There is considerable clinical evidence to support the conclusion that pregnancy does not increase the risk of thyroid malignancy or adversely influence the prognosis in patients who have thyroid carcinoma. Consequently, the decision to operate on a pregnant patient who has a solitary nodule should be based on the presence of clinical features suggesting malignancy, such as fixation of the gland, cervical lymphadenopathy, or the presence of a vocal cord paralysis.

Patients who have simple colloid goiters may experience enlargement, with pressure symptoms developing during pregnancy. This results from a decrease in the plasma iodine level secondary to increased renal clearance. Cunningham and Slaughter (57) noted enlargement during pregnancy in 13 of 18 patients with goiters.

In patients who have a multinodular goiter, a serum antithyroid antibody titer should be drawn to rule out Hashimoto's disease. Thyroid function tests will identify the approximately 30% of patients who have this disease and who become hypothyroid (60).

SUMMARY

Disorders of the head and neck arising in pregnancy have been reviewed according to the anatomic site of involvement.

In the ear there is an increased occurrence of eustachian tube dysfunction secondary to the edema of the mucosa of the upper respiratory tract. The incidence of facial paralysis is also greater in pregnant women; however, it carries a good prognosis, with spontaneous regression occurring postpartum in the majority of patients. No convincing evidence supports exacerbation of the hearing loss of otosclerosis or the vertigo of Meuniere's disease by pregnancy. Caution must be exercised in administering potentially ototoxic drugs to pregnant women because of the risk of transplacental transfer to the fetus.

Nasal obstruction commonly arises from hormonally induced congestion of the mucosa lining (rhinitis gravidarum). Rarely, a hemangioma or granuloma of pregnancy develops in the nose.

In the oral cavity, angiofibromatous lesions arise from the gingiva (pregnancy tumor), and giant cell reparative granulomas of the jaws show a pattern of accelerated growth in response to pregnancy.

Hoarseness may occur from dryness and crusting of the larynx (laryngopathia gravidarum). Unsuspected laryngeal edema may complicate obstetrical anesthesia by rendering intubation difficult at the time of delivery or in the immediate postpartum period.

REFERENCES

1. Arnold W, Niedermeyer HP, Altermatt HJ, Neubert WJ. Pathogenesis of otosclerosis. State of the art. HNO 1996;44:121–129.
2. Powers WH. Peripheral facial paralysis and systemic disease. Otolaryngol Clin North Am 1974;7:2, 398–399.
3. Nager FR. Pathology of the labyrinthine capsule and its clinical significance. In: Fowler EP, ed. Medicine of the Ear. New York: Thomas Nelson. 1947:260.
4. House HP. Personal communication, cited in Walsh TE. The effect of pregnancy on deafness due to otosclerosis. JAMA 1954;154: 1407–1409.
5. Walsh TE. The effect of pregnancy on deafness due to otosclerosis. JAMA 1954;154:1407–1409.
6. Gristwood RE, Venables WN. Pregnancy and otosclerosis. Clin Otolaryngol 1983;8:205–210.
7. Day KM. Personal communication, cited in Walsh TE. The effect of pregnancy on deafness due to otosclerosis. JAMA 1954;154: 1407–1409.
8. Sullivan J. Personal communication, cited in Walsh TE. The effect of pregnancy on deafness due to otosclerosis. JAMA 1954;154: 1407–1409.
9. Lindsay JR. Otosclerosis. In: Paparella MD, Shumrick DA, eds. Otolaryngology, 2nd ed. Philadelphia: WB Saunders, 1980:1619–1620.
10. Lederer FL, Tardy ME. Otorhinolaryngologic problems. In: Davis's gynecology and obstetrics. Hagerstown, MD: Harper & Row, 1976:1–7.
11. Uchide K, Suzuki N, Takiguchi T, Terada S, Inoue M. The possible effect of pregnancy on Meniere's disease. J Otorohinolaryngol Rel Spec 1997;59:292–295.
12. Derkay CS. Eustachian tube and nasal function during pregnancy. A prospective study. Otolaryngol Head Neck Surg 1988;99:558–566.
13. Robinson JR, Pou JW. Bell's palsy: a predisposition of pregnant women. Arch Otolaryngol 1972;95:125–129.
14. Pope TH, Kenan PD. Bell's palsy in pregnancy. Arch Otolaryngol 1969; 89:52–56.
15. Faris BD. Facial paralysis during pregnancy. Med Times 1955;83:185.
16. Ben-David Y, Tal J, Podoshin L, Fradis M, Sharf M, Pratt H, Faraggi D. Brain stem auditory evoked potentials: effects of ovarian steroids correlated with increased incidence of Bell's palsy in pregnancy. Otolaryngol Head Neck Surg 1995;113:32–35.
17. Quick CA. Chemical and drug effects on the inner ear. In: Paparella MM, Shumrick DA, eds. Otolaryngology, 2nd ed. Philadelphia: WB Saunders, 1980:1805–1827.
18. Naranbhai RC, Mathiassen W, Malan AF. Congenital tuberculosis localized to the ear. Arch Dis Child 1989;84:738–740.
19. Mortimer H, Wright RP, Collip JB. The effect of the administration of estrogenic hormones on the nasal mucosa of the monkey (*Macaca mulatta*). Can Med Assoc J 1936;35:503–513.
20. Mortimer H, Wright RP, Collip JB. The effect of estrogenic hormones on the nasal mucosa, their role in the naso-sexual relationship, and their significance in clinical rhinology. Can Med Assoc J 1936;35:615–621.
21. Mabry RL. Rhinitis of pregnancy. South Med J 1986;79:965–971.
22. Incaudo GA. Diagnosis and treatment of rhinitis during pregnancy and lactation. Clin Rev Allergy 1987;5:325–327.
23. Schatz M, Zeiger RS. Diagnosis and management of rhinitis during pregnancy. Allergy Proc 1988;9:545–554.
24. Goldman JL. Nasal complications. In: Rovinsky JJ, Guttmacher AF, eds. Medical, surgical and gynecologic complications of pregnancy, 2nd ed. Baltimore: Williams & Wilkins, 1965:226–230.
25. MacKenzie NJ. The physiological and pathological relations between the nose and the sexual apparatus of man. Bull Johns Hopkins Hosp 1898;9:10–16.
26. Proetz AW. Essays on the Applied Physiology of the Nose. St. Louis: Annals Publishing, 1941:320.
27. Hamano N, Terada N, Maesako K, et al. Expression of histamine receptors in nasal epithelial cells and endothelial cells—the effects of sex hormones. Int Arch Allergy Immunol 1998;115:220–227.
28. Ciprandi G, Liccardi G, D-Amato G, et al. Treatment of allergic diseases during pregnancy. J Invest Allergol Clin Immunol 1997;7: 557–565.
29. Settipane RA, Chafee FA, Settipane GA. Pollen immunotherapy during pregnancy: a long-term follow-up of offsprings. Allergy Proc 1988;9: 555–561.
30. Ash JE, Old JW. Hemangiomas of the nasal septum. Trans Am Acad Ophthalmol Otolaryngol 1950;54:350–356.
31. Fu YS, Perzin KH. Non-epithelial tumors of the nasal cavity, paranasal sinuses and nasopharynx. A clinico-pathologic study. 1. General features and vascular tumors. Cancer 1974;33:1275–1288.
32. Shalit JB, Smith GA, Francis D, Canalis RF. Nasal hemangioma of pregnancy. Ear Nose Throat J 1977;56:377–379.
33. Barter RH, Letterman GS, Schurter M. Hemangiomas in pregnancy. Am J Obstet Gynecol 1963;87:625–635.
34. McShane OP, Walsh MA. Nasal granuloma gravidarum. J Laryngol 1988;102:828–830.
35. Skau NK, Pilgaard P, Neilsen G. Granuloma gravidarum of the nasal mucous membranes. J Laryngol 1987;101:1286–1288.
36. Yan JH, Liao LS, Hy YH. Pregnancy and nasopharyngeal carcinoma. A prognostic evaluation of 27 patients. Int J Radiat Oncol Biol Phys 1984; 10:851–855.
37. Lindhe J, Branemark PI, Ludskcg J. Changes in vascular proliferation after local application of sex hormones. J Periodont Res 1967;2: 266–272.
38. Gridly MS. Gingival condition in pregnant women. Oral Surg 1954;7: 641–646.
39. Zarka FJ, Stark MM. Gingival tumors of pregnancy. Review of "pregnancy tumors" and a report of two cases. Obstet Gynecol 1956;8: 597–600.
40. Weir JC, Silverman SI, Cohen LA. Recurring oral pregnancy tumors. Obstet Gynecol 1979;54:358–360.
41. McGowan DA. Central giant cell tumor of the mandible occuring in pregnancy. Br J Oral Surg 1969;17:131–135.
42. Small GS, Rowe NH. A "true giant cell tumor" in the mandible. J Oral Surg 1975;33;296–301.
43. Littler BO. Central giant cell granuloma of the jaw—a hormonal influence. J Oral Surg 1979–1980;17:43–46.
44. Fechner RE, Fitz-Hugh GS, Pope TL. Extraordinary growth of giant cell reparative granuloma during pregnancy. Arch Otolaryngol 1984;110:116–119.
45. Arnold GE. Disorders of laryngeal function. In: Pararella MM, Shumrick DA, eds. Otolaryngology, 2nd ed. Philadelphia: WB Saunders, 1980:2479–2486.
46. Moir DD. Obstetric anaesthesia and analgesia. London: Bailliere Tindal, 1976:18.
47. Anonymous. Laryngeal oedema complicating obstetric anaesthesia. Anesthesia 1978;33:271–272.
48. Jouppila R, Jouppila P, Hollmen A. Laryngeal oedema as an obstetric anaesthesia complication. Case Reports. Acta Anaesth Scand 1980; 24:97–98.
49. Brock-Utne JG, Downing JW, Seedat F. Laryngeal oedema associated with preeclamptic toxaemia. Anesthesia 1977;32:556–558.
50. Peters M, Ryley D, Lockwood C. Hereditary angioedema and immunoglobulin A deficiency in pregnancy. Obstet Gynecol 1988;72: 454–455.
51. Biem J, Roy L, Halik J, Hoffstein V. Infectious mononucleosis complicated by necrotizing epiglottis, dysphagia and pneumonia. Chest 1989; 96:204–205.
52. Brandwein MS, Abramson AL, Shikowitz MJ. Supraglottic hemangioma during pregnancy. Obstet Gynecol 1987;96:450–453.
53. Mugliston TA, Sanewan S. Persistent cavernous haemangioma of the larynx—a pregnancy problem. J Laryngol 1985;99:1309–1311.
54. Dewhurst J. Integrated obstetrics and gynaecology for post-graduates, 3rd ed. Oxford, England: Blackwell, 1981:348–350.

55. Walker RP, Lawrence AM, Paloyan E. Nodular disease during pregnancy. Surg Clin North Am 1995;75:53–58.
56. Doherty CM, Shindo ML, Rice DH, Montero M, Mestman JH. Management of thyroid nodules during pregnancy. Laryngoscope 1995;105:251–255.
57. Cunningham MP, Slaughter DP. Surgical treatment of disease of the thyroid glands in pregnancy. Surg Gynecol Obstet 1970;131:486–488.
58. Rosvoll RV, Winship T. Thyroid carcinoma of pregnancy. Surg Gynecol Obstet 1965;121:1039–1042.
59. Hill GS, Clark RL, Wolf M. The effect of subsequent pregnancy on patients with thyroid carcinoma. Surg Gynecol Obstet 1966;122:1219–1222.
60. Burrow GN. The thyroid gland in pregnancy. Philadelphia: WB Saunders, 1972:113–132.

SECTION XI

Musculoskeletal and Connective Tissue Disorders

Cherry and Merkatz's Complications of Pregnancy,
Fifth Edition, edited by W. R. Cohen.

CHAPTER 36

Orthopedic Complications

Mark E. Pruzansky and Roger N. Levy

BACKACHE AND BIOMECHANICAL STRESSES

The most common orthopedic complaint in pregnancy is backache, generally in the lumbosacral area, but at times involving the dorsal spine and, less frequently, the cervical region. Its intensity can range from mild ache during the morning to agonizing low-back pain with sciatic radiation, and can develop with increasing severity during gestation or the puerperium.

Clinical Picture

Lumbosacral Spine

Antepartum. Low-back symptoms in the antepartum period are usually a consequence of mechanical postural alterations of pregnancy. These involve ligamentous and disc structures of the spinal column, in some instances requiring constant muscle strain to maintain balance. With enlargement of the uterus, the abdominal wall and contents are outwardly displaced and the abdominal musculature becomes distended (1). The actual effect of pregnancy on the anteroposterior curve of the lumbosacral spine and pelvic tilt is variable. Most observers describe an increase in lordosis associated with the forward tilt of the pelvis; however, flattening of the lumbar spine also may be encountered (Fig. 36-1) (2,3). Some degree of postural change is inevitable and occurs in association with alteration in weight distribution. Whatever the postural alteration in the lower back, an equivalent reverse compensatory curve must develop in the dorsal and cervical areas to maintain balance (Fig. 36-2) (4). Any change in the three-dimensional alignment of the normal spine reduces the biochemical efficiency of the muscles, ligaments, and discs. Paravertebral muscles fatigue more easily, which causes static structures such as ligaments and discs to absorb more stress. These soft tissues are strained beyond their limitations, resulting in local pain as well as sciatic symptoms referred to the lower extremities.

In multiparas, abdominal tone may be markedly decreased. This change permits greater anterior displacement of the abdominal contents and causes more imbalance. In the compensatory attempt to realign the spinal curvature to this altered mechanical need (resulting in cervical and lumbar lordosis and dorsal round back), the inherent posture to which the woman has become accustomed during her lifetime is disturbed. In young, healthy, well-toned women these relatively sudden changes may

M. E. Pruzansky: Department of Orthopaedic Surgery, Mount Sinai Medical School, Mount Sinai–NYU Medical Center, New York, NY 10029.

R. N. Levy: Private practice, New York, NY 10021.

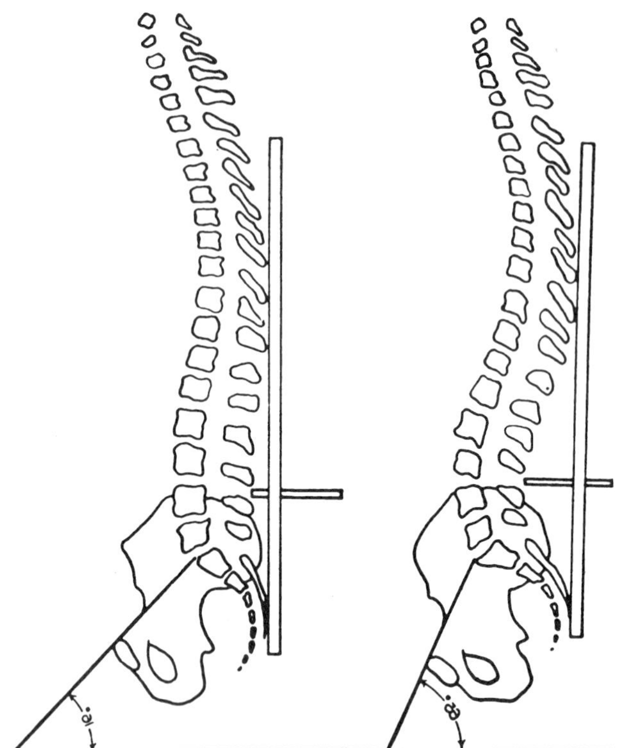

FIG. 36-1. The relationship of the degree of pelvic tilt and lumbar lordosis. The greater the pelvic tilt, the greater the degree of compensating lordosis and round back. (From Miller NF, Kretzchman NR. Posture of women. In: Davis C, Carter B, eds. Gynecology and obstetrics, Vol. 3. Hagerstown, MD: WF Prior, 1953.)

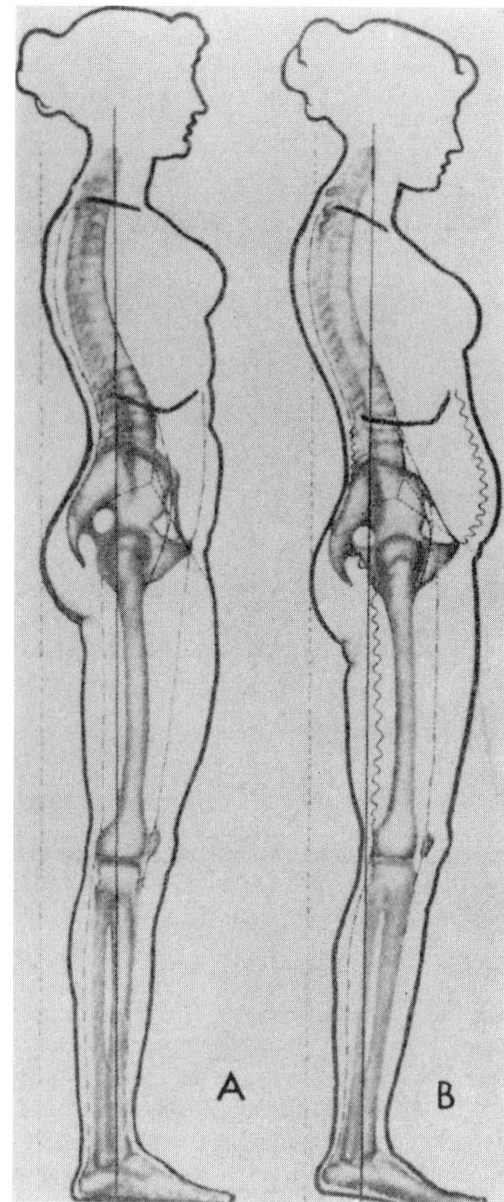

FIG. 36-2. Variations in posture. The normal posture **(A)** is associated with moderate lumbar lordosis and compensating dorsal round back. Increased round back is frequently associated with a lax and enlarging abdominal wall **(B)** as a cause of postural strain. (From Miller NF, Kretzchman NR. Posture of women. In: Davis C, Carter B, eds. Gynecology and obstetrics, Vol. 3. Hagerstown, MD: WF Prior, 1953.)

be easily tolerated. A poorly toned woman with a poor sense of balance will assume a strained, slouched posture with increasing lordosis and rounded back to maintain her equilibrium passively, rather than depend on dexterity and muscle agility. The additional weight borne by the lumbar spine and pelvis can create sufficient strain to produce low-back and radicular symptoms. Relaxin-induced ligamentous changes cause pubic symphysis and sacroiliac joint pain (5). Several biomechanical factors correlate with back pain: increased abdominal saggital and transverse diameters and increased lumbar lordosis (6).

A normal balanced spine in the vertical position requires minimal work from the paraspinal muscles. The electromyograph (EMG) demonstrates low-level activity from small contractions in response to appropriate messages to fine-tune spinal balance. Any changes in the normal weight distribution of the body cause muscular activity to increase, which adds to the axial compressive load placed on the spine. This occurs in pregnancy with the arms reaching forward and with standing hip flexion.

Low-back pain can be spinal or pelvic in origin. Posterior pelvic pain can be demonstrated by palpation and posterior pelvic compression. Although about half of all pregnant women experience lumbosacral pain, three fourths of those affected have pelvic pain, and the remainder have back pain (7). After delivery, back pain is more common and more intense, whereas during pregnancy, pelvic pain tends to predominate. Young age, multiparity, some preexisting physical and psychologic disorders, back pain with and without previous pregnancies, and heavy work all predispose to back pain (8–11). Exercise before and during pregnancy can reduce the incidence and intensity of back and posterior pelvic pain

(6,11). A nonelastic sacroiliac belt is usually helpful in reducing pelvic pain.

Postpartum. The cumulative strain on the low back is usually manifested in the postpartum period. During the second stage of labor, bearing-down efforts impose severe stresses on the lumbar intervertebral discs as well as the supporting structures. In addition, hormonal changes of pregnancy tend to weaken the spinal supports. Estrogen- and relaxin-induced ligamentous laxity makes these structures more vulnerable to repeated injury through minimal stress. Cesarean section may weaken the abdominal musculature and tend to increase pelvic tilt and compensatory lumbar lordosis. Return of muscle tone and healing of ligamentous structures usually lag far behind the demands placed on the mother in returning to a normal way of life, including the care of her children, which usually requires much stooping, bending, and lifting. This results in the common postpartum low backache. So frequently is it mentioned that many multiparous patients accept some degree of low-back pain as a normal aftermath of pregnancy, and the history obtained from women who seek advice for backache or sciatica usually discloses symptomatic periods following antecedent pregnancies. Most back pain disappears by 6 months postpartum, but physically heavy work can cause symptoms to persist (1).

Dorsal and Cervical Spine

The abdominal laxity, shifting of abdominal contents, and lumbar lordosis that produce the secondary round back of pregnancy, as well as a stooped posture and slouching of the shoulders, are frequently responsible for upper and mid-back fatigue and pain. The enlarging breasts add a further strain. Although cervical spine symptoms are not common, some patients complain of chronic fatigue of the neck, trapezius, and upper back muscles. This may imply underlying cervical disc degeneration but also can occur within the normal cervical spine and can be associated with radicular symptoms into the shoulders, upper extremities, chest, and head. An increasing dorsal round back necessitates compensatory cervical lordosis to permit the head to be held erect. For this reason a pregnant woman may complain of headaches, although other causes must of course be excluded.

Coccyx

Coccygodynia may be produced or aggravated by the postural changes described, with the added weight placed on the coccyx in sitting. This results in spraining of the sacrococcygeal joint in patients with problems of straight lower sacrococcygeal segments and in whom there is small buttock contour with little natural cushioning of the region.

Pathophysiology

Back pain can develop either during pregnancy or in the puerperium in a spine that falls well within the normal limits of architecture and posture. Pain, however, is especially prone to occur in the presence of preexisting abnormalities. In the absence of previous symptoms, in view of the inadvisability of x-ray studies during gestation, most of the abnormalities must remain occult. The presence of a hirsute patch over the lumbosacral spine is often a clue to an underlying bony abnormality. Postural alterations, such as scoliosis, excessive lordosis, and dorsum rotundum can be identified clinically (12). The same also is true of spondylolisthesis, the presence of which, in extreme form, is signaled by a short trunk and forward displacement of the lumbar spine on the sacrum, which produces a visible or probable "step" between adjacent low spinous processes. A transverse abdominal crease at the level of umbilicus may be present when hamstring tightness causes an upward rotation of the anterior pelvis (13). Straight leg raising causes regional or distally referred pain. Other intra- and extradural causes of spastic hamstring should be considered when this sign is present. Pregnancy does not cause progression of scoliosis or spondylolisthesis (14,15).

Calf claudication in the absence of peripheral vascular disease may be indicative of spinal stenosis syndrome. The pain is relieved by rest with the feet elevated as well as dependent. The diameter of the spinal canal may be narrowed owing to congenital malformation, exuberant osteophyte formation at the posterior joints, or thickened ligamenta flavae. Reduction in available intraspinal space predisposes the pregnant woman to this form of lumbar radiculopathy when ligamentous laxity and the additional physical stress of pregnancy supervene.

Idiopathic Scoliosis

A developmental condition of childhood or adolescence of unknown etiology, idiopathic scoliosis results in both angular and rotatory alterations of the normal spine curves. It is primarily a lateral deviation of the cervical, dorsal, dorsolumbar, or lumbar segment of the spine accompanied by rotation that results in a prominence of the pelvis, flank, or chest and asymmetry of the shoulders. Because idiopathic scoliosis is an affliction of skeletal growth, its progress usually ceases when full growth has been attained, on the average at about 16 years of age. The residual curvature, possible progression in adulthood, and compromised mobility remain as potential sources of back pain, especially during stressful times. In scoliosis cases, there is rarely additional risk for vaginal delivery or cardiorespiratory compromise to the mother or fetus (16), unless the spinal deformation is sufficiently severe to affect respiratory function.

Lordosis

Lordosis, or "hollow back," is associated with forward tilting of the pelvis and abdominal laxity and protrusion. The posture is usually slouched, with slight hip and knee flexion and compensating dorsal round back. Excessive strains are placed on the ligamentous structures of both the dorsal and lumbar segments of the spine. Abdominal obesity and pendulous, unsupported breasts aggravate the postural defect.

Although lordosis frequently is postural in nature, and can be corrected by exercise and training, it may be the result of underlying structural change. One of the most common is spondylolisthesis, in which a defect in the pars interarticularis in the posterior "hinge" element of the spine, usually between the fifth lumbar and the first sacral vertebra, permits the spinal column to be displaced forward on the sacrum, creating a hollow back (17). Frequently, spondylolisthesis or spondylolysis (presence of a defect without vertebral displacement) remains asymptomatic throughout life. The added strain of pregnancy may evoke symptoms for the first time.

Disc Degeneration

The shock absorber quality of the nucleus pulposus is a direct function of its normal state of health (18). Correlated with age and a lifetime of activities, the nucleus pulposus becomes scarred and fibrosed with diminished water content and, therefore, diminished buoyancy, so that the ligamentous structures, joints, and sometimes bone absorb the stress of motion or injury. This degeneration of the fourth and fifth lumbar interspace is not uncommon during the second and third decades of life, and often is the result of long-standing inflammation, trauma, or congenital developmental anomalies (19). Healed herniated discs as well as vertebral intrusions of disc substance (Schmorl's node) result in loss of material from the interspace and radiologic narrowing of the space. Disc degeneration is most commonly noted at the fourth lumbar interspace in cases of moderate congenital abnormality involving hemisacralization and limited mobility of the fifth lumbar vertebra. Normal low-back stresses, ordinarily equally shared between the fourth and fifth discs, then fall almost entirely on the fourth lumbar disc, resulting in premature degenerative changes. With this gradual diminution in the interspace height, there is often a forward or backward settling of one of the vertebral bodies on another. Together, disc narrowing and lysthesis result in increased mobility of the posterior facet joints, another potential source of symptoms. A concomitant narrowing of the neural canal or foramina at the points at which the nerves emerge from the spinal canal may produce radicular symptoms by mechanical irritation of the nerve root. There may be further encroachment on the neural canal by herniated disc material, thickened ligamenta flavae, or osteophytes that have formed in response to local instability. In the presence of preexisting disc degeneration, therefore, the additional stress produced by pregnancy may readily aggravate or produce back or radicular symptoms.

Disc Herniation

Herniation of the central nucleus pulposus through the confining annulus is common during the childbearing age. Often the result of injury, it is observed as frequently in the absence of known trauma (20–22). Apparently a complex group of mechanical and constitutional factors are responsible for disc herniation and predispose toward its occurrence during pregnancy. In instances of healed previous disc herniation, recurrence may occur through the same area of scarred annulus or at a completely different interspace level. Symptoms of acute early herniation before complete rupture has occurred are localized back pain and, frequently, a truncal list away from the site of impending disc rupture to relieve pressure on the injured tissue. This usually recovers with rest and adequate support. Rupture of the herniated disc is accompanied by dramatic relief of back pain and onset of sciatic radiculitis, muscle weakness (usually the dorsiflexors of the ankle or first toe), reflex changes (diminution of ankle or knee jerks), sensory disturbances (zone of hypesthesia over the involved nerve root pathway), or other manifestations of nerve root pressure such as limited straight leg-raising muscle atrophy and muscle weakness. Careful neurologic surveillance is necessary because of the ever-present possible differential diagnosis of spinal neoplasm that may require emergency surgery. Magnetic resonance imaging (MRI) analysis is an important adjunct in determining treatment. Occasionally, surgery is required for progressive back pain, urinary retention, and radiculopathy when conservative measures fail (23).

Dorsum Rotundum

The round shoulder habitus has a basic structural etiology. Scheuermann's disease, a common structural change, is characterized by alterations of the growth of vertebral ring apophyses at the superior and inferior borders of the vertebral bodies, which results in wedge formation and intervertebral disc narrowing in the dorsal spine. This type of fixed deformity, possibly the end result of vertebral collapse, osteoporosis, healed osteomyelitis, or tuberculosis, is irreversible and implies weakness and diminished reserve of the affected area. Secondary strains are placed on the lumbar and cervical areas, which must assume a compensatory position of hyperextension to a degree sufficient to balance the round back.

Postural dorsal round back itself may be a compensation for excessive lumbar lordosis, the result of heavy, unsupported breasts, or the residual effect of psychological factors in the adolescent girl who hid her growing breasts by assuming a more round-shouldered posture. This begins as a flexible curve but then progresses to a rigid deformity owing to secondary soft-tissue contractures and structural alterations in the vertebrae.

Preexisting Infection and Neoplasm

It is important to review carefully the prior history with particular reference to previous infections of the spine. The rare possibility of long-standing but silent osteomyelitis, either pyogenic or tuberculous, can be awakened by the biochemical changes of pregnancy. In cases of a positive history or clinical evidence of spinal infection, roentgenography of the spine is indicated except in very early gestation. When the suspect region is in the cervical or dorsal areas, shielding of the pelvis may be possible. The diagnosis of spinal infection must be diligently pursued because available therapy is both adequate and mandatory.

Neurofibromatosis type I in pregnant women often increases in severity during gestation. Changes in the size and number of fibromas can produce pain, paresthesias, and paresis about the spine and in the four extremities (24). The reader is referred to Snyder and Thomas's description of the care of the pregnant hemipelvectomy patient for details on their special care (25).

Summary

The mechanism of back pain in cervical and dorsal areas is usually muscle and ligamentous strain secondary to the excessive demands of maintaining postural balance in pregnancy (26). Joint strains and sprains cannot always be excluded. In the lumbar spine, the same conditions apply, but more frequently low-back pain, with and without radiation into the lower extremities, is attributable to disc derangement or deterioration, sometimes with retropulsion of disc material into the spinal canal, which causes pressure on the emerging roots of the cord or the cauda equina.

Supportive corsets are uncomfortable. A more tolerable alternative is a homemade reconstruction of a twelfth-century Japanese supporting corset (27). The Iwata Obi consists of 5 feet of 8-inch elastic cloth sewn to 10 feet of plain, folded cotton cloth that has been tapered 4 inches in its terminal to allow for tucking or pinning after it has been wrapped around the lower abdomen. In this way the supported pregnant belly places less strain on the back.

Prophylaxis and Therapy

Antepartum

Early recognition of basic postural defects, deformities, and preexisting musculoskeletal disease is essential in the presentation of orthopedic complications during pregnancy. Careful control of weight can be beneficial. A regimen of graduated exercises directed at strengthening abdominal musculature should be instituted early in pregnancy, especially in patients in whom back troubles are anticipated. Because x-ray studies of the low back are relatively contraindicated early in pregnancy, definitive diagnosis usually is not made during this period, and treatment is limited to palliation. MRI can be used when necessary. Much of the strain in the lower back can be eliminated by adhering to simple orthopedic principles. Proper rest and exercise are necessary along with firm mattress support at night. A half-inch plywood board beneath the mattress overcomes the sagging effect of the bedspring and affords more complete relaxation to the back during the sleeping hours, which permits the strain incurred during the day to heal. Avoidance of high heels (which in some instances may produce additional lordosis and increased imbalance) and elimination of stooping, forward bending, and lifting are essential. Carefully supervised postural exercises and elementary instructions in dynamic posture, which enable activities of daily living to be accomplished in a coordinated way that avoids back strain, may prevent disabilities later in pregnancy (28). Pain caused by fatigue in the cervical and dorsal spine may be relieved to some degree by various simple methods of home or office physiotherapy.

Proper posturing to balance the weight of the body symmetrically through the spine will reduce back strain (Fig. 36-2). When bending, the center of gravity must remain over the feet without simply shifting the buttocks backward and flexing the hips and lumbar spine (29). Squatting at the knees and hips is preferred. Choosing a well-designed chair in which to sit reduces fatigue by maintaining the center of gravity over the sitting base. A backrest inclined at 15 degrees preserves the normal S shape of the spine, whereas a too-vertical backrest will force the center of gravity forward and cause compensatory, increased paraspinal muscle activity.

Daily exercise, walking, and jogging have all been found helpful in reducing or alleviating the incidence and severity of backache in certain women. Strengthening specific muscle groups, especially abdominals and gluteals, lends additional support to the loaded spine. Williams' (30) flexion exercises are used often. Exercise must be tailored to the protuberance of the pregnant belly and to the endurance limits of the woman. Limits during the postnatal period can be more liberal. Back schools have been developed to evaluate all factors that contribute to a patient's low-back problem when relief is not obtained through basic conservative therapy. The multifactorial and interdisciplinary approach of these schools to treatment includes orthopedists, psychologists, and family counselors, when necessary (31).

Low-back pain may be caused by intrapelvic pathology aside from the imposition of a pregnant uterus.

Fibroid enlargement with increased strain around the uterosacral and cardinal ligaments as well as the low back can cause both referred and direct pain interpreted as arising in the lower back. Intraabdominal pathology (e.g., biliary, pancreatic, gastric, duodenal, appendiceal, intestinal, and tumors of the bone) may refer pain to the low back and should be considered in the evaluation of the lower back. Primary benign bone tumors can change histology and become a structurally weaker type that causes bone pain (32).

If spinal infection is diagnosed, treatment includes rest, supportive measures, antibiotic administration, and surgery when required (13). The choice and timing of specific antibiotics and antituberculous medications should be determined on an individual basis owing to potential teratogenesis. Aspiration or incision of the abscess is planned after consideration of the potential effects on the fetus of x-ray and general anesthesia. In cases of destructive and spine-destabilizing infection, therapeutic abortion may be recommended.

The acute, severe low-back pain of ligamentous or discogenic origin is effectively relieved only by absolute bed rest. The onset of these symptoms calls for abandonment of all exercises, because they invariably aggravate the pain, and adoption of a regimen of rest. Absolute bed rest in any comfortable position with the hips and knees in flexion in a supine or lateral decubitus position is usually most beneficial. Protracted back sprains, disc herniations, and radiculitis often can be forestalled by the investment of relatively short periods of absolute bed rest during an early stage. Gradual resumption of daily activities is begun after the acute symptoms have subsided. Avoidance of bending, lifting, and prolonged sitting in conjunction with a supervised exercise program will reduce the likelihood of a relapse.

Disc herniation may cause lower extremity motor weakness as well as pain. Bowel and bladder dysfunction are other ominous signs. Temporizing with conservative therapy beyond the first 4 months of pregnancy diminishes the possible harmful effect of diagnostic radiation and reduces the theoretical risks of the surgical procedure. However, the decision regarding surgery must be weighed against the risk of permanent neurologic damage to the mother.

Even when extremely severe back and radicular symptoms have not subsided after the first trimester, the chance of maintaining the pregnancy is excellent. Severe, disabling, progressive low-back derangement in women who have had several children may be an adequate indication to recommend sterilization to forestall the possibility of total disability or jeopardy to life or function that could result from further pregnancies.

Intrapartum

Delivery is a period of maximum physical exertion of the abdominal, hip, and pelvic musculature; maximum physical strain on the back, sacroiliac, and pelvic ligaments; and maximum relaxation of these ligaments, apparently on a hormonal basis. The lithotomy position or variants of it taken for delivery places additional strain on the back, pubic, and sacroiliac ligaments and, coupled with the increased intraabdominal pressure, results in extreme stresses being placed upon the disc structures in the lumbosacral area. Care should be taken to avoid sudden vigorous manipulations, and straining of these structures should be restricted, particularly in instances of known previous musculoskeletal symptoms or disease. In selected cases, delivery with the patient in the lateral Sims position may be indicated.

Epidural anesthesia can usually be safely attained in patients with previous spinal surgery (33). Patchy and failed blocks, multiple attempts, dural puncture, and low-back pain are complications that occur in more than one-half of these patients (34).

Exercise is physically and mentally important to the pregnant woman. Non–weight-bearing exercise (stationary bicycling) reduces blood glucose and may help to prevent or control gestational diabetes (35). When the level of exercise is commensurate with prepregnancy conditioning, there is no increase in the rate of spontaneous abortion (36).

Postpartum

Little thought is generally given to the rehabilitation of the mother after her discharge from the hospital. Because of diminished muscle tone, slow return of muscle power, and the clinical and subclinical effects of spraining the back structures, a well-designed postpartum regimen should be taught to the mother before discharge. This should incorporate the same principles used during pregnancy to avoid back strain. Most postpartum regimens provide for passive positions and occasional optional exercises for varying periods of time; few regimens call for 3 to 6 months of graduated resistance exercises designed to strengthen the abdominal, pelvic, and gluteal muscles to hasten the return of muscle power and posture to normal and to prevent postpartum back symptoms, which often result in permanent ligamentous or disc disability (30).

LOWER EXTREMITY PROBLEMS

With the exception of patients with preexisting abnormalities involving the lower extremities (e.g., degenerative disease of the hip, knee, or ankle from an old infection, deformity, or trauma), it is rare for any significant problem to arise in these areas.

Foot Pain

Because of the weight gain of pregnancy, foot pains may develop during the later months of gestation. Such symptoms occur frequently in the presence of preexisting abnormalities such as pes planus, pes equinus, metatarsus varus, hallux valgus, metatarsalgia, plantar neuroma, painful heels, plantar warts, corns, and other conditions (37). Therapy often is hampered by the presence of tight heel cords that result from wearing high-heeled shoes, in which most of the weight is thrown forward upon potentially painful conditions of the forefoot. As a result of this harmful practice, contractions of the Achilles tendon can reach the degree that the heel is unable to touch the ground when the patient is standing barefoot. Achilles tendonitis and posterior tibial tendonitis may result.

Therapy

Rest, relief from weight bearing, and shoe corrections, occasionally coupled with physiotherapy and hydrocortisone injections when symptoms are most acute, are the most effective therapy for chronic strains of the lower extremities caused by increased and altered weight bearing during pregnancy. In the cases of marked preexisting deformity, such as congenital dislocation of the hip, difficulties during pregnancy should be anticipated. Careful attention to the control of weight gain and a regimen of planned exercise with limited weight bearing to replace ordinary activity will reduce the difficulties in such a patient (38).

When heel cords are very tight, the sudden adoption of low-heeled shoes may produce calf and thigh pains as a result of sudden stretching of the gastrocnemius and soleus muscles. If the heel cords are only moderately tight, these symptoms may be avoided by gradually lowering the heel height down by 1/4 inch every 2 or 3 weeks, starting at the beginning of pregnancy. Only when the heel cord has been stretched to the point where low-heeled shoes can be worn with comfort can arch support and corrections be used to material advantage, because such supports are of minimal value in high-heeled shoes. For improved balance during pregnancy and for better distribution of weight, it is advisable to accustom the patient early in pregnancy to the lowest, broadest heel that is compatible with comfort.

Trauma: Antepartum

During the later stages of pregnancy, postural alterations and consequent awkwardness predispose the patient to minor traumas of the lower extremities. These may be treated in general as during the nonpregnant state.

Ankle Sprain

Ankle sprain is the most common lower extremity injury during pregnancy. The acute severe sprain is best treated initially by compression, ice, and elevation, followed by firm elastic, adhesive, or Unna's boot support when pain has subsided sufficiently to permit ambulation. Occasional recurrent sprain from actual tears of the lateral ligaments of the ankle may be prevented by the use of a ¼-inch outer heel and sole wedge with a broad, laterally flared heel. When an injury is to the mid-foot rather than the ankle, mild chip fractures of the cuboid bone or calcaneum may occur. These fractures are treated like sprains when the chip is small. Alternatively, when a significant portion of a joint is involved, a short-leg walking cast is applied.

Avulsion Fracture of the Base of the Fifth Metatarsal

This common injury is caused by sudden pull of the peroneus brevis muscle as the foot attempts to prevent the inevitable twist. Swelling, ecchymosis, and severe pain over the base of the fifth metatarsal results, with complete disability for several days. In most instances adhesive strapping or Unna's boot support is sufficient until the acute pain has subsided, and occasionally a light walking cast is necessary.

Small Toe Fractures

Small toe fractures commonly result from impact of a bare foot against a chair, table leg, or open door. If a deformity exists, manipulation under local anesthesia is a simple procedure. The most satisfactory splint for a contused or fractured small toe is a surface strapping, in which it is bound to the fourth toe for immobilization for a period of 3 weeks. Firm shoes serve as excellent splints for minor foot injuries of this type.

Knee Pain

Chondromalacia patella caused by malalignment is the most common cause of knee pain during pregnancy. Many women have lateral tilting of their patella as a result of any or all of the following: pes planus, loose medial retinacular ligament, tight lateral retinacular ligament, patella alta or baja, femoral anteversion, genu valgum, or back-knee deformity. Relaxin-induced ligamentous laxity and weight gain superimposed on the above anatomical factors can cause maltracking of the patella on the trochlear groove of the distal femur, producing knee pain. Ice, avoidance of high heels, squatting and kneeling, solely isometric quadriceps exercises, and knee braces usually are effective.

Hand and Wrist Pain

Carpal tunnel syndrome and de Quervain's tendonitis of the wrist commonly affect pregnancy and the puerperium (39,40). Compression of the median nerve of the wrist from idiopathic tenosynovitis of the nine flexors within the carpal tunnel usually responds to splinting. The burning pain, paresthesias, and weakness commonly disappear shortly after delivery. Occasionally the symptoms are so recalcitrant and unbearable that surgery under local anesthesia is performed. Inflammation of the long abductor and short thumb extensor produce a painful mass at the radial styloid, exacerbated by motion of the thumb. Treatment with a thumb spica splint ordinarily suffices until pregnancy and the rigors of early child-rearing have eased.

Hip Pain

Pain about the hip is usually musculoligamentous strain or referred from the back. Less commonly the pain is *de novo* from the joint itself. Transient osteoporosis of pregnancy can cause hip pain, which abates with rest and finally delivery (41–45). However, pathologic fractures can occur and are treated as surgical emergencies (42,46). Osteonecrosis of the femoral or humeral head responds to rest and non–weight bearing, but may require surgery to avoid progressive damage and degenerative arthritis of the hip joint (47,48).

PELVIS PROBLEMS

Fracture of the Pelvis

Direct trauma may fracture the pelvis during pregnancy as in the nonpregnant state. Most fractures involve the pubic or ischial rami, with little or no displacement of the fragments and no distortion of the pelvic architecture. Depending on the degree of comminution, a period of bed rest—up to 3 weeks—may be all that is necessary. A pelvic corset or the Iwata Obi Japanese maternity lumbosacral support may be used for a brief period for additional support as the patient becomes ambulatory. More severe fractures with displacement of fragments or sacroiliac derangement may require longer periods of bed rest, often with pelvic sling or tractional support. Alternatively, open reduction and internal fixation can be performed to reduce the likelihood of severe physical disabilities of the back and lower extremities (49,50). When marked disturbance of the pelvic architecture results, which when healed causes bony dystocia, cesarean section may be required.

Symphysial Separation

In late pregnancy the increased laxity of the pelvic ligamentous structures caused by relaxin and other hormones predisposes to traumatic damage with the head engaged in the pelvic inlet antepartum or during delivery. So pronounced can this combined ligamentous relaxation and pelvic strain become that one occasionally sees permanent diastasis of the pubic symphysis, with persistent symptoms caused by instability of the symphysis and the sacroiliac articulation (Fig. 36-3). The symptoms caused by the mild antepartum or postpartum symphysial diastasis usually can be controlled by a firm pelvic support and bed board. To reduce severe separations and permit ligamentous stabilization and healing, a period of absolute bed rest with a tight pelvic compression corset may be necessary after delivery. Continued use of a firm corset to provide tight pelvic compression for several months, in addition to the aforementioned precautions in the treatment of back sprains, is indicated. In traumatic cases, open reduction and internal fixation may be indicated (51–53).

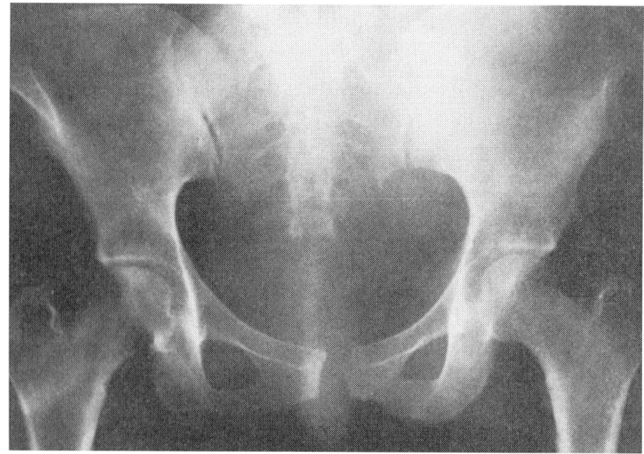

FIG. 36-3. Radiograph of the pelvis showing marked separation of the symphysis pubis resulting from pregnancy.

Seat Belts and Pregnancy

The mandatory construction of automobiles with seat belts has reduced the incidence and severity of personal injury. A lap belt is recommended despite the appearance of the "seat belt injury" as a pathologic entity. Flexion injuries of the lumbar spine include ligamentous strain of the supporting structures of the posterior elements, as well as the nonarticular, transverse Chance fracture.

The lap belt is most suited to the pregnant woman, unlike the shoulder harness, which leaves some doubt as to the wisdom of adding upward body restraint at the expense of increased intrauterine pressure and the risk of abruption. Rupture of the perforators arising from the intercostal arteries can occur with breast tissue laceration from seat belts (54). Intrauterine depressed skull fractures of the unborn fetus may be caused by compression of the fetal skull between the seat belt and the sacral promontory (55). However, the leading cause of fetal death in automobile accidents is still maternal death (56). During a collision a pregnant woman is vulnerable to head, neck, long bone, and visceral injuries. Seat belt restraint reduces both adult and fetal mortality.

Coccygeal and Sacrococcygeal Injuries

During delivery, a coccyx that is angled sharply anteriorly may obstruct easy passage of the fetus. Severe sprains of the sacrococcygeal joint and even fractures of the coccyx, with pain lasting many months, and often recurrently symptomatic, may result. Conservative measures such as local heat, bed rest, use of a doughnut cushion, upright sitting posture so that direct pressure on the coccyx is avoided, tight elastic support to cushion the buttocks over the injured areas, or hydrocortisone injections into the sprained coccygeal joint usually control symptoms. Coccygectomy is rarely necessary. Sacral rhizotomy (division of the roots of S4 and S5) gives lasting freedom from pain and coccygodynia, without distressing neurologic sequelae, but it is rarely indicated (57).

Traumatic Periostitis of the Ischium

Difficult forceps delivery may produce traumatic periostitis of the ischium or severe bruising of the overlying tissue. There is intense local pain, mainly on sitting, for several weeks to months. The condition is self-limiting and requires only symptomatic treatment.

DYSTOCIA DUE TO ORTHOPEDIC PROBLEMS

Some of the problems directly responsible for specific difficulty in labor and delivery are pelvic deformity, hip deformity, muscle weakness of the abdomen, and osteogenesis imperfecta.

Pelvic Deformity

A malformed pelvis, the result of developmental disease, rickets, previous fracture, or long-standing poliomyelitis, may preclude a normal delivery. The presence of musculoskeletal disease elsewhere in the body indicates the need for careful pelvimetry during the antepartum period. Pelvic examination early in the pregnancy also can detect benign osteochondromas of the pelvic wall and sacrum, malunion of old pelvic fractures and deformity, intrapelvic protrusion of the hip, and second-, third-, or fourth-degree spondylolisthesis, in which the lumbar spine has been displaced forward so that the fifth lumbar vertebra rests in front of the sacrum, narrowing the pelvic inlet. A long-standing limp suggests neuromuscular or musculoskeletal abnormalities, which, if present during growth, produce deformities of the pelvis.

Hip Deformity

Deformities of the hip, from congenital dislocation or subluxations, coxa vara, slipped epiphysis, coxa plana, osteomyelitis, and degenerative arthritis, are deformities associated with contracture, limitation of motion, or even ankylosis. The standard lithotomy position with stirrups is often impossible to assume. One option is to have assistants hold the patient's legs, particularly if the knee is ankylosed. Occasionally, the lateral Sims' position may be possible for delivery when the lithotomy position is not. General anesthesia is an important aid in those cases of coxalgia in which abduction of the thighs is insufficient for pelvic delivery. The increased morbility that anesthesia provides may allow sufficient space to make pelvic delivery feasible. Only infrequently is thigh abduction so restricted that cesarean section becomes necessary. By anticipating the obstetric implications of limited flexion and abduction of the hip, reconstructive hip surgery can be implemented prior to conception, making cesarean section unnecessary.

Muscle Weakness of the Abdomen

Poliomyelitis or muscular dystrophy may result in significant weakness of abdominal musculature, which makes the bearing-down process ineffective. Marked lordosis in patients often is caused by abdominal weakness, and its presence warrants abdominal muscle testing early in the pregnancy.

Osteogenesis Imperfecta

Osteogenesis imperfecta (58) is a disorder characterized by diffuse mesenchymal hyperplasia, which is manifested clinically by severe osteoporosis, blue sclerae, middle ear deafness (otosclerosis), and multiple early deformities secondary to repeated fractures. The disease is transmitted by a dominant autosomal gene and may arise spontaneously as a result of mutation; however, the gene may vary in expressivity. The condition presents clinically in two forms: the severe congenital neonatal form, which is usually compatible with life; and the latent form, which is diagnosed only in later life as it becomes evident that a person is subject to repeated bone fractures upon minimal trauma. Survival of women with osteogenesis imperfecta into their childbearing years is rare, but pregnancy in such women has been reported. Although many bony malformations can result from multiple fractures, the disease does not influence fertility or the course of pregnancy. Vaginal delivery has been accomplished when fractures have not previously involved the pelvic bones and the pelvic capacity has remained unimpaired. Where the pelvis is seriously distorted as a result of trauma, cesarean section is often necessary for delivery. Patients with osteogenesis imperfecta must be handled with care, particularly if anesthetized or sedated or otherwise helpless, lest fractures result from an injudicious, forceful lifting of the patient, spreading of the legs to lithotomy position, or other minimal bone stress.

REFERENCES

1. Miller NS, Kretzchman NR. Chapter 12. In: Davis C, Carter B, eds. Posture of women in gynecology and obstetrics. Vol. 3. Hagerstown, MD: WF Pryor, 1953.
2. Goldthwait JE, Brown LT, Swain AT, Kuhns JG. Essentials of body mechanics. In: Health and disease, 5th ed. Philadelphia: JB Lippincott, 1952.
3. Klar R. Wirbelsaule und Graviditat. Bonn: Kubens, 1936.
4. Phelps WL, Okitheth RJH, Doff CW. Diagnosis and treatment of postural defects, 2nd ed. Springfield, IL: Charles C Thomas, 1956.
5. MacLennan A, Nicolson R. Serum relaxin and pelvic pain of pregnancy. Lancet 1986;2:243–245.
6. Ostgaard HC, Zetherstrom G, Roos-Hansson E, Svanberg B. Reduction of back and posterior pelvic pain in pregnancy. Spine 1994;19: 894–900.
7. Ostgaard HC, Roos-Hansson E, Zetherstrom G. Regression of back and posterior pelvic pain after pregnancy. Spine 1996;21:2777–2780.
8. Ostgaard HC, Andersson GB, Karlsson K. Prevalence of back pain in pregnancy. Spine 1991;16:549–552.
9. Ostgaard HC, Andersson GB, Wennergren M. The impact of low back and pelvic pain in pregnancy on the pregnancy outcome. Acta Obstet Gynecol Scand 1991;70:21–24.
10. Ostgaard HC, Andersson GB. Previvous back pain and risk of developing back pain in a future pregnancy. Spine 1991;16:432–436.
11. Ostgaard HC. Assessment and treatment of low back pain in working pregnant women. Semin Perinatol 1996;20:61–19.
12. Steindler A. Diseases and deformities of the spine and thorax. St. Louis: CV Mosby, 1929.
13. Rothman R, Simeone S, Bernini P. Lumbar disk disease. In: The spine, 2nd ed. Philadelphia: WB Saunders, 1982.
14. Betz RR, Bunnell WP, Lambrecht-Mulier E, MacEwen GD. Scoliosis and pregnancy. J Bone Joint Surg 1987;69:90–96.
15. Saraste H. Spondylolysis and pregnancy—a risk analysis. Acta Obstet Gynecol Scand 1986;65:727–729.
16. To WW, Wong MW. Kyphoscoliosis complicating pregnancy. Int J Gynaecol Obstet 1996;55:123–128.
17. Caldwell EA. Spondylolisthesis. Ann Surg 1944;119:485.
18. Bradford HJ, Scurling RD. The intervertebral disc, 2nd ed. Springfield, IL: Charles C Thomas, 1947.
19. Lippman RK. Arthropathy due to adjacent inflammation. J Bone Joint Surg [Am] 1953;35:967.
20. JS. Ruptured intervertebral disc and sciatic pain. J Bone Joint Surg 1947;29:429.
21. Fridberg S. Low back and sciatic pain caused by intervertebral disc herniation. Acta Chir Scand 1941;85(suppl 64):1.
22. Minter WJ, Barr JS. Rupture of the intervertebral disk with involvement of the spinal cord. N Engl J Med 1934;211:210.
23. Garmel SH, Guzelian GA, D Alton JG, D'Alton ME. Lumbar disk disease in pregnancy. Obstet Gynecol 1997;89:821–822.
24. Ddugoff L, Sujansky E. Neurofibromatosis type 1 and pregnancy. Am J Med Genet 1996;66:7–10.
25. Snyder DJ, Thomas RL. Pregnancy complicated by hemipelvectomy: case presentations and review of the literature. Am J Perinatol 1989;6: 363–366.
26. Kendall HO, Kendall FP, Boynton DA. Posture and pain. Baltimore: Williams & Wilkins, 1952.
27. Weber HA, Budd FW, Curlin JP. Iwata obi (Japanese maternity lumbosacral support). Milit Med 1972;137:359–360.
28. Howorth MB. A textbook of orthopedics. Philadelphia: WB Saunders, 1952.
29. Ruge D, Wiltse L. Spinal disorders. Philadelphia: Lea & Febiger, 1977.
30. Williams PC. The Lumbosacral Spine. New York: McGraw-Hill, 1965.
31. White A. Back school and other conservative approaches to low back pain. St. Louis: CV Mosby, 1983.
32. Mintz MC, Dalinka MK, Schmidt R. Aneurysmal bone cyst arising in fibrous dysplasia during pregnancy. Radiology 1987;165:549–550.
33. Daley MD, Rolbin SH, Hew EM, Morningstar BA, Stewart JA. Epidural anesthesia for obstetrics after spinal surgery. Reg Anesth 1990;15:280–284.
34. Crosby ET, Halpern SH. Obstetric epidural anesthesia in patient with Harrington instrumentation. Can J Anaesth 1989;36:693–696.
35. Artal R, Masaki DI, Khodiguian N, Romen Y, Rutherford SE, Wisuell RA. Exercise prescription in pregnancy: weight-bearing vs non-weight-bearing exercises. Am J Obstet Gynecol 1989;161:1464–1469.
36. Clapp JF. The effects of maternal exercise on early pregnancy. Am J Obstet Gynecol 1989;161:1453–1957.
37. Lewin P. The foot and ankle, their injuries, diseases, deformities, and disabilities, 3rd ed. Philadelphia: Lea & Febiger, 1947.
38. Williams PC. Lesions of the lumbosacral spine. II. Chronic traumatic (postural) destruction of the lumbosacral intervertebral disc. J Bone Joint Surg 1937;19:690.
39. Schned ES. DeQuervain tenosynovitis in pregnant and postpartum women. Obstet Gynecol 1986;68:411–414.
40. Heckman JD, Sassard R. Musculoskeletal considerations in pregnancy. J Bone Joint Surg [Am] 1994;76:1720–1730.
41. Lose G, Lindholm P. Transient painful osteoporosis of the hip in pregnancy. Int J Gynaecol Obstet 1986;24:6–13.
42. Brodell JD, Burns Jr JE, Heiple KG. Transient osteoporosis of the hip of pregnancy. Two cases complicated by pathological fracture. J Bone Joint Surg [Am] 1989;71:1252–1257.
43. Fingeroth RJ. Successful operative treatment of a displaced subcapital fracture of the hip in transient osteoporosis of pregnancy. A case report and review of the literature. J Bone Joint Surg [Am] 1995;77:127–131.
44. Junk S, Ostrowski M, Kokoszczynski L. Transient osteoporosis of the hip in pregnancy complicated by femoral neck fracture: a case report. Acta Orthop Scand 1996;67:69–70.
45. Smith R, Athnasou NA, Ostlere SJ, Vipond SE. Pregnancy-associated osteoporosis. Q J Med 1995;88:865–878.
46. Pellici PM, Zolla-Pazner S, Rabban WN, Wilson PD. Osteonecrosis of the femoral head associated with pregnancy. Clin Orthop 1984;185: 59–63.
47. McGuigan L, Fleming A. Osteonecrosis of the humerus related to pregnancy. Ann Rheum Dis 1983;42:597–599.
48. Lausten GS. Osteonecrosis of the femoral head during pregnancy. Arch Orthop Trauma Surg 1991;110:214–215.
49. Yosipovitch Z, Goldberg I, Ventura E, Neri A. Open reduction of acetabular fracture in pregnancy. A case report. Clin Orthop 1992;282: 229–232.
50. Pals SD, Brown CW, Friermood TG. Open reduction and internal fixation of and acetabular fracture during pregnancy. J Orthop Trauma 1992;6:379–381.
51. Senechal PK. Symphysis pubis separation during childbirth. J Am Board Fam Pract 1994;7:141–144.
52. Luger EJ, Arbel R, Dekel S. Traumatic separation of the symphysis pubis during pregnancy: a case report. J Trauma 1995;38:255–256.
53. Scriven MW, Jones DA, McKnight L. The importance of pubic pain following childbirth: a clinical and ultrasonographic study of diastasis of the pubic symphysis. J R Soc Med 1995;88:28–30.
54. Murday AJ. Seat belt injury of the breast—a case report. Injury 1975; 14:276–277.
55. Garza-Mercado R. Intrauterine depressed skull fractures of the new born. Neurosurgery 1982;10:694–697.
56. Crosby W. Pathology of obstetric injuries in pregnant automobile-accident victims. In: Accident pathology, proceedings of an international conference. Washington, DC: US Government Printing Office, 1968.
57. Bohm E. Late results of sacral rhizotomy in coccygodynia. Acta Chir Scand 1962;123:6.
58. Cohn SL, Schreier R, Feld D. Osteogenesis imperfecta and pregnancy. Obstet Gynecol 1962;20:107.

Cherry and Merkatz's Complications of Pregnancy,
Fifth Edition, edited by W. R. Cohen.
Lippincott Williams & Wilkins, Philadelphia © 2000.

CHAPTER 37

Rheumatologic Diseases

John Meyerhoff

Rheumatologists treat a wide variety of diseases, ranging from infectious diseases such as Lyme disease, for which the etiology and treatment are well defined, to diseases such as rheumatoid arthritis, systemic lupus erythematosus, and scleroderma, for which the etiology is unknown and treatment varies dramatically from patient to patient. These latter diseases and others are often described as connective tissue diseases or autoimmune diseases in an attempt to bring some coherence to their classification.

As we learn more about these diseases, most of them have been demonstrated to be associated with the presence of autoantibodies. However, the exact role of these autoantibodies is not known and may vary from one disease to another. In all of these diseases, however, there are patients who have the clinical manifestations of the disease without the autoantibody. Depending on the disease, either a few or many individuals will have the autoantibody without having disease. This is particularly true, for example, when one considers that a positive antinuclear antibody (ANA) test result is not considered truly positive until the antibody is present in a dilution of 1:40. Positive rheumatoid factor test results increase in frequency as people age without a corresponding increase in the disease. Thus, it is clear that these autoantibodies are neither sufficient nor necessary for the development of the associated illness.

The exact mechanisms by which these autoantibodies cause disease is not known. Autoantibodies may attach directly to target cells, resulting in their destruction, as may occur with the thrombocytopenia and hemolytic anemia of lupus. The autoantibodies may form complexes with the target antigens and become deposited in organs that may be merely innocent bystanders, as in lupus nephritis. Antineuronal antibodies may bind to cells in the central nervous system and induce changes that result in seizures. Antiphospholipid antibodies may interfere in the proliferation of placental cells, leading to pregnancy failure.

Only recently has the medical investigation concerning pregnancy and rheumatologic disease moved out of the case report and the retrospective analysis stage. Moreover, many of these diseases occur so infrequently in women of childbearing age that collecting reasonable numbers of patients from which predictions and recommendations can be made is difficult. Only for rheumatoid arthritis, systemic lupus erythematosus (including antiphospholipid antibody syndrome), and scleroderma are prospective studies available, as opposed to collections of anecdotal case reports.

This chapter assumes that patients with known connective tissue diseases will be followed by their rheumatologist in conjunction with their obstetrician during pregnancy. It is also assumed that patients who develop features of these diseases during their pregnancy will be referred to a rheumatologist for definitive diagnosis. Classification criteria for many of the rheumatologic diseases have been developed and are available on the American College of Rheumatology web site at www.rheumatology.org.

RHEUMATOID ARTHRITIS

Rheumatoid arthritis is the most common cause of inflammatory arthritis. It is typically a chronic, additive, inflammatory polyarthritis involving the small joints of the hands, wrists, and the knees (1). It occurs more often in women then in men, with the average age of onset 35 years. It occurs in 1% to 2% of the population and is at least twice as common in women before menopause.

Over the past 20 years, there has been a dramatic change in the approach to the treatment of rheumatoid arthritis among rheumatologists. In the past patients were often tried initially on various nonsteroidal antiinflammatory drugs (NSAIDs) before being sequentially put on

J. Meyerhoff: Department of Medicine, Johns Hopkins University School of Medicine; Sinai Hospital of Baltimore, Baltimore, MD 21215.

one of the available second-line drugs: gold, antimalarials, or d-penicillamine. It is now clear that damage to the joints occurs early in the disease and that early control may require multiple second-line drugs at the same time. These second-line drugs are sometimes referred to as disease remittive, although they may be merely disease suppressive. In addition to the three mentioned above, more of these agents are now available. Methotrexate, sulfasalazine, azathioprine, and cyclosporine have all been approved for use in rheumatoid arthritis, and additional newer biologic therapies such as anti–tumor necrosis factor alpha may soon be available. Due to this change, obstetricians are more likely to see women whose rheumatoid arthritis is doing well on multiple medications and who want to become pregnant. It is not unusual to have a patient with rheumatoid arthritis on an NSAID, low-dose prednisone, methotrexate, and hydroxychloroquine to control the arthritis, and on calcium, multivitamins, folic acid, and alendronate to control the side effects of the disease and its treatment.

Fortunately, rheumatoid arthritis seems to have no deleterious effect on fertility or fetal outcome. As early as 1938, Hench reported from the Mayo Clinic that 90% of patients with chronic atrophic (infectious rheumatoid) arthritis improved during pregnancy (2). The investigation of the causes for this phenomenon was unsuccessful in its primary goal, but did lead to the discovery of corticosteroids and a Nobel prize. More recent studies have confirmed the amelioration of rheumatoid arthritis in pregnancy with rates of improvement ranging from 71% to 86% (3). The cause of this improvement remains elusive. A recent study suggested that maternal-fetal HLA DR/DQ incompatibilty is associated with improvement in the arthritis, whereas compatibility is not (4). If confirmed, this could allow one to make better decisions concerning the use of medications in patients wishing to become pregnant.

The only significant concern for those patients who go into remission during pregnancy may be for those with loss of motion in the hips and knees or replacement of these joints. This could lead to difficulty in positioning the patient for vaginal delivery. This should be obvious at the first prenatal pelvic examination.

Drug Therapy for Rheumatoid Arthritis During Pregnancy

The reduction in symptoms during pregnancy may allow for a reduction in medications. Most patients with rheumatoid arthritis are on NSAIDs, which have not been reported to be associated with birth defects. However, due to concern about bleeding and closure of the ductus arteriosus, it has generally been recommended that NSAIDs be discontinued during the third trimester. Because 95% of patients who had improved during pregnancy had reached maximum improvement by the seventh month (3), this should be possible.

Methotrexate has become a popular second-line drug for rheumatoid arthritis due to its rapid onset of action and long-term effectiveness. It is associated with fetal malformations and should generally not be used in pregnancy. Although there are reports of its use during the first and third trimester with some successful outcomes (5), its use in pregnancy in nonneoplastic conditions is contraindicated. It is listed in Pregnancy Category X by the U.S. Food and Drug Administration (FDA) (6). It should be discontinued at least 3 months prior to beginning attempting conception.

Unfortunately, it is difficult if not impossible to determine which patient has gone into remission and which patient's disease has merely been controlled. If a patient has had no difficulty becoming pregnant previously, a temporary increase in (or institution of) corticosteroids may control the arthritis until the amelioration due to pregnancy commences. If a patient's arthritis has been doing well for an extended period of time, it may be possible to discontinue the methotrexate.

Many patients will have a flare-up within a month after methotrexate is discontinued, particularly in the first several years of therapy. Alternatively, the patient can be switched to hydroxychloroquine or sulfasalazine. For patients requiring all three drugs for adequate control of their rheumatoid arthritis, azathioprine may be a safer alternative during pregnancy. However, because methotrexate may be the most effective of the second-line drugs, these substitutions may not be effective in controlling the disease.

Hydroxychloroquine and sulfasalazine are currently the other two most commonly used second-line drugs, with the former more common in the United States and the latter in Europe. Recent articles concerning small numbers of patients suggest that hydroxychloroquine is safe and can be continued throughout pregnancy (7,8). Even larger numbers of sulfasalazine-treated patients have been followed without complication (5). With both drugs this experience has been almost exclusively in conditions other than rheumatoid arthritis, but there is no reason to expect them to have a different effect in rheumatoid arthritis. Sulfasalazine is in FDA Category B (6).

For the remainder of the drugs used in rheumatoid arthritis there are more serious concerns or limited experience in pregnancy; these drugs are discussed at the end of the chapter.

SYSTEMIC LUPUS ERYTHEMATOSUS

Most of the literature addressing pregnancy in rheumatic diseases concerns patients with systemic lupus erythematosus and patients with the antiphospholipid antibody syndrome. This is due to the increased frequency of lupus in women of childbearing age, the deleterious effects of lupus and antiphospholipid antibody syndrome on pregnancy, and lack of an accepted effective approach to minimize these effects.

Systemic lupus erythematosus is a multisystem disorder with arthralgias and arthritis (rarely as deforming as rheumatoid arthritis) and mucocutaneous findings (malar rash, oral or nasal ulcers, and discoid skin lesions) being the most common manifestations (9). Over 95% of patients have a positive ANA test result; the sensitivity of this test allows for identification of almost all patients with lupus. Nevertheless, the prevalence of lupus has not been well defined (10). It is clearly more frequent in African-American women of childbearing age, with a prevalence of perhaps 1 in 250. Among white women of the same age, the prevalence is about 1 in 1,000. The disease occurs in Asian and Hispanic women with an incidence between those of blacks and whites. The average age of onset is 25 years.

The immune complexes that occur in lupus may involve antinuclear antibodies, anti-DNA antibodies, anti-Sm, anti-Ro, or other autoantibodies. Each of these autoantibodies has been reported to be associated with specific manifestations. Because the expression of lupus also may depend on the genetic makeup of the host, lupus should be regarded as a heterogeneous disease. The disease may range from mild joint, skin, and mucous membrane involvement only to severe disease with renal and central nervous system impairment.

The diagnosis of lupus should be considered in a patient who presents with symptoms that occur frequently in lupus (11). A detailed history and physical examination should be performed to look for those findings specific for lupus and that are unlikely to occur in similar conditions. Serologic testing for antinuclear and anti-DNA antibodies can be used to confirm the clinical diagnosis. Although the ANA test result is rarely positive in normal individuals, it is frequently positive in patients with conditions that can be confused with lupus. For example, approximately 50% of patients with rheumatoid arthritis will have a positive ANA test result, as will 90% of patients with scleroderma. About one third of patients with a first-degree relative with lupus will have a positive ANA test result (12). Anti–double-strand DNA antibodies are specific for lupus; a positive test result confirms the diagnosis. Unfortunately, only 50% of patients with otherwise documentable lupus have a positive assay; thus, a negative result does not rule out the disease. Patients with suggestive symptoms should be referred to a rheumatologist for evaluation.

Effect of Pregnancy on Lupus

One of the earliest reviews of lupus and pregnancy was published in 1955 (13). Turner and colleagues reviewed 10 cases of pregnancy in acute disseminated lupus erythematosus and five cases in subacute disease. At that time the 5-year survival of lupus was only 25%. Of the 10 acute cases, 5 of the women died 1 to 56 days after delivery, and only 1 of these 5 pregnancies was successful. Three of the remaining five women had a successful pregnancy, one had a stillbirth, and one had an induced abortion owing to maternal disease. During 7 of the 12 pregnancies (58%) the mothers were described as acutely ill during the pregnancy.

Over the subsequent 40 years lupus has become a much more commonly recognized disease, with a 5-year survival rate of over 95%. The outcome of pregnancy in lupus patients has improved greatly for the mothers; death during pregnancy is now rare. The frequency of successful pregnancy also has improved, but not to the same degree. Disease flares may be as common, but are probably less severe.

Since 1984 six prospective studies of lupus and pregnancy have been published (14–19). The results of these studies regarding the outcomes of fetus and mother are contradictory. Despite the use of well-defined criteria for lupus, the studies had methodologic differences and the study populations were heterogeneous with regard to socioeconomic status and race. In addition, lupus is rarely stable over a 1-year period. One of the studies reported 0.65 flare-ups per person-year in nonpregnant patients (17). This high background rate of flares makes these studies more difficult to interpret.

The prospective studies were split equally between those that reported an increase in flare-ups (16,17,19) and those that reported no worsening of lupus during pregnancy (14,15,18). Among patients who have recently had more active lupus there may indeed be an increase in flare-ups during pregnancy (19). Those studies that reported an increase in flare-ups during pregnancy may have included more patients whose disease was less well-controlled when they became pregnant (17).

The studies agree that flare-ups of lupus are common during pregnancy, with reported rates over 50% in five of the six studies. The flare-ups are generally mild (20), with only 11% having been characterized as severe in the Hopkins lupus cohort (17). In this group the patients tended to have less musculoskeletal and neurologic disease during flare-ups with pregnancy, and more renal and hematologic abnormalities than usually seen in nonpregnant women.

There is no agreement as to when flare-ups are most likely to occur, with wide discrepancies among studies having been reported. In a small series, Fraga and colleagues reported no flare-ups during the first trimester, but 43% among patients in the second trimester (21), whereas Mintz and colleagues reported 57% and 13% of flare-ups in the first and second trimesters, respectively (15). More detailed analyses of these issues have been published (22,23).

Nonlupus morbidity usually has not been considered in studies of these patients, but Petri reported increases in hypertension, diabetes, hyperglycemia, and cystitis in the Hopkins cohort in pregnancy (22).

Effect of Lupus on Pregnancy

There does not appear to be decreased fertility among patients with inactive, mild, or even moderate levels of lupus disease activity (24). There is, however, a clear increase in the frequency of fetal loss among patients with lupus. It has become clear over the past two decades that some of this is due to the presence of antiphospholipid antibodies, rather than to disease activity (20,22,25). Those antibodies may be most significant in lupus patients with recurrent pregnancy losses (26). The antibodies may be manifest as false-positive test results for syphilis, lupus anticoagulants, and anticardiolipin antibodies. Lupus anticoagulant is a misnomer because these antibodies occur in many diseases other than lupus. The anticoagulant activity is present only in *in vitro* assays and is associated with arterial and venous thromboses *in vivo* (27). Although most physicians use the activated partial thromboplastin time (aPTT) as the assay for an anticoagulant because of its universal availability, it may not be as predictive as other tests for anticoagulants, such as the Russell viper venom time (28). Not all the antiphospholipid antibodies are equally pathogenic. The presence of a lupus anticoagulant or high-titer immunoglobulin G (IgG) anticardiolipin antibody prior to pregnancy is most predictive of fetal loss (29). IgM and IgA anticardiolipin antibodies rarely are associated with increased fetal loss. Also, antiphospholipid antibodies associated with infections such as Lyme disease, human immunodeficiency virus, and syphilis do not appear to be pathogenic (30). In addition, low-titer IgG antibodies do not seem to be associated with adverse outcomes. The titer of these antibodies also fluctuates during pregnancy, but this fluctuation does not seen to have any predictive value (31).

Despite the attention this issue has received in the medical literature, it is important to remember that most patients with anticardiolipin antibodies and lupus anticoagulants in fact have successful pregnancies. Lima and colleagues reported on a group of 90 patients with lupus during pregnancy (20). Among the first pregnancies of each of these women, 73 were successful. There were approximately twice as many women with antiphospholipid antibody syndrome, anticardiolipin antibodies, and lupus anticoagulants among the successful pregnancies than among the failures. However, two thirds of those women with unsuccessful pregnancies had these features. The increase in fetal jeopardy associated with these antibodies seems to be associated with loss prior to week 20 of gestation and may be most closely associated with loss between weeks 13 and 20 (22). This may implicate involvement of the spiral artery as a crucial element in the pathogenesis of this process (27). Once a woman has had fetal loss during a pregnancy, the risk increases for future pregnancies. A fetal loss rate of up to 85% has been reported in women with high titer antibodies and previous fetal loss (30).

There is also an increase in preterm delivery in lupus patients, which may actually be more common than fetal loss. Like most of the literature concerning lupus and pregnancy, there is disagreement about the causes for this. The Hopkins experience suggests that disease activity, proteinuria, and dose of prednisone (22) are all risk factors, as is maternal hypertension and educational level (32). A study from the the St. Thomas Hospital in London found that disease activity and corticosteroid doses were not significant (20). Suspected intrauterine growth restriction (IUGR) was common in the latter study group, whereas premature rupture of membranes was more common in the Hopkins experience as indications for early delivery (33). Antiphospholipid antibodies do not seem to be associated with an increased risk of preterm birth (20).

Management of Lupus During Pregnancy

Management of pregnancy in patients with lupus begins with counseling patients regarding the risks of pregnancy. Ideally this should be done as preconceptional counseling so that the patient can make an informed decision about pregnancy and her disease can be optimally controlled before she becomes pregnant.

Unfortunately, as noted in the preceding paragraphs, it is difficult to give patients definitive answers. Pregnancy may or may not increase the risk of a flare-up and, although the flare-ups are often mild, they are occasionally severe. Patients should be counseled to try to conceive during periods of relative disease inactivity, because active lupus is strongly associated with prematurity and IUGR (rather than fetal loss). Inactivity of the disease may allow patients to reduce or discontinue some of their medications. Active or flaring renal disease is probably associated with higher rates of fetal complications and may make the recognition of preeclampsia difficult.

The presence of the antiphospholipid antibody syndrome (APS; arterial or venous thrombotic events, thrombocytopenia, or recurrent fetal loss, in association with a circulating anticoagulant or high-titer IgG anticardiolipin antibody) presents a particular challenge. Patients with a history of arterial thromboses should be strongly counseled not to become pregnant because of the significant risk of recurrent stroke (22). For those with venous thromboses who wish to become pregnant, pregnancy and the postpartum period may represent a particularly risky time for patients with the antiphospholipid antibodies. Perhaps half of all thromobotic events associated with these antibodies may occur during this period of time or during the use of combination oral contraceptives (34). Two prospective studies of pregnant patients with APS have reported rates of stroke and thromboses of 5% (35) and 12% (36), despite subcutaneous heparin in some cases. A retrospective study found that 30% of pregnancies were associated with venous thromboses during pregnancy or in the postpartum period (37). Eight patients in this study had deep venous thromboses on combination oral contraceptives or hormone replacement therapy. Active disease, hypertension, and hyperlipidemia may be as important as antiphospholipid antibodies as risk factors for thromboses in pregnant lupus patients (27) and need to be controlled before and during pregnancy. Patients with previous fetal loss should be counseled about the lack of well-controlled effective treatment trials and the risks of recommended treatments.

Antiphospholipid antibody syndrome can occur as a primary event (27,34). The same adverse outcomes that have been reported with APS in lupus also occur in primary APS. Because fetal loss, particularly in the first trimester, is a common event and primary APS represents only a small portion of patients with recurrent loss (38), screening all healthy pregnant women who do not have a history of thrombotic events for antiphospholipid antibodies is not warranted. After several first-trimester losses or a single second- or third-trimester fetal loss (27), and in otherwise healthy women with a history of thrombotic events, screening for these antibodies is appropriate.

Pregnancy is strongly contraindicated in patients who are on cyclophosphamide and methotrexate (6). Azathioprine is probably safer than other immunosuppressives (39,40). Other typically prescribed medications may be safer than generally appreciated and are not contraindicated during pregnancy. Hydroxychloroquine use during pregnancy does not seem to be associated with any increased risk of fetal malformation (7,8). Discontinuation of hydroxychloroquine is associated with flare-ups in one third of all lupus patients (41). Because active disease may be associated with adverse outcomes other than fetal loss (15,22) [although this is not a universal finding (23)], and because hydroxychloroquine also has some antithrombotic effects (27), it should not be discontinued because a patient is contemplating pregnancy. NSAIDs (42), particularly aspirin (43), also do not seem to be associated with any increased risk of birth defects and can probably be taken safely through the second trimester.

Certain blood tests should be performed to help counsel the patient, particularly if she is at high risk. Anti-Ro and anti-La antibodies are clearly associated with an increased risk of congenital heart block in the fetus (44). There are conflicting data regarding the value of screening for antiphospholipid antibodies in the nulliparous lupus patient without clinical evidence of antiphospholipid antibody syndrome. The St. Thomas Hospital experience showed an association between fetal loss in the first pregnancy with anticardiolpin antibodies (20). The data from the University of Pittsburgh showed increasing risk of all adverse outcomes (fetal loss, low birth weight, and complications) with the first, second, and third pregnancies associated with these antibodies, but the risk differential did not reach statistical significance (26).

Once a patient with lupus decides to become pregnant, she should be followed closely by both the rheumatologist and the obstetrician with visits occurring more frequently as the pregnancy progresses. When assessing a particular patient it is important to review critically the patient's symptoms and laboratory results. During pregnancy many of the effects of pregnancy on any woman can be confused with a flare-up of lupus. Low-back and pelvic pain, facial erythema, mild anemia, and carpal tunnel syndrome are all common symptoms and findings in pregnancy, but could be mistaken for symptoms of lupus (42). During pregnancy patients will develop a mild anemia due to an increase in plasma volume that is greater than the increase in red cell mass, and patients also may develop a relative thrombocytopenia during the third trimester.

The most difficult diagnostic issues revolve around the similar presentations of preeclampsia and a flare-up of lupus nephritis. The development of hypertension late in pregnancy should prompt particularly close monitoring. If such a patient develops other signs and symptoms of active lupus at this time, the diagnosis of a flare-up of lupus is obvious. In the absence of symptoms, cells and cellular casts in the urine (23) and decreasing C3 or CH50 (45) are all findings more suggestive of a lupus flare-up than of preeclampsia. Declining C3 values may be particularly predictive because they tend to increase during the last trimester of pregnancy in healthy patients and in preeclamptic patients (46). These studies should be performed on a regular basis during the pregnancy as part of routine disease monitoring, particularly in a patient with preexisting nephropathy, to establish a baseline in case hypertension develops. Calcium excretion below 195 mg per 24 hours is suggestive of preeclampsia, and some physicians recommend it be measured early in pregnancy in all lupus patients for a baseline in the event that hypertension develops (42).

Unfortunately, the prevention of fetal loss due to antiphospholipid antibody syndrome has proven to be difficult. This is reviewed in more detail by Weber and colleagues (27). Most of the studies have been in patients with primary APS. Steroids and low-dose aspirin (81–325 mg) have been a popular regimen with variable results. One rationale for the use of steroids is to try to reduce the level of circulating anticoagulants. As is true with almost every aspect of these reports, equal numbers of trials report an association or lack of an association between successful outcome and lower antibody titers. The use of steroids, particularly with increasing doses, has been associated with significant complications.

Different definitions for this syndrome based on the numbers of losses (two or more versus three or more), time of loss by either trimester or weeks, and the serologic assays used to define antiphospholipid antibodies have clouded the ability to interpret these studies. A large double-blind trial of prednisone and aspirin in 202 women without SLE was not successful in reducing fetal loss (47). The treatment also was associated with significant increases in premature births as well as maternal hypertension and diabetes. This study has been criticized for not using three or more losses as an entry criterion, as well as for including autoantibodies such as ANAs, rather than just antiphospholipid antibodies, as an entry criterion.

The complication rate related to the use of steroids and aspirin has led to the use of heparin for the prevention of fetal loss (35). This may prove to be an effective therapy, but the use of heparin has been associated with increased osteoporosis, which may result in fracture (27). Low molecular weight heparins may be less likely to cause this particular complication (48). However, one recent trial showed that heparin and low-dose aspirin was particularly successful compared with aspirin alone in preventing fetal loss without any increase in maternal complications (49).

Part of the answer for these women may depend on further classification of the placental pathology associated with fetal loss. One study suggested that women tend to experience recurrent loss owing to the same pathology each time (50). For example, in some patients with placental thromboses, anticoagulation is the most appropriate therapy; other patients with a more inflammatory process may do better with corticosteroids.

SCLERODERMA

Scleroderma is a disease characterized by changes in the skin resulting in bound-down skin and loss of range of motion in the involved parts of the body due to contractures in the soft tissues. Raynaud's phenomenon is the most common noncutaneous manifestation of scleroderma. Gastroesophageal reflux is also a common problem. More serious gastrointestinal involvement as well as cardiac and pulmonary disease may occur. Scleroderma renal crisis used to lead almost invariably to renal failure; nephrectomy was at times required to control blood pressure due to the inefficacy of the available drugs. With the release of captopril, the first angiotensin-converting enzyme (ACE) inhibitor, in the late 1970's, medical treatment of this dreaded complication was vastly improved.

Due to the rarity of this disease and its average onset at 43 years of age (51), there is a relative paucity of literature concerning pregnancy and scleroderma. There have been the usual case reports of adverse outcomes followed by retrospective studies and a prospective study (52). The results of these studies suggest that there is generally no increase in fetal loss. In the prospective study, patients with late diffuse scleroderma had an increase in fetal loss, but most of these patients were able to have a later successful pregnancy.

Scleroderma renal crisis (SRC) can present suddenly with malignant hypertension, proteinuria, and a microangiopathic hemolytic anemia. Because pregnancy may contribute to induction of renal crisis (53), patients should monitor their blood pressure three to five times a week. This is particularly true in patients with diffuse scleroderma of recent onset who are at greater risk for disease complications (54). Despite concerns about birth defects with ACE inhibitors, these drugs are the drugs of choice in SRC and should be started immediately with informed consent if a scleroderma patient's blood pressure increases.

Sclerodermatous skin changes in the extremities may pose a problem in positioning the patient at delivery. This should be obvious during prenatal examinations. At the time of delivery, care needs to be taken to keep patients warm because 90% of scleroderma patients have Raynaud's phenomenon. The delivery room should be kept warm and the patient should be kept as clothed as possible. Intravenous fluids should be warmed prior to infusion. Cesarean section is not contraindicated if the abdominal wall is involved with scleroderma, as long as the surgical repair is done well (54). A meticulously repaired episiotomy will heal better than an unplanned tear in these patients.

OTHER RHEUMATOLOGIC DISEASES

Primary Sjögren syndrome is the presence of symptoms of dryness (sicca syndrome) due to loss of secretions from the salivary and lacrimal glands. In addition to dry eyes and mouth, patients also may complain of dyspareunia and may have recurrent pulmonary infections due to loss of secretions in the bronchial tree. Secondary Sjögren syndrome occurs in rheumatoid arthritis, lupus, and scleroderma.

Two articles have included some data on pregnancies of patients with primary Sjögren syndrome. A Japanese report included 13 patients with primary Sjögren syndrome who had had 39 pregnancies (55). It is not clear how many of these occurred before the development of symptoms or diagnosis. Twenty-seven of the pregnancies were successful full-term deliveries, and one additional delivery was premature. There were only two spontaneous abortions, but nine artificial abortions (reasons not specified). These results were said not to be significantly different from those observed in the controls. A Finnish study reported an increased risk of fetal loss in primary Sjögren syndrome, but only eight of 55 pregnancies occurred after the onset of symptoms (56). Only one of these eight was not successful. These studies suggest that primary Sjögren syndrome is probably not associated with fetal complications.

Beyond case reports and collections of case reports, there is no reliable literature on the relationship of other rheumatologic diseases and pregnancy. The best advice is to enlist the services of an experienced rheumatologist and assume the pregnancy is a high-risk pregnancy, particularly in patients with a history of vasculitic disease.

DRUGS IN PREGNANCY

The use of NSAIDs, methotrexate, hydroxychloroquine, and sulfasalazine in pregnancy is discussed in the section on Rheumatoid Arthritis. Nonsteroidals and hydroxychloroquine are frequently used in SLE, whereas methotrexate is beginning to be used more as a steroid-sparing agent in lupus.

Corticosteroids, predominantly prednisone (category B), are used frequently in the rheumatologic diseases (6). Because it is metabolized by the placenta, less than 10% of the maternal dose is delivered to the fetus as prednisolone, the active form of the drug (5). Although cleft palates have been reported in rodents, they have not been reported in humans. It appears safe for use in pregnancy.

Azathioprine is in category D (6). The fetal liver lacks the enzyme to convert it to its active metabolites (5). It has not been associated with any consistent fetal abnormalities, although sporadic abnormalities have been reported with the use of azathioprine. Perhaps 40% of pregnancies are associated with IUGR. It has been used with relative safety in pregnant patients with renal allografts and lupus; but the risks of its use in pregnancy need to be discussed carefully with patients.

Cyclophosphamide is also a category D drug (6). It is estimated that 16% to 22% of pregnancies exposed to cyclophosphamide will produce offspring with congenital abnormalities (5). The drug should be discontinued at least 3 months prior to trying to conceive. Its most frequent use in rheumatologic diseases is as monthly pulses for nephritis and cerebral vasculitis in lupus and various vasculitides. Chronic oral cyclophosphamide is typically used in Wegener's granulomatosis, and occasionally in rheumatoid arthritis. Taken this way, it is associated with hemorrhagic cystitis and bladder cancer (5). Amenorrhea is associated with increasing age and increasing dose.

Cyclosporine, a category C drug (6), is effective in rheumatoid arthritis and systemic lupus; but its use has been limited by its renal toxicity and its previous availability only as a liquid. It has been approved for use in rheumatoid arthritis and is also available in a more convenient capsule form. Its use is associated with IUGR and prematurity in 40% of pregnancies (5). Birth defects have been reported, but experience with the drug is limited.

D-penicillamine is used in the treatment of rheumatoid arthritis, but it is used much less frequently than in the past. It is sometimes helpful to control the progression of scleroderma. It is teratogenic in rats when used at six times the human dose, although birth defects have been reported in human use (6). It should be used only when the risks outweigh the benefits. As noted above, hydroxychloroquine and sulfasalazine may be safer drugs. In addition, because penicillamine can cause proteinuria at any time during use, it may confuse the diagnostic process if proteinuria develops during pregnancy.

REFERENCES

1. Arnett FC, Edworthy S, Bloch DA, et al. The American Rheumatism Association 1987 revised criteria for the classification of rheumatoid arthritis. Arthritis Rheum 1988;31:315–324.
2. Hench PS. The ameliorating effect of pregnancy on chronic atrophic (infectious rheumatoid) arthritis, fibrositis and intermittent hydrarthrosis. Mayo Clin Proc 1938;13:161–167.
3. Nelson JD, Ostensen M. Pregnancy and rheumatoid arthritis. Rheum Dis Clin North Am 1997;23:195–212.
4. Nelson JL, Hughes KA, Smith AG, Nisperos BB, Branchaud AM, Hansen JA. Maternal-fetal disparity in HLA class II alloantigens and the pregnancy-induced amelioration of rheumatoid arthritis. N Engl J Med 1993;329:466–471.
5. Ramsey-Goldman R, Schilling E. Immunosupressive drug use during pregnancy. Rheum Dis Clin North Am 1997;23:149–167.
6. Physicians desk reference, 52nd ed. Montvale, NJ: Medical Economics, 1988.
7. Parke AL, Rothfield NF. Antimalarial drugs in pregnancy—the North American experience. Lupus 1996;5(suppl 1):67–69.
8. Buchanan NMM, Toubi E, Khamashta MA, Lima F, Kerslake S, Hughes GRV. Hydroxychloroquine and lupus pregnancy: review of a series of 36 cases. Ann Rheum Dis 1996;55:486–488.
9. Tan EM, Cohen AS, Fried JF, et al. The 1982 revised criteria for the classification of systemic lupus erythematosus. Arthritis Rheum 1982; 25:1271–1277.
10. Masi AT. Clinical epidemiologic perspective of systemic lupus erythematosus. In: Lawrence LS, Shulman LE, eds. Current topics in rheumatology. Epidemiology of the rheumatic diseases. New York: Gower, 1984.
11. Meyerhoff J. Systemic lupus erythematosus VII: making the diagnosis. Md State Med J 1984;33:42–45.
12. Richardson B, Epstein WV. Utility of the fluorescent antinuclear antibody test is a single patient. Ann Intern Med 1981;95:333–338.
13. Turner SJ, LeVine L, Rothman A. Lupus erythematosus and pregnancy. Am J Obstet Gynecol 1955;70:102–108.
14. Lockshin MD, Reinitz E, Druzin ML, Murrman M, Estes D. Lupus pregnancy. Case-control prospective study demonstrating absence of lupus exacerbation during or after pregnancy. Am J Med 1984;77: 893–898.
15. Mintz G, Niz J, Gutierrez G, Garcia-Alonso A, Karchmer S. Prospective study of prgnancy in systemic lupus erythematosus: results of a multidisciplinary approach. J Rheumatol 1986;13:732–739.
16. Wong KL, Chan FY, Lee CP. Outcome of pregnancy in patients with systemic lupus erythematosus: a prospective study. Arch Intern Med 1991;151:269–273.
17. Petri M, Howard D, Repke J. Frequency of lupus flare in pregnancy: the Hopkins Lupus Pregnancy Center experience. Arthritis Rheum 1991; 34:1538–1545.
18. Urowitz MB, Gladman DD, Farewell VT, Stewart J, McDonald J. Lupus and pregnancy studies. Arthritis Rheum 1993;36:1392–1397.
19. Ruiz-Irastorza G, Lima F, Alves J, et al. Increased rate of lupus flare during pregnancy and the puerperium. Br J Rheumatol 1996;35:133–138.
20. Lima F, Buchanan NMM, Khamashta MA, Kerslake S, Hughes GRV. Obstetric outcome in systemic lupus erythematosus. Semin Arthritis Rheum 1995;25:184–192.
21. Fraga A, Mintz G, Orozco J, Orozco JH. Sterility and fertility rates, fetal wastage, and maternal morbidity in systemic lupus erythematosus. J Rheumatol 1974;1:293–298.
22. Petri M. Hopkins Lupus Pregnancy Center: 1987 to 1996. Rheum Dis Clin North Am 1997;23:1–13.
23. Khamashta MA, Ruiz-Irastorza G, Hughes GRV. Systemic lupus erythematosus flares during pregnancy. Rheum Dis Clin North Am 1997; 23:15–30.

24. Munther A, Khamashta MD, Hughes GRV. Pregnancy in systemic lupus erythematosus. Curr Opin Rheum 1996;8:424–429.
25. Martinez-Rueda JO, Arce-Salinas CA, Kraus A, Alcocer-Varela J, Alarcon-Segovia D. Factors associated with fetal losses in severe systemic lupus erythematosus. Lupus 1996;5:113–119.
26. Ramsey-Goldman R, Kutzer JE, Kuller LH, Guzick D, Carpenter AB, Medsger TA. Pregnancy outcome and anti-cardiolipin antibody in women with systemic lupus erythematosus. Am J Epidmiol 1993;138: 1057–1069.
27. Petri M. Pathogenesis and treatment of the antiphospholipid antibody syndrome. Med Clin North Am 1997;81:151–177.
28. Petri M, Rheinschmidt M, Whiting-O Keefe Q, Hellmann D, Corash L. The frequency of lupus anticoagulant in systemic lupus erythematous. A study of sixty consecutive patients by activated partial thromboplastin time, Russell viper venom time, and anticardiolipin antibody test. Ann Intern Med 1987;106:524–531.
29. Lockshin MD, Qamar T, Druzin ML. Hazards of lupus pregnancy. J Rheumatol 1987;14(suppl 13):214–217.
30. Lockshin MD. Antiphospholipid antibody. Babies, blood clots, biology. JAMA 1997;277:1549–1551.
31. Lynch AM, Rutledge JH, Stephens JK, et al. Logitudinal measurement of anticardiolipin antibodies during normal pregnancy: a prospective study. Lupus 1995;4:365–369.
32. Petri M, Allbritton J. Fetal outcome of lupus pregnancy: a retrospective case-control study of the Hopkins Lupus Cohort. J Rheumatol 1993;20: 650–656.
33. Johnson MJ, Petri M, Witter FR, Repke JT. Evaluation of preterm delivery in a systemic lupus erythematosus pregnancy clinic. Obstet Gynecol 1995;86:396–399.
34. Welsch S, Branch DW. Antiphospholipid syndrome in pregnancy: obstetric concerns and treatment. Rheum Dis Clin North Am 1997;23: 71–84.
35. Branch DW, Silver RM, Blackwell JL, Reading JC, Scott JR. Outcome of treated pregnancies in women with antiphospholipid syndrome: an update of the Utah experience. Obstet Gynecol 1992;80:614–620.
36. Lima F, Khamashta MA, Buchanan NMM, Kerslake S, Hunt BJ, Hughes GRV. A study of sixty pregnancies in patients with the antiphospholipd syndrome. Clin Exp Rheumatol 1996;1:131–136.
37. Krnic-Barrie S, O Connor CR, Looney SW, Pierangeli SS, Harris EN. A retrospective review of 61 patients with antiphospholipid syndrome. Analysis of factors influencing recurrent thrombosis. Arch Intern Med 1997;157:2101–2108.
38. Lynch A, Silver R, Emlen W. Antiphospholipid antibodies in healthy pregnant women. Rheum Dis Clin North Am 1997;23:55–70.
39. Ramsey-Golden R, Schlling E. Immunosuppressive drug use during pregnancy. Rheum Dis Clin North Am 1997;23:149–167.
40. Ramsey-Goldman R, Mientus JM, Kutzer JE, Mulvihill JJ, Medsger TA. Pregnancy outcome in women with systemic lupus erythematosus treated with immunosuppressive drugs. J Rheumatol 1993;20:1152–1157.
41. The Canadian Hydroxycholoroquine Study Group. A randomized study of the effect of withdrawing hydroxychloroquine sulfate in systemic lupus erythematosus. N Engl J Med 1991;324:150–154.
42. Mascola MA, Repke JT, Obstetric management of the high-risk lupus patient. Rheum Dis Clin North Am 1997;23:119–132.
43. Sloane D, Siskind V, Heinonen OP, Monson RR, Kaufman DW, Shapiro S. Aspirin and congenital malformations. Lancet 1976;1:1373–1375.
44. Tseng C-E, Buyon JP. Neonatal lupus syndromes. Rheum Dis Clin North Am 1997;23:31–54.
45. Buyon JP, Tamerius J, Ordorica S, Young B, Abramson SB. Activation of the alternative complement pathway accompanies disease flares in systemic lupus erythematosus in pregnancy. Arthritis Rheum 1992;35: 55–61.
46. Buyon JP, Cronstein BN, Morris M, Tanner M, Weismann G. Serum complement values (C3 and C4) to differentiate between systemic lupus activity and pre-eclampsia. Am J Med 1986;81:194–200.
47. Laskin CA, Bombardier C, Hannah ME, et al. Prednisone and aspirin in women with autoantibodies and unexplained recurrent fetal loss. N Engl J Med 1997;337:148–153.
48. Nelson-Piercy C, Letsky EA, de Swiet M. Low-molecular-weight heparin for obstetric thromboprophylaxis: experience of sixty-nine pregnancies in sixty-one women at high risk. Am J Obstet Gynecol 1997;176:1062–1068.
49. Kutteh WH. Antiphopholipid antibody-associated recurrent pregnancy loss: treatment with heparin and low-dose aspirin is superior to low-dose aspirin alone. Am J Obstet Gynecol 1996;174:1584–1589.
50. Salafia CM Parke AL. Placental pathology in systemic lupus erythematosus and phospholipid antibody syndrome. Rheum Dis Clin North Am 1997;23:85–97.
51. Steen VD. Systemic sclerosis. Rheum Dis Clin North Am 1990;16: 641–654.
52. Steen VD, Brodeur M, Conte C. Prospective pregnancy (PG) study in women with systemic sclerosis (Ssc). Arthritis Rheum 1996;39(suppl): 151.
53. Traub YM, Shapiro AP, Rodnan GP, et al. Hypertension and renal failure (scleroderma renal crisis) in progressive systemic sclerosis: report of a 25 year experience with 68 cases. Medicine 1984;62:335–352.
54. Steen VD. Scleroderma and Pregnancy. Rheum Dis Clin North Am 1997;23:133–147.
55. Takaya M, Ichikawa Y, Shimizu H, Uchiyama M, Moriuchi J, Arimori S. Sjögren's syndrome and pregnancy. Tokai J Exp Clin Med 1991;16: 83–88.
56. Julkunen H, Kaaja R, Kurki P, Palosuo T, Friman C. Fetal outcome in women with primary Sjögren's syndrome. A retrospective case-control study. Clin Exp Rheum 1995:13:65–71.

SECTION XII

Dental Disorders

Cherry and Merkatz's Complications of Pregnancy,
Fifth Edition, edited by W. R. Cohen.
Lippincott Williams & Wilkins, Philadelphia © 2000.

CHAPTER 38

Dental Complications

Ronald E. Schneider, Andrew S. Kaplan, and Jack Klatell

The complex alterations of body physiology and chemistry that accompany pregnancy can affect the oral cavity and the dental apparatus. The extent of these changes is largely dependent on the previous health of the mouth and the thoroughness with which preventive measures have been employed before conception as well as during the stressful period of gestation.

Over the centuries, people's interest in pregnancy and childbirth has built up a mystique compounded of myth and conjecture about dental issues, intermixed with scientific facts gleaned from research. It was not so long ago that pregnant women were assured that they could expect to lose a tooth for every child. It also seemed reasonable that the nausea and vomiting of morning sickness and its attempted control with crackers or biscuits or other cariogenic foods would create an oral environment conducive to tooth decalcification and decay. Objective studies do not support this notion of inevitable tooth loss. However, there are some actual or potential dental and oral complications of pregnancy of which the physician, the dentist, and the patient should be aware. All concerned must cooperate to provide safe dental care to the expectant mother without harming the fetus.

R. E. Schneider, A.S. Kaplan, and J. Klatell: Mount Sinai School of Medicine, Mount Sinai Hospital, New York, NY.

CARIES, GINGIVITIS, AND PERIODONTAL DISEASE

The pregnant woman is subject to all the dental disorders that afflict other patients. The oral flora might be somewhat changed, as may some dietary routines, but the caries process is not significantly altered during pregnancy. The notion that pregnant women are more susceptible to tooth decay has not been borne out by research. Although minerals can be withdrawn from any part of the bony skeleton, the teeth are not generally affected. The mineral content of dentin (1,2) and enamel remain unchanged throughout pregnancy. Routine prevention and treatment of carious lesions must be performed as conscientiously for the pregnant as for the nonpregnant patient (3). Daily rinses with sodium fluoride and chlorhexidine have been effective in caries prevention (4). Recent studies suggest that the benefits of improved oral health and reduced cariogenic oral flora in the mother also result in better oral heath in their children (5–8).

It has long been known that the endocrine system affects the gingiva and periodontal tissues. The relationship of pregnancy to changes in these tissues has been studied in great detail (9–14). The gingival changes most commonly seen in pregnant women are referred to as pregnancy gingivitis. The changes are first seen in the second month of pregnancy and peak in the middle of the last trimester. Although the gingivitis will frequently disappear spontaneously after parturition, this condition can remain for up to 6 months after delivery. It has been reported that between 30% and 100% (15) of pregnant women are affected by this condition. The discrepancies in these statistics can be attributed to variations in research methodology and clinical judgment in identifying affected women.

Pregnancy gingivitis manifests as marginal inflammation of the attached gingiva and the interdental papillae. The tissues appear smooth, shiny, and swollen and are bright to bluish red in color (Fig. 38-1). They are compressible and have a strong tendency to bleed with probing or with brushing. Accompanying these changes, there might be increases in tooth mobility, in gingival crevicular fluid, and in periodontal pocket depth (10,12,15). These changes are generally painless and are usually accompanied by the accumulation of plaque and calculus. The tooth mobility is normally transient (15).

This form of gingivitis appears to be hormone modulated, an exaggerated response to local factors, such as oral deposits, plaque, and calculus (9,10). Hormones can interfere with mechanisms of action that respond to inflammatory challenges, such as the production of interleukin (12). The condition varies with the adequacy of local therapy and the hormonal changes experienced throughout the course of pregnancy. Meticulous oral hygiene can either prevent or markedly minimize the occurrence of pregnancy gingivitis. The obstetrician should encourage the patient to seek dental advice and to practice conscientious oral hygiene. Patients prone to this problem might need to use hygiene aids, such as an interdental stimulator or an oral irrigation device in addition to the routine use of a toothbrush and dental floss.

If the patient shows signs of gingivitis in the early stages of pregnancy, she might best be treated by the dentist with scaling and curettage. This treatment removes local irritants that cannot be removed with a toothbrush, thereby decreasing the local factors contributing to the exaggerated inflammatory changes. The gingival tissues can be very sensitive to this type of manipulation, and local anesthetic is sometimes needed. Methods to prevent or treat pregnancy gingivitis should be initiated at the earliest possible opportunity. Waiting until the termination of pregnancy risks permanent periodontal destruction (11,15,16). Explaining the nature of this process to the patient will usually result in better home care.

PREGNANCY TUMOR

A second pathologic gingival condition arising during pregnancy is the angiogranuloma, or pregnancy tumor. This localized enlargement appears in 3% to 5% of pregnant women (17), generally between the third and ninth months of pregnancy, and gradually increases in size. After delivery, these lesions tend to regress, but they can persist as a scarred epulis or fibroma. As is the case with pregnancy gingivitis, the cause is thought to be an intensified reaction to local irritation due to the effects of hormonal change.

Pregnancy tumors most frequently appear on the gingiva and, in particular, tend to originate between the teeth in the interdental papillae (Fig. 38-2). They might also be present on the tongue, palate, buccal mucosa, and lips (17). The clinical manifestation is a soft, flattened, pedunculated mass that is deep red in color, with a smooth surface. The lesion is usually painless unless its size or location interferes with chewing, swallowing, or speaking, in which case painful ulceration may ensue. On histologic

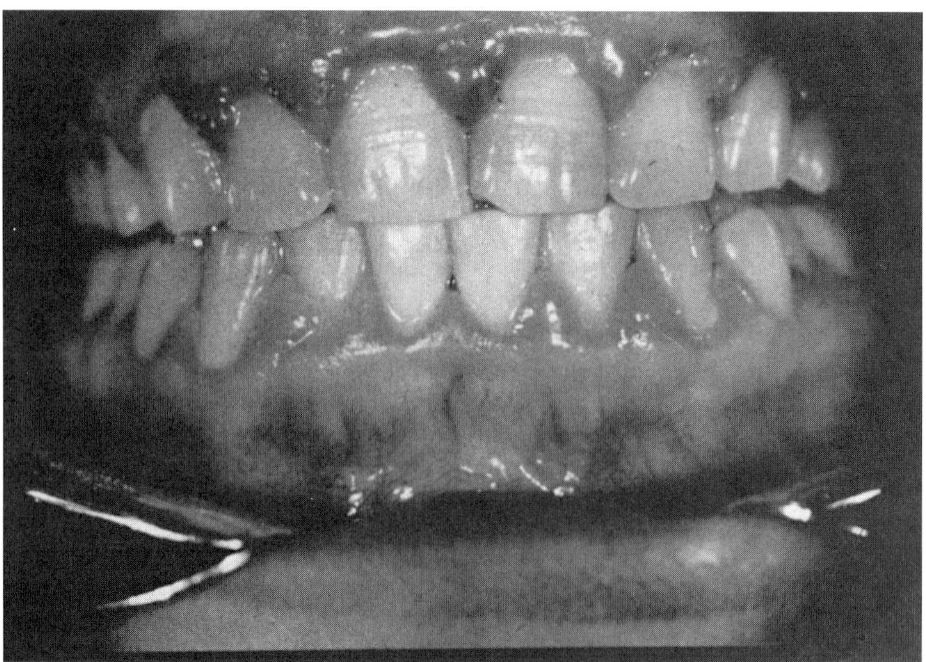

FIG. 38-1. Pregnancy gingivitis. Note the inflammation of interdental and marginal gingiva.

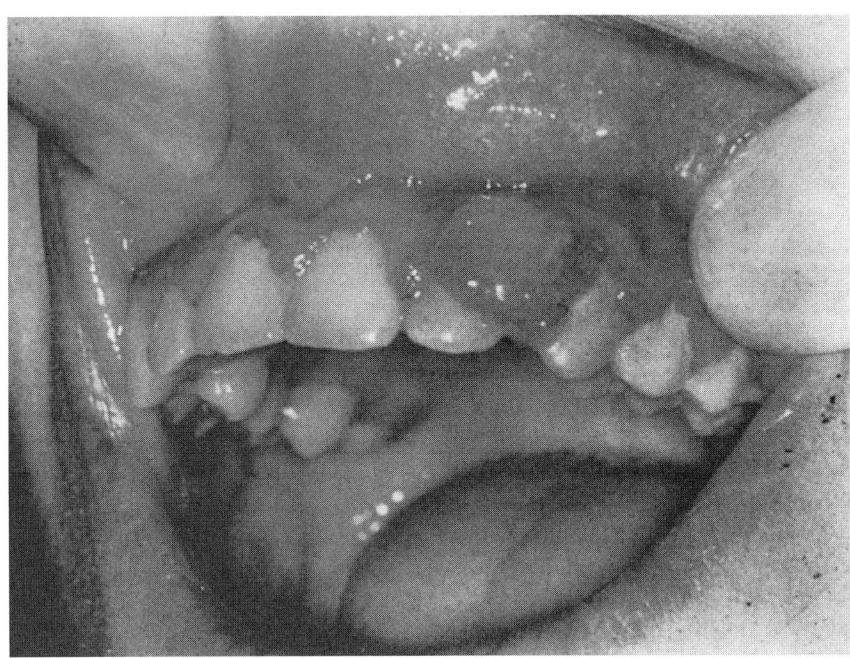

FIG. 38-2. Pregnancy tumor.

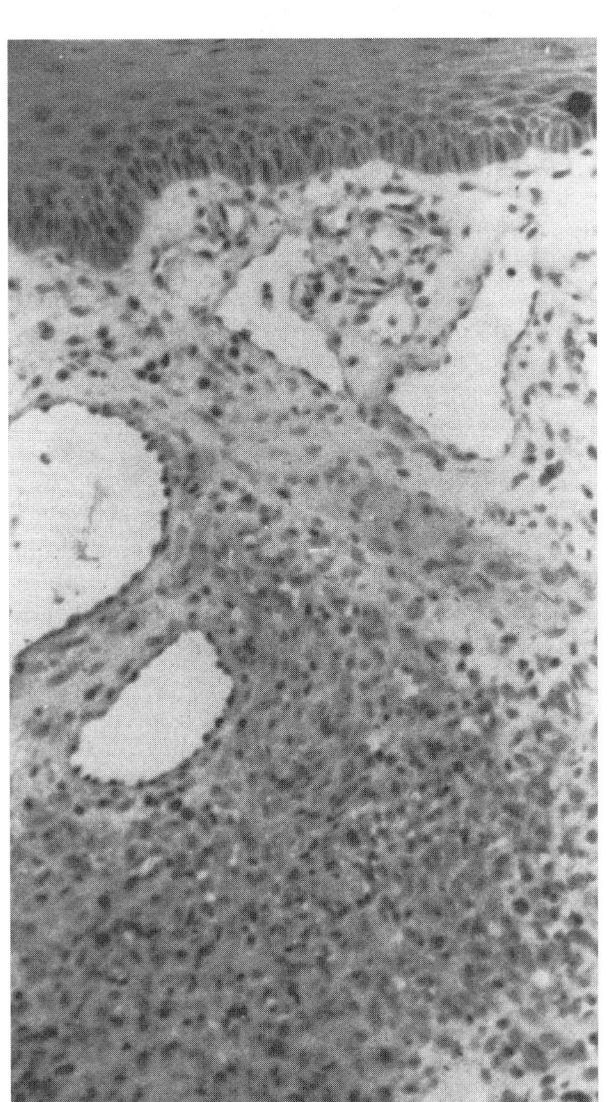

FIG. 38-3. Histologic section of a pregnancy tumor.

examination, the pregnancy tumor resembles a pyogenic granuloma (Fig. 38-3). The raised mass has a central area of connective tissue rich in thin-walled blood vessels and covered by a zone of stratified squamous epithelium. An acute inflammatory infiltrate is present only in those cases that are mechanically traumatized, in which case the epithelium might also be ulcerated.

Pregnancy tumors can be minimized by fastidious oral hygiene, and patients should be instructed in such hygiene and encouraged to work at it. Once tumors have occurred, the areas should be scaled and curetted to remove local irritants. Local anesthesia can be used. Should the pregnancy tumor be large and a continuing source of pain or infection owing to its interference with masticatory function, surgical removal is indicated. The patient should be warned of possible recurrence.

DENTAL TREATMENT CONSIDERATIONS

There are several issues to consider when addressing the risks and benefits of rendering dental care during pregnancy. Treatment might expose the mother to pain, stress, ionizing radiation, or medications. Delaying treatment could risk pain, infection, or even loss of teeth. In general, most elective dental procedures should be postponed until the second trimester, but the potential benefit of delaying any exposure of the fetus to risk is weighed against the risks of delaying the treatment. There is no significant problem with delaying many routine dental procedures, such as repair of small carious lesions, but some conditions require estimations of how rapidly the disease process will progress in order to make the best judgment about the timing of therapy. Guessing incorrectly about the progression rate can risk irreversible damage to the structures of the oral cavity or change a routine treatment into a more complicated one. The patient's obstetrician should be consulted to determine whether there are any special considerations or risks with regard to a particular patient.

Because treatment is usually performed with the patient seated or reclining in the dental chair, the dentist should be aware that pregnant women undergoing treatment can manifest symptoms of the supine hypotensive syndrome, particularly during the third trimester (18). This syndrome is generally evidenced by a loss of consciousness due to the pressure of the gravid uterus on the great vessels, causing poor venous return to the heart. Prevention and treatment are to turn the patient on her side, thus reestablishing venous return. The supine hypotensive syndrome occurs in approximately 10% of pregnant women during the third trimester. Even for those women who do not become manifestly hypotensive, lying supine can result in reduced uterine blood flow and potential fetal jeopardy. Thus, the supine position should always be avoided during dental work in the second half of pregnancy. Placing a wedge under the patient's right hip when she is reclining in the chair will usually serve to obviate this problem. Short appointments should be encouraged whenever possible (19).

Dental Radiography

The dentist always attempts to minimize exposure of patients to the ionizing radiation from dental radiography. The standards for radiographic evaluation have evolved to reflect this principle. Faster film speeds, higher beam energies, dental radiographic and panoramic machines with beam collimation, and the routine use of lead aprons all have contributed to less exposure for all dental patients. The two main concerns are risk when genetic tissues are exposed to radiation and risks to the somatic tissues (20). The uterine exposure for a full mouth series of radiographs is estimated to be less than 0.01 μ Gy, far less than the dose thought to be the threshold for risk of mental retardation (19,20). It is rare for a full mouth series to be taken in the pregnant patient.

A typical examination using one to four periapical radiographs or a panoramic radiograph would reduce the exposure to 75% less than the full mouth series. Using proper methods, the risk to the fetus is considered to be nonexistent. The use of old equipment with short cones, not using a lead apron, and poor positioning could raise that risk (21). Diagnostic radiography is an important aspect of evaluation and treatment planning. Expert panels of representatives from all areas of dentistry under the sponsorship of the Food and Drug Administration have stated that the recommendations for radiographic guidelines do not need to be altered for the pregnant patient (22,23).

For the pregnant patient who is also a dental health care worker, the concern is for repeated exposure over time. Maximum doses have been calculated for the pregnant and nonpregnant dental health care worker. The maximum permissible dose for the pregnant health care worker is one-tenth of the normal dose recommended for nonpregnant dental health care workers. Proper radiation safety precautions, such as shielding, barriers, and periodic equipment testing should always be followed (22).

Medications

There is always a concern that drugs or other chemical substances taken by the mother will affect the fetus. Although one could eliminate all risks by avoiding all drugs, the pregnant dental patient is still likely to need medications for treatment. Local anesthetic agents are commonly used for either routine dental care or for management of dental emergencies. There are many areas of the country where patients are seen by their dentist only in the context of an emergency, usually a toothache or an abscess. Treatment of these problems generally requires antibiotic therapy and, frequently, analgesics. Although they are rarely necessary, nitrous oxide or other anesthetic agents might also be used.

Local Anesthesia

For most patients, dental treatment is difficult to tolerate without a local anesthetic. Fortunately, in the volumes and concentrations used in dentistry, local anesthetics are very safe (24). At normal doses, no adverse reactions have been reported with lidocaine (Xylocaine) or mepivacaine (Carbocaine) alone and in combination with epinephrine. Schneider and Webster (25) have shown no statistically significant increase in complications in pregnant women who received surgical treatment using local anesthesia. Nevertheless, the dentist must be careful to use solutions with minimal amounts of vasoconstrictor injected slowly and after careful aspiration. With these safeguards, local anesthesia offers little risk to the pregnant patient. Accidental intravenous injection of epinephrine can diminish uterine blood flow; local anesthetics should be used without epinephrine when clinically feasible.

Nitrous Oxide and Anesthetic Agents

There are circumstances in which the inhalation agent nitrous oxide or other anesthetic agents are considered for the treatment of dental problems. There are dental phobic patients who have great difficulty facing even routine dental treatment without some antianxiety aid. For most of these dental phobics, the anxiety does not abate with pregnancy. There are also conditions, such as dental abscesses or prolonged toothaches, in which local anesthesia is not fully effective. Nitrous oxide is commonly available in dental offices and has been extensively and effectively used to facilitate dental treatment. It is generally considered safe, particularly with short procedures. There is no respiratory depression, and supplemental oxygen is automatically delivered with nitrous oxide. The risks of chronic exposure are generally more of a concern than the use for a single short procedure. It has been suggested that nitrous oxide is a factor in spontaneous abortions in health care workers chronically exposed.

Nitrous oxide can be very effective for anxiety management and somewhat effective for mild pain, particularly when there is an anxiety component. It has limited use in the management of moderately to severely painful procedures. For those painful procedures in which local anesthesia is not a viable option, sedation or general anesthesia might be necessary. Most studies support the safety of modern general anesthetic and sedative agents (26) in pregnant women (see Chapter 55).

Analgesic Therapy

With its low risk of side effect or complication, acetaminophen has been a mainstay of analgesic therapy for the pregnant patient. There are dental conditions, such as toothaches, in which pain is poorly controlled with acetaminophen. Short courses of narcotics are used effectively in these circumstances. Although some studies have suggested that malformations are associated with codeine use in early pregnancy in animals (27), the acetaminophen with codeine preparation remains a popular short-term pain medication for dental problems and probably carries negligible risk to the pregnancy. Oxycodone and hydrocodone preparations can also be used (19,28). There is concern that the narcotic can produce respiratory depression in the neonate if taken close to the time of delivery. It should be noted that most of these complications are dose and frequency dependent (29).

Antibiotic Therapy

Penicillin, clindamycin, and erythromycin are the most frequently used antibiotics for treatment of infections of dental origin. Fortunately, no serious adverse effects of penicillin or clindamycin have been reported (19), except for allergic reactions and the risk of pseudomembranous colitis. Erythromycin estiolate is less effective than either penicillin or clindamycin for most dental infections and is associated with potential hepatotoxicity. Streptomycin can lead to hearing loss in the fetus, and its use should be avoided. Other aminoglycosides are preferable if such coverage is necessary. If substantial amounts of tetracycline are administered to a pregnant woman during the second or third trimester, the developing deciduous teeth of the child can be discolored. Depending on the dosage (1), the teeth will appear yellowish to brownish-gray. While such teeth are structurally strong, the cosmetic detriment is significant.

Fluoride Supplementation

The effect of fluorides in reducing dental decay is well known (8,30). It might be reasoned that if a woman takes fluoride supplements during pregnancy and if the fluoride passes the placental barrier, it might impart resistance to dental caries to the baby. Research has generally supported this contention (4,5,27), but it is still a matter of debate. Fluoride-supplemented drinking water alone provides little exposure of the fetal teeth to fluoride (5). Supplementing during pregnancy with 1 mg/day by tablet will cause the developing deciduous teeth to acquire greater mineralization and an increased fluoride concentration in the hard tissues. At doses above 1 mg/day, the amniotic levels increase to near that of the maternal plasma (31). A greater concern is the rise of fluorosis (21) as the result of oversupplementation, usually because of a combination of fluoride drops and community fluoride-supplemented water supplies. It is not considered a health risk because there is no functional compromise of the teeth, but the discoloration of the teeth is a concern for children and parents.

REFERENCES

1. Dargiff DA, Karsham M. Effect of pregnancy on the chemical composition of human dentin. J Dent Res 1943;2:266.
2. Deakins M, Looby J. Effects of pregnancy on the mineral content of human teeth. Am J Obstet Gynecol 1943:6:265.
3. Brambilla E, Felloni A, Gaagliani M, Malerba A, Garcia-Godoy F, Strohmenger L. Caries prevention during pregnancy: results of a 30-month study. J Am Dent Assoc 1998;129:871–877.
4. Driscoll WS, Nowjack-Raymer R, Selwitz RH, Li SH, Heifetz SB. A comparison of the caries preventive effects of fluoride mouthrinsing, fluoride tablets, and both procedures combined: final results after eight years. J Public Health Dent 1992;52:111–116.
5. Glen FB, Glenn WD, Duncan RC. Fluoride tablet supplementation during pregnancy for caries immunity: a study of the offspring produced. Am J Obstet Gynecol 1982;143:560–564.
6. Gunay H, Dmoch-Bockhorn K, Gunay Y, Geurtsen W. Effect on caries experience of a long-term preventive program for mothers and children starting during pregnancy. Clin Oral Invest 1998;2(3):137–142.
7. Kohler B, Andreen I. Influence of caries-preventive measures in mothers on cariogenic bacteria and caries experience in their children. Arch Oral Biol 1994;39:907–911.
8. Tenovuo J, Hakkinen P, Paunio P, Emilson CG. Effects of chlorhexidine-fluoride gel treatments in mothers on the establishment of mutans streptococci in primary teeth and the development of dental caries in children. Caries Res 1992;26:275–280.
9. Grant D, Stern J, Listgarten M (eds). The epidemiology, etiology, and public health aspects of periodontal disease. In: Periodontics. St. Louis: CV Mosby, 1988:229, 332–335.
10. Jensen J, Lilijmark W, Bloomquist C. The effect of female sex hormones on subgingival plaque. J Periodontol 1981;52:599–602.
11. Kinnby B, Matsson L, Astedt B. Aggravation of gingival inflammatory symptoms during pregnancy associated with the concentration of plasminogen activator inhibitor type 2 (PAI-2) in gingival fluid. J Periodontal Res 1996;31:271–277.
12. Lapp CA, Thomas ME, Lewis JB. Modulation by progesterone of interleukin-6 production by gingival fibroblasts. J Periodontol 1995;66: 279–285.
13. Michelberger D, Matthews D. Periodontal manifestations of systemic diseases and their management. J Can Dent Assoc 1996;62:313–314, 317–321.
14. Raber-Durlacher JE, van Steenbergen TJ, Van der Velden U, de Graaff J, Abraham Inpijn L. Experimental gingivitis during pregnancy and post-partum: clinical, endocrinological, and microbiological aspects. J Clin Periodontol 1994;21:549–558.

15. Cohen W, Friedman L, Shapiro J, Kyle C. A longitudinal investigation of the periodontal changes during pregnancy. J Periodontol 1969; 40:563–570.
16. Littner M, Kaffe I, Tamse A, Moskona D. Management of the pregnant patient. Quintessence Int 1984;2(Report 22281):1–5.
17. Hatziotis JC. The incidence of pregnancy tumors and their probable relation to the embryo's sex. J Periodontol 1972;43:447–448.
18. Howard B, Goodson J, Mengert W. Supine hypotensive syndrome in late pregnancy. Obstet Gynecol 1953;1:371.
19. Pradel E. The pregnant oral and maxillofacial surgery patient. In: Oral Maxillofac Surg Clin North Am 19;10:471–489.
20. Langlais RP, Langland OE. Risks from dental radiation in 1995. Calif Dental Assn J 1995;23:33–39.
21. Serman NJ, Singer S. Exposure of the pregnant patient to ionizing radiation. Ann Dent 1994;53:13–15.
22. National Council on Radiation Protection and Measurements. Ionizing radiation exposure of the population of the United States. NCRP report no. 93. Bethesda: NCRP, 1987.
23. White SC. 1992 assessment of radiation risk from dental radiography. Dentomaxillofac Radiol 1992;21:118–126.
24. Wasylko L, Matsui D, Dykxhoorn SM, Rieder MJ, Weinberg S. A review of common dental treatments during pregnancy: implications for patients and dental personnel. J Can Dent Assoc 1998;64: 434–439.
25. Schneider S, Webster G. Maternal and fetal hazards of surgery during pregnancy. Am J Obstet Gynecol 1965;92:891.
26. Beilin Y, Bodian CA, Mukherjee T, et al. The use of propofol, nitrous oxide or isoflurane does not affect the reproductive success rate following gamete intrafallopian transfer (GIFT): a multicenter pilot trail/survey Anesthesiology 1999;90:36–41.
27. Williams J, Price CJ, Sleet RB, et al. Codeine: developmental toxicity in hamsters and mice. Fundam Appl Toxicol 1991;16(3):401–413.
28. Lawrenz DR, Whitley BD, Helfrick JF. Consideration in the management of maxillofacial infection in the pregnant patient, J Oral Maxillofac Surg 1996;54:474–485.
29. Delzer D, Povant D. Pregnancy and side effects of analgesics. Gen Dent 1981;29:49–51.
30. Whitford GM. Changing patterns of fluoride intake: dietary fluoride supplements. Workshop on Changing Patterns of Fluoride Intake. Chapel Hill, University of North Carolina. J Dent Res 1992;71:1249–1254.
31. Brambilla E, Belluomo G, Malerba A, Buscaglia M, Strohmenger L. Oral administration of fluoride in pregnant women, and the relation between concentration in maternal plasma and in amniotic fluid. Arch Oral Biol 1994;39:991–994.

SECTION XIII

Malignant Disease

Cherry and Merkatz's Complications of Pregnancy,
Fifth Edition, edited by W. R. Cohen.
Lippincott Williams & Wilkins, Philadelphia © 2000.

CHAPTER 39

Genital Cancers

Fouad A. Abbas

The tragic coincidence of genital malignancy and pregnancy places special demands on the health care team. In dealing with pregnancy and cancers, there are many important factors to consider to ensure that the medical and emotional needs of afflicted patients and their families are met. Obstetric patients are younger than most cancer patients. Moreover, there are two patients to consider in medical decision making (mother and the fetus), and the medical and ethical issues vary depending on the trimester of pregnancy in which the malignancy is detected.

Treatment of the malignancy may jeopardize the fetus, and this raises ethical and moral dilemmas. One such dilemma involves weighing the need for delaying treatment until the fetus can be safely delivered against the need for immediate treatment of the patient that could jeopardize the fetus. Certainly, proper management of these patients requires a body of specialized knowledge in oncology and obstetrics, and often requires a team approach to address all pertinent issues adequately.

Treatments for these malignancies may involve radiation and chemotherapy, which have recognized (but possibly also many unknown) effects on the fetus. Data on chemotherapy in pregnancy are scant. Chemotherapy given in the early first trimester of pregnancy has the potential to result in spontaneous abortion or teratogenesis (1). It is at times difficult to determine whether the incidence of these events is greater than the background rates of congenital anomalies and pregnancy loss (2).

Decisions about surgery in pregnancy involve determining which trimester would be optimum for such intervention. For instance, compared with the first few months of gestation, the second trimester carries a reduced abortion rate in response to surgery, and the uterus is of a size that the adnexal and pelvic structures can be readily exposed as required for the appropriate surgical procedure (3). During most of pregnancy a relatively relaxed gastroesophageal sphincter can increase the risk of aspiration under anesthetic. Positioning of the patient is important, especially in the third trimester, when the inferior vena cava and aorta may be occluded by the enlarged uterus if the patient is supine. This can result in maternal hypotension, reduced uterine blood flow, and fetal hypoxemia. Therefore, it is recommended that during surgery in the abdomen a wedge be placed under the right hip to push the uterus to the left and off the great vessels of the abdomen.

Malignancies of the vulva, vagina, or cervix are usually detected during the first prenatal visit because these diseases are often identified either by a Papanicolaou (pap) smear or direct inspection. Ovarian malignancies, however, are more occult and are usually detected by ultrasonography. Often this occurs serendipitously when ultrasonographic examination is performed to evaluate a

F. A. Abbas: Division of Gynecologic Oncology, Sinai Hospital of Baltimore, Baltimore, MD 21215.

uterus that seems larger than expected for the gestational age of the pregnancy. Once there is suspicion of malignancy, the appropriate workup and tissue diagnosis are important. This chapter will describe the current concepts governing the treatment of female genital cancers during pregnancy.

The estimated incidence of all maternal cancers complicating pregnancy is about 1 in 100 (4). Rarely there is metastasis of a maternal tumor to the fetus, primarily from melanoma (5).

CERVICAL NEOPLASIA

Overall, the cervical cancer rate in gestation is about 1.2 cases per 10,000 pregnancies. Pregnancy is a complication in about 3% of patients with cervical cancer (6). The incidence of diagnosis of invasive cervical cancer in pregnancy has decreased since the 1960's, and the overall survival is similar to that of patients who are not pregnant; therefore, standard treatment should be used (7). The rate of cervical dysplasia, however, is much higher than it was in the 1960's. This reflects the overall increase in dysplasia that is being picked up with cervical pap smears. In addition, the Bethesda system has made reporting pap smear results much more uniform across laboratories. The technique of preparing the pap smear for evaluation is changing in that more of these are being processed through a thin-layer technique (8). Although this is a technical improvement, it has resulted in detection of more dysplasia, and more pregnant patients are thus diagnosed.

The clinician is usually confronted initially with a pregnant patient with an abnormal pap smear result, and investigation of this may lead to the detection of the cervical malignancy. However, the initial cervical smear result may be normal, and she may present with signs of advanced cervical cancer later during her pregnancy, such as foul-smelling discharge, flank tenderness, or postcoital bleeding. These symptoms are usually attributable to obstetric problems such as round ligament pain, vaginitis, increasing vaginal discharge of pregnancy, cervical eversion, or rupture of membranes. It is important, however, to keep in mind that these may be symptoms and signs of cervical cancer and the patient needs to be examined with the cervix visualized as well as palpated. A repeat cervical smear may also need to be performed depending on the patient's previous cytologic results, or how concerning her symptoms are. Obviously, if a visible lesion is seen, one should not rely on the cytologic smear to determine whether or not there is a malignancy; in such cases cervical biopsy needs to be performed.

The preliminary evaluation of the pregnant woman with an abnormal pap smear is very similar to that of the nonpregnant patient (Fig. 39-1). In fact, the pregnant patient has overall a prognosis similar to the nonpregnant patient with cervical neoplasia (9). The workup involves a careful examination of the vulva and vagina with a bimanual examination of the paracervical tissues. On colposcopic examination the entire transformation zone will need to be seen, which is actually made easier by pregnancy because of the normal cervical eversion that occurs when patients are pregnant, moving the transformation zone onto the surface of the portio vaginalis. Any lesions need to be seen in their entirety so that a determination can be made of whether or not to evaluate the cervical canal. Suspicious areas should be examined via biopsy in pregnancy.

Clinicians are often uneasy about sampling the cervix of pregnant patients because of the increased vascularity and consequent risk of bleeding. A liberal amount of Monsel solution may need to be applied. Surgical 2×2-inch sponges are useful to absorb the bleeding caused by the biopsy. A vaginal pack should also be close at hand in case the bleeding becomes excessive. Despite the risks, most cervical biopsies during pregnancy are uneventful, and when a visible lesion is seen it must be sampled. If a pap smear result is consistent with a high-grade squamous intraepithelial lesion, a colposcopically directed biopsy is usually performed. If the pap smear shows only a mild abnormality and no lesion is found on colposcopy, then the biopsy can be postponed until after delivery. An endocervical curettage is not usually performed in pregnancy because of the fear of rupturing membranes or causing bleeding difficult to control. Colposcopy can be done safely in any of the trimesters of pregnancy and should not be delayed for obstetric reasons if there is suspicion of an invasive lesion (10).

If the pregnant patient's initial pap smear shows atypical squamous cells of undetermined significance (ASCUS), she should have this smear repeated in 2 or 3 months (see Fig. 39-1). If a second smear shows ASCUS, or another abnormality, the patient should undergo colposcopy with biopsies as necessary. If the initial pap smear shows a low-grade squamous intraepithelial lesion, the patient should undergo colposcopy and directed biopsy as needed, without waiting to repeat a pap smear. If the findings on colposcopy or biopsy show no higher grade lesion than suggested by the smear, the patient can be followed by pap smears taken approximately every 3 months during her pregnancy. The management of these low-grade lesions is controversial. Some experts advocate that patients with squamous atypia or low-grade dysplasia need not undergo a colposcopic examination and manage the situation conservatively, with serial pap smears (11). In such cases if a repeat smear shows a higher grade lesion, colposcopy needs to be performed.

Under any circumstances, approximately 6 weeks after the patient delivers, a colposcopy should be performed to determine if any of the dysplasia has persisted (see Fig. 39-1) (12). It is not uncommon for patients to have a vaginal delivery and have pap smear results subsequently return to normal. It is thought that perhaps the delivery disrupts the dysplastic cells as the cervix dilates. How-

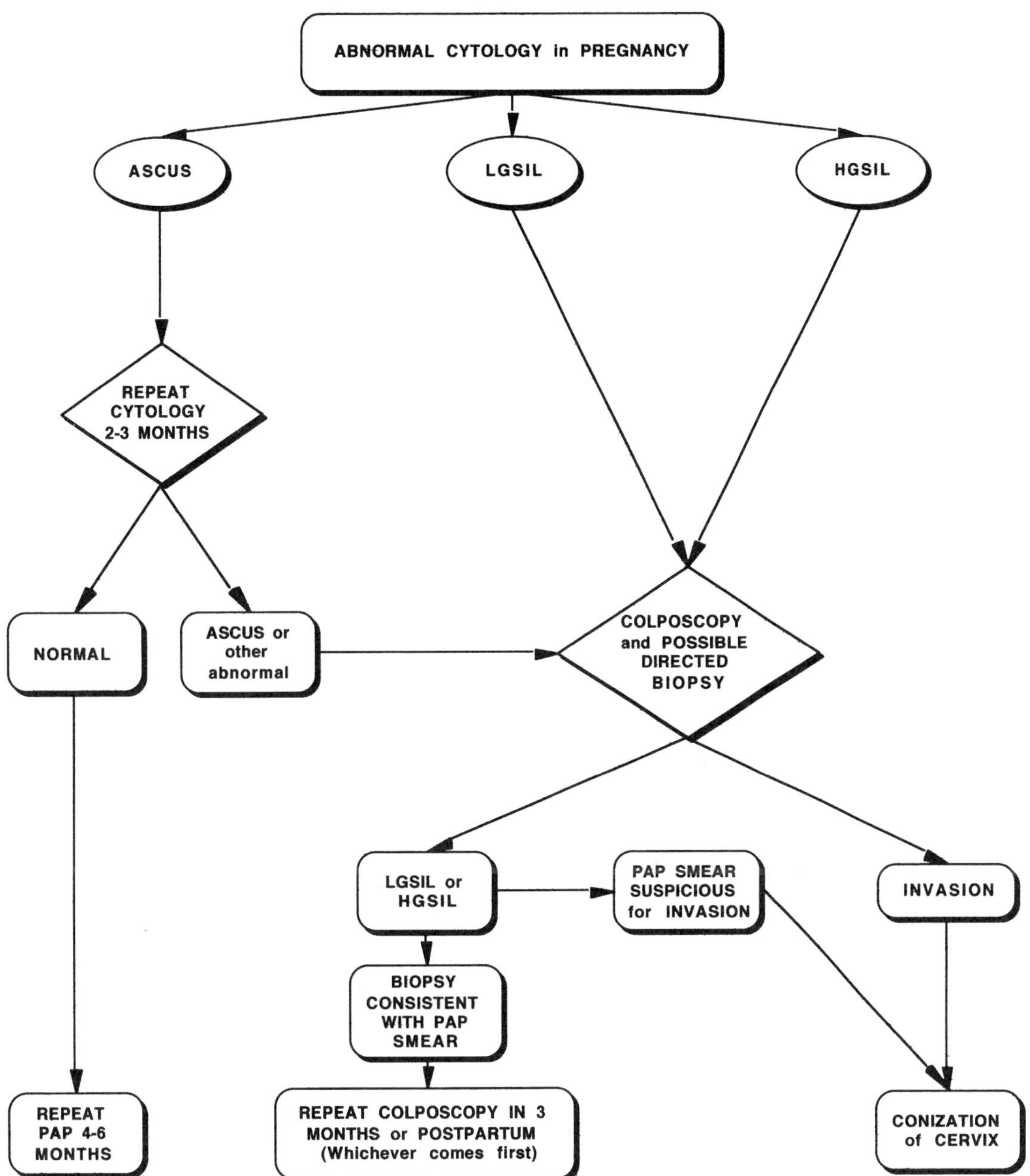

FIG. 39-1. Schema for evaluation of abnormal cytology in pregnancy.

ever, a recent report on carcinoma *in situ* in pregnant patients showed that there was an 80% persistence of disease after delivery. Hence, the higher the grade of dysplasia, the higher the chances of persistence (13). If the pap smear returns as a high-grade lesion after delivery, the patient needs to have a colposcopy with appropriate biopsies. For the low-grade or ASCUS pap smear in pregnancy, it also has been suggested that colposcopy need not be performed at all. However, the inclusion criteria of this study were quite liberal, and their good results may have been attributable to selection bias (14).

The advent of human papillomavirus (HPV) testing potentially has a useful place in pregnancy. There are not a lot of data published on HPV testing with abnormal pap smears in pregnancy, but this approach has the potential to decrease the number of procedures necessary to follow a pregnant patient who has an abnormal pap smear result, thereby reducing risks and inconvenience. HPV testing has been reported to decrease the need for referrals for colposcopy (15). The idea of HPV testing is to determine whether viral markers exist in abnormal pap smears. If the serologic types of HPV that are of concern in the genesis of cervical cancer (i.e., 16, 18, 31, 32, or 35) are present, that patient needs to have further testing, such as colposcopy with biopsies. If the HPV test shows no viral markers, the patient can forego colposcopy and be followed conservatively because the likelihood of progression to cervical malignancy is remote. This form of follow-up has not been subjected to large-scale evaluation, but it appears to be a rational method of following patients without the inherent fear that she harbors an undetected cervical malignancy. Over 95% of cervical squamous cancers have the designated high-risk HPV types. Viral load may play a role in the progression of disease or recurrence. It has been suggested that patients with persistent HPV DNA after conization of the cervix have a higher risk of recurrence of cervical dysplasia, but this finding has been difficult to reproduce (16).

There is controversy about what to do if the pap smear result is suspicious for an invasive lesion and the biopsy indicates a high-grade squamous intraepithelial lesion. In this case, the patient and the clinician need to consider cone biopsy as a definitive diagnostic (and sometimes therapeutic) test, which can be performed during pregnancy. It does have its own risks, but when the need arises to rule out invasive disease it should be seriously considered. There are methods for performing a prophylactic cervical cerclage when the cone excision is performed during pregnancy. I favor the sharp conization approach instead of loop electrode excision procedure (LEEP) because of the unknown effect of the monopolar electrocautery on the pregnancy. At times electrocautery may be necessary to control the bleeding that occurs at cone biopsy, but Monsel's solution is usually sufficient. LEEP excision of the cervix has been used in pregnancy and has been reported in a series. There was significant morbidity, with preterm labors and the need for blood transfusions, and the technique did not consistently produce diagnostic specimens that were very helpful. The conclusion was that LEEP excision of the cervix during pregnancy, although possible, may be limited in its effectiveness (17).

A time-tested and reliable approach to gestational conization described by Villa Santa (18) involves placement of a cerclage-type suture prior to the conization, thereby providing control of the cervical arteries at the time of cone biopsy. A no. 1 polyglycolic acid suture can be used for this procedure, thereby eliminating the need for later suture removal. A purse-string suture is placed around the cervix (in a manner similar to a McDonald cerclage), which when tightened gives control of bleeding from branches of the descending cervical branches of the uterine arteries. This technique decreases the amount of bleeding and allows an adequate specimen to be obtained, even when the cone specimen needs to be extensive.

If a microinvasive lesion is found and the margins are negative on the conization, the patient has the option of continuing the pregnancy without concern. However, if the margins are involved, a much more cautionary approach needs to be followed. If a lesion has invaded more than 3 mm below the epithelial basement membrane or there is lymphatic or vascular involvement, more treatment is necessary. This situation obviously has to be approached with particular compassion for a patient who is pregnant and may need to make difficult decisions about the fate of her pregnancy. Standard therapy for cervical cancer in pregnancy has a good outcome overall, and a delay in treatment, especially in patients with stage I typical squamous lesions, seems not to play a large role in overall survival, at least with a median delay of 144 days (16). In the delay of therapy, some researchers have used neoadjuvant chemotherapy to treat patients with advanced cervical cancer with a strong desire to preserve their pregnancy (19). It is unclear how effective this is because most of these are case reports rather than analyzable series (20). Other types of cervical cancer, such as small cell carcinoma, have been reported with progression to death 2 months after diagnosis (21).

Several pregnant women who were seen on our service declined treatment for cervical cancer because they did not want to reduce their probability of the pregnancy going to term. Their wishes in this regard were taken into consideration because data show that women who delay the treatment of the cervical squamous cancer until delivery or at least until maturity of the fetus do not decrease their survival. In villoglandular carcinomas of the cervix, the overall impact on survival is also seemingly not lessened by delay of diagnosis (22). Although there have generally been good outcomes after delay of treatment of cervical cancer in pregnant patients, there have been reported cases of tumor that was apparently seeded to the episiotomy site during delivery. A microinvasive adenocarcinoma of the cervix implanted in an episiotomy scar, with a fatal outcome (23). This situation has a poor prognosis. Three of the four patients reported by Cliby and colleagues died (24). Vaginal delivery does not seem to affect the natural history of early cervical cancers, and there is therefore no benefit to cesarean delivery in such patients.

If the patient is in the third trimester when the need for surgery is identified, fetal lung maturity can be determined by amniotic fluid analysis. When the fetal risks related to delivery are deemed acceptable, the patient can undergo a cesarean section with a radical hysterectomy and bilateral pelvic and paraaortic lymphadenectomy (25). During pregnancy, some researchers have reported an increased rate of bleeding, but most have shown that this is a reasonable procedure to perform and there is no need for delay until after the patient recovers from delivery. This approach is appropriate for patients with stage IB or IIA carcinoma of the cervix. However, more advanced stages of cervical cancer in pregnancy are treated with external beam radiation therapy followed after delivery by brachytherapy. Radiation therapy of cervical malignancies in pregnancy seems to have similar outcomes to those of patients who are not radiated (26).

If the patient is in her first trimester, the pregnancy is usually injured irrevocably and aborts before 40 Gy is delivered by external beam radiation (27). If spontaneous abortion does not occur, it is advised that a curettage be performed. If the patient has carcinoma of the cervix of any stage and undergoes cesarean delivery, palpation of the pelvic and paraaortic lymph nodes should be performed to see if any are enlarged. (Cesarean delivery should not be performed, however, solely for this purpose.) If so, these should be removed. If the paraaortic nodes are positive, the patient will need to have a therapeutic radiation field to include them. Magnetic resonance imaging (MRI) is superior to computerized tomography in detailing the extent of the cervical malignancy (27). The ovaries can be moved outside of the pelvis and sutured either retroperitoneally near the kidney or intraperitoneally out of the radiation field. Hemoclips can mark the location of the ovaries to guide the radiation therapist in avoiding them. This can potentially spare the patient an artificial menopause and the need for hormone replacement therapy.

It is important not to delay investigation of any form of abnormal bleeding in the pregnant patient, and, although it is not common, the possibility of a cervical or even an endocervical malignancy needs to be considered. A repeat pap smear is helpful, and a normal result is reassuring when bleeding originates from the cervix; but a visible lesion on the cervix should always be examined via biopsy. Overall, patients with cervical cancer in pregnancy have a good outcome because most of them are in the early stages when detected by pap smear. Cure rates for cervical cancer in pregnancy are about the same as patients who are not pregnant (28), with an 83% to 90% overall cure rate of stage I and cumulative 5-year survival in stage IB of 83%. Survival is 60% to 80% in stage II, with that in stage III falling below 50% (29).

OVARIAN CANCER

With the advent and liberal use of ultrasonography in pregnancy for determining gestational age and identifying fetal anomalies, it is common for women to be diagnosed with ovarian enlargement in the first and second trimester. Most such ovarian masses are physiologic in nature (most commonly corpus luteum cysts) and usually disappear by 12 to 14 weeks. Ovarian cancer associated with pregnancy is uncommon, reported in approximately 1 in 25,000 pregnancies (30).

When an ovarian mass is diagnosed in pregnancy, it is important that it be followed for resolution by serial clinical examination and sonography. Most cysts smaller than 6 cm resolve spontaneously. Patients have a low incidence of torsion while pregnant when followed by ultrasonography (31). The goal of following masses is to determine which are possibly malignant and when intervention is appropriate. Also, the risk of dystocia can be significant with an ovarian mass (32).

When a patient undergoes surgery in the first trimester and requires removal of an ovary, or a corpus luteum cyst, she should be given progestational supplementation in the form of 100 mg progesterone in oil intramuscularly or as vaginal suppositories on a daily basis to support the pregnancy until the placenta takes over progesterone production by around 12 to 14 weeks (33). Under ideal conditions, the patient should undergo surgery at around 18 weeks (34). The uterus is small enough then that the adnexa can be easily reached by the surgeon, but the pregnancy is advanced enough so that miscarriage in response to surgery is less likely, and adverse fetal effects of medication are of less concern than in the first trimester.

In imaging studies, the ominous signs that suggest the presence of a malignant neoplasm include septations, internal or external excrescences, and ascites. Although computerized tomography scanning can be used for imaging in pregnancy, it is not the ideal modality, except perhaps to evaluate upper abdominal disease, such as to rule out liver metastases or other upper abdominal problems. Computerized tomography can determine if there is a mass in the pelvis and often reveals pelvic adenopathy, but because the uterus is distended it may confuse interpretation. MRI has been used with fairly good success to determine whether the patient who is pregnant has a malignancy or not (35). A cyst larger than 6 to 8 cm that is persistent during the first and second trimester should be considered for surgical intervention. The risk of malignancy is about 5%, slightly lower than in the nonpregnant population for the reproductive age group (36). Approximately 25% of adnexal masses that are found during pregnancy are larger than 10 cm at the time of diagnosis (37). There is an increased risk of malignancy with larger cysts, especially over 10 cm (38). Obviously, solid components and papillations are worrisome as well. The rate of loss of fetuses perioperitively for pelvic mass during pregnancy ranges from 10% to 25%, depending on the nature of the surgery, gestational age, and comorbidities (39).

The most common ovarian cysts found during gestation, other than those that arise from the corpus luteum, are mature cystic teratomas. These are easily identified by ultrasonography. MRI in pregnancy also has proved to be a good tool for identifying these tumors. They contain fat, and the sonographic diagnosis is nearly always correct because of their characteristic appearance. These tumors can usually be followed without surgery during pregnancy, unless they are very large.

Of the malignant ovarian tumors that occur in reproductive-age women, the most common is the dysgerminoma (40), which is generally a solid tumor, a characteristic that can be detected on ultrasonography. Several studies have shown that in germ cell malignancies the outcomes after chemotherapy are usually good. However, immature teratomas and endodermal sinus tumors also occur and have a much worse prognosis (41). Usually dysgerminomas are modest in size, but they can be quite large (42). Other tumors, such as serous cystadenomas measuring 25×35 cm, have been reported (43).

Although tumor markers can be useful in nonpregnant women to predict whether an ovarian mass is malignant, CA125 is not useful during early pregnancy because there is normally an elevation of the serum CA125 during the first trimester (44). This is physiologic, peaks around 10 weeks, and then subsides to a normal nonpregnant value during the second and third trimesters (45,46). The serum CA125 level will become elevated again during delivery (47). Tumor markers are most helpful in dysgerminomas, in which the serum lactate dehydrogenase and CA125 may be useful (48). When the maternal serum alpha-fetoprotein (AFP) level is markedly elevated in the presence of an ovarian mass and there is no obstetric explanation for the high AFP level, the possibility of an endodermal sinus tumor should be considered.

At the time of surgical exploration of the abdomen in the third trimester, the patient should be in the left lateral tilt position, thereby keeping the uterus off the aorta and inferior vena cava. The uterus is not large enough to impinge on the great vessels of the abdomen when the patient undergoes surgery at around 18 weeks, so maternal position is at that time less of a consideration. However, a large pelvic mass can cause aortocaval compression in much the same way as can a full-term pregnant uterus. Early in pregnancy, laparoscopy can be an option for evaluation of a pelvic mass (49).

Upon exploration, excision of the cyst or of the adnexae with frozen section diagnosis should be used as guidance for further decision making. If a dysgerminoma is found, it should be staged with a unilateral pelvic and paraaortic lymphadenectomy. With the uterus being 18 weeks or larger in size, a pelvic lymphadenectomy is at times difficult to perform and may not be feasible. However, these tumors have a predilection for lymph node metastases, and adjuvant therapy would be important if extraovarian disease is found. Every effort should be made to perform an adequate lymph node dissection. Stage I dysgerminoma can be followed with no adjuvant therapy (50).

An immature teratoma, if a grade I, should be staged. A grade I immature teratoma that is found to have extraovarian disease will need to have chemotherapy. If confined to the ovary, no further therapy is necessary. Other grades of immature teratoma do not need a full staging because they will all need chemotherapy. Removal of gross extraovarian disease is necessary.

Endodermal sinus tumors are usually very vascular, and there is often obvious malignancy outside the ovary or there is a rupture of the tumor capsule. They require an adnexectomy and removal of any large extraovarian tumor masses. However, no extensive staging is necessary because these patients all will require chemotherapy (51).

The discovery of a tumor of low malignant potential is not uncommon in pregnancy because these neoplasms are most common in young women. Most low malignant potential tumors behave in a benign fashion, and once diagnosed at laparotomy and excised, they require omentectomy and (if no disease is found in the omentum) nothing further during pregnancy (52). It is unusual that the frozen section diagnosis in these cases is changed. The overall 10-year survival rate of patients with these tumors has been high, in the range of 95% to 97% (53). Therefore, most oncologists feel it is not necessary to be aggressive in the therapy of these tumors. The most recent National Institutes of Health consensus conference (54) supported conservative management for treatment of low malignant potential tumors. However, surgical debulking for serous low malignant potential tumors has been reported in pregnancy (55).

The risks and options to be weighed prior to the patient being taken to surgery include risk of premature delivery, harm to the fetus, or discovery of an invasive malignancy. It is very important to follow the patient for rupture of membranes or premature labor immediately following surgery. In one study most of the ovarian tumors that were found were benign and the patients frequently had perioperative complications (56). This makes consideration of conservative management even more important.

The determination of whether surgery for ovarian cancer should include hysterectomy or a bilateral (as opposed to unilateral) salpingoophorectomy needs to be individualized, and the wishes of the patient must be known prior to exploration. Sometimes, however, patients present with an acute abdomen secondary to torsion and it is not possible to be sure what the patient's desires are. In this situation the most conservative approach with a unilateral adnexectomy should be followed, with a limited staging (57). If frozen section diagnosis is not definitive, then it is better not to remove any of the organs other than the ovary or ovarian mass, or to do a unilateral salpingoophorectomy and wait for permanent histologic sections before determining what the optimal treatment should be. The patient can be brought back to surgery if necessary. Although that is an unpleasant prospect for the patient and adds further risk for the pregnancy, it is preferable to performing unnecessarily extensive surgery for disease that was over-read on frozen section.

At times the patient may be found to have a tumor of the ovary unexpectedly at the time of cesarean section. This pathology can be managed with logic. At times it is obvious that a malignancy is present. In such cases, surgical staging would be appropriate because the stage of the disease will determine outcome and follow-up therapy. If the obstetrician does not have the expertise to perform the staging, cannot obtain any help to do so, or even if the incision is not large enough for the staging, or the patient is unstable for various reasons, it is prudent to perform peritoneal washings, remove the affected ovary, abandon the procedure, and allow the patient to recover. A general inspection and palpation of the pelvic tissues is important (58). The staging can be performed at a later time.

Ovarian tumors that enlarge and are found to be of metastatic origin have been reported in pregnancy. Krukenberg tumors are metastatic ovarian masses in patients with a primary gastrointestinal malignancy. They have been reported in pregnancy with outcomes ranging from early death to prolonged disease-free survival (59–61). Virilization associated with these tumors has been reported. The treatment of these tumors includes removing the ovarian metastasis and possibly the originating source tumor, such as the stomach or the colon, if these are the only places where there is evidence of disease.

The risks of chemotherapy during pregnancy have been addressed in Chapters 7 and 40. Several studies have shown that in germ cell malignancies the outcomes of chemotherapy are usually good (62). The possibility of damage to the fetus needs always to be weighed against the benefits and risks of postponing chemotherapy or of pregnancy termination. There are no reported congenital abnormalities due to cisplatinum given in the first trimester. Although most oncologists will hold cisplatinum until delivery, this is the most commonly used medication in ovarian malignancies, and cisplatinum has been used during gestation (63,64). There are no useful data concerning taxol and topotecan use in pregnancy because these are much newer agents. If necessary, these can probably be given in the second and third trimester with relative safety. Breastfeeding is contraindicated when a patient is receiving chemotherapeutic agents because some of these, such as cytoxan, are present in high levels in breast milk (65). Individualization with patient preference is important in coming to an optimal decision for both the patient and her physicians.

VULVAR AND VAGINAL CANCER

Vulvar and vaginal cancer are rare in pregnancy because most patients with these malignancies are elderly. However, vulvar dysplasia has a bimodal age distribution and can be encountered in pregnancy. If a vulvar lesion is identified by inspection and a biopsy makes the diagnosis of vulvar dysplasia, this can be followed conservatively in pregnancy. The reason one need not do extensive resection in vulvar dysplasia is because this requires anesthesia, and the time element of delaying treatment until the patient delivers is usually reasonable. The dysplasia will not become a malignancy in such a short period of time and can simply be followed very closely. Sometimes these biopsy results show either an early form of vulvar epithelial malignancy or perhaps another neoplastic process altogether, such as vulvar sarcoma (66). Although the latter is rare, this occasionally occurs during pregnancy and the pathologic confirmation is straightforward. Because no series of a meaningful size has been reported, management is individualized, usually involving resection and follow-up chemotherapy.

Vulvar squamous cell cancers in pregnancy are also rare. There are several case reports describing these malignancies during pregnancy. Patients were treated with radical vulvectomy and bilateral inguinal lymphadenectomy, standard surgical therapy, during their pregnancies. The pregnancies were not terminated. With lymph node metastasis, radiation therapy was given after delivery by cesarean section (67–69). Vulvar sarcomas also have been reported during gestation. These seemed to have a more indolent course than carcinomas, with local recurrences common, but infrequent distant metastases. Resection should be performed during pregnancy, and radiation therapy and chemotherapy can follow after delivery (70–72).

Esoteric tumors of the vulva during pregnancy also have been reported, including desmoid tumor of the vulva and vulvar syringoma (73). Vulvar cancers and granular cell tumors have been reported to arise in an episiotomy site (74). Individualized therapy is necessary in these cases because there is no standard treatment, but it is safe to say that resection and any form of diagnostic surgical procedure that needs to be performed can be done safely in pregnancy (73,75).

Vaginal malignancies are almost unheard of during pregnancy and are usually a consequence of cervical or other malignancies having metastasized to the vagina. These are usually identified by visual inspection or by an abnormal pap smear followed by colposcopy and biopsy. There has been a reported case of antepartum hemorrhage, initially thought to be due to placenta previa, found to be caused by adenocarcinoma in the vagina. There was excessive blood loss and packing was used to control the hemorrhage (76). The patient went into preterm labor and was delivered by cesarean section, which was followed by radiation therapy. Malignant melanoma of the vagina with a good outcome also has been described. A 3-cm pedunculated lesion was found with a Breslow stage II, with no recurrence at 24 months (77).

ENDOMETRIAL CANCER

Endometrial cancer is a rare event in young women of childbearing age (78). It accounts for approximately 2.9% of cases occurring in women under age 40. Nevertheless, there have been two reported cases of endometrial cancer around the time of pregnancy, one in the early seventh gestational week after a therapeutic abortion, and one within 7 months after childbirth with poor prognosis with positive periaortic and pelvic lymph nodes and metastasis with demise. Persistent vaginal bleeding was the complaint in both cases (79,80).

REFERENCES

1. Nicholson H. Cytotoxic drugs in pregnancy. J Obstet Gynecol Br Commonw 1968;73:307–312.
2. Kalter H, Warkany J. Congenital malformations. N Engl J Med 1983; 308:424–431:491–497.
3. Jubb E. Primary ovarian carcinoma in pregnancy. Am J Obstet Gynecol 1963;85:345.
4. Donegan WL. Cancer and pregnancy. CA Cancer J Clin 1983;33: 194–214.
5. Potter JF, Schoenemann M. Metastasis of maternal cancer to the placenta and fetus. Cancer 1970;25:380–388.
6. Nevin J, Soeters R, Dehaech K, Bloch B, Van Wyk L. Cervical carcinoma associated with pregnancy. Obstet Gynecol Surv 1995:50: 228–239.
7. Hopkins M, Morley G. Cervical cancer in pregnancy. Obstet Gynecol 1992;80:9–13.
8. Papillo JL, Zarka MA, St. John TL. Evaluation of the ThinPrep pap test in clinical practice. Acta Cytol 1998;42:203–208.
9. van der Nange N, Weverling G, Ketting BW, Ankum WA, Samlal R, Lammes LB. Prognosis of cervical cancer associated with pregnancy in matched cohort study. Obstet Gynecol 1995;85:1022–1026.
10. Madej JG Jr. Colposcopy monitoring in pregnancy complicated by CIN and early cervical cancer. Eur J Gynaec Oncol 1996;17:59–65.
11. Jain AG, Higgins RV, Boyle MJ. Management of low-grade squamous intraepithelial lesions during pregnancy. Am J Obstet Gynecol 1977; 177:298–302.
12. LaPolla JP, O'Niell C, Wetrich D. Colposcopic management of abnormal cervical cytology in pregnancy. J Reprod Med 1988;33:301–306.
13. Coppola A, Sorosky J, Casper R, Anderson B, Buller RE. The clinical course of cervical carcinoma in situ diagnosed during pregnancy. Gynecol Oncol 1997;67:162–165.
14. Jain AG, Higgins RV, Boyle MJ. Management of low-grade squamous intraepithelial lesions during pregnancy. Am J Obstet Gynecol 1997; 177:298–302.
15. Cox JT, Lorincz AT, Schiffman MH, Sherman ME, Cullen A, Kurman RJ. Human papillomavirus testing by hybrid capture appears to be useful in triaging women with a cytologic diagnosis of atypical squamous cells of undetermined significance. Am J Obstet Gynecol 1995;172: 946–954.
16. Chua KL, Hjerpe A. Human papillomavirus analysis as a prognostic marker following conization of the cervix uteri. Gynecol Oncol 1997; 66:108–113.
17. Robinson WR, Webb S, Tirpack J, Degefu S, O'Quinn AG. Management of cervical intraepithelial neoplasia during pregnancy with LOOP excision. Gynecol Oncol 1997;64:153–155.
18. VillaSanta U. Instruments and methods: hemostatic "cerclage" after knife conization of the cervix. Obstet Gynecol 1973;42:299–301.
19. Duggan B, Muderspach L, Roman L, Curtain JP, 'de Ablaing G III, Morrow CP. Cervical cancer in pregnancy: reporting on planned delay in therapy. Obstet Gynecol 1993;82:598–602.
20. Tewari K, Cappuccini F, Gambino A, Hokler, MF, Pecorelli S, DiSala PJ. Neoadjuvant chemotherapy in the treatment of locally advanced cervical carcinoma in pregnancy: a report of two cases and review of issues specific to the management of cervical carcinoma in pregnancy including delay of therapy. Cancer 1998;82:1529–1534.
21. Chang DH, Hsueh S, Soong YK. Small cell carcinoma of the uterine cervix with neurosecretory granules associated with pregnancy. A case report. J Reprod Med 1994;39:537–540.
22. Hertu J. Villaglandular adenocarcinoma of the cervix: a case report. Obstet Gynecol 1995;85:906–908.
23. Van Den Broek NR, Lopes A, Ansink AD, Monaghan JM. "Microinvasive" adenocarcinoma of the cervix implanting in an episiotomy scar. A case report. Gynecol Oncol 1995;59:297–299.
24. Cliby W, Dodson M, Podratz K. Cervical cancer complicated by pregnancy: episiotomy site recurrences following vaginal delivery. Obstet Gynecol 1994;84:179–182.
25. Monk BJ, Montz FJ. Invasive cervical cancer complicating intrauterine pregnant: treatment with radical hyserectomy. Obstet Gynecol 1992;80: 199–203.
26. Sood AK, Sorosky JY, Mayr N, et al. Radiotherapeutic management of cervical carcinoma that complicates pregnancy. Cancer 1997;80: 1073–1078.
27. Cobby M, Browning J, Jones A, Whipp E, Gaddard P. Magnetic resonance imaging, computerized tomography, and endosonography in the local staging of carcinoma of the cervix. Br J Radiol 1993;63:673–679.
28. Hopkins MP, Morley GW. The prognosis and management of cervical cancer associated with pregnancy. Obstet Gynecol 1992;80:9–13.
29. Baltzer J, Regenbrecht ME, Kopcke W, Zander J. Carcinoma of the cervix in pregnancy. Int J Obstet Gynecol 1990;31:317–323.
30. Chung A, Birnbaum S. Ovarian cancer associated with pregnancy. Obstet Gynecol 1973;41:211–214.
31. Hogston P, Lilford RJ. Ultrasound study of ovarian cysts in pregnancy; prevelance and significance. Br J Obstet Gynaecol 1986;93:625–628.
32. Beischer NA, Buttry BW, Fortune DW, Macafee CAJ. Growth and malignancy of ovarian tumors in pregnancy. Aust N Z J Obstet Gynaecol 1971;8:208–214.
33. Goebelsmann U. Endocrinology of Pregnancy. In: Mishel D, Davajan V, ed. Infertility, contraception, and reproductive endocrinology, 2nd ed. Oradell, NJ: Medical Economics Books, 1986:113.
34. Hess LW, Peaceman A, O'Brien WF, Winkel CA, Cruikshank DW, Morrison JC. Adnexal mass occurring with intrauterine pregnancy: report of 54 patients requiring laparotomy for definitive management. Am J Obstet Gynecol 1988;158:1029–1034.
35. Curtis M, Hopkins M, Zarlingo T, Martino C, Graciansky-Lengyl M, Jenison E. Ovarian cancer in pregnancy. Obstet Gynecol 1983;82: 833–836.
36. Roberts JA. Management of gynecological tumors during pregnancy. Clin Perinatol 1983;10:369–382.
37. Tawa K. Ovarian tumors in pregnancy. Am J Obstet Gynecol 1964;90: 511–515.
38. Thornton JG, Wells M. Ovarian cysts in pregnancy: does ultrasound make traditional management inappropriate? Obstet Gynecol 1987;69: 717–721.
39. Katz VL, Watson WJ, Hansen WF, Washington JL. Massive ovarian tumor complicating pregnancy: a case report. J Reprod Med 1993;38: 907–910.
40. Karlen JR, Akbari A, Cook WA. Dysgerminomas associated with pregnancy. Obstet Gynecol 1979;53:330–335.
41. Malone JM, Gershenson DM, Creasy RK, Kavanagh JJ, Silva EG, Stringer CA. Endodermal sinus tumors of the ovary associated with pregnancy. Obstet Gynecol 1986;68(suppl):86–89.
42. Karlen JR, Assadollah A, Cook W. Dysgerminoma associated with pregnancy. Obstet Gynecol 1979;53:330–335.
43. Hunt MG, Martin NJ Jr, Martin RW, Meeks GR, Wiser WL, Morrison JC. Ovarian tumors. Am J Perinatol 1989;6:412–417.
44. Ocer F, Bese T, Saridogan E, Aydinli K, Asu T. The prognostic significance of maternal CA125 measurement in threatened abortion. Eur J Obstet Gynecol Repro Biol 1992;46:137–142.
45. Seki K, Kikuchi Y, Uesato T, Kato K. Increased serum CA125 levels during the first trimester of pregnancy. Acta Obstet Gynecol Scand 1986;65:583–585.
46. Itashi K, Inaba N, Fukazawa I, Takamizawa H. Immunoradiometrical measurement of tissue polypeptide antigen TPA, and cancer antigen CA125 in pregnancy and delivery. Arch Gynecol Obstet 1988;243: 191–197.
47. Lelle RJ, Henkel E, Leinemann D, Goeschen K. Measurement of CEA, TPA, Neopterin, CA125, CA153, and CA199 in sera of pregnant women, umbilical cord blood, and amniotic fluid. Gynecol Obstet Invest 1987;27:137–142.
48. Altarus MM, Goldberg GL, Levine W, Darge Bloch, Smith JA. The value of cancer antigen CA125 as a tumor marker in malignant germ cell tumors of the ovary. Gynecol Oncol 1986;25:150–159.
49. Guerrieri JP, Thomas RL. Open laparoscopy for an adnexal mass in pregnancy. J Reprod Med 1994:39;129–130.
50. Buller RE, Darrow V, Manetta A, Porto M, Desai PJ. Conservative surgical management of dysgerminoma concomitant with pregnancy. Obstet Gynecol 1992;79:887–890.
51. Kim DS, Park MI. Maternal and fetal survival following surgery and chemotherapy for endodermal sinus tumor of the ovary during pregnancy: a case report. Obstet Gynecol 1989;73:503–507.
52. Mooney J, Sylva E, Tornos C, Gershenson D. Unusual features of neoplasms of low malignant potential during pregnancy. Gynecol Oncol 1997;65:30–35.
53. Trimble CL, Trimble EL. Management of epithelial ovarian tumors of low malignant potential. Gynecol Oncol 1994;55(suppl):52–61.

54. Ovarian Cancer: Screening, Treatment, and Followup. NIH Consensus Statement April 5–7, 1994;12:1–30.
55. Tewari K, Brewer C, Cappuccini F, Macri C, Rogers LW, Berman ML. Advanced stage small cell carcinoma of the ovary in pregnancy: long-term survival after surgical debulking and multiagent chemotherapy. Gynecol Oncol 1997;66:531–534.
56. Platek D, Henderson CE, Goldberg GL. Management of patients for adnexal mass in pregnancy. Am J Obstet Gynecol 1995;173:1236–1240.
57. Schwartz PE. Cancer in pregnancy. In: Gusberg S, Shingleton H, Depp G, eds. Female genital cancers. New York: Churchill Livingstone, 1988: 725–736.
58. Antonelli NM, Dotters DJ, Katz VL, Kuller JA. Cancer in pregnancy: a review of the literature. Part I. Obstet Gynecol Surv 1996;51:125–142.
59. Cheng CY, Chen TY, Lin CK, Tsao SM, Shih IF, Shy SW. Krukenberg tumor in pregnancy with delivery of a normal baby: a case report. Chin Med J (Taipei) 1994;54:424–427.
60. De Palma P, Wronski M, Bifernino V, Bovani I. Krukenberg tumor in pregnancy with virilization. A case report. Eur J Gynaecol Oncol 1995; 16:59–64.
61. Mackey JR, Hugh J, Smylie M. Krukenberg tumor complicated by pregnancy. A case report. Gynecol Oncol 1996;61:153–155.
62. Sorosky JI, Sood AK, Buckers TE. The use of chemotherapeutic agents during pregnancy. Obstet Gynecol Clin North Am 1997;24:591–599.
63. King LA, Nevin PC, Willliams PP, Carson LF. Treatment of advanced epithelial ovarian carcinoma in pregnancy with cisplatinum-based chemotherapy. Gynecol Oncol 1991;41:78–80.
64. Malfinato J, Goldkrand JW. Cisplatinum combination chemotherapy during pregnancy for advanced epithelial cancer. Obstet Gynecol 1990; 75:545–547.
65. Durodola J. Administration of cyclophosphamide during late pregnancy and early lactation. J Natl Med Assn 1979;71:165.
66. Lupi G, Jin R, Clemente C. Malignant rhabdoid tumor of the vulva: a case report and review of the literature. Tumori 1996;82:93–95.
67. Gitsch G, van Eijkeren M, Hacker NF. Surgical therapy of vulvar cancer in pregnancy. Gynecol Oncol 1995;56:312–315.
68. Moore DH, Fowler WC Jr, Currie JL, Walton LA. Squamous cell carcinoma of the vulva in pregnancy. Gynecol Oncol 1991;41:74–77.
69. Regan MA, Rosenzweig BA. Vulvar carcinoma in pregnancy: a case report and literature review. Am J Perinatol 1993;10:334–335.
70. Kuller JA, Zucker PK, Peng TC. Vulvar leiomyosarcoma in pregnancy. Am J Obstet Gynecol 1990;162:164–166.
71. Fried-Oginski W, Lovecchio JL, Farahani G, Smitari T. Malignant mysoid sarcoma of the Bartholin gland in pregnancy. Am J Obstet Gynecol 1995;173:1633–1635.
72. Nielsen GP, Rosenberg AE, Koerner FC, Young RH, Scully RE. Smooth-muscle tumors of the vulva. A clinicopathological study of 25 cases and review of the literature. Am J Surg Pathol 1996;20:779–793.
73. Allen MV, Novotny DB. Desmoid tumor of the vulva associated with pregnancy. Arch Pathol Labor Med 1997;121:512–514.
74. Murcia JM, Idoate M, Laparte C, Baldonado C. Granular cell tumor of vulva on episiotomy site. Gynecol Oncol 1994;53:248–250.
75. Turan C, Ugur M, Kutluay I, et al. Vulvar syringoma exacerbated during pregancy. Eur J Obstet Gynecol Reprod Biol 1996;64:141–142.
76. Malhotra D, Malhotra S, Nijhawan R. Adenocarcinoma of the vagina in pregnancy. Int J Gynaecol Obstet 1993;43:198–199.
77. Zarcone R, Cardone G, Bellini P, Cardone A. Malignant melanoma of the vagina in pregnancy: description of a clinical case. Panminerva Med 1995;37:166–167.
78. Crissmann JD, Azoury RS, Barnes AE, Schellhass HF. Endometrial cancer in women forty years of age or younger. Obstet Gynecol 1981; 57:699–704.
79. Kodama J, Roshinouchi M, Miyagi Y, et al. Advanced endometrial cancer detected at 7 months after childbirth. Gynecol Oncol 1997;54: 501–506.
80. Kovacs AG, Cserni G. Endometrial adenocarcinoma in early pregnancy. Gynecol Obstet Invest 1996;41:70–72.

Cherry and Merkatz's Complications of Pregnancy,
Fifth Edition, edited by W. R. Cohen.
Lippincott Williams & Wilkins, Philadelphia © 2000.

CHAPTER 40

Nongenital Malignancies

Gina M. Villani and Gary L. Goldberg

Cancer is one of the leading causes of nonaccidental death in the United States among women 15 to 34 years of age, and it accounts for approximately 19% of the mortality in the group (1). In women 35 to 54 years of age, cancer accounts for 41% of all deaths (2). An estimated 1 in 1,000 women will be affected by cancer in some form while pregnant (2). The malignant neoplasms occurring during pregnancy are those most frequently seen in young women, that is, lymphoma, leukemia, melanoma, breast cancer, and cancers of the thyroid, cervix, ovary, and colon. There is no evidence that pregnancy results in an increased rate of malignancy; in fact, it may actually be less than in a matched nonpregnant population. Haas identified 355 cases of women 15 to 44 years of age who were pregnant at the time of their cancer diagnosis from 1970 to 1979 (3). Extrapolating from female population cancer rates, 555.8 cases were expected during this time period. Significantly less than the expected ratio occurred, and he postulated that underreporting or decreased fertility in women with neoplastic disease may be responsible for this lower incidence of cancer in pregnancy.

Few situations in medicine present as great a clinical dilemma as that of pregnancy complicated by a malignancy. Several management issues must be addressed when dealing with these patients. Will the disease or the treatment affect the fetus adversely? Will the pregnancy alter the natural history or prognosis of the disease? Is termination of pregnancy indicated? What are the long-term sequelae of *in utero* exposure to chemotherapeutic agents? What effect will the disease and its treatment have on subsequent fertility and pregnancy?

G. M. Villani, Department of Medicine, and G. L. Goldberg, Department of Obstetrics and Gynecology, Albert Einstein College of Medicine, Bronx, NY 10461.

This chapter will discuss acute leukemia, breast cancer, melanoma, Hodgkin's disease, and non-Hodgkin's lymphoma (NHL) in pregnancy because these are among the most common nongenital malignancies encountered during gestation. It is essential that the obstetrician-gynecologist be familiar with these disorders so that they can be recognized and diagnosed early, when they may be curable. Some pertinent generalizations regarding the use of chemotherapy and radiation in pregnancy are presented prior to describing the individual cancers.

CHEMOTHERAPY IN THE PREGNANT PATIENT

Little information is available concerning the use of chemotherapeutic agents in pregnant women with cancer. Prospective randomized trials have not been performed in this unique patient population and are unlikely to be performed in the future. Data from animal studies are difficult to extrapolate to humans because species differences exist with regard to the pharmacokinetics and pharmacodynamics of antineoplastic agents as well as to teratogenic risks. For these reasons most of the data concerning chemotherapy in pregnancy come from case reports and literature reviews. Although many reports suggest that chemotherapy can be administered safely during pregnancy, antineoplastic agents have been associated with both immediate and delayed effects on the fetus (4,5). Immediate effects include fetal death, abortion, premature birth, low birth weight, and organ toxicity, including bone marrow suppression (4,5). Putative long-term effects include carcinogenesis, growth and mental retardation, sterility, and teratogenesis in future generations (6–8). Given the low therapeutic index of antineoplastic agents, only clinicians familiar with the alteration in drug metabolism that occurs during pregnancy should be involved in the treatment of these patients.

PHARMOCOKINETIC ALTERATIONS IN PREGNANCY

Drug absorption, distribution, metabolism, and excretion are all affected by the physiologic changes that occur during pregnancy. In pregnancy, total body water increases by up to 8 L and plasma volume by 50% (9). The amniotic fluid acts as a third space for water-soluble drugs, leading to an increase in the apparent volume of distribution. The implication of these changes is a decrease in the peak concentration of a drug, prolongation of the half-life, and the retardation of drug elimination, unless metabolism or excretion is increased. The development of a third space leads to prolonged exposure to water-soluble drugs, resulting in potential maternal and fetal toxicity.

Plasma albumin levels decrease during pregnancy, with an overall reduction in plasma proteins (10). This may lead to an increase in the unbound active fraction of drugs, altering their activity. Drug metabolism and excretion are modified during pregnancy. Glomerular filtration rate and creatinine clearance are increased and lead to rapid removal of drugs that are cleared by the kidney (11). Drug metabolism by the liver may be enhanced or delayed. The mixed oxidative function system is faster in pregnant patients; thus, drugs metabolized by this mechanism are cleared more rapidly (12). Increased drug clearance can dramatically reduce the therapeutic efficacy of a drug. Fetal exposure is an important factor in determining fetal risk. Chemotherapeutic agents may cross the placenta from mother to fetus. The diffusion across the placenta is dependent on the molecular weight, plasma protein binding, lipophilicity, and state of ionization (10,11,13). Agents that cross the placenta readily are those with a low molecular weight and low protein binding, and those that are lipophilic and nonionized. These are characteristics of most chemotherapeutic agents. The dose, route of administration, and schedule of a drug are additional factors that determine fetal exposure (14), which does not necessarily imply fetal toxicity. Fetal toxicity may be more related to the trimester of exposure, mechanism of action of the drug, and frequency and duration of exposure. Although modifications in drug dosing and administration for the pregnant patient have not been defined, several general recommendations can be made:

1. When possible, exposure to chemotherapeutic agents should be avoided during the first trimester, especially during weeks 3 to 12.
2. High-dose, long-term therapy should be avoided.
3. Agents known to cause birth defects, such as folic acid antagonists and certain alkylating agents, are contraindicated, especially in the first trimester.
4. Drugs that can accumulate in third space compartments, such as methotrexate, should be avoided.
5. The intraperitoneal route may allow direct transuterine absorption and is contraindicated.
6. Breastfeeding should be discouraged in any patient receiving chemotherapy because many agents penetrate into breast milk.

RADIATION EFFECTS

The evaluation of radiation effects is minimally affected by species differences in absorption, metabolism, and placentation, making radiation embryology experiments in mammals reasonably helpful in predicting human reproductive effects. Mouse and rat embryos irradiated during the preimplantation stage rarely develop malformations, regardless of the dose administered (15). During this same period, however, the embryo is most sensitive to the lethal effects of ionizing radiation. One hundred fifty rad absorbed in the first day of gestation in the rat will kill approximately 70% of embryos exposed (15). Embryos that survive will develop normally. It thus appears that radiation will either kill the preimplanted embryo or allow it to develop unharmed.

During organogenesis in the rodent, equivalent to days 18 to 36 in humans, irradiation has its greatest teratogenic risk (16). Mice exposed to irradiation during this period have demonstrated developmental abnormalities such as cerebral and cerebellar hypoplasia and microcephaly, cleft palate, and evisceration (16). During the second and third trimesters in humans, radiation exposure is much less likely to produce congenital abnormalities (17). Those that occur usually involve the central nervous system because these tissues continue to differentiate throughout gestation. For a given dose of radiation, malformations are five times less likely to occur at this time than during organogenesis.

Fetal growth restriction may occur due to exposure to ionizing radiation *in utero*. Animal studies indicate that prior to implantation the embryo is resistant to the growth-retarding effects of radiation. After implantation, intrauterine growth retardation can result from radiation exposure delivered at any time during gestation (18). Animals irradiated during the period of organogenesis developed the most severe growth retardation; those irradiated at any stage of gestation with less than 25 rad did not appear to be affected.

Controlled human data on the effects of *in utero* radiation exposure are limited. However, there are numerous reports of unintentional damage to embryos and fetuses from maternal radiation. As with animals, the effects of ionizing radiation on a developing fetus can be lethal, cause growth and developmental abnormalities, or have no apparent effect, depending on the dose delivered and the stage of pregnancy at which the exposure occurs.

LETHALITY OF RADIATION IN EARLY PREGNANCY

Most information on the effects of *in utero* exposure comes from studies of children exposed prenatally to radiation released from the atomic bombs dropped in Japan at the close of World War II. Yamazaki studied 30 mothers who themselves had signs of radiation damage and who had received doses between 1 and 10 Gy (19). In this group, most of whom were exposed early in their pregnancy, there were 23% fetal deaths and 26.1% deaths in neonates and children born to these women. A second group of women, with signs of minor radiation sickness, who had received a dose of 1 Gy was also studied. Fetal deaths among this second cohort were 9%, compared with a 5.9% fetal death rate in the nonirradiated control group.

MALFORMATIONS INDUCED BY RADIATION

Miller and colleagues (20) also studied Japanese women exposed to doses of 1 to 9 Gy during weeks 6 to 11 of pregnancy and noted an 11% incidence of microcephaly and mental retardation in their offspring. It must be kept in mind that malformations in these children occurred as a result of a single-dose exposure. Similar doses over a more protracted period would be expected to have less of an effect. Debakan studied 26 women who had received pelvimetric irradiation and correlated gestational age with dose and fetal damage (21). At 2.5 Gy, more than 50% of infants exposed between the third and tenth weeks developed mental retardation, microcephaly, cataracts, retinal degeneration, and skeletal and genital abnormalities. Radiation exposure between 12 and 20 weeks resulted in stunted growth, mental retardation, and microcephaly. Radiation exposure after 20 weeks was not associated with any gross malformations. It appears that exposure during the fetal period of gestation (from 8 weeks to term) is less likely to produce congenital abnormalities than during organogenesis. After 30 weeks' gestation, radiation-induced congenital defects are rare. Dermal erythema and hematologic depression have been noted in these infants. The American College of Radiology concludes that the risk of malformation is not increased if the fetus was exposed to less than 0.05 Gy (22). Brent has extensively reviewed the world literature and regards a dose of 0.1 Gy as a practical threshold value below which the risk of teratogenesis has not been demonstrated to be increased at any stage of gestation (17).

DIAGNOSTIC RADIATION EXPOSURE

The estimated fetal dose from many commonly used radiologic diagnostic procedures is less than 0.01 Gy, and they are generally considered safe (23). Lymphangiography and computerized tomography of the abdomen and pelvis may expose the fetus to much larger doses (0.05–0.1 Gy) and should if possible not be used in a pregnant patient. Ultrasonography and magnetic resonance imaging (MRI) do not use ionizing radiation. Although there have been no documented adverse fetal effects reported from MRI, the National Radiological Protection Board arbitrarily advises against its use in the first trimester (24). Nuclear studies are performed by tagging a chemical agent with a radioisotope. Technetium 99m is used for brain, bone, renal, and cardiovascular scintography. In general this isotope results in fetal exposure of less than 0.05 Gy (25).

ACUTE LEUKEMIA

Definition

The acute leukemias are a heterogeneous group of neoplasms affecting uncommitted or partially committed hematopoietic stem cells (26). These cancers are a clonal proliferation of a single hematopoietic cell. The acute leukemias have been divided into myeloid and lymphoid subclasses. In 1976 a uniform classification system based on the morphologic characteristics of the leukemic cells was developed (27). This French-American-British classification (FAB) system subdivided the myeloid leukemias into seven and the lymphoid leukemias into three distinct divisions, permitting comparisons of clinical presentation and treatment results among these groups. With the advent of flow cytometry and chromosomal banding techniques, the acute leukemias have been further characterized. Karotyping can provide valuable prognostic information.

Incidence

Leukemia develops in 3.5 individuals per 100,000 per year in the United States and Western Europe (1,28). Leukemia associated with pregnancy is uncommon and occurs in only 1 per 100,000 pregnancies annually (3,29,30). There are only 350 reported cases of leukemia in the modern literature pertaining to pregnant women (5,30–32).

Etiology

Environmental factors may play a role in the genesis of acute leukemia. Benzene, a ubiquitous natural product used as a solvent in many industrial processes, is absorbed through the skin and lungs and can accumulate in body fat. The link between benzene exposure and the development of acute leukemia was established by the observations of Astoy (33) in Turkish factory workers and confirmed by a long-term study of rubber plant workers in Ohio (34). Induction of acute leukemia by other chemicals is not as firmly established.

Reviews on the leukemogenic effects of antineoplastic drugs have been published (35,36). Secondary or therapy-related leukemias have occurred in patients treated for lymphoma, as well as for carcinoma of the breast, gastrointestinal tract, ovary, and lung, suggesting that the major risk does not lie within the primary disease but is a consequence of treatment. The latency period for the development of these leukemias ranges from 2 to 20 years (37). Therapy-related leukemias are commonly associated with characteristic chromosomal abnormalities such as deletions within chromosomes 5 and 7, and are refractory to conventional therapy (38,39).

The leukemogenic effects of ionizing radiation were recognized after the atomic bombing of Hiroshima and Nagasaki in 1945 (40). Studies of low-dose radiation exposure have yielded equivocal results, and the question of a threshold relationship between irradiation and leukemic induction remains controversial (41,42).

Cigarette smoking also has been implicated in the induction of leukemia. Studies from the American Cancer Society have demonstrated an increased incidence of acute myeloid leukemia in smokers (43).

Clinical Presentation

Most early reports of pregnancy and acute leukemia described women in whom leukemia was diagnosed during pregnancy. Prior to the introduction of intensive chemotherapy, case reports of women with acute leukemia becoming pregnant were rare, given the extremely poor prognosis of such patients. In recent years, however, there have been increasing reports of patients with a previous diagnosis of leukemia becoming pregnant (44,45). Many of these women were receiving chemotherapy at the time of conception, suggesting that the ovaries may not suffer irreversible damage from treatment. Indeed, the results of a large retrospective cohort study of fertility in 2,283 survivors of cancer in childhood and adolescence demonstrated that previous treatment with nonalkylating agents resulted in no apparent decrease in fertility in either sex (46). Prior exposure to alkylating agents reduced fertility by 33%. Alkylating agents are not part of the therapeutic armamentarium for acute leukemia, and as the number of children and adults with acute leukemia who become long-term survivors increases, so too will the number of pregnancies in this population. Juarez and colleagues reported on 10 cases of pregnancy and acute leukemia. Of these 10 patients, 3 had a diagnosis of acute leukemia at the time of pregnancy (44). Two were in complete remission, and remission had not been achieved in the other. All were receiving cytostatic drugs at the time of conception. Pizzuto and colleagues reported on nine cases of pregnancy-associated leukemia (45). Three patients from his series had a diagnosis of leukemia prior to pregnancy.

There is no available evidence suggesting that pregnancy itself alters the incidence, natural history, or prognosis of acute leukemia. Therefore, the clinical presentation of pregnant patients would not be expected to differ from that of nonpregnant women. A review of 72 newly diagnosed cases of acute leukemia complicating pregnancy revealed that leukemias occurred more frequently in the later stages of gestation (32). Sixteen (22%) were diagnosed during the first trimester, 26 (36%) during the second trimester, and 30 (42%) during the third trimester.

The most common complaint among patients with acute leukemia is nonspecific malaise or fatigue, usually present for several months prior to diagnosis. Anemia may cause pallor and weakness. In the Juarez series, 5 of the 10 patients presented with symptoms of anemia as their initial complaint (44). Fever is common and is often associated with sweats. Hemorrhagic signs and symptoms such as easy bruisability, petechiae, and epistaxis are related to thrombocytopenia and, occasionally, disseminated intravascular coagulation. Weight loss, if it occurs, is usually not severe. Lymphadenopathy has been reported in acute myelogenous leukemia (AML), but occurs more commonly in acute lymphatic leukemia (ALL). Skin infiltration manifested by a violaceous rash can be seen in patients with a monocytic component, as can infiltration of the gums. Rarely, central nervous system disease can occur at the time of presentation and is associated with headache or cranial nerve palsies. More commonly, central nervous system disease occurs at relapse. Pulmonary symptoms may arise in patients with infections related to neutropenia. Perirectal abscess is not uncommon; however, rectal examination should be performed with caution in patients with profound neutropenia.

The hyperleukocytosis syndrome is a hematologic emergency that can be fatal (47). It usually occurs when the white cell count, composed mainly of immature cells and blasts, exceeds 100,000 per mm^2. This increased cell number and size can seriously affect flow in the circulation of the brain and lung, leading to stasis in microvascular beds. The clinical manifestations of pulmonary leukostasis include acute respiratory distress and hypoxemia, and may be impossible to distinguish from infection. Sudden death due to intracranial hemorrhage can complicate central nervous system leukostasis. Retinal vein distention, fundal hemorrhages, and papilledema may be found on physical examination. Emergent cranial radiation is required. Leukopheresis is used to lower the white blood cell count rapidly while chemotherapy is initiated without delay.

Laboratory Findings

The leukocyte count is elevated at presentation in more than half of all patients with acute leukemia. Leukemic blasts are usually identifiable in the peripheral smear. Aleukemic leukemia (no blasts in the peripheral blood) has been described, but is rare. Neutropenia occurs in most patients. A normochromic anemia with nucleated blood cells is common. Thrombocytopenia may be severe; thrombocytosis is rare. Disseminated intravascular coagulation with hypofibrinogenemia occurs more commonly in AML than in ALL, particularly in acute promyelocytic leukemia, the M3 variant. Hyperuricemia is seen in many patients with AML at presentation. Acute tumor lysis syndrome is associated with tumors with a high growth rate and a rapid cell turnover, as occurs in acute leukemia (48).

Patients develop hyperuricemia, hyperkalemia, hyperphosphatemia, and hypocalcemia as these ions are released from tumor cells. Tumor lysis syndrome may occur spontaneously or upon treatment with cytotoxic agents. Vigorous hydration, alkalinization of the urine, allopurinol to increase excretion of uric acid, and meticulous monitoring of serum levels of pertinent solutes can prevent renal failure and death from hyperkalemia.

Diagnosis

The diagnosis of acute leukemia is not difficult and should be suspected in a pregnant patient with an elevated blood leukocyte count, anemia out of proportion to that commonly seen in pregnancy, and thrombocytopenia. Review of the peripheral smear demonstrates immature cells. Bone marrow biopsy and aspirate will disclose a marrow that is replaced by blasts. Immunophenotyping and cytogenetic analysis should be performed to classify the leukemia further and to provide prognostic information.

Treatment

The diagnosis of acute leukemia complicating pregnancy demands immediate attention to the maternal disease for two reasons: the only hope for cure is immediate aggressive treatment; and the median duration of survival without treatment is 2 months, insufficient time for fetal maturation in most cases. The goal of therapy is achievement of complete remission, marked by a return to normal of the peripheral blood counts and absence of leukemic cells in the bone marrow. Partial remission, defined as some evidence of residual disease, has not resulted in prolongation of life. Management of acute leukemia requires induction of remission followed by some form of postremission therapy. Leukemia treatment must be intense and prolonged in order to be successful.

Most of the available information on the use of chemotherapeutic agents during pregnancy comes from case reports and small uncontrolled studies of women with acute leukemia. Drugs used to treat acute leukemia include the antimetabolites, the anthracyclines, and the vinca alkaloids. The administration of antineoplastic drugs during the first trimester of pregnancy may have disastrous effects. Treatment during the first few weeks after conception often results in spontaneous abortion. Later in the first trimester, major congenital malformations may occur. Of 139 patients treated with single agent chemotherapy early in pregnancy, 17% of fetuses developed major malformations (48). Among 30 women who received combination chemotherapy during this same pregnancy period, a 23% rate of malformations was reported (49). Once organogenesis is complete, the risk of teratogenicity decreases dramatically, as evidenced by a study of 131 pregnant patients treated with either single-agent or combination chemotherapy during the second and third trimesters (12). The incidence of fetal anomalies was only 1.5%. Unfortunately, if good results are to be achieved, the initiation of treatment for a pregnant patient with acute leukemia cannot be delayed until after the completion of the first trimester.

Antimetabolites such as methotrexate, aminopterin, and cytarabine interfere with the synthesis of DNA and RNA. Some of the antimetabolites are unequivocably teratogenic. Aminopterin, commonly used in the past for leukemic induction therapy, was administered to 52 first-trimester pregnant patients and resulted in a 19% incidence of congenital anomalies (50) including cranial dysostosis, micrognathia, irregular external ears, and cleft palate. This constellation of symptoms has been termed the aminopterin syndrome. Newer, more effective agents have replaced aminopterin in the treatment of acute leukemia. Cytarabine (Ara C), a nucleoside analogue, in combination with an anthracycline is now standard induction therapy for acute leukemia. Cytarabine has been administered safely in the second and third trimester of pregnancy (45,51). Fetal anomalies have been associated with its use during the first 8 weeks of gestation (52). Caliguiri and Mayer reviewed the literature concerning the treatment of acute leukemia during pregnancy (32). They reported 32 cases of patients who received cytarabine alone or in combination with an anthracycline or vinca alkaloid. These 32 pregnancies resulted in 18 normal infants, 2 congenital malformations, 1 fetal death, and 5 therapeutic abortions.

The anthracycline antibiotics (doxorubicin and daunorubicin) are potent inhibitors of DNA synthesis. Transplacental passage of these drugs has been examined, and results are conflicting. Roboz and colleagues reported that neither doxorubicin nor its metabolites could be detected in amniotic fluid 4 and 16 hours after administration to a pregnant woman (53). D'Incalci and colleagues reported that although they could not detect amniotic fluid doxorubicin concentrations, they could find concentrations of almost 10 times the maternal level in the liver, kidney, and lung of a 17 week fetus (54). Thus, the anthracyclines probably do cross the placenta; however, this class of compounds is considered relatively safe for the pregnant cancer patient. A variety of case reports describe normal infants born to mothers receiving anthracyclines for the treatment of leukemia (45,55–57). The long-term effects of these drugs have not been fully studied. In adults and children, treatment with anthracyclines has resulted in cardiac toxicity, which may manifest as congestive heart failure many years after treatment. To date there are no reports of late cardiac toxicity in the children of patients treated for leukemia during pregnancy.

The vinca alkaloids include vinblastine and vincristine. These agents are antimitotic and inhibit microtubule formation, leading to cell cycle arrest in metaphase. Little is known about the pharmacokinetics of these agents in the pregnant patient. They are metabolized by the liver, the majority of the drug being eliminated in the feces, with a small fraction being excreted by the kidney. In the nonpregnant patient the volume of distribution is large (approximately 97 L/m^2) (14). This may be increased significantly in the pregnant patient, raising the question of whether modified dosing is necessary. Vinblastine has been used in all trimesters of pregnancy without producing teratogenic effects (14). Vincristine also has not been directly associated with teratogenic effects. In fact, the only reports of teratogenic effects following the application of the vinca alkaloids have involved concomitant therapy with procarbazine or nitrogen mustard (58,59).

Chemotherapy for acute leukemia causes prolonged marrow aplasia in the mother, requiring aggressive supportive care. There have been reports of babies born with transient pancytopenia when their mothers received chemotherapy close to the time of delivery (45). Reynoso and colleagues reported cytopenias in 33% of fetuses of mothers treated within a month of delivery (5). Peripheral blood counts returned to normal in most within several weeks. There were, however, fetal deaths from neutropenia-induced sepsis. Whenever possible, chemotherapy should be withheld for several weeks prior to delivery.

Long-term Outcome of Fetuses Exposed to Antileukemic Therapy

The outcomes of 14 children whose mothers were treated for acute leukemia during pregnancy were reported by Aviles and Niz (31). Fifty-eight percent were exposed during the first trimester. No late side effects were found among these children when examined for growth and development, school performance, and neurologic function. In a later report by the same authors, 43 children born to mothers with a variety of hematologic neoplasms treated with various chemotherapeutic agents during pregnancy were evaluated (60). Forty-four percent of these children were exposed during the first trimester. All were found to be normal when examined 3 to 19 years following exposure.

Course of Leukemia During Delivery and Postpartum

Information on pregnancy outcomes of leukemic women is scant. Most case reviews and reports focus on the outcome of the fetus. Patients with acute leukemia appear to tolerate delivery well; however, many live only a short time following delivery. Most of these women die of progressive disease with sepsis and bleeding (61). A recent report found the median length of survival among 58 patients to be 16 months after delivery (5). Lloyd (62) observed that the course of leukemia is worsened following delivery and postulated that the sudden decrease in serum corticosteroid levels that occurs shortly after delivery could be responsible for this apparent exacerbation. This has prompted some clinicians to recommend administration of steroids in the postpartum period.

Excess bleeding postpartum occurs in approximately 20% of leukemic patients (29,63). Platelets and fibrinogen should be administered if bleeding occurs. Some researchers believe that bleeding during delivery in the thrombocyopenic patient develops in areas of injury because bleeding from the delivery itself is largely controlled by uterine contraction (64). Vaginal delivery appears to be the safest mode of delivery. Episiotomy should be avoided because infectious complications are common. In the Juarez study (44), four patients developed infections at the episiotomy site, one of whom died from sepsis.

In summary, acute leukemia is a disease that requires intense prolonged treatment with potent antineoplastic agents. When it occurs during pregnancy it must be treated in the same manner as in the nonpregnant patient. Aggressive supportive care must accompany the antileukemic therapy. Fetuses of women treated during gestation generally do quite well if their exposure to cytotoxic drugs occurred after the first trimester. Regrettably, only 20% of all patients with acute leukemia are long-term survivors, and the outlook for pregnant patients is equally grim.

PREGNANCY-ASSOCIATED BREAST CANCER

Definition

Traditionally, pregnancy-associated breast cancer is defined as a cancer diagnosed during pregnancy or within 1 year postpartum. The problem of pregnancy and breast cancer has gained increasing attention over the past several years because more women are becoming pregnant for the first time in their thirties and forties, and the incidence of breast cancer increases with advancing age and with age at first pregnancy. In addition, there has been an increase in breast cancer incidence in all age groups over the past decade, which has become a major public health concern (65).

Etiology

In a review prepared for the Breast Cancer Task Force (66), MacMahon and colleagues defined risk factors for human breast cancer. The major predictors of risk included age, geographic location, age at first birth, ovarian activity (i.e., ovulation), history of benign breast disease, and familial breast cancer history. One of the earliest known features of the epidemiology of breast cancer is the inverse relationship of risk with parity. A collaborative study performed in the early 1970's among seven areas with divergent breast cancer rates further refined this relationship. McMahon and colleagues summarized those findings as follows:

1. Breast cancer risk increases with increasing age at which a woman bears her first full-term child.
2. To be protective, pregnancy must occur before 30 years of age.
3. The protective effect is essentially limited to the first birth.
4. Protection is exerted only by a full-term pregnancy; abortion was associated with an increased risk.
5. The protection conveyed by early first birth is manifested at all subsequent ages.

If pregnancy confers some level of protection, how then can breast cancer occur during pregnancy? It has been postulated that during the decade after menarche etiologic factors for the development of breast cancer are operational (66). Pregnancy has a "trigger" effect that, when it occurs in a younger woman, produces either a permanent and positive change in the factors responsible for high risk of development of breast cancer, or changes the breast tissue, making it less susceptible to transformation. The older a woman is when she first becomes pregnant, the more likely she is to have transformed cells already present within the breast at the time of pregnancy. Stimulation of breast tissue during the extraordinary qualitative and quantitative changes in hormone balance that accompany pregnancy may promote these preexisting tumor cells.

Incidence

Wallack et al. reviewed 32 series of pregnancy-associated breast cancer that occurred during the past several decades and reported an incidence of 0.02% to 3.8% (67). A diagnosis of breast cancer occurs in 1 in 10,000 to 1 in 3,000 pregnancies (68), making it and cervical cancer the most common malignancies to occur in pregnancy. In Wallack's review, the average age of patients was between 32 and 38 years. The youngest reported patient was a 16-year-old with widely metastatic breast cancer that complicated her pregnancy (69).

Clinical Manifestations

The most common clinical presentation of breast cancer in the pregnant and nonpregnant patient is a palpable lump (70). Pregnant women present on average with a more advanced stage of disease than their nonpregnant counterparts. In a series from the Princess Margaret Hospital in London, of the 154 patients diagnosed with breast cancer during pregnancy, only 10% were found to have tumors less than 2 cm in diameter and 50% had positive nodes (70). In a similar study from Memorial Sloan-Kettering Cancer Center, seven of 63 cases of pregnancy-associated breast cancer were found to be inoperable at presentation (71). Two patients had distant metastasis, two had signs of local inoperability such as skin metastases or supraclavicular nodal involvement, and three had both distant metastases and signs of advanced local disease. In this same study, breast tumors tended to be larger in pregnant patients. Only 30% of pregnant patients had tumors measuring less than 2 cm, compared with 50% of their nonpregnant controls. Zemlickis and colleagues (72) compared 118 patients with pregnancy-associated breast cancer to 269 nonpregnant controls. Pregnant patients had a significantly lower chance of having stage I disease and were in fact 2.5 times more likely to have distant metastases. King and colleagues studied 63 pregnant patients treated at the Mayo Clinic between 1950 and 1980 and evaluated their clinical presentation (73). Sixty of these patients presented with an asymptomatic breast mass. Three had bloody nipple discharge. The primary tumor was located in the upper outer quadrant in the majority of patients; 90% were within the lateral portion of the breast. Consistent with other studies, their patients tended to present with more advanced tumors, and 8 of these 63 were found to have stage IV disease at presentation.

Debate continues as to whether patients with pregnancy-associated breast cancer present with more advanced disease because of a delay in diagnosis or because the intensified hormonal milieu of pregnancy results in a more aggressive disease. A report by Westberg and colleagues found that pregnant or lactating patients wait an average of 6 months before consulting a physician, and that physicians wait an average of 3 months before performing a biopsy (74). In the Memorial Hospital study of 63 referred patients, fewer than 20% had disease diagnosed and treated during pregnancy. Over 50% of these patients were diagnosed and treated 12 weeks after delivery for a mass noted during pregnancy.

Obstetrician-gynecologists have a major role in screening for breast cancer. A complete breast examination is a mandatory part of the first prenatal visit. As pregnancy progresses, the breasts become more nodular and increase in firmness, making a subtle mass more difficult to detect. Unlike the situation with menstruating females, there is no role for observation in a pregnant patient in whom a breast mass is palpated. Although there is virtually no ionizing radiation delivered to the fetus with abdominal shielding, mammography should not be performed routinely. The increased water content of the breasts makes mammographic detection of breast lesions difficult and inaccurate (75). Ultrasonography of the breast can safely differentiate solid from cystic lesions. Fine needle aspiration can also discern solid from cystic lesions, but due to the hyperproliferation that occurs during pregnancy, aspirate cytology has a high false-positive rate (76). Core needle biopsy may miss the lesion. As with nonpregnant patients, excisional breast biopsy is necessary for definitive diagnosis and should be performed by an experienced surgeon. Excisional biopsy imparts no significant risk to the mother or fetus. Local anesthesia is safer, although general anesthesia is not contraindicated. Byrd and colleagues (77) reported on 134 pregnant patients undergoing general anesthesia for breast biopsy and found only one fetal death, which occurred in an older patient who did not know that she was pregnant at the time of the procedure. Special consideration should be taken for the lactating patient. Milk provides an excellent culture medium, making infection in these patients more common. Milk fistula is not an uncommon complication, especially in centrally located biopsies. Therefore patients should cease lactating before a biopsy is performed. Bromocriptine can be used to stop lactation when necessary.

Evaluation of Metastatic Disease

Before definitive surgery is undertaken for invasive breast cancer, an evaluation for metastatic disease should be completed. As with the nonpregnant female, this evaluation must be thoughtful and individualized. In the nonpregnant asymptomatic patient preoperative screening usually includes a chest roentgenogram and a radionuclide bone scan. If positive, curative surgery is no longer feasible. Additional diagnostic tests are performed as clinically indicated; for example, computerized tomography of the head for patients with neurologic symptoms. In the pregnant patient, radiologic examinations should be performed only when there is a high index of suspicion for distant metastases. In patients with small tumors and a low risk of metastatic disease, these preoperative evaluations have a low diagnostic yield. On the contrary, in patients with large breast masses and a high probability of distant disease, the risk of possible radiation exposure to the fetus is justified.

Treatment

Surgery and Radiation for Local Disease

Local treatment for breast cancer involves either modified radical mastectomy with axillary node dissection or lumpectomy with axillary dissection followed by external beam radiation (Fig. 40-1). The usual course of 5,000 cGy of breast irradiation following lumpectomy can expose a fetus to approximately 10 cGy, if delivered early in the pregnancy, and to as high as 200 cGy later in the pregnancy (78). Typically the fetus receives several tenths of a percent to several percent of the total breast dose. Most of this radiation reaches the fetus by internal scatter and cannot be avoided by shielding. The exact amount of radiation the fetus receives depends on the distance of the fetus from the center of the field, the field size, and the energy source used to deliver the radiation (79). Literature on patients who have received breast irradiation during pregnancy is scant. In addition to safety concerns, it is not certain that the same excellent results in terms of local control enjoyed by nonpregnant patients after lumpectomy and breast irradiation are achieved in the pregnant patient. The pregnant or lactating woman's breast is not physiologically or anatomically equivalent to the nonpregnant breast. For these reasons, many clinicians consider modified radical mastectomy the surgical treatment of choice in order to lower the need for postoperative radiation. However, the option of breast-preserving surgery should be offered to the pregnant patient. If lumpectomy is desired, radiation should be delayed until after delivery. Stage III patients also may require radiation after mastectomy because their risk of chest wall and axillary recurrence is high. Radiation in this group of patients also should be delayed until the postpartum period. If local recurrence occurs during the course of the pregnancy, the nodule should be completely excised and radiation should be deferred until after delivery.

Adjuvant Chemotherapy

Adjuvant chemotherapy with a combination of agents has become the standard of care for premenopausal women with axillary nodal involvement (80). In addition, lymph node–negative patients with tumors larger than 1 cm also appear to benefit from systemic therapy (81). Adjuvant chemotherapy in nonpregnant women can reduce the risk of recurrence and death by approximately 25% (80). Studies have indicated that if a benefit in disease-free survival is to result from adjuvant chemotherapy, it will become evident within the first few years of follow-up, with the advantage likely to result from the first few cycles of treatment. Given this information, most clinicians administer a short course of intensive chemotherapy within weeks following surgery (82).

Data on the effects of *in utero* exposure to chemotherapy come primarily from treatment of women with pregnancy-associated leukemia and lymphoma. Although information regarding drug safety can be extrapolated from these studies, there are additional concerns when dealing with adjuvant therapy for the pregnant patient, namely, whether to treat and when to treat. As tumor size and number of involved nodes increase, so too does the risk of recurrence and death, as well as the benefit gained from adjuvant chemotherapy. The decision to treat must be based on the individual's risk of recurrence and expected benefit from therapy. The pregnant patient in her first trimester presents the greatest treatment dilemma. Many chemotherapeutic agents are potentially teratogenic when administered early in pregnancy, and it is generally recommended from the perspective of fetal safety that treatment be withheld until after the first trimester. However, the benefits of adjuvant therapy may be lost if there is a substantial delay. Clearly, decisions pertaining to when to treat also must be individualized. If chemotherapy is given in the first trimester, the CMF

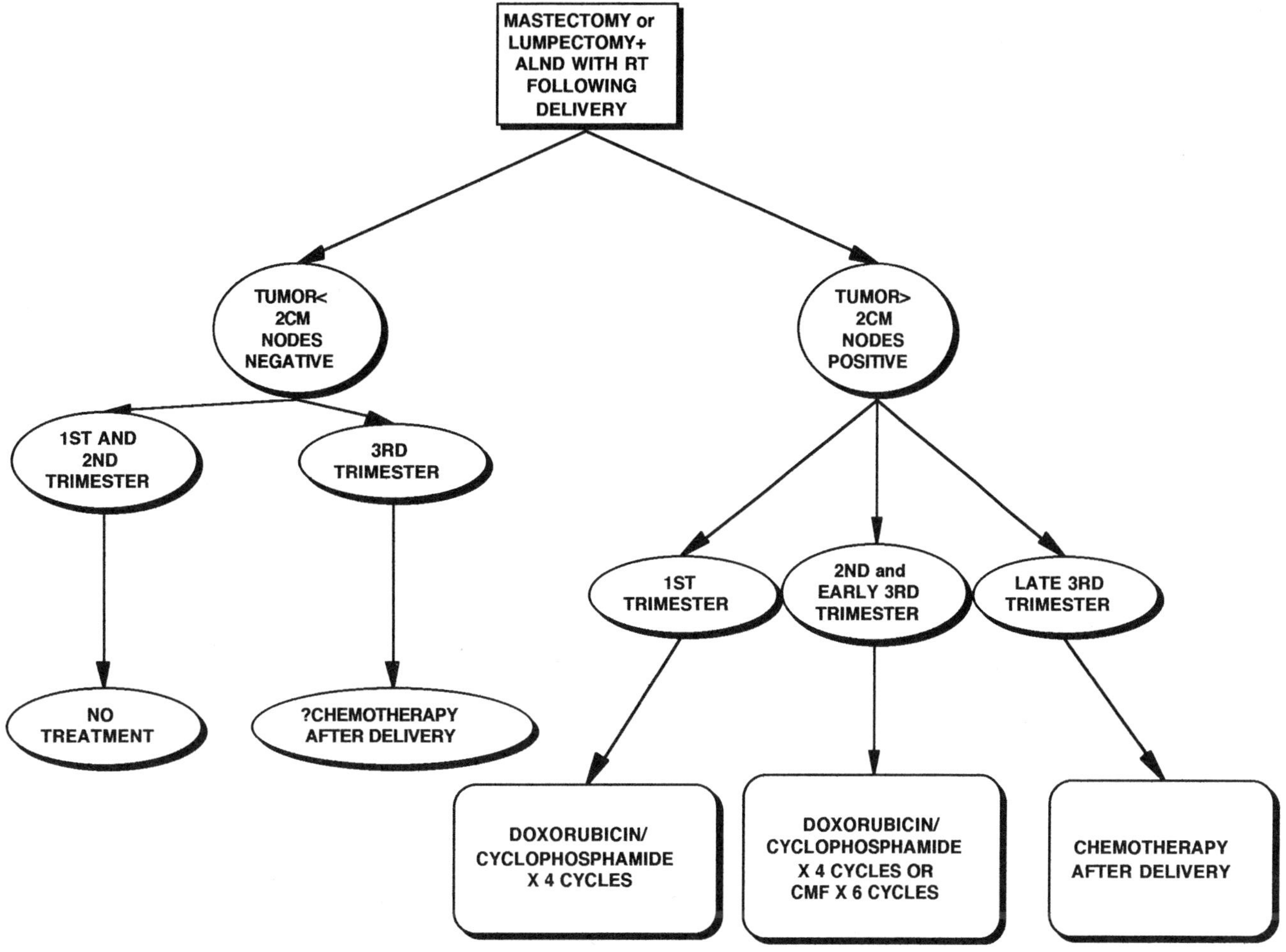

FIG. 40-1. Breast cancer: adjuvant therapy.

[cyclophosphamide, methotrexate, and 5-fluorouracil (5-FU)] regimen should be avoided. Methotrexate and 5-FU are inhibitors of both DNA and RNA synthesis and are teratogenic in early pregnancy (50,83). Most investigators consider doxorubicin and cyclophosphamide a safer drug regimen when given in the first trimester. This combination is administered every 3 weeks for a total of four cycles, and has equal efficacy to six cycles of CMF (82). In the second and third trimester patients may receive either regimen with low risk of fetal harm, although some researchers recommend that methotrexate not be given at any stage of pregnancy (84). Women in their third trimester should in most cases have delivery induced prior to initiating treatment.

Treatment of Metastatic Disease

The treatment of metastatic breast cancer is palliative. The response rates to chemotherapy can be as high as 50% to 70%, yet complete remission occurs in only approximately 10%, with a median duration of response of 3 to 6 months and a median survival of 18 to 24 months (85). Although the risks of chemotherapy and radiation are the same as those for patients receiving adjuvant therapy, the benefits in terms of prolongation of survival are small. The decision to treat a pregnant patient with metastatic breast cancer should be made on an individual basis. Combination chemotherapy consisting of doxorubicin and cyclophosphamide or CMF are the most commonly used regimens for metastatic disease and can effectively palliate symptoms in the majority of patients. Patients with uncontrolled pain or rapidly progressive visceral disease may be candidates for antineoplastic therapy. Newer agents such as the taxanes (paclitaxel and docetaxel), navelbine (a vinca alkaloid), and gemcitabine (a purine analogue) have shown improvement in response rates in the nonpregnant patient. Whether this will translate into an improvement in survival remains to be seen. No data are presently available concerning the use of these agents in pregnant patients and as such they cannot be advocated. Patients with metastatic disease should be monitored for signs and symptoms of cord compression and hypercalcemia, which are common occurrences in these clinical circumstances and require urgent medical attention.

Prognosis

In the past the prognosis of pregnancy-associated breast cancer was considered dismal. Early investigators believed that breast cancer during pregnancy was a distinct disease from that occurring in the nonpregnant patient. In 1943 Haagensen and Stout reported on 20 pregnant patients in whom breast cancer occurred (86), none of which was cured following radical mastectomy. Their article concluded that there was no justification for surgery in the pregnant patient. Subsequently several investigators reported a high incidence of positive nodes in pregnant patients (71–73). In order to assess the influence of pregnancy on the prognosis of breast cancer, one must review studies in which patients were matched for stage. This point is exemplified by a report from Peters and Meakins (87). When compared with a group of 1,992 premenopausal breast cancer patients, their study group of 271 pregnant females had a significantly lower 5-year survival rate. However, when matched for age and stage, there was no difference in 5- and 10-year survival rates between controls and study patients. Similarly, Nugent and O'Connell reported on 176 patients with breast cancer treated between 1970 and 1980 (88). Nineteen (11%) had cancer during pregnancy. Although there was a trend toward a higher stage in the study patients, overall survival was identical when matched for stage and age. An additional study from Memorial Sloan-Kettering reported on 56 pregnant patients who underwent radical or modified radical mastectomy (71). These cases were compared with 166 nonpregnant controls of similar age. When matched for stage, the 5- and 10-year survival rates were nearly identical. Among patients with negative nodes, the 5- and 10-year survival rates for both groups was 82% and 77%, respectively. Among the node-positive patients, the 5-year survival rates were 47% in the pregnancy-associated group and 59% in nonpregnant women. The 10-year survival rates were 25% and 41%, respectively, not statistically significantly different. Only one recent controlled study from Norway demonstrated a worse prognosis for the pregnant patient when matched for stage (71). In this study only 3 of 20 patients were alive after 4 years. The reasons for this disparate result are not clear.

It appears that overall, pregnancy-associated breast cancer does have a worse outcome despite equivalent survivals when matched stage for stage. It is the association with a more advanced stage of disease at presentation that portends a worse prognosis. Whether early detection can alter this fact remains to be seen.

Safety of Subsequent Pregnancy after Breast Cancer

An important and related issue involves the question of safety of pregnancy after a diagnosis of breast cancer. Hormonal events and changes have been shown to have an effect on the development of breast cancer. For a woman who has survived breast cancer, the issue is not only that of a second primary, but that of dormant micrometastases stimulated by the hormonal changes that occur during pregnancy. Several published studies report no detrimental effects of subsequent pregnancy. For example, Harvey and colleagues described 41 patients who became pregnant following a diagnosis of breast cancer (89). Even among the node-positive patients there appeared to be no increase in recurrence of the disease. A 1986 French study reported no difference in survival in breast cancer survivors who subsequently became pregnant (90). Another study from Memorial Sloan-Kettering of 16 patients whom became pregnant after mastectomy also found no difference in the 10-year survival rate (91). Unfortunately, a good survival in a highly selected group of patients does not prove or disprove the safety of pregnancy after a diagnosis of breast cancer. Petrek critically reviewed the Memorial study (92). She assumed that 7% of breast cancer patients under 40 become pregnant and concluded that to have adequate statistical power this study should have reported on at least 450 patients. Although it is tempting to conclude from the published reports that pregnancy after breast cancer is safe, the effect of pregnancy on tumor recurrence remains unclear. Most clinicians recommend that a patient should delay childbearing for at least 2 years because disease usually manifests within this time frame in those patients with aggressive disease and a poor prognosis.

MALIGNANT MELANOMA

Definition

Malignant melanoma is an increasingly common neoplasm that originates from normal melanocytes found within the skin. These melanocytes, which rarely proliferate in normal skin, are somehow transformed to become highly aggressive and often fatal tumors.

Etiology

The precise etiology of malignant melanoma remains unknown. There is little doubt nevertheless that it is the result of multiple genetic and environmental influences. Ultraviolet radiation (specifically ultraviolet B) has been implicated in the genesis of melanoma (93). The development and progression of the disease depends not only on ultraviolet exposure but on the individual's genotype, phenotype, and immunocompetence (93,94). Familial melanomas account for 8% to 12% of all cases (95). Recently, a germline mutation within the p21 region of chromosome 9 has been linked to these familial cases (95). Alterations in chromosomes 1, 6, 7, 10, and 11 also have been found to occur in melanoma lesions (96,97). The possible influence of reproductive or hormonal factors on the pathogenesis of melanoma has intrigued scientists and clinicians for decades. Compared with men, female patients tend to have more favorable lesions with regard to site, thickness, and stage (98,99). Melanoma in women tends to metastasize more slowly, and survival after the detection of metastatic disease is significantly longer in women than in men (99,100). Although melanoma is not considered a hormone-responsive disease, this circumstantial evidence suggests that endocrine factors may influence its behavior and prognosis. No association between risk of melanoma and age at menarche or duration of reproductive years has been found. Several retrospective studies have attempted to assess the protective effects of pregnancy (100–102). In a recent review of pregnancy and melanoma, the researchers concluded that there was no convincing evidence for a protective effect of pregnancy on the subsequent development of melanoma (103). Present molecular and clinical research on melanoma is aimed at deciphering the plethora of molecular and biochemical alterations that lead to the malignant phenotype.

Incidence

Melanoma incidence has increased 500% since the 1930's and affects approximately 32,000 individuals in the United States each year (104). By the year 2000 it is predicted that 1 in 75 individuals will develop melanoma in their lifetime (105). High-risk populations have been defined and include individuals with fair complexions and a propensity to sunburn, as well as individuals with numerous common nevi, a history of dysplastic nevi, and concomitant diseases such as immunodeficiency, immunosuppression, and xeroderma pigmentosum. The association of pregnancy with melanoma is fortunately uncommon, with an incidence of 0.14 to 2.8 cases per 1,000 births (106). Melanoma accounts for 8% of all malignancies diagnosed during pregnancy (107).

Clinical Presentation

Melanomas may be located on any part of the body, but in women the lesions are found most commonly on the lower extremities. If melanoma is discovered when it is a thin lesion, it is curable by wide local excision. All clinicians should familiarize themselves with the ABCD's of early diagnosis:

A = asymmetry of the lesion.
B = border irregularity.
C = color variation.
D = diameter greater than 6 mm.

Preexisting nevi may enlarge and become darker during pregnancy. Although the impression that nevi undergo malignant transformation more frequently during pregnancy has not been substantiated, the clinician should not hesitate to obtain an excisional biopsy sample of any lesion in which a change in size, configuration, or color occurs.

Microstaging of melanoma has important prognostic implications. Microstaging can be done by the Breslow staging method (108), which measures the thickness of the lesion, or Clark staging (109), which uses the depth of penetration of the malignant cells into the dermal layers and subcutaneous fat. Tumor thickness appears to be a more accurate and reproducible prognostic indicator. The American Joint Committee on Cancer has developed a uniform staging system based on tumor thickness, nodal metastases, and distant spread (110).

The presence of ulceration is an adverse prognostic sign independent of tumor stage. Reintgen and colleagues from Duke University examined 58 pregnant patients with stage I melanoma, 43 patients with stage I melanoma who became pregnant within 5 years of the diagnosis, and a control group of patients 15 to 44 years of age with stage I melanoma who were not pregnant either at diagnosis or within 5 years (111). Among the 58 pregnant women, median tumor thickness was 1.90 ± 0.39 mm. Superficial spreading melanoma was the dominant histologic type. Twenty percent of these patients had ulceration. Tumor thickness, level of invasion, and ulceration were significantly greater in the pregnant patients than in the control groups. In a retrospective review by Colbourn and colleagues, 103 patients were grouped into those diagnosed with melanoma during pregnancy, those in whom a diagnosis was made after their last pregnancy, and those with no history of pregnancy. Cases were analyzed as to stage, site of primary, depth of invasion, history of a preexisting nevus, family history, and outcome. They found no differences among the three groups with regard to any of these clinical parameters. Travers and colleagues studied 45 patients with melanoma diagnosed during pregnancy or within 1 year postpartum and compared them with a group of 420 controls (112). They found a statistically significant difference in tumor thickness between the two groups. Melanoma associated with pregnancy had a median tumor thickness of 2.28 mm compared with 1.22 mm in the control group. Surprisingly, survival among the two groups was similar.

From these recent reports it appears that in comparison with nonpregnant women, pregnant patients have no difference in the location or histologic type of their tumors, or in the presence of preexisting nevi. However, they may have greater tumor thickness. This increased thickness may be related to a delay in diagnosis. Travers and colleagues noted that 37% of his pregnant patients were diagnosed within 3 months of delivery. Medical records for many of these patients indicated that the patient had been advised to wait until after delivery to undergo excisional biopsy of the suspicious lesion.

Treatment

Surgery is the only effective treatment for malignant melanoma and, once a diagnosis is made, should be performed without delay. Control of the primary lesion requires wide local excision with at least a 1-cm margin of surrounding normal tissue (113). Regional lymph nodes are the most common site of metastatic disease; surgical excision of involved nodes can therefore provide regional disease control and is of prognostic significance. Therapeutic lymph node dissection involves removal of clinically demonstrable nodes. Elective lymph node dissection (ELND) involves resection of nonpalpable regional nodes in an attempt to decrease local recurrence and improve on disease-free survival because of the high risk of occult metastatic disease. Slingluff and colleagues examined 100 women with pregnancy-associated melanoma (114). The site of first metastasis was nodal in 70% and cutaneous in 13%. Among this group of patients only 50% were alive after 10 years. They noted a significantly higher incidence of nodal metastases in the study group and suggested that ELND be considered in the pregnant patients with melanoma. His approach remains unsubstantiated and controversial. Sentinel node biopsy uses intraoperative lymphatic mapping to identify the "sentinel" or first node to which the melanoma spreads. This node is removed and examined pathologically. If metastases have occurred to the sentinel node, all regional nodes are removed. If the sentinel node is negative, no further dissection is required. Sentinel node biopsy and lymphatic mapping is presently investigative and should be performed only in the context of a clinical trial.

Adjuvant Therapy for Malignant Melanoma

Patients who have deep primary melanoma (>4 mm) or melanoma metastatic to regional lymph nodes have a high risk of relapse and a mortality rate of 50% to 90% (115). In the past no adjuvant therapy had been shown to have an impact on relapse-free and overall survival. In 1996 Kirkwood and colleagues published the results of a large cooperative group trial examining the effects of alpha interferon as adjuvant therapy for patients with deep or regionally metastatic melanoma (116). They concluded that treatment with maximally tolerated doses of interferon alpha-2b resulted in a significantly prolonged relapse-free survival and a prolonged overall survival. However, interferon therapy is not currently approved for use during pregnancy. Pons and colleagues reported two cases of women who received alpha interferon prior to elective abortion (117) and found undetectable levels in fetal blood or amniotic fluid. Ruggiero reported a normal pregnancy outcome in a woman treated inadvertently with alpha interferon in her first trimester for hepatitis C infection (118). Until more information becomes available, adjuvant interferon cannot be recommended for pregnant patients at high risk for recurrence. However, because the patients in the Kirkwood trial received therapy for a total of 52 weeks, it may be advantageous to initiate treatment after delivery in patients who present late in pregnancy. Whether a prolonged interval between the time of resection and initiation of adjuvant therapy will mitigate the beneficial effects of interferon is not known.

Therapy for Metastatic Disease

Melanoma can metastasize to any organ or tissue in the body. Clinical evaluation often underestimates the extent of spread, and the majority of patients die with disseminated disease involving multiple organ sites. Patients with metastatic disease have an overall median survival of about 6 months (119). Treatment of metastatic melanoma is palliative and symptomatic only. Few chemotherapeutic agents have demonstrated activity against melanoma. Dacarbazine, the nitrosoureas, and cisplatinum appear to have the most activity, although these drugs either alone or in combination have produced response rates of only 10% to 20% (119). Additionally, there is a paucity of information available on the use of these drugs during pregnancy. Because they are of questionable benefit in the nonpregnant patient, their use in the pregnant patient with metastatic melanoma cannot be recommended.

Prognosis of Pregnant Patients with Melanoma

A number of case series and uncontrolled studies have suggested that pregnancy may worsen the prognosis of malignant melanoma. The first was published in 1951 by Pack and Scharnnagel, who reviewed 1,050 patients with melanoma (120), 10 of whom were diagnosed during pregnancy. Of these 10 patients, half died within 3 years of diagnosis, leading these investigators to conclude that melanomas grow and metastasize rapidly during pregnancy. In addition, they recommended that women with melanoma should avoid pregnancy for at least 3 to 5 years after the initial diagnosis. In 1983 Sutherland identified 18 patients with melanoma diagnosed during pregnancy and compared them with 12 unmatched nonpregnant subjects (121). Tumor thickness was unknown for most patients. After 5 years of follow-up, 4 of the pregnant patients were alive compared with 10 from the nonpregnant group. Although these groups were not directly comparable, Sutherland concluded that pregnant melanoma patients had a disproportionately higher mortality rate. To draw meaningful conclusions about the prognosis of pregnancy-associated melanoma, one must evaluate studies that include a control group of nonpregnant women of childbearing age; provide information regarding tumor stage, thickness, and location; and have long-term follow-up data. In one such study, Reitgen reported on 58 pregnant patients with stage I melanoma (111). The control group consisted of 585 stage I patients 14 to 55 years of age who either were not pregnant at the time of diagnosis or were pregnant within 5 years of the diagnosis. Information regarding tumor thickness was available for most patients, and the pregnant patients had significantly thicker tumors. There was no statistically significant difference in actuarial survival between study subjects and controls, despite a significantly shorter disease-free interval in the study group. In a matched control study,

Slingluff and colleagues found a similar trend (114). They too noted a significantly shorter disease-free interval in the pregnant cases, but no difference in the overall survival rate.

In 1989 McManamny reviewed 23 pregnant patients with stage I melanoma and compared them with 243 age-matched controls (122). In this study there was no difference in overall survival or disease-free survival between the two groups. Tumor thickness also was greater for pregnant patients, and the investigators concluded that pregnancy appears to have no influence on survival from melanoma. Controlled studies by Wong and colleagues (123) and MacKie and colleagues (124) also found no difference in disease-free or overall survival in the pregnant patients with melanoma. Wong noted a higher frequency of head, neck, and trunk lesions within the study group, which tend to have a poorer prognosis.

In conclusion, it has been suggested that pregnancy may affect the prognosis of malignant melanoma. However, inferences from retrospective, nonrandomized studies have led to this belief. Although pregnancy-associated melanomas may be thicker and may be associated with a shorter disease-free interval, five controlled studies have failed to confirm pregnancy as a significant adverse prognostic indicator. Care must be taken in interpreting these data because the size of the study samples may be too small to draw firm conclusions. In addition, these studies included mostly patients with stage I disease, and no conclusions can therefore be made regarding patients with a higher stage of melanoma at presentation.

HODGKIN DISEASE

Definition

Hodgkin disease is a unique hematologic malignancy first described by Thomas Hodgkin in 1832 (125). It has a distinct histopathologic appearance and is defined by the presence in the affected tissues of Reed-Sternberg giant cells, thought to represent the malignant cell line, in a background of inflammatory cells and lymphocytes. Although Reed-Sternberg cells are necessary for the diagnosis, they are not specific and can occur in other conditions.

Incidence

Hodgkin disease compromises approximately 40% of all lymphomas and has a bimodal distribution centering around ages 25 and 75 years (126). Because it is often a disease of younger people, it is not uncommon to find Hodgkin disease associated with pregnancy. It is estimated that one third of women with Hodgkin disease are pregnant or have delivered within 1 year of diagnosis (127,128). Its incidence during pregnancy has been reported to range from 1 in 1,000 to 1 in 6,000 pregnancies (128,129).

Etiology

The etiology of Hodgkin disease is not known. There is a 2.5 times higher risk of developing the disease among persons without siblings when compared with those with four or more (130). Clustering among communities has been described, and improved living conditions are associated with a higher incidence (131). These observations have led many researchers to conclude that an infectious childhood disease with a delayed adult exposure may be etiologic (130,131). Epstein-Barr virus has been associated with a subset of patients with the disease (132). There is no known influence of hormonal factors on the development of Hodgkin disease, although an epidemiologic study from Norway concluded that there was a lower incidence of Hodgkin's disease in women of high parity (133). In a case control study Zwitter and colleagues attempted to evaluate the role of pregnancy in the pathogenesis and clinical course of Hodgkin disease (134). They could not confirm the protective effects of pregnancy for the risk of Hodgkin disease.

Pathophysiology

Hodgkin lymphoma is subclassified histopathologically into four distinct categories. Lymphocyte predominant has the most favorable prognosis and is frequently asymptomatic at presentation. The nodular sclerosis variant occurs in young women, making it the most likely subtype to occur during pregnancy. Among 17 pregnant patients with Hodgkin disease reported by Gelb and colleagues, 13 had the nodular sclerosis type (135). In a similar study by Jacobs and colleagues, of 15 pregnant patients, all had a diagnosis of nodular sclerosis (136). The mixed cellularity pattern occurs in middle-aged individuals and usually manifests as systemic disease. The lymphocyte-depleted type has the least favorable prognosis and usually occurs in elderly men with advanced disease. It is rarely seen in pregnancy.

Clinical Presentation

Most women with Hodgkin disease present with an asymptomatic enlarging mass. Lymphadenopathy usually occurs first in the neck and progresses in an orderly and predictable fashion from one lymph node group to the next. The nodes are rubbery and nontender and are detected on routine physical examination or by the patient. Gelb examined the clinical characteristics of 15 patients with Hodgkin disease occurring during pregnancy (135). The median patient age in his study was 27 years. No patient presented with stage I disease (involvement of one lymph node region). Nine patients had stage II disease (involvement of at least two lymph node regions on the same side of the diaphragm). Four patients had stage III disease (involvement of lymph node regions on both sides of the diaphragm) and two had stage IV disease (involvement of one or more extralymphatic sites). Gestational age at diagnosis ranged from 3 to 30 weeks. The Jacobs study reported a similar stage distribution among their 136 patients, with the majority presenting with stage II disease. Staging in these two reports involved clinical staging only, raising the possibility that some patients may have been understaged. Unexplained fever, night sweats, and weight loss are usually manifestations of late disease and portend a worse prognosis. These "B" symptoms occur often in pregnancy-associated Hodgkin disease. Pruritus is also a prevalent complaint and has no prognostic significance. Pulmonary involvement, hepatic complications, and superior vena cava syndrome can occur, but these are rare manifestations.

Laboratory Findings

Anemia is the most common hematologic abnormality found at diagnosis. In most cases the anemia is mild and normochromic and normocytic. The leukocyte count may be increased; leukopenia is uncommon. Lymphopenia occurs in approximately one third of patients with Hodgkin disease. These hematologic abnormalities do not reflect the extent of the disease. Platelet counts are usually normal. When they are low, bone marrow involvement is likely. Bone marrow biopsy reveals Hodgkin disease in only 9% of patients at the time of diagnosis (131). Granulomas and lymphoid aggregates may be seen in the marrow and do not signify marrow involvement. An elevated sedimentation rate is common in Hodgkin disease and can be helpful in following disease activity. Studies of the immune system in patients with Hodgkin disease reveal a defect in cellular immunity that persists for several years following treatment.

Staging of the Pregnant Patient

Lymphomas are clinically staged using the medical history, physical examination, hemogram, biochemical tests, bone marrow biopsy results, and radiologic studies (Fig. 40-2). Traditonally Hodgkin disease has been surgically staged by exploratory laparotomy and splenectomy. Patients with intraabdominal disease were treated with chemotherapy, whereas those with stage I and II disease received radiation therapy. As the long-term toxicity of radiation therapy has become more clearly defined, clinicians are now treating early stage disease with chemotherapeutic agents, making meticulous surgical staging unnecessary. Nonpregnant patients are routinely staged with computerized tomography and, where available, lymphangiography. The effects of ionizing radiation have been discussed previously. A chest x-ray with abdominal shielding should be performed as part of the staging procedure in the pregnant patient. A single image abdominal film 24 hours after injection for a lymphangiogram is considered safe and can aid in the evaluation of the paraaortic nodes (137). Computerized tomography is not recommended for staging during pregnancy (129). Sonography, although not used as part of standard staging, may be a practical alternative. MRI also does not expose the fetus to ionizing radiation and is helpful in evaluating disease in the abdomen and the pelvis. MRI of the chest can evaluate the hilar, mediastinal, and paratracheal nodes. Surgery per se is not contraindicated during pregnancy, yet most investigators do not advocate staging laparotomy in the pregnant patient.

Treatment

The management of Hodgkin disease in the pregnant patient is complex and must be individualized. However, some generalizations regarding treatment can be made. In 1981 Jacobs and colleagues reported on 15 pregnant patients with Hodgkin disease (136). Based on their experience and a review of the available literature, they made treatment recommendations that are still followed by most clinicians. A schema for treatment based on their work is outlined in Fig. 40-2 and summarized as follows:

1. Patients with stage I, IIA, or IIB supradiaphragmatic disease in their second or third trimester should be observed and treated following delivery. Delivery should be induced as soon as the fetus has achieved pulmonary maturity.
2. Patients who have stage I, IIA, or IIB supradiaphragmatic disease that is rapidly growing or who have severe systemic symptoms should be treated with radiation therapy with a modified dose and field.
3. Patients with stage I, IIA, or IIB and stage III or IV subdiaphragmatic disease in their second or third trimester should have treatment delayed as above unless they have severe systemic symptoms or rapidly growing disease, or the tumor is impinging on vital structures of the mother or fetus.
4. Patients with stage III or IV disease who have major disease of concern above the diaphragm should have low-dose radiation to those supradiaphragmatic areas of concern.
5. Chemotherapy is indicated for subdiaphragmatic disease that requires treatment.

In 1986 investigators at Memorial Hospital published their experience with 17 pregnant patients with Hodgkin disease (137). Six underwent voluntary abortion. Seven were treated with limited supradiaphragmatic radiation to disease sites, followed by complete staging and further

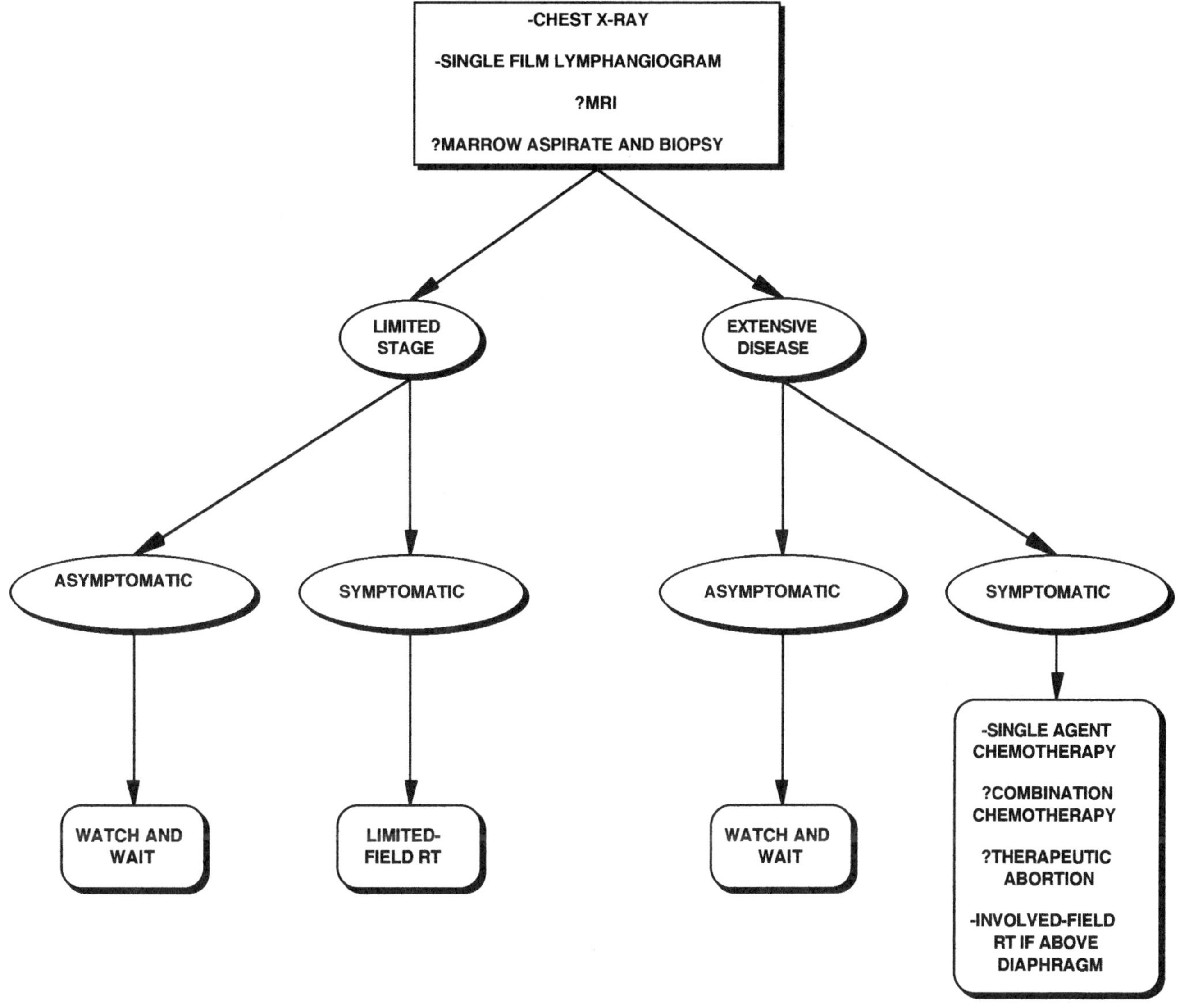

FIG. 40-2. Hodgkin disease: staging evaluation.

therapy postpartum. Total doses of radiation received during pregnancy ranged from 18 to 20 cGy. These investigators also advocated modification of radiation dose and field when delivered to the pregnant patient.

Woo and colleagues studied 775 women with a diagnosis of Hodgkin disease, 25 (3.2%) of whom were pregnant at diagnosis (79). Prior to treatment six women in their first trimester had a therapeutic abortion and three patients in their third trimester delivered at term. The remaining 16 patients were treated with 40 cGy to either the neck, neck and mediastinum, or full mantle depending on their sites of disease. The majority of patients had clinical stage IIA disease. These patients were evaluated for outcome of pregnancy and for whether any of their children developed congenital malformations or subsequent malignancies. Estimated time of gestation at the initiation of treatment ranged from 6 to 32 weeks. All 16 patients delivered normal full-term babies. Estimated radiation doses to the mid-plane of the fetus ranged from 1.4 to 13.6 cGy. Only one patient developed a treatment-related complication of incomplete transverse myelitis. The researchers concluded that 40 cGy could be safely administered to pregnant patients and that radiobiologic principles suggest that delays of several months between treatments may be less effective than continuous treatment and that split course treatment of the pregnant patient with Hodgkin disease may be disadvantageous.

Curative chemotherapy regimens for the nonpregnant patient with Hodgkin disease include combinations of drugs such as nitrogen mustard, vinca alkaloids, dacarbazine and procarbazine, doxorubicin, bleomycin, and prednisone. Estimated survival rates are between 70% and 90% for stage I and II patients (138). Although there does not appear to be an increased risk of congenital defects in women exposed to certain chemotherapeutic agents during the second and third trimesters, some researchers feel that combination regimens should be avoided unless the patient has poor prognostic features (129,135,136,139–141). Single-agent vinblastine may be used to control disease until after delivery, at which time additional drugs can be given (142). In the Memorial Hospital study one patient who presented at 18 weeks' gestation was treated to term with vinblastine without untoward effects (139). Jacobs also recommended single-agent vinblastine when treatment with chemotherapy becomes necessary (136). Extrapolating from the leukemic data, it appears that the anthracyclins can also be given when chemotherapy is indicated in pregnancy.

Maternal and Fetal Outcomes Following Treatment for Hodgkin Disease

Lishner and colleagues reported a case–control study of 48 pregnant patients with Hodgkin disease seen at the Princess Margaret Hospital (143). The effects of Hodgkin disease on the course and survival of these patients was studied and compared with nonpregnant controls matched for age and stage at presentation. Among these 48 patients there were 40 deliveries (two of which were stillborn), 5 miscarriages, and 4 induced abortions. No differences were found between babies born to women with Hodgkin disease and controls with regard to birth weight, gestational age, or method of delivery. One child was born with hydrocephaly. Her mother had received combination chemotherapy during the first trimester. When compared with the general population, the total number of stillbirths among the patients with Hodgkin disease was not statistically different. With regard to the effects of pregnancy on the outcome of Hodgkin disease, the authors failed to detect a statistically significant difference in survival among cases and controls. They concluded that Hodgkin disease occurring in pregnancy did not have a more adverse outcome than in nonpregnant patients. Pregnant women did not present with a higher stage of disease, and pregnancy did not change the biology of the tumor or postpone diagnosis.

In the study by Woo and colleagues, 12 patients remained disease free for 1 to 31 years (79). Four developed relapsed disease, two of whom died despite salvage therapy. The 10-year disease-free survival rate in this study was 71%, which was comparable with that of nonpregnant patients. They too found that the outcome of Hodgkin disease was not affected adversely by pregnancy. All offspring were physically and mentally normal, and none developed a malignancy during the time of follow-up.

Aviles reported on the outcome of fetuses born to mothers with Hodgkin disease (60). He followed 14 cases of mothers treated with chemotherapy during pregnancy, including 5 cases of women who received treatment during the first trimester. All infants were normal and without evidence of congenital abnormalities. These children have been followed for a mean of 10 years and have not been found to differ from controls and siblings in IQ, immune function, hematologic studies, and cytogenetics. Swerdlow and colleagues followed the reproductive outcome of 340 patients with Hodgkin disease treated between 1970 and 1991 (144). They did not find an increase in the number of stillbirths, low birth weight, or congenital abnormalities among 49 offspring studied. Chromosomal analysis was performed on 45 of these children, and all were normal except one child with Down syndrome.

Role of Induced Abortion

The role of induced abortion in pregnant women with Hodgkin disease remains controversial; however, most experts would agree with the following guidelines based on the fetal risks of therapy:

1. In early pregnancy (first trimester), abortion should be considered, especially when delay of treatment to later in the pregnancy is unacceptable
2. Abortion should be strongly considered by patients who become pregnant while receiving treatment, especially patients who have been treated with greater than 0.010 Gy to the pelvis or have received teratogenic chemotherapy.
3. Patients with subdiaphragmatic disease, visceral disease, or systemic symptoms or those with bulky mediastinal disease who require combined modality treatment and are in the first or second trimester should consider terminating the pregnancy.

NON-HODGKIN LYMPHOMA

Definition

The NHLs are a heterogeneous group of neoplasms that have in common a clonal proliferation of T- or B-lymphocytes. One of the more confusing and controversial areas concerning the NHLs is the classification of these disorders. Several schemas have been devised since the original description by Thomas Hodgkin in 1832. The Working Formulation was created as a means to provide a mophologic classification with clinical relevance. This classification divides the NHLs into three broad categories: the low-grade, the intermediate, and the high-grade lymphomas. An updated classification system named the REAL (Revised European American Classification of Lymphoid Malignancy) classification also has been devised (145). Most pregnancy-associated lymphomas are of the intermediate and high-grade types. The low-grade lymphomas are typically a disease of older patients and will not be discussed in this review.

Etiology

The NHLs serve as a model for understanding cancer as a genetic disease. Many cytogenetic abnormalities have been found to underly the NHLs. Viruses such as Epstein-Barr virus and the human T-lymphotropic virus type 1 (HTLV-1) may have a pathogenic role. Immunodeficiency states such as severe combined immunodeficiency, common variable immunodeficiency, organ transplantation, and acquired immunodeficiency syndrome increase the risk of developing NHL. Patients with autoimmune disorders (systemic lupus erythematosis, rheumatoid arthritis, and angioblastic lymphadenopathy) are also at an increased risk of developing lymphoma, suggesting that immune dysregulation plays a major role in the development of this disease.

Incidence

Lymphoid neoplasms have a variable worldwide distribution. The NHLs are more common in men than in women, with a ratio between 1.5 and 3.5:1 (146). Lymphomas are more common in adults than in children and have a steady increase in incidence from childhood through 80 years of age. More than 40,000 new cases per year will be diagnosed in the United States in the 1990's, and the incidence of NHL is increasing (147). The prevalence of NHL occurring during pregnancy is not known. Ward and Weiss reviewed the literature from 1937 to 1989 and could find only 75 cases of lymphoma previously diagnosed in a patient who became pregnant, who was newly diagnosed during pregnancy, or who was diagnosed postpartum with the onset of the disease having occurred during pregnancy (148).

Staging Evaluation in the Pregnant Patient

The staging system of NHLs is identical to that of Hodgkin lymphoma. The NHLs tend to be widely disseminated at the time of diagnosis. Local therapy is rarely indicated in this group of disorders, making surgical staging and lymphangiogram unnecessary. B symptoms such as fever, night sweats, and weight loss carry less predictive value than they do in Hodgkin lymphoma. Bone marrow biopsy and aspirate and cerbrospinal fluid cytology are an essential part of the evaluation of disease extent in the intermediate and high-grade lymphomas because these are areas commonly involved with disease.

Clinical Presentation

Patients with NHL typically present with a higher stage of disease than patients with Hodgkin disease. This is also true for patients with pregnancy-associated NHL. NHL in pregnancy is typically associated with an aggressive histology. Most reported cases involve either a diffuse large cell lymphoma or a Burkitt's type. Gelb and colleagues reported on 12 cases of NHL in pregnancy (135). Most of these patients had stage III or IV disease at diagnosis. Two cases presented with a periuterine mass. One patient had facial weakness attributed to cranial nerve involvement. Steiner-Salz and colleagues described six cases of pregnancy-associated NHL (149). Five of the six had stage IV disease. One patient presented with gastrointestinal bleeding secondary to involvement of the stomach. One had tracheal compression from a mediastinal mass, and a third had obstructive jaundice from enlarged porta hepatis nodes. All had markedly elevated lactate dehydrogenase levels, reflecting a high tumor burden. Falkson and colleagues reported a case of NHL in a 26-year-old pregnant woman who required emergent tracheostomy because the disease had infiltrated the trachea, great vessels, and thyroid gland, resulting in respiratory obstruction and decompensation (150). In addition, these researchers reviewed 13 previously reported cases, 11 of which were large cell lymphoma, one Burkitt lymphoma, and one of diffuse mixed histology. Only one of these 13 patients was successfully treated.

Burkitt lymphoma presenting in pregnancy typically pursues a rapidly progressive and fatal course. Breast and ovarian involvement are common. Jones and colleagues presented a case of a 17-year-old primigravida at 15 weeks gestation who developed bluish discoloration and enlargement of both breasts and died within 7 days (151). Autopsy revealed complete replacement of all normal breast tissue with Burkitt lymphoma. They reported on five other cases of Burkitt lymphoma in association with pregnancy. In all, the clinical presentation was fulminant, with massive unilateral or bilateral breast enlargement. Breast involvement by Burkitt lymphoma in the nonpregnant patient is uncommon.

Treatment

Unlike Hodgkin disease, the combination of NHL and pregnancy carries a grim prognosis. Few women with NHL have delivered live infants, and most have died with progressive disease prior to delivery or shortly after therapeutic abortion. In 1977 Ortega reported the first case of pregnancy-associated NHL successfully treated with combination chemotherapy (152), raising the possibility that some of these patients may be salvaged. Weiss and Ward reviewed 45 cases of NHL in pregnancy (148). Twenty-one of them received no treatment, seven underwent some form of surgery, four were treated with radiation alone, and the remainder were treated with either single-agent or combination chemotherapy. Twenty-eight patients died and 17 infants survived.

Given the rarity of the NHLs in pregnancy, there is no consensus on the most appropriate management of these patients. It appears that if the disease is detected early in pregnancy, immediate initiation of chemotherapy is required for the survival of the mother and fetus. If the diagnosis occurs close to term, one may wait for delivery and initiate therapy immediately postpartum. In the event of progressive disease or in the case of Burkitt lymphoma, therapy should not be delayed. Active chemotherapeutic agents include the anthracyclines, the vinca alkaloids, cyclophosphamide, vincristine, and prednisone. In the rare case of localized disease, radiation therapy may be employed and can be used in advanced disease as a temporizing measure. Some investigators have reported a rapid deterioration postpartum. The frequency of this event is unclear.

In summary, NHL in association with pregnancy is a rare occurrence. In pregnancy these lymphomas usually are characterized by an aggressive histology and advanced stage. NHL in pregnancy commonly results in the death of the mother. Treatment must be individualized. It appears that the only hope for an improved outcome is prompt intensive combination chemotherapy.

REFERENCES

1. Wingo PA, Tong T, Bolden S. Cancer Statistics. CA Cancer J Clin 1995;45:8–30.
2. Donegan WL. Cancer and Pregnancy. CA Cancer J Clin 1983;33: 194–214.
3. Haas JF. Pregnancy in association with newly diagnosed cancer: a population-based epidemiologic assessment. Int J Cancer 1984;34: 229–235.
4. Zemlickis D, Lishner M, Degendorfer P, Panzarella T, Sutcliffe SB, Koren G. Fetal outcome after in utero exposure to cancer chemotherapy. Ann Intern Med 1992;152:573–576.
5. Reynoso EE, Shepard FA, Messner HA, Farquharson HA, Garvey MB, Baker MA. Acute leukemia during pregnancy: the Toronto Leukemia Study Group Experience with long term follow-up of children exposed in utero to chematherapeutic agents. J Clin Oncol 1987;5: 1098–1106.
6. Blatt J, Mulvihill JJ, Ziegler JL, Young RL, Poplack DG. Pregnancy outcome following cancer chemotherapy. Am J Med 1980;69: 828–832.
7. Sweet DL Jr, Kinzie J. Consequences of radiotherapy and antineoplastic therapy for the fetus. J Reprod Med 1976;17:241–246.
8. Barber HR. Fetal and neonatal effects of cytotoxic agents. Obstet Gynecol 1981;58:415–475.
9. Pirani BK, Campbell DM, MacGillivray I. Plasma volume in normal first pregnancy. J Obstet Gynecol Br Commonw 1973;80:884–887.
10. Mucklow SC. The fate of drugs during pregnancy. Clin Obstet Gynecol 1986;13:161–175.
11. Redmond GP. Physiological changes during pregnancy and their implications for pharmacological treatment. Clin Invest Med 1985;8: 317–322.
12. Doll DC, Ringenburg Q, Yarbro JW. Management of cancer during pregnancy. Arch Intern Med 1988;148:2058–2064.
13. Zenk KE. An overview of perinatal clinical pharmacology. Clin Lab Med 1981;1:361–375.
14. Wiebe VJ, Sipila PE. Pharmacology of antineoplastic agents in pregnancy. Crit Rev Oncol Hematol 1994;16:75–112.
15. Brent RL, Bolden BT. The indirect effects of irradiation on embryonic development III. The contribution of ovarian irradiation, uterine irradiation, oviduct irradiation, and zygote irradiation to fetal mortality and growth retardation in the rat. Radiat Res 1967;30:759–773.
16. Russell LB. X-ray induced developmental abnormalities in the mouse and their use in analysis of embryological patterns. J Exp Zool 1950; 114:545.
17. Brent RL. The effect of embryonic and fetal exposure to x-ray, microwaves and ultrasound: counseling the pregnant and non-pregnant patient about these risks. Semin Oncol 1989;16:347–368.
18. Konerman C. Postimplantation defects in development. Adv Radiat Biol 1987;155.
19. Yamazaki J, Wright S, Wright P. Outcome of pregnancy in women exposed to the atomic bomb in Nagasaki. Am J Dis Child 1954;87:448.
20. Miller RW. Delayed radiation effects in atomic bomb survivors. Science 1969;166:569–574.
21. Dekaban AS. Abnormalities in children exposed to x-radiation during various stages of gestation: tentative timetable of radiation injury to the human fetus. I. J Nucl Med 1968;9:471–477.
22. Hammerman-Jacobsen K. Therapeutic abortion on account of x-ray examination during pregnancy. Dan Med Bull 1959;6:113.
23. American College of Obstetricians and Gynecologists. Committee Opinion Guidelines for diagnostic imaging during pregnancy. Int J Gynecol Obstet 1995;51:288–291.
24. Garden AS, Griffiths RD, Weindling AM, Martin PA. Fast-scan magnetic resonance imaging in fetal visualization. Am J Obstet Gynecol 1991;164:1190–1196.
25. Twickler DM. Diagnostic imaging in pregnancy. In: Williams Obstetrics, 19th ed. Norwalk, CT: Appleton & Lange, 1993:981–989.
26. Butturini A, Gale RP. Relationship between clonality and transformation in acute leukemia. Leukoc Res 1991;15:1.
27. Bennett JM, Catovsky D, Daniel MT, et al. Proposals for the classification of acute leukaemias. Br J Haematol 1976;33:451–458.
28. Hernandez TA, Land KJ, McKenna RW. Leukemias, myeloma and other lymphoreticular neoplasms. Cancer 1995;75:381–394.
29. Yahia C, Hyman GA, Phillips JL. Acute leukemia and pregnancy. Obstet Gynecol Surv 1958;13:1–21.
30. McLain CR. Leukemia in pregnancy. Clin Obstet Gynecol 1974;17: 185–94.
31. Aviles A, Niz J. Long-term follow-up of children born to mothers with acute leukemia during pregnancy. Med Pediatr Oncol 1988;16:3–6.
32. Caliguri MA, Mayer RJ. Pregnancy and leukemia. Semin Oncol 1989; 16:388–396.
33. Aksoy M. Hematotoxicity and carcinogenesis of benzene. Environ Health Perspect 1989;82:193–197.
34. Rinsky RA, Smith AB, Hornung R, Filoon TG, Young RJ, Okun AH, Landrigan PJ. Benzene and leukemia: an epidemiologic risk assessment. N Engl J Med 1987;316:1044–1050.
35. Thirman MJ, Larson RA. Therapy related myeloid leukemia. Hematol Oncol Clin North Am 1996;10:293–320.
36. Appelbaum FR, Le beau MM, Willman CL. Secondary Leukemia American Society of Hematology. Educational Program, December 7, 1996, Orlando, FL.
37. Pedersen-Bjergaard J, Philip P, Mortensen BT, et al. Acute nonlymphocytic leukemia, preleukemia and myeloproliferative syndrome secondary to treatment of other malignant diseases: clinical and cytogenetic characteristics and results of in vitro culture of bone marrow and HLA typing. Blood 1981;57:712–723.
38. Michels JD, McKenna RW, Arthur DC, Brunning RD. Therapy related acute myeloid leukemia and myelodysplastic syndrome: a clinical and morphologic study of 65 cases. Blood 1985;65:1364–1372.
39. Pedersen-Bjergaard J, Philip P, Larsen SO, Jensen G, Byrsting K. Chromosomal aberrations and prognostic factors in therapy related myelodysplasia and acute non lymphocytic leukemia. Blood 1990;76: 1083–1091.
40. Sandler DP. Epidemiology and etiology of acute leukemia: an update. Leukemia 1992;6:3–5.
41. Committee on the Biological Effects of Ionizing Radiation. The effects on populations of exposure to low levels of ionizing radiation: 1980. Washington, DC: National Academy Press, 1980.
42. Land CE. Estimating cancer risks from low of doses of ionizing radiation. Science 1980;209:1197–1203.
43. Garfinkel L, Boffetta P. Association between smoking and leukemia in two American Cancer Society prospective studies. Cancer 1990;65: 2356–2360.
44. Juarez S, Cuadrado-Pastor JM, Felin J, Gonzalez-Baron M, Ordonez, Montero JM. Association of leukemia and pregnancy: clinical and obstetric aspects. Am J Clin Oncol 1988;11:159–165.
45. Pizzuto J, Aviles A, Noriega L, Niz J, Morales M, Romero F. Treatment of acute leukemia during pregnancy: presentation of nine cases. Cancer Treat Rep 1980;64:679–683.
46. Byrne J, Mulvihill JJ, Myers MH, et al. Effects of treatment on fertility in long term survivors of childhood and adolescent cancer. N Engl J Med 1987;317:1315–1321.

47. Dutcher JP. Hyperleukocytosis in leukemia: an emergency. In: Dutcher JP, Wiernik HP, eds. Handbook of hematologic and oncologic emergencies. New York: Plenum, 1987:103–111.
48. Marcus SL, Einzig AI. Acute tumor lysis syndrome. In: Dutcher JP, Wiernik PH, eds. Handbook of hematologic and oncologic emergencies. New York: Plenum, 1987:9–15.
49. Katler H, Warkany J. Congenital malformations. N Engl J Med 1983; 308:424–431, 491–497.
50. Milunsky A, Graef JW, Gaynor MF Jr. Methotrexate-induced congenital malformations. J Pediatr 1968;72:790–795.
51. Durie DGM, Giles HR. Successful treatment of acute leukemia during pregnancy. Combination therapy in the third trimester. Arch Intern Med 1977;137:90–91.
52. Wagner VM, Hill JS, Weaver D, Baehner RL. Congenital abnormalities in baby born to cytarabuse treated mother. Lancet 1980;2:98–99.
53. Roboz J, Gleicher N, Wu K, Chanihian P, Kerenyi T, Holland J. Does doxorubicin cross the placenta? Lancet 1979;2:1382–1383.
54. Incalci M, Broggini M, Buscaglia M, Pardi G. Transplacental passage of doxorubicin. Lancet 1983;1:75.
55. Cantini E, Yanes B. Acute myelogenous leukemia in pregnancy. South Med J 1984;77:1050–1052.
56. Doney KC, Kraemer KG, Shepard TH. Combination chemotherapy for myelocytic leukemia in pregnancy. Cancer Treat Rep 1979;6e: 369–371.
57. Newcomb M, Balducci L, Thigpen JT, Morrison FS. Acute leukemia in pregnancy. Successful delivery after cytarabine and doxorubicin. JAMA 1978;239:2691–2692.
58. Thomas PR, Blochem D, Peckman MJ. The investigation and management of Hodgkin's disease in the pregnant patient. Cancer 1976; 38:1443–1451.
59. Mennutti MT, Shepard TH, Mellman WJ. Fetal renal malformation following treatment of Hodgkin's disease during pregnancy. Obstet Gynecol 1975;46:194–196.
60. Aviles A, Diaz Maqueo J, Talavera A. Growth and development of children of mothers treated with chemotherapy during pregnancy: current status of 43 children. Am J Hematol 1991;36:243–248.
61. Lilleyman JS, Hill AS, Anderton KJ. Consequences of acute myelogenous leukemia in early pregnancy. Cancer 1977;40:1300–1303.
62. Lloyd HO. Acute Leukemia complicated by pregnancy. JAMA 1961; 178:1140–1143.
63. Frenkel RP, Meyers MC. Acute leukemia and pregnancy. Ann Intern Med 1960;53:656–671.
64. Heys RF. Steroid therapy for idiopathic thrombocytopenic purpura during pregnancy. Obstet Gynecol 1966;28:532–542.
65. Harris J, Morrow M, Norton L. Malignant tumors of the breast. In: DeVita VT, Hellman S, Rosenbert S, eds. Cancer principles and practice of oncology. Philadelphia: Lippincott-Raven, 1996.
66. MacMahon B, Cole P, Brown J. Etiology of human breast cancer: a review. J Natl Cancer Inst 1973;50:21–42.
67. Wallack MK, Wolf JA Jr, Bedwinek J, et al. Gestational carcinoma of the female breast. Curr Prob Cancer 1983;7:1–58.
68. Anderson JM. Mammary cancers and pregnancy. Br Med J 1979;1: 1124–1127.
69. Richards SR, Chang F, Moynihan V, O'Shaughnessy R. Metastatic breast cancer complicating pregnancy. A case report. J Reprod Med 1984;29:211–213.
70. Clark RM, Chua T. Breast cancer and pregnancy: the ultimate challenge. Clin Oncol 1989;1:11–18.
71. Petrek JA , Dukoff R, Rogatko A. Prognosis of pregnancy-associated breast cancer. Cancer 1991;67:869–872.
72. Zemlickis D, Lishner M, Degendorfer P, et al. Maternal and fetal outcome after breast cancer in pregnancy. Am J Obstet Gynecol 1992; 166:781–787.
73. King RM, Welch JS, Martin JK Jr, Coullam CB. Carcinoma of the breast associated with pregnancy. Surg Gynecol Obstet 1985;160: 228–232.
74. Westberg SV. Prognosis of breast cancer for pregnant and nursing women. Acta Obstet Gynecol Scand 1946;25(suppl 4).
75. Hoeffken N, Lanyi M, eds. Mammography. Philadelphia: WB Saunders, 1977.
76. Finley JL, Silverman JF, Lannin DR. Fine needle aspiration cytology of breast masses in pregnant and lactating women. Diagn Cytopathol 1989;5:255–259.
77. Byrd BF, Bayer DS, Robertson JC, Stephenson SE. Treatment of breast tumors associated with pregnancy and lactation. Ann Surg 1962;155:940–947.
78. Petrek JA. Breast cancer during pregnancy. Cancer 1994;74(suppl): 518–527.
79. Woo SY, Fuller LM, Cundiff JH. Radiotherapy during pregnancy for clinical stages IA-IIA Hodgkin's disease. Int J Radiat Oncol 1992;23: 407–412.
80. Early Breast Cancer Trialists Collaborative Group. Systemic treatment of early breast cancer by cytotoxic, systemic or immune therapy. 133 randomized trails involving 31,000 recurrences and 24,000 deaths among 75,000 women. Lancet 1992;339:1–15.
81. Early Breast Cancer Trialists Collaborative Group. Effects of adjuvant tamoxifen and of cytotoxic therapy on mortality in early breast cancer. An overview of 61 randomized trials among 28,896 women. N Engl J Med 1988;319:1681–1692.
82. Tancini G, Bonadonna G, Valagussa P, Merchini S, Veronesi U. Adjuvant CMF in breast cancer: Comparative 5 year results of 12 versus 6 cycles. J Clin Oncol 1983;1:2–10.
83. Stephens JD, Golbus MS, Miller TR, Wilber RR, Epstein CJ. Multiple congenital anomalies in a fetus exposed to 5-fluorouracil during the first trimester. Am J Obstet Gynecol 1980;137:747–749.
84. Fisher B, Brown AM, Dimitrov NV, et al. Two months of doxorubicin and cyclophosphamide with and without interval reinduction therapy compared with 6 months of cyclophosphamide, methotrexate and fluorouracil in positive node breast cancer patients with tamoxifen unresponsive tumors: results from NSABP-15. J Clin Oncol 1990;8: 1483–1496.
85. Henderson CI. Chemotherapy for metastatic disease. In: Harris J, Hellman S, Henderson CI, eds. Philadelphia: JB Lippincott, 1991: 608.
86. Haagensen CD, Stout AP. Carcinoma of the breast: criteria of operability. Ann Surg 1943;118:859–870.
87. Peters MV, Meakins JW. The influence of pregnancy in carcinoma of the breast. Prog Clin Cancer 1965;1:471–506.
88. Nugent P, O'Connell TX. Breast cancer and pregnancy. Arch Surg 1983;120:1221–1224.
89. Harvey JC, Rosen PP, Ashikari R, Robbins GF, Kinne DW. The effect of pregnancy on the prognosis of carcinoma of the breast follow radial mastectomy. Surg Gynecol Obstet 1981;153:723–725.
90. Mignot L, Morvan F, Berdah J, et al. Grossesses apres cancer du sein traité. Résultats d une étude cas-temoins. Presse Med 1986;15: 1961–1964.
91. Ariel IM, Kempner R. The prognosis of patients who became pregnant after mastectomy for breast cancer. Int Surg 1989;74:185–187.
92. Petrek JA. Pregnancy safety after breast cancer. Cancer 1994; 24(suppl):528–531.
93. Elwood JM, Koh HK. Etiology, epidemiology, risk factors and public health issues of melanoma. Curr Opin Oncol 1994;6:179–187.
94. Armstrong BK, Kricker A. Cutaneous melanoma. Cancer Surv 1994; 19:219–240.
95. Greene MH, Praumeni JF Jr. The hereditary variant of malignant melanoma. In: Clark WJ, Goldman LI, Mastrangelo MJ, eds. Human malignant melanoma. New York: Grune & Stratton, 1979:139–167.
96. Albino AP, Fountain JW. The molecular genetics of malignant melanoma. In: Nathansin L, ed. Treatment and research; basic and clinical aspects of malignant melanoma. Boston: Martinus Nijhoff, 1993: 201–255.
97. Fountain JW, Bale JJ, Houseman DF, Dracopoli NC. Genetics of melanoma. In: Franks LM, ed. Cancer surveys: advances and prospects in clinical, epidemiological and laboratory oncology. Vol. 9. London: Oxford University Press, 1990:645–671.
98. Blois MS, Sagebiel RW, Abrabanel RM, Caldwell TM, Tuttle MS. Malignant melanoma of the skin I: The association of tumor depth and type and pattern of sex, age and site with survival. Cancer 1983;52: 1330–1341.
99. Rampen FH, Mulder JH. Malignant melanoma: an androgen dependent tumour? Lancet 1980;1:562–564.
100. Shaw HM, McGovern VJ, Milton GW, Farago GA, McCarthy PH. The female superiority in survival in clinical stage II cutaneous malignant melanoma. Cancer 1981;49:1941–1944.
101. Lederman JS, Sober AJ. Effect of prior pregnancy on melanoma survival. Arch Dermatol 1984;121:716.
102. Bork K, Brauninger W. Prior pregnancy and melanoma survival. Arch Dermatol 1986;122:1097.

103. Colbourn DS, Nathanson L, Bellkos R. Pregnancy and malignant melanoma. Semin Oncol 1989;16:377.
104. Deaths from melanoma—United States 1973–1982. MMWR 1993; 44:337–343.
105. Koh HK. Cutaneous melanoma. N Engl J Med 1991;325:171–182.
106. Shaw HM, Milton GW, Farago G, McCarthy WH. Endocrine influences on survival from malignant melanoma. Cancer 1978;42: 669–667.
107. Potter JF, Schoeneman M. Metastasis of maternal cancer to the placenta and fetus. Cancer 1970;25:380–388.
108. Breslow A. Thickness, cross sectional area and depth of invasion in the prognosis of cutaneous melanoma. Ann Surg 1970;172:902–908.
109. Johnson OK, Emrich LJ, Karakousis CP, Rao U, Greco WR. Comparison of prognostic factors for survival and recurrence in malignant melanoma of the skin, clinical stage I. Cancer 1985;55:1107–1117.
110. Beahrs OH, Meyers MH. Manual for staging of cancer, American Joint Committee on Cancer. Philadelphia: JB Lippincott, 1983:117.
111. Reintgen D, McCarty KS, Vollmer R, Cox E, Seigler HF. Malignant melanoma and pregnancy. Cancer 1985;55:1340–1344.
112. Travers RL, Sober AJ, Berwick M, Mihm MC Jr, Barnhill RL, Duncan LM. Increased thickness of pregnancy associated melanoma. Br J Derm 1995;132:876–883.
113. Veronesi U, Cascinelli N, Adamus J, et al. Thin stage 1 primary cutaneous malignant melanoma. Comparison of excision with margins of 1 or 3 cm. N Engl J Med 1988;318:1159–1162.
114. Slingluff CL Jr, Reintgen DS, Vollmer RT, Seigler HF. Malignant melanoma arising during pregnancy. A study of 100 patients. Ann Surg 1990;211:552–557.
115. Coit D, Sauven P, Brennan M. Prognosis of thick cutaneous melanoma of the trunk and extremity. Arch Surg 1990;125:322–326.
116. Kirkwood JM, Strawderman MH, Ernstoff MS, et al. Interferon Alpha-2b adjuvant therapy of high risk resected cutaneous melanoma. The Eastern Cooperative Oncology Group Trial EST 1684. J Clin Oncol 1996;14:7–17.
117. Pons JC, Lebon P, Freyman R, Delfraissy JF. Pharmacokinetics of interferon-alpha in pregnant women and fetoplacental passage. Fetal Diagn Ther 1995;10:7–10.
118. Ruggiero G, Andreana A, Zampino R. Normal pregnancy under inadvertent alpha-interferon therapy for chronic hepatitis C. J Hepatol 1996;24:646.
119. Ryan L, Kramar A, Borden E. Prognostic factors in metastatic melanoma. Cancer 1993;71:2995–3005.
120. Pack GT, Scharngel TM. The prognosis for malignant melanoma in the pregnant woman. Cancer 1951;4:324–334.
121. Sutherland CM, Loutfi A, Mather FJ, Carter RD, Krementz ET. Effects of pregnancy on malignant melanoma. Surg Obstet Gynecol 1983;157:433–436.
122. McManany DS, Moss AL, Pocock PV, Briggs JC. Melanoma and pregnancy: a long-term follow-up. Br J Obstet Gynecol 1989;96: 1419–1423.
123. Wong JH, Strens EE, Kopald KH, Nizze JA, Morton DL. Prognostic significance of pregnancy in stage I melanoma. Arch Surg 1989;124: 1227–1231.
124. MacKie RM, Bufalino R, Morabito A, Sutherland C, Cascinelli N. Lack of effect of pregnancy on outcome of melanoma. Lancet 1991; 337:653–655.
125. Hodgkin T. On some morbid appearances of the absorbent glands and spleen. Med Chir Trans 1832;17:68–114.
126. Cole P, MacMahon B, Aisenberg A. Mortality from Hodgkin's disease in the United States. Evidence for the multiple-aetiology hypothesis. Lancet 1968;2:1371–1376.
127. Steward HL, Monto RW. Hodgkin's disease and pregnancy. Am J Obstet Gynecol 1952;63:570–578.
128. Riva HL, Anderson PS, Grady JW. Pregnancy and Hodgkin's disease: a report of eight cases. Am J Obstet Gynecol 1953:66:866–870.
129. Sadural E, Smith LG Jr. Hematologic malignancies during pregnancy. Clin Obstet Gynecol 1995;38:535–546.
130. Vianna J, Greenwald P, Davies JN. Extended epidemic of Hodgkin's disease in high school students. Lancet 1971;1:1209–1211.
131. Eyre HJ. Hodgkin's disease. In: Lee CR, Tithell T, Foerster J, Athens J, Lukens J, eds. Wintrobe's clinical hematology. Philadelphia: Lea & Febiger, 1993:2054–2081.
132. Staal SP, Ambinder R, Berchorner WE, Hayward GS, Mann R. A survey of Epstein Barr DNA in lymphoid tissue. Frequent detection in Hodgkin's disease. Am J Clin Pathol 1989;91:1–5.
133. Kravdal O, Hansen S. Hodgkin's disease: the protective effects of childbearing. Int J Cancer 1993;55:909–914.
134. Zwitter M, Zakelj MP, Kosmelj K. A case-control study of Hodgkin's disease and pregnancy. Br J Cancer 1996;73:246–251.
135. Gelb AB, van de Rijn M, Warnke R, Kamel OW. Pregnancy-associated lymphomas. A clinicopathologic study. Cancer 1996;78:304–310.
136. Jacobs C, Donaldson SS, Rosenberg SA, Kadanlt S. Management of the pregnant patient with Hodgkin's disease. Ann Intern Med 1981; 95:669–675.
137. Thomas PR, Biochem D, Peckham MJ. The investigation and management of Hodgkin's disease in the pregnant patient. Cancer 1976; 38:1443–1451.
138. DeVita VT, Serpick AA, Carbone PP. Combination chemotherapy in the treatment of advanced Hodgkin's disease. Ann Intern Med 1970; 73:881–895.
139. Nisce LZ, Tome MA, He S, Lee BS 3d, Kutchner GJ. Management of co-existing Hodgkin's disease and pregnancy. Am J Clin Oncol 1986; 9:146–151.
140. Ward FT, Weiss RB. Lymphoma and pregnancy. Semin Oncol 1989; 16:397–409.
141. O'Dell RF. Leukemia and lymphoma complicating pregnancy. Clin Obstet Gynecol 1979;22:859–870.
142. Armstrong JG, Dyke RW, Fouts PJ, Jansen CJ. Delivery of a normal infant during the course of oral vinblastine sulfate therapy for Hodgkin's disease. Ann Intern Med 1964;61:106–107.
143. Lishner M, Zemlickis D, Degendorfer P, Panzarella T, Sutcliffe SB, Koren G. Maternal and fetal outcome following Hodgkin's disease in pregnancy. Br J Cancer 1992;65:114.
144. Swerdlow AJ, Jacobs PA, Marks A, et al. Fertility, reproductive outcomes and health of offspring, of patients treated for Hodgkin's disease: an investigation including chromosome examinations. Br J Cancer 1996;74:291–296.
145. Harris NL, Jaffe ES, Stern H, et al. Lymphoma classification proposal: clarification. 1995;85:857–860.
146. Shipp MA, Mauch PM, Harris NL. Non-Hodgkin's lymphoma. In: DeVita VT, Hellman S, Rosenberg S, eds. Cancer principles and practice of oncology, 5th ed. Philadelphia: Lippincott-Raven, 1997: 2165–2220.
147. Boring CC, Squires TS, Tong T. Cancer statistics 1991. CA Cancer J Clin 1991;41:19–36.
148. Ward FT, Weiss RB. Lymphoma and pregnancy. Semin Oncol 1989; 16:397–409.
149. Steiner-Salz D, Yahalom J, Samuelov A, Polliack A. Non-Hodgkin's lymphoma associated with pregnancy. Cancer 1985;56:2087–2091.
150. Falkson HC, Simson IW, Falkson G. Non-Hodgkin's lymphoma in pregnancy. Cancer 1980;45:1679–1682.
151. Jones DE, D'Avignon MB, Lawrence R, Latshaw RF. Burkitt's Lymphoma obstetric and gynecologic aspects. Obstet Gynecol 1980;56: 533–536.
152. Ortega J. Multiple agent chemotherapy including bleomycin of non-Hodgkin's lymphoma during pregnancy. Cancer 1977;40:2829–2835.

SECTION XIV

Integumental Disorders

Cherry and Merkatz's Complications of Pregnancy,
Fifth Edition, edited by W. R. Cohen.
Lippincott Williams & Wilkins, Philadelphia © 2000.

CHAPTER 41

Dermatologic Disorders

Warren Dotz and Brian Berman

The skin and its appendages undergo many changes during pregnancy and the postpartum period. In this chapter, these changes are considered in three categories: (a) changes in otherwise normal skin resulting from altered physiology, (b) diseases specifically associated with pregnancy, and (c) pregnancy-induced changes in primary cutaneous diseases and systemic diseases involving the skin.

CUTANEOUS CHANGES RESULTING FROM ALTERED PHYSIOLOGY

Pigmentation

Hyperpigmentation

Hyperpigmentation, although variable in degree, is seen in 90% of pregnant women (1). Although the mechanism has not been fully elucidated, elevated serum levels of estrogens and possibly melanocyte-stimulating hormone (MSH) as well as progesterone are suggested as causes. Hyperpigmentation is evident early in pregnancy and is more marked in dark-skinned women. Pigmentation is more pronounced in naturally pigmented areas, such as the areolae, perineum, vulva, and umbilicus. The linea nigra, a dark line extending from the pubis vertically to the umbilicus, and areas susceptible to friction, including the axillae and inner thighs, also may darken (Fig. 41-1). In addition, freckles, nevi, pigmentary demarcation lines, and scars may darken during gestation (2,3). Scars developing a few months before or during pregnancy will become more pigmented than older scars (4). Most of these pigmentary changes regress postpartum.

Melasma

Melasma, "the mask of pregnancy," has been reported in 70% of pregnant women (5) and in 5% to 34% of nonpregnant women taking oral contraceptives (6–8). The onset of melasma usually occurs during the second half of pregnancy. It is more common in dark-haired, dark-complexioned white women. There is often a genetic predisposition. The term *melasma* is derived from the Greek word *melas* meaning "black"(9). *Chloasma* is a term that has been used synonymously with melasma and is derived from the Greek word *chloazein*, meaning "to turn green." Therefore, the brown–black hyperpigmentation in this condition most properly should be designated as melasma.

Melasma (Fig. 41-2) consists of blotchy, irregular, light to dark brown hyperpigmentation that occurs in three clinical patterns: centrofacial, malar, and mandibular (10). The *centrofacial pattern* is the most common and involves the cheeks, forehead, upper lip, nose, or chin. The *malar pattern* is localized to the cheek and nasal regions. The *mandibular pattern* implies involvement of the ramus of the mandible and neck. Melasma may result from excessive

W. Dotz: Private Practice, Berkeley, CA 94705.
B. Berman: Departments of Dermatology, Cutaneous Surgery, and Internal Medicine, University of Miami/Jackson Memorial Medical Center, Miami, FL 33136.

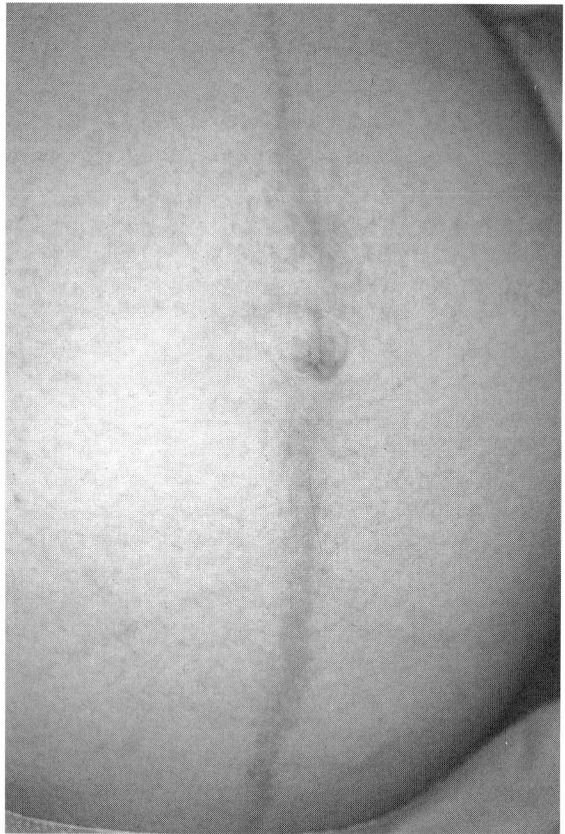

FIG. 41-1. The linea nigra extends vertically from the pubis to the umbilicus.

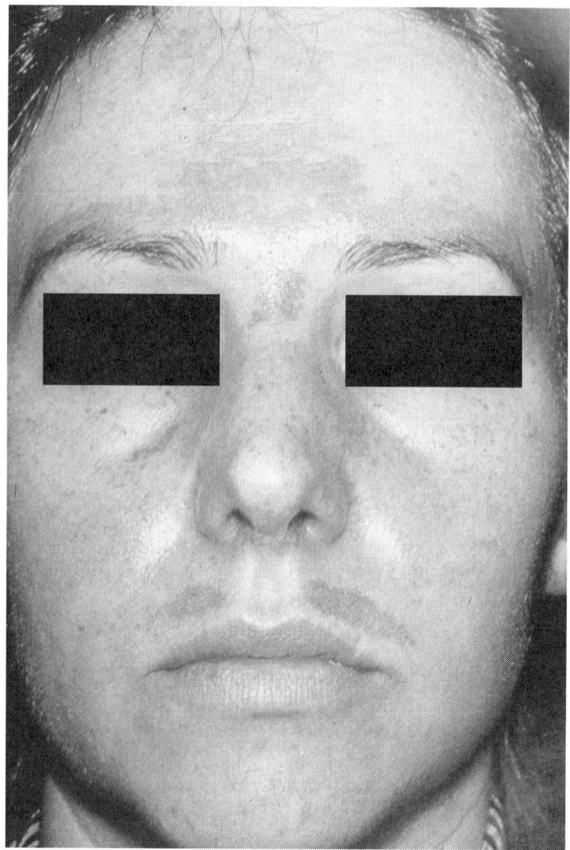

FIG. 41-2. Melasma, the mask of pregnancy, distributed in a centrofacial pattern.

melanin deposition in either the basal and suprabasal layers of the epidermis or within macrophages (melanophages) in the dermis. Histologically, it can be classified into epidermal, dermal, or mixed-type pigmentation based on the site of pigment deposition (10). Clinically, epidermal melasma is more responsive to bleaching creams.

The causal factors in melasma include pregnancy, oral contraceptives, genetic and racial predisposition, cosmetics, nutrition, hepatic disease, and parasitosis (10). Although MSH, progesterone, and estrogen have been reported to be increased in the third trimester of pregnancy, they have not been found to be consistently elevated in melasma (11).

Many women who develop melasma after taking oral contraceptives have had this condition previously during pregnancy. Resnick (8) reported 61 cases of melasma in women taking oral contraceptives, 52 (87%) of whom had melanoderma during a previous pregnancy. In most cases, gestational melasma will regress postpartum; however, pigmentation caused by oral contraceptives is frequently persistent. In patients who develop impressive melasma during pregnancy, nonhormonal methods of contraception should be considered.

Melasma often disappears within a year of delivery (12), but one study showed a persistence in 30% of cases after 10 years (13). Sunlight is considered necessary for the development of melasma, and in women with a melasma tendency, excessive solar exposure during pregnancy leads to marked pigmentation. Also, sun exposure postpartum can exacerbate the darkening of preexisting melasma. Conscientious use of broad-spectrum sunscreens should be advocated to patients who are at risk of developing melasma. With persistent treatment for weeks to months, melasma with pigmentation confined to the epidermis may respond to nightly applications of bleaching creams containing 2% to 5% hydroquinone. Tretinoin 0.05% or glycolic acid can be used additionally to increase epidermal penetration and the efficacy of the hydroquinone, the efficacy of which is caused by the inhibition of one or more steps in the melanin synthesis pathway. It also affects the formation, melanization, and degradation of intracellular melanosomes, eventually leading to necrosis of whole melanocytes. Hydroquinone is considered a category C drug; so generally it is offered to patients postpartum or after nursing. In our experience, hydroquinone therapy is only partially effective in most patients who have epidermal melasma. Dermal types of melasma of many years duration respond poorly, or not at all. Recently, azelaic acid 20%, currently used in the United States as a topical treatment for acne, has shown promising results in the treatment of melasma. This category B medication was shown to be superior to 2% hydroquinone and as effective as 4%

hydroquinone. Tretinoin 0.05% appears to enhance the effect of azelaic acid. The effect of azelaic acid may be attributed to its ability to inhibit the energy production or DNA synthesis of hyperactive melanocytes and partially to its antityrosinase activity. Dermal types of melasma also respond poorly to this alternative topical therapy (14).

Hair

The growth of hair occurs in a cyclic fashion in three phases: *anagen* (the growing phase), *catagen* (the transition phase), and *telogen* (the resting phase). When a hair approaches the end of its growing phase, involutional changes occur in the follicle, and a resting telogen club-shaped hair is formed. This hair remains in the follicle until it is displaced by a new hair. The effects of pregnancy on scalp hair are most noticeable to the patient during the postpartum period, but they reflect an altered physiology that commences with pregnancy. In the first trimester, telogen counts are within the normal range, with mean values between 15% and 20% of all scalp hairs. Thereafter, the number of telogen hairs decreases and may be reduced to 10% of the scalp hair during the second and third trimesters, indicating that many hair follicles that normally would have come to the end of their growing phase continue to grow until the end of pregnancy (1).

Postpartum Telogen Effluvium

Telogen effluvium is the shedding of club hairs following the precipitate shift from anagen follicles into telogen and is a process that may be regarded as a response of the follicle to physiologic changes during systemic stresses (15). Postpartum telogen effluvium probably is caused by the withdrawal of factors that have prevented the normal entry of hairs into the catagen and telogen phases. Following pregnancy, most hair follicles enter the telogen phase, which lasts approximately 3 months. When follicles reactivate, telogen club hairs are readily shed.

Postpartum telogen effluvium is probably universal but is most often subclinical. Patients note abnormal hair loss during the third month postpartum. Most patients are conscious of abnormal shedding when they wash or comb their hair. Although the distribution of hair loss is diffuse, in more severely affected cases, more marked hair loss along the anterior margin of the scalp is noted. Telogen effluvium lasts from 3 to 6 months.

As in all cases of telogen effluvium, the shedding of hair actually heralds regrowth, and the patient soon becomes reassured by observing many new hairs. Excessive brushing and braiding and the use of chemical hair preparations are not desirable and should be discontinued until new hair regrowth occurs. Reassurance is the best approach. Patients should be reassured that after 3 to 6 months of hair loss the hair density will return to normal.

Diffuse thinning of hair in postpartum women should not always be attributed to the gravid state. Excessive mechanical traction, especially from braids, metal brushes, hair rollers, cold waves, and hair straighteners, as well as diffuse alopecia areata, seborrheic dermatitis, collagen vascular disease, thyroid disease, iron deficiency anemia, and trichotillomania, also should be considered in the differential diagnosis.

Hirsutism

Many pregnant women develop some degree of hirsutism. It generally starts early in pregnancy and is usually more noticeable in women who have preexisting abundant body hair or dark hair. Hair growth is most pronounced on the face but also may involve the arms, legs, and back. Occasionally, there is new growth of suprapubic hair in the midline of the abdomen, assuming a male pattern of distribution. A possible causative factor is the placental secretion of androgens, corticotropins, and gonadotropins (16). Hirsutism of pregnancy usually disappears or diminishes within 2 to 6 months postpartum but may recur with subsequent pregnancies. More severe degrees of hirsutism are unusual and, if accompanied by evidence for masculinization, should prompt consideration for an abnormal androgen source.

Nails

Diverse nail changes may occur during pregnancy, although none is unique to the gravid state. The most common onychodystrophies seen during pregnancy are transverse grooving (Beau's lines), brittleness, and distal onycholysis (4). The pathogenesis of those changes and their relationship to pregnancy are unclear. Increased adrenal and pituitary activity may result in accelerated nail growth.

Beau's lines are transverse grooves in the nail plate caused by temporary impairment of nail plate formation by the nail matrix. They are sequelae of systemic physical stresses in susceptible persons. Beau's lines usually become visible several weeks after the period of stress as the nail returns to normal growth. Usually, they are seen during the puerperium and may reappear during subsequent pregnancies.

Brittle nails and *onycholysis* (distal separation of nail plate from nail bed) also occur in pregnant women. When these changes are observed, other causes of onychodystrophy (psoriasis, onychomycosis, lichen planus, cosmetic nail preparations) should be eliminated before attributing them to pregnancy. Nails should be kept short if they are brittle or susceptible to onycholysis.

Vascular Changes

Vascular changes of pregnancy include vasomotor instability, congestion, and vessel proliferation. Congestion of the vasculature of the vestibule and vagina appears early in gestation and is a diagnostic sign of pregnancy itself (*Jacquemier-Chadwick sign*).

Nonpitting edema of the eyelid, face, and extremities is a feature of at least 50% of all pregnancies and results from increased water content of the dermis. Vasomotor instability also may account for such symptoms and signs as pallor, facial flushing, hot and cold sensation, and *cutis marmorata* of the legs, a transitory mottling of the skin occurring on exposure to cold.

Edema and hyperemia of the gums leading to marginal gingivitis occur in 80% of pregnant women (17). Proliferations of capillaries within the hypertrophied gingiva can result in granuloma gravidarum.

Vascular Spiders

Vascular spiders (spider telangiectasia, spider angiomas) commonly develop in pregnancy and have been reported in 67% of white patients and in 11% of blacks (Fig. 41-3) (18). Vascular spiders first appear between the second and fifth months of pregnancy. There is a tendency for spiders to increase in size and number throughout pregnancy. Circulating estrogens are believed to be the cause of vascular spiders (18).

Vascular spiders are recognized as stellate, 0.5 to 2.0 cm diameter macules with a central red punctum and blanchable radiating small vessels. Vascular spiders are most common on the face, trunk, arms, and hands. About 75% of patients with vascular spiders in the ninth month of pregnancy lose them by the seventh week after delivery. Ten percent of these women show persistence of these spiders after pregnancy (18). Recurrences and enlargement during subsequent pregnancies can occur.

Treatment should be avoided during pregnancy because many vascular spiders do regress postpartum. Opaque cosmetic makeup can be used to camouflage lesions. For insistent patients or persistent lesions, low-voltage electrodesiccation or galvanic current can be applied with a fine needle to involute spiders. The pulsed dye laser, copper vapor laser, and diode-pumped yttrium aluminum garnet (YAG) laser also have been used to yield satisfactory cosmetic results (19).

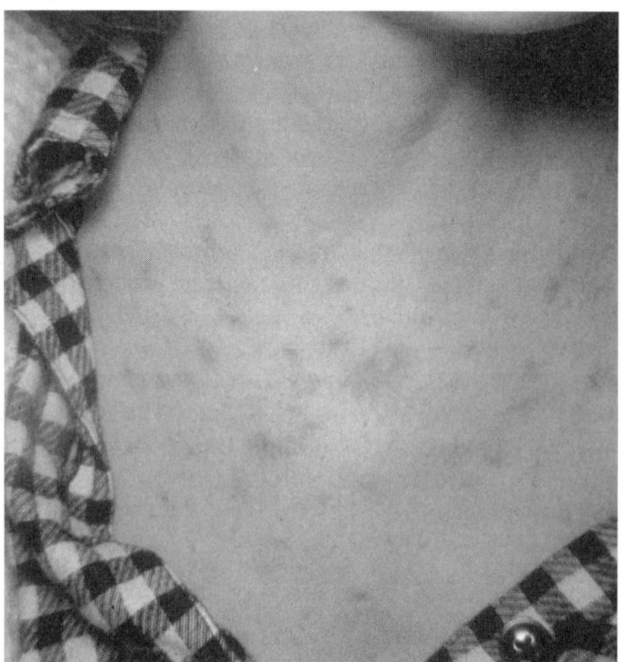

FIG. 41-3. Vascular spiders commonly develop during pregnancy.

Palmar Erythema

Palmar erythema is seen in nearly two thirds of pregnant white women and in one third of blacks, generally developing in those in whom vascular spiders are present (14). The incidence increases progressively during pregnancy and declines during the puerperium. Palmar erythema may occur in two forms: a red area sharply demarcated from normal skin or a diffuse mottled patch on the palmar surface. Even though this condition resembles "liver palms," liver disease need not be present when this condition is observed.

Varicosities

Varicosities, most frequently the saphenous, vulvar, and hemorrhoidal veins, appear in 40% of pregnant women (1). They are a result of increased venous pressure in the femoral and pelvic vessels caused by a gravid uterus. A familial tendency for varicose veins is also important. Varicosities tend to regress after delivery, but often they do not regress completely. Thrombosis occurs in fewer than 10% of pregnancies (1). Hemorrhoidal varicosities are also common and may cause pain and bleeding.

Dermatographism

Dermatographism and urticaria are common in the last half of pregnancy. Generalized urticaria may occur as a result of pregnancy, but the physician should rule out other causes, such as drug-induced reactions (20).

Cutaneous Glands

Eccrine gland sweating increases during pregnancy. The cause of this altered glandular activity is uncertain. Beginning with the third month of pregnancy, secretion of thyroid hormone increases, which might may account for the hyperhydrosis, warmth, and erythema of the skin (14). The increased weight during pregnancy also may play a role. Paradoxically, palmar sweating is decreased during pregnancy (21). Excessive sweating may lead to several clinical manifestations, the most common of which are miliaria and intertrigo.

Miliaria

Miliaria (prickly heat, heat rash) is the consequence of poral occlusion that results from and further causes eccrine sweat retention within the stratum corneum. Commonly affected areas are the back and sides of the trunk, the abdomen, buttocks, thighs, and the antecubital and popliteal fossae. Sites of friction, especially where clothing rubs, often are involved. Lesions consist of pinpoint, pruritic, erythematous papulovesicles.

The treatment of miliaria is to supply a cool environment to reduce humidity and to increase the evaporation rate. Clothing should be light, nonconstricting, and absorbent; wool, nylon, and synthetic fibers should be avoided. The application of occlusive and oily ointments should be restricted to prevent further poral plugging. Mild cases may respond to absorbent dusting powders, such as talcum or cellulose-based absorbent powder. A lotion containing 4% salicylic acid in 95% alcohol or calamine lotion with or without 0.25% menthol may be effective. Soothing, cooling baths containing colloidal oatmeal also may be beneficial.

Intertrigo

Intertrigo is a condition that occurs in areas of skin surfaces in apposition, such as the groin and axilla as well as abdominal, inguinal, and inframammary folds. Heat, moisture, and sweat retention cause maceration and irritation, primarily on a mechanical basis. The skin in these areas may look glazed and red in mild cases and may proceed to denudation and erosion. Secondary bacterial and *Candida albicans* overgrowth may perpetuate the lesions.

Hygienic care of the involved area is sufficient for the treatment of mild cases of intertrigo. Environmental changes to promote drying and to aerate the body folds are essential. The living and working areas should be cool and dry. Air conditioning or fans will help. Clothing should be light and nonocclusive. Intertriginous areas should be washed at least twice daily, and all soap should be completely rinsed off. An absorbent, starch-free talc or cellulose-containing powder should be applied liberally. In severe cases of intertrigo, when oozing and erosion are present, application of Burow's solution compresses (aluminum acetate in water, 1:40 dilution) to exudative areas three to four times daily will help to clean and dry exudative surfaces. Bland lotions or creams may be soothing and drying. Initially, a hydrocortisone or hydrocortisone–antibiotic lotion or cream can be applied to reduce inflammation and burning. Fluorinated steroids should be avoided because their prolonged use may lead to intertriginous striae and cutaneous atrophy.

Apocrine gland activity during pregnancy decreases. *Fox-Fordyce* disease, a condition caused by apocrine sweat retention, is comparable to miliaria of the eccrine glands and improves during pregnancy. This improvement is most pronounced in the last trimester (1). *Hidradenitis suppurativa*, a disease of apocrine sweat glands marked by tender and draining cysts, also may improve during pregnancy.

Sebaceous gland activity generally increases in the third trimester of pregnancy (see section on Acne). During gestation, sebaceous glands on the areolae of the breast enlarge and appear as small brown papules called *Montgomery's tubercles*, which usually persist after the pregnancy.

DEGENERATIVE CHANGES

Striae Gravidarum

Striae gravidarum (striae distensa, striae albicantes, striae atrophicae) occur to some degree in approximately 90% of pregnant women (1), and there often is a familial tendency (22). Striae usually develop in the sixth and seventh months of pregnancy. The striae are thin, narrow, irregular, linear bands of atrophy occurring on the abdomen, sacral area, breast, thighs, and axillae. Initially, striae may be pink or purplish but later progress to become silvery white or brown with a loosely wrinkled surface (Fig. 41-4).

Striae gravidarum probably are induced by several factors (23). Increased abdominal girth during pregnancy will initiate stretch, an essential condition for the development of the striae. A significant association seems to exist between the occurrence of striae and heavier infants as well as heavier or obese mothers (24). The state of the dermal collagen and elastin appears to be another important determinant. Although some authors have attributed striae simply to stretching and thinning of the dermal connective tissue, there is histologic evidence that dermal scarring plays a role in striae formation. In such a scenario, dermal collagen ruptures and separates, and the intervening gap is filled with newly synthesized, densely packed horizontal collagen bundles (10). It is also possible that one or more of the hormones of pregnancy, particularly the corticosteroids, may alter and weaken the connective tissue.

There is no effective way to prevent striae. Davey found that abdominal wall striae were significantly less common when the skin had been massaged with olive oil (24). There is some controversy as to whether striae can be prevented in this way. *Tretinoin*, a derivative of vitamin A and a category C topical medication, has been used in the treatment of acne for two decades. Besides its epi-

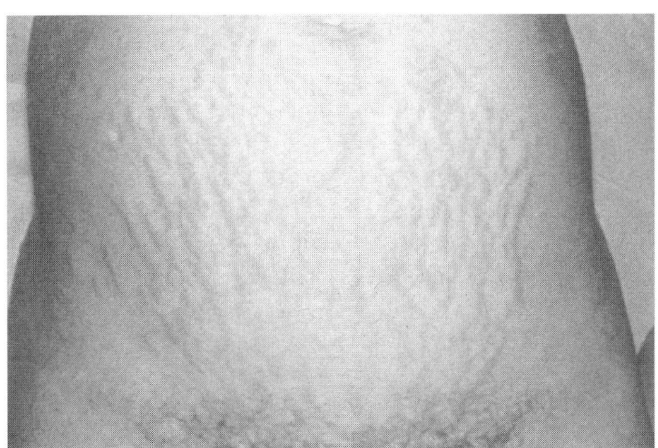

FIG. 41-4. Striae gravidarum initially may be pink or purple but later become silvery white or brown.

dermal effects, this medication has an effect on dermal fibroblasts and collagen formation. On this basis, Elson treated 20 patients with tretinoin cream 0.1% for 12 weeks (25). Of the 16 patients who completed the study, 10 of whom had striae gravidarum, all but one had improved clinically; some patients had complete clearing. Additional studies also have reported some clinical benefits of topical tretinoin cream on striae; however, it is by no means clear that the treatment of striae gravidarum with topical tretinoin is effective. Schoelch and associates reported a double-blind, randomized study in which patients served as their own control. Fifteen patients who had developed striae from their first pregnancy and were within 6 months postpartum, were studied by applying tretinoin cream 0.1% to one half of their abdomen and a placebo to the other half. After 4 months of treatment, the tretinoin cream had not affected the clinical improvement of the striae (26). The pulse dye laser also has been used in the treatment of striae, with some reports of moderate improvement of skin elasticity and depression (27). Patients should be told that, once formed, striae are permanent but to expect a gradual cosmetic improvement over several years whereby the striae will become flesh colored or even hypopigmented.

SKIN DISEASES SPECIFICALLY ASSOCIATED WITH PREGNANCY

A small group of dermatoses occur predominantly if not exclusively during pregnancy and the puerperium. Four of these conditions have a firm clinical, histologic, or laboratory basis and stand out as distinct entities: pruritus gravidarum, pruritic urticarial papules and plaques of pregnancy, herpes gestationis, and impetigo herpetiformis. Although the dermatoses of pregnancy are considered unique to gestation and the postpartum period, overall, pregnant patients are not more affected by skin disease than persons in the general population (1,28).

PRURITUS

One of the most frequent cutaneous disturbances of pregnancy is pruritus. Itching occurs to some extent in approximately 17% of pregnant patients (1). This subjective symptom may seem out of proportion to the visible changes on the skin. Pruritus in the absence of a skin eruption may be generalized or localized to the abdominal, vulvar, or perianal areas. Pruritus also may be an associated symptom of many of the dermatoses of pregnancy, or it may be the result of any of the numerous causes of pruritus that occur in the nonpregnant state.

Generalized Pruritus

Pruritus gravidarum is a condition marked by intense generalized pruritus in the absence of a primary cutaneous eruption. It is generally considered to be the result of a mild anicteric cholestasis resulting from disturbances of bilirubin excretion caused by the effects of estrogens and progestins (29).

Incidence

The incidence of pruritus gravidarum is reported to be 0.02% to 2.4% worldwide; however, higher rates have been reported from Chile (14%) and Scandinavia (3%) (30).

Clinical Presentation

Pruritus gravidarum begins in the third trimester in two thirds of cases. Pruritus tends to be intermittent at first, often limited to the abdomen, trunk, or extremities. It eventually becomes constant and generalized. Excoriations, particularly on the abdomen, frequently are produced by scratching. Symptoms clear within a few days after delivery but tend to recur in subsequent pregnancies or following oral contraceptive use (31). If the disorder progresses to cholestatic jaundice, icterus eventually may become detectable within 2 to 4 weeks after the onset of pruritus. The liver may become enlarged and tender, the urine darkens, and stools become clay colored.

Laboratory Findings

Liver function tests are helpful only in severe cases. The serum level of direct bilirubin may be normal or slightly increased and rarely exceeds 8 mg per deciliter. Mild to moderate transaminase elevations may be found.

The most marked laboratory abnormality found in patients with significant obstetric cholestasis is the serum concentration of bile acids. Bile acids are cleared incompletely by the liver and accumulate in the plasma of women with cholestasis. Levels are typically much greater than in normal pregnancy, and total bile acids may be elevated 10- to 100-fold. The most abnormal elevation of the individual bile acids is that of cholic acid. In fact, the measurement of cholic acid conjugates provides the most sensitive test for the diagnosis of obstetric cholestasis (32). Other factors also may be involved in the pruritus of this condition, because there is not always a direct correlation with bile acid levels. Lunzer and colleagues (32) studied serial plasma levels of the glycine conjugate of cholic acid, cholylglycine, during midpregnancy in 297 women. They observed a threefold elevation as pregnancy progressed. About 10% of these women had an abrupt rise of cholylglycine beginning in the third trimester, and one half had sustained pruritus until delivery. About 20% of those with normally elevated cholylglycine levels had significant pruritus as well, however. In rare instances, a liver biopsy may be required to substantiate the diagnosis and is as safe in pregnant women as in nonpregnant women (33).

Histology

Because there are no primary skin lesions in pruritus gravidarum, cutaneous histology has not been reported in pertinent reviews. Liver biopsy reveals nonspecific cholestasis with widely dilated, enlarged bile canaliculi, staining of parenchyma with bile pigments, and little to no inflammatory response (34). The abnormalities are completely reversible; they do not lead to any permanent functional or structural hepatic damage.

Pathophysiology

The pruritus in pruritus gravidarum is caused by the elevated concentration of bile acids in the skin. The increase in serum bile acids during pregnancy is related to a decreased capacity for hepatic excretion of organic anions such as bilirubin, bile acids, and sulfobromophthalein. In the genetically susceptible person, physiologic concentrations of estrogens and progestins are believed to interfere with hepatic excretion of bile acids. Synthetic agents in oral contraceptives also have been shown to induce decreased hepatic function in women who developed cholestasis in earlier pregnancies (35). There is evidence that the susceptibility to pruritus gravidarum may be an autosomal dominantly inherited condition.

Prognosis

Pruritus gravidarum subsides rapidly postpartum but may recur with variable severity in subsequent pregnancies or with the use of estrogen-containing medications. Restoration of normal liver function and structure may lag behind improved symptoms by several weeks. Maternal morbidity is limited to the inconvenience caused by pruritus. The question of fetal prognosis is more controversial. The fetus usually suffers no ill effects. Some data suggest, however, a significantly higher incidence of premature labor, low-birth-weight infants, and postpartum hemorrhage in pregnancies complicated by severe frank obstetric cholestasis (35,36). Pregnancy complicated only by pruritus may be associated with a tendency toward earlier delivery and meconium staining of amniotic fluid, features that can be considered less serious variations of those encountered with maternal jaundice (35,37).

Treatment

Mild forms of pruritus gravidarum can be treated with bland antipruritic preparations. More severe cases may require ion-exchange resins, such as cholestyramine, which bind bile acids in the intestine. Cholestyramine is a nonresorbable resin and is thus harmless to the fetus (38). It usually relieves pruritus within 2 weeks. Dosages of 12 to 16 g daily cause infrequent side effects. The adverse side effects include constipation, nausea, heartburn, skin eruptions, hyperchloremic acidosis, and malabsorption of calcium or fat-soluble vitamins. Profuse bleeding at delivery and an increased prothrombin time because of vitamin K deficiency have been reported (32, 39). Prothrombin time should be measured periodically to evaluate vitamin K requirements when cholestyramine is prescribed. When vitamin supplementation is administered, vitamins should be given within 1 hour before to 4 hours after the administration of cholestyramine (39). Although cholestyramine has been reported to be effective, some clinicians have found only marginal improvement with this therapy. Apparently, some patients will need to take medication for prolonged periods to experience relief. Hirvioja and colleagues reported prompt relief of pruritus in ten women given dexamethasone, 12 mg daily, for 7 days. They postulated that associated diminished estrogen synthesis caused relief of pruritus as well as lowered serum hepatic enzyme levels (40).

Localized Pruritus

Abdominal pruritus, a localized pruritus of the abdomen, occurs with higher incidence in the second half of pregnancy as the abdomen becomes distended. Kasdon, in a study of 365 pregnant patients, first described localized pruritus of the abdomen unrelated to specific dermatosis or itching elsewhere on the body (4). It occurred with sufficient severity to cause complaints in 17.8% of patients. It was most severe at night, with peak incidence occurring in warm, humid summer months, suggesting that warm weather and irritation from clothing may be factors. Although no clear relationship was found between the development of striae gravidarum and pruritus, patients who have marked striae tend to have more severe pruritus than those who have only mild striae. No clear correlation with cleanliness or neuropsychiatric disease could be made, although anxiety, fatigue, and discomfort near term may play a role. Abdominal pruritus also may herald the onset of herpes gestationis and pruritic urticarial papules and plaques of pregnancy.

Pruritus ani et vulvae, although beginning on the same basis as abdominal pruritus, has local factors that usually predominate to intensify the itching because of the numerous fine sensory nerve endings in this area. Vaginitis from bacteria, yeast, trichomonas, or *C. albicans* must be considered in the differential diagnosis along with varicosities, intestinal parasites, and fungal infections as well as psoriatic, seborrheic, contact, or atopic dermatoses. When no causal agent is found, a psychogenic basis for the pruritus must be considered. Affected areas show maceration, edema, excoriations, or fissuring.

Prurigo Gestationis

Prurigo gestationis, first reported by Besnier and colleagues in 1904, was described clinically by Nurse in 1962 as "early onset prurigo of pregnancy"(41,42).

Incidence

Prurigo gestationis occurs in approximately 1 in 300 pregnancies.

Clinical Presentation

Onset can occur between the fourth and ninth months of gestation but usually presents between 25 and 30 weeks of gestation. As a rule, prurigo gestationis occurs earlier in pregnancies than pruritic urticarial papules and plaques of pregnancy. Lesions consist of small, red, grouped papules that are excoriated and crusted. Papules usually are distributed on the exterior surfaces of the extremities, shoulders, and abdomen but may become widespread in severe cases. The eruption clears rapidly after delivery and may leave postinflammatory pigmentary changes. There is no apparent tendency to recur in subsequent pregnancies.

Histology

Histologic evaluation has demonstrated epidermal parakeratosis and acanthosis, frequently accompanied by full-thickness excoriation with serous crusting. The dermis shows a perivascular lymphocytic infiltrate and occasional localized areas of fibroplasia. Both direct and indirect immunofluorescent studies are negative.

Pathophysiology

Holmes and Black (43) noted in their study of eight patients that four had an atopic diathesis. The propensity of atopic persons to develop prurigo papules as a result of scratching is well recognized. These authors suggested that prurigo gestationis may be a papular neurodermatitis secondary to the pruritus gravidarum that occurs in women who have atopic eczema or an atopic diathesis.

Prognosis

No maternal or fetal complications have been reported (44).

Pruritic Urticarial Papules and Plaques of Pregnancy

Pruritic urticarial papules and plaques of pregnancy (PUPPP) was first described by Lawley and colleagues in 1979 (45). A critical review of the literature suggests that considerable overlap exists between PUPPP and several other eruptions that have been described to occur during pregnancy, including toxemic rash of pregnancy, late-onset prurigo of pregnancy, and toxic erythema of pregnancy (42,46,47). Holmes and Black suggested the term *polymorphic eruption of pregnancy* as a more accurate name that would include these entities as well as PUPPP (43). The designation *polymorphous eruption of pregnancy* (PEP) can be further categorized into three subtypes: a group with mainly urticarial plaques and papules; a group with nonurticarial erythema, papules, and vesicles; and a third group, a combination of the first two. In recent years, therefore, the dermatologic and obstetric literature has contained several reports that attach two names (PUPPP and PEP) to what actually is one disease.

Incidence

Many cases of PUPPP have been reported since its initial description (45,48–52). Aside from pruritus gravidarum, which has no clinical lesions, it is the most common dermatosis related to pregnancy (45,53). Estimates of the incidence of PUPPP vary from 1 in 120 to 1 in 240 pregnancies (43).

Clinical Presentation

The skin eruption usually begins in the third trimester, after the 34th week. The most frequent week of onset is the 39th week (52). Occasionally, PUPPP will develop in the immediate postpartum period. Generally, PUPPP is a disease of the first pregnancy, and most patients do not experience a recurrence in subsequent pregnancies (48,52). The lesions consist of pruritic erythematous papules that coalesce to form urticarial plaques (Fig. 41-5). Papules may be surrounded by a pale halo and may blanch easily on pressure. Although pruritus is a major symptom of PUPPP, excoriations are rare. The eruption almost always begins on the abdomen, particularly in the abdominal striae (Fig. 41-6) (52,54). Lesions then spread

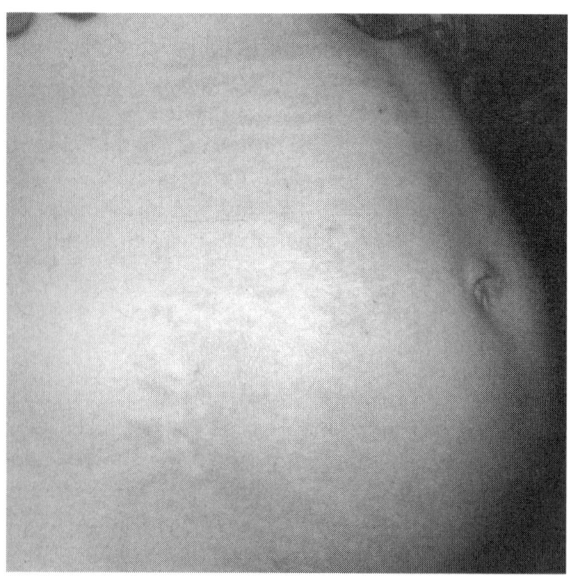

FIG. 41-5. Pruritic urticarial papules and plaques of pregnancy often present as erythematous urticarial papules and plaques on the abdomen.

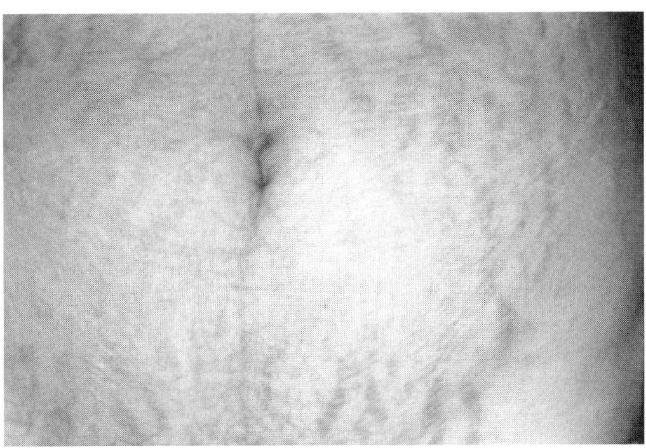

FIG. 41-6. Pruritic urticarial papules and plaques of pregnancy often appear in abdominal striae.

over the next several days to involve the buttocks, waistline, thighs, lower thorax, lower back, and upper inner arms. The face usually is spared as well as the hands and feet and mucous membranes. The eruption generally clears within several weeks after delivery. No laboratory abnormalities have been detected, and the pathophysiology is unknown.

Histology

Two histologic patterns have been described: a *superficial pattern* that consists of perivascular lymphohistocytic infiltration associated with some edema of the papillary dermis with local spongiosis, parakeratosis, and crusts in the epidermis; and a *deep pattern* that is marked by an uninvolved epidermis and perivascular and interstitial infiltrates in the mid and deep dermis (45). The papillary dermis may be edematous, and some eosinophils may be present in the infiltrate. Immunofluorescent studies are consistently negative (43).

Prognosis

The importance of recognizing PUPPP is to distinguish it from herpes gestationis, which is more rare and may be associated with fetal morbidity and mortality, whereas PUPPP is not. In cases of early nonbullous urticarial herpes gestationis, the clinical appearance of both diseases can be similar. Although PUPPP may resemble herpes gestationis, there are no vesicles or bullae. Histologic and immunofluorescence examinations can be helpful in distinguishing between the two disorders. There is no evidence that perinatal morbidity is increased.

Treatment

Pruritus is the major complaint of patients who have PUPPP, and almost all describe it to be severe enough to interfere with sleep. Despite intense pruritus, excoriations are rare. Most patients respond to topical corticosteroid creams of mid to high potency. Difficult cases may require a brief, tapering course of systemic corticosteroids. In general, PUPPP seems to be a self-limiting disorder in which corticosteroids provide symptomatic relief and hasten resolution of lesions.

Herpes Gestationis

Herpes gestationis is a rare, pruritic, recurrent urticarial and vesicobullous skin disease of pregnancy and the puerperium. Diagnosis rests on a distinctive clinical presentation and specific histopathologic and immunopathologic findings. Despite what its name implies, it is not a viral-induced illness. Herpes gestationis bears a close clinical and immunopathologic resemblance to bullous pemphigoid, an autoimmune disease of elderly people. On this basis, a number of researchers have proposed that herpes gestationis be renamed *pemphigoid gestationis* (43).

Incidence

The incidence of herpes gestationis has been estimated as 1 in 4,000 to 60,000 pregnancies (38,55,56).

Clinical Presentation

By definition, herpes gestationis is restricted to women of childbearing age. Onset of the disease is anywhere from the first trimester of pregnancy to the first 5 days of the postpartum period, but it is most common during the second trimester (57). It may begin with a prodrome of malaise, fever, nausea, headache, and alternating hot and cold sensations. Burning and severe pruritus may precede the eruption by several days. The earliest skin lesions are erythematous edematous papules and plaques with an urticarial quality. These plaques may assume circinate configurations and have a predilection for the trunk, especially the abdomen, and in particular the umbilical area (Fig. 41-7). Within days, papules, vesicles, and tense bullae develop. Target lesions like those of erythema multiforme sometimes appear. The eruption has a predilection for the abdomen, buttocks, back, forearm, palms, and soles. In 90% of patients, it begins in the periumbilical area. The mucous membranes are uncommon sites for lesions. Bilateral symmetry is not a constant feature, and lesions may spread centrifugally. With rupture of the bullae of vesicles, denuded areas become covered with a brownish yellow or hemorrhagic crust. Bacterial infection and excoriations may be present. Resolution of lesions leaves little or transient hyperpigmentation, but deep excoriations may leave scars. Transverse pitting and grooving of finger and toe nails may be observed corresponding to onset of the eruption.

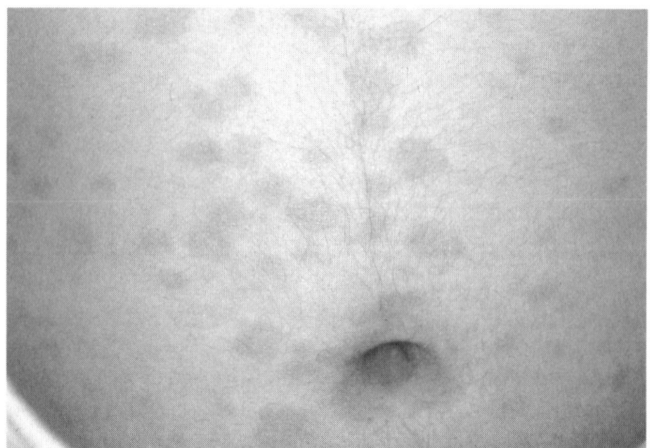

FIG. 41-7. Herpes gestationis often presents with periumbilical plaques.

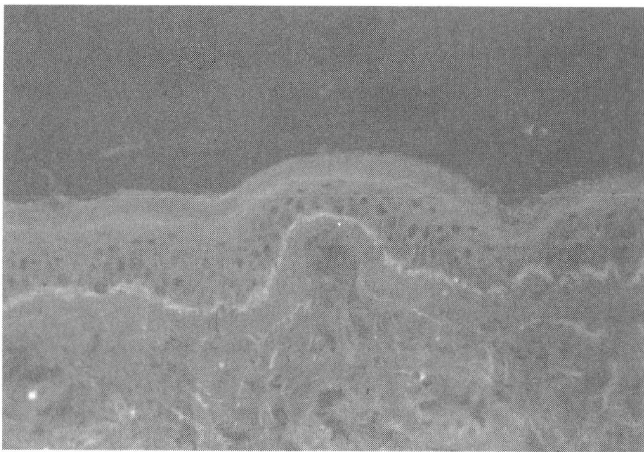

FIG. 41-8. Herpes gestationis direct immunofluorescence reveals diffuse linear deposition of C3 along the basement membrane zone. (Courtesy of R. Valenzuela, M.D., Ph.D.)

The clinical course of herpes gestationis is one of recurring crops of blisters, which, if untreated, usually resolve within a few days to 3 months postpartum. The dermatosis may wane in late pregnancy and wax again in the immediate postpartum period. Cases have been reported that have spontaneously resolved during pregnancy or that have lasted as long as 2 years after delivery (58).

Histology

Histologically, the urticarial lesions of herpes gestationis are characterized by a moderately dense, perivascular, mixed inflammatory cell infiltrate of lymphocytes, histiocytes, and eosinophils around the vessels of the superficial and deep dermal plexuses, with papillary dermal edema, spongiosis, and focal necrosis of basal cells over the tips of the dermal papillae (57). Eosinophils may be found in spongiotic foci within the epidermis. Neutrophils may be present in the dermal infiltrate in small numbers. Bullous lesions are the result of subepidermal separation, with the basal lamina forming the floor of the blister (59). Eosinophils usually are found within blister fluid. The presence of eosinophils, the most constant histologic feature of herpes gestationis, is seen in nearly every case (43).

Direct immunofluorescence of lesions of herpes gestationis reveals the third component of complement to be deposited at the dermal–epidermal junction in a linear pattern. The linear deposition of C3 along the basement membrane zone appears in lesional, perilesional, and uninvolved skin when examined with direct immunofluorescence (Fig. 41-8). Ten percent of patients have immunoglobulin G (IgG) deposits at the dermal–epidermal junction visible on direct immunofluorescence.

Immunoelectron microscopy has demonstrated a fairly uniform deposition of reaction products throughout the lamina lucida that contrasts only slightly with the findings in bullous pemphigoid. The events leading to these findings may occur by the generation of IgG antibody reacting against the basement membrane zone of the skin. The antigen apparently is a component of the lamina lucida and may be identical to the antigen of bullous pemphigoid. Because there is so much more C3 than IgG present at the basement membrane zone, C3 is detectable by direct immunofluorescence, whereas IgG usually is not. Fewer than 20% of patients have circulating skin-reactive IgG antibodies, as detected by routine indirect immunofluorescence (60).

Herpes gestationis factor is present in the sera of most patients and can induce exogenous complement (C3) to be deposited at the basement membrane zone of normal skin or mucous membranes. It is detectable by a technique called *complement indirect immunofluorescence*. Recent studies have shown that herpes gestationis factor is probably an IgG antibody, but usually it is not demonstrable on routine direct immunofluorescence and is not demonstrable in the sera of all patient with herpes gestationis (61). Herpes gestationis factor titers, although clearly playing a major role in the cause of the disease, correlate poorly with disease activity.

Pathophysiology

The similarity between herpes gestationis and bullous pemphigoid strongly suggests that the autoantibody for herpes gestationis may be induced by placental antigens that cross-react with the skin. Experimental support for this hypothesis exists. Ortonne and colleagues, using complement-fixing immunofluorescence and immune electron microscopy, showed that herpes gestationis factor could bind to the basement membrane zone of the amnion and chorion laeve of the placenta (62). Kelly and colleagues demonstrated that antibody binds to the amnion and to the umbilical cord (63). Illustrating the fact that herpes gestationis and bullous pemphigoid may have common pathogenic determinants is the clinical report of two patients who initially presented with clinicopathologic features of herpes gestationis but subsequently bullous pemphigoid evolved (64).

Eosinophils also seem to play an important role in herpes gestationis, because there often is striking tissue eosinophilia and serum eosinophilia in patients who have herpes gestationis. Products of eosinophil degranulation in lesional skin suggest their role in the tissue damage in herpes gestationis.

Differential Diagnosis

Herpes gestationis can be differentiated easily from the other dermatoses of pregnancy because it is the only condition that produces bullae. Early urticarial lesions may resemble PUPPP. Some clinicians suggest performing immunofluorescent biopsy in all cases of presumed PUPPP to rule out the slight possibility of herpes gestationis (56). They point to the occurrence of urticarial herpes gestationis without blisters during one pregnancy followed by typical bullous disease during subsequent pregnancies. The predictive power of immunofluorescence in such cases would be important. Others point out the rarity of herpes gestationis compared with PUPPP and suggest that routine immunofluorescence would not be worthwhile. Herpes gestationis must be differentiated from other bullous diseases that can occur coincidentally during pregnancy: bullous pemphigoid, pemphigus, dermatitis herpetiformis, bullous drug eruption, and erythema multiforme.

Treatment

Therapeutic goals include controlling maternal blister formation and pruritus and lessening the risks for fetal complications. Treatment of mild cases may require only antihistamines and topical steroids, but most patients will require the use of systemic corticosteroids. The preferred treatment for more severe disease is prednisone 40 to 60 mg daily in divided doses, which may be tapered and modified to an alternate-days schedule once clearing is achieved. Difficult cases unresponsive to oral corticosteroids may require immunosuppressive agents such as azathioprine, which should not be given during pregnancy without weighing risk versus benefit. Whenever possible, the use of azathioprine in pregnant patients should be avoided. Plasmapheresis has been used successfully in herpes gestationis as well. Postpartum flareups, which are not uncommon, often require aggressive therapy.

Course and Prognosis

Herpes gestationis is a disease of exacerbations and remissions. Clearing generally occurs within 3 months of delivery. Exacerbations have occurred before normal menses and following the use of progesterone-containing oral contraceptives (65). The disease usually occurs in subsequent pregnancies, with a tendency for earlier onset and more severe manifestations. Maternal prognosis, in the absence of secondary infection or steroid therapy side effects, is usually excellent. There appears to be an inherited predisposition to the disease. Specifically, there is a marked increased incidence of human leukocyte antigen (HLA)-DR3 antigens in affected women. For example, whereas more than half of women with herpes gestationis have these antigens, they are found in only 3% of unaffected women. These antigens also are associated with Graves disease, Hashimoto's thyroiditis, Addison's disease, type I diabetes mellitus, and systemic lupus erythematosus. Shornick reported that 11% of 75 women with herpes gestationis also had Graves disease (56).

The question of whether herpes gestationis is associated with significant fetal morbidity and mortality has been debated. Although reports describe an increased incidence of preterm delivery and small-for-gestational-age infants, increased perinatal mortality was not found. Neonatal skin lesions similar to those of the mother have been reported to develop in 5% to 10% of neonates (66). These vesicobullous lesions are mild and usually clear spontaneously within weeks. C3 complement deposited at the basement membrane of the newborn skin and herpes gestationis factor in cord serum have been described (67–69).

Impetigo Herpetiformis

Impetigo herpetiformis is a rare but serious generalized pustular eruption that resembles pustular psoriasis. Although originally described by von Hebra in 1872 as a disease specific for pregnancy, impetigo herpetiformis subsequently was reported in nonpregnant women and men (70). Hypoparathyroidism and hypocalcemia frequently are associated with impetigo herpetiformis, regardless of whether the patient is pregnant.

Incidence

Impetigo herpetiformis is a rare entity, with just more than 100 reported cases in the world literature (1,70).

Clinical Presentation

Onset of the disease in pregnant women is from late in the first trimester to the end of the third trimester. Peak incidence occurs in the last 3 months of gestation. Impetigo herpetiformis affects pregnant women who usually have no personal or family history of psoriasis. The disease usually recurs with every successive pregnancy, developing earlier and with increasing severity.

Cutaneous lesions begin as irregular patches or slightly raised plaques of erythema, on the margin of which later appear superficial white or greenish sterile pustules. These areas of involvement gradually enlarge by peripheral extension of the annular pustular margin, whereas the more central areas are rapidly broken down, becoming denuded or crusted. The eruption may become confluent so that in severe cases the entire skin surface (except the hands, feet, and face) may be covered with active pustules or older crusted lesions.

Usually cutaneous lesions first involve the intertriginous regions, such as the groin, axillae, inframammary folds, gluteal crease, and umbilicus. In flexural areas, moist vegetating plaques may resemble pemphigus vegetans. Lesions generally heal without scarring, although postinflammatory hyperpigmentation is seen regularly. Subungual pustules may cause onycholysis. Mucous membrane lesions have been reported to involve the oral and esophageal mucosa. These pustules leave painful erosions arranged in a circinate pattern.

Pruritus is not usually a problem. Severe constitutional symptoms are present in most cases and include fever, chills, nausea, vomiting, and diarrhea. Delirium, tetany, and convulsions may occur and are frequent in cases associated with hypocalcemia.

Histology

The histology of impetigo herpetiformis is in many respects identical to that of pustular psoriasis. The characteristic lesion is the spongiform pustule of Kogoj, a spongelike cavity containing a collection of neutrophils in the epidermis. Pierard and colleagues found histologic differences from pustular psoriasis in the following respects: The pustules did not show any tendency to confluence, and they contained both neutrophils and mononuclear cells that had abundant cytoplasm and large, irregularly shaped nuclei (71). Parakeratosis, with regular elongation of rete ridges and migration of mononuclear cells from dermal capillaries into the epidermis also is seen.

Laboratory

Leukocytosis and an elevated erythrocyte sedimentation rate are seen during severe exacerbations. Bacterial culture of pus from the lesions or peripheral blood are negative, provided no superinfection is present. Some patients have hypocalcemia secondary to hypoparathyroidism.

Pathophysiology

It is unclear whether impetigo herpetiformis is a variant of pustular psoriasis triggered by the metabolic state of pregnancy or a disease *sui generis*. Those who consider impetigo herpetiformis a true dermatosis of pregnancy point out that affected patients are free of the skin disorder between pregnancies and have no manifestations or history of psoriasis, whereas most patients with pustular psoriasis, whether pregnant or not, have had preexisting typical or atypical psoriasis.

Differential Diagnosis

Impetigo herpetiformis must be differentiated from other pustular conditions such as pustular psoriasis, candidiasis, subcorneal pustular dermatosis, impetigo, miliaria, dermatitis herpetiformis, and herpes gestationis.

Treatment

Termination of pregnancy is usually the cure for impetigo herpetiformis. Lotem and colleagues reported a case in which improvement after delivery failed to occur until complete removal of all pregnancy products was established (72). Corticosteroids are the treatment of choice, but most clinicians report only moderate responses. In classic pustular psoriasis, systemic corticosteroids have an immediate therapeutic effect. Fluid and electrolyte balance should be maintained and hypocalcemia corrected if it is present.

Course and Prognosis

Before the use of corticosteroids and antibiotics, a gloomy maternal prognosis was common. Maternal mortality is now rare, but stillbirth and placental insufficiency still may occur, even when the disease appears to be controlled by the use of corticosteroids. The disease remits promptly postpartum, usually without residual psoriatic plaques, but it may recur in successive pregnancies.

Papular Dermatitis of Pregnancy

Papular dermatitis of pregnancy (PDP) was described by Spangler and colleagues in 1962 (73). It has since received attention because of the authors' contention of increased fetal risk. Subsequent analysis of this report revealed that fetal mortality data were overestimated and were presented in a way that precluded valid reassessment (43). The initial report may have included severe cases of prurigo gestationis or PUPPP. We include PDP in this chapter but question its separate classification as a dermatosis of pregnancy; however, the reader should be aware that we are uncertain whether it is a discrete clinical entity.

Incidence

The syndrome is uncommon and was estimated by Spangler and Emerson to have an incidence of 1 per 2,500 pregnancies (74).

Clinical Presentation

Onset has been reported as occurring from the first to the last month of pregnancy. It is characterized by generalized, intensely pruritic papules involving all areas of the body, and it may involve the face and scalp. Individual lesions are 3 to 5 mm soft, erythematous edematous papules topped by slightly firmer acuminate papules. These are often scratched off, leaving a hemorrhagic crust. Lesions appear gradually rather than in crops so that three to eight lesions may appear daily while older lesions heal in 7 to 10 days with slight hyperpigmentation and no true scarring. Delivery abruptly terminates the eruption, and lesions clear within 2 days. The dermatitis tends to recur in subsequent pregnancies.

Laboratory Findings

In 12 patients studied by Spangler and Emerson, urinary chorionic gonadotropin levels were greatly increased during the last trimester (74). Low urinary estriol, low plasma hydrocortisone, and reduced plasma hydrocortisone half-life also were reported. Intradermal skin tests to the placental extracts of patients with PDP are positive. Similar tests with normal placental material are negative. Histopathology has not been reported.

Pathophysiology

The results of intradermal testing with placental extracts suggest a sensitization phenomenon. The eruption improves abruptly after delivery. The one exception to this pattern occurred when the dermatitis persisted for 6 weeks postpartum, after which time a placental fragment retained in the uterus was discovered. The rash subsequently disappeared after curettage.

Prognosis

Although no maternal complications have occurred, controversy surrounds the disease because of the 27% incidence of fetal stillbirths and spontaneous abortions reported by Spangler and associates in their initial study. This prognosis has made dermatologists reluctant to diagnose prurigo eruptions as PDP. Review of Spangler's data by Winton reveals that the 27% incidence of fetal death included all pregnancies of the initial study group, regardless of the presence of PDP (54). When only those pregnancies associated with the rash were considered, the incidence of fetal death was considerably lower (12.5%).

Treatment

Spangler and Emerson found that diethylstilbesterol (DES) in doses of 1,000 to 2,500 mg per day controlled the disease (74). The subsequent discovery of vaginal carcinoma in the offspring of mothers given DES during pregnancy led to avoidance of this therapy. Systemic corticosteroids are usually effective; however, doses up to 100 mg per day may be required to control the disease and reduce fetal loss to 12% or less (1,74). Topical corticosteroids may control the eruption and should be the first line of treatment.

DERMATOLOGIC THERAPY

The evaluation of generalized pruritus in a pregnant woman is extremely difficult. Coincidental causes of pruritus and rash must be excluded by history, physical examination, and appropriate laboratory testing. Pruritic conditions such as scabies, pediculosis, insect bites, urticaria, drug eruptions, diabetes, xerosis, atopic and nummular dermatitis, or neurodermatitis should be considered. The incidence of urticaria, dermatographism, and erythema multiforme appear to be increased in pregnancy. Some women develop dyshydrotic dermatitis *de novo,* whereas many others experience flareups of atopic eczema and other types of dermatitis, especially near term in hot weather. Knowledge of the patient's emotional state is necessary when determining whether a psychogenic basis for pruritus exists when no causal factor is found.

Nonspecific generalized pruritus occurring in pregnancy is managed best by conventional dermatologic therapy. The value of simple measures should not be underestimated because often such measures are effective in alleviating the most distressing symptoms.

Irritants such as rough or tight clothing, drying soaps, and adverse climatic factors should be avoided whenever possible. Colloidal oatmeal baths containing oil are soothing and antipruritic. After bathing, an antipruritic emollient cream or lotion is applied and repeated as often as necessary. Menthol (0.25%) may be added as a cooling antipruritic. Phenol should be avoided because it is readily absorbed through the skin in concentrations high enough to induce nephrotoxocity, with the possibility of subsequent fetal toxicity (38).

Topical steroids carry the same indications for pregnant women as for nonpregnant patients. Repeated applications of potent fluorinated steroids to large inflamed or denuded areas may lead to adrenal suppression, manifestations of hypercortism, and cutaneous atrophy or striae.

Antihistamines are sometimes effective for both their antipruritic and sedative effects. Diphenhydramine, cyproheptadine, loratidine, and cimetidine have been designated as category B antihistamines (75). Insufficient data are available regarding hydroxyzine, which is relatively contraindicated for pregnancy. Astemizole, terfenadine, and fexofenadine are considered category C medications.

Although the use of systemic corticosteroids in pregnancy has been the subject of much controversy, studies of human subjects have failed to demonstrate teratogenic activity. Cleft palate has been caused in offspring of pregnant rabbits treated with pharmacologic doses of steroids (6,76). The judicious use of steroids does not appear to be harmful in human pregnancy, and numerous reports attest to the relative lack of fetal hazards from corticosteroid therapy, particularly when given in short courses near term (77). Because of the possibility of premature delivery and rare transient fetal adrenal suppression, the risks and benefits of systemic steroid therapy should be considered carefully (1,78). The drugs should be withheld in the first trimester, and the dosage and duration should be the minimum consistent with required therapeutic effect (54,79–81).

The physician must be aware of potential effects on the fetus of drugs given the mother. Placental maternal–fetal transfer of substances is established by the fifth week of gestation. Drugs that are used in dermatologic therapeutics and are known or possible teratogenic agents include isotretinoin, etretinate, methotrexate, cyclophosphamide, nitrogen mustard, and azathioprine (38). Drugs that may affect fetal and newborn development adversely include tetracycline and podophyllin (38). A good general rule is to avoid drugs in pregnancy except when demanded for comfort or survival.

CHANGES THAT PREGNANCY INDUCES IN DERMATOLOGIC DISEASES

Cutaneous Tumors Influenced by Pregnancy

Granuloma Gravidarum

Granuloma gravidarum (pyogenic granuloma of pregnancy) is a gingival lesion that usually appears early in pregnancy. This vascular tumor of the gingiva usually is associated with extensive gingivitis and apparently is influenced by hormonal factors associated with pregnancy. The prevalence of granuloma gravidarum is estimated to approach 2% of all pregnancies (2,82,83).

The lesions appear as red or purple tumors ranging from 1 mm to several centimeters in diameter. They usually arise from the gingival papilla between adjacent teeth, although they can originate from the buccal or lingual surfaces of the marginal gingiva. Histologically, granuloma gravidarum is indistinguishable from pyogenic granulomas. The lesions are composed of granulation tissue covered with stratified squamous epithelium. The connective tissue and granulation tissue are infiltrated with lymphocytes, plasma cells, polymorphonuclear leukocytes, and histiocytes. Generally, these tumors are not treated until the termination of pregnancy. Postpartum shrinkage of lesions may occur, making surgical intervention unnecessary (54).

Cutaneous Hemangiomas

Cutaneous hemangiomas can develop and enlarge during pregnancy (4). In view of the effects of gestational hormones on vascular structures, the association of pregnancy with the spontaneous development of hemangioma, hemangioendothelioma, and glomus tumor is not surprising (54). Vascular tumors generally arise in the second or third trimesters, increase in size, and regress after delivery (4). Large hemangiomas resulting in arteriovenous shunting have been reported with subsequent high-output cardiac failure (54). These lesions regress postpartum only partially, tending to enlarge again in subsequent pregnancies (4). Small lesions need not be treated if they are cosmetically acceptable, but they may be treated by electrodesiccation or laser therapy after delivery.

Eruptive Xanthomas

Eruptive xanthomas may occur during pregnancy in association with hypertriglyceridemia. The added stimulus of increased estrogens during pregnancy may play a role in the elevation of triglycerides. Complications include severe pancreatitis, which can result in adult respiratory distress syndrome and fetal loss (84). Treatment consists of dietary restriction, cholestyramine, and nicotinic acid.

Molluscum Fibrosum Gravidarum

Molluscum fibrosum gravidarum (skin tag, acrochordon) is characterized by small, fleshy, pinhead- to pea-sized, pedunculated cutaneous tags that are seen most frequently around the front and sides of the neck, on the upper chest, within inframammary areas, and in the axillae. These lesions appear during the later months of pregnancy and commonly persist after delivery, sometimes presenting a cosmetic problem (4). The lesions are soft fibromas and histologically consist of a core of normal connective tissue covered with epidermis.

Miscellaneous Dermal Tumors

During pregnancy, dermatofibromas commonly develop. It also has been reported that leiomyomas can grow or become painful and that keloids can grow more rapidly.

Neurofibromatosis

Von Recklinghausen neurofibromatosis (NF) is an autosomal dominantly inherited disorder with a markedly variable expression (85). This disease may be inherited from a person who has NF, or it may be the result of a new, spontaneous mutation in the developing fetus. Each child of an affected parent has a 50% chance of inheriting the disease and of developing some stigmata of NF. NF is relatively common, with a frequency of about 1 in 3,000 births.

Cafe au lait spots are present in more than 99% of patients who have NF. Crowe and colleagues designated the presence of six or more cafe au lait spots larger than 1.5 cm in diameter as a diagnostic criterion for NF in their study (86). This number has come to represent the baseline for establishing the diagnosis under other circumstances as well (87).

Neurofibromas virtually always involve the skin but may occur in deeper peripheral nerves and nerve roots in or on viscera and blood vessels innervated by the autonomic system. Neurofibromas of the skin and elsewhere increase in size and number in both sexes at puberty and, in most cases among women, during pregnancy (88,89). Although there is no specific explanation for this feature, the accumulation of intercellular glycosaminoglycans has been suggested as the cause, as has the stimulation of neurofibroma growth by sex steroids, directly by or through mediation of nerve-growth factor (90,91). Lesions may show a complete or partial regression following delivery (88).

Some reported cases typify the serious effects that pregnancy can have on patients who have NF as a result of enlargement of neurofibromas (88,89,92). Ansari and Nagamani described a patient who had large NF lesions that enlarged greatly during the latter part of pregnancy as the result of massive hemorrhage within the tumors (88). In addition, the patient developed partial paralysis of the lower extremities either because of the enlargement of a preexisting intraspinal lesion or because of the development of new intraspinal neurofibromas.

Vascular changes with subsequent hypertension in NF is well documented, albeit rare, because most patients who have NF are free of hypertension (93). The association of NF and hypertension during pregnancy was reported by Swapp and Main (94), who reported 24 pregnancies in 11 women who had NF. Ten of these patients developed hypertension. In five women, lesions of NF appeared for the first time during pregnancy. In the others, cafe au lait macules and neurofibromas increased in size and number, and the nodules regressed considerably after delivery. The authors postulated that patients who have NF did not expand their intravascular space adequately because of diseased arterioles (atrophy of media and elastic layer) and, therefore, could not accommodate the increased plasma volume, red cell mass, and cardiac output of pregnancy, thus inducing hypertension. Jarvis and Crompton, in a study of 27 pregnancies of 10 patients who had NF, could not confirm a higher incidence of hypertension (89). Two cases of spontaneous hemothorax caused by vessel rupture have been reported (95). Ansari and Nagamani suggested that there is an increased incidence of abortion and stillbirth in NF; however, this finding has not been confirmed in other studies (54,88).

MELANOCYTIC NEVI AND MELANOMA

During pregnancy, there may be increased growth and darkening of existing melanocytic nevi, with occasional production of new, small, flat, brown ones. Fortunately, most of these lesions are benign and do not require treatment. Those of sufficient cosmetic and diagnostic concern should be excised completely and examined histologically.

The influence of pregnancy on melanoma is a controversial topic. Malignant melanoma not infrequently presents during the active reproductive years of women, and the effects of pregnancy on the course of the disease can be of considerable concern. The estimated incidence of malignant melanoma ranges from 0.14 to 2.8 cases per 1,000 deliveries, making it one of the most frequent cancers occurring during pregnancy (96).

Although melanoma is not generally regarded as hormone dependent, circumstantial evidence suggests that endocrine factors may have a bearing on the tumor's biologic behavior. Case reports of rapidly growing tumors, the appearance of multiple primary tumors, and malignant transformation of congenital and dysplastic nevi during pregnancy point toward an unfavorable impact of estrogens on melanoma, especially coupled with observed instances of the regression of metastases after delivery (97,98). It has been demonstrated that estrogen can bind to melanoma cells in a nonspecific manner. Feucht and colleagues identified a specific estrogen-binding protein in three human melanoma cell lines. Chronic exposure to estradiol resulted in slowed tumor growth, suggesting that estradiol may have indirect effects on melanoma cells in addition to its receptor-mediated effects (99). Shaw and colleagues, in a retrospective study of 938 women who had melanoma, found that endocrine influences in patients who have melanoma may be implicated in tumor formation and metastasis as well as in the distribution of the anatomic site of the primary lesion (100). They found no adverse effect on the survival rate among 17 patients who were pregnant at diagnosis of their melanoma. They also noted that patients not exposed to high circulating levels of endogenous or exogenous estrogens (e.g., nulliparous women and postmenopausal women) generally had more widespread disease initially and a lower 5-year survival rate than women who were exposed to high levels of endogenous or exogenous estrogens. These findings led the authors to suggest that estrogens may play a protective role in the development and progression of melanoma. Multiparity seems to confer a protective effect. The demonstration of an increased amount of melanocyte-stimulating substance in the blood and urine of pregnant women heightened the clinical suspicion of an adverse hormonal influence, although a direct association between MSH and melanoma was not found (101,102). George and colleagues, in a study of 115 cases of pregnancy coinciding with melanoma, failed to substantiate this impression and found no statistically significant difference in prognosis compared with a control group of 330 nonpregnant women who had melanoma (103). Other studies have substantiated these findings (104).

In 1975 Shiu and colleagues retrospectively reviewed 251 surgically treated cases of cutaneous melanoma in women of childbearing age (105). This study revealed a statistically significant difference in prognosis of melanoma in some patients with associated pregnancy, depending on the clinical stage of the disease. No statistical difference in disease-free survival at 5 years could be demonstrated between nulliparous, parous, nonpregnant, and pregnant women who had melanoma. For stage II melanoma, however, a significantly lower survival rate was observed for pregnant patients (29%) and parous women who had experienced activation (ulceration, bleeding, itching, scaling, elevation) of the lesion in a previous pregnancy (22%) compared with nulliparous patients (55%) and others in the parous group (51%). The authors suggested that a lack of deleterious effects of pregnancy on stage I melanoma could be explained by the probable total surgical eradication compared with stage II melanoma, in which occult foci could carry a potential for recrudescence stimulated by pregnancy. Melanomas occurring on the trunk also were found in greater frequency among pregnant patients (105).

Slingluff and Seigler studied 100 patients diagnosed with melanoma during pregnancy; mean follow-up was 6.8 years. Compared with a nonpregnant female population with melanoma, there was a significantly shorter disease-free interval for the pregnant group, with nodal metastases developing in 48% of the pregnant patients and in only 26% of the nonpregnant patients at 10-year follow-up. Thus, pregnancy at diagnosis of malignant melanoma was significantly associated with the development of metastatic disease (106).

Despite all the evidence, no conclusive data exist to support the belief that pregnancy has inevitable adverse effects on malignant melanomas. Until such data are available, it is wise to deal with each case individually with the knowledge that there have been cases in which, directly or indirectly, pregnancy did or did not affect the course of the neoplasm adversely. Therapeutic abortion, oophorectomy, adrenalectomy, or hypophysectomy are not advocated because no evidence exists to show that these measures improve the outcome of melanoma. The disease should be treated the same way in nonpregnant and pregnant patients (107).

Observations made in the study by Shiu and colleagues suggest that, for stage II melanoma, pregnancy may be hazardous, even after treatment, to patients with melanoma (105). It has been suggested that patients wait 2 to 3 years after a diagnosis of melanoma before attempting pregnancy because most recurrences develop thicker tumors within 3 years of diagnosis. For patients who have had activation of a lesion in a previous gestation, it seems wise to counsel against subsequent pregnancies. Likewise, the use of oral contraceptives in these patients would not be recommended until the cellular effects of estrogen and progesterone on melanoma are better understood. Two of four studies comparing oral contraceptive use in women who had melanoma and in those who did not found that the melanoma group had significantly greater use than the women who did not use them (108,109).

The best approach to melanoma is prevention. Prenatal examination of the mother should include a survey of all pigmented nevi at the first antenatal examination. Careful observation should be made of changes in size, alteration in uniformity or intensity of pigmentation, ulceration, pain, or bleeding at the site of any nevus. Attention should be given to irregular borders; elevations; shading of red, white, or blue; and, especially, changes in a preexisting pigmented lesion. Special evaluation should be given to lesions on the trunk, palms, soles, and vulvar area. Development of a new mole adjacent to one already present may be another indication of possible malignancy. All suspicious lesions should be examined by an experienced dermatologist, and a biopsy should be performed and sent for histopathological analysis.

The treatment of primary melanoma is surgical excision with wide margins. Elective lymph-node dissection is controversial. Metastatic disease has been resistant to many forms of therapy. Dacarbazine is the agent of choice for the initial treatment of metastatic disease; however, maternal salvage must be balanced against fetal risks. In some instances, early delivery of the infant may be necessary so that chemotherapy can be used as palliative therapy (94). Metastatic lesions to the fetus and placenta occur rarely. Gross and microscopic examination of the placenta should be performed for all pregnant patients diagnosed with malignant melanoma.

Carcinoid Tumors

Carcinoid tumors are rare; however, 22 cases associated with pregnancy have been reported. Most were appendiceal in origin and did not cause problems for either mother or fetus. The presence of metastatic disease with resulting carcinoid syndrome may cause serious maternal and fetal complications and even fetal death (110). Cutaneous manifestations of carcinoid syndrome include transient flushing affecting the face and upper extremities and a persistent erythema with or without telangiectases. Less common manifestations include scleroderma-like changes, pigment anomalies, and a pellagra-like dermatitis (111).

Cutaneous T-Cell Lymphoma

Cutaneous T-cell lymphoma (CTCL) may flare during pregnancy with the development of secondarily infected eczematous lesions and the appearance of new infiltrated plaques (112). Treatment of CTCL during pregnancy with cytotoxic agents is contraindicated, especially during the first trimester. Mechlorethamine is also contraindicated, because it can cause fetal malformations.

INFECTIOUS DERMATOLOGIC DISEASE INFLUENCED BY PREGNANCY

Condylomata Acuminata

Condylomata acuminata (genital warts) are fleshy verrucae that occur at mucocutaneous junctions and intertriginous areas (the mucosal surface of the female genitalia, the glans and shaft of the penis, and in perianal area) as soft, flesh-colored, pedunculated or polypoid nodules. In some patients, particularly young women, these lesions multiply and coalesce into large cauliflower-like masses. Condylomata acuminata are caused by a papilloma virus antigenically related to the agents for common skin warts (verruca vulgaris) and may be transmitted by sexual contact ("venereal warts") or may be associated with other forms of verrucae. Condylomata acuminata must be differentiated from the moist, wide-based 1- to 3-cm plaquelike papular or nodular lesions of secondary syphilis (condyloma lata) that occur in similar anatomic sites.

Pregnancy acts as a stimulus to the growth or enlargement, sometimes to massive size, of condylomata acuminata (112–117). There is no widely accepted explanation for the propensity of these lesions to enlarge during pregnancy. Suggested influences include increased vascularity, increased perineal moisture, and stimulation by elevated estrogen levels. Spontaneous resolution of warts may occur after pregnancy (114). Severe hemorrhage, an extended febrile course, sepsis, and even death have been reported as results of massive condylomata acuminata of the vulva complicating labor (113). If a cesarean section is not to be performed, surgical removal may be required to avoid a vaginal delivery through large, partially necrotic and infected condylomata. Surgical treatment of large vascular condylomata should not be attempted when the risks of removal are greater than the risks of cesarean section.

The inadequacies and danger of conservative therapy of larger growths through the traditional practice of applying 25% podophyllin are well described (118,119). Therapy with this agent during pregnancy is contraindicated, because it has been associated with premature labor and fetal death following absorption of the antimitotic resin into the maternal circulation. Podophyllin can produce bizarre histologic forms of epithelial cells that can be indistinguishable from those of squamous cell carcinoma; thus, biopsies of the cervix and vulva should be done before treatment is instituted. Fluorouracil creams, imiquimod cream, and alpha-interferon are generally contraindicated in pregnancy.

Massive lesions are best treated by electrodesiccation and curettage or by laser therapy with the patient under general or spinal anesthesia (120). Surgical removal of large warts in pregnant women is difficult because the lesions are highly vascular, and hemostasis often is difficult to achieve. Postoperative vulvar edema is the most common complication, but it responds rapidly to supportive therapy. Associated vaginitis should be treated vigorously, and systemic antibiotics should be used to treat infected lesions before therapy is begun. Cryosurgery, although sometimes effective for small lesions, generally is not useful in lesions massive enough to require therapy during pregnancy (120,121). Carbon dioxide laser photocoagulation and vaporization resulted in 80% of patients being cured after a single treatment, and a 91% cure rate was achieved with multiple treatments (122). Trichloroacetic acid is one of the treatments of choice because it is not absorbed systemically and it denatures on contact with tissue. Electrocautery also can be used safely during pregnancy; however, care must be exercised to avoid excess tissue destruction, which may result in scarring (123).

The strongest evidence implicating human papilloma virus (HPV) infections in the pathogenesis of genital tract malignancies comes from investigations of human tissues using molecular hybridization techniques. Beckmann and colleagues tested 32 women with a history of multicentric squamous cell carcinoma of the anogenital region for the presence of HPV; they used the polymerase chain reaction (PCR) or DNA hybridization technique (124). In 28 of 32 women, HPV was detected at all sites (most frequently types 6, 16, and 33); 245 women with vulvar condylomata were studied over a 4-year period. Eighteen patients were diagnosed with vulvar intraepithelial neoplasia, grade 3, and four patients were diagnosed with invasive carcinoma (123). It is important, therefore, to biopsy genital condyloma, because it is not possible to differentiate clinically between benign and malignant lesions.

Recurrent Respiratory Papillomatosis

Recurrent respiratory papillomatosis (RRP) can develop as a result of perinatal transmission of HPV transmitted via neonatal aspiration of vaginal secretions during vaginal delivery (125). Neonates appear to be at greater risk of HPV infection in the oropharyngeal tract than in the genital region. HPV types 6 and 11 are the primary types that have been detected in RRP. A report by Cook and colleagues associated maternal genital warts with the development of infant laryngeal papillomas in nine patients and suggested that the virus of genital warts (papilloma virus types 6 and 11) may be acquired at birth by neonates who subsequently develop papillomas of the larynx (126). Seventy-two women were tested during the third trimester and again during labor before delivery for the presence of HPV DNA in exfoliated cervical cells. These results were compared with swabs from the oropharyngeal cavity and genitalia of neonates 24 to 72 hours after delivery. Eighteen percent (13/72) of the mothers were HPV positive, and 2.8% (2/72) of the neonates tested positive for HPV from oropharyngeal secretions, supporting the hypothesis that RRP may develop as a result of perinatal vertical transmission of HPV. Prepartum treatment of HPV lesions may not protect against the neonatal acquisition of HPV.

Complications of RRP can be severe or fatal and include hoarseness, airway obstruction, and recurrent disease (127). There is a prolonged latency period between infection and clinically obvious lesions, making the true incidence of RRP difficult to estimate. The incidence in the pediatric population is thought to be seven new cases of RRP annually per million persons. Adult-onset disease constitutes up to 40% of all RRP cases (123).

Candidiasis

Monilial Vaginitis and Vulvitis

Monilial vaginitis and vulvitis occur 10 to 20 times more frequently during pregnancy, and the neonates of affected women are susceptible to developing candidiasis (4,5). Pregnancy seems to predispose to monilial vaginitis, perhaps because of the effect of glycosuria on vaginal acidity and the altered hormonal milieu in which elevated estrogen levels favor the growth of *C. albicans* (23,128). It has been estimated that 25% of pregnant women suffer from candidal vulvovaginitis and that up to 50% of their offspring show clinical signs of mucocutaneous candidiasis (129). Possibly for the same reason, monilial vaginitis appears more frequently in women who take estrogens for contraceptive purposes or for the treatment of endometriosis (128). Broad-spectrum antibiotics that radically alter the bacterial flora of the vagina also predispose to monilial infection.

Acute vulvitis resulting from infection by *C. albicans* sometimes accompanies primary monilial vaginal infections but also may occur after secondary monilial colonization of macerated lesions of intertrigo and pruritus ani et vulvae. Candidal vulvitis presents with itching, burning, soreness, and painful micturition and is associated with a thick, creamy white vaginal discharge. Typically, a beefy red, moist erythema of the vaginal mucous membranes exists, and the vulval skin is flecked with a curdy white discharge. There may be spread onto the perineum, perianal region, gluteal folds, and upper inner aspects of the thighs. In extensive involvement, subcorneal pustules may be seen at the periphery of the fringed irregular margin of the moist areas.

Diagnosis is established by the clinical signs and symptoms and by demonstration of the pseudohyphae by potassium hydroxide (KOH) microscopic examination and yeast culture.

Treatment consists of the use of vaginal suppositories that contain nystatin (100,000 U), deposited high in the vagina by means of an applicator (twice daily for 2 weeks and then nightly for an additional 2 weeks) or clotrimazole vaginal tablets inserted at bedtime for 3 to 7 days (130). Clotrimazole has not been studied during the first trimester; however, its use during the second and third trimesters of pregnancy has not been associated with ill effects.

Inflammatory vulvar and perineal lesions can be compressed three to five times daily with water or Burow's solution (1:30 dilution) or oilated oatmeal baths to cool and soothe as well as to remove irritant endotoxin produced by *C. albicans*. After compressing and thorough drying, a nystatin cream or powder or a steroid-nystatin cream is applied to the affected areas. Clotrimazole and miconazole creams also are effective topically; however, only when they are considered essential to the welfare of the patient should they be used in the first trimester of pregnancy (131). The safety of oral ketoconazole during pregnancy has not been studied, and lowered testosterone levels have been associated with its use in high doses. In severe cases, gentian violet (0.25%) may be applied; however, it tends to be messy and will stain clothing, linen, and skin. For further control of vulvar pruritus, an antipruritic cream or lotion may be necessary. Conditions leading to moisture and maceration must be eliminated. Air conditioning, drying of the groin using a fan or blow dryer, and wearing loose clothing may be necessary. After lesions resolve, application of a starch-free drying powder or nystatin powder should be continued.

Neonatal Candidosis

Neonatal candidosis is acquired by an infected birth canal. Skin lesions appear as a diaper dermatitis or oral thrush sometime after the first week of life. Presumably, the organisms are acquired during passage through an infected birth canal or by contact with the mother during the early postpartum period (132).

Congenital Cutaneous Candidiasis

Congenital cutaneous candidiasis (CCC) is due to ascending infection of fetal skin by candidal organisms in the birth canal. Infection can occur through intact membranes and yet is facilitated by subclinical rupture of the membranes (133). Whyte and colleagues reported a high percentage (94%) of prematurity in infants infected with *Candida* (134). Prematurity may enhance the possibility of systemic spread of *Candida* before or after birth (129).

The eruption is noted at birth or within 12 hours after delivery but may appear when the infant is between 2 and 7 days of age (135). The eruption is diffuse and may involve the trunk, neck, face, and extremities. Different evolutionary stages may coexist in the same area of the body, even at birth, and pass through macular, papular, vesicular, and pustular phases. Bulla formation also may occur, and the palms and soles are frequently involved. Desquamation is a prominent feature in the recuperative period (135). Some infants may present with respiratory distress, hepatosplenomegaly, or clinical signs of sepsis during the first 2 days of life (82). The lesions of CCC last 5 to 20 days and usually are characterized by an absence of constitutional signs and a normal white blood cell and platelet count; however, asymptomatic systemic dissemination may occur (82,135). Fatal outcome has been reported in infected neonates with low birth weight and signs of respiratory distress (136).

CCC is diagnosed by a careful history of maternal infection, fungal culture, and direct KOH examination from the pustules. This condition does not appear to be related to maternal age, parity, type of delivery, or duration of labor.

Trichomonal Vagnitis and Vulvitis

Trichomonal vaginitis and vulvitis are more prevalent among pregnant women than nonpregnant women (137, 138). Prenatal infection with *Trichomonas vaginalis*, however, does not appear to be associated with any serious maternal or fetal abnormalities, although few well-controlled prospective studies have been reported (5). Girls born to women who harbor *T. vaginalis* can develop symptomatic or asymptomatic vaginal infections with this organism following delivery.

The classic finding in trichomonal vaginitis is a reddened vaginal mucosa associated with a copious greenish yellow, frothy discharge that has an associated unpleasant odor. The patient usually complains of a vaginal discharge, vulvar irritation, itching, and dyspareunia. Urinary frequency and dysuria are common. The appearance of the cervix often gives the clue to the diagnosis because it may have a red, speckled "strawberry" appearance resulting from small punctate hemorrhages on the portio and adjacent vagina. In pregnancy, a yellow discharge with an offensive odor is not necessarily attributable to trichomonal infection; in some circumstances, vaginal moniliasis has a similar appearance, although the two conditions often coexist. Although the trichomonal infection affects primarily the vagina, the profuse watery discharge often causes maceration and irritation of the vulva.

Diagnosis is made easily by microscopic examination of a drop of the discharge in isotonic saline. The organisms are motile, pear shaped, and flagellate. The treatment of pregnant women who have trichomoniasis is controversial because there is concern about the safety during pregnancy of metronidazole therapy, the drug of choice in uncomplicated cases. Metronidazole therapy should be avoided in the first trimester because of evidence of its carcinogenicity in experimental animals and mutagenicity in bacteria; however, uncontrolled studies in which metronidazole was administered to pregnant women infected with *T. vaginalis* have not associated metronidazole with congenital malformations or untoward events (139–141). Because metronidazole does cross the placenta, delaying therapy until late pregnancy should be considered if the patient's symptoms permit. Pregnant patients might be treated better with vaginal inserts, because lower serum levels are achieved with them than with oral therapy. Initial treatment may be attempted with acidifying douches, reserving metronidazole for more recalcitrant infections.

Metronidazole is administered orally in doses of 250 mg three times daily for 7 to 10 days or as a single oral dose of 2.0 g. Vaginal tablets of this compound are also available but are less effective. Douches may be used for temporary relief of vaginal symptoms, but they have little effect in eliminating the organism. Sexual partners should be treated simultaneously to reduce the failure rate resulting from exongenous reinfection.

Treatment of trichomonal vulvitis includes wet compresses with Burow's solution (1:30) three to four times daily and application of antipruritic or low-potency steroid creams. Methods to achieve local dryness will help promote relief of vulvar symptoms.

Chlamydia trachomatis Infection

Chlamydia trachomatis, the most prevalent sexually transmitted disease, comprises several serotypes, some causing blinding trachomas and others causing lymphogranuloma venereum (LGV) and a mucopurulent cervicitis/salpingitis. Chlamydial infections have been associated with preterm delivery, intrauterine growth retardation, premature rupture of the membranes, and increased perinatal mortality (142,143). Conjunctivitis and pneumonia are the most frequent complications of infants infected with *Chlamydia* during birth. Conjunctivitis occurs in 18% to 50% of neonates born to infected mothers; pneumonia occurs in 11% to 18% of neonates (142,143). LGV infection can present with painful inguinal adenopathy, which is unilateral in 60% of the cases. Patients may present with periproctitis with fever, constipation, tenesmus, thin stools, and perianal pruritus. Later complications include esthiomene, with genital scarring and vulvar lymphedema, chronic fistulae, and draining abscesses. Pharmacologic treatment of choice for *Chlamydia* during pregnancy is erythromycin base 500 mg orally four times a day for 7 days.

Leprosy

Leprosy worsens in more than one third of patients during pregnancy or during the initial 6 months of lactation, with a concomitant increase in the number and viability of the leprae bacilli in slit-skin smears, the appearance of new lesions, the extension of old lesions, or the development of erythema in tuberculoid lesions (144,145). Patients may relapse despite being formerly under good control with chemotherapy, and subclinical disease may become clinically apparent during pregnancy. The reactional states of leprosy are greatly influenced by pregnancy. The type 1 reaction occurs with greater frequency during the first trimester, subsides until delivery, and increases again. This reaction is associated with the reversal phenomenon. The type 2 lepra reaction increases in frequency during the second and third trimesters and during the first 9 months of lactation. Hypersensitivity reactions (i.e., erythema nodosum leprosum) may develop from the third trimester through the first 15 months postpartum, and the clinical state may deteriorate (1,145,146). Cutaneous involvement during gestation is common, and nerve involvement is seen often postpartum.

Leprosy may have severe effects on the fetus, causing low birth weight and small placentas, which may account for the high incidence of infant mortality (147). Leprosy patients of childbearing age should be warned against pregnancy during the years when their leprosy is active. If leprosy is diagnosed during pregnancy or if pregnancy occurs during treatment, the patient can be assured that transplacental infection does not occur. The infant will be free of leprosy at birth, and there will be no need to separate the infant from his or her mother unless the mother has bacilli in skin smears when the birth takes place, which is possible in lepromatous leprosy. In such a case, the infant should be removed at birth and returned to maternal care only after living bacilli have disappeared from slit- skin smears.

Dapsone is the treatment of choice for uncomplicated cases of leprosy (148); however, drug resistance may occur. Thalidomide suppresses reactional states but is contraindicated in pregnancy because of its teratogenic effects. Clofazimine may be effective in dapsone-resistant cases and may suppress reactional states (146,148), but its use is limited by its side effects, and it has been associated with unexplained neonatal deaths. The current recommendation is that clofazimine not be used before the second trimester (145).

MISCELLANEOUS DERMATOLOGIC DISEASES INFLUENCED BY OR AFFECTING PREGNANCY

Antiphospholipid Syndrome and Lupus Anticoagulant

Antiphospholipid syndrome (APS) is defined by the presence of antiphospholipid antibody or lupus anticoagulant, usually in high titer and associated with all or some of the following clinical events: recurrent fetal losses, recurrent thromboses, and thrombocytopenia. Primary antiphospholipid syndrome often occurs in patients with systemic lupus erythematosus (SLE) who have antiphospholipid antibodies and may experience occlusive vascular disease, neurologic disease, or false-positive results of a syphilis test. The presence of the antibody alone does not define APS: Associated clinical events must occur. The lupus anticoagulant (LA) is an immunoglobulin acquired by some patients with SLE. The LA prolongs phospholipid-dependent coagulation times and is paradoxically associated with an increased risk of thrombotic episodes (149).

Livido reticularis is often a cutaneous marker for APS. Less common cutaneous manifestations include distal acral ischemia and necrosis, blue-toe syndrome, splinter hemorrhages, porcelain-white scars, and superficial thrombophlebitis (150). Patients may develop neurologic syndromes, renal hypertension, pulmonary thrombosis, endocrinopathies, cardiac manifestations, and hemolytic anemia.

In one study, 23 mothers with APS and their 29 newborn infants were compared with controls. All the women with APS were receiving therapeutic regimens, including prednisone, low-dose aspirin, and heparin. Neonatal complications in this study included hyperbilirubinemia, respiratory distress syndrome, bronchopulmonary dysplasia, necrotizing enterocolitis, intraventricular hemorrhage, sepsis, coarctation of the aorta, hypothyroidism, hypoglycemia, and one death. They found no increase in the overall rate of neonatal complications (151).

A retrospective review of the obstetric histories of 43 women with the LA recorded 162 pregnancy losses and only 20 (12%) surviving infants (36,149). Pollard and colleagues reported that 13 of 28 women with APS developed preeclampsia and subsequent preterm delivery. They concluded that complications seen in neonates of women with APS resulted from prematurity rather than from maternal APS or its treatments. Three quarters of the infants born to the women in this study were growing and developing normally at the time of childhood follow-up (152).

Systemic Lupus Erythematosus

SLE is a common disease; the female-to-male incidence ratio is 10:1. Its frequent occurrence in women of childbearing age makes the occurrence of SLE and pregnancy an important clinical problem. Little consensus exists as to whether pregnancy adversely affects the course of SLE or vice versa and whether the maternal or fetal outcome is compromised. Nevertheless, an increasing number of reports have determined that the outcome is more favorable than formerly believed (145,152). Pregnancy is tolerated best by mothers who have been in remission for 3 months before conception and who do not have significant nephropathy or cardiac disease (153).

Patients who develop SLE for the first time during pregnancy have a higher frequency of severe manifestations, including fever, heart failure, renal disease, lymphadenopathy, abdominal pain with jaundice, and pancreatitis. These patients may experience postpartum remission, however, and successful subsequent pregnancy may occur in approximately two thirds of the cases (145,153).

Pregnancy can incite exacerbation of SLE in as many as 38% of patients anytime from the first month of pregnancy to 8 weeks postpartum (54,154). Women with SLE have an increased incidence of abortion, two to four times normal, as well as premature births, which occur in 16% to 37% of pregnancies (145,155). Recent findings contrast with previous studies that reported a high frequency of flares of SLE and lupus nephritis during gestation or the postpartum period, with subsequent postpartum maternal mortality ranging between 50% and 82% (11, 156–159). Postpartum manifestations such as rash, arthritis, and fever were reported in 31% of patients who received no glucocorticoids during pregnancy and the postpartum period and in 9.5% of those who did receive glucocorticoids (152).

In cases in which maternal SSA/Ro antibodies are present, neonates may develop the neonatal lupus syndrome, with congenital heart block, liver and hematologic abnormalities, and skin lesions (160). The SS-A antigen is present in fetal skin and heart tissue (161). Most infants do not have significant titers of antinuclear antibodies. Approximately 50% of mothers of infants with neonatal lupus have signs of SLE, subacute cutaneous lupus erythematosus, or the Sicca syndrome. The remaining 50% of women are at greater risk of developing autoimmune disease in the future.

Skin lesions in NLE are transient and are usually present at birth or appear shortly thereafter. They appear clinically as well-demarcated, scaly annular plaques with a predilection for the periorbital and facial region. Late sequelae include telangiectases and atrophy, especially around the temples and scalp. Infants rarely have both skin and cardiac lesions. Infants with skin lesions and systemic features other than heart block show little evidence of disease after the age of 1 year. The risk of recurrence in later pregnancies is 25% (162). Treatment is usually not necessary, and sun protection is advisable.

Scleroderma

Scleroderma affects women during their reproductive years and if it is uncomplicated by renal disease, does not affect pregnancy adversely (54,163,164). In general, with the exception of renal disease, pregnancy does not alter the course of scleroderma, and fetal outcome is relatively unaffected (165). Steen and colleagues compared 48 women with age- and race-matched controls and found no differences in the frequencies of miscarriage or perinatal death (166); however, preterm births occurred slightly more frequently, and there were more small full-term infants. Ballou and associates reviewed the obstetric histories of 19 women with systemic sclerosis and did follow-up on two women in whom three pregnancies occurred (167). Maternal complications included hypertension in two of these three pregnancies and congestive heart failure during one. There were two premature deliveries, and all three infants survived.

The pregnancies of scleroderma patients who have preexisting renal involvement or of those in whom renal involvement develops during pregnancy, however, have been adversely affected (168–173). Women with early rapidly progressive, diffuse skin thickening should avoid becoming pregnant, because they are at a higher risk of developing renal crisis.

Dermatomyositis/Polymyositis

The peak incidence of dermatomyositis (DM) occurs during the reproductive years with twice as many cases reported in women than in men. Although there is a paucity of data concerning the outcome of pregnancy in this disease, DM is potentially harmful to both mother and fetus (174). The disease may manifest itself first in pregnancy; high fetal mortality (46%) prematurity and neonatal death have been reported (175). A facial rash or proximal muscle weakness may occur in 50% of affected patients, and fetal loss can occur in more than 50% of the cases due to abortion, stillbirth, or premature neonatal death. Eighteen women with dermatomyositis/polymyositis (DM/PM) had a total of 77 pregnancies before disease onset (174); of these, seven (9%) ended in abortion, and two (2.5%) ended in perinatal death. Three premature infants survived. There were 10 pregnancies in seven women with active disease at the time of pregnancy; three (30%) ended in abortion, three of the remainder ended in perinatal death (25%), and half the infants were born prematurely. The total fetal loss was 11.5% before and 55% after the onset of DM/PM. King and Chow noted a more favorable outcome in three patients with five successful pregnancies complicated by DM. They concluded that women with disease in remission may have successful pregnancies, and if exacerbation occurs, treatment with corticosteroids can minimize fetal loss (175). Pregnancy should be avoided during active DM but not necessarily during remission. Pharmacologic control of disease activity, usually through administration of prednisone, is associated with a more successful pregnancy. Surviving children of patients with DM/PM are not affected by the illness (145).

Erythema Nodosum

Reports of erythema nodosum occurring in pregnant (176,177) and lactating (178) women as well as in women taking oral contraceptives (136,177,179) lend support to a contributory role of estrogen in the pathogenesis of this disease. Erythema nodosum is characterized by painful, nonsuppurative red cutaneous nodules that usually occur over the extensor surfaces of the extremities. Lesions are sometimes associated with fever, swelling of the legs, and arthralgias. Individual nodules last several weeks before disappearing spontaneously. New lesions appear while old ones are resolving, and the entire course of the disease may last weeks to months.

Drug reactions (e.g., sulfonamides, anovulatories, penicillin), infections (e.g., streptococcal, mycobacterial, fungal), sarcoidosis, and inflammatory bowel diseases are causative factors and should be excluded. Diagnosis usually can be made clinically and confirmed histologically. Lesions associated with pregnancy tend to resolve spontaneously and may recur with subsequent oral contraceptive therapy. Bed rest with elevation of the legs will reduce pain and edema gradually, and analgesics may relieve arthralgias. In chronic or recurrent cases unresponsive to supportive therapy, intralesional injection of a corticosteroid suspension may cause involution of treated lesions. A 1- to 2-week course of oral corticosteroids also may be effective. There is an association between pregnancy and erythema nodosum; it may occur with consecutive pregnancies (180). It appears as though female hormones may influence the onset of erythema nodosum because it occurs predominantly during the years after menarche and before menopause.

Erythema Multiforme

Pregnancy is one of the many causes of erythema multiforme. Erythema multiforme is an acute, usually self-limiting, frequently recurrent, and distinctive morphologic mucocutaneous reaction that is a hypersensitivity response involving immune complex formation to numerous factors. The exact mechanism involved in pregnancy remains unexplained. Characteristically, there are symmetric polymorphous skin lesions (macules, papules, urticaria, bullae) that range in color from bright red to dusky purple. Development of iris or target lesions is seen most often on the hands and consists of a central vesicle or livid erythema surrounded by a pale ring and then by a concentric red ring. Iris lesions are characteristic of erythema multiforme but need not be present to make the diagnosis clinically.

Sites of predilection include the oral mucosa, palms and soles, distal extremities, extensor surfaces, and face. Burning and itching are the chief complaints. At times, only mucous membranes of the lip, mouth, pharynx, or vagina may be involved. These lesions may progress to denuded raw ulcerations that become crusted, tender, and painful and may interfere with nutrition if they involve the upper alimentary tract.

In severely affected persons, there is widespread cutaneous, mucosal and ocular involvement with large bullae. This severe mucocutaneous bullous form of the disease is frequently designated *erythema multiforme bullosum*, or Stevens-Johnson syndrome. The mild form of erythema multiforme heals spontaneously within 2 to 3 weeks; the severe form, with widespread mucosal involvement, may last 6 to 8 weeks and is a life-threatening disease.

A pregnant patient who develops erythema multiforme requires a workup to rule out other causal agents. Antecedent infection (e.g., herpetic, streptococcal, mycoplasma, deep fungal, viral hepatitis), drug administration (e.g., penicillin, barbiturates, sulfonamides), or illness occurring up to 3 weeks before the rash appears should be investigated.

Specific therapy is possible when a specific cause is found. Local treatment consists of measures to minimize burning and pruritus. Bullae may be drained, but the blister roof should be left intact. Open wet compresses for erosive, denuded, or bullous lesions can be used to clean involved areas. Antihistamines may decrease pruritus. General supportive measures and systemic steroid therapy may be required in episodes of severe involvement. Prednisone given in a short-term, tapering course may be effective; however, its effectiveness and the appropriateness of its use is controversial.

Pemphigus Vulgaris

Pemphigus vulgaris (PV), pemphigus foliaceus, and pemphigus vegetans may occur during pregnancy for the first time or may be exacerbated by pregnancy. The onset of pemphigus vulgaris during pregnancy is uncommon; few cases have been reported (4,181,182). Pemphigus vulgaris is characterized by bullae appearing on apparently normal skin and mucous membranes. At first, the bullae are tense but soon become flaccid and rupture to form erosions and raw surfaces that ooze and bleed easily. Lateral traction on normal skin may cause the epidermis to shear off and is called a positive *Nikolsky's sign*. Pemphigus usually manifests itself with lesions first appearing in the mouth as well as on the groin, scalp, face, neck, axillae, and genitals. Healing occurs without scarring and there may be postinflammatory hyperpigmentation. Involvement of the periumbilical area is a characteristic feature. Although the precise cause of pemphigus is unknown, an autoimmune mechanism is clearly fundamental. Intercellular antibodies are demonstrable throughout the epidermis or the oral epithelium, and circulating intercellular antibodies are present in the serum in most cases.

The pemphigus IgG antibodies are thought to be transplacentally transferred, because they have been demonstrated in fetal plasma and are deposited intercellularly in fetal skin (183). Active maternal PV skin lesions during pregnancy are not obligatory for the transfer of pemphigus antibodies to the infant. Maternal indirect immunofluorescence antibodies do not appear to influence fetal outcome (184). The course of the disease tends to be chronic and not affected by pregnancy, with the pregnancy terminating normally in most instances. Samitz and colleagues reported a case of pemphigus vulgaris that began before conception (182). The disease was mild in the first and last trimesters but became aggravated in the midtrimester and immediately after parturition. This variation in severity was attributed to the effects of varying adrenocortical activity during the different trimesters. A stillborn infant with pemphigus-like skin lesions, direct immunofluorescence findings, and circulating pemphigus antibodies (indirect immunofluorescence findings) has been reported in a case in which the mother developed a recurrence of pemphigus in the third trimester of pregnancy (183,185). Pregnant women with PV may experience intrauterine death despite careful antepartum monitoring (183). Erosions may occur on the infant's skin, and a gradually healing skin lesion correlates with a decrease in their circulating pemphigus antibodies. There is usually a complete disappearance of the skin lesions by 6 weeks of age (184).

The trauma of vaginal delivery can cause an exacerbation of vulvovaginal and perineal erosions, which can result in secondary infection and significant morbidity for the patient. Poor wound healing may occur and also may be seen at the site of cesarean section. Vaginal delivery is recommended with careful fetal monitoring (186).

Clinically, pemphigus can resemble herpes gestationis and may be differentiated by skin biopsy and immunofluorescence studies. The causes for stillbirths in 4 of 29 pregnancies complicated by pemphigus were unknown; however, the high dose of prednisone required or the use of azathioprine may have been be contributory as well as intercurrent infection or placental insufficiency (181). Blistering disease of the fetus is unlikely to be the sole cause of death.

High-dose steroids have been the treatment of choice for PV during pregnancy and are relatively safe. Doses greater than 160 mg daily may be required for initial control, with subsequent tapering (145). Choices of drug therapy are limited due to the possible teratogenic effects of drugs such as cyclophosphamide, azathioprine, gold and methotrexate. Pemphigus titers may be helpful in assessing and controlling disease activity (187). Plasmapheresis should be considered in severe cases or in patients with high titers.

Psoriasis

Pregnancy and parturition have an influence on psoriasis that is not predictable (4). Gruneberg claimed that, as a rule, this influence is a favorable one (188). Localized forms of psoriasis are most refractory, whereas generalized forms tend to improve. In another study, Church reviewed the effect of pregnancy on psoriasis in 43 women (67). During pregnancy, 33% of patients had clearing of their psoriasis, 21% displayed worsening, and 14% showed no change. In 44%, parturition was accompanied by exacerbation. Farber and Nall (189) noted that 32% of 1,018 patients surveyed reported improvement of their psoriasis during pregnancy, whereas 18% claimed that their disease worsened and 50% reported no change. Fluxes in hormones, such as cortisol, may play an important role in those flareups and improvements. It appears that there is a definite tendency toward remission or improvement of psoriasis during pregnancy. The use of oral and topical retinoid derivatives in the treatment of psoriasis is contraindicated during pregnancy.

Acrodermatitis Enteropathica

Acrodermatitis enteropathica can be exacerbated by pregnancy, with a measurable decline in serum zinc concentrations beginning early in gestation as a result of increased fetal demand for zinc and the effects of estrogens (190). Some patients may be diagnosed for the first time with the disease during pregnancy. The skin manifestations may be mild during puberty, and diarrhea may be slight or absent. During the late first trimester or second trimester, the disease progressively worsens until delivery and then rapidly clears postpartum.

Most pregnancies produce normal offspring; however, there have been isolated reports of achondroplastic dwarfism, anencephaly, and neonatal death associated with untreated maternal acrodermatitis enteropathica (191,192). These reports, coupled with the known teratogenic effects of zinc deficiency in mice, make it essential to diagnose and treat acrodermatitis enteropathica properly during pregnancy (145). Treatment with zinc, with monitoring of serum zinc levels, is effective in preventing adverse fetal outcome.

Androluteoma Syndrome of Pregnancy

Rarely, a persistent corpus luteum can produce excess androgens and cause severe abnormalities in both the mother and fetus. The mother can become masculinized with hypertrichosis, seborrhea, papulopustular acne, and a deep voice. Female fetuses may be born with signs of masculinization. Diagnosis is based on ultrasonic identification of the tumor in the ovary and by excess blood levels of androgens. Surgical removal of the androgen-producing corpus luteum during pregnancy is curative (193).

Hereditary Angioedema

Hereditary angioedema (HAE) is an autosomal dominant disease marked by a deficiency or dysfunction of the serum protein inhibitor of the first complement component, the C1 esterase inhibitor (C1-1NH) (194). Clinically, the illness is characterized by intermittent episodes of edema that may affect the limbs, face, pharynx, and vulva and may cause abdominal pain. Often antecedent minor trauma or dental manipulation is identified as the precipitating factor. Endogenous hormones may play a role in the precipitation of attacks. Gelfand and colleagues noted that attacks were more prevalent during menstrual periods in 5 of 12 female patients (195). Androgen administration has been associated with prompt and prolonged remission. Danazol, a synthetic androgenic steroid with minimal virilizing effects, has been used to prevent attacks with good success. Danazol suppresses ovulation in women and increases serum levels of C1 esterase inhibition in both men and women who have the disorder. In view of the hormonal influence on the disease, it is not surprising that pregnancy would have a definite effect on the clinical severity of HAE. Among 25 pregnancies of 10 women, significantly fewer or no attacks occurred during the last two trimesters (195). There were no episodes of angioedema at delivery, despite the significant tissue trauma associated with childbirth. The fetal outcome of pregnancy in women who have HAE would be expected to be normal. The possibility that female fetuses can become virilized as a result of maternal danazol therapy must be considered; the drug should not be used in pregnancy.

Ehlers-Danlos Syndrome

There are at least 10 variants of Ehlers-Danlos syndrome. Type I (classic or gravis) and type IV (ecchymotic or arterial) are the most likely to cause complications during pregnancy (145,191). Type I is inherited in an autosomal dominant fashion so that an affected mother will have a 50% chance of having an affected child. Pregnancy in Ehlers-Danlos syndrome type I involves risks for both mother and fetus. During pregnancy, affected mothers may buise more easily; develop abdominal wall, inguinal, umbilical, and femoral hernias; and develop varicosities of the leg and vulva (196,197). Pregnant women with either type are susceptible to poor wound healing, wound dehiscence, uterine lacerations, and bladder and uterine prolapse (198,199) as well as severe postpartum hemorrhage and formation of perineal hematomas. Patients commonly develop papyraceous scars, and, perhaps as a result of the fragility of the fetal membranes, prematurity is common. Ainsworth and colleagues found a miscarriage rate of 60% among 151 women with type I Ehlers-Danlos syndrome. Premature rupture of the membranes, uterine prolapse, and cervical tears were common complications (200). Type IV (ecchymotic or arterial) is similar to type I, but rupture of the aorta, pulmonary, and other major arteries as well as the uterus and bowel are more common, leading to a maternal death rate of nearly 25% (201). Type II (mitis) has a more favorable outcome of pregnancy with normal vaginal delivery. Episiotomy sites and cesarean incisions may heal slowly and may extend spontaneously. All sutures should remain at least twice the usual time to prevent wound dehiscence. Previous cesarean scars also may rupture during labor, and cesarean section should be avoided if possible. Spontaneous rupture of the intact uterus has not been reported. Forceps should be used with caution (196). Interestingly, women who have Ehlers-Danlos syndrome apparently do not develop striae gravidarum.

Managing the pregnant patient with Ehlers-Danlos syndrome is difficult. Complications are most likely to occur during labor, parturition, or postpartum (201). Pregnancies frequently terminate prematurely, either because of premature rupture of the fetal membranes (if the child is affected) or because of lax cervical tissues (incompetent cervix). Rapid effacement and dilation of the cervix may lead not only to premature but also to precipitate delivery. Cesarean section may not result in fewer complications than vaginal delivery. The clinician should consider early termination of pregnancy if ultrasonic examination of the aortic root reveals more than a 20% enlargement above baseline or a diameter greater than 4 cm (202).

Pseudoxanthoma Elasticum

Pseudoxanthoma elasticum (PXE), inherited in both autosomal dominant and recessive forms, is a syndrome that affects the gastrointestinal system, eyes, heart, vascular system, and skin. Cutaneous changes progressively develop in the second decade around the neck, axillary folds, umbilicus, genitals, face, and antecubital fossae. The ocular hallmark of PXE is the finding of angioid streaks, often preceding the infiltrative yellow, lax, redundant plaques and patches on the skin. Complications in pregnant women include gastrointestinal hemorrhage with massive hematemesis. Biopsy of the gastric mucosa shows degeneration of the elastic fibers in medium-sized arteries and the formation of microaneurysms. Other complications in pregnancy include epistaxis and congestive heart failure with ventricular arrhythmias (203). Hematuria, angina, mitral valve prolapse, hypertension, and intermittent claudication may occur in all patients with PXE. It is thought that pregnancy may aggravate the vascular effects of the disease; thus, careful monitoring of blood pressure to decrease the risk of hemorrhage is necessary. There is no proven fetal risk in PXE, although intrauterine growth retardation associated with placental abnormalities has been reported (204).

Marfan Syndrome

Marfan syndrome is adversely affected by pregnancy (1). The life-threatening cardiovascular complication seen in Marfan syndrome is cystic medial necrosis of the wall of the aorta, which predisposes to aneurysm formation. Aortic aneurysms as well as dissection and rupture of aortic aneurysms occur with increased frequency during pregnancy (205–208). The most stressful period for the aorta is the third trimester. Although no explanation for the increased susceptibility to vascular aneurysm is available, increased circulating estrogen levels and increased cardiac output may play a role. Women who have Marfan syndrome do not seem to be more susceptible to problems related to cesarean section and apparently have normal wound healing. Hernias and striae gravidarum occur more frequently during pregnancy in Marfan syndrome.

Porphyrias

From reported clinical experience and the literature review concerning pregnancy in the acute porphyrias, the general consensus is that the disease worsens during pregnancy. Zimmerman and colleagues noted a high incidence of prematurity and spontaneous abortion coinciding with acute exacerbations of porphyria; however, most premature infants survived the neonatal period (209). A study by Brodie and colleagues revealed a 13% fetal loss rate in 95 pregnancies of women with acute intermittent porphyria (210). Infants born to mothers who experience an acute attack during pregnancy had significantly lower birth weights compared with infants born to asymptomatic mothers with acute intermittent porphyria. It is unclear whether there is a permanent effect on the newborn.

Porphyria Cutanea Tarda (PCT)

Cutaneous porphyrias (PCT, erythropoietic protoporphyria, and erythropoietic porphyria) during pregnancy are of far less concern than the acute porphyria. The use of oral contraceptives exposes a group of predisposed young women to the risk of developing PCT. Estrogens, iron, and alcohol adversely effect PCT; however, there have been case reports of patients with successful pregnancies, suggesting that endogenous estrogens may not be harmful (211). In comparison, other reports demonstrate a clear worsening of disease during pregnancy with increased plasma and urine porphyrin levels. Lamon and colleagues measured serum iron, iron-binding capacity, and urine porphyrin levels during gestation. They noted a physiologic increase in serum estrogen and a high rate of porphyrin excretion coinciding with clinical exacerbation of skin fragility during the first trimester (212). As fetal iron requirements increased later in pregnancy, the skin disease improved and a concomitant decrease in serum iron and urinary porphyrins occurred, supporting the tendency of pregnancy to worsen PCT. The maternal loss of iron to the fetus could be therapeutic as a result of increased blood volume and hemodilution. Fetal morbidity and erythrodontia were not seen in the two offspring of women who had PCT (213). The use of iron supplementation could possibly exacerbate underlying PCT, and chloroquine use should be avoided because of reported birth defects including mental retardation, neurosensory hearing loss, and neonatal convulsions (214). Phlebotomy treatment during pregnancy has been used successfully to control PCT (138,215).

Erythropoietic Protoporphyria

Five women who had erythropoietic protoporphyria (EPP) were monitored by Schmidt and colleagues; these patients showed marked decrease or disappearance of their cutaneous symptoms during pregnancy (216). No information has been reported on the outcome of gestation or on fetal effects.

Congenital Erythropoietic Porphyria

The small number of reports of pregnancy in women with congenital erythropoietic porphyria (CEP) reflects the rarity of this autosomal recessive disease. Affected patients have a shortened life span and severe cutaneous disfigurement. Offspring of persons who have CEP invariably would be obligate heterozygotes. Townes reported on one woman with CEP who experienced a normal uncomplicated pregnancy and delivery (217).

Gingivitis of Pregnancy

Marginal gingivitis develops in about 80% of pregnant women and may progress to severe gingivitis with the development of granuloma gravidarum (2). Gingival changes usually occur toward the end of the first trimester with the development of inflammation and hypertrophy. Increased gingival reactivity to local irritation is maintained throughout pregnancy, although the most discomfort occurs during the third and fourth months. Management involves rigorous oral hygiene and mouth care. If inflammation is severe, the use of antiseptic mouth washes (e.g., hydrogen peroxide) is recommended.

Acne

Although sebaceous gland activity generally increases in the third trimester of pregnancy, the effect of pregnancy on acne is variable (218). Even when estrogen levels are high, sebum production does not diminish. Although the influence of increased circulating estrogen is beneficial in many patients, others may develop acne for the first time or have exacerbations of preexisting acne while pregnant. Some women recurrently develop acne during pregnancy with subsequent clearing after parturition. Proper dermatologic care should be afforded the pregnant patient who has acne to minimize scarring. Refractory cases should be referred to a dermatologist.

The use of systemic tetracycline therapy in pregnant patients is contraindicated and may produce discoloration of the teeth in their offspring. The period of greatest danger to the teeth during pregnancy extends from midtrimester to parturition. Tetracyclines also can be deposited in the skeleton of the human fetus, reversibly decreasing bone growth rate in premature infants. Oral erythromycin appears to be safe for the pregnant patient and fetus; however, there are no studies on erythromycin administration for periods lasting longer than 6 weeks during pregnancy. Systemic isotretinoin, a synthetic retinoid used to treat severe cystic acne, is contraindicated in pregnant patients because it can cause severe human birth defects. Pregnancy must be ruled out before initiating isotretinoin therapy in patients at risk for pregnancy. Two forms of effective contraception should be used for at least 1 month before and during isotretinoin therapy and 1 month after discontinuation of isotretinoin therapy or until a normal menstrual period occurs.

There have been no reports of abnormal offspring born to mothers who used topical acne therapies; however, in light of increased intrauterine death and skeletal abnormalities in the offspring of animals treated topically with tretinoin (all transretinoic acid), the decision to use topical tretinoin during pregnancy should be made following a thorough discussion of potential risks and benefits.

REFERENCES

1. Scoggins RB. Skin changes and diseases in pregnancy. In: Fitzpatrick TB, Eisen AZ, Wolff K, Freedberg IM, Austen KF, eds. Dermatology in general medicine. New York: McGraw-Hill, 1979;1363–1370.
2. Demis DJ. Clinical dermatology, vol 2. New York: Harper & Row, 1975:1–9.
3. Vasquez M, Ibanez MI, Sanchez JL. Pigmentary demarcation lines during pregnancy. Cutis 1986;38:263–266.
4. Peck SM, Rovinsky IK, Guttmacher, AF. The medical, surgical, and gynecologic complications of pregnancy, 2nd ed. Baltimore: Williams & Wilkins, 1964:619–646.
5. Rook A, Wilkinson DS, Ebling FJG. Textbook of dermatology, 3rd ed. Oxford: Blackwell, 1979:220–224.
6. Esoda ECJ. Chloasma from progestational oral contraceptives. Arch Dermatol 1963;87:486.
7. McKenzie AW. Skin disorders in pregnancy. Practioner 1971;206: 773–780.
8. Resnick S. Melasma induced by oral contraceptive drugs. JAMA 1967;199:95–99.
9. Leider M, Rosenblum M. A Dictionary of Dermatologic Words, Terms and Phrases. New York, McGraw-Hill, 1968, pp 90, 278.
10. Sanchez NP, Pathak MA, Sato S, Fitzpatrick TB, Sanchez JL, Mihm MC. Melasma: a clinical, light microscopic, ultrastructural, and immunofluorescent study. J Am Acad Dermatol 1981;4:698–710.
11. Zelenick JS. Endocrine physiology of pregnancy. Clin Obstet Gynecol 1964;8:534–541.
12. Hellreich PD. The skin changes of pregnancy. Cutis 1974;13:82–86.
13. Shizume K, Lerner AB. Determination of melanocyte stimulating hormone in urine and blood. J Clin Endocrinol 1954;14:1491–1510.
14. Breathnach AS. Melanin hyperpigmentation of skin: melasma, topical treatment with azelaic acid and other therapies. Cutis 1996;57:36–45.
15. Kligman AM. Pathologic dynamics of human hair loss. Arch Dermatol 1961;83:175.
16. Behrman HT. Diagnosis and management of hirsutism. JAMA 1960; 172:1924.
17. Cumings K, Derbes VJ. Dermatosis associated with pregnancy. Cutis 1967;3:120–125.
18. Bean WB. Vascular spiders and related lesions of the skin. Springfield, IL: Charles C Thomas, 1958:59–78.
19. Goldman MP, Bennett R. Treatment of telangiectasia. J Am Acad Dermatol 1987;17:167–182.
20. Bianchi P. Nature and significance of dermatographic variations in pregnancy and the puerperium. Riv Ital Ginecol 1949;32:285.
21. Wong RC, Ellis CN. Physiologic skin changes of pregnancy. J Am Acad Dermatol 1984;10:929–939.
22. Wade TR, Wade SL, Jones HE. Skin changes and diseases associated with pregnancy. Obstet Gynecol 1978;52:233–242.
23. Porter PS, Lyle JS. Yeast vulvovaginitis due to oral contraceptives. Arch Dermatol 1966;93:402–403.
24. Davey CMH. Factors associated with the occurrence of striae gravidarum. J Obstet Gynaecol Br Commonw 1972;79:1113–1114.
25. Elson ML. Treatment of striae distensae with topical tretinoin. J Dermatol Surg Oncol 1990; 16:267–270.
26. Schoelch SB. AAD San Francisco Poster Exhibit 1997.
27. Fox JL. Pulse dye laser eliminates stretch marks. Cosm Derm 1997; 10:51–52.
28. Crawford GM, Leeper RW. Disease of the skin in pregnancy. Arch Dermatol Syphilol 1950;61:753.
29. Hozbach RT. Jaundice in pregnancy. Am J Med 1976;61:367–376.
30. Itching in pregnancy [Editorial]. BMJ 1975;3:608.
31. Haemmerli UP. Jaundice during pregnancy. Acta Med Scand 1966; (Suppl)179:444.
32. Lutz EE, Margolis AT. Obstetric hepatosis: treatment with cholestyramine and interim response to steroids. Obstet Gynecol 1969;33: 64–71.
33. Lunzer M, Barnes P, Byth K, O'Halloran M. Serum bile acid concentrations during pregnancy and their relationship to obstetric cholestasis. Gastroenterology 1986;91:825–829.
34. Bynum TE. Hepatic and gastrointestinal disorders in pregnancy. Med Clin North Am 1977;61:129–138.
35. Johnston MB, Baskett TF. Obstetric cholestasis: a 14 year review. Am J Obstet Gynecol 1979;133:299–301.
36. Adlercruetz H, Svanborg A, Anberg A. Recurrent jaundice in pregnancy: a study of estrogens and their conjugates in late pregnancy. Am J Med 1970;49:630.
37. Ferhoff A. Itching in pregnancy. Acta Med Scand 1974;196:402–410.
38. Sasseville D, Wilkinson RD, Schrader JY. Dermatoses of pregnancy. Int J Dermatol 1981;20:223–241.
39. Noguera X, Puig L, de Moragas JM. Prurigo gravidarum. Cutis 1987; 39:437–440.
40. Hirvioja JL, Tuimala R, Vuori J. Treatment of intrahepatic cholestasis of pregnancy by dexamethasone. Br J Obstet Gynaecol 1992;99:109.
41. Besnier E, Brocq L, Jacquet L. La pratique dermatologique. Paris: Masson, 19:74.
42. Nurse DS. Prurigo of pregnancy. Aust J Dermatol 1968;9:258–267.
43. Holmes RC, Black MM. The specific dermatoses of pregnancy. J Am Acad Dermatol 1983;8:403–412.
44. Costello MJ. Eruptions of pregnancy. NY State J Med 1941;41: 849–55.
45. Lawley TS, Hertz KC, Wade TR, Ackerman AB, Katz SI. Pruritic urticarial papules and plaques of pregnancy. JAMA 1979;241: 1696–1699.
46. Bourne G. Toxemic rash of pregnancy. Proc R Soc Med 1962;55:462.
47. Holmes RC, Black MM, Dann J, James DCO, Bhogal B. A comparative study of toxic erythema of pregnancy and herpes gestationis. Br J Dermatol 1982;106:499–510.
48. Ahmed AR, Kaplan R. PUPPP. J Am Acad Dermatol 1981;4:679–681.
49. Stoller HE. Pruritic urticarial papules and plaques of pregnancy. JAMA 1980;243:2156.
50. Schwartz RA, Hansen RC, Lynch PJ. PUPPP. Cutis 1981;27:425–432.
51. Uhlin SR. PUPPP: involvement of mother and infant. Arch Dermatol 1981;117:3;238–239.
52. Yancey KB, Hall RP, Lawley TJ. Pruritic urticarial papules and plaques of pregnancy: clinical experience in twenty-five patients. J Am Acad Dermatol 1984;10:473–480.
53. Alcalay J, Wolf JE. Pruritic urticarial papules and plaques of pregnancy: the enigma and the confusion [Editorial]. J Am Acad Dermatol 1988;19:1115–1116.
54. Winton WB. Dermatoses of pregnancy. J Am Acad Dermatol 1982;6:977–998.
55. Russell B, Thorne NA. Herpes gestationis. Br J Dermatol 1957;69: 339–357.
56. Shornick JK. Herpes gestationis. J Am Acad Dermatol 1987;17: 539–556.
57. Lim HW, Bystryn JC. Bullous disease. Clin Obstet Gynecol 1978;21: 1007–1022.
58. Hertz KC, Katz SI, Maize J. Herpes gestationis: a clinicopathologic study. Arch Dermatol 1976;112:1543–1548.
59. Yaoita H, Gullino M, Katz SI. Herpes gestationis: ultrastructure and ultrastructural localization of *in vivo*-bound complement. J Invest Dermatol 1976;66:383–388.
60. Dahl MV. Clinical immunodermatology. Chicago: Year Book, 1981; 153–155.
61. Katz SI, Hertz KC, Yaoita H. Herpes gestationis: immunopathology and characterization of the HG factor. J Clin Invest 1976;57: 1434–1441.
62. Ortonne JP, Hsi BL, Verrando P, Bernerd F, Pautrat G, Pisani A, Yeh CJ. Herpes gestationis factor reacts with the amniotic epithelial basement membrane. Br J Dermatol 1987;117:147–154.
63. Kelly SE, Bhogal BS, Wojnarowska F, Black MM. Expression of a pemphigoid gestationis-related antigen by human placenta. Br J Dermatol 1988;118:605–611.
64. Jenkins RE, Jones SA, Black MM. Conversion of pemphigoid gestationis to bullous pemphigoid—two refractory cases highlighting the association. Br J Dermatol 1996;135:595–598.
65. Morgan JK. Herpes gestationis influenced by an oral contraceptive. Br J Dermatol 1968;7:456–458.
66. Chorzelski TP, Jabonski S, Beutner EH. Herpes gestationis with identical lesions in the newborn. Arch Dermatol 1976;112:1129–1131.
67. Church R. The prospect of psoriasis. Br J Dermatol 1958;70:139.
68. Kolodny KC. Herpes gestationis, a new assessment of incidence, diagnosis, and fetal prognosis. Am J Obstet Gynecol 1969;104:39–45.

69. Lawley TJ, Stingle G, Katz SI. Fetal and maternal risk factors in herpes gestationis. Arch Dermatol 1978;114:552–555.
70. Sauer GC, Geha BJ. Impetigo herpetiformis. Arch Dermatol 1961;83: 119–126.
71. Pierard GE, Pierard-Franchimont CP, dela Brassine M. Impetigo herpetiformis and pustular psoriasis during pregnancy. Am J Dermatopathol 1983;3:215–220.
72. Lotem M, Katzenelson V, Rotem A, Hod M, Sandbank M. Impetigo herpetiformis: a variant of pustular psoriasis or a separate entity? J Am Acad Dermatol 1989;20:338–341.
73. Spangler AS, Reddy W, Bardawil WA, et al. Papular dermatitis of pregnancy. JAMA 1962;181:577–581.
74. Spangler AS, Emerson K Jr. Estrogen levels and estrogen therapy in papular dermatitis of pregnancy. Am J Obstet Gynecol 1971;110: 534–537.
75. Heinonen OP, Slone D, Shapiro S. Birth Defects and Drugs in Pregnancy. Littleton, MA: Publishing Sciences Group, 1977:287–389.
76. Fraser FC, Walker BE, Fainstat TD. The experimental production of cleft palate with cortisone and other hormones. J Cell Comp Physiol 1954;(Suppl)42:237.
77. Greenberger P, Patterson R. Safety of therapy for allergic symptoms of pregnancy. Ann Intern Med 1978;89:234–237.
78. Schatz M, Patterson R, Zeitz S, O Rourke J, Melam H. Corticosteroid therapy for the pregnant asthmatic patient. JAMA 1975;233:804–807.
79. Corticosteroids and the fetus [Editorial]. Lancet 1976;1:74.
80. Peterson R, Imperato-McGinley J. Cortisol metabolism in the perinatal period. In: New MI, Fiser RH, eds. Diabetes and other endocrine disorders during pregnancy and the newborn. New York: Alan R Liss, 1976:141–172.
81. Villee DB. Reply: what risk to fetus from maternal steroid therapy. JAMA 1974;230:1202.
82. Atlas of tumor pathology. Washington, DC: Armed Forces Institute of Pathology, 1964:186–187.
83. McCarthy PL, Shklar G. Disease of the oral mucosa. New York: McGraw-Hill, 1964.
84. Jaber PW, Wilson BB, Johns DW, Cooper PH, Ferguson JE. Eruptive xanthomas during pregnancy. J Am Acad Dermatol 1992;27:300–302.
85. Ricardi VM. Medical progress: Von Recklinghausen neurofibromatosis. N Engl J Med 1981;305:1617–2166.
86. Crowe FW, Schull WJ, Neel JV. A clinical, pathological, and genetic study of multiple neurofibromatosis. Springfield, IL: Charles C Thomas, 1956:
87. Rosenbaum L, Paley SS. Neurofibromatosis. NY J Med 1955;35:1350.
88. Ansari AH, Nagamani M. Pregnancy and neurofibromatosis. Obstet Gynecol 1976;47 (Suppl):255–295.
89. Jarvis GT, Crompton AC. Neurofibromatosis and pregnancy. Br J Obstet Gynecol 1978;85:844–846.
90. Bolande RP. Neurofibromatosis—the quintessential neurocristopathy: pathogenic concepts and relationships. Adv Neurol 1981;29:67–75.
91. Perez-Polo JR, Hall K, Livingston K, Westlund K. Steroid induction of nerve growth factor synthesis in cell culture. Life Sci 1977;21: 1535–1544.
92. Strange HH. Recklinghausen's disease and pregnancy. Zentralbl Gynakol 1951;73:1787.
93. Cornell SH, Kirkendall WB. Neurofibromatosis of the renal artery, an unusual case of hypertension. Radiology 1967;88:24.
94. Swapp GH, Main RA. Neurofibromatosis in pregnancy. Br J Dermatol 1973;88:431–435.
95. Brade DB, Bolan JC. Neurofibromatosis and spontaneous hemothorax in pregnancy: Two case reports. Obstet Gynecol 1984;63(Suppl): 35–38.
96. Wong DJ, Strassner HT. Melanoma in pregnancy. Clin Obstet Gynecol 1990;33:782–789.
97. Riberti C, Marola G, Bertoni A. Malignant melanoma: the adverse effect of pregnancy. Br J Plast Surg 1981;34:338–339.
98. Schwartz BK, Zashin SJ, Spencer SK, Mills LE, Sober AJ. Pregnancy and hormonal influences on malignant melanoma. J Dermatol Surg Oncol 1987;13:276–281.
99. Feucht KA, Walker MJ, DasGupta TK, Beattie CW. Effects of 17 Beta-estradiol on the growth of estrogen receptor positive human melanoma in vitro and in athymic mice. Cancer Res 1988;48:7093–7101.
100. Shaw HM, Milton GW, Farago G, McCarthy WH . Endocrine influence on survival from malignant melanoma. Cancer 1978;42:669–677.
101. Ances IG, Pomerantz SH. Serum concentrations of beta-melanocyte stimulating hormone in human pregnancy. Am J Obstet Gynecol 1974;119:1062–1068.
102. Dahlberg B. Melanocyte stimulating substances in the urine of pregnant women. Acta Endocrinol (Suppl)1961;60.
103. George PA, Fortner JG, Pack GT. Melanoma with pregnancy. Cancer 1960;13:854–859.
104. White LP, Lindon G, Breslow L, et al. Studies on melanoma: The effect of pregnancy on survival in human melanoma. JAMA 1961; 177:235.
105. Shiu MH, Schottenfield D, Maclean MB, Fortner JG . Adverse effect of pregnancy on melanoma: a reappraisal. Cancer 1976;37:181–187.
106. Slingluff CL, Seigler HF. Malignant melanoma and pregnancy. Ann Plast Surg 1992;28:95–99.
107. Sober AJ, Fitzpatrick TB, Mihm MC. Primary melanoma of the skin: Recognition and management. J Am Acad Dermatol 1980;2:179–197.
108. Adam SA, Sheaves JK, Wright NH, Mosser G, Harris RW, Vessey MP. A case-control study of the possible association between oral contraceptives and malignant melanoma. Br J Cancer 1981;44:45–50.
109. Holly EA, Weiss NS, Liff JM. Cutaneous melanoma in relation to exogenous hormones and reproductive factors. J Natl Cancer Inst 1983;70:827–831.
110. Gough IR, Stitz RW. Metastatic carcinoid tumour: stability throughout pregnancy. Aust N Z J Surg 1991;61:960–962.
111. Andreev VC. Skin manifestations of visceral cancer. Curr Probl Dermatol 1978.
112. Benschine FW. Massive condylomata acuminata of vulva complicating labor. Am J Obstet Gynecol 1941;42:338.
113. Vonderheid EC, Dellatorre DL, Van Scott EJ. Prolonged remission of tumor-stage mycosis fungoides by topical immunotherapy. Arch Dermatol 1981;117:586–589.
114. Footer W. Spontaneous postpartum disappearance of massive condylomata of the vulva. Am J Obstet Gynecol 1944;48:266.
115. Garoner HL, Kaufman RH. Condyloma acuminata. Clin Obstet Gynecol 1965;8:938–45.
116. Gortlay RL, Krembs MA. Vulvar condylomata complicating labor. Obstet Gynecol 1954;4:67.
117. Powell LC. Condyloma acuminatum. Clin Obstet Gynecol 1972; 15:448.
118. Graber EA, Barber HRK, O'Rouke JJ. Simple surgical treatment for condyloma acuminata of the vulva. Obstet Gynecol 1967;29:247–250.
119. Ostergard DR, Townsend DE. The treatment of vulva condyloma acuminata by cryosurgery—a preliminary report. Cryobiology 1969; 5:340–342.
120. Young RL, Acosta AA, Kaufman RH. The treatment of large condylomata acuminata complicating pregnancy. Obstet Gynecol 1973;41: 65–73.
121. Matsunaga J, Berman A, Bhatia NN. Genital condylomata acuminata in pregnancy: effectiveness, safety and pregnancy outcome following cryotherapy. Br J Obstet Gynaecol 1987;94:168–172.
122. Calkins JW, Masterson BT, Magrina JF. Management of condylomata acuminata with the carbon dioxide laser. Obstet Gynecol 1982;59: 105–108.
123. Osborne NG, Adelson MD. Herpes simplex and human papillomavirus genital infections: controversy over obstetric management. Clin Obstet Gynecol 1990;33:801–811.
124. Beckmann AM, Acker R, Christiansen AE, Sherman KJ. Human papillomavirus infection in women with multicentric squamous cell neoplasia. Am J Obstet Gynecol 1991;165:1431–1437.
125. Smith EM, Johnson SR, Cripe TP, Pignatari S, Turek L. Perinatal vertical transmission of human papillomavirus and subsequent development of respiratory tract papillomatosus. Ann Otol Rhinol Laryngol 1991;100:479–483.
126. Cook TA, Cohn AM, Brunschwig JP, Butel JS, Rawls WE. Wart viruses and laryngeal papillomas. Lancet 1973;1:782.
127. Sedlacek TV, Lindheim S, Eder C, et al. Mechanism for human papillomavirus transmission at birth. Am J Obstet Gynecol 1989;161: 55–59.
128. Danforth DN. Obstetrics and gynecology, 3rd ed. New York: Harper & Row, 1977:873.
129. Almeida Santos L, Beceiro J, Hernandez R, et al. Congenital cutaneous candidiasis: report of four cases and review of the literature. Eur J Pediatr 1991;150:336–338.
130. Arndt KA. Manual of dermatologic therapeutics, 2nd ed. Boston: Little, Brown and Company, 1978:118–126.

131. Wallenburg HCS, Wladimiroff JW. Recurrences of vulvovaginal candidiasis during pregnancy. Obstet Gynecol 1976;48:491–494.
132. McCormick WM. Management of sexually transmissible infections during pregnancy. Clin Obstet Gynecol 1975;18:57–71.
133. Broberg A, Thiringer K. Congenital cutaneous candidiasis. Int J Dermatol 1989;18:464–465.
134. Whyte RK, Hussain Z, deSa D. Antenatal infections with candida species. Arch Dis Child 1982;57:528–535.
135. Rudolph N, Tariq AA, Reale MR, Goldberg PK, Kozinn PJ. Congenital cutaneous candidiasis. Arch Dermatol 1977;113:1101–1103.
136. Matz MH. Erythema nodosum and contraceptive medication. N Engl J Med 1967;276:351–352.
137. Brown MT. Trichomoniasis. Practitioner 1972;209:639.
138. Rajka G. Pregnancy and porphyria cutanea tarda. Acta Dermatol Venerol (Stockh) 1984;64:444–445.
139. Peterson WF, Stauch JE, Ryder CD. Metronidazole in pregnancy. Am J Obstet Gynecol 1966;94:393.
140. Robbie MO, Sweet RL. Metronidazole use in obstetrics and gynecology: a review. Am J Obstet Gynecol 1983;145:865–881.
141. Rodin P, Hass G. Metronidazole and pregnancy. Br J Vener Dis 1966; 42:210–212.
142. Blackburn LS. Effective treatment of chlamydia trachomatis infection during pregnancy to prevent perinatal and infant complications. Nurse Pract 1992;17:56–60.
143. Sweet RL, Landers DV, Walker C, Schachter J. *Chlamydia trachomatis* infection and pregnancy outcome. Am J Obstet Gynecol 1987;156: 824–833.
144. Duncan ME, Pearson JMH, Ridley DS, Melsom R, Bjune G. Pregnancy and leprosy: the consequences of alterations of cell-mediated and humoral immunity during pregnancy and lactation. Int J Lepr Other Mycobact Dis 1982;50:425–435.
145. Winton GB. Skin diseases aggravated by pregnancy. J Am Acad Dermatol 1989;20:1–13.
146. Duncan ME, Pearson JMH. The association of pregnancy and leprosy III, Erythema nodosum leprosum in pregnancy and lactation. Lepr Rev 1984;55:129–142.
147. Duncan ME. Babies of mothers with leprosy have small placentas, low birth weights and grow slowly. Br J Obstet Gynaecol 1980;87:471–479.
148. Kahn G. Dapsone is safe during pregnancy [Letter]. J Am Acad Dermatol 1985;13:838–839.
149. Branch DW, Scott JR, Kochenour NK, Hershgold E. Obstetric complications associated with the lupus anticoagulant. N Engl J Med 1985;313:1322–1326.
150. Lubbe WF, Butler WS, Palmer SJ, Liggins GC. Lupus anticoagulant and pregnancy. Br J Obstet Gynecol 1984;92:357–363.
151. Petri M. Antiphospholipid antibodies: lupus anticoagulant and anticardiolipin antibody. In Mackie RM, Provost T, eds. Current Problems in Dermatology. Vol IV. Mosby-Year Book, Inc., St. Louis, MO 1992.
152. Pollard JK, Scott JR, Branch DW. Outcome of children born to women treated during pregnancy for the antiphospholipid syndrome. Obstet Gynecol 1992;80:365–368.
153. Barnett EV. The influence of pregnancy, on the systemic manifestations of systemic lupus erythematosus. Ann Intern Med 1981;94:667–677.
154. Hyslett JP, Reece EA. Systemic lupus in pregnancy. Clin Perinatol 1985;12:539–550.
155. McGee CD, Makowski EL. Systemic lupus erythematosus in pregnancy. Obstet Gynecol 1970;107:1008–1012.
156. Mchugh NJ, Reilly PA, Mchugh LA. Pregnancy outcome and autoantibodies in connective tissue disease. J Rheumatol 1989;16:42–46.
157. Swaak AJG. Pregnancy in systemic lupus erythematosus. Neth J Med 1984;27:84–89.
158. Syrop CH, Varner MW. Systemic lupus erythematosus. Clin Obstet Gynecol 1983;26:547–557.
159. Bear R. Pregnancy and lupus nephritis. Obstet Gynecol 1976;47: 715–718.
160. Zulman JI, Talal N, Hoffman GS, Epstein WV. Problems associated with the management of pregnancies in patients with systemic lupus erythematosus. J Rheumatol 1980;7:37–49.
161. Lee LA, Harmon CE, Huff JC, Norris DA, Weston WL. The demonstration of SS-A/Ro antigen in human tissues and in neonatal and adult skin. J Invest Dermatol 1985;85:143–146.
162. Horowitz GM, Hankins GDV. Cutaneous manifestations of collagen vascular disease in pregnancy. Clin Obstet Gynecol 1990;33:759–766.
163. Dubois EL. Questions and answers: Raynaud phenomenon in pregnancy. JAMA 1975;233:283.
164. Winkelman RK. Scleroderma and pregnancy. Clin Obstet Gynecol 1965;8:280.
165. Johnson TR, Banner EA, Winkelmann RK. Scleroderma and pregnancy. Obstet Gynecol 1964;23:467–69.
166. Steen VD, Conte C, Day N, Ramsey-Goldman R, Medsger TA. Pregnancy in women with systemic sclerosis. Arthritis Rheum 1989;32: 151–157.
167. Ballou SP, Morley JJ, Kushner I. Pregnancy and systemic sclerosis. Arthritis Rheum 1984;27:295–298.
168. Stenever MA, Ng ABP. Scleroderma of the uterus and cervix. Am J Obstet Gynecol 1970;107:965–966.
169. Cook WA. Letter and reply: Raynaud's phenomenon in pregnancy. JAMA 1976;235:145–146.
170. Karlen JR, Cook WA. Renal scleroderma and pregnancy. Obstet Gynecol 1974;44:349–354.
171. Black CM. Systemic sclerosis and pregnancy. Baillieres Clin Rheumatol 1990;7:105–124.
172. Mor-Yosef S, Navot D, Rabinowitz R, Schenker JG. Collagen diseases in pregnancy. Obstet Gynecol Surv 1984;30:67–84.
173. Wilson AG, Kirby JD. Successful pregnancy in a woman with systemic sclerosis while taking nifedipine. Ann Rheum Dis 1990;49: 51–52.
174. Gutierrez G, Dagnino R, Mintz G. Polymyositis/dermatomyositis and pregnancy. Arthritis Rheum 1984;27:291–294.
175. King CR, Chow S. Dermatomyositis and pregnancy. Obstet Gynecol 1985;66:589–592.
176. Bombardieri S, Munno OD, DiPunzio C, Parero G. Erythema nodosum associated with pregnancy and oral contraceptives. BMJ 1977;1:1509–1510.
177. Salvatore MA, Lyn PJ. Erythema nodosum, estrogens and pregnancy. Arch Dermatol 1980;116:557–558.
178. Gordon H. Erythema nodosum: a review of 115 cases. Br J Dermatol 1961;73:393–409.
179. Holcomb F. Erythema nodosum associated with the use of oral contraception. Obstet Gynecol 1965;25:156–157.
180. Bartelsmeyer JA, Petrie RH. Erythema nodosum, estrogens and pregnancy. Clin Obstet Gynecol 1990;33:777–781.
181. Ross MG, Kanet B, Frieder R, Gurevitch A, Hayashi R. Pemphigus in pregnancy: a reevaluation of fetal risk. Am J Obstet Gynecol 1986; 155:30–33.
182. Samitz MH, Greenberg MS, Coletti JM. Pemphigus in association with pregnancy: observations of the effect of corticotrophin and cortisone on pemphigus, pregnancy and infant. AMA Arch Dermatol Syphilol 1953;67:10.
183. Wasserstrum N, Laros RK. Transplacental transmission of pemphigus. JAMA 1983;249:1480–1482.
184. Merlob P, Metzger A, Hazaz B, Pogorin H, Reisner SH. Neonatal pemphigus vulgaris. Pediatrics 1986;78:1102–1105.
185. Green D, Maize JC. Maternal pemphigus vulgaris with in vivo bound antibodies in the stillborn fetus. J Am Acad Dermatol 1982;7: 388–392.
186. Goldberg NS, DeFeo C, Kirshenbaum N. Pemphigus vulgaris and pregnancy: Risk factors and recommendations. J Am Acad Dermatol 1993;28:877–879.
187. Hayashi RH. Bullous dermatoses and prurigo of pregnancy. Clin Obstet Gynecol 1990;33:746–53.
188. Gruneberg T. Psoriasis and pregnancy. Hautarzt 1952;3:155.
189. Farber EM, Nall ML. The natural history of psoriasis in 5,600 patients. Dermatologia 1974;148:1–18.
190. Bronson DM, Barsky R, Barsky S. Acrodermatitis enteropathica: recognition at long last during recurrence in a pregnancy. J Am Acad Dermatol 1983;9:140–144.
191. Schulman JD, Simpson JL. Genetic disease in pregnancy. New York: Academic Press, 1981:2–83.
192. Hambidge KM, Neldner KH, Walravens PA. Zinc, acrodermatitis enteropathica and congenital malformations. Lancet 1975;1:577–578.
193. Zander J, Mickan H, Holzmann K, Lohe KJ. Androluteoma syndrome in pregnancy. Am J Obstet Gynecol 1978;130:170–177.
194. Frank MM, Gelfand JA, Atkinson JP. Hereditary angioedema. Ann Intern Med 1976;89:580–593.
195. Gelfand JA, Atkinson JP. Hereditary angioedema: the clinical syndrome and its management. Ann Intern Med 1976;84:580–593.
196. Beighton P. The Ehlers-Danlos syndrome. London: Heinemann, 1970.
197. Samuel MA, Schwartz ML, Meister MM. The Ehlers Danlos syndrome. US Armed Forces Med J 1953;4:737.

198. Rivera-Alsina ME, Kwan P, Zavisca FG, Hopkins S, Abouleish E. Complications of the Ehlers-Danlos syndrome in pregnancy, a case report. J Reprod Med 1984;29:757–759.
199. McKusick VA. Heritable disorders of connective tissue, 4th ed. St. Louis: CV Mosby, 1972.
200. Ainsworth SR, Aulicino PL. A survey of patients with Ehlers-Danlos syndrome. Clin Orthop 1993;286:250–255.
201. Rudd NL, Nimrod C, Holbrook KA, Byers PH. Pregnancy complications in type IV Ehlers-Danlos syndrome. Lancet 1983;1:50–53.
202. Hammerschmidt DE, Arneson MA, Larson SL, VanTassel RA, McKenna JL. Maternal Ehlers-Danlos syndrome type X: successful management of pregnancy and parturition. JAMA 1982;248: 1487–1488.
203. Berde C, Willis DC, Sandberg EC. Pregnancy in women with pseudoxanthoma elasticum. Obstet Gynecol Surv 1983;38:339–344.
204. Broekhuizen FF, Hamilton PR. PXE and intrauterine growth retardation. Am J Obstet Gynecol 1984;148:112–114.
205. Mandel W, Evans EW, Walford RL. Dissecting aortic aneurysm during pregnancy. N Engl J Med 1954;251:1059–1061.
206. Cava EF, Drier RL. The Marfan syndrome in pregnancy: a case report. Trans Pacific Coast Obstet Gynecol Soc 1970;38:129–133.
207. Elias S, Berkowitz RL. The Marfan syndrome and pregnancy. Obstet Gynecol 1976;47:338–361.
208. Hirst AE, Johns VJ, Kime SW. Dissecting aneurysm of the aorta: a review of 505 cases. Medicine 1958;37:270–279.
209. Zimmerman TS, McMillin JM, Watson CJ. Onset of manifestations of hepatic porphyria in relation to the influence of female sex hormones. Arch Intern Med 1966;118:229–240.
210. Brodie MJ, Moore MR, Thompson GG, Goldberg A, Low RA. Pregnancy and the acute porphyrias. J Obstet Gynecol Br Commonw 1977;84:726–731.
211. Marks R. Porphyria cutanea tarda. Arch Dermatol 1982;118:452.
212. Lamon JM, Frykholm BC. Pregnancy and PCT. Genet Clin Johns Hopkins Hosp 1979;145:235–237.
213. Lamon JM, Frykholm BC, Hess RA, Tschudy DP. Hematin therapy for acute porphyria. Medicine 1979;58:252–269.
214. Tanenbaum L, Tuffanelli DL. Antimalarial agents: chloroquine, hydroxychloroquine, and quinacrine. Arch Dermatol 1980;116:587–591.
215. Baxi LV, Rubeo TJ, Katz B, Harber LC. Porphyria cutanea tarda and pregnancy. Am J Obstet Gynecol 1983;146:333–334.
216. Schmidt H, Snitker G, Thomsen K, Lintrup J . Erythropoietic protoporphyria. Arch Dermatol 1974;110:58–64.
217. Townes PL. Transplacentally acquired erythrodontia. J Pediatr 1965; 67:600–602.
218. Plewig G, Kligman AM. Acne morphogenesis and treatment. Berlin, Springer-Verlag, 1975:33.

SECTION XV

Infectious Diseases

Cherry and Merkatz's Complications of Pregnancy,
Fifth Edition, edited by W. R. Cohen.
Lippincott Williams & Wilkins, Philadelphia © 2000.

CHAPTER 42

Sexually Transmitted Diseases

David A. Baker

Sexually transmitted diseases (STDs) are common medical complications of pregnancy, especially in certain socioeconomic populations and in those with a high incidence of drug abuse and prostitution. The incidence of specific infections varies widely; chlamydial infection is the most common, followed by genital herpes, human papillomavirus (HPV) infection, gonorrhea, and syphilis. The first prenatal visit provides a unique opportunity to screen for a variety of these infections. Many state codes or health department rules provide for mandatory screening for STDs during pregnancy. In addition to screening, the health care provider needs to provide proper educational support and to know the latest and pregnancy-appropriate treatments for these infections. Identification and treatment of the pregnant woman with an STD prevent the significant risks to her and her fetus or newborn and, in addition, allow for partner notification and treatment.

This chapter presents the most common STDs, except for human immunodeficiency virus (HIV), which is discussed in Chapter 43. The most recent recommendations from the treatment schedules provided by the Centers for Disease Control and Prevention (CDC) are incorporated into this chapter.

D. A. Baker: Department of Obstetrics and Gynecology, Division of Maternal–Fetal Medicine, State University of New York at Stony Brook, Stony Brook, NY 11794-8091.

GENITAL HERPES VIRUS INFECTION

Genital herpes simplex virus (HSV) infections have increased significantly in the United States (1) (Fig. 42-1) over the last few years. Many women of childbearing age are being infected, which poses a risk of maternal transmission of this virus to the fetus or newborn. Therefore, the health care provider must be able to recognize and properly manage this infection during pregnancy.

Incidence

Approximately 45 million Americans aged older than 12 years are infected with genital herpes (2), making it one of the most common viral STDs. Women acquire this infection in their late teens and early 20's. About 30% of the female population in the United States are infected with HSV-2 as determined by the use of sensitive HSV type-specific antibodies (2).

HSV type 1 (HSV-1) or type 2 (HSV-2) virus can infect the female genital tract; in the United States, most genital infection is caused by HSV-2. Initial infection of the female genital tract can present with clinical disease, or it can be subclinical (3). Genital infection with HSV is associated with risk factors that increase the chance for other STDs, including years of sexual activity, episodes of other genital infections, and multiple sex partners (4). Of the 1,500 to 2,000 newborn infants in the United

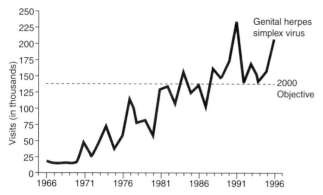

FIG. 42-1. Genital herpes simplex virus infections: initial visits to physicians' offices: United States, 1966–1996 and the Healthy People year 2000 objective. (From ref 1.).

States who contract neonatal herpes each year, most are born of mothers who do not know they are infected with genital herpes and shed the virus without lesions or symptoms (5,6).

Etiology

Two types of HSV can be identified and are designated types 1 and 2 (HSV-1 and HSV-2). Although there are differences between the type 1 and 2 viruses, they share some antigenic components; so there are cross-reacting antibodies capable of neutralizing the heterologous virus type (7).

Early childhood is the time when initial contact with HSV-1 occurs, with fewer than one in ten of these infections showing clinical signs. HSV-1 is the causative agent for most nongenital herpetic lesions, whereas HSV-2 is recovered predominantly from the genital tract. Sexual transmission is the primary mode of HSV-2 transmission (4).

Presentation of Infection

Primary Infection

Primary genital infection resulting from HSV usually is associated with significant symptoms but may be asymptomatic. In primary infection, lesions occur throughout the perineum and cervix, with an incubation period between 2 and 14 days. Multiple sites and larger areas usually are involved compared with recurrent disease, which is generally limited to one site. Local and systemic symptoms result from virus replication in the sites of lymphatic drainage (7). In a nonpregnant population of women after primary infection, subclinical cervical and vulvar shedding is more frequent than initially reported (8,9).

Nonprimary First Episode

Prior HSV-1 infection does not fully protect a patient from initial infection with HSV-2 in the genital tract. It may be difficult, based solely on clinical findings and patient symptoms, for a physician to differentiate a primary versus a nonprimary first episode of disease (10).

Recurrent Infection

After a symptomatic primary genital infection (11), almost all patients will experience recurrent disease. Usually, one to three lesions recur at the same anatomic site as the primary lesion.

Subclinical Shedding

This viral STD is difficult to control and prevent because shedding of virus without any symptoms or signs of clinical lesions can occur (*subclinical shedding*). Subclinical shedding of virus lasts an average of 1.5 days, and the quantity of virus is lower than when a visible lesion is present. A susceptible sexual partner or newborn can nevertheless acquire this virus during times of subclinical shedding (9,12–14).

Diagnosis

Direct staining and viral isolation in tissue culture are the most common ways in which HSV genital infections are diagnosed. Staining tests have a maximum sensitivity of 60% to 70% when dealing with clinical lesions. Isolation of virus by cell culture remains the standard and the most sensitive test for the detection of infectious herpes virus from clinical specimens. More sensitive techniques such as polymerase chain reaction (PCR) and hybridization methods currently are restricted to research laboratories (15).

Because of the frequent presence of cross-reacting antibodies to the heterologous virus, serologic testing is of relatively limited value. Currently available serologic tests that identify antibody to genital herpes infection cannot distinguish infection between HSV types 1 and type 2. Enzyme-linked immunosorbent assay (ELISA) and Western blot serological assays that are type specific are currently under development (16).

Transmission

Sexual and Direct Contact

Direct genital-to-genital contact is the most common source of genital HSV transmission to women (3). The virus also can be spread by direct contact with a person who is infected and has a lesion or is shedding virus asymptomatically from the genital tract, oral cavity, or other body site.

During Delivery

Several studies have demonstrated and calculated estimates of symptomatic and asymptomatic viral shedding in women who are in labor. It is estimated that culture techniques could demonstrate the presence of HSV in the genital tract of 3 per 1,000 gravid women at term. Cultures from pregnant women who have a history of recurrent genital herpes show an asymptomatic shedding rate for HSV-2 between 0.65% to 3.03% of pregnant women studied (17). The prevalence of asymptomatic reactivation is increased to between 2.3% and 14% of pregnant women who have a history of genital herpes when serial specimens for culture are obtained (18). It is estimated that one infant in 350 live births is delivered through a birth canal harboring infectious HSV virus, and yet the incidence of disseminated herpetic infection of the newborn is extremely low (i.e., 1:20,000 deliveries). Estimated risks of infection for an infant born to a mother with genital herpes have been reported: primary genital herpes, 30% to 50% (17); active recurrent genital herpes at the time of delivery, 4% to 8% (19,20); subclinical shedding, 0.3 to 3% (15,17).

Management of Pregnant Women

Antenatal

Conflicting studies address the risk to the fetus of maternal primary genital HSV infection occurring in the first trimester. An increased rate of abortion was reported in one study (17) but was not confirmed in a more recent analysis (21). Hematogenous dissemination of HSV to the conceptus may occur with true primary genital infection. Congenital herpetic infection has been reported as being associated with a variety of anomalies (22–25).

Antiviral therapy is recommended for pregnant patients with primary HSV infection during their pregnancy. It is unknown whether maternal antiviral therapy alters or prevents disease in the fetus. The focus of such therapy is to reduce viral shedding and to speed healing of lesions. The study by Koelle and colleagues (9) in nonpregnant women raises the concern of continued viral shedding and the suggestion that suppressive therapy for the duration of the pregnancy should be considered.

An increased rate of preterm delivery and increased risk of herpes virus transmission to the newborn have been reported with primary infection in the second or third trimester (17). Asymptomatic primary genital herpes infection near term, which poses a significant diagnostic problem, may be the cause of many cases of neonatal herpes (21).

Partner of the Pregnant Woman

Much acquisition of genital herpes is asymptomatic (26), and about one in ten pregnant women is at risk of contracting primary HSV-2 infection from their HSV-2-seropositive husbands (27). Hensleigh and colleagues (28) demonstrated the difficulty in distinguishing between primary and secondary herpetic infection in pregnancy. Only one of 23 women with clinical illnesses consistent with primary genital herpes virus simplex infections had serologically verified primary infection.

Antiviral Therapy for Genital Herpes in Pregnancy

Although many effective and safe treatment options are available for patients with genital herpes (29), none has received approval for use in pregnancy by the U.S. Food and Drug Administration (FDA). These compounds are nucleoside analogues that selectively inhibit viral replication and possess a high safety profile. The FDA has approved acyclovir, valacyclovir, and famciclovir for the treatment of primary genital herpes, for treatment of episodes of recurrent disease, and for daily treatment for suppression of outbreaks of recurrent genital herpes in nonpregnant women.

The first marketed purine nucleoside analogue with activity against HSV-1 and HSV-2 was acyclovir (30–33). The drug is safe, and it has few side effects (34) but poor oral absorption. Valacyclovir is acyclovir with a valine ester, and it has better bioavailability. Famciclovir is a prodrug of penciclovir. Bioavailability is good, but less information is available about clinical long-term use than for other agents. Several reports have shown the safety of acyclovir use in pregnancy (35–37). Even use in the first trimester of pregnancy did not demonstrate any increased risk to the developing fetus.

Pharmacokinetics in the Fetus and Newborn

After oral or intravenous administration, acyclovir readily crosses the placenta, is concentrated in amniotic fluid (38), and has a concentration of drug in the umbilical cord blood 1.3 times the maternal serum concentration.

Effectiveness of Antiviral Therapy

Cesarean delivery, which has many disadvantages, is a directed therapy against HSV maternal-to-newborn transmission (20,21). Antiviral prophylactic therapy of the mother to prevent maternal symptomatic and subclinical viral shedding during the intrapartum period is receiving attention as a means to reduce transmission and the need for cesarean section (37,39). The use of antiviral medication in the last few weeks of pregnancy to suppress recurrent disease also is being studied. An early description of five women treated with oral acyclovir suggested that antiviral therapy did not prevent subclinical viral shedding in one of the mothers, and viral transmission to one of the newborns occurred (39). A newer study did show a significant reduction in cesarean delivery but showed no increase in subclinical shedding. Use of antiviral medication in the last 4 weeks of pregnancy would be the most cost-effective approach (40).

Systemic HSV infections, herpes of the lung, herpes of the liver, and herpes encephalitis have responded to antiviral therapy, which has been life saving to mother and fetus (35,41,42).

Delivery Management

Cesarean section is unwarranted for prevention of neonatal herpes in the presence of recurrent maternal genital herpes because of the low incidence of serious consequences of this disease (43). Newer information, however, shows the problems involved in preventing neonatal herpes. Primary infection near term may be a critical factor for HSV disease of the newborn (21); but current recommendations are to deliver by cesarean section if an active herpetic lesion is present when the pregnant woman is in labor. Neonatal infection occurs in only 5% to 8% of infants whose mother had an active herpetic lesion during labor. Cesarean delivery increases costs as well as the morbidity and mortality of the mother and should be done only in well-defined clinical situations.

Several reports suggest that neonatal infection may result from the use of fetal-monitoring scalp electrodes (44–46). Generally, external ultrasound transducers should be used in lieu of direct electrodes in any patient in whom shedding of HSV is suspected.

The use of viral cultures during labor of the mother and of the newborn after birth have been reported in an effort to identify at-risk infants. This strategy is not effective because cultures are costly and there is poor correlation between a positive culture and newborn disease (19,14). A history of genital herpes without visible lesions certainly does not justify cesarean delivery (47). Without lesions in the intrapartum period, the probability of neonatal disease appears to be exceedingly low.

Breastfeeding

In rare situations, breastfeeding during the immediate postpartum period has been implicated in causing neonatal HSV-1 and HSV-2 infections (48,49). Transmission has occurred from a recurrent herpetic lesion on the nipple. Care should be taken to examine the breast for any signs of herpetic lesions, which are in any event a rare finding. If such lesions are absent, breastfeeding is acceptable. Having recurrent HSV lesions elsewhere does not contraindicate nursing as long as scrupulous care is taken to avoid transfer of the virus, which often includes covering the lesions with a dressing and frequent and thorough hand washing by the nursing mother.

Special Clinical Situations

Systemic Maternal Herpetic Infection and Pregnancy

Fulminant hepatitis after primary herpes is rare but is associated with a maternal mortality rate of 43% (50,51). The third trimester is when the disease occurs, often after a viral-like illness in association with genital or oral lesions. It is usually anicteric, and herpetic hepatitis should be included in the differential diagnosis of any hepatic dysfunction in the third trimester (41,42).

Hospital-acquired Neonatal Herpetic Infection

The mother may not be the only source for the newborn to acquire HSV (52,53). Hospital staff as well as family members and friends may inoculate the newborn with HSV, causing severe disease, most commonly from HSV-1.

HSV in Dysmature Gestation

An uncommon and difficult-to-manage situation is that of an immature gestation in conjunction with documented rupture of the fetal membranes and active maternal genital HSV. Systemic antiviral therapy can be considered and should be followed by oral antiviral therapy. Corticosteroids to accelerate pulmonary maturity in this kind of case should be considered experimental (54) because of concerns that the steroids could lead to exacerbation of the infection and risk of vertical transmission.

HSV in a HIV-positive Mother

Hitti and colleagues (55) reported that HIV-positive pregnant women have a significantly higher infection rate with HSV-2 compared with HIV-negative women. It is still uncertain whether an HIV-positive mother has a greater chance of transmitting HSV to her newborn.

HUMAN PAPILLOMAVIRUS INFECTION

Condylomata acuminata, or genital warts, usually are caused by nonmalignant types of human papillomavirus (HPV). Types 6 and 11 cause most external lesions and can produce warts, most likely transmitted by the mother, in the larynx of newborns. Many other HPV types infect the lower genital tract of women and may appear for the first time during pregnancy (56). Cancer risk is determined by viral type and usually is associated with infection with type 16 and 18 (56,57). After infection, HPV may cause clinical disease or may be subclinical in many patients. Because of gestational alterations in immune function and high levels of estrogen and progesterone, HPV disease may first present in pregnancy from a previously acquired infection or recent infection. Laryngeal papillomatosis in children caused by HPV types 6 and 11 is rare in the United States. The exact mode of transmission is still unknown. One small study from Taiwan indicated that the virus may be transmitted transplacentally (58).

In the pregnant woman, HPV disease may progress and prove difficult to manage. It must be remembered that such disease usually will regress postpartum. Treatment in pregnancy should be reserved for patients who show symptoms or who have proven dysplastic disease that in the view of the physician requires therapy before delivery.

Treatment

Treatment should be aimed at limiting the infection and preventing complications of bowel and bladder function as well as bleeding and secondary infection. Care directed to individual hygiene is important in preventing complications and for delaying therapy until after delivery. No therapy has been shown to decrease the small chance of HPV transmission to the newborn. Therefore, therapy should be directed toward medical problems of the pregnant woman. Imiquimod, interferon, podophyllin, podofilox, and 5-fluorouracil are contraindicated for use in pregnancy (57,59). Laser therapy, cryotherapy, and topical trichloroacetic acid have been used in pregnancy with variable success rates and outcomes (60–63). Therapy for large-volume disease is reserved for selected patients and is performed around 32 to 34 weeks' gestation. Reports suggest high recurrence rates in patients treated in the second trimester. Cesarean section is reserved for women with extensive genital warts in whom there is concern about obstructed labor or significant perineal hemorrhage.

Neonatal Infection

Infection of the newborn larynx with HPV and subsequent laryngeal papilloma is rare, occurring in 1 in 10,000 pregnancies (64). The true vocal cords are involved, and HPV-6 and HPV-11 are the predominant viral type isolated from these lesions (65). Although it has been assumed that cesarean delivery in the presence of maternal HPV will prevent this infection, one study clearly demonstrated that even with abdominal delivery the infant was infected (64). Positive findings of HPV DNA in samples of oral swabs from children born to mothers with genital HPV infection suggest that passage of this virus to the newborn is common, but clinical disease is rare (66).

HEPATITIS B INFECTION

Maternal transmission of hepatitis B virus (HBV) to the newborn is one of the most efficient and common ways in which HBV is spread (see Chapter 45). HBV can produce short-term and long-term severe sequelae in the newborn period and beyond. In most cases, immune globulin and a safe and effective vaccine can prevent fetal infection and its serious consequences.

Etiology

A small DNA virus produces this infection with a well-defined antigen–antibody response. Hepatitis B surface antigen (HBsAg) can be identified in serum 1 to 2 months after exposure to HBV and persists for varied periods. Hepatitis B surface antibody (HBsAb) develops after a resolved infection and is responsible for long-term immunity.

Antibody to core antigen (HBcAb) develops in all HBV infections and is a marker for long-term past exposure to this virus. Hepatitis B e antigen (HBeAg) may be detected in samples from persons who have acute or chronic HBV infection. HBeAg correlates with viral replication and high infectivity. The presence of antibody to e antigen (HBeAb) correlates with the loss of replicating virus and with lower infectivity (67).

Epidemiology

HBV is transmitted via contact with blood, sexual activity, and vertical transmission from mothers to newborns (68). Newborns are at risk of infection if the mother has acute HBV infection during the third trimester or is a chronic carrier. Depending on the antigen and antibody status of the mother, perinatal transmission can be high (70% to 90% if the mother is HBsAg positive and HBeAg positive; 25% if the mother is positive only for HBsAg; 10% to 15% if the mother is HBsAg positive and HBeAb positive) (69).

The HBV carrier is the most important factor in HBV transmission. A person who is HBsAg positive on at least two occasions at least 6 months apart is defined as a carrier. A person positive for HBsAg is potentially infectious, with the degree of infectivity best correlated with HBeAg positivity. The chance of developing the carrier state varies inversely with the age at which infection occurs. Therefore, vertical infection produces a high degree of carriers (up to 90% of infected infants), whereas only 6% to 10% of acutely infected adults become carriers (70).

Diagnosis

Serologic tests for the HBV antigens (HBsAg and HBeAg) and for antibodies to HBsAg, HBcAg, and

TABLE 42-1. *Identification of clinical hepatitis B infection by serological markers*

Stage	HBsAG	HbeAg	HBsAb	HBeAb	HBcAb
Acute infection	+	+	–	–	+ or –
Chronic carrier*					
Low	+	–	–	+	+
Moderate	+	–	–	–	+
High	+	+	–	–	+
Past infection	–	–	+ or –	+ or –	+
Post vaccination	–	–	+	–	–

HBsAG, hepatitis B surface antigen; HbeAg, hepatitis B e antigen; HBsAb, hepatitis B surface antibody; HBeAb, antibody to e antigen; HBcAb, antibody to core antigen.

*Low, moderate, high refer to the degree of infection.

HBeAg have allowed for precise diagnosis of this infection. Table 42-1 lists the common serologic patterns of HBV infection. By evaluating the clinical presentation and then determining the serologic pattern, the specific stage of hepatitis B infection can be determined (67).

Symptoms have gradual onset and may present as a flulike illness, along with fatigue, anorexia, nausea, and vomiting. Other clinical presentations of this infection may be myalgia, malaise, headache, and pharyngitis. Jaundice with a low-grade fever may occur. The severity of the disease is directly correlated with signs and symptoms. In 10% to 20% of patients, signs of hepatomegaly, splenomegaly, and lymphadenopathy may appear. Jaundice can persist for 4 to 6 weeks; symptoms resolve slowly. Most patients have complete recovery; however, as noted, the chronic carrier state will develop in some infected patients (67).

Treatment

No specific therapy for acute HBV is available, aside from supportive care. New therapies such as interferon for the chronic carrier state have been tested with some success. Their appropriateness during pregnancy is unclear.

Prevention

Health-care workers should be considered at high risk and should receive hepatitis B vaccine. The most common source of health care provider infection is the asymptomatic hospital patient who gives no history of HBV exposure and has not been screened for it. Both active and passive immunization for HBV is available and is highly effective and safe. The vaccine is based on developing an immune response to HBsAg, the surface antigen, which is the natural protective antibody against infection (71).

Prevention of Perinatal Transmission

HbsAg screening should be part of routine prenatal testing as recommended by the CDC and the American College of Obstetricians and Gynecologists. Part of prenatal care should be to alert women at greatest risk for contacting HBV who should be counseled about vaccination. Assessment of liver function is recommended for women who test positive for HbsAg, as is evaluation of family members (72–78).

The infant's health care provider must be notified about the maternal HbsAg-positive status and the baby should receive hepatitis B immune globulin (HBIG) and vaccine after birth. This therapy is 85% to 95% effective in preventing development of the HBV chronic carrier state in the newborn. Table 42-2 shows the recommended schedule of HBV immunoprophylaxis to prevent perinatal transmission. In addition, the CDC recommends uni-

TABLE 42-2. *Recommended schedule of hepatitis B immunoprophylaxis to prevent perinatal transmission of hepatitis B virus infection*

	Vaccine dose[a]	Age of infant
Infant born to mother known to be HBsAG positive	First	Birth (within 12 hr)
	HBIG[b]	Birth (within 12 hr)
	Second	1 mo
	Third	6 mo
Infant born to mother not screened for HBsAG[c]	First	Birth (within 12 hr)
	HBIG[b]	If mother is found to be HBsAg positive, administer dose to infant as soon as possible, not later than 1 wk after birth
	Second	1–2 months[d]
	Third	6 months[e]

HBsAG, hepatitis B surface antigen; HBIG, hepatitis B immune globulin.

[a]See Table 43-1 for appropriate vaccine dose.

[b]Hepatitis B immune globulin (HBIG) 0.5 mL administered intramuscularly at a site different from that used for vaccine.

[c]First dose=dose for infant of HBsAG-positive mother (see Table 43-1). If mother is found to be HBsAG positive, continue that dose; if mother is found to be HBsAG negative, use appropriate dose from Table 43-1.

[d]Infants of women who are HBsAG negative can be vaccinated at 2 mo of age.

[e]If four-dose schedule (engerix-B) is used, the third dose is administered at 2 mo of age and the fourth dose at 12 to 18 mo.

versal vaccination of all infants born to HbsAg-negative mothers (74).

Sequelae

Because infected newborns have a higher rate of becoming chronic carriers of HBV, prevention of HBV vertical transmission can make a major impact on the long-term health of this newborn and has important public health implications. One quarter of these carriers will die of primary hepatocellular carcinoma or cirrhosis. In addition, these infants have had acute disease, and fatal fulminant hepatitis from the vertical transmission of this virus occurs (67).

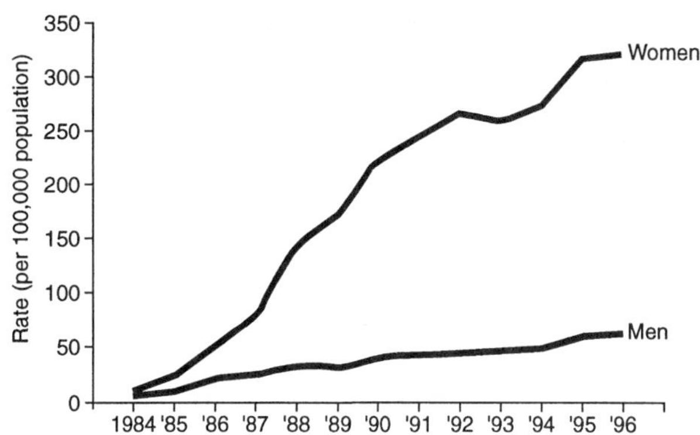

FIG. 42-3. Chlamydia—rates by gender: United States, 1984–1996. (From ref 1.)

CHLAMYDIAL INFECTIONS

Chlamydia trachomatis is the most common STD in the United States (Fig. 42-2) (1) and has a higher incidence in women than in men (Fig. 42-3) (1). The age group most affected for women is between 15 and 29 years, the age when the pregnancy rate is the highest (Fig. 42-4) (1). The most commonly encountered strains are those that attach only to columnar or transitional cell epithelium and cause cervical infection.

Etiology, Diagnosis, and Results of Infection

The organism needs a cell to grow and reproduce. It is therefore classified as an intracellular organism, but it is not a virus. After a short incubation period (7–21 days), this infection can produce specific symptoms, but most women are asymptomatic (79). Symptoms of infection, such as dysuria and frequency, may mimic those of a urinary tract infection. *Chlamydia* can produce a mucopurulent cervicitis (80). Positive cervical cultures for *Chlamydia* in pregnant populations have been reported to range from 2% to 24% (81), depending on socioeconomic and demographic characteristics of the population. Most laboratory tests for *Chlamydia* rely on antigen detection, and not on actual culture and isolation of the organism. Advances in diagnosis have been made using PCR and ligase chain reaction (LCR) assays (82–84), which have extremely high levels of sensitivity and specificity (greater than 95%) and can be used to test the introital area from pregnant women and urine. Paavonen (85) showed that adolescence, being single, use of oral contraceptives, and having a new sex partner are factors associated with chlamydial infection.

The CDC (59) recommends *C trachomatis* diagnostic testing at the first prenatal visit for all pregnant women and again in the third trimester for high-risk patients. Prenatal screening and treatment of pregnant women can prevent chlamydial infection among neonates (59). The American College of Obstetricians and Gynecologists has taken a different approach. It recommends targeted screening of high-risk populations (86).

Infection, Pregnancy Outcome, and the Newborn

Vertical transmission in infected women is common and is associated with neonatal conjunctivitis and pneumonia (87–89). Neonatal ocular prophylaxis with silver

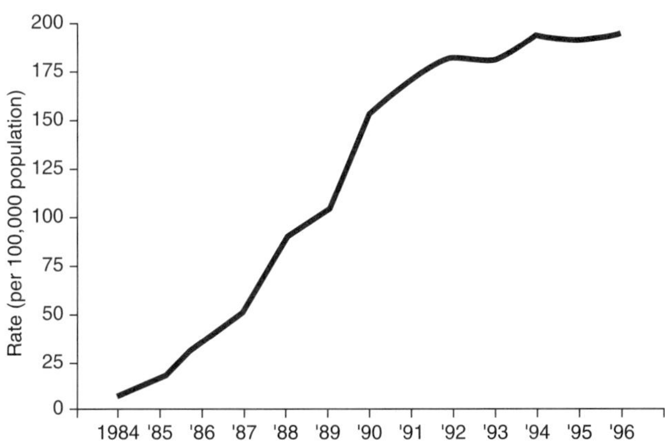

FIG. 42-2. Chlamydia—reported rates: United States, 1984–1996. (From ref 1.)

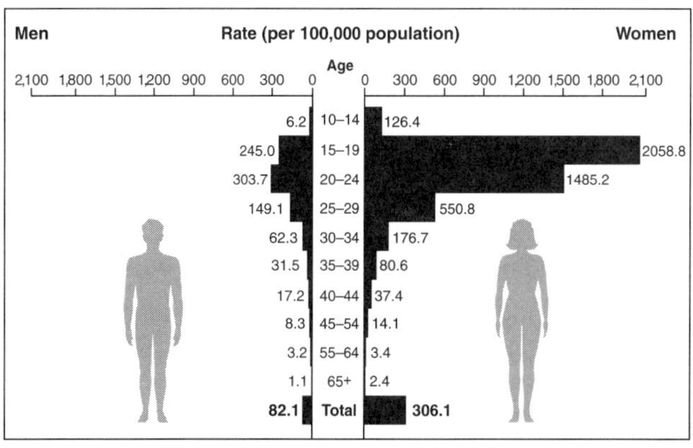

FIG. 42-4. Chlamydia—age- and gender-specific rates: United States, 1996. (From ref 1.)

TABLE 42-3. *Treatment of sexually transmitted diseases in pregnancy*

Organism	Primary regimen	Alternative regimen
N. gonorrhea[a]	Ceftriaxone 125 mg i.m.	Spectinomycin 2.0 g 1 i.m.
C. trachomatis	Erythromycin base 500 mg p.o. q.i.d. × 7 days or Amoxicillin 500 mg p.o. t.i.d. × 7 d	Azithromycin 1g p.o. Erythromycin base 250 mg p.o. q.i.d. × 14 d
T. pallidum		
Primary infection	Benzathine penicillin G 2.4 million U i.m., one dose	
Secondary infection	Benzathine penicillin G 2.4 million U i.m., one dose	
Early latent	Benzathine penicillin G 2.4 million U i.m., one dose	
Late latent[b] or tertiary	Benzathine penicillin G 2.4 million U × 3 doses @ weekly intervals	
Neurosyphilis	Aqueous penicillin G 3–4 million U i.v. q 4 hr × 14 d	

i.m., intramuscularly; p.o., orally; t.i.d., three times a day; q.i.d., four times a day; i.v., intravenous.
[a]Uncomplicated local infections of cervix, urethra, rectum, or pharynx.
[b]Applies to latent syphilis of unknown duration.
[c]Patients allergic to penicillin should be desensitized and treated with penicillin.
Adapted from *1998 Guidelines for Treatment of Sexually Transmitted Diseases,* Center for Disease Control and Prevention, Atlanta, GA.

nitrate solution or antibiotic ointments does not prevent perinatal transmission of *Chlamydia* (89).

The specific adverse outcomes of chlamydial infection on pregnancy still require further study. Some studies suggest that infection during pregnancy increases the risk of premature delivery (90–94); however, study design and the possibility of concurrent bacterial vaginosis (not tested for in most available studies) open the results of these studies to question. Perhaps it is only acute or recently acquired infection documented by testing for chlamydial IgM antibody, that increases the risk for these adverse outcomes (85,95,96). In addition to concerns about the newborn, chlamydial infection has been associated with an increased risk of postpartum and postabortion endometritis (85,97).

Treatment

The CDC recently published recommendations for treatment of chlamydial infection in pregnant women (Table 42-3) (59). The preferred approach is erythromycin base or amoxicillin administered for a week. Although azithromycin, 1 g orally in a single dose, is listed as an alternative regimen, it has the advantage of one-dose therapy with increased patient compliance, and it can be used as a provider-observed aproach (98). Repeat antigen testing as a test of cure is recommended three weeks following therapy.

SYPHILIS

Incidence, Etiology, and Pregnancy Outcome

After a resurgence of this disease in the United States in the early 1990's, the incidence of this infection continued to decline along with the number of cases of congenital disease (Fig. 42-5) (1). Although it can occur in anyone, the groups with the highest incidence are isolated high-risk populations: those associated with HIV, drug abuse (particularly crack cocaine), and lack of prenatal care (99). Syphilis is caused by the spirochete *Treponema pallidum,* which is spread to the fetus through the mother's bloodstream. Syphilis acquired during pregnancy can produce serious problems in the fetus and newborn, including preterm labor, fetal death, and neonatal infection (100). Congenital infection with syphilis is a readily preventable disease.

Clinical Manifestations

Pregnancy has no effect on the clinical course of syphilis (99). Primary syphilis with the presence of a chancre occurs 10 to 90 days after infection (average, 21 days) (101). After 1 to 6 weeks, the chancre heals. Depending on its location, it may not be noticed by the pregnant patient. The next stage of the disease, secondary infection, occurs 6 to 8 weeks after healing of the chancre, and presents as a skin rash, the characteristics of which can be highly vari-

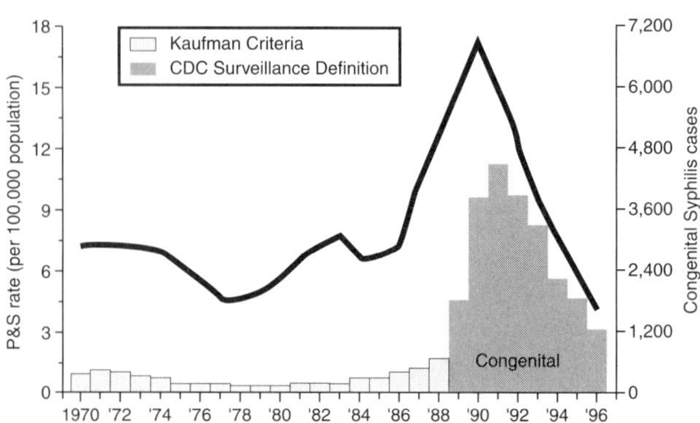

FIG. 42-5. Congenital syphilis. Reported cases for infants aged younger than 1 year and rates of primary and secondary syphilis among women: United States, 1970–1996. (From ref 1.)

able. This rash heals spontaneously within 1 to 3 months. This stage is the most contagious to the fetus because of large numbers of circulating spirochtes in the maternal circulation and increased chance of fetal infection. Early latent and late latent syphilis follows, the distinction depending on whether the initial infection was 1 year in duration or longer. Both periods can produce fetal infection (80). Teritiary syphilis follows if there is no treatment. Neurosyphilis can occur during any stage of this infection.

Diagnosis

With a pregnant population, serologic testing is the way in which this infection is identified. All women should be screened serologically for syphilis during the early stages of pregnancy, and many state health departments mandate retesting one or more times during gestion. The Venereal Disease Research Laboratoay (VDRL) slide test or the rapid plasma reagin (PPR) test is used. If positive, these tests are followed by more specific tests, such as a fluorescent treponemal antibody test (FTA-ABS) or the microhemagglutination assay for antibodies to *Treponema pallidum*. Repeat testing at 28 weeks' gestation and at delivery for women at high risk for syphilis should be considered (59). Testing may need to be done monthly in high-risk populations. *In utero* diagnosis of syphilis has been performed by using culture and serologic studies on amniotic fluid obtained by transabdominal amniocentesis (102,103).

Treatment, Complications, and Follow-up

Pregnant women with a serologically confirmed diagnosis of syphilis require HIV testing, because there is increased risk of being HIV positive if a diagnosis of syphilis is made (59). In addition, in the evaluation of the pregnant patient, consideration to performing a lumbar puncture should be based on the following: neurologic symptoms in a patient with latent syphilis of longer than 1 year's duration; initial titers of 1:32 or greater; HIV infection; and treatment failures (after 3 months, the nontreponemal test titer does not decline fourfold). If the patient declines cerebrospinal evaluation, consideration to treat for neurosyphilis must be entertained.

Treatment of syphilis in pregnancy relies on the use of penicillin because it is the only proven treatment for fetal infection (59). In pregnant women allergic to penicillin, desensitization and penicillin treatment are the therapy of choice (59).

Penicillin therapy in pregnancy can carry a risk of preterm labor and fetal distress (99) when, after treatment in primary syphilis and secondary infection, a Jarisch-Herxheimer reaction is precipitated (101). Warning signs and a detailed explanation of what to expect need to be given to pregnant women treated in the second half of pregnancy. Systemic symptoms with fever, chills, myalgia, headache, tachycardia, hyperventilation, and vasodilation have been observed (101).

It must be made clear to the patient that reports suggest that despite adequate maternal therapy closely following recommended guidelines, the risk of fetal demise or evidence of congenital neonatal infection still may exist. Most such reports are of women treated in the late third trimester who carry a diagnosis of secondary syphilis.

Documentation of declining nontreponemal titers is a useful indication of appropriate therapy. Careful and continued follow-up of the pregnant woman needs to be provided to ensure adequate therapy to mother and fetus (59).

GONORRHEA

Etiology, Diagnosis, and Coinfections

Neisseria gonorrhea is a gram-negative bacteria often found intracellularly *in vivo* and characterized as a diplococcus. The incubation period is short, and usually symptoms occur within 5 days after infection; but incubation may be as long as 2 weeks (104). The incidence has declined recently in the United States, and data suggest that infection affects men and women at the same rates (1). The incidence varies according to socioeconomic and marital status, race, and the presence or absence of a previous STD infection (105). The prevalence in pregnancy has been reported to range from 1% to 80% (106). In about 40% of infected pregnant women, there is concomitant chlamydial infection (107).

Gonococcal infections usually are limited to the lower genital tract in nonpregnant women (80). A differing pattern of gonorrhea infection is seen in pregnancy. A higher incidence of disseminated disease occurs during pregnancy, with rare cases of acute salpingitis occurring in the first trimester (104).

Pregnancy Outcome

Pregnancy complications have been reported in women infected with this organism. There is an increased incidence of preterm delivery, prematurely ruptured membranes, chorioamnionitis, and postpartum infection (90, 104,108,109). The relative risk of preterm delivery in a woman infected with gonorrhea is two to five times greater than in controls (110).

Current guidelines recommend screening at the first prenatal visit, before an induced abortion and before any special procedures performed during pregnancy. In high-risk populations, the CDC (59) recommend that a repeat culture be obtained after 28 weeks.

Treatment

Quinolones and tetracyclines should not be used to treat gonorrhea in pregnancy. The drug of choice is one dose of an oral cephalosporin. For pregnant women who are unable to take or are allergic to cephalosporins, alternative therapy of spectinomycin 2 g intramuscularly in a single dose is available (59).

Simultaneous treatment for chlamydial infections is necessary because of the high incidence of coinfection. Test of cure by culture is recommended in pregnancy. In addition, in high-risk populations and in regions with a high incidence of gonorrhea, repeat screening in late pregnancy should be considered for women treated earlier during pregnancy (86). Treatment of sexual contacts is mandatory to ensure that reinfection does not occur and thus jeopordize the pregnancy.

Treatment of disseminated gonococcal infections should be performed initially in a hospital setting with the use of intravenous antibiotics as recommended by the CDC (59). Intravenous medication should be continued for 24 to 48 hours, at which time with improvement the patient can be placed on oral medication as recommended in pregnancy.

Neonatal ophthalmic prophylaxis is recommended for all newborns to reduce significantly the risk of developing ophthalmia neonatorum caused by gonorrhea. Current guidelines are to use silver nitrate 1% aqueous solution, erythromycin (0.5%), or tetracycline 1% ointments in a single application (59).

REFERENCES

1. Centers for Disease Control. Division of STD Prevention. Sexually transmitted disease surveillance 1996 Atlanta, GA. 1997;5–32.
2. Fleming DT, McQuillan GM, Johnson RE, et al. Herpes simplex virus type 2 in the United States 1976 to 1994. N Engl J Med 1997;337: 1105–1111.
3. Mertz GJ, Schmidt D, Jourden JL, et al. Frequency of acquisition of first-episode genital infection with herpes simplex virus from symptomatic and asymptomatic source contacts. Sex Transm Dis 1985; 12:33–39.
4. Mertz GJ, Benedetti J, Ashley R, Selke SA, Corey L. Risk factors for the sexual transmission of genital herpes. Ann Intern Med 1992; 16:197–202.
5. Prober CG, Corey L, Brown ZA, et al. The management of pregnancies complicated by genital infections with herpes simplex virus. Clin Infect Dis 1992;15:1031–1038.
6. Frenkel LM, Garratty EM, Shen JP, Wheeler N, Clark O, Bryson YJ. Clinical reactivation of herpes simplex virus type 2 infection inseropositive pregnant women with no history of genital herpes. Ann Intern Med 1993;118:414–418.
7. Corey L, Spear PG. Infections with herpes simplex viruses. N Engl J Med 1986;314:686–749.
8. Benedetti J, Corey L, Ashley R. Recurrence rate in genital herpes after symptomatic first-episode infection. Ann Intern Med 1994;121: 847–854.
9. Koelle DM, Benedetti J, Langenberg A, Corey L. Asymptomatic reactivation of herpes simplex virus in women after the first episode of genital herpes. Ann Intern Med 1992;116:433–437.
10. Mertz GJ. Epidemiology of genital herpes infections. Infect Dis Clin North Am 1993;7:825.
11. Hirsch MS. Herpes simplex virus. In: Mandell JE, Bennet JE, Dolin R, et al., eds. Principles and practice of infectious diseases, 4th ed. New York: Churchill Livingstone, 1995:1336–1345.
12. Brock BV, Selke S, Benedetti J, Douglas JM Jr, Corey L. Frequency of asymptomatic shedding of herpes simplex virus in women with genital herpes. JAMA 1990;263:418–420.
13. Wald A, Zeh J, Selke S, Ashley RL, Corey L. Virologic characteristics of subclinical and symptomatic genital herpes infections. N Engl J Med 1995;333:771–775.
14. Prober CG. Herpetic vaginitis in 1993. Clin Obstet Gynecol 1993;36: 177–187.
15. Scott LL, Hollier LM, Dias K. Perinatal herpesvirus infections. Infect Dis Clin North Am 1997;11:27–53.
16. Woods GL. Update on laboratory diagnosis of sexually transmitted diseases. Clin Lab Med 1995;15:665–684.
17. Brown ZA, Benedetti J, Ashley R, et al. Neonatal herpes simplex virus infection in relation to asymptomatic maternal infection at the time of labor. N Engl J Med 1991;324:1247–1252.
18. Cone RW, Hobson AC, Brown ZA, et al. Frequent detection of genital herpes simplex virus DNA by polymerase chain reaction among pregnant women. JAMA 1994;272:792–796.
19. Arvin AM, Hensleigh PA, Prober CG, et al. Failure of antepartum maternal cultures to predict the infant's risk of exposure to herpes simplex virus at delivery. N Engl J Med 1986;315:796–800.
20. Prober CG, Sullender WM, Yasukawa LL, Au DS, Yeager AS, Arvin AM. Low risk of herpes simplex virus infections in neonates exposed to the virus at the time of vaginal delivery to mothers with recurrent genital herpes simplex virus infections. N Engl J Med 1987;316: 240–244.
21. Brown ZA, Selke S, Zeh J, et al. The acquisition of herpes simplex virus during pregnancy. N Engl J Med 1997;337:509–515.
22. Brown ZA, Ashley R, Douglas J, Keilly M, Corey L. Neonatal herpes simplex virus infection: relapse after initial therapy and transmission from a mother with an asymptomatic genital herpes infection and erythema multiforme. Pediatr Infect Dis J 1987;6:1057–1061.
23. Altshuler G. Pathogenesis of congenital herpesvirus infection: case report including a description of the placenta. Dis Child 1984; 127:427.
24. Chalhub EG, Baenziger J, Feigen RD, Middlecamp JN, Shackelford GD. Congenital herpes simplex type 2 infection with extensive hepatic calcification, bone lesions and cataracts: complete postmortem examination. Dev Med Child Neurol 1977;19:527–534.
25. Monif GRG, Kellner KR, Donnelly WH Jr. Congenital infection due to herpes simplex type 11 virus. Am J Obstet Gynecol 1985;152: 1000–1002.
26. Mertz GJ, Coombs RW, Ashley RI, et al. Transmission of genital herpes in couples with one symptomatic and one asymptomatic partner: a prospective study. J Infect Dis 1988;157:169–177.
27. Kulhanjian JA, Soroush V, Au DS, et al. Identification of women at unsuspected risk of primary infection with herpes simplex virus type 2 during pregnancy. N Engl J Med 1992;326:916–920.
28. Hensleigh PA, Andrews WW, Brown Z, Greenspoon J, Yasukawa L, Prober CG. Genital herpes during pregnancy: Inability to distinguish primary and recurrent infections clinically. Obstet Gynecol 1997;89: 891–895.
29. Lavoie SL, Kaplowitz LG. Management of genital herpes infections. Semin Dermatol 1994;13:248–255.
30. Reichman RC, Badger GJ, Mertz GJ, et al. Treatment of recurrent genital herpes simplex virus infections with oral acyclovir. JAMA 1984;251:22103–22107.
31. Nielsen AE, Aasen T, Halsos AM, et al. Efficacy of oral acyclovir in the treatment of initial and recurrent genital herpes. Lancet 1982; 2:571–573.
32. Kaplowitz LG, Baker D, Gelb L, et al., and the Acyclovir Study Group. Prolonged continuous acyclovir treatment of normal adults with frequently recurring genital herpes simplex virus infection. JAMA 1991;256:747–751.
33. Goldberg LH, Kaufman R, Kurtz TO, et al. Long-term suppression of recurrent genital herpes with acyclovir. Arch Dermatol 1993;129: 582–587.
34. Fife KH, Crumpacker CS, Mertz GJ, I-lill El, Boone GS, and the Acyclovir Study Group. Recurrence and resistance patterns of herpes simplex virus following cessation of >6 years of chronic suppression with acyclovir. J Infect Dis 1994;169:1338–1341.
35. Brown ZA, Baker DA. Acyclovir therapy during pregnancy. Obstet Gynecol 1989;79:526–531.
36. Centers for Disease Control and Prevention. Pregnancy outcomes following systemic acyclovir exposure. June 1, 1984–June 30, 1993. MMWR Morb Mortal Wkly Rep 1993;42:806–809.
37. Scott LL, Sanchez PJ, Jackson GL, Zeray F, Wendel GD. Acyclovir suppression to prevent cesarean delivery after first episode genital herpes. Obstet Gynecol 1996;87:69–73.

38. Frenkel LM, Brown ZA, Bryson YJ, et al. Pharmacokinetics of acyclovir in the term human pregnancy and neonate. Am J Obstet Gynecol 1991;164:569–576.
39. Haddad J, Langer B, Adtruc D, Messer J, Lokiec F. Oral acyclovir and recurrent genital herpes during pregnancy. Obstet Gynecol 1993; 82:102–104.
40. Randolph AG, Hartshorn BS, Washington AE. Acyclovir prophylaxis in late pregnancy to prevent neonatal herpes: a cost effectiveness analysis. Obstet Gynecol 1996;88:603–610.
41. Grover L, Kane J, Kravitz J, Cruz A. Systemic acyclovir in pregnancy: a case report. Obstet Gynecol 1985;65:284–287.
42. Lagrew DC Jr, Furlow TG, Hager WD, Yarrish RL. Disseminated herpes simplex virus infection in pregnancy: successful treatment with acyclovir. JAMA 1984;252:2058–2059.
43. Randolph AG, Washington E, Prober CG. Cesarean delivery for women presenting with genital herpes lesions: efficacy, risks and costs. JAMA 1993;270:77–82.
44. Amann ST, Fagnart RJ, Chartrand SA, Monif GRG. Herpes simplex infection with short-term use of a fetal scalp electrode. J Reprod Med 1992;37:372–374.
45. Golden SM, Merenstein GB, Todd WA, Hill JM. Disseninated herpes simplex neonatorum: a complication of fetal monitoring. Am J Obstet Gynecol 1977;129:917–918.
46. Goldkrand JW. Intrapartum inoculation of herpes simplex virus by fetal scalp electrode. Obstet Gynecol 1982;59:163.
47. Roberts SW, Cox SM, DAX J, Wendel GD Jr, Leveno KJ. Genital herpes during pregnancy: no lesions, no cesarean. Obstet Gynecol 1995; 85:261–264.
48. Dunkle LM, Schmidt RR, O Connor DM. Neonatal herpes simplex infection possibly acquired via maternal breast milk. Pediatrics 1979; 63:250–251.
49. Kibrick S. Herpes simplex virus in breast milk. Pediatrics 1979; 64:390.
50. Goyert GL, Bottoms SF, Sokol FJ. Anicteric presentation of fatal herpetic hepatitis in pregnancy. Obstet Gynecol 1985;65:585–585.
51. Klein NA, Mabie WC, Shaver DC, et al. Herpes simplex virus hepatitis in pregnancy: two patients successfully treated with acyclovir. Gastroenterology 1991;100:239–244.
52. Hammerberg O, Watts J, Chernesky M, Luchsinger I, Rawls W. An outbreak of herpes simplex virus type 1 in an intensive care nursery. Pediatr Infect Dis 1983;2:290–294.
53. Douglas JM, Schmidt O, Corey L. Acquisition of neonatal HSV-1 infection from a paternal source contact. J Pediatr 1983;103:908–910.
54. Major C, Towers C, Lewis D, Asrat T. Expectant management of patients with both preterm premature rupture of membranes and genital herpes. Am J Obstet Gynecol 1991;164:248.
55. Hitti J, Watts H, Burchett SK, et al. Herpes simplex virus seropositivity and reactivation at delivery among pregnant women infected with human immunodeficiency virus-1. Am J Obstet Gynecol 1997;177: 540–554.
56. Ferenczy A. Epidemiology and clinical pathophysiology of condylomata acuminata. Am J Obstet Gynecol 1995;172:1331–1339.
57. American College of Obstetricians and Gynecologists. Genital human papillomavirus infections. Technical Bulletin no. 193, June 1994a.
58. Tseng CJ, Lin CY, Wang RL, et al. Possible transplacental transmission of human papillomaviruses. Am J Obstet Gynecol 1992;169: 35–40.
59. Centers For Disease Control. 1998 Guidelines for treatment of sexually transmitted diseases. MMWR Morb Mortal Wkly Rep 1998;47: 1–116, 1998.
60. Ferenczy A. HPV-associated lesions in pregnancy and their clinical complications. Clin Obstet Gynecol 1989;32:191–199.
61. Ferenczy A. Treating genital condylomata during pregnancy with the carbon dioxide laser. Am J Obstet Gynecol 1984;148:9–12.
62. Bergman A, Bhatia NN, Broen EM. Cryotherapy for treatment of genital condyloma during pregnancy. J Reprod Med 1984;29:432–435.
63. Schwartz DB, Greenberg MD, Daoud Y, Reid R. Genital condylomas in pregnancy: use of trichloroacetic acid and laser therapy. Am J Obstet Gynecol 1988;158:1407–1416.
64. Shah K, Kashima H, Polk BF, Shah F, Abbey H, Abramson A. Rarity of cesarean delivery in cases of juvende-onset respiratory papillomatosis. Obstet Gynecol 1986;68:795–799.
65. Abramson AL. Steinberg BM, Winkler B. Laryngeal papillomatosis: clinical histopathologic and molecular studies. Laryngoscope 1987; 97:678–685.
66. Puranen M, Yliskoski M, Saarikoski S, Syrjanen K, Syrjanen S. Vertical transmission of human papillomavirus from infected mothers to their newborn babies and persistence of the virus in childhood. Am J Obstet Gynecol 1996;174:694–699.
67. Dinstag JL, Wants JR, Koff RS. Acute hepatitis. In: Braunwald E, Isselbacher KJ, Petersdorf RG, et al., eds. Harrison's principles of internal medicine. New York: McGraw-Hill, 1987:1325–1335.
68. Jonas MM, Reddy RK, DeMedina M, Schiff ER. Hepatitis B infection in a large municipal obstetrical population: characterization and prevention of perinatal transmission. Am J Gastroenterol 1990;85: 277–280.
69. Beasley RP, Hwang LY, Lee GC, et al. Prevention of perinatally transmitted hepatitis B virus infections with hepatitis B immune globulin and hepatitis B vaccine. Lancet 1983;2:1099–1102.
70. Summers PR, Viswas MJ, Pastorek JG, Permoll ML, Smith LG, Bean BE. The pregnant hepatitis B carrier: evidence favoring comprehensive antepartum screening. Obstet Gynecol 1987;69:701–704.
71. Centers for Disease Control and Prevention. Protection against viral hepatitis: recommendations of the Immunization Practices Advisory Committee. MMWR Morb Mortal Wkly Rep 1990;39:1–26.
72. ACOG Committee Opinion Guidelines for Hepatitis Virus Screening and Vaccination During Pregnancy, vol III, American College of Obstetrics and Gynecologists, Washington DC, 1992:1.
73. Arevato JA, Washington E. Cost effectiveness of prenatal screening immunization for hepatitis B. JAMA 1988;259:365–369.
74. Centers for Disease Control and Prevention. Hepatits B virus: a comprehensive strategy for elimination of transmission in the United States through universal childhood vaccination. MMWR Morb Mortall Wkly Rep 1991;40:1–25.
75. Centers for Disease Control and Prevention. Prevention of perinatal transmission of hepatitis B virus: prenatal screening for all pregnant women for hepatitis B surface antigen. MMWR Morb Mortal Wkly Rep 1988;37:341–346.
76. Jonas MM, Schiff ER, O'Sullivan MJ, et al. Failure of Centers for Disease Control criteria to identify hepatitis B infection in a large municipal obstetrical population. Ann Intern Med 1987;107:335–337.
77. Koretz RL. Universal perinatal hepatitis B testing: is it cost-effective? Obstet Gynecol 1989;74:808–814.
78. Petermann S. Ernest JM. Intrapartum hepatitis B screening. Am J Obstet Gynecol 1995;173:369–373.
79. Smith L, Lauver D, Gray P. Sexually transmitted diseases. In: Fogel C, Lauver D, eds. Sexual health promotion. Philadelphia: WB Saunders, 1990:459–484.
80. Lichtman R, Duran P. Sexually transmitted diseases. In: Lichtman R, Papera S, eds. Gynecology well-woman care. Norwalk, CT: Appleton & Lange, 1990:203–222.
81. Rettig P. Perinatal infections with *Chlamydia trachomatis*. Clin Perinatol 1988;15:321–350.
82. Witkin SS, Inglis SR, Polaneczky M. Detection of *Chlamydia trachomatis* and *Trichomonas vaginalis* by polymerase chain reaction in introital specimens from 165–167 pregnant women. Am J Obstet Gynecol 1996;175:409–167.
83. Gossack JP, Beebe JL. Use of DNA purification kits for polymerase chain reaction testing of Gen-Probe *Chlamydia trachomates* PACE 2 specimens. Sex Transm Dis 1998;25:265–271.
84. van Doomum GJ, Buimer M, Prins M, et al. Detection of chlamydia-trachomatis infection in urine samples from men and women by ligase chain reaction. J Clin Microbiol 1995;33:2042–2047.
85. Paavonen J. Chlamydial infections in pregnancy. In: Mead P, Hager W, eds. Infection protocols for obstetrics and gynecology. Montvale, NJ: Medical Economics, 1992:33–37.
86. American College of Obstetricians and Gynecologists. Gonorrhea and chlamydial screening. Technical Bulletin no. 190, March 1994b.
87. Hammerschlag MR, Cununings C, Roblin PM, Williams TH, Delke I. Efficacy of neonatal ocular prophylaxis for the prevention of chlamydial and gonococcal conjunctivitis. N Engl J Med 1989;320:769–772.
88. Schachter J, Grossman M, Sweet RL, Holt J, Jordan C, Bishop E. Prospective study of perinatal transmission of *Chlamydia trachomatis*. JAMA 1986;255:3374–3377.
89. McGregor JA, French JI. *Chlamydia trachomatis* infection during pregnancy. Am J Obstet Gynecol 1991;164:1782–1789.
90. Alger LS, Lovchik JC, Hebel JR, Blackmon LR, Crenshaw MC. The association of *Chlamydia trachomatis*, *Neisseria gonorroheae*, and group B streptococci with preterm rupture of the membranes and pregnancy outcome. Am J Obstet Gynecol 1988;159:397–404.

91. Claman P, Toye B, Peeling RW, Jessamine P, Belcher J. Serologic evidence of *Chlamydia tracbomatis* infection and risk of preterm birth. Can Med Assoc J 1995;153:259–262.
92. Gravett MG, Nelson HP, DeRouen T, Critchlow C, Eschenbach DA, Holmes KK. Independent associations of bacterial vaginosis and Chlamydia trachomatis infection with adverse pregnancy outcome. JAMA 1988;256:1899–1903.
93. Martius J, Krohn MA, Hdlier SL, Stamm WE, Holmes KK, Eschenbach DA. Relationships of vaginal *Lactobacillus* species, cervical *Chlamydia trachomatis*, and bacterial vaginosis to preterm birth. Obstet Gynecol 1988;71:89–95.
94. Ngassa PC, Egbe JA. Maternal genital *Chlamydia trachomatis* infection and the risk of preterm labor. Int J Gynecol Obstet 1994;47:241–246.
95. Berman SM, Harrison HR, Boyce WT, Haffner WJJ, Lewis M, Arthur JB. Low birth weight, prematurity, and postpartum endometritis. JAMA 1987;257:1189–1194.
96. Sweet RL, Landers CV, Walker C, Schachter J. *Chlamydia trachomatis* infection and pregnancy outcome. Am J Obstet Gynecol 1987;156: 824–833.
97. Hoyme UB, Kiviat N, Eschenbach DA: The microbiology and treatment of late postpartum endometritis. Obstet Gynecol 1986;68: 226–232.
98. Mercer L. The diagnosis and treatment of chlamydia infections. Proceedings from Telenet, New York, NY, April 7, 1994.
99. Sanchez PJ. Wendel GD. Syphilis in pregnancy. Clin Perinatol 1997; 24:71–88.
100. Wendel GD. Gestational and congenital syphilis. Clin Perinatol 1988; 15:287–303.
101. Crane M. The diagnosis and management of maternal and congenital syphilis. J Nurse Midwifery 1992;37:4–5.
102. Wendel GD, Maberry MC, Christmas JT, Goldberg MS, Norgard MV. Examination of amniotic fluid in diagnosing congenital syphilis with fetal death. Obstet Gynecol 1989;74:967–970.
103. Wendel GD, Sanchez PJ, Peters MT, Harstad TW, Potter LL, Norgard MV. Identification of *Treponema pallidum* in amniotic fluid and fetal blood from pregnancies complicated by congenital syphilis. Obstet Gynecol 1991;78:890–895.
104. Morales W. Gonococcal infections in pregnancy. In: Mead P, Hager W, eds. Infection protocols for obstetrics and gynecology, Montvale, NJ: Medical Economics Publishing, 1992:42–46.
105. Launders D. Uncomplicated anogenital gonorrhea. In: Mead P, Hager W, eds. Infection protocols for obstetrics and gynecology. Montvale NJ: Medical Economics Publishing, 1992:165–169.
106. Wendel PJ, Wendel GD. Sexually transmitted disease in pregnancy. Semin Perinatol 1993;17:443–451.
107. Christmas JT, Wendel GD, Bawdon RE, Farris R, Cartwright G, Little BB. Concomitant infection with Neisseria gonorrhoeae and Chlamydia trachomatis in pregnancy. Obstet Gynecol 1989;74:295–298.
108. Fogel C, Lauver D. Sexual promotion. Philadelphia: WB Saunders Company, 1990:22–65.
109. Elliott B, Brunham RC, Laga M, et al. Maternal gonococcal infection as a preventable risk factor for low birth rate. J Infect Dis 1990;161: 531–536.
110. Goldenberg RL, Andrews WW, Yuan AC, MacKay HT, St Louis ME. Sexually transmitted diseases and adverse outcomes of pregnancy. Clin Perinatol 1997;24:23–41.

Cherry and Merkatz's Complications of Pregnancy,
Fifth Edition, edited by W. R. Cohen.
Lippincott Williams & Wilkins, Philadelphia © 2000.

CHAPTER 43

Human Immunodeficiency Virus Infection

Nancy A. Hueppchen, Jean R. Anderson, and Harold E. Fox

Since recognition of the first case of human immunodeficiency virus (HIV) infection in a pregnant woman in 1982, the prevalence of HIV among reproductive-aged women has increased faster than in any other segment of the population. Fortunately, the armamentarium the obstetrician has available to treat the HIV-infected parturient and reduce transmission to the fetus also is growing rapidly. This chapter describes the epidemiologic trends of HIV in reproductive-aged women, the biology and natural history of the virus, the effect of HIV on pregnancy outcome, the effect of pregnancy on the disease, and factors associated with perinatal transmission. Management of the HIV-infected parturient, including antiretroviral (ARV) therapy and future strategies to reduce vertical transmission, are discussed. Any review of the literature concerning HIV infection and ARV therapy may become outdated rapidly. Tools to assist the obstetrician in keeping abreast of current issues in the management of HIV-affected pregnancies also is discussed.

EPIDEMIOLOGY

It is estimated that worldwide, in 1996, 21.8 million adults and children were infected with HIV, a more than twofold increase since 1990. Nearly nine million of infected persons (42%) were female. The World Health Organization (WHO) estimates that three million women will die with acquired immunodeficiency syndrome (AIDS) by the year 2000. The vast majority of the 1.5 million children with HIV worldwide are thought to have been infected perinatally. AIDS has become a leading cause of death in urban areas in sub-Saharan Africa, Europe, and the United States (1,2).

N. A. Hueppchen, J. R. Anderson and H. E. Fox: Department of Obstetrics and Gynecology, The Johns Hopkins School of Medicine, The Johns Hopkins Hospital, Baltimore, MD 21287–1201.

Whereas 86% of HIV-infected persons live in sub-Saharan Africa and south and southeast Asia, an estimated one million Americans are living with HIV. In 1991 in the United States, an estimated 1.7 per 1,000 childbearing women were HIV infected, with greater prevalence among black and Hispanic women (1). The seroprevalence among adolescent parturients in one southeastern U.S. inner-city population was as high as 4.7 per 1,000 (3). The National AIDS Surveillance system monitors cases of AIDS, which represents late-stage HIV infection, at the local and state health department levels. These statistics then are compiled by the Centers for Disease Control and Prevention (CDC) and published in the HIV/AIDS Surveillance Reports. In the United States, the incidence of AIDS has increased three times faster for women than for any other segment of the population. In 1996 in the United States, 71,704 cases of AIDS were reported, 19% of whom were women, compared with 7% reported in 1985. Women constitute 19% of all cumulative cases of AIDS in the United States, with 24% of all patients aged under the age of 25 years. AIDS is now the third leading cause of death for U.S. women aged 25 to 44 years, and fully 80% of female AIDS cases are women in their reproductive years (aged 15 to 44 years). More than 50% of new AIDS cases in the United States in 1995 were black women (1,4,5).

The primary risk factors for HIV exposure in women are injection drug abuse (IDU) and heterosexual contact; blood transfusion and occupational exposure play lesser roles. Statistically, more AIDS cases are attributed to IDU, but heterosexual transmission probably is underestimated. If the patient reports a history of IDU, the CDC assigns the transmission to the IDU category, regardless of sexual exposure history. Furthermore, transmission patterns have changed, and current AIDS statistics are actually a window to the past in that they represent transmission patterns of perhaps a decade ago, when these women were infected. There is also a secondary link

TABLE 43-1. *Pregnancy rates among ethnic groups in HIV-infected women*

Ethnic group	Pregnancy	Rate
White	102/835	12%
Black	400/2,313	17%
Hispanic	59/713	8%
Asian	0/10	0%
Native American	8/27	30%

between non-IDU and HIV infection, most likely through sexual contact. In a case–control study of pregnant adolescents in 1992, reported use of crack cocaine was 19.6% in the HIV-infected group versus 8.2% in the control group (3). Over the last decade, heterosexual transmission of HIV in women in the form of exchange of sex for money or drugs and multiple partners has increased by 146%. Male-to-female transmission appears to be more efficient than female-to-male transmission. The practice of receptive anal intercourse also makes transmission more likely, probably because the columnar epithelium of the rectum carries CD4 receptors and the rectal mucosa is more fragile and easily traumatized. Ulcerative genital lesions and other sexually transmitted diseases (STDs) increase the likelihood of acquiring HIV infection from a sexual contact.

Recent estimates nationwide indicate that approximately 1.7 per 1,000 live births occur in HIV-positive women (1). A 1996 study found the incidence of pregnancy at entry into the study group among HIV-positive women to be 14% with a large variance among ethnic groups (Table 43-1). Three percent of this population carried a diagnosis of AIDS, and 77% were aged younger than 25 years. Enrollees in the study had an annual pregnancy rate of 5.8%, and 12% chose to have more than one pregnancy despite their HIV status (6). More than 90% of pediatric cases of AIDS are secondary to perinatal transmission, and an estimated 12,000 U.S. children are currently living with HIV infection (1). Furthermore, 45% of children born to HIV-infected mothers are not living with a biological parent, largely because of the death or disability of the mother (7). Worldwide, it is estimated that five to ten million children may be orphaned by the year 2000 because of AIDS (2).

VIROLOGY

HIV is an RNA retrovirus that uses reverse transcriptase to transcribe DNA from RNA to replicate. The viral capsid consists of a major capsid protein (p24), a nucleocapsid protein (p7/p9), a single-stranded RNA genome, and three viral enzymes (protease, reverse transcriptase, and integrase). The capsid is coated with a matrix protein, which in turn is surrounded by the viral envelope. A lipid bilayer and protein complex combine to form the viral envelope (Fig. 43-1). An outer envelope protein, gp120, binds to CD4, allowing viral entry into host cells. A transmembrane protein, gp41, promotes fusion of the viral envelope with the host cell membrane (8).

After the viral envelope fuses with the CD4 receptor sites on the host cell membrane, the reverse transcriptase transcribes the genomic RNA into double-stranded DNA, or what is known as the *provirus* (Fig. 43-2). The provirus then is incorporated into the host genome, where it is replicated by cellular DNA-dependent RNA transcriptases into new viral RNA genome particles. Viral envelope proteins are synthesized in a similar fashion. Viral core proteins are assembled and processed by viral proteases in the cytoplasm. The envelope glycoproteins are synthesized in the endoplasmic reticulum and processed by cellular proteases. The new virions are assembled at the plasma membrane on release from the host cell (8). The life cycle of the virus is 2.6 days, representing the time from infection of one cell to the infection of another cell by the new progeny (9).

On the average, one billion virion particles are produced daily. Genetic diversity of the HIV genome is based on this high rate of production combined with an error-prone reverse transcriptase. These properties are believed to be largely responsible for the generation, under selective pressure, of resistance to antiretroviral therapy. The HIV isolates are divided into groups M and O. Group M, with ten serotypes (A–J), is the most common; subtype B is predominant in the United States and western Europe. Group O, along with several other group M subtypes, is found mainly in Africa (8). The genetic and replication characteristics of HIV have significant implications for vaccine development.

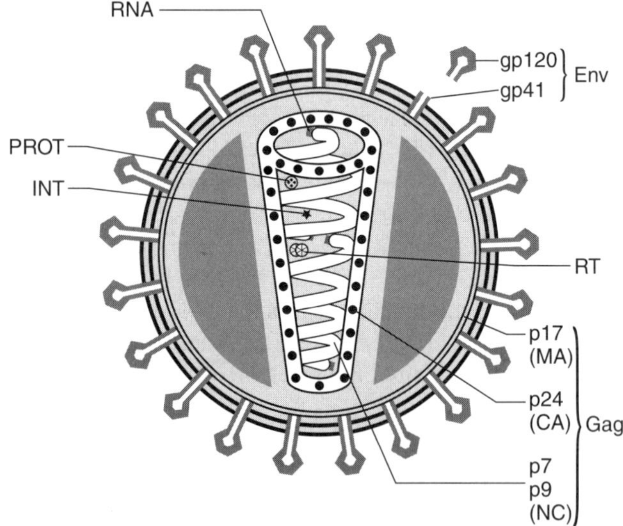

FIG. 43-1. Schematic of an HIV virion. (From ref. 8.)

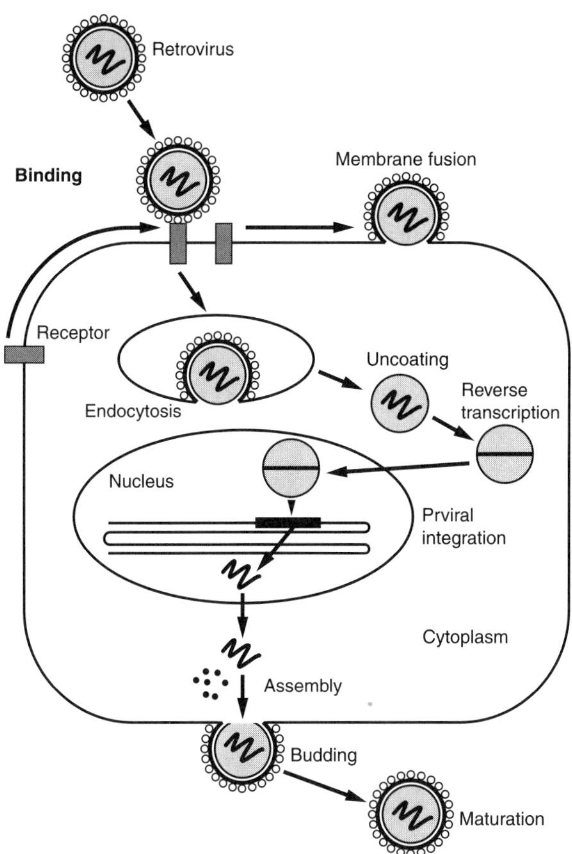

FIG. 43-2. Schematic of HIV replication. (From ref. 8.)

TABLE 43-2. *Top 10 AIDS-defining conditions in women*

1	*Pneumocystis carinii* pneumonia
2	HIV-wasting syndrome
3	Esophageal candidiasis
4	HIV encephalitis
5	HSV
6	Toxoplasmosis encephalitis
7	MAC
8	Extrapulmonary cryptococcosis
9	CMV-disseminated infection
10	CMV retinopathy

AIDS, acquired immunodeficiency virus; CMV, cytomegalovirus; HIV, human immunodeficiency virus; HSV, herpes simples virus; MAC, *Mycobacterium avium* complex.

NATURAL HISTORY OF THE DISEASE

When HIV transmission occurs, a viremia ensues and the virus is widely disseminated, largely to lymphoid tissues. The virus is trophic for CD4 T-lymphocytes in particular, which constitute more than 60% of the T-cell population. In nearly all infected persons, HIV infection leads to progressive destruction of CD4 T-lymphocytes as well as other immune cells expressing cell-surface CD4 receptors. This process results ultimately in profound immunosuppression (4,10).

Primary HIV infection occurs 2 to 4 weeks after exposure and is characterized by a variety of nonspecific symptoms: fever, adenopathy, pharyngitis, rash, myalgias, diarrhea, headache, nausea and vomiting, hepatosplenomegaly, and thrush. Symptomatic primary HIV infection is reported in 50% to 90% of patients. During this time, the HIV-specific immune response is generated. Both cellular and humoral immune responses appear to contribute to the downregulation of viral replication. At the time of seroconversion, approximately 6 to 12 weeks after transmission, there is generally a reduction of viral burden and apparent clinical recovery (4,10).

A period of clinical latency follows. The virus appears to be sequestered in lymphoid tissue. Generalized lymphadenopathy may or may not be present. The duration of latency may be a decade or longer. With currently available combination antiretroviral therapy, it is anticipated that this period will be increased (4).

Early symptomatic HIV infection may include conditions such as thrush, persistent vaginal candidiasis, peripheral neuropathy, cervical dysplasia, idiopathic thrombocytopenic purpura, and listeriosis and is associated with an increased viral burden. AIDS is diagnosed in the presence of an AIDS indicator condition or a CD4 count below 200/mm^3. The top ten indicator conditions for women are listed in Table 43-2. Advanced HIV infection applies to patients with CD4 counts below 50/mm^3, and their median survival is 12 to 18 months (4). Figure 43-3 illustrates the immunologic and virologic natural history of HIV disease, with correlation to clinical course of the infection (9).

Replication occurs at all stages of infection. Measurement of plasma HIV RNA is a reflection of replication rate. The magnitude of HIV replication determines the rate of disease progression. Viral burden and CD4 cell count are the most significant predictors of progression (11). Age is another variable associated with risk of progression. Median survival from seroconversion to AIDS

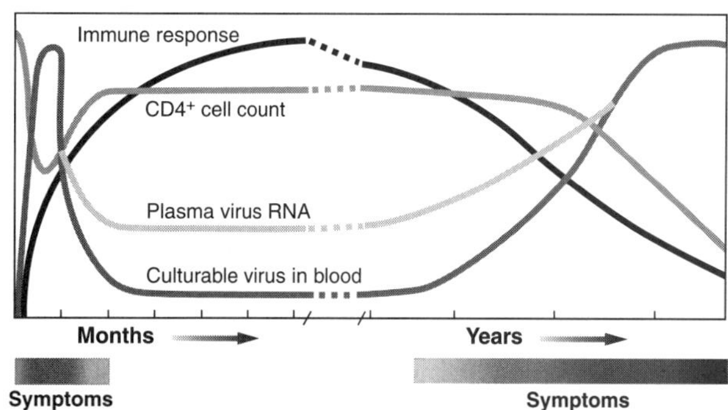

FIG. 43-3. Schematic of the natural history of HIV infection. (From ref. 9.)

in a 16- to 24-year-old patient is 15 years, whereas the median time to AIDS for a person aged 35 years or older is 6 years (12). Although the data used to describe the natural history of HIV infection are derived largely from studies involving HIV infection in male patients, most studies of the role of gender have not found significant differences between HIV-infected men and women when controlled for access to antiretroviral therapy (13).

LABORATORY DIAGNOSIS AND ASSESSMENT

HIV infection can be documented by detecting antibody to the virus, viral p24 antigen, nucleic acid-based tests (viral RNA or proviral DNA), or viral culture. The standard assay for HIV antibody is the enzyme-linked immunosorbent assay (ELISA), which, if positive, then is confirmed by the Western blot technique. The Western blot is declared positive if at least two of the following bands are present: p24 (viral capsid protein), gp41, or gp120/160 (viral envelope glycoproteins). During the window between infection and seroconversion, these assays may be negative and infection may not be recognized; however, once antibody to HIV is present, it persists for life (14). Persons with negative testing but ongoing risk behaviors should have periodic retesting (and ongoing counseling). The CDC evaluated 1,400 clinical laboratories in 1989 and found the combination of ELISA and Western blot to be highly accurate, with a sensitivity of 99.3% and a specificity of 99.7% (15). The results are reported as positive, negative, or indeterminate. An indeterminate result is a positive ELISA with only a single band on Western blot, most commonly in the p24 region. Causes of indeterminate results include cross-reacting alloantibodies from pregnancy or antibodies from other viral illnesses, early seroconversion, depleted antibodies with advanced infection, previous blood transfusion or transplant, or concurrent autoimmune diseases (4).

Normal values for CD4 cell counts range from 800 to 1,050/mm^3. CD4 counts are used to assess the stage of HIV infection and assist in making therapeutic decisions about ARV therapy and prophylaxis for opportunistic infections (OIs). In the past, CD4 counts also were used as a primary indicator of response to therapy. The rate of disease progression to AIDS is faster with a steeper decline in CD4 counts. Other factors that influence CD4 count include diurnal variations, intercurrent illness, and corticosteroids as well as significant interlaboratory variation (4,11).

The viral load is a measure of the HIV RNA circulating in plasma, determined by polymerase chain reaction (PCR). Viral load should be checked in a clinically stable state (i.e., no recent intercurrent illness or immunization). Viral load is useful in predicting disease progression and monitoring therapeutic efficacy. An increase is seen with progressive disease, failing therapy, and active intercurrent illness (9). During the period of acute infection, levels may not accurately predict the patient's risk of progression because of the high rate of initial viral replication; however, plasma HIV RNA levels stabilize after about 6 months and become more predictive of disease progression. Two specimens drawn 1 to 2 weeks apart are used to establish an initial baseline. With initiation of an effective ARV therapy, the viral load declines, reaching a nadir following approximately 8 weeks of therapy (16,17). A study of 209 HIV-infected patients demonstrated viral load to be a better predictor of progression to AIDS than CD4 count (11). There appears to be no viral load threshold above or below which transmission of the virus always or never occurs (18). Measurement of p24 antigen as an indicator of viral burden has been used, but it lacks adequate sensitivity and the correlation with clinical status that is seen with PCR RNA.

EFFECT OF PREGNANCY ON HIV

Prospective studies of pregnant women who are both HIV noninfected and infected demonstrated a decline in the CD4 count during pregnancy and immediately postpartum of approximately 100/mm^3 (19–21). As a result of the increase in blood volume in pregnancy, the absolute CD4 count may be diluted; thus, the percent of CD4 may be more accurate in pregnancy. In asymptomatic persons, when controlled for IDU, no discernable effect of pregnancy was noted on early progression of HIV disease (22). A prospective cohort study by Hocke and colleagues in 1995 compared the rate of disease progression in a group of HIV-positive pregnant women and a group of HIV-positive nonpregnant women matched for CD4 count, age, and year of HIV diagnosis. No acceleration of disease was noted in the pregnant group compared with the nonpregnant cohort (23). Mayaux and colleagues studied 320 HIV-infected women who did not receive ARV therapy during pregnancy. No significant variation occurred in viral load during pregnancy, although postpartum values were slightly lower than the first two trimesters of pregnancy (24).

EFFECT OF HIV ON PREGNANCY

Studies in the United States and Europe showed no significant impact of HIV infection on pregnancy course or perinatal outcome when controlled for IDU. Alger and colleagues, however, reported a significant reduction in reported risk behaviors during pregnancy (25). Birth weights of HIV-positive and HIV-negative infants were similar in the European Collaborative Study (26). A case–controlled study of HIV-infected women undergoing cesarean sections and their noninfected controls revealed no difference in the incidence of postpartum infections when matched for lifestyle-associated risk factors (parity, history of IDU, STDs, tobacco and alcohol use) (27). Another study of 693 women (of whom 82 were HIV positive) showed a small but significant decrease in birth weight standardized for gestational age in infants born to HIV-infected women. The clinical significance of this effect is questionable because it was less than the effect of smoking (28). Studies in developing countries demonstrated an increased incidence of preterm labor, chorioamnionitis, and postpartum endometritis; results concerning growth retardation, however, were conflicting (29,30).

PERINATAL TRANSMISSION

Pediatric HIV-1 infection is the result of vertical transmission in nearly all cases in the United States. Perinatal transmission accounts for 1.2% of AIDS cases overall, and in fiscal year 1996, it accounted for 0.9% of new AIDS cases. From 1978 through 1993, the CDC reported that 14,920 HIV-infected infants were born in the United States; 5,330 infants developed AIDS; and 2,580 infants died of the disease. The number of new cases of pediatric AIDS peaked in 1992 but declined by 26% by 1995 (31,32). The AIDS Clinical Trial Group (ACTG) 076 study was a randomized, placebo-controlled clinical trial that found the risk of perinatal transmission to be decreased from 22.6% to 7.6% when ZDV (zidovudine; azidothymidine, AZT) was administered antenatally, intrapartum, and to the neonate (33,34). The HIV-infected women entered in this intent-to-treat trial were ZDV-naïve and had CD4 counts higher than 200/mm^3. ACTG 185, a clinical trial evaluating the efficacy of HIV immunoglobin (HVIG) versus IVIG in HIV-infected pregnant women with CD4 counts below 500/mm^3 and who also were receiving ZDV during pregnancy was unable to detect any effect of HVIG or IVIG in decreasing the transmission rate. The study, however, confirmed the efficacy of ZDV in more advanced disease and with prior ZDV use. An unexpectedly low transmission rate of 4.8% was noted in the presence of ZDV therapy, and the study was terminated (35). Significant cost savings also are realized with a decrease in perinatal transmission of HIV. Mauskopf and colleagues performed a cost analysis for a population in which the incidence of HIV infection among pregnant women was 4.6 per 1,000. When ZDV therapy was instituted during pregnancy, the authors calculated the treatment (ZDV administration) costs as $104,502 for 100 HIV-positive women and their newborns. These costs were offset by the $1,701,333 savings (treatment of pediatric HIV) associated with the decrease in the pediatric infection rate (36).

To develop further successful prevention strategies, the timing and mechanisms of transmission must be delineated as well as factors influencing these mechanisms. Evidence suggests that transmission may occur during pregnancy, during labor, or in the postpartum period.

HIV has been demonstrated in first-trimester placental tissue (37,38). HIV p24 antigen has been found in fetal blood samples obtained by cordocentesis before second-trimester terminations (39). Wolinsky and colleagues determined that the dominant viral strains found in some infants represented strains that are more dominant in the maternal circulation early in pregnancy. These same strains were only minor variants in the mother at delivery (40). The absence of a dysmorphic syndrome or congenital anomalies suggests that a large proportion of perinatal infection occurs late in pregnancy or intrapartum (26). In women who have more advanced HIV disease, *in utero* transmission may play a relatively greater role than in women with early infection (41).

Studies of HIV-infected women who are not breastfeeding and their newborns have suggested that 50% to 70% of transmission likely occurs late *in utero* or intrapartum, with 30% to 50% of the cord bloods culture positive for HIV (42,43). Postpartum, HIV can be detected in breast milk, and case reports and small series have documented transmission by breastfeeding women who seroconverted after receiving HIV-positive blood transfusions in the immediate postpartum period. Van de Perre estimated the attributable risk of transmission from breastfeeding in women who seroconverted postpartum at 26%. The attributable risk of transmission in breastfeeding mothers who were infected before pregnancy is estimated at 14% (44). Many publications have described variables associated with increased (or decreased) risk of perinatal transmission. Discussion of these variables is divided into the categories of *viral* and *immunologic* factors, *maternal* factors, *obstetric* factors, and *fetal* factors.

Viral and Immunologic Factors

The course of HIV infection shows a great deal of variability, depending on the individual patient's antiviral immune response, target cell susceptibility, viral strain characteristics, and viral burden. Likewise, perinatal transmission is affected by these same variables. Selection, depending on the biologic features of the virus, may play a role in determining which viral strains are transmitted and when transmission occurs in pregnancy (40). Kliks and colleagues studied a cohort of 52 HIV-positive women and their infants and found that factors correlating with vertical transmission included rapid replication of HIV in human peripheral monocytes, T-cell line trophism, and resistance to neutralization by antibodies. This resistance is attributed to HIV strain variation, with rapid viral growth capability of certain strains. Several studies have correlated an increased risk of transmission with high levels of viral capsid p24 antigenemia and IgG antibodies to viral envelope protein gp160. Decreased risk of transmission has been limited to IgG antibodies to viral envelope protein gp 120; however, other investigators failed to find a protective effect of epitope-specific antibodies to gp120 (45–50).

High viral load and low CD4 counts correlate with enhanced vertical transmission (51–55). Dickover and colleagues, in a study of 95 pregnancies, found transmission in 15 of 19 women who had a viral load greater than 50,000 copies per milliliter ($p<0.001$), and no transmission in 63 women with a viral load less than 20,000 copies per milliliter (56). These findings suggest that the use of ARV drugs, which markedly decrease viral burden, may reduce perinatal transmission by this mechanism. In Sperling's most recent analysis of data from ACTG 076, ZDV was effective regardless of baseline CD4 or HIV-1 RNA level (34). The decrease in viral load with ZDV therapy in pregnancy accounted for only about 13% of the effect of ZDV treatment in reducing vertical transmission. There is no CD4 count above which, or viral load below which, transmission has not been reported to occur.

Perinatal transmission also may occur in HIV-indeterminate women (57). In the presence of acute infection, seroconversion may not be complete, whereas in advanced clinical disease the immune system may no longer be capable of mounting a detectable immune response. In both situations, the viral load is generally high.

Maternal Factors

Maternal features associated with a higher frequency of vertical transmission may act by altering maternal immune response (58). Factors that have been studied include maternal anemia and fever, coinfections (e.g., other STDs), IDU, tobacco use, and vitamin A deficiency. Maternal age and ethnicity do not appear to influence the risk of transmission. The Women and Infants Transmission Study (WITS) was a prospective, multicenter natural history study of 530 HIV-positive mothers and their infants. Hard drug use was identified in 42% of this population through self-reporting or urine toxicology. After adjustment for positive maternal HIV cultures at delivery, CD4 percentage, and gestational age, there was significantly greater transmission with drug use in women whose membranes were ruptured for more than 4 hours. In addition, cocaine use correlated significantly with a positive maternal HIV culture at delivery (59). Burns and colleagues found that tobacco smokers with CD4 percentages less than 20% had a relative risk (RR) of transmission equal to 3.30 (CI, 1.46–7.44) compared with nonsmokers (60). Vitamin A plays a role in immunity and maintenance of mucosal surfaces; thus, a deficiency may impair T-cell function and make mucous membranes more permeable. These effects also may be important in the function and integrity of the fetal and maternal placental surfaces. Vitamin A deficiency has been associated with an increased risk of perinatal transmission of HIV (61).

Obstetric Factors

Because late gestation and the intrapartum period are critical times in vertical transmission, mechanisms of transmission may involve maternal-fetal hemorrhage, placental transfer, ascending infection, and direct mucocutaneous contact between fetal and maternal blood and secretions. Several intrapartum events have been correlated with a risk of transmission, including mode of delivery, duration of labor, procedures increasing the potential for mixing of maternal and fetal blood, and the presence of concurrent maternal infectious diseases (51,62). Placental abruption and inflammation, such as with chorioamnionitis, have been linked with increased transmission, presumably as a result of interruption of the maternal-fetal interface (54,63). Invasive fetal monitoring, prolonged rupture of membranes, and vaginal laceration or episiotomy all carry a theoretic risk for increased fetal exposure to maternal blood and mucous membrane secretions. Vacuum or forceps delivery in a prolonged second stage of labor may offer some protection from prolonged exposure. First-born, vaginally delivered twins with greater exposure to maternal blood and genital secretions have increased risk of infection (64). One study revealed that 33% of HIV-positive women shed the virus in genital secretions and the likelihood of genital tract viral shedding increased in pregnancy (OR, 4.5; CI, 1.2–16.3) (65).

Prospective multicenter cohort studies have attempted to correlate risk of transmission with events during labor and delivery. The French perinatal cohorts found invasive procedures, preterm delivery, premature rupture of membranes, hemorrhage in labor, and bloody amniotic fluid all to be significantly associated with increased vertical transmission (66). Higher frequency of transmission in the WITS cohort was observed with rupture of membranes greater than 4 hours (25% versus 14% if less than 4 hours) (55). Mode of delivery was not related to risk of transmission in either study. The European Collaborative Study reported a protective effect against transmission of HIV among infants delivered by cesarean rather than a vaginal delivery, whereas neither the French Pediatric HIV Infection Study Group nor the WITS were able to demonstrate a significant difference in the transmission rate associated with mode of delivery.

Fetal and Newborn Factors

Although an estimated 50% of vertical transmission occurs intrapartum, a significant proportion of these infants will lack detectable virus at birth but can be diagnosed at 3 to 6 months of age. There seems to be a relative insensitivity of testing at birth, perhaps because of an immature immune response, small viral inoculum, slow growth of the virus before birth, or sequestration of the virus in fetal tissues (42,67). Potential fetal factors in transmission include gestational age at exposure, genetic susceptibility, and the maturity of fetal organ systems (particularly the immune barrier of the gastrointestinal system). Prematurity is associated with a transmission odds ratio of 3.8 in infants born before 34 weeks of gestation (53).

Neonates acquire maternal antibody passively and may test positve for HIV up to 18 months after birth (32). Newer methods of testing—PCR and p24 antigen assays—as well as HIV culture make diagnosis possible in almost 50% of infected infants at birth. All infants born to HIV-positive mothers should receive ZDV therapy (2 mg/kg every 6 hours) for the first 6 weeks of life, beginning within 12 hours after birth.

In perinatally infected infants, 30% to 50% will have positive PCR or HIV cultures at birth. Early onset of symptoms and rapid progression of disease occur in 20% to 30% of cases. The rate of progression is associated with viral load at birth, which tends to be high at birth (median, 219,000 copies/mL) and decline gradually over the first 2 years of life. In infants with early onset of disease, the viral load at birth is much higher (median, 724,000 copies/mL) (68).

ANTEPARTUM MANAGEMENT

Prenatal Counseling and Screening

Following the encouraging results of ACTG 076 and the knowledge that perinatal transmission could be reduced by approximately two thirds, the U.S. Public Health Service recommended that all women of childbearing age be offered HIV counseling and voluntary testing (14). Prepregnancy counseling and testing empower women to make appropriate reproductive decisions. The American College of Obstetricians and Gynecologists (ACOG) agrees and now advocates mandatory counseling and offering volunteer testing as part of routine prenatal care. Interestingly, a study in 1996 examining the familiarity and attitudes of physicians toward HIV testing in pregnant women revealed that two thirds favored mandatory testing and more than 90% favored public health reporting. Physician practice patterns varied by the type of practice environment and the seroprevalence in their geographic areas. Sixty percent acknowledged having no personal experience with the disease, and 10% to 20% admitted providing no counseling or testing (69). A universal approach to counseling and testing should be offered to avoid discrimination based on geographic or ethnic groups. With appropriate counseling in an inner-city clinic population, most women choose testing (70). Although this approach necessitates greater financial resources initially, the use of new therapies to reduce HIV morbidity in women and infants ultimately is cost effective (14). Any screening program should be prepared to address the negative psychosocial sequelae of women identified as HIV positive during pregnancy. Studies indicate that HIV-positive parturients experience greater health care discrimination, personal isolation, psychologic difficulties, and lower perceived overall quality of life (71,72).

Pretest counseling should include the risks and benefits of HIV testing, allowing the woman to make an informed decision before giving consent to testing (69, 73). The patient should be informed of HIV transmission routes, risk behaviors, and other factors associated with HIV infection, such as multiple sexual partners, IDU, non-IDU and alcohol abuse, history of cervical dysplasia or STDs, blood transfusion before 1985, and occupational exposure. The prevalence of HIV seropositivity may be increased in women with late or no prenatal care because of their desire to avoid being stigmatized or lifestyle disorganization associated with their at-risk behaviors. Women should be encouraged to learn their HIV status and to adopt behaviors that prevent transmission of HIV infection. A discussion of perinatal transmission and the benefits of ZDV therapy for the fetus also must address the benefits of early diagnosis and treatment of the mother. An explanation of the testing process includes what the result will mean as well as the psychosocial aspects of a positive result. Once adequate counseling has taken place, the patient is given a written consent form on which to document her decision to accept or decline testing. Currently, 41 states require informed consent to perform HIV testing (4).

Posttest counseling for women with negative results needs to address the possibility of incorrect results caused by the window period that precedes seroconversion. Further testing may be necessary if the patient admits recent risk behaviors. Risk-reduction behaviors should be reinforced. Counseling topics for a positive result should include an explanation of the natural history of HIV, current therapies, strategies for prevention of perinatal transmission, as well as a plan for resource referrals. Confidentiality is an important concern and should be addressed in detail. The patient should be encouraged to confide in her health care providers and to disclose to sexual or needle-sharing partners as well as to identify a social support system. She should understand that optimum management of her pregnancy embraces a team approach involving the patient, her obstetrician, an HIV specialist, and a social worker. Review of behaviors to optimize her general health is essential. A full evaluation to determine stage of disease, to assess the risk of transmission and long-term prognosis, and to determine that appropriate ARV and prophylactic therapy is performed. Appropriate follow-up for the patient's children, partner, and families should be facilitated (14).

Prenatal Care

Management of the HIV-infected pregnant women encompasses not only routine prenatal care but also treatment of HIV and strategies to prevent perinatal transmission. Early in the pregnancy, information concerning reproductive options should be provided, although HIV positivity seems to have little effect on reproductive decision making (74). Stressing compliance with prenatal visits was shown to decrease the odds of small-for-gestational-age infants by 43% in one large HIV-positive cohort (75). Frequency of prenatal visits should be increased with more advanced disease. Ongoing assessment for potential signs and symptoms of HIV infection should be part of each visit and should include looking for evidence of discrimination, domestic violence, substance abuse, psychological problems, and homelessness. The initial history and examination should strive to uncover HIV-associated problems, including anemia, cervical dysplasia, STDs, and OIs. Pneumococcal, hepatitis B, and influenza vaccines may be given because these are not live virus preparations. A transient vaccine-associated HIV viremia can be seen following immunization.

Prenatal fetal screening tests, such as ultrasound and maternal serum triple screen, may be offered; however, the HIV-positve mother must realize that abnormal findings may make invasive diagnostic testing an issue. Chorionic villus sampling, amniocentesis, and percutaneous umbilical blood sampling (PUBS) still may be considered for certain indications (potentially lethal conditions, for example). The patient should be counseled that no current data exist to estimate the risk of transmission associated with invasive procedures or to distinguish this risk from earlier fetal infection. Logically, the least invasive option is the most appropriate. One study of HIV-positive parturients undergoing PUBS before second-trimester termination found p24 antigen in 38% of amniotic fluid samples and 23% of fetal serum samples (39). *In utero* sampling carries a risk for fetal inoculation with HIV from maternal blood. The estimated risk of subsequent seroconversion from needlestick exposure in an adult is approximately one in 300; a similar theoretic risk of fetal inoculation with maternal HIV-infected blood is postulated (76). Currently, the recommendation is to avoid invasive prenatal diagnostic techniques in HIV-positive women except in the rarest of circumstances.

In addition to routine prenatal laboratory tests, the HIV-infected parturient requires monitoring of her disease to guide therapeutic decisions. CD4 counts or percent and viral loads are obtained every trimester and 4 weeks after alteration of the patient's ARV regimen. If CD4 counts fall below 200/mm^3, OI prophylaxis for *Pneumocystis carinii* pneumonia (PCP) should be instituted. Below 50/mm^3, an ophthalmology consult is encouraged because of increased risk for cytomegalovirus (CMV) retinitis. The viral load is measured by HIV RNA PCR, and the lower limit of detection in current tests is 400 copies per milliliter. The viral load is used for disease staging and to monitor response to ARV therapy. It is a more powerful prognostic indicator than the CD4 count (4,9). Complete blood counts, including mean cell volume, should be monitored, because myelosuppression is the major toxicity with ZDV treatment. If ZDV is taken on a regular basis, the patient likely will develop macrocytosis, which is often used as a surrogate to monitor compliance with ZDV. Other laboratory studies may be indicated, depending on the use of other therapies and their potential toxicities. A PPD is placed; anergy testing is not recommended routinely, although in patients with CD4 counts less than 200/mm^3, 75% of patients are anergic (14). A urine toxicology is obtained if the patient is a known or suspected substance abuser, and hepatitis C testing is done if she (or her partner) has a history of IDU. Toxoplasmosis and CMV serology should be considered in patients with low CD4 counts (<100/mm^3) or advanced clinical disease.

Antiretroviral Therapy

The area of ARV therapy is expanding rapidlly, with combination drug therapy becoming the standard for treatment of HIV infection (Table 43-3). Both the U.S. Public Health Service (USPHS) and ACOG agree that women should receive optimal ARV therapy regardless of pregnancy status (73,77). Recommendations concerning choice of drugs are affected by pharmacokinetic considerations and potential effects on the fetus and newborn. The goal of combination ARV therapy is to suppress HIV replication to undetectable levels, thereby delaying or preventing the emergence of drug-resistant viral variants and to preserve immune function. To avoid selection of ARV-resistant strains, compliance with optimum schedules and dosages of the drugs is necessary. The emergence of drug-resistant variants during pregnancy may reduce the ability to treat maternal disease adequately and may limit future treatment options. Currently, combination ARV therapy should be considered in pregnancy if the CD4 count is less than 500/mm^3, the viral load is greater than 10,000 copies per milliliter, or clinically symptomatic HIV disease is present. Currently, there is a lack of studies of these new agents in pregnancy.

The obstetrician and patient may consider delaying initiation of new drug treatments until 14 weeks, after the first trimester and greatest risk for teratogenicity. If the patient is already on ARV therapy, this therapy should generally be continued as interruption may cause a rebound in viral burden with potential increased risk to both mother and fetus. For current information on toxicity and teratogenicity, physicians and patients may contact the Antiretroviral Pregnancy Registry, which has been established in collaboration with Bristol-Meyers Squibb Co., Glaxo-Wellcome, Inc., Hoffmann-La Roche

TABLE 43-3. *Antiretroviral therapy*

Drug	Pregnancy category	Usual dose	Side effects	Clinical trials
Nucleoside analogs				
Zidovudine (ZDV, AZT)	B	200 mg t.i.d. or 300 mg b.i.d.	Bone marrow suppression, GI intolerance, HA, insomnia	ACTG 076
Didanosine (ddI)	B	>60 kg 200 mg b.i.d. <60 kg 125 mg b.i.d.	Pancreatitis, peripheral neuropathy	ACTG 249
Dideoxycitide (ddC)	C	0.75 mg t.i.d.	Peripheral neuropathy, stomatitis, apthous ulcers, pancreatitis	
Stavudine (d4T)	C	>60 kg 40 mg b.i.d. <60 kg 30 mg b.i.d.	Peripheral neuropathy	ACTG 332
Lamivudine (3TC)	C	150 mg b.i.d.	Minimal toxicity, HA, nausea	
Protease inhibitors				
Saquinavir	B	600 mg t.i.d. with high-fat meal (begin 300 mg b.i.d. and escalate gradually over 1st 14 d)	GI intolerance, HA, diarrhea	
Ritonavir	B	600 mg t.i.d. with food (begin 300 mg b.i.d. and escalate gradually over 1st 14 d)	GI intolerance, paresthesias, taste perversion, elevated triglycerides, elevated transaminases	ACTG 354
Indinavir	C	800 mg t.i.d. (empty stomach)	GI intolerance, nephrolithiasis, elevated indirect bili (?neonatal hyperbilirubinemia)	ACTG 358
Nelfinavir	B	750 mg t.i.d. (with food)	Diarrhea	ACTG 353
Nonnucleoside transcriptase inhibitors				
Nevirapine	C	200 mg q.d. × 14 d, then 200 mg b.i.d.	Rash, hepatitis, fever, nausea, HA	ACTG 250, 316
Delaviridine	C	400 mg t.i.d. (empty stomach)	Rash, fever	

GI, gastrointestinal; b.i.d., twice a day; t.i.d. three times a day; q.i.d., four times a day; HA, headache; q.d., each day.

Inc., and Merck and Co. (Table 43-4) (78). The registry has an advisory committee of CDC and National Institutes of Health (NIH) representatives as well as clinicians. Physicians who are prescribing any ARV in pregnancy are encouraged to report these cases to the registry. Patient assistance programs are available for those lacking prescription insurance plans through local and state funds and the Ryan White program (4).

The efficacy of ZDV (a nucleoside analog) in preventing perinatal transmission of HIV was established by the ACTG 076 protocol, a double-blinded, placebo-controlled clinical trial that included antepartum, intrapartum, and neonatal treatment (33). Analysis of 402 mother–infant pairs noted a significant reduction in transmission, from 22.6% in the placebo group to 7.6% in the ZDV group ($p<0.001$). This trial was confined to asymptomatic patients with CD4 counts greater than 200/mm^3, in the second or third trimester, and without previous ARV therapy. No significant differences in toxicity or side effects were found between placebo and ZDV recipients, except for mild anemia in infants exposed to ZDV. The neonatal anemia resolved spontaneously after discontinuation of the drug and did not require transfusion. Congenital anomalies did not occur at a risk higher than expected in the general population. Further review of the ACTG 076 data revealed that maternal viral load correlated with perinatal transmission in women receiving placebo; however, the reduction in viral load accounted for less than 17% of ZDV effectiveness in decreasing perinatal transmission. The effectiveness of ZDV in reducing the risk of transmission occurred regardless of the initial maternal viral load or CD4 levels. Other possible mechanisms of ZDV effectiveness include prophylaxis of the infant either before or after exposure. There is no threshold above which transmission always occurs; conversely, there is no threshold below which transmission never occurs (34,79). The maximal effect of ZDV therapy on viral load is noted after 8 to 16 weeks of treatment. A study using oral antenatal ZDV therapy alone (only one component of the

TABLE 43-4. *Antiretroviral pregnancy registry*

Phone	(800) 722-9292 ext 3-8465
FAX	(919) 315-8981

ACTG 076 study) in patients with CD4 counts less than 200/mm^3 also demonstrated a decreased transmission rate of 5.5% (80). Similarly, other observational studies of ZDV use in populations not included in the ACTG 076 study (CD4 less than 200/mm^3, prior ARV use) or using only a part of the 076 study regimen have shown significant reductions in perinatal transmission of HIV. Even if suspicion of ZDV resistance exists (i.e., prior failure of ZDV-containing regimen or prolonged treatment with ZDV), there still may be a role for ZDV in reducing perinatal transmission. Transfer of viral escape mutants to the fetus has been demonstrated, suggesting that ZDV-susceptible virus may be transmitted even if the predominant maternal strain is resistant.

Data exist that show reduced efficacy of many ARV regimens among patients with previous ZDV therapy, raising concern regarding the use of monotherapy during pregnancy (81). As noted previously, if the CD4 count is less than 500/mm^3, the viral load greater than 10,000 copies per milliliter, or there is clinically symptomatic HIV disease, it is now recommended that combination ARV therapy be given during pregnancy (77). Combinations of ARV therapy are more effective in decreasing the viral load, increasing the CD4 count, and reducing the emergence of viral resistance. If strict adherence to dosing regimens is not followed, resistance still may develop. Treatment with combination ARV therapy during pregnancy is used to ensure appropriate therapy for the mother during pregnancy (Table 43-5) (78). ZDV should be added or substituted as part of the regimen because it is the only ARV agent proven to reduce perinatal transmission at this time. If the CD4 count is greater than 500/mm^3 and the viral load is less than 10,000 copies/milliliter, ZDV alone may be considered because the likelihood of resistance developing over the course of pregnancy in this scenario is thought to be low.

TABLE 43-5. *Antiretroviral pregnancy registry committee consensus*

For the following therapies the calculation of the frequency of birth defects in the prospective registry is not possible because of the small number of reports.

- Didanosine
- Indinavir
- Lamivudine
- Saquinavir
- Stavudine
- Zalcitabine
- Didanosine, indinavir, lamivudine, saquinavir, stavudine, and zalcitabine in combination with and without zidovudine

To date, the registry findings on zidovudine monotherapy do not show an increase in the number of birth defects among the prospective reports compared with what would be expected based on rates in the general population. In addition, there is no pattern of defects among prospective and retrospective reports. These findings should provide some assurance when counseling women regarding prenatal exposure.

Currently available ARV agents fall into three categories: nucleoside analogs, nonnucleoside reverse transcriptase inhibitors, and protease inhibitors (see Table 43-3). Choice of specific drugs depends on prior therapy and response, other medications, and known or suspected risks and benefits from use during pregnancy (i.e., maternal or fetal toxicity and side effects). New drugs also are becoming available rapidly. For these reasons, consultation with a clinician with infectious disease expertise is important to ensure that the therapy chosen for each specific patient conforms to the most current guidelines and recommendations (4,41).

Prophylaxis for Opportunistic Infections

In the United States, the major cause of morbidity and mortality among AIDS patients is OI. The CDC made recommendations for primary and secondary prophylactic regimens in immunocompromised patients, including pregnant AIDS patients (Table 43-6). The most commonly encountered OI is PCP. Trimethoprim-sulfamethoxazole (TMP-SMX) is recommended for prophylaxis when the CD4 count is less than 200/mm^3. Daily TMP-SMX is not well tolerated by 30% to 50% of HIV-infected patients; however, many will respond to a decreased dosing regimen (three times weekly). The theoretic concerns of kernicterus in the newborn resulting from maternal sulfonamide therapy have not been realized in clinical practice. Alternative choices for PCP prophylaxis include dapsone or aerosolized pentamidine. Pentamidine is more costly, and this form of dosing may not achieve maximal lung distribution during pregnancy, but it has the advantage of once-a-month dosing. Primary prophylaxis also is recommended for toxoplasmosis, *Mycobacterium avium* complex, CMV, and tuberculosis according to the indications outlined in Table 43-6. The benefit of prophylaxis of these infections during pregnancy is believed to outweigh possible risks to the fetus (4,73,82).

Immunotherapy

Both active and passive forms of immunization are under investigation as methods of perinatal HIV transmission prophylaxis. Recombinant envelope vaccines have been shown to induce long-lasting humoral and cell-mediated immunity. Theoretically, the vaccine may induce passive immunity in the fetus. In studies thus far, a minimum of three doses monthly for 3 months has been required to develop significant neutralizing antibody in uninfected adults. No significant teratogenic effects have been reported in animal testing (83).

Although studies correlating maternal antibody with transmission are conflicting, many have shown a trend toward decreased transmission rates with increased mater-

TABLE 43-6. *Opportunistic infection prophylaxis*

Pathogen	Antibiotic Regimen	Pregnancy category	Indication
Pneumocystic carinii	TMP-SMX DS tablet q.d.	B	$CD_4 < 200/mm^3$ or H/O previous infection or unexplained fever >2 wk
Toxoplasma gondii	TMP-SMX DS tablet q.d.	B	$CD_4 < 100/mm^3$ and IgG antibody to toxoplasma
Mycobacterium avium complex	Azithromycin 1200 mg q/wk	A	$CD_4 < 50/mm^3$
Cytomegalovirus	Gancyclovir 1 g t.i.d.	C	$CD_4 < 50/mm^3$ and CMV antibody positivity
Mycobacterium tuberculosis	Isoniazid 300 mg q.d. plus pyridoxine 500 mg q.d. for 12 mo	A	PPD reaction >5 mm and negative CXR or prior positive PPD without treatment or contact with active TB case

CMV, cytomegalovirus; CXR, chest x-ray; PPD, purified protein derivative; q.d., each day; q.w.k., each week; TMP-SMXDS, trimethoprim sulfamethoxazole, double strength; TB, tuberculosis; H/O, history of.

nal antibody to HIV envelope proteins. Hyperimmune anti-HIV immunoglobulin (HIVIG) has undergone Phase I testing and was found to cross the placenta; high p24 antibody titers were found in newborns. The short-term safety of HIVIG was confirmed. Unfortunately, the preliminary results of PACTG 185 (see section on perinatal transmission) show no increased efficacy of HIVIG over IVIG in decreasing transmission in patients already taking ZDV in pregnancy (35,84). Enrollment in this study was halted because of a lower than expected transmission rate (4.8%), which would require significantly greater enrollment than initially calculated, making the study unfeasible.

INTRAPARTUM MANAGEMENT

Intrapartum monitoring of the fetus should avoid techniques that enhance exposure to maternal blood or genital secretions and may increase risk of perinatal transmission, such as use of fetal scalp electrodes, fetal scalp blood sampling, and artificial rupture of membranes (ROM) (4). Active management of labor and use of vacuum or forceps to shorten the second stage may be appropriate to decrease exposure time to maternal blood and genital secretions, but these measures have not been proved. In the WITS, ROM for more than 4 hours was significantly associated with increased risk of vertical transmission, particularly in patients with low CD4 counts (55). Vaginal deliveries with obstetric complications (placental abruption, placenta previa, maternal hemorrhage, premature rupture of membranes, and prolonged labor) also have been associated with an increased risk of transmission. Other studies, however, have shown no association with the duration of labor or the mode of delivery (63,85).

Current recommendations for intrapartum prophylaxis of HIV transmission include the use of intravenous ZDV during labor and delivery. A loading dose of 2 mg per kilogram is given at presentation in labor, followed by a continuous infusion of 1 mg per kilogram each hour until delivery and neonatal ZDV therapy for the infant (77). A study with oral ZDV during labor is ongoing, using a 400-mg loading dose with 200 mg every 4 hours until delivery (4). In developing countries, ARV therapy is generally not available, and there is a need to identify low-cost methods of reducing risk of intrapartum transmission. Vaginal lavage with 0.25% chlorhexidine on admission and every 4 hours until delivery did not result in a statistically significant reduction in transmission rates in one study; however, vaginal lavage, possibly with other agents, deserves further study (86). For updates on management and prevention of perinatal HIV transmission, physicians can refer to the CDC internet site at www.cdc.gov in the Division of HIV/AIDS Prevention.

Cesarean section in HIV-infected parturients should be performed for standard obstetric indications only, and not for the purpose of reducing vertical transmission at the current time. An estimated 40% to 80% of perinatal transmission occurs late in the third trimester or intrapartum (87). An observational study of 115 twin sets revealed greater infant HIV infection rates among first-born twins and among those delivered vaginally. Twin A was infected at a rate of 35% with vaginal delivery and 16% with cesarean section. Twin B was infected at a rate of 15% with vaginal delivery and 8% with cesarean section (64). The results of the European Collaborative Study published in 1994 showed a 17.6% transmission rate among vaginally delivered infants and an 11.7% rate among those delivered by cesarean section. The crude odds ratio of infection was 0.6 after elective cesarean section in HIV-infected pregnant women. The protective effect of cesarean section was thought to be more marked in advanced disease; however, this study estimated that it would require 12 elective cesarean sections to prevent transmission to one infant (88). In 1996, Ho-Hsiung Lin and colleagues reported that the lowest rate of mother-to-fetus microtransfusion occurred with elective cesarean section (89). A metanalysis of more than 900 cases documented significant protective effect of cesarean section, whereas individual studies did not show significance.

Most of the individual studies did not control for potential confounders. The analysis estimated that one would need to do 16 cesarean sections to prevent one case of perinatal transmission (90). A review of observational studies including more than 3,000 infants born to HIV-positive mothers did not justify routine cesarean section (91). Finally, the most recent report by Simpson and colleagues documented no association between mode of delivery and transmission rate (80). Most of these studies occurred before the routine use of ZDV prophylaxis. Furthermore, any potential benefit from cesarean section must be weighed against the increased risk to the mother from the operative procedure. There is currently an ongoing European prospective randomized trial of planned cesarean section versus vaginal delivery in HIV-infected parturients. This study should address this issue more definitively.

The placenta may play a role in intrapartum as well as antenatal vertical transmission of HIV to the fetus. CD4 receptors for HIV-1 have been documented in both first-trimester and term placentas, suggesting that the placenta is susceptible to infection and may be a conduit for transmission to the fetus. Most of the cells with CD4 receptors were found nested in the placental stroma and a few on the chorionic villi (37). Placentas of HIV-infected women at term exhibited significantly more chorionitis histopathologically than HIV-negative placentas ($p<0.01$). These findings suggest a potential mechanism for transmission, with chorionitis facilitating entry of the virus into fetal tissues by interfering with the normal placental barrier (92). The obvious question arises as to whether prophylactic antibiotics against chorioamnionitis would have any benefit in decreasing fetal HIV infection. Of interest, ZDV also is known to have bactericidal effects, particularly on gram-negative *Enterobacteria* species. This effect occurs when phosphorylated ZDV is incorporated in the bacterial DNA chain and prematurely terminates bacterial DNA synthesis.

Strategies to alter the viral burden during the intrapartum period and decrease the risk of fetal exposure to maternal blood and mucous membranes have been studied. Probably the largest impact is the result of ACTG 076 and subsequent treatment antepartum, intrapartum, and neonatally with ZDV. Theoretically, ARV therapy would decrease the viral burden available for any of the above routes of transmission (33,34).

POSTPARTUM MANAGEMENT

Free HIV virus and proviral DNA have been found in breast milk. Breastfeeding in the postpartum period is known to confer an additional risk for perinatal transmission of HIV infection to the neonate. A metanalysis of prospective studies revealed the transmission risk from breastfeeding by a mother with HIV infection acquired during or before pregnancy to be an additional 14%. The attributable risk of transmission for breastfeeding mothers acquiring HIV infection while lactating, with seroconversion postpartum, is 29% (32,53).

Evidence for maternal–infant transmission following postpartum seroconversion was illustrated in a prospective cohort of 212 Rwandan mother–infant pairs. All mothers were HIV negative at delivery, breastfed their infants, and had follow-up for 16 months. Of the mothers who seroconverted during lactation, 56% of their infants became HIV positive. The high transmission rate is linked to the increased viral burden found in early HIV infection. Nevertheless, breastfeeding still is considered desirable in developing countries with poor sanitation and hygiene where diarrheal diseases and respiratory infections remain the major causes of morbidity and mortality; and safe alternatives to breastfeeding do not exist. In developed countries, these pathogens are comparatively less important, and suitable breast milk substitutes are available. Breastfeeding by the HIV-positive mother in these countries is not recommended (44,93–95).

The routine postpartum follow-up should consist of all the usual components, including a Papanicolaou (Pap) smear. If the patient is newly diagnosed with HIV, the Pap smear should be repeated at 6 months and then annually, because immunocompromised women are at increased risk for cervical dysplasia. Reproductive counseling encompasses issues related to future fertility and contraception. Even if the partner also is infected with HIV, the use of condoms should be encouraged to prevent transmission of other STDs. General behaviors to prevent transmission of HIV to other household members should be reviewed (for example, avoid sharing of razors and contact with bodily fluids).

A study of recently pregnant HIV-positive women in an indigent urban population assessed the use of health care for themselves and their infants. Most infants received adequate health care using immunization status as a measure of care. Only 45% of these same women reported seeking HIV-related health care for themselves over the 3-year postpartum period, however. Factors associated with adherence to HIV care included the HIV-infection status of the infant and lack of drug use or incarceration (96). Appropriate follow-up medical care for both mother and infant is essential. Combination ARV therapy and OI prophylaxis should continue if indicated. Immunologic and virologic monitoring should begin 6 to 8 weeks postpartum. Follow-up testing and ZDV treatment of the newborn should be emphasized. As part of the ACTG 076 protocol, the infant receives ZDV syrup beginning 8 to 12 hours after birth, 2 mg per kilogram every 6 hours for 6 weeks. It is also important to encourage testing of other children born after 1977 (2,14). Social service referrals are focused on the needs of the patient and her family and are especially important in the face of advanced disease because HIV-infected mothers are often the sole caregivers for their children (7,97).

HIV AND HEALTH CARE WORKERS

Seroconversion of health care workers has been documented from both needlestick and mucous membrane exposures to HIV-infected body fluids. Universal precautions should be encouraged in obstetric procedures whether or not the patient is known to be infected. Orientation to proper technique should include protective eye shields, double-gloving, avoidance of mouth suction for DeLee suction devices, and proper handling of needles and sharp instruments. The effectiveness of postexposure prophylaxis (PEP) with ZDV was shown to decrease the risk of seroconversion by 79% in a retrospective, case–control study (98). Current recommendations for PEP include combination ARV therapy with triage to a two- or three-drug regimen based on risk of exposure. HIV serology should be obtained in the exposed individual before prophylactic treatment and then at 6 weeks, 3 months, and 6 months after exposure. An exposure at high risk for seroconversion, for example, would be a deep puncture with a hollow needle from an HIV-infected patient. PEP would include ZDV (200 mg three times daily), 3TC (150 mg twice daily), and indinavir (800 mg three times daily) or nelfinavir (750 mg three times daily) taken orally for 4 weeks. A low-risk exposure might occur as a splash of blood from an HIV-infected patient to the eye or a puncture with a solid needle. PEP would include ZDV (200 mg three times daily) and 3TC (150 mg twice daily), again taken orally for 4 weeks (73,99). Prophylaxis should begin within 1 hour of exposure. The National Clinicians Postexposure Hotline is available to assist with management of PEP (888-448-4911).

FUTURE DIRECTIONS

With the advent of combination ARV therapy and new drugs on the horizon and the ability to monitor viral replication, persons who have HIV are living longer and healthier lives, although the possibility of a cure is still remote. Strategies being investigated to reduce perinatal HIV transmission include reduction of maternal viral burden with combination ARV treatment or passive or active immunization; reduction of viral exposure with cesarean section or vaginal lavage; reducing secondary risk factors, such as using antibiotics to decrease the incidence of chorioamnionitis or induction and augmentation of labor to shorten duration of ruptured membranes; enhancing immunity with cytokines, interleukins, and immune cell transplants; and enhancing resistance to infection with gene therapy. When developing any of these interventions, maternal and fetal safety, cost of therapy, and technical difficulty of administration must be considered (86). Unfortunately, access to many, if not most, of these therapies will be beyond the reach of women around the world who most need them.

REFERENCES

1. XI International Conference on AIDS. The status and trends of the global HIV/AIDS pandemic. 1–32.
2. Quinn TC. Global burden of the HIV pandemic. Lancet 1996;348: 99–106.
3. Lindsay MK, Johnson N, Peterson HB, Willis S, Williams TT, Klein L. Human immunodeficiency virus infection among inner-city adolescent parturients undergoing routine voluntary screening, July 1987 to March 1991. Am J Obstet Gynecol 1992;167:1096–1098.
4. Bartlett JG. Management of HIV infection. Baltimore: Port City Press, 1998:1–25,31–34,67,117–119,220,258–261.
5. Wortley PM, Fleming PL. AIDS in women in the US: recent trends. JAMA 1997;278:911–916.
6. Chu SY, Hanson DL, Jones JL. Pregnancy rates among women infected with human immunodeficiency virus. Obstet Gynecol 1996;87: 195–198.
7. Caldwell MB, Fleming PJ, Oxtoby MJ. Estimation of the number of AIDS orphans in US. Pediatrics 1992;90:482.
8. Barre-Sinoussi F. HIV as the cause of AIDS. Lancet 1996;348:31–35.
9. Saag MS, Holodniy M, Kuritzkes DR, et al. HIV viral load markers in clinical preactice. Nat Med 1996;2:625–629.
10. Fauci AS, Pantaleo G, Stanley S, Weissman D. Immunopathogenic mechanisms of HIV infection. Ann Intern Med 1996;124:654–663.
11. Mellors JW, Rinaldo CR, Gupta P. Prognosis in HIV-1 infection predicted by the quantity of virus in plasma. Science 1996;272:1167–1170.
12. Mariotto AB, Mariotti S, Pezzoti P, Rezzo G, Verdecchia A. Estimation of the acquired immunodeficiency syndrome incubation period in intravenous drug users: a comparison with male homosexuals. Am J Epidemiol 1992;135:428–437.
13. Chaisson RE, Keruly JC, Moore RD. Race, sex, drug use, and progression of HIV disease. N Engl J Med 1995;333:751–756.
14. Interpretation and use of the Western blot assay for serodiagnosis of HIV type 1 infections. MMWR Morb Mortal Wkly Rep 1989;38:1–7.
15. USPHS recommendations for HIV counselling and voluntary testing for pregnant women. MMWR Morb Mortal Wkly Rep 1995;44:1–15.
16. Hughes MD, Johnson VA, Hirsch MS, et al. Monitoring plasma HIV-1 RNA levels in addition to CD4- lymphocyte count improves assessment of antiretroviral therapeutic response. ACTG 241 Protocol Virology Substudy Team. Ann Intern Med 1997;126:929–938.
17. Landesman SH, Burns D. Quantifying HIV (editorial). JAMA 1996; 275:640–641
18. Cao Y, Krogstad P, Korber BT, et al. Maternal HIV-1 viral load and vertical transmission of infection: the Ariel Project for the prevention of HIV transmission from mother to infant. Nat Med 1997;3:549–552.
19. Burns DN, Nourjah P, Minkoff H, et al. Changes in CD4 and CD8 cell levels during pregnancy and post partum in women seropositive and seronegative for human immunodeficiency virus-1. Am J Obstet Gynecol 1996;174:1461–1468.
20. Johnstons FD, Naurjah P, Minkoff H, et al. Lymphocyte subpopulations in early human pregnancy. Obstet Gynecol 1994;83:941–946.
21. Brettle RP, Raeb GM, Ross A, Fielding KL, Gore SM, Bird AG. HIV infection in women: immunological markers and the influence of pregnancy. AIDS 1995;9:1177–1184.
22. Ahmad N, Baroudy BM, Baker RC, Chappey C. Genetic analysis of HIV-1 envelope V3 region isolates from mothers and infants after perinatal transmission. J Virol 1995;69:1001–1012.
23. Hocke C, Morlat P, Chene G, Dequae L, Dabis F. Prospective cohort study of the effect of pregnancy on the progression of human immunodeficiency virus infection. Obstet Gynecol 1995;86:886–891.
24. Mayaux MJ, Dussaix E, Isopet J, et al. Maternal virus load during pregnancy and mother-to-child transmission of HIV-1: the French perinatal cohort studies. SEROGEST Cohort Group. J Infect Dis 1997;175: 172–175.
25. Alger LS, Farley JJ, Robinson BA, Hines SE, Berchin JM, Johnson SP. Interactions of human immunodeficiency virus infection and pregnancy. Obstet Gynecol 1993;82:787–796.

26. Anonymous. Perinatal findings in children born to HIV-infected mothers. The European Collaborative Study. Br J Obstet Gynecol 1994;101: 136–141.
27. Hanna G, Hueppchen N, Kriebs J. Post-cesarean febrile morbidity in HIV-infected patients. Am J Obstet Gynecol 1997;176:S59 (Abst 180).
28. Johnstone FD, Raab GM, Hamilton BA. The effect of human immunodeficiency virus infection and drug use on birth characteristics. Obstet Gynecol 1996;88:321–326.
29. Ryder RW, Temmerman M. The effect of HIV-1 infection during pregnancy and the perinatal period on maternal and child health in Africa. AIDS 1991;5:S75–S85.
30. Temmerman M, Ephantus NC, Ndinya-Achola J, et al. Maternal HIV-1 infection and pregnancy outcome. Obstet Gynecol 1994;83:495–501.
31. Davis SF, Byers RH Jr, Lindegren ML, Caldwell MB, Karon JM, Gwinn M. Prevalence and incidence of vertically acquired HIV infection in the United States. JAMA 1995;274:952–884.
32. AIDS Among Children United States, 1996. MMWR Morb Mortal Wkly Rep 1996;45:1005–1010.
33. Connor EM, Sperling RS, Gelber R, et al. Reduction of maternal-infant transmission of HIV-1 with zidovudine treatment. N Engl J Med 1994; 331:1173–1180.
34. Sperling RS, Shapiro DE, Coombs RW, et al. Maternal viral load, zidovudine treatment, and the rusk of transmission of human immunodeficiency virus type 1 from mother to infant. N Engl J Med 1996; 335:1621–1629.
35. Mofenson L. PACTG Protocol 185 Executive summary presented at the Workshop on ARV Therapy to Reduce the Risk of Perinatal Transmission, May 1997; National Institutes of Health, Washington, D.C. pp1–5.
36. Mauskopf JA, Paul JE, Wichman DS, White AD, Tilson HH. Economic impact of treatment of HIV-positive pregnant women and their newborns with zidovudine: implications for HIV screening. JAMA 1996; 276:132–138.
37. Maury W, Potts SJ, Rabson AB. HIV-1 infection of first-trimester and term human placental tissue: a possible mode of maternal-fetal transmission. J Infect Dis 1989;160:583–588.
38. Lewis SH, Reynolds-Kohler C, Fox HE, Nelson JA. HIV-1 in trophoblastic and villous Hofbauer cells, and haematological precursors in eight-week fetuses. Lancet 1990;335:565–568.
39. Viscarello RR, Cullen MT, DeGennaro NJ, Hobbins JC. Fetal blood sampling in human immunodeficiency virus-seropositive women before elective midtrimester termination of prenancy. Am J Obstet Gynecol 1992;167:1075–1079.
40. Wolinsky SM, Wike CM, Korber BT, et al. Selective transmission of human immunodeficiency virus type-1 variants from mothers to infants. Science 1992;255:1134–1137.
41. Newell ML. Working towards a European strategy for intervention to reduce vertical transmission of HIV. Br J Obstet Gynecol 1994;101: 192–196.
42. Dickover RE, Dillon M, Leung KM, et al. Early prognostic indicators in primary perinatal human immunodeficiency virus type 1 infection: importance of viral RNA and the timing of transmission on long-term outcome. J Infect Dis 1998;178:375–387.
43. Bryson YJ, Dillon M, Garratty E, et al. The role of timing of HIV on maternal-fetal transmission HIV phenotype on onset of symptoms in vertically infected infants. Presented at the IX International Conference on AIDS; June, 1993; Berlin, Germany.
44. Van de Perre P. Postnatal transmission of human immunodeficiency virus type 1: the breast-feeding dilemma. Am J Obstet Gynecol 1995; 173:483–487.
45. Goedert JJ, Mendez H, Drummond JE, et al. Mother-to-infant transmission of human immunodeficiency virus type 1: association with prematurity or low anti-gp120. Lancet 1989;2:1351–1354.
46. Ugen KE, Goederf JJ, Boyer J, et al. Reactivity of maternal sera with glycoprotein 120 and 41 peptides from HIV type I. Vertical transmission of human immunodeficiency virus infection. J Clin Invest 1992; 89:1923–1930.
47. Goedert JJ, Dublin S. Perinatal transmission of HIV-1: associations with maternal anti-HIV serological reactivity. Mothers and Infants Cohort Study and the HIV-1 Perinatal Serology Working Group. AIDS Res Hum Retroviruses 1994;10:1125–1134.
48. Mann DL, Hamlin-Green G, Willoughby A, Landesman SH, Goedert JJ. Immunoglobulin class and subclass antibodies to HIV proteins in maternal serum: association with perinatal transmission. J Acquir Immune Defic Syndr Hum Retrovirol 1994;7:617–622.
49. Rossi P, Moschese V, Broliden PA, et al. Presence of maternal antibodies to human immunodeficiency virus1 envelope glycoprotein gp120 epitopes correlates with the uninfected status of children born to seropositive mothers. Proc Natl Acad Sci U S A 1989;86:8055–8058.
50. Parekh BS, Shaffer N, Pau CP, et al. Lack of correlation between maternal antibodies to V3 loop peptides of gp120 and perinatal HIV-1 transmission. AIDS 1991;5:1179–1184.
51. St. Louis ME, Kamenga M, Brown C, et al. Risk for perinatal HIV-1 transmission according to maternal immunologic, virologic, and placental factors. JAMA 1993;269:2853–2859.
52. Tibaldi C, Tovo PA, Ziarati N, et al. Asymptomatic women at high risk of vertical HIV-1 transmission to their fetuses. Br J Obstet Gynecol 1993;100:334–337.
53. European Collaborative Study. Risk factors for mother-to-child transmisssion of HIV-1. Lancet 1992;339:1007–1012.
54. Temmerman M, Nyongo AO, Bwayo J, Fransen K, Coppens M, Piot P. Risk factors for mother-to-child transmission of human immunodeficiency virus-1 infection. Am J Obstet Gynecol 1995;172:700–705.
55. Landesman SH, Ralish LA, Burns DN, et al. Obstetrical factors and the transmission of human immunodeficiency virus type 1 from mother to child. N Engl J Med 1996;334:1617–1623.
56. Dickover RE, Garratty EM, Herman SA, et al. Identification of levels of maternal HIV-1 RNA associated with risk of perinatal transmission: effect of maternal zidovudine treatment on viral load. JAMA 1996;275: 599–605.
57. Johnson JP. Vertical transmission of human immunodeficiency virus from seronegative or indeterminate mothers. Am J Dis Child 1991;145: 1239–1241.
58. Anderson JR. Perinatal human immunodeficiency virus transmission. Postgrad Obstet Gynecol 1995;15:1–5.
59. Rodriguez EM, Mofenson LM, Chang BH, et al. Association of maternal drug use during pregnancy with maternal HIV culture positivity and perinatal HIV transmission. AIDS 1996;10:273–282.
60. Burns DN, Landesman S, Muenz LR, et al. Cigarette smoking, premature rupture of membranes, and vertical transmission of HIV-1 among women with low CD4 levels. J Acquir Immune Defic Syndr Hum Retrovirol 1994;7:718–726.
61. Semba RD, Miotti PG, Chiphangwi JD, et al. Maternal vitamin A deficiency and mother-to-child transmission of HIV-1. Lancet 1994;343: 1593–1597.
62. European Collaborative Study. Mother-to-child transmission of HIV infection. Lancet 1988;296:1039–1042.
63. Kuhn L, Stein ZA, Thomas PA, Singh T, Tsai WY. Maternal-infant HIV transmission and circumstances of delivery. Am J Public Health 1994; 84:1110–1113.
64. Duliege A, Amos CI, Felton S, Biggar RJ, Joedert JJ. Birth order, delivery route, and concordance in the transmission of human immunodeficiency virus type 1 from mothers to twins. J Pediatr 1995;126:625–631.
65. Clemetson DB, Moss GB, Willerford DM, et al. Detection of HIV DNA in cervical and vaginal secretions. JAMA 1993;269:2860–2864.
66. Mandelbrot L, Mayaux MJ, Bongain A, et al. Obstetric factors and mother-to-child transmission of human immunodeficiency virus type 1: the French perinatal cohorts. Am J Obstet Gynecol 1996;175: 661–667.
67. Bryson YJ, Luzuriaga K, Sullivan J, Wara D. Proposed definitions for in utero versus intrapartum transmission of HIV-1. N Engl J Med 1993; 327:1246–1247.
68. Shearer WT, Quinn TC, LaRussa P, et al. Viral load and disease progression in infants infected with human innumodeficiency virus type 1. N Engl J Med 1997;336:1337–1342.
69. Segal AI. Physician attitudes toward human immunodeficiency virus testing in pregnancy. Am J Obstet Gynecol 1996;174:1750–1756.
70. Cozen W, Mascola L, Enguidanos R, et al. Screening for HIV and hepatitis B in LA County prenatal clinics: a demonstration project. J Acquir Immune Defic Syndr Hum Retrovirol 1993;6:95–98.
71. Larrabee KD, Monga M, Eriksen N, Helfagott A. Quality of life assessment in pregnant women with the human immunodeficiency virus. Obstet Gynecol 1996;88:1016–1020.
72. Lester P, Partridge JC, Chesney MA, Cooke M. The consequences of a postive prenatal HIV antibody test for women. J Acquir Immune Defic Syndr Hum Retrovirol 1995;10:341–349.
73. ACOG Educational Bulletin. HIV infections in pregnancy. No. 232; January, 1997.
74. Sunderland A, Minkoff H, Handte J, Moroso G, Landesman S. The impact of HIV serostatus on reproductive decisions of women. Obstet Gynecol 1992;79:1027–1031.

75. Turner BJ, McKee LJ, Silverman NS, Hauck NW, Fanning TR, Markson LE. Prenatal care and birth outcomes of a cohort of HIV-infected women. J Acquir Immune Defic Syndr Hum Retrovirol 1996;12:259–267.
76. Valente P, Sever JL. In utero diagnosis of congenital infections by direct fetal sampling. Isr J Med Sci 1994;30:414–420.
77. United States Public Health Service task force recommendations for use of antiretroviral drugs in pregnant women infected with HIV-1 for maternal health and for reducing perinatal HIV-1 transmission in the United States. MMWR 1998;47:1–26.
78. Antiretroviral pregnancy registry for ddI, IDV, 3TC, SQV, d4t, ddC, and ZDV. Interim Report, 1 January 1989 through 30 June 1997. A Collaborative Project Managed by Bristol Myers Squibb Co., Glaxo Wellcome, and Hoffman-La Roche, Inc. Research Triangle Park, NC 1997.
79. Matheson PB, Weedon J, Cappelli M, et al. Comparison of methods of estimating the mother-to-child transmission rate of human immunodeficiency virus type 1. Am J Epidemiol 1995;142:714–718.
80. Simpson BJ, Shaprio ED, Andiman WA. Reduction in the risk of vertical transmission of HIV-1 associated with treatment of pregnant women with orally administered zidovudine alone. J Acquir Immune Defic Syndr Hum Retrovirol 1997;14:145–152.
81. Minkoff H, Augenbraun M. Antiretroviral therapy for pregnant women. Am J Obstet Gynecol 1997;176:478–489.
82. 1997 USPHS/IDSA guidelines for the prevention of opportunistic infections in persons infected with HIV. MMWR Morb Mortal Wkly Rep 1997;46:1–46.
83. Consensus Workshop II. Strategies for prevention of perinatal transmission of HIV infection. J Acquir Immune Defic Syndr Hum Retrovirol 1995;8:161–175.
84. Lambert, JS, Mofenson LM, Fletcher CV, et al. Safety and pharmacokinetics of hyperimmune anti-human immunodeficiency virus (HIV) immunoglobulin administered to HIV-infected pregnant women and their newborns. J Infect Dis 1997;175:283–291.
85. Minkoff H, Burns DN, Landesman S, et al. The relationship of the duration of ruptured membranes to vertical transmission of human immunodeficiency virus. Am J Obstet Gynecol 1995;173:585–589.
86. Biggar RJ, Miotti PG, Taha TE, et al. Perinatal intervention trial in Africa: effect of a birth canal cleansing intervention to prevent HIV transmission. Lancet 1996;347:1647–1650.
87. Minkoff H, Mofenson LM. The role of obstetric interventions in the prevention of pediatric human immunodeficiency virus infection. Am J Obstet Gynecol 1994;171:1167–1175.
88. Newell ML, Lin HH, Kao JH, et al. Caesarean section and risk of vertical transmission of HIV-1 infection. Lancet 1994;343:1464–1467.
89. Lin HH, Kao JH, Hsu HY, Mizokami M, Hirano K, Chen DS. Least microtransfusion from mother to fetus in elective cesarean delivery. Obstet Gynecol 1996;87:244–248.
90. Villari P, Spino C, Chalmers TC, Lau J, Sacks HS. Cesarean section to reduce perinaal transmission of HIV. A metaanalysis. Online J Curr Clin Trials 1993;Doc no. 74.
91. Dunn DT, Newell ML, Mayaux MJ, et al. Mode of delivery and vertical transmission of HIV-1: A review of prospective studies. J Acquir Immune Defic Syndr Hum Retrovirol 1994;7:1064–1066.
92. Chandwani S, Greco MA, Mittal K, Antonine C, Krasinski K, Borkowsky W. Pathology and human immunodeficiency virus expression in placentas of seropositive women. J Infect Dis 1991;163: 1134–1138.
93. Oxtoby MJ. Human immunodeficiency virus and other viruses in human milk: placing the issues in broader perspective. Pediatr Infect Dis J 1988;7:825–835.
94. Ruff AJ, Coberly J, Halsey NA, et al. Prevalence of HIV-1 DNA and p24 antigen in breast milk and correlation with maternal factors. J Acquir Immune Defic Syndr Hum Retrovirol 1994;7:68–73.
95. Van de Perre P, Simonon A, Msellati P, et al. Postnatal transmission of human immunodeficiency virus type 1 from mother to infant. N Engl J Med 1991;325:593–598.
96. Butz AM, Hutton N, Joyner M, et al. HIV-infected women and infants. Social and health factors impeding utilization of health care. J Nurse Midwifery 1993;38:103–109.
97. Schable B, Diaz T, Chu SY, et al. Who are the primary caregivers of children born to HIV-infected mothers? Pediatrics 1995;95:511–515.
98. Case–control study of HIV seroconversion in health-care workers after percutaneous exposure to HIV-infected blood France, United Kingdom, and United States, January 1988–August 1994. MMWR Morb Mortal Wkly Rep 1995;44:929–933.
99. Update: provisional PHS recommendations for chemoprophylaxis after exposure to HIV. MMWR Morb Mortal Wkly Rep 1996;45:468–472.

Cherry and Merkatz's Complications of Pregnancy,
Fifth Edition, edited by W. R. Cohen.
Lippincott Williams & Wilkins, Philadelphia © 2000.

CHAPTER 44

Parasitic Infections

Babill Stray-Pedersen

Parasitic infections are common throughout the world, but most gynecologists treating pregnant women are inexperienced in the diagnosis and treatment of these diseases. However, due to an increasing frequency of international travel and immigration of people from tropical areas and developing countries, physicians are being confronted more and more with foreign parasitic infections such as malaria and schistosomiasis. Other infections, such as giardiasis and amebiasis, may cause epidemics in both developing and industrialized countries. Renewed interest in infections such as toxoplasmosis is partly attributable to today's advances in prenatal diagnosis and new understanding of the effect of therapy.

Parasitic infections may affect fertility and pregnancy outcome in several ways:

1. The infecting organism may cause anatomic or functional changes in the genital tract, so that conception or implantation does not occur.
2. The parasitic infection may be severe enough to affect maternal health adversely during pregnancy, sometimes to a point where termination of pregnancy is required.
3. The parasites may infect and cross the placenta to produce adverse effects such as abortion, stillbirth, intrauterine growth restriction, and fetal or congenital infection.

If infection occurs during pregnancy or immediately prior to pregnancy, the effect on maternal health and the developing fetus is dependent on the type of parasitic infection, the natural immunity to the infection, and the parasitic load. Diagnosis is often based on a high index of suspicion due to having traveled to or from an endemic area or to the presence of certain diseases in the local community.

B. Stray-Pedersen: Department of Obstetrics and Gynecology, University of Oslo, National Hospital, 0027, Oslo, Norway.

The gynecologist should be familiar with the mode of transmission, clinical manifestations, diagnosis, and effect on pregnancy of the most common parasites. The decision to treat a parasitic infection in a pregnant mother is difficult, but should be based on the knowledge of the associated maternal and fetal morbidity and mortality of that disease and the toxic effect of the antiparasitic drug on the developing fetus.

This chapter addresses the more important parasitic infections that the gynecologist may encounter. For more extensive information, the reader is referred to textbooks on tropical medicine and parasitology.

MALARIA

Malaria is one of the most prevalent and serious infectious diseases occurring in tropical and subtropical areas. The disease infects probably more than 300 million individuals every year, leading to at least 3 million deaths (1). Mortality and morbidity are greatest in children, pregnant women, and travelers. Approximately 1,000 cases of malaria occur in the United States yearly, half in returning travelers (2). Pregnant women should therefore be informed of the risk of malaria if traveling to malaria-infected areas (Fig. 44-1) (3).

Transmission

The transmission of malaria occurs through the bite of a mosquito, but the infection also can be acquired from blood transfusion. Following the bite of an infected mosquito, the sporozoites of *Plasmodium* enter the blood of the victim and are transported to the liver, where they invade the hepatocytes and immediately start to multiply, creating up to 4,000 daughter merozoites. Within 1 to 2 weeks the hepatocytes rupture and thousands of merozoites are released into the bloodstream, where they invade the erythrocytes. Within the red blood cells a cycle

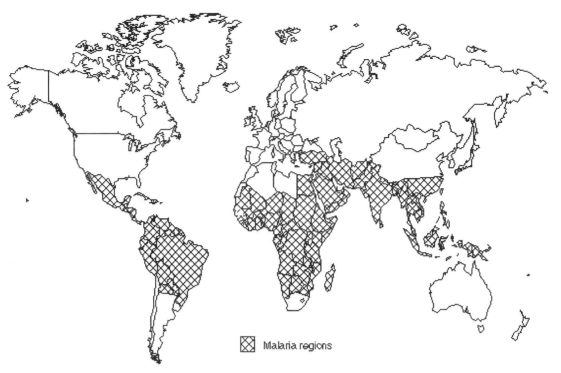

FIG. 45-1. Malaria regions in the world. From Preventing Malaria in Travelers. CDC Web site. Available at http://aepo–xdv–www.epo.cdc.gov.

of growth and multiplication starts, which eventually leads to the destruction of the erythrocytes; thereafter, new release and new invasion occurs (erythrocytic or clinical phase). The cycle of reproduction leading to rupture of red blood cells requires 48 hours for *Plasmodium vivax* and *P. falciparum*, the latter causing the most severe infection and serious complications (4).

Clinical Manifestation

The clinical picture of malaria is highly variable. Some patients have few symptoms, and others may develop a rapidly fatal course. The pattern of fever and other symptoms in primary infections is not typical and may mimic that of other febrile diseases (4,5). The state of host immunity plays a major role; thus, a high level of suspicion is required to diagnose malaria. During the initial period, the patient suffers from a low-grade fever with random peaks. After several days, cyclical fever—the hallmark of malaria—may occur. After 1 to 2 hours of feeling cold, the hot phase commences with rising temperature and warm, dry skin. Other symptoms, such as headache and aches and pains elsewhere over the body, are common. These fevers are coincident with the rupture of erythrocytes and release of parasites in the circulation.

Untreated patients with malaria may have attacks for weeks until spontaneous recovery generally occurs (4). Occasionally the clinical picture may progress with severe rapidity and lead to major complications and death. All serious infections are caused by *P. falciparum*, which, if untreated, may cause cerebral malaria, anemia, and kidney failure (5,6). Rupture of infected erythrocytes leads to anemia and hemoglobinuria, the severity of which depends on the parasitic load. Malarial patients often demonstrate abnormal chronic normocytic hemolytic anemia, leukopenia, and thrombocytopenia (7). They usually have hepatosplenomegaly.

Diagnosis

The blood smear is the cornerstone of diagnosis. Examination of thick and thin peripheral blood films, which are best stained with Giemsa, will reveal malaria parasites (4). Repeated smears should be examined before the patient is declared negative. In order to confirm or exclude the diagnosis of malaria by classic methods, a new smear should be examined every 8 hours for up to 3 days. The degree of parasitemia should be assessed to exclude drug resistance, and follow-up smears should be reexamined after the institution of treatment (4,5). In the smear the malaria parasites are always intracellular, with blue cytoplasm and a red chromatin dot.

The dangerous *P. falciparum* should be differentiated from the other forms. When initial specification cannot be determined, treatment must be for falciparum (8). Today alternative diagnostic techniques with even greater sensitivity and specificity are available for diagnosis of *P. falciparum*. This includes enzyme-linked immunosorbent assay (ELISA) for a parasitic antigen, as well as amplification of the parasite DNA using polymerase chain reaction (PCR) (4).

Malaria in Pregnancy

Malaria has an impact on the pregnant woman, her placenta, her fetus, and the newborn. In endemic areas the frequency and severity of falciparum malaria are greater during pregnancy; parasitemia and malaria attacks are 4 to 12 times more common (5,6,9). In some regions more than 50% of pregnant women may be parasitemic and have clinical manifestations. The susceptibility to infection and severity of disease are determined in part by the prepregnancy immune status (5). Pregnancy enhances susceptibility and clinical severity of falciparum malaria in women both with and without preexisting immunity (6). Several hypotheses to explain this have been suggested, such as depressed cell-mediated immunity, increased cortisol levels, altered immune function of the spleen, and immune evasion by parasites.

Complications

The following complications are common in pregnancies affected by malaria:

Anemia

In endemic areas, severe anemia in pregnancy is the major antenatal problem responsible for a large portion of maternal morbidity and even mortality, due to an increased danger of fatal hemorrhage (5,7). Levels of haptoglobin in pregnant women with malaria are often low, indicating active hemolysis. The malaria-induced anemia is usually normochromic and normocytic, with hemoglobin levels below 7 g/dL. The mechanisms are complex and include hemolysis, hyperferritinemia, bone marrow dyserythropoiesis, and iron or folic acid deficiency. The hematocrit concentrations should be monitored, and blood should be transfused if the hematocrit level falls below 20% (7). Otherwise at this stage of anemia there is also a high risk of acute right heart failure in labor, and if not treated before, the patient should be transfused slowly with packed cells and given furosemide. Prophylactic iron supplementation is advised during pregnancy, especially in malaria-endemic areas. However, caution should be exercised because iron overload may increase host susceptibility to malaria (4).

Cerebral Malaria

This condition is particularly common in pregnant women with falciparum malaria, and the rate of mortality during pregnancy is considerably higher than in the general patient population (5,6). Altered consciousness, confusion, seizure, focal neurologic findings, and coma are the main features, and if left untreated, the situation may lead to death. In cerebral malaria, fever is common, while hypertension is unusual, thus distinguishing the condition from eclampsia (7).

Hypoglycemia

Severe falciparum malaria may lead to hypoglycemia in pregnant women. Treatment with quinine will exacerbate this. Abnormal behavior, sweating, or loss of consciousness, particularly in a patient receiving quinine, should be considered to be due to hypoglycemia until proven otherwise (7,9).

Acute Pulmonary Edema

In pregnancy the blood volume increases significantly. Additional fluid overload, hyperparasitemia, and renal failure are important predisposing factors for developing pulmonary edema. The basic pathogenetic mechanism is capillary leakage. Infusions given during labor greatly increase the risk of pulmonary edema. If the condition develops, the patient should be sat upright immediately and given a high concentration of oxygen and intravenous diuretics (7). Pulmonary edema may develop even several days after institution of antimalarial drugs.

Preterm Labor

Falciparum malaria in nonimmune pregnant women commonly induces uterine contractions, which may give rise to preterm labor (5,10). The frequency and intensity of the contractions appear to be related to the height of fever. Hyperthermia also may cause fetal distress in late pregnancy, especially in anemic women. In these patients preterm labor and fetal distress are associated with poor neonatal prognosis.

Fetal Complications

Preterm birth and placental insufficiency are the main threats (10). Placental parasitemia is common, especially in primigravidas living in endemic areas. Parasites have been observed in placental blood smears even if absent from peripheral blood. Pathologic changes include the presence of malarial pigment in different cells of the placenta. There is trophoblastic damage with focal necrosis, loss of microvilli, and irregular thickening of the basement membrane. These changes are directly correlated to the level of the placental parasitemia. Clinically, these changes may lead to decreased nutrition and oxygen exchange between the mother and fetus, and reduced hormone secretion by the placenta. The placental weight is reduced and the fetus may suffer from intrauterine growth restriction, low birth weight, and sometimes stillbirth.

Maternal hypoglycemia may cause fetal brain damage. The malaria-associated fever, dehydration, and anemia may add to the fetal distress and also induce premature labor. Low birth weight in the premature baby is without question the main problem and is most frequent in primigravidas in high endemic areas (6). In areas with sporadic and seasonal transmission, the effect of malaria is extended to subsequent pregnancies as well.

Congenital Malaria

Fortunately, the incidence of congenital malaria is low, even in endemic areas, considering the large number of women who have malaria in pregnancy. Placental involvement has been found in 30% to 50% of pregnancies, whereas the incidence of symptomatic congenital malaria is estimated to be 0.1% to 0.3% in immune mothers and maximally 10% in nonimmune mothers in endemic areas (2,6,7). On examination of umbilical cord blood, however, almost 1 of 10 newborns has demonstrable parasitemia at birth. The parasite may infect the fetus *in utero* or may be acquired as a result of close contact between maternal and fetal blood during delivery. Transfer of antimalarial immunoglobulin G has some protective effect on the fetus and the newborn in the first month after delivery. In true congenital malaria the neonate presents with fever, hepatosplenomegaly, jaundice, and anemia within 5 days after birth (5,11).

Neonatally Acquired Malaria

The condition is much more common than congenital malaria, but it is difficult to distinguish mother-child infection from vector-transmitted malaria.

Treatment

Pregnant Women

The treatment regimens for malaria in pregnant women are similar to those in nonpregnant patients. Clinical episodes of malaria in nonimmune pregnant women should be treated immediately. The same applies to severe and complicated malaria (3,8,12). In areas of endemic malaria, women are assumed to be infected before pregnancy. The World Health Organization (WHO) recommends that these women receive an initial loading dose of an antimalarial drug, followed by regular chemoprophylaxis (3). Chemoprophylaxis also should be provided for travelers to these areas. All studies show that malaria treatment during pregnancy is beneficial to the maternal-fetal unit (12,13). The prophylaxis is associated with protection from illness in the mother with a reduced number of malarial attacks, as well as a reduction in antenatal parasitemia. There are also some suggestions that prophylaxis may be associated with higher mean birth rate, especially in primigravidae. According to the Cochrane Review (13) there are too few treatment studies with adequate total sample size to draw any firm conclusion about obstetric complications and maternal and fetal morbidity and mortality. A program to prevent anemia, including iron and folate supplementation together with antimalarial drugs, might have more power to detect effects on anemia and prenatal outcome (13).

Recommendations for the treatment of malaria vary in different areas of the world (3). The changing patterns of drug resistance, mainly to falciparum malaria, necessitate constant reviews. Treatment in different areas should be tailored by those who are familiar with the disease and the epidemiology of drug resistance in that area (1,4).

Chloroquine is the mainstay of malaria treatment and prophylaxis. The usual prophylactic regimen for travelers is chloroquine phosphate 300 mg orally once per week, or 5 mg/kg weekly beginning 1 to 2 weeks prior to departure and continuing for 4 weeks after leaving the epidemic area. The use of mosquito netting and insect repellent is also crucial to any preventive program (3). The dosage of chloroquine for severe malaria is 10 mg/kg infused over 8 hours, followed by three doses of 5 mg/kg over 8 hours, for a total of 25 mg/kg within 32 hours (3).

Chloroquine has been used for many years to pregnant women and is considered safe (14). However, surprisingly few data have been published on its safety in pregnancy, especially on adverse outcome following exposure during the first trimester. Between 1965 and 1994, 24 reports of congenital abnormalities associated with chloroquine use during early pregnancy were reported to WHO (15). In only 4 cases was chloroquine administered at a dosage used for prophylaxis or therapy. Fear of potential toxicity has limited antimalarial drug use in pregnancy (11,15). Except for the tetracyclines, there is no evidence to suggest that at standard dosage any of the antimalarial drugs used today is teratogenic (3,14). Standard dosage of chloroquine does not increase the risk of abortion or preterm delivery (15).

Fansidar is a combination of sulphadoxine and pyrimethamine. Currently it is used mainly for the self-treatment of travelers until they are able to seek medical care. It is safe to use in pregnancy, especially with the addition of folinic acid to ensure against folic acid depletion.

In an increasing number of areas worldwide chloroquine resistant *P. falciparum* is appearing (1,3). *Mefloquine* is considered the drug of choice in these areas. It is safe during the second and third trimester, but data on teratogenicity in the first trimester are lacking (14–16). The regimen is usually mefloquine (Larinam) (Roche) 250 mg orally once per week. *Proguanil* (Paludrine) (Zeneca) 200 mg orally once per day in combination with weekly chloroquine is an alternative regimen in resistant areas, especially in the first trimester.

Short-term travelers to chloroquine- or mefloquine-resistant areas can use doxycycline 100 mg daily (3). Prophylaxis usually should begin 1 day prior to travel and can be continued for 4 weeks after departure from the endemic area. Doxycycline is a tetracycline and is thus contraindicated in pregnancy (14,16).

Lactating Women

A mother breastfeeding her baby can use the same antimalarial drugs that are recommended in pregnancy (3,16). The concentration of the drug in breast milk is minimal. However, if mothers travel with their newborn babies to malarious areas, the infants should be given additional prophylaxis (chloroquine or proguanil) because their concentrations in breast milk are not protective. As a general recommendation, babies or young children should not be taken to a malarious area unless absolutely necessary. If they must be in these areas, special precautions should be taken to protect them against mosquito bites.

Traveling During Pregnancy

Women who are pregnant or likely to become pregnant should avoid traveling to malarious endemic areas, especially where the chloroquine-resistant strains are dominant (3). When travel is unavoidable, chloroquine is recommended as prophylaxis. A combination with proguanil is used in resistant-strain areas, especially during the first 3 months of pregnancy. Thereafter, mefloquine is recommended (3,16).

In areas of Thailand and Cambodia, *P. falciparum* infections do not respond to chloroquine or fansidar, and mefloquine treatment failures are reported in more than 50% (1,3). In these situations doxycycline chemoprophylaxis is recommended, along with vigorous use of personal protection procedures. Because pregnant women should avoid long use of doxycycline, it is strongly advised that women should avoid entering these malarious areas. Other malaria prevention strategies include avoidance of being outside in rural areas during the evening and night hours and the use of mosquito repellents, bednets, and anti-mosquito spray. If women using malaria prophylaxis find that they have conceived, none of the presented prophylactic drugs, including doxycycline, is considered as indication to consider pregnancy termination (14). Malaria we hope will one day be eradicated by effective vaccination.

TOXOPLASMOSIS

Human infection with *Toxoplasma gondii* occurs worldwide. The frequency varies greatly depending on geographic location, socioeconomic status, and dietary habits. The infection is usually benign and asymptomatic in children and adults but can lead to severe complications if it occurs in an immunocompromised patient or in a developing fetus (17,18).

Transmission

Toxoplasma gondii is a parasite that exists in three forms: as a tachyzoite, oocyst, or tissue cyst (17). The cat represents the host and reservoir. The parasites reproduce within the cat's intestine to form oocysts, which are shed in millions in the feces for 1 to 3 weeks. The oocysts become infectious after 1 to 5 days and may remain so for years. Infected cats develop immunity, but on reinfection they may excrete oocysts again. After infection in humans, parasitemia occurs and the tachyzoites may invade different organs throughout the body. The immune response with development of antibodies leads to formation of tissue cysts that contain thousands of parasites. These cysts may persist in a dormant state in skeletal or heart muscles, brain, or eye for years, but may reactivate if the immune system becomes compromised.

Toxoplasma tissue cysts are frequently found in pork and lamb, rarely in beef or chicken. Freezing below –12°C or cooking until the meat changes color (66°C) renders the parasites nonviable. The oocysts are also destroyed by freezing or exposure to dry heat and boiling water, but they are resistant to the usual detergents (17).

Human infection results from digestion of raw meat containing tissue cysts or from contact with cat feces directly or by eating contaminated fruit or vegetables (18). Cat owners have an increased risk of infection, as do people working in gardens or children playing in soil where cats may have buried their infected feces. Human-to-human transmission may occur in pregnant women where the fetus may become infected during primary maternal infection.

Clinical Manifestation

Primary infection with *T. gondii* is usually asymptomatic, or the mild symptoms are ignored. The incubation period varies between 4 and 21 days. Vague flulike symptoms such as fatigue, headache, and fever may appear together with nuchal lymphadenopathy. The condition may resemble the common cold, influenza, or infectious mononucleosis (18). In my own series of studies one third of the infected pregnant women had enlarged lymph nodes unrecognized by the doctor.

Epidemiology

The prevalence of toxoplasma antibodies varies according to age and geographic area (Fig. 44-2). Seropositivity is highest in areas with warm, moist climates, where the survival of the oocysts is good, and lower in cold regions and high altitudes. In Central and Southern Europe, Africa, and South America and Asia more than 50% of the population is infected (17,18). In France, where many people prefer minimally cooked and raw meat, the prevalence is especially high. In Europe

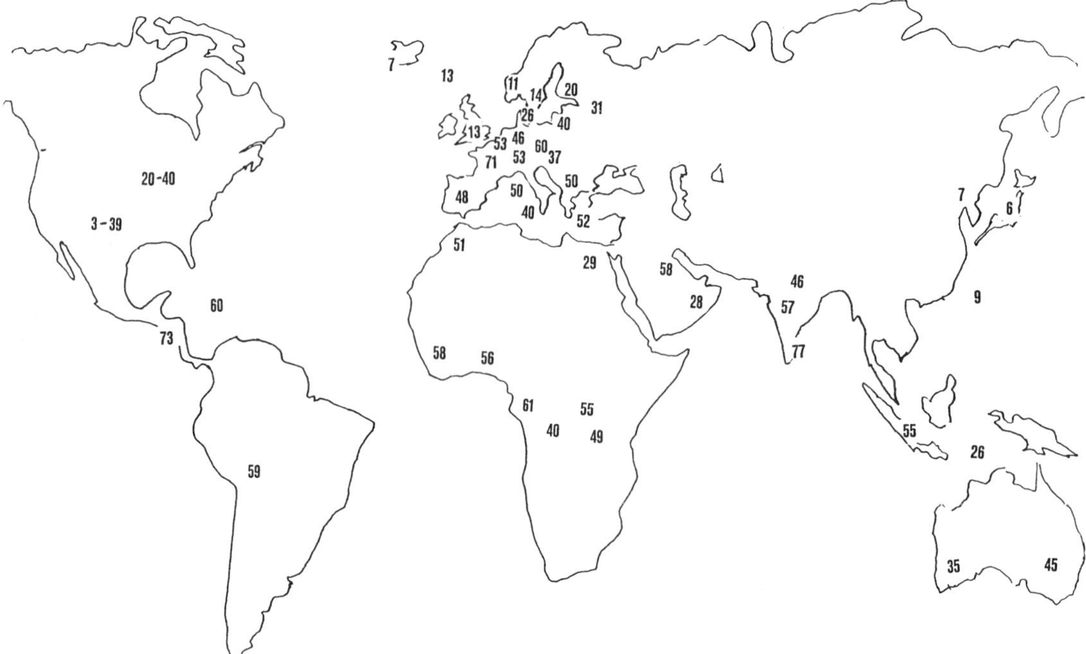

FIG. 44-2. The prevalence of *Toxoplasma* antibodies among pregnant women in the world.

and the United States, a decrease in seropositivity has been observed over the past 20 years. These changes may be ascribed to an increased consumption of instant or ready-cooked food and to the more common use of home freezers for food storage (18).

The frequency of *Toxoplasma* infection in pregnancy depends on the number of uninfected (seronegative) women of childbearing age in the population and on the infection risks. The estimated infection incidence per 1,000 women varies from 1 to 8 in Europe and United States (17–19). The incidence of congenital infection is underreported in areas without screening programs because less than 10% of infected infants have symptoms at birth. U.S. estimations indicate that congenital infection occurs in 1 in 1,000 (0.1%) to 1 in 8,000 (0.013%) live births (19).

Effect on Pregnancy

Primary infection with *T. gondii* acquired during pregnancy causes congenital disease in nearly half of the cases (17,18). During maternal parasitemia, the organisms infect the placenta and then the fetus. The vertical transmission rate increases from 6% to 80%, with increasing gestational age (17–21). The severity of the fetal infection, however, shows a gradient in the reverse direction. Acquisition early in pregnancy may cause miscarriage or severe sequelae resulting in hydrocephalus, chorioretinitis, or mental retardation (17–21). Infection occurring in the latter part of pregnancy most often causes subclinical infection not apparent at birth. Nearly all symptomatic neonates suffer long-term neurologic or ophthalmologic sequelae. But many of the asymptomatic neonates also develop complications later in life (17,22). It has been observed that 50% of untreated infants suffer from chorioretinitis, leading to severe impairment of vision, whereas hearing deficits and developmental delay have been recorded in 10% to 30% of these infected infants (18,23).

Diagnosis

The diagnosis of *Toxoplasma* infection depends either on identification of parasites in body fluids and tissues or on detection of specific antibodies. The *Toxoplasma* IgM antibodies appear within the first week of infection, reach a peak at 1 month, and decrease thereafter; but in some individuals IgM may remain detectable for years after primary infection.

In pregnancy the diagnostic challenge lies in differentiating between the primary maternal infection, which may cause fetal infection, and past latent infection, which is without importance. In the fetus and neonate, the challenge is to identify infected cases at an early stage.

Pregnant Women

The most reliable indication of primary maternal infection is *Toxoplasma*–IgG seroconversion confirmed by the presence of specific IgM and low IgG avidity (24,25). Without this latter test, ascertaining the exact timing of the infection may be difficult, especially determining if the infection has occurred before or after conception in the cases in which the first blood sample is drawn in the first half of pregnancy. The use of both IgG and IgM tests is required, whereas supplementary tests should include IgA or IgG avidity. A single positive IgM test in early pregnancy is no indication for termination of pregnancy. A new sample has to be collected after 2 to 3 weeks in order to confirm recent infection (24,25).

Prenatal Diagnosis

Whenever primary infection in pregnancy is identified or suspected, it is urgent to know if the infection has passed on to the fetus. The definitive diagnosis of fetal infection relies on the identification of parasites in the fetus or fetal material or on the demonstration of specific IgM antibodies in fetal blood (17,18,24). The detection of IgM depends on the gestational age. IgM is demonstrated in less than 10% of the infected fetuses in the fifth gestational month. The detection rate increases up to the time of delivery, but never exceeds 60% (1). Today the PCR technique for identification of the *Toxoplasma* antigen in amniotic fluid has an excellent sensitivity; thus, amniocentesis rather than cordocentesis is recommended in infected pregnancies (24).

If fetal infection is diagnosed in early pregnancy, therapeutic abortion is an option when ultrasound scans have shown abnormalities such as hydrocephalus or brain necrosis (17). If the pregnancy is continued, drug treatment should be initiated immediately in order to limit the effects of fetal infection (18).

Infants

Clinical signs of congenital toxoplasmosis in newborns are rare and nonspecific. The diagnosis must be made based on laboratory confirmation, such as demonstration of parasites from blood or body tissues obtained within the first 6 months of life; positive specific IgM or IgA, which are demonstrated in approximately two thirds of the cases; or persistently positive IgG beyond the first year of life (18,24). In some infected treated infants, however, the therapy has had the result that toxoplasma IgG antibodies are not detectable at the end of treatment; but antibodies may appear later (24).

If the mother is untreated, and material from the delivery is collected, parasites can be isolated from the placenta in nearly 90% of the infected offspring. In many areas neonatal screening for specific IgG and IgM has been initiated (19,26). By this strategy infection in the fetus cannot be modified, so it is of importance that treatment of the newborn is initiated as soon as the diagnosis is confirmed.

Treatment

Pregnant Women

Antiparasitic treatment is today offered to every woman when primary infection is discovered (27,28). The aim is to prevent fetal infection if it has not already occurred and to treat and reduce tissue damage in an already infected fetus. Pyrimethamine (25 mg per day) combined with sulphonamides (3 g per day) and folinic acid (5 mg twice a week) is the combination of choice for primarily infected mothers (17). The macrolide spiramycin (3 g per day) is another alternative used in Europe (27). Newer drugs such as azithromycin have been tried with some success on pregnant women (Table 44-1) (29).

In France spiramycin has been used since the early 1970's and parasites have been detected less frequently in the placentas of spiramycin-treated mothers (19%) than in untreated mothers (50%) (20,30). A significant reduction in the number of infected infants of the treated (23%) versus untreated (61%) mothers also was noted. However, the percentage of babies with clinical disease was the same in both groups. It was concluded that spiramycin reduced the incidence of fetal infection but had little effect on an already infected fetus (20). Later studies have shown that pyrimethamine-sulfadiazine treatment in pregnancy is more effective in eradication of parasites from placenta (30) and also leads to a significant reduction in the number of severely affected babies and a shift to less severe and subclinical forms of disease (31). A recent multicenter European study (21) investigated 144 seroconverting mothers, of whom 119 received prenatal treatment, although 25 were not treated at all. Prenatal antiparasitic treatment had no impact on the fetomaternal transmission rate but demonstrated a significant beneficial effect on sequelae and especially on severe sequelae in the infant at 1 year of age. Early start of treatment in pregnancy resulted in a significant reduction in the number of severely infected infants. The majority of these women were treated with spiramycin (21).

A combination of pyrimethamine combined with the long-acting sulfonamide sulphadoxine (Fansidar) has been used with good effect (18). The benefit is that this drug can be given once a week (serum half-life 8 days).

Antiparasitic treatment should be offered to every woman with a primary infection. Initially spiramycin should be administered until the status of the fetus is settled by prenatal diagnosis. If the fetus is infected, pyrimethamine-sulfadiazine-folinic acid should be offered in a three weekly course. These drugs are safe in pregnancy (14). Alternative treatment is pyrimethamine-sulphadoxine (Fansidar) (Roche) two tablets every week until term (27).

Infants

Every case of congenital toxoplasmosis should be treated whether or not the infant displays clinical manifestations in the newborn period (17). Treatment should be instituted as soon as possible after birth and given for

TABLE 44-1. *Treatment of Toxoplasma infection in pregnant women and newborn infants*

Drugs	Adults	Newborn
Spiramycin	3 g=9 MIU/day	50–100 mg/kg/day
or		
Pyrimethamine (P)	25 mg/day*	1 mg/kg/day
Sulfadiazine (S)	50–100 mg/day*	100 mg/kg/day
or		
Fansidar	2 tablets/week	1 tablet/20 kg/wk
During pyrimethamine therapy		
Folinic acid	5 mg twice weekly	5 mg twice weekly
Blood cell counts (platelets, white cells) every 1–2 wk		
If ocular or CNS toxoplasmosis, corticosteroids		1–2 mg/kg/day
Indications		
Pregnant women with acquired infection		
Before conception	No need for treatment	
Suspected cases	Spiramycin	
Proven cases		
1st trimester	Spiramycin continuously	
2nd, 3rd trimester	P + S (3 wk) + Spiramycin (3 wk)	
Evidence of fetal infection	P + S (3 wk), then Spiramycin (3–6 wk). Repeat until delivery.	
Newborns with congenital infection		
Suspected infection	Spiramycin until diagnosis	
Subclinical congenital infection	P + S (4 wk) + Spiramycin (4–6 wk) Repeat until 12 months of age	
Overt congenital infections	P + S (6–12 mo)	

*Use double this for a loading dose.

a minimum of 6 months, usually 1 year. Therapy beyond 12 months is only recommended in cases where the infection is still active. In infants with symptomatic congenital toxoplasmosis, prospective studies from the United States using pyrimethamine-sulfadiazine continuously for a year showed a striking beneficial effect in the ophthalmologic follow-up and neurodevelopmental outcome (32,33). The key question is whether or not treatment is necessary for subclinical newborns with no symptoms. Controlled trials with long prospective follow-up do not exist (27). However, there is historical evidence that early treatment protects against development of late ocular lesions (17). Pyrimethamine and sulfadiazine treatment has proven more effective than spiramycin alone.

The guidelines of today are that symptomatic infants should be treated for at least 1 year with pyrimethamine-sulfadiazine (17,18). If active chorioretinitis or cerebral infection exists, corticosteroids should be added. In asymptomatic cases spiramycin is recommended during the first months of life; thereafter, 4-week courses of pyrimethamine-sulfadiazine alternating with 6-week courses of spiramycin are given. In France and Switzerland Fansidar (one tablet per 20 kg body weight orally) is given every week during the first year (27).

After 30 years of experience, the optimum schedules and duration of therapy in pregnancy and newborns remains unknown. Future international multicenter studies with long-term follow-up observations are needed to provide sufficient data.

Prevention

Primary Prevention

Seronegative pregnant women should be educated in how to reduce the risk of acquiring *Toxoplasma* infection. A prospective case–control study in Norway (34)—a country with a *Toxoplasma* antibody prevalence in pregnant women of 11%—identified the following factors to be independently associated with an increased risk of infection: eating of raw or undercooked mutton or pork, especially minced meat products; eating of unwashed raw vegetables or fruit; infrequent washing of the kitchen knife; and cleaning of the cat litter box (34). In addition, traveling to areas with a higher frequency of infection was identified as an appreciable risk factor. Seronegative persons at risk should thus be informed of these simple dietetic and hygienic measures (17–19). In fact, educational programs in which pregnant women received information have been shown to be effective in reducing primary infection (35).

Secondary Prevention

The need for systematic serologic screening in pregnancy is controversial (17–19). In Europe, France, Austria, and Belgium, antenatal screening is performed routinely at least three times in pregnancy. In other areas, neonatal screening is offered as an alternative (Denmark and some parts of the United States) (26). Whether systematic screening should be introduced depends on factors like the infection risk in the area and the effect of treatment. Stray-Pedersen and Jenum (36) concluded that screening is of economic benefit when the incidence of maternal toxoplasmosis is 1 to 1.5 per 1,000.

AMEBIASIS

Amebiasis is an ulcerative and inflammatory disease of the colon, caused by *Entamoeba histolytica.* The protozoan is spread throughout the world with a frequency parallel to the level of sanitation and personal hygiene within the community. The organism infects 3% to 5% of the population in temperate climates (including the United States), and up to 40% of those in tropical areas (12,37). Epidemics and severe disease are seen in certain parts of Central and South America, the West Coast of Africa, and Southeast Asia (1,37). Pregnant women traveling to these areas are at highest risk and should be advised that they could easily be exposed and subsequently infected. The disease is not rare, but seldom thought about, and should not be overlooked in women presenting with abdominal pain and diarrhea.

Transmission

Entamoeba histolytica exists in two forms: the motile trophozoite and the cyst. The trophozoites dwell in the lumen and the wall of the colon; they encyst and are excreted in the stool. In moist environments the cysts can survive for weeks. They are highly resistant and survive gastric acid and chlorine at concentrations found in drinking water (37). Sometimes the trophozoites may invade the mucosal wall of the colon and cause the characteristic ulcer of amebiasis, whereas outside the body this form degenerates within minutes; the cysts are therefore the main reason for the extensive prevalence of the infection throughout the world. Individuals are infected though fecal contamination of water and vegetables, or through direct oral or fecal contact with an infected person.

Clinical Presentation

Infections in 75% of the cases are asymptomatic or mild, but the condition may convert to symptomatic disease or severe dysentery at any time (37). Patients often complain of intestinal irritation characterized by crampy abdominal pain, with or without diarrhea. The stool is usually liquid, but not bloody. On physical examination, abdominal tenderness may be present. In cases with extensive invasive disease, the picture is severe, with frequent bloody diarrhea, abdominal and upper right quadrant pain, hepatomegaly, and fever. The mortality rate may be as high as 9% during acute attacks of dysentery, twice as high in women than in men. In extreme cases, the patient may present with an acute abdomen, secondary to bowel perforation and amebic peritonitis. Amebic liver abscess is observed in some patients (37,38).

Diagnosis

Diagnosis of intestinal amebiasis is based on identifying *E. histolytica* in the stool (37). The presence of trophozoites or cysts confirms the diagnosis. Stool specimens should be examined fresh, and multiple samples may be necessary. Specimens collected by endoscopy and examined immediately for motile erythrocyte-containing ameba provide the most reliable diagnosis. Ultrasonography or computed tomography may be used to image liver abscesses (2).

Serologic determination of antibodies to *E. histolytica* should be performed in individuals suspected of having inflammatory bowel disease. Up to 75% of patients with invasive intestinal amebiasis have a positive serology, but the symptoms should have been present for more than 1 week before testing (12,37). Newer methods for antigen detection in serum and feces have made it possible to diagnose the infection before the antibody response has occurred.

Effect on Pregnancy

Amebiasis during pregnancy may be more severe than in nonpregnant women (38,39). Acute exacerbation of the disease and more prominent symptoms are observed in pregnancy. Abioye reported that two thirds of the fatal cases of the amebiasis in females occurred in association with pregnancy (40). This more fulminant course of amebiasis associated with pregnancy has been thought to be attributable to the increase in circulating cholesterol, which is a growth substrate requirement of the organisms (38–40). Malnutrition and anemia may also increase susceptibility. The frequency of liver abscesses, however, is less in pregnancy, which is thought to be a consequence of a protective effect of estrogen (37).

There is no evidence that *E. histolytica* is associated with intrauterine fetal infection (37–40). Obviously, a pregnant woman with acute dysentery who develops dehydration and persistent nutritional deprivation can have a fetus with intrauterine growth restriction. Likewise, an acute febrile illness, regardless of etiology, can lead to premature labor or premature rupture of the membranes. Even if transplacental transmission is not described, the newborn infant born to a mother with amebiasis is at risk of being infected at the time of delivery, or during the neonatal period through person-to-person transmission, usually from its mother.

Prevention

Eradicating fecal contamination of food and water prevents amebic infection (1,37). The most commonly contaminated foods are fresh ground vegetables. Water is the prime source for the spread of the infection. Chlorination of the water does not kill the parasites, but boiling is good enough. Vegetables should be treated with a strong detergent soap and then soaked in acetic acid or vinegar for 10 to 15 minutes. Pregnant women in endemic areas should boil water used for drinking and for cleaning food, or they should use bottled water.

Treatment

Pregnant women with amebiasis should be treated because of the increased risk of severe disease (2,12). Therapy consists of relief of symptoms, and replacement of fluid, electrolytes, and blood, combined with eradication of the organisms. No drug currently available is active against the amebic cyst (16). The antimicrobial therapy is thus directed against the trophozoitic stage.

Asymptomatic cases should be treated with paromomycin, an oral aminoglycoside that is an effective luminal amebicide and the drug of choice, given as 30 mg/kg/day in three divided doses for 5 to 10 days (16). Paromomycin is poorly absorbed from the gastrointestinal tract and thus considered safe to use in pregnancy for the intestinal infection (14). Another effective intraluminal drug is diloxanide furoate, also poorly absorbed, but no data on possible teratogenic effects are available (14). Metronidazole (750 mg three times daily for 10 days) is an alternative choice in pregnancy. This drug is regarded as safe for pregnant women because no teratogenic effect in humans has been documented (14,16).

Symptomatic dysentery should be treated for 10 days with two agents: paromomycin or diloxanide furoate combined with metronidazole (37). Tetracycline (250 mg orally three times daily) or erythromycin (500 mg orally four times daily) is also effective in combination with one of the intraluminal drugs (16). In cases with extraintestinal disease including hepatic abscess, the treatment of choice is metronidazole followed by paromomycin or diloxanide furoate (37–38).

GIARDIASIS

Giardia lamblia is the leading parasitic cause of diarrhea in travelers, but water-borne outbreaks also occur in industrialized countries. Giardiasis is found throughout the world, with an average incidence of 7% (1,41). High prevalence rates are found in areas of poor sanitation and among populations unable to maintain adequate personal hygiene. Areas of increased risk include Southeast and South Asia, West and Central Africa, South America, Mexico, Korea, and the former Soviet Union (2,12,41). Large-scale epidemics of giardiasis have occurred in the United States, where *G. lamblia* has been isolated from 3% to 9% of stool specimens (41).

Transmission

Giardia lamblia, like *E. histolytica,* has a trophozoitic and cystic stage and inhabits the intestine. Infection in humans is initiated after ingestion of the cystic form. The organism remains in the duodenum and upper jejunum. The trophozoites attach to the intestinal epithelial surface by means of powerful sucking disks. When the trophozoites pass through the colon, encystation occurs and the cysts are excreted from the body. The cysts are resistant and may remain viable and infectious in water for longer than 3 months. Acquisition of *G. lamblia* requires oral ingestion of fecally contaminated water. Person-to-person transmission is frequent in day-care centers and among male homosexuals (41).

Clinical Presentation

Diarrhea, abdominal cramps, and nausea are the most common symptoms of giardiasis (41). Characteristically, giardiasis presents with sudden onset of explosive, watery, fowl-smelling diarrhea. Most cases last for several weeks and may lead to weight loss and dehydration. However, not everyone infected has symptoms.

Diagnosis

All patients with prolonged diarrhea should be considered for giardiasis. The traditional method of diagnosis is a stool examination for trophozoites or cysts. Newer antigen detection methods such as the immunofluorescent assay (IFA) or the ELISA are also available (41). The stool may be examined either fresh or after preservation. The trophozoites or cysts can easily be detected. Sometimes samples are collected from the duodenum by endoscopy or the string test is performed: the patient swallows a gelatin capsule attached to a string, which is left in place for 6 hours. The string is then retrieved and examined for the presence of organisms. Serologic testing for *Giardia* antibodies has been useful in epidemiologic studies. *Giardia* IgG antibodies remain elevated for a long time, whereas *Giardia* IgM antibodies can be used to differentiate current from previous infection. A PCR method to identify *Giardia* antigen in the stool is also available (12,41). The sensitivity and specificity is superior to the stool examination for parasites.

Effect on Pregnancy

Maternal giardiasis does not directly affect the fetus (2,42). However, significant malabsorption and nutritional deprivation may impair fertility and adversely affect pregnancy. Three cases of severe giardiasis in pregnant women have been described, which suggest that the disease may be more severe in pregnancy with significant weight loss and disability (42).

Prevention

Proper handling and treatment of water used for communities and good personal hygiene is important. Chlorinating alone may be sufficient to kill *G. lamblia* cysts (41). For traveling women, water should be brought to boil for at least 10 minutes (3). Avoiding oral-genital sex can decrease transmission.

Treatment

Pregnant women should receive therapy only if severely symptomatic because the infection may be self-limited in many persons (41,42). The treatment of choice may be paromomycin for up to 10 days or metronidazole 250 mg three times daily for 7 days (16).

INFECTION WITH HELMINTHES

Helminthes (worms) infect humans all over the world, especially in tropical regions (1). Disease and morbidity related to these infections are basically a function of the number of worms in the body. Two major groups of parasitic helminthes are considered: roundworms, including hookworm, roundworm, and pinworm; and flatworms or flukes, including schistosomiasis.

Hookworm

Hookworm is caused by infection of the small intestine with *Ancylostoma duodenalis* or *Necator americanus,* which is found in the Southeastern United States (43).

Transmission

In the life cycle of the hookworm, eggs are discharged in stool and hatch and live in the soil. A person can be infected by walking barefoot through a field contaminated by human feces because the larvae can penetrate the skin. The larvae reach the lungs through the lymphatic vessels and blood stream. Then they climb the respiratory tract and are swallowed. About a week after penetrating the skin they reach the intestine, where they attach to the mucus tissue in the jejunum and secrete an anticoagulant which causes bleeding. Hookworm infections often begin in childhood but reach the highest peak of incidence in young adults (43).

Clinical Presentation

The symptoms may include fever, coughing, and wheezing when the larva migrates through the lungs, and then pain in the upper abdomen (43). Iron deficiency anemia and low levels of protein in the blood can result from intestinal bleeding. Diagnosis of hookworm disease depends on demonstration of eggs in direct fecal smears.

Effect on Pregnancy

Little attention has been directed to hookworm infections in pregnancy. Hookworm can cause severe anemia because of iron deficiency due to chronic blood loss. In severe cases (hemoglobin <7.0 g/L), the risk of perinatal maternal and child morbidity increases up to 500-fold (2,44). Anemia due to maternal deficiency affects the fetus, causes restricted intrauterine growth, and reduces the fetal ability to absorb iron provided by the mother. Hookworm infection without anemia or malnutrition does not require treatment in pregnancy (16,44). Replacement of iron, vitamins, and protein is often sufficient. However, if the nutritional support is not adequate, specific hookworm treatment is necessary. Mebendazole is the drug of choice in nonpregnant patients, in a dose of 100 mg twice daily for 3 days (16,44). In rats the drug is teratogenic, but no reports of human teratogenicity have been published (14). One review recommended mebendazole therapy when treatment is indicated (44). Pyrantel pamoate is another recommended antihookworm drug for pregnant patients, in a dose of 11 mg/kg daily for 3 days (16).

Roundworm

Ascariasis is the most common helminthic infection of humans, with an estimated 1 billion cases worldwide (1, 43). Transmission of ascariasis is usually hand to mouth. The infection is asymptomatic in the overwhelming majority of cases, but it can cause serious and fatal disease. Occasionally worms obstruct the appendix, the biliary tract, or the pancreatic duct. The migration of larvae through the lungs can cause fever, coughing, and wheezing. Tuboovarian abscesses also have been described (2).

The diagnosis of ascariasis is made by demonstrating ascaris eggs in the stools or by seeing larva in sputum or gastric aspirates (43). During pregnancy pyrantel pamoate (11 mg/kg in one dose) is recommended therapy (16). Piperacine citrate is an alternative drug. Treatment in early pregnancy should be given only to mothers with heavy worm infections. However, lightly infected mothers should be treated immediately before or after delivery because of the risk of neonatal infection.

Pinworm

Infection with pinworm (*Enterobius vermicularis*) is the most common parasite in children and families who live in the temperate climates (43,45). At least one of five children and up to 90% of the children in institutions have pinworms.

Transmission

The parasite is a small (1 cm in length) white thread-like worm inhabiting the cecum and adjacent bowel.

Infection usually occurs in a two-step process (43). Eggs are first transferred from the area around the anus to clothing, bedding, and toys. Then the eggs are transferred often from the fingers to the mouth of another person who swallows them. Eggs also can be inhaled from the air and then swallowed. People can reinfect themselves. Pinworms mature in the lower intestine within 2 to 6 weeks. The female worms migrate to the area around the anus, usually at night, to deposit their eggs. Eggs can survive outside the body for as long as 3 weeks at normal room temperature (43).

Diagnosis is made by finding the worms; they can be seen by the naked eye and look like white threads. If an adhesive tape is pressed against the perianal region early in the morning, the eggs and worms on the tape can be identified. This can be done at home by the parent. The tape can be folded down on its self-sticking side and taken to the doctor for evaluation.

Clinical Presentation

Perianal and perineal pruritus, local itching, and restless sleep are common complaints. Pinworms have been noted to migrate into the genital tract, producing vaginitis and on occasion pelvic inflammatory disease (45). Appendicitis also has been described. It has been suggested that pregnancy may exacerbate symptoms of vaginitis or pruritus vulvae from pinworms. No congenital infection has been described (45).

Treatment

Mebendazole (Vermox) (Fanssen-Cilag) in a single dose of 100 mg is the drug of choice in nonpregnant patients (16). A 1986 review (44) also recommended mebendazole for pregnant women, whereas another review (45) recommended piperazine. Pyrantel (1 g single dose) has become the preferred drug of some clinicians (2,16), whereas others feel that it is contraindicated because no human studies exist (12,14). When the child in a family has pinworms, usually all the family members must take the medicine because reinfection within the family is common.

Schistosomiasis

Schistosomiasis is the second most prevalent tropical disease (following malaria). Two hundred million people are infected worldwide, of whom 20 million are severely ill (1). In the United States nearly half a million individuals are affected, all with imported infections from endemic areas (46).

Transmission

Human blood flukes have a complex life cycle that involves a freshwater snail as an intermediate host (46). Two forms of the human disease exist: *Schistosoma haematobium* produces urinary illness, whereas *S. mansoni* causes intestinal disease. The snail host determines the geographic distribution. *S. mansoni* exists in Africa, Arabia, the Caribbean, and South America. *S. haematobium* is found in North Africa, the Middle East, and India. Humans are the definitive hosts of the parasite, and after infection eggs are excreted in human feces (*S. mansoni*) or urine (*S. haematobium*). Eggs hatch in fresh water, where they release ciliated forms that can invade snails. Multiplication occurs inside the snail, and free-swimming infectious larval parasites are released that can penetrate the human skin within 2 minutes of contact. People are thus infected after contact with infected water.

Clinical Manifestations

Acute schistosomiasis is frequently associated with a dermatitis or swimmer's itch, which may be prominent within 24 hours after the infection (46). A pruritic papular skin rash may appear in the area of acquisition. Thereafter, the organisms may spread systemically.

Infections with *S. haematobium* are characterized by hematuria during the acute phase, whereas the chronic stage is associated with polyposis and malignant changes in the bladder. The female genital tract may be infected with eggs of *S. mansoni* and *S. haematobium* (47). Acute and chronic inflammation of the fallopian tubes often leads to the development of salpingitis, infertility, and ectopic pregnancies. The vulvar regions are often the predominant place for eggs and lesions in young women (48). Otherwise lesions in the cervix and vagina, especially ulcerative lesions, may bleed easily upon contact and are usually painful with coitus. These lesions may play a role in facilitating human immunodeficiency virus (HIV) transmission from infected men to uninfected women especially, since HIV in semen may have easy access to the deeper vaginal cell layers in women with genital schistosomiasis (1,47–49). Untreated individuals may continue to carry the disease for several years, with different intervals having been noted before reactivation. Caution is therefore indicated in patients returning from endemic areas who manifest unusual symptoms (46).

Effect on Pregnancy

Schistosomiasis in pregnancy may affect the placenta and fetus (46–48). There is no evidence today that pregnancy accelerates the development or increases the severity of the disease in the mother. The frequency of placental infection is high in endemic areas, but the severity is usually mild. Furthermore, there is no evidence that placental schistosomiasis is associated with growth retardation or preterm delivery (2,12,47). However, in a mother with ulcerative lesions, the risk of primary HIV infection in pregnancy is increased.

Diagnosis

Laboratory diagnosis rests on the finding of eggs in either stool, urine, or tissue biopsies. Serologic tests using immunodiagnostic methods with purified worm antigens are used to screen travelers and immigrants from endemic areas (46). However, these tests are unable to distinguish between new and old infections. Assays for detecting antigens against adult worms have become available that are useful for distinguishing active from inactive infections. It should be stressed that schistosomiasis should always be suspected in patients with characteristic clinical findings or ulcerated lesions of the genital tract with a history of travel to an endemic area.

Treatment

Praziquantel is a new broad-spectrum antihelminthic agent that is effective against all human species of schistosomes (16,46). This drug causes spastic paralysis and damage to the worms. The recommended dose depends on the parasites involved. Both *S. haematobium* and *S. mansoni* require 40 mg/kg in 1 day (16,44,46). There are no data on toxicity of this drug to the human fetus, but it has been found to be safe in pregnant animals (14). Other possible therapeutic agents include metrifonate, which is specifically given for *S. haematobium* infection (16). If other drugs have to be used, it is recommended to withhold treatment in pregnant women until after delivery, due to possible fetal toxicity (29).

INFECTIONS WITH ECTOPARASITES

An ectoparasite is an organism that lives on or in the skin. Two different common conditions, which occur worldwide, are presented.

Scabies

Human scabies is a highly contagious infestation caused by the itch mite, *Sarcoptes scabiei,* a parasite that burrows into and resides and reproduces in human skin. Scabies occurs in all races and social classes, but especially among people with crowded living conditions (50). The disease is spread by close and prolonged person-to-person contact, sexual or nonsexual. It can be transferred by sharing beds or clothes, although the risk of spread from contaminated bed linen or clothing is small. Live mites can be found in dust samples from homes of infected persons. Studies suggest that the female mite can survive off a human host for up to 2 days (50).

Clinical Presentation

Intense itching is the usual manifestation. The characteristic involvement includes finger webs and flexor side of the wrists, elbows, axillae, breast, genitals, and buttocks. The itching is usually worse at night. For pruritus to occur, sensitization to *Sarcoptes scabiei* must occur. Among persons with their first infection, sensitization takes several weeks to develop, and itching starts long after the infestation. After reinfestation, however, pruritus may occur within 24 hours (49,50). Scabies is often called the great imitator because the patient may present with a variety of lesions, imitating several dermatologic disorders, such as eczema, acute impetigo, insect bites, and dermatitis herpetiformis.

Diagnosis

The diagnosis may be suspected in women with the characteristic skin lesions or burrows of scabies (50). The organism may be seen as a tiny brown and white speck at the inner end of the burrow. Microscopic examination may confirm the diagnosis if the mite eggs or fecal pellets are identified, but this may be difficult.

Treatment

Correct application of an effective scabicide to the patient, her sexual contacts, and family members is important. Lindane (1%) lotion or cream is highly effective against scabies and has been the treatment of choice for many years (2,16,49,50). It should be applied thinly on dried skin to all areas of the body from the neck down and washed off thoroughly after 8 hours. Small amounts are absorbed through intact skin and mucus membranes; therefore, care should be taken when the patient is pregnant, even though no reports linking the use of this drug with toxic or congenital defects have been published (14). In animal studies no teratogenic effect has been reported in animals receiving 10 times the human dose. However, seizures have been reported when lindane was used by persons with extensive dermatitis, or when the drug has been applied after a bath, which increases the systemic absorption (49). Lindane resistance has been reported in some areas of the world, including the United States. The Centers for Disease Control and Prevention thus recommend that pregnant and lactating women be treated with permetrin (5%) (49). This is a cream that is also effective and safe for use in smaller children. No adequate controlled studies have been performed, but the drug is poorly absorbed through the skin and is therefore less likely than lindane to cause systemic side effects. One application is usually curative.

Pregnant women can also be treated with crotamiton (10%) cream or lotion (Eurax) (Squibb) (12). It should be applied to the entire body from the neck down nightly for two consecutive nights and washed off 24 hours after the second application. Another treatment comprises 6% sulfurs in petrolatum applied nightly for 3 days; however, allergic reactions have been described with this approach.

It is important that not only the women, but also the household members and close contacts, be treated at the same time. Bedding and clothing should be decontaminated (machine washed, and machine dried using the hot cycle or dry cleaned) or removed from body contact for at least 72 hours. Fumigation of living areas is not necessary (49).

Follow-up

Lesions and pruritus may persist for several weeks, even though the mites and eggs have been killed. Retreatment after 1 week for patients who are still symptomatic is often recommended, whereas some authorities recommend retreatment only if live mites can be observed (50). Patients who are not responding to the recommended treatment should be retreated with an alternative regimen. Lindane treatment should be reserved for difficult cases.

Lice

Lice infection is of medical importance not only because it is a significant cutaneous disease, but also because lice may serve as a vector for infectious diseases such as epidemic typhus and relapsing fever (1,50). Three different entities exist: *Body lice* are rarely seen in those with good personal hygiene, who change their clothes frequently. *Head lice* can affect persons from all social and economic backgrounds and infestations can often reach epidemic proportions, especially among schoolchildren. Head lice are transferred by close personal contact and possibly by sharing of hats, combs and brushes. *Pubic lice* (*Pediculosis pubis*) are considered a sexually transmitted parasite requiring close body or sexual contacts (49). About one third of the patients have other sexually transmitted diseases, and the infection is more common in women than in men. Pregnancy is not a predisposing factor.

Clinical Presentation

Pubic lice generally affect the pubic and perineal areas. The typical lesion results from the attachment of numerous nits (eggs) to the pubic hair. Dermatitis may result from scratching in response to the intense pruritus believed to be due to allergic sensitization. The time from the exposure to the onset of pruritus is usually 30 days, the time it takes for sensitization to the lice to occur (50).

Diagnosis

Pediculus pubis is diagnosed by identification of nits attached to the hair shaft by use of a magnifying glass. Microscopic examination with the identification of typical adult crab lice from a plucked hair may be possible.

Treatment

Pregnant women should be treated with pyrethrins with piperonyl butoxide applied to the affected area and washed off after 10 minutes (16,44,50). This drug is only effective against lice and not against scabies. No reports of its use in pregnancy have been published, but topical absorption is poor, so the potential toxicity should be minimal (14). Lindane also may be used (see the section on Scabies), but should be reserved for resistant or difficult cases. Lindane shampoo is applied for 4 minutes, then washed off (12).

Another alternative is permethrin (1%) cream rinse applied to the affected area and washed off after 10 minutes. Following all treatments, combing of infected areas with a fine-toothed comb facilitates removal of remaining lice and nits.

Retreatment is indicated after 1 week if lice or eggs are observed. Clothing or bed linen that may have been contaminated within the preceding 2 days should be washed and dried on the hot cycle or dry cleaned. In special cases with prolonged itching, antihistamine may be given to eradicate the pruritus, whereas if secondary bacterial infections have occurred, systemic antibiotics covering *Staphylococcus aureus* should be given (50).

REFERENCES

1. World Health Organization 1998. The World Health Report. Geneva, Switzerland: World Health Organization, 1998:1–149.
2. Sweet RL, Gibbs RS, eds. Parasitic diseases in pregnancy. In: Infectious diseases of the female genital tract. Baltimore: Williams & Wilkins, 1995:617–654.
3. World Health Organization. International travel and health. Geneva, Switzerland: World Health Organization, 1997:1–97.
4. Krogstad DJ. *Plasmodium* species (Malaria). In: Mandel GL, Benetts JE, Dolin R, eds. Principle and practice of infectious diseases, 4th ed. New York: Churchill Livingstone, 1995:2415–2427
5. Mutabingwa TK. Malaria and pregnancy: epidemiology, pathophysiology and control options. Acta Trop 1994;57:239–254.
6. Silver HM. Malarial infection during pregnancy. Infect Dis Clin North Am 1997;11:99–107.
7. Nathwani D, Currie PF, Douglas JG, Green ST, Smith NC. *Plasmodium falciparum* malaria in pregnancy:a review. Br J Obstet Gynaecol 1992; 99:118–121.
8. Stekeete RW, Wirima JJ, Slutsker L, Khoromana CO, Heymann DL, Breman JG. Malaria treatment and prevention in pregnancy: indications for use and adverse events associated with use of chloroquine or mefloquine. Am J Trop Med Hyg 1996;55(suppl):50–56.
9. Santiso R. Effects of chronic parasitosis on women's health. Int J Gynaecol Obstet 1997;58:129–136.
10. Stekeete RW, Wirima JJ, Hightower AW, Slutsker L, Heymann DL, Breman JG. The effect of malaria and malaria prevention in pregnancy of offspring birthweight, prematurity, and intrauterine growth retardation in rural Malawi. Am J Trop Med Hyg 1996;55(suppl):33–41.
11. Gilstrap LC, Faro S, eds. Infections in pregnancy, 2nd ed. New York: Wiley-Liss, 1997:1–345.
12. Garner P, Rabin B. A review of randomized controlled trials of routine antimalarial drug prophylaxis during pregnancy in endemic malarious areas. Bull World Health Org 1994;72:89–99.
13. Gülmezoglu AM, Garner P. Interventions to prevent malaria during pregnancy in endemic malarious areas. In: Garner P, Gelband H, Olliaro P, Salinar R, Volmin J, Wilkonson D, eds. Infectious diseases module of the Cochrane Database of Systematic Reviews. The Cochrane Collaboration, Issue 4. Oxford, England, 1997.
14. Briggs GG, Freeman RK, Yaffe SJ, eds. Drugs in pregnancy and lactation, 4th ed. Baltimore: Williams & Wilkins, 1994.

15. Phillips-Howard PA, Wood D. The safety of antimalarial drugs in pregnancy. Drug Safety 1996;14:131–135.
16. Bawdon R. Antibiotics, antifungal, antiparasite and antiviral drugs. In: Pastorec JG, ed. Obstetric and Gynecologic Infectious Diseases, 2nd ed. New York: Raven, 1994:677–699.
17. Remington JS, McLeod R, Desmonts G. Toxoplasmosis. In: Remington JS, Klein JO, eds. Infectious diseases of the fetus and newborn infant, 4th ed. Philadelphia: WB Saunders, 1995:140–267.
18. Stray-Pedersen B. Toxoplasmosis in pregnancy. Baillieres Clin Obstet Gynaecol 1993;17:107–137.
19. Wong S-Y, Remington JS. Toxoplasmosis in pregnancy. Clin Infect Dis 1994;18:853–862.
20. Desmonts G, Couvreur J. Congenital toxoplasmosis. A prospective study of 378 pregnancies. N Engl J Med 1974;290:1110–1116.
21. Foulon W, Villena I, Stray-Pedersen B, et al. Treatment of toxoplasmosis during pregnancy: impact on fetal transmission and children's sequelae: a multicenter study. Am J Obstet Gynecol 1999 (in press).
22. Wilson CB, Remington JS, Stagno S, Reynolds DW. Development of adverse sequelae in children born with subclinical *Toxoplasma* infection. Pediatrics 1980;66:767–774.
23. Roberts T, Frenkel JK. Estimating income losses and other preventable costs caused by congenital toxoplasmosis in people in the United States. J Am Vet Med Assn 1990;196:249–256.
24. Lebech M, Joynson DHM, Seitz HM, et al. Classification system and case definitions of *Toxoplasma gondii* infection in immunocompetent pregnant women and their congenitally infected offspring. Eur J Clin Microbiol Infect Dis 1996;15:799–805.
25. Jenum PA, Stray-Pedersen B, Guindersen AG. Improved diagnosis of primary *Toxoplasma gondii* infection in early pregnancy by determination of antitoxoplasma immunoglobulin G avidity. J Clin Microbiol 1997;35:1972–1977.
26. Guerina NG, Ho-Wen H, Meissner HC, et al. Neonatal serologic screening and early treatment for congenital *Toxoplasma gondii* infection. N Engl J Med 1994;330:1858–1863.
27. Stray-Pedersen B. Treatment of toxoplasmosis in mother and child. Scand J Infect Dis 1992;84(suppl):23–31.
28. McCabe RE, Oster S. Current recommendations and future prospects in the treatment of toxoplasmosis. Drugs 1998;38:973–987.
29. Stray-Pedersen B and The European Research Network of Congenital Toxoplasmosis Treatment Group. Azitromycin levels in placental tissue, amniotic tissue and blood. In: Abstracts of the 36th interscience conference on antimicrobial agents and chemotherapy (ICAAC). American Society for Microbiology, 1996:13.
30. Desmonts G, Couvreur J. Toxoplasmose congenitale. Etude prospective del'issue de la grossesse chez 542 femmes atteintes de toxoplasmose acquise en cours de gestation. Ann Pediatr 1994;31:805–809.
31. Hohlfeld J, Daffos F, Thulliez P. Fetal toxoplasmosis: outcome of pregnancy and infant follow-up after in utero treatment. J Pediatr 1989;115: 765–769.
32. McAuley J, Boyer KM, Patel D, et al. Early and longitudinal evaluations of treated infants and children and untreated historical patients with congenital toxoplasmosis: The Chicago Collaborative Treatment Trial. Clin Infect Dis 1994;18:38–72.
33. McGee T, Wolters C, Stein L, et al. Absence of sensorineural hearing loss in treated infants and children with congenital toxoplasmosis. Otolaryngology 1992;106:75–80.
34. Kapperud G, Jenum PA, Stray-Pedersen B, Melby KK, Eskild A, Eng J. Risk factors for Toxoplasma gondii infection in pregnancy. Am J Epidemiol 1996;144:405–412.
35. Foulon W, Naessens A, Derde MP. Evaluation of the possibilities for preventing congenital toxoplasmosis. Am J Perinatol 1994;11:57–62.
36. Stray-Pedersen B, Jenum PA. Economic evaluation of preventive programmes against congenital toxoplasmosis. Scand J Infect Dis 1992; 84(suppl):86–92.
37. Ravdin JI. Amebiasis. Clin Infect Dis 1995;20:1453–1466.
38. Reinhardt MC. Effect of parasitic infections in pregnant women. Perinatal infection. Ciba Found Symp 1980;77:149–170.
39. Armon PJ. Amoebiasis in pregnancy and the puerperium. Br J Obstet Gynecol 1978;85:264–268.
40. Abioye AA. Fatal amoebic colitis in pregnancy and the puerperium: a new clinico-pathological entity. J Trop Med Hyg 1973;76:97–100.
41. Hill D. *Giardia lamblia.* In: Mandel GL, Benetts JE, Dolin R, eds. Principles and practice of infectious diseases, 4th ed. New York: Churchill Livingstone, 1995:2487–2493.
42. Kreutner A, Del Bene VE, Amstey MS. Giardiasis in pregnancy. Am J Obstet Gynecol 1981;140:895–899.
43. Mahmoud AAF. Intestinal nematodes. In: Mandel GL, Benetts JE, Dolin R, eds. Principle and practice of infectious diseases, 4th ed. New York: Churchill Livingstone, 1995:2526–2533.
44. Ellis CJ. Antiparasitic agents in pregnancy. Clin Obstet Gynecol 1986; 13:269–275.
45. Leach FN. Management of threadworm infestation during pregnancy. Arch Dis Child 1990;65:399–400.
46. Mahmoud AAF. Trematodes (schistosomiasis) and other flukes. In: Mandel GL, Benetts JE, Dolin R, eds. Principles and practice of infectious diseases, 4th ed. New York: Churchill Livingstone, 1995: 2538–2544.
47. Feldmeier H, Poggensee G, Krantz I. Female genital schistosomiasis. New challenges and a gender perspective. Trop Geogr Med 1995;47 (suppl 2):1–16.
48. Feldmeier H, Krantz I, Poggensee G. Female genital schistosomiasis: a neglected risk for transmission of HIV. Trans R Soc Trop Med Hyg 1995;89:237–242.
49. Centers for Disease Control and Prevention. 1998 Guidelines for treatment of sexually transmitted diseases. MMWR 1998;47:1–118.
50. Wilson BB. Ectoparasites. In: Mandel GL, Benetts JE, Dolin R, eds. Principle and practice of infectious diseases, 4th ed. New York: Churchill Livingstone, 1995:2559–2564.

Cherry and Merkatz's Complications of Pregnancy,
Fifth Edition, edited by W. R. Cohen.
Lippincott Williams & Wilkins, Philadelphia © 2000.

CHAPTER 45

Common Viral Infections

Lindsay Staubus Alger

CYTOMEGALOVIRUS

Definition

Human cytomegalovirus (CMV) is responsible for cytomegalic inclusion disease, a condition characterized by greatly enlarged cells that contain intranuclear and cytoplasmic inclusions. Although cells with the pathognomonic owl's eye appearance were first described by Ribbert in 1881, the virus was not isolated until 1956 and the nomenclature *cytomegalovirus* was not proposed until 1960 (1). CMV is a double-stranded DNA virus and is the largest member of the herpesvirus family. It shares with other herpes viruses the properties of latency and reactivation. Human CMV is host specific and infects only humans. The virus has existed since ancient times, and this long-standing, successful host–parasite relationship has permitted the evolution of multiple different strains. CMV is of particular concern to the obstetrician because it is now recognized as the most common cause of intrauterine infection resulting in congenital disease.

Incidence

CMV infection is ubiquitous in all populations, infecting the majority of the world's people at some point in their lives. Disease occurrence is sporadic rather than epidemic. There is no seasonal variation, and climate does not affect the prevalence of disease (2). The prevalence of CMV antibody increases with age (3). However, the age of acquisition is influenced by socioeconomic status, ethnic background, social and sexual practices, geography, and child-care setting (2,4). CMV seropositivity is more prevalent among women of lower socioeconomic strata, those with multiple sexual partners, those who have had many pregnancies, or those who attended day-care facilities in childhood (5).

Among women of childbearing age in the United States, 40% to 60% of middle to high socioeconomic status women are seropositive compared with 80% of those of low socioeconomic status (4,6). Despite greater baseline seropositivity, women of lower socioeconomic status are more likely to seroconvert—6% per year versus 2% per year—placing them at greater risk for seroconverting during pregnancy (6). On average, primary infection with CMV occurs in a little over 1% (0.7%–4.1%) of pregnancies (2–4,6,7). The resulting risk of transmission to the fetus is about 40% (6).

Unlike rubella or *Toxoplasma* infection, where preexisting maternal immunity is essentially protective against vertical transmission, maternal antibody does not protect the fetus from intrauterine CMV infection. Depending on socioeconomic status, a previously infected woman has up to a 2% risk of delivering a congenitally infected infant (8–10). Evidence suggests that worldwide, congenital infection is more often the result of maternal virus reactivation than primary maternal infection (6). It is estimated that infection occurs in approximately 1% of all births (0.2%–2.2%) and that 40,000 infected infants are born annually in the United States (3,11,12). Of these, 7,000 to 8,000 infants either die or develop significant sequelae.

Pathogenesis

Cytomegalovirus is not highly contagious; spread requires close contact with infected secretions. Common modes of acquisition include sexual contact, breastfeeding, transfer of virus in saliva to hands and toys in the day-care setting, and poor hand-washing practices by care providers after contact with infected secretions. The most common source for primary CMV infection during

L. S. Alger: Department of Obstetrics, Gynecology, and Reproductive Sciences, University of Maryland School of Medicine, University of Maryland Medical Systems, Baltimore, Maryland 21210.

pregnancy is an intrafamilial source, frequently a young CMV-infected child who has been in day care (13–15). Overall, 25% of children in day care under the age of 3 years excrete CMV (16). Infected children can shed virus in their saliva and urine for up to 2 years. When CMV is introduced into the home, 50% of susceptible women will seroconvert (17).

Once infected, the host does not eradicate the virus, and latent CMV remains in many tissues. Recurrent excretion of CMV in asymptomatic women is a common occurrence. CMV can be cultured from urine, the cervix, or breast milk in 2% to 28% of pregnant women (18). Possible mechanisms to explain this include reinfection with a different strain of virus; low-grade chronic infection that periodically achieves detectable levels of excretion; and latent infection reactivated by external stimuli or when the individual is immunosuppressed. In this regard, pregnancy is a mild immunosuppressant.

In most cases of primary infection, intrauterine infection is thought to result from maternal viremia, subsequent placental infection, and then hematogenous dissemination to the fetus. The virus then replicates in fetal renal tubular epithelium and is excreted into the amniotic fluid. This process may take weeks to months. Alternatively, after virus spreads to the placenta, infected amniocytes may be swallowed by the fetus, permitting replication in the oropharynx. Placental infection can be present without fetal infection. Ascending infection from the cervix across intact membranes also may occur. Isolation of the virus from the cervix or urine is a poor predictor of the risk of intrauterine infection. Possible mechanisms of transmission for recurrent infection include reinfection with a different strain of CMV; migration of infected leukocytes across the placenta; reactivation of infection locally within the endometrium; and ascending infection via the cervical canal as a result of lower genital tract virus shedding. Infection also may be acquired intrapartum following exposure to infected genital tract secretions or postpartum by ingesting virus-containing breast milk. Of infants breastfed by seropositive mothers for over 1 month, 40% to 60% will become infected (19).

Transmission occurs with equal frequency in all trimesters, but infection is more virulent when it occurs early in pregnancy (6,20). In each trimester there is roughly a 40% chance of transmission following a primary infection, but most adverse outcomes are the result of infection prior to 20 weeks' gestation. When infection occurs in the third trimester, infants are generally asymptomatic at birth. Although prior maternal immunity does not prevent fetal infection, it dramatically reduces the severity of infection. Almost all cases of an infant symptomatic at birth result from primary maternal infection. The virus is not teratogenic in the strict sense, rather, fetal damage most likely results from cell death, vasculitis resulting in ischemia, and immune system mechanisms. Malformations such as congenital heart defects or cataracts are rarely seen.

Preconceptional Counseling

Two groups of women are candidates for preconceptional counseling: women of unknown serostatus whose jobs may involve contact with CMV-infected individuals, and women who have previously delivered an affected infant and are concerned about the chances of infection in subsequent pregnancies. Included in the first group are health care personnel, such as pediatric or nursery nurses and physicians. However, studies show that health care workers are not at increased risk of seroconversion during pregnancy, most likely because of the appropriate use of gloves and hand-washing practices (21–24). Therefore, there is no greater reason to perform pre- or postconceptional serologic screening for these women than for the general population. Assuming a woman is not already seropositive, continued use of appropriate body fluid precautions should prevent seroconversion. CMV is readily inactivated by soaps, detergents, and alcohol. Women do not need to change work assignments in an attempt to avoid exposure to CMV-excreting patients. Adler and colleagues reported that pregnant women are sufficiently motivated to adhere to proper sanitation and hygiene practices that they can successfully prevent seroconversion (25). After receiving instructions on risk reduction measures, none of the 14 pregnant women with a child under the age of 3 years who was shedding virus seroconverted during pregnancy, compared with 8 of 17 nonpregnant control patients who received no instructions in proper hygiene.

The only occupation known to carry an increased risk of CMV infection is that of day-care worker; gloves typically are not used in this setting. Adler found that the annual seroconversion rate was five times as high for day-care workers as for the general age-matched population (11% versus 2.2%) (16). These women should be instructed regarding the benefits of frequent hand washing and the use of gloves when handling diapers or respiratory tract secretions. There are no standard guidelines that recommend preconceptional testing in this latter group, but determining serostatus just prior to pregnancy would permit the detection of seroconversion in early pregnancy.

With regard to the second group, there is no evidence that the risk of vertical transmission is increased for women with one affected offspring above that for seropositive women in general. This group can be reassured that the chance of delivering an infected infant is relatively small. [Although most researchers cite a risk of under 2%, investigations using polymerase chain reaction (PCR) or testing for avidity of IgG antibodies indicate the risk may be much greater, as high as 6%–10%

(26,27).] Should infection occur, the neonate is anticipated to be asymptomatic at birth with only a low risk of long-term sequelae. Overall, the risk of delivering a child with clinically apparent sequelae is approximately 0.2%. There are currently no prophylactic measures that can be taken to prevent transmission, and prenatal diagnosis is impractical.

Clinical Manifestations

Cytomegalovirus infection is well-tolerated in the immunocompetent adult, and over 90% of primary infections are asymptomatic and, thus, undetected. The severity of the disease is unaffected by pregnancy. Occasionally, patients will develop a febrile illness mimicking mononucleosis, with malaise, myalgias, fatigue, lymphadenopathy, and a mild sore throat. Hepatosplenomegaly is rarely seen. Laboratory findings consistent with acute CMV infection include a lymphocytosis with atypical lymphocytes (or sometimes lymphopenia), thrombocytopenia, abnormal liver function tests, and positive cultures for CMV from urine, saliva, blood, or the lower genital tract. Recurrent infection is almost always asymptomatic.

An increase in the rate of spontaneous abortions and late pregnancy loss in women developing a primary CMV infection has not been proven. Rates are generally similar to those observed in uninfected women and those infected prior to pregnancy. Congenital CMV infection has been associated with an increased likelihood of premature rupture of membranes and preterm delivery (28).

Clinical Manifestations in the Fetus and Infant

Symptoms in the newborn depend on whether the infection originates *in utero* or intrapartum and whether the mother is already seropositive at the time of conception. CMV infection acquired intrapartum does not result in permanent sequelae (except occasionally in the very-low-birth-weight infant). Virus may be excreted for 2 years, but these infants develop normally. Thus, cesarean section in order to avoid intrapartum fetal exposure is not justified.

Infections acquired *in utero* are of much greater concern, especially when the mother develops a primary CMV infection during early pregnancy. In only 10% of congenital infections is the infant symptomatic at birth (6,7). Findings in these infants are shown in Table 45-1 (29,30). Chorioretinitis lesions caused by CMV cannot be differentiated from those caused by toxoplasmosis, but rarely progress postnatally and soon become inactive. Optic atrophy, hydrocephalus, hemolytic anemia, or, rarely, pneumonitis also may be apparent. There is no convincing evidence that CMV is a teratogen, but an increased incidence of inguinal hernias has been reported in males and there are case reports of anomalies of the first branchial arch. Congenital CMV infection is also associated with defective tooth enamel (31). This defect is characterized by yellowish discoloration and soft, opaque enamel that chips away from dentin. The defect mainly involves primary dentition, and affected teeth tend to wear down rapidly.

Fetal effects of CMV infection may be manifested on ultrasonographic examination. Findings compatible with, but not specific to, CMV infection include intrauterine growth restriction, oligohydramnios or polyhydramnios, microcephaly or hydrocephaly, ascites, pleural effusions, nonimmune hydrops, intracranial calcifications, hyperechoic bowel, hepatomegaly, and intrahepatic calcifications. Cerebral calcifications are characteristically distributed in the periventricular subependymal region. Their presence indicates that the child will have at least moderate, if not severe, mental retardation (28). Sonographic abnormalities typically become apparent late in pregnancy and are insufficiently specific to allow confident diagnosis of *in utero* CMV infection. At times, findings such as pleural effusions or ascites will resolve spontaneously. The absence of findings does not preclude fetal damage.

The prognosis for infants symptomatic at birth is poor; the mortality rate is 25% (2,6,32). Of the survivors, 90% develop permanent sequelae, predominantly neurologic. Sensorineural hearing loss, frequently bilateral, is the most common handicap; CMV is a major cause of childhood deafness (33). The hearing loss typically does not become apparent until after the first year of life. In most

TABLE 45-1. *Features of congenital CMV infection in decreasing order of frequency*

Abnormality	%
Elevated liver enzymes	83
Thrombocytopenia (<100×10^3/mm^3)	77
Petechiae	76
Conjugated hyperbilirubinemia (>4 mg/dL)	69
Jaundice	67
Hepatosplenomegaly	60
Sensorineural hearing loss	58
Mental retardation (IQ <70)	55
Microcephaly	52
Small for gestational age	48
Increased cerebrospinal fluid protein (>120 mg/dL)	46
Prematurity	34
Lethargy/hypotonia	27
Inguinal hernia	26
Seizures	23
Chorioretinitis	18

From Stagno S, Pass RF, Dworsky ME, Alford CA. Congenital and perinatal cytomegalovirus infection. Semin Perinatol 1983;7:30–42; and Boppana S, Pass RF, Britt WS, Stagno S, Alford CA. Symptomatic congenital cytomegalovirus infection: neonatal morbidity and mortality. Pediatr Infect Dis J 1992;11:93–99 (29,30).

cases the onset of hearing impairment is noted by 2 to 3 years of age, but, on occasion, may not be detected until after age 8. Mental retardation, seizures, paresis, spastic diplegia, expressive language delays, learning disabilities, and visual motor dysfunction also can develop in infants symptomatic at birth. The tetrad of findings considered to be characteristic of CMV is mental retardation, cerebral calcifications, microcephaly, and chorioretinitis.

Congenitally infected infants who are asymptomatic at birth following maternal primary infection generally do well, but 5% to 15% will develop abnormalities, usually within the first 2 years of life (29,33). These infants are at risk for hearing loss, learning disabilities, mental retardation, behavioral difficulties, microcephaly, and motor defects (34). The hearing impairment is bilateral in almost 40% of cases and can interfere with learning and communication. The conclusion of a small study by Conboy and colleagues—who prospectively compared 18 asymptomatic, congenitally infected school-aged children with normal hearing with 18 uninfected controls—was that children with normal hearing are not at increased risk of developing mental deficits as a result of CMV (35).

Preexisting maternal antibody does not prevent a reactivation or recurrence of infection during pregnancy, nor does it prevent fetal transmission. Congenital CMV infection has been documented in consecutive pregnancies as much as 3 years apart. Virus isolated from serially infected siblings has been shown to be identical by restriction endonuclease analysis (36). However, with rare exceptions, infants are asymptomatic at birth following recurrent infection and are less likely to develop long-term sequelae than after a primary infection (10,37,38). In one series of 56 infants, sensorineural hearing loss ultimately developed in 5% of children, but it was always unilateral (38). Overall, the risk of mild sequelae in children of mothers with recurrent infection was 8%. There were no instances of mental retardation. Thus, the maternal immune response provides a measure of protection. Although present information indicates that most of these children are normal intellectually, it has yet to be resolved to what degree they may be at increased risk for learning disabilities. Significantly immunocompromised women, such as those with human immunodeficiency virus (HIV) infection, may deliver severely affected infants despite previous CMV immunity.

Diagnosis

Maternal

In most cases, maternal CMV infection is asymptomatic and the diagnosis is not suspected. When symptoms do occur, they are generally mild and nonspecific; the possibility of CMV infection is not considered. In the immunocompetent, nonpregnant adult, it is unnecessary to make a diagnosis of CMV infection because it does not influence treatment and is not cost effective. However, the potential to identify fetal infection *in utero* and to perhaps prevent delivery of an affected neonate has prompted some patients and physicians to screen for acute CMV infection during pregnancy.

Screening usually involves a serologic test to detect IgG antibody, such as the enzyme linked immunosorbent assay (ELISA), indirect fluorescent antibody, indirect hemagglutination, and complement fixation tests. The sensitivity and specificity of these tests varies and should be taken into account when interpreting results. ELISA (or a modification of the ELISA) is the preferred method and has replaced complement fixation, which is less sensitive and specific (39). If the test is positive, this does not differentiate previous infection from current or recent infection. Demonstration of seroconversion is the best documentation of a primary infection, but few patients have serologic testing performed prior to conception as a basis for comparison. A fourfold increase in titer between paired samples of the screening specimen and a follow-up sample drawn 3 to 4 weeks later also supports recent infection.

Many clinicians rely upon testing for CMV-specific IgM antibody to determine whether there has been recent infection. Unfortunately, IgM may persist for up to 18 months after a primary infection, and it may be present during recurrent infections as well (40). A single positive IgM test result should be confirmed using a different assay before proceeding with further investigation. A negative test result also may require follow-up because it may take up to 4 weeks for the titer to increase. Overall, the sensitivity and specificity of IgM antibody testing for CMV infection are 75% (41). Capture-ELISA techniques, which control for the presence of rheumatoid factor, improve accuracy. At present, in the absence of seroconversion, there is no reliable method for determining whether a pregnant woman has had a primary infection during pregnancy. In this regard, testing for CMV IgG antibody avidity before and after urea denaturation may prove useful. In acute infection the IgG antibody produced has low affinity for CMV antigens, whereas with reactivation or reinfection, the antibody present has high avidity. Studies have confirmed that the great majority of women with IgM antibodies detected in the first serologic test available during pregnancy actually have been infected at least 3 months prior to pregnancy (27,42). Antibody avidity testing is not yet widely available.

Viral isolation from urine, saliva, or blood samples in human fibroblast cultures accurately identifies infection, but requires 2 to 6 weeks to produce results. Recent modifications of conventional tissue culture techniques using monoclonal antibodies against the early antigen of CMV allow detection in as little as 24 hours with only a modest decrease in sensitivity (43). However, viral isolation does not differentiate between acute and recurrent infection, and a single sample from an infected individual may test negative. Therefore, its use is reserved for fetal or neonatal diagnosis.

Prenatal

Prenatal diagnosis is possible, but requires invasive techniques. Experience is still relatively limited and is based on case reports and small series of patients with presumed primary infection. Many of these patients were referred because of known fetal abnormalities, which may have biased results (26,44–54). Investigators have used amniocentesis, cordocentesis, or a combination of these techniques to obtain amniotic fluid or fetal blood samples for analysis.

Fetal blood culture has such low sensitivity that it cannot be recommended. The presence of CMV-specific IgM antibody in fetal blood can be used to diagnose infection, but it is generally not present until after 20 weeks' gestation and may be absent even in late gestation, despite congenital infection. A false-positive case has also been reported (51). Abnormal results on nonspecific tests such as thrombocytopenia, anemia, or elevated liver transaminases are only suggestive of infection. However, when infection is confirmed by other means, such abnormal results suggest that the fetus is affected and at risk for serious sequelae (47,52).

Analysis of amniotic fluid by viral culture or PCR is more accurate and less risky. If amniotic fluid tests positive, the fetus can be assumed to be infected and excreting virus into the urine. By using two sets of primers to amplify two different CMV genes, PCR sensitivity has improved such that it is more sensitive than viral culture. Donner and colleagues investigated 36 at-risk fetuses and were able to detect the presence of virus by PCR in amniotic fluid containing low quantities of virus for which culture results were negative (53). Infection was subsequently confirmed in these infants. Although the sensitivity of PCR was 100% and there were no false-positive results when patients were sampled beyond 21 weeks' gestation, the sensitivity of PCR before 21 weeks was only 45.4%. Culture was even less accurate, with a sensitivity of 18.2%. Thus, amniotic fluid sampling should be deferred until at least 21 weeks' gestation and at least 4 weeks after maternal serologic diagnosis (55). If the need to determine fetal infection prior to this time is compelling, and an amniocentesis is done, a negative result cannot exclude intrauterine infection and a repeat sample should be obtained 4 to 8 weeks later. It can take from weeks to months for transplacental transmission to occur. Thus, false-negative results can occur at any time of gestation. Contamination of the sample with even small amounts of maternal blood can lead to false-positive results. To date there is no evidence to suggest that amniocentesis can introduce an infection to the fetus, although this remains theoretically possible. Although amniotic fluid analysis can be used to detect fetal infection, it cannot be used to predict to what degree the fetus is affected or to determine a prognosis.

Neonatal

Congenital CMV infections should be suspected in any newborn exhibiting signs of congenital infection or whose mother has had a possible primary infection during pregnancy. Virus isolation from urine, saliva, or cord blood in tissue culture during the first 2 weeks of life has been the most effective diagnostic technique. IgM serology is also of value, but is not as sensitive and cannot be relied upon as the sole technique. PCR methodology continues to improve and has been used successfully to detect CMV in neonates. It requires only a small sample, and infectious virus is not necessary (56). It can provide results comparable with or even superior to tissue culture techniques. A positive PCR test result on neonatal cerebrospinal fluid indicates that the infant is at high risk for abnormal neurologic development.

Management

Maternal screening for primary CMV infection is currently not recommended (42,57,58) for several reasons. To be of use, documentation of seronegativity would require serial samples in the first half of pregnancy to exclude seroconversion. There is no evidence that this practice is cost effective. Instruction regarding hygiene and sanitation practices that decrease rates of primary infection can be given to all patients and do not require knowledge of a woman's serostatus. No vaccine is available. Available serologic testing for primary infection is of questionable accuracy. CMV-specific IgM tests have not been evaluated as screening tools. IgM is present for several months (typically 8 but as long as 18 months) after an acute infection and may be present during reactivation as well. Detection of IgM antibody is suggestive of, but does not confirm, an acute infection, nor does failure to detect IgM entirely exclude infection. All other tests, including PCR, have even lower sensitivity and specificity for diagnosing acute maternal infection. A woman who is seropositive must make the difficult decision as to whether to proceed with additional testing to determine if the fetus is infected, which usually involves invasive procedures with their associated small, but finite, risks of fetal-maternal injury or pregnancy loss. This decision is made more difficult by the knowledge that she cannot be sure that her fetus is at risk (her infection may antedate pregnancy), and that even if at risk, the majority of infants will not be infected (Fig. 45-1). Because fewer than 25% of infected fetuses will be affected (i.e., symptomatic at birth or develop subsequent disabilities), it is difficult to advise a patient how to proceed if fetal infection is documented. There is currently no therapy available to prevent fetal damage, and

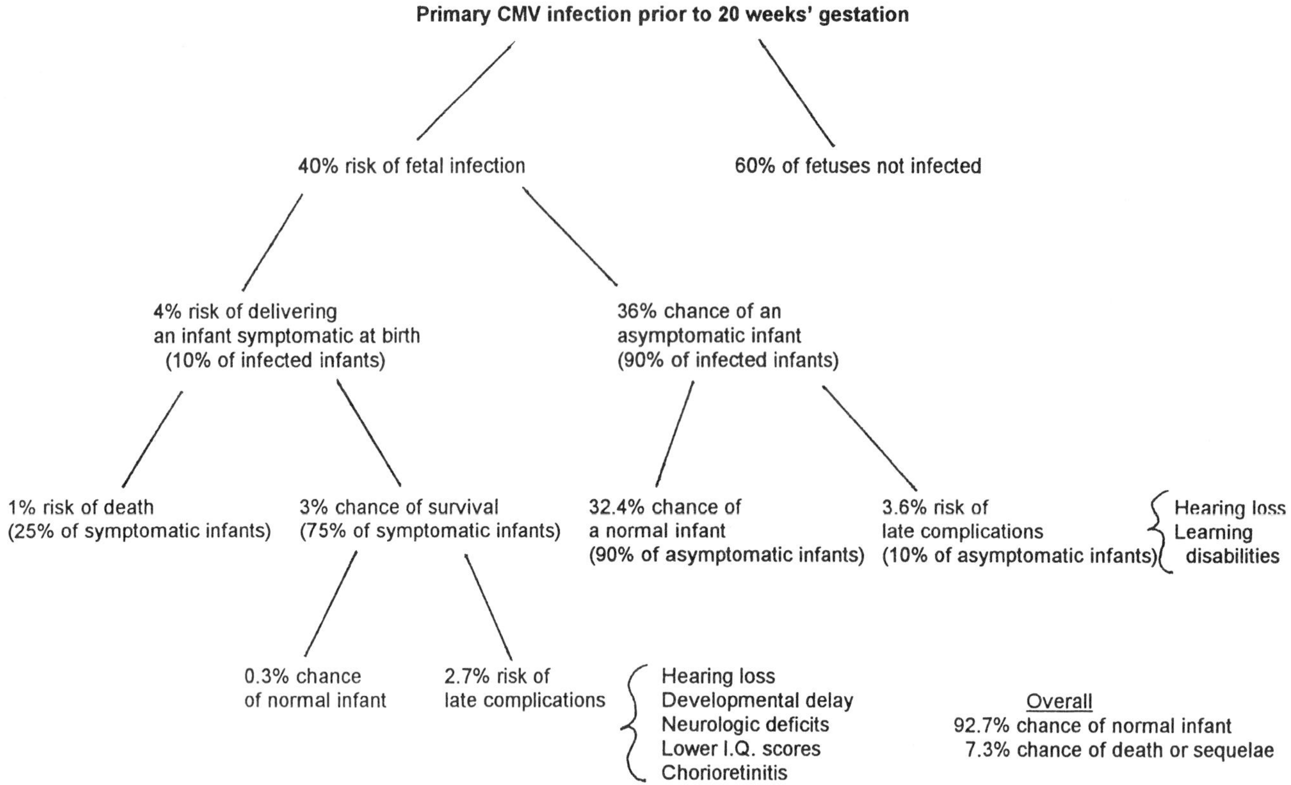

FIG. 45-1. Risk of delivering an affected infant for women with primary CMV infection during pregnancy.

pregnancy termination is the only alternative to expectant management.

On occasion, a woman with a known exposure may present with an acute illness consistent with primary CMV, which is subsequently confirmed by seroconversion. Alternatively, she may present with a positive serology for IgM obtained because the patient felt her occupation placed her at risk. In these situations, a thorough discussion of the risks and benefits of additional testing is warranted. Possible management options are presented in Figure 45-2. Options include pregnancy termination, expectant management, or an attempt to determine whether the fetus is affected using ultrasonography or amniocentesis.

There is insufficient information on which to base recommendations regarding termination of pregnancy after a primary infection in the first half of gestation. At least 90% of aborted fetuses would have developed normally; the patient must decide what is an acceptable risk. She must decide whether she is willing to undergo the risks of an invasive procedure or to proceed with pregnancy termination on the basis of nondefinitive information regarding neonatal prognosis. If a woman chooses to proceed with amniocentesis, the option of a cordocentesis to obtain fetal blood at the same time may be discussed, but it is uncertain whether enough additional information would be obtained to justify the increased risk and cost associated with this procedure. On occasion a patient with normal ultrasonographic but positive amniotic fluid PCR results may decide whether or not to continue a pregnancy based on the results of fetal liver enzyme and complete blood count. *In utero* treatment of the fetus with antiviral therapy such as ganciclovir or foscarnet is theoretically possible. Ganciclovir has been used with some success in neonates who have CMV infection (59), but considerable drug toxicity can be encountered. In animal models, ganciclovir is mutagenic, teratogenic, and carcinogenic. Nicolini and colleagues were unable to prevent a fetus from becoming infected by using cordocentesis to administer ganciclovir (54). Its use must be considered investigational. At delivery, a cord blood sample can be obtained and set aside for use by the neonatologist for diagnosing congenital CMV. There are no data to indicate how long conception should be delayed after a primary infection.

Prevention

In addition to using hygienic measures to prevent primary infection, other methods of possibly preventing fetal infection or damage include administration of hyperimmune globulin and vaccination. To date there are no controlled studies to support the use of passive immunization with hyperimmune plasma or globulin after primary infection. Vaccine trials using CMV surface glycoproteins rather than live, attenuated virus are currently

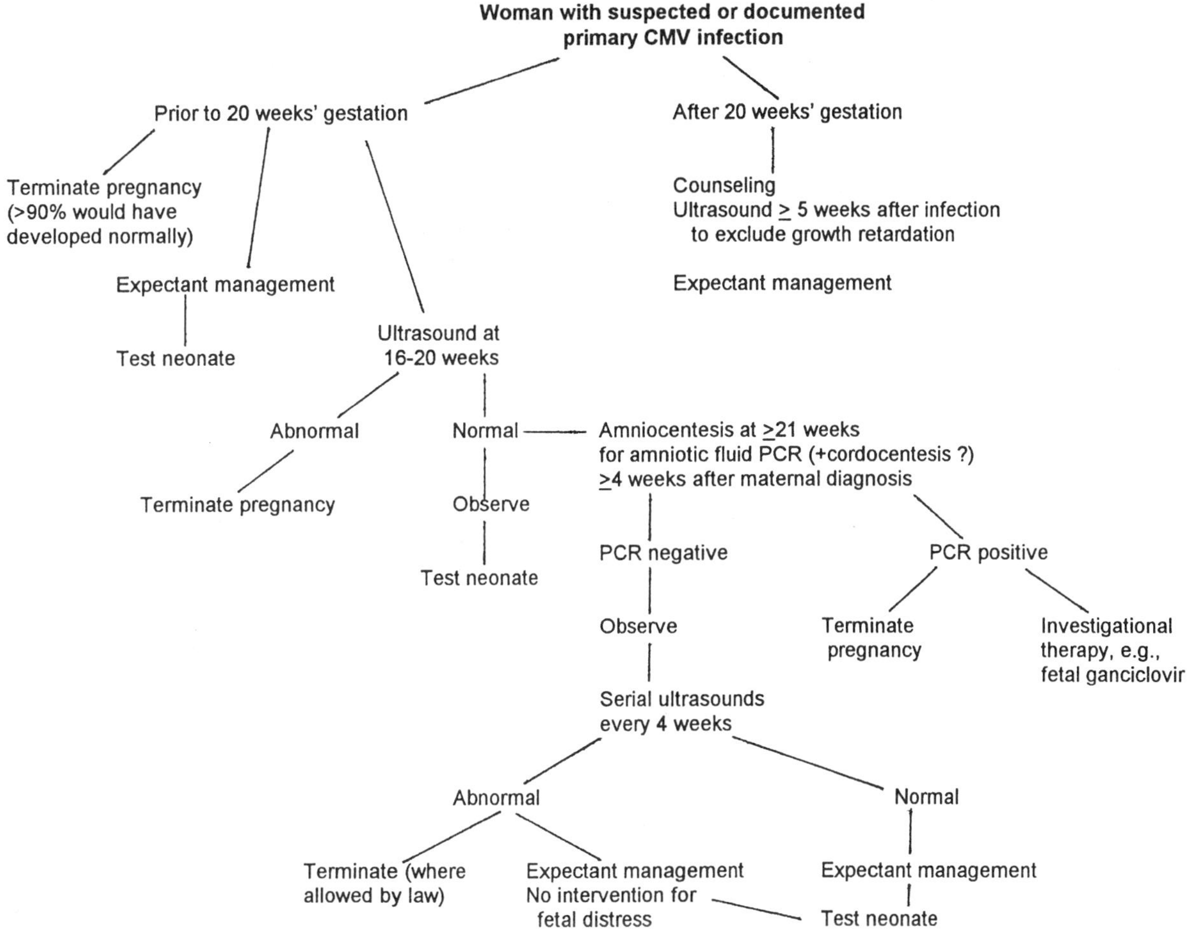

FIG. 45-2. Management options for women with presumed primary CMV infection.

being conducted (60). Such vaccines avoid the possibility of reactivation of the vaccine virus during pregnancy or any oncogenic potential. However, these vaccines are not available for general use. Maternal infection may result if a seronegative woman receives blood products from a seropositive donor. If transfusion is necessary during pregnancy, seronegative blood should be used whenever possible if the woman is known to be seronegative. If her serostatus is unknown, consideration should be given to using seronegative blood during the first two trimesters.

VARICELLA-ZOSTER VIRUS

Definition

The varicella-zoster virus (VZV) is a DNA herpes virus responsible for two illnesses. Primary infection results in chickenpox and its associated complications of varicella pneumonia, hepatitis, and encephalitis. Reactivation of latent virus results in zoster (shingles) and complications such as postherpetic neuralgia and ophthalmic zoster with central nervous system involvement (61). When primary infection occurs during pregnancy, the virus may rarely be transmitted to the fetus, resulting in defects known as the congenital varicella syndrome. Maternal chickenpox within 5 days before and 2 days after delivery can cause severe disease and death in the newborn.

Incidence

The virus is highly contagious and most children are exposed before adolescence. Fewer than 10% of cases occur in patients over the age of 15, but almost 25% of the fatal cases belong to this age group (62). In temperate climates, at least 90% of women of childbearing age are immune, but because of the prevalence of the virus in the community, it is possible for a susceptible woman to come into contact with an infected individual during her pregnancy, particularly if she has young children. In household settings, attack rates of up to 90% have been reported following infection of one member of the family (63). Still, chickenpox in pregnancy is uncommon, occurring in 1 to 7 per 10,000 pregnancies or an estimated 3,000 to 10,000 cases annually in the United States (64,65). The recent introduction of the OKA vaccine is expected to reduce greatly the possibility of maternal infection in much the same way that the rubella vaccine has reduced congenital rubella in developed countries (66).

Pathogenesis

Varicella-zoster virus is transmitted by infected respiratory secretions and contact with skin lesions. An individual is infectious from 2 days prior to the onset of lesions until the lesions have crusted 6 to 10 days later (66). The incubation period is 10 to 21 days (mean 15 days), which permits administration of passive immune globulin within the first 4 days of exposure to prevent, or at least ameliorate, infection. After initial replication in the nasopharynx, the virus is seeded to the reticuloendothelial cells during a transient primary viremia. VZV is then disseminated by mononuclear cells to the skin and sometimes to other organs.

Following the initial infection, the virus becomes dormant in dorsal root ganglia. An intact immune system is required to maintain latency of the virus; episodic, asymptomatic replication of the virus occurs associated with periodic increases in VZV-specific IgM antibodies (61). Cellular immunity is also essential. As the host ages and the cellular immune response diminishes, the incidence of herpes zoster increases (61). Similarly, infants who have been infected *in utero* or in early infancy may develop an inadequate response due to an immature immune system and are at increased risk for zoster (67). Although pregnancy may influence the maternal immune response, zoster is rare in pregnant women and does not affect the fetus (68–71). The virus is confined to the nerve roots of a specific ganglion and neither systemic nor transplacental spread occurs.

Clinical Manifestations

Following infection, a prodrome of fever, malaise, headache, and anorexia may precede the onset of rash by 1 to 2 days. Prodromal symptoms are more prominent in adults than in children. The rash presents as pruritic macules on the trunk, face, and scalp and spreads centripetally to involve the extremities. Over the course of a week to 10 days, the lesions progress to papules, vesicles, pustules, and finally crusted lesions (66). Lesions may become secondarily infected with bacteria and cause a local cellulitis; most resolve without producing scarring. Although typically there are 250 to 500 lesions, in some cases there may be fewer than 10. In this situation, the diagnosis may be missed, accounting for why some patients who deny a history of chickenpox are found to be immune. If fever is present, it lasts only 1 to 3 days. In addition to the skin, the organ systems most commonly involved are the lungs and liver, but any system may be involved.

The most common serious complication in adults is pneumonia; 30% to 50% of adults with acute varicella may develop pneumonia, although this is probably an overestimation because adverse outcomes are more likely to be reported (72,73). Debate persists regarding whether pregnancy predisposes to the development of pneumonia or increases its severity (74,75). Pneumonia does appear to be more common in the second half of pregnancy, with most deaths having occurred in the third trimester (73, 76,77). This may be related to altered immune function or physiologic changes in pulmonary function induced by pregnancy.

Pneumonia presents several days after the onset of the rash and is preceded by a dry cough. Symptoms may remain mild or progress to tachypnea, shortness of breath, chest tightness or pain, hemoptysis, and cyanosis. Typically, diffuse, nodular peribronchial infiltrates are seen on radiographs (74). Pneumonia is often life threatening; up to 40% of gravidas died prior to the use of antiviral chemotherapy and advanced pulmonary care (73). Infrequent complications of VZV infection include cerebellar ataxia, encephalitis (which may progress to coma), arthritis, nephritis, pericarditis, and myocarditis (78). Reye syndrome is generally limited to those under age 15 and has become rare since its relationship to the use of aspirin became apparent.

Infected gravidas are more likely to experience preterm labor and delivery, perhaps due to the production of inflammatory mediators (73,79). There does not seem to be an increased risk of spontaneous abortion (70,80). Although there have been reported cases of placental abruption, there is no evidence that this complication occurs with greater frequency than in the general population.

Effects on the Fetus and Neonate

Congenital Varicella Syndrome

Women with primary VZV infection during pregnancy can transmit the virus to the fetus in up to 25% of cases, but the infection is usually asymptomatic (70,81,82). However, some of these asymptomatic infants will subsequently develop herpes zoster during infancy, reflecting failure of the immature immune system to prevent reactivation of latent virus (67). Transplacental infection resulting in birth defects or stillbirth was first described in 1947, but occurs uncommonly (65,68,70,79,83–88). The incidence of congenital anomalies is so low that studies have been unable to demonstrate a statistically significant increase associated with maternal varicella (64). Findings associated with the congenital varicella syndrome include cutaneous scars and cicatricial lesions of the extremities in 70% of cases, limb hypoplasia, malformed or absent digits, muscle atrophy, cataracts, microophthalmia, Horner syndrome, and chorioretinitis.

The skin lesions are in a dermatomal distribution with limb hypoplasia arising distal to the skin involvement (Fig. 45-3). This prompted one group of investigators to postulate that the congenital varicella syndrome is not due to fetal varicella, but to the development of herpes zoster *in utero* (89). About half of affected neonates have neurologic involvement evidenced by cerebral calcifications, cortical atrophy, bowel or bladder sphincter dysfunction, and psychomotor retardation.

Transmission can occur at any gestational age, but symptomatic cases are largely confined to the first half of pregnancy, typically between 8 and 20 weeks' gestation. Rarely, the congenital varicella syndrome may follow late second-trimester infections (90,91). The combined results of seven studies that prospectively followed over 1,100 women with varicella during the first 20 weeks of pregnancy revealed that of the 1,092 liveborn infants studied, 10 infants had the congenital varicella syndrome (65,68,70,79,81,87,92) (Table 45-2). The risk of embryopathy was 0.9%. If suspected cases among those pregnancies that ended in spontaneous abortion, therapeutic abortion, or intrauterine death are included, the risk was 13 of 1,175 (1.1%). Confining the analysis to the first trimester, the average risk derived from the combined results of five prospective studies was 0.6% (5 of 675 liveborn infants). This may represent an overestimation of risk during the first trimester because some of these infants did not have serologic confirmation of congenital infection and the abnormalities reported were sometimes minor (e.g., horizontal nystagmus). None of the 518 infants whose mothers were infected after 20 weeks' gestation were affected, although these infants remained at risk for developing zoster in infancy. The risk of embryopathy appears to be fairly uniform for the first 20 weeks of gestation, but the above results suggest that it is somewhat greater when maternal infection occurs in the early second trimester (13 to 20 weeks) (68).

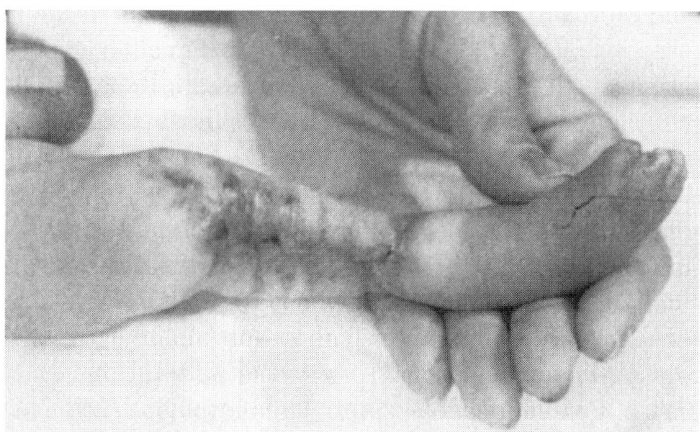

FIG. 45-3. Atrophy of the right lower extremity with bony defects and cutaneous scarring in a neonate with congenital varicella syndrome. (From Paryami SG, Arvin AM. Intrauterine infection with varicella-zoster virus after maternal varicella. N Engl J Med 1986;314:1542–1546.)

TABLE 45-2. *Frequency of the congenital varicella syndrome in live-born infants in relation to the gestational age when maternal infection occurred*

Study	Fetal risk (no. infected/no. liveborn)		
	1st trimester	Prior to 20 weeks[a]	after 20 weeks
Paryani, 1986 (70)	1/11	—	0/16[b]
Balducci, 1992 (65)	0/36	—	—
Jones, 1994 (87)	1/110	2/156	0/13[b]
Pastuszak, 1994 (79)	1/49	1/86	0/14
Enders, 1994 (68)	1/469	7/816	0/475
Liesnard, 1994 (81)	—	0/17	—
Dufour, 1996 (92)	—	0/17	—
Total	5/675 (0.6%)	10/1092 (0.9%)	0/518

[a]First trimester + second trimester < 20 weeks' gestation.
[b]Third trimester only.

Perinatal Varicella

Women who develop varicella within 5 days prior to or 2 days following delivery will not have sufficient time to produce antibodies that can cross the placenta to protect the fetus and newborn. Near the time of delivery, 25% to 50% of maternal infections will result in fetal infections manifested during the first 10 days of life (66,70). These infants are at risk for developing life-threatening systemic disease. If untreated, the mortality rate can exceed 30% (93). If maternal infection occurs between 3 weeks and 5 days before delivery, perinatal chickenpox may occur and the neonate may develop skin lesions, but the infection is not serious due to protection from transplacental passage of maternal antibody. Mothers who develop symptoms more than 2 days after delivery may infect their newborns postnatally (usually via respiratory secretions), but the illness is usually mild.

Laboratory Findings and Diagnosis

The lesions of varicella are sufficiently characteristic that the diagnosis of chickenpox is usually established based on clinical findings. If there is doubt, viral isolation in human tissue culture can yield results in 3 to 4 days from a sample of fluid or scrapings obtained from the base of a new vesicle (61). However, viral cultivation is difficult and is not widely available. Multinucleated giant cells and epithelial cells containing eosinophilic intranuclear inclusions can be seen in samples from the base of vesicular lesions or sputum from patients with varicella pneumonia. Commercial antigen detection tests using a monoclonal antibody to VZV that is conjugated to fluorescein are also available. Alternatively, PCR technology is now offered in some research laboratories, although there is no commercial test available. The white blood cell count in patients with uncomplicated chickenpox or zoster is normal. If there is hepatic involvement, liver enzyme elevations may be present. A mononuclear pleocytosis can be found in the cerebrospinal fluid in patients with encephalitis or zoster involving the cranial nerves.

Serologic testing is used both to document seroconversion and, hence, confirm primary infection and to determine whether a patient is susceptible to infection (94–97). Antibody to VZV develops within 2 weeks of onset of varicella and persists for years (98). The four tests most frequently used are ELISA, fluorescent antibody to VZV membrane antigen (FAMA), radioimmunoassay (RIA), and latex agglutination (LA). Complement fixation testing is unreliable for determining immune status because titers decline rapidly and may be undetectable after 1 year (66). Although FAMA and RIA are sensitive tests, they are time consuming and unsuitable for most diagnostic laboratories. The ELISA and LA tests are readily available and both are highly sensitive and specific (95,97).

To make the diagnosis of congenital varicella syndrome, the following criteria have been suggested:

1. Clinical, serologic, or virologic confirmation of maternal VZV infection during pregnancy
2. Skin lesions on the infant corresponding to a dermatome distribution
3. Immunologic confirmation of intrauterine VZV infection (persistence of IgG antibody, identification of IgM specific antibody) or the development of herpes zoster in the first few months of life without preceding chickenpox (99).

Varicella zoster virus has been detected using PCR on tissue samples from stillborn infants with the congenital varicella syndrome in the research setting (100,101), but has not been isolated in cell cultures from any affected infant, suggesting that fetal infection is not persistent.

Preconceptional Counseling

Women presenting for preconceptional counseling or their first obstetric visit should be routinely queried regarding a previous history of varicella infection (102). A positive history can be accepted as evidence of immunity; the chance of nonimmunity in this scenario is less than 3% (66). Women without a history of chickenpox should be tested serologically for the presence of VZV-specific IgG antibody. Serologic testing is cost effective (103,104)—studies indicate that 50% to 80% of patients who deny previous infection are actually immune, whereas over 90% of those who are uncertain of their past history are immune (105–107). However, the number of susceptible adults in the United States appears to be increasing due to immigration from tropical countries where childhood varicella infection is less common (108).

Nonpregnant patients who are seronegative should be immunized using two doses of live, attenuated varicella vaccine 4 to 8 weeks apart (66). In adults the seroconversion rate is 99% after two doses. The vaccine is well tolerated, but a sparse generalized maculopapular or vesicular rash can occur within 1 month in about 5% of vaccinees. Vaccination greatly reduces, but does not eliminate, the chance of contracting varicella. However, illnesses associated with vaccine failure are significantly attenuated, and most patients are afebrile. Transmission of vaccine virus from healthy vaccinees to others is rare, but has been reported. A case report has described transmission of vaccine virus from a healthy 12-month-old infant to his pregnant mother (109). She had an elective abortion at 7 to 8 weeks' gestation; examination of the fetal tissue showed no evidence of virus. The vaccine should not be given to immunosuppressed women such as those infected with HIV. However, varicella vaccine use in other family members is not contraindicated.

Pregnancy is a contraindication for vaccination, and it is recommended that conception be avoided for 1 month after each dose of vaccine. To date, there are no reports of fetal damage as a consequence of inadvertent vaccination during, or in the 3 months preceding, pregnancy. A registry has been established by Merck & Co., Inc. in collaboration with the Centers for Disease Control and Prevention (CDC) to follow outcomes of such pregnancies (110). Women whose nonimmune status is first discovered during pregnancy should avoid exposure to infected persons and receive varicella vaccine postpartum. Vaccination should be delayed for 5 months if the patient has received peripartum blood, plasma, or immunoglobulin. Most live vaccines either have not been demonstrated to be secreted in breast milk; if secreted, they produce asymptomatic infection. Breastfeeding is not considered a contraindication to VZV vaccination (66).

Treatment

Women who present following exposure to varicella may be managed as outlined in Figure 45-4. Those who give a history of prior chickenpox can be reassured that they are not at risk. It is not cost effective to perform serologic screening. Repeat varicella in immune women during pregnancy has been described, but it is extremely rare and there are no reports of either congenital varicella or varicella pneumonia in this scenario (111).

If the woman denies having had chickenpox and confirmatory serologic testing was not performed previously, it should be performed immediately. The presence of VZV-specific IgG antibody within a week of exposure reflects prior immunity. If the woman has no antibody, administration of varicella-zoster immune globu-

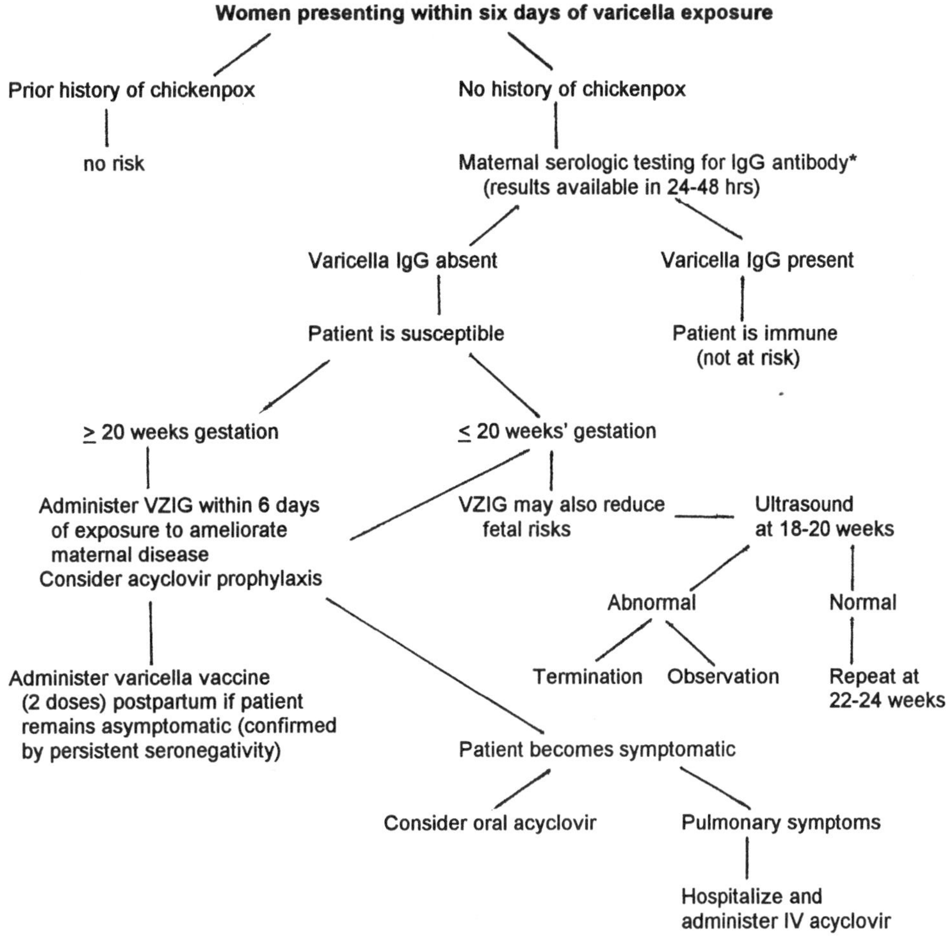

FIG. 45-4. Management options for women exposed to varicella during pregnancy.

lin (VZIG) will ameliorate, if not prevent, the clinical features of varicella (66,68,71). Recent studies using acyclovir prophylaxis for household contacts of varicella suggest that oral acyclovir reduces the rate of clinical varicella by at least two thirds (86,112), but there have been no studies in pregnant women, and VZIG remains the agent of choice. Ideally, VZIG should be given within 96 hours of exposure (113). Although its administration is generally not recommended after 6 days (144 hours) (114), the United Kingdom Health Departments suggest that VZIG may provide some benefit even if given up to 10 days postexposure (115). If serologic tests to confirm susceptibility cannot be completed within 96 hours of exposure, VZIG should be given prophylactically, but it should be remembered that VZIG is costly and in short supply. It has no role once symptoms appear. The recommended dose is 625 units (five vials) intramuscularly for women weighing over 100 pounds and four vials if under this weight (66). The use of VZIG can prolong the incubation period of varicella to as long as 35 days.

There is evidence to suggest that VZIG may also reduce the risk of fetal infection. In a series of 97 women who developed varicella despite the administration of VZIG, there were no cases of congenital varicella syndrome. Only one infant (1%) had detectable VZV-specific IgM, a significantly lower rate than for the offspring of untreated women (12%) (68).

A woman who develops clinical chickenpox may be observed as an outpatient and receive supportive care with antipruritic and analgesic agents. She should be watched closely for evidence of disseminated disease, particularly respiratory involvement, and instructed to report for evaluation at the first sign of coughing or shortness of breath. Many experts recommend treating all infected gravidas with acyclovir (a pregnancy category C drug) within the first 24 hours of rash onset to reduce the chance of developing a pneumonia or other serious complication (116). Studies in adolescents and adults have demonstrated a significant reduction of days of fever, time to crusting, and time out of school or work in patients treated within the first 24 to 48 hours (117–119). Acyclovir has been used safely in thousands of women during pregnancy, but there are no data from controlled studies to support its use in uncomplicated varicella infections. There also is no evidence that acyclovir influences the incidence or severity of fetal infection, although therapeutic levels are achieved in the fetus. If elected, the oral dosage is 800 mg, five times daily; acyclovir is less active against VZV than against herpes simplex, and larger doses are required (120). Oral famciclovir has similar efficacy but is less well studied in pregnancy (121).

Acyclovir should be given to all women with infection involving organs other than the skin. In particular, there is considerable evidence that treatment of varicella pneumonia with intravenous acyclovir significantly improves outcomes (73,76,77,122). In a series of 21 patients treated with acyclovir, only three patients (14%) died, compared with 36% of untreated historic controls (73). The recommended dose of acyclovir is 10 to 15 mg/kg every 8 hours intravenously for 7 days. Patients with varicella pneumonia need to be treated aggressively; as many as half will require ventilatory support. In severe cases, acute respiratory distress syndrome develops and has required extracorporeal membrane oxygenation (122).

Herpes zoster requires no specific treatment in pregnancy. It is not associated with adverse fetal or maternal outcomes, which would justify the routine use of acyclovir, with one exception. Patients with lesions on the forehead or tip of the nose may develop ophthalmic zoster, which can result in serious central nervous system involvement, coma, and death. Acyclovir should be initiated immediately in all patients with zoster involving the ophthalmic branch of the trigeminal nerve to reduce the risk of these, and serious ocular, complications.

Management of the Fetus and Neonate

The congenital varicella syndrome is sufficiently rare that, in contrast to perinatal rubella infection, termination cannot be routinely recommended at any time during gestation. Prenatal diagnosis using PCR on amniotic fluid (123), chorionic villi (124), or fetal tissue (100) or using serologic testing of fetal blood (125) can indicate whether there has been fetal infection, but not whether the fetus has the congenital varicella syndrome. Ultrasonography has been used to identify correctly some infected fetuses (126). The presence of certain sonographic abnormalities (ascites, hydrops, liver calcifications) does not preclude a favorable outcome (123). However, the presence of a limb abnormality is associated with a poor prognosis (50% are brain damaged or die) and some patients choose pregnancy termination in this situation. Abnormalities typically are not apparent until several weeks after maternal infection but are often observed by 20 weeks' gestation. Reported findings include polyhydramnios, hydrops, hydrocephaly, microcephaly, limb abnormalities and hepatic calcifications (Fig. 45-5). A baseline scan obtained at 18 to 20 weeks' gestation and repeated at 22 to 24 weeks' gestation may permit identification of the most seriously infected fetuses without the risks associated with invasive testing. Unfortunately, the scan can be normal with a severely affected fetus.

To avoid severe varicella of the newborn, delivery should be delayed until 5 to 7 days after the onset of maternal illness to allow passive transfer of antibody. If contractions begin during this window and the patient presents while in early labor, consideration may be given to the use of tocolytic agents to delay labor and delivery. If delay is impossible, 125 units VZIG should be administered immediately to the newborn (66,127). Treatment with VZIG is only 50% effective in preventing the disease, although it may decrease the overall severity (128). Fatal neonatal varicella has been reported despite the appropriate use of VZIG, leading some researchers to recommend doubling the dose (129,130). Direct contact between the newborn and maternal lesions should be avoided, but breastfeeding is permissible in the absence of vesicles on the nipple or the immediately surrounding area (131).

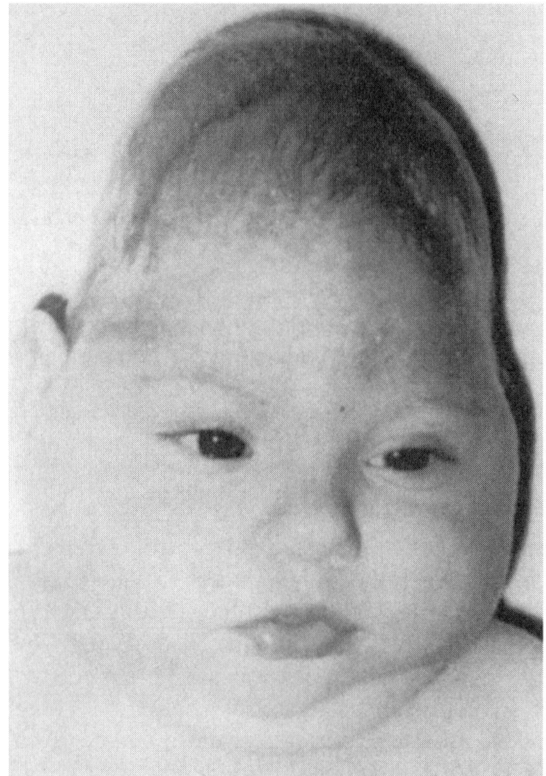

FIG. 45-5. Patient with congenital varicella syndrome at 5 months of age demonstrating severe microcephaly. (From Scheffer IE, Baraitser M, Brett EM. Severe microcephaly associated with congenital varicella infection. Dev Med Child Neurol 1991;33:916–920.)

PARVOVIRUS B19

Definition

Parvovirus B19 is a small, single-stranded DNA virus that is the only known pathogenic parvovirus in humans. It was discovered serendipitously in 1974 when Cossart and colleagues found a serum parvovirus-like particle while evaluating serum samples for hepatitis B surface antigen (132). It is responsible for erythema infectiosum (EI), or fifth disease, a common childhood illness, and aplastic crises in patients with sickle cell anemia. Most importantly for the obstetrician, maternal parvovirus infection has been linked to the development of nonimmune hydrops and fetal death (133–136). By adulthood, at least 50% of women in the United States are immune, having been infected as children most often between the ages of 4 and 11 years (137–140). The virus is spread primarily by the respiratory route, but also can be transmitted by hand-to-mouth contact with infected secretions or by the administration of infected blood products. In temperate climates, infections are most common from late winter to early summer, peaking from March to May (138). The virus is highly contagious, and epidemics occur every 4 to 5 years.

Incidence

In women of childbearing age, B19 seroconversion occurs at an annual rate of 1.4%, which is equivalent to a 1.1% risk of seroconversion during pregnancy when adjusted for the normal duration of gestation (141). During epidemics, the rate is much higher. The type and extent of exposure determines the risk of maternal acquisition. For example, Adler and colleagues found that in the absence of an epidemic, the annual seroconversion rates were 0.42% for hospital workers and 2.93% for school employees (142). However, during epidemics, attack rates for workers with close contact with elementary school–aged children were 20% to 30% (143). Fifty percent of nonimmune household members will become infected when exposed to an infected member of the family (144).

Pathogenesis

Following entry into the host through mucosal surfaces, there is a period of viremia and dissemination of the virus to the erythroid progenitor cells and the bone marrow. Subsequent development of a rash or arthropathy coincides with the production of anti-B19 IgM and IgG antibodies, suggesting an immune-complex disease as the basis for these symptoms. Parvovirus B19 has a predilection for the hematopoietic system, where it binds to a specific cellular receptor, erythrocyte P antigen. In addition to erythroid progenitor cells, it infects endothelial cells and the myocardium. To a lesser degree, leukocyte and megakaryocyte lines may be affected. Acute anemia can occur in normal patients infected with B19, but there is usually sufficient hematopoietic reserve that symptoms do not occur (145). However, in patients with underlying chronic hemolytic processes such as thalassemia or sickle cell disease, a transient aplastic crisis may result (146). Severe anemia, decreased reticulocytosis, and absent erythroid precursors in bone marrow are prominent features of this condition. Occasionally this process progresses to death.

Pregnancy does not adversely affect the course of parvovirus infection. Conversely, infection sometimes may have a profound effect on the course of pregnancy. In most cases, the virus is not passed to the fetus, and the pregnancy continues undisturbed. In one fourth to one third of cases, the virus is transmitted transplacentally to the fetus without detrimental effect (147,148). Unfortunately, in up to 5% of maternal infections, fetal transmission results in transient aplastic crisis, high-output failure, hydrops, and fetal death (147,149–152). The fetus has a rapidly expanding red blood cell volume and a shortened red blood cell life span (153). The fetus thus quickly becomes anemic if erythrocyte production abruptly stops. Infection of the fetal myocardium results in myocarditis, which predisposes to the development of heart failure (154,155). Parvovirus B19 may be responsible for 10% to 15% of all cases of nonimmune hydrops (156,157).

Fetal loss can occur at any time during gestation, even at term (158), but the second-trimester fetus is particularly vulnerable (148,152). Hematopoiesis does not play as great a role in fetal development during the first trimester, and a statistically significant increase in early spontaneous abortions has not been demonstrated (148). During the early second trimester, the fetus is unable to produce its own IgM antibodies, and transplacental transport of maternal protective antibody is minimal. In a recent prospective study, 93% of the fetal deaths occurred before 20 weeks' gestation (148).

Clinical Manifestations

Parvovirus has a relatively short incubation period of 5 to 14 days. EI is the most common clinically distinct manifestation of infection. In children, EI is often associated with fever, headache, coryza, and gastrointestinal symptoms (diarrhea and nausea). This is followed in 2 to 5 days by the classic, red, slapped-cheek facial rash. Within 1 to 4 days, an erythematous, maculopapular rash may appear on the trunk and limbs, and occasionally involves the soles and palms. Rash is frequently pruritic and may recur in subsequent weeks after stress, exercise, or exposure to heat or cold. In adults, at least half of infections are asymptomatic (159). However, when carefully followed prospectively, only 33% of 52 infected women were entirely asymptomatic (140). In symptomatic cases a nonspecific prodromal illness is followed only occasionally by the facial rash, which may last just a few hours. The rash, and hence the disease, is even more likely to go unrecognized in black patients (144). Joint symptoms occur uncommonly in children, but approximately 50% to 80% of adult women develop polyarthropathy, particularly in the hands, wrists, ankles, and knees (159). Pain, stiffness, and swelling usually last 1 to 3 weeks, but may persist for months. The symptoms can sometimes be confused with those of Lyme disease. Transient, acute anemia has been described in normal patients infected with B19; in immunosuppressed patients, however, chronic transfusion-dependent anemia may result.

In general, the course of pregnancy is unaffected by parvovirus infection. The incidences of preterm labor and delivery do not appear to be increased (148). Pregnancy-induced hypertension and preeclampsia have been described in association with maternal B19 infection and fetal hydrops (135,160–162). It has yet to be determined whether this represents an increased risk for these conditions compared with uninfected women. In one case, maternal preeclampsia resolved following spontaneous resolution of the fetal hydrops (160).

Fetal Manifestations

Parvovirus B19 has not been documented to be teratogenic (148,163–165). There are occasional reports of fetal abnormalities following maternal infection; ocular structural abnormalities were described in an 11-week embryo from a therapeutic abortion (166), and a case of multiple defects, including bilateral cleft lip, micrognathia, and webbed joints, was reported in a 17-week fetus (167). Such reports do not represent any specific pattern of abnormalities, and they do not exceed the expected frequency of congenital anomalies for a normal population. A case report of a child who developed encephalitis and permanent neurologic sequelae following EI raises the possibility that this could occur *in utero* (168). Indeed, a preliminary report describing three infants with severe central nervous system abnormalities including cerebral atrophy, ventricular enlargement, cranial calcifications, delayed myelination, and developmental delays after maternal B19 infection suggests that this concern may be real (169). Two additional infants with hydrocephalus have been reported, emphasizing the need for additional studies to determine the role of infection in causing fetal damage (170).

The risk of fetal growth restriction may be slightly increased (148,171). In one study, the birth weight of 11 of 142 live-born infants (8%) was less than the third percentile for gestational age (148). Additional series are needed to confirm this. If hydrops develops, this may be seen on ultrasonographic examination along with poly- or oligohydramnios. At birth, laxity of the abdominal wall has been found as a consequence of hydrops (160,172). Residual pleural or ascitic fluid can compromise pulmonary function. Most infants do well, and in general, follow-up of neonates has failed to detect developmental abnormalities. Occasionally infection persists after birth and can result in a chronic anemia and hypogammaglobulinemia that may necessitate blood transfusions and is poorly responsive to immunoglobulin therapy (156,173).

Diagnosis

Diagnosis based on clinical characteristics is often inaccurate, and culture techniques are not often useful because the period of viremia is brief, lasting only 1 to 3 days (174). The clinical manifestations of rash and joint pain in patients with EI are secondary to immune complex formation; hence, patients do not come to medical attention until after the period of viremia (156). Diagnosis is best made using serologic testing for specific IgG and IgM antibodies. IgM antibodies start to appear within 10 to 12 days of inoculation, just before the onset of symptoms (174). IgG antibodies appear about 2 weeks after inoculation and persist for years. IgG antibodies provide protective immunity; second infections with B19 have not been documented in immunocompetent individuals.

A woman exposed to EI should undergo immediate serologic testing using an ELISA for specific IgG and IgM. Detectable IgG in the absence of IgM antibody indicates prior immunity. A woman who has neither IgG nor IgM antibodies is at risk and should be retested after 3 weeks to determine whether seroconversion (and thus an acute infection) has occurred. A patient who has IgM antibodies but is IgG negative is presumed to have acquired infection within the past week, although false-positive IgM results are possible (175) and some patients never mount an IgG response (176). If both IgG and IgM are present on initial testing, the patient usually has been infected within the preceding 6 months, but specific IgM may be detected for up to 10 months in some patients (177). The exact timing of infection cannot be determined precisely. Immunocompromised women may not mount an antibody response to the virus, and PCR testing may be necessary to determine infection.

Fetal blood obtained at cordocentesis can be analyzed for B19-specific IgM, B19 DNA (using a PCR assay), or characteristic nuclear clearing and inclusions in nucleated red blood cells (154,178–181). B19 IgM determinations are relatively insensitive. IgM production is frequently not present until after 22 weeks' gestation, and most fetuses at risk for hydrops are seronegative. Unlike the adult, the fetus is incapable of mounting a brisk antibody response until relatively late in gestation. Therefore, it may be possible to recover virus in fetal blood for relatively long periods using PCR techniques (178,179). PCR also can be performed on amniotic fluid and appears to be the most sensitive and accurate means of testing for antenatal infection (178). Histologic examination of fetal blood or tissue is not reliable because findings are often absent in cases in which infection is documented by other techniques, whereas nuclear clearing may be seen in cases in which the fetus is known to be uninfected (182).

Management

Erythema infectiosum usually requires no treatment, and specific pharmacotherapy for parvovirus is unavailable. There are three clinical scenarios for which the obstetrician must make management decisions (Fig. 45-6):

1. The asymptomatic patient who presents with recent exposure to an infected individual should undergo immediate serologic testing to establish her immune status. While awaiting the results of testing, the woman may be informed that she has less than a 1% risk of fetal death after a major exposure and that her fetus is not otherwise at any significant risk for an adverse outcome.
2. A woman who presents with acute, symptomatic maternal B19 infection should also undergo serologic testing because B19 infection may be mimicked by other viral infections. IgM is detectable in more than 90% of cases of EI by the onset of rash. IgG is usually present within 1 week of the onset of illness (174).
3. A woman may present with a hydropic fetus, but deny any prior history of exposure or symptomatic illness. Absence of B19 IgG generally excludes parvovirus as the etiology, but the absence of IgM does not exclude recent infection. In some women, IgM may no longer be produced by the time hydrops is detected. Rarely, maternal serum may be negative for any specific anti-B19 antibodies despite positive fetal specimens (171,178).

If acute infection is confirmed by the test results, weekly sonograms over an 8-week period to search for early signs of fetal hydrops has been suggested (151). Most fetal losses occur within 6 weeks of onset of maternal symptoms, although fetal death occasionally occurs as late as 12 weeks or more after infection (151,172,183). In two series that used serial sonograms, none of 91 fetuses surveyed developed hydrops, suggesting that the yield may be insufficient to justify routine use (140,151). In most cases it is not necessary to determine whether the fetus has been infected to manage appropriately a pregnant woman who has been exposed to, or infected with, parvovirus B19. Invasive testing can be avoided. The

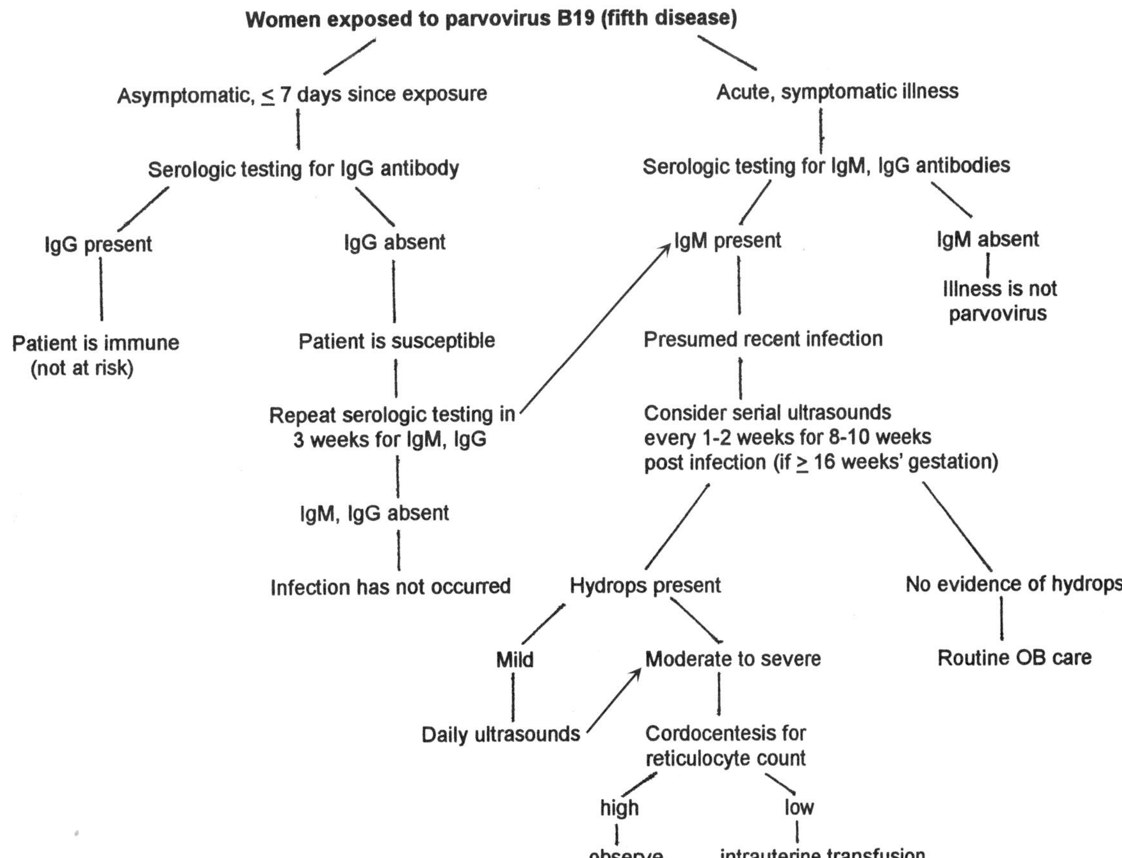

FIG. 45-6. Management options for women exposed to parvovirus B19 during pregnancy.

pregnancy can be evaluated for intracranial anatomy, evidence of placental thickening, and alterations in amniotic fluid volume, as well as for fetal skin and scalp edema, ascites, and pleural or pericardial effusions. If there is no evidence of hydrops, the pregnancy is expected to proceed uneventfully.

In several reports, an elevated maternal serum alphafetoprotein (MSAFP) level has antedated the development of hydrops by as long as 4 to 6 weeks (184,185). Some investigators have suggested that monitoring of MSAFP may predict those fetuses at highest risk. The sensitivity of MSAFP testing is unknown. Most laboratories have not established normal values for pregnancies less than 14 or more than 22 weeks' gestation, and MSAFP levels may be elevated for other reasons. A normal value may provide some reassurance but does not eliminate the need for surveillance; levels may be normal even when fetal disease is present (172). Conversely, an elevated MSAFP without other evidence of B19 infection is not an indication for B19-specific testing (186).

If hydrops develops, daily ultrasonographic monitoring is appropriate for following mild cases for evidence of deterioration in status. For moderate to severe hydrops, fetal blood sampling can be used to determine the hemoglobin, platelet count, and reticulocyte count. If the reticulocyte count is high, marrow aplasia is already in the resolution stage, and hydrops should resolve without therapy. The severely anemic fetus with a low reticulocyte count may benefit from an immediate transfusion. If feasible, intrauterine blood transfusion may be life-saving, particularly in pregnancies of less than 22 weeks' gestation. In a randomized, retrospective series of 38 hydropic fetuses, 12 of whom received intrauterine transfusions and 26 of whom did not, the odds of death for those who received blood was significantly less (odds ratio 0.14, 95% confidence interval 0.02–0.096) (187). However, one fourth of the transfused fetuses died despite this intervention. It is also possible for severe hydrops to resolve spontaneously over a period of 4 to 6 weeks without transfusion (160,172, 188). Thus, it is difficult to determine which fetuses will benefit from transfusion. Complications following cordocentesis include posttransfusion bleeding secondary to parvovirus-induced thrombocytopenia (180).

Digitalization may assist recovery if myocarditis plays a prominent role, but currently there are no guidelines for the use of digoxin in this setting. Maternal administration of high-dose intravenous immunoglobulin (IVIG) has been proposed as an alternative to fetal transfusion. It has been effective in treating serious or persistent parvovirus B19 infections in immunocompromised children (189). A case report has described its successful use to treat a hydropic fetus. Fetal anemia, ascites, and pericardial effusion, as well as signs of severe preeclampsia in the mother, resolved after a single infusion of IVIG, 25 g at 25 weeks' gestation (190). Placental passage of IgG is dependent on gestational age and unpredictable. Additional studies are necessary to determine the efficacy of this approach.

Prevention

Universal antenatal screening for parvovirus B19 is not recommended. A vaccine is currently under development and should be in human trials soon. In the interim, little can be done to prevent maternal infection. During periods when B19 is known to be present in the community, hand washing before eating or after contact with respiratory or other secretions should reduce the risk of infection. Theoretically, IVIG is a good source of neutralizing antibodies because much of the adult population has been infected previously. Administration of IVIG might be effective for postexposure prophylaxis because this method has worked in the canine model (191). There are no reports on the use of IVIG for prophylaxis in pregnant women. Avoiding exposure to infected individuals is desirable. However, during endemic periods, the occupational risk of fetal death due to B19 infection for a woman of unknown serologic status is so low (between 1:500 and 1:4,000) that serologic screening and temporary reassignment of nonimmune employees to non–child-care positions is considered unjustified (140,142). Similar rates of seroconversion have been found among nonimmune health care workers exposed to infected patients and those not exposed to infected patients (192). During epidemic periods, infection rates may be 5- to 20-fold higher. Although unproved, screening and temporary transfer of seronegative women working in day-care or elementary school settings may be appropriate; however, once an epidemic is in progress, exposure will likely have already occurred. Unfortunately, there is no good method of preventing exposure to the source of most maternal B19 infections, one's own school-age children.

RUBELLA

Definition

Rubella (German measles) first caught the attention of obstetricians in 1941 when Gregg, an Australian ophthalmologist, found an association between maternal rubella and congenital cataracts (193). This was the first convincing evidence that infection could be a cause of birth defects. In addition to cataracts, the major anomalies linked to rubella are heart disease and deafness, but mental retardation, growth restriction, and a variety of other abnormalities involving almost every organ system have been reported. Rubella also may result in spontaneous abortions and stillbirth. The development and widespread use of effective vaccines have made eradication of this disease a practical goal. Unfortunately, although the frequency of maternal rubella has declined to record low levels, cases of congenital rubella syndrome (CRS) are still occasionally reported.

Incidence

Rubella is an RNA virus belonging to the togavirus family. The disease occurs worldwide and is usually seen in late winter and spring; peak attack rates prevail March through May. Widespread immunization has disrupted the previous 6- to 9-year epidemic cycle. In 1996, only 238 cases of rubella were reported the CDC in the United States; yet, according to serologic surveys, 6% to 11% of women of childbearing age remain nonimmune (194). Rubella is contagious, although less so than measles, and outbreaks still occur among young adults in settings where people work or live in close proximity, such as hospitals or college dormitories.

Pathogenesis

Rubella is spread via expectorated respiratory droplets, which infect the new host's respiratory tract. The virus subsequently disseminates to other tissues through the blood stream. In adults, viremia develops a week before and subsides within a few days after the onset of rash. The rash of rubella coincides with the development of antibodies and is immunologically mediated. The incubation period is 12 to 23 days, with a mean of 18 days. There are no convincing data to support the contention that pregnant women are at greater risk of serious complications.

Maternal viremia may result in placental seeding and spread to the fetus, but the fetus may entirely escape infection. It is unclear what factors permit infection of only one fetus in a set of identical twins (195). The pathogenesis of the cellular and tissue damage seen in congenital rubella is also uncertain because only a small number of cells are infected, cytopathic effect is uncommon in tissue culture, and inflammation is minimal. Proposed mechanisms include vascular insufficiency, interference with cell mitosis, chromosomal breaks, and immunologic responses (196–199). Fetal infection is characterized by its chronicity and persistence after birth. Congenitally infected infants may excrete virus in respiratory secretions and urine for up to 2 years.

Despite the development of antibodies and cell-mediated immunity following primary infection or vaccination, asymptomatic reinfection is common upon reexposure to rubella, but rarely results in viremia (200,201). Fetal infection has occurred in this setting, so although extremely unlikely, rubella-immune women can deliver an infant with CRS (202–212).

Clinical Manifestations

In adults, infection is usually subclinical or mild, although it can be more severe than in children (213,214). Asymptomatic women cannot be reassured that they are at any less risk of delivering an anomalous infant than women experiencing a rash (215). A prodrome of malaise, headache, low-grade fever, anorexia, coryza, sore throat, cough, and conjunctivitis precedes the onset of rash by 1 to 5 days. Posterior auricular, cervical, and suboccipital lymphadenopathy is typically present. The maculopapular rash begins on the face and spreads downward over the body over 1 to 2 days. It may be pruritic and lasts 2 to 5 days. One third of adult women develop transient arthralgias but frank arthritis is uncommon (216). The fingers, wrists and knees are the most commonly involved joints. Symptoms usually resolve within 2 weeks, and chronic arthritis is extremely rare. Other complications of rubella include thrombocytopenia (1 of every 3000 patients) with or without hemorrhage, encephalitis (1 per 6000 cases), myocarditis, Guillain-Barré syndrome, mild hepatitis, optic neuritis, and bone marrow aplasia (213,217–220).

Fetal Manifestations

Rubella infection can cause fetal death, resulting in spontaneous abortion or stillbirth; can result in congenital defects apparent at birth or upon subsequent development; or may have no clinically detectable effect (221). In one series, two thirds of infected infants had subclinical infections (222). However, among those followed longitudinally, 71% developed manifestations in the first 5 years of life. The most common permanent abnormalities seen in CRS are hearing loss, mental retardation, cardiac malformations, and ophthalmic defects (223). Deafness occurs in 80% of CRS children and may be the only finding. The most common cardiac lesions are patent ductus arteriosis, pulmonary artery stenosis, and pulmonary valvular stenosis. A salt and pepper retinopathy, secondary to altered growth of the pigmentary layer of the retina, and cataracts are the two most frequent ocular findings. Mental retardation, motor retardation, and microcephaly can occur and are related to acute meningoencephalitis. Endocrine abnormalities may present as late-onset manifestations of CRS. Insulin-dependent diabetes mellitus develops in 20% of patients by age 35 (224–226). As a consequence of autoimmune mechanisms, thyroid dysfunction—either hyperthyroidism, hypothyroidism, or thyroiditis—is reported in 5% of individuals (224–227). Other late complications include glaucoma, hypertension, autism, and, rarely, a progressive, ultimately fatal panencephalitis (225). Transient abnormalities, which may be present at birth but spontaneously resolve, include hepatosplenomegaly, adenopathy, jaundice, thrombocytopenia, petechiae, blueberry muffin spots (bluish-red lesions of dermal erythropoiesis), rash, hemolytic anemia, interstitial pneumonia, and myocarditis.

Diagnosis and Laboratory Findings

Diagnosis of rubella on clinical grounds can be difficult. Many cases are asymptomatic, and other viral diseases may mimic rubella (roseola, parvovirus B19, modified measles, and enteroviral infections). The majority of clinically suspected cases of rubella are not confirmed by serologic evaluation (228). Isolation of rubella in cell culture is both costly and difficult; with the exception of diagnosing congenital rubella in the neonate, it is not commonly done. The diagnosis is best made using serologic testing, usually an ELISA for specific IgG and IgM antibodies.

Diagnosis is straightforward if the woman is known to be susceptible and if a serum sample obtained 4 or more weeks after exposure is ELISA positive. If the woman's immune status is unknown but the first specimen is obtained within 10 days of exposure and has detectable antibody, the patient can be assumed to have preexisting immunity. If she presents later, but still within 4 weeks of exposure, a fourfold or greater increase in antibodies in paired acute and convalescent phase serum taken 2 to 3 weeks apart is diagnostic. A single high titer is insufficiently specific to diagnose recent infection because it may be present in 15% of the normal population (229). Rubella-specific IgM is also considered diagnostic, but unfortunately false-positive results can occur in response to parvovirus B19 (230) or Epstein-Barr virus (EBV) (231). Low levels of IgM may persist for many months in some patients after natural infection (232). It may be present with reinfection as well (200,214,229,232). False-negative results may occur because IgM may disappear in less than 4 to 5 weeks.

If the first sample is taken more than 7 days after rash onset, titers may have already peaked, preventing detection of a significant increase in antibodies. Because passive hemagglutination (PHA) antibodies appear later, a high titer on ELISA with little or no PHA antibody is consistent with recent infection. If exposure occurred more than 5 weeks previously or if onset of rash was noted more than 3 weeks previously, and an initial titer is positive, diagnosis can be complicated. Although conclusive determination of the timing of infection may be impossible, IgG avidity testing may help to differentiate recent from long-ago infection (233,234). The patient should be counseled regarding the uncertainties in determining her degree of risk for CRS.

Management and Counseling

There is no specific treatment for rubella, but symptomatic relief can be provided with antipyretics and analgesics. Postexposure prophylaxis with immunoglobulin does not prevent infection or viremia. Women have delivered infants with CRS despite receiving immunoglobulin shortly after exposure. Thus, immunoglobulin is not routinely recommended, but might be considered for those women exposed to rubella in the first 16 weeks of gestation who under no circumstances would terminate their pregnancy. The suggested dose is 20 mL.

Prenatal diagnosis of congenital rubella has been performed using a variety of techniques, but must still be considered investigational. Techniques include amniocentesis to evaluate fluid for the presence of virus; cordocentesis to search for virus, rubella-specific antibodies, and interferon; and chorionic villous sampling to test for viral RNA with nucleic acid hybridization (235–240). Recently, PCR technology has been applied to placental tissue, amniotic fluid, and fetal blood (241,242). False-negative and false-positive results can occur, and a true positive result does not indicate to what degree the fetus is affected (243). Instead, management of the pregnant woman with rubella is based on accurate confirmation of primary infection, as discussed above, and proper counseling regarding the possible types of congenital defects and their likelihood of occurrence in order to aid the woman in her decision of whether to terminate her pregnancy.

The most important factor influencing the manifestations of infection is gestational age at the time of infection. Fetal infection may occur at any stage of pregnancy, but fetal damage is more likely to occur in early gestation. Miller and colleagues prospectively followed 1,016 women with confirmed rubella during pregnancy, 407 of whom continued their pregnancies to term (244). Of 258 children evaluated, 45% were congenitally infected. When infection occurred prior to 11 weeks, 90% (9 of 10) were infected; at 11 to 14 weeks, 67% (16 of 24) were infected. There was a continuous decline in infection rates, reaching a nadir in the late second trimester (25%, or 8 of 32). In the third trimester, infection rates steadily increased as term approached (overall 53%, or 34 of 64).

Cardiac defects and deafness occurred in all of the infants infected prior to 10 weeks; deafness was the sole defect at 11 to 16 weeks, occurring in 37% (11 of 30). No defects were found in 63 children infected after 16 weeks, but some of those infected in the third trimester were growth restricted. Peckham and colleagues observed no abnormalities after 20 weeks' gestation (245,246), and Monroe and colleagues also found that the risk of deafness is small when infection occurs after the 16th week (247). Based on the experience of Miller and colleagues, patients can be informed that the risk of congenital defects after maternal infection is 90% before the 11th week, 33% during weeks 11 and 12, and 18% from weeks 13 to 16 (244). Similarly, when children were followed to 6 to 8 years of age, Peckham's group found the risk of abnormalities with first-trimester infection was 82%. No studies have documented congenital defects when maternal infection occurred after 20 weeks' gestation.

More problematic is how to counsel appropriately pregnant women with known immunity who are exposed to rubella. Reinfection following vaccination or natural infection can occur, resulting in viremia and IgM antibody production (200,201). However, the IgM titers are low level. There are also over 20 reported cases of congenital infection and CRS following maternal reinfection (202–212). This has prompted some authorities to recommend that all women exposed to rubella undergo serologic testing to exclude reinfection (201,202,248). However, only one case has been reported from North America (212), the serologic diagnosis of reinfection is not always accurate, and the degree of risk to the fetus is uncertain. The risk does appear to be much less than after primary infection. Two prospective studies examining the outcomes of maternal reinfection found no cases of fetal infection among 41 pregnancies that continued to term (200,215). Some cases of apparent reinfection may actually represent primary infection in a woman with a previous false-positive rubella serologic test result. For this reason, it is recommended that women be tested for rubella antibodies in every pregnancy (249). Until additional information on risk or reliable prenatal diagnosis is available, it is best to inform such a woman that she is at low risk for reinfection, her fetus is at low risk for CRS, and pregnancy termination is unwarranted.

All pregnant women should be tested for rubella antibodies at the first prenatal visit. Those who are nonimmune should be vaccinated postpartum prior to hospital discharge. Over one third of the reported cases of congenital rubella in the United States during recent years have occurred in second or subsequent pregnancies and thus were theoretically preventable by appropriate screening and postpartum immunization. The RA27/3 rubella vaccine induces seroconversion in over 95% of recipients. Although joint pain occurs in up to 25% of adult female vaccinees, the vaccine is generally well tolerated and does not appear to have long-term adverse effects. Slater and colleagues compared 485 women vaccinated postpartum with 493 matched controls and found no association between the vaccine and the subsequent development of arthritis (250). The vaccine causes no problem in women with preexisting immunity, so if there is a question regarding a patient's immune status, it is best to proceed with vaccination, usually by administering the trivalent mumps-measles-rubella (MMR) vaccine. Breastfeeding is not contraindicated, although the neonate may seroconvert. Rubella vaccine should not be given 3 months prior to or during pregnancy because of the theoretical risk of CRS. However, even though fetal infection has been described (251), there are no reports of CRS in over 600 cases of inadvertent maternal immunization. Therapeutic abortion is not recommended. Patients who receive blood products or immunoglobulin in late pregnancy or intrapartum should still receive the vaccine postpartum but may not develop an adequate immune response. These women should be tested at least 3 months later to confirm rubella immunity (252,253).

MEASLES (RUBEOLA)

Definition and Incidence

Measles is the most contagious of the childhood exanthematous diseases (254). It is a member of the paromyxovirus family and is closely related to the virus causing canine distemper. Measles occurs worldwide, but it is seen less frequently in pregnant women than is chickenpox or mumps. Before development of the MMR vaccine, 99% of adults were immune and the reported incidence was only 0.4 to 0.6 cases of measles per 10,000 pregnancies (64,255). The incidence is even lower since implementation of vaccine programs, but mini-epidemics of measles still occur. After a record low of 1,497 cases in 1983, over 27,000 cases of measles were reported to the CDC in 1990. Of these, 40% occurred in individuals of reproductive age (256). By 1993, partly due to emphasis on administering two doses of vaccine, only 312 cases were reported (257).

Today, despite the upward shift in age distribution, measles is usually seen in preschool children who have not yet been vaccinated. However, half of the cases reported in school children occur regardless of prior vaccination due to primary vaccine failure, which occurs in about 5% of individuals. Infection rates are highest among low socioeconomic populations and environments characterized by crowding (including boarding schools); thus, nonimmune adult women are more likely to be found in rural or isolated communities. Measles is seen most frequently in the winter and spring, peaking between March and May.

Pathogenesis

Measles is transmitted by expelled respiratory secretions or, occasionally, by articles that have been contaminated by secretions. The virus gains entry through respiratory epithelium of the nose and oropharynx, initiates a viremia by which it spreads to the reticuloendothelial system, infects white blood cells, and subsequently disseminates to the skin, respiratory tract, intestines, and other organs. Characteristic multinucleated giant cells with inclusion bodies are seen. Damage to the respiratory tract facilitates secondary bacterial infections such as pneumonia and otitis media. Infection and destruction of lymphocytes results in lymphopenia and transient impaired cellular immunity. Patients who already have deficient cellular immunity, such as those with AIDS, are at risk for severe measles. Protein deficiency is also associated with an increased incidence of complications and death.

Viremia precedes the onset of symptoms by several days. Patients are contagious from 2 to 3 days preceding symptom onset until 4 days after the rash appears, although viremia may persist until day 7 of the rash (258). The mean incubation period is 10 days to onset of symptoms (range 8–13 days) and 14 days to onset of rash. Measles antigens have been demonstrated in skin lesions, but it is the reaction of the immune system to the virus in endothelial cells of skin and mucosal capillaries that causes the rash and pathognomonic Koplik spots. In severely immunocompromised women, measles may not be accompanied by a rash. Measles encephalitis is characterized by focal hemorrhage, congestion, and perivascular demyelination, but the virus is rarely isolated from cerebrospinal fluid.

Clinical Manifestation

Measles begins with a prodrome of fever, malaise, and respiratory symptoms: coryza, conjunctivitis, cough, and sneezing. At the end of the prodrome, and prior to the onset of the rash, Koplik spots appear. These are tiny (1–2 mm), slightly raised white spots with surrounding erythema, typically located on the buccal mucosa adjacent to the second molars. They may be extensive and involve the lips and inner eyelids as well. Once the rash begins, the spots soon disappear. The nonpruritic, erythematous, maculopapular rash begins at the hairline and on the neck behind the ears. It spreads to the trunk and upper extremities followed by the lower extremities, including the palms and soles, and may become confluent. By the fourth day, the rash starts to fade in the order of its appearance. Bronchitis, sinusitis, diarrhea, vomiting, lymphadenopathy, and splenomegaly are also common findings.

The most common serious complication is pneumonia, seen in at least 3% of young adults. Although primarily of viral origin, pneumonia may be due to bacterial superinfection with streptococci, pneumococci, *Haemophilus influenzae,* or staphylococci (259). Encephalitis with headache, drowsiness, coma, or seizures occurs in only 1 per 1,000 cases (260), but encephalographic abnormalities without symptoms are seen more frequently. Encephalitis may result in permanent sequelae such as mental impairment or seizures; it is fatal in 10% of patients. Subacute sclerosing panencephalitis is more common among children but it is almost never seen today. Other reported complications include hepatitis, appendicitis, mesenteric adenitis, nephritis, myocarditis, and thrombocytopenic purpura (261). The morbidity rate varies with different populations and is influenced by age (increased risk in the old or very young), socioeconomic status, nutrition, and medical care. In the United States, the case:fatality ratio is between 1:1,000 and 1:10,000 cases.

Maternal Effects

Most pregnant women tolerate measles well (262,263), but there is some evidence, although not definitive, to suggest that measles is more severe in pregnant than nonpregnant women (264–268). Christensen and colleagues investigated an epidemic in a previously unexposed population in Greenland and found that pregnant women were at least three times as likely to die from their infections (mortality 4.8% versus 1.0% in nonpregnant women) (265). Heart failure with pulmonary edema was observed more frequently. Respiratory complications requiring ventilatory support and higher rates of measles-related hospitalization also have been reported (265–268).

Fetal Effects

Higher rates of preterm labor and birth of an appropriately grown fetus have been described in association with gestational measles (255,262,263,265–269). In the series reported by Eberhart-Phillips and colleagues, of 6,614 cases of measles, 58 occurred in pregnant women (267). Eighteen of these pregnancies (31%) ended prematurely and three others (5%) were induced abortions. All but 2 of the 18 pregnancies that delivered early did so within 2 weeks of the onset of rash. Siegel and Fuerst identified low birth weight in 10 of 60 infants (16.7%) born to infected mothers compared with 2 of 62 matched controls (3.3%) (255). Fetal death *in utero* also has been reported. Interestingly, in one case involving a fetus at 25 weeks' gestation, there was no evidence of virus in the fetus, although virus was present in syncytial trophoblast cells of the placenta and in the decidua (270). The investigator suggested that fetal death was the result of placental damage and consequent hypoxia. A significant increase in the rate of abortion has not been demonstrated, but there are multiple reports of spontaneous abortions temporally related to maternal measles (263,265–267).

Although measles can cross the placenta, this does not appear to occur frequently. There is no convincing evidence that the measles virus causes congenital anomalies (85,262,265,269,271). Information is sparse because infection during the first trimester is rare. Case reports of a variety of anomalies reveal no particular pattern. Denominator figures are unavailable, and documentation that the maternal illness was measles rather than another viral disease is often not provided. A small prospective trial found no increase in congenital malformations (85). Aaby and colleagues have reported an increased perinatal mortality rate among children of mothers exposed to measles during pregnancy in Guinea-Bassau. There are no reports of such an association in the United States (272). Recent reports have raised the possibility that *in utero* exposure to the measles virus may predispose to the subsequent development of Crohn's disease later in life (273), but a subsequent study refuted these findings (274).

Neonatal Effects

Maternal infection just before delivery does not result in fetal and, hence, congenital infection, in the majority of cases (262,264). In the Greenland epidemic in 1951 (265) and a series reported from Los Angeles from 1988 to 1991 (267), there were no cases of congenital measles diagnosed among 37 newborns whose mothers had measles within 2 weeks of delivery. When congenital infection does occur, it can result in a spectrum of illness ranging from mild disease to death (usually from pneumonia). The current mortality rate is not known but is certainly less than 32%, the rate derived from reports antedating the use of immunoglobulin prophylaxis and antibiotics (275). Premature infants are at higher risk than term infants.

Diagnosis and Laboratory Findings

The clinical diagnosis of measles is reasonably reliable especially if Koplik spots are seen. Siegel and Hirshman reported serologic confirmation of clinically suspected measles in 40 of 41 cases (276). If there is doubt, exfoliated cells from respiratory secretions or the urinary tract can be examined by immunofluorescent staining for measles antigen or microscopically for multinucleated giant cells. ELISA for IgM and IgG antibodies is the most useful serologic test for diagnosing acute infection or verifying immunity even though antibodies are not present until 1 to 2 days after the rash appears.

Treatment

Pregnant women who are susceptible to measles and are exposed to the disease should receive postexposure prophylaxis with immunoglobulin within 6 days. The dose is 0.25 mL/kg intramuscularly, not to exceed 15 mL (277). In some women, immunoglobulin may prolong the incubation interval without preventing infection. All newborns delivered of mothers with active measles in the 6 days preceding delivery also should be given immunoglobulin. Susceptible women should receive the MMR vaccine postpartum prior to hospital discharge. Vaccination should be deferred for 6 months after the receipt of immunoglobulin or blood transfusion. It does not need to be delayed if Rh immune globulin is given (277). Women who have previously received inactivated virus vaccine (available between 1963 and 1967) should be considered nonimmune and receive a dose of live vaccine. Women born before 1957 are considered immune. Although there have been no reports of congenital anomalies resulting from vaccine administration, the vaccine should not be given during pregnancy. Inadvertent vaccination or measles infection during pregnancy is not an indication for pregnancy termination.

Therapy for measles in pregnancy is largely supportive. Immunoglobulin is of no value in established disease. Prophylactic antibiotics are not warranted, but bacterial superinfections should be treated with appropriate agents. Ribavirin is effective against measles *in vitro,* and aerosolized ribavirin therapy has been offered to pregnant patients beyond 20 weeks' gestation with life-threatening disease; however, no definitive clinical benefit has been demonstrated (266). High-dose vitamin A therapy is of potential benefit in children with severe measles. It has not been tried in pregnancy, and high doses of vitamin A in the first trimester have been associated with birth defects. Pregnant women should be informed of the risk of preterm labor, and oral hydration is encouraged. There is no indication for attempting diagnosis of *in utero* infection.

MUMPS

Definition and Incidence

Mumps is a paramyxovirus responsible for a contagious disease most notable for prominent swelling of the parotid glands. Mumps occurs worldwide and in the absence of immunization has a peak incidence in late winter to early spring. Historically, mumps was principally a disease of childhood occurring most frequently between the ages of 5 and 15 years. The majority of women of childbearing age were immune, and mumps in pregnancy was uncommon. Prospective studies estimated the incidence to be 0.8 to 10 cases per 10,000 pregnancies (85,278). Since the widespread implementation of vaccine programs using the MMR vaccine, the disease has become exceedingly rare in pregnancy.

Pathogenesis

Mumps is transmitted by expelled respiratory droplets, saliva, and fomites. It is less contagious than measles or chickenpox. The virus initially replicates in upper respiratory tract epithelium, which is followed by viremia. Virus spreads to glandular tissues (parotids, other salivary glands, occasionally the pancreas) and frequently the central nervous system. The incubation period from exposure to onset of parotitis can be anywhere from 7 to 23 days, but usually is 14 to 18 days. Early in the illness, the virus can be recovered from saliva, throat swabs, and urine, as well as from cerebrospinal fluid in women with meningitis. The virus is present less often in blood and milk (279). It persists longest in urine, sometimes for up to 2 weeks.

Clinical Manifestations

Up to half of mumps infections in pregnancy are subclinical (280). When symptoms occur, a short prodrome of fever, malaise, myalgias, and anorexia precedes the onset of parotitis by approximately 24 hours. Swelling may be delayed for up to a week, or may not occur at all. It is usually bilateral. The submaxillary glands are affected less often, and the sublingual glands are rarely involved. These glands are not affected in the absence of parotid gland disease. Aseptic meningitis can occur in 5% to 25% of cases; pleocytosis of the cerebrospinal fluid is seen in up to 50% of clinically apparent mumps (275). Rarely, cranial nerve involvement can result in permanent sequelae such as deafness. Other complications of mumps in women include oophoritis, mastitis, thyroiditis, myocarditis, pancreatitis, nephritis, and arthritis. Mumps is no more virulent in pregnant women than in other adults, and the illness is usually benign (280–283). Death is rare, with only a single case reported in the literature (284).

Fetal Effects

The incidence of spontaneous abortion is increased among women who develop mumps in the first trimester (85,281,283,285). Siegel and colleagues found that 9 of 33 (27%) first trimester pregnancies ended in fetal death following mumps compared with 13% of controls (80). The majority of these deaths occurred within 2 weeks of the onset of maternal disease. Kurtz and colleagues were able to isolate virus from a 10-week fetus spontaneously aborted 4 days after the mother became symptomatic with mumps (286). The incidence of low birth weight and prematurity are unaffected by maternal mumps (255).

The mumps virus can cross the placenta. In 1855, Homans described a case of a woman who delivered 3 days after developing clinical mumps. Her newborn developed unilateral parotitis the following day (287). In animals, mumps can produce congenital malformations, including cataracts, myocardial necrosis, and stenosis of the aqueduct of Sylvius. In humans, there are multiple reports of sporadic anomalies following antenatal mumps, although no data have been provided regarding the incidence of anomalies in matched controls, nor has *in utero* infection been confirmed virologically or serologically in the infants (288–293). Malformations described have included hydrocephalus, spina bifida, intestinal atresia, imperforate anus, chorioretinitis and optic atrophy, cataracts, urogenital anomalies, and skin lesions. However, the only controlled, prospective study found no difference in the frequency of birth defects between children of infected mothers and those of uninfected women (2 of 117 versus 2 of 123) (85). None of the 24 children whose mothers had mumps in the first trimester had any anomalies. Similarly, a retrospective study by Manson and colleagues found no increase in congenital malformations among 501 infected women compared with a control group (294).

There has been considerable debate as to whether mumps is a cause of endocardial fibroelastosis in the neonate. This condition, characterized by generalized subendocardial thickening, was first linked to mumps in 1963, when Noren and colleagues noted that affected neonates demonstrated delayed hypersensitivity to mumps on skin testing (295). Two other groups of investigators confirmed these findings (296,297). However, most of these infants lacked humoral antibodies to mumps, and in no case was the virus isolated. Although it has been postulated that *in utero* infection in the presence of an immature immune system may result in split immunologic reactivity, a cellular response in the absence of a humoral response, this phenomenon has not been seen with other viral infections. In addition, other investigators have found no relationship between endocardial fibroelastosis and positive skin tests (298–301). Skin testing is relatively nonspecific, and patients are typically only weakly reactive to mumps antigens, which may represent cross-reactivity to another virus. It is unlikely that the controversy will be resolved anytime soon. The incidence of endocardial fibroelastosis was always low and began declining before the development of the mumps vaccine; since introduction of the vaccine, both maternal mumps and endocardial fibroelastosis are rare. The diagnosis has not been made antenatally.

Neonatal mumps is extremely uncommon, even when the mother develops mumps immediately before or after delivery (302,303). Despite the lack of maternally derived antibodies, the majority of infants do not become infected (280,285,303). When infection does occur, it is often asymptomatic or mild; typical mumps occurs in less than 10% of cases (303). Serious complications have developed only rarely (302–305). Three newborns developed viral pneumonia severe enough to require mechanical ventilation. One of these infants died due to pneumothoraces and a pneumopericardium. Another neonate developed thrombocytopenia, which resolved with conservative management (303).

Diagnosis and Laboratory Abnormalities

The diagnosis is usually made based on clinical findings, but this can be inaccurate, even in the presence of parotid swelling. Mumps virus is readily cultured in a variety of host cell systems, including rhesus monkey kidney cells and human embryonic lung fibroblasts. Serologic testing using commercially available ELISA kits is more practical for determining both susceptibility and, in the presence of specific IgM, acute infection. Other laboratory tests, such as a complete blood count, may be altered by mumps infection, but in no predictable or characteristic fashion.

Treatment

Most women of childbearing age should have received the live attenuated mumps vaccine prior to conception. However, the clinical efficacy of the vaccine ranges from 75% to 95%, and sporadic cases of mumps can occur. Treatment is symptomatic using antipyretics, analgesics, and local application of heat or cold to any swelling in the submandibular area. Mastitis may be treated with ice packs and a breast binder.

Mumps immunoglobulin is of no proven value in either the treatment or prevention of disease and is no longer commercially available. No antiviral drugs are effective against mumps. Vaccine is contraindicated during pregnancy, but women without a history of vaccination should receive vaccine postpartum. Although virus has been isolated from milk (306), breastfeeding is permitted in women who receive vaccine or who develop peripartum mumps (307). Neither inadvertent vaccination nor clinical mumps during early pregnancy is an indication for pregnancy termination or antenatal surveillance.

ENTEROVIRUSES

Definition

Enteroviruses are small single-stranded RNA viruses that are members of the picornavirus family. Although named for their ability to multiply in the gastrointestinal tract, they are not a common cause of gastroenteritis. There are four main groups and almost 70 different serotypes: the polioviruses, group A and B coxsackieviruses, the echoviruses, and more recently discovered serotypes now classified as enteroviruses. For example, hepatitis A virus has now been classified as enterovirus type 72. All four groups may cause neonatal disease. Enteroviruses have a worldwide distribution, but are more common in socioeconomically depressed areas (308,309). For example, enteroviruses have been recovered from flies, which may facilitate spread where sanitation is poor (310). Eighty percent to 90% of infections occur in children under 17 years of age.

Infection is asymptomatic in the majority of patients. In symptomatic patients, the most common clinical manifestation of enteroviral infection is a nonspecific febrile illness with malaise, headache, and, sometimes, upper respiratory symptoms, nausea, or vomiting. More severe manifestations of enteroviral infection include exanthems, hand-foot-and-mouth disease, acute hemorrhagic conjunctivitis, herpangina and lymphonodular pharyngitis, aseptic meningitis, paralysis including Guillain-Barré syndrome, myocarditis, pericarditis, pleurodynia, and pneumonia. However, there are no reports of increased susceptibility or greater disease severity during pregnancy. Serious illness is seen most frequently in neonates or adolescents and adults. Enterovirus infections can occur at any time of the year but in temperate climates are most common during the summer and fall (311).

Incidence

The risk of enteroviral infection during pregnancy depends on multiple factors, including time of year, prevalence of viruses in the community, prior maternal immunity to these viruses, exposure to young children, and socioeconomic status, but is quite high in all populations. Infection with group B coxsackieviruses occurred in 9% of 198 women studied by the NIH Collaborative Perinatal Project during the course of their pregnancies (312). Cherry and colleagues found that seroconversion to enteroviruses during peak enterovirus season occurred in one fourth of 55 women followed prospectively during the final weeks of pregnancy (313). None of these women delivered infants with severe infection. In general, enterovirus infections in late pregnancy are common but rarely cause significant maternal or neonatal morbidity (311).

Pathogenesis

Enteroviruses are spread by the fecal-oral, oral-oral, and respiratory routes. Swimming pools may serve as a source of infection during the summer (314). Infection is initiated in the pharynx and lower gastrointestinal tract and quickly spreads to regional lymph nodes. The incubation period for most enteroviruses ranges from 2 to 14 days, and is usually less than a week. Infection is cytolytic, resulting in cell death and release of more virus. Maternal viremia occurs commonly during enteroviral infections, usually from the third to the seventh day of infection, and results in secondary organ involvement. Many tissues are susceptible, including the myocardium, central nervous system, liver, spleen, pancreas, and adrenals. Placental infection may result, and active virus has been recovered from the placenta (315). However, fetal infection can occur without histologic evidence of placental disease, even though it is believed that such infections are the result of hematogenous dissemination from the involved placenta. Fetal infection also may result from the ingestion of amniotic fluid containing virus, leading to infection of the oropharynx, lungs, and gastrointestinal tract. The onset of antibody production halts the maternal viremia and leads to recovery, although fecal shedding may persist for months. Immunity against the specific serotype involved appears to be lifelong.

In general, fetal enteroviral infection is uncommon (316). However, neonatal infection occurs in a significant proportion of infants delivered of infected women. Cherry and colleagues found that 29% of mothers (4 of 14) with peripartum echovirus or coxsackievirus infection transmitted the infection to the infant (313). Modlin and colleagues reported that four of seven women excreting echovirus 11 during labor transmitted the virus within 3 days of giving birth (317). The actual route of transmission is unknown, but vaginal delivery is not a prerequisite (311). Virus is present in maternal blood, vaginal and cervical secretions, stool, and respiratory secretions (318,319). Studies in suckling mice have confirmed the generally held belief that enterovirus infections in the fetus and neonate are more severe than in older individuals, although the mechanisms underlying this increased vulnerability are incompletely understood (320,321).

Poliovirus

Poliomyelitis, the first enteroviral disease to be recognized, has essentially been eradicated in developed countries and is unlikely ever to be encountered by an obstetrician in the United States. The only cases of poliomyelitis in the United States are due to live virus vaccine and may result when a person who has not received a full course of vaccine comes in close contact with a recent vaccinee. However, poliovirus remains endemic in some countries. Infection in pregnancy can cause abortion, stillbirth, or neonatal infection, or may be completely asymptomatic (322–330). Siegel and Greenberg found that 46.7% of cases (14 of 30) of first-trimester poliomyelitis resulted in fetal death (325). Spontaneous abortion occurred in 13.2% of 325 pregnancies affected by polio in Horn's series (322). An increased risk of low birth weight (322,331), particularly following maternal infection early in pregnancy, and an increase in prematurity associated with maternal paralytic poliomyelitis (325), also have been reported.

Transplacental transmission of the virus to the fetus, which causes congenital disease and, at times, paralysis, has been observed on many occasions (326–330). In most cases of neonatal paralytic poliomyelitis, maternal disease occurred just before or at the time of delivery. There is no evidence that polioviruses are teratogenic or that pregnancy termination improves maternal outcome. Viremia also occurs after oral polio vaccine administration and virus likely crosses transplacentally. Fetal infection has never been documented, and a woman who inadvertently receives vaccine during pregnancy should be reassured. However, a case of monoparesis resulting from neonatal infection with a vaccine-type poliovirus has been reported (332). The probable source of infection was another child who had received live oral poliovirus vaccine.

Coxsackievirus

Despite the finding that both group A and B coxsackieviruses can cross the placenta and infect the fetus (315, 333–338), this has been reported only rarely for coxsackieviruses A; group A viruses generally do not cause significant perinatal disease. There is no conclusive evidence linking coxsackievirus infection with spontaneous abortion or preterm labor and delivery. However, Axelsson and colleagues found a significantly higher incidence of coxsackie B virus–specific IgM among women with first-trimester miscarriages than among control women (339). Occasional stillbirths have been described, but these are sufficiently rare that it has not been possible to determine whether the infection was causal (315,337).

There have been several reports, none definitive, suggesting a relationship between coxsackieviruses and congenital anomalies. In a large prospective study of 22,935 women, Brown and Karunas found a correlation between maternal infection with coxsackieviruses B2, B3, B4, and A9 and neonatal urogenital anomalies such as hypospadius and cryptorchidism (340). Coxsackievirus A9 was also associated with gastrointestinal anomalies, and the coxsackieviruses B1 to B5 were associated with congenital heart disease. There was no correlation between symptomatic maternal disease and serologic evidence of infection in the neonate. Importantly, there was no seasonal variation in the births of infants with these specific defects, and this brings into question the validity of the study. Gauntt and colleagues suggested that there may be an association between coxsackievirus B and severe central nervous system defects based on their study of ventricular fluid from affected newborns (341). However, this has not been confirmed by others. There have been additional sporadic case reports of infected women delivering children with congenital malformations; nevertheless, a cause-and-effect relationship has not been established (335). There have been reports of an association between maternal coxsackievirus B (and other enterovirus) infection during pregnancy and early-onset childhood insulin-dependent diabetes mellitus as a result of slowly progressive pancreatic beta-cell damage (342,343).

Congenital coxsackievirus infection within 48 hours of birth occurs rarely. More commonly, neonatal disease is acquired from the mother, nursing personnel, or infected babies in the nursery. These infections can be severe, resulting in myocarditis, meningitis, or meningoencephalitis. Coxsackievirus B myocarditis is frequently rapidly progressive, resulting in circulatory failure, respiratory distress, and death. Of the 45 infants studied by Kibrick, only 12 survived (344). Both coxsackievirus and echovirus infections can cause a sepsislike picture with disseminated intravascular coagulation and shock.

Echoviruses

Echoviruses cross the placenta (318,345–348) relatively infrequently (313,349,350). Although there are occasional case reports of adverse pregnancy outcome in infected gravidas, there is no evidence suggesting that maternal echovirus infections are a frequent cause of spontaneous abortion, premature delivery, or congenital anomalies (340,351–353). Late stillbirth has been described in association with maternal echovirus (354–357), but virus is rarely isolated from the fetus (354) and has been cultured from the amniotic fluid in only one case (356). Neonatal infection can result in fever, rash, meningitis, encephalitis, severe vomiting, diarrhea and dehydration, pneumonitis, otitis media, and splenomegaly. Fatal cases are usually attributable to massive hepatic necrosis, often with accompanying necrosis of the adrenal glands, myocardium, and acute tubular necrosis of the kidney (318,346,358,359). Echovirus 11 appears to be particularly virulent, accounting for approximately 70% of serious neonatal disease (360).

Maternal infection late in pregnancy may sometimes present with fever and lower abdominal pain, which has been incorrectly diagnosed as placental abruption or appendicitis, resulting in an emergency cesarean section (311). These symptoms may be manifestations of mesenteric adenitis (318).

Diagnosis

The majority of infections in women are asymptomatic and do not result in fetal abnormalities. When symptoms do occur, they may be nonspecific and, given the large number of possible serotypes, serologic testing can be costly, time consuming, and of little clinical use. Thus, outside of a research setting, definitive diagnosis is infrequently made. If necessary, the diagnosis can be made within 1 week by isolation of enterovirus in cell culture from throat or stool samples. PCR provides more rapid results and can detect over 92% of the human serotypes with a single pair of PCR primers. PCR is more sensitive than culture and highly specific, but is not universally available (361).

Treatment

Most enteroviral infections are mild, resolve spontaneously, and do not require specific therapy. Care is supportive because there are no chemotherapeutic agents available to treat enteroviral illness. Rarely, intensive supportive care may be necessary for women with cardiac, hepatic, or central nervous system involvement. In specific instances of serious disease in immunodeficient adults or neonates with severe infection, intravenous or intrathecal immunoglobulin containing high titers of antibody has been used with some success. Optimal dosing regimens have not been determined, however (362, 363). Good hand-washing practices will reduce the chance of acquiring infection during pregnancy. Poliovirus vaccines should not be administered during pregnancy unless immediate protection is needed, in which case enhanced-potency inactivated poliovirus vaccine (IPV-e) can be given. IPV-e is preferred in susceptible adults because there is a lower risk of paralysis than with the oral vaccine.

INFLUENZA VIRUS

Definition

The term "influenza" was first used in the fifteenth century following an epidemic in Italy attributed to the effects of the stars (364). Before antibiotics became available, influenza was a potentially serious infection in pregnancy due to secondary infections with bacterial pneumonia. Morbidity and mortality were higher for pregnant women, as seen in the pandemic of 1918, which resulted in a 27% mortality rate (365). During the 1957 pandemic of Asian influenza, half of all women who died in Minnesota were pregnant (366). Pregnant women may not be more likely to contract influenza or develop pneumonia, but if they do, the pneumonia appears to be more severe. Today death from influenza still occurs, although rarely. Influenza is a concern mostly because of its economic toll due to hospitalization, visits to health care providers, and high rates of work and school absenteeism.

Influenza viruses are single-stranded RNA viruses that belong to the orthomyxovirus family. There are three antigenically different types of influenza virus, types A, B, and C, determined by their nuclear material. Type A is the most common and virulent in adults; it is responsible for the majority of epidemics. All influenza viruses have an envelope that is covered with surface projections consisting of glycoproteins possessing either hemagglutinin (H) or neuraminidase (N) activity. There are multiple different antigenic subtypes of the H and N surface antigens with different amino acid sequences. A defining characteristic of influenza virus is the propensity to undergo frequent alterations in antigenicity, referred to as antigenic drift or shift, depending on whether the variation is minor or major. Antigenic drift results in enough change to permit new influenza epidemics each year. With antigenic shift, there is little or no serologic relationship between the old and new virus. Such major antigenic changes occur at 10- to 30-year intervals; the population lacks immunity, and a pandemic occurs.

Pathogenesis

Influenza is spread via virus-laden aerosol droplets, which result when an infected person coughs or sneezes. The virus is inhaled and attaches to, replicates in, and then destroys cells in the trachea and bronchi. In the northern hemisphere infection most often occurs between November and April, when people are more likely to remain in closed environments. The incubation period is usually 2 days (range 1–4 days).

Clinical Manifestations

Influenza presents with abrupt onset of fever (usually 101° to 102°F), myalgias, headache, rhinorrhea, dry cough, sore throat, weakness, and malaise. Only 50% of patients develop these classic symptoms. Gastrointestinal symptoms are uncommon in adults. Systemic symptoms typically last only 3 days, and most patients recover within a week. The most serious complication of influenza is pneumonia, either viral pneumonia as a direct result of influenza or secondary bacterial pneumonia. Viral pneumonia is rare in pregnant women, but is potentially fatal. It is characterized by paroxysms of coughing, shortness of breath, scant sputum, and hypoxia. Lung tissue becomes edematous with intraalveolar hemorrhage, thickening of alveolar septae, and hyaline membrane formation. An infiltrate may be seen on chest x-ray. Bacterial pneumonia is much more frequent with *Streptococcus pneumoniae, Staphylococcus aureus, Klebsiella,* or *Haemophilus influenzae* often the responsible organism. Women with chronic pulmonary or cardiac conditions may have exacerbations of their disease. Myocarditis has rarely been reported with influenza.

Fetal Effects

Viremia is uncommon during influenza infections; the virus has never been isolated from blood. Nevertheless, influenza virus does cross the placenta in an unknown proportion of infected gravidas. Reports of confirmed transplacental passage are rare (367,368). Monif and colleagues could not document fetal infection in any of eight infants born to women who had influenza A/Hong Kong in the second or third trimester (369). Even with infections severe enough to result in maternal death, transplacental passage may not occur (370). Intraamniotic infection on occasion may mimic bacterial amniotic fluid infection and result in uterine tenderness and preterm contractions (368).

Whether fetal infection can cause congenital anomalies has never been completely resolved. Initial reports, which relied on patient recall or did not include serologic confirmation of infection, noted an increased risk for congenital anomalies, such as neural tube defects and cardiac anomalies, among infants born to mothers with a history of antenatal influenza (371–375). Since maternal hyperthermia has been associated with birth defects, the increased risk cited in these reports may have been unrelated to fetal infection per se. Another possibility is that greater use of nonprescription drugs by infected women may have had adverse fetal effects. Other data, including the Collaborative Perinatal Research Study, have not revealed any association between influenza and congenital anomalies (376–379). Similarly, there has been controversy regarding whether maternal influenza predisposes to the development of childhood leukemia or adult schizophrenia in offspring (380,381). What can be said is that the vast majority of women contracting influenza during pregnancy have normal obstetric outcomes; the influenza virus does not cause a consistent congenital syndrome; if there is a risk of malformation, it is small; and maternal infection has little influence on fetal growth, prematurity, or stillbirth. Because infection of the newborn is possible if the mother contracts disease peripartum, and may cause considerable morbidity, consideration should be given to delaying delivery until maternal symptoms have resolved and transplacental passage of protective antibody has occurred.

Diagnosis

In most cases, the diagnosis can be made on the basis of history and clinical findings. Virus can be cultured from nasopharyngeal swabs obtained early in the course of infection, and a serologic diagnosis can be made using complement fixation or hemagglutination inhibition tests on acute and convalescent specimens taken 2 to 3 weeks apart. Results usually do not influence treatment; hence, these tests are not cost effective. If pneumonia is suspected, a chest x-ray and sputum culture are appropriate.

Treatment

Therapy for uncomplicated influenza infection is supportive, consisting of antipyretics (acetaminophen), analgesics, oral fluid, and bed rest. Aspirin is best avoided in adolescents because of its association with Reye syndrome. If pneumonia develops, the patient should be promptly hospitalized and started on broad-spectrum antibiotic coverage to treat or prevent bacterial superinfection. Respiratory support may be necessary. Amantadine hydrochloride and rimantadine hydrochloride interfere with the replication cycle of type A influenza. Both agents are 70% to 90% effective in preventing illness if started immediately after exposure and may hasten recovery for women who are already symptomatic, but they are ineffective against type B influenza. Both drugs are listed as pregnancy category C. Amantadine is teratogenic and embryotoxic in animals. Until there is more information regarding safety in humans, it is prudent to avoid the use of these drugs in gravidas with uncomplicated infections. However, influenza pneumonia can be life-threatening, and the use of amantadine in pregnant women exhibiting respiratory failure is justified. Kirshon and colleagues reported successful treatment of such a patient at 33 weeks' gestation using a combination of oral amantadine and ribavirin inhalation therapy (382). Ribavirin exhibits activity against several respiratory viruses, including influenza virus types A and B, respiratory syncytial virus, and the parainfluenza viruses.

Prophylaxis

The administration of inactivated virus vaccine is the most practical and effective method of preventing infection in pregnancy. Pregnancy in the otherwise healthy woman is not a significant risk factor for developing complications of influenza. However, the vaccine is safe for pregnant women, and the Advisory Committee on Immunization Practices recommends that it be offered to all women who will be in the second or third trimester during the influenza season (383). It is estimated that one to two hospitalizations can be prevented for every 1,000 pregnant women vaccinated. The optimal time to vaccinate is in October and November, just before the flu season begins. Mounting an effective antibody response can take up to 14 days. Although, ideally, vaccination should be delayed until after the first trimester, in patients with chronic medical conditions that increase risk, delay is inadvisable if the flu season has begun. Women infected with HIV will increase their viral loads for a period of 2 weeks following influenza vaccination.

It is unknown whether this increases the risk of vertical transmission of HIV.

EPSTEIN-BARR VIRUS

Definition and Incidence

Epstein-Barr virus is another member of the human herpesvirus family and shares the property of latent and persistent infection for the lifetime of the host. The virus was first discovered in 1964 by electron microscopy of Burkitt's lymphoma tumor cells (384), although it is best known as the cause of infectious mononucleosis. EBV is a lymphotropic virus that selectively infects B-lymphocytes. Two different EBV strains, A and B, have been identified in humans, with different geographic distributions. In most women, the A strain predominates in peripheral B cells, but patients with AIDS have increased rates with type B virus. Most women of childbearing age have already been asymptomatically infected in childhood. Primary EBV infection in pregnancy is uncommon because less than 5% of pregnant women are susceptible (7,385–387) In prospective evaluations of over 12,000 pregnant women, only 3 seroconverted (388).

Pathogenesis

Epstein-Barr virus is transmitted predominantly through saliva and only occasionally through blood. It affects mature epithelial cells of the oropharynx and salivary gland ducts, as well as the cervix. The full replication cycle occurs at these sites, and infectious virus is released into secretions. Chronic viral replication persists in these sites throughout the lifetime of the host. EBV has the ability to transform B cells such that they grow continuously as lymphoblastoid cell lines that secrete immunoglobulins. Although infected B cells are rapidly destroyed by the immunocompetent host, the pool is continuously replenished as circulating B cells pass through chronically infected oropharyngeal epithelium and are transformed. EBV has been implicated in the pathogenesis of Burkitt's lymphoma, nasopharyngeal carcinoma, Hodgkin's disease, and X-linked lymphoproliferative syndrome.

Antibodies are produced against several EBV antigens at different times during the course of infection. These antibodies help bring the initial infection under control even though they do not entirely eliminate the virus or episodes of reactivation. Soon after infection, women form IgG and IgM antibodies to EBV viral capsid antigen (VCA) and early antigen (EA). Levels of EA antibody decrease rapidly and are usually undetectable after 6 months. If EA antibody is detected at later times after an acute infection, it is thought to result from EBV reactivation. Antibodies to EBV-associated nuclear antigen (EBNA) develop 3 to 4 weeks, or even months, after primary infection and persist for life, along with VCA-IgG antibodies.

Clinical Manifestations

The majority of primary EBV infections are subclinical, with adults being more likely than children to develop symptoms. Most symptoms are due to the immune reactions of the host. Infectious mononucleosis is the only known primary disease caused by EBV. In young adults the incubation period is 5 to 7 weeks. A prodromal phase lasting 3 to 5 days and consisting of nonspecific complaints such as malaise, headache, and fever is followed by the characteristic triad of fever, sore throat, and cervical lymphadenopathy. Hepatosplenomegaly also may be present. The illness usually resolves within 2 to 4 weeks but can last for several months. EBV has been implicated as one cause of the controversial chronic fatigue syndrome. Infrequent complications include myocarditis, nephritis, upper airway obstruction, necrotizing epiglottitis, Guillain-Barré syndrome, Bell's palsy, meningoencephalitis, hematologic abnormalities (anemia, thrombocytopenia, neutropenia), splenic rupture, and even death (389,390).

Fetal Effects

Transplacental passage of EBV occurs rarely given that maternal seroconversion is itself rare. Several investigators have been unable to document serologic or virologic evidence of *in utero* infection even in offspring of women with serologically proven infectious mononucleosis or primary asymptomatic EBV infection in early pregnancy (391–395). However, transplacental passage has been confirmed infrequently in case reports (396,397). Joncas and colleagues described an infant with coexistent CMV and EBV infection in whom IgM antibody to EBV was present at birth (396). The abnormalities demonstrated by the infant (microcephaly, periventricular calcifications, hepatosplenomegaly) were also compatible with CMV effects.

There have been isolated reports of birth defects after maternal primary EBV infection. No samples, however, were taken from any of these infants to confirm infection (386,391,398–401). In general, rather than a characteristic syndrome, there is a variety of abnormalities. Because early reports implicated EBV as a cause of congenital heart disease, Tallqvist and colleagues compared the incidence of EBV antibodies in children 6 to 23 months of age with congenital heart disease to that of normal age-matched controls (402). They were unable to show any increase, suggesting that EBV does not cause, or is an uncommon cause of, cardiac defects.

There are only two reports of infants with congenital abnormalities in whom *in utero* EBV infection is reasonably well documented. Goldberg and colleagues described a male infant hypotonic at birth with micrognathia, bilateral cataracts, thrombocytopenia, and metaphyseal lucencies (397). The infant's serologic profile at 22 days of age was consistent with recent infection. Weaver and colleagues described an infant with extrahepatic bile duct atresia who was EBV-IgM seropositive at 3 weeks of age (403). Because EBV can be detected in the maternal cervix by DNA hybridization (404), it is possible that both of these cases represent intrapartum acquisition of EBV, with the defects being unrelated to EBV infection. In summary, there is no conclusive evidence that EBV causes birth defects.

Previously infected women may experience reactivation of EBV during pregnancy; indeed, this phenomenon is more common in pregnant than nonpregnant women (387,405,406). EA antibodies have been detected in 37% to 55% of pregnant women. The fetal consequences of reactivation are uncertain. Icart and Didier found that the presence of EA antibody in the first 3 months of pregnancy was associated with fetal death, congenital defects, prematurity, and fetal growth restriction (407). No virologic or serologic studies were conducted on the offspring of these women, so the role of EBV in these adverse outcomes is uncertain. Fleisher and Bolognese did not find a greater risk for any of these parameters associated with reactivation in their study population (387). Recently, Meyohas and colleagues used nested PCRs and found two neonates, from among 67 seropositive mothers, who were PCR positive at less than 1 week of age (408). Both mothers were also PCR positive, and both infants were healthy. This suggests that vertical transmission is possible in previously infected women, and that maternal antibody is generally protective. In addition, epidemiologic studies indicate that transplacental passage of maternal antibody will prevent infection in infants up to 6 months of age (409). Seroconversion prior to 1 year is rare in developed countries.

Laboratory Abnormalities and Diagnosis

Epstein-Barr virus cannot be isolated directly in tissue culture, so laboratory diagnosis of EBV infection is based on the detection of heterophil antibodies. Their presence is considered diagnostic of primary infection, although there are occasional false-positive results. EBV-specific serology can be used to evaluate women with a negative heterophil antibody test result. Primary or recent infection is diagnosed by detecting VCA-IgM antibodies, or IgG antibodies to VCA and EA but not to EBNA. Lymphocyte transformation assays, DNA hybridization, and PCR are not widely available and are usually limited to research studies.

Management

A woman who comes in contact with an individual with infectious mononucleosis is most likely already immune. Serologic testing is unnecessary because no effective prophylaxis is available. Testing can be done if the woman needs to know her serologic status in order to determine if intimate contact with the individual should be avoided. Treatment of infectious mononucleosis is symptomatic. Corticosteroids are used only for treating complications such as airway obstruction or severe hematologic abnormalities. Pregnancy termination is not warranted, and there does not appear to be a need for increased fetal surveillance. Breastfeeding is safe; it is not a source of early infection in the neonate (410). No vaccine is available.

ADENOVIRUS

Human adenoviruses are double-stranded DNA viruses belonging to the genus *Mastadenovirus,* which consists of at least 47 serotypes. The replicating virus is capable of establishing latent infection in lymphoid cells and is also responsible for cell lysis. Infection is common in infancy and childhood, and nearly all adults possess serum antibody against multiple serotypes. Infection can occur throughout the year, most commonly in the fall to spring. Adenoviruses are transmitted by inhalation of infected respiratory secretions or by the fecal-oral route. Following infection, type-specific antibody production protects only against infection with the same serotype.

In adults, the most frequent clinical presentation following infection is an acute respiratory illness characterized by a sore throat, gradually rising fever, and cough. Coryza and regional lymphadenopathy are also common. Although the pharynx and tonsils are injected and edematous, there is little or no exudate. On occasion, pneumonia may develop, and this is more likely in immunosuppressed patients in whom the virus may become disseminated. Adenoviruses also have been associated with acute diarrheal disease, hemorrhagic cystitis, and epidemic keratoconjunctivitis, all of which are more common in children. Reports of neonatal infection are rare, but fatal obliterative bronchiolitis and necrotizing pneumonitis have been described (411–414).

The virus can be transmitted transplacentally to the fetus in various animal models (415,416), and there is some evidence to suggest that this can happen in human pregnancies (411,412,417). Adenovirus has been isolated from a newborn with a congenital pleural effusion (418). Towbin and colleagues treated a fetus at 29 weeks' gestation with digoxin for adenoviral myocarditis (419). Ultrasonography showed that the fetus had massive ascites, scalp and skin edema, and pleural and pericardial effusions. Using PCR, these investigators were able to demonstrate identical adenoviral DNA in fetal, neonatal, and maternal blood, as well as in the placenta. This is consistent with recent evidence provided by PCR analysis of children with myocarditis, which supports the possibility that adenovirus is a common etiologic agent (420,421).

Both of the above infants survived, and subsequently did well, but perinatal adenovirus infections are often fatal.

In a review of 13 reported neonatal adenoviral infections, 11 (85%) were fatal (5). All 13 cases followed vaginal delivery; prolonged rupture of the membranes was seen more frequently than expected; the gestational age of 7 of the infants was equal to or less than 36 weeks; and almost half of the mothers had symptoms consistent with a viral syndrome peripartum. This suggested to the researchers the possibility of an ascending infection or one acquired from the birth canal during delivery. Adenovirus is known to infect the female genital tract, and this pathogen has been detected in routine cervical cytology smears (422). Montone and colleagues reported a case of neonatal adenovirus infection in a 25-week preterm infant whose delivery followed 4 days of ruptured membranes (414). *In situ* hybridization of neonatal samples and a cervical smear taken 6 weeks prior to delivery confirmed the presence of adenovirus.

Recently, PCR analysis was performed on a variety of samples from 303 fetuses considered to be at risk for intrauterine viral infection based on ultrasonographic findings (nonimmune hydrops, fetal pleural effusions, stuck twin, ventriculomegaly, fetal calcifications, myocarditis, poly- or oligohydramnios, intrauterine growth restriction, or maternal exposure to virus) (423). In total, viral genomes were found in 41% of fetuses. Adenovirus was the most commonly encountered virus, present in 24% of fetuses compared with 2% of the control group. Adenovirus was amplified from 33% (30 of 91) of those with nonimmune hydrops, 37% (8 of 22) of those with intrauterine growth restriction, and 50% (6 of 12) of those with myocarditis. McLean and colleagues found no amplification of viral genome using PCR to evaluate 243 amniotic fluid specimens from low-risk pregnancies (424). Although preliminary, these results suggest a causative role for adenovirus in fetal pathology.

It is difficult to differentiate adenoviral infections from those caused by a number of other viral agents on clinical grounds. Definitive diagnosis requires viral isolation by culture, immunofluorescence or other immunologic techniques, PCR, or serologic techniques such as an ELISA. Treatment is supportive because no antiviral agents have proven useful. Live vaccines have been developed against adenoviruses types 4 and 7 and have been used in military recruit populations, but they are not administered to the general population or during pregnancy.

REFERENCES

1. Weller TH, Hanshaw JB, Scott DE. Serologic differentiation of viruses responsible for cytomegalic inclusion disease. Virology 1960;12: 130–132.
2. Demmler GJ. Summary of a workshop on surveillance for congenital cytomegalovirus disease. Rev Infect Dis 1991;13:315–329.
3. Alford C, Britt W. Cytomegalovirus. In: Fields BN, Snipes DM, Chanock RM, et al., eds. Virology, 2nd ed. New York: Raven, 1990: 1981–2010.
4. Yow MD, Williamson DW, Leeds LJ, et al. Epidemiologic characteristics of cytomegalovirus infection in mothers and infants. Am J Obstet Gynecol 1988;158:1189–1195.
5. Chandler SH, Holmes KK, Wentworth BB, et al. The epidemiology of cytomegaloviral infection in women attending a sexually transmitted disease clinic. J Infect Dis 1985;152:597–604.
6. Stagno S, Pass RF, Cloud G, et al. Primary cytomegalovirus infection in pregnancy: incidence, transmission to fetus and clinical outcome. JAMA 1986;256:1904–1908.
7. Hunter K, Stagno S, Capps E, Smith RJ. Prenatal screening of pregnant women for infections caused by cytomegalovirus, Epstein-Barr virus, herpesvirus, rubella, and *Toxoplasma gondii.* Am J Obstet Gynecol 1983;145:269–273.
8. Stagno S, Reynolds DW, Huang ES, Thames SD, Smith RJ, Alford CA. Congenital cytomegalovirus infection: occurrence in an immune population. N Engl J Med 1977;296:1254–1258.
9. Schopfer K, Lauber E, Krech U. Congenital cytomegalovirus infection in newborn infants of mothers infected before pregnancy. Arch Dis Child 1978;53:536–539.
10. Rutter D, Griffiths P, Trompeter RS. Cytomegalic inclusion disease after recurrent maternal infection. Lancet 1985;2:1182.
11. Yow MD. Congenital cytomegalovirus disease: a NOW problem. J Infect Dis 1989;159:163–167.
12. Hanshaw JB. Congenital cytomegalovirus infection: a 15 year prospective study. J Infect Dis 1971;123:555–556.
13. Pass RF, Little EA, Stagno S, Britt WJ, Alford CA. Young children as a probable source of maternal and congenital cytomegalovirus infection. N Engl J Med 1987;316:1366–1370.
14. Pass RF, Hutto C. Group day care and cytomegalovirus infections of mothers and children. Rev Infect Dis 1986;8:599–605.
15. Adler SP. Molecular epidemiology of cytomegalovirus: viral transmission among children attending a day care center, their parents and care takers. J Pediatr 1988;112:366–372.
16. Adler SP. Cytomegalovirus transmission and child day care. Adv Pediatr Infect Dis 1992;7:109–122.
17. Taber LH, Frank AL, Yow MD, Bagley A. Acquisition of cytomegaloviral infection in families with young children: a serological study. J Infect Dis 1985;151:948–952.
18. Sweet RL, Gibbs RS. Perinatal Infections. In: Infectious diseases of the female genital tract, 3rd ed. Baltimore: Williams & Wilkins, 1995: 465–528.
19. Stagno S, Cloud GA. Working parents: the impact of day care and breast-feeding on cytomegalovirus infections in offspring. Proc Natl Acad Sci U S A 1994;91:2384–2389.
20. Monif GRG, Egan EA, Held B, Eitzman DV. The correlation of maternal cytomegalovirus infection during varying stages of gestation and neonatal involvement. J Pediatr 1972;80:17–20.
21. Dworsky ME, Welch K, Cassady G, Stagno S. Occupational risk for primary cytomegalovirus infection among pediatric health care workers. N Engl J Med 1983;309:950–953.
22. Flowers RH, Torner JC, Farr BM. Primary cytomegalovirus infection in pediatric nurses: a meta-analysis. Infect Control Hosp Epidemiol 1988;9:491–496.
23. Balfour CL, Balfour HH. Cytomegalovirus is not an occupational risk for nurses in renal transplant and neonatal units. Results of a prospective surveillance study. JAMA 1986;256:1909–1914.
24. Balcarek KB, Bagley R, Cloud GA, Pass RF. Cytomegalovirus infection among employees of a children s hospital: no evidence for increased risk with patient care. JAMA 1990;263:840–844.
25. Adler SP, Finney JW, Manganello AM, Best AM. Prevention of child-to-mother transmission of cytomegalovirus by changing behaviors: a randomized controlled trial. Pediatr Infect Dis J 1996;15:240–246.
26. Kyriazopoulou V, Bonds J, Frantzidou F, et al. Prenatal diagnosis of fetal cytomegalovirus infection in seropositive pregnant women. Eur J Obstet Gynecol Reprod Biol 1996;69:91–95.
27. Ruellan-Eugene G, Barjot P, Campet M, et al. Evaluation of virological procedures to detect fetal human cytomegalovirus infection: avidity of IgG antibodies, virus detection in amniotic fluid and maternal serum. J Med Virol 1996;50:9–15.
28. Toma P, Magnano GM, Mezzano P, Lazzini F, Bonacci W, Serra G. Cerebral ultrasound images in prenatal cytomegalovirus infection. Neuroradiology 1989;31:278–279.
29. Stagno S, Pass RF, Dworsky ME, Alford CA. Congenital and perinatal cytomegalovirus infection. Semin Perinatol 1983;7:30–42.
30. Boppana S, Pass RF, Britt WS, Stagno S, Alford CA. Symptomatic

congenital cytomegalovirus infection: neonatal morbidity and mortality. Pediatr Infect Dis J 1992;11:93–99.
31. Stagno S, Pass RF, Thomas JP. Defects of tooth structure in congenital cytomegalovirus infection. Pediatrics 1982;69:646–648.
32. Pass RF, Stagno S, Meyers GJ, Alford CA. Outcome of symptomatic congenital cytomegalovirus infection: results of long-term longitudinal follow-up. Pediatrics 1980;66:758–762.
33. Hanshaw JB, Scheiner AP, Moxley AW, Gaer L, Abel V, Scheiner B. School failure and deafness after silent congenital cytomegalovirus infection. N Engl J Med 1976;295:468–470.
34. Reynolds DW, Stagno S, Stubbs KG, et al. Inapparent congenital cytomegalovirus infection with elevated cord IgM levels: causal relation with auditory and mental deficiency. N Engl J Med 1974;290: 291–296.
35. Conboy TJ, Pass PF, Stagno S, et al. Intellectual development in school-aged children with asymptomatic congenital cytomegalovirus infection. Pediatrics 1986;77:801–806.
36. Stagno S, Pass RF, Dworsky ME, Alford CA Jr. Maternal cytomegalovirus infection and perinatal transmission. Clin Obstet Gynecol 1982;25:563–576.
37. Morris DJ, Sims D, Chiswick M, Das VK, Newton VE. Symptomatic congenital cytomegalovirus infection after maternal recurrent infection. Pediatr Infect Dis J 1994;13:61–64.
38. Fowler KB, Stagno S, Pass RF, Britt WJ, Ball TJ, Alford CA. The outcome of congenital cytomegalovirus infection in relation to maternal antibody status. N Engl J Med 1992;326:663–667.
39. Landini MP, Mach M. Detection of antibodies specific for human cytomegalovirus. Is it diagnostically useful? When and how? Scand J Infect Dis 1995;99(suppl):18–23.
40. McGowan KL, Hodinka RL. Laboratory diagnosis of fetal infections. Clin Lab Med 1992;12:523–552.
41. Stagno S, Tinker MK, Elrod C, Fuccillo DA, Cloud G, O'Beirne AJ. Immunoglobulin M antibodies detected by enzyme-linked immunoabsorbent assay and radioimmunoassay in the diagnosis of cytomegalovirus infections in pregnant women and newborn infants. J Clin Microbiol 1985;21:930–935.
42. Schoub BD, Johnson S, McAnerney JM, et al. Is antenatal screening for rubella and cytomegalovirus justified? S Afr Med J 1993;83: 108–110.
43. Gleaves CA, Smith TF, Shuster EA, Pearson GR. Rapid detection of cytomegalovirus in MRC-5 cells innoculated with urine specimens by using low-speed centrifugation and monoclonal antibody to an early antigen. J Clin Microbiol 1984;19:917–919.
44. Grosse C, Weiner CP. Prenatal diagnosis of congenital cytomegalovirus infection: two decades later. Am J Obstet Gynecol 1990;163: 447–450.
45. Meisel RI, Alvarez M, Lynch L, Chitkara U, Emanuel DJ, Berkowitz RL. Fetal cytomegalovirus infection: a case report. Am J Obstet Gynecol 1990;162:663–664.
46. Lynch L, Daffos F, Emanuel D, et al. Prenatal diagnosis of fetal cytomegalovirus infection. Am J Obstet Gynecol 1991;165:714–718.
47. Hohlfeld P, Vial Y, Maillard-Brignon C, Vaudaux B, Fawer C-L. Cytomegalovirus fetal infection: prenatal diagnosis. Obstet Gynecol 1991; 78:615–618.
48. Skvorc-Ranko R, Lavoie H, St. Denis P, et al. Intrauterine diagnosis of cytomegalovirus and rubella infections by amniocentesis. Can Med Assoc J 1991;145:649–654.
49. Lamy ME, Mulongo KN, Gadisseux JF, Lyon G, Gaudy V, VanLierde M. Prenatal diagnosis of fetal cytomegalovirus infection. Am J Obstet Gynecol 1992;166:91–94.
50. Weber B, Opp M, Born HJ, Langenbeck U, Doerr HW. Laboratory diagnosis of congenital cytomegalovirus infection using polymerase chain reaction and shell vial culture. Infection 1992;20:155–157.
51. Hogge WA, Buffone GJ, Hogge JS. Prenatal diagnosis of cytomegalovirus (CMV) infection: a preliminary report. Prenat Diagn 1993;13: 131–136.
52. Donner C, Liesnard C, Content J, Busine A, Aderca J, Rodesch F. Prenatal diagnosis of 52 pregnancies at risk for congenital cytomegalovirus infection. Obstet Gynecol 1993;82:481–486.
53. Donner C, Liesnard C, Brancart F, Rodesch F. Accuracy of amniotic fluid testing before 21 weeks gestation in prenatal diagnosis of congenital cytomegalovirus infection. Prenat Diagn 1994;14:1055–1059.
54. Nicolini U, Kustermann A, Tassis B, et al. Prenatal diagnosis of congenital human cytomegalovirus infection. Prenat Diagn 1994;14: 903–906.
55. Catanzarite V, Danker WM. Prenatal diagnosis of congenital cytomegalovirus infection: false negative amniocentesis at 20 weeks gestation. Prenat Diagn 1993;13:1021–1025.
56. Demmler GJ, Buffone GJ, Schimbor CM, May RA. Detection of cytomegalovirus in urine from newborns by using polymerase chain reaction DNA amplification. J Infect Dis 1988;158:1177–1184.
57. Hagay ZJ, Biran G, Ornoy A, Reece EA. Congenital cytomegalovirus infection: a long-standing problem still seeking a solution. Am J Obstet Gynecol 1996;174:241–245.
58. Pass RF. Commentary: is there a role for prenatal diagnosis of congenital cytomegalovirus infection? Pediatr Infect Dis 1992;11: 608–609.
59. Stronati M, Revello MG, Cerbo RM, Furione M, Rondini G, Gernai G. Ganciclovir therapy of congenital human cytomegalovirus hepatitis. Acta Paediatr 1995;84:340–341.
60. Adler SP. Current prospects for immunization against cytomegalovirus disease. Infect Agents Dis 1996;5:29–35.
61. Weller TH. Varicella and herpes zoster—changing concepts of the natural history, control, and importance of a not-so-benign virus. N Engl J Med 1983;309:1362–1368.
62. Preblud SR. Varicella. Complications and costs. Pediatrics 1986;78: 728–735.
63. Ross AH, Lenchner E, Reitman G. Modification of chickenpox in family contacts by administration of gamma globulin. N Engl J Med 1962;267:369–376.
64. Sever J, White LR. Intrauterine viral infections. Ann Rev Med 1968; 19:471–486.
65. Balducci I, Rodis JF, Rosengren S, Vintzileos AM, Spivey G, Vosseller C. Pregnancy outcome following first trimester varicella infection. Obstet Gynecol 1992;79:5–6.
66. Prevention of varicella: recommendations of the advisory committee on immunization practices (ACIP). MMWR 1996;45(RR-11):1–36.
67. Brunell PA, Kotchmar GS. Zoster in infancy: failure to maintain virus latency following intrauterine infection. J Pediatr 1981;98:71–73.
68. Enders G, Miller E, Cradock-Watson J, Bolley I, Ridehalgh M. Consequences of varicella and herpes zoster in pregnancy: prospective study of 1739 cases. Lancet 1994;343:1547–1550.
69. Brazin SA, Simkovich JW, Johnson WT. Herpes zoster during pregnancy. Obstet Gynecol 1979;53:175–181.
70. Paryani SG, Arvin AM. Intrauterine infection with varicella-zoster virus after maternal varicella. N Eng J Med 1986;314:1542–1546.
71. Enders G. Management of varicella-zoster contact and infection in pregnancy using a standardized varicella-zoster ELISA test. Postgrad Med J 1985;61:23–30.
72. Triebwasser JH, Harris RE, Bryant RE, Rhoades ER. Varicella pneumonia in adults. Medicine 1967;46:409–423.
73. Smego RA, Asperilla MO. Use of acyclovir for varicella pneumonia during pregnancy. Obstet Gynecol 1991;78:1112–1116.
74. Harris RE, Rhodes ER. Varicella pneumonia complicating pregnancy. Report of a case and review of the literature. Obstet Gynecol 1965;25: 734–740.
75. Esmonde TF, Herdman G, Anderson G. Chickenpox pneumonia: an association with pregnancy. Thorax 1989;44:812–815.
76. Broussard RC, Payne K, George RB. Treatment with acyclovir of varicella pneumonia in pregnancy. Chest 1991;99:1045–1047.
77. Cox SM, Cunningham FG, Luby J. Management of varicella pneumonia complicating pregnancy. Am J Perinatol 1990;7:300–301.
78. Guess HA, Broughton DD, Melton LJ, Kurland LT. Population-based studies of varicella complications. Pediatrics 1986;78(suppl):723–727.
79. Pastuszak AL, Levy M, Schick B, et al. Outcome after maternal varicella infection in the first 20 weeks of pregnancy. N Engl J Med 1994; 330:901–905.
80. Siegel M, Fuerst RT, Peress NS. Comparative fetal mortality in maternal virus diseases: a prospective study on rubella, measles, mumps, chickenpox and hepatitis. N Engl J Med 1966;274:768–771.
81. Liesnard C, Donner C, Brancart F, Rodesch F. Varicella in pregnancy. Lancet 1994;344:950–951.
82. Stagno S, Whitley RJ. Herpesvirus infections of pregnancy. II. Herpes simplex virus and varicella zoster virus infections. N Engl J Med 1985;313:1327–1330.
83. La Foret EG, Lynch CL. Multiple congenital defects following maternal varicella. N Engl J Med 1947;236:534–536.
84. Connan L, Ayoubi J, Icart J, Halasz A, Thene M, Berrebi A. Intrauterine fetal death following maternal varicella infection. Eur J Obstet Gynecol Repr Biol 1996;68:205–207.

85. Siegel M. Congenital malformations following chickenpox, measles, mumps, and hepatitis. Results of a cohort study. JAMA 1973;226: 1521–1524.
86. Huang Y-C, Lin T-Y, Chiu C-T. Acyclovir prophylaxis of varicella after household exposure. Pediatr Infect Dis J 1995;14:152–154.
87. Jones KL, Johnson KA, Chambers CD. Offspring of women infected with varicella during pregnancy: a prospective study. Teratology 1994; 49:29–32.
88. Kustermann A, Zoppini C, Tassis B, Della Morte M, Colucci G, Nicolini U. Prenatal diagnosis of congenital varicella infection. Prenat Diagn 1996;16:71–74.
89. Higa K, Dan K, Manabe H. Varicella-zoster virus infections during pregnancy: hypothesis concerning the mechanisms of congenital malformations. Obstet Gynecol 1987;69:214–222.
90. Salzman MB, Sood SK. Congenital anomalies resulting from maternal varicella at 25 1/2 weeks of gestation. Pediatr Infec Dis J 1992; 11:504–505.
91. Bai PVA, John TJ. Congenital skin ulcers following varicella in late pregnancy. J Pediatr 1979;94:65–67.
92. Dufour P, deBievre P, Vinatier D, et al. Varicella and pregnancy. Eur J Obstet Gynaecol Reprod Biol 1996;66:119–123.
93. Meyer JD. Congenital varicella in term infants: risk reconsidered. J Infect Dis 1974;129:215–217.
94. La Russa P, Steinberg S, Waithe E, Hanna B, Holzman P. Comparison of five assays for antibody to varicella-zoster virus and the fluorescence-antibody-to-membrane antigen test. J Clin Microbiol 1987;25: 2059–2062.
95. Wreghitt TG, Tedder RS, Nagington J, Ferns RB. Antibody assays for varicella virus: comparison of competitive enzyme-linked immunosorbant assay (ELISA), competitive radioimmunoassay (RIA), complement fixation, and indirect immuno-fluorescence assays. J Med Virol 1984;13:361–370.
96. Bogger-Goren S, Baba K, Hurley P, Yabruuchi H, Takahashi M, Ogra PL. Antibody response to varicella-zoster virus after natural or vaccine-induced infection. J Infect Dis 1982;146:260–265.
97. Gershon AA, La Russa PS, Steinberg SP. Detection of antibody to varicella zoster virus using the latex agglutination assay. Clin Diagn Virol 1994;2:271–278.
98. Cradock-Watson JE, Ridehalgh MKS, Bourne MS. Specific immunoglobulin responses after varicella and herpes zoster. J Hyg (London) 1979;82:319–336.
99. Alkalay AL, Pomerance JJ, Rimoin DL. Fetal varicella syndrome. J Pediatr 1987;111:320–323.
100. Puchhammer-Stockl E, Kunz C, Wagner G, Enders G. Detection of varicella zoster virus (VZV) DNA in fetal tissue by polymerase chain reaction. J Perinat Med 1994;22:65–69.
101. Sauerbrei A, Muller D, Eichhorn U, Wutzler P. Detection of varicella-zoster virus in congenital varicella syndrome: a case report. Obstet Gynecol 1996;89:687–689.
102. Seidman DS, Stevenson DK, Arvin AM. Varicella vaccine in pregnancy [Editorial]. Br Med J 1996;313:701–702.
103. Rouse DJ, Gardner M, Allen SJ, Goldenberg RL. Management of the presumed susceptible varicella (chickenpox)-exposed gravida: a cost effectiveness/cost-benefit analysis. Obstet Gynecol 1996;87:932–936.
104. Lieu TA, Finkler LJ, Sorel ME, Black SB, Shinefield HR. Cost effectiveness of varicella serotesting vs presumptive vaccination of school-age children and adolescents. Pediatrics 1995;95:632–638.
105. Shehab ZM, Brunell PA. Susceptibility of hospital personnel to varicella-zoster virus. J Infect Dis 1984;150:786–787.
106. McGregor JA, Mark S, Crawford GP, Levin MJ. Varicella zoster antibody testing in the case of pregnant women exposed to varicella. Am J Obstet Gynecol 1987;157:281–284.
107. Silverman N, Ewing SH, Todi N, Montgomery OC. Maternal varicella as a predictor of varicella immune status. J Perinatol 1996;16: 35–38.
108. Longfield JN, Winn RE, Gibson RL, Juchau SV, Hoffman PV. Varicella outbreak in army recruits from Puerto Rico. Varicella susceptibility in a population from the tropics. Arch Intern Med 1990;150: 970–973.
109. Salzman MB, Sharrar RG, Steinberg S, LaRussa P. Transmission of varicella-vaccine virus from a healthy 12-month-old child to his pregnant mother. J Pediatr 1997;131:151–154.
110. Establishment of VARVAX pregnancy registry. From the Centers for Disease Control and Prevention. JAMA 1996;275:1073.
111. Martin KA, Junker AK, Thomas EE, Van Allen MI, Friedman JM. Occurrence of chickenpox during pregnancy in women seropositive for varicella-zoster virus. J Infect Dis 1994;170:991–995.
112. Suga S, Yoshikawa T, Ozaki T, Asano Y. Effect of oral acyclovir against primary and secondary viremia in incubation period of varicella. Arch Dis Child 1993;69:639–643.
113. Zaia JA, Levin MJ, Preblud SR, et al. Evaluation of varicella-zoster immune globulin: protection of immunosuppressed children after household exposure to varicella. J Infect Dis 1983;147:737–743.
114. Chapman S, Duff P. Varicella in pregnancy. Semin Perinatol 1993;17: 403–409.
115. Venkatesan P. Chickenpox in pregnancy: how dangerous? Practitioner 1996;240:256–259.
116. Kesson AM, Grimwood K, Burgess MA, et al. Acyclovir for the prevention and treatment of varicella zoster in children, adolescents and pregnancy. J Paediatr Child Health 1996;32:211–217.
117. Feder HM Jr. Treatment of adult chickenpox with oral acyclovir. Arch Intern Med 1990;150:2061–2065.
118. Balfour HH, Rotbart HA, Feldman S, et al. Acyclovir treatment of varicella in otherwise healthy adolescents. J Pediatr 1992;120: 627–633.
119. Wallace WR, Bowler WA, Murray NB, Brodine SK, Oldfield EC III. Treatment of adult varicella with oral acylovir. Ann Intern Med 1992; 117:358–363.
120. Hirsch MS, Swartz MD. Antiviral agents. N Engl J Med 1980;302: 949–953.
121. Famciclovir for herpes zoster. Med Lett Drugs Ther 1994;36:97–98.
122. Clark GPM, Dobson PM, Thickett A, Turner NM. Chickenpox pneumonia, its complications and mangement: a report of three cases, including the use of extracorporeal membrane oxygenation. Anaesthesia 1991;46:376–380.
123. Lecuru F, Taurelle R, Bernard J-P, et al. Varicella zoster virus infection during pregnancy: the limits of prenatal diagnosis. Eur J Obstet Gynecol Reprod Biol 1994;56:67–68.
124. Isada NB, Paar DP, Johnson MP, Evans MI, Holzgreve W, Straus SE. In utero diagnosis of congenital varicella virus infection by chorionic villus sampling and polymerase chain reaction. Am J Obstet Gynecol 1991;165:1727–1730.
125. Cuthbertson G, Weiner CP, Giller RH, Grose C. Clinical and laboratory observations. Prenatal diagnosis of second trimester congenital varicella syndrome by virus specific immunoglobulin M. J Pediatr 1987;111:592–595.
126. Pretorius DH, Hayward I, Jones KL, Stamm E. Sonographic evaluation of pregnancies with maternal varicella infection. J Ultrasound Med 1992;11:459–463.
127. Miller E, Cradock-Watson JE, Ridehalgh MKS. Outcome in newborn babies given anti–varicella-zoster immunoglobulin after perinatal maternal infection with varicella-zoster virus. Lancet 1989;2: 371–373.
128. Hanngren K, Grandien M, Granstrom G. Effect of zoster immunoglobulin for varicella prophylaxis in the newborn. Scand J Infect Dis 1985;17:343–347.
129. Bakshi SS, Miller TC, Kaplan M, Hammerschlag MR, Prince A, Gershon AA. Failure of varicella-zoster immunoglobulin in modification of severe congenital varicella. Pediatr Infect Dis 1986;5:699–702.
130. Holland P, Isaacs D, Moxon ER. Fatal neonatal varicella infection. Lancet 1986;2:1156.
131. Frederick IB, White RJ, Braddock SW. Excretion of varicella-herpes zoster virus in breast milk. Am J Obstet Gynecol 1986;154: 1116–1117.
132. Cossart YE, Field AM, Cant B, Widdows D. Parvovirus-like particles in human sera. Lancet 1975;I:72–73.
133. Brown T, Anand A, Ritchie LD, Clewley JP, Reid TMS. Intrauterine parvovirus infection associated with hydrops fetalis. Lancet 1984;2: 1033–1034.
134. Knott PD, Welpy GAC, Anderson MJ. Serologically proved intrauterine infection with parvovirus. Br Med J 1984;289:1660.
135. Anand A, Gray ES, Brown T, Clewley JP, Cohen BJ. Human parvovirus infection in pregnancy and hydrops fetalis. N Engl J Med 1987;316:183–186.
136. Centers for Disease Control. Risks associated with human parvovirus B19 infections. MMWR 1988;38:81–87.
137. Anderson LJ. Role of parvovirus B19 in human disease. Pediatr Infect Dis J 1987;6:711–718.
138. Anderson MJ, Cohen BJ. Human parvovirus B19 infections in United Kingdom 1984–86. Lancet 1987;1:738–739.

139. Cohen BJ, Buckley MM. The prevalence of antibody to human parvovirus B19 in England and Wales. J Med Microbiol 1988;25:151–153.
140. Harger JH, Adler SP, Koch WC, Harger GF. Prospective evaluation of 618 pregnant women exposed to parvovirus B-19: risks and symptoms. Obstet Gynecol 1998;91:413–420.
141. Koch WC, Adler SP. Human parvovirus B19 infections in women of childbearing age and within families. Pediatr Infect Dis J 1989;8: 83–87.
142. Adler SP, Manganello A-MA, Koch WC, Hempfling SH, Best AM. Risk of human parvovirus B19 infections among school and hospital employees during endemic periods. J Infect Dis 1993;168:361–368.
143. Gillespie SM, Cartter ML, Asch S, et al. Occupational risk of human parvovirus B19 infection for school and day-care personnel during an outbreak of erythema infectiosum. JAMA 1990;263:2061–2065.
144. Chorba T, Coccia P, Holman RC, et al. The role of parvovirus B19 in aplastic crisis and erythema infectiosum (fifth disease). J Infect Dis 1986;154:383–393.
145. Hamon MD, Newland AC, Anderson MJ. Severe aplastic anemia after parvovirus infection in the absence of underlying haemolytic anemia. J Clin Pathol 1988;41:1242.
146. Sergent GR, Goldstein AR. B19 virus infection and aplastic crisis. In: Pattison JR, ed. Parvoviruses and human disease. Boca Raton, FL: CRC Press, 1988:85.
147. Gratecos E, Torres P-J, Vidal J, et al. The incidence of human parvovirus B19 infection during pregnancy and its impact on perinatal outcome. J Infect Dis 1995;171:1360–1363.
148. Public Health Laboratory Service Working Party on Fifth Disease. Prospective study of human parvovirus (B19) infection in pregnancy. Br Med J 1990;300:1166–1170.
149. Guidozzi F, Ballot D, Rothberg AD. Human B19 parvovirus infection in an obstetric population: a prospective study determining fetal outcome. J Reprod Med 1994;39:36–38.
150. Kinney JS, Anderson LJ, Farrar J, et al. Risk of adverse outcomes of pregnancy after human parvovirus B19 infection. J Infect Dis 1988; 157:663–667.
151. Rodis JF, Quinn DL, Gary GW, et al. Management and outcomes of pregnancies complicated by human B19 parvovirus infection: a prospective study. Am J Obstet Gynecol 1990;163:1168–1171.
152. Torok TJ, Anderson LJ, Gary GW, et al. Reproductive outcomes following human parvovirus B19 infection in pregnancy [Abstract 374]. In: Program and Abstracts of the 31st Interscience Conference on Antimicrobial Agents and Chemotherapy for Microbiology, 1991:328.
153. Gray ES, Davidson RJC, Anand A. Human parvovirus and fetal anemia. Lancet 1987;1:1144.
154. Naides SJ, Weiner CP. Antenatal diagnosis and palliative treatment of nonimmune hydrops fetalis secondary to fetal parvovirus B19 infection. Prenat Diagn 1989;9:105–114.
155. Porter HJ, Quantrill AM, Fleming KA. B19 parvovirus infection of myocardial cells. Lancet 1988;1:535–536.
156. Brown KE, Young NS, Liu JM. Molecular, cellular and clinical aspects of parvovirus B19 infection. Crit Rev Oncol Hematol 1994; 16:1–31.
157. Jordan JA. Identification of human parvovirus B19 infection in idiopathic nonimmune hydrops fetalis. Am J Obstet Gynecol 1996;174: 37–42.
158. Hadi HA, Easley KO, Finley J. Clinical significance of human parvovirus B19 infection in pregnancy. Am J Perinatol 1994;11:398–400.
159. Woolf AD, Campion GV, Chishick A, et al. Clinical manifestations of human parvovirus B19 in adults. Arch Intern Med 1989;149: 1153–1156.
160. Humphrey W, Magon M, O'Shaughnessy R. Severe nonimmune hydrops secondary to parvovirus B19 infection: spontaneous reversal in utero and survival of a term infant. Obstet Gynecol 1991;78: 900–902.
161. Pryde PG, Nugent CE, Pridjian G, Barr M Jr, Faix RG. Spontaneous resolution of nonimmune hydrops fetalis secondary to human parvovirus B19 infection. Obstet Gynecol 1992;79:859–861.
162. Morey AL, Keeling JW, Porter HJ, Fleming KA. Clinical and histopathogical features of parvovirus B19 infection in the human fetus. Br J Obstet Gynaecol 1992;99:566–574.
163. Mortimer PP, Cohen BJ, Buckley MM, Cradock-Watson JE, Burkhardt F, Schilt V. Human parvovirus and the fetus [Letter]. Lancet 1985;2:1012.
164. Kinney JS, Anderson LJ, Farrar J, Strikas RA, Kumar IL, Kliegman RM. Risk of adverse outcomes of pregnancy after human parvovirus B19 infection. J Infect Dis 1988;157:663–667.
165. Ager EA, Chin TDY, Poland JD. Epidemic erythema infectiousum. N Engl J Med 1966;275:1326–1331.
166. Weiland HT, Vermeij-Keers C, Salimans MMM, Fleuren GJ, Verweg RA, Anderson MJ. Parvovirus B19 associated with fetal abnormality. Lancet 1987;1:682–683.
167. Tiessen RG, Van Elsacker-Niele AMV, Vermeij-Keers C, Oepkes D, van Roosmalen J, Gorsira MC. A fetus with a parvovirus B19 infection and congenital anomalies. Prenat Diagn 1994;14:173–176.
168. Hall CB, Horner FA. Encephalopathy with erythema infectiosum. Am J Dis Child 1997;131:65–67.
169. Conry JA, Torok T, Andrews PI. Perinatal encephalopathy secondary to in utero human parvovirus B19 (HPV) infection [Abstract 7365]. Neurology 1993;43(suppl):A346.
170. Katz VL, McCoy MC, Kuller JA, Hansen WF. An association between fetal parvovirus B19 infection and fetal anomalies: a report of two cases. Am J Perinatol 1996;13:43–45.
171. Weiner CP, Naides SJ. Fetal survival after human parvovirus B19 infection: spectrum of intrauterine response in a twin gestation. Am J Perinatol 1992;9:66–68.
172. Sheikh AU, Ernest JM, O'Shea M. Long-term outcome in fetal hydrops from parvovirus B19 infection. Am J Obstet Gynecol 1992; 167:337–341.
173. Koch WC, Adler SP, Harger J. Intrauterine parvovirus B19 infection may cause an asymptomatic or recurrent postnatal infection. Pediatr Infect Dis J 1993;12:747–750.
174. Anderson MJ, Higgins PG, Davis LR, et al. Experimental parvoviral infection in humans. J Infect Dis 1985;152:257–265.
175. Basetse HR, Baker EF, Steele AD, Lecatsas G. Possible false-positive results for parvovirus B19 IgM antibodies. S Afr Med J 1993;83;441.
176. Sergeant GR, Sergeant BE, Thomas PW, Anderson MJ, Patou G, Pattison JR. Human parvovirus infection in homozygous sickle cell disease. Lancet 1993;341:1237–1240.
177. Rao SP, Miller ST, Cohen BJ. Transient aplastic crisis in patients with sickle cell disease: B19 parvovirus studies during a 7-year period. Am J Dis Child 1992;146:1328–1330.
178. Torok TJ, Wang Q-Y, Gary GW Jr, Yang CF, Finch TM, Anderson LJ. Prenatal diagnosis of intrauterine infection with parvovirus B19 by the polymerase chain reaction technique. Clin Infect Dis 1992;14: 149–155.
179. Yamakawa Y, Oka H, Hori S, Arai T, Izumi R. Detection of human parvovirus B19 DNA by nested polymerase chain reaction. Obstet Gynecol 1995;86:126–129.
180. Peters M, Nicolaides K. Cordocentesis for the diagnosis and treatment of human fetal parvovirus infection. Obstet Gynecol 1990;75:501–504.
181. Kovacs BW, Carlson DE, Shahbakrami B, Platt L. Prenatal diagnosis of human parvovirus B19 infection in nonimmune hydrops fetalis by polymerase chain reaction. Am J Obstet Gynecol 1996;167:461–466.
182. Rogers BB, Singer DB, Mak SK, Gary GW, Fikrig MK, McMillan PN. Detection of human parvovirus B19 in early spontaneous abortuses using serology, histology, electron microscopy, in situ hybridization, and the polymerase chain reaction. Obstet Gynecol 1993;81:402–408.
183. Rodis JF, Hovick TJ, Quinn DL, Rosengren SS, Tattersall P. Human parvovirus infection in pregnancy. Obstet Gynecol 1988;72:733–738.
184. Bernstein IM, Capeless EL. Elevated maternal serum alphafetoprotein and hydrops fetalis in association with fetal parvovirus B19 infection. Obstet Gynecol 1989;74:456–457.
185. Carrington D, Gilmore DH, Wittle MJ, et al. Maternal serum alphafetoprotein: A marker of fetal aplastic crisis during intrauterine human parvovirus infection. Lancet 1987;1:433–435.
186. Johnson DR, Fisher RA, Helwick JJ, Murray DL, Patterson MJ, Downes FP. Screening maternal serum alphafetoprotein levels and human parvovirus antibodies. Prenat Diagn 1994;14:455–458.
187. Fairley CK, Smoleniec JS, Caul OE, Miller E. Observational study of effect of intrauterine transfusions on outcome of fetal hydrops after parvovirus B19 infection. Lancet 1995;346:1335–1337.
188. Faure JM, Giacalone PL, Deschamps F, Boulot P. Nonimmune hydrops fetalis caused by intrauterine human parvovirus B19 infection: a case of spontaneous reversal in utero. Fetal Diagn Ther 1997; 12:66–67.
189. Kurtzman GJ, Cohen B, Meyers P, Amunullah A, Young N. Persistent B19 parvovirus infection as a cause of severe chronic anemia in children with acute lymphocytic leukemia. Lancet 1988;2:1159–1162.

190. Selbing A, Josefsson A, Dahle LO, Lindgren R. Parvovirus B19 infection during pregnancy treated with high-dose intravenous gammaglobulin. Lancet 1995;345:660–661.
191. Schwartz TF, Roggendorf M, Hottentrager B, Modrows S, Deinhardt F, Middleldorp J. Immunoglobulins in the prophylaxis of parvovirus B19 infection. J Infect Dis 1990;162:1214.
192. Ray SM, Erdman DD, Berschling JD, Cooper JE, Torok TJ, Blumberg HM. Nosocomial exposure to parvovirus B19: low risk of transmission to healthcare workers. Infect Control Hosp Epidemiol 1997;18: 109–114.
193. Gregg NM. Congenital cataract following German measles in the mother. Trans Ophthalmol Soc Aust 1941;3:35–46.
194. Rubella and pregnancy. ACOG Technical Bulletin Number 171, 1992.
195. Forrester RM, Lees VT, Watson GH. Rubella syndrome: escape of a twin. Br Med J 1966;1:1403.
196. Tondury G, Smith DW. Fetal rubella pathology. J Pediatr 1966;68: 867–879.
197. Chang TH, Moorhead PS, Boue JG, Plotkin SA, Hoskins JM. Chromosome studies of human cells infected in utero and in vitro with rubella virus. Proc Soc Exp Biol Med 1966;122:236–243.
198. Coyle PK, Wolinsky JS, Buimovici-Klein E, Moucha R, Cooper LZ. Rubella-specific immune complexes after congenital infection and vaccination. Infect Immun 1982;36:498–503.
199. Verder H, Dickmeiss E, Haahr S, et al. Late-onset rubella syndrome: coexistence of immune complex disease and defective cytotoxic effector cell function. Clin Exp Immunol 1986;63:367–375.
200. Morgan-Capner P, Hodgson J, Hambling MH, et al. Detection of rubella-specific IgM in subclinical rubella reinfection in pregnancy. Lancet 1985;1:244–246.
201. Grangeot-Keros L. Rubella and pregnancy. Pathol Biol 1992;40: 706–710.
202. Robinson J, Lemay M, Vaudry WL. Congenital rubella after anticipated maternal immunity: two cases and a review of the literature. Pediatr Infect Dis J 1994;13:812–815.
203. Best JM, Benatvala JE, Morgan-Capner P, Miller E. Fetal infection after maternal reinfection with rubella: criteria for defining reinfection. Br Med J 1989;299:773–775.
204. Gilbert J, Kudesia G. Fetal infection after maternal reinfection with rubella. Br Med J 1989;299:1217.
205. Das BD, Lakhani P, Kurtz JB, et al. Congenital rubella after previous maternal immunity. Arch Dis Child 1990;65:545–546.
206. Partridge JW, Flewett TH, Whitehead JEM. Congenital rubella affecting an infant whose mother had rubella antibodies before conception. Br Med J (Clin Res) 1981;282:187–188.
207. Enders G, Calm A, Schaub J. Rubella embryopathy after previous maternal vaccination. Infection 1984;12:96–98.
208. Hornstein L, Levy U, Fogel A. Clinical rubella with virus transmission to the fetus in a pregnant woman considered to be immune. N Engl J Med 1988;319:1415–1416.
209. Bott LM, Eizenberg DH. Congenital rubella after successful vaccination. Med J Aust 1982;1:514–515.
210. Saule H, Enders G, Zeller J, Bernsau U. Congenital rubella infection after previous immunity of the mother. Eur J Pediatr 1988;147: 195–196.
211. Morgan-Capner P, Miller E, Vurdien JE, Ramsay MEB. Outcome of pregnancy after maternal reinfection with rubella. Commun Dis Rep 1991;1:R57–R59.
212. Barfield W, Gardner R, Lett S, Johnsen C. Congenital rubella reinfection in a mother with anti-cardiolipin and anti-platelet antibodies. Pediatr Infect Dis J 1997;16:249–251.
213. Cherry JD. Rubella. In: Feigin RD, Cherry JD, eds. Textbook of pediatric infectious disease, 3rd ed. Philadelphia: WB Saunders, 1992: 1792.
214. Cooper LZ, Preblud SR, Alford CA. Rubella. In: Infectious diseases of the fetus and newborn infant, 4th ed. Philadelphia: WB Saunders, 1995:286.
215. Cradock-Watson JE, Ridehalgh MKS, Anderson MJ, Pattison JR. Outcome of asymptomatic infection with rubella virus during pregnancy. J Hyg 1981;87:147–154.
216. Smith CA, Petty RE, Tingle AJ. Rubella virus and arthritis. Rheum Dis Clin North Am 1987;13:265–274.
217. Townsend JJ, Baringer JR, Wolinsky JS, et al. Progressive rubella panencephalitis. Late onset after congenital rubella. N Engl J Med 1975;292:990–993.
218. Fujimoto T, Katoh C, Hayakawa H, Yokota M, Kimura E. Two cases of rubella infection with cardiac involvement. Jpn Heart J 1979;20: 227–235.
219. Saeed AA, Lange LS. Guillain-Barre syndrome after rubella. Postgrad Med J 1978;54:333–334.
220. Connolly JH, Hutchinson WM, Allen LV, et al. Carotid artery thrombosis, encephalitis, myelitis and optic neuritis associated with rubella virus infections. Brain 1975;98:583–594.
221. Menser MA, Forrest JM. Rubella—high incidence of defects in children considered normal at birth. Med J Aust 1974;1:123–126.
222. Schiff GM, Sutherland J, Light I. Congenital rubella. Symposium of Vienna. September 2–3, 1970. Stuttgart: George Thieme Verlag, 1971: 31.
223. South MA, Sever JL. Teratogen update: the congenital rubella syndrome. Teratology 1985;31:297–307.
224. Floret D, Rosenberg D, Hage GN, Monnet P. Hyperthyroidism, diabetes mellitus and the congenital rubella syndrome. Acta Paediatr Scand 1980;69:259–261.
225. Sever JL, South MA, Shaver KA. Delayed manifestations of congenital rubella. Rev Infect Dis 1985;7(suppl 1):164–169.
226. Shaver KA, Boughman JA, Nance WE. Congenital rubella syndrome and diabetes: a review of epidemiologic, genetic, and immunologic factors. Am Ann Deaf 1985;130:526–532.
227. Hanid TK. Hypothyroidism in congenital rubella. Lancet 1976;2: 854.
228. Shirley JA, Revill S, Cohen BJ, Buckley MM. Serological study of rubella-like illnesses. J Med Virol 1987;21:369–379.
229. Grangeot-Keros L, Nicolas JC, Bricout F, Pillot J. Rubella reinfection and the fetus. N Engl J Med 1985;313:1547.
230. Kurtz JB, Anderson MJ. Cross reactions in rubella and parvovirus specific IgM tests. Lancet 1985;2:1356.
231. Morgan-Capner P, Tedder RS, Mace JE. Rubella-specific IgM reactivity in sera from cases of infectious mononucleosis. J Hyg 1983;90: 407–413.
232. Pattison JR, Dane DS, Mace JE. Persistence of specific IgM after natural infection with rubella virus. Lancet 1975;1:185–187.
233. Hedman K, Seppala I. Recent rubella virus infection indicated by a low avidity of specific IgG. J Clin Immunol 1988;8:214–221.
234. Rousseau S, Hedman K. Rubella infection and reinfection distinguished by avidity of IgG. Lancet 1988;1:1108–1109.
235. Levin MJ, Oxman MN, Moore MG, Daniels JB, Scheer K. Diagnosis of congenital rubella in utero. N Engl J Med 1974;290:1187–1188.
236. Cederqvist LL, Zervoudakis IA, Ewool LC, Senterfit LB. Prenatal diagnosis of congenital rubella. Br Med J 1977;276:615.
237. Daffos F, Forestier F, Grangeot-Keros L, et al. Prenatal diagnosis of congenital rubella. Lancet 1984;2:1–3.
238. Lebon P, Daffos F, Checoury A, Grangeot-Keros L. Presence of an acid-labile alpha-interferon in sera from fetuses and children with congenital rubella. J Clin Microbiol 1985;21:775–778.
239. Grangeot-Keros L, Pillot J, Daffos F, Forrestier F. Prenatal and postnatal production of IgM and IgA antibodies to rubella virus studied by antibody capture immunoassay. J Infect Dis 1988;158:138–143.
240. Ho-Terry L, Terry GM. Londesborough P, Rees KR, Wielard F, Dennisen A. Diagnosis of fetal rubella infection by nucleic acid hybridization. J Med Virol 1988;24;175–182.
241. Bosma TJ, Corbett KM, Eckstein MB, et al. Use of PCR for prenatal and postnatal diagnosis of congenital rubella. J Clin Microbiol 1995; 33:2881–2887.
242. Tanemura M, Suzumori K, Yagami Y, Katow S. Diagnosis of fetal rubella infection with reverse transcription and nested polymerase chain reaction: a study of 34 cases diagnosed in fetuses. Am J Obstet Gynecol 1996;174:578–582.
243. Enders G, Jonatha W. Prenatal diagnosis of intra-uterine rubella. Infection 1987;15:162–164.
244. Miller E, Craddock-Watson JE, Pollock TM. Consequences of confirmed congenital rubella at successive stages of pregnancy. Lancet 1982;2:781–784.
245. Peckham C. Congenital rubella in the United Kingdom before 1970: the prevaccine era. Rev Infect Dis 1985;7(suppl 1):11–16.
246. Peckham CS. Clinical and laboratory study of children exposed in utero to maternal rubella. Arch Dis Child 1972;47:571–577.
247. Munro ND, Sheppard S, Smithells RW, Holzel H, Jones G. Temporal relations between maternal rubella and congenital defects. Lancet 1987;2:201–204.

248. Miller E. Rubella reinfection. Arch Dis Child 1990;65:820–821.
249. Morgan-Capner P. Diagnosing rubella. Br Med J 1989;299:338–339.
250. Slater PE, Ben-Zvi T, Fogel A, Ehrenfeld M, Ever-Hadani S. Absence of an association between rubella vaccination and arthritis in underimmune postpartum women. Vaccine 1995;13:1529–1532.
251. Centers for Disease Control. Rubella vaccination during pregnancy—United States, 1971–1988. MMWR 1989;38:289–293.
252. Centers for Disease Control. Update: Vaccine side effects, adverse reactions, contraindicated precautions. Recommendations of the Advisory Committee on Practices (AICP). MMWR 1996;45(RR-12):1–35.
253. Siber GR, Werner BC, Halsey NA. Interference of immune globulin with measles and rubella immunization. J Pediatr 1993;122:204–211.
254. Hope-Simpson RE. Infectiousness of communicable diseases in the household (measles, mumps, and chickenpox). Lancet 1952;2:549–554.
255. Siegel M, Fuerst HT. Low birth weight and maternal virus diseases. A prospective study of rubella, measles, mumps, chickenpox and hepatitis. JAMA 1966;197:680–684.
256. Centers for Disease Control. Summary—cases of specified notifiable diseases, United States. MMWR 1991;39:936.
257. Watson BM, Laufer DS, Kuter BJ, Staehle B, White CJ, Starr SE. Safety and immunogenicity of a combined live attenuated measles, mumps, rubella, and varicella vaccine (MMR(II)V) in healthy children. J Infect Dis 1996;173:731–734.
258. Forthal DN, Aarnaes S, Blanching J, de la Maza L, Tilles JG. Degree and length of viremia in adults with measles. J Infect Dis 1992;166:421–424.
259. Gremillion DH, Crawford GE. Measles pneumonia in young adults. An analysis of 106 cases. Am J Med 1981;71:539–542.
260. LaBoccetta AC, Tornay AS. Measles encephalitis. Report of 61 cases. Am J Dis Child 1964;107:247–255.
261. Gavish D, Kleinman Y, Morag A, Chajek-Shaul T. Hepatitis and jaundice associated with measles in young adults. An analysis of 65 cases. Arch Intern Med 1983;143:644–647.
262. Dyer I. Measles complicating pregnancy. Report of twenty-four cases with three instances of congenital measles. South Med J 1940;33:601–604.
263. Packer AD. The influence of maternal measles (morbilli) on the unborn child. Med J Aust 1950;1:835–838.
264. Grenhill JP. Acute (extragenital) infections in pregnancy, labor, and the puerperium. Am J Obstet Gynecol 1933;25:760–772.
265. Christensen PE, Schmidt H, Bang HO, Andersen V, Jordal B, Jensen O. An epidemic of measles in Southern Greenland, 1951. Measles in virgin soil. II. The epidemic proper. Acta Med Scand 1953;144:430–449.
266. Atmar RL, Englund JA, Hammill H. Complications of measles during pregnancy. Clin Infect Dis 1992;14:217–226.
267. Eberhart-Phillips JE, Frederick PD, Baron RC, Mascola L. Measles in pregnancy: a descriptive study of 58 cases. Obstet Gynecol 1993;82:792–801.
268. Stein SJ, Greenspoon JS. Rubeola during pregnancy. Obstet Gynecol 1991;78:925–929.
269. Gazala E, Karplus M, Liberman JR, Sarov I. The effect of maternal measles on the fetus. Pediatr Infect Dis J 1985;4:203–204.
270. Moroi K, Saito S, Kurata T, Sata T, Yanagida M. Fetal death associated with measles virus infection of the placenta. Am J Obstet Gynecol 1991;164:1107–1108.
271. Jespersen CS, Littauer J, Sagild U. Measles as a cause of fetal defects: a retrospective study of ten measles epidemics in Greenland. Acta Paediatr Scand 1977;66:367–378.
272. Aaby P, Bukh J, Lisse IM, Seim E, deSilva MC. Increased perinatal mortality among children of mothers exposed to measles during pregnancy. Lancet 1988;1:516–519.
273. Ekbom A, Daszak P, Kraaz W, Wakefield AJ. Crohn's disease after in-utero measles virus exposure. Lancet 1996;348:515–517.
274. Nielsen LL, Nielsen NM, Melbye M, Soderman M, Jacoken M, Aaby P. Exposure to measles in utero and Crohn's disease: Danish register study. Br Med J 1998;316:196–197.
275. Gershon AA. Chickenpox, measles and mumps. In: Remington JS, Klein JO, eds. Infectious diseases of the fetus and newborn infant, 4th ed. Philadelphia: WB Saunders, 1995.
276. Siegel D, Hirshman SZ. Hepatic dysfunction in acute measles infection in adults. Arch Intern Med 1977;137:1178–1179.
277. ACIP Task Force on Adult Immunization and Infectious Diseases Society of America. Guide of adult immunization, 2nd ed. Philadelphia: American College of Physicians, 1990:63–119.
278. Sever J, White LR. Intrauterine viral infections. Ann Rev Med 1968;19:471–486.
279. Lennette E. Laboratory diagnosis of viral infections, 2nd ed. New York: Marcel Dekker, 1992:549.
280. Philip RN, Reinhard KR, Lackman DB. Observations on a mumps epidemic in a virgin population. Am J Epidemiol 1959;69:91–111.
281. Schwartz HA. Mumps in pregnancy. Am J Obstet Gynecol 1950;60:875–876.
282. Hardy JB. Viral infections in pregnancy. A review. Am J Obstet Gynecol 1965;93:1052–1065.
283. Bowers D. Mumps during pregnancy. West J Surg Obstet Gynecol 1953;61:72–73.
284. Dutta PC. A fatal case of pregnancy complicated with mumps. J Obstet Gynecol Br Emp 1935;42:869–870.
285. Hyatt H. Relationship of maternal mumps to congenital defects and fetal deaths, and to maternal morbidity and mortality. Am Pract Diagn Treat 1961;12:359–363.
286. Kurtz J, Tomlinson A, Pearson J. Mumps virus isolated from a fetus. Br Med J Clin Res Ed 1982;284:471.
287. Homans A. Mumps in a pregnant woman. Premature labor, followed by the appearance of the same disease in the infant, twenty-four hours after its birth. Am J Med Sci 1855;29:56.
288. Swan C. Congenital malformations associated with rubella and other virus infections. In: Banks HS, ed. Modern practice in infectious fevers. Vol. 2. New York: PB Hoeber, 1951:528–552.
289. Greenberg MW, Beilly JS. Congenital defects in the infant following mumps during pregnancy. Am J Obstet Gynecol 1949;57:805–806.
290. Siddall RS. Epidemic parotitis in late pregnancy. Am J Obstet Gynecol 1937;33:524–525.
291. Holowach J, Thurston DL, Becker B. Congenital defects in infants following mumps during pregnancy. A review of the literature and a report of chorioretinitis due to fetal infection. J Pediatr 1957;50:689–694.
292. Grenwall H, Selander P. Some virus diseases during pregnancy and their effect on the fetus. Nord Med 1948;37:409–415.
293. Baumann B, Danon L, Weitz R, Schonfeld T, Nitzam M. Unilateral hydrocephalus due to obstruction of the foramen of Monro: another complication of intrauterine mumps infection. Eur J Pediatr 1982;139:158–159.
294. Manson MM, Logan WDP, Loy RM. Rubella and other virus infections during pregnancy. Rep Public Health Med Subj No. 101. London: Her Majesty's Stationary Office, 1960.
295. Noren GR, Adams P Jr, Anderson RC. Positive skin test reactivity to mumps virus antigen in endocardial fibroelastosis. J Pediatr 1963;62:604–606.
296. Shone JD, Munoz AS, Manning JA, Keith JD. The mumps antigen skin test in endocardial fibroelastosis. Pediatrics 1966;37:423–429.
297. Vosburgh JB, Diehl AM, Liu C, Lauer RM, Fabiyi A. Relationship of mumps to endocardial fibroelastosis. Am J Dis Child 1965;109:69–73.
298. Gersony WM, Katz SL, Nadas AS. Endocardial fibroelastosis and the mumps virus. Pediatrics 1966;37:430–434.
299. Guneroth WG. Endocardial fibroelastosis and mumps. Pediatrics 1966;38:309.
300. Nahmias AJ, Armstrong G. Mumps virus and endocardial fibroelastosis. N Engl J Med 1966;275:1448–1449.
301. Chen S-C, Thompson MW, Rose V. Endocardial fibroelastosis: family studies with special reference to counseling. J Pediatr 1971;79:385–392.
302. Jones JF, Ray G, Fulginiti VA. Perinatal mumps infection. J Pediatr 1980;96:912–914.
303. Lacour M, Maherzi M, Vienny H, Suter S. Thrombocytopenia in a case of neonatal mumps infection: Evidence for further clinical presentations. Eur J Pediatr 1993;152:739–741.
304. Reman O, Freymuth F, Laloum D, Bonte JF. Neonatal distress due to mumps. Arch Dis Child 1986;61:80–81.
305. Groenendaal F, Rothbarth PH, van den Anker JN, Spritzer R. Congenital mumps pneumonia: a rare cause of neonatal respiratory distress. Acta Paediatr Scand 1990;79:1252–1254.
306. Kilham L. Mumps virus in human milk and in milk of infected monkey. JAMA 1951;146:1231–1232.
307. Sterner G, Grandien M. Mumps in pregnancy at term. Scand J Infect Dis Suppl 1990;71:36–38.

308. Kalter SS. A serological survey of antibodies to selected enteroviruses. Bull WHO 1962;26:759–763.
309. Fox JP. Epidemiological aspects of coxsackie and ECHO virus infections in tropical areas. Am J Public Health 1964;54:1134–1142.
310. Downey TW. Poliovirus and flies: studies on the epidemiology of enteroviruses in an urban area. Yale J Biol Med 1963;35:341.
311. Modlin JF. Perinatal echovirus and group B coxsackie virus infections. Clin Perinatol 1988;15:233–246.
312. Sever JL, Huekner RJ, Castellano GA, Bell JA. Serologic diagnosis en masse with multiple antigens. Am Rev Respir Dis 1963;88: 342–349.
313. Cherry JD, Soriano F, Jahn CL. Search for perinatal viral infection. A prospective, clinical, virologic and serologic study. Am J Dis Child 1968;116:245–250.
314. Keswick BH, Gerba CP, Goyal SM. Occurrence of enteroviruses in community swimming pools. Am J Public Health 1981;71:1026–1030.
315. Batcup G, Holt P, Hambling MH, Gerlis LM, Glass MR. Placental and fetal pathology in coxsackie virus A9 infection: a case report. Histopathology 1985;9:1227–1235.
316. Amstey MS, Miller RK, Menegus MA, diSant Agnese PA. Enterovirus in pregnant women and the perfused placenta. Am J Obstet Gynecol 1988;158:775–782.
317. Modlin JF, Polk BF, Horton P, Etkind P, Crane E, Spiliotes A. Perinatal echovirus 11 infection: risk of transmission during a community outbreak. N Engl J Med 1981;205:368–371.
318. Jones MJ, Kolb M, Votava HJ, Johnson RL, Smith TF. Intrauterine echovirus type II infection. Mayo Clin Proc 1980;55:509–512.
319. Reyes MP, Ostrea EM, Roskamp J, Lerner AM. Disseminated neonatal echovirus 11 disease following antenatal maternal infection with a virus-positive cervix and virus-negative gastrointestinal tract. J Med Virol 1983;12:155–159.
320. Heineberg H, Gold E, Robbins FC. Differences in interferon content in tissues of mice of varius ages infected with coxsackie B1 virus. Proc Soc Exp Biol Med 1964;115:947–953.
321. Teisner B, Haahr S. Poikilothermia and susceptibility of suckling mice to coxsackie B1 virus. Nature 1974;247:568.
322. Horn P. Poliomyelitis in pregnancy. A twenty-year report from Los Angeles County, California. Obstet Gynecol 1955;6:121–137.
323. Bowers VM Jr, Danforth DN. The significance of poliomyelitis during pregnancy—an analysis of the literature and presentation of twenty-four new cases. Am J Obstet Gynecol 1953;65:34–39.
324. Anderson GW, Anderson G, Skaar A, Samdler F. Poliomyelitis in pregnancy. Am J Hyg 1952;55:127–139.
325. Siegel M, Greenberg M. Poliomyelitis in pregnancy. Effect on fetus and newborn infant. J Pediatr 1956;49:280–288.
326. Bates T. Poliomyelitis in pregnancy, fetus, and newborn. Am J Dis Child 1955;90:189–195.
327. Carter HM. Congenital poliomyelitis. Obstet Gynecol 1956;8:373.
328. Schaeffer M, Fox MJ, Li CP. Intrauterine poliomyelitis infection. JAMA 1954;155:248–250.
329. Elliott GB, McAllister JE, Alberta C. Fetal poliomyelitis. Am J Obstet Gynecol 1956;72:896–902.
330. Wyatt HV. Poliomyelitis in the fetus and the newborn. A comment on the new understanding of the pathogenesis. Clin Pediatr 1979;18: 33–38.
331. Aycock WL. Acute poliomyelitis in pregnancy: its occurrence according to month of pregnancy and sex of fetus. N Engl J Med 1946;235: 160–161.
332. Bergeisen GH, Bauman RJ, Gilmore RL. Neonatal paralytic poliomyelitis. Arch Neurol 1986;43:192–194.
333. Kibrick S, Benirschke K. Acute septic myocarditis and meningoencephalitis in the newborn child infected with coxsackie virus group B, type 3. N Engl J Med 1956;255:883–884.
334. Brightman VJ, Scott TFM, Westphal M, Boggs TR. An outbreak of coxsackie B-5 virus infection in the newborn nursery. J Pediatr 1966; 69:179–192.
335. Makower H, Skurska Z, Halazinska L. On transplacental infection with coxsackie virus. Tex Rep Biol Med 1958;16:346–354.
336. Basso NGS, Fonseca MEF, Garcia AGP, Zuardi JAT, Silva MR, Outani H. Enterovirus isolation from foetal and placental tissues. Acta Virol 1990;34:49–57.
337. Bates HR. Coxsackie virus B3 calcific pancarditis and hydrops fetalis. Am J Obstet Gynecol 1970;106:629–630.
338. Benirschke K, Pendleton ME. Coxsackie virus infection. An important complication of pregnancy. Obstet Gynecol 1958;12:305–309.
339. Axelsson C, Bondestam K, Frisk G, Bergstrom S, Diderholm H. Coxsackie B virus infections in women with miscarriage. J Med Virol 1993;39:282–285.
340. Brown GC, Karunas RS. Relationship of congenital anomalies and maternal infection with selected enteroviruses. Am J Epidemiol 1972; 95:207–217.
341. Gauntt CJ, Gudvangen RJ, Brans YW, Marlin AE. Coxsackie virus group B antibodies in the ventricular fluid of infants with severe anatomic defects in the central nervous system. Pediatrics 1985;76: 64–68.
342. Hyoty H, Hiltunen M, Knip M, et al. A prospective study of the role of coxsackie B and other enterovirus infections in the pathogenesis of IDDM. Diabetes 1995;44:652–657.
343. Dahlquist G, Frisk G, Ivarsson SA, Svanberg L, Forsgren M, Diderholm H. Indications that maternal coxsackie B virus infection during pregnancy is a risk factor for childhood-onset IDDM. Diabetologia 1995;38:1371–1373.
344. Kibrick S. Viral infections of the fetus and newborn. Perspect Virol 1961;2:140–159.
345. Berkovich S, Smithwood EM. Transplacental infection due to ECHO virus type 22. J Pediatr 1968;72:94–96.
346. Philip AGS, Larsen EJ. Overwhelming neonatal infection with ECHO 19 virus. J Pediatr 1973;82:391–397.
347. Nielsen JL, Berryman GK, Hankins GD. Intrauterine fetal death and the isolation of echovirus 27 from amniotic fluid. J Infect Dis 1988; 158:501–502.
348. Toce SS, Kennan WJ. Congenital echovirus 11 pneumonia in association with pulmonary hypertension. Pediatr Infect Dis J 1988;7:360–362.
349. Moscovici C, Maisel J. Intestinal viruses of newborn and older prematures. Am J Dis Child 1961;101:771–777.
350. Eichenwald HF, Kostevalov O. Immunologic responses of premature and full-term infants to infection with certain viruses. Pediatrics 1960; 25:829.
351. Landesman JB, Grist NR, Ross CAC. Echo 9 virus infection and congenital malformations. Br J Prev Soc Med 1964;18:152–156.
352. Rantasalo I, Penttinen K, Saxen L, Ojala A. Echo 9 virus antibody status after an epidemic period and the possible teratogenic effect of the infection. Ann Paediatr Fenn 1960;6:175–184.
353. Kleinman H, Prince JT, Mathey WE, Rosenfield AB, Bearman JE, Syverton JT. ECHO 9 virus infection and congenital abnormalities: a negative report. Pediatrics 1962;29:261–269.
354. Garcia AG, Basso NG, Fonseca ME, Gutani HN, Congenital echo virus infection—morphological and virological study of fetal and placental tissue. J Pathol 1990;160:123–127.
355. Freedman PS. Echovirus 11 infection and intrauterine death. Lancet 1979;1:96–97.
356. Skeels MR, Williams JJ, Ricker FM. Perinatal echovirus infection [Letter]. N Engl J Med 1981;305:1529.
357. Johansson ME, Holmstrom S, Abebo A, Jacobson B, Eman G, Samuelson A, Wirgart BZ. Intrauterine fetal death due to echovirus II. Scand J Infect Dis 1991;24:381–385.
358. Hughes JR, Hanover NH, Wilfert CM, Moore M, Benirschke K, Hoyos-Guevara E. Echovirus 14 infection associated with fatal neonatal hepatic necrosis. Am J Dis Child 1972;123:61–67.
359. Georgieff MK, Johnson DE, Thompson TR, Belani K, Ferrieri P. Fulminant hepatic necrosis in an infant with perinaally acquired echovirus 21 infection. Pediatr Infect Dis 1987;6:71–73.
360. Magnius L, Sterner G, Enocksson E. Infections with echoviruses and coxsackie viruses in late pregnancy. Scand J Infect Dis Suppl 1990;71: 53–57.
361. Abzug MJ, Loeffelholz M, Rotbart HA. Diagnosis of neonatal enterovirus infection by polymerase chain reaction. J Pediatr 1995; 126:447–450.
362. Abzug MJ, Keyserling HL, Lee ML. Neonatal enterovirus infection: virology, serology, and use of intravenous immune globulin. Clin Infect Dis 1995;20:1201–1206.
363. Johnston JM, Overall JM Jr. Intravenous immunoglobulin in disseminated neonatal echovirus 11 infection. Pediatr Infec Dis J 1989;8: 254–256.
364. LaForce FM, Nichol KL, Cox NJ. Influenza: virology, epidemiology, disease, and prevention. Am J Prev Med 1994;10(suppl):31–44.

365. Harris JW. Influenza occurring in pregnant women. A statistical study of thirteen hundred and fifty cases. JAMA 1919;72:978–980.
366. Freeman DW, Barno A. Deaths from Asian influenza associated with pregnancy. Am J Obstet Gynecol 1959;78:1172–1175.
367. Yawn DH, Pyeatte JC, Joseph JM, Eichler SL, Garcia-Bunuel R. Transplacental transfer of influenza virus. JAMA 1971;216:1022–1023.
368. McGregor JA, Burns JC, Levin MJ, Burlington B, Meiklejohn G. Transplacental passage of influenza A/Bangkok (H_3N_2) mimicking amniotic fluid infection syndrome. Am J Obstet Gynecol 1984;149: 856–859.
369. Monif GR, Sowards DL, Eitzman DV. Serologic and immunologic evaluation of neonates following maternal influenza during the second and third trimesters of gestation. Am J Obstet Gynecol 1972;114: 239–242.
370. Ramphal R, Donnelly WH, Small PA Jr. Fatal influenzal pneumonia in pregnancy: failure to demonstrate transplacental transmission of influenza virus. Am J Obstet Gynecol 1980;138:347–348.
371. Coffey VP, Jessop WJE. Congenital abnormalities. Ir J Med Sci 1955; 349:30–48.
372. Coffey VP, Jessop WJE. Maternal influenza and congenital deformities. A prospective study. Lancet 1959;2:935–938.
373. Hardy JMB, Azarowicz EN, Mannini A, Medearis DN, Cooke RE. The effect of Asian influenza on the outcome of pregnancy. Baltimore 1957–1958. Am J Public Health 1961;51:1182–1188.
374. Hakosalo J, Saxen L. Influenza epidemic and congenital defects. Lancet 1971;2:1346–1347.
375. Warrell MJ, Tobin OH, Wald NJ. Examination for influenza IgA and IgM antibodies in pregnancies associated with fetal neural-tube defects. J Med Microbiol 1981;14:159–162.
376. Leck I. Incidence of malformations following influenza epidemics. Br J Prev Soc Med 1963;17:70–80.
377. Wilson MG, Stein AM. Teratogenic effects of Asian influenza. JAMA 1969;210:336–337.
378. Korones SB, Todaro J, Roane JA, Sever JL. Maternal virus infection after the first trimester of pregnancy and status of offspring to 4 years of age in a predominantly Negro population. J Pediatr 1970;77: 245–251.
379. Doll R, Hill AB, Jakula J. Asian influenza in pregnancy and congenital defects. Br J Prev Soc Med 1960;14:167–172.
380. MacKenzie JS, Houghton M. Influenza infections during pregnancy: association with congenital malformations and with subsequent neoplasms in children, and potential hazards of live virus vaccines. Bacteriol Rev 1974;38:356–370.
381. Wright P, Takei N, Rifkin L, Murray RM. Maternal influenza, obstetric complications and schizophrenia. Am J Psychiatry 1995;152: 1714–1720.
382. Kirshon B, Faro S, Zurawin RK, Samo TC, Carpenter RJ. Favorable outcomes after treatment with amantadine and ribavirin in a pregnancy complicated by influenza pneumonia. J Reprod Med 1988;33: 399–401.
383. Centers for Disease Control and Prevention. Prevention and control of influenza. Recommendations of the Advisory Committee on Immunization Practices (ACIP). MMWR 1997;46(RR-9).
384. Epstein MA, Achong BG, Barr YM. Virus particles in cultured lymphoblasts from Burkitt's malignant lymphoma. Lancet 1964;1: 252–253.
385. Le CT, Chang RS, Lipson MH. Epstein-Barr virus infections during pregnancy: a prospective study and review of the literature. Am J Dis Child 1983;137:466–468.
386. Gervais F, Joncas JH. Seroepidemiology in various population groups of the greater Montreal area. Comp Immunol Microbiol Infect Dis 1979;2:207–212.
387. Fleisher G, Bolgnese R. Persistent Epstein-Barr virus infection and pregnancy. J Infect Dis 1983;147:982–986.
388. Stagno S, Whitley RJ. Herpesvirus infections of pregnancy. Part I. Cytomegalovirus and Epstein-Barr virus infections. N Engl J Med 1985;313:1270–1274.
389. Biem J, Roy L, Halik J, Hoffstein V. Infectious mononucleosis complicated by necrotizing epiglottitis, dysphagia, and pneumonia. Chest 1989;96:204–205.
390. Penman HG. Fatal infectious mononucleosis: a critical review. J Clin Pathol 1970;23:765–771.
391. Fleisher G, Bolognese R. Epstein-Barr virus infection in pregnancy. A prospective study. J Pediatr 1984;104:374–379.
392. Fleisher G, Bolognese R. Seroepidemiology of Epstein-Barr virus in pregnant women. J Infect Dis 1982;145:537–541.
393. Joncas J, Boucher J, Granger-Julien M, Filion C. Epstein-Barr virus infections in the neonatal period and in childhood. Can Med Assoc J 1974;110:33–37.
394. Chang RS, Blakenship W. Spontaneous in vitro transformation of leukocytes from a neonate. Proc Soc Exp Biol Med 1973;144:337–339.
395. Chang RS, Seto DSY. Perinatal infection by Epstein-Barr virus. Lancet 1979;2:201.
396. Joncas JH, Alfieri C, Leyritz-Wills M, et al. Simultaneous congenital infection with Epstein-Barr virus and cytomegalovirus. N Engl J Med 1981;304:1399–1403.
397. Goldberg GN, Fulginiti VA, Ray CG, et al. In utero Epstein-Barr virus (infectious mononucleosis) infection. JAMA 1981;246:1579–1581.
398. Brown ZA, Stenchover MA. Infectious mononucleosis and congenital anomalies. Am J Obstet Gynecol 1978;131:108–109.
399. Leary DC, Welt LC, Beckett RS. Infectious mononucleosis complicating pregnancy with fatal congenital anomaly of infant. Am J Obstet Gynecol 1949;57:381–384.
400. Visintine AM, Gerber P, Nahmias AJ. Leukocyte transforming agent (Epstein-Barr virus) in newborn infants and older individuals. J Pediatr 1976;89:571–575.
401. Icart J, Didier J, Dalens M, Chabanon G, Boulays A. Prospective study of Epstein-Barr virus (EBV) infection during pregnancy. Biomedicine 1981;34:160–163.
402. Tallqvist H, Henle W, Klemola E, et al. Antibodies to Epstein-Barr virus at the ages of 6 to 23 months in children with congenital heart disease. Scand J Infect Dis 1973;5:159–161.
403. Weaver LT, Nelson R, Bell TM. The association of extrahepatic bile duct atresia and neonatal Epstein-Barr virus infection. Acta Paediatr Scand 1984;73:155–157.
404. Sixbey JW, Limon SM, Pagano JS. A second site for Epstein-Barr virus shedding: the uterine cervix. Lancet 1986;2:1122–1124.
405. Costa S, Barrasso R, Terzano P, Zerbini M, Carpi C, Musiani M. Detection of active Epstein-Barr infection in pregnant women. Eur J Clin Microbiol 1985;4:335–336.
406. Meyohas M, Merechal V, Parnet-Mathieu F, Gaha S, Jacob I, Nicolas JC. Detection of Epstein-Barr virus transactivator (Zebra) antibodies in serum from pregnant women. J Viral Dis 1992;1:73–77.
407. Icart J, Didier J. Infections due to Epstein-Barr virus during pregnancy. J Infect Dis 1981;143:499.
408. Meyohas MC, Marechal V, Desire N, Bouillie J, Frottier J, Nicolas JC. Study of mother-to-child Epstein-Barr virus transmission by means of nested PCRs. J Virol 1996;70:6816–6819.
409. Biggar RJ, Henle W, Fleisher G, Bocker J, Lenette ET, Henle G. Primary Epstein-Barr virus infections in African infants. I. Decline of maternal antibodies and time of infection. Int J Cancer 22: 239–243.
410. Kusuhara K, Takabayashi A, Ueda K, et al. Breast milk is not a significant source for early Epstein-Barr virus or human herpes 6 infection in infants: a seroepidemiologic study in 2 endemic areas of human T-cell lymphotropic virus type I in Japan. Microbiol Immunol 1997;41:309–312.
411. Angella JJ, Connor JD. Neonatal infection caused by adenovirus type 7. J Pediatr 1968;72:474–478.
412. Matsuoka T, Naito T, Kubota Y, et al. Disseminated adenovirus (type 19) infection in a neonate: rapid detection of the infection by immunofluorescence. Act Paediatr Scand 1990;79:568–571.
413. Abzug MJ, Levin MJ. Neonatal adenoviral infection: four patients and review of the literature. Pediatrics 1991;87:890–896.
414. Montone KT, Furth EE, Pietra GG, Gupta PK. Neonatal adenovirus infection: a case report with in situ hybridization confirmation of ascending intrauterine infection. Diagn Cytopathol 1995;12:341–344.
415. Belak S, Rusavi M. In utero adenoviral infection of sheep. Vet Microbiol 1986;12:87–91.
416. Narita M, Imada T, Fukusho A. Pathologic changes caused by transplacental infection with an adenovirus-like agent in pigs. Am J Vet Res 1984;46:1126–1129.
417. Sun CJ, Duara S. Fatal adenovirus pneumonia in two newborn infants, one case caused by adenovirus type 30. Pediatr Pathol 1985;4: 247–255.
418. Meyer K, Girgis N, McGavey V. Adenovirus associated with congenital pleural effusion. J Pediatr 1985;107;433–435.
419. Towbin JA, Griffin LD, Martin AB, et al. Intrauterine adenoviral

myocarditis presenting as nonimmune hydrops fetalis: diagnosis by polymerase chain reaction. Pediatr Infect Dis J 1994;13:144–150.
420. Martin AB, Zhang YH, Griffin LD, et al. Evaluation of acute and chronic myocarditis by polymerase chain reaction (PCR) in children. Am J Cardiol 1992;70:563.
421. Towbin JA, Ni J, Demmler G, Martin A, Kearney D, Bricker JT. Evidence for adenovirus as a common cause of myocarditis in children using polymerase chain reaction (PCR). Pediatr Res 1993;33: 27A.
422. Gupta PK. Microbiology, inflammation, and viral infections. In: Bibbo M, ed. Comprehensive cytology. Philadelphia: WB Saunders, 1991: 115–151.
423. Van den Veyver IB, Ni J, Bowles N, et al. Detection of intrauterine viral infection using the polymerase chain reaction. Mol Genet Metab 1998;63:85–95.
424. McLean LK, Chehab FF, Goldberg JD. Detection of viral deoxyribonucleic acid in the amniotic fluid of low-risk pregnancies by polymerase chain reaction. Am J Obstet Gynecol 1995;173:1282–1286.

Cherry and Merkatz's Complications of Pregnancy,
Fifth Edition, edited by W. R. Cohen.
Lippincott Williams & Wilkins, Philadelphia © 2000.

CHAPTER 46

Bacterial Infections

Glenn S. Hammer

The anatomic, physiologic, and immunologic alterations of pregnancy pose special risks of infection for both mother and fetus. This chapter discusses the pathogenesis and therapy of certain bacterial diseases that are of particular concern in the pregnant patient. Practical guidelines will be provided for common therapeutic dilemmas.

INCREASED SUSCEPTIBILITY TO INFECTION DURING PREGNANCY AND DELIVERY

Pregnancy engenders an increased susceptibility to a wide variety of infective processes, which may be more severe than in the nonpregnant patient. The contribution of the anatomic and hormonal changes that occur during pregnancy as well as the risks from the process of labor and delivery are easy to understand. For example, there is an increased frequency of cystitis and a high risk of ascending pyelonephritis during pregnancy. This increase is explained, in part, by the anatomic consequences of an enlarging uterus compressing the bladder and ureters at the pelvic brim in association with hormonal alterations in vescicoureteral smooth muscle tone. These factors contribute to the development of ureteral dilatation, increases in residual urine volume, and vescicoureteral reflux, with a consequent increase in the risk of ascending urinary tract infection. Labor and delivery pose additional risks from urethral catheterization and urethral trauma. Intraamniotic infection, endometritis, pelvic peritonitis, and abdominal wound infections have their pathogenesis in the bacterial contamination of the uterine contents from prior endocervical infection, premature rupture of the membranes, and cesarean section as well as normal labor and delivery. Aspiration pneumonia arising from events at the time of delivery (Mendelssohn syndrome) is a result of the patient's dependent position, increased pressure on the diaphragm, and suppression of normal cough and gag reflexes from pain medication and anesthesia.

G. S. Hammer: New York, NY 10128.

More difficult to understand are the increased incidence and severity of a variety of bacterial, fungal, protozoan, and viral diseases during pregnancy. These diseases include brucellosis, listeriosis, salmonellosis, tuberculosis, histoplasmosis, coccidioidomycosis, coxsackievirus infection, hepatitis A and E, influenza, poliomyelitis, rubella, and smallpox. Investigations point to alterations in cellular and humoral defense mechanisms, which likely arise from the necessity that the mother not immunologically reject her growing fetus, which bears an assortment of foreign antigens.

Cell-mediated immune function is impaired during pregnancy (1). Alterations of maternal immune function appear to be related to hormonal changes and the induction of suppressor cells in the fetus that mute maternal, cell-mediated immune responses. This correlates well with the type of infections that are described in pregnancy.

During pregnancy, hydrocortisone levels are elevated threefold to sevenfold over their baseline, nonpregnant levels. Olding and Oldstone showed that fetal cord blood lymphocytes inhibit the proliferation of maternal lymphocytes (2). Similar findings in mice were described by Bassett and associates (3). Morito and colleagues demonstrated that fetal suppressor cells elaborate soluble factors that inhibit both T-and B-cell function of adult lymphocytes (4). *In vitro* studies demonstrated that alpha-fetoprotein is capable of direct activation of suppressor cells (5). In humans, chorionic gonadotrophin has been shown to induce suppressor cells *in vitro* (6). Sridama et al. reported significant decreases in T-helper lymphocytes during pregnancy, which did not normalize until the third to fifth postpartum month (7).

ANTIMICROBIAL AGENTS

Use in Pregnancy

With the use of any drug in pregnancy, an overriding concern is the question of safety for both the mother and developing fetus. Adequate human data from controlled trials are generally not available. For most agents, data from animal studies are not strictly applicable to humans. Therefore, recommendations for antibiotic use in pregnancy are based on long-term clinical experience and the absence of reports of adverse effects on fetal development.

Virtually all antimicrobial agents cross the placenta (8,9). A long history of safe use in pregnancy indicates that penicillins, cephalosporins, most macrolides (erythromycins), and the lincomycins are unlikely to affect fetal development adversely. One erythromycin derivative, the estolate ester (Ilosone), should be avoided during pregnancy because it can cause cholestatic jaundice. In addition, in a study of pregnant women treated for genital mycoplasma infection, this agent was associated with elevations of serum aminotransferases in 9.9% of patients (10). Clarithromycin, the 6-methoxy derivative of erythromycin, should be avoided because of possible teratogenicity (11).

The tetracyclines are contraindicated in pregnancy. These agents are chemically complexed by calcium and deposited in fetal teeth and long bones, producing permanent staining and hypoplasia of the deciduous teeth and stunting of long-bone growth (12). Calcification of the deciduous teeth begins in the 12th week. These adverse effects of tetracyclines are most prominent in the last trimester. Furthermore, tetracyclines have been reported to produce acute fatty liver necrosis, pancreatitis, and possibly renal damage in the mother. The risk is greatest in the last trimester and with parenteral administration (13,14).

Sulfonamides are generally safe during pregnancy, but they should be avoided at or near term. These drugs cross the placenta extremely well and displace bilirubin from albumin binding sites in fetal blood. This is of little consequence *in utero* because excess free bilirubin is cleared through the placenta and metabolized by the maternal liver. The neonatal liver, however, cannot metabolize bilirubin normally. Sulfonamides administered at parturition have been reported to produce a 10-fold increase in the incidence of kernicterus in premature infants, frequently at bilirubin levels below 15 mg/100 mL (15). It should also be remembered that sulfonamides are secreted in breast milk and can produce a hemolytic anemia in nursing children with glucose 6-phosphate dehydrogenase (G6PD) deficiency.

Trimethoprim-sulfamethoxazole (Bactrim, Septra) has been commonly used in pregnancy; however, concerns have been expressed about the risks of the trimethoprim component of this agent during pregnancy because trimethoprim is a folic acid antagonist. Although data have not shown an increase in fetal malformations compared with sulfonamides alone (16), in rats high doses have proved teratogenic (17).

Chloramphenicol, like the sulfonamides, is contraindicated at or near term. The hepatic glucuronyl transferase is poorly developed in the neonate. This enzyme is responsible for the normal metabolism of chloramphenicol to an inactive, nontoxic glucuronide derivative. Neonates, particularly premature infants, given normal doses of chloramphenicol may manifest a disease process known as "gray baby syndrome." Mortality may reach 40% as a result of cardiovascular collapse (18).

The mutagenic potential of some of the reduction products of metronidazole and its safety in pregnancy are of concern. Metronidazole is known to produce chromosomal alterations in bacteria; one of its minor metabolites, acetamide, is a proven rat hepatic carcinogen (19). In high doses, metronidazole resulted in an excess of pulmonary tumors and malignant lymphomas in mice and mammary tumors in rats but not in hamsters (20,21).

Only one of nine studies in a variety of animal models has shown any evidence of teratogenicity for metronidazole. Only two of six studies of maternal trichomoniasis suggest an increase in human teratogenic risk (19). Two clinical studies are reassuring. In a review from the Mayo Clinic, follow-up for a mean of 10 years of 771 women treated for vaginal trichomonas infections failed to reveal any increase in the incidence of cancer (22). Another study of pregnant women who were similarly treated for vaginal trichomonas infections also failed to reveal any increase in prematurity or fetal abnormalities (23). Nevertheless, it would be prudent to minimize the use of this agent in pregnancy and lactating women. The drug reaches significant concentrations in human milk.

Streptomycin and kanamycin have produced congenital deafness in children born to mothers treated with prolonged courses of these drugs for tuberculosis (24). This problem has not been reported with other aminoglycosides, such as gentamicin and tobramycin, which may be because these latter agents are used most commonly for short courses of therapy for serious bacterial infections. Nevertheless, the potential for fetal ototoxicity exists. Alternative agents to aminoglycosides are available for the therapy of most cases of tuberculosis. The newer broad-spectrum penicillins, third- and fourth-generation cephalosporins, monbactams, and carbapenams are excellent alternatives to aminoglycosides for serious gram-negative infections. When necessary for the therapy of serious gram-negative infections, the use of these agents should be limited and drug levels carefully monitored.

The quinolones are presently contraindicated in pregnancy. In animal studies, this group of antibiotics interfered with fetal cartilage formation. When used in children with cystic fibrosis, quinolones have been used with varying reports of joint and tendon toxicity; in one European study, 14% of children with cystic fibrosis treated with pefloxacin developed arthralgias or arthritis (25).

For these same reasons, quinolones should be avoided in nursing mothers as well.

Pharmacology of Antimicrobial Agents in Pregnancy

The physiologic changes that accompany pregnancy may alter drug pharmacology by significant increases in plasma volume, renal blood flow, and glomerular filtration rate. The last of these may be increased by as much as 50% over baseline by the third trimester. These changes will lead to reductions of drug levels because of their increased volume of distribution and enhanced renal clearance.

Philipson et al., in crossover studies of the pharmacokinetics of ampicillin, cephradine, and cefuroxime in pregnant women, compared with studies in the same women after pregnancy, demonstrated 30% to 50% reductions in plasma antibiotic levels and significantly shorter half-lives of these antibiotics during pregnancy (26–28). Zaskie et al. had similar findings with gentamicin (29). Studies of hepatically metabolized agents suggest that there is an increase in the liver's capacity to metabolize these drugs as well (30). Therefore, in pregnant women, larger doses of most antibiotics may be necessary, particularly for life-threatening infections.

General Uses

Penicillins

Penicillin G is active against most streptococci including *S pneumoniae*, *S pyogenes* (group A), *S agalactiae* (group B), *Enterococcus* species, *N menigitidis*, most strains of *N gonorrhoeae*, most anaerobic organisms, including *Clostridium* species, *Actinomycetes* species, most oral *Bacteroides* species, and *Fusobacterium* species. The *Bacteroides fragilis* group is resistant. The vast majority of clinical isolates of *Staphylococcus aureus* presently produce beta-lactamase and are therefore resistant to penicillin G. Many hospital-acquired staphylococcal strains are also resistant to the beta-lactamase–resistant penicillins (methicillin, oxacillin, and nafcillin) and must be treated with vancomycin. Alarmingly, an increasing percentage (currently 10%–15%) of pneumococcal strains have become relatively and occasionally absolutely resistant to penicillin. Vancomycin and several quinolones are reliably active against these strains. In the near future, penicillin is unlikely to remain a reliable agent for pneumococcal pneumonia.

Ampicillin and amoxicillin retain all the activity of penicillin G with an extended spectrum that includes the gram-negative bacilli *E coli* and *Proteus mirabilis* and beta-lactamase–negative *Haemophilus influenzae*. With widespread use, resistance to ampicillin has grown. Currently, 25% of *E coli* 15% of *Proteus* species and 25% to 30% of *H influenzae* are resistant. Ampicillin remains the drug of choice for listeriosis.

Ampicillin-sulbactam (Unasyn) consists of a 2:1 ratio of ampicillin and the beta-lactamase inhibitor sulbactam. The latter extends the spectrum of ampicillin to include beta-lactamase–producing *S aureus* and *H influenzae*, *Klebsiella* species, indole-negative *Proteus* species (Morganellae), and *B fragilis*. Indeed, the antimicrobial activity spectrum of ampicillin–sulbactam closely resembles that of the second-generation cephalosporin derivatives cefoxitin and cefotetan. Amoxicillin–clavulanic acid (Augmentin) is an equivalent oral agent.

The extended-spectrum penicillin derivatives include the carboxy-penicillin derivatives carbenicillin, ticarcillin, and ticarcillin-clavulanic acid (Timentin) as well as the ureidopenicillin derivatives azlocillin, mezlocillin, piperacillin, and piperacillin–tazobactam (Zosyn). These are active against most gram-negative bacilli. In general, the ureidopenicillins are more active than the carboxy derivatives against most gram-negative bacilli, in particular *P aeruginosa* and *Klebsiella* species and are as active as ampicillin against *Enterococcus* species; however, they are not as active as the third-generation cephalosporins against most gram-negative organisms. The addition of beta-lactamase inhibitors to ticarcillin as ticarcillin–clavulanic acid (Timentin) and to piperacillin as piperacillin–tazobactam (Zosyn) further improves the gram-negative spectrum of these agents and adds reliable coverage for methicillin sensitive *S aureus* and anaerobic bacteria, including *B fragilis*.

Carbenicillin and ticarcillin are rarely used now. As divalent cations containing two sodium groups, these agents can cause electrolyte disturbances such as hypernatremia, hypokalemia, and salt and water retention, leading to edema and congestive heart failure. Their alpha-carboxy-penicillin causes interference with platelet function. These agents have been associated with clinical bleeding. The ureidopenicillins are monosodium salts and have substantially less effect on platelet function. For these reasons and their improved antimicrobial spectrum, piperacillin and piperacillin–tazobactam have become the drugs of choice from this group. The latter is a superb choice for the therapy of serious, hospital acquired, intraabdominal and pelvic infections.

Cephalosporins

First-generation cephalosporins (e.g., cefazolin) have a good spectrum of activity against gram-positive and gram-negative bacteria, including beta-lactamase–producing staphylococci, streptococci, *E coli*, *Klebsiella* species, and *Proteus mirabilis*. Importantly, *Enterococcus* species are highly resistant to most cephalosporins.

The second-generation cephalosporins include cefamandole, cefuroxime, cefoxitin, and cefotetan. The latter two agents are technically cephamycins because of the addition of a 7-methoxy group, but they are so close in chemical structure that they are conceptually included with the second-generation cephalosporins. Cefamandole and cefuroxime are similar agents. They are superior to first-generation cephalosporins against *E coli*, *Klebsiella* species, and indole-negative *Proteus* species and are active against beta-lactamase–producing strains of *H influenzae*. The cephamycins are less active against gram-positive organisms but have good activity against anaerobes, including *B fragilis*. They are similar in their antimicrobial spectra to ampicillin-sulbactam (Unasyn). By comparison, the cephamycins provide more reliable coverage against *Klebsiella* species, but they lack any activity against the enterococci. All are excellent choices for uncomplicated intraabdominal and pelvic infections. Cefotetan has the advantage of a long serum half-life, approximately 3.5 hours, permitting twice-daily dosing.

The third-generation cephalosporins are significantly more active against the *Enterobacteriaceae* and *Pseudomonas* species. Cefotaxime, ceftizoxime, and ceftriaxone have nearly the activity of first- and second-generation agents against gram-positive organisms, but they are significantly more active against the *Enterobacteriaceae*, including *Morganella* and *Serratia* species. These three agents differ primarily in their pharmacokinetics. Ceftriaxone has the longest serum half-life of this group, 6 to 8 hours, and can be dosed once daily in most clinical situations. Ceftizoxime, like the second-generation agents cefoxitin and cefotetan, possesses significant activity against penicillin-resistant anaerobes; however, clinical studies are conflicting as to whether it is the clinical equal of these second-generation agents for anaerobic infections.

Ceftazidime and cefoperazone have excellent activity against *Pseudomonas aeruginosa*. Overall, ceftazidime has the best activity against gram-negative bacteria, but it has significantly poorer activity against gram-positive organisms. Cefoperazone is somewhat less active than the other agents of this class against some members of the *Enterobacteriaceae* but maintains good gram-positive activity and excellent activity against *P aeruginosa*. It has the most balanced spectrum of activity of any agent in this group. In addition, it also has the advantage of a dual excretion pathway. Unlike most cephalosporins, dosing does not have to be modified in the presence of renal failure.

Moxalactam is technically an oxycephem derivative, but it is usually classed with the third-generation cephalosporins. It has a similar spectrum of activity to ceftazidime, but it has superior anaerobic activity. This drug has fallen out of favor because of serious bleeding complications associated with its use. Cephalosporins, such as moxalactam with a methylthiotetrazole group at the three position of the cephalosporin molecule, have been associated with prolonged prothrombin times through interference with the hepatic synthesis of vitamin-K-dependent clotting factors. These derivatives also can produce disulfiram-like reactions to alcohol. Other cephalosporins with these characteristics are cefamandole, cefotetan, cefmetazole, and cefoperazone.

The latest extended spectrum cephalosporins to be developed, cefepime and cefpirome, have been referred to as "fourth-generation cephalosporins." They are more resistant to the broad-spectrum beta-lactamases of gram-negative bacteria. As bipolar zwitterions, they are able to penetrate the outer membrane of gram-negative bacteria more easily. They are superior to ceftazidime in their activity against *Enterobacteriaceae* and *P aeruginosa* and yet maintain acceptable gram-positive activity.

As with the penicillins, the major side effects of cephalosporins are hypersensitivity reactions. Antibodies that develop in patients experiencing allergic reactions to penicillin-based drugs may cross-react with cephalosporins. Consequently, 5% to 10% of patients who are allergic to penicillin may develop hypersensitivity reactions when treated with cephalosporins. This is of more concern in patients with a history of an immunoglobulin E (IgE) type of allergic reaction to penicillin. These patients are most at risk for an anaphylactic reaction. Patients with a history of less serious reactions to penicillins most often can be given cephalosporins safely. In situations where the history is unclear, patients can be skin tested before cephalosporin administration.

Monobactams and Carbapenems

Monobactams are beta-lactam agents that lack a secondary thiazole or dihydrothiazine ring structure. Aztreonam is the only clinically available monobactam antibiotic. Its antimicrobial spectrum is limited to *Enterobacteriaceae* and *P aeruginosa*, against which its activity is roughly equivalent to that of ceftazidime. It has no gram-positive or anaerobic activity. Consequently, this agent is used most often in combination with other agents.

Antibodies directed against penicillins and cephalosporins tend not to cross-react with aztreonam. Therefore, this agent may be used in place of a third generation cephalosporin in patients with a history of a major penicillin allergy.

Imipenem and meropenem are the two clinically available carbapenem antibiotics. Carbapenems are beta-lactam antibiotics in which the sulfur atom of the five-member thiazole ring of penicillin is replaced by a carbon atom. These agents are remarkable in that they are highly active against most bacterial species, including anaerobes. They are also active against most third generation cephalosporin-resistant gram-negatives. Exceptions are the non-aeruginosa pseudomonad species, *P cepacia* and *P maltophilia*, methicillin-resistant *S aureus* and *Enterococcus faecium*.

Aminoglycosides

The aminoglycosides, once the mainstay in the armamentarium against serious gram-negative infections, have been largely replaced by the safer extended-spectrum penicillins, third-generation cephalosporins, monobactams, carbapenams, and fluoroquinolones. Because of their narrow toxic–therapeutic window, nephrotoxicity, and ototoxicity, they have become distinctly second-line agents. On occasion, however, aminoglycosides may be the only viable agents active against hospital-acquired, multiply resistant, gram-negative infections for use in patients who are allergic to multiple other antibiotics and for their synergistic activity in the therapy of enterococcal endocarditis (31).

Currently available aminoglycosides include gentamicin, tobramycin, netilmicin, and amikacin. They have a broad range of activity against most gram-negative organisms, amikacin being the most active of the group. An energy- and oxygen-dependent transport system is required for these agents to cross the outer membrane of gram-negative rods. They are, therefore, devoid of anaerobic activity.

Neomycin is too toxic for parenteral use. It is also inappropriate to use this agent for irrigation of the abdominal cavity because it is well absorbed by this route. It is used in topical medications and oral bowel preparations, where it is safe because of minimal systemic absorption. For similar reasons, paromomycin (Humatin) is marketed only as an oral agent, principally to treat intestinal amebic infections.

Rather than dosing these agents at the traditional 8- to 12-hour intervals, it has become popular to administer them in large, single daily doses (32). Extended dosing intervals are possible because these agents exhibit concentration dependent bactericidal activity and prolonged postantibiotic effects on bacterial regrowth. Because of longer renal washout times, once-daily aminoglycoside (ODA) dosing may be less nephrotoxic. Efficacy is equivalent. Only trough aminoglycoside levels remain relevant. Peak levels obviously will appear to be high with ODA using standard criteria. Other antibiotics that demonstrate long postantibiotic effects and concentration-dependent bacterial killing are the quinolones and metronidazole.

Quinolones

The quinolones are synthetic antimicrobial agents that are related to nalidixic acid. Fluorination and chemical modifications have produced a class of drugs that are up to 100-fold more active than nalidixic acid. They act by interfering with bacterial DNA synthesis through inhibition of the bacterial enzyme DNA gyrase, which is necessary for DNA supercoiling. Ciprofloxacin ofloxacin, levofloxacin, and trovafloxacin are the members of this group of drugs that are available for intravenous use. They are well absorbed after oral administration, thereby permitting the treatment of serious gram-negative infections by the oral route. These agents are broadly active against a wide variety of gram-negative organisms. Ciprofloxacin is significantly less active against gram-positive bacteria. With the exception of trovafloxacin, most have little activity against anaerobic organisms.

Levofloxacin is the L-isomer of ofloxacin and is twofold to fourfold more active than the parent compound. Trovafloxacin is a novel naphthyridone quinolone that has enhanced activity against gram-positive and anaerobic organisms. Both are highly active against penicillin-resistant pneumococci.

As discussed above, the quinolones are contraindicated in pregnancy and children. In animals, these agents have produced articular cartilage lesions in weight-bearing joints and fetal wastage.

Macrolides, Lincomycins, and Chloramphenicol

Erythromycin, the parent macrolide antibiotic, is one of the oldest and safest antibiotics in clinical use. Clarithromycin and the azalide derivative, azithromycin, are newer macrolide derivatives with some increase in potency but with significantly improved gastrointestinal tolerance. These agents are well suited for the therapy of a variety of upper and lower respiratory tract infections, genital diseases, and certain gastrointestinal illnesses. They are active against most streptococci, 75% of staphylococci, *T pallidum*, *Mycoplasma pneumoniae, Legionella* species, pneumonic and genital *Chlamydia* strains, and *Campylobacter jejuni*. The newer derivatives have enhanced activity against *Haemophilus* and *Moraxella* species. Clarithromycin is active against *H pylori*. Unfortunately, this agent is rated as a pregnancy category C drug because, at high doses, it has been found to be teratogenic in rats and mice. Azithromycin carries a pregnancy category B rating.

Clindamycin, 7-chlorolincocin, is the preferred lincomycin derivative. The parent drug, lincomycin, is only of historic interest. Clindamycin is notable for its excellent activity against anaerobic organisms. *Clostridium perfringens* and *Peptococci* may be resistant, however, rendering this agent unreliable in the therapy of gas gangrene. The aerobic spectrum of clindamycin is limited to gram-positive bacteria, including *S aureus*. Methicillin-resistant staphylococci and enterococci are generally resistant. Clindamycin has no aerobic gram-negative activity. This agent carries the highest risk for the complication of pseudomembranous colitis of any antibiotic.

Chloramphenicol has an extended spectrum of activity against a wide variety of gram-positive, gram-negative, and most anaerobic bacteria. It diffuses well into virtually all body cavities, including the central nervous system and abscess fluids; however, because of the potential for serious bone marrow toxicity, chloramphenicol should be used only in highly selected clinical situations. In the United States, it is no longer available for oral administration.

Metronidazole is a nitroimidazole derivative, which is active against most anaerobic bacteria, including *B fragilis* and *C difficile*. *P acnes* and some anaerobic gram-positive cocci are resistant. *Gardnerella vaginalis*, *Helicobacter pylori,* and the protozoan agents *Trichomonas vaginalis* and *Entamoeba histolytica* are also susceptible. Metronidazole, clindamycin, chloramphenicol, the penicillin beta-lactamase inhibitor combinations (ampicillin–sulbactam, ticarcillin–clavulanate, and piperacillin–tazobactam), and the carbapenam derivatives have the best anaerobic spectrums of currently available antibiotics.

Glycopeptides

Vancomycin and the investigational agent teichoplanin are glycopeptide derivatives. With the exception of *Neisseria* species, these agents have an exclusively gram-positive spectrum of activity. Vancomycin is most often used in the therapy of suspected or proven infections with methicillin-resistant *S aureus* and in serious staphylococcal and enterococcal infections in patients with a history of major penicillin allergy. Reversible nephrotoxicity, which was previously common with the original impure preparations, is now unusual. Ototoxicity can be avoided by maintaining peak serum concentrations below 30 µg/mL. Administration of vancomycin may be complicated by phlebitis and nonallergic flushing reactions resulting from histamine release (red-man syndrome) unless the drug is properly diluted and given by slow infusion. Primary allergic reactions in patients not previously treated with vancomycin are distinctly rare.

PUERPERAL INFECTIONS

Intraamniotic infection

Intraamniotc infection is also referred to as amnionitis, and chorioamnionitis. It should be suspected whenever a maternal temperature of 100°F or higher develops during labor and delivery. Maternal or fetal tachycardia and leukocytosis are common and support the diagnosis; however, the maternal white blood cell count is normally elevated in labor and rises with the duration of normal labor and delivery (33). Uterine tenderness and a foul odor to the amniotic fluid may occur but are inconsistent findings.

Inflammation of the chorionic membranes is demonstrable on pathology in 11% to 16% of deliveries (34), and viable bacteria in low numbers can be found in the amniotic fluid in 10% of women at term with intact membranes (35). Clinically recognized infection, however, occurs much less frequently, in 0.5% to 2% of all deliveries. Intraamniotic infection accounts for 10% to 40% of peripartum febrile morbidity and is associated with 20% to 40% of cases of neonatal sepsis and pneumonia (36).

Intraamniotic infection most often develops as a result of ascending bacterial colonization from the cervix. Risk factors include ruptured membranes, long duration of labor, frequent cervical examinations, obstetric manipulations, use of internal fetal monitoring devices, low parity, preterm labor, meconium staining, and the presence of bacterial vaginosis (37–39). The bacteriology of intraamniotic infections reflects the vaginal microflora, from which it is felt to originate. Gibbs and colleagues performed a quantitative bacteriologic case–control study of the amniotic fluid from 52 women with amnionitis (34). Specimens were collected via an intrauterine catheter that demonstrated higher bacterial counts in the amniotic fluid of the infected group; 80.5% had counts greater than 100 colony forming units per milliliter versus 31% in the control group. Polymicrobial infection was common. The bacteria isolated in the infected group were more virulent than those in the control group. These included aerobic and anaerobic streptococci, including group B streptococci and Enterococci, *E coli,* and anaerobic gram-negative bacilli, such as *Bacteroides bivius* and *fragilis*, *Fusobacteria* species, and *Gardnerella vaginalis.* Lactobacilli, micrococci, anaerobic gram-negative cocci, and non-spore-forming, gram-positive bacilli, and so-called low-virulence organisms, were much less common. Subsequent studies by Sperling et al. demonstrated the high frequency of isolation of *Ureaplasma urealyticum* and *Mycoplasma hominis* in intraamniotic infections, 47% and 30%, respectively (39). *Chlamydia trachomatis*, a cause of cervicitis and late postpartum endometritis and associated with premature births, has not been associated with intrapartum fevers (40).

Endometritis

Endometritis is the most common cause of fever in the puerperium. Sweet and Ledger reported an overall incidence of 3.8%, but the rate was seven times higher following cesarean section (41). Endometritis may progress from previous intraamniotic infection. It can extend through the myometrium to the parametrial tissues, resulting in salpingitis, parametrial pelvic abscess, septicemia, and pelvic thrombophlebitis. Patients with endometritis are generally sicker than those with intraamniotic infection. High fevers, lower abdominal pain, uterine tenderness, and leukocytosis are more consistent findings.

The bacteriology and secondary risk factors for endometritis are similar to those for intraamniotic infection. Green and Sarubbi found that antecedent labor, obesity, general anesthesia, and anemia were independently associated with post-cesarean section febrile morbidity

(42). Group A streptococci, the organism responsible for the epidemics of childbed fever described by Holmes and Semmelweiss, was isolated in only 7% of patients reported by Gibbs's group (43) Bacteremia has been reported in 10% to 20% of cases. Facultative gram-negative rods and anaerobes account for a disproportionate percentage of the bacteremias (44). Enterococcal superinfection has been described in up to 25% of patients who have received cephalosporin prophylaxis for cesarean section (45).

The therapy of intraamniotic infections and postpartum endometritis is similar. DiZerega et al. demonstrated the importance of covering for penicillin-resistant anaerobes in pelvic infections (46). They performed a controlled trial of clindamycin and gentamicin versus penicillin and gentamicin in 200 women with endometritis following cesarean section. A poor clinical outcome was observed in 29% of the penicillin group but in only 5% of the clindamycin-treated patients. Classic "triple antibiotic" regimens, consisting of clindamycin or metronidazole, ampicillin, and gentamicin, have been replaced with single-drug regimens such as ampicillin-sulbactam (Unasyn) and cefoxitin or its clinical equivalent, cefotetan. The anti-pseudomonas coverage of the extended-spectrum penicillins piperacillin–tazobactam (Zosyn) and ticarcillin–clavulanic acid (Timentin), third-generation cephalosporins, and the penams imipenam and meropenam are generally not needed. After being afebrile for 48 to 72 hours, most patients may be switched to oral ampicillin-clavulanic acid (Augmentin). If the patient is not breastfeeding, the quinolone of choice would be trovafloxacin because of its activity against anaerobes and mycoplasma agents.

Antibiotic treatment failure should suggest the presence of a deep wound infection, pelvic abscess, ovarian vein thrombophlebitis, drug fever, or unusually resistant bacteriology. The last of these may be suggested by recent antimicrobial therapy prior to delivery. Treatment failure on non-penicillin regimens should raise the question of enterococcal superinfection, which is commonly found in endometritis following cephalosporin prophylaxis for cesarean section (45). Endometritis occurring days to weeks after delivery may be from infection with *C trachomatis*, which will not respond well to beta-lactam agents. Cervical cultures are helpful in establishing a specific bacteriologic diagnosis. Macrolides, tetracyclines, or the newer quinolones are the drugs of choice.

Listeriosis

Listeria monocytogenes is a facultative anaerobic, small, pleomorphic, gram-positive, non-spore-forming, catalase-positive, bacillus with characteristic tumbling motility and "ground glass" beta-hemolysis on sheep blood agar. It must be differentiated from diphtheroids and group A streptococci. *Listeria* is ubiquitous in nature and has been isolated from soil, dust, streams, and the gastrointestinal tract of a variety of mammals, birds, reptiles, fish, and insects (47). Ingestion from food sources and invasion through the gastrointestinal tract are thought to be the mechanisms of human infection. The organism can be isolated from the stools of 1% of normal, healthy people, where it can persist for several weeks (48).

Listeria causes a meningoencephalitis (circling disease) and septic abortion in ungulates. Bacteremia and meningitis characterize most human infections; but localized cerebritis, brain abscess, endocarditis, osteomyelitis, empyema, and cellulitis also have been described. Pregnant women account for 27% of human cases (49). Most of the remainder of cases occur in immunosuppressed persons, particularly those with underlying hematologic diseases and patients with organ transplants or who are receiving long-term corticosteroid therapy. *Listeria* infection is the most common cause of meningitis in patients with cancer (50).

Most human cases occur in urban environments without a history of animal contact. In an outbreak in Manitoba, Canada, Schlech et al. found infection to be related to the ingestion of raw vegetable products, notably coleslaw (51). Local farmers were fertilizing their cabbage fields with raw manure from their sheep herds. In a multihospital outbreak in the Boston area, Ho et al. also incriminated the consumption of lettuce and raw vegetables as the vehicle for infection in immunosuppressed patients (52). Cold storage of contaminated agricultural products may enhance the growth of *Listeria*, just as cold-enrichment laboratory techniques aid in the laboratory isolation of the organism from mixed bacterial populations (53). Other patients have been infected from contaminated meats and unpasteurized milk (47).

Infection may occur anytime during pregnancy, but it is most common in the third trimester, during maximal immune suppression. The diagnosis of maternal listeriosis may be suspected only after delivery of a stillbirth or congenitally infected child (granulomatosis infantiseptica). It should be suspected in any pregnant woman with unexplained fever. The disease may mimic a "flulike" syndrome with fever, myalgia, back pain, and headache. Meningitis is inexplicably rare in pregnant women (49). An antecedent diarrheal illness is common. Fever may begin with the onset of labor, which is often premature. There is often evidence of intraamniotic infection. In 22% of cases, perinatal listeriosis results in stillbirth or neonatal death (49). The clinical diagnosis is confirmed by isolation of the organism from blood, amniotic fluid, the products of conception, or cultures or postmortem examination of the newborn.

Early treatment may prevent fetal infection and fetal death. Zervoudakis and Cederquist reported the successful treatment of a 33-year-old woman who developed *Listeria* bacteremia in her 20th week of gestation (54). They reviewed six similar cases documenting a 71% survival of normal infants, more than double the 29% survival rate when the diagnosis is established only after the birth of an infected infant.

Neonatal infection most commonly presents with sepsis and prematurity, most likely from infection acquired *in utero*. In contrast, full-term children with perinatal infection developing in the first month, but after the third to fifth day of life, characteristically present with meningitis and have a better prognosis. Their infection is likely acquired from passage through the birth canal.

There is some controversy over whether *L monocytogenes* is a cause of repeated abortions from chronic colonization of the female genital tract. Rappaport et al. isolated Listeria from the cervix of 25 of 34 patients with a history of repeated abortions (55). Three of the patients with positive cultures rapidly aborted. Eight were treated with antibiotics and proceeded to term. Ansbacher et al. were able to isolate the organism from only one of 72 chronic aborters (56). A number of other workers (57–59) found no evidence of listeriosis in more than 700 habitual aborters. Bottone and Sierra analyzed these discrepant data and suggested that earlier reports linking *Listeria* to recurrent abortion may have been flawed by poor bacteriologic methods (53). At present, *Listeria* is not considered a cause of repeated abortions in humans.

High-dose intravenous penicillin G, 20 to 24 million units per day, or ampicillin, 12 g per day, for 10 to 21 days is the therapy of choice for listeriosis in pregnancy. Aminoglycosides act synergistically with penicillins *in vitro* and *in vivo* animal models of infection (60–62). The addition of gentamicin is recommended in severe infections and in the rare cases of listeria endocarditis.

Patients allergic to penicillin present a therapeutic dilemma. *Listeria* is susceptible to chloramphenicol, erythromycin, tetracycline, trimethoprim-sulfamethoxazole, and vancomycin. Tetracycline is contraindicated in pregnancy. Erythromycin and chloramphenicol have high failure and relapse rates (63,64). Vancomycin has been used successfully in a few patients, but one patient developed *Listeria* meningitis while receiving the drug (65).

Trimethoprim-sulfamethoxazole is bactericidal for Listeria and has proved effective in a limited number of patients (66). It can be used in the postpartum patient allergic to penicillin. In the antepartum situation, one must decide whether the benefits of the drug outweigh its risks. One may have to consider desensitization and therapy with a penicillin compound.

SYSTEMIC INFECTIONS

Lyme Borreliosis

Lyme borreliosis, Lyme disease, or Lyme arthritis is a multisystem illness caused by the spirochetal organism *Borrelia burgdorferi*. It was first described in 1977 by Steere et al. as occurring in children in Lyme, Connecticut, who suffered from a peculiar form of recurrent, asymmetric, nondestructive, oligoarticular arthritis of large joints, particularly the knee (67). It is now the most common arthropod-borne illness in the United States (68) and is epidemic along the Atlantic coast from Massachusetts to Maryland, in Wisconsin and Minnesota in the midwest, and in California and Oregon in the west.

B burgdorferi is a fastidious, microaerophilic bacterium that is closely related to the *Leptospirae* and *Treponemae*. The agent is transmitted by Ixodes ticks, *Ixodes scapularis* in the northeast and midwest, *I pacificus* in the west, *I ricinus* in Europe, and *I persulcatus* in Asia (69). Humans are most commonly infected in the spring and early summer after being bitten by the tiny nymph forms of infected ticks.

Lyme disease, like syphilis, has several clinical stages. After an incubation period of 3 to 30 days, the primary phase of Lyme disease may begin with the characteristic skin lesion, erythema chronicum migrans (ECM). The latter typically starts as an erythematous papule or macule that slowly enlarges, usually with central clearing, to form an irregular red ring that may grow as large as 20 to 30 cm in diameter. A central bite mark, which may be necrotic, vesicular, or secondarily infected may or may not be present at the time of diagnosis. This stage can be accompanied by "flulike" constitutional symptoms of fever, headache, and myalgias. This phase lasts from days to weeks and may be followed by disseminated multiple secondary ECM-like lesions.

The second stage of Lyme disease may present with cranial nerve palsies, most commonly unilateral or bilateral Bell's palsies, meningitis, or carditis. The incubation of symptomatic secondary disease is usually 1 to 3 months after inoculation. The organism can be isolated from the bloodstream as well as from infected tissues. Transplacental transmission may occur at this time.

Late Lyme disease develops an average of 6 months after infection in about 60% of untreated patients. Most often, this will manifest as intermittent attacks of an asymmetric, oligoarticular, nondestructive arthritis, most commonly the knee. The number of patients experiencing such recurrences decreases by 10% to 20% per year, but after several years, about 10% of patients may be left suffering from a chronic destructive arthritis that does not respond to antibiotic therapy. At this point, the disease has presumably evolved to an autoimmune disease. Of the chronic arthritic patients, 89% test positive for human leukocyte antigen (HLA)-DR4 and HLA-DR2 specificities (70).

Late Lyme disease also may produce a variety of syndromes involving the central or peripheral nervous system. These syndromes include a progressive encephalomyelitis, dementia, demyelinating syndromes resembling multiple sclerosis, neuropathies, and radicular pain syndromes. A keratitis that is similar to syphilitic keratitis and an unusual skin disease, acrodermatitis chronica atrophica, have been described.

Two infants born to mothers who developed ECM during their first trimester have been reported to have died of congenital disease within the first 48 hours of life (71). One was born at 35 weeks' gestation to a mother who had ECM during the second month of her pregnancy and was not treated. The infant died after 39 hours of life from congestive heart failure secondary to multiple congenital abnormalities of the heart and aorta. Spirochetes were identified in the spleen, renal tubules, and bone marrow but not in the heart of the fetus. A teratogenic effect of fetal infection was postulated to have accounted for the cardiovascular abnormalities. The second case was of a full-term infant born to a woman who had ECM during the second month of her pregnancy and had been treated with a 7-day course of oral penicillin. The infant died after 23 hours of life of respiratory distress and cerebral and cerebellar edema. Spirochetes were identified in the brain and liver of the fetus at postmortem examination.

Markowitz et al. (72) reviewed 19 cases of Lyme disease occurring in pregnancy, all but two of whom had ECM. Five (26%) of the cases were associated with adverse outcomes: prematurity, cortical blindness with developmental delay, intrauterine fetal death, syndactyly, and rash. No significant difference in outcome was seen based on the trimester of onset, the presence or absence of systemic manifestations of Lyme disease versus ECM alone, or maternal treatment with antibiotics. All the congenital outcomes were different; so no conclusions could be drawn about the association of maternal Lyme disease with an adverse outcome other than the fact that an adverse outcome seemed to occur more frequently than expected.

Williams et al. (73), in a prospective study of 463 infants from endemic and nonendemic areas, could find no association of congenital malformations with the presence of detectable antibody to *B burgdorferi* in infant cord blood. Thus, although it has been documented that maternal Lyme disease may result in severe congenital infection and neonatal death in sporadic cases, the incidence of severe embryonal or fetal infection must be quite low.

Pregnant women who develop Lyme disease should be treated with amoxicillin, 500 mg orally three or four times daily, with or without probenecid, for 10 to 30 days, depending on the stage and severity of disease and the rate of clinical response. Myocardial involvement and neurological disease other than isolated facial palsies or peripheral neuropathies also should be treated with high-dose parenteral penicillin or ceftriaxone (69). Dattwyler et al. (74) have demonstrated the superiority of ceftriaxone to penicillin in late chronic disease. They had a 50% treatment failure rate in the high-dose penicillin group compared with a 10% failure rate in the ceftriaxone-treated group.

Therapeutic options are limited in patients with a history of serious allergic reactions to penicillin. Erythromycin is very active against *B bergdorferi in vitro*, but it is not as effective as either penicillin or tetracycline *in vivo* (75). Azithromycin, which is active *in vitro*, is similarly inferior. The tetracyclines, of course, must be avoided in pregnancy.

URINARY TRACT INFECTIONS

The incidence of bacteriuria during pregnancy ranges from 4% to 6.9%, similar to the rate among nonpregnant women (76). There is no relation to the duration of pregnancy, but the incidence increases with gravidity (77). Women from lower socioeconomic groups are three times more likely to be bacteriuric than women from middle and upper income brackets (78). If urine cultures are initially sterile, it is rare for infection to develop later during pregnancy (79).

Bacteriuric pregnant women are about three times as likely as their nonpregnant counterparts to become symptomatic (80). Acute pyelonephritis may develop in as many as 25% to 35% of untreated bacteriuric pregnant women (76). The risk is greatest in the last trimester and can be largely prevented with early recognition and therapy.

The increased susceptibility to symptomatic urinary tract infection is related to the anatomic and physiologic alterations that take place during pregnancy. Hundley et al., in a study published in 1935 that is unlikely to be repeated, performed intravenous urograms on normal pregnant women and demonstrated that pyelocaliectasis and upper ureteral dilatation (hydroureter) are normal findings in the last trimester of pregnancy. The ureteral dilatation extended to the pelvic brim and was more marked on the right side. This condition was thought to result from hormonal relaxation of ureteral smooth muscle with decreased peristalsis (81). The resultant increase in upper tract, residual urine volume has been estimated to be as much as 200 mL, thereby predisposing to infection (82). Additionally, there is evidence to suggest that estrogens may enhance the pathogenicity of *E coli* (83).

Infection of the urinary tract is a common cause of puerperal fever. Sweet and Ledger found a 4.4% incidence in their large review of 6,436 patients (41). Undoubtedly, urethral trauma, bladder catheterization, difficulty voiding from local and general anesthesia, as well as pain medication contribute to this problem.

PUERPERAL BREAST ABSCESSES

Nonlactating breast abscesses are uncommon. In the puerperium, breast abscesses tend to occur in the setting of epidemics of staphylococcal infections involving the newborn infant and nursery (84). Pathogenic staphylococci initially colonize the nasopharynx of the newborn, leading to a high rate of colonization of the milk and ducts of the nursing mothers (85). Maternal infection may develop from 10 to 14 days postpartum (86).

Patients present with fever, breast pain, and local induration. *S aureus* is the offending pathogen in the vast majority of cases, which can be confirmed on culture and gram stain of breast milk. If discovered early, infection may resolve with oral anti-staphylococcal penicillins and warm soaks. Once suppuration develops, incision and drainage are usually necessary (87). Breastfeeding should be continued or the infected breast emptied with a pump if the infant is reluctant to feed from it until the infection resolves.

FUNGAL INFECTIONS

Candidiasis

Disseminated candidiasis during pregnancy is almost always an iatrogenic disease. Hospitalization, surgery, broad-spectrum antibiotics, central monitoring catheters, and parenteral nutrition predispose all patients, regardless of whether they are pregnant, to disseminated yeast infection. For life-threatening fungal infections during pregnancy, amphotericin B is preferred to fluconazole because of documented teratogenetic effects with prolonged high-dose therapy. Pursley et al. reported three cases of congenital abnormalities in women being treated for coccidioidomycosis with 400 to 800 mg per day of fluconazole for at least 3 months (88). The teratogenic effects of fluconazole appear to be dose and duration dependent (89). Short-course, low-dose therapy, as used for vaginal candidiasis, has not been found to be harmful (90).

Coccidioidomycosis

Coccidioides immitis is a dimorphic fungus found in the soil of arid regions of the Western Hemisphere, including the southeastern United States, northern Mexico, California, and the plains of Argentina. Disease is acquired by inhalation of the highly infective fungal arthrospores during hot, dry, dusty seasons. In most cases, infection produces an acute self-limited "flulike" illness that may be associated with erythema nodosum. Progressive pulmonary or disseminated disease develops in about 1% of cases. The risk is dependent on the presence of underlying diseases (such as diabetes), immunosuppression, and ethnic background. Mexicans, blacks, and Filipinos are, respectively, 3.4, 13.7, and 175.5 times as likely to develop disseminated disease as whites and 5, 23.3 and 191.4 times as likely to die of their illness (91).

Coccidioidomycosis is a particular hazard in pregnancy. Pregnancy increases the risk of progressive disseminated disease for white women to levels customarily expected among blacks. This risk is progressive with the duration of pregnancy. In Harris's series 7 of 22 patients who acquired their disease in the second or third trimesters developed disseminated disease, whereas only 4 of 26 patients who acquired coccidioidomycosis before or during the first trimester developed disseminated disease (92).

Dissemination may involve any organ system. Rare cases of pelvic granuloma and congenital infection have been described. The major risk, however, is to the life of the mother. Because of the magnitude of the risk, prophylactic therapy of pregnant women has been recommended (91). Patients with pulmonary symptoms lasting more than 2 weeks or with high or rapidly rising complement fixation antibody tiers should receive amphotericin B.

Other Fungal Diseases

Disseminated histoplasmosis and blastomycosis are uncommon infections in pregnancy. They are mostly limited to endemic geographic areas. Dermatophyte infections are treated topically.

REFERENCES

1. Thompson SE III, Dretler RH. Epidemiology an treatment of chlamydial infections in pregnant women and infants. Rev Infect Dis 1982;4(Suppl):S747–S757.
2. Olding LB, Oldstone MBA. Lymphocytes from human newborns abrogate mitoses of their mother's lymphocytes. Nature 1974;249:161–162
3. Bassett M, Coons TA, Wallis W, Goldberg EH, Williams RC Jr. Suppression of stimulation of mixed leukocyte culture by newborn splenic lymphocytes in the mouse. J Immunol 1977;119:1855–1857.
4. Morito T, Bankhurst AD, Williams RJ Jr. Studies of human cord blood and adult lymphocyte interaction using *in vitro* immunoglobulin production. J Clin Invest 1979;64:990–995.
5. Murgita RA, Goidl EA, Kontiainen S, Wigzell H. Alpha-fetoprotein induces suppressor T cells *in vitro*. Nature 1977;267:257–259.
6. Fuchs T, Hammarstrom L, Smith CIE, Brundin J. *In vitro* induction of human suppressor T cells by a chorionic gonadotropin preparation. J Reprod Immunol 1981;3:75–84.
7. Sridama V, Pacini F, Yang SL, Moawad A, Reilly M, DeGroot LJ. Decreased levels of helper T cells: a possible cause of immune deficiency in pregnancy. N Engl J Med 1982;307:352–356.
8. Charles D. Dynamics of antibiotic transfer from mother to fetus. Semin Perinatol 1977;1:89–100.
9. Charles D, MacAulay M. Use of antibiotics in obstetric practice. Clin Obstet Gynecol 1970;13:255–271.
10. McCormack WM, George H, Donner A, et al. Hepatotoxicity of erythromycin estolate during pregnancy. Antimicrob Agents Chemother 1977;12:630–635.
11. The Medical Letter. Drugs for parasitic infections. Med Lett Drugs Ther 1995;37:99–108.
12. Kline AH, Blatter RJ, Lunin M. Transplacental effect of tetracyclines on teeth. JAMA 1964;188:178–180.
13. Schultz JC, Adamson JS, Workman WW. Fatal liver disease after intravenous administration of tetracycline in high doseage. N Engl J Med 1963;269:999–1004.
14. Taylor W, Sabbath LD. Adverse effects of antimicrobial agents. In: Kagen BM, ed. Antimicrobial therapy, 2nd ed. Philadelphia: WB Saunders, 1974:423–424.
15. Silverman WA, Anderson DH, Blanc WA, et al. A difference in mortality rate and incidence of kernicterus among premature infants allotted to two prophylactic antibacterial regimens. Pediatrics 1956;18: 614–625.
16. Brumfitt W, Purcell R. Trimethoprim-sulfamethoxazole in the treatment of bacteriuria in women. J Infect Dis 1973;128(Suppl): S657–S663.
17. Burroughs-Wellcome. Information for investigators for trimethoprim-

sulfamethoxazole. Medical Department, Burroughs-Welcome, Research Triangle Park, NC (undated).
18. Weiss CF, Glazko AJ, WestonJK. Chloramphenicol in the newborn infant: a physiologic explanation of its toxicity when given in excessive doses. N Engl J Med 1960;262:787–794.
19. Lossick JG. Treatment of *Trichomonas vaginalis* infection. Rev Infect Dis 1982;4(Suppl):801–818.
20. Finegold M. Metronidazole. Ann Intern Med 1980;93:585–587.
21. Goldman P. Metronidazole. N Engl J Med 1980;303:1212–1218.
22. Beard CM, Noller KL, O'Fallon WM, Kurland LT, Dahlin DC. Cancer after exposure to metronidazole. Mayo Clin Proc 1988;63:147–153.
23. Robbie MO, Sweet RL. Metronidazole use in obstetrics and gynecology: a review. Am J Obstet Gynecol 1983;145:865–881.
24. Robinson GC, Cambon KG. Hearing loss in infants of tuberculous mothers treated with streptomycin during pregnancy. N Engl J Med 1964;271:949–951.
25. Pertuiset E, Lenoir G, Jehanne M, Douchain F, Guillot M, Menkes CJ. Tolérance articulaire de la pefloxacine et de l'ofloxacine chez les enfants et adolescents atteints de mucoviscidose. Rev Rheum 1969;56:735–740.
26. Philipson A. Pharmacokinetics of ampicillin during pregnancy. J Infect Dis 1977;136:370–376.
27. Philipson A, Stiernstedt G. Pharmacokinetics of cephradine in pregnancy: current chemotherapy and infectious disease. Proceedings of the 11th ICC and the 19th ICAAC. Washington DC: American Society for Microbiology, 1980;1172–1174.
28. Philipson A, Stiernstedt G. Pharmacokinetics of cefuroxime in pregnancy. Am J Obstet Gynecol 1982;142:823–828.
29. Zaske DE, Cipolle RJ, Strate RG, Malo JW, Koszalka MF Jr. Rapid gentamicin elimination in obstetric patients. Obstet Gynecol 1980;56:559–564.
30. Philipson A. The use of antibiotics in pregnancy. J Antimicrob Chemother 1983;12:101–102.
31. Edson RS, Terrell CL. The aminoglycosides. Mayo Clin Proc 1991;66:1158–1164.
32. Blam ME, Hammer GS. Extended-interval dosing of aminoglycosides. Mt Sinai J Med 1997;386–391.
33. Acker DB, Johnson MP, Sachs BP, Friedman EA. The leukocyte count in labor. Am J Obstet Gynecol 1985;153:737–739.
34. Gibbs RS, Blanco JD, StClair PJ, Castaneda YS. Quantitative bacteriology of amniotic fluid from women with clinical intraamniotic infection at term. J Infect Dis 1982;145:1–8.
35. Prevedourakis CN, Strigou-Charalabis E, Kaskarelis DB. Bacterial invasion of the amniotic cavity during pregnancy and labor. Obstet Gynecol 1971;37:459–461.
36. Newton ER. Chorioamnionitis and intraamniotic infections. Clin Obstet Gynecol 1993;36:795–808.
37. Newton ER, Prihoda TJ, Gibbs RS. Logistic regression analysis of risk factors for intra-amniotic infection. Obstet Gynecol 1989;73:571–575.
38. Soper DE, Mayhall CG, Dalton HP. Risk factors for intraamniotic infection: A prospective epidemiologic study. Am J Obstet Gynecol 1989;161:562–566.
39. Sperling RS, Newton E, Gibbs RS. Intraamniotic infection in low-birth-weight infants. J Infect Dis 1988;157:113–117.
40. Wager GP, Martin DH, Koutsky L, et al. Pueperal infectious morbidity: relationship to route of delivery and to antepartum *Chlamydia trachomatis* infection. Am J Obstet Gynecol 1980;138:1028–1037.
41. Sweet RL, Ledger WJ. Pueperal infectious morbidity: a two year review. Am J Obstet Gynecol 1973;117:1093–1100.
42. Green SL, Sarubbi FA. Risk factors associated with post cesarean section febrile morbidity. Obstet Gynecol 1977;49:686–690.
43. Gibbs RS, O'Dell TN, MacGregor RR, Schwarz RH, Morton H. Pueperal endometritis: a prospective microbiologic study. Am J Obstet Gynecol 1975;121:919–925.
44. Ledger WJ, Norman M, Gee C, Lewis W. Bacteremia on an obstetric-gynecological service. Am J Obstet Gynecol 1975;121:205–212.
45. Gibbs RS, StClair PJ, Castillo MS, Castaneda YS. Bacteriologic effects of antibiotic prophylaxis in high-risk cesarean section. Obstet Gynecol 1981;57:277–282.
46. DiZerega G, Yonekura L, Roy S, Nakamura RM, Ledger WJ. A comparison of clindamycin-gentamicin and penicillin-gentamicin in the treatment of post-cesarean section endometritis. Am J Obstet Gynecol 1979;134:238–242.
47. Armstrong D. *Listeria monocytogenes*. In: Mandell GL, Bennett JE, Dolin R, eds. Principles and practice of infectious diseases, 4th ed. New York: Churchill Livingstone, 1995;1880–1889.
48. Bojsen-Moller J. Human listeriosis, diagnostic epidemiological and clinical studies. Acta Path Microbiol Scand 1972;229(Suppl):1–157.
49. Lorber B. Listeriosis. Clin Infect Dis 1997;24:1–11.
50. Chernick NL, Armstrong D, Posner JB. Central nervous system infections in patients with cancer: changing patterns. Cancer 1977;40: 268–274.
51. Schlech WF, Lavigne PM, Bartolussi RA. Epidemic listeriosis: evidence for transmission by food. N Engl J Med 1983;308:203–206.
52. Ho JL, Shands KN, Friedland G. A multitrospital outbreak of type 4b *Listeria monocytogenes* infection. The 21st Interscience Conference of Antimicrobial Agents and Chemotherapy. Chicago, Nov 4–6, 1981;No. 632.
53. Bottone EJ, Sierra MF. *Listeria* monocytogenes: another look at the "Cinderella among pathogenic bacteria." Mt Sinai Med J 1977;44: 42–59.
54. Zervoudakis IA, Cederquist LL. Effect of *Listeria monocytogenes* septicemia during pregnancy on the offspring. Am J Obstet Gynecol 1977;129:465–467.
55. Rappaport F, Rabinowitz M, Toaff R, et al. Genital listeriosis as a cause of repeated abortion. Lancet 1960;1:1273–1275.
56. Ansbacher R, Borchardt KA, Hannegan MW, Boyson WA. Clinical investigation of *Listeria monocytogenes* as a possible cause of human fetal wastage. Am J Obstet Gynecol 1966;94:386–390.
57. Lawler FE, Wood WS, King S, et al. *Listeria monocytogenes* as a cause of fetal loss. Am J Obstet Gynecol 1964;89:915–923.
58. Macnaughton MC. *Listeria monocytogenes* in abortion. Lancet 1962;2: 484–486.
59. Rabau E, David A. *Listeria monocytogenes* in abortion. J Obstet Gynecol Br Commonw 1963;70:481–482.
60. Edmiston CE Jr, Gordon R. Evaluation of gentamicin and penicillin as a synergistic combination in experimental murine listeriosis. Antimicrob Agents Chemother 1979;16:862–863.
61. Scheld WM, Fletcher DD, Fink FN, Sande MA. Response to therapy in an experimental rabbit model of meningitis due to *Listeria monocytogenes*. J Infect Dis 1979;140:287–294.
62. Wiggins GL, Albritton WL, Feeley JC. Antibiotic susceptibility of clinical isolates of *Listeria moncytogenes*. Antimicrob Agents Chemother 1978;13:854–860.
63. Cherubin CE, Marr JS, Sierra MF, Becker S. *Listeria* and gram-negative bacillary meningitis in New York City, 1972–1979: frequent causes of meningitis in adults. Am J Med 1981;71:199–209.
64. Stamm AM, Dismukes WE, Simmons BP, et al. Listeriosis in renal transplant recipients: report of an outbreak and review of 102 cases. Rev Infect Dis 1982;4:665–682.
65. Baldassarre JS, Ingerman MJ, Nansteel J, Santoro J. Development of *Listeria meningitis* during vancomycin therapy: a case report (letter). J Infect Dis 1991;164:221–222.
66. Scheer MS, Hirschman SZ. Oral and ambulatory therapy of listeria bacteremia and meningitis with trimethoprim-sulfamethoxazole. Mt Sinai J Med 1982;49:411–414.
67. Steere AC, Malawista SE, Snydman DR, et al. Lyme arthritis: an epidemic of olioarticular arthritis in children and adults in three Connecticut communities. Arthritis Rheum 1977;20:7–17.
68. Centers for Disease Control. Lyme disease—Connecticut. MMWR Morb Mortal Wkly Rep 1988;37:1–3.
69. Steere AC. Lyme disease. N Engl J Med 1989;321:586–596.
70. Steere AC, Dwyer E, Winchester R. Association of chronic lyme arthritis with HLA-DR4 and HLA DR2 alleles. N Engl J Med 1990;323: 219–223.
71. Schlesinger PA, Duray PH, Burke BA, Steere AC, Stillman AT. Maternal-fetal transmission of the Lyme disease spirochete, *Borrelia burgdorferi*. Ann Intern Med 1985;103:67–68.
72. Markowitz LE, Steere AC, Benach JL, Slade JD, Broone CV. Lyme disease during pregnancy. JAMA 1986;255:3394–3396.
73. Williams CL, Benach JL, Curran AS, et al. Lyme disease during pregnancy: a cord blood survey. Ann NY Acad Sci 1988;539:504–506.
74. Dattwyler RJ, Halperin JJ, Volkman DJ, Luft BJ. Treatment of late Lyme borreliosis—randamized comparison of ceftriaxone and penicillin. Lancet 1988;1:1191–1194.
75. Steere AC, Hutchinson GJ, Rahn DW, et al. Treatment of the early manifestations of Lyme disease. Ann Intern Med 1983;99:22–26.
76. Stamey TA. Urinary tract infections in women. In: Pathogenesis and

treatment of urinary tract infections. Baltimore: Williams & Wilkins, 1980:122–209.
77. Savage WE, Hajj SN, Kass EH. Demographic and prognostic characteristics of bacteriura in pregnancy. Medicine 1967;46:385–407.
78. Turck M, Goffe BS, Petersdorf RG. Bacteriuria of pregnancy: relation to socioeconomic factors. N Engl J Med 1962;266:857–60.
79. McFadyen IR, Erkyn SJ, Gardner NHN, et al. Bacteriuria in pregnancy. J Obstet Gynecol Br Commonw 1973;80:385–405.
80. Gaymans R, Haverkorn MJ, Valkenburg H, Goslings WR. A prospective study of urinary tract infections in a Dutch general practice. Lancet 1976;2:674–677.
81. Hundley JM Jr, Walton HJ, Hibbotts JT, et al. Physiologic changes occurring in the urinary tract during pregnancy. Am J Obstet Gynecol 1935;30:625–669.
82. Lindheimer MD, Katz AI. The kidney in pregnancy. N Engl J Med 1970;283:1095–1097.
83. Harle EMJ, Bullen JJ, Thomson DA. Influence of estrogen on experimental pyelonephritis caused by *Escherichia coli*. Lancet 1975;2: 283–286.
84. Sherman AJ. Pueperal breast abscess; I. Report of an outbreak at Philadelphia General Hospital. Obstet Gynecol 1956;7:268–273.
85. Duncan JT, Wlaker J. *Staphylococcus aureus* in the milk of nursing mothers and the alimentary canal of their infants. Journal of Hygiene 1942;42:474–484.
86. Smith MHD, Teele DW. Tuberculosis. In: Remington JS, Klein JO, eds. Infectious diseases of the fetus and newborn infant. Philadelphia: WB Saunders, 1995;1074–1086.
87. Ekland DA, Zeigler MG. Abscess in the nonlactating breast. Arch Surg 1973;107:398–401.
88. Pursley TJ, Blomquist IK, Abraham J, Andersen HF, Bentley JA. Fluconazole-induced congenital anomalies in three infants. Clin Infect Dis 1996;22:336–340.
89. King CT, Rogers PD, Cleary JD, Chaptman SW. Antifungal therapy during pregnancy. Clin Infect Dis 1998;27:1151–1160.
90. Inman W, Pearce G, Wilton L. Safety of fluconazole in the treatment of vaginal candidiasis: a prescription-event monitoring study, with special reference to the outcome of pregnancy. Eur J Clin Pharmacol 1994;46: 115–118.
91. Drutz DJ, Catanzero A. Coccidioidomycosis. Am J Respir Dis 1978; 117:559–85, 727–771.
92. Harris RE. Coccidiodomycosis complicating pregnancy: report of 3 cases and review of the literature. Obstet Gynecol 1966;28:401–405.

Cherry and Merkatz's Complications of Pregnancy,
Fifth Edition, edited by W. R. Cohen.
Lippincott Williams & Wilkins, Philadelphia © 2000.

CHAPTER 47

Vaginitis

Martin S. Goldstein

Most pregnant women have vaginal discharges that are either physiologic or pathologic. The challenge to the clinician is to separate the vaginal infections with potentially serious import for pregnancy from annoying but not serious abnormal secretions, irritations, and pruritis. Infectious vaginitis is usually a result of yeast, *Trichomonas vaginalis,* bacterial vaginosis (BV), gonorrhea, *Chlamydia trachomatis, Mycoplasma,* group B *Streptococcus* (GBS), or herpes. Normal vaginal secretions consist of water, electrolytes, epithelial cells, microbial organisms, fatty acids, and carbohydrate compounds (1). Many microorganisms are present in vaginal fluids, in concentrations that range from rare organisms to those with a colony count as high as 10^9 colony forming units per milliliter of fluid (2). The concentration of anaerobic bacteria is usually five times that of aerobic organisms. The most prevalent organisms in the vagina are lactobacilli, streptococci, *Staphylococcus epidermidis, Gardenerella vaginalis,* and *Escherichia coli.* Anaerobic species frequently isolated include peptostreptococci, anaerobic lactobacilli, and *Bacteroides.*

Vaginal pH, glycogen content, and amount of secretion influence the quantity and type of organisms present in the vagina. Lactobacilli restrict the growth of other organisms by producing lactic acid and thus maintaining a low pH. These bacteria also produce hydrogen peroxide, which is toxic to anerobes. The normal vaginal bacterial population assists in inhibiting the growth of pathologic vaginal organisms. If the normal vaginal ecosystem is altered, there is a greater chance of pathogenic organisms proliferating. Complaints of vaginitis should be evaluated at the initial pregnancy visit. The challenge of treating vaginitis in pregnancy is in the need to make accurate diagnoses and treat correctly. True infections (some of which can have a dangerous effect on gestation) must be separated and distinguished from the exaggeration of physiologic discharge by pregnancy. Infection with BV, chlamydia, trichomonads, or GBS have been associated with septic abortion, premature rupture of membranes (PROM), and premature delivery. Sexually transmissible infections that do not appear to have a deleterious effect on pregnancy include pediculosis pubis, scabies, molluscum contagiosum, chancroid, granuloma inguinale, and lymphogranuloma venereum.

Neisseria gonorrhoeae and *Chlamydia trachomatis* should be screened for at the first prenatal visit and again in the third trimester in high-risk groups. *Chlamydia* is prevalent in all population groups and warrants initial screening, which is more than is recommended by the Centers for Disease Control and Prevention (CDC) guidelines (3) of screening for *Chlamydia* in the third trimester. If a patient is positive for gonorrhea or *Chlamydia*, she and her partner should be treated and tested for cure. Culture tests for *N. gonorrhoeae* are accurate, but DNA probes and enzyme immunoassays are not fully reliable. These tests are not 100% sensitive for chlamydia. Polymerase chain reaction (PCR) and ligase chain reaction are more sensitive and offer vaginal introitus and urine screening rather than cervical screening in the third trimester (4).

CHLAMYDIA

The cervix is the most common site infected by *C. trachomatis. Chlamydia* does not cause vaginitis, but the cervix may be eroded, have a mucopurulent discharge, or appear normal. The discharge may be perceived by the patient to be vaginal in origin. Neonates born to women with *Chlamydia* infection have a significant likelihood of acquiring inclusion conjunctivitis during delivery. Twenty-five percent to 50% of exposed infants will develop conjunctivitis in the first 2 weeks of life, and 10% to 20% will develop pneumonia within 3 to 4 months after birth if not treated earlier (5,6). *Chlamydia* infection in early pregnancy is associated with premature delivery (7) and premature rupture of membranes

M. S. Goldstein: Department of Obstetrics and Gynecology, Mount Sinai School of Medicine, New York, New York 10128.

(PROM). An increased incidence of late-onset endometritis following vaginal delivery and severe pelvic infection after cesarean section has been reported when *C. trachomatis* has been diagnosed at the initial prenatal visit (8). A single oral dose of 1 g of azithromycin is effective in the treatment of *Chlamydia* in pregnancy.

TRICHOMONIASIS

Trichomonas vaginalis is a sexually transmitted anerobic parasite. Symptoms include a copious yellow-gray or greenish foul-smelling discharge. The prevalence of the organism as diagnosed by positive cultures ranges from 3% to 15% of asymptomatic women in private practice settings to 13% to 23% of clinic patients (9). Trichomoniasis may be more prevalent among pregnant women. The causative protozoan primarily infects the urogenital tract, with extragenital infection being unusual. *T. vaginalis* as a cause of amnionitis, PROM, prematurity, and postpartum endometritis has been postulated since 1931 but not proved (8,10). These complications have been disputed by many who feel that *T. vaginalis* is not associated with serious maternal or fetal effects and has no influence on prematurity, amnionitis, and pyrexia. Recent studies have shown that *T. vaginalis* is associated with increased risk of preterm and low-birth-weight infants either independent of or associated with gonorrhea, *Chlamydia* infection, and bacterial vaginoses (11,12). Female infants born to mothers with *T. vaginalis* may develop symptomatic or asymptomatic vaginal infections following delivery (13).

The diagnosis of trichomoniasis can be made by Papanicolaou (pap) smear or a wet smear microscopic evaluation of vaginal secretions mixed with warm saline. Dyes such as 0.1% safranin 0, 1% brilliant cresyl blue, or aqueous fluorescein can be used to counterstain the organism. Such wet preparation evaluations have been estimated to be 30% to 75% sensitive in diagnosing trichomoniasis. Trichomonads can be cultured using liquid or semisolid media (14). Culture techniques are more sensitive than wet smears and pap smears. PCR is the most sensitive diagnostic test for trichomoniasis. Introital samples tested by PCR can detect evidence of organisms with 95% sensitivity and 100% specificity (4).

Trichomonas infection is accepted to be a sexually transmitted disease. The organism has been shown to survive on wet sponges for several hours and in urine for more than 24 hours (15). It is possible that transmission can occur through communal bathing, hot tubs, shared douche equipment, bath towels, and swim suits. The incubation period for trichomoniasis is between 4 and 28 days. The organism flourishes at a pH of 6.0 to 6.5. Symptoms and severity of an infection correlate with the number of organisms present in vaginal secretions. Symptoms are rarely present if the presence of trichomonads is not confirmed by a wet smear microscopic examination.

The accepted treatment regimen for trichomoniasis is a single oral 2g dose of metronidazole. Sexual partners must be treated simultaneously for treatment to be effective. Resistant strains may require repeat treatment at higher dose regimens. Vaginal metronidazole is not an effective treatment alternative. Metronidazole crosses the placenta (16) and can be found in fetal tissue, cord blood, and amniotic fluid in high concentrations. Metronidazole concentration in breast milk is comparable with serum levels. Metronidazole has been shown not to be teratogenic in mice, rats, and guinea pigs; however, it is mutagenic for bacteria and carcinogenic in mice after long-term use (17). Carcinogenicity has never been reported in humans (18). A recent metaanalysis regarding safety of metronidazole in pregnancy concluded that metronidazole does not appear to be associated with an increased teratogenic risk (19). Current recommendation is for the use of metronidazole after the first trimester. A single 2g dose of metronidazole can be used during lactation coupled with temporary cessation of breastfeeding.

VULVOVAGINAL CANDIDIASES

Candida albicans can be isolated in small numbers in 25% to 50% of healthy women (20). It causes between 80% and 90% of vaginal fungal infections. *Candida tropicalis, Candida pseudotropicalis, Candida krusei,* and *Torulopsis glabrata* are sometimes isolated from women whose conditions have not responded to therapy and who have had recurrences of signs and symptoms of yeast infections. Symptoms are present when the *Candida* organism is present in a high concentration. Pregnancy is a common predisposing factor for *Candida* infection. As many as 15% to 20% of pregnant women demonstrate symptomatic *Candida* infections in the later stages of pregnancy. These symptoms may include vulvar pruritis, vulvar erythema, and labial edema. Excoriations from scratching are frequently present. The odorless candidal discharge is white, floccular, and viscous. The pH is usually less than 4.5, with lactobacilli present in the discharge. There is no amine odor, nor are there white blood cells, trichomonads, or clue cells detectable in the discharge. A diagnosis can be confirmed by the presence of mycelia and spores in a microscopic coverslip preparation of vaginal discharge in a 10% to 20% potassium hydroxide solution. *Candida* can be recovered from the stool and oral cavities of a large number of women with yeast infections.

Infants born to women with a *C. albicans* infection in either the vaginal or gastrointestinal tracts may develop an oral fungal infection (thrush), a fungal dermatitis in the diaper area, or both. Severe intrauterine and perinatal infections with *C. albicans* have been reported but are extremely rare. Recurrent infections should be evaluated to confirm the presence of candidal infections. Cultures can confirm the presence of yeast and whether a species other than *C. albicans* is present. Repetitive positive *C. albicans* cultures suggest reinfection from a gastrointestinal reservoir or recurrent sexual transmission.

Cellular immunity is needed for a host response to candidiases. Patients with depressed cellular immunity due to pregnancy or immunosupressive therapy are predisposed to candidiases. Therapy in pregnancy is directed at patient comfort, prevention of secondary infections, and protection against neonatal fungal infections. Elimination of *Candida* during pregnancy may not be possible. Most *C. albicans* infections respond to clotrimazole or miconazole administered vaginally. Non-albicans species may be resistant to the over-the-counter antifungals and may require agents such as terconazole, butoconazole, ticonazole, ketoconazole, and fluconazole. Fluconazole is an approved oral antiyeast agent. The effectiveness of oral agents may be due to the elimination of the rectal reservoir of yeast. First-trimester exposure to fluconazole does not appear to increase the prevalence of miscarriages, congenital anomalies, and low-birth-weight infants (12).

BACTERIAL VAGINOSIS

Bacterial vaginosis is a polymicrobial syndrome including *Gardnerella vaginalis, Bacteroides* species, *Peptostreptococcus* species, *Mycoplasma hominis,* and *Enterobacteriaceae.* There is usually an overgrowth of several bacterial species with the absence of inflammatory cells. Patients with symptomatic infections present with a homogeneous, gray-white watery discharge that adheres to the vaginal mucosa and has a foul fishy odor. The discharge has a pH above 4.5 with a prominent amine odor when mixed with a 10% KOH solution (whiff test). The odor is caused by putrescene and cadaverene, which are bacterial metabolites. It is more noticeable after coitus when the pH of seminal fluid increases the volatility of the metabolites. *G. vaginalis* is often found accompanying an overgrowth of anaerobic bacteria. Amine and ammonia production by these anaerobes raises vaginal pH, allowing *G. vaginalis* to proliferate. If lactobacillus is present with the discharge, the patient is usually asymptomatic. Microscopic evidence of epithelial cells with a stippled or granulated appearance has diagnostic importance. These are referred to as clue cells. The clue cell may be covered by a tiny (0.4–0.7×1–3 μm) pleomorphic, gram-negative *Coccobacillus* adherent to the cell surface. Cultures can document the presence of *G. vaginalis*, which can be recovered from 40% of asymptomatic women (21).

Bacterial vaginosis has been associated with preterm delivery, low-birth-weight infants, preterm prelabor membrane rupture, late miscarriages, chorioamnionitis at delivery, and postpartum endometritis (22–24). The presence of BV at 28 weeks' gestation is strongly associated with an increase in spontaneous preterm birth (22). Women with prior preterm delivery, first-trimester bleeding, and multiple infections who have BV are at increased risk for complications in pregnancy and should be screened and treated for BV in the first trimester or at the initial visit. Patients with vaginitis during pregnancy should be screened and treated for BV. The consequences of preterm delivery are costly and devastating. The minimal cost for BV screening and treatment raises the issue of whether BV screening would be appropriate in asymptomatic pregnant women. A National Institutes of Health–funded randomized controlled trial of pregnant women with BV now underway should clarify this issue. Current treatment is oral clindamycin 300 mg twice daily for 7 days orally or metronidazole 500 mg twice daily for 7 days. Vaginal treatment, which may give symptomatic relief of vaginitis, is insufficient to prevent pregnancy complications of BV.

GROUP B STREPTOCOCCAL INFECTION

Group B steptococcal infection in pregnancy can lead to intrapartum transmission to the neonate, premature labor, PROM, and mid-trimester fetal loss. GBS should be screened for by urine culture at the initial prenatal visit. Vaginal and cervical cultures should be performed between 35 and 37 weeks of gestation in all pregnancies and in patients with preterm labor and PROM (25). Although GBS can probably cause clinical vaginitis, it is usually an asymptomatic colonizer of the lower genital tract. Although heavy GBS colonization at 23 to 26 weeks' gestation is associated with an increased risk of delivering a preterm infant, cervicovaginal colonization at 23 to 26 weeks' gestation is not a reliable predictor of GBS sepsis in neonates. Only colonization at birth is strongly associated with neonatal sepsis (26). Neonatal infections at birth in women colonized with GBS at term are more prevalent with PROM (27).

Group B streptococcal bacteriuria should be treated. A Danish study reduced the rates of prematurity considerably by looking for GBS bacteriuria in pregnancy and treating with oral penicillin when they found it (27). Asymptomatic colonization of the vagina requires treatment during labor to reduce the risk of newborn infection.

GENITAL *MYCOPLASMA* INFECTIONS

Mycoplasma hominis and *Ureaplasma urealyticum* are organisms frequently found in the lower genital tract of sexually active women. Colonization rates increase with the numbers of sexual partners. The isolation by culture by these organisms does not define a pathologic situation. Genital mycoplasmas have been found in up to 33% of newborns, the organisms presumably having been acquired during passage through the birth canal (26). No convincing evidence exists that *M. hominis* or *U. urealyticum* in the vagina is associated with poor pregnancy outcome for the mother or the infant. The presence of *M.*

hominis in the cervix is associated with higher levels of trichomoniasis and BV and by proxy with the negative effects on pregnancy of these organisms of postabortal infections, postcesarean infection, preterm labor, prematurity, and PROM.

Symptomatic complaints related to vulvovaginitis and cervicitis in pregnancy must be carefully evaluated and treated. Patients should be screened and treated for bacteriuria at the first prenatal visit. Sexually transmitted organisms, including *N. gonorrhoeae*, *C. trachomatis*, and *T. vaginalis* should be screened for at the first visit, at exposure to a new sexual partner, and in the third trimester in high-risk populations. BV should be diagnosed and treated in symptomatic women or if risk factors for premature delivery are present. Oral antibiotic therapy should be prescribed in the first 24 weeks, with tests of cure and retreatment if required. With a program of screening and evaluating and treating patient complaints of irritation and discharge during pregnancy, we can treat symptomatic vaginitis and diagnose more severe conditions before they lead to severe fetal and maternal morbidity.

REFERENCES

1. Huggins GR, Preti G. Vaginal odors and secretions. Clin Obstet Gynecol 1981;24:355–377.
2. Levison ME, Trestman L, Quash R, Sladowski C, Floro CN. Quantitative bacteriology of the vaginal flora in vaginitis. Am J Obstet Gynecol 1979;133:139–144.
3. Centers for Disease Control and Prevention. 1998 Guidelines for treatment of sexually transmitted diseases. MMWR 1998;47(RR-1): 81–111.
4. Witkin SS, Inglis SR, Polaneczky M. Detection of *Chlamydia trachomatis* and *Trichomonas vaginalis* by polymerase chain reaction in introital specimens from pregnant women. Am J Obstet Gynecol 1996; 175:165–167.
5. Frommell GT, Rottenberg R, Wang SP, McIntosh K. Chlamydial infection of mothers and their infants. J Pediatr 1979;95:28–32.
6. Schachter J, Grossman M, Holt J, Goodner E, Sweet R, Mills J. Prospective study of chlamydial infections in neonates. Lancet 1979;2: 377–380.
7. Sweet RL, Landers DV, Walker C, Schachter J. Chlamydia trachomatis infection and pregnancy outcome. Am J Obstet Gynecol 1987;156: 824–833.
8. Cytryn A, Sen P, Haingsub R, et al. Severe pelvic infection of *Chlamydia trachomatis* after cesarian section. JAMA 1982;247:1732–1734.
9. Rein MF, Chabel TA. Trichomoniasis, candidiasis and the minor venereal diseases. Clin Obstet Gynecol 1975;18:73–88.
10. Jirovec O, Petru M. Trichomonas vaginalis and trichomoniases. Adv Parasitol 1968;6:117–188.
11. Hillier SL, Nugent RP, Eschenbach DA, et al. Association between bacterial vaginosis and preterm delivery of a low birth weight infant. N Engl J Med 1995;333:1737–1742.
12. Mastroiacovo P, Mazzone T, Botto LD, et al. Prospective assessment of pregnancy outcomes after first trimester exposure to fluconazole. Am J Obstet Gynecol 1996;175;1645–1650.
13. Bramley M. Study of female babies of women entering confinement with vaginal trichomoniases. Br J Vener Dis 1976;52:58–62.
14. Diamond LS. The establishment of various trichomonads of animals and man in axenic culture. J Parasitol 1957;43:488–490.
15. Brown D, Kaufman RH. Vulvovaginitis. In: Glass RH, ed. Office gynecology. Baltimore: Williams & Wilkins, 1981:34.
16. Amon I, Amon K, Franke G, Mohr C. Pharmacokinetics of metronidazole in pregnant women. Chemotherapy 1981;27:73–79.
17. Roe JFC. A critical appraisal of the toxicology of metronidazole. In: Phillip I, Collier J, eds. Metronidazole proceedings, Geneva, Switzerland, 1979. New York: Academic, 1979:215–222.
18. Beard CM, Noller KL, O'Fallon WM, Kurland LT, Dockerty MB. Lack of evidence for cancer due to the use of metronidazole. N Engl J Med 1979;301:519–522.
19. Burtin P, Taddio A, Ariburnu O, Einarson TR, Koren G. Safety of metronidazole in pregnancy: a meta analysis. Am J Obstet Gynecol 1995;172:525–529.
20. Drake TE, Maibach HI. Candida and cadidiases, part 1, 2. Postgrad Med 1973;53:83–120.
21. Spiegel CA, Amsel R, Eschenbach D, Schoenknecht F, Holmes KK. Anaerobic bacteria in non specific vaginitis. N Engl J Med 1980;303: 601–607.
22. Meis PJ, Goldenberg RL, Mercer B, et al. The preterm prediction study: significance of vaginal infections. Am J Obstet Gynecol 1995;173: 1231–1235.
23. Newton ER, Piper J. Bacterial vaginoses and intraamniotic infection. Am J Obstet Gynecol 1997;176:672–677.
24. McGregor J, French JL, Parker R, et al. Prevention of premature birth by screening for common genital infections: results of a prospective controlled evaluation. Am J Obstet Gynecol 1995;173:157–167.
25. Simpson AJ, Mawn JA, Heard SR. Assessment of two methods for rapid intrapartum detection of vaginal group B streptococcal colonisation. J Clin Pathol 1994;47:752–755.
26. Regan JA, Klebanoff MS, Nugent RP, et al. Colonization with group B streptococci in pregnancy and adverse outcome. Am J Obstet Gynecol 1996;174:1354–1360.
27. Itakura A, Kurauchi O, Morikawa S, Matsuzawa K, Mizutami S, Tomoda Y. A prospective study on the relationship between intrapartum maternal GBS concentration and signs of infection in neonates. J Obstet Gynaecol Res 1996;22:101–105.

General Considerations

Cherry and Merkatz's Complications of Pregnancy,
Fifth Edition, edited by W. R. Cohen.
Lippincott Williams & Wilkins, Philadelphia © 2000.

CHAPTER 48

Principles of Critical Care

Pamela S. Lewis and Jan M. Lanouette

A broad spectrum of conditions in the pregnant patient can warrant intensive care. These conditions include pathophysiologic processes seen commonly in the nonpregnant patient, such as pulmonary embolism and sepsis, as well as processes encountered uniquely in the pregnant patient, such as preeclampsia and anaphylactoid syndrome of pregnancy (amniotic fluid embolism). This chapter highlights those situations in which the physiology of pregnancy can alter intensive care approaches and treatment and focuses on the modifications that need to be made in critical care medicine when diagnosing and treating the critically ill pregnant patient. While there are maternal–fetal medicine specialists who have formal training in critical care, most obstetric patients in need of intensive care are co-managed by perinatologists and intensive care specialists.

CARDIOVASCULAR PHYSIOLOGY

The pregnant woman experiences dramatic hemodynamic alterations during the antepartum and intrapartum periods. They are addressed in detail in Chapters 12 and 14. These adaptations result from maternal–fetal interactions, begin shortly after conception, and continue throughout pregnancy. These physiologic alterations need to be considered when treating the critically ill obstetric patient, because they can affect diagnostic and therapeutic decision making profoundly.

Pregnancy can be thought of as a natural volume-overload state resulting from renal sodium and water retention, with a shift of fluid from the intravascular to the extravascular space. There is an increase in urinary sodium excretion caused by an enhanced glomerular filtration rate and high progesterone levels. This rise is counterbalanced by sodium-sparing mechanisms, predominantly through amplified mineralocorticoid activity (1). Plasma volume and red cell mass both increase during pregnancy. The maternal plasma volume rises by as much as 11% by the seventh week of pregnancy (2). This increase reaches a plateau at about 32 weeks and remains stable until delivery (3) (Fig. 48-1). During the course of normal gestation, blood volume enlarges 40% to 50% and is accompanied by an increase in heart rate and cardiac output (CO) of 18% and 50%, respectively (4,5). The increase in blood volume is positively correlated with the number of fetuses present (5). The relatively greater rise in plasma volume compared with that of red cell mass accounts for the maternal anemia that is seen in pregnancy despite an adequate intake of iron (6).

Arterial blood pressure generally declines in pregnancy beginning in the first 8 weeks of gestation (7). Systolic blood pressure remains relatively stable throughout pregnancy, whereas diastolic blood pressure decreases 5 to 10 mm Hg at 28 weeks and then returns to nonpregnant levels closer to term (8). In pregnancy, blood pressure measured

P. S. Lewis and J. M. Lanouette: Division of Maternal-Fetal Medicine, Sinai Hospital of Baltimore, Baltimore, MD 21215.

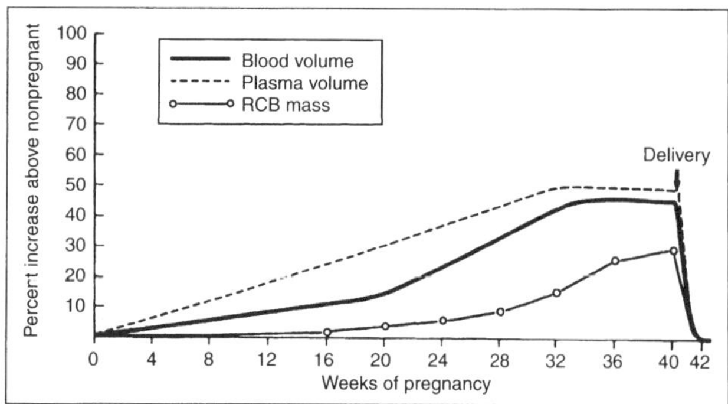

FIG. 48-1. Blood volume changes during pregnancy. (From Scott DE. Anemia during pregnancy. Obstet Gynecol Annu 1972;1:219.)

in the lateral decubitus position is usually the lowest, whereas that in the supine position is usually the highest; this may not hold true in situations in which there is significant aortocaval compression in the supine position.

The physician treating the postpartum obstetric patient needs to be aware of the immediate and dramatic hemodynamic changes in the puerperium. Ueland and Hansen (9) measured hemodynamic parameters in 13 postpartum women and found a 71% increase in stroke volume and a 59% increase in CO by 10 minutes after delivery. After 1 hour, the stroke volume was still 67% above baseline, and the CO was 49% above baseline. When measured 4 to 5 days after delivery, CO remains elevated by as much as 18% to 29% above prelabor values. The return of CO to nonpregnant values occurs about 2 to 4 weeks postpartum (10).

Chesley and colleagues reported a 2-L decline in the sodium space compartment, along with a 3-kg weight loss within the first week after delivery (11). This postpartum diuresis usually comes about between the second and fifth day and provides a means by which the extracellular fluid accumulated during pregnancy can be lost. If this mobilization of fluid occurs when the renal mechanisms do not allow for diuresis, the patient is at risk of pulmonary edema. Indeed, pulmonary edema in perigestional women usually develops in the postpartum period.

During pregnancy, illness severe enough to require intensive care admission often also requires the information derived from invasive monitoring for treatment. These basic hemodynamic changes need to be considered when using invasive monitoring in pregnancy.

CENTRAL VENOUS PRESSURE MONITORING

The technique of central venous pressure (CVP) assessment consists of measuring pressure via fluid-filled tubing placed into the superior vena cava or right atrium and linked to a fluid manometer or an electronic transducer. Central venous catheters can be inserted in any of several access sites, including the internal jugular, external jugular, femoral, and subclavian veins or peripheral veins in the arm. In obstetrics, the most common means of central catheterization is by internal jugular or subclavian cannulation. The latter is effected by either the infraclavicular or the supraclavicular approach. The pregnant patient is positioned in the same way as the nonpregnant patient, that is, in the Trendelenberg position with the head lowered 15 degrees, the shoulders depressed caudally, and the head turned away from the site of puncture. The catheter is inserted as it would be in a nonpregnant patient.

There are no special considerations when using CVP readings in pregnant women, aside from the possible difficulty in identifying the zero reference point, which should be the right mid-atrium. CVP readings should not be made in the supine position in pregnant women in their third trimester, because vena caval compression will cause false readings. Women should be in the lateral position or on their backs with lateral uterine displacement induced by a wedge under one hip. After the central venous catheter has been inserted and secured, a portable chest radiograph should be obtained to verify proper placement of the catheter tip in the superior vena cava. The most common complication of percutaneous central venipuncture is pneumothorax, with a reported incidence between 3% and 6% (12). Less common complications include arterial puncture or cannulation, hemothorax, thrombosis, embolism, local infection, and cardiac arrhythmia.

Central venous pressure monitoring has undergone a reappraisal since the introduction of the Swan-Ganz catheter. In patients without cardiopulmonary dysfunction, the CVP is generally an accurate reflection of left atrial pressure. In many common critical care conditions, however, the CVP might be elevated for reasons independent of volume status, making this measurement an inaccurate predictor of left ventricular filling pressures. This is especially true in patients with pulmonary or cardiac disease and applies to some critical care conditions specific to pregnancy. For example, the CVP has been shown to be inconsistent in the hemodynamic assessment of patients with amniotic fluid embolism (13) and severe preeclampsia (14,15). For these reasons, when central hemodynamic monitoring is indicated, the Swan-Ganz catheter, which provides much more data, is usually used.

Swan-Ganz Catheter

First introduced by Swan and Ganz in the early 1970's (16), the flow-directed pulmonary artery catheter has found widespread use in medical and surgical intensive care. The original catheter had a double-lumen, radiopaque, balloon-tipped design. Modifications now incorporated in the catheter include a third lumen opening into the right atrium and a thermistor to measure CO. Other available additions include a fiber-optic channel to measure mixed venous oxygen saturation and cardiac pacing wires. The Swan-Ganz catheter is capable of directly

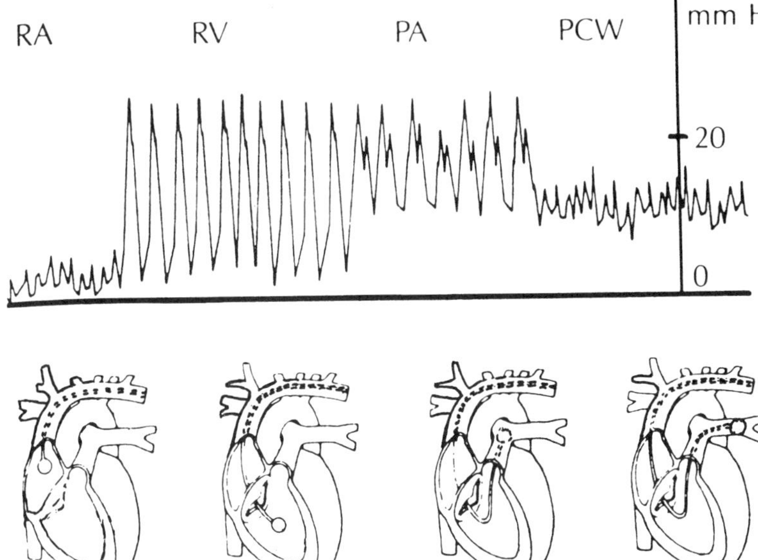

FIG. 48-2. Pressure waves in relation to catheter position from the right atrium to the right ventricle to the pulmonary artery to the pulmonary capillary wedge position. (From Dizon CT, Barash PG. The value of monitoring pulmonary artery pressure in clinical practice. Conn Med 1977;41:622.)

measuring pulmonary artery pressure, pulmonary capillary wedge pressure (PCWP), and right atrial pressure. The mixed venous oxygen concentration can be continuously measured by reflection spectrophotometry, and CO is determined intermittently by thermodilution.

Insertion is accomplished by threading the catheter into the superior vena cava from any of several accessible veins. The balloon is then inflated. Characteristic oscilloscopic pressure waveforms are used to establish the catheter's location as it is being advanced. (Fig. 48-2). Inflation of the balloon assists in positioning of the catheter because it is carried through the right heart chambers by normal blood flow patterns. Once it is in the pulmonary artery, a characteristic arterial waveform is seen, and when the balloon wedges itself into a distal portion of the artery, the pulmonary artery and a characteristic pulmonary capillary wedge trace are visible on the oscilloscope. In this position the balloon occludes the lumen of the artery and exposes the catheter tip (which is distal to the balloon) to pressures of the pulmonary venous circulation.

Assuming there is no obstruction between the pulmonary veins and the left ventricle, the catheter lumen is thus able to reflect left ventricular end diastolic pressure, a good measure of preload. Once a pulmonary artery catheter is placed, confirmation of its location in the pulmonary artery should be made immediately by chest radiography. This will also allow the operator to assess evidence of pneumothorax. When the catheter is in place, pulmonary artery pressures can be continuously monitored with the balloon deflated, and PCWPs can be determined intermittently by inflating the balloon. The most common complication in pulmonary artery catheterization in obstetrics and gynecology is premature ventricular contractions, with an incidence of 27%. Other, less common complications include arterial puncture, superficial cellulitis, and pneumothorax (4).

When using a pulmonary artery catheter in obstetrics, the operator needs to be familiar with the normal hemodynamic changes seen in pregnancy (Table 48-1) as well as the hemodynamic changes seen in specific complications of pregnancy, such as preeclampsia. Clinical conditions for which invasive monitoring is potentially indicated in obstetrics are listed in Table 48-2. Clark and associates investigated the most common indications for pulmonary artery catheterization in obstetrics, which included severe preeclampsia, rheumatic or congenital

TABLE 48-1. *Hemodynamic measures*

Parameter	Nonpregnant	Pregnant
Cardiac output (L/min)	4.3 ± 0.9	6.2 ± 1.0
Heart rate (beats/min)	71 ± 10	83 ± 10
Systemic vascular resistance (dyne × cm × sec^{-5})	1,530 ± 520	1,210 ± 266
Pulmonary vascular resistance (dyne × cm × sec^{-5})	119 ± 47	78 ± 22
Colloid oncotic pressure (mm Hg)	20.8 ± 1.0	18.0 ± 1.5
Colloid oncotic pressure—pulmonary capillary wedge pressure (mm Hg)	14.5 ± 2.5	10.5 ± 2.7
Mean arterial pressure (mm Hg)	86.4 ± 7.5	90.3 ± 5.8
Pulmonary capillary wedge pressure (mm Hg)	6.3 ± 2.1	7.5 ± 1.8
Central venous pressure (mm Hg)	3.7 ± 2.6	3.6 ± 2.5
Left ventricular stroke work index (g × min × min^{-2})	41 ± 8	48 ± 6

Values are mean ± standard deviation.

TABLE 48-2. *Indications for invasive hemodynamic monitoring*

Sepsis with refractory hypotension or oliguria
Unexplained or refractory pulmonary edema, heart failure, or oliguria
Severe pregnancy-induced hypertension with pulmonary edema or persistent oliguria
Intrapartum or intraoperative cardiovascular decompensation
Massive blood and volume loss or replacement
Shock, regardless of origin, refractory to standard therapies
Adult respiratory distress syndrome
Chronic conditions, especially when associated with labor or major surgery
New York Heart Association Class III or IV cardiac disease
Peripartum or perioperative coronary artery disease
Severe valvular heart disease

TABLE 48-3. *Hemodynamic characteristics of severe preeclampsia*

Preload
Systemic (pulmonary capillary wedge pressure): variable but usually low
Pulmonary (central venous pressure): low to normal
Afterload
Systemic (systemic vascular resistance): usually elevated
Pulmonary (pulmonary vascular resistance): normal
Contractility
Systemic (left ventricular stroke work index): vast majority elevated
Heart rate
Normal

heart disease, septic shock, adult respiratory distress syndrome (ARDS), and amniotic fluid embolism (4).

HEMODYNAMIC CONSIDERATIONS FOR SPECIFIC CONDITIONS

Preeclampsia

Few studies have documented baseline hemodynamic profiles in women with preeclampsia who have undergone no pretreatment with vasodilators or intravenous fluid before Swan-Ganz catheter placement. Groenendijk and co-workers studied 10 such women before any treatment, and their hemodynamic profiles were suggestive of a hypovolemic, vasoconstricted, low-output state (17). Another group of researchers examined 87 untreated patients with preeclampsia and came to the same conclusion (18). In contrast, Cotton and colleagues studied five untreated women with severe preeclampsia and found that these patients had profiles that indicated a high-output, mildly vasoconstricted state (19). In all likelihood, preeclampsia represents an overall vasoconstrictive condition. The hemodynamic profile can be influenced by underlying disease processes such as chronic hypertension, duration and severity of illness, and various therapeutic methods. A summation of hemodynamic characteristics observed in severe preeclampsia is provided in Table 48-3.

In light of the fact that there seem to be a variety of hemodynamic states in preeclampsia, simplification of management of patients with oliguric preeclampsia was proposed by Clark and co-workers by dividing this population into clinical groups (15). Oliguria was defined as urine output less than 30 mL per hour for three consecutive hours, with failure to improve after a 300 to 500 mL intravenous fluid bolus. The first group consisted of patients with intravascular volume depletion. Their hemodynamic profiles showed a low to low-normal PCWP, moderately increased systemic vascular resistance (SVR), and hyperdynamic left ventricular function. This group responded to intravenous hydration with an increase in PCWP and CO, a decrease in SVR, and resolution of the oliguria. The second group comprised patients whose profiles indicated renal arteriospasm. These patients had normal to increased PCWP and CO and normal SVR. Oliguria in these women responded to intravenous hydralazine and nitroglycerin. The third group, which consisted of one patient, had a hemodynamic profile suggestive of generalized vasospasm, leading to reduced CO, elevated PCWP and SVR, and depressed left ventricular function. The recommended treatment for this category was afterload reduction with hydralazine (15,20).

Mitral Stenosis

Patients with New York Heart Association class III or IV cardiac disease pose a challenge for obstetric management during labor and in the immediate postpartum period. Clark and associates studied eight patients with mitral stenosis and proposed optimal treatment for these patients by studying their hemodynamic profiles. This descriptive study reported that intrapartum preload reduction using diuretics in anticipation of postpartum fluid shifts helped avoid postpartum pulmonary edema. They recommend the predelivery capillary wedge pressure be at or below 14 mm Hg. Other recommendations included propranolol for any patient with tachycardia and epidural anesthesia for labor. All eight patients in this study were delivered vaginally, with no need for midforceps delivery (21).

Anaphylactoid Syndrome of Pregnancy

Since examination of the national registry of amniotic fluid embolism in 1995, it has been proposed that amniotic fluid embolism be more accurately named anaphylactoid syndrome of pregnancy (22). There are only a few published reports that describe the hemodynamic changes associated with amniotic fluid embolism in humans. Animal studies have consistently reported profound pulmonary hypertension and acute cor pulmonale; however, more recent data from humans acquired using central monitoring have shown that left ventricular failure is the only hemodynamic abnormality consistently observed (13).

A biphasic pattern of hemodynamic disturbance in amniotic fluid embolism has been postulated. Specifically, the initial response is one of intense vasospasm, producing severe pulmonary hypertension and profound hypoxia. Although the initial insult is severe, it appears to be transient and accounts for the deaths of perhaps 50% of patients from amniotic fluid embolism. When patients survive the initial injury, the second phase is left ventricular failure, variable elevation of pulmonary artery pressure, and return of normal right ventricular function. There is often pulmonary edema in conjunction with moderate elevation of PCWP, suggesting a component of noncardiogenic pulmonary edema as well. The left ventricular compromise may be the direct effect of a toxic component of amniotic fluid on the myocardium or of the initial profound hypoxia.

Treatment of patients should begin with the highest oxygenation possible during the initial phase of respiratory insult and placement of a pulmonary artery catheter for central hemodynamic assessment. Inotropic support is recommended, with agents such as dopamine or dobutamine (13). There is an abysmal maternal and perinatal outcome seen with amniotic fluid embolism, with one review reporting that 85% of patients either died or survived with permanent neurologic injury (22).

NONINVASIVE HEMODYNAMIC MONITORING

It is a widely held opinion that a Swan-Ganz catheter provides more accurate hemodynamic measurements than noncentral methods, and it is generally preferred over these approaches (23). However, several noninvasive methods have been investigated and are worth reporting, because in some circumstances they can provide useful clinical information without the risks associated with catheterization of the central circulations.

Electrical impedance cardiography is a noninvasive method of determining CO. Variations in thoracic electrical impedance caused by changes in aortic blood flow are measured using four skin electrodes attached to the patient's chest and connected to an impedance cardiograph. This technology has been studied in nonpregnant patients (24,25) and in pregnancy (26) and appears to correlate well with thermodilution methods; however, it is not widely used in critical care obstetrics. It might be more useful for following trends in CO than for determining absolute levels.

Another noninvasive approach to obtaining CO is the Doppler technique. Using A-mode ultrasound, the operator measures the area of the aortic root, and, with continuous Doppler, the velocity of blood flow in the aorta is determined. These measurements can be used in an equation to determine stroke volume, and CO can then be calculated (27). This approach has been shown to provide readings comparable to thermodilution methods (28). Despite the reported accuracy of this noninvasive technique, it also is not widely used in critical care obstetrics.

ARTERIAL ACCESS

Arterial cannulation is often helpful in treating the critically ill pregnant patient. The arterial line affords several benefits, such as access for repeated arterial samples and blood samples in general and the ability to monitor arterial blood pressure continuously. For safety reasons, the order of preference for arterial line placement site is radial, dorsalis pedis, femoral, axillary, and brachial; however, the femoral site can be difficult to access, especially in the obese gravid patient. The operator should have experience in choosing a site and testing for adequate collateral circulation. Beards and colleagues compared three arterial line insertion methods and found the classic Seldinger technique to be the most efficient and successful approach with the fewest complications. This method employs a separate guide wire to assist in threading the catheter, which is polyurethane rather than Teflon (29).

Using the arterial catheter to measure arterial blood pressure is optimal in critically ill patients, because many of the noninvasive methods can be inaccurate when the blood pressure is extremely low or high. The arterial line is most useful in patients who have low blood pressure or when use of vasoactive drugs requires frequent blood pressure evaluation. The physician must also always consider the positioning of the patient and attempt to measure the blood pressure consistently with the pregnant patient in the left lateral recumbent position or supine with a wedge under the right hip, to avoid any influence of aortocaval compression on the measurements.

PULMONARY PHYSIOLOGIC CHANGES

The pulmonary function of pregnant women reflects changes in the airway, thoracic cage, and respiratory drive. Alterations in the maternal airway, most pronounced in the third trimester, include mucosal hyperemia, edema, hypersecretion, and increased friability. There is widening of the anteroposterior and transverse diameters of the chest in pregnancy. In addition, the growing uterus produces upward displacement of the diaphragm up to 4 cm. Diaphragmatic function remains normal. Progesterone, acting with the increased carbon dioxide production from amplified oxygen consumption and an elevated metabolic rate, causes increased ventilation that begins in the first trimester and rises as much as 48% by the third trimester (30,31). Greater tidal volume results in increased minute ventilation. A summary of normal pulmonary function values in pregnant and nonpregnant women is provided in Table 48-4.

TABLE 48-4. *Respiratory function measures*

Term	Definition	Nonpregnant values	Pregnant values	Clinical significance in pregnancy
Tidal volume (V_T)	Amount of air moved in one normal respiratory cycle	450 mL	600 mL (increases up to 40%)	Reduces dose requirements for inhalation drugs
Respiratory rate (RR)	Number of respirations per minute	16/min	Changes very little	
Minute ventilation	Volume of air moved per minute: product of RR and V_T	7.2 L	9.6 L (increases up to 40% because of the increase in V_T)	Increases oxygen available for the fetus
Forced expiratory volume in 1 second (FEV_1)		Approximately 80%–85% of the vital capacity	Unchanged	Valuable to measure because there is no change due to pregnancy
Peak expiratory flow rate (PEFR)			Unchanged	Valuable to measure because there is no change due to pregnancy
Forced vital capacity (FVC)	Maximum amount of air that can be moved from maximum inspiration to maximum expiration	3.5 L	Unchanged	If over 1 L, pregnancy is usually well tolerated
Residual volume (RV)	Amount of air that remains in the lung at the end of a maximal expiration	1,000 mL	Decreases by ~200 mL to ~800 mL	Improves gas transfer from alveoli to blood

The increasing size of the uterus acts to decrease residual volume, functional residual capacity, and total lung capacity. Changes in lung volumes brought about by the enlarging uterus can also cause mild bibasilar atelectasis in the late third trimester. This might result in bibasilar rales on lung examination in a normal, asymptomatic patient. A phenomenon called dyspnea of pregnancy is also seen in approximately 75% of women by the third trimester. Although the source is unclear, it is thought to be due to heightened respiratory center sensitivity to carbon dioxide and hypoxia in some women.

With these alterations in mind, assessment of the pulmonary status of the pregnant patient shows normal arterial blood gas values that differ from those in the nonpregnant state (Table 48-5). The partial pressure of carbon dioxide is lower—28–32 mm Hg—and the partial pressure of oxygen (PO_2) is higher, generally more than 100 mm Hg. This is important to consider in evaluating the pregnant woman with respiratory distress who is being considered for intubation and assisted ventilation. Arterial carbon dioxide tensions that would be normal in a nonpregnant woman could reflect significant hypoventilation in pregnancy. Low partial pressure of oxygen can result from poor gas exchange as well as from inadequate ventilation. Hypoxia is present when the partial pressure of oxygen falls below 60 mm Hg or when the oxygen saturation falls below 90% (32). The physiologic anemia of pregnancy was described earlier. Oxygen delivery is maintained in spite of anemia because of the increase in maternal carbon dioxide. It is important for the intensive care specialist to realize this, because the pregnant patient relies more on CO for the maintenance of oxygenation than does the nonpregnant patient (33).

MECHANICAL VENTILATORY SUPPORT

Endotracheal intubation is performed for the same reasons in a pregnant as in a nonpregnant patient. There are several indications for initiating mechanical ventilation (Table 48-6) (34). Hypoxemia, meaning an arterial oxygen tension of <60 mm Hg on a 50% or greater fraction of inspired oxygen, and hypoventilation, meaning an arterial

TABLE 48-5. *Arterial blood gas values*

Parameter	Nonpregnant	Normal range—pregnant
pH	7.35–7.45	7.40–7.46
PO_2	85–100 mm Hg	87–106 mm Hg
PCO_2	32–45 mm Hg	26–32 mm Hg
HCO_3^-	22–30 mEq/L	18–21 mEq/L

PO_2, partial pressure of oxygen; PCO_2, partial pressure of carbon dioxide; HCO_3^-, serum bicarbonate concentration.

TABLE 48-6. *Indications for mechanical ventilation*

- Pulmonary hypoventilation
  - Apnea
  - Acute ventilatory failure
  - Impending acute ventilatory failure
- Hypoxia
- Airway control
- Increased work of breathing
- Nonphysiologic ventilatory management

TABLE 48-7. *Drugs for sedation and paralysis in mechanical ventilation*

Narcotics
Morphine
Fentanyl
Anxiolytics
Midazolam
Diazepam
Anesthetics
Propofol
Nondepolarizing muscle relaxants
Vercuronium
Pancuronium
Atracurium

partial pressure of carbon dioxide (Pa_{CO_2}) of >60 mm Hg, are two well-known indications for intubation. These parameters need to be considered with the entire clinical picture in mind and not as absolute indications for initiating mechanical ventilation. For example, a patient with chronic obstructive pulmonary disease might function with a relatively high Pa_{CO_2}; in such cases the change in Pa_{CO_2} rather than the absolute Pa_{CO_2} would be used to dictate when mechanical ventilation should be considered. Another example is the asthmatic patient. Given the usual respiratory alkalosis in pregnancy, a slight increase in such a patient's Pa_{CO_2} could indicate impending respiratory failure. Drugs used to sedate and paralyze the critically ill obstetric patient requiring intubation are similar to those used in nonpregnant patients. Table 48-7 lists commonly used agents in critical care obstetric patients (32).

ACUTE RESPIRATORY DISTRESS SYNDROME

The incidence of acute respiratory distress syndrome (ARDS), also known as adult respiratory distress syndrome, in pregnancy has been reported as 1 in 2,893 deliveries (35). Even though this complication is infrequent, the maternal and perinatal mortality rates associated with ARDS in pregnancy have been reported to be as high as 20% to 50% and 20% to 35%, respectively (35–38). ARDS can result from a variety of types of pulmonary injury, which include causes unique to obstetrics, such as preeclampsia, amnionitis-endometritis, tocolytic therapy, and obstetric hemorrhage, as well as causes unrelated to pregnancy.

The diagnosis of ARDS is usually made on clinical grounds. The patient will have dyspnea. Crackles are frequently heard on lung examination. There is an increased alveolar-arterial oxygen gradient, and supplemental inspired oxygen rarely raises the arterial PO_2 above 100 mm Hg. The chest radiograph characteristically shows diffuse interstitial infiltrates. The most important consideration in the differential diagnosis is cardiogenic pulmonary edema, which can be ruled out if the patient has a normal PCWP (39). The pulmonary artery catheter is used to assist in making the diagnosis, and a PCWP less than or equal to 18 mm Hg confirms the diagnosis (40,41) (Table 48-8). The pulmonary artery catheter also helps in managing fluid balance and inotropic therapy and can be used to calculate CO and obtain mixed venous blood gases. Oxygen delivery, oxygen consumption, and evaluation of any intrapulmonary shunt can then be estimated.

TABLE 48-8. *Criteria for diagnosis of ARDS*

Acute event
Noncardiogenic[a]
Chest radiograph with bilateral infiltrates
Pa_{O_2}/F_{IO_2} <200

ARDS, adult respiratory distress syndrome; Pa_{O_2}, partial pressure of oxygen, arterial; F_{IO_2}, fraction of inspired oxygen.

[a]If the pulmonary capillary wedge pressure is available, it should be below 19 mm Hg.

From Schuster DP. What is acute lung injury? What is ARDS? Chest 1995;107:1721–1726.

Therapy for ARDS is supportive. In the vast majority of cases intubation will be necessary for several reasons, primarily for mechanical ventilation. Several issues need to be considered when using mechanical ventilation in the ARDS patient so as to avoid further lung injury. Pulmonary compromise in ARDS is due to immune system activation in response to an event or injury. Pulmonary tissues are damaged, and an increase in pulmonary vascular permeability results. The lung injury in ARDS is diffuse but nonuniform. Consequently, ventilation in the ARDS-affected lung will occur in the unaffected or less-affected alveolar segments. Mechanical ventilation of ARDS patients usually involves a strategy to limit overdistension of these relatively unaffected alveoli.

The most straightforward method of achieving this goal is to reduce tidal volume. The use of lower tidal volumes, as low as 5 to 8 mL/kg, can aid in reducing pulmonary barotrauma (42). The respiratory rate must be increased in these instances, to maintain an appropriate minute volume. Limitation of peak plateau airway pressure to less than 35 to 40 cm water also can contribute to limiting barotrauma (43). Permissive hypercapnia has also been described as a method to prevent lung injury when ventilating a patient with ARDS. This technique reduces tidal volume, allows spontaneous breathing with synchronized intermittent mandatory ventilation, and disregards hypercapnia. It has been associated with improved outcomes (41). Extracorporeal carbon dioxide removal is an adjunctive therapy that has also been used in pregnancy (44,45). This method enables one to decrease ventilator parameters, such as tidal volume, positive end expiratory pressure, respiratory rate, and peak airway pressure, all of which serve to permit pulmonary recovery.

Because of the extremely poor prognosis with ARDS and its strong connection to infection, the use of broad-spectrum empiric antibiotics is reasonable (46). Other therapies include the use of dopamine to preserve renal perfusion and CO in these patients, who often require diuresis. In a patient with low SVR, phenylephrine or norepinephrine can be used to treat hypotension (39). In the pregnant patient, care must be taken not to compromise uterine perfusion, and continuous fetal heart rate monitoring is indicated.

The question of timing the delivery in a pregnant patient with ARDS is crucial. In some patients with ARDS the process causing the respiratory distress might dictate the need for delivery, for example, chorioamnionitis, preeclampsia, or amniotic fluid embolism. Whether delivery will be of net benefit to the mother in the course of ARDS is unresolved. Tomlinson and associates recommend that given the limited benefit of delivery on maternal respiratory status, along with the inherent risks of labor induction in this critically ill population, caution should be exercised in initiating the induction process. (47). Catanzarite and Willms indicated that delivery should be considered a therapeutic option if the maternal status continues to deteriorate despite standard treatment of ARDS (39).

COLLOID OSMOTIC PRESSURE

Colloid osmotic pressure defines the ability of the intravascular space to retain fluid due to the presence of large molecules that are unable to traverse the endothelial membrane and therefore establish a gradient, which we refer to as an osmotic gradient. Albumin and globulin are the major components in plasma that account for colloid osmotic pressure. Colloid osmotic pressure is intimately associated with hydrostatic pressure (PCWP) for the pulmonary circulation as modulators of water movement between the intravascular and interstitial spaces.

Oian et al. investigated colloid osmotic pressure in 10 normal pregnant patients in the first trimester and in 10 other healthy women in the third trimester. They found that pregnancy is associated with a moderate fall in plasma colloid osmotic pressure and a rise in hydrostatic pressure (48,49). Bungum et al., using the same methods, examined changes in osmotic pressure from 37 to 40 weeks' gestation to postpartum day 5. There was a significant increase in the colloid osmotic pressure both in plasma and in the interstitial fluid in the postpartum period, thought to be due to mobilization of fluid from the interstitium and increased albumin synthesis or transport of interstitial proteins back to the vascular compartment (50).

It is important to understand the relationship of colloid osmotic pressure and PCWP. Pulmonary edema becomes more likely with increasing PCWP. For example, in the context of normal colloid osmotic pressure, PCWP at about 18 mm Hg can be associated with evidence of early pulmonary congestion. PCWPs between 20 and 25 mm Hg are associated with more overt congestion, and patients with pressures above 25 mm Hg often have frank pulmonary edema. Based on Starling's equation, it would make sense that pulmonary edema would occur at a lower PCWP if the colloid osmotic pressure were reduced. In fact, Rackow and Weil observed that a colloid osmotic pressure to PCWP gradient of less than 4 mm Hg greatly enhanced the risk of pulmonary edema in critically ill nonpregnant patients (51). The same observation has been made in the obstetric population (14). This is highly relevant in treating the patient with pregnancy-induced hypertension. Colloid osmotic pressure at term and postpartum in patients with pregnancy-induced hypertension has been shown to be lower when compared with values in pregnant patients without pregnancy-induced hypertension (52). This makes these patients especially vulnerable to pulmonary edema; their fluid status should accordingly be managed very carefully.

FETAL CONSIDERATIONS

While the pregnant patient is in the intensive care unit, fetal surveillance should be undertaken by a perinatologist or obstetrician with critical care experience. One method of assessing fetal status is by continuous electronic fetal heart monitoring. It is not recommended that continuous fetal monitoring be instituted, however, if a fetus is not viable, which, in this context refers to the fetus's ability to survive if delivered. The gestational age at which a fetus is considered viable is constantly changing, but at present it is roughly 24 weeks. The obstetrician can ascertain the probable viability of the fetus using such information as the last menstrual period and fetal ultrasound data, including biometry and estimated fetal weight, to decide if continuous fetal monitoring is indicated. Even if delivery is not anticipated or desirable, fetal heart rate monitoring or other biophysical evaluations can sometimes help guide maternal therapy. For example, drugs that reduce uterine blood flow, such as diuretics or α-adrenergic agonists, should be used at the lowest dose that resolves the maternal problem and causes no alteration in fetal heart rate patterns or umbilical blood flow.

While stabilizing a critically ill pregnant patient with a viable fetus, the fetal heart tracing can be transiently nonreassuring. In these instances, an experienced obstetrician would need to decide whether action, such as delivery or further testing, was immediately required or if it would be more prudent to wait for the maternal status to improve. It should be borne in mind that hypothermia, whether due to environmental exposure or induced intentionally for cardiac or neurosurgery, can produce a persistent fetal bradycardia that resolves on warming. Also, almost all fetuses of mothers on cardiopulmonary bypass have bradycardias that do not seem to be a consequence of hypoxia.

Maternal arterial oxygenation can be continuously monitored using pulse oximetry. A maternal oxygen saturation of 95% or greater is considered optimal; below this level there is steep dropoff in the hemoglobin–oxygen dissociation curve, which might compromise the fetal oxygen supply. For this reason, obstetricians aim to keep maternal oxygen saturation above 95%. When the pregnant patient experiences cardiac arrest, timely delivery of the fetus can improve maternal status and neonatal outcome (see Chapter 12). Optimal outcome would be expected if delivery is accomplished within several minutes of absent circulation.

This time limit is based on primate studies that showed successful newborn resuscitation when complete asphyxia lasted no more that 3 minutes (53).

REFERENCES

1. Oparil S, Ehrlich EN, Lindheimer MD. Effect of progesterone on renal sodium handling in man: relation to aldosterone excretion and plasma renin activity. Clin Sci Mol Med 1975;49:139–147.
2. Clapp JF, Seaward BL, Sleamaker RH. Maternal physiologic adaptations to early human pregnancy. Am J Obstet Gynecol 1988;156: 1456–1460.
3. Scott DE. Anemia in pregnancy. Obstet Gynecol Ann 1972;1:219–244.
4. Clark SL, Horenstein JM, Phelan JP, Montag TW, Paul RH. Experience with the pulmonary artery catheter in obstetrics and gynecology. Am J Obstet Gynecol 1985;152:374–378.
5. Pritchard JA. Changes in the blood volume during pregnancy and delivery. Anesthesiology 1965;26:393.
6. Cavill I. Iron and erythropoiesis in normal subjects and in pregnancy. J Perinat Med 1995;23:47–50.
7. Capless EL, Clapp JF. Cardiovascular changes in early phase of pregnancy. Am J Obstet Gynecol 1989;161:1449–1453.
8. Wilson M, Morganti AA, Zervoudakis J, et al. Blood pressure, the renin–aldosterone system and sex steroids throughout normal pregnancy. Am J Med 1980;68:97–103.
9. Ueland K, Hansen JM. Maternal cardiovascular dynamics. III. Labor and delivery under local and caudal anesthesia. Am J Obstet Gynecol 1969;103:8–18.
10. Adams JQ, Alexander AM. Cardiovascular physiology in normal pregnancy: studies with dye-dilution technique. Am J Obstet Gynecol 1964;67:741–759.
11. Chesley LC, Valenti C, Uichano L. Alterations in body fluid compartments and exchangeable sodium in early puerperium. Am J Obstet Gynecol 1959;77:1054.
12. Helmkamp BF, Sanko SR. Supraclavicular central venous catheterization. Am J Obstet Gynecol 1985;153:751–754.
13. Clark SL, Montz FJ, Phelan JP. Hemodynamic alterations associated with amniotic fluid embolism: a reappraisal. Am J Obstet Gynecol 1985;151:617–621.
14. Cotton DB, Gonik B, Dorman K, Harrist R. Cardiovascular alterations in severe pregnancy-induced hypertension: relationship of central venous pressure to capillary wedge pressure. Am J Obstet Gynecol 1985;151:762–764.
15. Clark SL, Greenspoon JS, Aldahl D, Phelan JP. Severe preeclampsia with persistent oliguria: management of hemodynamic subsets. Am J Obstet Gynecol 1986;154:490–494.
16. Swan HJC, Ganz W, Forrester J, Marcus H, Diamond G, Chonette D. Catheterization of the heart in man with use of a flow-directed balloon-tipped catheter. N Engl J Med 1970:283:447–451.
17. Groenendijk R, Trimbos J, Wallenburg H. Hemodynamic measurements in preeclampsia: preliminary observations. Am J Obstet Gynecol 1984;150:232–236.
18. Visser W, Wallenburg H. Central hemodynamic observations in untreated preeclamptic patients. Hypertension 1991;17:1072–1077.
19. Cotton D, Gonik B, Dorman K. Cardiovascular alterations in severe pregnancy-induced hypertension: acute effects of intravenous magnesium sulfate. Am J Obstet Gynecol 1984:148:162–165.
20. Fox DB, Troiano NH, Graves CR. Use of the pulmonary artery catheter in severe preeclampsia: a review. Obstet Gynecol Surv 1996;51:684–695.
21. Clark SL, Phelan JP, Greenspoon J, Aldahl D, Horenstein J. Labor and delivery in the presence of mitral stenosis: central hemodynamic observations. Am J Obstet Gynecol 1985;152:984–988.
22. Clark SL, Hankins GDV, Dudley DA, Dildy GA, Porter TF. Amniotic fluid embolism: analysis of the national registry. Am J Obstet Gynecol 1995;172:1158–1169.
23. Nolan TE, Wakefield ML, Devoe LD. Invasive hemodynamic monitoring in obstetrics; a critical review of its indications, benefits, complications, and alternatives. Chest 1992;101:1429–1433.
24. Donovan KD, Dobb GJ, Woods WPD, Hockings BE. Comparison of transthoracic electrical impedance and thermodilution methods for measuring cardiac output. Crit Care Med 1986;14:1038–1044.
25. Judy WV, Langley FM, McCowen KD, Stinnett DM, Baker LE, Johnson PC. Comparative evaluation of the thoracic impedance and isotope dilution methods for measuring cardiac output. Aerospace Med 1969;40:532–536.
26. Masaki DI, Greenspoon JS, Ouzounian JG. Measurement of cardiac output in pregnancy by thoracic electrical bioimpedance and thermodilution. Am J Obstet Gynecol 1989;161:680–684.
27. Easterling TR, Watts DH, Schmucker BC, Benedetti TJ. Measurement of cardiac output during pregnancy: validation of Doppler technique and clinical observations in preeclampsia. Obstet Gynecol 1987;69:845–850.
28. Easterling TR, Carlson KL, Schmucker BS, Brateng DA, Benedetti TJ. Measurement of cardiac output in pregnancy by Doppler technique. Am J Perinatol 1990;7:220–222.
29. Beards SC, Doedens L, Jackson A, Lipman J. A comparison of arterial lines and insertion techniques in critically ill patients. Anesthesia 1994;49:968–973.
30. Cuggell DW, Frank NR, Gaensler EA. Pulmonary function in pregnancy. I. Serial observations in normal women. Am Rev Tuberc Pulmon Dis 1953;67:568.
31. Prowse CM, Gaensler EA. Respiratory and acid–base changes during pregnancy. Anesthesiology 1965;26:381.
32. Van Hook JW. Ventilator therapy and airway management. In: Clark SL, Cotton DD, Hankins GD, Phelan JP, eds. Critical care obstetrics, 3rd ed. Malden, Mass.: Blackwell Science, 1997:156–158.
33. Barron W, Lindheimer M. Medical disorders during pregnancy, 1st ed. St Louis: Mosby Year Book, 1991:234.
34. Slutsky AS. Consensus conference on mechanical ventilation—January 28–30, at Northbrook, Illinois, USA. Part 2. Int Care Med 1994;20: 150–162.
35. Mabie WC, Barton JR, Sibai BM. Adult respiratory distress syndrome in pregnancy. Am J Obstet Gynecol 1992;167:950–957.
36. Hankins GD, Nolan TE. Adult respiratory distress syndrome in obstetrics. Obstet Gynecol Clin North Am 1991;18:273–287.
37. Perry KG, Martin RW, Blake PG, Roberts WE, Martin JN. Maternal mortality associated with adult respiratory distress syndrome. South Med J 1998;91:441– 444.
38. Collop NA, Sahn SA. Critical illness in pregnancy: an analysis of 20 patients admitted to a medical intensive care unit. Chest 1993;103: 1548–1552.
39. Catanzarite VA, Willms D. Adult respiratory distress syndrome in pregnancy: report of three cases and review of the literature. Obstet Gynecol Surv 1997;52:381–392.
40. Mabie WC, Barton JR, Sibai BM. Adult respiratory distress syndrome in pregnancy. Am J Obstet Gynecol 1992;167:950–957.
41. Schuster DP. What is acute lung injury? What is ARDS? Chest 1995; 107:1721–1726.
42. Hickling KG, Henderson SJ, Jackson R. Low mortality associated with low volume pressure limited ventilation with permissive hypercapnia in severe adult respiratory distress syndrome. Int Care Med 1990;16: 372–377.
43. Van Hook JW. Acute respiratory distress syndrome in pregnancy. Semin Perinatol 1997;21:320–327.
44. Greenberg LR, Moore TR. Staphylococcal septicemia and adult respiratory distress syndrome in pregnancy treated with extracorporeal carbon dioxide removal. Obstet Gynecol 1995;86:657–660.
45. Abrams JH, Gilmour IJ, Kriett JM, et al. Low-frequency positive-pressure ventilation with extracorporeal carbon dioxide removal. Crit Care Med 1990;18:218–220.
46. Hankins GDV, Nolan TE. Adult respiratory distress syndrome in obstetrics. Obstet Gynecol Clin North Am 1991;18:273–287.
47. Tomlinson MW, Caruthers TJ, Whitty JE, Gonik B. Does delivery improve maternal condition in the respiratory-compromised gravida? Obstet Gynecol 1998;91:108–111.
48. Oain P, Maltau JM, Noddeland H, Fadnes HO. Oedema-preventing mechanisms in subcutaneous tissue of normal pregnant women. Br J Obstet Gynaecol 1985;92:1113–1119.
49. Oian P, Maltau JM. Calculated capillary hydrostatic pressure in normal pregnancy and preeclampsia. Am J Obstet Gynecol 1987;157:102–106.
50. Bungum L, Tollan A, Oian P. Antepartum to postpartum changes in transcapillary fluid balance. Br J Obstet Gynaecol 1990;97:838–842.
51. Rackow EC, Weil MH. Recent trends in diagnosis and management of septic shock. Curr Surg 1983;40:181–185.
52. Benedetti TJ, Carlson RW. Studies of colloid osmotic pressure in pregnancy-induced hypertension. Am J Obstet Gynecol 1979;135:308–311.
53. James LS. Emergencies in the delivery room. In: Behrman RE, ed. Neonatal–perinatal medicine: diseases of the fetus and infant, 2nd ed. St. Louis: Mosby, 1977:128–145.

Cherry and Merkatz's Complications of Pregnancy,
Fifth Edition, edited by W. R. Cohen.
Lippincott Williams & Wilkins, Philadelphia © 2000.

CHAPTER 49

Maternal Mortality and Severe Morbidity

Emile Papiernik and Hervé Fernandez

Improvements in obstetric techniques and in the organization of obstetric care have been successful in reducing maternal deaths and severe morbidity in developed countries. However, these changes have not benefited the majority of women whose deliveries are not attended by a skilled professional. In this chapter, we analyze the definitions of maternal mortality and severe morbidity, recount the history of the decline in maternal deaths in developed countries, review the current situation in developing nations, and describe the remaining problems and challenges in further reducing maternal risks.

DEFINITIONS

Maternal mortality is defined as the death of a woman while pregnant or within 42 days of termination of the pregnancy from any cause related to or aggravated by the pregnancy or its treatment, but not from accidental or incidental causes (1,2). According to the International Classification of Diseases (ICD), direct obstetric deaths are defined as those resulting from obstetric complications; from interventions, omissions, or incorrect treatment; or from a chain of events resulting from any of these factors. Indirect obstetric deaths are those resulting from preexisting disease or disease that develops during pregnancy and that is not due to direct obstetric factors but is aggravated by the physiologic effects of pregnancy (2).

There are problems with this definition because the distinction between direct and indirect causes is not always easy to establish. For example, suicide after childbirth, which could be directly related to childbirth, is classified as indirect. For this reason, the ICD committee also proposed the term "pregnancy-related deaths" to cover all deaths in women during pregnancy or after its termination, regardless of cause. In 1989, the ICD-10 (3) defined late maternal death as the death of a woman from direct or indirect obstetric causes more than 42 days but less than 1 year after termination of pregnancy. In this classification, pregnancy-related death is the death of a woman while pregnant or within 42 days of termination of pregnancy *regardless* of the cause of death, including accidental or incidental causes (Table 49-1) (4).

The enumeration of maternal deaths is difficult, since, for example, it is not always noted on the death certificate that a woman who dies from a severe complication in an intensive care unit is pregnant. Studies that have examined all deaths of women of reproductive age, and cross-checked with all available information for each case, find large numbers of deaths for which this information is missing. For example, in one U.S. collaborative study, the proportion of missing information about pregnancy status was between 20% and 75% among deaths that occurred in intensive care units (5). Other causes of death that are often misclassified on U.S. death certificates relate to ectopic pregnancy, gestational trophoblastic disease, and induced or spontaneous abortions (6,7).

More thorough studies of maternal mortality have made it possible to quantify this underregistration. In the United Kingdom, the system of confidential inquiries into maternal deaths overseen by the Royal College of Obstetricians and Gynaecologists has collected more cases of maternal deaths than those officially published by the Registrar General (Table 49-2). In France, a cross-check of death certificates with information about pregnancy status was done for all deaths of women ages 15 to 49 years from December 1988 to March 1989. A further analysis involved directly questioning the doctor who signed the death certificate. This study found underreporting of 50%, with a correction of 22 to 45 maternal deaths (8). Complete data were obtained from 89.7% of death certificates. Sixty-eight percent were not clearly identified as maternal

E. Papiernik: University René Descartes, Maternité de Port-Royal Paris, France; H. Fernandez: University Pierre et Marie Curie, Orsay-Paris, Hôpital Antoine Béclère, Clamart, France.

TABLE 49-1. *Effect of use of definitions on the maternal mortality ratio in Sweden, 1980–1988*

Definition	ICD	Number of deaths	Ratio
Maternal mortality	ICD 8	36	4.6
Maternal mortality	ICD 9	58	7.4
Pregnancy related mortality	ICD 10	64	8.1
Late maternal mortality	ICD 10	76	10.0
Pregnancy-related mortality, up to 1 year	ICD 10	140	26.2

ICD, International Classification of Diseases.
Data from Högberg U, Innala E, Sandström A. Maternal mortality in Sweden 1980–1988. Obstet Gynecol 1994;84: 240–244.

deaths. For 41%, the information about the pregnancy was on the certificate but was not registered. Finally, for 27%, information about pregnancy was not on the certificate but was available in medical records. Similar results were observed in the district of Nice (9).

The maternal mortality rate is generally expressed in relation to all live births. It has been proposed this denominator be modified to include all pregnancies, including ectopic pregnancies, spontaneous abortions, and legal terminations of pregnancy, because the risk of death is related to all pregnancies, whatever their duration. Furthermore, the number of live births does not include stillbirths and the number of births, because of multiple pregnancies, does not reflect the number of women at risk. Technically, the number of maternal deaths expressed as a proportion of total births is not a rate (since the denominator does not represent the group at risk of experiencing a maternal death). For this reason, many researchers refer to this statistic as the maternal mortality ratio.

Despite the logic of this approach, in many countries the number of live births is the only accurate and comparable denominator available, because stillbirths are not registered in a uniform way by gestational age. (A stillbirth might be registered at a threshold of 500 g, 1,000 g, 22 weeks, 24 weeks, or 28 weeks, whereas a live birth, in most developed countries, is enumerated after 22 weeks.) Moreover, the numbers of spontaneous abortions or ectopic pregnancies are not recorded. The number of legal pregnancy terminations is recorded in many countries, but the quality of this information is not always reliable.

Substandard care is a notion that is key to a discussion of maternal deaths, but it also needs to be defined carefully. Substandard care is used in the United Kingdom's reports of confidential inquires into maternal deaths to take into account not only failure in clinical care but also underlying factors that may have produced a low standard of care for the patient. This includes situations that result from the actions of the woman herself or her relatives, which might be outside the control of clinicians. It also takes into account the shortage of resources for staffing and facilities as well as administrative failure in the maternity units and backup services, such as the intensive care, anesthesiology, radiology, and pathology departments. "Substandard" in this context means that the care received or the care that was made available for the pregnant woman was below the standard that the authors considered should have been offered, given current medical knowledge. This definition is used for the remainder of this chapter.

HISTORICAL EVOLUTION OF MATERNAL MORTALITY IN DEVELOPED COUNTRIES

The rate of maternal deaths has been lowered remarkably in developed countries. This trend started during the nineteenth century. The best document describing the early decline of maternal deaths is a continuing Swedish data series that began to be documented in 1750 from church registries (10). This is a unique source, since it makes it possible to follow the evolution of maternal mortality over more than 200 years. Sweden was the only country in which cases of maternal death were enumerated over this time span. In most nations, the recording of maternal deaths as a public health measure or a marker of effectiveness of maternity care was introduced much later. The absence of reliable data is still a key problem in most developing countries; no national statistics on maternal deaths are available, and measurement relies on hospital sources and a few population studies, often carried out by outside teams of researchers (11).

If the Swedish figures are plotted on a semi-log scale (Fig. 49-1), we can better observe the pace of the decline. We also see that the decline can be separated into three

TABLE 49-2. *Comparison of two different sources for counting maternal deaths*

Years	1985–1987	1988–1990	1991–1993
Deliveries	2,268,766	2,360,309	2,315,204
Maternal deaths known by the Registrar General (n)	174	171	140
Rate per 100,000 births	7.7	7.2	6.0
Maternal deaths included in the confidential inquiry review system (n)	223	238	228
Rate per 100,000 births	9.8	10.1	9.8

Report on confidential inquiries into maternal deaths in England and Wales 1991–1993. London: HMSO, 1996 (23).

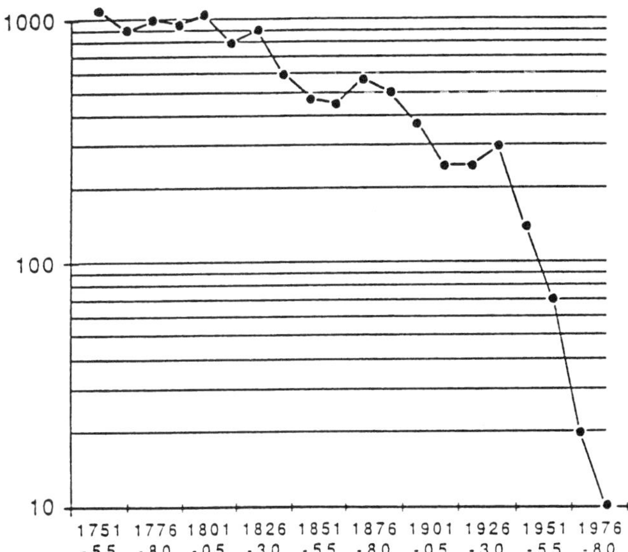

FIG. 49-1. Maternal deaths in Sweden, 1951–1980. The vertical axis shows maternal deaths per 100,000 live births. (From Högberg U, Joelsson J. The decline in maternal mortality in Sweden 1931–1980. Acta Obstet Gynecol Scand 1985;64:583–592.)

successive phases. In the first phase, from 1751 to 1800, no decline is evident. At this time there were about 1,000 deaths per 100,000 live births, a figure within the range observed in other countries in which no medical care was available to most women during pregnancy or delivery. During the second phase, up to 1930, a decline is observed to approximately 300 maternal deaths per 100,000 births. The halving of maternal deaths to 500 per 100,000 births had occurred by the years 1876–1880. Finally, in the third phase, the downward trend of maternal mortality accelerated, with a reduction by half almost every 10 years to 7 deaths per 100,000 births in 1976–1980.

Maternal mortality figures are available for England and Wales beginning with the 4-year period 1896–1900 (12). At that time, the rate was 469 deaths per 100,000 births. The evolution of maternal mortality progressed at the same low rate as in Sweden until it reached a figure of 341 deaths per 100,000 births in 1935. An accelerated pace of decline is then observed with a similar reduction by half or more every 10 years—145 in 1945, 50 in 1955, 19 in 1965 and 11 per 100,000 in 1975.

A higher rate of maternal deaths was noted in the year 1930 in the United States (13): 600 deaths per 100,000 births. In France at the same time, the ratio of maternal deaths to births was in the same range as observed in other European series, more than 200 deaths per 100,000 births in 1925–1929 (14). The proportion of women's deaths during their reproductive years related to pregnancy or delivery complications was about 30% before 1930 (15). In Sweden, this proportion was 12% in the 4-year period 1931–1935, declining to 4% in 1976–1980 and to 1% at the present time.

Major innovations in obstetric techniques are the principal reasons for the observed improvement in maternal outcome. However, the change in the organization of care offered to women during pregnancy and delivery has also played an important role. Progress was realized through better medical care for certain diseases, as witnessed by the reduction in maternal deaths within specific etiologic categories. A second major reason for progress has been the increasing emphasis on preventive medical care, leading to a reduction in the prevalence of certain complications of pregnancy.

The observed evolution of the decrease in maternal deaths in developed countries is also due to changes in economic and social factors, such as increases in income, education, and the status of women. While improvements in obstetric practice and the organization of health care played major roles in lessening maternal risk, it is difficult to identify selectively the distinct effects of the many factors that have contributed to better outcomes for pregnant women. Understanding this process better would be useful for devising strategies to limit maternal deaths in developing countries today.

This absence of progress from 1750 to 1800 in Swedish figures is surprising, because during those years, interest in the problem of maternal mortality was evident, obstetrics was taught in medical schools, and midwives were formally trained. Midwives and general practitioners were able to carry out some obstetric interventions, such as manual removal of the placenta or a forceps delivery. However, there are no available data from which one can assess the acceptance of new medical techniques in obstetrics, and we cannot measure the proportion of births for which a midwife was present. In those times, only rich and educated people called a midwife to attend a home birth.

The diffusion of knowledge and skills requisite for safe obstetric practice by midwives and general practitioners seems to be the best explanation for the progress in the decline in maternal deaths in the second phase, from 1800 to 1930. In the third phase, since 1930, two major modifications in obstetric care were introduced: (a) delivery in a maternity hospital instead of a home and (b) the introduction of cesarean section done for maternal indications. The modern technique of cesarean section, through the lower segment (instead of the classical cesarean section through the corpus uteri), became accepted in the 1920's but was not in widespread practice before the 1930's. These two changes were related, as access to cesarean section was obviously much more difficult if the delivery occurred at home rather than at a maternity hospital or clinic.

Large population data sets show that the risk of maternal death is strongly related to the proportion of births that occur in maternity units. This was established for 22 countries in North, South, and Central America by a study during the period 1972–1984 (16). This study contrasted the proportion of births in maternity units and the rate of maternal deaths in each country over the same time span. These countries fall into three broad groups. In some, less than 10% of deliveries took place in maternity units (Bolivia, Paraguay, Equador, Peru, Haiti, Guatemala). The rate of maternal deaths in this group ranged between 150 and 500 deaths per 100,000 births. At the other end of the distribution are countries where less than 10% of births took place at home (Argentina, Panama, Chile, Uruguay, Costa Rica, Cuba, United States, Puerto Rico, and Canada). In these nations, the rate of maternal death was below 100 per 100,000 births, the lowest figures being in the United States and Canada. The middle group is composed of those countries in which the proportion of home deliveries varied from 10% to 75% (Honduras, Colombia, Mexico, Nicaragua, El Salvador, Brazil, Venezuela). In these countries the rate of maternal death was close to the level of 100 per 100,000 births (Fig. 49–2).

This study showed that reductions in maternal mortality pass through two stages. In the first stage it is possible to lower the maternal death rate to about 100 per 100,000 births. This number can be attained when at least 10% of deliveries take place in maternity hospitals. The second stage, of reaching very low maternal mortality, is only noted when more than 90% of births take place in maternity hospitals or clinics. This is a very striking observation that explains how maternal deaths were reduced in developed countries. It is also an important point in terms of defining what advice should be given to developing countries. In other words, the data suggest that there is a need for access to specialized care in a maternity hospital if significant reductions in maternal deaths are to be realized. (Of course, the availability of specialized medical care and in-hospital birth can be a

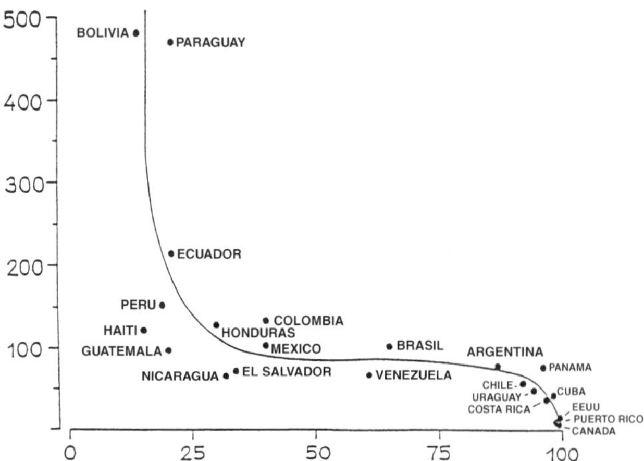

FIG. 49-2. The relationship between the proportion (%) of births that occur in a maternity hospital (x-axis) and the maternal mortality rate (y-axis, deaths per 1,000,000 live births). (From Schwartz ZR. Mortalidad materna y cobertura institucional para el pastro 22 paises de la Region las Americas. CLAP OPS, 1973-84, WHO FHE 1985.)

proxy for many of the social and economic advantages that accompany such amenities.)

In developed countries, the transition from home deliveries to institutional deliveries took place after World War II. Most births were home deliveries up to 1950, as shown by the following data from Sweden (10). The proportion of home deliveries in Sweden declined from 95% in 1916–1920 to 40% in 1936–1940, 5% in 1950–1955, and 0% in 1966–1970. This pattern has been followed in most developed countries. In England and Wales the rate of home deliveries was 33.4% in 1955, 26% in 1965, 3.2% in 1975, and 1.1% in 1981. The only important exception is the Netherlands, where for many years about half of the deliveries took place at home. Today, home deliveries are still common for women with low-risk pregnancies who do not request peridural analgesia; home deliveries now constitute approximately 30% of all deliveries in the Netherlands.

The advantage for women delivering in institutions has been that they can benefit from advances in obstetric care, perhaps most importantly the opportunity to have a cesarean section for obstructed labor. At first, indications for cesarean section were not related to fetal outcome; they were meant to reduce risks for the mother. Women accepted the offer of delivering in maternity hospitals and clinics when the improved safety became obvious to them. In England and Wales, the rate of cesarean section was 2.2% of all births in 1953, when 60.2% of those births took place in a hospital. During the transition from home deliveries to hospital deliveries, the risk of maternal death remained high for those women who decided to deliver at home, even if they could be transferred to the hospital (15). Similarly, in Sweden in 1961–1965, when 85% of all deliveries were in institutions, the rate of maternal deaths was low—only 10 per 100,000 births for women who were booked for hospital delivery. But the rate remained high, at 450 deaths per 100,000 births, for the 15% of women booked for home deliveries, even if a transfer to the hospital was possible in case of severe complications (10). Births in institutions also made it possible to provide blood transfusions, and one of the major advances of the 1950's was the organization of blood banks. Technological innovations in anesthesiology and emergency medicine underlie the improvements in maternal outcomes in the past 30 years.

In developing countries, most pregnant women do not have access to essential obstetric care, and this is the basic reason for the persisting high rate of maternal death. The importance of access to basic obstetric care for emergencies is underlined by a study of a local maternity ward in the city of Divo, in the Ivory Coast. In this hospital, which undertook about 5,000 deliveries a year, the maternity ward was run by midwives and a general practitioner without access to an operating theater. Women with complicated deliveries were transferred to the referral teaching hospital in Abidjan 250 km away, if the family was able to pay for the transport. In 1985, the maternity ward was upgraded by the addition of one obstetrician and one anesthesiologist. They were able to perform various operative interventions, including cesarean sections and hysterectomies. The hospital also organized a blood bank with blood donations from members of the patient's family and close friends.

Outcomes were compared in 1980, before the intervention, and in 1985, after the upgrading, and they were also compared with outcomes from two other local maternity wards of the same size that did not benefit from the presence of a surgical team. The number of women transferred from Divo to Abidjan during labor changed dramatically from 65 in 1980 to none in 1985. This number did not decline for the two control maternity wards. Moreover, the mortality rate decreased significantly, from 300 to 30 deaths per 100,000 births, that is, 1 maternal death per 2,954 births for women living in Divo. In addition, this maternity ward became a referral center for obstructed labor for women living within 250 km. This study illustrates that women did appreciate the importance of delivering in a maternity hospital, where essential obstetrical care was available, and that such care had a dramatic impact on mortality risk (17).

INFLUENCES ON MORTALITY TRENDS

The downward trend in maternal mortality shows important variations by type of disease. We first contrast the patterns in the reduction in maternal mortality by disease and then consider if the decrease in disease-specific mortality was due to the reduction in deaths for women with the disease (the case fatality ratio) or was related to a change in the prevalence of the disease among pregnant women.

The differential decline of maternal mortality by disease can be examined in Swedish data from 1931 to 1950, as shown in Table 49-3. This table lists the principal causes of death, such as puerperal infection, eclampsia, hemorrhage, and uterine rupture (10). The pace of progress is significantly different for these specific complications. Mortality rates for puerperal infection declined the fastest, with a reduction of 30% in the years 1931–1935 and 1936–1940 and a further decrease of 75% from 1936–1940 to 1941–1945. Surprisingly, this decline began before antibiotics became available; penicillin was used only after 1945 in Europe and sulfonamides only in the last years of the 1930s. Our explanation for this decline is that the management of labor according to medical principles became an accepted practice, and use of cesarean section in obstructed labors became possible. Similar patterns, showing a steep decrease in maternal deaths due to puerperal infection, were observed in England and Wales (12) and in France (14). Other causes of death did not evidence the same rapid reduction observed for infection. For deaths related to eclampsia, the reduction was only 50% from 1931 to 1950; for those due to hemorrhage, only 60%; and for those due to uterine rupture, only 35% during the same time span in Sweden (15).

Another way to measure advances in the management of severe complications of pregnancy and delivery is by the case fatality rate (cases of deaths/1,000 cases of the specific complication). Here also the Swedish figures show very different results related to specific diseases. The case fatality rate for eclampsia did not decline significantly from 1956 to 1980 in Sweden. There were 2.4 deaths per 1,000 eclampsia cases in 1956–1960 and 3.1 deaths per 1,000 cases in 1971–1980 (10). In contrast, maternal deaths from uterine rupture declined from 8.3 per 1,000 cases in 1956–1960 to 1.9 deaths per 1,000 in 1971–1980. For prenatal bleeding (placenta previa or abruptio placentae or other causes of severe prenatal bleeding) the case fatality rate decreased by a factor of 20, from 4 deaths per 1,000 cases in 1956–1960 to 0.2 deaths per 1,000 cases in 1971–1980 (10) (Table 49-4).

Trends in the incidence of each disease is the second component to consider in interpreting the reduction in overall disease-specific mortality rates. As shown in Table 49-5, using the Swedish data from 1956 to 1980, the incidence of obstetric complications has changed. For exam-

TABLE 49-3. *Historical evolution of the causes of maternal death*

Cause	Years			
	1931–1935	1936–1940	1941–1945	1946–1950
Infection	93.5	62.0	15.6	3.5
Elcampsia	51.2	50.7	38.2	26.4
Hemorrhage	17.9	20.1	11.9	5.9
Uterine rupture	20.6	35.7	26.0	13.2

[a]Maternal deaths per 100,000 births.

From Högberg U, Joelsson J. The decline in maternal mortality in Sweden 1931–1980. Acta Obstet Gynecol Scand 1985;64:583–592.

TABLE 49-4. *Case fatality ratio*

Cause	Years			
	1956–1960	1960–1965	1966–1970	1971–1980
Eclampsia	2.4	3.0	2.2	3.1
Prenatal bleeding (abruptio placentae and placenta previa)	4.0	1.0	2.0	0.2
Uterine rupture	8.3	1.8	1.7	1.9

[a]Risk of maternal death per 1,000 cases of specific complications.

From Högberg U, Joelsson J. The decline in maternal mortality in Sweden 1931–1980. Acta Obstet Gynecol Scand 1985;64:583–592.

TABLE 49-5. *Incidence of three maternal diseases in Sweden, 1956–1980a*

Cause	Years			
	1956–1960	1961–1965	1966–1970	1971–1980
Eclampsia	1.25	0.77	0.45	0.21
Prenatal bleeding (placenta previa and abruptio placentae)	7.9	7.6	5.3	8.1
Uterine rupture	0.34	0.58	0.42	0.25

From Högberg U, Joelsson J. The decline in maternal mortality in Sweden 1931–1980. Acta Obstet Gynecol Scand 1985;64:583–592.

ple, the incidence of eclampsia changed over the years from 1.25 cases per 1,000 births in 1956–1960 to 0.21 pcr 1,000 births in 1971–1980. However, the observed incidence of prenatal bleeding has remained constant (7.9 cases per 1,000 births in 1956–1960 versus 8.1 in 1971–1980), as has that of uterine rupture.

MATERNAL MORTALITY IN THE DEVELOPING WORLD

In many countries, women do not have access to maternity hospitals or to skilled professional help for delivery. The World Health Organization (WHO) estimates that 46% of the 140.7 million deliveries that occur annually worldwide take place in a health facility. Table 49-6 shows the major differences that exist among regions of the world, and Fig. 49-2 displays the relationship between the proportion of women who deliver in a maternity hospital and the maternal mortality rate (16,18). In Europe and the United States, nearly all of the roughly 2.5 million births take place in a health facility; in contrast, of the 30,730,000 annual deliveries in Africa, only 36% are in a health facility. Within these regional aggregated figures, there are great disparities by country, as shown in Table 49-7, which presents institutional delivery rates in individual countries in eastern, south-central, and southeastern Asia. These rates vary from 5% in Afghanistan and Bangladesh to 100% in North or South Korea, Hong Kong, or Singapore.

It is notable that economic development is not synonymous with a high rate of institutional deliveries. In fact, some low-income countries have a high rate of births in health facilities. This is the case in Sri Lanka, Tadzhikistan, and Uzbekistan, where more than 90% of all deliveries occur in health facilities. There are striking differences in institutional deliveries between the large nations of Southeast Asia, such as China with 51% and India with 26%. On the other end of the distribution are Pakistan (13%), Afghanistan (5%), and Bangladesh (5%), countries in which maternal mortality is high. Delivering in a health facility does not imply that these women have access to essential obstetric care. Health facilities range from institutions with operating theaters, blood banks, obstetricians, and anesthesiologists to maternity wards where trained midwives do the deliveries but in which a cesarean section is not possible.

TABLE 49-6. *Estimated proportion of pregnant women delivering in a health facility*

Area	Deliveries (thousands)	Proportion of deliveries in a health facility
World	140,470	46
Asia	83,410	37
Africa	30,730	36
Latin America and the Caribbean	12,000	71
Oceania	230	52
Europe	8,330	97
North America	4,290	99

From World Health Organization. Coverage of maternity care, a listing of available information—Geneva, Switzerland. Maternal and newborn health, safe motherhood. WHO/RHT/MSM/96–28, 1997.

TABLE 49-7. *Estimated proportion of deliveries in a health facility in Asia*

Area	Deliveries (thousands)	Deliveries in health facilities (%)
Eastern Asia		
China	21,700	51
North Korea	540	100
Hong Kong	60	100
Mongolia	70	97
Republic of Korea	740	99
Southcentral Asia		
Afghanistan	1,800	5
Bangladesh	4,200	5
Bhutan	26,000	26
India	2,000	65
Iran	340	95
Kasakstan	n.a	n.a
Maldives	833	6
Nepal	5,510	13
Pakistan	350	94
Sri Lanka	240	92
Tadjikistan	120	90
Uzbekistan	700	90
Brunei Darassalam	10	10
Cambodia	23	30
East Timor	n.a.	n.a.
Indonesia	4,722	18
Lao	144	7
Malaysia	520	90
Myanmar	1,485	n.a.
Philippines	2,214	28
Singapore	40	99
Thailand	1,155	n.a.
Vietnam	2,200	70

From World Health Organization. Coverage of maternity care, a listing of available information—Geneva, Switzerland. Maternal and newborn health safe motherhood. WHO/RHT/MSM/96–28, 1997. n.a., not available.

The real question to be asked is whether women have access to what can be called essential obstetrical services, for example, cesarean section or blood transfusions. This information is not available from most developing countries. The WHO collects information on whether a person trained in midwifery is present during the delivery in a health facility or at home. These data show that such coverage is low. The lack of access to basic obstetric care explains in large measure why the number of annual maternal deaths in the world remains so disturbingly high—500,000 to 600,000 maternal deaths per year, most of them in the developing world. Moreover, there are few data covering the severe maternal handicapping conditions that result from obstructed labor, such as vesicovaginal fistulas or nerve injury.

The WHO has only recently taken the step of proposing the organization of essential obstetric service at the first-referral level, meaning at the nearest available hospital. Previous WHO efforts were devoted to the training of traditional birth attendants. Although that approach proved effective in improving some infant outcomes, it did not have an effect on reducing maternal deaths. The only manifest success of the policy of distributing a "clean delivery set" to traditional birth attendants is the reduction of umbilical tetanus of the newborn. Transport to a referral hospital has been proposed as a solution for obstetric emergencies. But in cases of obstetric hemorrhage, there is often not enough time, and the severity of the situation does not allow transport in many cases. The major reason for referral is obstructed labor, but for many women the obstacles are great and often insurmountable because of the long distances to referral hospitals and lack of vehicles and money.

Organization and development of essential obstetric services in poor countries require a strong political will, but such services are unfortunately not often considered a national priority. For such a policy to succeed, it will take considerable effort to organize first-referral level hospitals, to train the midwives and doctors, to persuade them to serve in these places, and to pay for these services. The lack of organized obstetric care also creates obvious deficiencies in basic prenatal care. The latter has not been successful in achieving its objectives, such as the prevention of anemia by iron supplementation, early awareness of high blood pressure or proteinuria, and the recognition of risk factors for dysfunctional labor, such as a height below 150 cm or very young maternal age (19).

International health organizations have not generally given very serious consideration to the importance of decreasing maternal deaths. In spite of the marketing of the Safe Motherhood Initiative by WHO (see below), and despite several international conferences on this subject, it is clear that more money is devoted to special programs for reproduction, which help initiate contraception in many countries, than to policies for reducing maternal deaths. Indirectly, of course, lessening the number of pregnancies per mother does lower the risk of maternal death.

TABLE 49-8. *Age, parity, and risk of eclampsia, obstructed labor, and vesicovaginal fistulas*

	Nulliparas (yr)		Multiparas (yr)	
Age	<15	17–19	20–29	≥30
n	466	1,961	2,366	2,210
Eclampsia (%)	16.7	4.9	0.5	0.3
Obstructed labor (%)	27.3	7.9	4.1	7.1
Vesicovaginal fistulas (%)	1.7	0.3	0.1	0.5

From Harrison KA, Rossiter CE. Maternal mortality. A survey of 22,774 consecutive hospital births in Zaria, northern Nigeria. Br J Obstet Gynaecol 1985; [suppl 6]: 100–119.

The International Federation of Gynecologists and Obstetricians has for many years had a committee on maternal mortality that has advocated better obstetric care for women. The success of any attempts to improve the status of the problem is clearly related to the efforts devoted by governments and politicians to the development and support of programs to lower the rate of maternal deaths. In developing countries, high rates of maternal deaths are related to the cultural status of women. While the underlying reason for excess maternal mortality is global poverty, the societal acceptance of this common fate of women of childbearing age reflects traditional cultural beliefs, illiteracy, and ignorance.

The considerable adverse effects of some social mores, such as early marriage and teenage pregnancy, on maternal death and risks are not often considered. For example, the risks of eclampsia, obstructed labor, and vesicovaginal fistulas are much higher for women giving birth at less than 15 years of age (20) (Table 49-8). Women in developing countries are also at greater risk because of growth stunting from poor childhood nutrition and repeated infections. High parity and inadequate contraceptive use also contribute to the risks of maternal death (21).

In the most afflicted areas, no prophylactic action is taken against anemia, hypertension goes unrecognized, and neglect in labor leads to obstruction, uterine rupture, obstetric fistulas, and fetal and or neonatal deaths. A comparison between Nigeria and Botswana illustrates these facts. In Nigeria, there are 200 deaths per 100,000 live births in a country were a high proportion of girls are effectively enrolled in secondary education (109 girls per 100 boys). In Botswana the level of maternal deaths is 1,000 per 100,000 births, and the proportion of girls enrolled in secondary schools is only 48 per 100 boys (21).

CURRENT CHALLENGES IN DEVELOPED COUNTRIES

In developed countries, a remarkable effort has been exerted by professional organizations of obstetricians and anesthesiologists directed toward the reduction of maternal deaths (5–7). In England and Wales, obstetricians and anesthesiologists set up a specific inquiry system for maternal deaths based on confidentiality. This approach has made it possible to acquire a better understanding of the causes of maternal mortality. The reports of these inquires, each covering a 3-year time span, have been issued since 1957 and have had a tremendous impact by defining and identifying substandard care and limiting avoidable deaths.

The proposed improvements in quality of care originating from the analysis of these maternal deaths have related to developing appropriate clinical protocols as well as to improving the organization of care. The conclusions of these reports are sent to all obstetric departments and are also used for state or regional strategic decision making concerning maternal care by the United Kingdom National Health Service. The value of these confidential reports is due in great measure to the large population base for the inquiries, which covered all of England and Wales beginning in 1957 and, more recently, the entire United Kingdom. Also, the definitions of the causes of death have remained constant, allowing for meaningful comparisons over this period of time.

The most recent report cited the rate for maternal deaths among women 15 to 44 years, in order to contrast the proportion of maternal deaths with other causes of deaths of women at the same age, as shown in Table 49-9. This presentation illustrates the relatively rapid decline in maternal deaths from 1973 to 1993. The proportion of deaths that were the direct result of childbearing is given in Table 49-10. These figures can be compared with results from other countries. The rate per total pregnancies cannot be compared with results in other countries, however, since most countries do not include pregnancies not ending in a live birth in the denominator. The most common cause of death is thrombosis, and the second is hypertensive disorders of pregnancy. Deaths related to antepartum and postpartum bleeding rank fourth. The latter ranking is found only in countries where there is an organized effort to lower the rate of maternal deaths, such as in Sweden, but not in countries where such a policy does not exist, as in France. In countries in which the transition from high rates of maternal death to lower rates has occurred over a short period of time, obstetric hemorrhage has been noted as the cause of maternal death that is most easily diminished.

TABLE 49-9. *Maternal deaths compared to all causes of women's death, ages 15–44*

Years	Deaths from all causes (Rate per one million women)	Maternal deaths (Rate per one million women)	Percentage due to maternal deaths
1973–1975	807.9	9.0	1.1
1976–1978	763.2	7.5	1.0
1979–1981	697.2	6.6	1.0
1982–1984	641.7	4.7	0.7
1985–1987	622.5	4.2	0.7
1988–1990	625.9	4.1	0.7
1991–1993	605.6	3.8	0.6

From DHSS. Report on confidential inquiries into maternal deaths in England and Wales 1991–1993. London: HMSO, 1996 (23).

TABLE 49-10. *Cause of direct maternal deaths*[a]

Cause of death	N	%	Rate
Thrombosis (thromboembolism)	35 (5)	27	13.0
Hypertensive disorders of pregnancy	20	15.5	8.6
Early pregnancy deaths (abortion and ectopic pregnancy)	18 (8)	14	7.0
Ante- and postpartum hemorrhage	15	11.6	6.5
Genital sepsis, excluding abortion	9	7	3.9
Amniotic fluid embolism	10	7.8	4.3
Genital tract trauma	4	3.1	1.7
Other	10	7.8	4.3
All direct	129	100.0	55.7

[a]Rate per 1,000,000 births—United Kingdom 1991–1993 (total births; 2,315,204).

From DHSS. Report on confidential inquiries into maternal deaths in England and Wales 1991–1993. London: HMSO, 1996 (8).

In France, fatal hemorrhage remains the principal cause of maternal mortality. A specific inquiry was implemented to look at maternal outcomes in France by studying the reasons that pregnant women or those who had just given birth were admitted to intensive care units (22). Two regions of France participated on a population basis (Nord Pas de Calais and Lorraine), with 435 women admitted to intensive care units and 13 maternal deaths. As shown in Table 49-11, women were admitted to intensive care units

TABLE 49-11. *Admissions to intensive care in two French regions (Nord Pas de Calais and Lorraine) by major cause and case fatality rate*

Cause		Admission to ICU N	Deaths n	Case fatality rate
Hypertensive	(Total)	114	6	5.3
Preeclampsia		61	0	
Eclampsia		41	4	
HELLP		11	1	
Stroke		1	1	
Hemorrhage	(Total)	87	5	5.7
Abortion		6	0	
Ectopic		9	0	
Antepartum		1	0	
Uterine rupture		4	1	
Postpartum		67	4	
Thromboembolism	(Total)	54	2	3.9
Abortion		3	0	
Amniotic fluid embolism		2	1	
Pulmonary embolus		24	0	
Venous Thrombosis		25	1	

From Bouvier-Colles MH, Salanave B, Ancel Y, et al. and the regional teams for the survey. Obstetrical patients treated in intensive care units and maternal mortality. Eur J Obstet Gynecol Reprod Biol 1996;65:121–125.

HELLP, the syndrome of hemolytic anemia, elevated liver enzymes, and low platelet count.

TABLE 49-12. *Reasons for admission to an intensive care unit (percentage) by cause and type of maternity hospital*

Cause	Teaching hospital	Large public hospital	Small public hospital	Small private hospital
High blood pressure	35.8	25.0	20.0	18.0
Hemorrhage	11.7	23.4	30.0	26.2
Thromboembolism	9.9	13.7	15.0	18.0
Obstetrical cause	9.3	12.9	20.0	21.3
Indirect	24.7	15.3	5.0	4.9
Other	8.6	9.7	10.0	11.5

$p < 0.001$ among hospital levels for all causes.

From Bouvier-Colles MH, Salanave B, Ancel Y, et al. and the regional teams for the survey. Obstetrical patients treated in intensive care units and maternal mortality. Eur J Obstet Gynecol Reprod Biol 1996;65:121–125.

primarily for complications of high blood pressure, hemorrhage, and thromboembolism. The reasons for admission were different and depended on the level of hospital or clinic at which the woman sought care initially (Table 49-12). Moreover, the study found (Table 49-13) that small public hospitals and small private maternity clinics transferred these women only in severe cases, and, thus, severity at intensive care unit admission is significantly different by level of initial care (Table 49-13). Adjusted odds ratios show the importance of this difference in management. This study showed how the organization of obstetric care in France, characterized by the presence of many small units in public and private hospitals, is a factor affecting maternal safety. Large units are organized in such a way that an intensive care facility is nearby.

The diseases for which the decision is made to transfer to intensive care on such services are less severe than in units that have no proximate intensive care unit. This study also showed that the risk of death was related to the size of the unit, after standardization for disease severity. This fact will be important in the current debate about the organization of obstetric care in France, where small maternity units have very active supporters among consumers. These discussions about the size of maternity units often do not focus on safety or economic issues, but on the political reasons for defending proximity of maternal care to small communities.

TABLE 49-13. *Proportion of high-severity index cases of maternal conditions among pregnant or delivered women admitted to an intensive care unit by level of care of initial hospital*

Initial hospital	N	Percentage high severity	Crude OR (95% CI)
Teaching	102	8.8	1
Large public	98	12.2	1.4 (0.6–3.6)
Small public	51	15.7	1.9 (0.7–5.3)
Small private	72	26.4	3.7 (1.6–8.8)

From Ancel PY, Bouvier-Colles MH, Bréart G, Vernoux N, Salanave B, and the maternal morbidity study group. Does health care organization play a role? J. Perinat Med, 1998; 26:354–364.

OR, odds ratio; CI, confidence interval.

The challenges to improving maternal safety in developed countries can be illustrated by a review of the deaths in the most recent reports of the confidential inquiries of the United Kingdom (23). These cases show that quality of care in many situations is associated with the risk of maternal death; however, they also underline the complexity of achieving quality obstetric management for unforeseen emergencies. For instance, cases of placenta previa, particularly in patients with an existing uterine scar, can be associated with uncontrollable hemorrhage at delivery, and cesarean hysterectomy may be necessary. The analysis of deaths from this cause concluded that the presence of a consultant (a senior obstetrician) at operation is essential, that all units where a birth occurs should have a blood bank on site, and that a protocol is needed for managing massive hemorrhage, with appropriate training of teams for these rare events.

In the 3 years from 1991 to 1993 in the United Kingdom, antepartum and postpartum hemorrhage was the cause of death in 15 women. In 11 of these cases, the care was considered to be appropriate. In four cases, placenta previa–related deaths were judged to be associated with substandard care. In one, even though a cesarean section was performed by a senior registrar, blood loss was underestimated, and replacement blood was delivered late because of the distance to the blood bank. In two cases the diagnosis of placenta previa was not made by routine ultrasound, and in one of these cases, the woman had had a cesarean section for a previous delivery. In these two cases, the appropriate decision was made to do a cesarean section because of bleeding. At the time of operation, placenta previa accreta was recognized, but it had invaded the bladder and was inadequately treated; no immediate decision was made to do a hysterectomy. In the last case, a woman experienced bleeding but was told that it was slow and was not advised to go to hospital. When a neighbor called, a midwife came to the home and found the woman had collapsed and was unconscious.

Care is often inadequate in the context of hypertensive complications of pregnancy. Among deaths related to high blood pressure, there was evidence of suboptimal care in 16 of 20 deaths in 1991–1993, associated with failure to take prompt action and inadequate consultant involvement. The recommendations for ensuring better quality of care for these situations are that an obstetrician with specialized knowledge should put together a team in every obstetric unit to formulate and update preeclampsia and eclampsia protocols and should be available to give advice in difficult cases. Furthermore,there should be links with a regional consultant who has a special interest in the management of these cases. On occasion, such advice might mean referral of the case. In none of the 20 cases in the study was there any evidence that advice had been sought from a regional consultant, despite repeated recommendations to do so. In 10 of 11 cases of eclampsia, the first seizure occurred in the hospital. Magnesium sulfate was not used in any of these cases despite the fact magnesium sulfate has been found to be superior to diazepam and phenytoin. Since magnesium sulfate treatment is not without danger, however, the recommendation was that it should be introduced in those units not using it only after appropriate training.

Delay in appropriate treatment was confirmed in several cases. In one case the delay was caused by a shortage of neonatal facilities, and the condition of the woman deteriorated rapidly. In a second case, the delay was related to the fact that the woman was not seen by a consultant despite the presence of massive proteinuria and high blood pressure. Fatal eclampsia resulted. In a third case a planned emergency cesarean section was canceled because the fetus died *in utero*, and, despite deteriorating preeclampsia, labor was induced. It lasted for 26 hours, during which circulatory overload developed, and death occurred from adult respiratory distress syndrome.

Delay in delivery also occurred in an effort to gain fetal maturity in three cases. One patient suspected of being in preterm labor was admitted with a twin pregnancy at 30 weeks, having had 2+ proteinuria and hypertension for 3 days. For 3 days corticoids and ritodrine were administered, with inadequate monitoring of blood pressure and fluid volume. The patient had an eclamptic fit and died of cerebral hemorrhage. Another delay occurred in treating a woman admitted at 26 weeks' gestation with a blood pressure of 170/100 and 5.8 g of proteinuria. She was transferred to the intensive care unit, where hypoxia and oliguria developed. Disseminated intravascular coagulation ensued, and the woman died of multiple organ failure. The decision to transfer to the intensive care unit and not to deliver the baby was inappropriate despite the very early gestation.

Another patient was admitted to the hospital at 29 weeks with severe preeclampsia and was treated with labetalol. She was also given corticoids. The preeclampsia continued to deteriorate without any additional action, and fatal eclampsia resulted 5 days later, when her blood pressure suddenly increased despite treatment. As these detailed examples show, progress in reducing maternal mortality is still possible in developed countries where obstetric care is available. A careful organization of audits to identify failures in the current system can help improve outcomes for all women (24).

THE SAFE MOTHERHOOD INITIATIVE

Launched in 1987 by more than a hundred representatives of international organizations, health specialists, experts in development, and decision makers from more than 45 countries, the Safe Motherhood Initiative has just celebrated its tenth anniversary (25). The initiative led to the first real universal mobilization in favor of safe motherhood. It was born of the awareness that developed in the early 1980's of the enormous extent of maternal morbidity and mortality in developing nations (25–29) and the recognition, admittedly late, that health professionals—and obstetrician-gynecologists, in particular—had paid little attention to this tragedy (30,31).

Ten years later, the initial objective to reduce the number of maternal deaths by at least half within a decade is far from realized. Unknown territory barely a generation ago (32), the scope and the details of maternal morbidity and mortality in developing countries are now better understood, and there has been a remarkable proliferation of scientific publications on the subject since the mid-1980's. Ambitious projects, including the Safe Motherhood Initiative, were launched all over the world; the World Bank multiplied the number of projects it funded in this area by ten between 1987 and 1993 (33), and the number of organizations financing programs related to safe motherhood exceeded 50 by 1992 (34). The most important advance might be that the very concept of maternal mortality prevention has changed. We know better today what can really improve the health of mothers, and we are beginning to see how to implement truly effective strategies in developing countries.

According to the latest estimates of the WHO and UNICEF (35), 585,000 women still die every year from complications of pregnancy or delivery, that is, nearly 80,000 more than in the mid-1980's (36–38). Obstetric disorders continue to constitute the leading cause of death (nearly 16%) among women of childbearing age, far ahead of tuberculosis, suicide, war injuries, traffic accidents, or AIDS (39). Moreover, more than 40% of pregnant women, that is, at least 60 million people across the world, suffer from obstetric disorders that are not immediately lethal (vesicovaginal fistulas, chronic kidney disorders, sterility, etc.) (40–41). Although progress has been recorded in northern Africa, eastern Asia, and Latin America, maternal mortality remains 100 times higher in sub-Saharan Africa than in Europe. It is in Africa that the situation today is most disquieting, even though the majority of maternal deaths (55%) still occur in Asia, where 60% of worldwide births also occur. In many countries of eastern, central, and western Africa, maternal mortality is increasing and surpasses, sometimes by a wide margin, 1,000 per 100,000 live births (35).

A 1995 study at the Burkina Faso national hospital center in Ouagadougou (42) reported a maternal mortality rate of more than 4,100 per 100,000 live births. This number substantially exceeds the findings of the most catastrophic of the hospital surveys previously conducted in Africa and illustrates the gravity of the situation. The principal causes of maternal morbidity and mortality in developing countries seem hardly to have changed over the past 10 years: hemorrhage, dystocia, eclampsia, infections, and complications of abortion underlie most maternal deaths (42–46), although it is now clearer that the consequences of illegal abortions are substantially underestimated. Far from narrowing, the extraordinary disparity between the levels of maternal mortality in industrialized countries and developing countries that aroused indignation and then mobilization in the mid-1980's seems to have increased. A woman today runs a risk a thousand times greater of dying from pregnancy or childbirth complications if she lives in Africa than if she is a Swiss or Norwegian citizen.

THE SAFE MOTHERHOOD INITIATIVE OVER TIME

The Safe Motherhood Initiative has not stopped provoking reaction and reflections from public health professionals and participants in international health cooperative efforts; indeed, it has increased them. As a consequence, approaches to the prevention of maternal morbidity and mortality have changed markedly over the past 10 years. It has become clear that socioeconomic factors should be considered separately and that the prevention of maternal mortality is, above all, a public health issue based on family planning and on the accessibility of high-quality obstetric care during pregnancy and childbirth. This change of view is based in part on the historical lessons showing that maternal mortality rates have been reduced in the industrialized nations since the beginning of the nineteenth century not because of economic growth but by the diffusion and professionalization of obstetric care (43). Supporting this view are studies of women in extremist religious communities in the United States who, although they are well nourished, well educated, and relatively well off economically, have maternal mortality rates more than one hundred times higher than the national mean, close to those recorded in the poorest of developing countries (47).

The relationship between discrimination against women and maternal morbidity and mortality has also been called into question. The good maternal health record of such countries as Saudi Arabia, Iran, and Algeria—where the maternal mortality rates are, respectively, 100, 120, and 80 per 100,000 live births—shows that despite persistent sexual discrimination some progress has been made in reducing mortality through improved obstetric care.

Nevertheless, respect for women's rights is an explicit and principal stake of Safe Motherhood, intended to restore to more than a half million women every year their right to life.

In 1987, family planning was considered one of the surest solutions for limiting maternal mortality in developing countries. At least some of the sponsors of the initiative considered that most maternal deaths resulted from unwanted or at least unnecessary pregnancies. This conviction was based on observations showing particularly high mortality rates among adolescents, grand multiparas, and women older than 35 years (47) and on the fact that approximately one-fourth of deaths occurred during abortions, most illegal and performed in unsanitary, unhealthy conditions.

Here, too, reality has proved to be more complex than expected. Experience has shown that the increased prevalence of contraceptive use in a community can result in as much as a 30% reduction in the maternal mortality rate. Limiting the number of pregnancies lessens the number of possible complications and thus the number of maternal deaths, but family planning does not modify a woman's risk of dying once she is pregnant. Moreover, most maternal deaths occur during or after wanted pregnancies. Taking into account these elements, together with the risks of sexually transmitted diseases and AIDS in developing countries, the widespread distribution of contraceptives is no longer considered the surest method of diminishing maternal mortality.

Prenatal Care

The relevance of the concept of high-risk pregnancy was challenged at the beginning of the 1990's. Indeed, most complications of childbirth arise in the context of low-risk pregnancies (48). In truth, this fact has long been known. An article by F. Neon Reynolds in a 1934 issue of the *Lancet* pointed out that more than 80% of maternal deaths were due to complications for which no prenatal screening was possible: puerperal sepsis, postpartum hemorrhage, and shock—and it is somewhat surprising that it took as long as it did for doubts to be voiced about the validity of the risk approach in obstetrics (49).

Consequently, the role and objectives of prenatal care in strategies for preventing maternal mortality have had to be revised. Some researchers have even recommended a complete renunciation of prenatal care (50). The most widely accepted attitude, however, considers that the most certainly useful acts in the course of prenatal care are the prescription of iron and folate supplements, malaria prophylaxis, tetanus vaccinations, and, when possible, the treatment of pregnancy-related hypertension (51). All authors agree, however, that prenatal care has no value unless the professionals who provide it have available the necessary equipment and, most important, the potential for appropriate and effective referral in case of complications. Whatever the multiple factors that affect the progress of a pregnancy when complications arise, it is ultimately obstetric intervention that can prevent maternal morbidity and mortality. The efficacy of the intervention, which is often surgical, depends on its timeliness. Geographic accessibility to a referral institution where basic obstetric care is available is the primary factor determining the mother's survival (52).

From a public health viewpoint, the principal problem is how best to determine needs and, in particular, the minimum cesarean rate necessary for avoiding maternal and perinatal deaths and grave complications. The rates most often reported in the literature are on the order of at least 5%, while those observed in most developing countries range, at best, between 1% and 2% (53,54). The objective then is to establish sufficient obstetric coverage to make up the deficit in interventions, in both urban and rural areas. With this perspective, programs for preventing maternal morbidity and mortality aim to decentralize the basic obstetric interventions, such as the cesarean, to the level of district hospitals. Such a strategy requires that these establishments have a minimum level of equipment (water, electricity, surgical supplies) and a level of competence that can be maintained only with the practice of at least one cesarean per week. Such health structures must cover, on average, 30,000 to 50,000 people, in a zone with a radius of 10 to 30 km. In rural zones where the population density is low and residences are widely dispersed, it might be necessary to develop strategies based on means of communication and on emergency evacuations.

Today, more than ever, the solution is in the hands of obstetricians. To reduce maternal morbidity and mortality, basic obstetrics must be accessible to all populations. This means that women, wherever they live, must be able to undergo medical and surgical procedures that are likely to save their lives in the case of obstetric complications. If health authorities do not encourage and support the training of obstetricians and their maintenance in primary care hospitals by guaranteeing them motivating working conditions and a satisfactory salary, and if obstetricians do not become conscious of the fact that their primary mission is to provide basic obstetric services (55,58), then the Safe Motherhood Initiative may well remain an orphan for the next 10 years.

CONCLUSION

An organized effort to lower the maternal death rate and limit severe maternal morbidity can be successful with low-tech methods in most developing countries. The history of the success of this policy in developed countries has been presented to show that the means needed for such a policy are affordable (57), if the political will to address this question is present and if the welfare of women is a real goal for the society. In developed societies, major technological and organizational changes have dramatically transformed the risks associated with childbirth in our lifetimes (58). Avoidable deaths still occur, however; continued vigilance is necessary to provide quality obstetric care for all women.

REFERENCES

1. Hughes EC (ed): Obstetrics–Gynecologic Terminology. Philadelphia, F.A. Davis, 1972.
2. ICD 9 CM Code Book. Reston, Va.: St. Anthony Publishing, 1997.
3. Fortney JA. Implications of the ICD-10 definitions related to deaths in pregnancy, childhood, and puerperium. World Health Stat Q 1990;3: 246–248.
4. Högberg U, Innala E, Sandström A. Maternal mortality in Sweden 1980–1988. Obstet Gynecol 1994;84:240–244.
5. Rochat RW, Koonin LM, Atrash HK, Jewett JF. Maternal mortality in the United States: report from the maternal mortality collaborative. Obstet Gynecol 1988;72:91–97.
6. Lawsen HW, Frye A, Atrash HK, Smith JC, Schulman HB, Ramick M. Abortion mortality in the United States 1972 through 1987. Am J Obstet Gynecol 1994;171:1365–1372.
7. Jacob S, Bloebaum L, Shah G, Warner MW. Maternal mortality in Utah. Obstet Gynecol 1998;91:187–191.
8. Bouvier-Colles MH, Varnoux N, Costes P, Hatton F. Mortalité maternelle en France: fréquence et raisons de sa sous-estimation dans les statistiques de causes médicales de décès. J Gynecol Obstet Biol Reprod (Paris) 1991;20:885–891.
9. Huss M, Bongain A, Bertrandy M, Hofman P, Grimaud D, Gillet JY. Mortalité maternelle à Nice: resultats d'une enquate de gype "Ramos" à parter des registres de decès du Centre Hospitalier Universitaire à Nice, 1986–1993. J Gynecol Obstet Biol Reprod (Paris) 1996;25:636–644.
10. Högberg U, Joelsson J. The decline in maternal mortality in Sweden 1931–1980. Acta Obstet Gynecol Scand 1985;64:583–592.
11. Papiernik E. La réduction de la mortalité maternelle: analyse historique. In: Bouyer J, Bréart G, Delecourt M, eds. Réduire la mortalité maternelle dans les pays en développement. Paris: INSERM, 1989:31–54.
12. Charlton HR, Veliz R. Maternal mortality. Br Med J 1985;292:295–301.
13. Ryan G. La mortalité périnatale et maternelle aux Etats Unis. Union Med Can 1984;113:572–576.
14. Vallin J, Mesle F. Les causes des décès en France de 1925 à 1978. Volume I. Paris: INSSE EDIT, 1982.
15. Högberg U. Secular trends in maternal mortality in Sweden from 1750 to 1980. Bull World Health Organ 1986;64:7984–7986.
16. Schwart R. Mortalidad materna y cobertura institucional para el pastro 22 paises de la Region las Americas. CLAP OPS, 1973–84, WHO FHE, 1985.
17. Berardi JC, Richard A, Djanhan Y, Papiernik E. Evaluation du bénéfice de l'installation d'une structure obstétrico-chirurgicale décentralisée en terme de réduction de la mortalité maternelle et des transferts en Côte d Ivoire. Med d'Afrique Noire 1989;364:280–287.
18. World Health Organization. Coverage of maternity care, a listing of available information—Geneva, Switzerland: maternal and newborn health-safe motherhood. WHO/RHT/MSM/96.28, 1997.
19. Harrison KA, Rossiter CE. Maternal mortality: a survey of 22,774 consecutive hospital births in Zaria, northern Nigeria. Br J Obstet Gynaecol 1985;[Suppl 6]:100–119.
20. Harrison KA. Childbearing, health and social priorities: a survey of 22,774 hospital births in Zaria, northern Nigeria. Br J Obstet Gynaecol 1985;91(Suppl 5):13–22, 61–80, 86–99, 100–105.
21. Harrisson KA. The importance of the educated healthy women in Africa. Lancet 1997;349:644–647.
22. Bouvier-Colles MH, Salanave B, Ancel Y, et al. and the regional teams for the survey. Obstetrical patients treated in intensive care units and maternal mortality. Eur J Obstet Gynecol Reprod Biol 1996; 65:121–125.
23. Department of Health Report on confidential inquiries into maternal deaths in the United Kingdom. 1991–1993. London: HMSO, 1996;32–47.
24. Ancel PY, Bouvier-Colles MH, Bréart G, Vernoux N, Salanave B, and the maternal morbidity study group. Does health care organization play a role? J Perinat Med 1998;26:354–364.
25. Starrs A. Preventing the tragedy of maternal deaths: report on the International Safe Motherhood Conference, Nairobi (February, 1987). Edited by The World Bank, 1987:56.
26. Mahler H. Maternal and child health: report by the Director General, presented at the 32nd World Health Assembly, Geneva, 1979.

27. Reference 27 deleted in text.
28. OMS. Les femmes, la santé et le développement: rapport du Directeur Général, Genève, 1985:38.
29. OMS. Prevention of maternal mortality: report of a WHO interregional meeting, Geneva, 1985:23.
30. Mahler H. The Safe Motherhood Initiative: a call to action. Lancet 1987;1:668–670.
31. Rosenfield A, Maine D. Maternal mortality: a neglected tragedy. Where is the M in MCH? Lancet 1985:2:83–85.
32. Rochat RW. Maternal mortality in the United States of America. World Health Stat Q 1981;34:2–13.
33. Tinker A, Koblinsky MA. Vers une maternité sans risque. Washington, D.C.: World Bank, 1993:95.
34. OMS Directory of funding sources for safe motherhood projects. WHO/FHE/MSM/95.2.
35. OMS and UNICEF. Revised 1990 estimates of maternal mortality: a new approach. Geneva: WHO/FRH/MSM/96.11, 1996:16.
36. Boerma JT. The magnitude of the maternal mortality problem in sub-Saharan Africa. Soc Sci Med 1997;24:551–558.
37. Royston E, Lopez A. De l'evaluation de la mortalité maternelle. Rapp Trimest Statsit Sanit Mond Genève 1987;40:214–224.
38. Abou Zahr C, Royston E. Maternal mortality: a global factbook. Geneva: Division of Family Health—WHO, 1991.
39. Murray CH, Lopez A. Mortality by cause for eight regions of the world: Global Burden of Disease Study. Lancet 1997;349:1269–1276.
40. Koblinsky M, Campbell O, Harlow S. Mother and more: a broader perspective on women's health. In: Koblinsky M, Timyan J, Gay J, eds. The health of women: a global perspective. Boulder, Colo.: Westview Press, 1992.
41. Glazener C, Abdalla M, Stroud P, Naji S, Templeton A, Russell IT. Postnatal maternal morbidity: extent, causes, prevention and treatment. Br J Obstet Gynaecol 1995;102:282–287.
42. Lankoandé J, Sondo B, Ouedraogo C, Ouedraogo A, Kone B. La mortalité maternelle au centre hospitalier national de Ouagadougou (Burkina Faso): à propos de 123 cas colligés en 1995. Rev Epidemiol Santé Publique 1997;45:174–176.
43. Berg C, Atrash H, Koonin L, Tucker M. Pregnancy-related mortality in the United States, 1987–1990. Obstet Gynecol 1996;88:11–167.
44. Harrison KA. Childbearing, health and social priorities: a survey of 22,774 consecutive hospital births in Zaria, northern Nigeria. Br J Obstet Gynaecol 1985;93(Suppl 5):1–119.
45. Harrison KA. Family planning and maternal mortality in the third world. Lancet 1986;2:1441.
46. Harrison KA. Maternal mortality in developing countries. Br J Obstet Gynaecol 1989;96:1–3.
47. Kaunitz A, Spence C, Danielson TS, Rochat RW, Grimes DH. Perinatal and maternal mortality in a religious group avoiding obstetrical care. Am J Obstet Gynecol 1984;50:826–831.
48. Winikoff B. The effects of birth spacing on child and maternal health. Stud Fam Plann 1983;14:213–245.
49. McDonagh M. Is antenatal care effective in reducing maternal morbidity and mortality? Health Pol Plann 1996;11:1–15.
50. Maine D. Safe motherhood programs: options and issues. New York: Center for Population and Family Health, Columbia University, 1991:59.
51. Rooney C. Antenatal care and maternal health: How effective is it? A review of evidence, 4th ed. Geneva: WHO/MSM/92, 1992.
52. Oaklye A. The capture womb: a history of the medical care of pregnant women. Oxford: Blackwell, 1984.
53. Fortney J. Antenatal risk screening and scoring: a new look. Int J Gynecol Obstet 1995;50:53–58.
54. Fernandez H, Djanhan Y, Papiernik E. Mortalité maternelle par hémorragie dans les pays en développement: quelle politique proposer? J Gynecol Obstet Biol Reprod (Paris) 1998;17:687–692.
55. Fernandez H, Cosson M, Papiernik E. Obstétrique essentielle. Paris: Editions Parallèles, 1996:276.
56. Fernandez H. Hemorragies obstétricales. In: Bouvier-Colles MH, Varnoux N, Bréart G, eds. Les morts maternelles en France, Paris: INSERM, 1994:51–62.
57. Jougl E, Ducimetière P, Bouvier-Colles MJ, Hatton F. Relation entre le niveau de développement du système de soins et le niveau de mortalité établis selon les départements français. Rev Epidemiol Santé Publique 1987;35:365–377.
58. Schmitermaker NWE, Bennbroek Gravenhorst J, Van Geign HP, Dekker GA, Van Dougen PWJ. Maternal mortality and its prevention. Eur J Obstet Gynecol Reprod Biol 1991;42:31–35.

Cherry and Merkatz's Complications of Pregnancy,
Fifth Edition, edited by W. R. Cohen.
Lippincott Williams & Wilkins, Philadelphia © 2000.

CHAPTER 50

Surgical Considerations

Clifford Roberts Wheeless, Jr.

I heard Nicholas Eastman of the Johns Hopkins Hospital say on numerous occasions, "Take the disease out of the pregnancy, not the pregnancy out of the disease." In fact, the list of medical and surgical disorders that require removing the pregnancy prior to fetal viability is shrinking as medical science advances. Except for those diseases that threaten the integrity of the placenta and thus the viability of the fetus, the pregnancy should be continued if that is the wish of the mother (1). Nevertheless, the notion of removing disease from the pregnant patient is often the source of general fear and concern by surgeons. The pregnant uterus is foreign territory to most surgeons not trained in obstetrics and gynecology, and they are often uncomfortable operating on pregnant women. Many surgeons feel that if they could get the pregnant uterus out of the way they would know how to manage the woman's problem. A more logical approach would be to continue the pregnancy and alter the surgical techniques to accommodate the pregnancy, rather than terminating the pregnancy prior to fetal viability.

The emphasis of this chapter will be on modifying surgical technique to allow the fetus to remain in the uterus until viability is probable. There are certain situations in which this may not be possible, but it should be the goal of modern surgery involving the pregnant woman.

UNSTABLE PATIENTS

The approach to the pregnant unstable patient should be the same as the approach to any unstable patient. Maintenance of an open airway and ventilation should be the first priority. If respiration is severely compromised from any cause the patient should be ventilated with an Ambu bag and face mask, using an oral airway until an endotracheal tube can be inserted and connected to a mechanical ventilator. If the upper jaw is unstable or if the anatomy of the neck is unusual there should be no hesitancy to perform a tracheostomy. The new needle kit tracheostomies (Cook Cath Corp, Spencer, IN) are ideal for an emergency procedure. After respiration is ensured, cardiac function must be stabilized, concomitant with attempts to normalize intravascular volume. Large-bore silastic lines should be inserted into the superior vena cava. Internal jugular or subclavian vein routes are preferred when the need for large fluid volumes exists. A long central line also can be inserted into an arm vein and threaded into the chest. If subclavian or cephalic veins are not available, the femoral vein can be used when massive trauma or blood loss is present. All too often the unstable pregnant patient is compromised by the use of small-gauge needles inserted into veins on the back of her hand or forearm. All unstable surgical patients require large volumes of intravenous fluid and monitoring lines inserted through large needles. Renal output should be monitored through drainage of the bladder with a Foley catheter. The patient's vascular space should be expanded with blood, crystalloids, or colloids as required to achieve an osmotic pressure approaching 300 mOsm/kg H_20. Expansion of the vascular space will increase cardiac preload. Swan-Ganz catheter measurements should approximate a central venous pressure of 9 to 11 mm Hg, a pulmonary wedge pressure of 13 mm Hg, and a cardiac index of 4.5 L/min. The urine output should be maintained at no less than 50 mL/h. The infusion of crystalloids alone will not always achieve the above goals. When a pregnant patient has lost a significant volume of blood, it should be replaced with blood products as soon as they are available. Colloids of various types (plasminate, hispan, and total parenteral nutrition) raise the vascular osmotic pressure and draw in fluids from the third space, thus expanding the intravascular space, which in turn improves venous return and cardiac output (2,3). The normal blood volume of a pregnant patient at term is approx-

C. R. Wheeless, Jr.: Department of Obstetrics and Gynecology, Institute for Special Pelvic Surgery, Sinai Hospital of Baltimore, Baltimore, Maryland 21215.

imately 30% to 40% greater than that of the nonpregnant patient. Although this serves the woman well for the initial phases of acute hemorrhage, she will often require blood transfusion if she has lost significant volumes of blood (4). Hypovolemia and anemia can compromise fetal oxygenation, even if the mother is tolerant of them.

Penetrating Trauma

Preoperative care of the seriously ill surgical patient is best served with one physician in charge. He or she should determine which of the traumatized organs has priority and thus establish the order of the treatment plan (e.g., penetrating thoracoabdominal wounds would have priority over a fracture of the femur).

The amniotic sac filled with fluid surrounding the fetus offers a zone of protection from penetrating high-velocity missile wounds. The experience of the American Hospital in Beirut, Lebanon, during their civil war was that numerous gunshot wounds to the pregnant abdomen could be treated with conservative expectant management of the fetus and mother while concentrating on stabilization of the mother. In their experience, this approach, even with fetal bone fracture, had a better outcome than emergency evacuation of an immature fetus by cesarean section. The unstable pregnant mother should have priority over the fetus in a treatment plan, unless the chances of maternal survival are nil (5).

STABLE PATIENTS

The preoperative care of the hemodynamically stable pregnant patient has a similar focus. The first priority is the respiratory tract. Pregnant patients scheduled for elective surgery who smoke should discontinue smoking several weeks prior to their procedure. Pulmonary disorders such as asthma or chronic bronchitis should be medically treated prior to surgery to optimize the patient's condition (6). Blood volume is usually not a problem in the stable pregnant patient. Autologous transfusion with the patient's own blood that can be stored 2 weeks prior to cesarean section or elective abdominal surgery is possible. Under any circumstances, the pregnant patient should have sufficient intravenous access lines inserted prior to surgery. Except for elective complicated cesarean sections, it is usually wise to advance large-bore intravenous catheters into the superior vena cava through the subclavian or the external jugular vein approach if significant blood loss is probable.

A Foley catheter should be inserted into the bladder to monitor urine output, which should generally be maintained at about 50 mL/h. We do not recommend preoperative ureteral stents, even for cesarean radical hysterectomy. Most gynecologic pelvic surgeons are adequately trained to identify the ureter even in the pregnant patient. Ureteral stents are a source of ureteral trauma and infection (7).

A home bowel preparation 2 days before surgery with a clear liquid diet, laxative, and magnesium citrate is adequate. It is especially important to avoid volume depletion (and its potential adverse effects on uterine blood flow) in pregnant women undergoing preoperative bowel preparation at home (8).

In the simple elective cesarean section, preoperative bowel preparation is not necessary. However, if one contemplates cesarean section hysterectomy, it is a distinct advantage to the patient to have the bowel prepared in the event an enterotomy is necessary. In the hospital we prepare the patient's intestine with 4 L of a preparation such as GoLytely (Braintree Laboratories, Inc., Braintree, MA). Obviously, in patients with acute appendicitis or bowel obstruction, preparation of the bowel would not apply.

HEMORRHAGE CONTROL

Hemorrhage in a pregnant patient in any trimester can be one of the most frightening and disturbing events to her obstetrician. In this section we will focus on antepartum, intrapartum, and postpartum hemorrhage (see Chapter 51).

Antepartum Hemorrhage

Hemorrhage from cervical punch biopsies and cervical conization can be surprisingly extensive. Indeed, some obstetricians postpone study of cervical neoplasia in the pregnant patient because of the fear of hemorrhage, an approach that can prove disastrous if an advanced or a rapidly progressive cervical lesion is present.

Colposcopically directed biopsy of the cervix is the safest technique for study of abnormal Papanicolaou smears in a pregnant patient. Directed biopsy allows for precise, accurate sampling of the most suspicious area on the cervix. Control of bleeding from the cervical biopsy site can frequently be accomplished with silver nitrate solution placed on the biopsy site using a wooden applicator stick. In addition, a regular tampon that has had the distal portion soaked in Monsel's jelly or solution and applied to the cervix will control most bleeding. Suturing of the pregnant patient's cervix to control bleeding is rarely necessary.

Conization of the cervix has a greater chance for severe bleeding in pregnant patients. Senior gynecologic oncology consultation should be made prior to any pregnant patient having a cold knife or electrosurgical cervical conization. This is especially true in the third trimester, when bleeding from this procedure can be very difficult to control. Before attempting the conization, it should be determined whether the conization will make a difference in the management of the patient in the third trimester, particularly if there is no grossly visible lesion of her cervix. Pregnant patients with early carcinoma of the cervix (carcinoma *in situ* or stage IA-1 or IA-2) may be allowed to deliver vaginally, with cesarean section reserved for the usual obstetric indications. Carcinoma of the cervix stage IB-1 or IB-2 lesions can usually be diagnosed with a simple colposcopically directed biopsy. The need for cone biopsy should be rare (9).

If information derived from a cone biopsy will make a significant difference in management, it can be performed with a low risk of hemorrhage by performing a cervical cerclage. Usually a McDonald purse-string suture suffices with a 2-0 monofilament suture on a gastrointestinal needle preceding the cone. When the cerclage suture is tied after the cone has been performed, bleeding is controlled in most cases (10).

Blunt and penetrating trauma can be a source of severe hemorrhage in the prepartum patient. Blunt trauma to the abdominal wall can produce abruptio placentae. This often is noted after automobile accidents, even when the pregnant patient is wearing the standard seat belt. The patient should be prepared for immediate cesarean section if fetal monitoring indicates a compromised fetus (11).

Penetrating injury from bullets and knifes may not be associated with the high fetal morbidity and mortality as previously thought. The American University in Beirut, Lebanon, reported their experience during their civil war with high-velocity rifle wounds in which the mother was observed and stabilized. Their hypothesis was that intervention would produce a premature fetus that would not survive because of prematurity. Thus, pregnant women with penetrating wounds to the abdominal wall and uterus were treated by stabilization of the mother and constant monitoring of the fetus. The uterus in the third trimester with its amniotic sac filled with amniotic fluid was protective to the fetus and the mother's abdominal organs. Overall, cardiovascular, respiratory, and renal stabilization in a surgical intensive care unit with fetal monitoring and serial magnetic resonance images were the best method for management of rifle and hand gun wounds to the abdomen of the pregnant patient (12). First- and second-trimester patients should be managed similarly to nonpregnant patients with penetrating wounds to the abdomen (13).

Intrapartum Hemorrhage

The major contributors to intrapartum hemorrhage are the products of conception, abdominal pregnancy, laceration of the uterine artery and vein, and extension of uterine lacerations into branches of the hypogastric veins.

Unrecognized lacerations of the uterine artery and vein at the time of low cervical transverse incision can be a source of severe postpartum hemorrhage. The branches of the hypogastric vein can be torn more easily than the branches of the hypogastric artery. Lacerated hypogastric veins can retract into the fat of the lateral extent of the cardinal ligament and are the source of many severe postpartum hemorrhages. The primary management of a lacerated uterine artery or vein should obviously be to identify, clamp, and ligate the vessel. If the obstetrician/gynecologist is trained in radical pelvic surgery and the development of the paravesical and pararectal spaces as required in the performance of a radical Wertheim hysterectomy, the branches of the hypogastric vein can be controlled by clamping the lateral extent of the cardinal ligament (Figs. 50-1 and 50-2). Ligation of the anterior division of the hypogastric artery will reduce the pulse pressure in the uterine artery and may give a window of opportunity for clotting in the vessels located within the walls of the pregnant uterus. Because of the copious collateral circulation in the pelvis, ligation of the anterior division of the hypogastric artery alone may not control hemorrhage from the lacerated retracted branches of the hypogastric veins.

When intrapartum hemorrhage from this source cannot be controlled and the lateral cardinal ligaments cannot be exposed by developing the paravesical and pararectal spaces, it may be efficacious to perform a cesarean hysterectomy. Removal of the postpartum uterus will gain exposure to the bleeding branches of the hypogastric veins in the lateral extent of the cardinal ligament. To avoid a hysterectomy, it may be helpful to pack the lateral pelvic walls and vagina in order to compress the blood

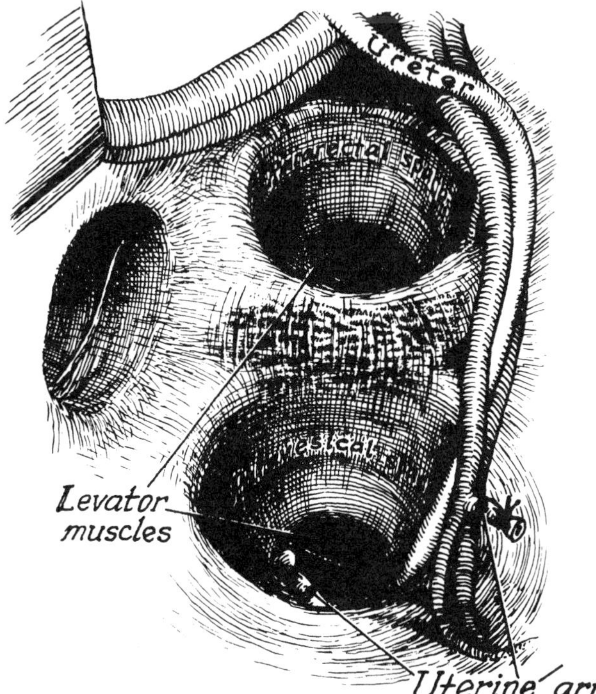

FIG. 50-1. The paravesical space and pararectal space. The branches of the hypogastric artery and veins are located within the cardinal ligament between these spaces. The uterine artery has been ligated just distal to its origin from the hypogastric artery. (From Wheeless CR Jr. Atlas of pelvic surgery. Baltimore: Williams & Wilkins, 1997.)

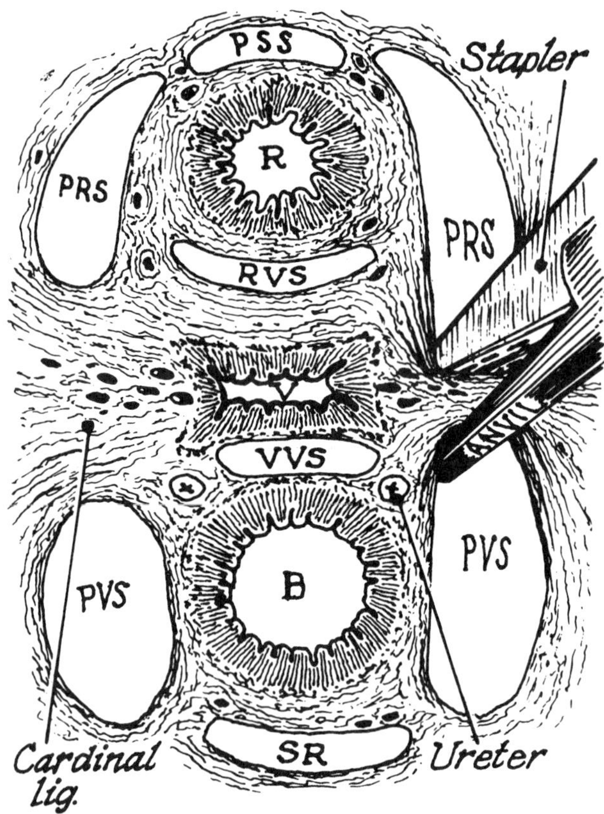

FIG. 50-2. Drawing of the spaces in the pelvis. The lateral extent of the cardinal ligament contains the hypogastric veins. *PSS*, presacral space; *PRS*, pararectal space; *RVS*, rectovaginal space; *VVS*, vesicovaginal space; *PRS*, paravesical space; *SR*, space of Retzius; *B*, bladder; *R*, rectum. (From Wheeless CR Jr. Atlas of pelvic surgery. Baltimore: Williams & Wilkins, 1997.)

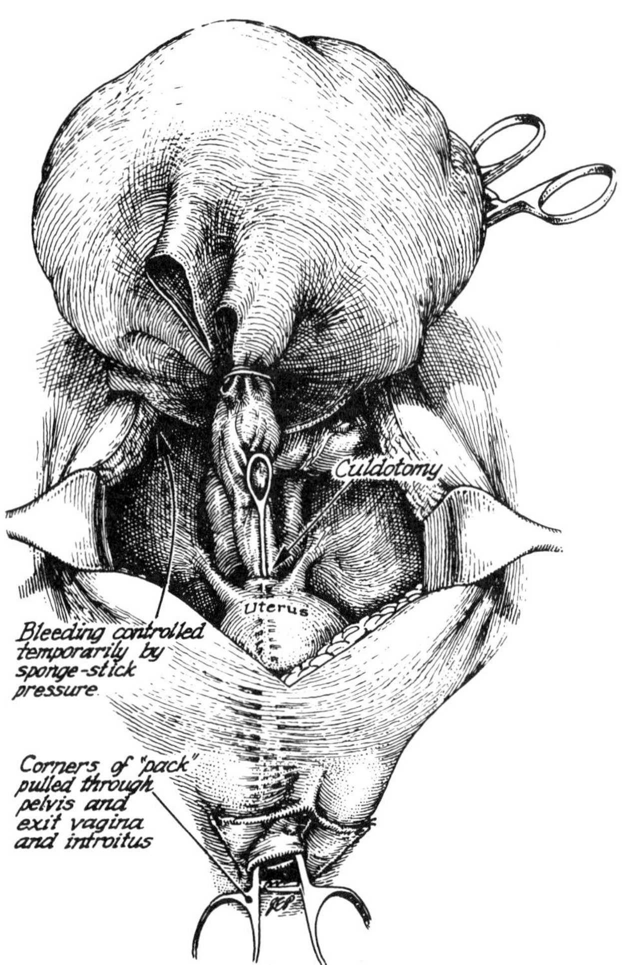

FIG. 50-3. A parachute pack placed in the pelvis and exteriorized through the vagina can be helpful in exerting pressure to control bleeding from branches of the hypogastric vessels. (From Wheeless CR Jr. Atlas of pelvic surgery. Baltimore: Williams & Wilkins, 1997.)

vessels within the cardinal ligament and stop bleeding. This should be done with very large bulky packs that are capable of producing enough pressure on the branches of the hypogastric vein to control bleeding (14). The use of the so-called parachute pack is quite efficacious (Fig. 50-3). Several laparotomy pads are inserted into the center of one opened laparotomy pad to achieve a parachute-shaped structure with a diameter of 12 to 14 cm or more. The ends of the open pack are folded over to fashion the shape of a parachute. A large suture is tied at the bottom of the ball structure on the parachute. The strings of the parachute representing the ends of the pack can be brought through a colpotomy by inserting a large sponge forceps up the vagina and perforating the cul-de-sac. The strings of the pack are pulled through the vagina. The pack, together with the postpartum uterus, represent a major tamponade on the branches of the hypogastric vessels within the cardinal ligament. A strong line or rope is tied around the strings of the pack exiting the vaginal introitus. The rope is draped over a pulley at the foot of the bed, and a 5-pound weight placed on the rope. The abdominal wall should be closed only with the skin using towel clips. The patient should be transported to the surgical intensive care unit. All the vital parameters for observation of a patient in hemorrhagic shock are monitored and corrected. The patient's temperature, blood pressure, pulse, respiration, hematocrit, acidosis, magnesium, potassium, and renal output should be appropriately monitored and brought into normal range. After 48 hours the patient should be returned to the operating room, the abdomen reopened, the parachute pack removed, and the pelvis thoroughly irrigated. The hemorrhage is usually controlled. At this time the fascia can be closed with a running monofilament delayed synthetic absorbable suture, the skin should be closed, and monitoring should continue in the surgical intensive care unit (15).

A source of dramatic intrapartum hemorrhage in the pregnant patient is that from abdominal pregnancies. The placentas are frequently located in many parts of the lower abdomen (Fig. 50-4) (4). When the fetus is removed, the traumatic removal of the placentas at the time

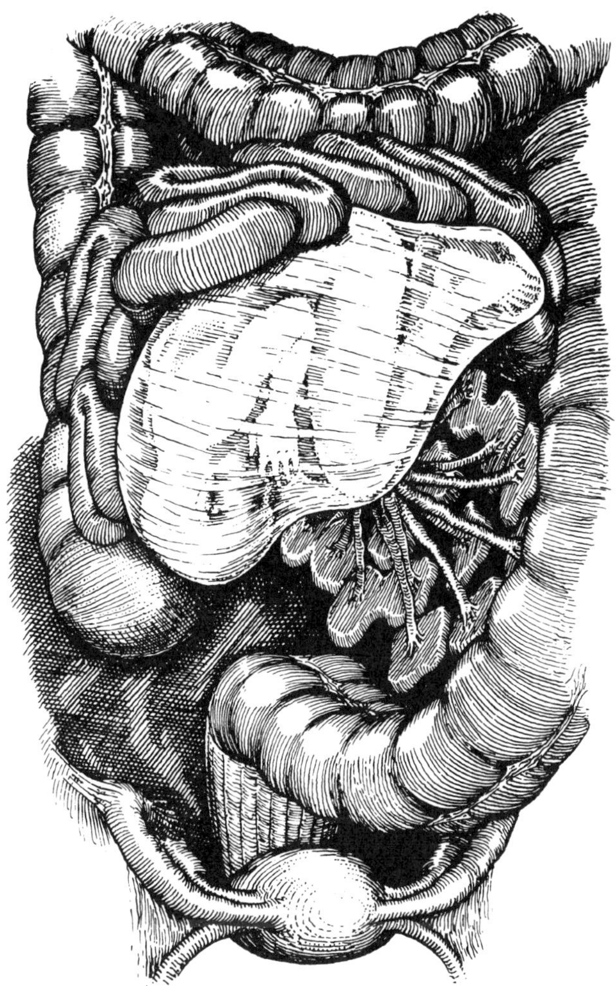

FIG. 50-4. Abdominal pregnancy with multiple placentas implanted on sites within the abdominal cavity. (From Wheeless CR Jr. Atlas of pelvic surgery. Baltimore: Williams & Wilkins, 1997.)

of laparotomy by inexperienced surgeons can result in maternal mortality attributable to hemorrhage. The best policy is to remove the fetus, ligate and tie the cord, close the abdomen, and treat the patient postpartum with chemotherapy appropriate for gestational trophoblastic disease (16,17). Some patients develop intraabdominal abscesses several months postpartum. These can usually be drained by the interventional radiologist with needle aspiration inserted under fluoroscopic control. This should be attempted prior to a surgical approach. Chemotherapy drugs normally used in gestational trophoblastic neoplasia, such as methotrexate or VP16, are a reasonable alternative to eliminate placental tissue and may obviate the need to control intraperitoneal hemorrhage caused by removal of the placenta in an abdominal pregnancy (16), a task that can be extremely difficult.

If the abdominal pregnancy placenta is removed and bleeding occurs that is not readily controlled, control of hemorrhage is best obtained by large bulky packing. If the entire abdominal cavity can be packed, the abdominal wall skin (not rectus fascia) is closed (14). The patient can be taken to the surgical intensive care unit as noted above for 48 hours (15). In most instances the hemorrhage will be under control. Furthermore, after packing and therapy in the surgical intensive care unit, one is taking a patient back to the operating room for the second look who is stable, and senior surgical expertise can be on hand if the packs have not properly controlled the hemorrhage.

Postpartum Hemorrhage

The most common cause of postpartum hemorrhage is uterine atony associated with retained portions of the placenta. When postpartum hemorrhage is severe and attempts to control it with the standard techniques are unsuccessful, lacerations of the uterine artery or vein or of hypogastric veins should be considered, especially if the delivery has been by cesarean section. Branches of the hypogastric vein can be lacerated without the knowledge of the obstetrician. The patient is noted to have heavy hemorrhage in the obstetrical recovery room both vaginally and even intraabdominally. We have found that closed suction drains, such as Jackson-Pratt and Hemovacs, placed in the abdominal cavity are poor indicators of the presence of intraabdominal hemorrhage. They were not designed for evacuation of large clots. If the patient becomes unstable with alteration in her vital signs, a decrease in urinary output, and distention of the abdomen, she must be returned to the operating room for reexploration. If the bleeding is coming from a source in the lateral pelvic wall, it is probably from lacerations of the branches of the hypogastric veins. The surgical development of the paravesical and pararectal spaces will allow a direct approach to the branches of the hypogastric veins, and they may be clamped and tied en masse, as done in performing a radical Wertheim hysterectomy (see Figs. 50-1 and 50-2). If this approach fails and the patient continues to bleed and becomes unstable with hypothermia, metabolic acidosis, and disseminated intravascular coagulation, it is best to pack the pelvis with a parachute pack as noted above, with the ends of the parachute pack exteriorized through a colpotomy in the pouch of Douglas. The ends of the pack are placed on tension with a 5-pound weight hanging over the end of the patient's bed (see Fig. 50-3). In most cases the extensive packing, which is removed after 48 hours, should control hemorrhage, often making hysterectomy unnecessary.

Another source of postpartum hemorrhage has its etiology from deep lacerations of the vaginal wall. The branches of the hypogastric vein, especially the pudendal branches, are involved. Suturing the vaginal mucosa in these cases is rarely successful for controlling hemorrhage. Extensive packing with large packs in the vagina may work; but if this fails to control bleeding, a laparotomy should be performed, and the branches of the hypogastric vein clamped and tied from the abdominal approach.

In cases of attempted control of hemorrhage in the pelvis in the pregnant patient, a postoperative intravenous pyelogram is often useful to ensure that the ureters have not been sutured or injured in the process of trying to control hemorrhage.

Postpartum episiotomy hemorrhage with the resultant hematoma should be controlled by reopening the episiotomy, evacuating the hematoma, and ligating any bleeding noted from branches of the pudendal vessels. The issue of resuture of the episiotomy versus packing remains a controversial one. I feel that if the hematoma has been evacuated and the bleeding points controlled, it is safe to resuture the episiotomy. The wound will heal faster and the patient will have more comfort than allowing an episiotomy to granulate from its base to the skin.

ABDOMINAL INCISIONS

Incision options in the pregnant patient are determined by the length of gestation as well as the expected procedure and the patient's medical condition and body habitus. Understanding the alterations in anatomy as the uterus enlarges is important in making good decisions about what incisions to use (18). We shall consider incision options in four groups: first, second, and third trimester, and thoracoabdominal. Closure of these incisions will be discussed in the latter part of this section, including the engineering science and the chemistry of modern suture available for surgical wound closure.

In the first trimester, the anatomy of the intraabdominal contents is, from a surgical point of view, not significantly different from that of the nonpregnant patient. In such patients with acute appendicitis, a McBurney incision is still possible in most cases (19). The problem with this approach derives from uncertainty regarding the source of the patient's abdominal symptoms. Although acute appendicitis may be addressed readily through this incision, a twisted ovarian cyst or some other problem may not be. Therefore, an incision that offers a wide exposure to the organs of the lower abdomen and pelvis is preferred in these patients. Most experienced gynecologic surgeons would elect a lower midline abdominal incision. However, a transverse Pfannenstiel incision (maintaining the option of conversion to a Maylard incision) is adequate for most surgery in the lower abdomen and pelvis. A Maylard incision can present difficulties if the etiology of the patient's problem is found to be in the upper abdomen. In a situation in which a Pfannenstiel incision has been made and surgical pathology is located in organs in the upper abdomen, the Pfannenstiel incision should be closed rather than extending it to a Maylard incision. A proper midline incision extended above the umbilicus should then be made in order to deal with the upper abdominal surgical problems.

In the second trimester of pregnancy the uterus is enlarged to such a size that a midline incision is the proper choice for an acute surgical abdomen (19). The paramedian incision, usually made on the right, is a reasonable alternative to the midline approach. There are few patients with surgical problems in the abdomen that cannot be operated upon through a midline incision. It can be extended around the umbilicus if necessary. By the second trimester of pregnancy the cecum and appendix are at the same transverse level as the umbilicus and can be best managed with an upper midline or paramedian incision. The same is true for gallbladder, kidney, upper gastrointestinal tract, and liver problems.

There is no role for incisions in the lower abdomen during the third trimester of pregnancy, unless a cesarean section is to be part of the surgery or the urinary bladder needs to be approached. If a third-trimester gestation is to be maintained after the surgery, an upper abdominal midline incision is preferable. On occasion, hepatobiliary or renal lesions are approached via subcostal transverse incisions.

Rarely, thoracic or thoracoabdominal incisions are necessary in the pregnant woman (e.g., for management of blunt or penetrating trauma). For patients requiring cardiac surgery in pregnancy, a median sternotomy incision without abdominal exposure allows exposure to the heart. Entry into the thoracic cavity require a chest tube connected to water seal drainage be placed prior to closure of the incision.

The technique of closure of abdominal incisions has changed in the last decade of surgery. Application of mechanical engineering principles to study of abdominal wall closure has directed much of this change (20). In addition, the chemistry, textile engineering, and mechanics of modern suture have changed. There is virtually no role for nonsynthetic suture in this era of surgery. Catgut, silk, and cotton are all sutures whose proper place should be on the shelves of the medical historical society. There are two general types of suture that carry scientific efficacy in contemporary surgery: permanent synthetic and absorbable synthetic (21).

Polygalactide (L-lactide) chemistry has evolved toward making all sutures monofilament. Use of woven sutures of any type (synthetic or natural) increases the risk of bacteria invading the weave of the suture, which can act like a wick. Their use should be discouraged, particularly in wounds that have a high probability of contamination, such as those encountered in surgery of the uterus and vagina.

Permanent sutures of monofilament nylon and polypropylene, and synthetic absorbable sutures (designed with various rates of hydrolysis and absorption) are the most useful materials for most surgery. The polygalactide L-lactide chemistry determines the speed of the hydrolysis of the suture material once it is placed in tissue. The time the suture has been in the wound and its chemical composition determine the degree of its tensile strength in tissue per unit of time. The major advantage of synthetic absorbable sutures is that they dissolve by chemical hydrolysis rather than by phagocytosis. Phagocytosis is associated with an inflammatory reaction and a zone of necrosis that surrounds catgut, silk, or cotton sutures when they are used. This has implications for the integrity and ultimate strength of the wound. Ideally, rather than trade names for synthetic absorbable suture made from polygolactide L-lactide, they should have a large printed number on the package of the suture indicating the number of days this suture will take to hydrolyze to 50% of its tensile strength. If one studies the physiology and chemistry of wound closure, it would be ideal to have available 7-, 28-, 42-, and 65-day sutures. The hydrolysis of these sutures would match the chemistry and physiology of the anticipated collagen synthesis and the physics of the collagen fibril matrix formation in the wound.

Wounds in the pregnant uterus are best closed using monofilament synthetic absorbable suture that hydrolyzes to 50% of its tensile strength in 28 days. Sutures such as monofilament Byosin (U.S. Surgical Corp., Norwalk, CT) and Monocryl (Ethicon Corp., Somerville, NJ) are ideal for closure of the cesarean section uterine wound. Sutures for ligation of large pelvic vessels need more time for hydrolysis to the 50% tensile strength than do sutures required for closing a myometrial incision. Large vessels in the pelvis can be safely and adequately ligated with suture that hydrolyzes to its 50% tensile strength level in 42 days, such as Vicryl (Ethicon Corp.), Polysorb (U.S. Surgical), and Dexon (Davis & Geck Corp., Pearl River, NY). Suture for closing the fascia, muscle, and peritoneal layers of the abdominal wall should be a delayed synthetic absorbable suture such as PDS (Polydioxanone) (Ethicon, Inc.) or Maxon (Davis & Geck).

Concepts of the best technique for closure of the abdominal wall have undergone changes during recent years. The most scientifically acceptable closure from a mechanical engineering point of view is the single-layer closure of fascia, muscle, and peritoneum, referred to as the running mass closure (Fig. 50-5) (21). These sutures should be placed 3 to 4 cm from the margin of the anterior fascia and include the rectus abdominis muscle, posterior rectus fascia, and the peritoneum. They should be placed 2 to 3 cm apart along the length of the wound. This technique allows this type of suture to give with the motion of stress from coughing, respiration, and vomiting. A suture that is fixed and has no alternative to motion is more likely to tear the fascia and muscle of the wound. There are those who still prefer the running Smead-Jones suture, but it has the disadvantage of not allowing enough elasticity in the suture line to accommodate stress. There is probably little role for interrupted sutures in the closure of the abdominal wall in pregnant or nonpregnant patients.

In contaminated skin wounds such as those used to treat a ruptured appendix, ruptured colon, penetrating trauma to the bowel with fecal spillage, and severe endometritis, the skin has traditionally been left open after closure of the fascia. A delayed closure is made 5 to 7 days later. Rarely is this technique indicated in today's surgery with modern suture and surgical technique. Contaminated skin and subcutaneous fat are best excised, and the wound thoroughly irrigated and closed primarily. A small percentage of these wounds will develop a wound abscess; but it seems unfair to subject large numbers of women to the discomfort and inconvenience of a delayed wound closure for a 1% to 2% wound abscess rate. It is rare in today's surgery for so-called stay sutures to be used. These through-and-through abdominal wall sutures were previously recommended for all wounds with an increased risk of separation. Currently, wounds at risk for dehiscence are best closed after the required intraabdominal surgery with a running mass closure using large (no. 0 or 1) monofilament delayed synthetic absorbable suture such as PDS or Maxon. Alternatively, a nonabsorbable monofilament material of similar caliber can be used.

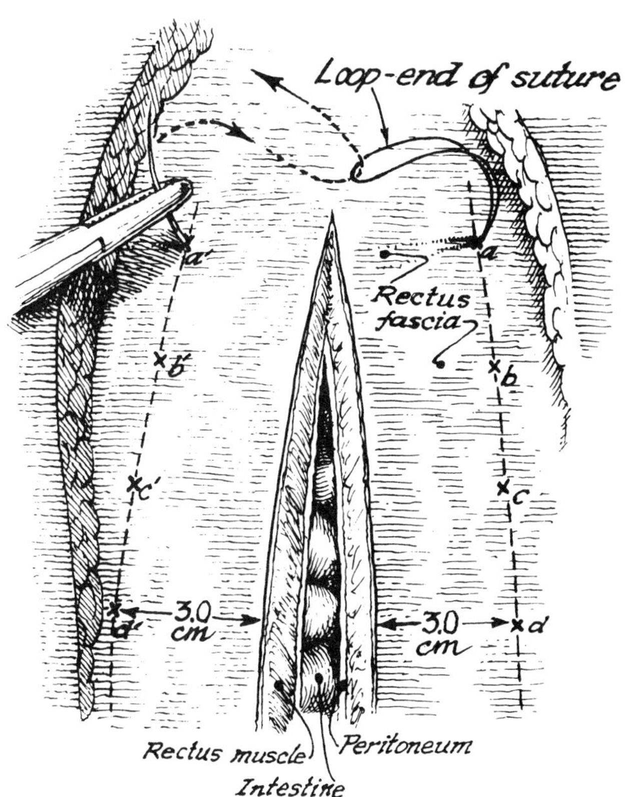

FIG. 50-5. Fascial closure with the mass running technique. The suture includes anterior rectus fascia, parectal peritoneum, and all intervening layers. (From Wheeless CR Jr. Atlas of pelvic surgery. Baltimore: Williams & Wilkins, 1997.)

The majority of obstetric wounds in the uterus and vagina can be closed with synthetic absorbable monofilament suture (not delayed), such as Byosin or Monocryl. These sutures make an excellent closure of lacerations and incisions in the vagina.

Dressings

Surgical dressings can be considered in two categories: biocclusive film dressings and traditional gauze dressings. Biocclusive film dressings consist of a synthetic sheet of clear polymer with adhesive on one side. They cover the entire incision and can remain in place for as long as needed. The biocclusive dressings have the disadvantage that if fluid drains from the wound it may disrupt the biocclusive dressing and dislodge it. The second type of dressing is traditional gauze, held in place with tape. Tape is manufactured with different chemical compositions to accommodate the patient's possible allergies.

Wounds requiring frequent dressing changes may benefit from Montgomery straps. Traditionally these are wide bands of adhesive tape fixed to the skin on both sides of the incision with an undercoating of tincture of Benzoin solution. They have umbilical cord tape tied across the bands to hold the gauze dressing over the incision in place. The umbilical tape is easily untied when access to the incision is required.

There are schools of surgical thought about wound care that vary from insistence on using no dressing at all to the use of newer spray occlusive dressings made of chemical polymers. Whether dressings of any kind clearly promote healing of surgical abdominal wounds is not clear. Dressings do serve to protect the wound for 3 to 4 days as a cushion to keep clothing and bed linens from irritating the incision and causing pain. They do not keep bacteria out of the sutured wound.

Draining wounds are best covered with modern ostomy appliance bags of various sizes and shapes that can be cut to custom fit the wound, rather than with gauze dressings. Fluid from the wound can be collected in the ostomy bag for laboratory analysis, and this approach prevents wound fluid from contact with the patient's skin.

Drains

Drains required for surgical procedures in the pregnant patient should generally consist of closed suction drains. There is no useful role for the Penrose-type drain or other open drains in contemporary surgery. The Jackson-Pratt and Hemovac suction drains serve most purposes. There is a controversy as to the need for drains after pelvic and lower abdominal surgical procedures. Several prospective, randomized studies have shown that no drainage has the same result as the use of closed suction drains. Obviously this does not apply to abscesses. They require closed suction drains placed in the abscess cavity after initial surgical drainage. Anastomoses of the bladder to the ureter or primary ureteral anastomoses need closed suction drainage to prevent the formation of an intraperitoneal uroma.

Urinary Tract Catheterization

There are few data confirming the effectiveness of prophylactic placement of ureteral stents prior to surgery in the pelvis or lower abdomen. It is far more efficacious to dissect out the ureter rather than depend on the ability of the surgeon to palpate a stent within the ureter. In some situations the stent could contribute to the risk of ureteral injury.

Catheters in the urinary bladder continue to be a source of controversy. Catheters placed for the convenience of the patient and nursing staff should be avoided. It is far better to have patients mobilized from their beds to void on bedside toilets or in the bathroom than to place an indwelling catheter for simple convenience. Catheters are indicated to decompress the bladder to prevent stretching of suture lines in the bladder wall and thus allow proper wound healing. The length of time that catheters remain in the bladder depends on the size of the wound in the bladder wall. Simple 1- to 2-cm bladder wall incisions suitably repaired usually need no Foley catheter drainage at all. This assumes that the patient will have no urinary retention from temporary detrusor malfunction. When the bladder is temporarily nonfunctional secondary to malfunctioning of the neuromyoreceptor site, a catheter is efficacious. This can be an indwelling Foley catheter or periodic straight "in and out" catheterization of the bladder every 4 to 6 hours. The latter, if done properly, may confer less risk of urinary tract infection.

The placement of a suprapubic catheter drainage tube has the advantage of being more hygienic then a transurethral catheter, and it allows the catheter to be clamped to ascertain when the detrusor muscle has regained its function. At that time the suprapubic catheter can be removed.

Stomas

Stomas result from exteriorization of the bowel on the abdominal wall for temporary or permanent drainage of feces or urine (22). Those stomas required for antepartum surgery and stomas placed in the early postpartum period may require different positions upon the abdominal wall than those placed in nonpregnant women. It is difficult for a patient to reach a stoma that is over the horizon of her abdominal wall. In general, the antepartum stoma should be placed high on the abdominal wall so that the ostomy appliance can be applied easily by the patient even when the pregnancy reaches term. Postpartum stomas can be placed in the optimal site that has been selected in consultation between the enterostomal therapist and the surgeon.

The surgeon has three choices for colostomy stomas in pregnant women: loop, end, and double-barrel colostomy (Figs. 50-6 and 50-7). The differences among these three colostomies is determined by the volume of "spill-over"

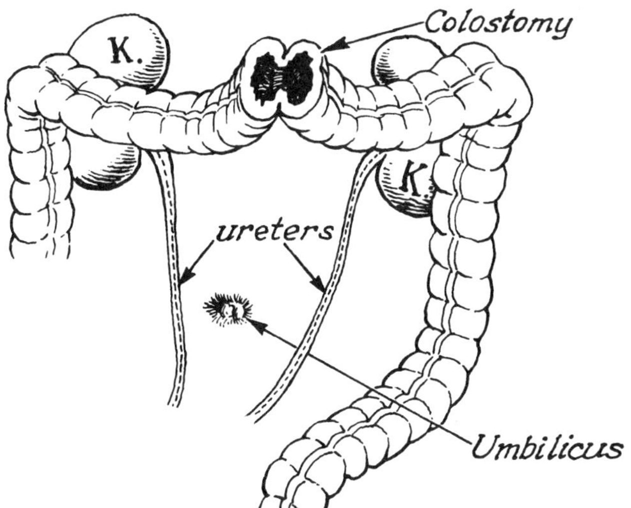

FIG. 50-6. A loop colostomy. (From Wheeless CR Jr. Atlas of pelvic surgery. Baltimore: Williams & Wilkins, 1997.)

of feces the surgeon thinks is compatible with the patient's intraabdominal pathology, the ease of reversing the colostomy in the future, and the need for a mucous fistula if there is obstruction of the colon between the colostomy and anus. Loop colostomies can be made quickly and safely for pregnant women in the second and third trimester when performed upon the transverse colon. The descending colon in the second and third trimesters is not easily accessible. An end colostomy with a Hartmann pouch may be needed if the spill-over from the afferent bowel stoma to the efferent bowel (as will occur in a loop colostomy) is not desirable. In most cases, the loop colostomy is sufficient for the needs of the pregnant patient. It also offers the advantage for closure of the colostomy postpartum after the colon-rectal problem has been treated. End colostomy is desirable when the colostomy is to be permanent. In the pregnant patient, after the first trimester, the low-end colostomy is rarely possible to perform because of the enlarging uterus.

In antepartum surgical patients who need diversion of the fecal stream and in whom bowel preparation has not taken place, a loop colostomy can be performed, and maturing of the colostomy delayed for 2 days until the peritoneum around it has sealed. The anterior wall of the colostomy can be matured on the second day. The rod under the posterior wall of a loop colostomy can be removed on the fifth postoperative day if needed. Modern colostomy appliances are available with a small rod that fits the ring of the appliance. This allows the rod to be left in longer, until wound healing has been completed (22). In prepartum as well as postpartum patients who have had the advantage of a mechanical and antibiotic bowel preparation the stoma can be matured at the time of surgery. Urostomy stomas are generally placed on the patient's right upper quadrant and colostomy stomas on the patient's left upper quadrant after the second trimester of pregnancy. The urostomy stoma is best exteriorized as a so-called "rose-bud" stoma, in which the intestine is sutured back upon itself. The stoma rises above the skin for approximately 2 cm. This allows the appliance bag to fit around the stoma so there is little leakage of urine onto the skin.

Postpartum stomas can generally be placed in the same areas as in the nonpregnant patient. Usually the colostomy stoma is in the patient's left abdominal wall at a level that avoids her waistline. The urostomy stoma is placed slightly below the level of the umbilicus on a point between the anterior superior iliac spine and the umbilicus (23). This can vary with obese patients. The site for placement of the stoma should be chosen in consultation with the enterostomal therapy nurse.

The only indication for a double-barrel colostomy with wide separation of the afferent and efferent stomas by a skin bridge is a condition in which the overflow and spillage of fecal material from the afferent to efferent

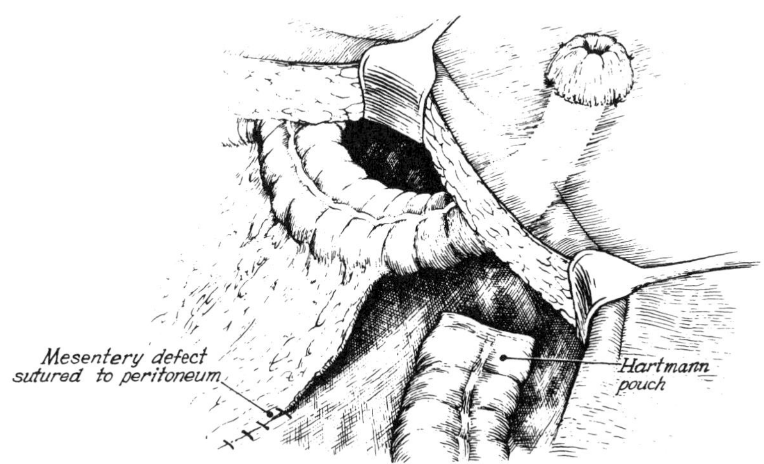

FIG. 50-7. A drawing of an end colostomy. The proximal segment of the descenting colon is used to form the stoma. The distal segment is closed as a Hartmann pouch. (From Wheeless CR Jr. Atlas of pelvic surgery. Baltimore: Williams & Wilkins, 1997.)

stoma must be almost zero, yet you need a decompression mucous fistula from the efferent stoma to relieve mucous pressure proximal to colonic obstructive disease. This is needed for obstructions in the lower rectum. The double-barrel stoma allows less spill-over than the loop colostomy and yet provides a mucous fistula to prevent development of a mucus-filled tumor in the colon or rectum (24).

Wound Infections

Prophylaxis against wound infection starts with adherence to the principle of surgery that the environment of the wound must be protected and improved. Tissues in the abdomen and pelvis have an oxidation-reduction potential that can be measured in millivolts. The normal oxidation-reduction potential in the female pelvis is approximately 150 mV. Trauma to the pelvic structures initiates a process of lowering the oxidation-reduction potential from 150 positive mV down toward 90 positive mV, at which point a clinical infection is inevitable. Bacteria in pelvic surgical wounds often originate from the vagina, which is normally colonized by bacteria. Reducing the volume of bacteria in the vagina potentially improves the environment of the surgical wound if the vagina is to be open to the surgical field, such as in cesarean section. When the wound has a smaller burden of organisms, there is more oxygen in the wound, less carbon dioxide, and fewer enzymes from tissue necrosis caused by bacteria. Reduced bacterial contamination results in a pH near 7.4, high oxidation-reduction potential, and therefore reduced chance of clinical infection (25).

Prophylactic preoperative antibiotics have been proven effective in many situations, but are not a panacea (26–28). Other features of wound care such as delicate handling of tissue, small bites of tissue in clamps, meticulous hemostasis, and proper irrigation of the wound all play a role in prophylaxis against wound infections.

The preparation of the skin prior to surgery in pregnant women serves a similar purpose. The bacterial colonization of the skin should be reduced to as small a volume as possible. This is performed in two steps: mechanical scrubbing of the skin, followed by application of antiseptic. In cesarean section, simply painting the skin with an organic iodine solution (e.g., Betadine; Clinipad Corporation, Guilford, CT) without prior scrubbing is sufficient for most cases. There are even commercial products available that have Betadine impregnated into the adhesive of a bioocclusive dressing that, when simply applied to the skin, can reduce the bacterial count in the wound environment. Shaving of the abdominal skin should be avoided. It produces multiple microlacerations that become a habitat for bacteria and promote wound infection. Excess hair can be cut without shaving. If shaving the skin is necessary, it should be done in the operating room just prior to surgery.

Postpartum wound infections in the pregnant patient generally involve postpartum endometritis, abdominal wall wound infections, and infected episiotomy incisions. The incidence of postpartum endometritis has been reduced as a consequence of the widespread use of preoperative prophylactic antibiotics (29). There are a variety of antibiotics that have demonstrable efficacy as prophylaxis against endometritis. They all function in the same manner. They reduce the volume of bacteria normally found in the vagina and, to a lesser degree, the bacteria that live on the skin. Patients who have as part of their labor more manipulation through the vagina, such as multiple pelvic examinations, stripping of membranes, amniotomy, insertion of uterine pressure catheters, attachment of scalp electrodes, or performance of blood scalp sampling, have greater contamination of the endometrium than do patients who have a simple repeat cesarean section at term prior to labor. The level of reduction of endometritis by prophylactic antibiotics is inversely related to the presence of the above factors.

The cardinal rule of prophylactic antibiotics is the same whether operating from a contaminated to a sterile area of the body or going from a sterile area into a contaminated one. It is essential that the antibiotic be started 30 minutes before the incision is made. This point is especially important and often overlooked in cesarean section patients. If one waits until the umbilical cord is clamped and then administers the antibiotic, most authorities feel there is less efficacy of the antibiotic on the incidence of postpartum endometritis then if antibiotic is given prior to clamping the cord (30). This fact needs to be thoroughly understood by the obstetricians and pediatricians taking care of the mother and infant.

Wound infections in abdominal wall incisions are diagnosed by the classic findings of erythema, tenderness, and fluctuance under the skin. Incision and drainage is the treatment of choice. The length of the drainage incision in these patients is not as important as previously thought. It is not uncommon for physicians to open the entire incision if a wound abscess is suspected. This has little demonstrable efficacy. After a small area of the wound is opened, the pus may be drained, a culture for aerobic and anaerobic bacteria taken, and the wound irrigated copiously with normal saline. Placement of antibiotics or iodine in the saline wash has not been shown to be necessary. The wound can be gently packed with a saline or Dakin's solution-soaked gauze. The traditional technique of packing wet-to-dry dressings has a long history in the surgical sciences and remains the procedure of choice. Whether antibiotics are necessary after incision and drainage of a local abscess without systemic spread of the infection remains controversial. The antibiotics, if they are given, should be guided by the cultures and sensitivities; but most patients recover who have had incision, drainage, and irrigation of their wounds. Antibiotics should definitely be given when there is evidence of a systemic infection. The infected wound should be allowed to heal by secondary intention and granulate from the fascia to the skin. There is an occasional indication for excising the granulating wound and suturing it primarily.

DEHISCENCE

Dehiscence must be differentiated from dehiscence with evisceration (Fig. 50-8). The morbidity and mortality are dramatically different, evisceration conferring greatly increased risk. The first sign of dehiscence is the leakage of peritoneal fluid through the skin closure. When serosanguinous drainage is noted, the diagnosis of dehiscence should be entertained. The wound should be opened and explored with a finger covered with a sterile glove. If there is separation of the fascia, the patient should be returned to the operating room and the fascial defect closed. If the wound is not infected and only sterile serosanguineous fluid is coming from the dehiscence in the skin, the superficial portions of the wound can be resutured at the time of fascial reclosure (31).

The etiology of dehiscence is multiple. Even when surgical closure technique has been good, separation of the rectus fascial closure can result from mechanical stress from excessive postoperative coughing, sneezing, and vomiting. Wound factors, particularly infection, may play an important part in failure of closure of the fascia wound. Systemic factors resulting in increased risk of poor wound closure are diabetes mellitus, corticosteroid therapy, and inflammatory bowel disease. Occasionally, wound dehiscence occurs in the absence of any predisposing factor.

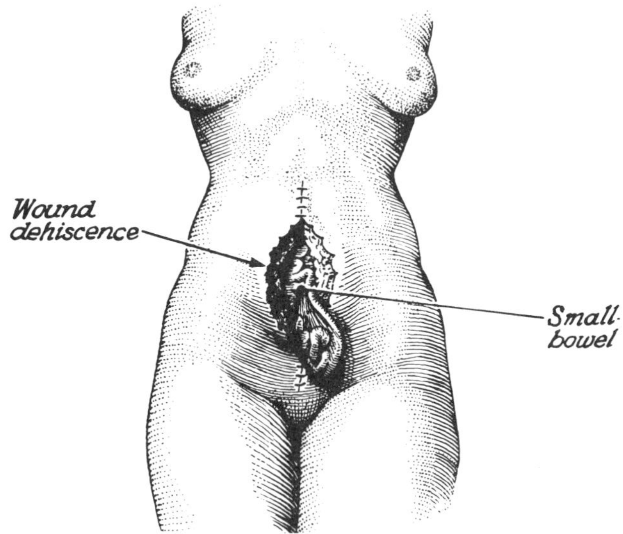

FIG. 50-8. Abdominal wound evisceration. (From Wheeless CR Jr. Atlas of pelvic surgery. Baltimore: Williams & Wilkins, 1997.)

Evisceration occurs in a small percentage of patients who have dehiscence. Poor surgical technique and suture selection are among the multiple causes of dehiscence leading to evisceration. The emergency treatment of evisceration starts at the bedside. The intestines should be replaced in the abdominal cavity using a sterile technique. The abdominal wound is covered with sterile saline-dampened towels. The patient is sedated with codeine to prevent further coughing and repeat evisceration while she is taken to the operating room promptly.

After examination under general anesthesia, all sutures and necrotic tissue should be excised. There are two acceptable techniques for closure of dehiscence with evisceration. The traditional technique has been the placement of wide stay sutures through all layers of the abdominal wall with a large monofilament material such as nylon or prolene. Stay sutures should enter the skin, and penetrate the subcutaneous fat, rectus fascia, rectus muscle, and abdominal parietal peritoneum and exit through the same layers on the opposite side. The entire abdominal wall is closed, with the portion of each suture on the surface of the abdominal wall threaded through a red rubber catheter to soften the effect of such a large suture upon the skin (32).

A contemporary acceptable technique for management of dehiscence is the standard running mass closure described above. Permanent suture such as nylon or prolene or delayed synthetic absorbable suture such as PDS and Maxon can be used. There is a trend toward the use of this technique of a running mass suture with delayed synthetic absorbable material. It is unacceptable to leave a dehiscence in the fascia to be covered only by skin. An incisional hernia or recurrent evisceration is inevitable.

Necrotizing Fascitis

Necrotizing fasciitis can be a terribly traumatic postoperative, postpartum event. It is a psychological as well as a medical disease, a catastrophe to the obstetric patient, her family, nurses, and obstetrician. It is essential that the diagnosis be made quickly and accurately. Radical debridement of the entire infected area must be performed. There is no role for conservative therapy such as incision, drainage, and antibiotics. The cause of necrotizing fasciitis is anaerobic streptococcal bacteria, frequently combined with *Clostridium*. These infections in pregnant patients are usually secondary to infected episiotomy incisions, traumatic lacerations of the vulva, trauma to the lower abdominal wall from seat belts in automobile accidents, and infected cesarean wounds. They spread rapidly. The typical picture is a patient whose is febrile with an obvious crepitant infection on the vulva and mons pubis or lower abdomen. Antibiotics alone are ineffective (33,34).

If rapid surgical attention is not performed in necrotizing fasciitis, the patient will not survive. Most cases of necrotizing fasciitis involving the labia or a cesarean incision will require a vulvectomy with resection of the abdominal wall from the mons pubis up to the umbilicus. Obviously this type of radical resection in a postpartum woman is a psychological disaster for everyone. After the surgical resection, aggressive surgical intensive care unit therapy should be instituted. The wound should be inspected on an hourly basis. If signs or symptoms of additional necrotizing fasciitis surrounding the large area of resection of the lower abdominal wound are noted, the patient should be taken back to the operating room and additional tissue resected.

These wounds can never be closed primarily. After the infectious process has been completed, the wounds may be grafted with split-thickness skin grafts or possibly covered with rotation flaps in areas where they are available.

GASTROINTESTINAL INJURIES

Gastrointestinal injuries in the pregnant woman in the third trimester are rare. Bowel perforation at the time of cesarean section occurs on occasion. In the third trimester the most common entry into the gastrointestinal tract is the fourth-degree tear of the rectum and anus at delivery. Repair of the fourth-degree tear should reconstruct the anal mucosa, vagina, superficial transverse peronei muscle, anal sphincter muscle, and perineal body. This repair should be executed with monofilament synthetic absorbable suture. The most common cause of failure of repair of fourth-degree tears is wound infection. Other contributors to wound repair failure can be diabetes, inflammatory bowel disease, and smoking. In some instances it may be a consequence of poor surgical technique. The wound failure can result in incontinence of feces and flatus, and most cases are associated with severe entrance dyspareunia (35).

Even penetrating missile wounds into the abdominal wall in the third trimester that injure the gastrointestinal tract are unusual. The largest reported series is from the American University Hospital in Beirut (5). The term pregnant uterus, with its large sac of amniotic fluid, serves as a barrier for the fetus and the mother from gunshot wounds.

In the first and second trimester, gunshot and stab wounds may result in perforation of the gastrointestinal tract more often than in the third trimester. The uterus is smaller in size and there is more intestine exposed to the abdominal wall (5). Surgical enterotomy associated with treatment of acute appendicitis, cholecystitis, and ovarian cyst is more common in the first and second trimester than in the third trimester. When enterotomy occurs, the most common site is the terminal ileum. Approximately 85% of enterotomies associated with obstetric and gynecologic problems occur in the terminal ileum. The transverse and rectosigmoid colon account for the remaining 15% of gastrointestinal injuries.

Perforating injuries from sharp objects to the small and large bowel are best managed by exploratory laparotomy and simple closure of the penetrating wounds. High-velocity missile wounds from firearms require wide resection of the damaged bowel tissue. The missile entering the wound destroys cells in the bowel proportionately to the velocity, and tissue injury may occur at a considerable distance from the perforation. This is why simple closure of the perforation site is not an acceptable technique (36).

Colostomy or ileostomy following resection and closure of intestinal perforations is rarely indicated. Most series of reported perforated bowel wounds have demonstrated that more morbidity and mortality is associated with a protective diverting colostomy or ileostomy than with primary closure of the intestinal wound, copious lavage of the abdominal cavity, placement of the patient on broad-spectrum antibiotics, and not draining the abdominal cavity (37). In the rare case of a perforating injury to the rectosigmoid colon in the late second and third trimester, surgical access to the enterotomy may be difficult without delivery of the fetus (12). The most efficacious procedure would often be rough suture closure of the colonic wound and a protective loop diverting colostomy of the transverse colon. Adequate exposure for a proper anastomosis of the penetrating wound in the lower colon would be difficult because of the third-trimester pregnant uterus, and the fetus may be judged too premature for delivery.

The proper technique for closure of a penetrating wound of the bowel by a sharp instrument (knife, scalpel, scissors, etc.) is the closure of the enterotomy either with sutures or one of the surgical stapling instruments (Fig. 50-9), cleansing of all fecal material from the abdomen by multiple washings with saline, closure of the abdomen without drains or colostomy, and placement of the patient on antibiotics chosen with the fetus in mind. The same is true for penetrating wounds of the small intestine or stomach.

Postoperative care for gastrointestinal tract injuries in pregnancy may require total parenteral nutrition. Generally an 1,800-calorie diet diluted to 1 calorie/mL is useful; but more calories may be necessary depending on the stage of pregnancy. A balance between protein, carbohydrates, fat, and trace elements is needed. An excellent nutritional technique after gastrointestinal surgery is the

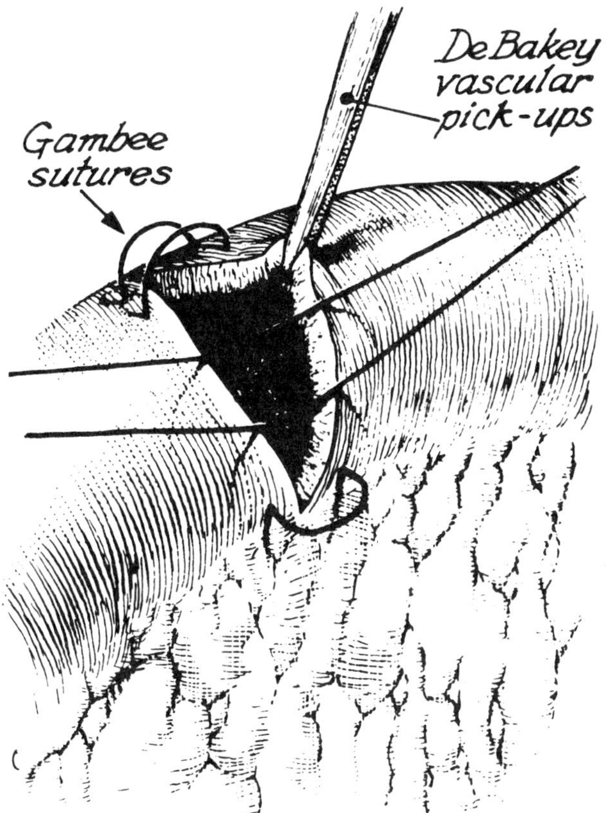

FIG. 50-9. Gambee suture closure of an enterotomy. (From Wheeless CR Jr. Atlas of pelvic surgery. Baltimore: Williams & Wilkins, 1997.)

utilization of enteral feedings beyond the ligament of Treitz in the jejunum. A standard enteral nutrition formula with 1 calorie/mL that includes ample amounts of glutamine and arginine per day will stimulate the brush border of the mucosa in the small bowel, thus aiding in protection from sepsis from the intestinal organisms crossing the mucosa. Intestinal bacteria have the ability to cross injured bowel mucosa and enter the vasculature. Patients fed only with total parenteral nutrition need the branched-chain amino acids glutamine and arginine. Enteral feeding can be performed immediately after gastrointestinal surgery in most cases (38).

GENITOURINARY INJURIES

Genitourinary injuries in the pregnant woman are most commonly injuries to the bladder at the time of cesarean section. The ureters can be injured at cesarean hysterectomy, by blunt and sharp trauma. Sometimes clamping the uterine artery and vein to control postpartum hemorrhage may result in accidental crushing of the ureter.

When the bladder is dissected caudally with blunt dissection using a sponge stick or the surgeon's finger, the bladder can be torn. The proper method for dissecting the bladder from the cervix is sharp dissection with scissors. This will minimize risk of injury.

When the bladder has been lacerated, the cystotomy wound should be closed in two layers with synthetic monofilament absorbable suture, such as Monocryl (Fig. 50-10). A Foley catheter should be inserted transurethrally into the bladder until the incision has properly sealed and detrusor muscle function has been restored. During cesarean section hysterectomy, the possibility of injury to the bladder and ureters is considerable. The ureter is usually injured at the junction of the uterine artery and ureter or near the infundibulopelvic ligament when the adnexae are removed. The ureters should be repaired over a ureteral stent (Fig. 50-11). The stent should be left in place for 2 weeks, then removed with a cystoscope (39). It is efficacious to drain ureteral anastomoses with a closed-suction drain such as a Jackson-Pratt.

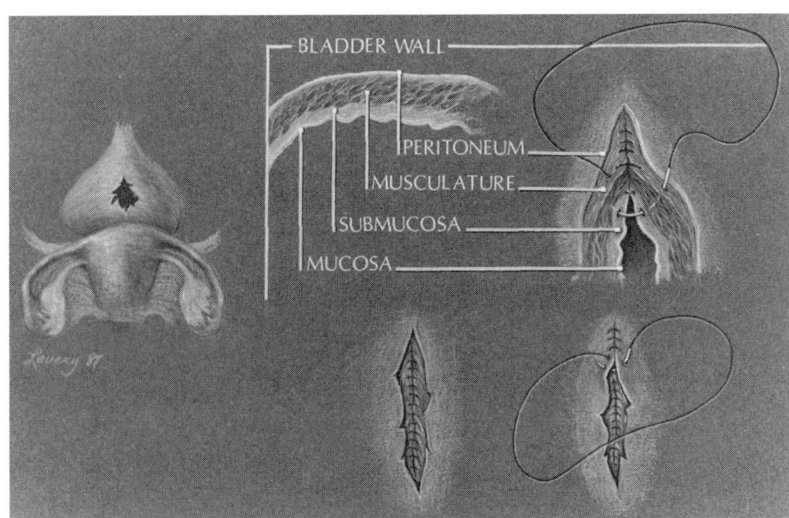

FIG. 50-10. Suture closure of a cystotomy. (From Wheeless CR Jr. Atlas of pelvic surgery. Baltimore: Williams & Wilkins, 1997.)

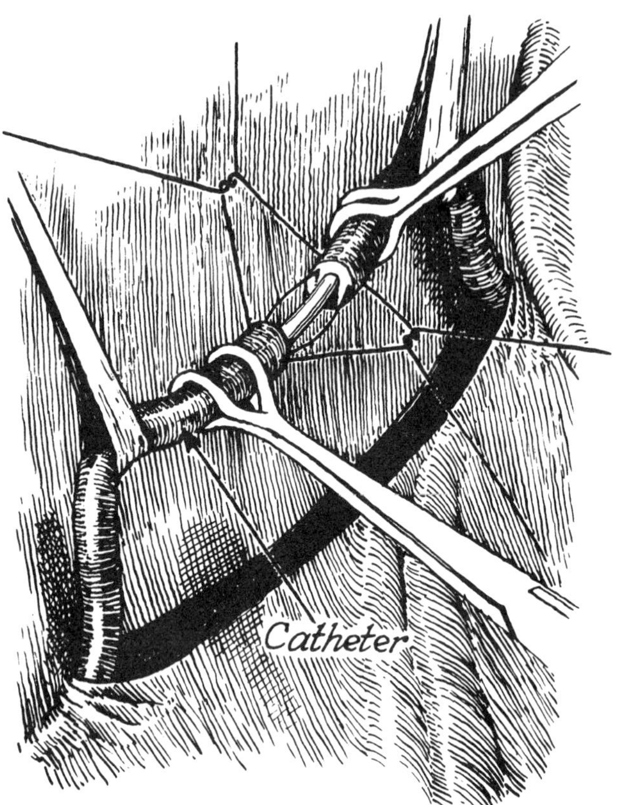

FIG. 50-11. A ureteral stent is in place in preparation for anastomosis. (From Wheeless CR Jr. Atlas of pelvic surgery. Baltimore: Williams & Wilkins, 1997.)

POSTOPERATIVE CARE

Postoperative care in the pregnant or postpartum patient centers around the respiratory, cardiovascular, and renal systems. The respiratory rate must be monitored by the staff in the recovery room. The patient should not be extubated until she can breathe on her own. The magnesium level is very important for proper breathing. In a patient with a magnesium level below 1.0 mg/dL, the magnesium should be replaced by intravenous infusion until a proper level of 1.8 to 2.0 mg/dL has been achieved. Low levels of magnesium are common after prolonged surgery. There will be a tendency toward metabolic acidosis in these patients. Respiratory acidosis and alkalosis are rare in postoperative pregnant patients. Metabolic acidosis is more common and should be treated in part by increasing the plasma oncotic pressure, by expanding the vascular space with colloids as well as crystalloids. If the urinary output is adequate (greater than 50 mL/h), most postpartum patients will self-correct their metabolic acidosis through their kidneys and, to a lesser extent, from respiration. Transfusion is an important consideration, and blood loss of over 500 mL should be replaced if there is any hint of instability in the patient. However, multiple blood transfusions in obstetric patients are probably unnecessary unless there is demonstrable vascular instability.

Pregnant patients with nonmetastatic gestational trophoblastic neoplasia (hydatidiform mole) should be monitored for the special problem of pulmonary edema associated with anemia and rapid blood transfusion. This phenomenon is well recognized, but the exact etiology is not known.

The bladder in postpartum patients should be carefully monitored for urinary retention and failure to void. This can occur even if there has been no surgery performed on the bladder. The technique of periodic "in and out" catheterization by a straight catheter is preferable to an indwelling Foley catheter.

The etiology of postoperative fever can be identified in most cases using the axiom of the five W's. These W's stand for wonder drugs, wind, wound, walking, and water. Ninety percent of postpartum operative sepsis can be identified using the 5 W's. The first W stands for the allergic reaction to "wonder drugs." Eosinophilia in the white blood cell count is a helpful finding in making the diagnosis of a drug reaction. "Walking" reminds the physician to search for deep vein thrombophlebitis of the legs or pelvis. It is a common finding in postoperative pregnant patients. "Water" stands for urinary tract infection, and "wound" for endometritis or a wound infection in the abdominal wall incision. "Wind" is the last W. The most common source of fever in the immediate postoperative period is atelectasis.

Surgical considerations in the pregnant patient are vital if the future health and quality of life in mother and fetus are to be maintained. Fortunately, most parturitions are vaginal births and do not require operative surgery. Abdominal gastrointestinal and urologic surgery is rarely undertaken in the pregnant patient except when indicated owing to trauma, appendicitis, and cholecystitis. This makes the consideration of surgical problems more important because they are not common and not prominent in the obstetrician's mind. The general axiom noted previously should be followed, to "take the disease out of the pregnancy rather than the pregnancy out of the disease."

REFERENCES

1. Samuels P, Landon MB. Medical Complications. In: Gabbe SG, Niebyl JR, Simpson JL, eds. Obstetrics. Normal and problem pregnancies. New York: Churchill Livingstone, 1986.
2. Cogan MG. Fluid & electrolytes: Physiology and pathophysiology. New York: Appleton & Lange, 1991.
3. Schrier RW. Body fluid volume regulation in health and disease: a unifying hypothesis. Ann Intern Med 1990;113:155–159.
4. Henricks CH, Quilligan EJ. Cardiac output during labor. Am J Obstet Gynecol 1956;71:953.
5. Awwad JT, Azar GB, Seoud MA, Mroueh AM, Karam KS. High-velocity penetrating wounds of the gravid uterus: review of 16 years of civil war. Obstet Gynecol 1994;83:259–264.
6. Bartlett RH. Special problems in perioperative care (VII): pulmonary insufficiency. In: Wilmore DW, Cheung LY, Harken AH, et al., eds. New York: Scientific American Surgery, 1996.
7. Thompson JD. Operative injuries to the ureter: prevention, recognition, and management. In: Thompson JD, Rock JA, eds. TeLinde's operative gynecology, 7th ed. Philadelphia: JB Lippincott, 1992:1135–1174.

8. Handelsman JC, Zieler S, Coleman J, Dooley W, Walrath JM. Experience with ambulatory preoperative bowel preparation at The Johns Hopkins Hospital. Arch Surg 1993;128:441–444.
9. DiSaia JP, Creasman WT. Cancer in Pregnancy. In: DiSaia JP, Creasman WT, eds. Clinical gynecologic oncology, 4th ed. St. Louis; Mosby-Year Book, 1993:533–581.
10. Wheeless CR. Atlas of pelvic Surgery, 3rd ed., Baltimore: Williams & Wilkins, 1997.
11. Plauche WC. Rupture of the uterus. In: Nichols DH, ed. Gynecologic and obstetric surgery. St. Louis: Mosby-Year Book, 1993:1135–1146.
12. Buchsbaum HJ, ed. Penetrating injury of the abdomen: trauma in pregnancy. Philadelphia: WB Saunders, 1979:82.
13. Pearlman MD, Tintinalli JE. Evaluation and treatment of the gravida and fetus following trauma during pregnancy. Obstet Gynecol Clin North Am 1991;18:371–381.
14. Wheeless CR. Atlas of pelvic surgery, 3rd ed. Baltimore: Williams & Wilkins, 1997.
15. Cue JI, Cryer HG, Miller FB, Richardson JD, Polk HC. Packing and planned re-exploration for hepatic and retroperitoneal hemorrhage: critical refinements of a useful technique. J Trauma 1990;30:1007–1011.
16. Rock JA, Damario MA. Ectopic Pregnancy. In: Rock JA, Thompson JD, eds. TeLinde's operative gynecology, 8th ed. Philadelphia: Lippincott-Raven, 1997:501–528.
17. Strafford JC, Ragan WD. Abdominal pregnancy. Review of current management. Obstet Gynecol 1977;50:548–552.
18. Ball TL, Nichols DH. Penetrating wounds of the pregnant uterus and fetus. In: Ball TL, Nichols DH, eds. Obstetrical and gynecology surgery. St. Louis: Mosby, 1993:1163–1166.
19. Thompson JD, Warshaw JS. The vermiform appendix in relation to gynecology. In: Rock JA, Thompson JD, eds. TeLinde's operative gynecology, 8th ed. Philadelphia: Lippincott-Raven, 1997:1267–1287.
20. Lewis RT, Wiegand FM. Natural history of vertical abdominal parietal closure: Prolene versus Dexon. Can J Surg 1989;32:196–200.
21. Lipscomb GH, Ling FR. Wound healing, suture material, and surgical instrumentation. In: Rock JA, Thompson JD, eds. TeLinde's operative gynecology, 8th ed. Philadelphia: Lippincott-Raven, 1997: 263–281.
22. Abrams JS. Abdominal stomas: indications, operative technique and patient care. Boston: John Wright PSG, 1984:1–157.
23. Barwin BN, Harley JMG. Ileostomy in Pregnancy. Br J Clin Pract 1944;20:256–258.
24. Wheeless CR. Recent advances in surgical reconstruction of the gynecologic cancer patient. Curr Opin Obstet Gynecol 1992;4:91–101.
25. Sanders WE. Principles of antimicrobial therapy. In: Monif RG, ed. Infectious diseases in obstetrics and gynecology, 2nd ed. Philadelphia: Harper & Row, 1982.
26. Allen JL, Rampone JF, Wheeless CR. Use of prophylactic antibiotics in elective major gynecologic operations. Obstet Gynecol 1972;39:218–224.
27. Ledger WJ. Antimicrobial agents. In: Ledger WJ, ed. Infection in the female. Philadelphia: Lea & Febiger, 1977:94–126.
28. Hoeprich PD. Current principles of antibiotic therapy. Obstet Gynecol 1980;55(suppl):121S–127S.
29. Chang PL, Newton ER. Predictors of antibiotic prophylactic failure in post-cesarean endometritis. Obstet Gynecol 1992;80:117–122.
30. Cunningham FG, Leveno KJ, DePalma RT, Roark M, Rosenfeld CR. Perioperative antimicrobials for cesarean delivery: before or after cord clamping? Obstet Gynecol 1983;62:151–154.
31. Helmkamp BF. Abdominal wound dehiscence. Am J Obstet Gynecol 1977;128:803–807.
32. Rollins RA, Corcoran JJ, Gibbs CE. Treatment of gynecologic wound complications. Obstet Gynecol 1966;28:268–270.
33. Owen J, Andrews WW. Wound complications after cesarean sections. Clin Obstet Gynecol 1994;37:842–855.
34. Ramin SM, Ramus RM, Little BB. Early repair of episiotomy dehiscence associated with infection. Am J Obstet Gynecol 1992;167:1104–1107.
35. Wheeless CR. Ten steps to avoid fecal incontinence secondary to fourth degree obstetrical tear. Obstet Gynecol Surv 1998;53:131–132.
36. Thompson BH, Wheeless CR. Gastrointestinal complications of laparoscopy sterilization. Obstet Gynecol 1973;41:669–676.
37. Chappuis CW, Frey DJ, Dietzen CD, Panetta TP, Buechter KJ, Cohn I Jr. Management of penetrating colon injuries. A prospective randomized trial. Ann Surg 1991;213:492–497.
38. Moore FA, Feliciano DV, Andrassy RJ, et al. Early enteral feeding compared with parental, reduces postoperative septic complications: results of meta-analysis. Ann Surg 1992;216:172–183.
39. Clark SL, Yeh SY, Phelan JP, Bruce S, Paul RH. Emergency hysterectomy for obstetric hemorrhage. Obstet Gynecol 1984;64:376–380.

Cherry and Merkatz's Complications of Pregnancy,
Fifth Edition, edited by W. R. Cohen.

CHAPTER 51

Postpartum Hemorrhage and Hemorrhagic Shock

Wayne R. Cohen

The third stage of labor and the puerperium are normally associated with some uterine bleeding. Excessive blood loss occurs in 2% to 10% of deliveries (1,2), but severe hemorrhage probably develops in about 1% of all pregnancies (3). Nevertheless, serious postpartum hemorrhage is a major contributor to maternal mortality and morbidity (see Chapter 49) (4–6). All obstetricians should be aware of how to manage this potentially lethal complication.

Postpartum hemorrhage is generally categorized as acute (developing within the first 24 hours after delivery) or delayed (evolving between 1 day and 6 weeks postpartum). The definition of acute postpartum hemorrhage is elusive because clinical estimates of blood loss are notoriously inaccurate and the range of bleeding after normal delivery is quite broad. Generally, postpartum blood loss in excess of 500 mL is considered abnormal. Investigators who have used carefully controlled techniques to estimate blood loss at birth suggest that during vaginal delivery it is generally not more than 500 mL to 1,000 mL and that the average loss at cesarean section is about 1,000 mL (7,8). Late postpartum hemorrhage is even more difficult to define, because quantitation of normal blood loss in the late puerperium has not been documented. Nevertheless, it is reasonable to assume that any bleeding over and above the light spotting that characterizes lochia after the first postpartum week should be considered abnormal.

Several obstetric features predispose to postpartum hemorrhage (Table 51-1). Advanced maternal age and parity and a history of puerperal hemorrhage in a previous pregnancy are risk factors. If a third-stage complication arose in the previous pregnancy, there is at least a 20% likelihood of one occurring in subsequent gestations (9). Conditions that result in uterine overdistension (e.g., polyhydramnios, multiple gestation, and fetal macrosomia) are also predisposing factors, as are those that interfere with uterine contractility (e.g., chorioamnionitis, tocolytic drugs, leiomyomata, and uterine inversion). Many acquired or inherited coagulation abnormalities result in an increased likelihood of excessive postpartum bleeding (2,10). Both prolonged and precipitate labors are risk factors, as are diseases that have the potential to diminish smooth-muscle contractility.

Forceps delivery and cesarean section can both result in excessive blood loss from intentional (large episiotomy, uterine incision) or unanticipated (laceration) trauma to the birth canal. Operative intervention during a very long second stage of labor accounts for the increased risk of postpartum hemorrhage reported in those situations (11). The presence of factors that generally predispose to antepartum hemorrhage, such as placenta previa

TABLE 51-1. *Risk factors for postpartum hemorrhage*

Obstetric factors	Maternal factors
Cesarean section	Inherited coagulopathy
Instrumental delivery	Previous postpartum hemorrhage
Chorioamnionitis	Uterine malformations
Dysfunctional labor	Grand multiparity
Oxytocin administration	Myotonic dystrophy
Birth canal injury	Dermatomyositis
Prolonged third stage	Anticoagulant/antiplatelet drugs
Placenta previa	Distended bladder
Placenta accreta	Uterine arteriovenous malformations
Multiple gestation	Acquired coagulopathy
Leiomyomata uteri	
Hydramnios	
Tocolytic drug use	
Inhalation anesthesia	
Low-lying placenta	
Placental anomalies	
Uterine inversion	

W. R. Cohen: Sinai Hospital of Baltimore, Baltimore, MD.

and abruptio placentae, are also associated with postpartum hemorrhage.

When any of these risk factors is known to exist, the obstetrician should make certain preparations in anticipation of excess immediate postpartum blood loss. Plans for delivery in an institution with the resources and personnel to deal with serious hemorrhage and an active pharmacologic approach to minimizing blood loss during and after the third stage of labor are important (12–14). These preparations can minimize the risk of postpartum hemorrhage and result in its efficient management if it occurs. Unfortunately, hemorrhage cannot be always predicted or avoided. At least two-thirds of cases of postpartum hemorrhage develop in the absence of predisposing factors.

ACUTE POSTPARTUM HEMORRHAGE

The most commom sources of postpartum hemorrhage are genital tract trauma, uterine atony, and retained placental tissue. Less often, coagulation abnormalities cause or contribute to hemorrhage. A thorough and systematic inspection of the cervix, vagina, labia, and perineum should be done after every delivery, even if there is no obvious hemorrhage. Much subsequent trouble can be avoided by detection and proper repair of lacerations of the lower genital tract before the patient leaves the delivery room. Injuries to the cervix and vagina are most common after dysfunctional labor or operative vaginal delivery, but they can occur under any circumstances.

Uterine rupture is an unusual, but obviously very serious cause of postpartum bleeding. Although many patients with rupture have initial symptoms of abdominal pain and obvious signs of massive hemorrhage, uterine scars can sometimes dehisce relatively silently, with initially minimal bleeding and symptoms. An exploration of the uterine cavity should be performed when possible in patients who deliver with risk factors for uterine rupture; lack of any apparent signs does not, however, completely exclude the diagnosis of rupture, because small discontinuities in the uterine wall are not always detectable.

Retained Placenta

Retained secundines can take several forms, from complete retention of the attached or separated placenta to fragments of cotyledons or membranes that remain stubbornly behind after placental expulsion. When allowed to evolve spontaneously, placental delivery usually occurs within 15 minutes of birth, and only 2% to 3% of placentas remain unexpelled after 30 minutes. Some form of intervention should thus generally occur after 30 minutes of the third stage of labor (1,12); nevertheless, one report (15) suggests that the normal third stage might be considered to take even longer.

When the placenta fails to deliver promptly, it has usually separated, and a contracted lower uterine segment prevents complete expulsion. Sometimes the placental cake separates from the uterine wall, but adherence of membranes to the surrounding decidua can prevent expulsion (16). In other circumstances, normal separation of the placenta does not occur. For unexplained reasons, unusually broad, flat placentas or those with excessive lobulation often do not separate after delivery, but failure to separate can happen even when the placenta appears to be completely normal. The possibility of placenta accreta should always be considered. In the absence of this feared complication, the placenta can generally be readily cleaved from the uterine wall by the examiner.

Some authorities recommend the use of oxytocin for a retained placenta, and this approach would be salutary in circumstances in which delayed separation is attributable to inadequate contractility. This technique seems reasonable, because the normal third stage is probably accompanied by a release of endogenous oxytocin (17); however, the administration of such a uterotonic can make subsequent manual exploration of the uterus quite difficult.

Manual extraction of the placenta must always be done carefully, to ensure that placental tissue is removed completely, that the patient's discomfort is minimized, and that no trauma is induced in the birth canal. On rare occasions, even uterine rupture can result from careless attempts at placental removal. Often minimal analgesia or anesthesia is all that is required, but at times uterine relaxant anesthesia or a β-mimetic drug is necessary to allow sufficient myometrial relaxation for entry of the examining hand. It is surprisingly easy to perforate a uterus thus relaxed, and the exploration must be done with utmost care. Whenever there is even the remotest suspicion of placenta accreta, the obstetrician should ensure that blood will be promptly available for transfusion.

Another maneuver to encourage separation of a retained placenta has been described. Injection of oxytocin into the umbilical vein can expedite placental delivery in both the normal (18) and prolonged (19) third stage. The required dose is between 20 and 100 U of oxytocin. The true efficacy and risks of this approach are as yet uncertain.

Placenta Accreta

Placenta accreta is a condition in which the trophoblast implants without the layer of decidua basalis that is normally interposed between it and the muscular uterine wall. Thus, the placenta attaches directly to or even invades the myometrium. The definitive diagnosis of placenta accreta can be made only on histologic examination, but the problem should be presumed to exist whenever a distinct cleavage plane cannot be developed between the placenta and the uterine wall. Various degrees of placenta accreta occur in about 1 in 2,500 deliveries (20). This results in failure of the placenta to separate after delivery, and attempts to identify a cleavage plane during manual removal can produce considerable hemorrhage. When the entire placental bed is adherent, no discrete plane of separation can be found. Sometimes only focal areas are involved in the abnormal implantation, and these tend to result in the most severe hemorrhage as stubborn attempts to remove adherent portions of the placenta are made. Hysterectomy is usually necessary and should be considered standard therapy, but on occasion it can be avoided if the accreta is focal, blood loss is not excessive, and bleeding is controllable by other measures (21). Anecdotal cases of treatment of retained placenta accreta with methotrexate have appeared (22). The efficacy and safety of this approach have yet to be determined.

There is an association between placenta accreta and placenta previa, especially when the latter condition overlies the site of previous uterine incision. About 5% to 10% of patients with placenta previa have placenta accreta. Implantation over a hysterotomy scar increases that risk threefold (20). The dramatic increase in the number of cesarean sections performed during the past 20 years will undoubtedly increase the frequency with which placenta accreta is encountered. One study suggested that the incidence of placenta accreta during pregnancy in a patient with three or more previous cesarean sections is more than 50% (21); another found that in a group of 711 patients who became pregnant after previous cesarean section, there were 10 cases (1.4%) of catastrophic hemorrhage, including 7 cases of placenta previa (23). When the placenta invades anteriorly into the bladder, bleeding can be particularly pernicious (24). When placenta percreta is suspected on ultrasound examination, the surgeon should be prepared to deal with (or preferably to avoid) massive hemorrhage.

Ultrasound findings that suggest various degrees of placenta accreta include absence of the normal hypoechoic space between the placenta and the uterine wall and large atypical vessels within or extending through the myometrial wall. The sensitivity and specificity of these findings are yet to be determined. When they are present, they strongly suggest abnormal placentation; when they are absent, placenta accreta can still exist. Magnetic resonance imaging might prove useful (25), but current experience with this approach for diagnosis of placenta accreta is limited.

Several surgical options should be considered if placenta accreta (especially percreta) is suspected. The chosen approach needs to be tailored to the specific clinical situation. The uterine incision should be planned to avoid the placental site. After delivery of the fetus, a thorough assessment of the situation should be made. If the diagnosis is certain and hysterectomy is planned, begin the procedure without disturbing the placental site. Consider ligation of the internal iliac arteries before hysterectomy is begun, especially if placenta percreta exists. If it is necessary to attempt removal of the placenta, do so gingerly and do not persist if a separating plane is not readily identified. Above all, be sure that blood for transfusion is available and that venous access is adequate. Blood loss in these situations can be stunningly rapid and profuse. The surgeon should be capable of dealing promptly with exsanguinating hemorrhage.

Uterine Atony

When the normal mechanism for uterine contraction after delivery of the fetus and placenta is disordered, severe bleeding can result. Uterine atony accounts for the vast majority of cases of postpartum hemorrhage (26) and for about 40% of hysterectomies done for obstetric hemorrhage (27). An overdistended uterus, dysfunctional labor, use of oxytocin, leiomyomata, and uterine infection all appear to predispose to uterine atony, although it can occur in the absence of any risk factors. When the likelihood of atony is increased or when there is a history of third-stage problems in previous pregnancies, the use of oxytocin immediately after placental delivery is important, as is gentle massage of the uterine fundus.

Initial pharmacotherapy of uterine atony should be intravenous oxytocin infusion, at a rate of at least 50 mU/min (Fig. 51-1). This should be combined with manual uterine stimulation, because sometimes massage of the uterus will provoke contraction. In addition, compression of an atonic uterus might slow bleeding while one awaits the benefits of drug therapy. Uterine compression is readily accomplished when the abdomen is opened at cesarean section. Placing one hand in the pouch of Douglas and wrapping the fingers firmly about the lower uterine segment and broad ligaments might provide a degree of uterine artery constriction while the other hand compresses the fundus directly. When the abdomen is closed, the uterus should be anteflexed, and compressed by the examiner with one hand in the patient's vagina and the other on the abdominal wall.

Failure of hemorrhage to respond readily to uterine massage and to oxytocin administration should prompt reevaluation of the birth canal to rule out lacerations as the source of hemorrhage. Uterine exploration should be done with a gauze-covered hand or large curette. Even if the delivered placenta appears to be intact, retained fragments or accessory lobes are surprisingly common. Uterine rupture can sometimes be diagnosed in this fashion as well. Moreover, curettage sometimes provokes uterine contractions even if no retained placental tissue is removed. Anesthesia will be necessary for uterine exploration or curettage, and it is necessary to carefully communicate with the anesthesiologist regarding the need to avoid uterine relaxant agents.

Administration of an ergot derivative, such as ergonovine or ergometrine, can be considered when oxytocin and uterine compression are ineffective. Intramuscular

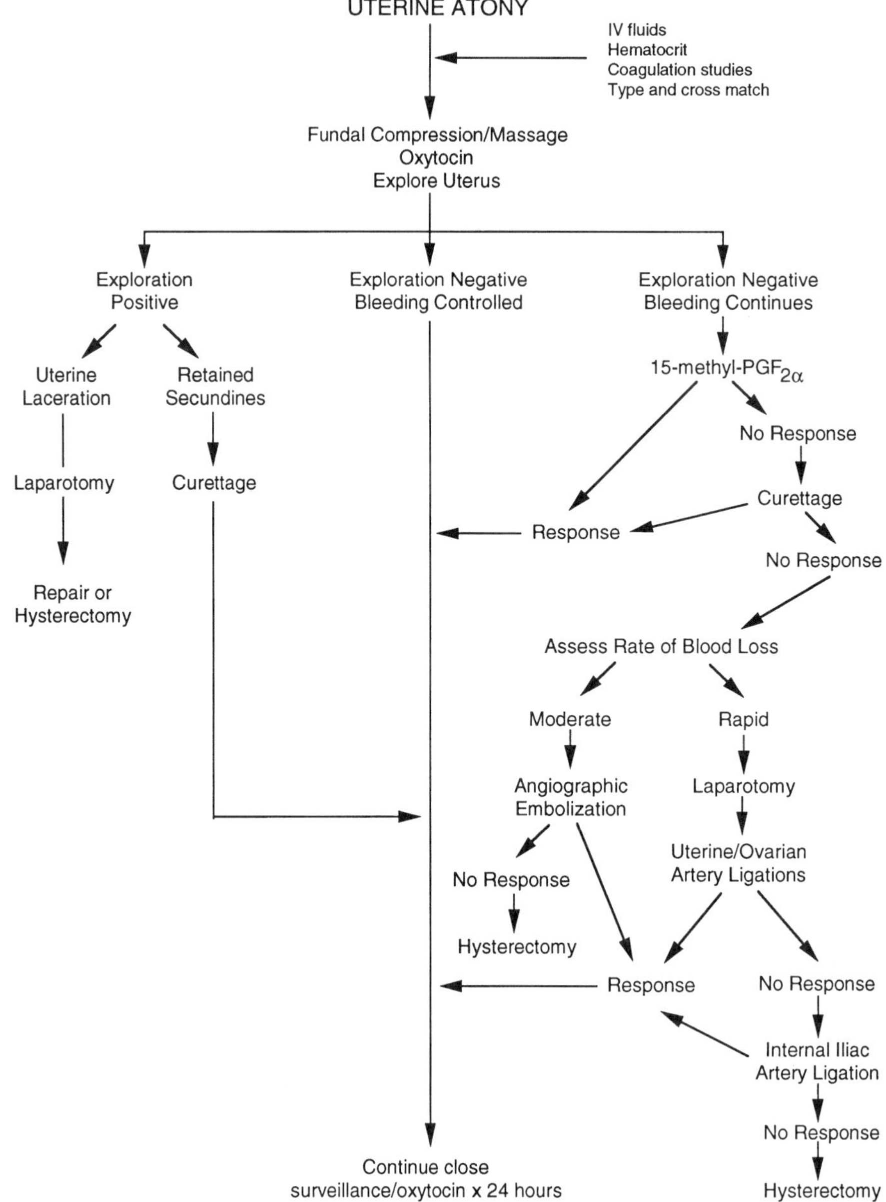

FIG. 51-1. Algorithm for the systematic management of hemorrhage from uterine atony.

administration does not cause the marked rise in blood pressure that sometimes develops when these drugs are given intravenously; however, absorption from muscle can be unpredictable, especially when peripheral perfusion is diminished in hypotensive patients. Ergot derivatives should probably not be used if the patient is hypertensive or otherwise hemodynamically unstable. Moreover, reports of coronary artery spasm (28) are disturbing, and ergot derivatives, once a standard of obstetric care, are being used less frequently.

If bleeding continues after massage, curettage, and oxytocin infusion and the uterus remains atonic, further pharmacologic therapy is indicated. The development of a 15-methylated analogue of prostaglandin $F_{2\alpha}$ ($PGF_{2\alpha}$) has added a new dimension to the management of severe postpartum hemorrhage, and use of this drug has largely supplanted that of ergot derivatives. This prostaglandin, carboprost tromethamine, has been approved for injection into skeletal muscle, although intramyometrial administration is also effective. The drug is more potent and has a longer duration of action than its parent compound. Results of several studies suggest that 60% to 85% of patients with uterine atony unresponsive to standard therapy can be treated successfully with 15-methyl $PGF_{2\alpha}$ (29,30). Most patients who have responded have done so after one or two doses of 250 μg intramuscularly. Repeated injections can be made at 15- to 90-minute intervals, depending on need. In one study in which intramyometrial injection was used (31), a second dose was given within 5 minutes of the first, without adverse reaction. Blood levels peak 15 to 60 minutes after intramuscular injection, and sometimes therapeutic effects are not observed until this amount of time has passed.

Side effects of 15-methyl $PGF_{2\alpha}$ include a 10% to 25% incidence of gastrointestinal symptoms and about a 5% incidence of pyrexia. Hypertension develops rarely. The drug is contraindicated in women with cardiovascular or pulmonary disease, because of its potential hypertensive and bronchoconstrictor effects. One report cited arterial desaturation associated with carboprost therapy, possibly a consequence of increased intrapulmonary shunting (32). While the significance and prevalence of this problem remain to be determined, it must be emphasized that the potential for serious side effects of the drug exists, despite its considerable advantages. Patients who receive carboprost should be monitored carefully.

If massage, curettage, and uterotonic therapy are to no avail, surgical or angiographic treatment should be considered. There are still advocates of uterine packing (33), and it can work. It is infrequently helpful, however, and carries considerable risks, not the least of which is providing a false sense of security as hemorrhage continues unobserved. Another pharmacologic alternative has been suggested to avoid the need for surgery. The intramyometrial injection of vasopressin (5 IU in 19 mL normal saline) at the placental site has been reported to control otherwise intractable uterine bleeding after cesarean section in several patients (34). Prolonged manual uterine compression can be lifesaving (35), as can aortic compression (36,37). The latter procedure is obviously readily accomplished at laparotomy, but in most patients it is possible to effect through the closed abdomen by exerting pressure with a fist over the distal aorta. Disappearance of femoral pulses indicates that the maneuver has been successful, and it might be useful as a temporizing measure while preparations are made for more definitive therapy.

Reports of successful uterine tamponade with the esophageal balloon of a Sengstaken-Blakemore tube (as an alternative to packing) have appeared (38), as have reports of cases in which intrauterine prostaglandins (39) or intravenous antifibrinolytic agents were used (38,40). The true efficacy and risks of these therapies are unknown.

Other Causes

Heavy uterine bleeding can sometimes occur in the absence of uterine atony and without genital trauma or evidence of a coagulation disorder. This bleeding typically stems from the lower uterine segment, particularly if it has been the site of placental implantation. Bleeding from the lower segment can persist despite good fundal contraction, perhaps because the lower segment is thinner and inherently less able to provide sufficient contractility for hemostasis in the floridly vascular placental bed. Bleeding from discrete areas in the cervical canal or corpus or fundus of the uterus can also happen in the context of a contracted uterus (41,42). The cause and the source of such bleeding are usually difficult to define. Local suture ligation is sometimes effective, but therapy must often be directed at reduction of overall uterine blood flow.

Puerperal hemorrhage also derives from surgical complications of cesarean section. Extensions of the uterine incision into the vascular broad ligament or other portions of the uterus can result in considerable hemorrhage. In addition, cesarean delivery often accompanies other factors that predispose to postpartum hemorrhage, such as placenta previa, abruptio placentae, or prolonged labor. When surgical misadventures occur, they should be treated in the standard manner. The approach to placenta accreta or atony is simplified somewhat when either of these problems develops at cesarean section, because the doctor does not have to make the reluctant decision to intervene surgically, as he or she would after a vaginal delivery.

DELAYED POSTPARTUM HEMORRHAGE

Excessive bleeding after the first postpartum day is caused by the same factors that contribute to acute puerperal hemorrhage. Delayed bleeding is most common in the first 2 weeks after delivery, with a peak incidence at 7 days (43). It is more common in primiparas than in multiparas and is very frequently associated with retained placental fragments. Perhaps this persistent trophoblast somehow results in subinvolution of the placental site and loss or recanalization of thrombi that formed after delivery (44). The management principles for this kind of bleeding are the same as those for acute postpartum hemorrhage, but prompt uterine curettage should be the mainstay of therapy.

SELECTIVE ANGIOGRAPHY

When persistent postpartum uterine bleeding has not responded to the standard therapies outlined here and is sufficiently slow such that the patient is hemodynamically stable and can tolerate a 1- to 2-hour period until bleeding is controlled, angiography should be considered before surgical intervention (45,46). If skilled personnel and facilities for selective abdominal angiography and arterial embolization are available, the risks of surgery and anesthesia can be avoided and the need for hysterectomy minimized. During the procedure, a catheter is advanced into the abdominal aorta, generally after insertion into a femoral artery, and an aortogram is taken to locate the distal bleeding site. The catheter is then advanced into the offending vessels, and blood flow is stopped by embolization.

Typically, small particles of gelatin sponge or a specially designed stainless steel coil wrapped with Dacron is used (47). Alternatively, infusion of vasopressin has been employed, to effect an overall reduction in pelvic blood flow (41). If specific distal bleeding branches cannot be identified, the anterior division of each internal iliac artery can be embolized. If bleeding continues, or even if angiography has been preceded by surgical internal iliac artery ligation, feeding collateral branches can sometimes be individually identified and embolized successfully (48). Angiography is also of considerable use for postpartum hemorrhage from vulvar or vaginal trauma. Sometimes the extensive hematoma formation that accompanies these birth injuries makes surgical therapy difficult or impossible (49).

SURGICAL THERAPY

When more conservative approaches to puerperal hemorrhage fail, surgery must be performed. The operative approaches to control serious bleeding are either vaso-occlusive or extirpative; the former are performed in an effort to avoid hysterectomy and its consequences. Reduction of uterine blood flow by selective ligation of pelvic arteries allows endogenous hemostatic mechanisms to cope with the problem.

Ligation of the uterine artery logically ought to contribute significantly to the control of uterine hemorrhage. Ligation of the uterine artery within the broad ligament was suggested by Waters (50) as a tool for management of postpartum hemorrhage. O'Leary and O'Leary (51) emphasized the utility of this procedure and described a simple, rapid, and safe approach for ligation of the ascending branch of the uterine artery adjacent to the lateral border of the uterus. This kind of vascular ligation should generally be done as a primary procedure in the operative treatment of postpartum hemorrhage, because it is readily accomplished and is unlikely to cause complications. In addition, interruption of the ovarian arterial contribution to uterine blood flow is straightforward and should be performed along with uterine artery ligation. This often overlooked step is important because ovarian arterial flow can make a considerable contribution to total uterine flow during pregnancy (52).

Control of ovarian arterial inflow can be accomplished by locating the ovarian arteries in the mesovarium and ligating them near the utero-ovarian ligament (53). Alternatively, a large encompassing suture ligature can be placed around the utero-ovarian ligament and the artery. If the latter approach is used, special care must be taken to avoid compromising the fallopian tube or injuring the adjacent large venous anastomoses between the uterine and ovarian vessels. The surgeon should avoid interrupting the ovarian vessels more proximally in the infundibulopelvic ligament; if hysterectomy proves necessary, the consequent devascularization will result in loss of the ovaries.

If combined ascending uterine and ovarian artery ligation, which can be accomplished within a very few minutes, is not successful in controlling uterine hemorrhage, ligation of the internal iliac arteries can be attempted. This procedure for controlling massive pelvic hemorrhage was probably first described by Baumgartner in 1888 (54). Although internal iliac ligation obviates the need for hysterectomy in only about half of the cases in which it is attempted (55,56), it is a useful procedure in many circumstances and might make more extensive and time-consuming extirpative surgery unnecessary (57).

The effect of internal artery ligation is primarily ipsilateral, and such ligation functions to control hemorrhage primarily by decreasing pulse pressure and blood flow dramatically in the pelvis (58). Once the pulsatile quality of the arterial circulation is dampened markedly, hemostasis is achieved more readily. Generally, bilateral ligation should be performed, but a unilateral approach might be sufficient, if the bleeding source is known to be localized on one side. Controversy exists about whether the artery should be ligated near its origin or distal to the takeoff of its posterior division so as to reduce the risk of gluteal ischemia. Such ischemia would be rare indeed in reproductive-age women, and proximal ligation has the advantage of reducing pelvic blood flow in those patients whose internal pudendal or obturator arteries arise from the posterior division of the internal iliac artery (58). The collateral arterial circulation of the pelvis is so extensive that uterine blood flow remains adequate to support normal pregnancy even after ligation of both internal iliac and both ovarian arteries (59,60).

A thorough knowledge of pelvic anatomy and the ability to deal with its potential complications are prerequisites for the surgeon performing internal iliac artery ligation (Fig. 51-2). A physician unfamiliar with retroperitoneal dissection in this area or with the management of the most serious risk of the operation (large vessel injury, most commonly to the iliac veins) can do more harm than good by attempts to ligate the arteries. It is useful to have a special set of surgical instruments designated for iliac artery ligation available in the delivery room. Without question, the safety of the procedure is enhanced if suitable instrumentation and suture material are at hand for the procedure and for control of complications.

A large postpartum uterus can make exposure of the operative field difficult. The surgeon should not hesitate to make a skin incision sufficiently large to allow proper verification of anatomic landmarks. A vertical midline lower abdominal or a Maylard incision makes access to the iliac bifurcation easy. The area can also be approached retroperitoneally with bilateral inguinal incisions. Although it is rapid and reasonable to take this approach in some circumstances, the route is of limited value when the ligation is to be done for puerperal hemorrhage. No access to the ovarian blood supply is afforded, and if hysterectomy becomes necessary, another incision would be required. If a Pfannensteil incision has already been made for cesarean section, exposure will be

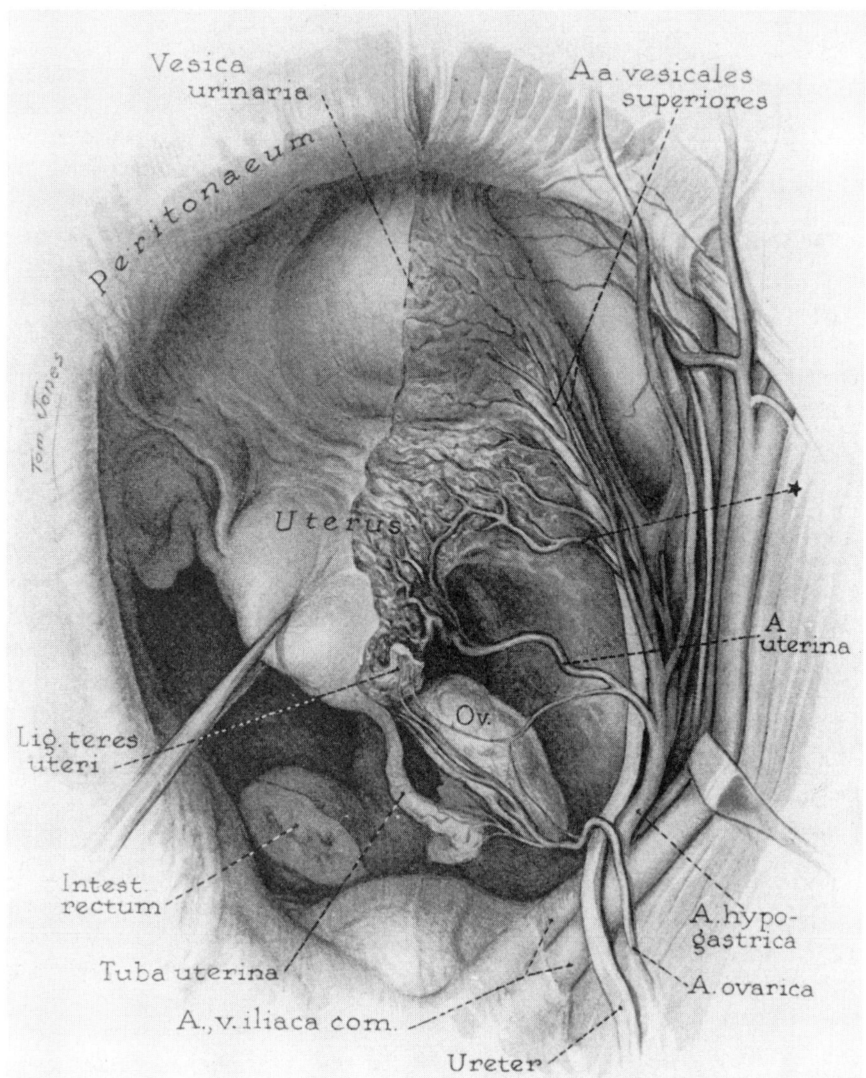

FIG. 51-2. The relationship of the internal iliac and distal ovarian artery. Of particular surgical importance are the proximity of the ureter and the large fragile external iliac vein, which lies between the external and internal iliac arteries. A thorough knowledge of this anatomy is necessary to treat postpartum hemorrhage surgically. (From Curtis AH, Anson BJ, Ashley FL, Jones T. The blood vessels of the female pelvis in relation to gynecologic surgery. Surg Gynecol Obstet 1942;75:421–423.)

difficult. The rectus muscles should be cut transversely to provide sufficient space.

The internal iliac vessels can be approached by several different routes, and the surgeon should be able to adapt his or her approach to the situation at hand. The presence of an extensive retroperitoneal hematoma can make the dissection of this area particularly difficult and potentially hazardous. The most fail-safe approach to the internal iliac artery is to open the anterior portion of the pararectal space (61,62).

First, the parietal peritoneum is incised over the surface of the psoas major muscle, a landmark easily identified. By reflecting the cut edge of the peritoneum medially, the external iliac artery will be pinpointed lying along the anteromedial border of the muscle. Usually the genitofemoral nerve is found lateral to the artery on the surface of the muscle. The nerve must not be injured. Gentle traction on the medial peritoneal flap and blunt dissection between the external iliac vessels laterally and the infundibulopelvic ligament medially will expose the ureter, which must be gently pulled out of harm's way. A retractor placed in the cephalic angle of the peritoneal incision will be helpful in this regard. A similar retractor placed in the lower pole of the incision allows the surgeon a clear view of the anterior surface of the external iliac artery, and dissection should take place cephalad along this artery until the bifurcation is reached. The internal iliac artery is directed posteriorly from this point, and dissection should continue on its anterior surface for a distance of approximately 1 to 2 cm. It is important to maintain the plane of dissection over the anterior surface of the arteries in order to avoid injury to the underlying external and internal iliac veins, which are quite fragile and easily torn. The external iliac vein is particularly vulnerable, lying posteromedial to its companion artery. Often the vein is obscured by areolar and lymphatic tissue, and the surgeon must be aware of its location.

A ligature should be carefully placed around the internal iliac artery. The best instruments for obtaining a plane beneath the artery are a long right-angle clamp or a blunt Deschamps needle holder. Use of absorbable suture allows subsequent recanalization of vessels (63), but even if permanent suture is used, uterine blood flow eventually returns to normal. There is no need to divide the ligated artery. If bilateral ligation of uterine, ovarian, and internal iliac arteries does not result in sufficient abatement of uterine bleeding, hysterectomy is the only remaining recourse. Although total hysterectomy is generally preferred, this is a situation in which supracervical hysterectomy is often sufficient therapy and might even be preferable when the patient is hemodynamically unstable and operating time must be minimized.

Hysterectomy is performed in the standard fashion. The tissue edema of pregnancy sometimes facilitates identification of dissection planes. Difficulty may be encountered in removing the cervix, especially when considerable dilatation has been reached before delivery, making the cervix very difficult to distinguish. A vertical incision made in the lower uterine segment can be helpful in this aspect of the operation. This allows one to palpate or to identify the cervix visually and determine the appropriate level for the vaginal incision. Care must be taken to ensure both that the entire cervix is removed and that the vagina is not foreshortened unnecessarily.

Other surgical techniques for control of postpartum uterine hemorrhage have been described. The B-Lynch technique (64) places sutures around the uterus that provide fundal compression. Segmental resection of isolated hypotonic areas of the uterus has also been reported (65). The effectiveness and applicability of these approaches is still undetermined. For diffuse bleeding in the pelvis (usually after hysterectomy) that cannot be controlled surgically, application of fibrin glue (66,67) or placement of a large pack (68) can be helpful.

The psychosocial consequences of hysterectomy done in the wake of unexpected puerperal hemorrhage should not be underestimated. Although hysterectomy is performed as a lifesaving procedure in the face of postpartum hemorrhage, many women have understandable difficulty coping with this disastrous event at a time when they anticipated a normal obstetric experience. They can feel betrayed by their own bodies and their physician, and the obstetrician must be especially sensitive to the emotional needs of the patient in such circumstances. Special care should be taken to provide a thorough understanding of the situation and appropriate counseling.

UTERINE INVERSION

Acute puerperal uterine inversion is an uncommon cause of severe postpartum hemorrhage and shock. The patient generally complains of pelvic or uterine pain, and bleeding can be sudden and profuse (69–71). The inverted fundus often is found at the introitus or is discovered on routine examination of the cervix after delivery. Inversion is sometimes iatrogenic, the result of overzealous traction on the umbilical cord during the third stage of labor. Some cases are the consequence of uterine atony, but most develop without apparent cause or provocation. Prompt replacement of the fundus is important, to minimize bleeding and to prevent or reduce hypotension; such hypotension is sometimes out of proportion to the blood loss, perhaps as the result of a vasovagal response to visceral stimulation.

The traditional approach to this problem has been to replace the fundal inversion under general anesthesia using a method similar to that described by Johnson (72). With uterine relaxant anesthesia, the palm of the hand is placed over the dome of the inverted fundus, and the uterus is elevated into the abdominal cavity. Firm and persistent pressure at the uterine-cervical junction by the examining hand puts tension on the uterine supporting ligaments, and in 3 to 5 minutes, the fundus usually begins to recede. If this maneuver fails, laparotomy and surgical reversion are advocated. Fortunately, surgery is rarely necessary; neither is general anesthesia always required, particularly if modern obstetric drugs are used.

When the inversion is diagnosed, a tocolytic drug can be given to relax the uterus. Beta-mimetic drugs are a reasonable form of therapy (73,74), but magnesium sulfate might be more advantageous in this particular situation (75). Beta-mimetic drugs can potentiate hypotension if the patient is volume depleted, a side effect that might be less serious with magnesium sulfate. Once the uterus is relaxed, the Johnson maneuver can be used and the fundus replaced with relative ease. After the inversion has been corrected, 15-methyl $PGF_{2\alpha}$ is given to induce firm myometrial contraction and to prevent reinversion, which otherwise often ensues.

HYPOVOLEMIC SHOCK

Every obstetric unit should be prepared to deal with unanticipated massive hemorrhage and its consequences. When blood loss is excessive, a syndrome of hypovolemic shock occurs, which is characterized by inadequate blood flow to vital organs. The clinical and biochemical features of shock are well documented (76).

Pathophysiology of Shock

As intravascular volume is lost during hemorrhage, evidence of tissue hypoperfusion is seen. Sympathoadrenal activity increases in an attempt to maintain cardiac output and, as cardiac output falls, to defend the blood pressure. This increase in vascular resistance is relatively selective, redistributing the available cardiac output preferentially to the heart and brain at the expense of lower-priority vascular beds, such as those of the skin and viscera. This explains why patients have tachycardia and pale, cool skin and why clinically measured systemic arterial pressure does not always reflect global tissue perfusion.

This redistribution of cardiac output probably serves to maintain oxygen delivery to tissues when supplies are limited (77,78). It is of particular importance in pregnancy in that uterine blood flow is not autoregulated, as is that of the heart and brain. Consequently, intervillous space perfusion is usually an early casualty of hemorrhagic shock during gestation. It is therefore of special importance to avoid aortocaval compression by the uterus when maternal blood volume is diminished.

Hypoperfusion results in increased anaerobic metabolism and lactic acidosis. In compensation, tissue extraction of oxygen is enhanced by increased red cell levels of 2,3-diphosphoglycerate and a consequent shift of the oxyhemoglobin dissociation curve to the right.

As part of these compensatory responses to volume loss, autonomic reflexes and circulatory catecholamines serve to increase heart rate, myocardial contractility, and sympathetic tone in some vascular beds. The overall high total peripheral resistance might actually be reflected initially by increased diastolic blood pressure. As hemorrhage becomes increasingly severe, stroke volume and blood pressure fall. Heart rate may continue to rise in an attempt to maintain cardiac output, but eventually all these compensatory responses fail.

If the shock state continues, sympathoadrenal mechanisms are no longer able to protect the blood pressure, and effects of circulating vasodilating substances supervene. In ischemic tissue beds a systemic inflammatory response sequence develops progressively. At this point, the process is almost inevitably irreversible, even if volume and red cell deficits are corrected (79). Metabolically, a catabolic state develops during shock. Catecholamines prompt glycogenolysis and lipolysis, suppress insulin release, and activate the renin–angiotensin system. Anxiety, restlessness, and diaphoresis are clinical manifestations of these sympathoadrenal effects. Cellular changes evolve as well (80).

Normally, the negative charge of the cell membrane allows it to serve as a semipermeable barrier that governs the homeostatic transfer of water and solutes between the intracellular and extracellular environments. Early in response to hemorrhage, membrane polarization changes lead to intracellular edema, as sodium and water move from the extracellular space. Consequent derangements in metabolism contribute to declines in tissue pH and enhanced lactate concentration. The mediators of these changes in membrane permeability and the homeostatic responses to them are understood only incompletely. It is possible that many factors play a role, the influence of each of which is probably determined by the patient's nutritional status and the hormonal response to hemorrhage. As noted, catecholamine and cortisol are released during hemorrhage. Circulating shock protein can cause cell membrane depolarization, as can platelet activating factor, leukotrienes, and thromboxane A_2.

This change in membrane potential is one of the critical factors in shock that leads to metabolic destabilization and, eventually, death. From the clinical perspective it is important to realize that the membrane changes probably begin before the appearance of systemic hypotension and can be reversed (at least up to a point) by replacement of extracellular fluid (80). Sometimes, especially after long periods of shock, irreversible hypotension persists, despite adequate volume repletion and establishment of hemostasis.

The pathophysiologic changes described here translate into three clinical phases of hemorrhagic shock: compensated, uncompensated but reversible, and irreversible (79). In compensated shock the blood volume deficit is usually relatively mild, less than 20%. Orthostatic changes in pulse and blood pressure might be present, and a redistribution of cardiac output takes place, denying some flow to organs relatively resistant to ischemia, such as skin, bone, and skeletal muscle. With a loss of 20% to 40% of intravascular volume, supine hypotension ensues. Regional reductions in organ blood flow result in oliguria and lactic acidosis. With even greater volume deficits, there is markedly diminished perfusion of brain and heart; metabolic acidosis becomes profound; tachypnea, agitation, or obtundation are evident, and the process is no longer reversible.

Changes in pulmonary function can also develop in shock states, and they require careful medical management (81). There is an increase in intrapulmonary arteriovenous shunting, often a marked augmentation of the work of breathing, and other factors that suggest impairment of lung compliance. This is probably related to increases in pulmonary interstitial sodium and water and lead, in the worst instance, to respiratory failure and adult respiratory distress syndrome.

Treatment of Shock

Therapy is geared toward supplying the cells of the shock patient with sufficient substrates and oxygen to attenuate the metabolic derangements caused by reduced perfusion that can ultimately lead to permanent damage (Table 51-2). Consequently, the overriding principle of therapy is to identify hypovolemia promptly and begin rapid fluid replacement while attempts are made to control the source of the bleeding. Also important are the recognition and treatment of the secondary manifestations of hypoperfusion, including hypoxia, acidosis, respiratory failure, and coagulopathy. The most common error in the treatment of obstetric hemorrhage is the fail-

TABLE 51-2. *Management of hemorrhagic shock*

Provide adequate ventilation and oxygenation
Establish wide-bore intravenous access
Obtain blood for lab analysis (complete blood count, electrolytes, type and cross-match, renal function, coagulation tests)
Control hemorrhage as soon as possible
Infuse crystalloid
Prepare red cell transfusion
Monitor hemodynamic function

ure to respond promptly to blood loss with adequate volume replacement and definitive medical and surgical therapy to stem the bleeding. The threshold of irreversible shock can be rapidly traversed by the patient; it is then too late to help her.

Equivolumetric replacement of blood loss is generally not sufficient therapy for shock from acute hemorrhage because fluid losses into the extravascular space must also be replaced. Initial fluid resuscitation should consist of large quantities of crystalloid solution. A balanced salt solution, such as Ringer's lactate, is better than physiologic saline solutions when large volumes are transfused, because less iatrogenic acidosis will result; the lactate is advantageously metabolized to bicarbonate if the liver is adequately perfused. Aggressive fluid replacement must be tempered by the risk of pulmonary edema, to which the shock patient is susceptible. Postpartum, the patient can be particularly vulnerable to this risk, because of the fall in colloid osmotic pressure that follows delivery.

Crystalloid solutions are the mainstay of therapy for volume deficits. While there are advocates of colloids for initial volume resuscitation, salt solutions are much less expensive and carry no risk of infection transmission or other adverse effects. In fact, most data suggest that patients treated with crystalloids have a survival advantage over those who receive colloids (82,83). When colloid is deemed necessary, hetastarch (5% hydroxyethyl starch) has become popular, because it is relatively inexpensive and remains in the plasma longer than albumin. All colloids will tend to draw water from the already depleted interstitial space during hypovolemic shock, which may not be desirable.

Comprehensive monitoring of patients with massive blood loss is vital to ensure optimal outcome. Placement of a central venous pressure catheter is helpful in monitoring fluid replacement, but a Swan-Ganz pulmonary artery catheter might be necessary to guide therapy optimally, particularly if the patient does not respond to initial therapy, if there is clinical evidence of pulmonary congestion, or if urine flow is persistently low (84). Be aware that percutaneous access to subclavian or internal jugular veins can be difficult in a hypovolemic patient, and the risk of hemothorax or pneumothorax is probably higher than normal. The cardiac rhythm should be monitored continuously and urine output and blood pressure measured frequently. It is sometimes appropriate to place an indwelling arterial catheter for continuous blood pressure monitoring. Once initial volume deficits have been treated, blood replacement with cross-matched packed red blood cells can be accomplished. (In urgent situations type-specific blood that has not been cross-matched, or even universal donor O-negative blood with low antibody titers to red cell antigens, could be necessary.)

The goal of initial fluid resuscitation is not to return the blood pressure to normal; tissue perfusion usually becomes adequate in advance of this. The urine output and central venous pressure are used to determine the adequacy of circulating volume. (The central venous pressure is usually a reflection of right atrial filling pressure, but it could be an inaccurate indicator when the patient has cardiac or pulmonary compromise. As noted, in those circumstances a Swan-Ganz catheter is preferable.) The urine output should be maintained at least at 0.5 mL/kg per hour and the central venous pressure at 4 to 8 cm water. Repletion of red cell mass should target a hemoglobin concentration of 10 to 12 g/dL. This level usually achieves a balance between the need to provide more oxygen-carrying capacity and the higher cardiac work required by the increased blood viscosity at high hemoglobin levels. Excess heat loss should be reduced with warm blankets or mechanical devices designed to help maintain body temperature in patients during surgery. Hypothermia can be provoked by multiple transfusions; for this reason, a blood warmer should be used as necessary (Table 51-3).

Electrolyte imbalance is common in hemorrhagic shock and could require attention. Hypokalemia is not unusual; it is probably one consequence of the dramatic increase in sympathoadrenal activity that accompanies hemorrhagic shock. Catecholamines cause potassium to be transported intracellularly. This is a transient phenomenon that will self-correct if perfusion is restored. Treatment is generally not required unless the serum potassium is profoundly low (<2.5 mEq/L) or cardiac arrhythmias are present.

Hypocalcemia is seen often in patients treated with multiple blood product transfusions, because the citrate anticoagulant chelates calcium. In addition, shock can result in failure of sarcolemmal ATP-dependent ion pumps that cannot export calcium from cells. The high

TABLE 51-3. *Complications of massive transfusion*

Hypothermia
Hyperkalemia
Hypocalcemia
Coagulopathy
2,3-DPG depletion
Jaundice
Infection
Alloimmunization
Transfusion reactions

intracellular calcium level disrupts ATP synthesis and myocardial contractility, among other things. Treatment is generally necessary if ionized calcium levels fall below about 1.5 mEq/L or if electrocardiographic changes (Q-T interval lengthening) manifest. Similarly, hypomagnesemia occurs and replacement should occur when serum levels reach 1.5 mEq/L or cardiac rhythm is disturbed.

Although systemic acidosis is detrimental to many aspects of metabolism and cardiac function, treatment of metabolic acidosis in hemorrhagic shock is the subject of controversy. Therapy aimed at improving perfusion is the best route to reversing acidosis. When it is obdurate and severe, acidosis can impede the process of hemodynamic hemostasis. Sodium bicarbonate can be used, but THAM (tris [hydroxymethyl] aminomethane) has theoretical advantages related to the fact that it buffers intracellular pH. Usually 5 to 10 mg/kg are given over 10 to 15 minutes. THAM can cause vasodilation and thus should be avoided in the early resuscitative treatment of hemorrhagic shock.

When very large volumes of fluid and blood are replaced, dilution of clotting factors can occur; moreover, severe shock might provoke true disseminated intravascular coagulation. This condition should be treated by blood and blood component replacement. Fresh-frozen plasma and, in particular, cryoprecipitate are the most concentrated sources of fibrinogen available and should be used early in hypofibrinogenemic states. Platelet concentrates can also be useful. Disseminated intravascular coagulation will generally not improve in these circumstances until the source of bleeding is controlled and peripheral tissue perfusion is restored.

The prophylactic use of platelets and fresh-frozen plasma in patients receiving multiple red cell transfusions is probably not necessary (85–87), unless the patient has generalized bleeding attributable to coagulopathy. Fresh-frozen plasma comes in units of 200 to 250 mL. Each unit will increase all clotting factors by about 2% to 3% in a patient with disseminated intravascular coagulation. A unit contains 500 mg of fibrinogen. Cryoprecipitate might be more useful if large amounts of fibrinogen need to be administered rapidly; each 20-mL unit contains 250 mg of fibrinogen and about 80 units of factors VIII and XIII and von Willebrand factor. As a generalization, 1 unit per 5 kg body weight will provide a plasma fibrinogen level of at least 100 mg/dL.

Platelet concentrates are prepared as 40-mL units containing about 5.5×10^{10} platelets. If type-specific platelets are not available, those from a D-positive donor can sensitize a D-negative recipient, because the platelet concentrates contain a few red blood cells. Sensitization can be prevented in such circumstances by administration of Rh-immune globulin. The usual dose of platelets is 1 unit per 10 kg body weight. Each unit will raise the platelet count by 5,000 to 10,000/mm^3. Blood component doses must be tailored to the extant clinical situation.

A new product, solvent-detergent-treated plasma, is now available. It differs from fresh-frozen plasma in having been treated to inactivate lipid-enveloped viruses, including HIV and hepatitis B and C viruses. Elimination of transmission of these viruses is obviously desirable, but the new product is considerably more expensive than fresh-frozen plasma. Another product with similar benefits but lower cost, called delayed release plasma, will soon be available as well.

Successful treatment of exsanguinating postpartum hemorrhage depends on efficient collaboration among all members of the patient care team. The obstetrician, nurses, anesthesiologist, and other consultants must coordinate their efforts to recognize excessive bleeding promptly, provide vigorous intravascular volume replacement, identify the source of the bleeding, and treat its secondary complications. Appropriate and timely intervention will usually result in a gratifying outcome.

REFERENCES

1. Fliegner JR, Hibbard BM. Active management of the third stage of labour. Br Med J 1966;2:622–623.
2. Gilbert L, Porter W, Brown VA. Postpartum hemorrhage: a continuing problem. Br J Obstet Gynaecol 1987;94:67.
3. Stones RW, Paterson CM, Saunders NS. Risk factors for major obstetric hemorrhage. Eur J Obstet Gynecol Reprod Biol 1993;48:15–18.
4. Fliegner JR. Third stage management: How important is it? Med J Aust 1978;2:190.
5. Berg CJ, Atrash HK, Koonin LM, Tucker M. Pregnancy-related mortality in the United States, 1987–1990. Obstet Gynecol 1996;88:161–167.
6. Fernandez H, Djanhan Y, Papiernik E. Mortalité maternelle par hémorrragie dans les pays en voie de développement: quelle politique proposer? J Gynecol Obstet Biol Reprod 1988;17:687–692.
7. Gahres EE, Albert SM, Dodek SM. Intrapartum blood loss measured with Cr^{51}-tagged erythrocytes. Obstet Gynecol 1962;19:455–462.
8. Pritchard JA. Changes in the blood volume during pregnancy and delivery. Anesthesiology 1965;26:393–399.
9. Dewhurst CJ, Dutton WAW. Recurrent abnormalities of the third stage of labor. Lancet 1957;2:764–767.
10. Reece EA, Fox HE, Rapoport F. Factor VIII inhibitor: a cause of severe postpartum hemorrhage. Am J Obstet Gynecol 1982;144:985–987.
11. Cohen WR. Influence of the duration of second stage labor on perinatal outcome and puerperal morbidity. Obstet Gynecol 1977;49:226–269.
12. Prendiville WJ. The prevention of post partum haemorrhage: optimising routine management of the third stage of labour. Eur J Obstet Gynecol 1996;69:19–24.
13. Nordström L, Fogelstein K, Fridman G, Larsson A, Rydhstroem H. Routine oxytocin in the third stage of labour: a placebo controlled randomised trial. Br J Obstet Gynaecol 1997;104:781–786.
14. Soriano D, Dulitzki M, Schiff E, Barkai G, Mashiach S, Seidman DS. A prospective cohort study of oxytocin plus ergometrine compared with oxytocin alone for prevention of postpartum haemorrhage. Br J Obstet Gynaecol 1996;103:1068–1073.
15. Prendiville WJ, Harding JE, Elbourne DR, Stirrat GM. The Bristol third stage trial: active versus physiological management of third stage of labor. Br Med J 1988;297:1295–1300.
16. Leff M. Management of the third and fourth stage of labor. Surg Gynecol Obstet 1939;68:224–229.
17. Thornton S, Davison JM, Baylis PH. Plasma oxytocin during third stage of labor: comparison of natural and active management. Br Med J 1988:297.
18. Wilken-Jensen C, Strom V, Nielsen MD, Rosenkilde-Gram B. Removing a retained placenta by oxytocin: a controlled study. Am J Obstet Gynecol 1989;161:155–156.
19. Reddy VV, Carey JC. Effect of umbilical vein oxytocin on puerperal blood loss and length of the third stage of labor. Am J Obstet Gynecol 1989;160:206–208.

20. Miller DA, Chollet JA, Goodwin TM. Clinical risk factors for placenta previa–placenta accreta. Am J Obstet Gynecol 1997;177:210–214.
21. Read A, Cotton DB, Miller FC. Placenta accreta: changing clinical aspects and outcome. Obstet Gynecol 1980;56:31–34.
22. Lagro RS, Price FV, Hill LM, Caritis SN. Nonsurgical management of placenta percreta: a case report. Obstet Gynecol 1994;83:847–849.
23. Chazotte C, Cohen WR. Catastrophic complications of previous cesarean section. Am J Obstet Gynecol 1990;163:738–742.
24. Leaphart WL, Schapiro H, Broome J, Welander CE, Bernstein IM. Placenta previa percreta with bladder invasion. Obstet Gynecol 1997;89: 834–835.
25. Thorp JM, Councell RB, Sandridge DA, et al. Antepartum diagnosis of placenta previa percreta by magnetic resonance imaging. Obstet Gynecol 1992;80:506–508.
26. Weeks LR, O'Toole DM. Postpartum hemorrhage: a five-year study at Queen of Angels Hospital. Am J Obstet Gynecol 1956;71:45–50.
27. Clark SL, Yeh S-Y, Phelan JP, Bruce S, Paul RH. Emergency hysterectomy for obstetric hemorrhage. Obstet Gynecol 1984;64:376–380.
28. Taylor GJ, Cohen B. Ergonovine-induced coronary artery spasm and myocardial infarction after normal delivery. Obstet Gynecol 1985;66: 821–822.
29. Hayashi RH, Castillo MS, Noah ML. Management of severe postpartum hemorrhage with a prostaglandin $F_2\alpha$ analogue. Obstet Gynecol 1984;63:806–808.
30. Toppozada M, El-Bossaty M, El-Rahman HA, El-Din AHS. Control of intractable atonic postpartum hemorrhage by 15-methyl prostaglandin $F_2\alpha$. Obstet Gynecol 1981;58:327–330.
31. Bruce SL, Paul RH, Van Dorsten JP. Control of postpartum uterine atony by intramyometrial prostaglandin. Obstet Gynecol 1982;59: 47S–50S.
32. Hankins GDV, Berryman GK, Scott RT Jr, Hood D. Maternal arterial desaturation with 15-methyl prostaglandin F_2 alpha for uterine atony. Obstet Gynecol 1988;72:367–370.
33. Hester JD. Postpartum hemorrhage and reevaluation of uterine packing. Obstet Gynecol 1975;45:501 504.
34. Lurie S, Appleman Z, Katz Z. Subendometrial vasopressin to control intractable placental bleeding. Lancet 1997;349:698.
35. Kovavisarch E, Kosolkittiwong S. Bimanual uterine compression as a major technique in controlling severe postpartum hemorrhage from uterine atony. J Med Assoc Thai 1997;80:266–269.
36. Keogh J, Tsokas N. Aortic compression in massive postpartum hemorrhage—an old but lifesaving technique. Aust N Z J Obstet Gynaecol 1997;37:237–238.
37. Riley DP, Burgess RW. External abdominal aortic compression: a study of a resuscitation maneuvre for postpartum hemorrhage. Anaesth Intensive Care 1994;22:571–575.
38. Chan C, Razui K, Tham KF, Arulkumaran S. The use of a Sengstaken-Blakemore tube to control post-partum hemorrhage. Int J Gynecol Obstet 1997;58:251–252.
39. Barrington JW, Roberts A. The use of gemeprost suppositories to arrest postpartum haemorrhage. Br J Obstet Gynaceol 1993;100:691–692.
40. Alok K, Hagen P, Webb JB. Tranexamic acid in the management of postpartum haemorrhage. Br J Obstet Gynaecol 1996;103:1250–1251.
41. Sacks B, Palestrandt A, Cohen WR. Internal iliac artery vasopressin infusion for postpartum hemorrhage. Am J Obstet Gynecol 1982;143: 601–603.
42. Schuitemaker NEW, Mackenzie MR. Postpartum hemorrhage due to a laceration in the endocervical canal: three case reports. Eur J Obstet Gynecol Reprod Biol 1989;30:183–185.
43. Thorsteinsson VT, Kempers RD. Delayed postpartum bleeding. Am J Obstet Gynecol 1970;107:565–571.
44. deBrux J, Solal R. Hémorragies incoercibles tardives du post-partum par prétendue subinvolution des vaiseaux de l'insertion placentaire. Gynecol Pratique 1972;23:111–115.
45. Brown BJ, Heaston DK, Poulson AM, Gabert HA, Mineau DE, Miller FJ Jr. Uncontrollable postpartum bleeding: a new approach to hemostasis through angiographic arterial embolization. Obstet Gynecol 1979;54:361–364.
46. Duggan PM, Jamieson MG, Wattie WJ. Intractable postpartum hemorrhage managed by angiographic embolization: case report and review. Aust N Z J Obstet Gynaecol 1991;31:229–234.
47. Well I. Internal iliac artery embolization in the management of pelvic bleeding. Clin Radiol 1996;51:825–827.
48. Pais SO, Glickman M, Schwartz P, Pingoud E, Berkowitz R. Embolization of pelvic arteries for control of postpartum hemorrhage. Obstet Gynecol 1980;55:754–758.
49. Chin HG, Scott DR, Resnik R, Davis GB, Lurie AL. Angiographic embolization of intractable puerperal hematomas. Am J Obstet Gynecol 1989;160:434–438.
50. Waters EG. Surgical management of postpartum hemorrhage with particular reference to ligation of uterine arteries. Am J Obstet Gynecol 1952;64:1143–1148.
51. O'Leary JL, O'Leary JA. Uterine artery ligation for control of post cesarean section hemorrhage. Obstet Gynecol 1974;43:849–853.
52. Fernstrom I. Arteriography of the uterine artery: its value in the diagnosis of uterine fibromyoma, tubal pregnancy, adnexal tumor, and placental site localization in cases of intra-uterine pregnancy. Acta Radiol Suppl 1955;22:1–128.
53. Cruikshank SH, Stoelk EM. Surgical control of pelvic hemorrhage: method of bilateral ovarian artery ligation. Am J Obstet Gynecol 1983;147:724 725.
54. Smith DC, Wyatt JF. Embolization of the hypogastric arteries in the control of massive vaginal hemorrhage. Obstet Gynecol 1977;49:317—322.
55. Clark SL, Phelan JP, Yeh S-Y, Bruce SR, Paul RH. Hypogastric artery ligation for obstetric hemorrhage. Obstet Gynecol 1985;66:353–356.
56. Evans S, McShane P. The efficacy of internal iliac artery ligation in obstetric hemorrhage. Surg Gynecol Obstet 1985;160:250.
57. Likeman RK. The boldest procedure possible for checking the bleeding: a new look at an old operation, and a series of 13 cases from an Australian hospital. Aust N Z J Obstet Gynaecol 1992;32:256–262.
58. Burchell RC. Physiology of internal iliac artery ligation. J Obstet Gynaecol Br Commonw 1968;75:642–651.
59. Shafiroff BGP, Grillo EB, Baron H. Bilateral ligation of the hypogastric arteries. Am J Surg 1959;98:34–40.
60. Mengert WF, Burchell RC, Blumstein RW, Daskal JL. Pregnancy after bilateral ligation of the internal iliac and ovarian arteries. Obstet Gynecol 1969;34:664.
61. Cohen WR. The third stage and postpartum hemorrhage. In: Cohen WR, Acker DB, Friedman EA, eds. Management of labor. Rockville, Md.: Aspen, 1989:61–76.
62. Knapp RC, Donahue VC, Friedman EA. Dissection of paravesical and pararectal spaces in pelvic operations. Surg Gynecol Obstet 1973;137: 758–762.
63. Dubay ML, Holshauser CA, Burchell RC. Internal iliac artery ligation for postpartum hemorrhage: recanalization of vessels. Am J Obstet Gynecol 1980;136:689–691.
64. B-Lynch C, Coker A, Lawal A, Abu J, Cowen MJ. The B-Lynch surgical technique for the control of massive postpartum haemorrhage: an alternative to hysterectomy? Five cases reported. Br J Obstet Gynaecol 1997;104:372–375.
65. McGuinness TB, Jackson JR, Schnapf DJ. Conservative surgical management of placental implantation site hemorrhage. Obstet Gynecol 1993;81:830–831.
66. Malviya VK, Deppe G. Control of intraoperative hemorrhage in gynecology with the use of fibrin glue. Obstet Gynecol 1989;73:284–286.
67. Kram HB, Nathan RC, Stafford FJ, Fleming AW, Shoemaker WC. Fibrin glue achieves hemostasis in patients with coagulation disorders. Arch Surg 1989;124:385–387.
68. Cassels JW Jr, Greenberg H, Otterson WN. Pelvic tamponade in puerperal hemorrhage. J Reprod Med 1985;30:689–692.
69. Bell JE, Wilson GF, Wilson LA. Puerperal inversion of the uterus. Am J Obstet Gynecol 1953;66:767–780.
70. Watson P, Besch N, Bowes WA Jr. Management of acute and subacute puerperal inversion of the uterus. Obstet Gynecol 1980;55:12–16.
71. Rasmussen OB. Puerperal inversion of the uterus. Acta Obstet Gynecol Scand 1992;71:558–559.
72. Johnson AB. A new concept in the replacement of the inverted uterus and a report of nine cases. Am J Obstet Gynecol 1949;57:557–562.
73. Kovacs BW, DeVore GR. Management of acute and subacute puerperal uterine inversion with terbutaline sulfate. Am J Obstet Gynecol 1984;150:784–786.
74. Thiery M, Delbeke L. Acute puerperal uterine inversion: two-step management with a β-mimetic and a prostaglandin. Am J Obstet Gynecol 1985;153:891–892.
75. Catanzarite VA, Moffitt KD, Baker ML, Awadalla SG, Argubright KF, Perkins RP. New approaches to the management of acute puerperal uterine inversion. Obstet Gynecol 1986;68:75–105.

76. MacLean LD. Shock. Br Med Bull 1988;44:437–452.
77. Schlichtig R, Kramer DJ, Pinsky MR. Flow redistribution during progressive hemorrhage is a determinant of critical O_2 delivery. J Appl Physiol 1991;70:169–178.
78. Hemmer M. Regional blood flow and hemorrhage. How far do the protective mechanisms go? Intensive Care Med 1996;20:1006–1008.
79. Shoemaker WC, Peitzman AB, Bellamy R, et al. Resuscitation from severe hemorrhage. Crit Care Med 1996;24[Suppl]:512–523.
80. Barber AE, Shires GT. Cell damage after shock. New Horizons 1996; 4:161–167.
81. Moss GS, Saletta JD. Traumatic shock in man. N Engl J Med 1974;290: 724–726.
82. Domsky MF, Wilson RF. Hemodynamic resuscitation. Crit Care Clin 1993;10:715–726.
83. Velanovich V. Crystalloid versus colloid fluid resuscitation: a meta-analysis of mortality. Surgery 1989;105:65.
84. Harrison E, Cohen WR. Critical care of the parturient. In: Cohen WR, Acker DB, Friedman EA, eds. Management of labor. Rockville, Md.: Aspen, 1989:479–513.
85. Harrigan C, Lucas CE, Ledgerwood AM, Walz DA, Mammem AF. Serial changes in primary hemostasis after massive transfusion. Surgery 1985;98:836–844.
86. Martin DJ, Lucas CE, Ledgerwood AM, Hochsner J, McGonigal MD, Grabow D. Fresh frozen plasma supplement to massive red blood cell transfusion. Ann Surg 1985;202:505–511.
87. Reed RL, Heimbach DM, Counts RB, et al. Prophylactic platelet administration during massive transfusion: a prospective, randomized, double-blind clinical study. Ann Surg 1986;203:40–48.

Cherry and Merkatz's Complications of Pregnancy,
Fifth Edition, edited by W. R. Cohen.
Lippincott Williams & Wilkins, Philadelphia © 2000.

CHAPTER 52

Sepsis

Steven M. Hollenberg and Virginia S. Kelly

Septic shock is a response to infection resulting in peripheral circulatory decompensation with failure to maintain adequate tissue and cellular perfusion. Septic shock is a form of distributive shock and is characterized by a high cardiac output and a low systemic vascular resistance. A classification of shock based on the underlying causes of abnormal tissue perfusion is shown in Table 52-1, and the pathogenesis of different forms of shock is shown in Figure 52-1. In hypovolemic, cardiogenic, and extracardiac obstructive shock, decreased tissue perfusion results from inadequate cardiac output. In patients with distributive shock, both hypotension resulting from decreased systemic vascular resistance and maldistribution of blood flow in the microcirculation compromise tissue perfusion.

The overall incidence of bacteremia in obstetric patients has been documented infrequently but is estimated at 0.75%. In the setting of acute chorioamnionitis, pyelonephritis, or postpartum endometritis, the incidence is approximately 5% to 10%. Ledger and colleagues estimated that only 4% of those with bacteremia develop septic shock, substantially less than the 20% to 50% incidence in hospitalized nonpregnant patients (1). The low incidence of obstetric septic shock probably reflects the general good health of this relatively young population, whose age, lack of underlying chronic disease, and general immunocompetence allow them to tolerate bacteremia fairly well. Nonetheless, although septic shock is uncommon in pregnant patients, sepsis accounts for about 20% of maternal deaths, and may involve a catastrophic outcome for the fetus (2). This chapter reviews aspects of sepsis pertinent to the practicing obstetrician, with particular emphasis on pathophysiology, microbiology, diagnosis, and treatment of septic shock.

S.M. Hollenberg: Sections of Cardiology and Critical Care Medicine, Rush-Presbyterian-St. Luke's Medical Center, Chicago, IL 60612.

V.S. Kelly: Department of Obstetrics and Gynecology, Northwestern University School of Medicine, Chicago, IL 60611.

PATHOGENESIS

Sepsis is the systemic response to the presence in the bloodstream of pathogenic microorganisms or their byproducts. This systemic response is characterized by hyperthermia or hypothermia, tachycardia, tachypnea, and either leukocytosis or leukopenia. Definitions of sepsis, sepsis syndrome, and septic shock are listed in Table 52-2. Septic shock refers to sepsis-induced hypotension, along with hypoperfusion, which may be manifested by lactic acidosis, oliguria, or altered mental status, as well as by organ dysfunction. Septic shock carries a mortality of 30% to 70% and is the most common cause of death in many critical care units (3). Sepsis is caused most often by gram-negative bacteria, but can be produced by gram-positive organisms, fungi, *Rickettsia,* protozoa, and viruses. The hemodynamic syndrome of septic shock is similar, however, regardless of the etiologic infectious agent (4).

Pregnant patients may be predisposed to develop sepsis because pregnancy is a state of altered immune competence; maternal immune hyporesponsiveness allows for tolerance of paternal antigens in fetoplacental tissue (5). Studies suggesting increased susceptibility to septic shock in pregnancy come largely from animal models. Beller and colleagues (6) compared the effect of injecting *Escherichia coli* endotoxin in pregnant and nonpregnant pigs; pregnant animals died significantly more quickly, had a more pronounced metabolic acidosis, and had decreased uterine tissue oxygenation compared with nonpregnant controls.

Septic shock is characterized clinically by a high cardiac output and a low systemic vascular resistance. Early studies, which reported a low cardiac output (7,8), were performed before the advent of the pulmonary artery catheter and before aggressive fluid repletion was routine, so hypovolemia may have decreased cardiac output in some of the patients. Subsequent studies in which fluid was given have demonstrated that early in the course of

TABLE 52-1. *Classification of forms of shock*

Cardiogenic shock
- Myopathic
  - Acute myocardial infarction
  - Dilated cardiomyopathy
  - Myocardial depression in septic shock
- Mechanical
  - Mitral regurgitation
  - Ventricular septal defect
  - Ventricular aneurysm
  - LV outflow tract obstruction (aortic stenosis, hypertrophic cardiomyopathy)
- Arrhythmic

Extracardiac obstructive shock
- Pericardial tamponade
- Pulmonary embolism (massive)
- Severe pulmonary hypertension (primary or Eisenmenger)
- Constrictive pericarditis
- Coarctation of the aorta

Hypovolemic shock
- Hemorrhage
- Fluid depletion

Distributive shock
- Septic shock
- Toxic products (drug overdose)
- Anaphylaxis
- Neurogenic shock
- Endocrinologic shock

Modified from Hollenberg SM, Parrillo JE. In: Shires GT, Barie PL (eds). *Surgical intensive care.* New York: Little, Brown, 1993.

septic shock, in patients who have received aggressive volume replacement, the cardiac output is almost always high or normal (9,10). The hemodynamics of sepsis in 10 pregnancies complicated by septic shock were reviewed by Lee and colleagues (5). Hypotension was associated with elevated cardiac index (4.6±1.9 L/min/m^2) and decreased systemic vascular resistance in all cases. Mabie and colleagues reviewed 18 cases of septic shock during gestation and found a similar elevation of cardiac index, more prominent in the 11 survivors (mean 4.7 L/min/m^2) than in the 7 nonsurvivors (mean 3.2 L/min/m^2) (11).

Thus, as opposed to other forms of shock in which low cardiac output leads to decreased organ and tissue perfusion, in septic shock, tissue hypoperfusion results from abnormal shunting of a normal or increased cardiac output. In addition to shunting, in some septic patients, despite adequate organ blood flow, a mediator-induced metabolic block exists at the tissue level, preventing adequate utilization of oxygen and other nutrients. Lactate accumulates because cells are unable to use oxidative metabolic pathways normally. Thus, in these patients, blood flow through large vessels to tissues is adequate, but abnormalities of microvascular flow or an inability of cells to use nutrients leads to widespread cellular dysfunction and progressive shock.

Septic shock usually begins with a nidus of infection that releases microorganisms into the bloodstream (Fig. 52-2). Toxic effects can result from the organisms themselves, from components such as endotoxin (the lipopolysaccharide associated with the outer membrane of gram-negative bacteria) or from elaboration of exotoxins (12). The most important pathologic effects of these organisms and toxins may result from stimulation of the release of massive quantities of endogenous inflammatory mediators (12). Endotoxin is a potent trigger for release of cytokines, most notably the interleukins and tumor necrosis factor (TNF), which amplify the systemic response to endotoxin by stimulating neutrophils, endothelial cells, and platelets and by causing the release of other mediators, such as platelet activating factor, arachidonic acid metabolites, complement, kinins, histamine, and endorphins (13).

The effects of these mediators can be divided into two broad categories: effects on the peripheral vasculature and effects on the heart. Both exogenous and endogenous

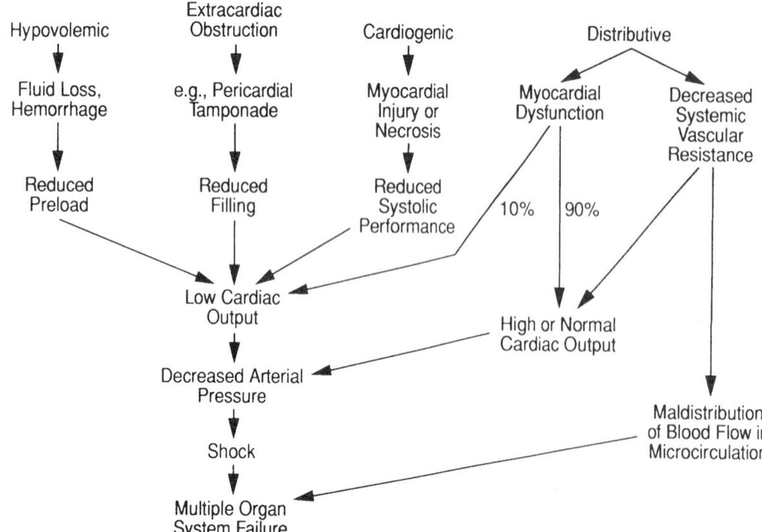

FIG. 52-1. Pathogenesis of different forms of shock. For hypovolemic, extracardiac obstructive, and cardiogenic forms of shock, hypotension and shock are caused by a low cardiac output. In septic shock, however, low cardiac output leads to shock in less than 10% of patients. The majority of patients with sepsis have a high or normal cardiac output, and shock is caused by peripheral vasodilation with decreased systemic vascular resistance. (From Parrillo JE. Mechanisms of disease: pathogenetic mechanisms of septic shock. N Engl J Med 1993;328:20.)

TABLE 52-2. *Definitions of SIRS, sepsis, severe sepsis, and septic shock*

Systemic inflammatory response syndrome (SIRS)
- Systemic response to infection, manifested by two or more of the following:
  - Hyperthermia (T>38°C) or hypothermia (T<36°C)
  - Tachycardia (HR>90)
  - Tachypnea (RR>20 of Pa_{CO_2}<32 mm Hg)
  - Leukocytosis (WBC>12,000/mm^3) or leukopenia (WBC<4,000/mm^3)

Sepsis
- Clinical evidence of infection, with a systemic response to infection, as defined by SIRS criteria

Severe sepsis
- Sepsis with evidence of organ dysfunction, evidenced by hypoperfusion, oliguria, lactic acidosis, hypoxemia (Pa_{O_2}/FI_{O_2}<280)

Septic shock
- Severe sepsis with hypotension (systolic blood pressure <90 mm Hg or >40 mm Hg decrease from baseline)

Modified from Bone R et al. Definitions for sepsis and organ failure and guidelines for the use of innovative therapies in sepsis. Chest 1992;101:1644–1655.

mediators have been shown to mediate peripheral vasodilation in sepsis. Administration of small doses of endotoxin to normal volunteers causes a decrease in arterial pressure, an increase in cardiac output, and a decrease in systemic vascular resistance similar to changes seen in sepsis (14). Similar vasodilation with increased cardiac output occurs after administration of TNF, interleukin-1 (IL-1), or IL-2 (13,15–17). A pivotal mediator of vasodilation in response to cytokines is nitric oxide, which is formed from arginine by the enzyme nitric oxide synthase (18). Endotoxin, TNF, and interleukins can stimulate inducible nitric oxide synthase in macrophages and vascular smooth muscle cells, with release of large amounts of this vasodilator molecule (19,20).

Other potential vasodilatory mechanisms in septic shock include activation of the kinin system, with release of the vasodilators bradykinin and histamine (21). Activation of phospholipase A_2 in sepsis can lead to formation of vasodilatory and proinflammatory prostaglandins, as well as to release of leukotrienes, which increase vascular permeability and promote neutrophil aggregation (22).

Although patients with septic shock have high cardiac outputs, left and right ventricular ejection fractions are reduced (23,24). Dilation of the ventricles allows normal stroke volumes to be maintained despite the depression of myocardial contractility, and tachycardia results in an elevated cardiac output. Septic patients also manifest a decreased ventricular stroke work response to volume infusion, further indicating depressed myocardial performance (25). The mechanisms responsible have not been completely clarified; it appears that cytokines, particularly TNF and IL-1, play an important role, possibly through generation of nitric oxide (26,27). Decreased myocardial responsiveness to catecholamines and diastolic dysfunction also may contribute to myocardial dysfunction in sepsis.

Endotoxin also can activate the intrinsic coagulation cascade along with the fibrinolytic system (28,29); this can lead to deposition of fibrin microaggregates in the microvasculature, obstructing flow and exacerbating tissue hypoxia. Increased fibrinolytic activity may cause cir-

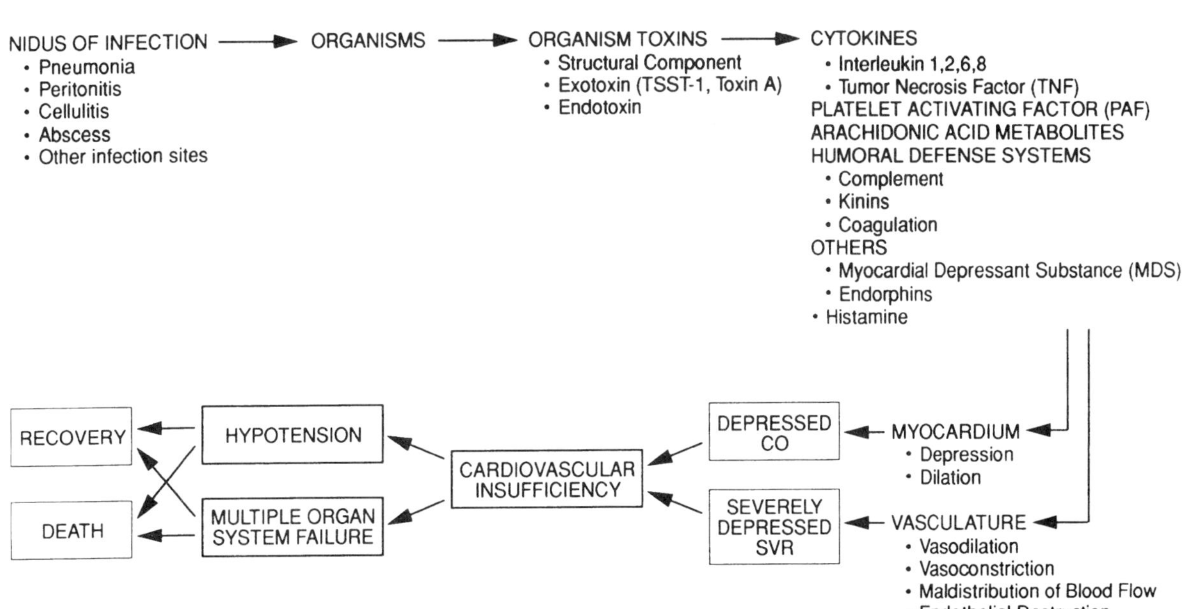

FIG. 52-2. Pathogenesis of septic shock. In the bloodstream, invading microorganisms or their products induce the release of endogenous mediators that have effects on the myocardium and the vasculature. These effects produce circulatory insufficiency, with hypotension and multiple organ system failure.

culating fibrin split products to inhibit coagulation. The development of microthrombi along with clotting abnormalities and consumption of clotting factors is seen clinically as disseminated intravascular coagulation (DIC).

Tumor necrosis factor and the interleukins activate both endothelial cells and neutrophils, leading to neutrophil aggregation and further microcirculatory insufficiency (30,31). Severe infection also activates the complement system, probably via the alternate complement pathway; endotoxin may be responsible for this activation (29). The complement components C5a and C3a are anaphylatoxins that can activate mast cells to release histamine, prostaglandins, leukotrienes, and other mediators. Complement activation also aggregates neutrophils, which may lead to endothelial cell dysfunction and damage (32). TNF can also stimulate the extrinsic coagulation cascade by inciting expression of tissue factor on the surface of monocytes and endothelial cells, initiating a process that may result in DIC (33).

Cellular dysfunction in sepsis is the final outcome of a process with multiple stimuli. In early shock, compensatory mechanisms are activated in an attempt to restore pressure and flow to vital organs. When these compensatory mechanisms begin to fail, damage to cellular membranes, leakage of lysosomal enzymes, and reductions in cellular energy stores occur and may result in cell death. Once a sufficiently large number of cells from vital organs have reached this stage, shock can become irreversible, and death can occur despite eradication of the underlying septic focus. This concept of irreversibility is useful because it emphasizes the need to prevent the progression of shock.

The transition from reversible cellular dysfunction to irreversible cellular damage in sepsis may relate to the development of a self-amplifying and self-sustaining inflammatory process (34). This inflammatory process occurs in response to the infectious stimulus and is of vital importance in host defense. If the inflammatory stimulus is sufficiently severe or prolonged, however, cellular autocrine and paracrine responses can lead to the development of positive feedback loops, with massive and sustained cytokine release, tissue damage, and cellular injury (34). Accumulated injuries within a cell can reach a threshold at which self-destruction occurs.

About half of the patients who succumb to septic shock die of multiple organ system failure. Most of the remaining patients have progressive hypotension with low systemic vascular resistance refractory to pressor agents; death from myocardial failure is rare (12).

ORGAN DYSFUNCTION IN SEPSIS

The clinical presentation of shock varies because each organ system is affected differently, depending on the severity of the perfusion deficit, the underlying cause, and prior organ dysfunction. If circulatory failure persists and sufficient cellular dysfunction occurs, dysfunction of multiple organ systems results. Multiple organ failure may be fatal, even without massive cell death, if cellular dysfunction is severe enough to interfere with organ function in a manner incompatible with life.

Cardiovascular

The principal pathophysiologic abnormalities in sepsis result from vascular dysfunction, and include peripheral vasodilatation and increased capillary permeability. Capillary leak can cause relative hypovolemia early in the course of sepsis, but after aggressive fluid repletion, vasodilation predominates, almost always accompanied by increased cardiac output. This vasodilation occurs despite elevated levels of endogenous catecholamines (35) and can be refractory to exogenously administered vasopressors (36). As noted previously, septic shock is associated with high cardiac output and reduced ventricular ejection fractions.

Pulmonary

Sepsis is the most frequent factor predisposing to the development of the adult respiratory distress syndrome (ARDS), and the two combined confer a mortality rate approaching 80% (37). Pulmonary dysfunction in sepsis can result from direct toxic effects of endotoxin and other cytokines or from cytokine-mediated increases in neutrophil chemotaxis. Activation of inflammatory cells and release of mediators causes acute lung injury. This lung injury causes decreased compliance, impaired gas exchange, and shunting of blood through unventilated areas. The clinical consequence of this injury, severe hypoxemia with bilateral pulmonary infiltrates in the setting of normal filling pressures, constitutes ARDS. The work of breathing increases, with increased respiratory muscle oxygen requirements in the setting of tissue hypoperfusion. Respiratory muscle fatigue and ventilatory failure can ensue, requiring mechanical ventilation. The pathologic hallmarks of early ARDS are neutrophil-fibrin aggregates within the pulmonary microvasculature. With progression, there is extension of inflammation into the interstitium and alveoli and exudation of proteinaceous fluid into the alveolar space. Consolidation and fibrosis are seen in the end stages.

Renal

Renal perfusion is compromised in sepsis, due not only to diminished effective circulating volume and hypotension, but also in part because blood flow is directed preferentially toward the heart and brain and away from the kidney. Increased afferent arteriolar tone compensates initially for decreased renal blood flow and maintains glomerular perfusion. When this compensatory mechanism fails, reduction in renal cortical blood flow can lead to oliguria, acute tubular necrosis, and renal failure (4). Associated insults, such as nephrotoxic drugs or intravenous contrast medium, can exacerbate renal injury in sepsis, and their use should be monitored extremely carefully. Another potential mechanism of renal damage associated with sepsis involves immune complex deposition and the development of interstitial nephritis.

Neurologic

Patients with sepsis can develop obtundation or confusion. The etiology is multifactorial; hypoperfusion, hypoxemia, acid-base abnormalities, and electrolyte disturbances all contribute. When mean arterial pressure remains very low for long periods of time, compensation for hypoperfusion by cerebral autoregulation can fail, and critical cerebral hypoperfusion can lead to ischemic injury (4).

Liver and Gastrointestinal Tract

Hepatic injury results from hypoperfusion, often complicated in septic shock by activation of Kuppfer cells and release of cytokines. Derangements of metabolic function of the liver include impairment of both synthesis and detoxification. Phagocytic clearance within the hepatic reticuloendothelial system is also impaired. Increased serum levels of transaminases, lactic dehydrogenase, and bilirubin reflect hepatic parenchymal injury. Decreased levels of albumin and clotting factors indicate decreased synthetic capability. Dramatic increases in transaminases can be seen with profound hypoxemia or hypotension (shock liver); these are transient states and resolve rapidly with reperfusion (4). In septic shock, intrahepatic cholestasis can be present, with marked increases in bilirubin and only modest increases in transaminases; these changes may reflect dysfunction of bile canaliculi due to bacterial toxins.

Splanchnic blood flow is compromised in shock as cardiac output is diverted elsewhere. Intestinal ischemia may occur, and injury may be further exacerbated by subsequent release of oxygen radicals during reperfusion following resuscitation. It has been hypothesized that ischemia/reperfusion injury may compromise the integrity of the intestinal mucosal barrier, leading to translocation of bacterial toxins, although this has not been demonstrated conclusively in patients. Splanchnic hypoperfusion can also lead to stress ulceration, ileus, and malabsorption; acalculous cholecystitis occasionally occurs.

Hematologic System

Sequestration of white cells at sites of inflammation or in the reticuloendothelial system can lead to depression of circulating leukocyte counts initially, but marked leukocytosis usually follows. The hematocrit may be elevated due to hemoconcentration or decreased due to hemolysis or hemorrhage. Abnormalities of coagulation are frequent in septic shock. Activation of the coagulation cascade within the microvasculature can cause DIC, which leads to thrombocytopenia, microangiopathic hemolytic anemia, decreased fibrinogen, and circulating fibrin split products. Thrombocytopenia in sepsis also can occur in the absence of DIC, in which case it is usually immunologically mediated.

Pregnancy-Specific Complications

The specific effects of maternal sepsis in pregnancy appear to result from altered uteroplacental blood flow (38,39). Morishima and colleagues injected sublethal doses of endotoxin into four pregnant baboons and observed maternal tachycardia, hypotension, and acidosis, along with increased uterine activity. Fetal distress, manifested by decreased heart rate, developed prior to the onset of maternal hypotension, and all fetuses developed acidosis and died *in utero.* Abruptio placentae and cerebral hemorrhage were also seen in two cases. Fetal distress was attributable to the combination of maternal hypotension and shunting of flow away from the uterine vasculature (39). Of interest, studies in pregnant ewes suggest that the fetus itself appears to be somewhat resistant to the effects of endotoxin (40).

CLINICAL FEATURES

The initial symptoms of sepsis are nonspecific and include malaise, tachycardia, rigors, fever, and sometimes hypothermia. Although most septic patients have elevated white counts, some may present with leukopenia. Arterial blood gases may reveal metabolic acidosis, often with respiratory compensation; hypoxemia may indicate early ARDS. Tissue hypoperfusion and organ dysfunction in septic shock can be manifested by oliguria and a clouded sensorium. Because these signs and symptoms are nonspecific, the clinician must have a high index of suspicion, especially in patients at high risk for infection. Because septic shock is associated with a high rate of mortality once established and can progress to potentially lethal disease so rapidly, empiric therapy often must initiated when there is a strong likelihood of its presence, before the results of all planned diagnostic studies are available.

Another important issue in pregnant patients is the level of blood pressure at which shock is diagnosed. In the nonpregnant patient, a systolic blood pressure greater than 90 mm Hg or a mean arterial pressure greater than 60 mm Hg is usually needed to maintain adequate perfusion. In pregnant patients, however, lower blood pressures can be normal. Conversely, in women with pregnancy-induced hypertension, much higher blood pressures may be necessary to maintain adequate uteroplacental perfusion. In addition, the effects of a particular blood pressure on uteroplacental perfusion in any given patient cannot be generalized but are related to gestational age and placental condition (41). Therefore, shock in pregnancy is diagnosed on the basis of the entire clinical picture, including pulse, mental status, urine output, and fetal condition rather than relying solely on a given level of blood pressure (41).

Microbiology of Sepsis in Pregnancy

The female genitourinary tract is colonized with large numbers of aerobic and anaerobic bacteria, which can gain access to the bloodstream during labor or following delivery. Common obstetric conditions that place pregnant women at risk for bacteremia include antepartum pyelonephritis, prolonged rupture of fetal membranes, retained products of conception, chorioamnionitis, and postpartum endometritis (5). Other potential causes include septic abortion, intraamniotic infections, necrotizing fasciitis, and toxic shock syndrome (5). The most common organisms that cause septic shock in pregnancy are gram-negative aerobic bacilli, most prominently *E. coli*, which is found in about 50% of isolates from septic shock patients; *Klebsiella, Proteus,* and *Enterobacter* organisms are not infrequent (33). Most of the remaining cases are due to gram-positive aerobic organisms such as group A, B, and D streptococci, *Streptococcus pneumoniae*, and anaerobic bacteria such as *Bacteroides* species, *Fusobacterium,* and peptostreptococci. Approximately 20% of septic obstetric patients have a polymicrobial bacteremia (42). *Staphylococcus aureus* and *Clostridium* are unusual isolates, and are seen primarily in postoperative patients with wound infections (33).

TABLE 52-3. *Septic shock therapy*

Goal 1: Eradicate infection
Begin empiric antibiotics (broad coverage)
Attempt to identify source of infection
Remove focus of infection (remove foreign body, drain abscess)
Goal 2: Provide supportive care
Intensive care setting
Full-time critical care nurses, physicians, therapists, and technicians
Intraarterial monitoring
Accurate
Immediate beat-to-beat analysis
Frequent arterial blood gas sampling
Right heart catheterization
Confirmation of diagnosis
Accurate cardiac filling pressure and flow measurements
Monitor effects of therapy
Cardiac rhythm monitoring
Antiarrhythmic agents
Electrical cardioversion
Fluid resuscitation
Eliminate other causes of cardiovascular depression
Correct anemia, hypoxemia, acidosis, hypoglycemia, hypophosphatemia, hypocalcemia, hypoalbuminemia
If MAP <60 mm Hg, optimize preload
Volume expansion to PCWP 12–18 mm Hg
Crystalloids/albumin/synthetic colloids
Consider transfusion
Avoid pulmonary edema
Vasopressors
If MAP <60 mm Hg despite PCWP 12–18 mm Hg, begin pressors (see Table 54-4)
Goal 3: Neutralize toxins
Investigational therapy in humans
Corticosteroids
Monoclonal antibodies to endotoxin
Antibodies to tumor necrosis factor (TNF), soluble TNF receptors
Antibodies to IL-1, IL-1 receptor antagonist
Ibuprofen
Platelet activating factor antagonists
Nitric oxide synthase inhibition
Methylene blue (guanylate cyclase inhibition)

Modified from Natanson C, Hoffman WD. In: Parillo JE, ed. *Current therapy in critical care medicine.* Philadelphia: BC Decker, 1987.

THERAPY

Principles of Therapy

The critically ill septic obstetric patient requires an aggressive approach to optimize maternal and fetal outcome. Therapy of septic shock may be viewed as having three main components (Table 52-3). First, the nidus of infection must be identified and eliminated, using surgical drainage, antibiotic therapy, or both. Second, while the source of sepsis is being eradicated, adequate organ system perfusion and function must be maintained, guided by cardiovascular monitoring. A third general therapeutic goal is to interrupt the pathogenic sequence leading to septic shock.

Initial Measures

Management of septic shock entails balancing the need to initiate therapy before shock causes irreversible damage to vital organs against the need to perform the clinical assessment required to identify the source of sepsis. A practical approach is to make a rapid evaluation initially, based on a limited history, physical examination, and specific diagnostic procedures directed toward determining the cause and severity of shock. Initial assessments ordinarily include a chest x-ray, electrocardiogram, arterial blood gas, electrolytes, complete blood count, and other tests directed at specific questions raised by the initial examination. Right heart catheterization with a balloon-tipped, flow-directed (Swann-Ganz) catheter is frequently useful early in the course of the evaluation. As this initial evaluation is in progress, therapy should be initiated. After stabilization, a more comprehensive diagnostic evaluation should be undertaken, and the response to the initial therapeutic interventions should be assessed.

Eradication of Infection

Rapid institution of appropriate antibiotic therapy leads to improved survival, but the specific organisms causing sepsis are usually not known when the patient presents. Accordingly, a broad-spectrum antibiotic regimen should be chosen initially that will be effective against all the likely causative microorganisms given the patient's clinical presentation and the hospital's organism resistance patterns.

Because of the polymicrobial nature of obstetric infections, a combination of antibiotics is usually chosen as initial therapy. The combination of ampicillin, gentamicin, and clindamycin or metronidazole covers most of the possible gram-negative, gram-positive, and anaerobic bacteria. Aminoglycoside doses should be titrated by following peak and trough levels. Other acceptable regimens include broad-spectrum ureidopenicillins (mezlocillin, azlocillin, piperacillin), penicillins in combination with β-lactamase inhibitors (ticarcillin-clavulanic acid, ampicillin-sulbactam), or a cephalosporin combined with an aminoglycoside. Imipenem-cilastatin as a single agent can be considered as an alternative. Women with evidence of a serious wound infection or manifestations of toxic shock syndrome should receive coverage for *Staphylococcus aureus* with nafcillin or vancomycin. The choice of a particular regimen for empiric coverage should be made with an understanding of the sensitivity patterns of the organisms involved in pelvic infection in the physician's institution. The antibiotic coverage can be tailored after an organism is identified or a site of infection is determined.

After obtaining all the necessary cultures (blood, sputum, urine, cerebrospinal fluid when indicated, and sites of pus or loculated fluids) and beginning antibiotic treatment, the clinician should search intensely for sites of infection. In the postpartum septic patient who is worsening despite appropriate antibiotic therapy, a thorough search for an infected nidus is mandatory. Possible infected sites include retained products of conception, uterine microabscesses, pelvic abscess, necrotizing fasciitis from wound infection, and septic pelvic vein thrombosis. Ultrasonography can be helpful in an evaluation of retained products of conception, but if there is clinical suspicion that placental tissue may be remaining, prompt uterine curettage should be performed regardless of the ultrasonographic findings. Intravenous pyelography or renal ultrasonography may be useful in detecting upper tract obstruction due to pyelonephritis and perinephric or renal abscess. Abdominal ultrasonography or computed tomography can be useful in some cases, but negative results should not be overinterpreted; one recent series reported a sensitivity of only 48% and a specificity of 64% in identifying sources of sepsis in critically ill surgical patients (43). Careful clinical examination is important as well. Uterine microabscesses present clinically as a large, tender, boggy uterus, often with a dilated cervical os. Postsurgical wounds should be examined carefully. Subcutaneous crepitus or air should lead to suspicion of necrotizing fasciitis from streptococcal or clostridial infection. In advanced cases, gas may be demonstrable on radiographic studies.

Surgical Treatment

Surgical removal of infected tissue is vital to the achievement of a good outcome in septic patients. In the series of Lee and colleagues (5), 40% of septic obstetric patients required surgical removal of infected products of conception. If chorioamnionitis is present in the septic patient, prompt delivery is the treatment of choice. The route of delivery depends on the clinical picture. Immediate delivery in the face of maternal cardiovascular collapse may increase the risk of both maternal and fetal mortality. However, if the mother fails to improve after initial resuscitative efforts, consideration should be given to immediate cesarean section. If the mother's status improves with therapy, and there is no evidence of fetal compromise, vaginal delivery is preferred, provided it can be achieved expeditiously (within 12 to 18 hours) (33). Necrotizing fasciitis requires extensive surgical debridement. Adjunctive therapy with hyperbaric oxygen may be useful in some cases. Septic pelvic vein thrombosis usually responds to heparin and antibiotics, but operative intervention may occasionally be necessary in cases with septic emboli or persistent sepsis. Patients with evidence of intraabdominal infections that remain unresponsive to therapy may require exploratory laparotomy for definitive treatment, with consideration of hysterectomy if an intrauterine or endometrial source is suspected.

Supportive Measures

An initial priority in managing septic shock must be to maintain a reasonable mean arterial pressure to keep the patient alive. Then, while the source of sepsis is being eradicated, adequate organ system perfusion and function must be maintained, to keep the patient's organs alive. This entails supportive care aimed at reversing cardiovascular and pulmonary pathophysiology, blood flow abnormalities, and metabolic derangements, with careful monitoring of hemodynamic profiles, oxygenation, and metabolic parameters.

Patients with septic shock should be treated in an intensive care unit. Retrospective studies have shown that survival increases significantly when patients with septic shock are treated by full-time critical care physicians and nurses using the technology available in modern intensive care units (12). Continuous electrocardiographic monitoring should be performed for detection of rhythm disturbances. Frequent measurements of blood gases, serum electrolytes, complete blood counts, and coagulation parameters should be performed to follow the patient's progress and to monitor the effects of therapy. Serum calcium, phosphorus, and magnesium should be checked as well, because substantial reductions in these ions can be associated with depression of myocardial and respiratory muscle function. The frequency of measurements should be based on the clinical course and the perceived need to assess responses to therapy (4).

Pulmonary function should be monitored using continuous pulse oximetry and intermittent arterial blood gas analysis. Maternal Pa_{O_2} should be maintained above 60 mm Hg, using assisted ventilation and positive end-expiratory pressure. Below this level, further decreases in maternal Pa_{O_2} may result in drastic reductions in fetal oxygen saturation and fetal hypoxia (41). Conversely, because the fetus functions on the steep portion of its oxygen dissociation curve, small increases in maternal Pa_{O_2} may produce important enhancements in fetal oxygen saturation (41).

Hemodynamic Monitoring

The introduction of the arterial cannula and the pulmonary artery catheter has revolutionized the diagnosis and treatment of most forms of shock, including septic shock. Such monitoring makes it possible to give large quantities of fluids and potent vasopressor and inotropic agents safely to critically ill patients. In shock states, estimation of blood pressure using a cuff is commonly inaccurate, and use of an arterial cannula provides a more appropriate measurement of intraarterial pressure. These catheters also allow beat-to-beat analysis so that decisions regarding therapy can be based on immediate and reproducible blood pressure information.

The different categories of shock (see Table 52-1) have different hemodynamic profiles (Table 52-4). That of septic shock is characterized by decreased arterial pressure with normal or increased cardiac output and de-

TABLE 52-4. *Use of right heart catheterization to diagnose the etiology of shock*

Diagnosis	Pulmonary capillary wedge pressure	CO	Miscellaneous comments
Cardiogenic shock			
Cardiogenic shock due to myocardial dysfunction	⇑⇑	⇓⇓	Usually occurs with evidence of extensive myocardial infarction (>40% of LV infarcted), severe cardiomyopathy, or myocarditis
Cardiogenic shock due to mechanical defects			
Acute ventricular septal defect	⇑	LVCO ⇓⇓ and RVCO > LVCO	Predominant shunt is left to right, pulmonary blood flow is greater than systemic blood flow: oxygen "step-up" occurs at RV level
Acute mitral regurgitation	⇑⇑	Forward CO ⇓⇓	V waves in pulmonary capillary wedge pressure tracing
Right ventricular infarction	normal or ⇓	⇓⇓	Elevated RA and RV filling pressures with low or normal pulmonary capillary wedge pressures
Extracardiac obstructive forms of shock			
Pericardial tamponade	⇑	⇓ or ⇓⇓	RA mean, RV end-diastolic pulmonary capillary wedge mean pressures are elevated and within 5 mm Hg of one another
Massive pulmonary embolism	Normal or ⇓	⇓⇓	Usual finding is elevated right-sided pressures
Hypovolemic shock	⇓⇓	⇓⇓	
Distributive forms of shock			
Septic shock	⇓ or normal	⇑ or normal, rarely ⇓	
Anaphylactic shock	⇓ or normal	⇑ or normal	

Systemic vascular resistance is increased, initially, in all forms of shock except distributive shock, in which it is usually reduced.

Modified from Hollenberg SM, Parrillo JE. In: Shires GT, Barie PL, eds. *Surgical intensive care.* New York: Little, Brown, 1993.

⇑⇑ or ⇓⇓ designates a moderate to severe increase or decrease; ⇑ or ⇓ designates a mild to moderate increase or decrease. CO, cardiac output; RA, right atrium; RV, right ventricle; LV, left ventricle.

creased systemic vascular resistance. Although the principal cause of shock in sepsis is marked vasodilation of peripheral resistance arteries, other hemodynamic abnormalities can be contributory. These abnormalities include reversible cardiac dysfunction (which is usually compensated by ventricular dilation to maintain stroke volume and cardiac output at normal levels), maldistribution of blood flow, and relative hypovolemia as a result of capillary leakage and venodilation. The practical import of this is that although patients with mild hypovolemic shock may be treated successfully with simple fluid replacement, right-sided heart catheterization is usually necessary to provide a diagnostic hemodynamic assessment in patients with moderate or severe shock. In addition, because hemodynamics can change rapidly in sepsis, and because noninvasive evaluation is frequently incorrect in estimating filling pressures and cardiac output, pulmonary artery catheterization is often useful for monitoring the response to therapy.

It is important to interpret the hemodynamic parameters in light of the normal alterations encountered in the pregnant patient. These include an increase in cardiac output of approximately 30%, a decrease in systemic vascular resistance, and an increase in arterial pH by 0.05 units (33).

Volume Infusion

Because septic shock is accompanied by fever and diffuse capillary leakage, most septic patients present with an inadequate preload. Volume resuscitation represents the best initial therapy for treatment of hypotension in sepsis. As an initial goal for fluid support, we recommend a mean arterial pressure of more than 60 mm Hg. Below this level, coronary, renal, and central nervous system blood flow may be reduced as autoregulation is compromised.

Volume administration is best guided by monitoring both left ventricular filling pressure [as estimated by pulmonary capillary wedge pressure (PCWP)] and ventricular performance (measured by thermodilution assessment of cardiac output). We recommend aiming for a PCWP of 12 to 18 mm Hg. Studies in critically ill patients have suggested that 12 mm Hg is the optimal wedge pressure in sepsis because cardiac performance was enhanced up to but not beyond this point (44). In studies of patients with cardiogenic shock, however, cardiac performance was optimized at wedge pressures of 15 to 18 mm Hg. Above 20 mm Hg, interstitial or alveolar pulmonary edema can occur. To maintain optimal ventricular performance and avoid pulmonary edema, we try to maintain a PCWP of 12 to 18 mm Hg.

The type of fluid administered is probably less important than the rapidity with which fluid resuscitation is achieved and the use of physiologic endpoints to evaluate the response to therapy and adjust accordingly (45). Crystalloids are safe and inexpensive and are usually used for initial resuscitation. Albumin and synthetic colloids are more rapid volume expanders, but are more expensive, and capillary permeability to albumin increases in septic shock. No convincing benefit has been demonstrated from administration of colloids rather than crystalloids for fluid repletion despite numerous studies (46,47). We begin resuscitation with rapid infusion of crystalloid solutions at 500 to 2,000 mL/h. If the serum albumin level is very low (<2 g/dL), infusion of 25% albumin may be used to increase intravascular oncotic pressure.

Whether to transfuse red blood cells remains a clinical decision based on the scenario at hand. Although studies suggest that oxygen delivery is optimal at a blood hemoglobin level greater than 10 g/dL, patients without intercurrent illness may tolerate lower levels without difficulty (48). This is clearly true in uncomplicated pregnancies, in which the combination of the physiologic anemia of pregnancy and peripartum blood loss lowers hematocrit, usually without presenting clinical problems. In anemic critically ill patients, however, blood transfusion may provide clinically important increases in oxygen delivery. Transfusion should be considered in patients with severe ongoing hemodynamic instability, and especially in critically ill patients with ongoing blood loss.

Vasopressor Therapy

Maintaining uterine blood flow is an important consideration in the critically ill pregnant patient. Near term, uterine blood flow accounts for almost 10% of maternal cardiac output, and the uterine arteries have little autoregulatory capability (41). Thus, compensatory vasoconstriction in a hypotensive mother tends to shunt blood away from the uterus, resulting in potential fetal oxygen deprivation (41). Vasopressor therapy can exacerbate this tendency. This emphasizes the importance of aggressive fluid resuscitation to achieve adequate intravascular volume. Nonetheless, the initial goal is to stabilize the mother, and if fluid therapy alone fails to restore adequate arterial pressure and organ perfusion, therapy with vasopressor agents should be initiated. The most commonly used vasopressors and their effects on the heart and the peripheral vasculature are listed in Table 52-5.

Initially, we infuse dopamine at a low dosage (1–5 μg/kg/min). This dosage has mild positive inotropic and chronotropic effects and usually increases blood pressure. At low dosages of 1 to 3 μg/kg/min, dopamine increases renal and splanchnic blood flow through an action on dopaminergic receptors (49). If low doses of dopamine do not increase mean arterial pressure to more than 60 mm Hg, we use higher dosages, up to a maximum of 20 μg/kg/min. At these dosages, the vasoconstrictive effects of dopamine are predominant. Adverse effects of dopamine include tachycardia, atrial arrhythmias, ventricular arrhythmias, and the precipitation of angina (49). These effects usually end within minutes after discontinuation of the dopamine infusion.

TABLE 52-5. *Commonly used vasopressor agents (relative potency*)*

Agent	Dose	Cardiac (heart rate)	Peripheral vasculature			
			Contractility	Vasoconstriction	Vasodilation	Dopaminergic
Dopamine	1–4 µg/kg/min	1+	1+	0	1+	4+
	4–20 µg/kg/min	2+	2-3+	2-3+	0	2+
Norepinephrine	2–40 µg/min	1+	2+	4+	0	0
Dobutamine	2–20 µg/kg/min	1-2+	3-4+	0	2+	0
Isoproterenol	1–4 µg/min	4+	4+	0	4+	0
Epinephrine	1–20 µg/min	4+	4+	4+	3+	0
Phenylephrine	20–200 µg/min	0	0	3+	0	0

The 1 to 4+ scoring system is an arbitrary system to allow a judgment of comparative potency among these vasopressor agents.

Adapted from JE Parrillo, *Major Issues in Critical Care Medicine,* JE Parrillo, SM Ayres, (eds), Baltimore, Williams & Wilkins, 1984.

If high dosages of dopamine fail to achieve an adequate increase in blood pressure, or produce arrhythmias, we recommend use of norepinephrine, a more powerful vasoconstrictor with less tendency to produce tachycardia. Norepinephrine infusion is started at 2 µg/min, and increased as necessary; most patients respond to dosages of 2 to 10 µg/min (49). The vasoconstrictive effects of norepinephrine can decrease blood flow to and produce ischemia in peripheral vascular beds, but the alternative is inadequate perfusion of vital organs. With norepinephrine infusions, we commonly give low dosages of dopamine (1–2 µg/kg/min), based on animal studies suggesting that dopamine can increase renal blood flow even in conjunction with high doses of norepinephrine (50).

In patients with serious tachyarrhythmias, phenylephrine can be substituted for norepinephrine, although its vasoconstrictive properties are more modest. In those rare cases in which a patient with a low cardiac output does not respond well to dopamine or norepinephrine, dobutamine or epinephrine may be used. Epinephrine, however, is highly arrhythmogenic and can produce myocardial ischemia. Dobutamine is a good inotropic agent, but has vasodilatory effects that can decrease systemic vascular resistance and blood pressure (49).

Septic patients are hypermetabolic and may require higher levels of oxygen delivery to maintain oxidative metabolism. In addition, because tissue hypoperfusion in sepsis results in part from abnormal shunting of cardiac output, some clinicians have hypothesized that increasing cardiac output to very high, supranormal levels may be beneficial (51,52). Oxygen delivery appears to be proportional to oxygen consumption up to very high levels of delivery in sepsis (53). However, use of inotropic agents to achieve such supranormal cardiac outputs has not been shown to be beneficial in controlled trials (54,55).

Neutralization of Toxins

A third general therapeutic goal is to interrupt the pathogenic sequence leading to septic shock. Several multicenter trials have documented that early corticosteroid therapy fails to improve either morbidity or mortality in septic shock (56–58). Newer therapies have focused on inhibition of the mediators felt to be involved in the pathogenesis of septic shock. Trials of human and mouse monoclonal antibodies to endotoxin, the pathogenetic component of the cell wall of gram-negative bacteria, have failed to show decreased mortality in septic patients (59–62). The inflammatory cytokines TNF and IL-1 play an important role in mediating the systemic and hemodynamic manifestations of septic shock. Antibodies to TNF and soluble TNF receptors, and to IL-1, and IL-1 receptor antagonists have been protective in animal models of sepsis. Clinical trials of cytokine inhibitors in sepsis, however, which include trials of anti-TNF antibodies, IL-1 receptor antagonists, and soluble TNF receptors, have not demonstrated a significant reduction in mortality in septic patients (63).

The cyclooxygenase inhibitor ibuprofen reduced eicosanoid metabolites and led to more rapid resolution of shock in a small trial of patients with sepsis syndrome (64). In a larger randomized, double-blinded trial of ibuprofen in septic patients, the drug reduced fever, tachycardia, oxygen consumption, and lactic acidosis; however, it did not prevent the development of shock or the acute respiratory distress syndrome, and no mortality benefit was seen (65).

Nitric oxide plays an important role in sepsis-induced hypotension, and use of nitric oxide synthase inhibitors is theoretically attractive because they would be expected to affect most prominently those vascular beds with the most abundant overproduction of nitric oxide (36). Despite these theoretical advantages, other considerations would suggest the potential for detrimental effects of nitric oxide synthase inhibitors in sepsis. Nitric oxide synthase inhibitors have been shown to increase systemic vascular resistance and blood pressure in two small trials of hypotensive septic patients, but cardiac output was decreased (66,67). Nitric oxide is an important modulator of both vascular permeability and leukocyte adherence

(68), and nitric oxide synthase inhibition increases microvascular leakage and potentiates endotoxin-induced hepatic damage (69). Further trials will be necessary to clarify the most appropriate role for nitric oxide synthase inhibitors in sepsis.

These disappointing results suggest that inhibition of mediators of sepsis may be a two-edged sword: although antagonizing elements in the sepsis cascade may help interrupt the inflammatory spiral and ameliorate toxic effects of cytokines, these mediators are a crucial component of host defense against infection (63). More thorough study of the pathogenesis of sepsis and identification of the subgroups of patients most likely to benefit from antimediator therapy will be the challenges for the future.

REFERENCES

1. Ledger WJ, Norman M, Gee C, Lewis W. Bacteremia on an obstetric-gynecologic service. Am J Obstet Gynecol 1975;121:205–212.
2. Gibbs CE, Locke WE. Maternal deaths in Texas, 1969 to 1973. A report of 501 consecutive maternal deaths from the Texas Medical Association's Committee on Maternal Health. Am J Obstet Gynecol 1976;126: 687–692.
3. Cunnion RE, Parrillo JE. Myocardial dysfunction in sepsis. Recent insights. Chest 1989;95:941–945.
4. Hollenberg SM, Parrillo JE. Shock. In: Fauci AS, Braunwald E, Isselbacher KJ, et al., eds. Harrison's principles of internal medicine. New York: McGraw-Hill, 1997:214–222.
5. Lee W, Clark SL, Cotton DB, Gonik B, Phelan J, Faro S, Giebel R. Septic shock during pregnancy. Am J Obstet Gynecol 1988;159:410.
6. Beller FK, Schmidt EH, Holzgreve W, Hauss J. Septicemia during pregnancy: a study in different species of experimental animals. Am J Obstet Gynecol 1985;151:967–75.
7. Wilson RF, Thal AP, Kindling PH, Grifka T, Ackerman E. Hemodynamic measurements in septic shock. Arch Surg 1965;91:121–129.
8. Udhoji VN, Weil MH. Hemodynamic and metabolic studies on shock associated with bacteremia. Observations on 16 patients. Ann Intern Med 1965;62:966–978.
9. Parker MM, Shelhamer JH, Natanson C, Alling DW, Parrillo JE. Serial cardiovascular variables in survivors and nonsurvivors of human septic shock: heart rate as an early predictor of prognosis. Crit Care Med 1987;15:923–929.
10. Parrillo JE, Parker MM, Natanson C, et al. Septic shock in humans: advances in the understanding of pathogenesis, cardiovascular dysfunction, and therapy. Ann Intern Med 1990;113:227–242.
11. Mabie WC, Barton JR, Sibai BM. Septic shock in pregnancy. Obstet Gynecol 1997;90:553–561.
12. Parrillo JE. Pathogenetic mechanisms of septic shock. N Engl J Med 1993;328:1471–1477.
13. Billiau A, Vandekerckhove F. Cytokines and their interactions with other inflammatory mediators in the pathogenesis of sepsis and septic shock. Eur J Clin Invest 1991;21:559–573.
14. Suffredini AF, Fromm RE, Parker MM, et al. The cardiovascular response of normal humans to the administration of endotoxin. N Engl J Med 1989;321:280–287.
15. Natanson C, Eichenholz PW, Danner RL, et al. Endotoxin and tumor necrosis factor challenges in dogs simulate the cardiovascular profile of human septic shock. J Exp Med 1989;169:823–832.
16. Tracey KJ. Tumor necrosis factor (cachectin) in the biology of septic shock syndrome. Circ Shock 1991;35:123–128.
17. Ognibene FP, Rosenberg SA, Lotze M, et al. Interleukin-2 administration causes reversible hemodynamic changes and left ventricular dysfunction similar to those seen in septic shock. Chest 1988;94: 750–754.
18. Nathan C, Xie QW. Nitric oxide synthases: roles, tolls, and controls. Cell 1994;78:915–918.
19. Marletta MA. Nitric oxide synthase structure and mechanism. J Biol Chem 1993;268:12231–12234.
20. Dinerman JL, Lowenstein CJ, Snyder SH. Molecular mechanisms of nitric oxide regulation. Potential relevance to cardiovascular disease. Circ Res 1993;73:217–222.
21. Robinson JA, Klodnycky ML, Loeb HS, Racic MR, Gunnar RM. Endotoxin, prekallikrein, complement and systemic vascular resistance. Am J Med 1975;59:61–67.
22. Vadas P, Pruzanski W. Induction of group II phospholipase A2 expression and pathogenesis of the sepsis syndrome. Circ Shock 1993;39: 160–167.
23. Parker MM, Shelhamer JH, Bacharach SL, et al. Profound but reversible myocardial depression in patients with septic shock. Ann Intern Med 1984;100:483–490.
24. Parker MM, McCarthy K, Ognibene FP, Parrillo JE. Right ventricular dysfunction and dilatation, similar to left ventricular changes, characterize the cardiac depression of septic shock in humans. Chest 1990;97: 126–131.
25. Ognibene FP, Parker MM, Natanson C, Shelhamer JH, Parrillo JE. Depressed left ventricular performance. Response to volume infusion in patients with sepsis and septic shock. Chest 1988;93:903–910.
26. Hollenberg SM, Cunnion RE, Lawrence M, Kelly JL, Parrillo JE. Tumor necrosis factor depresses myocardial cell function: results using an in vitro assay of myocyte performance. Clin Res 1989;37:528A.
27. Balligand J-L, Unhureanu D, Kelly RA, et al. Abnormal contractile function due to induction of nitric oxide synthesis in rat cardiac myocytes follows exposure to activated macrophage-conditioned medium. J Clin Invest 1993;91:2314–2319.
28. Suffredini AS, Harpel PC, Parrillo JE. Promotion and subsequent inhibition of plasminogen activation after administration of intravenous endotoxin to normal subjects. N Engl J Med 1989;320:1165–1172.
29. Moore KL, Andreoli SP, Esmon NL, Esmon CT, Bang NU. Endotoxin enhances tissue factor and suppresses thrombomodulin expression of human vascular endothelium in vitro. J Clin Invest 1987;79:124–130.
30. Springer T. Adhesion receptors of the immune system. Nature 1990; 346:425–434.
31. Pober JS, Cotran RS. Cytokines and endothelial cell biology. Physiol Rev 1990;70:427–451.
32. Jacob HS, Craddock PR, Hammerschmidt DE, Modlow CF. Complement-induced granulocyte aggregation. An unsuspected mechanism of disease. N Engl J Med 1980;302:789–794.
33. Yancey MK, Duff P. Acute hypotension related to sepsis in the obstetric patient. Obstet Gynecol Clin North Am 1995;22:91–109.
34. Bone RC. The pathogenesis of sepsis. Ann Intern Med 1991;115: 457–469.
35. Chernow B, Rainey TR, Lake CR. Endogenous and exogenous catecholamines in critical care medicine. Crit Care Med 1982;10:409–416.
36. Hollenberg SM, Cunnion RE. Endothelial and vascular smooth muscle function in sepsis. J Crit Care 1994;9:262–280.
37. Bernsten A, Sibbald WJ. Acute lung injury in septic shock. Crit Care Clin 1989;5:49–79.
38. American College of Obstetricians and Gynecologists. Septic shock. ACOG technical bulletin no. 204. Washington, DC: 1995.
39. Morishima HO, Niemann WH, James LS. Effects of endotoxin on the pregnant baboon and fetus. Am J Obstet Gynecol 1978;131:899–902.
40. Bech-Jansen P, Schmidt EH, Holzgreve W, Hauss J. Circulatory shock in pregnant sheep. I. Effects of endotoxin on uteroplacental and fetal umbilical circulation. Am J Obstet Gynecol 1972;112:1084–1094.
41. Clark SL. Shock in the pregnant patient. Semin Perinatol 1990;14:52–58.
42. Monif GR, Baer H. Polymicrobial bacteremia in obstetric patients. Obstet Gynecol 1976;48:167–169.
43. Norwood SH, Civetta JM. Abdominal CT scanning in critically ill surgical patients. Ann Surg 1985;202:166–175.
44. Packman MJ, Rackow EC. Optimum left heart filling pressure during fluid resuscitation of patients with hypovolemic and septic shock. Crit Care Med 1983;11:165–169.
45. Brar R, Hollenberg SM. The technique of fluid resuscitation. J Crit Illness 1996;11:539–549,550–555,672–683.
46. Velanovich V. Crystalloid versus colloid fluid resuscitation: a meta-analysis of mortality. Surgery 1989;105:65–71.
47. Bisonni RS, Holtgrave DR, Lawler F, Marley DS. Colloids versus crystalloids in fluid resuscitation: an analysis of randomized controlled trials. J Fam Pract 1991;32:387–390.
48. Consensus Conference. Perioperative red blood cell transfusion. JAMA 1988;260:2700–2703.
49. Hollenberg SM, Parrillo JE. Pharmacologic circulatory support. In: Shires GT, Barie PL, eds. Surgical critical care. New York: Little, Brown, 1993:417–451.

50. Schaer GL, Fink MP, Parrillo JE. Norepinephrine alone versus norepinephrine plus low-dose dopamine: enhanced renal blood flow with combination pressor therapy. Crit Care Med 1985;13:492–496.
51. Shoemaker WC, Appel PL, Kram HB. Role of oxygen debt in the development of organ failure sepsis, and death in high-risk surgical patients. Chest 1992;102:208–215.
52. Tuchschmidt J, Fried J, Astiz M, Rackow E. Elevation of cardiac output and oxygen delivery improves outcome in septic shock. Chest 1992; 102:216–220.
53. Fiddian-Green RG, Haglund U, Gutierrez G, Shoemaker WC. Goals for the resuscitation of shock. Crit Care Med 1993;21(suppl):25–31.
54. Hayes MA, Timmins AC, Yau EHS, Palazzo M, Hinds CJ, Watson D. Elevation of systemic oxygen delivery in the treatment of critically ill patients. N Engl J Med 1994;330:1717–1722.
55. Gattinoni L, Brazzi L, Pelosi P, et al. A trial of goal-oriented hemodynamic therapy in critically ill patients. N Engl J Med 1995;333: 1025–1032.
56. Sprung CL, Caralis PV, Marcial EH, et al. The effects of high-dose corticosteroids in patients with septic shock. A prospective, controlled study. N Engl J Med 1984;11:1137–1143.
57. Group VASSCS. Effect of high-dose glucocorticoid therapy on mortality in patients with clinical signs of systemic sepsis. N Engl J Med 1987;317:659–656.
58. Bone RC, Fisher CJ, Clemmer TP, Slotman GJ, Metz CA, Balk RA. A controlled clinical trial of high-dose methylprenisolone in the treatment of severe sepsis and septic shock. N Engl J Med 1987;317:653–658.
59. Ziegler EJ, Fisher CJ Jr, Sprung CL, et al. Treatment of gram-negative bacteremia and septic shock with HA-1A human monoclonal antibody against endotoxin. A randomized, double-blind, placebo-controlled trial. N Engl J Med 1991;324:429–436.
60. McCloskey RV, Straube RC, Sanders C, Smith SM, Smith CR, Group. CTS. Treatment of septic shock with human monoclonal antibody HA-1A. Ann Intern Med 1994;121:1–5.
61. Greenman RL, Schein RMH, Martin MA, et al. A controlled clinical trial of E5 murine monoclonal IgM antibody to endotoxin in the treatment of gram-negative sepsis. JAMA 1991;266:1097–1102.
62. Bone RC, Balk RA, Fein AM, et al. A second large controlled clinical study of E5, a monoclonal antibody to endotoxin: results of a prospective, multicenter, randomized, controlled trial. Crit Care Med 1995;23: 994–1006.
63. Suffredini AF. Current prospects for the treatment of clinical sepsis. Crit Care Med 1994;22(suppl):12–18.
64. Bernard GR, Reines HD, Halushka PV, et al. Prostacyclin and thromboxane A2 formation is increased in human sepsis syndrome. Effects of cyclooxygenase inhibition. Am Rev Respir Dis 1991;144:1095–1101.
65. Bernard GR, Wheeler AP, Russell JA, et al. The effects of ibuprofen on the physiology and survival of patients with sepsis. The Ibuprofen in Sepsis Study Group. N Engl J Med 1997;336:912–918.
66. Lorente JA, Landin L, De Pablo R, Renes E, Liste D. L-arginine pathway in the sepsis syndrome. Crit Care Med 1993;21:1287–1295.
67. Petros A, Lamb G, Leone A, Moncada S, Bennett D, Vallance P. Effects of a nitric oxide synthase inhibitor in humans with septic shock. Cardiovasc Res 1995;28:34–39.
68. Kubes P, Suzuki M, Granger DN. Nitric oxide: an endogenous modulator of leukocyte adhesion. Proc Natl Acad Sci U S A 1991;88: 4651–4655.
69. Harbrecht BG, Billiar TR, Stadler J, et al. Inhibition of nitric oxide synthesis during endotoxemia promotes intrahepatic thrombosis and an oxygen radical-mediated hepatic injury. J Leukoc Biol 1992;52: 390–394.

Cherry and Merkatz's Complications of Pregnancy,
Fifth Edition, edited by W. R. Cohen.
Lippincott Williams & Wilkins, Philadelphia © 2000.

CHAPTER 53

Pregnancy in Women with Disabilities

Sandra Welner

PSYCHOSOCIAL ASPECTS OF THE CARE OF PREGNANT WOMEN WITH DISABILITIES

There were 28 million women with disabilities in this country as of 1990 (1). Of these 28 million women, approximately 14 million are of reproductive age. Certainly the year 2000 census will reflect even higher numbers as people with disabilities become more visible, more active, and more willing to be included in demographic information–gathering activities. Such women are becoming more vocal and more empowered in the knowledge that they have the right to expect to be treated like any other woman when they seek medical care. Unfortunately, stereotypes still exist about the right of women with disabilities to become pregnant, stay pregnant, and take care of children (2). There are many societal attitudes that label those with physical impairments as disabled. This term implies a lack of capability, independence, and competence. A more accurate descriptor might be "differently abled." This term recognizes that those with physical limitations might have difficulties in some areas, but in other areas they might excel.

Because the traditional view of the disabled is that they are less than able, society frequently concludes that women with disabilities should not be parents. This attitude denies the obvious fact that living life as a disabled woman by definition necessitates the development and incorporation of patience and many creative, adaptive strategies to manage daily life (3). Part of the parenting role—and indeed any new challenge that individuals face—requires exactly such flexibility, strengths, and coping strategies. Thus, women with disabilities, when confronted with unexpected complications or roadblocks, will likely have developed finely tuned methods for dealing with and circumventing these obstacles to achieve positive outcomes.

S. Welner: Georgetown University School of Medicine, Washington DC.

Unfortunately, many obstetricians have not had much exposure to disability in their training and may view the disabled pregnant woman as one who is not fit to maintain her pregnancy. Thus, many stories abound in the disability literature of obstetricians recommending that otherwise healthy women with disabilities terminate pregnancy solely on the basis of their physical impairment (4). Although some disabilities are hereditary, others are not, and it behooves the clinician to understand these differences. For example, counseling a pregnant woman with cerebral palsy (CP) to terminate pregnancy because her child might inherit CP shows a lack of understanding of the origin of the disorder. It is also critical for the clinician not to make a judgment as to whether a disability is too severe for the pregnancy to continue. Some inherited disabilities do not result in a greater incidence of cognitive disturbance among offspring and might be linked only to mild physical disabilities. It is important for the clinician first to develop a rapport with a couple, because if a woman herself has an inherited disorder and she is counseled to terminate pregnancy, the message she is receiving is that perhaps her own conception should have been terminated as well (4).

Attitudinal barriers by physicians can also present obstacles for women seeking prenatal care. Reports from women with disabilities that they have been refused prenatal care are commonplace. Flimsy excuses are offered frequently. For example, a woman with deafness who had even provided her own sign language interpreter was still refused prenatal care and was given the unsubstantiated reason that her deafness would put her at high risk of complications and that she should seek a specialist (4a). During medical training, early exposure to disabled patients, and not just those from institutions, is critical in helping enlighten providers that disabled individuals are just like any other patients but might have unique challenges that require different treatment approaches. The acceptance of the disabled and the understanding that they are not a burden or an oddity can go far in integrating this population into mainstream medical practice.

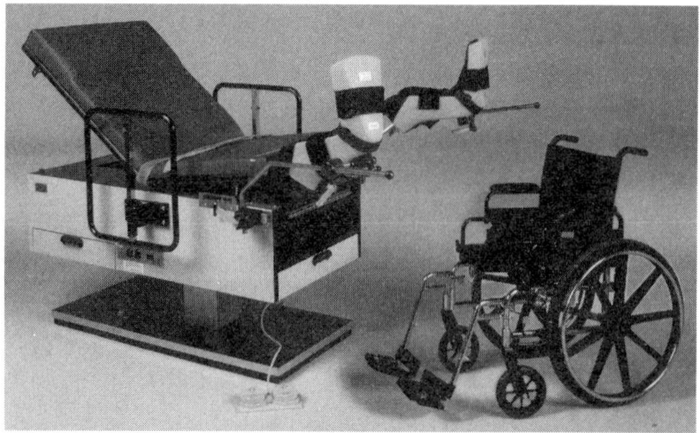

FIG. 53-1. Universally accessible examination table (U.S. patent number 5507050).

There are many structural barriers in medical offices for pregnant women with disabilities. In addition to a lack of accessible examination tables, platform scales for weighing patients are often available only in shipping and loading docks, if at all. Having to be weighed in this setting clearly can be somewhat humiliating and cumbersome for women. Platform scales are available for purchase and would overcome this problem. Unfortunately, when such equipment is not available, physicians may be forced to rely on inaccurate assessments to estimate weight. It is important to identify early in pregnancy where accessible facilities are located so that the individual can be weighed regularly and accurately.

Further examples relating to physical inaccessibility abound, including reports by patients that they have been refused care because they require extra help from office staff and more lengthy appointment times. Compliance with the Americans with Disabilities Act should have resolved the issue of architectural barriers within medical offices (5), but inaccessible equipment and facilities are still commonly encountered. A wheelchair-accessible examination table could facilitate transfers and reduce the amount of time required to maneuver the patient on and off the table, providing the added benefit of minimizing staff injury from lifting heavy patients (Fig. 53-1). This becomes increasingly critical as women progress in their pregnancy, where even the able-bodied can have difficulty with mobility.

Another critical component of compliance with the Americans with Disabilities Act that is harder to measure is discriminatory attitudes toward the disabled. This can be manifest by insensitive comments from staff members and office personnel. In-service training sessions can aid in improving understanding about disability issues, especially if people with disabilities are recruited to participate in this training (6).

PRENATAL CARE

Early prenatal care is one of the cornerstones of good maternal and fetal outcome. The access barriers described here could contribute to inadequate compliance with these essentials, leaving women vulnerable to many preventable complications. It is not uncommon for a woman with physical limitations, especially those affecting dexterity, to have diets poor in nutritional value. This could be an issue even before conception, since many diets high in processed foods are low in folic acid, high in sugar, and lacking in essential vitamins. Thus, it is important to intervene as early as possible to prevent related complications. Antepartum complications related to many disabling conditions include bowel and bladder changes, skin integrity problems, and mobility alterations. These issues can be successfully managed so that they do not progress to complications.

Medications Commonly Used by Women with Disabilities in Pregnancy

Women with disabling disorders frequently use medications to treat the symptoms and complications of their conditions. These typically include acute and chronic pain syndromes, excess muscle spasticity, urinary tract infections (UTIs), and neurogenic bladder-related incontinence.

Analgesics and Anti-inflammatory Agents

Analgesics regularly used by women with disabilities include acetaminophen, aspirin, and other nonsteroidal anti-inflammatory agents (NSAIDs). Steroidal agents are also frequently prescribed. Inhibition of prostaglandin synthesis in patients using acetaminophen is mild and quickly reversible; therefore, as the drug is metabolized, platelet function rapidly returns to baseline. There is no evidence of teratogenicity with acetaminophen use, and it is considered safe in all trimesters and in lactation for analgesic as well as antipyretic use (7).

Although it was postulated that there was a link between aspirin use in the first trimester and fetal anomalies, large controlled studies have failed to confirm this association. Low-dose (60–100 mg/day) aspirin use in the third trimester has not been linked to any specific adverse perinatal outcomes. Among the maternal risks with higher doses is increased bleeding, including postpartum hemorrhage. Adverse neonatal effects include elevated risk of subdural hematoma and intracranial hemorrhage. Consequently, it is often preferable to discontinue use of these agents in the third trimester (8).

Nonsteroidal anti-inflammatory agents often are used to control mild-to-moderate discomfort associated with many disabling conditions. These agents differ slightly in chemical composition, and some of them have been better studied in pregnancy than others. Among those that have been evaluated thoroughly and appear to be relatively safe are ibuprofen and diclofenic sodium (category B, except in the third trimester, when it is contraindicated). Other agents are less well studied and, for this reason, might be less suitable for use during pregnancy. Two examples of these are etodolac and nabumetone (category C except in the third trimester, when it is contraindicated). Use of NSAIDs during the second trimester appears to be acceptable; however, serious complications can arise with third-trimester administration. Accordingly, NSAIDs are contraindicated as a treatment option in the third trimester in most cases.

Complications from maternal use in the third trimester of agents that inhibit cyclo-oxygenase, including NSAIDs, consist of prolongation of gestation and labor, constriction of the ductus arteriosus, persistent fetal circulation, impairment of renal function in the neonate, and bleeding. Most of these adverse effects can be prevented by discontinuing NSAIDs 8 weeks before delivery. These agents are transferred into breast milk in small quantities and are felt to be safe for newborn infants (9).

Corticosteroids are often used by women with autoimmune diseases during pregnancy. There is evidence that these agents can be embryocidal or teratogenic in laboratory animals (category C), but this effect has not been documented in human fetuses. Nevertheless, they should be avoided, if at all possible, in the first trimester. Prednisone is the preferred form of corticosteroid, since it crosses the placenta relatively poorly (10). Dosages need to be adjusted intrapartum, to accommodate for the stress of delivery according to standard protocols (11).

Antibiotics

Many disabled women require antibiotic treatment during pregnancy, usually for the treatment or prevention of UTIs (12). Ampicillin and cephalosporins have wide acceptability and safety for use in all trimesters (7). Nitrofurantoin has a long track record of safe and effective use for the treatment of UTIs in pregnancy (13). There is limited concern about a theoretical risk of development of hemolytic anemia in the newborn who is exposed paripartum. Accordingly, in the third trimester it should probably be avoided (7).

Methenamine hippurate (Hiprex) is an agent often used on a long-term basis for its bacteriostatic properties in women with neurogenic bladders who use catheter devices. This practice should be discontinued during pregnancy, as methenamine has been poorly studied in gestation, and it is not known if adverse fetal effects can result from its administration. It is considered a category C drug in pregnancy. This product is excreted in breast milk and should be taken with caution.

The quinolone class of antibiotics has revolutionized options for outpatient therapy for UTIs for cases in which resistant strains of many types of common bacteria have evolved. These situations are typically encountered in women who have neurogenic bladder and frequently experience asymptomatic bacteriuria and also suffer from recurrent infections exacerbated by the use of catheter devices. Unfortunately, this class of antibiotics has been overprescribed and even occasionally offered as first-line therapy for UTIs in disabled patients. Even before obtaining culture and sensitivity results, it has been assumed that such patients harbor resistant bacterial strains. This is a potentially harmful practice. Quinolones should be used only if the bacteria has documented resistance to all other agents. Data concerning quinolone exposure in all trimesters have been collected from registries, and there has not been any clear evidence of any ill effects to the fetus. However, since studies are incomplete, this antibiotic is still considered category C and should be avoided if possible (13,14).

Trimethoprim-sulfamethoxazole is an antibiotic combination normally used to treat UTIs. Although there is no evidence of adverse effects from first-trimester exposure, third-trimester use should be avoided because of the tendency of the sulfa moiety to bind with circulating albumin, potentially leading to elevated levels of neonatal bilirubin (15).

Skeletal Muscle Antispasmodics and Muscle Relaxants

Spasticity is a common feature of neurologic conditions, especially multiple sclerosis, CP, and spinal cord injury (SCI). Women who have these disabling conditions frequently require medications to reduce excess spasticity, which can interfere with activities of daily living. Women are often treated long term with such agents, and, for this reason, their safety in pregnancy is of considerable interest. Agents most commonly used in the management of muscle spasticity include baclofen, gabapentin, and the benzodiazepines. All of these agents should be avoided in the first trimester if at all possible.

Studies regarding baclofen use in the first trimester have been inconclusive. An increased incidence of abdominal wall defects in laboratory animals given high doses of this agent has been reported, but this complication has not been documented in humans. It is therefore listed as category C in pregnancy. Even so, it has been widely used to treat spastic conditions in the second and third trimesters. It is increasingly popular to administer baclofen through the intrathecal route, especially in cases where excess spasticity is a chronic problem. Isolated case reports have documented the safety and efficacy of this method for treatment of spasticity in patients during labor. In these cases, painful stimuli can trigger many serious complications, including excess spasticity (16).

Botulinum toxin type A (category C) has been used to treat severe spasticity in patients who have such conditions as CP. There have been no studies of the effects of this agent during pregnancy in woman. It should be avoided (17). Gabapentin was first used as an anticonvulsant but has recently shown promise in the management of excess muscle spasticity. There have been few studies examining the effects of gabapentin in pregnancy (18). To date, there have been no reported cases of congenital anomalies in humans exposed to this agent during pregnancy. Administration of gabapentin in rodent fetuses has resulted in urinary tract anomalies, such as hydronephrosis and hydroureter, and a slightly increased risk of pregnancy loss in rabbits. Because it is considered a category C agent, women who are being treated successfully with this drug should be carefully counseled regarding its risk–benefit ratio. Gabapentin is excreted in breast milk in very limited quantities. Studies are still ongoing regarding the use of neurontin in pregnancy and lactation.

Benzodiazepines have been prescribed for many years to treat spasticity. Their use is becoming less popular because of the risk of addiction, and newer antispasmodic agents, such as baclofen and gabapentin, might relieve spasticity without these undesirable side effects. Nevertheless, some women with spastic conditions are still being treated with benzodiazepines and have difficulty changing medications because of addiction. In these patients, it is advisable to avoid first- and third-trimester use when possible. Some studies have reported congenital anomalies in fetuses after first-trimester exposure to benzodiazepines, including facial clefts and cardiac anomalies, but the best controlled studies do not support these findings. Benzodiazepines have been labeled category D and, if possible, are to be avoided by pregnant women in all circumstances. The use of these agents in the paripartum period has been linked to significant complications, including neonatal depression, poor suckling, apneic spells, and even withdrawal syndromes. Neonates exposed to benzodiazepines therefore require monitoring, and breast-feeding should be avoided, to limit further neonatal compromise (19).

Urinary Tract Agents

Bladder dysfunction is extremely common in many types of disabling conditions. Even women who were previously continent can become less so with the anatomic changes of the urinary tract as pregnancy progresses. Other women, such as those who have SCI or spina bifida (SB), live with neurogenic bladders. In this context, voiding difficulties can worsen during pregnancy. Other disabling conditions in which bladder antispasmodics are used include SCI, SB, CP, and multiple sclerosis. Many women with these conditions have received long-term treatment with bladder antispasmodics. Thus, discontinuing these agents during pregnancy might pose difficulties. Fortunately, there are bladder antispasmodics and analgesics that are category B, such as oxybutin chloride and phenazopyridine hydrochloride. For patients who have been using other bladder agents that are category C, such as dantrolene sodium and propantheline bromide, regimens should be adjusted, especially in the first trimester.

During pregnancy, urinary tract tone diminishes, leading to an increased incidence of reflux, urine stasis, bacteriuria, and even pyelonephritis (20). Some disabling conditions are inherently linked to exactly these complications, such as SCI, SB, and, in some cases, multiple sclerosis, CP, and other spastic disabilities. Use of prophylactic urinary antiseptics is the subject of controversy, and some researchers recommend limiting the routine use of these agents to lower the risk of development of resistant organisms. If a woman has documented recurrent UTIs, however, this strategy might need to be reevaluated (21). Pregnant women with neurologic disabilities also have a higher incidence of nephrolithiasis, and noninvasive monitoring, such as with renal ultrasounds, can be used to assess this condition (22). Simple measures, such as maintaining the urine at an acid pH and increasing fluid intake, might be helpful in this regard.

If a UTI is suspected, aggressive treatment must be instituted, especially in women with SB and SCI, in whom high incidences of pyelonephritis (23) and other complications have been reported. In the first trimester (weeks 4–8) a fever above 102.2°F (39°C) has been linked to a higher risk of congenital anomalies, such as neural tube defects (NTDs), microcephaly, and microphthalmia; therefore, prevention of UTIs and pyelonephritis as well as use of antipyretics, such as acetaminophen, can be especially critical during this stage of fetal development (24).

Bowel function can also be affected in pregnant women. High progesterone levels relax the smooth muscle of the intestines, resulting in increased constipation. For women with neurogenic bowel, this physiologic change can lead to new challenges in bowel management. In addition, many prenatal vitamins are constipating, which exacerbates the problem. It is important to maximize fluid intake and foods containing roughage and to avoid laxatives to aid evacuation (25).

Skin integrity can develop as a new problem for women who were previously capable of shifting position in their wheelchairs and lifting their weight when transferring from surface to surface. As weight distribution changes, these transfers can become more awkward and difficult, resulting in unrecognized damage to the insensate skin of a paralyzed woman. Additionally, she might require reevaluation in terms of wheelchair seating and cushioning, since alterations in body mass distribution can make her wheelchair less comfortable or pose problems with newly developed pressure areas. In patients who use wheelchairs, visits should always include inspection of the skin on the lower body.

Changes frequently develop in the posture and carriage of pregnant women owing to the different weight distribution posed by the protuberant abdomen. Women who have chronic back pain can experience worsening symptoms in pregnancy as the result of this new stress (26). Early in pregnancy and, when necessary, periodically throughout gestation, these women should consult with a physiatrist and a physical therapist about mobility aids, exercises, and alternative therapies that might relieve this discomfort. For those with balance and coordination difficulties, such as is seen in women with head injuries, multiple sclerosis, CP, and other disabling conditions, the change in center of gravity can be especially destabilizing and can lead to an increased risk of falls. Joint instability, which is seen in many pregnant women as a result of pregnancy hormone effects on connective tissue, can compound this problem (27). A physiatrist and a physical therapist should be consulted for evaluation of ambulation and recommendations of mobility aids that would best suit a particular woman's condition. It might be necessary for this evaluation to be repeated during the course of pregnancy, and a woman might need to change to more supportive ambulation aids toward the later stages.

CEREBRAL PALSY

There are approximately 250,000 women of all ages in the United States with CP (28). CP is a group of medical conditions characterized by nerve and muscle dysfunction resulting from damage *in utero* to the part of the brain that controls and coordinates muscular action. According to the location of the damage, varying disabilities can develop. The most common effects are lack of muscle coordination, involuntary tremors, and, occasionally, speech difficulties. The majority of individuals with CP have normal intellectual capacity (29). Defective development of brain cells before birth, injury during delivery, an accident, or infectious disease can all result in CP. The effects are permanent, and regular treatment is often necessary to prevent some of the resulting conditions from becoming more severe.

Prenatal Care

There is a paucity of literature discussing pregnancy in women with CP. In a survey of women with CP who experienced a pregnancy, there were several prominent issues surrounding their prenatal care. In the first trimester, increased abdominal muscle cramping was reported frequently. Also noted were sciatic pain, dislocated vertebrae, and backaches. Many women reported increased muscle spasticity and joint tightness, especially in the groin area. Additionally, difficulties with balance and ambulation became prominent as the pregnancy progressed into the second trimester, and considerable edema was often present. Patients noted exacerbation of the muscle spasticity observed in the first trimester, spreading to the thighs, back, and groin area. Back pain was common, and some women experienced sharp pain with fetal movements as well.

In the third trimester, overall activities were significantly impaired, from ambulation to transfers (e.g., from bed or toilet to wheelchair) to the execution of activities of daily living. Symptoms and findings that were worsening in the second trimester—such as back pain, edema, urinary frequency and incontinence, and skin problems—became even more noticeable and difficult to manage. UTIs and incontinence were more frequently reported in pregnant women with CP. Among the women in this survey there was an increased incidence of pyelonephritis in the third trimester. Worsening scoliosis contributed not only to more severe back pain but also to pulmonary dysfunction as the growing fetus limited diaphragmatic excursion (30,31).

Intrapartum Care

The intrapartum course of pregnant women with CP has also received little attention in the obstetric literature. Only one peer-reviewed journal article discusses issues pertaining to delivery in these women (32). The sample size was relatively small (28 patients), and, for this reason, it is difficult to generalize these findings to all pregnant women with CP. The article reported that 18% of pregnant women with CP experienced preeclampsia (34) versus 6% among the general population (32,33).

Among the study patients, there was a higher percentage of cesarean deliveries (32%) (32). This might have been the result of dystocia, fetal malpresentation, cephalopelvic disproportion, or the uneasiness of the obstetric staff in monitoring long labors in these women. Moreover, the women in the study sample had relatively mild-to-moderate CP, and this might have minimized abnormalities in their intrapartum course. The use of magnetic resonance pelvimetry in these patients in the third trimester might have been a helpful predictor of those who were unlikely to deliver successfully vaginally. This technique might be preferable to standard radiography and computed tomography scans, since there is less radiation exposure to the fetus (34).

Although the type of anesthesia was not mentioned in this discussion of the intrapartum treatment of patients, anecdotal reports support the safety of epidural anesthesia for use in children with CP. The anesthetic course must be individualized, since some women with CP have severe scoliosis, making the placement of epidural anesthesia challenging. Women with CP might also have micrognathia and other jaw deformities, making intubation for general anesthesia difficult. These issues must be taken into account during the prenatal period, and an anesthesia consult should be obtained (35).

NEURAL TUBE DEFECTS

Spina bifida is diagnosed in 2,000 neonates every year in the United States (36). In many infants, corrective surgery and adaptive technology have enabled these babies to grow up to be women who lead active lives, including, of course, motherhood. Women with SB do not necessarily give birth to offspring with SB, though the incidence is certainly higher (about 2%–4%) than among the general population (37). Consequently, women with SB should receive very comprehensive counseling before conception about adequate folate supplementation. The standard recommendation for primary prophylaxis of 400 mg folic acid per day, taken as a dietary supplement combined with food sources, may need to be exceeded for secondary prevention in women who have given birth to an affected infant (38). Prenatal testing with triple screen (39) (estriol, alphafetoprotein, and beta-human chorionic gonadotropin) can pick up many cases of NTDs as well as other anomalies. There have been a number of reported studies looking at the course of pregnancy in women with SB. There are a few recurrent issues that arise during the prenatal and intrapartum course of these women.

Women with SB are unique in that their disabilities arose at birth. Long-standing problems with fecal and bladder incontinence as well as recurrent UTIs have often resulted in the need to undergo surgical procedures, such as ileal conduits (urinary diversion) (40) and intestinal diversion (41). These procedures might have been done at a young age, resulting in intraabdominal adhesions (42).

Prenatal Care

In a study of pregnant women with SB, there was a higher risk of early pregnancy failure in the study population, with eight women experiencing one or more cases of this adverse outcome, totaling 17 episodes (43). Some complications are similar to those of women who have SCI and relate to issues of mobility and bowel and bladder changes. There have been a number of reports of increased incontinence, frequently resulting in vulvitis (44) as well as UTIs and pyelonephritis. The latter two are associated with the development of preterm labor (45). There have also been some case reports of renal function deterioration in pregnant women with SB (37). Abdominal pain has also been reported, possibly the result of intraperitoneal adhesions (43). There have been case reports of iromaru conduit obstruction (up to 10%) (40,46) during pregnancy, with shifting of the intraabdominal contents as the uterus expands.

Intrapartum Care

The presence of a contracted pelvis resulting in cephalopelvic disproportion and malpresentation has been reported in pregnant women with SB. There are very limited data on the intrapartum experiences of these women, including mode of anesthesia and method of delivery. In two small studies reviewing labor, six of nine pregnancies were delivered by cesarean section (45,47). As mentioned in the discussion of CP, magnetic resonance pelvimetry can help identify those patients with a contracted pelvis. The decision to perform cesarean section should be made for the usual obstetric reasons. Women with SB have poorly developed pelvic floor structures that could influence the progress of labor. Even without the effects of vaginal deliveries, they are at higher risk of pelvic prolapse. Indeed, a survey of 52 women with NTDs reported permanent loss in perineal muscle strength postpartum (48). This should be taken into account when deciding on the mode of delivery for a woman who has previously undergone vaginal delivery.

Cesarean section can be accompanied by unusual complications because of the aforementioned incidence of intraperitoneal adhesions in some women with NTDs, a consequence of ventriculoperitoneal shunting (46,49). Great care must be taken during cesarean section to avoid damaging intraperitoneal shunt structures, which are usually located in the right paracolic space but also can be present in other intraperitoneal locations, such as in the pleural space, cardiac atrium, ureter, stomach, and fallopian tube (47,50).

Anesthetic choices for women with NTDs have been described. Three case reports have discussed anesthesia of women with NTDs (51–53). The key factor in administering anesthesia to women with NTDs is to identify the level of the lesion, because attempting epidural anesthesia above this location is highly likely to result in a dural tap. A case report of this complication in a woman with SB occulta resulted in postural headache (52). Some women with SB have grossly deformed vertebral anatomy. Spinal anesthesia was successfully administered to one such patient intrapartum (53) An obstetric anesthesiologist should be consulted for advice about pain relief during labor for SB patients.

SPINAL CORD INJURY

Approximately 30,000 women in the United States have SCIs (54). With improved medical technology, these women can look forward to complete and rewarding lives. SCI is certainly not a contraindication to pregnancy, although many women with this disability have been discouraged from conceiving. It is sometimes difficult for others to realize that living life from the level of a wheelchair and dealing with issues surrounding paralysis, such as bowel and bladder routines, still leave time for an active life as a parent. Reports of successful pregnancy in hundreds of SCI mothers confirm the validity of this choice (4,55). That being said, regular and close monitoring through all stages of pregnancy is a critical factor in maximizing good maternal and neonatal outcome.

Prenatal Care

Many of the issues of prenatal care are similar to those described in the introductory section on prenatal care. The most common complications seen in women with SCI during the prenatal period include bacteriuria, UTIs, pyelonephritis, constipation (see section on prenatal care), anemia, breakdown in areas of insensate skin (usually in the buttocks and perineal area), vulvovaginitis, respiratory problems, preterm contractions, and autonomic dysreflexia.

Urinary tract complications are one of the most common difficulties encountered by women with SCIs during pregnancies. Indeed, there is a 5% to 10% incidence of bacteriuria, a 50% to 100% risk of UTIs, and a 30% likelihood that a woman with SCI will experience pyelonephritis during the course of her pregnancy (23). Accordingly, it is important to establish a routine of regular UTI monitoring early in the pregnancy. Prophylactic bacteriostatic agents, such as might be useful in cases in which a woman has more than one UTI during pregnancy, are indicated. Because the classic symptom of dysuria is often absent in this population, urine evaluation should not depend on the woman's complaints of such discomfort. Because bacteriuria is so common, it is important to evaluate the urinalysis for evidence of infection that the woman might not be able to recognize.

Many urinary anti-infectives are safe for use during pregnancy. Unfortunately, because of the nature of SCI, women typically harbor microorganisms resistant to standard antimicrobial agents. For this reason, it is prudent to obtain sensitivity results so as not to encourage this pattern. Nevertheless, resistant organisms will often be found in such patients, posing difficult treatment dilemmas. Quinolones are commonly used in nonpregnant women with SCIs who have resistant bacteria found on culture. Their use in pregnancy is usually discouraged if other options are available.

Pyelonephritis has been reported as a complication in up to 30% of pregnant women with SCI (23). Depending on the stage of pregnancy, different risks are present. In the first trimester, it is important to avoid high fever in the mother, which is potentially teratogenic. It should be noted that women with tetraplegia can have an impaired ability to mount a fever as a response to infection. Consequently, temperature elevation may not be a reliable method for detection of lower UTIs or pyelonephritis in these patients (56). This condition can be suspected if there are symptoms of autonomic activation (Table 53-1). In the second and third trimesters, bacteriuria and pyelonephritis are associated with uterine irritability and premature labor (57).

Anemia is an extremely common condition in all pregnant women; it develops in approximately 55% of all pregnancies (58). No figures are available for the incidence of anemia in women with SCI; however, it has been reported to occur more frequently than in the nondisabled population. Possible causes include a combination of anemia of chronic disease and hemodilution of pregnancy (59,60). In tetraplegic patients, blood pressure regulation can be impaired, and these patients might experience significant hypotension (61). Patients with both anemia and hypotension require especially careful monitoring. Additionally, anemia might predispose women to skin breakdown in areas of pressure; decubitus ulceration develops in up to 25% of pregnant women with SCI. Therefore, anemia as well as other nutritional deficits need to be monitored and corrected in pregnant SCI patients (59).

Monilial vulvovaginitis is prevalent in all pregnant women (62). When a woman is also a wheelchair user, the additive influences of poor ventilation, moisture, and pregnancy can cause these infections to be especially troublesome (63).

Immobilization is a risk factor for venous thrombosis. Because pregnancy is a hypercoagulable state (64), women with SCI, especially those with tetraplegia, might be at increased risk of venous thrombosis. Thromboprophylaxis should be considered an option on an individualized basis, depending on risk assessment (65).

Pregnancy influences pulmonary function through progesterone effects on the central nervous system and on smooth muscles in the airways. The tidal volume increases and accounts for the 40% increase in minute ventilation. The expiratory residual volume and the residual volume both decline by 20%. The functional residual capacity therefore also decreases by 20% (20). These changes related to pregnancy, as well as upward pressure on the diaphragm from the expanding uterus, can challenge women with tetraplegia who have preexisting compromised pulmonary capacity. They have a 20% risk of worsening pulmonary function during pregnancy (66).

Autonomic dysreflexia, also called autonomic hyperreflexia or dysreflexia, occurs in 85% of people with SCI (61). Women with thoracic SCI, or paraplegia, with spinal cord lesions above T6 are at risk of autonomic dysreflexia, and tetraplegic patients are at an even higher risk. In these

TABLE 53-1. *Autonomic dysreflexia in the prenatal period*

Cause	Painful stimuli from visceral organs resulting in activation of the autonomic nervous system
Manifestations	Diffuse muscle spasms commonly seen in the lower extremities
Symptoms and findings	Headache, labile hypertension, and autonomic nervous activity resulting in sweating and piloerection above the level of the lesion, cardiac arrhythmias, nasal stuffiness, facial flushing
Potential triggers	UTIs or blocked catheter, decubitus ulcers, severe constipation or fecal impaction, uterine irritability, fetal movement
Treatment	Identify and remove causative factors (speculum and kinked catheters), semisupine positioning, rapid-acting antihypertensive agents when necessary, treat infection (UTIs)

UTI, urinary tract infection.

From Atterbury JL, Groome LJ. Pregnancy in women with spinal cord injuries. Nurs Clin North Amer 1998;33:603–612; Colachis SC. Autonomic hyperreflexia with spinal cord injury. J Am Paraplegia Soc 1992;15:171–186.

women, varying degrees of stimuli to the autonomic nervous system can trigger symptoms of dysreflexia (Table 53-1). Women with tetraplegia might experience flushing and sweating and increased spasticity with fetal movement or Braxton Hicks contractions. More significant stimuli, such as uterine irritability or UTIs, can trigger dysreflexic symptoms in paraplegic women as well.

Intrapartum Care

Instructing a woman in a bowel management program before labor and delivery is helpful in minimizing embarrassing bowel accidents during labor and in identifying and removing impaction, which could be a trigger for dysreflexia. Intrapartum management of women with SCI includes ensuring adequate bladder drainage, monitoring for respiratory compromise, shifting position regularly (since breakdown of delicate skin can take place very rapidly), and cushioning legs during spasms to avoid damaging skin on the legs and feet during these involuntary movements. Management of pain from contractions, which frequently results in autonomic dysreflexia, is critical in preventing this condition. Autonomic dysreflexia, which occurs in approximately two-thirds of pregnant patients with spinal cord lesions above T6, is a response of the autonomic nervous system to noxious stimuli from visceral organs, such as the bowel, bladder, cervix, and uterus, all of which experience changes during labor and delivery. It is critical to institute early intervention to prevent autonomic dysreflexia, because serious or even fatal complications can ensue as the result of delay (Table 53-2). This can be effectively accomplished with the use of epidural anesthesia, which should be instituted at an early stage in the intrapartum period (60).

Agents most effective in treating autonomic dysreflexia–related hypertension must be fast acting and of short duration. Because this hypertension is paroxysmal and related to the painful stimulus of labor, blood pressure elevations will be seen to coincide with contractions (67) (Table 53-2). Examples of antihypertensives that have a rapid onset and relatively short duration of action include hydralazine and nifedipine. Antihypertensives that have prolonged action will have a sustained effect during the downslope of paroxysmal hypertension, leading to intrauterine hypoxia and fetal distress; for this reason, they should be avoided (61). Since induction of labor with oxytocin can quickly trigger autonomic dysreflexia, the decision to induce or augment labor with this agent must be accompanied by extremely careful monitoring; life-threatening consequences have been reported with its use (68).

Vaginal delivery is preferable; however, care should be taken to avoid an unattended delivery. There can be an increased incidence of such deliveries because of the diminished pelvic sensory input in response to the descent of the fetal head (57). This is especially critical because of the risk of autonomic dysreflexia. Maternal pushing efforts may be diminished; consequently, assisted delivery might be required (66). The decision to perform a cesarean section should be for obstetric indications only or if dysreflexia or respiratory compromise in tetraplegic patients cannot be controlled. Rates of cesarean delivery among women with SCI vary widely with different series

TABLE 53-2. *Autonomic dysreflexia versus preeclampsia*

	Autonomic dysreflexia	Preeclampsia
Cause	Painfull stimuli from visceral organs resulting in activation of the autonomic nervous system	Idiopathic—possible immunologic link
Manifestations	Diffuse muscle spasms commonly seen in the lower extremities, trace proteinurea from catheter or UTIs	Edema, hyperactive reflexes, proteinurea
Target vessels	Affects aorta, large blood vessels in brain	Affects small blood vessels in brain, eyes, kidneys, liver
Target muscles	Visceral smooth muscle	Skeletal muscles
Symptoms and findings	Headache, labile hypertension, autonomic nervous activity resulting in sweating and piloerection above the level of the lesion, vagus nerve–mediated cardiac arrhythmias, nasal stuffiness, facial flushing, pupillary dilation	Headache, steady hypertension
Link with contractions	Blood pressure normal between contractions, labile hypertension markedly higher during contractions	Steady hypertension—not related to contractions
Treatment	Epidural analgesia, rapid-acting short-duration antihypertensives, semisupine positioning	Magnesium sulfate, antihypertensives throughout labor
Worst scenario if mismanaged	Seizures, intracranial hemorrhage, coma	Kidney failure, blindness, seizures, stroke
Risk of death	Significant	Rare

UTI, urinary tract infection.

From Atterbury JL, Groome LJ. Pregnancy in women with spinal cord injuries. Nurs Clin North Am 1998;33(4):603–612; Colachis SC. Autonomic hyperreflexia with spinal cord injury. J Am Paraplegia Soc 1992;15(3):171–186.

(18%–67%) (69) and appear to be higher than those seen in the general population (70,71). Epidural anesthesia has been widely used for analgesia during labor and delivery as well as to control autonomic dysreflexia (72).

POSTPARTUM CARE

Postpartum issues for women with disabilities vary according to the disabling condition. UTIs are common in all women postpartum, but they can be a particular concern in women with neurogenic bladder. This complication should be investigated and treated promptly. Women with SCI who are at risk of dysreflexia should be monitored for urinary retention postpartum, because this could be a potential trigger. Those who are ambulatory might need to make frequent trips to the bathroom to void, which could be difficult because of unsteadiness and fatigue, putting them at risk of falls. The natural postpartum diuresus can put demands on patients who self-catheterize, since they might have to do this more frequently (73).

Poor episiotomy healing and deep vein thrombosis are other complications seen in the postpartum period. As stated earlier, anemia is common in pregnancy and can be compounded by blood loss during delivery, leading to decreased energy levels. Fatigue linked to the new demands of motherhood can also be compounded by physical limitations and increased energy expenditures required to accomplish parenting tasks. As mentioned previously, it is important to engage the expertise of the physical and occupational therapist during all stages of pregnancy, but the need for their input is especially critical during the postpartum period. Physical therapists can be helpful in demonstrating safer transfer techniques and ambulation methods to avoid injury when the mother is experiencing fatigue and unsteadiness. Occupational therapists can assist in troubleshooting and problem solving with the couple for issues such as positioning for breast feeding and changing diapers (74).

In addition, the woman and her partner, as well as family and friends, can readily adapt infant care equipment to be accessible and useful. Key components to success for the new mother in the neonatal period are a good support system, a sense of humor, and creativity. New mothers with disabilities frequently encounter prejudicial comments, which may be hurtful and erode their self-confidence. Armed with the support of family, friends, and the medical team, they can be empowered to educate society that they are indeed parents and good ones at that. Two main support systems are available for new parents with disabilities. Through the Looking Glass in Berkeley, California (telephone: (800) 644-2666; E-mail: TLG@lookingglass.org; Website: www.lookingglass.org) is an organization designed to facilitate independent parenting for all people with disabilities. They produce guidebooks, adaptive manuals, and catalogs of equipment designed to facilitate independent parenting for even the most severely limited women as well as a hotline for pressing questions. Another source available for parenting support is Diana Michelle's home page: The Internet's 1-Stop Resource for Parents with Disabilities (Website: http://ourworld.compuserve.com/homepages/Trish_and_John; E-mail: 74731.2325@compuserve.com), a support network for parents with disabilities established by a new mother with CP who had difficulty locating a peer network to discuss common experiences and share solutions to frequently encountered problems.

CONCLUSION

Caring for a pregnant woman with a physical disability can be a challenging and rewarding experience. When the clinician takes an interest in learning about the woman's disability and how her pregnancy is affecting her well-being, a coordinated interdisciplinary team can rally around the couple to maximize a good outcome.

ACKNOWLEDGMENTS

Dr. Welner acknowledges the assistance of Mr. Keith Gentile in the preparation of this manuscript and the guidance and support of her parents, Mr. Nick Welner and Mrs. Barbara Welner.

REFERENCES

1. McNeil JM. Americans with disabilities: 1994–1995. Curr Popul Rep Series P70–61. 1–18, 1997.
2. Nosek MA. Wellness among women with physical disabilities. In: Krotoski DM, Nosek MA, Turk MA, eds. Women with physical disabilities: achieving and maintaining health and well-being. Paul H. Brookes Publishing Co., Baltimore, 1996:17–33.
3. Rogers JG. Pregnancy and physical disabilities. In: Krotoski DM, Nosek MA, Turk MA, eds. Women with physical disabilities: achieving and maintaining health and well-being. Paul H. Brookes Publishing Co., Baltimore, 1996:101–108.
4. Rogers JG, Matsumura M. Mother to be: a guide to pregnancy and birth for women with disabilities; Demos (pub) 1991:51–91.

4a. American Health Lawyers Association. U.S. Court in the District of Columbia says obstetrician who refused to treat deaf woman violated the Rehabilitation Act and the DC Human Rights Law. Health Law Digest 1997;25:27–28.

5. Americans with Disabilities Act of 1990. 42 U.S.C. § 12101 et seq., 28 CFR part 36.
6. Fiduccia BW. Multiplying choices: improving access to reproductive health services for women with disabilities. Berkeley, Calif.: Berkeley Planning Associates, 1997.
7. Niebyl JR. Drugs and related areas in pregnancy. In: Sciarra JJ, ed. Gynecology and obstetrics. New York: Lippincott–Raven Publishers, 1992:2(100):6.
8. Ostensen M, Ramsey-Goldman R. Treatment of inflammatory rheumatic disorders in pregnancy. Drug Saf 1998;19:389–410.
9. Rayburn WF. Connective tissue disorders and pregnancy: recommendations for prescribing. J Reprod Med 1998;43:341–349.
10. Ostensen M, Ramsey-Goldman R. Treatment of inflammatory rheumatic disorders in pregnancy: What are the safest treatment options? Drug Saf 1998;19:389–410.
11. Holland EG, Taylor AT. Glucocorticoids in clinical practice. J Fam Pract 1991;32:512–519.
12. Bint AJ, Hill D. Bacteriuria of pregnancy: an update on significance, diagnosis and management. J Antimicrob Chemother 1994;33[Suppl A]:93–97.
13. Schaefer C, Amoura-Elefant E, Vial T, et al. Pregnancy outcome after prenatal quinolone exposure: evaluation of a case registry of the European Network of Teratology Information Services (ENTIS). Eur J Obstet Gynecol Reprod Biol 1996;69:83–89.
14. Loebstein R, Addis A, Ho E, et al. Pregnancy outcome following ges-

tational exposure to fluoroquinolones: a multicenter prospective controlled study. Antimicrob Agents Chemother 1998;42:1336–1339.
15. Czeizel A. A case-control analysis of the teratogenic effects of co-trimoxazole. Reprod Toxicol 1990;4:305–313.
16. Delhaas EM, Verhagen J. Pregnancy in a quadriplegic patient treated with continuous intrathecal baclofen infusion to manage her severe spasticity: case report. Paraplegia 1992;30:527–528.
17. Delisa JA, Gans BM, eds. Rehabilitation medicine: principles and practice, 3rd ed. New York: Lippincott–Raven Publishers, 1998;42:1052.
18. McLean MJ. Gabapentin. Epilepsia 1995;36:S73–S86.
19. McElhatton PR. The effects of benzodiazepine use during pregnancy and lactation. Reprod Toxicol 1994;8:461–475.
20. Baker ER. Physiologic adaptations to pregnancy. In: Carr PL, Freund KM, Somani S, eds. The medical care of women. Philadelphia: WB Saunders, 1995;32:298.
21. Harris RE. Urinary tract infections during pregnancy. In: Sciarra JJ, ed. Gynecology and obstetrics, vol. 3. New York: Lippincott–Raven Publishers, 1998:6–8.
22. Perkash I. Long-term urologic management of the patient with spinal cord injury. Urol Clin North Am 1993;20:423–434.
23. Atterbury JL, Groome LJ. Pregnancy in women with spinal cord injuries. Nurs Clin North Am 1998;33:603–612.
24. Jirasek JE. Prenatal development: growth, differentiation, and their disturbances. In: Sciarra JJ, ed. Gynecology and obstetrics. New York: Lippincott–Raven Publishers, 1998: 2(14):15.
25. Bonapace ES, Fisher RS. Constipation and diarrhea in pregnancy. Gastroenterol Clin North Am 1998;27:197–221.
26. Donaldson JO. The nervous system in pregnancy. In: Sciarra JJ, ed. Gynecology and obstetrics. New York: Lippincott–Raven Publishers, 1988:3(19):9.
27. Shrock P. Exercise and physical activity during pregnancy. In: Sciarra JJ, ed. Gynecology and obstetrics. New York: Lippincott–Raven Publishers, 1990:2(8):3.
28. Arcand M. CP and aging: proceedings. Wisconsin Council on Developmental Disabilities (pub) Jan 1996:10.
29. Kroll K, Klein EL. Enabling romance: a guide to love, sex, and relationships for the disabled. New York: Harmony Books, 1992:122.
30. Delisa JA, Gans BM, eds. Rehabilitation medicine: principles and practice, 3rd ed. New York: Lippincott–Raven Publishers, 1998:42:1052.
31. Rogers J, Matsumura M. Mother to be: a guide to pregnancy and birth for women with disabilities. New York: Demos, 1991:5–11.
32. Winch R, Bengtson L, McLaughlin J, Fitzsimmons J, Budden S. Women with cerebral palsy: obstetric experience and neonatal outcome. Dev Med Child Neurol 1993;35:974–982.
33. Lydakis C, Beevers DG, et al. Obstetric and neonatal outcome following chronic hypertension in pregnancy among different ethnic groups. Q J Med 1998;91:837–844.
34. Sporri S, Hanggi W, et al. Pelvimetry by magnetic resonance imaging as a diagnostic tool to evaluate dystocia. Obstet Gynecol 1997;89:902–908.
35. Burstein FD, Cohen SR, et al. Surgical therapy for severe refractory sleep apnea in infants and children: application of the airway zone concept. Plast Reconstr Surg 1995;96:34–41.
36. Yen IH, Khourg MJ, et al. The changing epidemiology of neural tube defects: United States. Am J Dis Child 1992;146:857–861.
37. Reitberg CC, Lindhout D. Adult patients with spina bifida cystica: genetic counselling, pregnancy and delivery. Eur J Obstet Gynecol Reprod Biol 1993;52:63–70.
38. Neuhouser ML, Beresford SA, et al. Absorption of dietary and supplemental folate in women with prior pregnancies with neural tube defects and controls. J Am Coll Nutr 1998;17:625–630.
39. Bahado-Singh RO, Oz U, Kovanci E, et al. New triple screen test for Down syndrome: combined urine analytes and serum AFP. J Mat Fetal Med 1998;7:111–114.
40. Mann WJ, Jones DE. Pregnancy complicated by maternal neural tube defect and an ileal conduit: a case report. J Reprod Med 1976;17: 399–341.
41. Christiansen J. Advances in the surgical management of anal incontinence. Baillieres Clin Gastroenterol 1992;6:43–57.
42. Khosrovi H, Kaufman HH, et al. Laparoscopic-assisted distal ventriculoperitoneal shunt placement. Surg Neurol 1998;49:127–134.
43. Bradley NK, Liakos AM, et al. Maternal shunt dependency: implications for obstetric care, neurosurgical management, and pregnancy outcomes and a review of selected literature. Neurosurgery 1998;43:448–460.
44. Farine D, Jackson U. Pregnancy complicated by maternal spina bifida: a report of two cases. J Reprod Med 1988;33:323–326.
45. Yamamoto M, Yamada K, et al. Pregnancy and delivery in patients with spina bifida: report of 5 cases. Nippon Hinyokika Gakkai Zasshi 1997; 88:1005–1012.
46. Powell B, Garvey M. Complications of maternal spina bifida. Ir J Med Sci 1984;153(1):20–21.
47. Richmond D, Zaharievski I, et al. Management of pregnancy in mothers with spina bifida. Eur J Obstet Gynecol Reprod Biol 1987;25: 341:5.
48. Dunne KB, Gingher N. A survey of the medical and functional status of members of the adult network of the SBAA. Washington, D.C.: Spina Bifida Association of America, 1988.
49. Lortat-Jacob S, Pierre-Kahn A, et al. Abdominal complications of ventriculo-peritoneal shunts in children. 65 cases. Chir Pediatr 1984;25: 17–21.
50. Ketoff JA, Klein RL, et al. Ventricular cholecystic shunts in children. J Pediatr Surg 1997;32:181–183.
51. Broome IJ. Spinal anaesthesia for caesarean section in a patient with spina bifida cystica. Anaesth Intensive Care 1989;17:377–379.
52. McGrady EM, Davis AG. Spina bifida occulta and epidural anaesthesia. Anaesthesia 1988;43:867–869.
53. Nuyten F, Gielen M. Spinal catheter anaesthesia for caesarean section in patient with spina bifida. Anaesthesia 1990;45:846–847.
54. Ficke R. 1992 Digest of data on persons with disabilities. Washington, D.C.: The National Institute of Disability and Rehabilitation Research, 1992.
55. Welner S, Badell A. The care of women with physical disabilities. In: Seltzer VL, Pearce WH, eds. Women's primary health care: office practice and procedures. 1995:731–736.
56. Mathias CJ, Frankel HL. Clinical manifestations of malfunctioning sympathetic mechanisms in tetraplegia. J Auton Nerv Syst 1983;7: 303–312.
57. Greenspoon JS, Paul RH. Paraplegia and quadriplegia: special considerations during pregnancy and labor and delivery. Am J Obstet Gynecol 1986;155:738.
58. Perry KG, Morrison JG. Anemia associated with pregnancy. In: Sciarra JJ, ed. Gynecology and obstetrics. New York: Lippincott–Raven Publishers, 1993;1.
59. Feyi-Waboso PA. An audit of five years' experience of pregnancy in spinal cord damaged women: a regional unit's experience and a review of the literature. Paraplegia 1992;30:631–635.
60. McGregor JA, Meeuwsen J. Autonomic hyperreflexia: a mortal danger for spinal cord–damaged women in labor. Am J Obstet Gynecol 1985;151:330–333.
61. Colachis SC. Autonomic hyperreflexia with spinal cord injury. J Am Paraplegia Soc 1992;15(3):171–186.
62. Weinstein L. New perspectives on vaginosis, vaginitis, and vagilitis. In: Sciarra JJ, ed. Gynecology and obstetrics. New York: Lippincott–Raven Publishers, 1994:3:6–8, 1998.
63. Welner SL. Caring for the woman with a disability. In: Wallis LA, ed. Textbook of women's health. New York: Lippincott–Raven Publishers, 1998:89.
64. Heffernan JJ. Thromboembolic complications of pregnancy and the puerperium. In: Carr PL, Freund KM, Somani S, eds. The medical care of women. Philadelphia: WB Saunders, 1995:376.
65. Bonnar J, Green R, et al. Inherited thrombophilia and pregnancy: the obstetric perspective. Semin Thromb Hemost 1998;24[Suppl 1]:49–53.
66. Baker ER, Cardenas DD, et al. Risks associated with pregnancy in spinal cord–injured women. Obstet Gynecol 1992;80:425.
67. Young BK, Katz M, et al. Pregnancy after spinal cord injury: altered maternal and fetal response to labor. Obstet Gynecol 1983;2:59–63.
68. Verduyn WH. Pregnancy and delivery in tetraplegic women. J Spinal Cord Med 1997;20:371–374.
69. Sipski ML, Alexander CJ. Spinal cord injury and sexual function. Gaithersburg, Md.: Aspen, 1997:169.
70. Jackson AB. Pregnancy and delivery. In: Krotoski DM, Nosek MA, Turk MA, eds. Women with physical disabilities: achieving and maintaining health and well-being. Paul H Brookes Publishing Co., Baltimore, 1996:7:91–99.
71. Westgren N, Hultling C, et al. Pregnancy and delivery in women with a traumatic spinal cord injury in Sweden, 1980–1991. Obstet Gynecol 1993;81:926–930.
72. Hambly PR, Marin B. Anaesthesia for chronic spinal cord lesion. Anaesthesia 1998;53:273–289.
73. Irons DW, Baylis PH. The metabolic clearance of atrial natriuretic peptide during human pregnancy. Am J Obstet Gynecol 1996;175:449–454.
74. Rogers J, Matsumura M. Mother to be: a guide to pregnancy and birth for women with disabilities. Demos, 1991:323–324.

Cherry and Merkatz's Complications of Pregnancy,
Fifth Edition, edited by W. R. Cohen.
Lippincott Williams & Wilkins, Philadelphia © 2000.

CHAPTER 54

Perinatal Outcome after *In Vitro* Fertilization

François Olivennes

The first pregnancy after *in vitro* fertilization (IVF) was obtained 20 years ago (1). Today IVF is used commonly as a treatment for infertile couples. Since the first birth after IVF, many scientific papers have been published on the technical aspects of the IVF procedure and on new technologies designed to enhance pregnancy rates, but few studies have addressed the issue of the perinatal outcome of IVF pregnancies.

Since the earliest use of assisted reproductive technologies, studies have demonstrated that the pregnancies obtained in infertile patients are at increased risk, as shown in papers published after the beginning of the use of gonadotropins (2,3) or soon after the first IVF births (4). The adverse perinatal outcomes were related to the high percentage of multiple pregnancies obtained with ovarian stimulation that resulted in multifollicular development and multiple embryo transfers. Multiple pregnancies are a significant public health problem considering the medical, social, and financial consequences of their perinatal complications (5,6). Multiple pregnancies are not the only factor involved in the increased rate of perinatal complications. Some studies also have found a high rate of adverse outcome in singleton pregnancies (7,8).

The major indicators of perinatal outcome are prematurity, birth weight, and perinatal mortality. The congenital malformation rate is also an important factor. The high rates of premature birth and of low-birth-weight infants resulting from IVF pregnancies were mentioned as early as 1985 by an Australian group (4) who analyzed 244 pregnancies, 22% of which were multiple births. The prematurity rate was 19% for singleton pregnancies, three times higher than the rate observed in the general population of Australia, and 33.4% for multiple births. The rate of infants with a birth weight below 2,500 g was 30% for all IVF pregnancies and 19% for singletons.

F. Olivennes: Department of Obstetric Gynecology, Antoine Béclère Hospital, Clamart, France 92140.

It is important to understand the way gestational age of IVF pregnancies is calculated. During IVF, the day of the egg retrieval and the day of the birth are known exactly, and the theoretic term is calculated by adding systematically 14 days to the difference between these two dates. This calculation assumes that ovulation occurs on day 14 of the cycle. In spontaneous pregnancies, the exact date of ovulation is not usually known, and the mean length of the first part of the cycle could be longer than 14 days. Spira and colleagues in 1985 showed that the length of the proliferative phase of 894 spontaneous menstrual cycles was 18.1±5.7 days (9). Estimation of the onset of pregnancy by ultrasound is not totally accurate, nor is estimation of gestational age based on the date of the last menstrual period (10). The modification of only 2 days in the calculation of term results in a slight reduction in the prematurity rate. We analyzed the data from 162 singleton pregnancies after IVF. The prematurity rate (<37 weeks) was 10.7% if 14 days were added to the date of the retrieval but only 7.5% or even 5.7% if 16 or 18 days were added, respectively, because many of the premature births took place between 36 and 37 weeks of amenorrhea (WA) (11). Thus, possible influences on the prematurity rate induced by the mode of calculation of the gestational age should be taken into account in the interpretation of IVF outcome data.

In collaboration with an epidemiology department (Unité INSERM U292, Kremlin Bicêtre, France), we organized one of the largest multicenter studies to evaluate the obstetric and pediatric complications after IVF. The outcome of all such pregnancies conceived in 11 IVF centers between 1987 and 1988 with a follow-up of the children until age 1 year was recorded (12). Complete information on the pregnancies and deliveries was obtained for 1,637 cases.

A total of 1,263 pregnancies with delivery after 25 WA were analyzed (Table 54-1). More than one quarter of all the pregnancies were multiple (23% twins and 4% triplets

TABLE 54-1. *Perinatal outcome of IVF pregnancies*

	Singleton	Twin	Triplets and greater	Total	*p* Value
Prematurity (%)[a]					
25–27 WA	0.3	2.8	1.8	1.0	
28–31 WA	1.8	2.8	16.1	2.6	
32–33 WA	0.8	8.3	25.0	3.6	
34–35 WA	3.6	13.8	17.9	6.6	
36 WA	5.7	16.2	23.2	8.9	
25–36 WA	12.2	43.8	83.9	22.7	<0.001
Birth weight					
mean g±SD	3095±561	2,363±532	1,927±52	2,719±697	<0.001
<1500 g[b]	1.6	5.9	18.8	4.9	<0.001
<2,500 g[b]	12.3	55.4	84.4	34.7	<0.001
SFGA (%)[b]	15.0	49.6	62.4	29.8	<0.001
Mortality (%)					
Perinatal[a]	18.6	34.4	81.9	30.6	<0.001
Neonatal (days 1–6)[b]	9.9	14.1	36.8	14.1	<0.05
Infant[b] (1 yr)	14.3	19.4	61.3	20.8	<0.001
Malformation (%)					
With induced abortions	1.86	3.09	2.92	2.40	NS
Without induced abortions	2.49	3.42	2.92	2.86	NS

IVF, *in vitro* fertilization; WA, weeks of amenorrhea; SFGA, Small for gestational age (birth weight below 10th percentile); NS, not significant.

[a]Based on all births.

[b]Based on live births only.

or more). Cesarean sections were done in 36% of the multiple pregnancy cases and in 28% of the cases for singleton pregnancies. The rate of singleton pregnancies (73%) was similar to that found in other studies in France (72%) (8), England (77%) (7), and the United States (77%) (13,14).

The overall rate of prematurity was high, with 22.7% of the children born before 37 WA. This rate was related mainly to the high proportion of multiple pregnancies. The prematurity rate increased according to the number of fetuses (12.2%, 43.8%, and 83.9%, respectively, for singleton, twins, and triplets); however, this prematurity rate was high even in the singleton pregnancies. These results were higher than those observed in the French national population: 5.6% for singleton and 35.5% for twin births (15). Comparison of our results to national data is possible only for singleton births and twins, because data on triplet births are extremely rare. Our own figures were slightly below those observed in the English study (respectively, 13%; 57%, and 95%) (7).

Most low-birth-weight infants came from multiple pregnancies; however, 12.3% of the singletons had a birth weight of less than 2,500 g, whereas the figure observed in the French national population was 5.2% (16). The rate of children with a birth weight below 1,500 g was four times higher than that found in the general French population (1.6% versus 0.4%) (16). This increase in the incidence of low birth weight also was observed in other studies (7); however, the high rate of prematurity, of course, plays a role in the number of infants with low birth weight. Therefore, we chose to analyze the small-for-gestational age infants measured to the 10th percentile of reference curves, which adjust the birth weight according to the duration of pregnancy. The rate of infants who were small for gestational age was also high: Almost 30% of all these infants were below the 10th percentile. This rate also increased in singleton pregnancies, in which 15% of newborns weighed less than the 10th percentile.

Perinatal mortality varied considerably, depending on the rank of the pregnancy. The mortality rate was four times higher for children originating from triplet births compared with that for singleton births. The rates of perinatal mortality were higher for singleton births than those observed in French national data for perinatal mortality (18.6% versus 12.3%) or for infant mortality (14.3% versus 9.7%) (15,16). In a study of 15,501 pregnancies, Bréart and colleagues (15) demonstrated that gestational age and birth weight are the main risk factors for perinatal mortality. Compared with birth occurring after 41 WA, the rate of perinatal mortality was four times higher for birth at 37 WA, 12 times that at 35 to 36 WA and 60 times that below 35 WA. When taking into account gestational age to analyze birth weight, the perinatal mortality was twofold higher at 37 WA, fourfold higher at 35 to 36 WA, and 12 times higher before 35 WA.

The malformation rate observed at birth in our IVF population did not differ from that observed in the general population (2.4% for all births and 2.86% if induced abortions were included). No specific type of malformation was observed. In the early days of IVF, few studies drew attention to a suspected increase in the rate of malformations in IVF pregnancies (17). This finding was not confirmed by the recent large studies.

The role played by induction of ovulation in the incidence of malformations has been the subject of many studies. Clomiphene citrate, the structure of which is similar to that of diethystilbestrol (DES), was incriminated early in some malformations (18). The gonadotropins also were suspected (19) and then excluded (20,21). In a recent review, Venn and colleagues concluded that there are no convincing data to show a link between clomiphene citrate and malformation, but optimal data clearly refuting this link are not available (22). Large series of IVF births have shown a global rate of malformations comparable to that of the general population (7,12,23). Shoham and colleagues (24), after analyzing most of the published studies available, concluded that the use of clomiphene, human menopausal gonadotropins (hMG), or the association of both with IVF or gamete intrafallopian transfer (GIFT) does not induce an increased rate of malformation.

The unique feature of our multicenter study is its low rate of patients lost to follow-up. We obtained information about 97% of the deliveries. This study of a large group of IVF pregnancies confirmed the high rate of adverse outcome observed in IVF pregnancies. Prematurity, low birth weight, intrauterine growth restriction, and perinatal mortality were higher than in the general French population, confirming the results of other international studies. We also have confirmed that, although most of these complications are related to multiple births, they also are found in singleton pregnancies.

MUTIPLE PREGNANCIES

Multiple pregnancies are the main risk factor for adverse outcome of IVF pregnancies. In our multicenter study, the rate of prematurity was four times higher in twins compared with singletons (12.2% versus 43.8%). In the last report on data collected from all French IVF centers, the prematurity rate in singletons was 9.1% and 42% for the 5,914 twins (23).

The rate of triple pregnancies in IVF is around 2.5% to 5%. This figure, however, is artificially reduced by the practice of embryo reduction. Triple pregnancies have a high rate of complications. In our multicenter study, the 56 triplet pregnancies had a 83.9% prematurity rate (<37 WA) and a 17.9% extreme prematurity rate (<31 WA).

Many studies have analyzed the results of small series of high-rank multiple pregnancies (25–31). All found a significant increase in adverse perinatal outcome. Although most IVF centers now try to avoid triple pregnancies, the risk of adverse outcome in twin pregnancy should not be ignored.

Twin Pregnancies

Twin pregnancies represent 20% to 25% of all pregnancies obtained by IVF (4,23,32,33). Few studies have been published on IVF twin pregnancies (7,12,30,34, 35–37), but all found an increased rate of prematurity and low birth weight compared with singleton births.

A total of 318 twin pregnancies were included in a study done in Antoine Béclère Hospital in France. Seventy-two pregnancies occurred after IVF and 82 after ovarian stimulation; 164 were spontaneous (36). Twin pregnancies obtained after embryo reduction were excluded from the study. The rates of complications, expressed with odd ratios, are presented in Table 54-2.

We found no significant differences among the three groups of patients in the incidence of high blood pressure, premature rupture of membranes, and threatened premature labor. We did not find differences in the global rates of cesarean section in the IVF group (54.2%), the stimulation group (41.5%), and spontaneous group (43.3%). Emergency cesarean sections were more frequent in the IVF group (30.5%) compared with the stimulation group (15.8%) and the spontaneous group (16.5%). The total prematurity rate did not differ in the IVF group (38.9%), the stimulation group (45.1%), and the spontaneous group (39.6%). Extreme prematurity (<31 WA) was

TABLE 54-2. *Obstetric and perinatal outcome of twin pregnancies*

	IVF (n=72)			Stimulation (n=82)			Spontaneous (n=168)	
	No. of patients	OR	CI (95%)	No. of patients	OR	CI (95%)	No. of patients	OR
HBP	11	0.77	(0.34–1.73)	19	1.29	(0.65–2.58)	31	1
PROM	9	1.66	(0.62–4.41)	5	0.75	(0.28–2.38)	13	1
TPL	38	1.29	(0.72–2.34)	44	1.34	(0.76–2.36)	76	1
Cesarean section	39	1.55	(0.85–2.81)	34	0.93	(0.52–1.64)	71	1
Prematurity								
<31 WA	6	1.77	(0.52–5.91)	4	1.00	(0.24–3.81)	8	1
32–35 WA	10	0.59	(0.26–1.35)	17	0.96	(0.48–1.94)	35	1
36 WA	12	1.29	(0.56–2.95)	16	1.56	(0.73–3.35)	22	1
Total	28	0.97	(0.53–1.78)	37	1.25	(0.71–2.22)	65	1

CI, confidence interval; HBP, high blood pressure; IVF, *in vitro* fertilization; OR, odds ratio; PROM, premature rupture of membranes; TPL threatened premature labor; WA, weeks of amenorrhea.

higher in the IVF group (8.3%) compared with the spontaneous or stimulation group (4.9%), but this difference was not significant. The rate of premature birth resulting from a medical decision was not different (13.9%, 17.9%, and 14.1%, respectively, for the IVF, stimulation, and spontaneous groups). The percentage of patients admitted to the hospital because of threatened premature labor was close to 50% in the three groups, comparable to that observed in other studies (35,37). The high rate of prematurity in the IVF group (39%) was also comparable to that found by others (8,12,35,32,37,30). In the study published by Tan and colleagues (34), the prematurity rate was higher (58%) but was similar to that found in the control population of spontaneous twin pregnancies. The results for birth weight, small-for-gestational-age delivery, and perinatal mortality are presented in Table 54-3.

The rate of intrauterine growth restriction (birth weight below the 10th percentile for gestational age) was not different among the groups (18%, 23%, and 23% for the IVF, stimulation, and spontaneous groups, respectively) and were comparable to those observed in other studies (8,12). Perinatal mortality also did not differ statistically in the IVF group (3.47%), stimulation group (3.05%), and spontaneous group (4.27%).

The fact that no differences were found among the three groups of patients might be influenced by the fact that the twin pregnancies after IVF or ovarian stimulation have an early diagnosis by ultrasound. This early diagnosis can induce modification in the activity of the patients and other aspects of management in early pregnancy. In fact, IVF patients had more visits during the first and second trimesters in our study compared with spontaneous pregnancies. Whether in fact this influenced outcome is unknown.

Twin pregnancies represent more than 20% of all IVF pregnancies. They often are presented as "a nice opportunity for a childless couple to have two children at one time." It is clear, however, that twin pregnancies have an increased risk of adverse perinatal outcome compared with singleton births, and this fact must be borne in mind by couples contemplating IVF and by the physicians who advise them.

Triplet Pregnancies

Because of their relative rarity, it is not possible to study a large population of triplet pregnancies and to analyze the related complications meaningfully. Moreover, adaptation of the number of embryos transferred and the practice of embryo reduction have reduced artificially the number of ongoing triplet pregnancies observed after IVF or ovarian stimulation. Because they are so rare (i.e., 1 in 10,000 births), a control group of spontaneous triplet pregnancies is impossible to obtain to determine whether IVF triplet pregnancies have a comparable outcome.

The rate of perinatal mortality observed in the large multicenter study described in this chapter speaks for itself: 18% for singleton births and 81.9% for triplets. Triplet prgnancies are clearly high-risk pregnancies.

Selective embryo reduction was proposed to avoid the adverse outcome of triplet and higher-order pregnancies (38). A consensus seems to exist to propose embryo reduction in case of quadruplet pregnancy and for all pregnancies of higher rank (38–42). With regard to triplet pregnancies, the decision remains controversial. Some studies found a clear amelioration of perinatal complications after reducing triplet pregnancies to twins (39,41,43), whereas others did not find a clear obstetric benefit (42,44).

We recently did a study in which we compared the evolution of the triplet pregnancies managed from the first trimester at Antoine Béclère hospital between 1993 and 1997 (unpublished data). The results of the 17 triplet pregnancies reduced to twins were compared with those of the 24 ongoing triplet pregnancies. No difference was found between the two groups in the incidence of threatened premature labor, premature rupture of membranes, high blood pressure, and spontaneous abortion. The duration of hospitalization before delivery was comparable in the two groups.

Table 54-4 presents the cesarean section rate, the prematurity rate, and the mean postpartum hospital stay for patients with triplets. Although the mean gestational age was comparable in the ongoing triplets and the reduced-to-twins group, the prematurity rate was considerably

TABLE 54-3. *Birth weight, small for gestational age and perinatal mortality in twins*

	IVF (n=144)			Stimulation (n=164)			Spontaneous (n=328)	
	No. of patients	OR	CI (95%)	No. of patients	OR	CI (95%)	No. of patients	
Birth weight (g)								
<1,500	11	1.51	(0.64–3.52)	10	1.20	(0.49–2.82)	17	1
<2500	71	1.09	(0.72–1.64)	88	1.29	(0.87–1.92)	155	1
SFGA	26	0.74	(0.44–1.25)	38	1.02	(0.64–1.62)	75	1
Perinatal mortality	5	0.81	(0.25–2.46)	5	0.71	(0.22–2.14)	14	1

IVF, *in vitro* fertilization; OR, odds ratio; SFGA, Small for gestational age.

TABLE 54-4. *Perinatal outcome of ongoing and reduced triplet pregnancies*

	Reduced		Ongoing	
	N=17	(%)	N=24	(%)
Gestational age (WA)	34.5±4.1		34.7±2.5	
Prematurity (<37 WA)	10	(62.5)	22	(95.6)[a]
Extreme prematurity (<33 WA)	2	(6.25)	0	(0)
Cesarean section	4	(23.5)	17	(70.8)[a]
Maternal hospitalization (days)	11.7±7.6		12.7±4.9	

WA, weeks of amenorrhea.
[a]$p<0.05$

higher in the ongoing triplets (95.6% versus 62.5%). The prematurity rate was higher in the reduced group, but the numbers are too small to allow statistical analysis. The cesarean delivery rate was higher in the ongoing triplets (70.8%) compared with the reduced pregnancies (23.5%).

Table 54-5 presents the birth weight, the length of hospitalization of neonates, and the mortality for these groups. A nonsignificant trend toward lower birth weight and a greater number of infants who were small for gestational age was seen in the unreduced triplets. A significantly higher percentage of hospitalized children was seen in the ongoing triplet group, but the length of hospitalization did not differ significantly.

Our results showed an increased proportion of complications (cesarean sections, prematurity, hospitalized neonates) in the ongoing triplet pregnancy group. Interestingly, apart from the cesarean rate, which could increase maternal morbidity, the other complications do not seem to compromise the well-being of the infants. The premature delivery occurs after 32 WA for most of them, a time after which pediatric sequelae are relatively low today (45). Of course, the small sample studied here limits the power of the comparison and specifically did not allow comparison of extreme prematurity and mortality. Other studies have not found an advantage to reduction of triplet pregnancies to twins (44). Table 54-6 presents the results of the major studies comparing ongoing and reduced triplet pregnancies (41,43,44,46,47).

TABLE 54-5. *Birth weight, neonatal hospitalization, and mortality for triplets*

	Reduced n (%)	Ongoing n (%)
Total fetuses	34	72
Intrauterine death	3 (8.9)	4 (5.5)
Live births	31 (91.1)	68 (94.5)
Mean weight (g)	2,207±523	1,996±494
Small for gestational age[b]	12 (38.7)	36 (52.9)
Hospitalized neonates (%)	21 (67.7)	59 (86.8)[a]
Hospitalization (days)	11.5+11.0	13.0+12.0
Perinatal mortality	1 (2.9)	1 (1.4)

[a]$p<0.05$.
[b]Live births only

Compared with other studies, our series of ongoing triplets had a low incidence of extreme prematurity (<32 WA). There are large variations in this rate in the groups of ongoing triplet pregnancies (0% in our series to 43% for Macones and colleagues), whereas this rate is comparable among the different series in the groups of reduced pregnancies. The perinatal results of ongoing triplet pregnancies determine the potential desirability of reducing triplets to twins.

The better perinatal outcome observed in our series confirms amelioration in the outcome of multiple births in recent years resulting from better obstetric management and progress in neonatal intensive care (48). Most previous studies included a longer study period, which could explain the differences, at least in part.

After reduction of multiple pregnancies, the outcome is not completely comparable to a spontaneous pregnancy of the same rank (49). Despite a diminution in the rate of abortion (50), a higher risk of premature birth seems to persist when comparing spontaneous twin pregnancies to twin pregnancies coming from embryo reduction (41,43). Among the different hypotheses to explain these observations, the residual fetal tissue left after the procedure may affect the remaining fetuses and seems to play a role in the production of membrane rupture (49,50). In a recent study, Lipitz and colleagues (51) did not find a significant difference in various outcomes between a group of reduced (to twins) triplet pregnancies compared with a group of spontaneous twins, except for a higher risk of premature rupture membrane after reduction.

These results led to a reexamination of the aim of embryo reduction in triplet pregnancies. The procedure might not confer significant obstetric advantages but still could modify the high rate of psychological and social complications related to triplet births (52,53). In view of the improved outlook for triplet pregnancies, the risk-to-benefit balance of reducing triplets to twins should be reevaluated, especially in light of the long-term psychological consequences of embryo reduction (54). The reduction of triplets to singletons is possible but could

TABLE 54-6. *Results of studies comparing ongoing and reduced pregnancies*

Authors and study period	Porreco et al. (44) 1991		Melgar et al. (41) 1987–1990		Macones et al. (43) 1988–1992		Lipitz et al. (47) 1984–1992		Boulot et al. (46) 1985–1991		Our series 1992–1995	
	T	R	T	R	T	R	T	R	T	R	T	R
No. of patients	11	13	20	5	14	47	106	34	48	32	24	17
Premat. (<26 WA)						0	25%	11.8%	6.3%	12.5%	4.2%	5.9%
Premat. (<32 WA)					43%	7%	23.8%	9.7%	15.5%	7.1%	0%	6.2%
Premat. (<37 WA)					93%	64%	91.7%	25.8%	91.1%	53.5%	95.6%	62.5%
Mean gestational age (WA±SD)	35.7± 2.5	35.5± 2.3	33.1	34.8	31.2± 4.9	35.6± 2.8	33.5± 3.6	36.7± 3.7	34.4± 2.3	36.7± 2.3	34.7± 2.5	34.5± 4.1
Mean weight (gr±SD)	2239	2227	1924	2305	1593	2279	1780± 470	2350± 670	1870± 450	2340± 460	1996± 496	2207± 523
I.U.D. %					47	10				55	89	
Perinatal mortality (%)			30	0	210	30	109	48	59	37.7	14	29
Neonatal mortality (%)							46	0	45.1	19	0	0
ICU			82%	20%	84.6%	36.3%					86.8	67.7

IUD, intrauterine death; ICU, intensive care unit admission; R, reduced; T, triplets; WA, weeks of amenorrhea; SD, standard deviation.

increase the likelihood of miscarriage and can be ethically more difficult to justify.

Clearly, it is better to prevent triplet pregnancies than to interrupt a medically assisted conception. Many factors influence the implantation rate in IVF, however, and most centers claim that it is therefore difficult to minimize the number of embryos transferred. Prevention of multiple pregnancies should nevertheless be the primary goal of IVF centers. In some countries—Germany, for example—the maximum number of embryos that can be transferred is strictly regulated. In the United States, this kind of regulation has been the subject of considerable recent debate (55,56). Competition among different IVF centers to obtain the best success rates can lead to good overall pregnancy rates but can include a multiple pregnancy rate that sometimes may be more than 50% related to the high number of embryos transferred.

In France, it is generally advised to transfer a maximum of three or four embryos, taking into account the patient's age. The progress in ovarian stimulation techniques and in the handling of gametes and embryos clearly has increased the implantation rate in some IVF teams, but the compromise between an acceptable multiple pregnancy rate and the success rate remains a clinical challenge. Some teams now advise that the transfer of a maximum of two embryos should be systematically proposed, because in selected indications this approach does not diminish the total pregnancy rate but reduces considerably the multiple pregnancy rate (57–61). Pregnancies of higher rank than triplets are not discussed because they are extremely rare and are reduced in most cases.

SINGLETON PREGNANCIES

If multiple pregnancies represent the major factor involved in the rate of complications of IVF, the results observed in singleton pregnancies can help to analyze the possible risk factors involved in the adverse perinatal outcome of IVF *per se*. Table 54-7 presents the results of the major studies on perinatal outcome of singleton pregnancies.

One of the major problems in comparing IVF results among various international studies is that definitions differ from one country to another. For example, it is difficult to compare prematurity rates because definitions of live birth differ. The limit is 20 WA in Australia (64) and in the United States (74) and 28 WA in England (7) or France. Birth weight sometimes is analyzed in absolute values or by taking into account gestational age. Most studies from all countries that perform IVF find a high rate of prematurity, small-for-gestational-age births, low birth weight, and perinatal mortality compared with the national data available or to the specific control group chosen for the study. The increased risk of complications in singletons should lead to an analysis of the potential risk factors.

RISK FACTORS OF ADVERSE OUTCOME

To analyze the rate of complications of IVF pregnancies, these pregnancies often are compared with spontaneous ones; however, the general population of spontaneous pregnancies do not necessarily constitute the perfect control group. IVF patients are different from

TABLE 54-7. *Results of studies on perinatal outcome of singleton pregnancies*

		No. of patients		Prematurity		<2,500 g		Hypotrophy (<10th percentile)		Perinatal mortality		
References	Country	IVF	Controls	IVF	Controls	IVF	Controls	IVF	Controls	IVF	Controls	Controls
Steptoe et al. (62)	England	263		12.2		6.8						
Austral.coll. (63)	Australia	108		19	6.2	19						General population
Saunders et al. (64)	Australia	1,046		17.8		15.9			35.4			
MRC (7)	England	843		13.0	6.0*	12.0	7.0*			11.7	10.7	General population
World coll. (65)	International	5,363		12.8		11.8						Absent
Rufat et al. (12)	France	916		12.2		12.3		15.0		18.6		Absent
Tan et al. (34)	England	494	978	14	8	14	7	16	10	24.7		Matched spontaneous pregnancies
Friedler et al. (66)	Israel	863		19.3		14.6	6.4			12.9	13.0	General population
Wang et al. (67)	Australia	465	21,547	16.0	6.2			16.3	10*			Matched spontaneous pregnancies
Tanbo et al. (68)	Norway	355	643	14.9	9.5	11.5	6.7	4.3	3.6	11.3	9.3	Matched spontaneous pregnancies
Fivnat 86.90 (1995) (8)	France	3,889	Absent	9.1				14.6		12.0		
Fivnat 91.95 (23)	France	9,432	Absent	9.1		10.5		14.4		12.9		
Mc Faul et al. (69)	England	79		13.0	7.0	16	6					General population
Gissler et al. (70)	Finland	746	188,381	11	4.5*					17.4	6.5	General population
Antoine et al. (71)	France	205		15						24.0		
Verlaenen et al. (72)	Belgium	140	140	11.4	1.4*	10	4.3			21.0	14	Matched spontaneous pregnancies
Tallo et al. (73)	USA	62	62	10	2.0	5.0	3.0	1.6	1.6			Matched spontaneous pregnancies

IVF, *in vitro* fertilization; MRC, Medical Research Council; *significantly different from IVF groups ($p<0.05$).

women with spontaneous pregnancies in many aspects: age, parity, infertility, socioeconomic class, and previous medical history, among others. All these factors could influence the rate of adverse outcome. In a metanalysis of all the controlled studies published on small-for-gestational-age and prematurity rates, Kramer (75) studied 895 articles published since 1970. The number of factors that could influence the duration of gestation and the birth weight are numerous. The author found 33 risk factors for small for gestational age and 37 for prematurity, the influence of which has been well demonstrated. From this study, it is interesting to analyze which factor could differentiate infertile patients. Concerning prematurity, for example, socioeconomic status, educational level, and alcohol and tobacco consumption could differ in these two populations. Some factors, such as the early and careful obstetric management of the pregnancy, could play a role in favor of IVF patients. Other factors play a role in the opposite direction. The medical history of miscarriage, the stress and anxiety, and maternal age are higher in IVF patients. A large study would be necessary to analyze each of these factors but cannot be done easily.

If the rate of complications observed in IVF pregnancies compared wih the rate in spontaneous pregnancies is important in guiding obstetric management, it should be understood that the responsibility of IVF *per se* for the occurrence of all adverse outcomes has not been demonstrated conclusively. Sample size is one of the major factors in limiting the validity of the available studies. Of course, a crucial paradox exists: A study in one center cannot reach the number of patients necessary to have a valid statistical analysis, and multicenter studies can be biased because of variations in obstetric management in the different centers. As an example, in the last world report on IVF centers (76), the rate of premature delivery (<37 WA) varied from 3.36% to 33.3% for singleton pregnancies and from 28.6% to 71.6% for twins. Risk factors involved in IVF complications can be classified in two categories: those related to the characteristics of the patients and those related to the technique itself.

Patient-related Factors

Infertility

A link between infertility, prematurity, and low birth weight was found in some studies (77–81) but not in others. Ghazi and colleagues (79), in one of the largest published studies, analyzed the Swedish birth registry from 1983 to 1986. Among 379,779 pregnancies, 7.8% occurred in infertile patients without any IVF treatment. The prematurity rate was 7.1% in patients with a history of infertility over 4 years, whereas it was only 5.4% in patients without a history of infertility ($p<0.001$). Berkowitz (77) found a risk of premature birth three times higher for patients with a history of infertility after taking into account the age of the patient and the rank of the pregnancy.

A relation also was found for low birth weight at the beginning of the use of ovulation induction (82,83). Many studies since then have confirmed an increase in the risk of low birth weight in infertile patients (79,84).

In the study by Ghazi and colleagues (79), the authors found a significant increase in the perinatal mortality rate in patients with an infertility history of more than 1 year; this difference was no longer significant when the patients were matched for age and parity. The high rate of prematurity and small-for-gestational-age infants in infertile patients largely explains the excess perinatal mortality found in these patients (15).

Maternal Age

IVF patients are on average older than patients with spontaneous pregnancies, and this fact often has been used to explain the adverse outcome observed in these patients. Since the 1950's, many studies have shown that pregnancies in older primigravidae are associated with a high risk of prematurity and low birth weight (85). The limit of 35 years usually used to define older patients is subjective, and some authors found a progressive increase in adverse outcome starting at the age of 25 years.

Recent studies on the subject show contradictory results (86–94). Most studies from the 1960's show a clear elevation of prematurity rate in older patients (95, 96). Studies of birth registers also show an increase in the prematurity rate with age, even when factors such as previous history of miscarriage, socioeconomic class, maternal pathology, or a history of infertility are taken into account (93,97,98). Nevertheless, many studies, generally done in one center on large numbers of patients, did not find a relation between age and prematurity (86,87, 89,91,99,100). Prysak and colleagues (94), in a retrospective study in three centers, compared the first births of a group of 890 women aged over 35 years with those of a group of 1,054 women aged from 25 to 29 years. They found a twofold higher risk of premature birth in the women aged over 35. Two recent large population studies also showed a clear increase in the prematurity rate related to age (93,98).

In terms of low birth weight, the studies in the literature are also contradictory. Older studies show an increase in the number of infants of low birth weight in older primigravidas (85,95,96). Some recent studies done on large samples confirm this increase in the risk of low birth weight infants (88,97); however, few confounding risk factors have been analyzed.

Studies done in one center, taking into account the different risk factors for low birth weight, do not show a clear relation between age and low birth weight (86,87, 89,91). Other studies, such as the one by Cnattingius and colleagues (92), found an increased risk of low birth weight for mothers older than 30 years, after matching for risks factors. Aldous and Edmonson (93) also showed a relation between age and low birth weight; however, these results should be interpreted carefully, because many studies analyze the birth weight and not the rate of small-for-gestational-age infants; therefore, the rate of prematurity could influence these results. Effects of advanced maternal age on the birth weight have been suggested by some authors to be related to modifications in uterine vascularity that accompany aging, leading to a decrease in the uterine-placental perfusion (101).

Other Risk Factors

Other risk factors often found in infertile patients could increase the likelihood of premature birth and low birth weight. For example, a medical history of spontaneous abortion or pregnancy termination could constitute a risk, although this subject is controversial (102). Anxiety was demonstrated to play a role in some studies (103) but not in others (104). The objective evaluation of anxiety is, of course, extremely difficult. Social and economic factors could influence adverse outcome, because infertile and IVF patients are usually of higher economic class (105). The influence of parity is also possible, but Berkowitz (77) and Kramer (75) showed that parity does not clearly influence the rate of prematurity. A relation between parity and prematurity was established more firmly in multiparous women, but they are rarely IVF patients.

Technical Factors

Role of Ovarian Stimulation

Some studies have drawn attention to the relation between ovulation induction and obstetric complications.

In 1968 Goldfarb and colleagues, in a study of 160 pregnancies obtained by using clomiphene citrate, showed an increase in the rate of premature births (106). The authors of these publications related the rate of prematurity to the high proportion of multiple births (2,3,21,107), and Karow and Payne found the same results (108). Adashi et al. (20) analyzed the risk factors in these patients in a prospective analysis of a group of patients with polycystic ovaries. They compared 86 pregnancies obtained using clomiphene citrate with 51 pregnancies obtained using ovarian resection. These authors did not observe any difference in the prematurity rate of these two groups of patients in singleton pregnancies.

Studies of the role of stimulation on the occurrence of the adverse perinatal outcome are difficult. A control group cannot be found easily, and treating fertile patients with stimulation drugs is impossible. Some studies comparing pregnancies in infertile patients with or without IVF could not find differences in these two groups (11,109,110). The role of ovarian stimulation itself, apart from its role in producing multiple pregnancies, deserves further study. One hypothesis could be that ovarian stimulation induces many ovulating follicles, which will lead to multiple corpora lutea and could result in an early pregnancy hormonal milieu different from that of spontaneous pregnancy.

Role of IVF Itself

Few studies have analyzed the role of IVF technique on the occurrence of pregnancy complications. Comparison between pregnancies obtained with IVF and those that resulted from other infertility treatments could be a model to answer this question. These patient groups usually have different types of infertility, however, and could differ by other factors. Most cases in both groups of patients are exposed to ovarian stimulation, the role of which therefore cannot be excluded.

Hill and colleagues (109) compared infertile patients treated with or without IVF and did not find significant difference for birth weight and gestational age in singleton pregnancies. Howe and colleagues (110) found no difference in prematurity between two groups of infertile patients treated with or without IVF.

In a study done in 1993 (111), we compared retrospectively 164 singleton pregnancies obtained after IVF in Antoine Béclère Hospital (Clamart, France), 263 pregnancies obtained after ovarian stimulation without IVF, and 5,096 spontaneous pregnancies delivered in our center during the same period. Table 54-8 shows the obstetric results from these three groups of patients.

We did not find any differences between the IVF group and the stimulation group for high blood pressure, threatened premature labor, premature rupture of the membranes, and cesarean section rate. The cesarean section rate was almost double in the group of IVF compared with the spontaneous pregnancy group (29% versus 14.7%).

TABLE 54-8. *Percent of patients with complications in three groups of pregnancies*

	IVF (n=162)	Ovarian stimulation (n=263)	Spontaneous (n=5,096)
High blood pressure	9.2	14.1[a]	9.7
Threatened premature labor	14.2	9.9	10.1
Premature rupture of membrane	2.5	1.5	1.2
Cesarean section	29.0[a]	21.7[a]	14.7

IVF, *in vitro* fertilization.
[a]Different from spontaneous group: $p<0.05$

Table 54-9 shows the prematurity rate and the small-for-gestational-age and perinatal mortality rates for this study. No significant difference was found between the IVF and the stimulation groups, but the proportion of premature births (<37 and 35 WA), low birth weight (<2,500 g) and small-for-gestational-age infants (<10th percentile) was higher in the IVF group compared with the spontaneous group. The extreme prematurity (<31 WA) was threefold higher in the IVF group compared with the spontaneous group; however, the number of patients was too low to attain statistical significance. The risk of perinatal mortality was also higher in the IVF and stimulation groups compared with the spontaneous group, but the small numbers make meaningful statistical analysis of this outcome impossible.

It seems clear that pregnancies obtained in infertile patients are exposed to a higher rate of perinatal compli-

TABLE 54-9. *Rates of prematurity, small for gestational age, and perinatal mortality*

Groups	IVF (n=162) (%)	Stimulation (n=263) (%)	Spontaneous (n=5,096) (%)
Prematurity (WA)			
<28	0.6	0	0.1
28–31	0.6	2.3[a]	0.3
32–35	3.1[a]	1.1	1.5
36	5.7[a]	2.7	2.5
Total <37	11.2[a]	6.1[a]	4.4
Total <35	4.3[a]	3.4	1.9
Total <31	1.2	2.3[a]	0.4
Birth weight (g)			
<2500	11.1[a]	6.5[a]	3.6
<1,500	0.6	2.3[a]	0.4
SFGA	11.2[a]	10.6[a]	5.9
Perinatal mortality	18.5/1000	11.4/1000	5.0/1000

[a]Different from spontaneous group: $p<0.05$.
IVF, *in vitro* fertilization; SFGA, birth weight below 10th percentile (small for gestational age); WA, weeks of amenorrhea.

cations, but the IVF technique does not clearly increase this risk. The fact that both groups are exposed to ovarian stimulation does not allow analysis of its role in perinatal outcome.

SPECIAL TECHNIQUES ASSOCIATED WITH *IN VITRO* FERTILIZATION

Studies of pregnancies obtained from frozen embryos do not show specific obstetric risks related to this procedure. Frydman and associates (112) did not find any perinatal abnormalities in a small group of 50 such pregnancies. Wada and colleagues (113) compared 232 pregnancies from frozen embryos with 763 pregnancies from fresh embryo transfers and did not find any difference in perinatal outcome. The largest study published was done by the French *in vitro* national registry (FIVNAT) (114) and compared 465 pregnancies from frozen embryos to 8,757 pregnancies from fresh embryo transfers. Prematurity and small-for-gestational-age rates were lower in the group of pregnancies originating from frozen embryos. In singleton pregnancies, the small-for-gestational-age rate was half that of the pregnancies from frozen embryos. Interestingly, the main difference in these patients is that ovarian stimulation is mild or even absent in frozen embryo replacement cycles.

The outcome of pregnancies obtained after oocyte donation was studied in small samples, and the authors generally did not find any enhancement of adverse outcome in those patients (115–119). The perinatal outcome does not seem to differ from the pregnancies obtained with IVF. One study (120), unfortunately done on a small sample matched for age, parity, and rank, compared 22 pregnancies obtained after oocyte donation to 22 IVF pregnancies. They found that rates of prematurity and low birth weight were smaller in the pregnancies obtained from oocyte donation.

Few data have been reported on the perinatal outcome of pregnancy obtained after intracytoplasmic sperm injection (ICSI). Wisanto and colleagues (121) reported the largest study of 424 pregnancies obtained by ICSI. A total of 29.1% of the pregnancies were twins, and 1.6% were triplets. The rate of prematurity was 7.6% for the singleton pregnancies. The overall rate of low birth weight was 28.9% for infants weighing less than 2,500 g and 4.7% for infants weighing less than 1,500 g. The perinatal mortality was 13.5 per 1,000 for singletons and 266 per 1,000 for triplets. The malformation rate was 3.3%. The data were comparable to the results in classic IVF pregnancies. Wennerholm and colleagues (122) reported the perinatal outcome of 175 births after ICSI. The overall prematurity rate was 17% and 9% for singletons. A total of 17% of the babies weighed less than 2,500 g and 2% less than 1,500 g. The perinatal mortality was 0.5%. These values were elevated compared with Swedish national data but appear to be better than those of classic IVF pregnancies. The ICSI techniques are too recent to have a clear understanding of their influence on perinatal outcome. In the case of male factors, women might be less concerned by all the risk factors observed in IVF.

CONCLUSION

All the data obtained in the different studies published on the perinatal outcome of IVF pregnancies found an increase in associated complications. A large proportion of these complications are related to the high percentage of multiple pregnancies, but these complications also are observed with a higher frequency in singleton pregnancies. Numerous risk factors could explain these results. Few prospective studies have included a matched control group to allow complete analysis of the different variables possibly involved. Age and parity may be important factors. The role of IVF itself has not been demonstrated convincingly, because studies comparing infertile patients treated by IVF and patients treated by ovarian stimulation without IVF found no difference between these groups.

Two factors deserve particular emphasis. The infertile status of IVF patients clearly plays a role in their risk of adverse outcome, and many studies have demonstrated an increase in the rate of prematurity and low birth weight in infertile patients. The effect of ovarian stimulation *per se* deserves further study, but such an approach will be hampered by the fact that a suitable control group is almost impossible to find.

The effect of the high rate of multiple pregnancies on outcome is obvious, and risks are generally proportional to the number of fetuses. Today embryo reduction often is proposed to patients with triplet and higher-rank IVF pregnancies. Important progress in the management of multiple pregnancies and in neonatal intensive care has changed the prognosis of premature infants considerably, and some authorities believe that embryo reduction may no longer have a clear obstetric justification in triplets if the management is accomplished in a tertiary care center. Embryo reduction still has potential benefits, however, such as the ability to diminish the postnatal complications of triplet births (social, psychologic, financial), that could be very important.

The main goal of IVF centers should be to diminish the rate of multiple pregnancies to reduce the complications observed in IVF pregnancies. All IVF pregnancies should be monitored with great care because they are often difficult to obtain and obviously are exposed to an increased risk of complications.

REFERENCES

1. Steptoe PC, Edwards RG. Birth after reimplantation of a human embryo [letter]. Lancet 1978;7:366.
2. Hack M, Brish M, Serr DM, Insler V, Lunenfeld B. Outcome of pregnancies after induced ovulation. JAMA 1970;211:791–797.
3. Tsapoulis AD, Zourlas PA, Comninos AC. Observation on 320 infertile patients treated with human gonadotropins. Fertil Steril 1978; 29:492–495.

4. Australian In Vitro Fertilization Collaborative Group. High incidence of preterm births and early losses in pregnancy after *in vitro* fertilization. BMJ 1985;291:1160–1163.
5. Levene MI, Wild J, Steer P. Higher multiple births and the modern management of infertility in Britain. Br J Obstet Gynaecol 1992;99: 607–613.
6. Tuppin P, Blondel B, Kaminski M. Trends in multiple deliveries and infertility treatments in France. Br J Obstet Gynaecol 1993;100: 383–385.
7. MRC working party on children conceived by I.V.F. Birth in Great Britain resulting from assisted conception 1978–87. BMJ 1990;300: 1229–1233.
8. FIVNAT (French *In Vitro* National). Pregnancies and births resulting from in vitro fertilization: French national registry, analysis of data 1986 to 1990. Fertil Steril 1995;64:746–756.
9. Spira A, Spira N, Papiernik-Berkauer E, Schwartz D. Pattern of menstrual cycles and incidence of congenital malformations. Early Hum Dev 1985;11:317–324.
10. Kramer MS, McLean FH, Boyd ME, Usher RH. The validity of gestational age estimation by menstrual dating in term, preterm, and postterm gestations. JAMA 1988;260:3306–3308.
11. Olivennes F, Rufat P, Andre B, Pourade A, Quiros MC, Frydman R. The increased risk of complication observed in singleton pregnancies resulting from *in-vitro*-fertilization (IVF) does not seem to be related to the IVF method itself. Hum Reprod 1993;8:1297–1300.
12. Rufat P, Olivennes F, De Mouzon J, Dehan M, Frydman R. Task force report on the outcome of pregnancies and children conceived by *in-vitro*-fertilization (France: 1987–1989). Fertil Steril 1994;61:324–330.
13. Medical Research International. Society for Assisted Reproduction Technology. The American Fertility Society. *In vitro* fertilization-embryo transfer (IVF-ET) in the United States: 1987 results from the national IVF-ET registry. Fertil Steril 1989;51:13–19.
14. Medical Research International. Society of Assisted Reproduction Technology. The American Fertility Society. *In vitro* fertilization/embryo transfer in the United States: 1989 results from the national IVF/ET registry. Fertil Steril 1991;55:14–23.
15. Bréart G, Blondel B, Kaminski M, Kabir M, Dargent Pare C, Tupin P. Mortalité et morbidité périnatales en France In: Tournaire M, ed. Mise jour en gynécologie et obstétrique. Paris: CNGOF-Vigot, 1991: 175–213.
16. Rumeau-Rouquette C, Du Mazaubrun C, Rabarizon Y. Naître en France-10 ans d'evolution. Paris: Doin Editeurs. Editions INSERM, 1984.
17. Lancaster P. Congenital malformations after IVF. Lancet 1987;2: 1392–1393.
18. Berman P. Congenital abnormalities associated with clomiphene ingestion. Lancet 1975;2:878.
19. Elbling L. Does gonadotropin-induced ovulation in mice cause malformations in the offspring? Nature 1973;246:37–39.
20. Adashi EY, Rock JA, Sapp KC, Martin EJ, Colston Wentz A, Seegar Jones G. Gestational outcome of clomiphene-related conceptions. Fertil Steril 1979;31:620–626.
21. Kurachi K, Aono T, Minagawa J, Miyake A. Congenital malformations of newborn infants after clomiphene induced ovulation. Fertil Steril 1983;40:187–189.
22. Venn A, Grad Dip Epid, Lumley J. Clomiphene citrate and pregnancy outcome. Aust N Z Obstet Gynecol 1994;34:56–66.
23. FIVNAT: Bilan FIVNAT 1996. Contracept Fertil Sex 1997;25: 499–502.
24. Shoham Z, Zosmer A, Insler V. Early miscarriage and fetal malformation after induction of ovulation by clomiphene citrate and/or human metropins. Fertil Steril 1991;55:1.
25. Feldberg D, Laufer N, Dicker D, Goldman JA, DeCherney A. Quadruplet pregnancy in IVF. Eur J Obstet Gynecol Reprod Biol 1986;23: 101–106.
26. Collins MS, Bleyl JA. Seventy-one quadruplet pregnancies: management and outcome. Am J Obstet Gynecol 1990;162:1384–1392.
27. Gonen R, Heymann E, Asztalos EV, et al. The outcome of triplet, quatruplet, and quintuplet pregnancies managed in a perinatal unit: obstetric, neonatal, and follow-up data. Am J Obstet Gynecol 1990; 162:454–459.
28. Kingsland CR, Steer CV, Pampiglione JS, Mason BA, Edwards RG, Campbell S. Outcome of triplet pregnancies resulting from IVF at Bourn Hallam 1984–1987. Eur J Obstet Gynecol Reprod Biol 1990; 34:197–203.
29. Lipitz S, Seidman DS, Alcalay M, Achiron R, Mashiach S, Reichman B. The effect of fertility drugs and *in vitro* methods on the outcome of 106 triplet pregnancies. Fertil Steril 1993;60:1031–1034.
30. Seoud MAF, Toner JP, Kruithoff C, Muasher SJ. Outcome of twin, triplet, and quadruplet *in vitro* fertilization pregnancies: the Norfolk experience. Fertil Steril 1992;57:1992.
31. Friedler S, Mordel N, Lipitz S, Mashiach S, Glezerman M, Laufer N. Perinatal outcome of triplet pregnancies following assisted reproduction. J Assist Reprod Genet 1994;11:459–462.
32. FIVNAT: Grossesses multiples. Contracept Fertil Sex 1995;23: 494–497.
33. Society For Reproductive Medicine. Assisted Reproductive Technology In The United States and Canada: 1994 results generated from the American Society for Reproductive Medicine/Society for Assisted Reproductive Technology Registry. Fertil Steril 1996;66:697–705.
34. Tan Sl, Doyle P, Campbell S, et al. Obstetric outcome of in vitro fertilization pregnancies compared with normally conceived pregnancies. Am J Obstet Gynecol 1992;167:778–784.
35. Brinsden PR, Rizk B. The obstetric outcome of assisted conception treatment. Assisted Reproduction Reviews 1992;2:116–125.
36. Olivennes F, Kadhel P, Rufat P, Fanchin R, Fernandez H, Frydman R. Perinatal outcome of twin pregnancies obtained after in vitro fertilization: comparison with twin pregnancies obtained spontaneously or after ovarian stimulation. Fertil Steril 1996;66:105–109.
37. Epelboin S, Blondeau MA. Grossesses multiples après procréation médicalement assistée: devenir obstétrical. Contracept Fertil Sex 1989;17:756–758.
38. Berkowitz Rl, Lynch L, Chitkara U, Wilkins IA, Mehalex KE, Alvarez E. Selective reduction of multifetal pregnancies in the first trimester. N Engl J Med 1988;318:1043–1047.
39. Vautier-Brouzes D, Lefebvre G. Selective reduction in multifetal pregnancies: technical and psychological aspects. Fertil Steril 1992;57: 1012–1016.
40. Lipitz S., Mashiach S, Seidman DS. Multifetal pregnancy reduction: the case for nondirective patient counselling. Hum Reprod 1994;9: 1978–1979.
41. Melgar CA, Rosenfeld DL, Rawlinson K, Greenberg M. Perinatal outcome after multifetal reduction to twins compared with nonreduced multiple gestations. Obstet Gynecol 1991;78:763–766.
42. Dommergues M, Nisand I, Mandelbrot L, Isfer E, Radunovic N, Dumez Y. Embryo reduction in multifetal pregnancies after infertility therapy: obstetrical risks and perinatal benefits are related to operative strategy. Fertil Steril 1991;55:805–811.
43. Macones GA, Schemmer G, Pritts E, Weinblatt V, Wapner RJ. Multifetal reduction of triplets to twins improves perintal outcome. Am J Obstet Gynecol 1993;169:982–986.
44. Porreco RP, Burke MS, Hendrix ML. Multifetal reduction of triplets and pregnancy outcome. Obstet Gynecol 1991;78:335–338.
45. Expertise Collective INSERM. Grande prématurité: Dépistage et prévention du risque. Paris: INSERM, 1997.
46. Boulot P, Hedon B, Pelliccia G, Peray P, Lafargues F, Viala JL. Effects of selective reduction in triplet gestation: a comparative study of cases managed with or without this procedure. Fertil Steril 1993;60: 497–503.
47. Lipitz S, Reichman B, Uval J, et al. A prospective comparison of the outcome of triplet pregnancies managed expectantly or by multifetal reduction to twins. Am J Obstet Gynecol 1994;170:874–879.
48. Albrecht JL, Tomich PG. The maternal and neonatal outcome of triplet gestations. Am J Obstet Gynecol 1996;174:1551–1556.
49. Evans MI, May M, Drugan A, Fletcher JC, Johnson MP, Sokol RJ. Selective termination : clinical experience and residual risks. Am J Obstet Gynecol 1990;162:1568–1572.
50. Berkowitz RL, Lynch L, Stone J, Alvarez M. The current status of multifetal pregnancy reduction. Am J Obstet Gynecol 1996;174: 1265–1272.
51. Lipitz S, Uval J, Achiron R, Schiff E, Lusky A, Reichman B. Outcome of twin pregnancies reduced from triplets compared with nonreduced twin gestations. Obstet Gynecol 1996;87:511–514.
52. Garel M, Blondel B. Assessment at 1 year of psychological consequences of having triplets. Hum Reprod 1992;7:729–732.
53. Garel M, Salobir C, Blondel B. Psychological consequences of having triplets: a 4-year follow-up study. Fertil Steril 1997;67:1162–1165.
54. Schreiner-Engel P, Walther VN, Mindes J, Lynch L, Berkowitz RL. First-trimester multifetal pregnancy reduction: acute and persistent psychologic reactions. Am J Obstet Gynecol 1995;172:541–547.

55. Alikani M, Wiemer K. Embryo number for transfer should not be strictly regulated. Fertil Steril 1997;68:782–783.
56. De Jonge, De Wolf DP. Embryo number for transfer should not be strictly regulated. Fertil Steril 1997;68:784–786.
57. Staessen C, Janssenswillen C, Van Den Abbeel E, Devroey P, Van Steirteghem ACV. Avoidance of triplet pregnancies by elective transfer of two good quality embryos. Hum Reprod 1993;8:1650–1653.
58. Devreker F, Englert Y. Implantation rates and embryo numbers. Debate: "Is it time to replace only two embryos?" Hum Reprod 1994;9:186.
59. Franco JG Jr. The risk of multifetal pregnancy. Debate: "Is it time to replace only two embryos?" Hum Reprod 1994;9:185–186.
60. Nijs M. Factors involved in replacing two or more embryos. Debate: "Is it time to replace only two embryos?" Hum Reprod 1994;9:185.
61. Walters DE. Is it time to replace only two embryos? Can pregnancy rates be maintained when two embryos are replaced in *in-vitro* fertilization. Hum Reprod 1994;9:184.
62. Steptoe PC, Edwards RG, Walters DE. Observation on 767 clinical pregnancies and 500 births after human in vitro fertilization. Hum Reprod 1986;1:89–94.
63. Australian *in Vitro* Fertilization Collaborative Group. *In Vitro* Fertilization and GIFT pregnancies in Australia and New Zealand, 1979–85. Med J Aust 1988;148:429–436.
64. Saunders DM, Lancaster PAL. The wider perinatal significance of the Australian in vitro fertilization data collection program. Am J Perinatol 1989;6:252–255.
65. Testart J, Plachot M, Mandelbaum J, Salat-Baroux J, Frydman R, Cohen J. World Colloborative Report on IVF-ET and GIFT: 1989 results. Hum Reprod 1992;2:362–369.
66. Friedler S, Mashiah S, Laufer N. Births in Israel resulting from *in vitro* fertilization/embryo transfer, 1982–1989: National registry of the Israeli association for fertility research. Hum Reprod 1992;7,8: 1159–1163.
67. Wang XJ, Clark AM, Kirby CA, et al. The obstetric outcome of singleton pregnancies following in-vitro fertilization/gamete intra-fallopian transfer. Hum Reprod 1994;9:141–146.
68. Tanbo T, Dale PO, Lunde O, Moe N, Abyholm T. Obstetric outcome in singleton pregnancies after assisted reproduction. Obstet Gynecol 1995;86:188–192.
69. Mcfaul PB, Patel N, Mills J. An audit of the obstetric outcome of 148 consecutive pregnancies from assisted conception: implications for neonatal services. Br J Obstet Gynecol 1993;100:820–825.
70. Gissler M, Silverio MM, Hemminiki E. *In-vitro* fertilization pregnancies and perinatal health in Finland 1991–1993. Hum Reprod 1995; 10:1856–1861.
71. Antoine JM, Gomes A, Uzan S, et al. Evolution au-delà du premier trimestre de 305 grossesses obtenues par fécondation *in vitro*. J Gynecol Obstet Biol Reprod 1990;19:901–907.
72. Verlaennen H, Cammu H, Derde MP, Amy JJ. Singleton pregnancy after *in vitro* fertilization: expectations and outcome. Obstet Gynecol 1995;86:906–910.
73. Tallo CP, Vohr B, Oh W, Rubin LP, Seifer DB, Haning RV Jr. Maternal and neonatal morbidity associated with *in vitro* fertilization. J Pediatr 1995;127:794–800.
74. Assisted Reproductive Technology In The United States And Canada. 1994 Results generated from the American Society For Reproductive Medicine/Society For Assisted Reproductive Technology Registry. Fertil Steril 1996;66:697–705.
75. Kramer M. Determinants of low birth weight: methodological assessment and meta-analysis. Bull WH0 1987;65:663–736.
76. World Collaborative Report On IVF. Preliminary data for 1995. J Assist Reprod Genet 1997;14(Suppl):251–265.
77. Berkowitz GS. An epidemiologic study of preterm delivery. Am J Epidemiol 1981;113:81–92.
78. Bhalla AK, Sarala G, Dhaliwa L. Pregnancy following infertility. Aust NZ J Obstet Gynaecol 1992;32:249–251.
79. Ghazi HA, Spielberger C, Kallen B. Delivery outcome after infertility-a registry study. Fertil Steril 1991;55:726–732.
80. Tuck SM, Yudkin PL, Turnbull AC. Pregnancy outcome in elderly primigravidae with and without a history of infertility. Br J Obstet Gynaecol 1988;95:230–237.
81. Varma TR, Patel RH. Outcome of pregnancy following investigation and treatment of infertility. Int J Gynecol Obstet 1987;25:113–120.
82. Wilson MG, Parmelee AH, Huggins MH. Prenatal history of infants with birth weights of 1500 g or less. J Pediatr 1963;6:1140–1148.
83. Funderburk S. Offspring of subfertile parents, a preliminary survey. Int J Fertil 1975;20:73–76.
84. Olsen J, Rachootin P, Schiodt AV. Alcohol use, conception time and birth weight. J Epidemiol Commun Health 1983;37:63–65.
85. Morrisson I. The elderly primigravida. Am J Obstet Gynecol 1975; 121:465–470.
86. Kirz DS, Dorchester W, Freeman RK. Advanced maternal age: the mature gravida. Am J Obstet Gynecol 1985;152:7–12.
87. Barkan SE, Bracken MB. Delayed chilbearing: no evidence for increased risk of low birth weight and preterm delivery. Am J Epidemiol 1987;125:101–109.
88. Lee KS, Ferguson RM, Corpuz M, Gartner LM. Maternal age and incidence of low birth weight at term: A population study. Am J Obstet Gynecol 1988;158:84–89.
89. Berkowitz GS, Skovron ML, Lapinski RH, Berkowitz RL. Delayed chilbearing and the outcome of pregnancy. N Engl J Med 1990;322: 659–664.
90. Van Noord-Zaadstra BM, Looman CW, Alsbach H, Habbema JD, Te Velde ER, Karbaat J. Delaying childbearing: effect of age on fecundity and outcome of pregnancy. BMJ 91;302:1361–1365.
91. Edge VL, Laros RK. Pregnancy outcome in nulliparous women aged 35 or older. Am J Obstet Gynecol 1993;168:1881–1885.
92. Cnattingius S, Berendes HW, Forman MR. Do delayed childbearers face increased risks of adverse pregnancy outcomes after the first birth? Obstet Gynecol 1993;81:512–516.
93. Aldous MB, Edmonson MB. Maternal age at first childbirth and risk of low birth weight and preterm delivery in Washington state. JAMA 1993;270,21:2574–2577.
94. Prysak M, Lorentz R, Kisly A. Pregnancy outcome in nulliparous women 35 years and older. Obstet Gynecol 1995;85:6570.
95. Israel SL, Deutschberger J. Relation of the mother's age to obstetric performance. Obstet Gynecol 1964;24:411–417.
96. Kane SH. Advancing age and the primigravida. Obstet Gynecol 1967; 29:409–413.
97. Forman MR, Meirik O, Berendes HW. Delayed childbearing in Sweden. JAMA 1984;252:3135–3139.
98. Cnattingius S, Forman MR, Berendes HW, Isotalo L. Delayed chilbearing and adverse perinatal outcome: a population based study. JAMA 1992;268:886–890.
99. Grimes DA, Gross GK. Pregnancy outcomes in black women aged 35 and older. Obstet Gynecol 1981;58:614–620.
100. Berkowitz GS, Kasl SV. The role of psychosocial factors in spontaneous preterm delivery. J Psychosom Res 1983;27:283–290.
101. Naeye RL. Maternal age, obstetric complications, and the outcome of pregnancy. Obstet Gynecol 1983;61:210–216.
102. WHO Task Force on Sequelae of Abortion. Gestation, birth-weight, and spontaneous abortion in pregnancy after induced abortion. Lancet 1979;20:142–145.
103. Wadhawa PD, Sandman CA, Porto M, Dunkel Schetter C, Garite TJ. The association between prenatal stress, infant birth weight and gestational age at birth: a prospective investigation. Am J Obstet Gynecol 1993;169:858–865.
104. Perkin MR, Bland JM, Peacock JL, Anderson HR. The effect of anxiety and depression during pregnancy on obstetric complications. Br J Obstet Gynecol 1993;100:629–634.
105. Mutale T, Creed F, Maresh M, Hunt L. Life events and low birth-weight—analysis by infants preterm and small for gestational age. Br J Obstet Gynecol 1991;98:166–172.
106. Goldfarb AF, Morales A, Rakoff AE, Protos P. Critical review of 160 Clomiphene-related pregnancies. Obstet Gynecol 1968;31:342–345.
107. Miyake A, Kurachi H, Wakimoto H, et al. Second pregnancy with spontaneous ovulation following clomiphene- or gonadotropin-induced pregnancy. Eur J Obstet Gynecol Reprod Biol 1988;27:1–5.
108. Karow WG, Payne SA. Pregnancy after clomiphene citrate treatment. Fertil Steril 1968;19:351–362.
109. Hill GA, Bryan S, Herbert CM, Shah DM, Wentz AC. Complications of pregnancy in infertile couples: routine treatment versus assisted reproduction. Obstet Gynecol 1990;75:790–794.
110. Howe RS, Sayegh RA, Durinzi KL, Tureck RW. Perinatal outcome of singleton pregnancies conceived by in vitro fertilization: a controlled study. J Perinatol 1990;10:261–266.
111. Olivennes F, Frydman R, Rufat P, De Mouzon J, Dehan M. How to halve the prematurity rates of in vitro fertilization pregnancies in 4 days. J Assist Reprod Genet 1992;9:406–407.

112. Frydman R, Forman R, Belaisch-Allart J, Hazout A, Fernandez H, Testart J. An obstetric analysis of fifty consecutive pregnancies after transfer of cryopreserved human embryos. Am J Obstet Gynecol 1989;160:209–213.
113. Wada I, Macnamee MC, Wick K, Bradfield JM, Brinsden PR. Birth characteristics and perinatal outcome of babies conceived from cryopreserved embryos. Hum Reprod 1994;9:543–546.
114. FIVNAT. Comparaison des grossesses issués de transferts d'embryons congelés aux grossesses issués de transferts d'embryons frais en fécondation *in vitro*. Contracept Fertil Sex 1994;22:287–291.
115. Serhal PF, Craft IL. Oocyte donation in 61 patients. Lancet 1989;1: 1185–1187.
116. Cornet D, Antoine JM, Casanova S, et al. Obstetric evolution of pregnancies obtained from donated oocytes. Fetal Diagn Ther 1992; 7:31–35.
117. Pados G, Camus M, Van Steirteghem AV, Bonduelle M, Devroey P. The evolution and outcome of pregnancies from oocyte donation. Hum Reprod 1994;9:538–542.
118. Blanchette H. Obstetric performance of patients after oocyte donation. Am J Obstet Gynecol 1993;168:1803–1809.
119. Applegarth L, Goldberg N, Cholst I, et al. Families created through ovum donation: preliminary investigation of obstetrical outcome and psychosocial adjustment. J Assist Reprod Genet 1995;12:574–580.
120. Friedman F, Copperman AB, Brodman ML, Shah D, Sandler B, Grunfeld L. Perinatal outcome after embryo transfer in ovum recipients—a comparison with standard *in vitro* fertilization. J Reprod Med 1996; 41:640–644.
121. Wisanto A, Bonduelle M, Camus M, et al. Obstetric outcome of 904 pregnancies after ICSI. Hum Reprod 1996;11:121–129.
122. Wennerholm UB, Haberger L, Nilsson L, Wennergren M, Wikland M, Bergh C. Obstetric and perinatal outcome of children conceived from cryopreserved embryos. Hum Reprod 1997;12:1819–1825.

Cherry and Merkatz's Complications of Pregnancy,
Fifth Edition, edited by W. R. Cohen.
Lippincott Williams & Wilkins, Philadelphia © 2000.

CHAPTER 55

Anesthesia: Principles and Techniques

Susan H. Kim-Lo, Christopher F. Ciliberto, and Richard M. Smiley

Between 1.6% and 2.2% of pregnant women undergo nonobstetric surgery during their gestation (1,2). Thus, 50,000 to 75,000 pregnant women in the United States require anesthesia and surgery annually, and this incidence is probably an underestimate because it does not consider early pregnancies unsuspected at the time of operation (3). A wide variety of operations are performed in pregnant women at different gestational ages. The types of operations include those directly related to pregnancy, such as cervical cerclage; those indirectly related to pregnancy, such as ovarian cystectomy; and those unrelated to gestation, such as appendectomy. In the largest single series concerning surgery and anesthesia during pregnancy, 42% of surgeries during pregnancy occurred during the first trimester, 35% during the second trimester, and 23% during the third (4).

This chapter reviews the physiologic and anatomic changes that affect anesthetic care during pregnancy and then discusses the effects of anesthetic drugs and perioperative events on the fetus and on pregnancy outcome. Anesthetic considerations for some specific types of surgery and medical diseases and complications are outlined. Although many of the principles and practices of anesthesia for pregnant women are derived from experience and the study of parturients, the primary focus of this chapter is on anesthetic management for surgical procedures during pregnancy.

PHYSIOLOGY OF PREGNANCY AND ANESTHETIC IMPLICATIONS

Physiologic changes resulting from pregnancy affect almost every organ system, and these alterations influence anesthetic management of pregnant women. Some anesthesiologists believe the physiologic alterations are significant enough that they classify healthy pregnant patients as an American Society of Anesthesiologists physical status 2 (a patient with a mild systemic disease) (5). The adaptive physiologic changes are partially hormonally mediated. Anatomic factors include adaptation to the low-pressure placental circulation and the mechanical compression of the gravid uterus, especially later in pregnancy (6–8). Certain physiologic alterations, including an increased metabolic rate, may increase the risk of specific anesthetic or surgical complications, especially in women with coexisting medical or surgical conditions. Finally, perhaps most obviously, anesthetic management will be affected by the nature of the surgical procedure, ranging from a simple peripheral operation, to a somewhat more involved laparoscopy, to a major endeavor such as complex cardiac surgery involving cardiopulmonary bypass.

Cardiovascular System

Pregnancy produces a relative hypervolemic and hyperdynamic state. As early as weeks 6 to 12 of pregnancy, both the plasma volume and the red cell volume begin to increase. By term, there is a 40% to 50% increase in plasma volume and a 25% to 40% increase in the total blood volume (9–12). Red cell volume increases less than plasma, resulting in the physiologic anemia of pregnancy. This hemodilution causes a decreased plasma protein concentration despite an increase in absolute amount. Thus, the free fraction of highly protein-bound drugs (e.g., bupivacaine) may be increased during pregnancy (12). Plasma levels of pseudocholinesterase, the enzyme involved in the metabolism of several anesthetic drugs, is decreased by about 25%, although this moderate decrease is usually clinically insignificant (13–16).

Cardiac output (CO) begins to rise in the first trimester, around the eighth week, as a result of an increase in both stroke volume and heart rate. CO increases, with an elevation of 50% from nonpregnant values by 30 to 34

S. H. Kim-Lo, C. F. Ciliberto, and R. M. Smiley: Department of Anesthesiology, Columbia Presbyterian Medical Center, New York, NY 10032.

weeks, and by as much as 80% to 100% in the immediate postpartum period (17). Many of these alterations occur surprisingly early in the pregnancy. Capeless and associates reported that by 8 weeks of gestation, 57% of the CO increase, 78% of the stroke volume increase, and 90% of the systemic vascular resistance decrease that will be present by 24 weeks already has occurred (18). There is also a redistribution of CO, with preference to organs such as the placenta, uterus, and skin. The uterine artery blood flow at term is at least 500 to 600 mL per minute; thus, an obstetric hemorrhage during the last trimester can be catastrophic (11).

Older studies suggested that CO decreases near term, but more recent studies suggest that the previous findings actually were detecting the effect of aortocaval compression (17,19,20). If aortocaval compression is prevented, no decrease in CO occurs in late pregnancy. As many as 10% of parturients at term may experience "supine hypotensive syndrome" as a result of positional compression. A radiographic study demonstrated that 90% of supine parturients at term had complete obstruction of the inferior vena cava (21).

Vascular resistance is decreased as a result of direct vasodilatation from the increased progesterone and possibly prostacyclin levels and the presence of a low-resistance circuit in the placenta (22). This lowered peripheral vascular resistance decreases the arterial blood pressure despite the increase in cardiac output. By the latter half of pregnancy, the blood pressure gradually recovers to normal or near normal nonpregnant values (6). In the already vasodilated state of pregnancy, further vascular relaxation resulting from vasodilating anesthetic agents, which include most commonly used agents, or from regional anesthetic techniques may adversely affect blood pressure and cardiac output, especially if aortocaval compression is also present.

Electrocardiographic (ECG) changes occur during pregnancy because of a shift in the position of the heart, resulting in possible left axis deviation, premature contractions, nonspecific ST-segment and T-wave changes, and an increased risk of supraventricular tachyarrhythmias (23). ECG signs of myocardial ischemia may be normal under some circumstances; a number of investigators have reported a high incidence of ST-segment depression and other "ischemic" findings in normal women undergoing cesarean sections in whom there has been no evidence of actual myocardial ischemia (24–26). Dyspnea, flow murmurs, a prominent third heart sound, peripheral edema, and even cardiomegaly may be detected in normal parturients.

Respiratory System

The pregnant patient lives with a compensated respiratory alkalosis. The diaphragm is displaced 3 to 4 cm upward, but the rib cage flares outward, resulting in minimal changes in vital capacity. Expiratory reserve volume, residual volume, and functional residual capacity (FRC) decrease, but a concomitant increase in inspiratory capacity and inspiratory reserve volume keeps total lung capacity unchanged (10,11). Tidal volume increases (140% of prepregnancy values by term), respiratory rate increases (115%), with a 25% increase in alveolar ventilation by 3 to 4 months and an increase of as much as 45% to 70% in minute ventilation by term (8). The partial pressure of oxygen in arterial blood ($PaCO_2$) decreases to 28 to 32 mm Hg, with a slight rise in pH to about 7.44. Increased renal bicarbonate excretion decreases renal buffer reserve, making the patient more susceptible to metabolic acidosis. The bicarbonate level decreases by about 4 mEq per liter to about 21 mEq per liter, and the PaO_2 is slightly increased to a mean of 105 mmHg, which decreases in the supine position.

The closing capacity (the lung volume at which small airway closure occurs) in the nonpregnant healthy patient is usually well below the FRC (the lung volume at end expiration); so small airways rarely close during normal spontaneous ventilation. During pregnancy, FRC decreases by about 20%, mostly as a result of anatomic factors, which puts the pregnant patient at increased risk of small-airway closure and atelectasis. Factors that lower FRC further, such as morbid obesity, supine positioning, or pulmonary disease, may result in arterial desaturation and hypoxemia. In the pregnant patient, apnea may decrease the partial pressure of oxygen in arterial blood (PaO_2) up to 150 torr in 1 minute (27). Hence, the speed of airway and ventilatory control is paramount during anesthetic induction and in emergency resuscitation situations.

Pulmonary vascular resistance is decreased as a result of vasodilatation of the pulmonary vascular smooth muscle. Pulmonary pressures are not altered significantly because vascular volume increases by roughly the same order of magnitude as resistance decreases. Pulmonary circulatory reserve is decreased in part because of a decrease in colloid osmotic pressure, leading to susceptibility to transudation of fluid and pulmonary edema in the obstetric patient. Perioperatively, fluid management should be monitored carefully, but a somewhat hypervolemic state is probably desirable to maintain uteroplacental perfusion while monitoring for any signs of pulmonary overflow.

The capillary engorgement of the nasopharynx and the oral airway mucosa, perioral edema, the weight gain of pregnancy, and the higher risk of hypoxemia for the reasons mentioned may lead to difficulties in airway management and an increase in respiratory complications in pregnant women (28). Both mask ventilation and intubation may be hindered. The incidence of failed intubation in the term pregnant population presenting for cesarean section is eight times higher than in the general population. The incidence of fatal failed intubation is 13 times that in the general population (29,30).

Gastrointestinal System

Pregnant patients are at increased risk for aspiration pneumonitis. The classic risk factors for this complication are shared by most pregnant women: an incompetent lower esophageal sphincter, low gastric pH, and gastric volume of 25 mL or more (31–33). During pregnancy, the stomach is pushed upward, and the pylorus is displaced posteriorly because of an enlarging uterus. Some studies suggest that gastric emptying is delayed during pregnancy, whereas several recent reports suggest that gastric emptying is little affected during most of pregnancy but is slowed by the pain and hormonal effects of labor and opioid medication (34–39). There is, however, an increased incidence of reflux esophagitis and heartburn among obstetric patients (40). What time during gestation these anatomic changes increase the aspiration risk of an anesthetic procedure is a controversial issue. Esophageal sphincter tone seems to be affected early in pregnancy, but the mechanical effects should be more apparent later. Many anesthesiologists would insist on intubation of any pregnant woman undergoing general anesthesia after the first trimester, whereas others believe that this step may not be mandatory until perhaps the late second trimester. Preoperatively, a nonparticulate antacid to neutralize gastric contents should be administered to any pregnant woman undergoing surgery because the risk of doing so is negligible. Many or most patients could receive metoclopramide to facilitate gastric emptying and to increase lower esophageal sphincter tone and perhaps histamine-2 receptor (H_2) blockers to decrease gastric volume and raise gastric pH.

Central Nervous System

Although the physiologic reasons are not completely understood, the anesthetic requirement during pregnancy is reduced for both general and regional techniques. The minimal alveolar concentration (MAC) or median effective dose (ED_{50}) for volatile agents is reduced by 25% to 40% as a result of hormonal and biochemical changes and elevated endogenous opiate levels (41–43). The effects of other sedative and hypnotic agents are probably similarly affected. The dose of local anesthetics required for a given level of spinal or epidural anesthesia is also decreased. Progesterone-related membrane alterations may be responsible for the reduced local anesthetic requirements as early as the first trimester (44). With progression of pregnancy, engorged epidural vessels decrease the volume of cerebral spinal fluid and the epidural space, further reducing the spinal and epidural anesthetic dose on an anatomic basis.

Hematologic System

Pregnancy is a hypercoagulable state, with a rate of thromboembolic complications as high as five to six times that of nonpregnant women (6). Estrogen increases protein production, including liver-synthesized clotting factors VII, VIII, IX, and X. Fibrinogen concentration increases by at least 20%. Hypercoagulability also is related to decreased concentrations of protein S and plasminogen. The concentration of antithrombin III, the main inhibitor of thrombin, is unchanged or only slightly decreased. Platelet turnover increases, but the platelet count usually remains within the low-normal range (45).

The physiologic anemia decreases oxygen-carrying capacity and raises the question about the proper time or hematocrit at which to commence transfusion, with little data to support any particular answer. There is a physiologic leukocytosis resulting from a demargination of mature leukocytes from the vascular endothelial lining.

Renal System

Renal blood flow and glomerular filtration rate (GFR) are markedly increased during pregnancy as a result of humoral and mechanical factors. Renal blood flow increases 60% to 80% above nonpregnancy levels by early midtrimester and decreases to about 40% above nonpregnant values by term (46). GFR increases 50% by weeks 10 to 16 and remains at this level until term. There is an increased clearance of creatinine, urea, and uric acid, resulting in decreased serum concentrations to about two thirds of the nonpregnant values. A value that would be normal in a nonpregnant woman may indicate markedly reduced renal function. Drugs with significant renal clearance may need to be administered at higher or more frequent doses to account for the increased clearance. The renal glucose threshold decreases, and proteinuria is common. Sodium excretion remains normal because of balanced effects of increased progesterone and aldosterone (47).

TERATOGENICITY AND DRUG EFFECTS ON THE FETUS

Exposure to anesthetic drugs during pregnancy may constitute a risk for teratogenicity, growth restriction, or early loss of the pregnancy by spontaneous abortion or preterm labor. Important factors are the stage of embryonic development at exposure, teratogenicity of the drug, and amount and duration of exposure. The most vulnerable time for teratogenic effects is during organogenesis. Days 13 through 55 of human gestation are the most critical in this regard, although many systems, especially the central nervous system, continue to develop for much longer. In the later stages of pregnancy, the adverse effects of drug exposure are most likely to lead to minor morphologic changes or functional abnormalities rather than gross structural anomalies (48). It is important to keep the emotional issue of drug-induced effects on pregnancy and fetal development in context and perspective; physiologic derangements such as infection, hypoxemia, hypotension, and severe anemia, which may occur in the woman being considered for surgery and anesthesia during pregnancy, may have more potential for teratogenesis than almost any possible medical or anesthetic therapy needed.

Most investigations of drug teratogenicity involve animal models or epidemiologic studies of chronic exposure. The duration of exposure to any drug in the perioperative period is limited, however, and the teratogenic potential of any agent should therefore be considered with this in mind. The U.S. Food and Drug Administration (FDA) has developed a system to categorize each specific drug. Categories range from category A, well-studied drugs that carry no risk; through B, C, and D, which are progressively less well studied or possibly risky; to category X, in which fetal risk has been clearly demonstrated (49). This classification system is of limited utility in aiding in drug choices for anesthesia, because most anesthetic and analgesic drugs are somewhere between the two extremes, and exposure is one time or limited in dose and duration. Few absolute recommendations can be made.

Opioids

Most of the major opioid agonists are category C drugs (risk cannot be ruled out, and human data are lacking). Morphine, meperidine, and hydromorphone have been associated with fetal resorption and malformations in rodents. The doses given, however, were orders of magnitude beyond the usual clinical range (50). Clinical experience strongly suggests that all these agents are safe when used in the limited perioperative period. In animals, fentanyl has not been shown to have teratogenic effects. This drug is used routinely for anesthesia during pregnancy and for labor analgesia at term, but there continue to be no published data regarding its safety in human pregnancy (51). Fentanyl can induce a loss of variability in the fetal heart rate tracing without fetal hypoxia, a property shared with most, if not all, opioids (52). There are conflicting reports about both sufentanil and alfentanil having either embryocidal effects in animals or no reproductive or teratogenic effects (53). Apparent teratogenic or other adverse effects of opioids in many small animal studies may well be mediated by their effects on maternal physiology, such as respiratory depression, and may not be relevant to the human clinical environment.

Benzodiazepines

Benzodiazepines have been implicated in a variety of birth defects ranging from spina bifida to cardiac abnormalities, but there is uncertainty about their teratogenic potential (54). The most often cited and controversial congenital anomaly is cleft palate. Although much has been written on this subject, several large, well-controlled studies have shown no association (55,56). Laegrid and associates recently described "behavioral teratogenicity" in an animal study, suggesting that *in utero* exposure to benzodiazepines (and, by inference, other sedative–hypnotics) could have the potential for long-term effects on behavior or memory (57). For all these reasons, many anesthesiologists tend to avoid using diazepam and other benzodiazepines during gestation, and the drug has been given a category D classification by the FDA. Midazolam is currently the most commonly used benzodiazapine in the perioperative setting, and it also has been given a category D classification. Limited animal studies suggest that both midazolam and lorazepam, another commonly used benzodiazepine, are neither embryotoxic nor teratogenic (58).

Local Anesthetics

Controversy exists in the literature on the issue of effects of local anesthetics on the neurobehavioral scores in the neonate after epidural analgesia during labor (59–61). Effects in the earlier stages of gestation have not been well studied, but there is much clinical experience. No noticeable adverse or teratogenic effects have been associated with the use of local anesthetics during pregnancy. Lidocaine is a category B drug; two other commonly used local anesthetics in obstetric anesthesia, bupivacaine and chloroprocaine, are category C, although it is likely their effects are similar and relatively benign. Bupivacaine, however, is known to cause more cardiac toxicity than the other commonly used local anesthetics. High blood concentrations of bupivacaine, such as those that occur when surgical epidural doses are inadvertently injected directly into the bloodstream, may result in therapy-resistant cardiac arrhythmias and cardiovascular collapse. This toxicity may be greater during pregnancy (62,63). All these local anesthetics have been used extensively at term and in preterm labor for both labor analgesia and cesarean anesthesia with excellent results, so any fetal effects of acute exposure must be minimal.

Muscle Relaxants

All conventionally used depolarizing and nondepolarizing muscle relaxants are large, positively charged molecules that do not cross the placenta to any significant degree, and there have been no reports of teratogenic effects when these drugs are administered to pregnant animals nor any studies suggesting that such drugs cause problems in human pregnancy. Sensitivity to these medications is mildly increased in pregnancy (64).

Inhaled Anesthetics

No evidence has been found to demonstrate that any of the volatile anesthetics used in clinical practice is teratogenic in humans. Nonetheless, it must be considered that it would take an impossibly large number of studied exposures to rule out any effect completely. As with most drugs during pregnancy, the data in animal studies are unclear and conflicting. The most important problem to consider, and a difficult one to resolve with small animal investigation, is that of the indirect effects of anesthetic exposure; hypoxia, hypotension, and even malnutrition from prolonged exposure to any anesthetic may and actually have resulted in adverse outcome.

Nitrous oxide (N_2O) is the most controversial inhalational anesthetic agent with regard to administration during pregnancy. N_2O inhibits DNA synthesis by oxidizing the cobalt ion in vitamin B_{12}, interfering with the synthetic pathway for methionine. In addition, N_2O interferes with the production of tetrahydrofolate from methyl tetrahydrofolate (65–67). The resulting changes in the activity of fetal methionine synthetase persist for 2 to 3 days (66). As recently as the late 1980's, it was common to recommend that any pregnant woman who was to receive N_2O as part of her anesthetic should receive folinic acid as a supplement to bypass pharmacologically the methionine step in DNA synthesis. Interestingly, the addition of a volatile anesthetic eliminated the teratogenic effects of N_2O in rats (65), suggesting that the N_2O effect responsible for its teratogenicity may not be its disruption of DNA synthesis but rather on uterine blood flow or activation of the stress response. At least one series has reported administration of N_2O to several hundred women for cervical cerclage in the first half of pregnancy without complication (68). The role of the administration of folinic acid to patients who are about to receive N_2O is unclear; we do not give folinic acid to pregnant women receiving N_2O at our institution.

Antiemetics

Effective antiemetics have long been sought for use in women during pregnancy. Antiemetic use during the perioperative period has increased as modern anesthetic practices have evolved. Metoclopramide is a dopamine antagonist that acts as a gastrointestinal prokinetic; it is frequently used to promote gastric emptying and increase lower esophageal sphincter tone, thereby decreasing the potential for regurgitation and aspiration during general anesthesia. It easily crosses the placenta, but it has not been shown to be teratogenic in ewes (69). No human studies of chronic or acute use of metoclopramide during pregnancy have been reported.

The histamine receptor antagonists cimetidine and ranitidine are both category B. These agents produce their clinical effects by selective and competitive H_2 receptor antagonism, which then blocks the histamine induction of H^+ secretion by gastric parietal cells. Although there are no reports of adverse outcomes after the use of these drugs either from long- or short-term use, the risk-to-benefit ratio in the first trimester is unclear. During the second and third trimesters, however, the ratio is almost certainly in favor of using these drugs when indicated in the perioperative period (70). Such use of these drugs is common, especially given the widespread, although possibly incorrect, opinion that gastric emptying is decreased after about week 10 of gestation.

Oral antacids are the third class of drugs used in what is often referred to as *triple aspiration precautions*. This group of medications carries with it the least amount of concern about teratogenicity; therefore, these drugs are the safest to administer at all times and chronically during gestation. The most important factor to be considered with the use of this class of drugs is differentiation between particulate and nonparticulate antacids. It is crucial to use nonparticulate antacids (e.g., sodium citrate) in the perioperative setting because of the risk associated with aspiration of particulate antacids.

MATERNAL AND FETAL OUTCOMES FROM SURGERY AND ANESTHESIA

The effects of surgery, surgical disease, and anesthesia on the unborn fetus have been addressed in several large retrospective studies over the past three decades. These studies examined the maternal and fetal outcomes after surgical procedures performed at various times during gestation. Many questions remain about the role each of these variables plays in the outcome of pregnancies complicated by the need for surgery. Even the largest of these retrospective reports is of inadequate size to answer questions confidently regarding optimal anesthetic technique or drugs.

In 1963, Smith examined more than 18,000 charts and found 67 women who had undergone nonobstetric surgery during pregnancy (71). He identified many of the major perioperative concerns that still exist today surrounding surgery during pregnancy. Approximately one third of these patients had general anesthesia for their procedures. The most common adverse outcome was fetal loss, which was strongly associated with the nature of the procedure; for example, four losses occurred in ten cases in which cervical cerclage was performed. The procedure associated with the next highest incidence of loss was appendectomy, with a 25% incidence (4 of 16). All other procedures had similar rates of pregnancy loss of about 5%. In this small group, no congenital anomalies were reported.

In 1965, Shnider and Webster reported on 147 cases and included the incidence of preterm labor, spontaneous abortion, and congenital anomalies (72). Underlying pathology and surgical procedure were highly associated with fetal loss and poor fetal outcome, especially low birth weight. The inclusion of cerclage cases makes the findings difficult to interpret. Again, no congenital anomalies were seen in their patients, but the sample was small. In contrast to a report on surgery during pregnancy from early in this century in which maternal mortality was 35% (73), Shnider's group reported no maternal mortality.

In 1980 Brodsky published the results of a questionnaire sent to female dental workers and the wives of dentists in an attempt to evaluate the effects of occupational exposure to N_2O along with exposure to surgical anesthesia in those of the group who happened to undergo surgery during pregnancy. There were 287 surgical procedures performed, 187 of which occurred in the first trimester; the other 100 procedures were performed in the second trimester. The spontaneous abortion rate was increased slightly, from 5% to 8% among those who had no occupational exposure to N_2O and an increase from 9% to 15% in women who had (or whose husbands had) exposure to N_2O. Congenital anomalies were not increased in any group. No information was given about the nature of any of the surgical procedures, and the study suffers from the likely existence of recall and retrieval bias.

Data from the provincial health system in Manitoba, Canada, provided one of the largest series of operations during pregnancy (74). Between 1971 and 1978, surgery was performed on 2,565 pregnant women in Manitoba. The report compared these women to matched controls. In this fairly large series, no evidence was found for an increased incidence of congenital anomalies in the group of women who underwent surgery during pregnancy. Overall, no increase occurred in the spontaneous abortion rate, but women who received general anesthesia had a slight but statistically significant increase compared with the group of women who had no surgery (risk ratio, 1.58). Women who had surgical procedures performed under local or spinal anesthesia did not have an increased risk of fetal loss. Only 46 women received a spinal anesthetic in this series. It is difficult to analyze separately the effect of general anesthesia on the incidence of spontaneous abortion, but it is likely that patients with more extensive surgical pathology required general anesthesia and the surgical pathology itself may have influenced pregnancy outcome.

The largest and most recent series to date was based on data from the Swedish national health system. Mazze and Källén reported on 5,405 surgical procedures performed between 1973 and 1981 (4). Cervical cerclages were not included in the analysis. Surgical procedures were performed at all stages of pregnancy; 2,252 cases occurred during the first trimester, 1,881 in the second trimester, and 1,272 in the third trimester. Slightly more than half of these cases were performed using general anesthesia, and nearly all patients who received general anesthesia received N_2O (98%). In only about 14% of these operations was regional anesthesia documented, whereas no anesthetic was defined in the remaining 32%. Reassuringly to anesthesiologists, surgeons, and patients, no increase in congenital anomalies was seen in this series. This report calmed much of the concern about the use of N_2O in the gravida at any gestational age. Low birth weight at delivery and neonatal death in the first week after birth were increased significantly in the surgical group compared with pregnancies in which no surgery was performed. Again, the impact of anesthesia *per se* compared with that of the surgical disease is difficult to separate.

These series, taken together, suggest that the risk of congenital anomalies resulting from anesthetic exposure and surgery, if it exists at all, is quite small. Overall, the risks of anesthesia and surgery during pregnancy are limited if the anesthetic is managed properly. Our ability to define the specific risks and advantages of particular anesthetic techniques or timing of surgical procedures is limited by the numbers of subjects that would be needed to have confidence in any specific conclusions.

GUIDELINES AND RECOMMENDATIONS

Unlike the situation at delivery, for which there is substantial evidence that regional anesthesia is safer than general anesthesia (75), there is no good evidence that any one anesthetic technique is preferable to another for other surgical procedures during pregnancy. Decisions must be made on a case-by-case basis, with surgical considerations a prominent factor in anesthetic choice. Nonetheless, many anesthesiologists and patients prefer local or regional anesthesia when they present for surgery during pregnancy, often because of fears, rational or not, about drug effects on the fetus or the pregnancy. If a regional technique is chosen for these reasons, it might be preferable to use spinal anesthesia rather than an epidural to limit the amount of drug exposure. If general anesthesia is chosen, it is reasonable to use at least a moderate dose of a volatile anesthetic agent, because these agents tend to decrease uterine tone and increase uterine blood flow. Whatever the anesthetic approach, attention to fluid volume and avoidance of hypotension are crucial. Other precautions similar to those taken at the time of cesarean section should be used, especially in the second and third trimesters. These precautions include antacid aspiration prophylaxis and cricoid pressure at the time of induction and intubation after early pregnancy. Maintenance of left uterine displacement is also important by the third trimester and sometimes forgotten outside the labor suite. Hyperventilation should be avoided unless clearly indicated.

Fetal heart rate (FHR) and uterine activity monitoring are controversial issues for the perioperative period. FHR can be monitored continuously as early as 16 weeks of gestation, but there is a question of what to do with this information perioperatively in the fetus that would not be viable, if delivered. Anesthesiology textbooks and review articles are fairly uniform in their recommendation in favor of aggressive fetal and uterine monitoring once it is possible, whereas much of the obstetric literature is more equivocal. It is the opinion of some authors that there is little to do at the time of surgery in response to any changes noted on these monitors; however, normalization of maternal blood pressure and adjustments to anesthetic levels and doses, removal of surgical equipment, tocolysis, and alteration of patient position and ventilatory patterns in women receiving general anesthesia all may be used to improve fetal condition if compromise is suspected. If FHR monitoring is performed in the operating suite, there must be an understanding of the effects of anesthetic agents on FHR; typically, a loss of variability is seen. When the fetus is viable and possible compromise is noted perioperatively, it is mandatory at least to obtain obstetric consultation to help determine the causes and to decide on treatment (e.g., surgical delivery, tocolysis, continued observation). We use FHR monitoring whenever it is possible to place the monitor outside the surgical field. Uterine tone also can be monitored by using external tocodynamometers. This monitoring should be continued (or instituted) postoperatively, because this is the time when the patient is most susceptible to the onset of uterine contractions. Adequate analgesia and intravascular volume may decrease the incidence of postoperative uterine contractions by attenuating maternal catecholamine release, but it must be kept in mind that analgesics may blunt the perception of pain associated with uterine activity.

SPECIFIC SURGICAL PROCEDURES

Gynecologic Surgery

Cervical cerclage is a common procedure and, *vide supra*, one that has the potential to confuse the issues when considering outcomes related to exposure of the gravida to surgery and anesthesia. Cervical incompetence itself is of course a risk factor for fetal loss and preterm delivery, resulting in low and very low birth weight neonates. It is also one of the few procedures performed during pregnancy and often is scheduled electively. This procedure allows patients to fast for at least 8 hours before surgery and avoids the need for full-aspiration precautions. In the United States, most such cases probably are performed with the patient under spinal anesthesia, thus limiting both drug exposure and recovery time.

Ovarian cysts occasionally require surgery during pregnancy. Specific considerations for this surgical procedure relate to the increased cardiac output to the adnexal region in pregnancy, with a potential for blood loss. If surgery is performed through a "minilaparotomy," regional or general anesthesia can be used; but if surgery is to be attempted laparoscopically, general anesthesia is preferred because of the chest and shoulder discomfort often associated with intraabdominal insufflation. These cases are often urgent, and patients are in a sufficient amount of pain to cause decreased gastric emptying. Triple-aspiration prophylaxis (e.g., nonparticulate antacid, H_2 blockers, metoclopramide) should be considered with any anesthetic technique in these patients. Maintaining uterine displacement may become more challenging when the abdomen is insufflated, and CO_2 concentration must be followed, at least by end-tidal gas monitoring, to avoid any harmful effects on uterine blood flow or fetal acid-base status.

Nongynecologic Surgery

The acute abdomen is a relatively common surgical emergency during pregnancy; both appendicitis and cholecystitis can occur. Although these procedures can be performed in an open fashion with the patient under regional anesthesia, laparoscopy is becoming more and more common. The potential benefits of decreased time to ambulation must be weighed against the potential risk of requiring general anesthesia for the procedure to be performed laparoscopically.

Neurosurgery

The pregnant woman who presents for surgery (or labor) with a central nervous system abnormality presents some unique issues to the anesthesiologist. Lesions significant enough to result in surgery during pregnancy often involve increased intracranial pressure (ICP). Perioperative management of increased ICP conflicts with the usual management of the pregnant woman. Hyperventilation, frequently necessary to decrease or prevent increases in ICP, may compromise uteroplacental blood flow and places the gravid patient at increased risk for aspiration if prolonged and aggressive mask ventilation is required before intubation (76). The need for hyperventilation must be weighed against the risk to the fetus. If hyperventilation is used, the fetal heart rate should be monitored. For the pregnant woman at term or in labor, the presence of increased ICP is a relative contraindication to regional anesthesia because epidural injections can acutely increase ICP (77) and lumbar puncture can (rarely) precipitate brainstem herniation. Many obstetric anesthesiologists, however, favor placement of an epidural for labor because the pain, stress, and expulsive efforts of labor will have detrimental effects on ICP. Contemporary perioperative management of neurosurgical patients sometimes involves maintaining mild to moderate hypothermia to decrease the cerebral metabolic rate and limit ischemic injury. Mild hypothermia is reasonably well tolerated by the fetus (78). Mannitol and furosemide are frequently given to decrease ICP and brain volume, but they may have adverse effects on circulating blood volume, blood pressure, and uteroplacental perfusion. Special monitoring during these procedures also may be prudent; somatosensory evoked potential monitoring or electroencephalogram can prove helpful in ensuring maternal safety with no effect on the fetus. Fetal hypothermia often is associated with a bradycardia that is not hypoxic in origin.

Cardiac surgery

Several series and case reports have demonstrated the relative safety of performing cardiac surgery with cardiopulmonary bypass (CPB) in pregnant women (79–81). The most common indication is valvular disease, when less invasive approaches (balloon valvotomy) have failed or are inappropriate. Maternal mortality has been as low as 3%, a rate that is similar to that of valvular surgery in the nonpregnant population, with fetal mortality about 20% (80). When such major intervention is warranted, the anesthetic management of these patients is not much different from the that in the nonpregnant patient with similar disease, but a few specific recommendations can be made. If surgery can be postponed without jeopardizing the mother, the late second trimester or early third trimester might be the best time for surgery because the period of increased cardiovascular demands later in gestation is avoided and the risk of premature labor may be less (82). On the other hand, if labor commences or delivery of the fetus becomes necessary intraoperatively or postoperatively, at this time in gestation, delivery of a significantly premature infant would result. Some suggest performing surgery later in the third trimester, with cesarean section electively performed after heparinization and the abdomen left open during the cardiac operation to allow continuous assessment of the uterus for hemorrhage (80).

No specific anesthetic drug regimen is preferred. Typical cardiac anesthesia with high doses of opioids combined with a moderate dose of volatile anesthetics is reasonable. Benzodiazepines, another mainstay of cardiac anesthesia, are controversial and could be avoided, although the evidence for the need for avoidance is weak (*vide supra*). Relatively high flows should be used on bypass to simulate the cardiac output of pregnancy, with high-normal pressures (about 70 mm Hg) maintained in an attempt to ensure adequate uterine perfusion. The operation should take place at normothermia or only mild hypothermia (32°C) if at all possible, because hypothermia below this level has been reported to result in a higher incidence of FHR abnormalities, cardiac arrest, and poor outcome (83).

Monitoring of FHR and uterine activity should be instituted and left uterine displacement maintained. Alterations in FHR have been treated with increasing flows on bypass, alteration of temperature, increasing oxygen content in maternal blood, or emergency delivery (84). CPB usually results in loss of variability on the FHR, but this event alone is not an indication for intervention. CPB also is associated with onset of uterine contractions, perhaps as a result of the release of prostaglandins (79). Vasopressor selection for blood pressure and cardiac support should be similar to that during cesarean section, with ephedrine as first choice, moderate doses of phenylephrine a second choice, and other agents depending on the cardiac physiology and clinical condition. Maternal cardiovascular and respiratory stability are probably the most important variables in fetal outcome. Simple maneuvers, such as left uterine displacement and avoidance of hyperventilation, are second nature to most obstetric anesthesiologists and should not be forgotten in the cardiac operating room. Even with all these precautions, some cases of poor fetal outcome and death have been reported (83).

ANESTHETIC IMPLICATIONS OF MEDICAL COMPLICATIONS AND DISEASE DURING PREGNANCY

Concurrent medical problems will affect anesthetic management strategies for pregnant women. We briefly outline some issues for common medical complications of pregnancy. Most of these conditions are discussed in detail elsewhere in this book; therefore, etiology, pathophysiology, and treatment are discussed only briefly herein, and specific anesthesia-related issues for each disease state are emphasized.

Cardiovascular Disease

With contemporary medical and surgical therapy, many women with significant structural or functional heart disease are surviving to childbearing age and electing to attempt pregnancy. The medical literature is replete with case reports and clinical investigations attesting to the success of anesthetic and medical strategies for the reduction of maternal morbidity and mortality in women with preconceptional cardiac lesions. Case reports and even series, however, tend to report successes in preference to failures. It is still probably appropriate to counsel women with severe disease such as pulmonary hypertension, coarctation of the aorta with involvement of the aortic root, and Marfan disease with aortic root widening against pregnancy (85–88). A patient with cardiac disease severe enough to warrant surgery during her pregnancy likely will have her anesthetic management based mostly on the particular cardiac lesion and condition. More commonly, patients with moderate to severe structural or functional cardiac disease present for obstetric and anesthetic management at term or in labor, and anesthetic management of such patients has been the subject of a recent review (89).

Arrhythmias

Cardiac arrhythmias are relatively common in pregnancy but rarely have medical, obstetric, or anesthetic implications (90). Life-threatening arrhythmias such as ventricular tachycardia or fibrillation may occur secondary to embolic phenomena, hypertensive disease, hemorrhage, or other complications. Although not strictly an anesthetic issue, the conduct of cardiopulmonary resuscitation (CPR) is somewhat modified in pregnancy. Rapid endotracheal intubation is essential, both for ventilation and oxygenation as in any resuscitation and to prevent aspiration of gastric contents. The apical lead for the application of defibrillating doses of energy should be placed more laterally than the customary placement for nonpregnant women (91). It is essential to maintain uterine displacement during CPR; aortocaval compression by the gravid uterus will diminish venous return, making CPR futile (92–94). If a cardiac arrest does not respond promptly to resuscitative efforts, a "perimortem" cesarean section usually should be performed 4 to 5 minutes into the resuscitation at the site of the arrest. This procedure can result in the delivery of a viable infant, and removal of the obstruction to venous return may increase the likelihood of maternal survival (95,96).

Valvular Disease

Mitral stenosis (MS) is the most common significant cardiac lesion seen in pregnancy. The objective with any patient with MS is to minimize left atrial pressure and to maximize left ventricular end-diastolic volume to facilitate movement of the cardiac output toward the periphery. Aortic stenosis is less common, but it shares some of the same management issues. The normal pregnancy-induced tachycardia, especially the further increases seen during labor, may be catastrophic in the parturient with MS, because the shortening of diastolic time with tachycardia leaves little time for blood to flow through the small mitral orifice. Tachycardia is similarly troublesome in aortic stenosis (AS), although it is somewhat better tolerated than in MS. Avoidance of atrial arrhythmias, especially rapid atrial fibrillation, is important with either stenotic lesion. In AS, new-onset atrial fibrillation can be devastating because the atrial contribution to filling of the hypertrophied, noncompliant left ventricle can be as high as 40%. Aggressive prevention or treatment of atrial fibrillation or other tachydysrhythmias with cardioversion or appropriate antiarrhythmic agents is mandatory.

The mainstay of the anesthetic management of labor for these patients is a carefully performed regional analgesia procedure, with attention to monitoring and maintenance of intravascular and intracardiac volume. Multiple case reports and series have demonstrated the beneficial role epidural (or presumably some forms of combined spinal–epidural) analgesia can have in patients with MS or AS (97,98). Although it appears logical that the obligate sympathetic block that is present with a labor or surgical epidural could be a problem in the case of valvular stenosis, with careful attention to fluid loading and appropriate monitoring, epidural analgesia is well tolerated and appears to improve the parturient's chance of a successful outcome. If these patients need surgical delivery, regional anesthesia is preferred, although some suggest general anesthesia with high-dose opioids (a classic "cardiac anesthetic") in the case of severe AS, where any decrease in arterial or venous tone could result in cardiovascular collapse. Arterial catheter placement seems reasonable in most of these patients, and the threshold for instituting full hemodynamic monitoring should be low, especially for surgical delivery. Tachycardia alone can increase pulmonary capillary wedge pressure significantly in both stenotic syndromes. Patients with severe aortic stenosis have a higher risk of developing ischemic complications as a result of left ventricular hypertrophy and increased myocardial work. Pulmonary edema is a possible complication of the requisite volume load for regional analgesia, but the parturient with MS or AS tolerates (and can be resuscitated from) mild fluid overload better than from hypovolemia.

Clinically significant regurgitant lesions of the mitral and aortic valve are rarely seen in pregnancy, although detectable tricuspid and, to a lesser extent, mitral and aortic insufficiency is present in many normal pregnancies (99). In general, patients with mitral and aortic regurgitation tolerate the hypervolemia and vasodilatation of pregnancy and regional analgesia and anesthesia rather well. An exception is the patient with aortic regurgitation and aortic root widening from Marfan's syndrome, in whom aggressive analgesia, beta-adrenergic blockade to prevent a hyperdynamic circulation, and vasodilatation to decrease blood pressure as much as possible are critical to decreasing aortic wall shear stress and the possibility of aortic rupture.

Neuromuscular Diseases

Myasthenia gravis

Myasthenia gravis (MG) is a chronic disease of autoimmune origin that affects the voluntary muscles, usually presenting with muscle weakness and fatigue that worsen with activity (100). Its incidence has been reported to range from 1:19,000 to 1:40,000, with a 3:1 preference for women, especially those aged between 20 and 30 years (101). This epidemiology makes MG one of the most common neuromuscular diseases in pregnant women. Immunoglobulin G (IgG) antibodies against acetylcholine receptors are found in 90% of patients (101). Treatment involves use of anticholinesterase drugs, other medications, and plasmapheresis. The course of MG during pregnancy is unpredictable. About a third of patients improve, another third worsen, and the other third show no change. Exacerbations occur more commonly during the first trimester and the postpartum period. As many as 30% of MG patients have a relapse postpartum. Maternal mortality has been reported to be about 4.5% (102). Many drugs commonly used during anesthesia can exacerbate symptoms of MG, the most obvious of which are the neuromuscular blocking agents that act as competitive antagonists at the acetylcholine receptor, but others include propranolol, quinidine, magnesium sulfate, ritodrine, terbutaline, and aminoglycoside antibiotics (100,101,103).

The major anesthetic concern is involvement of respiratory and bulbar muscles. Patients with ocular or mild generalized myasthenia or those who have well-controlled disease may do well with regional anesthetic techniques such as spinal or epidural anesthesia. When significant bulbar or respiratory compromise occurs, a high spinal or epidural anesthetic level may impair respiratory function, especially for the obstetric population, which is already at a higher risk for respiratory complications. General anesthesia with endotracheal intubation should be performed to protect the airway and ensure respiratory adequacy in patients with severe disease.

Myasthenic patients with respiratory involvement are more sensitive to narcotic-induced respiratory depression (100). Thiopental, ketamine, and propofol have been used uneventfully for the induction of anesthesia. Patients taking anticholinesterases have a reduced plasma cholinesterase activity, which can reduce metabolism of ester local anesthetics. The use of succinylcholine is controversial because the noninvolved muscles are resistant to depolarizing muscle relaxants and involved muscles are more sensitive to the drug. Also, the presence of anticholinesterases may prolong its duration of action significantly. These patients are extremely sensitive to nondepolarizing muscle relaxants as a result of the decreased number of receptors; typically, doses 5% to 20% of normal will result in surgical relaxation. The use of the newer, shorter-acting agents such as rocuronium appears to add a margin of safety, but monitoring the extent of muscle relaxation is mandatory because of the variability of responses to both classes of relaxant. It is often both possible and desirable to maintain anesthesia without the use of muscle relaxants. Some patients will not tolerate extubation after general anesthesia. The need for postoperative mechanical ventilation can be predicted by factors such as a 6-year or longer history of MG, a history of chronic respiratory disease, a pyridostigmine dose requirement greater than 750 mg per day, or a vital capacity less than 2.9 L (104).

Multiple Sclerosis

Multiple sclerosis is a chronic demyelinating disease of unclear etiology that affects the brain and the spinal cord. Its prevalence varies across different populations, with a noticeable geographic distribution (105,106). An incidence of less than 1 in 100,000 has been noted in equatorial areas, with 80 cases per 100,000 in Canada, northern Europe, and the northern United States. It is more common among women than men, with peak incidence in the childbearing ages of 20 to 35. The course is characterized by periods of exacerbations and remissions of variable neurologic disabilities over the years. During relapse, active demyelination occurs, especially in the periventricular white matter, and may resolve completely with restoration of myelin and neurologic function or result in gliosis and permanent destruction of axons (105). Stress, exhaustion, infection, and hyperpyrexia, known risk factors for multiple sclerosis relapses, often present peripartum.

Although the published data are limited, multiple sclerosis does not seem to increase anesthetic risks for obstetric patients undergoing general anesthesia. Baskett and Armstrong suggested that barbiturates are associated with relapse of multiple sclerosis (107), but many other authors refute this association (100,108,109). Regional anesthesia is controversial because of the theoretic neurotoxic effects of local anesthetics on demyelinated areas of the spinal cord. Diagnostic spinal taps are not associated with exacerbation of multiple sclerosis, but two studies suggest that spinal anesthesia might provoke relapse of multiple sclerosis (108,110). These studies involved a small number of relapses. One report with epidural anesthesia suggested minor exacerbations in two vaginal deliveries, perhaps related to the concentrations of local anesthetic used (111). Bader and colleagues suggest that higher concentrations of local anesthetics may affect the relapse rates (106). Theoretically, the risks of epidural anesthesia may be less than direct subarachnoid injection because of the lower concentrations of drug reaching the cerebrospinal fluid, spinal cord, and nerves. Thus, the usual clinical recommendation is to use epidural rather than spinal anesthesia when possible. The addition of opioids to epidural local anesthetics can reduce the total dose of local anesthetics administered, and neuraxial opioids have not been associated with exacerbation of multiple sclerosis.

Scoliosis

Idiopathic scoliosis is a developmental condition of childhood and adolescence. It results in a lateral deviation of the vertical axis of the spine, often with a rotatory component. Conditions associated with nonidiopathic scoliosis include myopathic disorders such as muscular dystrophy, neurologic disorders such as cerebral palsy, congenital vertebral anomalies, connective tissue disorders, osteochondrodystrophies, and infections. The incidence among adolescents between 12 and 14 years is 4% to 13%, with equal predominance between men and women for minor curvatures (<20 degrees) (112). Larger scoliotic curvatures are much less frequent, and they occur five to seven times more frequently in women than in men (112–114). Any alterations from normal spinal anatomy, whether from disease or surgical repair, obviously can affect regional anesthetic management. Management of a general anesthetic is affected if cardiopulmonary changes have occurred (115).

Scoliotic curves less than 25 to 30 degrees, stable curves before pregnancy, and surgically corrected curves do not seem to worsen during pregnancy (114,116). No specific alteration in anesthetic management may be needed for such patients, although technical aspects of regional anesthesia may be affected. In more severe cases with prior unstable curvatures, progression may occur during pregnancy with worsening back pain and cardiopulmonary impairment. Elevation of the diaphragm from an enlarging uterus and the scoliotic noncompliant rib cage can lower the FRC and closing capacity further, leading to a higher risk of hypoxemia and ventilation/perfusion mismatch.

Regional anesthesia may be used in severe thoracolumbar scoliosis, and it is not contraindicated even after corrective spinal instrumentation. Many anesthesiologists will attempt regional anesthesia in patients with scoliosis, even after spinal surgery, although success rates are lower than in patients with normal anatomy. When severe curvatures are present, placement of epidural catheters and even subarachnoid medication becomes more challenging, and a higher incidence of complications should be anticipated (115–117). Maldistribution of local anesthetic in the epidural space may result in uneven analgesia or anesthesia. The effects of standard local anesthetic doses are not always predictable, and hyperbaric spinal anesthetics may accumulate in dependent areas of the spinal column, resulting in unilateral blockade. Other concerns about epidural or spinal anesthesia include chronic back pain in many patients that later may be attributed to the anesthetic technique, patient refusal of a regional technique, and a higher potential for inadvertent dural puncture and its complications (113,115,118).

In women with significant pulmonary dysfunction secondary to scoliosis, a continuous epidural anesthetic may be a wiser choice than a spinal or a general anesthetic technique. The epidural allows more control of the anesthetic level, resulting in lesser hemodynamic and respiratory derangements. A continuous spinal anesthetic can be used in the same way but increases the risk of a postdural puncture headache. This condition may be difficult to treat because an epidural blood patch may be either difficult or impossible. Opioids should be used with caution to avoid respiratory compromise. If patients with severe curvatures display symptoms of arterial hypoxemia or have lung volumes less than 50% of predicted, an echocardiogram may be needed to evaluate cardiac, especially right ventricular, function. If significant right-sided cardiac dysfunction or pulmonary hypertension is present, regional anesthetic techniques might not be tolerated, mandating general anesthesia with appropriate invasive monitoring. These patients are at increased risk for postoperative assisted ventilation and major cardiovascular instability.

Spinal Cord Injuries

Spinal cord injuries can result from trauma, infections, tumors, or vascular lesions. There has been an improved survival of young victims, creating a new patient population who require obstetric anesthetic care. The anatomic location of the insult within the spinal cord will dictate the level of function. Patients with lesions below S2 will experience labor pain but will have relaxed perineal muscles. Injuries above T10 will result in paraplegia. These women, however, will not experience labor pain and are at a higher risk of preterm labor. Lesions above T6 will result in different levels of respiratory difficulties, and these patients are at risk for episodes of autonomic hyperreflexia (AH) (100).

AH, a potentially life-threatening complication of spinal cord injury, is particularly relevant to the perioperative and peripartum period. It involves an exaggerated sympathetic response to stimulation, often of visceral organs, with severe systolic hypertension from vasoconstriction below the level of injury. This response, unlikely with lesions below T7, appears to be due to afferent impulses entering the cord and initiating segmental reflexes that are not inhibited by higher centers (119). Bradycardia and vasodilatation occur above the level of the lesion because of reflex arcs involving the baroreceptors. Several afferent stimuli may trigger this reflex. Skin stimulation below the lesion, rectal or genital manipulation, bladder or cervical distention, fecal impaction, and hollow viscus contraction, including the uterus and the gut, are all potential triggers for AH. Patients with cord injuries have a greater pressor response to similar doses or concentrations of catecholamines than patients with intact spinal cords (109). Pregnancy may aggravate many of the physiologic problems of patients with spinal cord injuries. Pregnancy-related decreases in FRC and expiratory reserve volume may be exaggerated, placing paraplegic parturients at risk for additional pulmonary complications including atelectasis, pneumonia, impaired cough, and hypoxemia. These patients are also susceptible to development of deep vein thrombosis, urinary tract infections, decubitus ulcers, hypertension, and electrocardiographic changes.

Regional anesthesia may be the best way to block the autonomic hyperreflexic response from surgery (or labor), although performance of regional anesthesia in paraplegic or quadriplegic patients involves practical problems and may appear counterintuitive. Placement and control over the level of anesthesia can be difficult. Patients may not be optimally positioned for placement, and there is often a distortion of the spinal column. Whereas it may be difficult or impossible to assess the sensory level depending on the level of injury, the cephalad sensory level can be accurately estimated if the lesion is below the desired level. Spinal anesthesia can be and is used, but anesthesiologists tend to favor epidural anesthesia over spinal because it is more easily titrated. Alternative treatments for AH, such as vasodilators and adrenergic and ganglionic blockers, must be available if regional anesthesia is unsuccessful. An intraarterial catheter for continuous blood pressure control may be indicated because of baseline hemodynamic instability, an exaggerated response to catecholamines, and the risk of AH. If general anesthesia is necessary for the specified surgical procedure, aspiration prophylaxis is strongly recommended. A depolarizing muscle relaxant should be avoided for up to a year after the spinal cord injury because of the risk of severe, life-threatening hyperkalemia in response to succinylcholine (100). It is not clear when, if ever, nondepolarizing agents are once again safe.

Respiratory Disease—Asthma

Asthma is present in about 1% of pregnant patients, although this number may be a significant underestimation for certain subpopulations, such as pregnant teenagers, in whom the incidence is about 6.6% among 15- and 16-year-olds (120–123). As many as 15% of asthmatic parturients may require hospitalization for exacerbations during the course of pregnancy. However, the overall effect of pregnancy on asthma varies significantly. Some studies describe improvement of symptoms during pregnancy; others have suggested otherwise (120,122).

Anesthesia and surgery during pregnancy in the asthmatic woman raise special concerns. Aspiration risk is increased in pregnancy, and even a small aspiration may be disastrous in parturients with bronchospastic disease. These patients are already at higher risk for maternal and fetal hypoxemia. Fetal oxygenation may be endangered by maternal hypoxemia and especially by maternal alkalosis. Because of the emergent or urgent nature of many operations performed during pregnancy, stabilization of asthmatic symptoms may not be possible. For elective or semielective surgery, however, asthma should be controlled as well as possible to minimize risks of maternal and fetal morbidity and mortality.

Anesthetic management of the asthmatic patient, pregnant or not, depends to a large extent on current symptoms along with the history and nature of the disease. Patients with recurrent exacerbations during pregnancy or who are currently symptomatic may need to have their medical regimen intensified. If the surgical procedure is elective, it should be postponed and the exacerbation treated, including associated factors such as respiratory infections. Perioperatively, the anesthesiologist will aim to reduce or prevent any stimuli that may exacerbate a bronchospastic episode. Relieving anxiety, avoiding stimuli for hyperpnea, minimizing airway instrumentation and irritation, and providing modes of pain relief without respiratory depression are the components of perioperative management of the asthmatic patient. Regional anesthesia often is preferred, because one of the strongest stimuli for bronchospasm during the perioperative period is endotracheal intubation. A high sensory or motor blockade may cause abnormal sensation of respiration or create more difficulty in coughing and clearing secretions by affecting thoracic musculature or airway reflexes. Theoretically, the sympathetic blockade from high (thoracic) spinal or epidural anesthesia can result in bronchospasm from withdrawal of the bronchodilating sympathetic tone, but this is rarely if ever seen in clinical practice.

When general anesthesia is necessary because of the nature of the planned surgery, urgency of the procedure, or contraindication to regional anesthesia, the risks for pulmonary aspiration, bronchospasm, and inadequate oxygenation must be addressed. The awake or rapid sequence induction of anesthesia may not provide enough anesthesia or analgesia to prevent a bronchospastic reflex to endotracheal intubation. Ketamine, with its bronchodilator and intense analgesic properties, may be the induction agent of choice. Propofol induction also is less likely than thiopental to result in bronchospasm after intubation (124). Coadministration of lidocaine or rapid-acting opioids (fentanyl, sufentanil, alfentanil, or remifentanil) also may be helpful by decreasing airway reactivity to laryngoscopy. Most asthmatic patients should be pretreated with an inhaled beta-adrenergic agonist, and aspiration prophylaxis with at least a clear antacid is indicated. H_2 receptor blockers theoretically may provoke bronchospasm. Anesthesia usually is maintained by using relatively high concentrations of volatile agents with their associated bronchodilatory properties. The strategy for emergence from general anesthesia requires finding a balance between the risks of aspiration versus those of bronchospasm. Extubation with the patient fully awake will reduce the risk of aspiration, but it may induce bronchospasm. If aspiration is more than a theoretic risk (advanced pregnancy, recent oral intake), maintaining intubation until airway reflexes have returned is probably preferable because bronchospasm on emergence seems less common than with induction and intubation and is more treatable than aspiration.

Other medications used during pregnancy or during cesarean section may increase the risk of bronchospasm. Prostaglandin $F_{2\alpha}$ used for induction of labor and for treatment for uterine atony has bronchoconstricting effects, even in healthy patients. Ergot alkaloids rarely precipitate bronchospasm. Beta-adrenergic antagonists used at times to treat gestational or chronic hypertension in pregnant women may induce bronchospasm as well.

Endocrine Diseases

Diabetes

Pregnancy is associated with a progressive peripheral resistance to insulin at the postreceptor cellular level as a result of increases in counterregulatory hormones during pregnancy (125,126). Diabetes in pregnancy, its management, and its complications are covered extensively elsewhere in this book. The anesthetic management of women with gestational diabetes is affected primarily by their obstetric issues, especially fetal macrosomia, an increased incidence of cesarean section, and pregnancy-induced hypertension. We focus mainly on some of the anesthetic concerns in the smaller population of type I insulin-deficient (juvenile onset) diabetic women who become pregnant and then need surgery or anesthesia during pregnancy.

Studies of anesthetic management in pregnant diabetic patients are scarce. No data on the relationship between the complications of diabetes and responses to anesthetic agents or anesthetic outcomes in pregnant patients have been published (127). Management of diabetic parturients is based on extrapolations or deductions from studies of both nondiabetic pregnant patients and diabetic nonpregnant patients. Hypoglycemia and hyperglycemia are frequent complications of diabetes and its treatment and are of concern during anesthesia for surgery or labor. Detection can be delayed under general anesthesia. Frequent serum glucose monitoring is warranted intraoperatively. As with nonpregnant surgical patients, the basic rule is to monitor frequently in the perioperative (peripartum) period and to treat with insulin or glucose as needed.

Pregestational diabetic patients with severe autonomic neuropathy are at increased risk of pulmonary aspiration from gastroparesis and hemodynamic lability from autonomic cardiovascular dysfunction, including a risk of perioperative cardiorespiratory arrest. Signs such as early satiety, lack of sweating, and the lack of pulse rate changes with inspiration or orthostatic maneuvers may forewarn the anesthesiologist of the presence of significant autonomic disease. A difference between the maximum and minimum heart rate on deep inspiration of five or fewer beats per minute in diabetic patients suggests significant autonomic dysfunction (the normal difference is 15 beats per minute) (128,129).

No studies have been done comparing the safety and outcome of regional versus general anesthesia for nonobstetric surgery (or cesarean section for that matter) in pregnant women with diabetes. As in other patients, however, regional techniques have some theoretic advantages, including earlier detection of hypoglycemia as well as a lower risk of aspiration and attenuation of catecholamine responses. Aspiration prophylaxis with a nonparticulate antacid and metoclopramide should be provided, especially if gastroparesis is suspected. Autonomic cardiovascular dysfunction is predictive of hemodynamic lability and the need for vasopressor therapy during general anesthesia (130). These patients are susceptible to orthostatic hypotension and to marked hypotension from sympathetic blockade during spinal anesthesia. Because some diabetic parturients may suffer from chronic uteroplacental insufficiency, an epidural technique may be preferred because of its slower onset, which may allow more control over the level of sympathectomy. Aggressive intravenous hydration before a spinal or epidural procedure may lessen the hypotension, but maternal hyperglycemia is possible if the fluid administered contains dextrose.

Thyroid Diseases

Thyroid disorders during pregnancy are not always easy to diagnose because of the biochemical and physiologic changes of pregnancy, including the physiologic hypertrophy of the thyroid gland (131). Thyroid disorders are discussed in detail elsewhere in this book. This section concentrates on anesthetic concerns in the presence of thyroid abnormalities.

The main goal of preoperative management of hyperthyroid patients is to attempt to achieve the euthyroid state before scheduled surgery to minimize but not eliminate the risk of thyroid storm. *Thyroid storm*, which is a medical emergency, can be precipitated by many factors, among them surgery, childbirth, and emotional stress. If it occurs, rapid, aggressive, symptomatic treatment with beta-adrenergic blocking agents and other hypotensive agents is imperative. If emergency surgery is necessary in the presence of poorly controlled or newly diagnosed hyperthyroidism, patients can be prepared by oral propylthiouracil, intravenous glucocorticoids, sodium iodide, and beta-adrenergic blockers, with additional potent cardiovascular medications kept readily available (127).

Aside from concerns about a hyperdynamic circulatory state, other features of hyperthyroidism can interfere with the safe administration and conduct of an anesthetic. Airway obstruction from an enlarged gland is possible, as are respiratory muscle weakness and electrolyte abnormalities. Both regional and general anesthetic techniques have been safely administered to these patients. If general anesthesia is chosen, it is wise to avoid medications that may contribute to or worsen the hyperdynamic state, such as ketamine and atropine. Thiopental is a reasonable choice for induction; etomidate, a drug with few cardiovascular effects, is another option. The presence of exophthalmos necessitates careful eye protection to prevent corneal abrasions. If spinal or epidural anesthesia is chosen, omission of epinephrine is suggested.

The prevalence of hypothyroidism during pregnancy is about 0.3%. Depending on the severity and extent of the disease, parturients may present with cardiovascular dysfunction, including coronary artery disease, hypoxic ventilatory drive dysfunction, obstructive sleep apnea, coagulation abnormalities and anemia, electrolyte imbalances such as hyponatremia, and low glucocorticoid levels (127). No prospective, randomized studies have been done to suggest a superior anesthetic technique in patients with thyroid diseases, although some techniques may be preferred, depending on the patient's condition. As with hyperthyroidism, perhaps even more so, it is desirable to achieve euthyroid status before surgery because severe hypothyroidism combined with general anesthesia is a potent depressant of physiologic function. Hypothyroid patients may have an abnormal response to peripheral nerve stimulation, which complicates monitoring of muscle relaxation. Emergence and recovery of these patients from general anesthesia require close monitoring of temperature as well as cardiac and respiratory function.

Obesity

The prevalence of morbid obesity varies with the definition applied. One common measure of morbid obesity uses the body mass index (BMI), which is the weight in kilograms divided by the height in meters squared; in the United States, normal values range from 22 to 26, and morbid obesity is defined as BMI of 35 to 40. Anesthetic morbidity and mortality are increased with severe obesity (132–134).

The morbidly obese woman is at increased risk for developing diabetes, hypertension, gestational hypertension, thromboembolic events, and other surgical and anesthetic complications. Many of the physiologic changes of pregnancy are exaggerated by the similar changes induced by obesity. Oxygen consumption and CO_2 production increase linearly with weight gain. Ventilation–perfusion mismatch makes these patients more susceptible to hypoxemia, especially in the supine and Trendelenburg positions. These women may present with left ventricular hypertrophy and are susceptible to premature ventricular contractions. Hiatal hernias are more common, posing a risk for gastric regurgitation and pulmonary aspiration. When surgery is planned during pregnancy, cardiovascular and pulmonary status may need evaluation and optimization. If there are any questions regarding maternal ventilation, arterial blood gas analysis may be warranted. The need for special equipment, such as appropriate blood pressure cuff sizes and longer epidural and spinal needles, must be anticipated. Intravenous access may be technically more difficult. Pulmonary aspiration prophylaxis should be provided with nonparticulate antacid, H_2 receptor antagonist, and metoclopramide preoperatively in obese pregnant women.

As in many other conditions already described, regional anesthesia has several advantages: less respiratory depression and blood loss, fewer thromboembolic events, better hemodynamic stability, and, most importantly, less likelihood of an airway-related catastrophe. Because of the technical difficulty of placing spinal or epidural analgesia, general anesthesia may be the only alternative. There is a reported 20% incidence of failed epidural anesthesia in morbidly obese parturients (135). A large percentage of patients receiving labor analgesia may require replacement of epidural catheters for inadequate or misplaced epidurals. Hood and Dewan reported that only about 50% of initial epidurals resulted in successful labor analgesia (136). Spinal anesthesia is technically possible in most obese patients. Nevertheless, there are concerns of high spread of local anesthetic and hypotension when patients are placed supine after the procedure. The resulting sympathetic blockade combined with the decreased cardiac output resulting from aortocaval compression, which may be exaggerated in these patients, can cause profound hypotension. A high spinal anesthesia level involving respiratory muscle function and the effect of the supine position may be sufficient to cause significant hypoxemia in the morbidly obese patient. The anesthesiologist must be cognizant of the possibility of prolonged surgical time and the risk of surgery outlasting a spinal anesthetic. A continuous spinal anesthetic may be the best option if epidural placement is unsuccessful and the risk of general anesthesia is significant.

General anesthesia in morbidly obese parturients poses obvious concerns for the anesthesiologist. The consequences of an inability to intubate (aspiration or inadequate ventilation and oxygenation) are magnified and made more probable by both pregnancy and obesity. Obesity accentuates many of the anatomic changes of pregnancy. Large breasts, increased anteroposterior diameter of the chest, increased fat in the neck and shoulders, airway edema, and decreased chin-to-thyroid cartilage distance make positioning and intubation difficult in these patients. Of even more concern is that mask ventilation is likely to be ineffective if intubation fails. In the general obstetric population, between 1:300 and 1:750 attempted tracheal intubations will fail (136). Among 284 morbidly obese patients undergoing gastric bypass, a 2.4% prevalence of difficult intubations was noted among patients with 1.5 to 1.75 times the ideal body weight, with 7.3% prevalence among patients whose weight is more than 1.75 to 2 times ideal body weight (137). Nasal mucosal engorgement may lead to significant bleeding during attempted awake fiberoptic or blind nasal intubation. Obesity also impairs the proper placement of cricoid pressure.

Obesity alters the pharmacodynamics and pharmacokinetics of anesthetic agents. An increase in the volume of distribution prolongs the elimination half-lives of some drugs such as thiopental and some local anesthetics such as bupivacaine. Pseudocholinesterase activity may be increased in obese patients, but this is likely to be counteracted by the usual decrease seen during pregnancy. There is a prolonged effect of vecuronium but not of atracurium (138). The increased fat stores result in the accumulation of inhalation and intravenous drugs, maintaining their residual effects and possibly delaying emergence from anesthesia. Morbidly obese parturients' propensity for hypoxemia may not allow high nitrous oxide concentrations because they require high inspired oxygen concentrations. Vaughan and Wise reported that 77% of obese patients had a PaO_2 of less than 80 mm Hg with a fractional inspired oxygen (FiO_2) of 0.4 during surgery (139). The problem should be worsened by pregnancy. Intraoperative use of larger tidal volumes and positive end-expiratory pressure may improve oxygenation, at a cost of decreased cardiac output and possible impairment of uteroplacental blood flow.

During emergence from anesthesia, the risk of aspiration and the possibility of prolonged sedation from residual anesthetics must be considered. These obese women are at higher risk of postoperative hypoxemia and other pulmonary complications. Caution and close monitoring must be performed when postoperative analgesia is used (i.e., narcotics) by either intravenous or neuraxial routes, as a result of the higher risk of respiratory depression. These drugs, in general, need to be used cautiously in obese patients. Therapeutic strategies for dealing with the increased risk of venous thromboembolism in obese patients during the perioperative period must be used.

Hematologic Diseases

Hemoglobinopathies

The most common hemoglobinopathy in the United States is sickle cell disease (140–142). The prevalence of sickle cell trait (heterozygous, Hb A/S) is about 8% among adult American blacks. In Africa, this prevalence is as high as 20% to 40% (45). Patients with sickle trait are generally asymptomatic. Parturients with sickle cell disease (homozygous, Hb S/S) are susceptible to vasoocclusive events and may present with infarctive, aplastic, or sequestration crises or cerebrovascular accidents. They are at a higher risk for preterm labor, abruptio placentae, placenta previa, and gestational hypertension (140,143). Prophylactic transfusion therapy during pregnancy is no longer done on a routine basis. Koshy and colleagues demonstrated no difference in perinatal and maternal outcomes in a group of patients who received a prophylactic blood transfusion compared with a group who received "transfusion for emergency situations" (143). The incidence of painful crises was decreased, however, in the mothers who were transfused to maintain a hemoglobin level of about 10 g/dL.

The anesthetic management of parturients with sickle cell disease involves the maintenance of adequate intravascular volume, oxygenation, and temperature. Pregnant patients are already often in a relative hyperdynamic, hypervolemic state. Analgesia is essential, whether pain is due to a sickle crisis, surgery, or labor. Depending on the circumstances, either regional or general anesthesia may be acceptable. Hypotension from regional anesthesia is potentially a cause of localized ischemia, which theoretically can trigger a sickling episode. Maintenance of adequate oxygenation, ventilation, and hemodynamics and warming devices to maintain normothermia are the mainstays of therapy.

Coagulopathies

Pregnancy is a state of relative hypercoagulability. Parturients are, of course, not immune to coagulation disorders or to platelet abnormalities. For normal hemostasis to occur, intact vascular tissue with adequate quantities of normal functioning platelets and coagulation factors are necessary. In many conditions that can coexist with pregnancy, coagulation may be impaired. Gestational thrombocytopenia is an often incidental finding in healthy parturients with no evidence of bleeding histories or bleeding tendencies. Platelet counts tend to be above 75,000/mm^3 at delivery (144). The incidence of mild thrombocytopenia in pregnancy is 4.6% to 8.3% (140,144). More significant dysfunction of platelets or coagulation cascade is seen in autoimmune thrombocytopenic purpura, von Willebrand disease, the various factor deficiencies (140), in patients who are therapeutically anticoagulated with heparin or low-molecular weight heparin, and most commonly with severe preeclampsia and the HELLP syndrome (hemolysis, elevated liver enzymes, and low platelet count). The major specific anesthetic concern in these disorders is the risk of spinal-epidural hematoma after spinal or epidural anesthesia or analgesia.

Severe coagulopathy is a contraindication to spinal or epidural anesthesia. What constitutes severe coagulopathy is, however, a subject that is much in debate. Usually, the degree of impairment is unclear, and the anesthesiologist must weigh the risks and benefits of regional versus general anesthesia or epidural versus other labor analgesia in patients with clinical or laboratory coagulation abnormalities (145). The prothrombin time, activated partial thromboplastin time, and platelet counts are the most commonly performed tests before the performance of regional anesthesia. Although much has been written about how to assess the risk of bleeding in the neuraxis after anesthetic procedures, little is known (140). Recommendations for minimum platelet counts have ranged from 150,000/ mm^3 in the 1970's and 1980's to 75,000 to 100,000 now (140,146,147). The bleeding time, which was used in the past to assess platelet function, is no longer thought to be helpful (148,149). Although no absolute consensus and little solid evidence have been found, most anesthesiologists will perform regional anesthesia in patients with isolated laboratory abnormalities of the coagulation system, with no clinical evidence or history of bleeding and a stable platelet count of 80,000 to 100,000/mm^3. Healthy parturients with isolated gestational thrombocytopenia can be considered for regional anesthesia. Beilin and colleagues found no documentation of any neurologic complications from 30 parturients with platelet counts below 100,000/mm^3 who had received epidural anesthetics (147). Few published case reports of epidural hematomas in pregnant women have appeared, and none when any coagulopathy was or could have been identified (150–152). A large number and variety of pregnant women have been treated with aspirin for prevention or treatment of preeclampsia or other pregnancy complications, and such treatment alone does not appear to be a risk factor for the development of an epidural hematoma (153–156).

Clinical judgment is the most important tool in assessing the risks and in deciding the safest anesthetic for each individual patient. In a preeclamptic patient with severe airway edema, a difficult airway for intubation, a stable platelet count of about 100,000/mm^3, and no evidence of clinical coagulopathy, the morbidity and mortality risks of general anesthesia are probably much greater than the risk of epidural hematoma. Nevertheless, an extensive discussion with the patient about the risks and benefits should occur before the procedure. Using the minimally effective doses for analgesia or anesthesia, spinal or epidural routes may make diagnosis of a spinal–epidural hematoma more rapid and likely. Severe back pain, the development of bowel or bladder incontinence, recurrence of motor or sensory block with no additional medication, or an abnormally prolonged effect of the anesthetic all suggest the need for further evaluation using computed tomography or, preferably, magnetic resonance imaging. If necessary, decompressive laminectomy may restore or preserve neurologic function. The timing of any anesthetic or surgical procedures may be critical. If pharmacologic anticoagulation with heparin or low-molecular-weight heparin has occurred, reversal and normalization of coagulation with protamine, time, or both may be appropriate. Specific factor assays may be performed for coagulation disorders to assess adequate levels and govern appropriate therapies.

REFERENCES

1. Brodsky JB, Cohen EN, Brown BW Jr, Wu ML, Whitcher C. Surgery during pregnancy and fetal outcome. Am J Obstet Gynecol 1980;138: 1165–1167.
2. Cohen EN, Bellville JW, Brown BW Jr. Anesthesia, pregnancy, and miscarriage: a study of operating room nurses and anesthetists. Anesthesiology 1971;35:343–347.
3. Manley S, de Kelaita G, Joseph NJ, Salem MR, Heyman HJ. Preoperative pregnancy testing in ambulatory surgery: incidence and impact of positive results. Anesthesiology 1995;83:690–693.
4. Mazze RI, Källén B. Reproductive outcome after anesthesia and operation during pregnancy: a registry of 5405 cases. Am J Obstet Gynecol 1989;161:1178–1185.
5. Anonymous. Classification of physical status. Anesthesiology 1963; 24:111.
6. Barron WM. The pregnant surgical patient : medical evaluation and management. Ann Intern Med 1984;101:683–691.
7. Barron WM. Medical evaluation of the pregnant patient requiring nonobstetric surgery. Clin Perinatol 1985;12:481–496.
8. Cohen SE. Nonobstetric surgery during pregnancy. In: Chestnut DH, ed. Obstetric anesthesia: principles and practice. St Louis: Mosby-Year Book, 1994:273–293.
9. Lund CJ, Donovan JC. Blood volume during pregnancy. Significance of plasma and red cell volumes. Am J Obstet Gynecol 1967;98: 393–403.
10. Finster M. Surgical anaesthesia for the pregnant patient. Can J Anaesth 1988;35:S14–S17.
11. Gianopoulos JG. Establishing the criteria for anesthesia and other precautions for surgery during pregnancy. Surg Clin North Am 1995; 75:33–45.
12. Steinberg ES, Santos AC. Surgical anesthesia during pregnancy. Int Anesthesiol Clin 1990;28:58–66.
13. Weissman DB, Ehrenwerth J. Prolonged neuromuscular blockade in a parturient associated with succinylcholine. Anesth Analg 1983;62: 444–446.
14. Leighton BL, Cheek TG, Gross JB, et al. Succinylcholine pharmacodynamics in peripartum patients. Anesthesiology 1986;64:202–205.
15. Kuhnert BR, Philipson EH, Pimental R, Kuhnert PM. A prolonged chloroprocaine epidural block in a postpartum patient with abnormal pseudocholinesterase. Anesthesiology 1982;56:477–478.
16. Jatlow P, Barash PG, VanDyke C, Radding J, Byck R. Cocaine and succinylcholine sensitivity: a new caution. Anesth Analg 1979;58: 235–238.
17. Conklin KA. Physiologic changes of pregnancy. In: Chestnut DH, ed. Obstetric anesthesia: principles and practice. St Louis: Mosby-Year Book, Inc., 1994:17–42.
18. Capeless EL, Clapp JF. Cardiovascular changes in early phase of pregnancy. Am J Obstet Gynecol 1989;161:1449–1453.
19. Pritchard JA, Rowland RC. Blood volume changes in pregnancy and the puerperium. Am J Obstet Gynecol 1964;88:391–395.
20. Hamilton HFH. The cardiac output in normal pregnancy. J Obstet Gynaecol Br Commonw 1949;56:548–552.
21. Kerr MG, Scott DB, Samuel E. Studies of the inferior vena cava in late pregnancy. BMJ 1964;1:532–533.
22. Mone SM, Sanders SP, Colan SD. Control mechanisms for physiological hypertrophy of pregnancy. Circulation 1996;94:667–672.
23. Pedersen H, Finster M. Anesthetic risk in the pregnant surgical patient. Anesthesiology 1979;51:439–451.
24. Eisenach JC, Tuttle R, Stein A. Is ST segment depression of the electrocardiogram during cesarean section merely due to cardiac sympathetic block? Anesth Analg 1994;78:287–292.
25. Palmer CM, Norris MC, Giudici MC, Leighton BL, DeSimone CA. Incidence of electrocardiographic changes during cesarean delivery under regional anesthesia. Anesth Analg 1990;70:36-43.
26. Zakowski MI, Ramanathan S, Baratta JB, et al. Electrocardiographic changes during cesarean section: a cause for concern? Anesth Analg 1993;76:162–167.
27. Archer GWJ. Arterial oxygen tension during apnoea in parturient women. Br J Anaesth 1974;46:358–360.
28. Cheek TG, Gutsche BB. Maternal physiologic alterations during pregnancy. In: Shnider SM, Levinson G, eds. Anesthesia for obstetrics. 3rd ed. Baltimore, MD: Williams & Wilkins, 1993:3–17.
29. Rasmussen GE, Malinow AM. Toward reducing maternal mortality: the problem airway in obstetrics. Int Anesthesiol Clin 1994;32:83–101.
30. Glassenberg R. General anesthesia and maternal mortality. Semin Perinatol 1991;15:386–396.
31. Attia RR, Ebeid AM, Fischer JE, Goudsouzian NG. Maternal fetal and placental gastrin concentrations. Anaesthesia 1982;37:18–21.
32. Roberts RB, Shirley MA. The obstetrician's role in reducing the risk of aspiration pneumonitis: with particular reference to the use of oral antacids. Am J Obstet Gynecol 1976;124:611–617.
33. Roberts RB, Shirley MA. Reducing the risk of acid aspiration during cesarean section. Anesth Analg 1974;53:859–868.
34. Levy DM, Williams OA, Magides AD, Reilly CS. Gastric emptying is delayed at 8-12 weeks gestation. Br J Anaesth 1994;73:237–238.
35. Simpson KH, Stakes AF, Miller M. Pregnancy delays paracetamol absorption and gastric emptying in patients undergoing surgery. Br J Anaesth 1988;60:24–27.
36. Whitehead EM, Smith M, Dean Y, O'Sullivan G. An evaluation of

gastric emptying times in pregnancy and the puerperium. Anaesthesia 1993;48:53–57.
37. Dodds WJ, Dent J, Hogan W. Pregnancy and the lower esophageal sphincter. Gastroenterology 1978;74:1334–1336.
38. Macfie AG, Magides AD, Richmond MN, Reilly CS. Gastric emptying in pregnancy. Br J Anaesth 1991;67:54–57.
39. O Sullivan GM, Sutton AJ, Thompson SA, Carrie LE, Bullingham RE. Noninvasive measurement of gastric emptying in obstetric patients. Anesth Analg 1987;66:505–511.
40. Davison JS, Davison MC, Hay DM. Gastric emptying time in late pregnancy and labour. J Obstet Gynaecol Br CommonW 1970;77: 37–41.
41. Palahniuk RJ, Shnider SM, Eger EI II. Pregnancy decreases the requirement for inhaled anesthetic agents. Anesthesiology 1974; 41:82–83.
42. Lyrenas S, Nyberg F, Lindberg BO, Terenius L. Cerebrospinal fluid activity of dynorphin-converting enzyme at term pregnancy. Obstet Gynecol 1988;72:54–58.
43. Datta S, Hurley RJ, Naulty JS, et al. Plasma and cerebrospinal fluid progesterone concentrations in pregnant and nonpregnant women. Anesth Analg 1986;65:950–954.
44. Datta S, Lambert DH, Gregus J, Gissen AJ, Covino BG. Differential sensitivities of mammalian nerve fibers during pregnancy. Anesth Analg 1983;62:1070–1072.
45. Sayers MH, McArthur J, McDonald JS. The hematology of pregnancy. In: Bonica JJ, McDonald JS, eds. Principles and practice of obstetric analgesia and anesthesia. 2nd ed. Baltimore: Williams & Wilkins, 1995:1096–1119.
46. Davison JM, Dunlop W. Renal hemodynamics and tubular function in normal human pregnancy. Kidney Int 1980;18:152–161.
47. Delaney AG. Anesthesia in the pregnant woman. Clin Obstet Gynecol 1983;26:795–800.
48. Tuchmann-Duplessis H. The effects of teratogenic drugs. In: Phillipp EE, Barnes J, Newton M, eds. Scientific foundations of obstetrics and gynaecology. Philadelphia: FA Davis, 1970:636–648.
49. Anonymous. Physicians desk reference. 48th ed. Montvale, NJ: Medical Economics Data, 1994:2888.
50. Vincent RD. Anesthesia for the pregnant patient. Clin Obstet Gynecol 1994;37:256–273.
51. Fuginaga M,Stevenson JB, Mazze RI. Reproductive and teratogenic effects of fentanyl in Sprague-Dawley rats. Teratology 1986;34:51–57.
52. Johnson ES, Colley PS. Effects of nitrous oxide and fentanyl anesthesia on fetal heart-rate variability intra- and postoperatively. Anesthesiology 1980;52:429–430.
53. Fuginaga M, Mazze RI, Jackson EC, Baden JM. Reproductive and teratogenic effects of sufentanil and alfentanil in Sprague-Dawley rats. Anesth Analg 1988;67:166–169.
54. Bracken MB, Holford TR. Exposure to prescibed drugs in pregnancy and association with congenital malformations. Obstet Gynecol 1981; 58:336–344.
55. Rosenberg L, Mitchell AA, Parsells JL, Pashayan H, Louik C, Shapiro S. Lack of relation of oral clefts to diazepam use during pregnancy. N Engl J Med 1983;309:1282–1285.
56. Shiono PH, Mills JL. Oral clefts and diazepam use during pregnancy. N Engl J Med 1984;311:919–920.
57. Laegreid L, Hagberg G, Lundberg A. Neurodevelopment in late pregnancy after prenatal exposure to benzodiazepines—a prospective study. Neuropediatrics 1992;23:60–67.
58. Schläppi B. Safety aspects of midazolam. Br J Clin Pharmacol 1983; 16(Suppl 1):37S–41S.
59. Samsoon GLT, Young JRB. Difficult tracheal intubation: a retrospective study. Anaesthesia 1987;42:487–490.
60. Sepkoski CM, Lester BM, Ostheimer GW, Brazelton TB. The effects of maternal epidural anesthesia on the neonatal behavior during the first month. Dev Med Child Neurol 1992;34:1072–1080.
61. Scanlon JW, Brown WU, Weiss JB, Alper MH. Neurobehavioral response of newborn infants after maternal epidural anesthesia. Anesthesiology 1974;40:121–128.
62. Santos AC, Pedersen H, Harmon TW, Morishima HO, Finster M, Arthur GR, Covino BG. Does pregnancy alter the systemic toxicity of local anesthetics? Anesthesiology 1989;70:991–995.
63. Santos AC, Arthur GR, Wlody D, De Armas P, Morishima HO, Finster M. Comparative systemic toxicity of ropivacaine and bupivacaine in nonpregnant and pregnant ewes. Anesthesiology 1995;82:734–740.
64. Puhringer FK, Sparr HJ, Mitterschiffthaler G, Agoston S, Benzer A. Extended duration of action of rocuronium in postpartum patients. Anesth Analg 1997;84:352–354.
65. Fujinaga M, Baden JM, Yhap EO, Mazze RI. Reproductive and teratogenic effects of nitrous oxide, isoflurane, and their combination in Sprague-Dawley rats. Anesthesiology 1987;67:960–964.
66. Baden JM, Serra M, Mazze RI. Inhibition of fetal methionine synthase by nitrous oxide. Br J Anaesth 1984;56:523–526.
67. Baden JM, Rice SA, Serra M, Kelley M, Mazze R. Thymidine and methionine synthesis in pregnant rats exposed to nitrous oxide. Anesth Analg 1983;62:738–741.
68. Crawford JS, Lewis M. Nitrous oxide in early human pregnancy. Anaesthesia 1986;41:900–905.
69. Riggs KW, Rurak DW, Taylor SM, McErlane BA, McMorland GH, Axelson JE. Fetal and maternal placental and nonplacental clearances of metoclopramide in chronically instrumented pregnant sheep. J Pharm Sci 1990;79:1056–1061.
70. Lewis JH, Weingold AB, Committee on FDA-Related Matters, American College of Gastroenterology. The use of gastrointestinal drugs during pregnancy and lactation. Am J Gastroenterol 1985;80:912–923.
71. Smith BE. Fetal prognosis after anesthesia during gestation. Anesth Analg 1963;42:521–526.
72. Shnider SM, Webster GM. Maternal and fetal hazards of surgery during pregnancy. Am J Obstet Gynecol 1965;92:891–900.
73. Babler EA. Perforative appendicitis complicating pregnancy. J Amer Med Assn 1908;51:1310–1314.
74. Duncan PG, Pope WDB, Cohen MM, Greer N. Fetal risk of anesthesia and surgery during pregnancy. Anesthesiology 1986;64:790–794.
75. Hawkins JL, Koonin LM, Palmer SK, Gibbs CP. Anesthesia-related deaths during obstetric delivery in the United States, 1979–1990. Anesthesiology 1997;86:277–284.
76. Levinson G, Shnider SM, deLorimier AA, Steffenson JL. Effects of maternal hyperventilation on uterine blood flow and fetal oxygenation and acid-base status. Anesthesiology 1974;40:340–347.
77. Grocott HP, Mutch WAC. Epidural anesthesia and acutely increased intracranial pressure: lumbar epidural space hydrodynamics in a porcine model. Anesthesiology 1996;85:1086–1091.
78. Stånge K, Halldin M. Hypothermia in pregnancy. Anesthesiology 1983;58:460–461.
79. Pomini F, Mercogliano D, Cavalletti C, Caruso A, Pomini P. Cardiopulmonary bypass in pregnancy. Ann Thorac Surg 1996;61:259–268.
80. Parry AJ, Westaby S. Cardiopulmonary bypass during pregnancy. Ann Thorac Surg 1996;61:1865–1869.
81. Sullivan HJ. Valvular heart surgery during pregnancy. Surg Clin NA 1995;75:59–75.
82. Johnson MD, Saltzman DH. Cardiac disease. In: Datta S, ed. Anesthetic and obstetric management of high-risk pregnancy. 2nd ed. St. Louis: Mosby-Year Book, 1996:200–245.
83. Khandelwal M, Rasanen J, Ludormirski A, Addonizio P, Reece EA. Evaluation of fetal and uterine hemodynamics during maternal cardiopulmonary bypass. Obstet Gynecol 1996;88:667–671.
84. Chambers CE, Clark SL. Cardiac surgery during pregnancy. Clin Obstet Gynecol 1994;37:316–323.
85. Abdalla MY, Mostafa EED. Contraception after heart surgery. Contraception 1992;45:73–80.
86. Bhagwat AR, Engel PJ. Heart disease and pregnancy. Cardiol Clin 1995;13:163–178.
87. Hess DB, Hess LW. Management of cardiovascular disease in pregnancy. Obstet Gynecol Clin North Am 1992;19:679–695.
88. Sciscione AC, Callan NA. Pregnancy and contraception. Cardiol Clin 1993;11:701–709.
89. Ridley DM, Smiley RM. The parturient with cardiac disease. Anesthesiol Clin North Am 1998;16:419–440.
90. Page RL. Treatment of arrhythmias during pregnancy. Am Heart J 1995;130:871–876.
91. Anonymous. Cardiac disease in pregnancy. ACOG Technical Bulletin Number 168. Int J Gynecol Obstet 1993;41:298–306.
92. Anonymous. Guidelines for cardiopulmonary resuscitation and emergency cardiac care. Part IV. Special resuscitation situations. JAMA 1992;268:2242–2250.
93. Goodwin APL, Pearce AJ. The human wedge. Anaesthesia 1992;47: 433–434.
94. Lindsay SL, Hanson GC. Cardiac arrest in near-term pregnancy. Anaesthesia 1987;42:1074–1077.

95. Lopez-Zeno JA, Carlo WA, O'Grady JP, Fanaroff AA. Infant survival following delayed portmortem cesarean delivery. Obstet Gynecol 1990;76:991–992.
96. Katz VL, Dotters DJ, Droegemueller W. Perimortem cesarean delivery. Obstet Gynecol 1986;68:571–576.
97. Colclough GW, Ackerman WE, Walmsley PM, Hessel EA. Epidural anesthesia for a parturient with critical aortic stenosis. J Clin Anesth 1995;7:264–265.
98. Brian JE Jr, Seifen AB, Clark RB, Robertson DM, Quirk JG. Aortic stenosis, cesarean delivery, and epidural anesthesia. J Clin Anesth 1993;5:154–157.
99. Campos O, Andrade JL, Bocanegra J, et al. Physiologic multivalvular regurgitation during pregnancy: a longitudinal Doppler echocardiographic study. Int J Cardiol 1993;40:265–272.
100. Bader AM. Neurologic and neuromuscular disease. In: Chestnut DH, ed. Obstetric anesthesia: principles and practice. St Louis: Mosby-Year Book, 1994:920–941.
101. Rolbin SH, Levinson G, Shnider SM, Wright RG. Anesthetic considerations for myasthenia gravis and pregnancy. Anesth Analg 1978;57: 441–447.
102. Plauche WC. Myasthenia gravis. Clin Obstet Gynecol 1983;26: 592–604.
103. Catanzarite VA, McHargue AM, Sandberg EC, Dyson DC. Respiratory arrest during therapy for premature labor in a patient with myasthenia gravis. Obstet Gynecol 1984;64:819–822.
104. Leventhal SR, Orkin FK, Hirsh RA. Prediction of the need for postoperative mechanical ventilation in myasthenia gravis. Anesthesiology 1980;53:26–30.
105. Davis RK, Maslow AS. Multiple sclerosis in pregnancy: a review. Obstet Gynecol Surv 1992;47:290–296.
106. Bader AM, Hunt CO, Datta S, Naulty JS, Ostheimer GW. Anesthesia for the obstetric patient with multiple sclerosis. J Clin Anesth 1988; 1:21–24.
107. Baskett PJF, Armstrong R. Anaesthetic problems in multiple sclerosis: are certain agents contraindicated? Anaesthesia 1970;25:397–401.
108. Bamford C, Sibley W, Laguna J. Anesthesia in multiple sclerosis. Can J Neurol Sci 1978;5:41–44.
109. Hughes SC. Anesthesia for the pregnant patient with neuromuscular disorders. In: Shnider SM, Levinson G, eds. Anesthesia for obstetrics. 3rd ed. Baltimore: Williams & Wilkins, 1993:563–580.
110. Stenuit J, Marchand P. Sequalae of spinal anesthesia. Acta Neurol Belg 1968;68:626–635.
111. Warren TM, Datta S, Ostheimer GW. Lumbar epidural anesthesia in a patient with multiple sclerosis. Anesth Analg 1982;61:1022–1023.
112. Rogala EJ, Drummond DS, Gurr J. Scoliosis: incidence and natural history. A prospective epidemiological study. J Bone Joint Surg Am 1978;60:173–176.
113. Lee Y-SJ, Bundschu RH, Moffat EC, Lambrecht-Mulier E, MacEwen GD. Unintentional subdural block during labor epidural in a parturient with prior Harrington rod insertion for scoliosis: case report. Reg Anesth 1995;20:159–162.
114. Betz RR, Bunnell WP, Lambrecht-Mulier E, MacEwen GD. Scoliosis and pregnancy. J Bone Joint Surg Am 1987;69:90–96.
115. Daley MD, Rolbin SH, Morningstar BA, Stewart JA. Epidural anesthesia for obstetrics after spinal surgery. Reg Anesth 1990;15: 280–284.
116. Crosby ET. Musculoskeletal disorders. In: Chestnut DH, ed. Obstetric anesthesia: principles and practice. St Louis: Mosby-Year Book, 1994:904–919.
117. Moran DH, Johnson MD. Continuous spinal anesthesia with combined hyperbaric and isobaric bupivacaine in a patient with scoliosis. Anesth Analg 1990;70:445–447.
118. Schachner SM, Abram SE. Use of two epidural catheters to provide analgesia of unblocked segments in a patient with lumbar disc disease. Anesthesiology 1982;56:150–151.
119. Greenspoon JS, Paul RH. Paraplegia and quadriplegia: special considerations during pregnancy and labor and delivery. Am J Obstet Gynecol 1986;155:738–741.
120. Eisler EA. Anesthesia for the pregnant patient with asthma. In: Shnider SM, Levinson G, eds. Anesthesia for obstetrics. 3rd ed. Baltimore: Williams & Wilkins, 1993:525–538.
121. Lindeman KS. Respiratory disease. In: Chestnut DH, ed. Obstetric anesthesia: principles and practice. St Louis: Mosby-Year Book, 1994: 967–981.
122. Turner ES, Greenberger PA, Patterson R. Management of the pregnant asthmatic patient. Ann Intern Med 1980;6:905–918.
123. Schatz M, Zeiger RS, Harden KM, et al. The safety of inhaled β-agonist bronchodilators during pregnancy. J Allergy Clin Immunol 1988; 82:686–695.
124. Pizov R, Brown RH, Weiss YS, et al. Wheezing during induction of general anesthesia in patients with and without asthma: a randomized, blinded trial. Anesthesiology 1995;82:1111–1116.
125. Buchanan TA. Glucose metabolism during pregnancy: normal physiology and implications for diabetes mellitus. Isr J Med Sci 1991;27: 432–441.
126. Kuhl C. Insulin secretion and insulin resistance in pregnancy and gestational diabetes mellitus: implications for diagnosis and management. Diabetes 1991;40(Suppl 2):18–24.
127. Wissler RN. Endocrine disorders. In: Chestnut DH, ed. Obstetric anesthesia: principles and practice. St Louis: Mosby-Year Book, 1994: 780–814.
128. Roizen MF. Diseases of the endocrine system. In: Benumof JL, ed. Anesthesia and uncommon diseases. 4th ed. Philadelphia: WB Saunders, 1998:223–273.
129. Page MM, Watkins PJ. Cardiorespiratory arrest and diabetic autonomic neuropathy. Lancet 1978;1:14–16.
130. Burgos LG, Ebert TJ, Asiddao C, et al. Increased intraoperative cardiovascular morbidity in diabetics with autonomic neuropathy. Anesthesiology 1989;70:591–597.
131. Nolan TE, Hess LW, Hess DB, Morrison JC. Severe medical illness complicating cesarean section. Obstet Gynecol Clin North Am 1988; 15:697–717.
132. Douglas MJ, Flanagan ML, McMorland GH. Anaesthetic management of a complex morbidly obese parturient. Can J Anaesth 1991;8: 900–903.
133. Abrams B, Parker J. Overweight and pregnancy complications. Int J Obes Relat Metab Disord 1988;12:293–303.
134. Oberg B, Poulsen TD. Obesity: an anaesthetic challenge. Acta Anaesthesiol Scand 1996;40:191–200.
135. Buckley FP, Robinson NB, Simonowitz DA, Dellinger EP. Anaesthesia in the morbidly obese: a comparison of anaesthetic and analgesic regimens for upper abdominal surgery. Anaesthesia 1983;38:840–851.
136. Hood DD, Dewan DM. Anesthetic and obstetric outcome in morbidly obese parturients. Anesthesiology 1993;79:1210–1218.
137. Dewan D. Obesity. In: Chestnut DH, ed. Obstetric anesthesia: principles and practice. St Louis: Mosby-Year Book, 1994:942–955.
138. Weinstein JA, Matteo RS, Ornstein E, Schwartz AE, Goldstoff M, Thal G. Pharmacodynamics of vecuronium and atracurium in the obese surgical patient. Anesth Analg 1988;67:1149–1153.
139. Vaughan RW, Wise L. Intraoperative arterial oxygenation in obese patients. Ann Surg 1976;184:35–42.
140. Lechner RB. Hematologic and coagulation disorders. In: Chestnut DH, ed. Obstetric anesthesia: principles and practice. St Louis: Mosby-Year Book, 1994:815–832.
141. Rust OA, Perry KG Jr. Pregnancy complicated by sickle hemoglobinopathy. Clin Obstet Gynecol 1995;38:472–484.
142. Perry KG, Morrison JC. The diagnosis and management of hemoglobinopathies during pregnancy. Semin Perinatol 1990;14:90–102.
143. Koshy M, Burd L, Wallace D, Moawad A, Baron J. Prophylactic red-cell transfusions in pregnant patients with sickle cell disease: a randomized cooperative study. N Engl J Med 1988;319:1447–1452.
144. Paidas MJ, Haut MJ, Lockwood CJ. Platelet disorders in pregnancy: implications for mother and fetus. Mt Sinai J Med 1994;61:389–403.
145. Sage DJ. Epidurals, spinals and bleeding disorders in pregnancy: a review. Anaesth Intens Care 1990;18:319–326.
146. Rasmus KT, Rottman RL, Kotelko DM, Wright WC, Stone JJ, Rosenblatt RM. Unrecognized thrombocytopenia and regional anesthesia in parturients: a retrospective review. Obstet Gynecol 1989;73:943–946.
147. Beilin Y, Zahn J, Comerford M. Safe epidural analgesia in thirty parturients with platelet count between 69000 and 98000. Anesth Analg 1997;85:385–388.
148. Rodgers RPC, Levin J. A critical reappraisal of the bleeding time. Semin Thromb Hemost 1990;16:1–20.
149. Petersen P, Hayes TE, Arkin CF, et al. The preoperative bleeding time test lacks clinical benefit. Arch Surg 1998;133:134–139.
150. Ballin NC. Paraplegia following epidural analgesia. Anaesthesia 1981;36:952–953.
151. Lao TT, Halpern SH, MacDonald D. Spinal subdural haematoma in a

parturient after attempted epidural anaesthesia. Can J Anaesth 1993; 40:340–345.

152. Roscoe MWA, Barrington TW. Acute spinal subdural hematoma: a case report and review of the literature. Spine 1984;9:672–675.
153. Crowther MA, Burrows RF, Ginsberg J, Kelton JG. Thrombocytopenia in pregnancy: diagnosis, pathogenesis and management. Blood Rev 1996;10:8–16.
154. Orlikowski CE, Payne AJ, Moodley J, Rocke DA. Thrombelastography after aspirin ingestion in pregnant and non-pregnant subjects. Br J Anaesth 1992;69:159–161.
155. Sibai BM, Caritis SN, Thom E, Shaw K, McNellis D. Low-dose aspirin in nulliparous women: safety of continuous epidural block and correlation between bleeding time and maternal–neonatal bleeding complications. Am J Obstet Gynecol 1995;172:1553–1557.
156. Williams HD, Howard R, O Donnell N, Findley I. The effect of low dose aspirin on bleeding times. Anaesthesia 1993;48:331–333.

Cherry and Merkatz's Complications of Pregnancy,
Fifth Edition, edited by W. R. Cohen
Lippincott Williams & Wilkins, Philadelphia © 2000

CHAPTER 56

Clinical Laboratory Referent Values

Deborah Bowers and Robert E. Wenk

Clinical laboratory referent values for pregnancy are the expected test values in a population of pregnant patients who have no complicating illness. Generally, a referent range refers to the central 95% of values derived from a sample of otherwise normal pregnant women. Each referent range depends on several variables. *Preanalytical* variables include the method of specimen collection; the presence and type of anticoagulant or preservative; the method and duration of specimen preservation; and the state of the patient with respect to age, race, heredity, environment (e.g., altitude), duration of pregnancy, use of drugs, and others. *Analytical* variables include the method, operator, calibrators and instrument (with their attendant accuracy and precision), the type of specimen (e.g., serum versus plasma), and the substances in the specimen that interfere with the results. Aside from the variables listed, human error (e.g., clerical) must be considered in a clinical interpretation of results. Although interpretation is usually straightforward, there are times when the obstetrician should call the laboratory for a consultation with a laboratory-based technologist, scientist, or physician for assistance.

The referent ranges of frequently requested tests are tabulated in this chapter. Discussions of abnormal values or changes in laboratory values are found in the various chapters dealing with specific disorders.

Ranges are noted in both mass concentration and substance concentrations (i.e., Systeme Internationale, or SI units) because some physicians, laboratories, and countries have chosen to use one or the other set of units. Referent ranges appear first in mass concentrations for nonpregnant women. Conversion factors are given so that mass and substance concentrations of individual patient results can be interconverted and interpreted. Mass concentration units are given for pregnancy and are stratified for each trimester when they could be documented as changing with the duration of the pregnancy. If the literature affirmed that no change in referent ranges is known to occur during pregnancy, that has been specifically noted in the table. A list of useful references is appended.

D. Bowers: Department of Obstetrics and Gynecology, and R. E. Wenk: Department of Pathology, Sinai Hospital of Baltimore, Baltimore, MD 21215.

BIBLIOGRAPHY

General Topics

Alosachie IJ, Lad PM. Laboratory diagnosis in hypertension. J Clin Lab Anal 1994;8:293–308.

Christie RW, Marallo T. Experiences with conversion to Systeme Internationale units. N Engl J Med 1990;323:1075–1077.

Conn RB. Scientific medicine and Systeme Internationale units. Arch Pathol Lab Med 1987;111:16–19.

Cruikshank DP, Hays PM. Obstetrics: normal and problem pregnancies. 2nd ed. New York: Churchill Livingstone, 1991.

Gordon JP, Rydfors JT, Druzin ML, Tadid Y. Obstetrics, gynecology and infertility. 4th ed. Menlo Park: Scrub Hill Press, 1995.

Hytten FE, Leitch I. The physiology of human pregnancy. 2nd ed. Oxford: Blackwell, 1971.

Hytten FE, Lind T. Diagnostic indices in pregnancy. 1st ed. Basel: Ciba-Geigy, 1975.

Laros RK Jr. Implications of metric conversion. Obstet Gynecol 1980;56:646.

Lehmann HP. Metrication of clinical laboratory data in SI units. Am J Clin Pathol 1976;65:2–18.

Lind T: Maternal physiology. 1st ed. Washington DC: Council on Resident Education in Obstetrics and Gynecology, 1985.

Sasse EA. Determination of reference intervals in the clinical laboratory using the proposed guideline National Committee for Clinical Laboratory Standards C28-P. Arch Pathol Lab Med 1992;116:710–713.

Wallach J. Interpretation of diagnostic tests: a synopsis of laboratory medicine, 5th ed. Boston: Little, Brown and Company, 1992.

Chemistry

Bermes EW, Young DS. Tietz textbook of clinical chemistry. 2nd ed. Philadelphia: WB Saunders, 1994.

Boutourline-Young H, Boutourline-Young E. Alveolar carbon dioxide levels in pregnant, parturient and lactating subjects. J Obstet Gynaecol Br Emp 1956;63:509–528.

Kampmann J, Siersbaek-Nielsen K, Kristensen M, Hanseen JM. Rapid evaluation of creatinine clearance. Acta Med Scand 1974;196:517–520.

Lockitch G. Clinical biochemistry of pregnancy. Crit Rev Clin Lab Sci 1997;34:67–139.

TABLE 56-1. *Hematologic system*

Examination	Specimen	Referent Range (mass units)	Conversion Factor (SIU)	Referent Range (SIU)
Whole blood volume		55–75 mL/kg	—	—
Plasma volume		28–45 mL/kg	—	—
Total erythrocyte count	Whole blood	3.5–5.0 × 10^6/mm^3	1	3.5–5.0 × 10^{12}/L
Hemoglobin electrophoresis	Whole blood			
Hemoglobin A		>95%	—	
Hemoglobin A2		1.5–3.0%	—	
Hemoglobin F		<2%	—	
Hemoglobinopathies		*Clinical severity*	*Hemoglobin*	
Hemoglobin AS, AC		No symptoms	Referent range	
Hemoglobin SS		Mod/sev	6–9 g/dL	
Hemoglobin SC		Mild/mod	9–14 g/dL	
Hemoglobin S/B thalassemia +		Mild/mod	8–13 g/dL	
Hemoglobin S/B thalassemia o		Mild/sev	7–10 g/dL	
Beta thalassemia minor		Mild	10–12 g/dL	
Beta thalassemia major		Mod/sev	>6.5 g/dL	
Hemoglobin H Disease		Mod	7–10 g/dL	
Complete blood count	Whole blood			
Hemoglobin		11.5–15.5 g/dL	10	115–155 g/L
Hematocrit		33–43%	0.01	0.33–0.43
Mean corpuscular hemoglobin		27–33 pg	1	27–33 pg
Mean corpuscular volume		82–92 m^3	1	82–92 fL
Red cell distribution width (RDW)		11.5–14.5%	0.01	0.115–0.145
Reticulocytes		0.1–2.4%	10	1–24 × 10^{-3}/L
Total white blood cell count		3,200–9,800/mm^3	0.001	3.2–9.8 × 10^9/L
Neutrophils		3,000–5,800/mm^3	(53–62%)	—
Lymphocytes		1,500–3,000/mm^3	(24–33%)	—
% T4		38.2–57.6%	—	—
Total T4		605–1,240/cu mm^3	—	—
% T8		19.5–35.3%	—	—
Total T8		360,652/mm^3	—	—
T4/T8 ratio		1.1–2.6	—	—
Monocytes		280–500/mm^3	(4.2–12.4%)	—
Eosinophils		50–250/mm^3	(0.1–4.5%)	
Basophils		15–50/mm^3	(0–2%)	—
Platelets		150–450 × 10^3/mm^3	1	150–450 × 10^9/L
Carboxyhemoglobin		<5%	—	—
Methemoglobin		<3%	—	—
Coagulation studies	Plasma			
Prothrombin time		10–14 sec	—	—
Activated partial thromboplastin time		25–38 sec	—	—
Fibrin degradation products		0–10μg/mL	—	—
Fibrinogen		200–400 mg/dL	0.01	2.0–4.0 g/L
Bleeding time: Mielke modification		4.0–7.0 min	—	—
Clotting factors		values reported as % of normal		
Factor II (Prothrombin)		60–140%		0.60–1.40
Factor V		60–140%		0.60–1.40
Factor VII		70–130%		0.70–1.30
Factor VIII		50–200%		0.50–2.00
Factor IX		60–140%		0.60–1.40
Factor X (Stuart)		70–130%		0.70–1.30
Factor XI		60–140%		0.60–1.40
Factor XII (Hageman)		60–140%		0.60–1.40
Factor XIII		50–200%		0.50–2.00
Antithrombin III		—	—	—
Immunologic		21–30 mg/dL	10	210–300 mg/L
Functional		80–120%	0.01	0.8–1.2
Ferritin		20–120 ng/mL	1	20–120 μg/mL
Transferrin		240–480 mg/dL	0.01	2.4–4.8 g/L
Serum iron	Serum	60–160 μg/mL	0.1791	11–29 μmol/L
Iron binding capacity	Serum	250–460 μg/dL	0.1791	45–82 μmol/L
% Saturation		20%–50%	—	—
Vitamin B12	Serum	200–1,100 pg/mL	—	—
Folic acid	Serum	2.0–20.0 ng/mL	—	—
Sedimentation rate				
Wintrobe	Whole blood	0–15 mm/hr	1	0–15 mm/hr
Westergren	Whole blood	0–30 mm/hr	1	0–30 mm/hr

TABLE 56-1. *Continued.*

Examination	1st Trimester	2nd Trimester	3rd Trimester
Whole blood volume	77–81	84–93	94–99
Plasma volume	52–54	57–66	67–72
Total erythrocyte count	4.2–4.4	4.1–4.4	3.7–4.3
Hemoglobin **(Hgb)** ***Electrophoresis***			
Hgb A 55–60%	Hgb S or C 38–45%	Hgb A_2 1–3%	—
Hgb S 80–90%	Hgb F 2–20%	Hgb A_2 <3.6%	—
Hgb S 45–55%	Hgb C 45–55%	Hgb F <8%	—
Hgb S 55–75%	Hgb A 15–30%	Hgb F 1–20%	Hgb A_2 >3.6%
Hgb S 50–85%	Hgb F 2–30%	Hgb A_2 >3.6%	—
Hgb A 85–90%	Hgb A_2 3.5–7.5%	Hgb F 2–10%	—
Hgb F 90%	Hgb A_2 3–11%	—	—
Hgb A 60–80%	Hgb H 20–40%	—	—
Complete blood count			
Hemoglobin	11.5–12.7	10.5–12.5	10.9–13.5
Hematocrit	34.5–38.3	31.5–37.5	32.7–36
Mean corpuscular hemoglobin	29.3	—	28.8–30.3
Mean corpuscular volume	86	89–90	89–91
Red cell distribution width (RDW)	*Does not change in pregnancy*		
Reticulocytes	*Does not change in pregnancy*		
Total white blood cell count	5,100–9,900	5,400–11,400	5,600–12,200
Neutrophils	3,500–7,700	3,800–8,400	3,700–9,000
Lymphocytes	1,100–2,300	1,100–2,600	1,100–2,600
% T4	—	39.4–42.6%	39.8–41.8%
Total T4	—	788–1065	800–1040
% T8	—	25.4–27.8	25.9–27.9
Total T8	—	508–695	515–695
T4/T8 ratio	—	1.4–1.7	1.4–1.6
Monocytes	250–500	220–650	230–820
Eosinophils	70–800	70–870	40–70
Basophils	15–80	15–80	15–80
Platelets	253–397	243–353	203–353
Carboxyhemoglobin	—	—	—
Methemoglobin	—	—	—
Coagulation studies			
Prothrombin time	*Does not change in pregnancy*		
Activated partial thromboplastin time	*Does not change in pregnancy*		
Fibrin degradation products	4.0–9.2	4.1–12.3	7.1–20.9
Fibrinogen	200–286	286–415	250–500
Bleeding time: Mielke modification	*Does not change in pregnancy*		
Clotting factors			
Factor II (Prothrombin)	*Does not change in pregnancy*		
Factor V	*Elevated immediately postpartum*		
Factor VII	—	*increased up to ten fold*	*Increased up to ten fold*
Factor VIII	—	87–90	200
Factor IX	*Increased throughout pregnancy*		
Factor X (Stuart)	—	—	150–210
Factor XI	—	20	50–100
Factor XII (Hageman)	—	20–27	33
Factor XIII	—	—	35–75
Antithrombin III			
Immunologic	—	27–29	44–51
Functional	—	—	—
Ferritin	58–136.8	7.6–36.8	7.0–21.7
Transferrin	194.6–293.3	264.2–408.8	307.4–418.2
Serum iron	84–130	38.5–112.1	25–87
Iron binding capacity	358	—	—
% Saturation	33%	—	—
Vitamin B12	267–420	260–360	190–310
Folic acid	5.8–6.8	4.8–5.8	3.9–4.7
Sedimentation rate			
Wintrobe	*Increased throughout pregnancy*		
Westergren	*Increased throughout pregnancy*		

TABLE 56-2. *Chemical analyses*

Examination	Specimen	Referent range	Conversion factor (SIU)	Referent range (SIU)
Sodium	Serum	135–147 mEq/L	1	135–147 mmol/L
Potassium	Serum	3.5–5.0 mEq/L	1	3.5–5.0 mmol/L
Chloride	Serum	95–105 mEq/L	1	95–105 mmol/L
Bicarbonate	Serum	22–28 mEq/L	1	22–28 mmol/L
Calcium	Serum	8.8–10.0 mg/dL	0.2495	2.2–2.5 mmol/L
Ionized calcium	Serum	4.60–5.40 mg/dL	0.2495	1.15–1.35 mmol/L
Magnesium	Serum	1.8–3.0 mg/dL	0.4114	0.8–1.2 mmol/L
Phosphorus	Serum	2.5–5.0 mg/dL	0.3229	0.8–1.6 mmol/L
Serum urea nitrogen	Serum	8–18 mg/dL	0.357	3.0–6.5 mmol/L
Creatinine	Serum	0.6–1.2 mg/dL	88.4	50–110 mmol/L
Creatinine clearance	Serum, urine	75–125 mL/min	0.01667	1.24–2.08 mL/sec
Glucose	Plasma			
Fasting		70–110 mg/dL	0.05551	3.9–6.1 mmol/L
1 Hr/50g load		—	—	—
Hemoglobin A_1C	Plasma	4.4–6.4%	—	—
Alanine aminotransferase	Serum	0–35 U/L	1	0–35 U/L
Aspartate aminotransferase	Serum	0–35 U/L	1	0–35 U/L
Gamma-glutamyltransferase	Serum	0–30 U/L	1	0–30 U/L
Amylase	Serum	0–130 U/L	1	0–130 U/L
Lipase	Serum	30–190 U/L	1	30–190 U/L
Lactic dehydrogenase	Serum	340–670 U/L	1	340–670 U/L
Alkaline phosphatase	Serum	30–120 U/L	1	30–120 U/L
Uric acid	Serum	2.0–7.0 mg/dL	59.48	120–420 µmol/L
Bilirubin (total)	Serum	0.1–1.0 mg/dL	17.1	2–18 µmol/L
Bilirubin (conjugated)	Serum	0–0.2 mg/dL	17.1	0–4 µmol/L
Albumin	Serum	4.0–6.0 g/dL	10	40–60 g/dL
Total protein	Serum	6.0–8.0 g/dL	10	60–80 g/L
Cholesterol	Plasma	140–200 mg/dL	0.02586	3.62–5.20 mmol/L
High-density lipoproteins		33–80 mg/dL	0.02586	0.85–2.06 mmol/L
Low density lipoproteins		50–190 mg/dL	0.02586	1.29–4.91 mmol/L
Triglycerides		85–125 mg/dL	0.02586	2.2–3.2 mmol/L
Acetone	Serum	0.3–2.0 mg/dL	—	—
Ketones	Serum	Negative	—	—
Beta-hydroxybutyric acid	Serum	0.05–0.15 mmol/L	—	—
pH	Whole blood	7.35–7.45	—	—
$PaCO_2$		32–45 mm Hg	0.1333	>11.3 kPa
PaO_2		>85 mm Hg	0.1333	>11.3 kPa

Pitkin RM, Gebhardt MP. Serum calcium concentrations in human pregnancy. Am J Obstet Gynecol 1977;127:775–778.

Propp DA, Weber D, Ciesla ML. Reliability of urine dipsticks in emergency department patients. Ann Emerg Med 1989;18:560–563.

Simms EA, Krantz KE. Serial studies of renal function during pregnancy and the puerperium in normal women. J Clin Invest 1958;37:1764–1774.

Endocrine

Bishnoi A, Sachmechi I. Thyroid disease during pregnancy. Am Fam Physician 1996;53:215–220.

Buster JE, Chang J, Preston DL, et al. Interrelationships of circulating maternal steroid concentrations in third trimester pregnancies. II. C18 and C19 steroids: estradiol, estriol, dehydroepiandrosterone, dehydroepiandrosterone sulfate, delta 5-androstenediol, delta4-androstenedione, testosterone, and dihydrotestosterone. J Clin Endocrinol Metab 1979;48: 139–142.

Coustan DR. Screening and diagnosis of gestational diabetes. Semin Perinatol 1994;18:407–413.

Felig P, Lynch V. Starvation in human pregnancy: hypoglycemia, hypoinsulinemia and hyperketonemia. Science 1970;170:990–993.

Glinoer D, de Nayer P, Bourdoux P, et al. Regulation of maternal thyroid during pregnancy. J Clin Endocrinol Metab 1990;71:276–287.

Harada A, Hershman JM, Reed AW, et al. Comparision of thyroid stimulators and thyroid hormone concentrations in sera of pregnant women. J Clin Endocrinol Metab 1979;48:793–797.

Montoro MN. Management of hypothyroidism during pregnancy. Clin Obstet Gynecol 1997;40:65–80.

Olive D. The range of normal. Semin Reprod Endocrinol 1996;14:119–123.

Smikle CB, Sorem KA, Wians FH, Hankins GD. Measuring quantitative serum human chorionic gonadotropin variations in levels between kits. J Reprod Med 1995;40:439–442.

Hematology

Burns DN, Nourjah P, Minkoff H, et al. Changes in CD4-and CD8- cell levels during pregnancy and post partum in women seropositive and seronegative for immunodeficiency virus-1. Am J Obstet Gynecol 1996;174:1461–1468.

TABLE 56-2. *Continued.*

Examination	1st Trimester	2nd Trimester	3rd Trimester
Sodium	135–146	131–144	133–143
Potassium	3.2–5.2	3.2–4.7	3.2–4.5
Chloride	99–107	96–108	92–97
Bicarbonate	18–27	17–26.5	17.5–25
Calcium	9.71–10/29	9.15–8.77	8.95–9.22
Ionized calcium	*Does not change in pregnancy*		
Magnesium	1.3–2.2	1.1–1.9	1.1–1.8
Phosphorus	2.2–4.0	1.9–4.1	2.0–4.0
Serum urea nitrogen	2–5	2–5	2–6
Creatinine	0.3–0.7	0.3–0.7	0.5–0.6
Creatinine clearance	132–166	134–170	118–182
Glucose	—	—	—
Fasting	—	65–95	60–80
Challenge test (50g load, 1-hour)			<140mg/dL
Fasting	<105 mg/dL	0.05551	<5.83 mmol/L
60 min	<190 mg/dL	0.05551	<10.55 mmol/L
120 min	<165 mg/dL	0.05551	<9.16 mmol/L
180 min	<145 mg/dL	0.05551	<8.05 mmol/L
Hemoglobin A_1C	*Does not change in pregnancy*		
Alanine aminotransferase	*Does not change in pregnancy*		
Aspartate aminotransferase	*Does not change in pregnancy*		
Gamma-glutamyltransferase	*Does not change in pregnancy*		
Amylase	*Does not change in pregnancy*		
Lipase	35.3–44.5	—	15.5–21.7
Lactic dehydrogenase	220–500	250–520	220–620
Alkaline Phosphatase	20–110	30–130	120–320
Uric acid	2.4–3.6	2.6–3.8	2.5–5.9
Bilirubin (total)	*Does not change in pregnancy*		
Bilirubin (conjugated)	*Does not change in pregnancy*		
Albumin	3.1–4.9	2.6–4.3	2.3–4.2
Total protein	6.5–7.3	5.6–7.0	5.9–7.2
Cholesterol	110–250	145–295	168–256
High-density lipoproteins	48–90	48–97	48–97
Low-density lipoproteins	—	—	78–260
Triglycerides	25–90	70–200	130–415
Acetone	—	—	—
Ketones	*Does not change in pregnancy*		
Beta-hydroxybutyric acid	—	0.33–0.41	0.07–0.11
pH	—	7.40–7.44	7.40–7.44
$PaCO_2$	—	27–32	28–30
PaO_2	—	92–104	104–108

Burns ER, Lawrence C. Bleeding time: a guide to its diagnostic and clinical utility. Arch Pathol Lab Med 1989;113:1219–1224.

Henderson AH, Pugsley DS, Thomas DP. Fibrin degradation products in preeclamptic toxaemia and eclampsia. BMJ 1970;3:545–547.

Jackson SR, Carter JM. Platelet volume: laboratory measurement and clinical application. Blood Reviews 1993;7:104–113.

Kaneshige E. Serum ferritin as an assessment of iron stores and other hematologic parameters during pregnancy. Obstet Gynecol 1981;57:238–242.

Laros RK, Alger LS. Thromboembolism and pregnancy. Clin Obstet Gynecol 1979;22:871–888.

Lusher JM. Screening and diagnosis of coagulation disorders. Am J Obstet Gynecol 1996;175:778–783.

Macik BG, Ortel TL. Clinical and laboratory evaluation of the hypercoaguable states. Clin Chest Med 1995;16:375–387.

Magann EF, Martin JN Jr. The laboratory evaluation of hypertensive gravidas. Obstet Gynecol Surv 1995;50:138–145.

Mani S, Duffy TP. Anemia in pregnancy. Clin Perinatol 1995;22:593–607.

Mitchell GW Jr, McRipley RJ, Selvaraj RJ, Sbarra AJ. The role of the phagocyte in host-parasite interactions. IV. The phagocytic activity of leukocytes in pregnancy and its relationship to urinary tract infection. Am J Obstet Gynecol 1966;96:687–697.

Pitkin RM, Witte DL. Platelet and leukocyte counts in pregnancy. JAMA 1979;242:2696–2698.

Romslo I, Haram K, Sagen N, Augensen K. Iron requirement in normal pregnancy as assessed by serum ferritin, serum transferrin saturation, and erythrocyte protoporphyrin determinations. Br J Obstet Gynaecol 1983;90:101–107.

Scott DE. Anemia during pregnancy. Obstet Gynecol Ann 1972;1:219.

Temmerman M, Nagelkerke N, Bwayo J, Chomba EN, Piot P. HIV-1 and immunological changes during pregnancy: a comparison between HIV-1 seropositive and HIV-1 seronegative women in Nairobi, Kenya. AIDS 1995;9:1057–1060.

US Department of Health,CDC criteria for anemia in children and childbearing-aged women. MMWR Morb Mortal Wkly Rep 1989;38:400–407.

Waye JS, Eng B, Cai S, et al. Carrier detection and prenatal diagnosis of hemoglobinopathies in Ontario. Clin Invest Med 1993;16:358–371.

Woodfield DG, Cole SK, Allan AG, Cash JP. Serum fibrin degradation products throughout normal pregnancy. BMJ 1968;4:665–668.

TABLE 56-3. *Endocrine system*

Examination	Specimen	Referent range	Conversion factor (SIU)	Referent range (SIU)
Pituitary	Serum			
Prolactin		0–23 ng/mL	20	20–460 mIU/L
Follicle-stimulating hormone (FSH)				
Follicular phase		2.0–15.0 mIU/L	1	2.0–15.0 IU/L
FSH midcycle peak		20–50 mIU/L	1	20–50 IU/L
Luteinizing hormone				
Follicular phase		<30 mIU/L	1	<30 IU/L
LH mid-cycle peak		30–150 mIU/L	1	30–150 IU/L
Thyroid	Serum			
Thyroid stimulating hormone (TSH)		0.4–6.0 mIU/L		
Thyroxine binding globulin		12–28 μg/mL	12.87	150–360 nmol/L
Total thyroxine (T4)		4–11 μg/mL	12.87	51–142 nmol/L
Free thyroxine (FT4)		0.8–2.8 ng/dL	12.87	10–36 pmol/L
Total Triiodothyronine (T3)		80–220 ng/dL	0.01536	1.22–3.38 nmol/L
Triiodothyronine (T3) RIA		716 ng/dL		
Reverse Triiodothyronine (T3)		75–220 ng/dL	0.01536	1.2–3.4 nmol/L
T3 Resin Uptake		26–35%		
Adrenal	Plasma			
Adrenocortotropic hormone (ACTH)		<60 pg/mL	0.2202	<13.2 pmo/L
Cortisol		7–25 μg/mL	0.028	0.2–0.7 μmol/L
Aldosterone		1–21 ng/dL	10	100–200ng/L
Metanephrines	24 hr Urine	1.3mg/24 hrs.	—	—
Epinephrine	Plasma			—
Supine		<110 pg/mL	5.458	<600 pmol/L
Standing		<140 pg/mL	5.458	<764 pmol/L
Norepinephrine				—
Supine		70–750 pg/mL	0.0059	0.41–0.43 nmol/L
Standing		200–1700 pg/mL	0.0059	1.18–10.00 nmol/L
Ovary/placenta				
Quantitative hCG RIA	Plasma	—	—	—
2nd International System		<2.0 mIU/mL	—	—
Estradiol	Plasma			
Follicular phase		<0.1 ng/mL	—	—
Luteal phase		0.1–0.4 ng/mL	—	—
Estriol	Plasma	<0.01 ng/mL	—	—
Progesterone	Plasma	—	—	—
Follicular phase		<2 ng/mL	3.18	<6 nmol/L
Luteal phase		2–20 ng/mL	3.18	6–64 nmol/L
Androstendione		0.2–3.1 ng/mL	—	—
DHEA		2.0–5.2 ng/mL	—	—
DHEA-S		40–410 μg/L	—	—
Testosterone		<0.6 ng/mL	3.467	<2.0 nmol/L
Maternal serum alpha-fetoprotein (MsAFP)	Serum	<10 ng/mL	—	—
MsAFP in MoM (15–21 weeks EGA)	—	—	—	—

Fetus, Amniotic Fluid

Ashwood E. Standards of laboratory practice: evaluation of fetal lung maturity. Clin Chem 1997;43 211–214.

Gluck L, Kulovich MV, Borer RC Jr, Brenner DH, Anderson GG, Spellacy WN. Diagnosis of the respiratory distress syndrome by amniocentesis. Am J Obstet Gynecol 1971;109:440–445.

Gluck L, Kulovich MV, Borer RC Jr, Keidel WN. The interpretation and significance of the lecithin-sphingomylin ration in amniotic fluid. Am J Obstet Gynecol 1974;120:142–55.

Hobbins JL, Brock W, Speroff L, Anderson GC, Caldwell B. L-S ratio in predicting pulmonary maturity in utero. Obstet Gynecol 1972;39: 660–664.

Kulovich MV, Gluck L. The lung profile. II. Complicated pregnancy. Am J Obstet Gynecol 1979;135:64–70.

Moore TR, Cayne JE. The amniotic fluid index in normal human pregnancy. Am J Obstet Gynecol 1990;162:1168–1173.

Roberts NS, Dunn LK, Weiner S, Godmilow L, Miller R. Midtrimester amniocentesis: indications, technique, risks and potential for prenatal diagnosis. J Reprod Med 1983;28:167–168.

TABLE 56-3. *Continued.*

Examination	1st Trimester	2nd Trimester	3rd Trimester
Pituitary			
Prolactin	10.0–25	125–200	200–400
Follicle-stimulating hormone			
Pregnancy	—	11.2–15.6	—
Luteinizing hormone			
Pregnancy	9.4–16.2	7.3–14.9	5.1–10.1
Thyroid			
Thyroid stimulating hormone	0.5–1.5	0.9–1.3	1.2–1.6
Thyroxine binding globulin	35.4–41.4	39.7–45.7	53.2–59.2
Total thyroxine (T4)	9–16	10.4–14	1.2–10
Free thyroxine (FT4)	*Does not change in pregnancy*		
Total triiodothyronine (T3)	160–200	200–250	200–240
Triiodothyronine (T3) RIA	—	15.2–22.4	14.4–28.8
Reverse triiodothyronine (T3)	—	—	—
T3 resin uptake	—	—	<10%
Adrenal			
Adrenocortotropic hormone (ACTH)	24–88	23–107	20–60
Cortisol	7.0–25	21–55	25–60
Aldosterone	215–247	148–180	20–70
Metanephrines	*Does not change in pregnancy*		
Epinephrine	*Does not change in pregnancy*		
Norepinephrine	*Does not change in pregnancy*		
Ovary/placenta			
Quantitative hCG RIA			
2nd International System			
Wk 1	<30	—	—
Wk 2	30–100	—	—
Wk 3	100–1,000	—	—
Wk 4	1,000–10,000	—	—
Wk 5–12	30,000–100,000	10,000–30,000	5,000–15,000
Estradiol			
Pregnancy	0.18–3.5	7.3–17.9	3.4–37.2
Estriol	0.05	3.0–17	6.0–35
Progesterone			
Pregnancy	11.9–58.2	15.6–114.3	101.8–397.2
Androstendione	—	2.2–4.2	2.0–3.8
DHEA	—	3.3–4.2	2.8–5.5
DHEA-S		1,200–1,800 ng/mL	800–1000 μg/mL
Testosterone	—	0.7–1.8	0.55–2.0
Maternal serum alpha-fetoprotein (MsAFP)	—	20–50	30–80
MsAFP in MoM (15–21 wk GA)			
Increased risk of trisomy 21	—	<0.4 MoM	
Increased risk of NTD	—	>2.0 MoM	

GA, gestational age; MoM, multiples of median; NTD, neural tube defects

TABLE 56-4. *Urinary evaluations*

Examination	Specimen	Referent range	Conversion factor (SIU)	Referent range (SIU)
Volume		0.6–2.5 L/24 hr	—	—
Specific gravity		1.003–1.030	—	—
pH		4.6–8.0	—	—
Protein	24-Hour urine	<150 mg/24 hr	0.001	<0.15 g/24 hr
Glucose		<0.3 g/24 hr	—	—
Ketones: qualitative		negative	—	—
Leukocyte esterase: qualitative		negative	—	—
Renal plasma flow		408–552 mL/min	—	—
Glomerular filtration rate				
Creatinine clearance		72–121 mL/min	—	—
Inulin clearance		105–132 mL/min	—	—

TABLE 56-5. *Amniotic fluid examination*

Examination	Referent range	
Volume: amniotic fluid index (by ultrasound, mm)		
Alpha-fetoprotein	µg/mL	
Acetylcholinesterase	qualitative	
Urea	mg/dL	
Creatinine	mg/dL	
Glucose	mg/dL	
Total protein	g/L	
Evaluation of fetal lung maturity		
Lecithin/sphingomyelin ratio	Predictive of fetal lung maturity at	L/S > 2
Phosphatidylglycerol	Predictive of fetal lung maturity at	PG > 3%

TABLE 56-4. *Continued*

Examination	1st Trimester	2nd Trimester	3rd Trimester
Volume	0.975–1.825	1.038–1.864	1.057–1.965
Specific gravity	*Does not change in pregnancy*		
pH	*Does not change in pregnancy*		
Protein	<300 mg/24 hr	<300 mg/24 hr	<300 mg/24 hr
Glucose	0–0.2	0–0.7	0–1.0
Ketones—qualitative	negative	negative	negative
Leukocyte esterase: qualitative	negative	negative	negative
Renal plasma flow	700–985	611–1,170	600–846
Glomerular filtration rate			
Creatinine clearance	132–166	134–170	118–182
Inulin clearance	100–170	160–170	160–170

TABLE 56-5. *Continued*

	1st Trimester	2nd Trimester	3rd Trimester
Volume	59–103	79–228	94–248
pH	7.23	7.17	7.11
Alpha-fetoprotein	12.2–14.7	4.7–7.3	1.4–3.3
Acetylcholinesterase		Negative	
Urea	15–20	18–25	18–32
Creatinine	0.8–1.1	0.95–1.5	1.16–1.9
Glucose	43–65	24–60	13–44
Total protein	6.0–18	4.0–8.0	1.6–3.5
Evaluation of fetal lung maturity			
Lecithin	0.1–0.3 mg/dL	0.3–1.2 mg/dL	1.2–8.8 mg/dL
Sphingomyelin	0.3–0.6 mg/dL	0.6–2.8 mg/dL	1.2–2.8 mg/dL
Lecithin/Sphingomyelin ratio	0.5	0.5–0.7	0.7–4.0
Phosphatidylglycerol	0	0–3%	0–3%

Subject Index